Pediatric Hematology

THIRD EDITION

Pediatric Hematology

EDITED BY

Robert J. Arceci

King Fahd Professor of Pediatric Oncology
Kimmel Comprehensive Cancer Center at Johns Hopkins
Baltimore
Maryland
USA

Ian M. Hann

Professor of Paediatric Haematology and Oncology
Great Ormond Street Hospital for Children NHS Trust
London
UK

Owen P. Smith

Professor of Paediatric Haematology
Department of Paediatric Haematology/Oncology
Our Lady's Hospital for Sick Children
Crumlin
Dublin
Ireland

THIRD EDITION

FOREWORD BY

A. Victor Hoffbrand

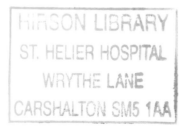
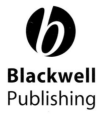

Blackwell
Publishing

© 1992, 1999 Harcourt Publishers Ltd
© 2006 by Blackwell Publishing Ltd

Blackwell Publishing, Inc., 350 Main Street, Malden, Massachusetts 02148-5020, USA
Blackwell Publishing Ltd, 9600 Garsington Road, Oxford OX4 2DQ, UK
Blackwell Publishing Asia Pty Ltd, 550 Swanston Street, Carlton, Victoria 3053, Australia

The right of the Authors to be identified as the Authors of this Work has been asserted in accordance with the Copyright, Designs and Patents Act 1988.

First published 1992
Second edition 1999
Third edition 2006

1   2006

Library of Congress Cataloging-in-Publication Data
Pediatric hematology / edited by Robert J. Arceci, Ian M. Hann, Owen
        P. Smith ; foreword by A. Victor Hoffbrand. — 3rd ed.
            p.   ;   cm.
        Includes bibliographical references and index.
        ISBN-13: 978-1-4051-3400-2 (alk. paper)
        ISBN-10: 1-4051-3400-3 (alk. paper)
        1. Pediatric hematology.   I. Arceci, Robert.   II. Hann, Ian M.
    III. Smith, Owen P.
        [DNLM: 1. Hematologic Diseases.   2. Child.   WS 300 P126 2006]
    RJ411.P35 2006
    618.92'15—dc22

2006010107

ISBN-13: 978-1-4051-3400-2
ISBN-10: 1-4051-3400-3

A catalogue record for this title is available from the British Library

Set in 9/12pt Palatino by Graphicraft Limited, Hong Kong
Printed and bound in India by Replika Press Pvt. Ltd, Haryana

Commissioning Editor: Maria Khan
Editorial Assistant: Victoria Pittman
Development Editor: Nick Morgan
Production Controller: Kate Charman

For further information on Blackwell Publishing, visit our website:
http://www.blackwellpublishing.com

Appreciation of Richard Frederick Stevens

Richard Stevens, better known to all his friends and colleagues as Dick, died in tragic circumstances in July 2003. As John Lilleyman's appreciation in the *Journal of the Royal College of Pathology* testified, Dick radiated warmth of character and was the best of company. Those of us who travelled with him to meetings were regaled with clinical conundrums, insight into the workings of railway timetables and delays in travel, and not a little in-depth knowledge of medical and musical history. This was frequently interspersed with clinical anecdotes and discussion on pediatric hemato-oncology problems. He was a national figure both in hemophilia and in acute leukemia management, particularly myeloid leukemia.

With Ian Hann he oversaw the AML 10 study, which produced the great leap forward in survival that we had all been waiting for since the 1970s. Dick wrote extremely well in his chosen subjects and in the previous editions of this text on leukemia and in the last edition on disorders of granulopoiesis and granulocyte function. His remarkable enthusiasm led to far too many calls on his time: as Clinical Director, Chairman of the local Trust Staff Medical Committee, Secretary to the National Childhood Leukaemia Working Party, and Secretary to the UK Haemophilia Doctors' Association and at the time of his disappearance he had just been elected President of the Manchester Paediatric Club.

His lectures always contained fascinating anecdotes on the topic in question. He became more and more respected as a historian. Those of us who knew him well and worked with him sadly miss him, his excellent company and his immensely friendly support. It can be said of very few of us that we make friends but no enemies. He fought for his patients, particularly at the difficult time which all hemophilia patients faced when recombinant factor VIII became available at a price that many in the Health Service were not willing to pay.

His death was an unpredictable tragedy. We are privileged to have known and worked with this very special man. He is truly a great loss to pediatric hematology in the UK and the world.

Appreciation of Anton H. Sutor

During the period of editing the current issue of this book, Professor Dr Anton H. Sutor, one of the leading scientists in pediatric hemostasis, passed away. We greatly appreciate his significant contributions to both clinical and laboratory research in pediatric hemostasis.

Born in Augsburg, Germany, Anton Sutor's early years studying medicine were in Freiburg, Berlin and Worcester (MA). During a fellowship at the Mayo Clinic in Rochester, Minnesota, 1967–1970, he began working in the field of pediatric hemostasis. He returned to Freiburg, and from 1977 to 1982 he held a position as an Associate Professor at the Department of Pediatric Hematology and Oncology in Münster. In 1982, he accepted the position of Professor of Pediatric Hematology and Hemostasis at the University of Freiburg.

Professor Sutor contributed significantly to pediatric hematology through his work on vitamin K, the genetics of thrombosis, the toxicity of heparin, and the pathophysiology of procoagulant and anticoagulant factors. During his last years, he focused on the pathophysiology and treatment of thrombocytosis and thrombocytopenia. He published over 100 articles in peer-reviewed journals and numerous textbook chapters, edited 16 textbooks, and organized many international meetings. He also earned various awards, including the Goedecke Research Award, the Alexander Schmidt Award of the German Society of Thrombosis and Hemostasis (GTH), and an award for excellence in teaching. He served as chair for the section on pediatric hemostasis in the GTH and as co-chairman of the International Society of Thrombosis and Haemostasis (ISTH). In 2000, Professor Sutor was president of the International Conference of this society in Freiburg, which was combined with a meeting of the Japanese Society of Pediatric Hemostasis.

Professor Sutor was very much honored by the international scientific community in pediatric hematology and oncology. He had excellent contacts with many international groups, particularly in Japan. Besides medicine, he had a passion for flying, skiing, and chamber music. His tremendous clinical and scientific work, his skills for teaching students and young fellows, and his lovely personality will be always remembered by us.

Contents

List of contributors, ix

Foreword, xii

Preface, xiii

Section 1: The Scientific Basis

1 Hematopoiesis: an introduction, 3
  Hugh J.M. Brady

Section 2: Marrow Failure Syndromes

2 Failure of red cell production, 11
  Sarah E. Ball

3 Inherited bone marrow failure syndromes, 30
  Yigal Dror

4 Acquired aplastic anemia, 64
  Juliana Teo and Yigal Dror

Section 3: Red Cell Disorders

5 Disorders of iron metabolism: iron deficiency, iron overload and the sideroblastic anemias, 79
  Andrew M. Will

6 Megaloblastic anemia and disorders of cobalamin and folate metabolism, 105
  Eric J. Werner

7 Nonimmune neonatal anemias, 130
  Brenda E.S. Gibson and Christina Halsey

8 Immune hemolytic anemias, 151
  Bertil Glader

9 Disorders of erythrocyte metabolism including porphyria, 171
  Lawrence Wolfe and Peter E. Manley

10 Sickle cell disease, 213
  Corrina McMahon

11 Hemoglobin variants and the rarer hemoglobin disorders, 231
  Andreas E. Kulozik

12 Red cell membrane abnormalities, 255
  Patrick G. Gallagher

13 Thalassemias, 281
  Nancy F. Olivieri and David J. Weatherall

Section 4: Granulocyte Disorders

14 Disorders of granulopoiesis and granulocyte function, 305
  Arian Laurence, Pratima Chowdary and Philip Ancliff

15 Histiocytic disorders, 340
  Amir H. Shahlaee and Robert J. Arceci

16 Acute myeloid leukemia, 360
  Leslie S. Kean, Robert J. Arceci and William G. Woods

17 Chronic myeloid leukemia, 384
  Irene A.G. Roberts and Inderjeet S. Dokal

18 Myelodysplastic syndromes, 405
  David K.H. Webb

Section 5: Lymphocyte Disorders

19 Primary and acquired immunodeficiency, 425
  Andrew R. Gennery, Adam H.R. Finn and Andrew J. Cant

20 Clinical features and therapy of lymphoblastic leukemia, 450
  Owen P. Smith and Ian M. Hann

21 Lymphomas, 482
  O.B. Eden and Ross Pinkerton

Section 6: Platelet Disorders

22 Inherited and congenital thrombocytopenia, 507
Owen P. Smith

23 Idiopathic thrombocytopenic purpura, 526
Paul Imbach

24 Thrombocytosis, 548
Christof Dame

25 Platelet function disorders, 562
Alan D. Michelson

Section 7: Coagulation Disorders

26 Hemophilia A and B, 585
Judith Smith and Owen P. Smith

27 von Willebrand disease, 598
David Lillicrap

28 Rare congenital hemorrhagic disorders, 608
Nigel S. Key and Margaret A. Heisel-Kurth

29 Acquired disorders of hemostasis, 624
Elizabeth A. Chalmers, Michael D. Williams and Angela Thomas

30 Bleeding in the neonate, 643
Elizabeth A. Chalmers

31 Thromboembolic complications in children, 672
Mary Bauman and M. Patricia Massicotte

Section 8: Supportive Therapy

32 Blood components and fractionated plasma products: preparation, indications and administration, 693
Nancy Robitaille and Heather A. Hume

33 Hazards of transfusion, 724
Naomi L.C. Luban and Edward C.C. Wong

34 Management of infection in children with bone marrow failure, 745
Subarna Chakravorty and Ian M. Hann

Section 9: Secondary Problems

35 Hematologic effects of systemic disease and nonhematopoietic tumors, 757
Angela Thomas

36 Lysosomal storage disorders, 778
Brad T. Tinkle and Gregory A. Grabowski

37 Reference values, 792
Paula S. Simpkin and Roderick F. Hinchliffe

Index, 811

List of contributors

Philip Ancliff
Consultant Haematologist, Camelia Botnar Laboratories, Great Ormond Street Hospital for Children, Great Ormond Street, London WC1N 3JH, UK

Robert J. Arceci
King Fahd Profesor of Pediatric Oncology, Johns Hopkins Oncology Center, 1650 Orleans Street, 2M51, Baltimore, MD 21231-1000, USA

Sarah E. Ball
Reader/Honorary Consultant in Paediatric Haematology, St George's Hospital Medical School, Cranmer Terrace, London SW17 0RE, UK

Mary Bauman
Advanced Practice Nurse Intern, Pediatric Thrombosis, Stollery Children's Hospital, University of Alberta, WMC 2C3, 8440 112 Street, Edmonton, Alberta, T6G 2B7, Canada

Hugh J.M. Brady
Head of Unit, Molecular Haematology and Cancer Biology Unit, Institute of Child Health, University College London, 30 Guilford Street, London WC1N 1EH, UK

Andrew J. Cant
Consultant in Paediatric Immunology and Infectious Diseases, Ward 23A, Paediatric Immunology and Infectious Diseases Unit, Newcastle General Hospital, Westgate Road, Newcastle Upon Tyne NE4 6BE, UK

Subarna Chakravorty
Specialist Registrar in Paediatric Haematology, Great Ormond Street Hospital for Children, Great Ormond Street, London WC1N 3JH, UK

Elizabeth A. Chalmers
Consultant Paediatric Haematologist, Department of Haematology, Royal Hospital for Sick Children, Yorkhill, Glasgow G3 8SJ, UK

Pratima Chowdary
SpR Haematology, Department of Haematology, University College Hospital, 235 Euston Road, London NW1 2BU, UK

Christof Dame
Assistant Professor, Department of Neonatology, Charite – University Medicine Berlin, Campus Virchow-Klinikum, Augustenburger Platz 1, D-13353 Berlin, Germany

Inderjeet S. Dokal
Department of Haematology, Commonwealth Building, 4th Floor, Imperial College Hammersmith Campus, Du Cane Road, London W12 0NN, UK

Yigal Dror
Director, Marrow Failure and Myelodysplasia Program, The Hospital for Sick Children, 555 University Avenue, Toronto, Ontario, M5G 1X8, Canada

O.B. Eden
Professor of Adolescent, Teenage and Young Adult Cancer, Paediatric, Adolescent and Young Adult Oncology Unit, Christie Hospital NHS Trust, University of Manchester, Manchester M20 4BX, UK

Adam H.R. Finn
Institute of Child Life and Health Clinical Sciences at South Bristol, UBHT Education Centre, Upper Maudlin Street, Bristol BS2 8AE, UK

Patrick G. Gallagher
Associate Professor, Department of Pediatrics, Yale University School of Medicine, 333 Cedar Street, New Haven, LCI 402, New Haven, CT 06520-8064, USA

Andrew R. Gennery
Watson Senior Lecturer in Paediatric Immunology and Bone Marrow Transplantation, Paediatric BMT Unit, Ward 23, Newcastle General Hospital, Westgate Road, Newcastle Upon Tyne NE4 6BE, UK

Brenda E.S. Gibson
Consultant Paediatric Haematologist, Department of
Haematology, Royal Hospital for Sick Children, Yorkhill,
Glasgow G3 8SJ, UK

Bertil Glader
Professor of Pediatrics (Hematology/Oncology), Stanford
University Medical Center, 300 Pasteur Drive, Stanford,
CA 94305-5208, USA

Gregory A. Grabowski
Professor and Director, Division and Program in Human
Genetics, Cincinnati Children's Hospital Medical Center,
3333 Burnet Avenue, Cincinnati, OH 45229-3039, USA

Christina Halsey
Leukaemia Research Fund (LRF) Clinical Research Fellow,
Division of Immunology, Infection and Inflammation,
Glasgow Biomedical Research Centre NHS Trust, 120
University Place, Glasgow G12 8TA, UK

Ian M. Hann
Professor of Haematology, Camelia Botnar Laboratories,
Great Ormond Street Hospital for Children NHS Trust,
Great Ormond Street, London WC1N 3JH, UK

Margaret A. Heisel-Kurth
Pediatric Hematology-Oncology, Minneapolis Childrens'
Hospitals and Clinics of Minnesota, and Hemophilia and
Thrombosis Center, Fairview-University Medical Center,
Minneapolis, MN, USA

Roderick F. Hinchliffe
Senior Chief Biomedical Scientist, Department of Paediatric
Haematology, Sheffield Children's NHS Trust, Western
Bank, Sheffield S10 2TH, UK

Heather A. Hume
Executive Medical Director, Transfusion Medicine Canadian
Blood Services, Associate Clinical Professor, Department of
Pediatrics, Université de Montréal, Montreal, Quebec, Canada

Paul Imbach
Paediatric Oncology/Haematology, University Children's
Hospital Basel, and Children's Hospital Aarau,
Roemergasse 8, CH-4005 Basel, Switzerland

Leslie S. Kean
AFLAC Cancer Center and Blood Disorders Service,
Children's Healthcare of Atlanta/Emory University, 1405
Clifton Road, Atlanta, GA 30322, USA

Nigel S. Key
Professor of Medicine, University of Minnesota Medical
School, MMC 480 Mayo Building, 420 Delaware Street SE,
Minneapolis, MN 55455, USA

Andreas E. Kulozik
Professor of Pediatrics, Universitätsklinik fuer Kinder- und
Jugendmedizin, Im Neuenheimer Feld 153, D-69120
Heidelberg, Germany

Arian Laurence
Haematology Registrar, University College Hospital
London, Grafton Way, London WC1E 6DB, UK

David Lillicrap
Professor, Department of Pathology and Molecular
Medicine, Richardson Laboratory, Queen's University,
88 Stuart Street, Kingston, Ontario K7L 3N6,
Canada

Naomi L.C. Luban
Chair, Laboratory Medicine and Pathology, and Director,
Transfusion Medicine/Donor Center, Children's National
Medical Center, 111 Michigan Avenue NW, Washington,
DC 20010, USA

Peter E. Manley
Division of Pediatric Hematology/Oncology, Hasbro
Children's Hospital, Brown University School of Medicine,
593 Eddy Street, Providence, RI 02903, USA

M. Patricia Massicotte
Professor of Pediatrics, University of Alberta Division
of Hematology and Cardiology, Stollery Children's
Hospital, 8440 112 Street, Edmonton, Alberta T6G 2B7
Canada

Corrina McMahon
Consultant Haematologist, Department of Paediatric
Haematology/Oncology, Our Lady's Hospital for Sick
Children, Crumlin, Dublin 2, Ireland

Alan D. Michelson
Director, Center for Platelet Function Studies, and Professor
of Pediatrics, Medicine and Pathology, Vice Chair for
Academic Affairs, Department of Pediatrics, University of
Massachusetts Medical School, 55 Lake Avenue North,
Worcester, MA 01655, USA

Nancy F. Olivieri
Professor of Pediatrics and Medicine, Toronto General
Hospital, 200 Elizabeth Street, Toronto, Ontario, Canada

Ross Pinkerton
Director of Cancer Services, Mater Hospitals, Raymond
Terrace, Brisbane, Queensland 4101, Australia

Irene A.G. Roberts
Professor of Paediatric Haematology, Departments
of Paediatrics and Haematology, St Mary's and
Hammersmith Hospitals, Imperial College London,
Commonwealth Building, 4th Floor, Du Cane Road,
London W12 0NN, UK

Nancy Robitaille
Medical Director, Blood Bank, Centre Hospitalier
Universitaire Sainte-Justine and Clinical Instructor,
Department of Pediatrics, Université de Montréal,
Montreal, Quebec, Canada

Amir H. Shahlaee
Assistant Professor of Pediatric Hematology and Oncology, University of Florida Health Science Center, Box 100296, Gainesville, FL 32610, USA

Paula S. Simpkin
Senior Biomedical Scientist, Haematology Laboratory, Sheffield Children's NHS Trust, Western Bank, Sheffield S10 2TH, UK

Judith Smith
Nurse Manager, National Centre Hereditary Coagulation Disorders, Dublin, Ireland

Owen P. Smith
Professor of Paediatric Haematology and Oncology, Department of Paediatric Haematology/Oncology, Our Lady's Hospital for Sick Children, Crumlin, Dublin 2, Ireland

Juliana Teo
Pediatric Hematologist, Division of Hematology/Oncology, The Hospital for Sick Children, 555 University Avenue, Toronto, Ontario, M5G 1X8, Canada

Angela Thomas
Consultant Paediatric Haematologist, Department of Haematology, Royal Hospital for Sick Children, Sciennes Road, Edinburgh EH9 1LF, UK

Brad T. Tinkle
Clinical Geneticist, Division of Human Genetics, Cincinnati Children's Hospital Medical Center, 3333 Burnet Avenue, Cincinnati, OH 45229, USA

Sir David J. Weatherall
Weatherall Institute of Molecular Medicine, John Radcliffe Hospital, Headington, Oxford OX3 9DS, UK

David K.H. Webb
Consultant Haematologist, Department of Haematology, Great Ormond Street Hospital for Children, Great Ormond Street, London WC1N 3JH, UK

Eric J. Werner
Professor of Pediatrics, and Director, Division of Pediatric Hematology/Oncology, Eastern Virginia Medical School, and Co-Director, Division of Pediatric Hematology/Oncology, Children's Specialty Group, Children's Hospital of the King's Daughters, 601 Children's Lane, Norfolk, VA 23507, USA

Andrew M. Will
Consultant Paediatric Haematologist, Royal Manchester Children's Hospital, Hospital Road, Pendlebury, Manchester M27 4HA, UK

Michael D. Williams
Consultant Paediatric Haematologist, Birmingham Children's Hospital, Steelhouse Lane, Birmingham B4 6NH, UK

Lawrence Wolfe
Division of Pediatric Hematology/Oncology, New England Medical Center, 750 Washington Street, Boston, MA 02111, USA

Edward C.C. Wong
Director of Hematology and Associate Director of Transfusion Medicine, Children's National Medical Center, 111 Michigan Avenue NW, Washington, DC 20010, USA

William G. Woods
Director, The Daniel P. Amos Children's Chair for AFLAC, Cancer Center and Blood Disorders Service, Children's Healthcare of Atlanta/Emory University, 1405 Clifton Road, Atlanta, GA 30322, USA

Foreword

It is a great honor for me to write the foreword for the Third Edition of this well established major textbook which deals with all aspects of blood diseases in infants and children. Pediatric hematology has led the world in the application of the new techniques of molecular biology to elucidate at a DNA level, the underlying defect in both inherited and acquired diseases. New discoveries have led to a better understanding of the etiology and clinical manifestations of these diseases and to substantial improvements in their prevention and management. Moreover, the study of rare genetic diseases in childhood has led to a major increase in knowledge of the normal physiological and biochemical processes of the human body. Advances in pediatric hematology have also had a major impact on treatment of many adult diseases. The use of combination chemotherapy for childhood lymphoblastic leukemia, for example, now achieves an impressive cure rate of approximately 85%, and has provided a model for chemotherapy of cancer in general.

Two of the Editors, Ian Hann, Great Ormond Street Hospital for Sick Children, London and Owen Smith, Our Lady's Hospital for Sick Children, Dublin were most impressive trainees in the Department of Haematology at the Royal Free Hospital. Together with Robert Arceci of Johns Hopkins Oncology Center, Baltimore, USA their combined expertise covers the whole range of benign and malignant disorders of the bone marrow as well as diseases of the immune and hemostatic systems. They are to be congratulated on assembling as authors such a distinguished team of international experts. The publishers have ensured clarity of the presentation of the text and produced beautiful diagrams. In the age of the internet and easy electronic access to information, a large text book has to justify its existence by being outstanding in all respects. The Third Edition of *Pediatric Hematology* meets these criteria. The Editors have succeeded in producing a book that is authoritative and up to date, describing in a comprehensive and lucid fashion one of the most rapidly advancing areas of medicine. It will be of great value to all working in the field of hematology and related areas of medicine, especially for those dealing with neonates, infants and children.

A. Victor Hoffbrand
DM, FRCP, FRCPath, DSc, FMedSci
Emeritus Professor of Haematology
Royal Free and University College School of Medicine
London

Preface

There is an old Chinese proverb that says "when you drink from the well, remember who dug it." To this end, the Third Edition of *Pediatric Hematology* owes its current form and substance to an original solo text of Dr. Michael Willoughby followed by the First Edition (c. 1992), edited by Drs. Lilleyman and Hann. The Second edition (c. 1999) was edited by Drs. Lilleyman, Hann and Blanchette. In addition, we are immensely indebted to all the authors of the chapters in the current edition. These individuals represent an extraordinary breadth and depth of experience of both scientific and practical experience. The authors also represent wide geographical as well as chronological ranges. We hope that both characteristics provide a balanced and a cutting edge tone to the content. We are also thankful for the good natured persistence and expertise of Nick Morgan from Blackwell Publishing Ltd, as well as the publication prowess of Kathy Auger project manager for Graphicraft Limited. Without them, this Third Edition could not have been made a reality.

The Third Edition has not succumbed to the often immense temptation of relentless expansion. The number of authors is similar to the previous edition and the total number of chapters has been condensed from 40 to 37. This was accomplished by combining some chapters, such as those on topics concerning the hematologic effects of systemic disease and nonhematologic tumors, as well as the chapters on erythrocyte metabolism and porphyria. We have also eliminated the chapters dedicated strictly to the pathology of acute myelogenous and lymphoblastic leukemia and have instead integrated the essential aspects of biology directly into the chapters on those respective topics. Instead of expansion, we have therefore tried to retain the comprehensive yet practical aspects of the content.

The organization of the Third Edition has remained true to previous editions. This straightforward organization presents an introductory chapter on the Holy Grail of Hematopoiesis followed by sections on Marrow Failure, disorders of the Red Blood Cell, the Granulocytic lineage, Lymphocytes and Platelets. These "cell lineage" directed sections are followed by a comprehensive series of chapters covering Coagulation, Supportive Therapy and Secondary Problems. The last section includes information on standard Reference Values.

The intended audience for Pediatric Hematology includes students, subspecialty trainees, pediatricians and established subspecialists in Pediatric Hematology/Oncology or other subspecialists who will see patients with these benign and malignant disorders of the blood. In addition, nursing specialists taking care of children and young adults with hematologic disorders will find this a practical reference.

At its very essence, a textbook like this is a labor of love including the intense and time consuming process of writing and editing. It is clearly not for fame, ego or money as our subspecialty is unlikely to significantly support any of these. Instead, it is a debt to be paid to the incredible history that precedes us as well as a hope for the future that will succeed us. There is still also a remarkable satisfaction with "turning a page" on where we've been, where we are and where we expect to be. The study of normal and abnormal blood formation remains both a clinically important and scientifically challenging field. We hope that Pediatric Hematology will help to chronicle this discipline while providing caretakers with information that improves the lives of their patients.

Robert J. Arceci, Ian M. Hann & Owen P. Smith

The Scientific Basis

1 Hematopoiesis: an introduction

Hugh J.M. Brady

All the cells of the hematopoietic system originate from pluripotent hematopoietic stem cells (HSCs). HSCs have the intrinsic capacity for self-renewal but are low in number and divide infrequently. Therefore, it is the committed progenitors that are responsible for initiating the large amount of cell proliferation required to maintain blood cell production. These multipotent progenitors, which are the immediate progeny of HSCs in bone marrow, do not have detectable self-renewal *in vivo*. The common lymphoid progenitor (CLP) develops into T and B cells (T and B lymphocytes) whereas the common myeloid progenitor (CMP) gives rise to erythrocytes, megakaryocytes, monocytes and granulocytes. Cells mature from the CMP through two intermediates, the megakaryocyte/erythrocyte progenitor (MEP) and the granulocyte/monocyte progenitor (GMP). However, recent work has suggested that the immediate progeny of HSCs may not be CLPs and CMPs exclusively.[1] An adult bone marrow population (termed LMPP, lymphoid primed multipotent progenitor) has been identified that has the potential to become both lymphoid and granulocyte/monocyte lineage cells but lacks the capacity to give rise to erythroid cells or megakaryocytes.

Lymphoid cells

T and NK cells

Mature circulating T cells are small cells with condensed chromatin in the nucleus and few cytoplasmic organelles. When T cells are activated upon exposure to antigen the volume of the T cells increases, the chromatin decondenses and the cytoplasm contains abundant mitochondria and endoplasmic reticulum. Circulating NK (natural killer) cells are large granular lymphocytes with abundant cytoplasmic granules containing molecules required for cytolysis. T cells are characterized by the surface expression of the T-cell

receptor (TCR) and CD3 complex, which is not found on NK cells. However, the two cell types share the expression of a large number of cell surface differentiation markers. Human NK cells are commonly defined by expression of the cell surface markers CD16 and CD56 although subpopulations of T cells also express these markers.

T cells can be divided into two subsets on the basis of their cell surface markers and function. CD4+ T-helper (Th) cells are required for the activation of other cells of the immune system (e.g., B cells and macrophages) and secretion of cytokines upon recognition of foreign antigens in the context of major histocompatibility complex (MHC) class II molecules. CD8+ cytotoxic T lymphocytes (CTL) recognize antigenic peptides in the context of MHC class I molecules and have two main functions, cytolysis and cytokine secretion. CTL and NK cells show great functional similarities. Both CTL and NK cells lyse their target using both perforin-based mechanisms and Fas–Fas ligand interactions. They also respond to the same cytokines both for proliferation and to increase cytolysis, and both produce a similar set of cytokines, namely interferon-γ (IFN-γ), granulocyte–macrophage colony-stimulating factor (GM-CSF), and tumor necrosis factor-α (TNF-α). However, the effector mechanisms of CTL and NK cells are triggered in distinct ways. Following recognition of the specific MHC class I–antigenic peptide complex, T cells proliferate. They also acquire their effector potential and are able to become memory T cells. NK cells can also interact with MHC class I molecules through specialized killer inhibitory receptors (KIR), and this recognition results in the inhibition of NK cell effector functions. The downregulation or absence of MHC class I molecules on target cells induces lysis by NK cells. Therefore, NK cells can eliminate cells that, due to lack of MHC class I molecules, evade CTL recognition. Complete or partial loss of MHC class I expression is a common consequence of viral infections and malignant transformations. NK cells are also able to participate in the adaptive immune response by expressing the CD16 receptor complex, which allows them to perform antibody-dependent cell-mediated cell killing of antibody-coated target cells.

Hematopoietic cells seem to originate independently both in the yolk sac[2] and in the aorta–gonad mesonephros (AGM) region[3] then migrate to the fetal liver, which is the major hematopoietic organ during fetal life. Precursors of T cells and mature NK cells can be identified in the fetal liver starting from as early as 6 weeks of gestation. A thymic rudiment of epithelial origin is formed by week 7, and by week 9 of gestation it is colonized by dendritic cells, macrophages, and thymic precursors. In the neonate, bone marrow becomes the major hematopoietic organ and is thought to be where NK cells develop, whereas the vast majority of T cells mature in the thymus. Some T cells can have an extrathymic differentiation in the gut mucosa or in the liver, but these cells differ from the thymic T cells in both phenotype and function. T-cell precursors proceed to differentiation and selection in the thymus. The immature precursors lack expression of the T-cell receptor (TCR), CD4 and CD8. The earliest thymic precursors are CD34+CD33+CD45RA+ and subsequently express CD7 and CD38 at the cell surface and CD3 intracellularly. These cells are still able to give rise to both T and NK cells. The T cells acquire the expression of CD1, CD2 and CD5 and the rearrangement of the TCRβ chain starts. At this stage, T-cell precursors for the TCRγδ T-cell lineage differentiate from TCRαβ-committed thymocytes. The rearranged TCRβ chain is expressed at the cell surface associated with a pre-TCRα (pTα) chain and CD3. Expression of the pre-TCR complex prevents further rearrangements at the TCRβ locus, controls the initiation of rearrangement of the TCRα chain, and is required for the expression of CD4 and CD8 molecules on the thymocytes.[4]

The rearrangement of TCR genes during early stages of thymocyte maturation allows the generation of a large number of immature T cells bearing a single specificity. Each TCR locus consists of variable (V), joining (J) and constant (C) region genes; TCRβ and TCRγ chain loci also contain diversity (D) segment genes.[5] When both TCRβ and TCRα loci are rearranged, thymocytes undergo selection. In positive selection, only thymocytes that recognize self MHC molecules become mature T cells: thymocytes that cannot interact with any self MHC molecule die by neglect; negative selection eliminates potentially self-reactive cells that have been generated during VDJ rearrangement. Greater than 98% of thymocytes are eliminated during selection. It is widely accepted that the strength of the interaction between TCR and peptide–MHC complexes as well as the amount of complexes are responsible for the selective events. If the signal is weak, the thymocytes can mature, but if the signal is too low, the thymocytes will die of neglect. A very strong signal leads the thymocytes to undergo programmed cell death and negative selection.

The identification of a T/NK bipotential precursor in the thymus indicates that NK cells can develop in the thymus although the thymus is not required for normal NK cell development and the main site of NK cell development is likely to be the bone marrow.[6]

Mature but naive T cells leave the thymus and migrate through the bloodstream into peripheral lymphoid organs where, upon exposure to antigen, T cells proliferate and differentiate into effector T cells. All mature T lymphocytes express the TCR–CD3 complex on their cell surface. TCRα and TCRβ chains have two immunoglobulin-like domains in the extracellular portion and a short intracellular domain. They are associated with the polypeptide chains of the CD3 complex, which contain immunoreceptor tyrosine-based activation motifs (ITAMs), which are responsible for the transduction of activating signals upon TCR engagement. The CD3 proteins are also required for the assembly and cell surface expression of TCR.

The activation of naive T cells in the lymph nodes requires two signals: cross-linking of the TCR (signal 1) and also co-stimulatory molecules such as CD28 (signal 2). Only professional antigen-presenting cells (APCs), such as macrophages, dendritic cells and B cells, express the CD28 ligands B7.1 (CD80) and B7.2 (CD86) on their surface together with MHC molecules.[7] Antigen recognition by naive T cells in the absence of costimulatory signals induces a state of anergy (i.e., signal 1 only). This mechanism helps to ensure tolerance of T cells to self antigens. CD8+ T cells are cytotoxic effectors while CD4+ T cells can differentiate into inflammatory T cells (Th1) or helper cells (Th2). Following activation, Th1 lymphocytes produce cytokines (IFN-γ, GM-CSF and TNF-α) that activate macrophages to more efficiently eliminate intracellular microorganisms. Th2 cells secrete a different set of cytokines – mainly interleukin-4, -5 and -6 (IL-4, -5 and -6) – that activate B cells to allow them to differentiate and produce antibodies.

Mature NK cells migrate from the bone marrow to the blood. All mature NK cells have a significant level of cell surface expression of adhesion molecules including three β₂ integrins (CD11a/b/c) and CD56. As many as 10% of NK cells express high levels of CD56 (CD56^{high}) and these cells also express both the high- and intermediate-affinity IL-2 receptors (IL-2R). The remaining NK cells have a lower expression of CD56 (CD56^{low}) and express only the intermediate-affinity IL-2R. The activation of CD56^{high} NK cells leads to increased proliferation and an increase in the cell killing effect, whereas activation of CD56^{low} NK cells only results in an enhancement of their cell killing effect. CD56^{high} NK cells resemble immature NK cells, with poor cell killing activity but high proliferative capacity, while CD56^{low} cells are more differentiated. T cells only recognize antigens presented by self MHC molecules, while NK cells are not dependent on MHC although their function is regulated by the MHC. Mature NK cells express KIR, which act as inhibitory receptors for MHC class I molecules, engagement of which transmits a negative signal that leads to the blocking of NK cell activation.[8]

B cells

B cells undergo most of their differentiation in the bone marrow and mature B cells express immunoglobulins which interact directly with antigenic epitopes. Surface immunoglobulins are part of the B cell receptor (BCR) analogous to the TCR on T cells. B cells differentiate in the fetal liver and then in the bone marrow during embryonic development.

Following birth, B-cell differentiation starts in the bone marrow and precursors derived from the hematopoietic stem cells become immature B cells. This stage of differentiation is antigen-independent and is required to generate the basic immunoglobulin repertoire, which is the result of multiple V–D–J gene rearrangements.[9] Immature B cells migrate to the secondary lymphoid organs, namely spleen, lymph nodes, tonsils, mucosa and gut-associated lymphoid tissue (GALT). The next stage of differentiation requires antigen encounter and a number of cell–cell interactions, principally T–B-cell cooperation. A second level of diversity is then generated from somatic mutations, and the final steps of differentiation, including isotype switching, lead to the emergence of plasma cells, which secrete antibodies, and memory B cells.

The B lineage derives from a precursor common to B, T and NK cells. The first steps of B-cell differentiation require interactions of the precursor cells with stromal cells, mediated by various cellular adhesion molecules. The VLA-4 integrin expressed on the cell surface interacts with stromal vascular cell adhesion molecule-1 (VCAM-1) and the resulting early pro-B cells express c-Kit, the receptor for the stem cell factor (SCF) produced by stromal cells. This triggers proliferation of pro-B cells. Late pro-B cells are stimulated by IL-7 produced by the stromal cells, which also activates proliferation of pre-B cells.

During differentiation the B cells are cycling and immunoglobulin gene rearrangements are taking place. CD34, expressed on hematopoietic stem cells, remains on early B-cell precursors and pro-B cells. Late pro-B cells are characterized by the coexpression of CD34 and CD19, which is a specific B-cell marker. CD10 is expressed up to the immature B-cell stage, and is expressed earlier than CD19.[10]

B-cell differentiation leads to the acquisition of the initial repertoire of immunoglobulins that are expressed as surface IgM (sIgM) on immature B cells. Immunoglobulins are made up of two heavy (H) chains and two light (L) chains (κ or λ). Depending upon the nature of the H chain, immunoglobulins exist as discrete isotypes, termed IgM, IgG, IgA, IgD and IgE, corresponding to the μ, γ, α, δ and ε heavy chains, respectively.[11] Each different isotype can be either cell surface or secreted immunoglobulins. When they are expressed at the surface of B cells, immunoglobulin molecules are associated with the Igα–Igβ heterodimer, encoded by the *mb1* and *B29* genes respectively, to form the B-cell receptor (BCR). Each of the H and L chains has a variable and a constant region. The variable regions of the H and L chains interact in the antibody-combining site leading to specific antigen recognition.

Immature B cells that express surface IgM are exposed to self antigen before leaving the bone marrow. Cross-linking of surface immunoglobulins by multivalent antigens results in clonal deletion by apoptosis. However, self antigens do not induce cell death of immature B cells but will induce an anergic state in which the cells still migrate to the peripheral lymphoid organs. At this point, cells that have encountered self antigen may also escape cell death or anergy by changing their specificity. This is achieved by "receptor editing", which allows the cells to replace one light chain by another one, or induces secondary rearrangement of both heavy and light chain loci. Negative selection of B cells has a threshold that still leaves a fraction of self-reactive cells entering the periphery.

When the immature B cells enter the periphery they colonize the secondary lymphoid organs and then recirculate. The final steps of B-cell differentiation then happen in the periphery and are antigen-dependent. Immature B cells emigrate from the bone marrow to the spleen to the bone marrow, as transitional T1 and T2 B cells. Transitional T2 cells will move on either to mature follicular or marginal zone B cells. Following antigen stimulation and T-cell help the activated B cells may differentiate into plasma cells and B memory cells, which are the final stages of B-cell differentiation.

Plasma cells are large cells that contain large amounts of endoplasmic reticulum and secrete immunoglobulins. After a primary stimulation, the first antibodies produced have the IgM isotype. However, some stimulated B cells can generate a germinal center where they interact with follicular dendritic cells. B cells divide rapidly, giving rise to clonal amplification in situ. They have blast-like morphology and are termed centroblasts, which form the dark zone of the germinal center. When centroblasts divide, they accumulate somatic mutations at a very high rate ($\sim 10^{-3}$).[12] These mutations are mostly localized in the variable regions of the heavy (V_H) and light (V_L) chains that interact with the antigen. The mechanism, known as somatic hypermutation and found only in B cells, considerably amplifies antibody diversity. Following these mutations, the range of affinities is much greater, and the germinal center permits the antigen to positively select the B cells that express the immunoglobulins with the highest affinities. The centroblasts then cease to divide and become small non-dividing centrocytes that accumulate in the light zone of the germinal center, where they interact with follicular dendritic cells.

Following antigenic stimulation, circulating antibodies belonging to the IgM isotype are produced initially, before being replaced by immunoglobulins of another isotype, usually IgG. This is known as isotype switching and is the consequence of a new type of gene rearrangement, which takes place in the germinal center. The light chain genes are not affected by isotype switching so the antigen recognition site remains unaffected. Isotype switching changes the Ig isotype without modifying the specificity of the antibody but gives an antibody a distinct biological function, which can alter its physiological role, for instance, to enable a more effective attack against certain pathogens, to ensure fetal protection through transplacental transfer, or to be present in certain secretions. Isotype switching requires interaction between T and B cells and dual molecular signals. One signal involves CD40 ligand (CD40L) found on Th cells and CD40 on B cells. The second signal is provided by the Th cell and is release of cytokine to act on the B cell. Depending upon the cytokine released, the switch mechanism will give rise to a certain isotype. For example, IL-4 favors a switch toward the IgE isotype, whereas transforming growth factor-β1 (TGF-β1) favors a switch to IgA.

Myeloid lineage

Phagocytic leukocytes

The inflammatory response requires the recruitment of a large number of phagocytic leukocytes, which are cells of the myeloid lineage, to sites of tissue damage or infection. The cells of the myeloid lineage originate in the bone marrow. Mature myeloid cells have a short lifespan and are incapable of cell division. Hence, large numbers of cells have to be produced each day. Monocytes, macrophages and neutrophils protect against microbial invasion. Usually, neutrophils are the more efficient phagocytic cells compared with monocytes and macrophages. However, in response to a large load of pathogens, mononuclear phagocytes are more effective. The antimicrobial capacity of macrophages can be enhanced upon activation by substances such as bacterial endotoxin. Activated cells can kill ingested microorganisms by generating toxic metabolites.

Both mononuclear phagocytes and neutrophils are able to phagocytose and kill bacteria in sites of infection. They move toward the sites of infection by chemotaxis in response to stimuli, which include complement and substances derived from bacteria, cells and connective tissue proteins.

Chemokines form a novel class of small (92–99 amino acids) chemotactic cytokines that have the ability to activate phagocytes as mediators of inflammation. There are two subfamilies, which are distinguished by the arrangement of the first two cysteine residues, resulting in the family of so-called C-X-C chemokines, in which either cysteine is separated by one amino acid, or the C-C chemokines, where they are adjacent. A third group, the C chemokines, have only one cysteine residue at this location. The C-C chemokines, which include the monocyte chemotactic proteins (McP-1, -2 and -3) predominantly stimulate monocytes, while the C-X-C chemokine family, consisting of interleukin-8 (IL-8) and a number of

related molecules (e.g., macrophage inflammatory protein-1α, MIP-1α), is mainly active on neutrophils. C chemokines include lymphotactin and eotaxin, which acts on eosinophils.[13]

Neutrophil production in the adult only occurs in the bone marrow. The polymorphonuclear neutrophils in the blood are fully differentiated cells that remain in circulation for only a few hours before migrating into the tissues. During infection, the numbers of neutrophils may increase 10–30-fold within hours, requiring the rapid release of mature cells into circulation from the bone marrow. Mature neutrophils remain for several days in the bone marrow and act as a store, but during infection as well as in response to treatment with granulocyte colony-stimulating factor (G-CSF), the marrow transit time can be significantly reduced. This allows rapid increase in circulating neutrophil numbers during infection.

Polymorphonuclear neutrophils play a crucial role in combating bacterial infections, their primary function being phagocytosis. Impaired neutrophil function or a reduction in their number are directly associated with an increased risk of infections, for example, bacterial sepsis in newborn infants and chronic bacterial infections in older children. The lack of function can result from congenital syndromes or from neutropenia induced by chemotherapy or following conditioning from stem cell transplantation. Neutrophils, eosinophils and basophils differentiate in the bone marrow and are then released into the peripheral circulation. The major function of eosinophils relates to hypersensitivity reactions and to mechanisms acting against the larval states of parasitic infections. Basophils and mast cells are capable of phagocytosis, but their major function stems from their high content of histamine, present in basophilic granules. Histamine is released from the granules in response to a variety of stimuli, including antigen exposure (IgE) in sensitized subjects, and certain cytokines (e.g., IL-3 and GM-CSF).

The mononuclear phagocyte system comprises monocytes, macrophages and their precursor cells, all derived from bone marrow.[14] The monocyte-macrophage lineage and neutrophils are derived from a common progenitor cell, the so-called colony-forming unit granulocyte-monocyte (CFU-GM). Monocytes derived from CFU-GM remain in the blood for approximately 12 hours before they migrate into the tissues, to become macrophages. The macrophages do not re-enter the circulation and have various roles in different tissues, for example as Kupffer cells in the liver or as alveolar macrophages in the lung.

In addition to their phagocytic functions, mononuclear phagocytes are required for the cellular and humoral immune responses. The presentation of antigen on MHC to T cells is preceded by phagocytosis and antigen processing by macrophages.[15] Mononuclear phagocytes act as antigen-presenting cells and, in particular, dendritic cells (which are a distinct cell type from macrophages) act as professional antigen-presenting cells. These cells also secrete IL-1, which enhances both T- and B-cell proliferation. Mononuclear phagocytes secrete a number of other soluble factors that promote the proliferation of other cell types. In addition to IL-1, macrophages are able to produce TNF-α as well as a number of myeloid colony-stimulating factors (i.e., G-CSF, GM-CSF) and macrophage colony-stimulating factor (M-CSF). They also produce factors that inhibit hematopoiesis (e.g., IFN-α and MIP-1α). Activated macrophages can recognize tumor cells in a manner independent of antigen recognition and subsequent cytotoxic activity requires cell-to-cell contact and a number of intracellular mediators, including nitric oxide (NO). Alternatively, mononuclear phagocytes may also recognize and kill antibody-coated tumor cells.

Dendritic cells (DC) are a subset of phagocytic leukocytes that are found at the sites of potential pathogen entry such as epithelial and mucosal surfaces.[16] Sentinel DC normally have an immature phenotype sampling the local environment for evidence of pathogens, tissue damage or inflammation. These immature DC are particularly effective at antigen capture, uptake and processing, but less efficient at antigen presentation. DC are rapidly activated in response to environmental stimuli that signal danger, such as microbial products and cytokines found at inflammatory sites. Activation initiates a coordinated sequence of processes that causes the DC to differentiate. Mature DC switch off their capacity to capture antigen, and increase the expression of antigen-presenting molecules (MHC molecule–peptide complexes and costimulatory molecules) on their cell surface.

At least two definable types of dendritic cells are found in the peripheral blood, where they account for less than 1% of mononuclear cells. These cells express CD4 and high levels of MHC II molecules, but most lack lineage markers. When isolated from blood, DC have an immature appearance and lack dendrites but after culture *in vitro* can stimulate T cells. One type of DC expresses myeloid markers such as CD11b, CD11c, CD13, CD33 and GM-CSFRα (CD116), as well as the MHC-like molecules CD1b/c/d, but shows little or no expression of IL-3Rα (CD123w), and such cells are often referred to as CD11c⁺ DCs. The other type of DC is referred to as myeloid or CD11c⁺ PBDC (Peripheral Blood Dendritic Cell) also known as plasmacytoid DC, and these express high levels of IL-3Rα, low levels of GM-CSFRα and low levels of the myeloid markers indicated above. The FLT3 ligand (FLT3L) has been shown to be the main cytokine responsible for the development of plasmacytoid DCs although G-CSF is required for mobilization from the bone marrow. The plasmacytoid DCs seem distinct from other DCs in that they do not act as sentinels but circulate in a manner driven mainly by inflammatory stimuli. They are likely not to be required for initiating immune responses but for modulating them. *In vitro* evidence has suggested that DCs are primarily lymphoid in origin. Bone marrow CD34⁺CD10⁺ Lin-precursors

with T-, B- and NK-cell potential can generate DC after culture with IL-1β, IL-7, GM-CSF, SCF and FLT3L. Putative lymphoid-derived DC may also be generated from CD34⁺ CD1a⁻ lymphoid-committed thymic precursors after culture with IL-7, TNF-α, SCF and FLT3L.

Erythroid cells

Erythropoiesis is the pathway that produces mature red blood cells from the hematopoietic stem cell.[17] During mammalian development, erythropoiesis takes place in the yolk sac, the fetal liver and finally the bone marrow. The earliest forms of committed erythroid progenitors have been detected by the formation of erythroid colonies after *in vitro* culture in methylcellulose, and are called burst-forming unit erythroid (BFU-E) and the colony-forming unit erythroid (CFU-E). BFU-E are the most immature hematopoietic cells committed to the erythroid lineage. These cells represent less than 0.2% of bone marrow hematopoietic cells, and only about one in three CFU-E make up about the same proportion of bone marrow hematopoietic cells, although most of them are cycling. CFU-E differentiate into the first readily morphologically identifiable cell of the erythroid lineage, the erythroblast, which is the last nucleated cell of the mammalian erythrocyte lineage. Enucleation of the late erythroblast gives rise to reticulocytes and finally red blood cells.

The formation of BFU-E in cell culture is regulated by erythropoietin (EPO) and other growth factors, including SCF, while the formation of CFU-E is highly dependent on low concentrations of EPO alone. EPO is necessary for erythroid differentiation until the late basophilic erythroblast stage, and then the erythroid cells are no longer dependent on EPO for final maturation. The development of the erythroid lineage is characterized by a precise pattern of erythroid gene expression, mainly regulated at the transcriptional level.

Functional analysis of erythroid-specific genes, such as the globin genes, the porphobilinogen deaminase gene, the glycophorin A and B genes and EPO receptor gene have shown the importance of a sequence 5′ A/T GATA A/G 3′, now called the GATA motif, in the regulated expression of these genes. The sequence is recognized by a family of transcription factors whose members are structurally defined by the presence of two highly conserved zinc fingers. The range of genes regulated by members of the GATA family extends well beyond hematopoietic cells, but two members of this family, GATA-1 and GATA-2, are expressed during erythropoiesis and play a major role in this hematopoietic lineage. GATA-1 expression is restricted to the erythroid, megakaryocyte and mast cell lineages. Deletion of the GATA-1 gene in mouse embryonic stem cells blocks differentiation at the proerythroblast stage of development, where the cells die by apoptosis,[18] and highlights the absolute requirement of GATA-1 transcription factor for red blood cell production. In addition to GATA-1, other transcription factors required for erythroid development have been identified of which the most significant is probably EKLF (erythroid Krüppel-like factor). The DNA-binding site for this factor is mutated in some patients with β-thalassemia and these mutations impair EKLF binding.[19] In addition, mice with the EKLF gene deleted die early in fetal development with a major thalassemia syndrome due to defective β-globin production.[20]

Megakaryocyte lineage cells

Platelets are enucleated cells that play an important role in hemostasis by their adhesion to the endothelium and by the release of the contents of their storage organelles following activation. Platelets are produced by the cytoplasmic fragmentation of their polyploid bone marrow precursors, the megakaryocytes, which are rare, accounting for less than 0.1% of cells in bone marrow.[21]

The megakaryocyte and erythroid lineages have many similarities in their differentiation pathways and in the regulation of their specific genes, and there is evidence for a bipotent progenitor common to the erythroid and megakaryocyte lineages. In the early stages of megakaryopoiesis, megakaryocyte progenitors are capable of proliferation and have the potential to give rise to megakaryocyte colonies *in vitro*. These cells undergo a variable number of cell divisions to differentiate into promegakaryoblasts, which begin to synthesize numerous platelet proteins and enter an endomitotic process (DNA replication without cytokinesis). This process induces a parallel increase in both nuclear and cytoplasmic volumes and gives rise to a cell containing a single multilobule nucleus. After three or so DNA replication cycles the volume of cytoplasm within the cell increases substantially and terminal cytoplasmic maturation occurs, leading to proplatelet formation and platelet production. Platelet production occurs through a highly regulated process of cytoplasmic fragmentation, with each successive stage having increased platelet production, and depends on the number of megakaryocytes, their sizes and the efficiency of platelet release. However, platelet shedding following cytoplasmic maturation does appear to be independent of polyploidization as platelet shedding can occur even in diploid cells. The majority of platelet shedding occurs directly in the circulation not in the bone marrow; mature megakaryocytes are detected in the circulation. When platelets are first released into the blood, they have a characteristic elongated shape and thereafter acquire their definitive shape in the circulation.

References

1. Adolfsson J, Mansson R, Buza-Vidas N *et al*. Identification of Flt3+ lympho-myeloid stem cells lacking erythro-megakaryocytic potential: a revised road map for adult blood lineage. *Cell* 2005; **121**: 295–306.
2. Yoder MC, Hiatt K, Dutt P, Mukherjee P, Bodine DM, Orlic D. Characterization of definitive lympho-haemopoietic stem cells in the day 9 murine yolk sac. *Immunity* 1997; **7**: 335–44.
3. Medvinsky A, Dzierzak E. Definitive hematopoiesis is autonomously initiated by the AGM region. *Cell* 1996; **86**: 897–906.
4. Malissen B, Ardouin L, Lin SY, Gillet A, Malissen M. Function of the CD3 subunits of the pre-TCR and TCR complexes during T cell development. *Adv Immunol* 1999; **72**: 103–48.
5. Nemazee D. Receptor selection in B and T lymphocytes. *Annu Rev Immunol* 2000; **18**: 19–51.
6. Sanchez MJ, Muench MO, Roncarolo MG, Lanier LL, Phillips JH. Identification of a common T/natural killer cell progenitor in human fetal thymus. *J Exp Med* 1994; **180**: 569–76.
7. Chen L. Co-inhibitory molecules of the B7-CD28 family in the control of T-cell immunity. *Nat Rev Immunol* 2004; **4**: 336–47.
8. Vilches C, Parham P. KIR: diverse, rapidly evolving receptors of innate and adaptive immunity. *Annu Rev Immunol* 2002; **20**: 217–51.
9. Martin F, Kearney JF. Selection in the mature B cell repertoire. *Curr Top Microbiol Immunol* 2000; **252**: 97–105.
10. Hardy RR, Hayakawa K. B cell development pathways. *Annu Rev Immunol* 2001; **19**: 595–621.
11. Harriman W, Volk H, Defranoux N, Wabl M. Immunoglobulin class switch recombination. *Annu Rev Immunol* 1993; **11**: 361–84.
12. Honjo T, Kinoshita K, Muramatsu M. Molecular mechanism of class switch recombination: linkage with somatic hypermutation. *Annu Rev Immunol* 2002; **20**: 165–96.
13. Rossi D, Zlotnik A. The biology of chemokines and their receptors. *Annu Rev Immunol* 2000; **18**: 217–42.
14. Dinauer MC. The phagocyte system and disorders of granulopoiesis and granulocyte function. In: Nathan DG, Orkins SH, Ginsburg D, Look AT (eds) *Nathan and Oski's Hematology of Infancy and Childhood*, 6th edn. Philadelphia: WB Saunders, 2003, pp. 923–1010.
15. Watts C. Capture and processing of exogenous antigens for presentation on MHC molecules. *Annu Rev Immunol* 1997; **15**: 821–50.
16. Banchereau J, Briere F, Caux C *et al*. Immunobiology of dendritic cells. *Annu Rev Immunol* 2000; **18**: 767–811.
17. Peschle C. Erythropoiesis. *Annu Rev Med* 1980; **31**: 303–14.
18. Orkin SH, Zon LI. Genetics of erythropoiesis: induced mutations in mice and zebrafish. *Annu Rev Genet* 1997; **31**: 33–60.
19. Feng WC, Southwood CM, Bieker JJ. Analyses of beta-thalassemia mutant DNA interactions with erythroid Kruppel-like factor (EKLF), an erythroid cell-specific transcription factor. *J Biol Chem* 1994; **269**: 1493–500.
20. Perkins AC, Sharpe AH, Orkin SH. Lethal beta-thalassaemia in mice lacking the erythroid CACCC-transcription factor EKLF. *Nature* 1995; **375**: 318–22.
21. Sims RB, Gewirtz AM. Human megakaryocytopoiesis. *Annu Rev Med* 1989; **40**: 213–24.

Marrow Failure Syndromes

2

Failure of red cell production

Sarah E. Ball

This chapter encompasses isolated red cell aplasia, and the congenital dyserythropoietic anemias, in which ineffective erythropoiesis is the predominant cause of anemia. Impaired red cell production in association with syndromes of global marrow failure is covered in Chapters 3 and 4. Thalassemia, in which ineffective erythropoiesis is also prominent, is discussed in Chapter 13.

Red cell aplasia

The three most important causes of pure red cell aplasia in childhood are:
- Diamond–Blackfan anemia (DBA; congenital red cell aplasia);
- transient erythroblastopenia of childhood (TEC);
- parvovirus B19-induced aplastic crisis on the background of chronic hemolysis.

Of these disorders, the chronic red cell aplasia of DBA and the self-limiting red cell aplasia of TEC are unique to early childhood, while an aplastic crisis may occur at any age. Acquired chronic pure red cell aplasia is much less common in children than in adults, but should be considered, especially in an older age group.

Diamond–Blackfan anemia

DBA, a congenital pure red cell aplasia presenting early in infancy, was first described in the 1930s.[1,2] The results of national registries have put the incidence of typical DBA at 4–7/million live births.[3–5] There is no apparent ethnic predominance, and both sexes are equally affected.

Clinical features

Age at presentation

Affected babies most commonly present at 2–3 months of age with symptoms of anemia, such as pallor or poor feeding.

Anemia is evident at birth in 25% of cases,[4,6] but fetal anemia leading to hydrops has only rarely been reported.[7–9] In the absence of associated physical anomalies or an unequivocal family history, the diagnosis of DBA should be accepted with caution in children over the age of 1 year. However, mildly affected individuals may be diagnosed as adults, for example, through family studies, or when anemia is exacerbated during pregnancy.[10–12]

Associated physical anomalies

These are present in up to 50% of children with DBA (Table 2.1), with a wide range of severity.[13–16] Craniofacial abnormalities are the commonest, with cleft or high arched palate, hypertelorism, and flat nasal bridge contributing to the typical DBA facies described by Cathie[17] (Fig. 2.1). Thumb abnormalities are present in 10–20% of affected children, ranging in severity from a flat thenar eminence to absent radii, including the classic triphalangeal thumb described by Aase and Smith.[18] Deafness is a relatively common feature, and other musculoskeletal, renal and cardiac abnormalities may also occur. Learning difficulties are relatively rare in DBA.

Table 2.1 Prevalence and pattern of physical anomalies in 65 children with Diamond–Blackfan anemia born in the UK over the 20-year period 1975–1994[4]

	Number (%)
Physical anomalies	
Any abnormality	38 (58)
Craniofacial (including cleft palate, typical facies, ophthalmic)	34 (52)
Thumb (including hypoplastic, bifid, triphalangeal)	12 (18)
Growth retardation	
Height below 3rd percentile for age	18 (28)
With associated physical anomalies	11 (17)
Isolated growth retardation	7 (10)

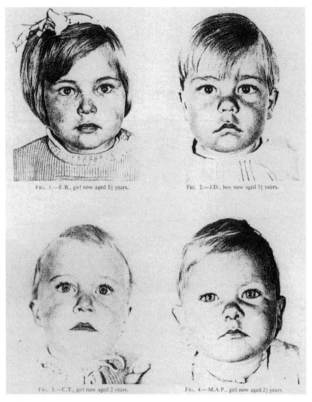

Fig. 2.1 Diamond–Blackfan anemia (DBA) facies: similarity in appearance between unrelated children with DBA. Reproduced with permission from Ref. 17.

Growth retardation

Over 60% of children reported in the UK DBA registry were below the 25th centile for height at the time of study, 28% being below the 3rd centile[4] (Table 2.1). Of affected children, 10–30% have low birthweight prior to the onset of anemia or starting steroid therapy,[4,5,19] and short stature is then likely to persist.[4] Short stature can therefore be considered to be part of the spectrum of physical anomalies, although the final height achieved by each affected individual will be influenced by other factors, notably steroids and iron overload. Growth hormone therapy has been reported to be of benefit in the management of impaired pubertal growth in DBA.[20–22]

Laboratory investigation of DBA

Red cell indices

The anemia at presentation may be normocytic or macrocytic. The mean corpuscular volume (MCV) is usually within the normal range for neonates,[15] while children presenting after the first few months are more likely to have macrocytosis. The anemia is, by definition, associated with reticulocytopenia. The white blood cell count is usually normal at presentation, and platelets are normal or raised. However, trilineage marrow failure may become evident with increasing age.[23–25] Fetal characteristics of red cells frequently persist after re-

sponse to therapy, in the form of raised MCV, high levels of fetal hemoglobin (HbF) and increased expression of i antigen.[26] These may be useful in the diagnosis of difficult cases, but are relatively nonspecific, and notably can occur during the recovery phase of TEC,[27] as discussed below.

Bone marrow findings

Bone marrow aspirate reveals a cellular marrow, with an isolated reduction in erythroid precursors, with normal myeloid and megakaryocytic differentiation.

Erythrocyte adenosine deaminase (eADA)

High eADA activity is present in a high proportion of patients with DBA.[28–34] eADA activity is not raised in normal cord blood,[31] nor in juvenile chronic myeloid leukaemia[28] despite the fetal pattern of erythropoiesis characteristic of that disorder.[35] However, eADA activity may also be high in other disorders, including leukemia and myelodysplastic syndromes,[36,37] and so cannot be considered a specific marker for DBA. Its measurement, however, may be useful in establishing family phenotypes for genetic studies as discussed further below.

Inheritance and genetics

There is a positive family history in 10–20% of babies presenting with DBA.[3–6] The pattern of inheritance is typically autosomal dominant,[33,34,38–41] although recessive inheritance has been inferred in families with parental consanguinity. There has been an increasing recognition that the phenotypic spectrum of DBA is broader than that of the classical presentation of severe red cell aplasia presenting in early infancy. It is now recognized that an isolated increase in eADA activity may be the only manifestation of DBA.[33,34] As a result, detailed family studies have revealed a higher proportion of cases of familial DBA than previously appreciated. For example, in a UK DBA Registry study, hematologic abnormalities, including raised eADA activity, were found in first-degree relatives of 31% of patients not previously considered to have familial DBA.[34] Inheritance was most consistent with an autosomal dominant pattern, with incomplete penetrance.

While there is no specific karyotypic abnormality associated with DBA, a *de novo* balanced t(X;19) translocation was described in a sporadic case of DBA.[42] Linkage was established to 19q in familial DBA,[43] although with evidence of genetic heterogeneity.[44,45] Analysis of the 19q breakpoint led to the identification of the gene encoding ribosomal protein S19 (*RPS19*) as the first DBA gene.[46] *RPS19* mutations have subsequently been identified in up to 25% of patients with DBA, both sporadic and familial.[34,47–51] Linkage studies have identified a possible second DBA locus on chromosome 8 in families without *RPS19* mutations, but there are also multiplex families in which DBA cosegregates with neither 8p nor 19q, showing that there must be at least three genes responsible for DBA.[52] Several studies have found that it is not possible to distinguish between patients with and without *RPS19* mutations on the basis of clinical phenotype.[34,47–51]

Pathogenesis

The typical clinical response to steroids in DBA was initially interpreted as reflecting an immune-mediated suppression of erythropoiesis, despite the general lack of efficacy of other immunosuppressive agents. However, there is no consistent *in vitro* evidence to support the existence of a humoral inhibitory agent,[53] nor of cell-mediated inhibition of erythropoiesis.[54] Observations interpreted as showing immune suppression of erythropoiesis in DBA[55–57] may in fact be attributable to transfusion-related alloimmunization.

The primary pathophysiology of DBA is now generally accepted to be due to an intrinsic defect in erythropoiesis. Strong support for this comes from the demonstration of impaired erythroid differentiation *in vitro* of enriched erythroid progenitor cells[58] and of purified CD34[+] cells[59] from patients with DBA. The success of stem cell transplantation in DBA[60] provides additional *in vivo* evidence for an intrinsic defect. Further important supportive evidence comes from the partial correction of the *in vitro* abnormality in erythroid maturation and proliferation by the induced expression of the wild-type *RPS19* gene in CD34[+] cells carrying an *RPS19* mutation.[61,62]

The timing and molecular basis of the erythroid defect have not yet been fully defined. Short-term erythroid colony assays have revealed a variable deficiency in burst-forming unit erythroid (BFU-E) and colony-forming unit erythroid (CFU-E)[63] in DBA,[53,64–66] with partial correction *in vitro* in response to IL-3 and to stem cell factor (kit ligand; SCF).[67–71] However, the *in vitro* response to IL-3 did not correlate with clinical efficacy in subsequent trials of recombinant IL-3.[72–75] In a two-phase liquid erythroid culture system,[76] it was observed that the pre-erythropoietin stage of erythroid commitment was intact,[77] while the erythropoietin-dependent phase of erythroid expansion and maturation was defective.

This could be partially corrected by steroids, although again with poor *in vivo–in vitro* correlation.[77]

RPS19 mutations might cause DBA by an effect on ribosomal function, whether by a global effect on translation, or by a more selective influence on the translation of a critical protein.[78] However, there is also increasing evidence that ribosomal proteins may also have extraribosomal functions.[79] The future identification of the gene responsible for linkage to 8p[52] will be an important step in the elucidation of the role of *RPS19* mutations in the as yet elusive pathogenesis of DBA.

Treatment

Steroids

Steroids remain the mainstay of treatment in DBA more than half a century after the original report of their efficacy.[80] Prednisolone is usually started at a dose of 2 mg/kg, to which up to 70% of patients show a good initial response in that they achieve transfusion-independence (Fig. 2.2).[4–6,13,19] An increase in reticulocytes is usually seen within 2 weeks, but a rise in hemoglobin may take up to 1 month. In some other cases, a transient reticulocytosis is seen, but transfusion-independence is not achieved.

In responders, the dose may then be gradually tapered to determine the minimum alternate-day dosage required for continuing transfusion independence. Hemoglobin levels of 8–9 g/dL are often the highest that can be achieved, but may be acceptable provided that growth and normal activity are not compromised. Macrocytosis and markers of fetal erythropoiesis generally persist during response to treatment.[4,19] The maintenance dose of prednisolone in steroid responders is highly variable, some children requiring extremely small doses. Steroids may be stopped completely in some cases, although there is usually a persistent mild macrocytic anemia with raised eADA activity. Steroid-independent remission with completely normal hematologic parameters including normal eADA suggests the original diagnosis may have been TEC rather than DBA.

Steroid therapy may have to be discontinued in responders

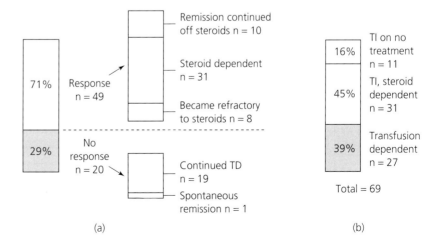

Fig. 2.2 Initial response to steroids (a) and subsequent treatment status (b) of 69 children with Diamond–Blackfan anemia born in the UK over the 20-year period 1975–1994.[4] TI, transfusion independent; TD, transfusion dependent.

in the presence of unacceptable side-effects, including growth suppression. Growth curves should be closely monitored, especially during periods of high growth velocity in infants and at puberty. A growth plateau may indicate that steroids should be interrupted and substituted with a short-term transfusion program. In babies, the need for relatively high doses and prolonged duration of steroid therapy should be balanced against the possible detrimental effect on growth and motor developmental milestones. It may be preferable to wait until the patient has reached the age of one year before initiating steroids. Delaying steroid therapy has the additional advantage of allowing immunization against chicken pox, which otherwise carries a risk of serious and potentially fatal complications as a consequence of long-term steroid therapy started before natural immunity has developed. Active immunization with attenuated varicella vaccine may be considered,[81] although varicella vaccine is not currently licensed in the UK. If the child is not immune, families should be advised to seek urgent medical attention following exposure to chickenpox, for treatment with aciclovir and/or varicella-zoster immunoglobulin.

Transfusion program

Of children and adults with DBA, 40–50% are dependent on long-term transfusion programs (Fig. 2.2), having failed to respond to steroids, having become refractory, or because of unacceptable steroid side-effects.[4–6,13,19] An immunization program against hepatitis B should therefore be initiated as soon as possible after diagnosis. Chelation therapy forms an essential part of a long-term transfusion program as iron overload contributes significantly to morbidity and mortality in this patient group (see Chapter 13).[5,15] Transfusion programs may also be associated with problems of venous access; two deaths reported by the French registry,[5] and one in the UK,[4] have been attributed to sepsis of indwelling central venous lines.

Megadose methylprednisolone

There have been anecdotal reports of response to extremely high doses of methylprednisolone in DBA.[82,83] However, a prospective study of oral megadose (100 mg/kg) methylprednisolone failed to demonstrate a clinically significant benefit.[84] The low chance of response and the significant risk of side-effects, including serious infection, preclude the routine use of megadose steroids in children who fail to respond to conventional doses.

Interleukin-3

Clinical trials of interleukin-3 (IL-3)[72–75] were prompted by the finding that IL-3 can enhance *in vitro* erythropoiesis. Combined results from 77 patients reported in the literature revealed a disappointingly low response rate of only 11%,[75] although IL-3 and steroid-independent remission persisted for longer than 3 years in at least two patients.[72,75] Further trials of IL-3 have not been attempted in view of the low chance of response, difficulties in obtaining recombinant IL-3 for clinical use, and increasing recognition of the long-term risk of acute myeloid leukemia (AML) in DBA.[15,85,86] Treatment with stem cell factor has not been attempted, despite an often striking *in vitro* response,[67–71] for similar reasons.

Prolactin

Pregnancy or the oral contraceptive pill may exacerbate the anemia of DBA,[10,11] and transfusions may be required during pregnancy in women who are normally steroid responsive. However, the anemia in one woman was found to remit during late pregnancy and for the duration of breastfeeding, a pattern suggestive of a prolactin effect.[87] She subsequently responded to metoclopramide, which had been selected because of its known side-effect of hyperprolactinemia. A pilot study suggested potential benefit of metoclopramide in a proportion of patients with DBA,[87] a finding which is being further tested in larger scale clinical trials.

Other therapies

Ciclosporin (cyclosporin),[88] erythropoietin,[89,90] intravenous immunoglobulin,[91] androgens or splenectomy have been used with some reports of success in anecdotal cases, but without consistent evidence of benefit. Prior splenectomy or androgen therapy were in fact associated with significantly worse survival in a follow-up study of patients treated at a single center over a 60-year period.[15] Splenectomy may still be indicated in the event of an increased transfusion requirement secondary to hypersplenism.

Spontaneous remission

The 20–30% incidence of "spontaneous remission" described in the literature includes individuals who require no therapy following an initial response to steroids,[4] and who probably represent the milder end of the phenotypic spectrum of DBA.[33,34] However, true spontaneous remission may occur in severe cases of DBA, even following several years of transfusion-dependence, albeit with persistent macrocytosis and high eADA. The true incidence is not known, but the UK Registry includes only one unequivocal example.

Bone marrow transplantation

Bone marrow transplantation (BMT) is potentially curative in DBA,[60,92–96] with 75–85% long-term survival reported following matched sibling donor BMT,[60,95,96] including successful outcome from cord-blood transplant.[97] BMT can therefore be considered an option for transfusion-dependent patients where there is a suitable donor, although BMT from other than matched sib donors carries a worse prognosis, and is not currently recommended.[60] The chance that a spontaneous remission may occur in DBA often influences the decision to undertake BMT in an individual case, but against this must be balanced the increased long-term risk of AML,[15,85,86] which is still apparent after spontaneous remission.[15] Risk stratification for BMT in thalassemia, which is significantly influenced by the degree of iron overload,[98] is probably equally applicable to DBA.

The existence of a mild or clinically silent DBA carrier phenotype[33,34] in the donor presents a particular hazard in sibling donor transplants,[99,100] unless the proband has an *RPS19* mutation, for which the donor can be tested. As a minimum, a potential family donor should be confirmed to have normal hemoglobin and MCV, and normal eADA activity, including the new baby in the case of sibling cord-blood transplantation.

Prognosis

Many adults with DBA who are stable on small doses of steroids or who achieve spontaneous remission are often lost to follow-up, and representative data on long-term prognosis are hard to collate. Prospective data derived from national registries will be particularly valuable in this context.

Janov *et al.*[15] analyzed 76 patients with DBA seen at Boston Children's Hospital over a 60-year period. The median survival for the entire group was 38 years, with a significantly worse prognosis for those treated before the routine use of steroids in 1960. Many deaths were directly or indirectly attributable to iron overload, a finding echoed in the data from the French DBA registry,[5] underscoring the need for adequate chelation in this group. AML developed in 4 of 76 of the Boston patients, 1 of whom had previously received radiotherapy, and a further patient developed aplastic anemia.[15] Aplastic anemia has also been reported in 2 of 132 French patients,[5] and neutropenia and thrombocytopenia are relatively common after the first decade.[25] There is thus evidence for progressive hemopoietic stem cell dysfunction, which is also reflected in the reduced *in vitro* cloning efficiency of myeloid progenitors in DBA with increasing patient age.[24] These long-term marrow complications further endorse the use of stem cell transplantation in this patient group.

Patients with DBA are probably also at increased risk of developing nonhemopoietic malignancies.[6,101–104] In particular, there have been reports of osteogenic sarcoma occurring at an unusually young age,[6,104] although determination of the actuarial risk will depend on representative population-based data generated by DBA registries.[6]

Transient erythroblastopenia of childhood

Transient erythroblastopenia of childhood (TEC) is an acquired, self-limiting red cell aplasia unique to childhood, which was recognized as a clinical entity in 1970.[105,106] One regional study in the UK of red cell aplasia in childhood over a 7-year period suggests an incidence of 5 per million per year.[107]

Clinical features

The usual presentation is a previously fit child up to the age of 5 years, with gradual onset of symptoms of anemia. The commonest age at presentation is 2 years, but TEC has also been described in infants under the age of 6 months.[108,109] TEC thus tends to present in an older age group than DBA, although there is some overlap. Boys and girls are equally affected, and there is no ethnic predominance. Unlike DBA, there are no associated physical anomalies, and affected children are generally of normal stature.[110] Transient neurologic abnormalities, including seizures and hemiparesis, have occasionally been described in association with otherwise typical TEC.[111–113]

Hematologic findings

The anemia of TEC is normochromic and normocytic and is characterized by reticulocytopenia, although macrocytosis may occur during recovery, and reticulocytosis may be noted if recovery has already started by the time of presentation. In one study, more than 25% of children with TEC were already in the recovery phase at the time of presentation.[114] Raised levels of HbF and expression of i antigen have been reported during recovery,[27] but eADA levels should be normal.[115]

There is a high incidence of neutropenia in TEC. In one study of 50 patients, 64% had a neutrophil count below $1.5 \times 10^9/L$, and in 28% this was below $1.0 \times 10^9/L$.[114] The platelet count is usually normal, although thrombocytopenia has been documented in some cases of TEC following parvovirus infection.[116,117]

Bone marrow examination reveals a normocellular marrow with erythroid hypoplasia; the presence of left-shifted erythropoiesis with apparent maturation arrest suggests early recovery. Myeloid maturation appears normal, despite the frequent association with neutropenia.

Serum lactate dehydrogenase, bilirubin and serum haptoglobin levels are normal in TEC. If there is evidence of hemolysis, the alternative diagnosis of an acute aplastic crisis on the background of a previously unrecognized hemolytic anemia should be considered.

Red cell enzyme activities tend to be low at the nadir of TEC,[118,119] consistent with an older red cell population in the absence of new red cell production. Similarly, glycosylated hemoglobin (HbA$_{1c}$) is likely to be raised.[120] It should be remarked that HbA1c levels will be influenced by recent transfusions. Although these tests might theoretically aid discrimination between acute erythroblastopenia and chronic hypoplastic anemia, in practice it is seldom necessary to do more than the basic investigations.

Etiology and pathophysiology

Many children give a history of an antecedent viral infection, and there have been varying reports of seasonality in TEC,[121,122] but no consistent pattern has emerged. Although viral serology may reveal evidence of recent infection, for example echovirus,[123] adenovirus or parainfluenza,[107] no specific candidate agent has been implicated. These findings do not suggest a direct viral etiology for TEC and are more consistent with a postviral process, presumably immune-mediated, analogous to childhood idiopathic thrombocytopenic purpura (ITP).[124] This is supported by *in vitro* culture results. Erythroid colony numbers may be normal or reduced, and serum inhibitors of erythroid colony formation have been detected in a high proportion of cases of TEC.[125–127] Cell-mediated suppression of erythroid colony formation has also been reported.[127,128]

Treatment and prognosis

Spontaneous, complete recovery of TEC usually occurs within 4–8 weeks of presentation and recurrence is rare.[129] A peak reticulocyte response is usually seen within a month of presentation, and some children will already have entered the recovery phase at the time of diagnosis.[114] A raised MCV and increased red cell distribution width (RDW) accompany the reticulocytosis, but after recovery the steady-state hemoglobin and red cell indices are normal. Any associated neutropenia also resolves and no complications due to infection have been reported. All reported cases with neurologic abnormalities recovered fully, with no neurologic sequelae.

Transfusion may be necessary at the nadir of TEC, but the decision to transfuse should be made on clinical grounds, rather than the hemoglobin level, given the gradual onset of anemia and predicted early recovery. There is no indication to treat TEC with steroids or intravenous immunoglobulin.

Differential diagnosis of TEC

Parvovirus infection
There is usually no serologic evidence of recent infection with parvovirus B19.[114] However, occasional cases of a TEC-like hypoplastic anemia have been reported following parvovirus infection. These tend to differ a little from typical TEC in that both thrombocytopenia and neutropenia may occur and the marrow may be hypocellular.[116,117] The pathogenesis of parvovirus-associated TEC might reflect direct marrow suppression, equivalent to the acute aplastic crisis of chronic hemolytic anemias, rather than sharing the probable immune-mediated process underlying TEC that follows other viral infections. Certainly, parvoviral infection of hematologically normal volunteers causes neutropenia and thrombocytopenia as well as reticulocytopenia.[130]

DBA spectrum
Transient anemia in childhood may be the only clinical manifestation of DBA in some individuals, as observed in families with incomplete penetrance and variable phenotype,[33,34] although eADA activity is usually persistently raised. This

may provide one explanation for the occurrence of TEC in more than one sibling,[131–133] which may otherwise be the effect of clustering.

Parvovirus-associated acute acquired red cell aplasia (aplastic crisis)

Transient erythroid hypoplasia caused by parvovirus infection underlies the aplastic crisis that may occur in hemolytic anemias, first recognized in association with hereditary spherocytosis (HS).[134] The presentation is usually that of an acute onset of symptoms of anemia in a child with a pre-existing hemolytic anemia, often with a febrile illness during the preceding week, but without exacerbation of jaundice. The duration of reticulocytopenia is generally 7–10 days, and this resolves with the emergence of an antibody response. Children are infectious during this time and therefore represent a risk to other children with hematologic or immunologic abnormalities. The risk to staff, especially early in pregnancy, should also be considered.[135]

Etiology and pathogenesis

An infectious etiology for the aplastic crisis in patients with an underlying hemolytic process was inferred from clustering of cases. The realization that the illness has a relatively well-defined pattern and usually occurs only once in each individual, suggested that a single infectious agent was largely responsible. Parvovirus B19 was first discovered in the serum of normal blood donors,[136] and was subsequently linked to aplastic crisis in sickle-cell anemia.[137,138] Although the majority of aplastic crises are attributable to parvovirus, in a small percentage of cases there is no evidence of B19 infection[139] and other infections may be responsible.

The red cell aplasia associated with parvovirus is the result of direct viral infection of the erythroid progenitor cell. The tropism of parvovirus B19 for erythroid cells, at all stages of maturation,[140] is explained by the identification of the erythrocyte P antigen (globoside) as the parvovirus receptor.[141] The virus inhibits erythroid colony formation,[142] and is cytotoxic for erythroid progenitor cells at the colony-forming unit erythroid (CFU-E) stage *in vitro*.[143]

Any event leading to an interruption of erythropoiesis, however short, is likely to cause profound anemia in the presence of a shortened red cell lifespan. Thus a precipitous, potentially fatal fall in hemoglobin may be sustained by children with a severe underlying hemolytic process, such as homozygous sickle-cell disease, in which the steady-state hemoglobin may be as low as 6–7 g/dL despite massive erythroid expansion. Alternatively, a period of erythroid hypoplasia may induce anemia on a background of otherwise well-compensated hemolysis, as in mild HS, and can be the event leading to the diagnosis of the hematologic disorder. The transient anemia is usually clinically inapparent when the red cell lifespan is normal.[144] However, parvovirus-induced acute exacerbation of anemia may also occur in nonhemolytic anemias, including iron deficiency,[145] and has been described in a patient with DBA.[146]

Hematologic features

The aplastic crisis is characterized by a decrease in hemoglobin in association with reticulocytopenia, but neutropenia and thrombocytopenia may also occur. Bone marrow aspirate, although rarely required for diagnosis, shows erythroid hypoplasia, often with characteristic giant basophilic proerythroblasts, which are up to 100 μm in diameter with prominent nucleoli.

Chronic parvovirus B19 infection

Parvovirus B19 infection in the absence of an effective antiviral immune response may cause prolonged rather than transient red cell aplasia.[147–152] This has been described in association with AIDS,[150] as well as in children with congenital immune deficiency disorders.[151] Hemophiliacs who are HIV-positive may be particularly vulnerable as parvovirus can persist in factor concentrates despite solvent-detergent treatment.[153] Severe chronic anemia may also result from parvovirus infection in children receiving chronic immunosuppressive therapy, including chemotherapy for acute lymphoblastic leukemia (ALL).[152] Chronic parvovirus infection may occur in the absence of other evidence for an immunocompromised state,[154] and should be considered as a cause of chronic acquired red cell aplasia even in the absence of other evidence for immune deficiency. Bone marrow aspirate may reveal the giant typical pronormoblasts. Viral serology is unreliable in the diagnosis of parvovirus-induced chronic red cell aplasia, as affected patients often fail to mount an antibody response.[149] The diagnosis may be confirmed by direct detection of parvovirus DNA in serum or bone marrow.[155]

Intravenous immunoglobulin can be effective in decreasing parvoviremia and restoring bone marrow erythroid activity,[156] although repeated courses may be necessary.

Chronic acquired red cell aplasia

Chronic acquired pure red cell aplasia (PRCA) is rare in children; in a regional study of 33 children with red cell aplasia, none had "adult-type" PRCA.[107] However, it should be considered, especially in older children without features of DBA, and in whom chronic parvoviremia has been excluded. When a diagnosis of PRCA is considered, appropriate investigations should be undertaken to exclude any underlying cause.

Chronic PRCA may be idiopathic in both children and adults, or associated with autoimmune, viral and neoplastic disorders, including acute lymphoblastic leukemia[157] and juvenile chronic arthritis.[158] Despite the classical association,[159] thymoma is relatively rare.[160] Many drugs have been associated with PRCA;[161] among those with particular relevance to pediatric practice are carbamazepine,[162,163] phenytoin,[164] and sodium valproate.[165] Resolution of the anemia usually follows withdrawal of the relevant drug.

The pathogenesis of chronic acquired PRCA is likely to be autoimmune. Both antibody-mediated[166,167] and cell-mediated[168–170] mechanisms of erythroid suppression have been demonstrated.[171] Red cell aplasia has been reported in some patients treated with recombinant human erythropoietin (epoetin), secondary to the development of antiepoetin antibodies, which cross-react with and thus neutralize endogenous erythropoietin.[172–175] This should be considered as a possible cause of PRCA, especially in children with chronic renal failure. Withdrawal of epoetin is not sufficient in this context, and immunosuppressive therapy is usually necessary.

Treatment of chronic PRCA is thus directed at the underlying cause, with the use of immunosuppression where appropriate. In idiopathic chronic PRCA the remission rate with steroids is of the order of 40%.[160] Ciclosporin and other forms of immunosuppressive therapy may be effective in patients who fail to respond to steroids.[160,176] The demonstration of normal colonies in clonogenic assays *in vitro* may be predictive of clinical response.[177,178] Plasmapheresis has been found to be effective in some cases,[179] providing further evidence for humoral-mediated suppression of erythropoiesis.

Differential diagnosis of red cell aplasia in childhood

DBA vs. TEC

Despite the difference in their typical age of onset of anemia, TEC may occur in the first year of life,[108,109] and DBA may present later than infancy.[4,33,34] The distinction between TEC and sporadic DBA is straightforward in the presence of a positive family history or characteristic physical anomalies, or if there is an *RPS19* mutation. Neutropenia at presentation is more consistent with a diagnosis of TEC.[114] Measurement of red cell ADA levels may be helpful, and persistence of anemia and macrocytosis in remission also favor the diagnosis of DBA,[118] although fetal characteristics of erythropoiesis in the form of raised MCV, high HbF and i antigen expression may also occur during the recovery phase of TEC.[27] When there is doubt it may be appropriate simply to observe the patient for a few months, rather than starting steroids immediately, as a response to steroids may be coincidental with the recovery of TEC, or reflect the likely immune-mediated red cell aplasia in TEC. A firm diagnosis of TEC is often only made retrospectively, after recovery of a normal blood count and normal red cell indices.

DBA vs. parvovirus B19

Parvovirus infection during pregnancy is associated with hydrops fetalis at all gestational ages,[180] while hydrops is a very rare presentation of DBA.[7–9] In addition, physical anomalies are an unlikely consequence of intrauterine parvovirus infection.[181] However, parvovirus infection should be excluded in a new case of presumed DBA by viral serology (IgM and IgG) in both mother and infant. As chronic red cell aplasia is more likely in the absence of an effective immune response to parvovirus,[149] polymerase chain reaction (PCR) amplification of viral nucleic acid from presentation bone marrow should also be performed.

DBA vs. chronic acquired PRCA

The distinction between late-presenting DBA and chronic acquired PRCA may be difficult in the absence of physical anomalies or a positive family history. Both may be associated with macrocytosis, but raised eADA activity would favor a diagnosis of DBA.

DBA vs. alloimmune erythroid hypoplasia

Maternal anti-Kell alloimmunization may result in profound fetal anemia, but with relative reticulocytopenia,[182] consistent with erythroid progenitor suppression.[183,184] This is analogous to the pure red cell aplasia that may occur after ABO-incompatible bone marrow transplantation, and which is probably mediated by residual recipient isohemagglutinins.[171,185] Maternal and infant blood group serology should therefore be included in the investigation of babies with presumed DBA who are anemic at birth.

DBA vs. other congenital syndromes of marrow failure
(see Chapter 3)

DBA and Fanconi anemia have an overlapping spectrum of physical anomalies,[186] and macrocytic anemia may be an early hematologic manifestation of Fanconi anemia.[187] In practice, the distinction is rarely difficult and is resolved by the demonstration of increased chromosome breakages in response to clastogenic agents in Fanconi anemia.[188] Neutropenia is a more consistent hematologic finding than anemia in children with Shwachman–Diamond syndrome, who will also have evidence of exocrine pancreatic dysfunction. The majority of patients with Shwachman–Diamond syndrome have mutations affecting the *SBDS* gene.[189,190] *SBDS* mutation analysis may therefore be useful in cases of uncertainty.

Congenital dyserythropoietic anemias

The congenital dyserythropoietic anemias (CDAs) are uncommon hereditary disorders of erythropoiesis in which there is chronic mild-to-moderate anemia on a background of erythroid hyperplasia and ineffective erythropoiesis,[191] associated with characteristic morphologic changes in the bone marrow.[192,193] The CDAs have been classified into three main types based on morphologic and serologic findings,[194,195] but there is clearly heterogeneity within the types, and many individual cases of CDA have been reported that do not fit into this classification.[193,195]

The ineffective erythropoiesis in CDAs is associated with intramedullary destruction of red cell precursors, with elevation of the serum bilirubin and lactic dehydrogenase (LDH). The serum haptoglobin is usually reduced. There is a marked tendency to increased iron absorption,[196] the consequence of expanded erythropoiesis, which can lead to iron overload and organ damage. Soluble transferrin receptor levels are likely to be raised, in the absence of iron deficiency, reflecting the degree of erythroid expansion in the presence of ineffective erythropoiesis.[197,198]

The management of an individual patient depends on the CDA subtype, the degree of anemia and the extent of iron loading. The majority of cases of CDA have a benign course, but severe variants may present as hydrops fetalis or neonatal jaundice and require exchange transfusion. In common with other disorders of red cell production, patients with even relatively mild CDA are susceptible to parvovirus-induced aplastic crisis.

The clinical and laboratory findings characterizing the three main types of CDA are described below and are summarized in Table 2.2.

Congenital dyserythropoietic anemia type I (CDA I)

Clinical features

There is usually mild anemia with slight icterus and a palpable spleen,[199,200] which may slowly enlarge with increasing age. Physical anomalies may be present, most typically in the form of skeletal abnormalities affecting the hands or feet, with syndactyly and absence of distal phalanges and nails.[201,202] Neurologic abnormalities have also been described.[203] Significant iron loading may occur, even in the presence of only mild anemia, and there is an increased risk of gallstones.

Laboratory findings

The hemoglobin is usually between 8 and 11 g/dL, but milder or more anemic cases may be seen. There is macrocytosis (MCV 95–120 fL), with striking anisocytosis and poikilocytosis on the blood film. Reticulocytes are reduced in number for the degree of anemia. Cabot rings, a thin circle of nuclear remnant within the circulating red cells that stains purple with Romanowsky stains, may be seen in CDA I, most conspicuously in splenectomized patients.[204,205] White cells

Table 2.2 Comparison of the three main types of congenital dyserythropoietic anemia

	CDA I	CDA II (HEMPAS)	CDA III
Inheritance	Autosomal recessive	Autosomal recessive	Autosomal dominant
Gene	*CDAN1* (15q)	Linkage to 20q, but genetic heterogeneity	Linkage to 15q in Swedish kindred
Associated anomalies	Syndactyly, absent distal phalanges, neurologic abnormalities	Uncommon, variable learning difficulties	Monoclonal gammopathies, retinal abnormalities
Anemia	Mild to moderate	Mild to moderate	Mild
Iron loading	High risk	High risk	Unusual
MCV	Increased	Slight increase	Normal or mild increase
Bilirubin	Increased	Increased	Normal or mild increase
Bone marrow morphology	Megaloblastic changes affecting early and late erythroblasts Internuclear bridging	Multinuclearity of intermediate and late erythroblasts	Gigantoblasts
Electron microscopy	Spongy chromatin ("Swiss cheese" appearance) Invagination of cytoplasm into nuclear region	Cisternae and "double membrane"	Nuclear clefts Autolytic areas in cytoplasm
Acidified serum lysis	Negative	Positive (selected sera)	Negative
Anti-i reaction	Negative	++	Variable
Treatment	α-Interferon, prevention of iron overload	Splenectomy, prevention of iron overload	Screen for monoclonal gammopathy, ophthalmic review

and platelets are normal in number, morphology and function. Unconjugated bilirubin is elevated, usually 2–3 times normal, and serum LDH is raised.[200] The acidified serum lysis test is negative and the expression of i and I antigens on the red cell surface is within the normal adult range. HbF levels are usually within the normal range or only slightly raised (0.5–2.0%), although occasional individuals with higher levels (up to 6.0%) may be found.

The characteristic features of CDA I are apparent on the bone marrow aspirate, which is generally hypercellular with erythroid hyperplasia. Both early and late erythroblasts are characterized by anomalies of nuclear division with, most characteristically, incompletely separated normoblasts connected by an internuclear bridge.[206] Abnormalities of nuclear chromatin condensation may make the erythropoietic changes appear megaloblastic, but giant myeloid cells and hyperlobulated megakaryocytes are absent. Iron staining may show increased storage iron and sideroblasts, but ringed sideroblasts are not a usual feature of CDA I.[196]

Electron microscopy

Electron microscopy of erythroblasts in CDA I typically shows a spongy appearance of heterochromatin (so-called "Swiss cheese" appearance), increased nuclear pore size and invaginations of the nucleus resulting in cytoplasm with some hemoglobin intruding into the nuclear region. These changes are not apparent in very early erythroblasts.[206,207]

Inheritance and genetics

CDA I is inherited as an autosomal recessive disorder.[199,208] The gene responsible for CDA I in a large Bedouin kindred was localized to chromosome 15,[208] 20 and subsequently identified as *CDAN1*.[209] Mutations affecting *CDAN1* have also been identified in unrelated CDA I patients. *CDAN1* encodes codanin-1, but its function and role in normal erythropoiesis and in the pathogenesis of CDA I have yet to be elucidated.

Management of CDA I

The majority of patients with CDA I have a mild anemia, which requires no specific treatment. However, progressive iron loading can occur, even in patients who are transfusion-independent, and regular monitoring is essential. Chelation therapy may be indicated.

Occasionally, patients may become more anemic as they get older, possibly because of progressive enlargement of the spleen and pooling of red cells. Splenectomy has been successful in ameliorating the anemia in some of these patients, but it is not generally recommended in CDA I.

Interferon-α (IFN-α) was found by chance to improve the anemia in a patient with CDA I being treated for transfusion-acquired hepatitis C infection. Erythrokinetic studies demonstrated a reduction of the ineffective erythropoiesis, and there was an improvement in the morphologic abnormalities seen on electron microscopy.[210] IFN-α has subsequently been used with beneficial effect in other cases of CDA I,[211] with no apparent loss of effect on prolonged treatment.[212] It is not clear whether IFN-α therapy might also prevent iron loading in nonanemic patients with CDA I. While IFN-α has been used successfully to treat severe CDA I presenting in infancy,[213] there remain concerns about neurologic side-effects, especially in very young children.[214,219] The mechanism of action of IFN-α in this context is not known, although lymphoblastoid cell lines generated from patients with CDA I, but not other types of CDA, have been shown to produce low levels of IFN-α.[220]

Congenital dyserythropoietic anemia type II

Clinical features

CDA II, or hereditary erythroblastic multinuclearity with positive acidified serum test (HEMPAS),[221] is commoner than CDA I, and has been described in most ethnic groups. Associated physical abnormalities may be present, although less common than in CDA I. Learning difficulties probably represent the most consistently reported nonhematologic manifestations.[222] There is a broad spectrum in the clinical presentation of CDA II. The majority of patients have mild-to-moderate anemia with jaundice and splenomegaly.

Like hereditary spherocytosis,[223,224] the anemia of CDA II is more severe in infancy. Anemia is present from birth in 23% of affected babies, and neonatal jaundice to the extent of requiring treatment is common. Over 30% of patients reported to the International CDA II Registry required transfusions during the first year of life, although only 5 of 88 remained transfusion dependent.[225] Severely affected children may have considerable medullary hyperplasia leading to facial deformities, analogous to those seen in β-thalassemia. Extramedullary hemopoiesis may occasionally occur.[222] In less severely affected individuals, jaundice may be the only clinical finding. Gallstones are common, presenting at a young age.[222] Of the different types of CDA, CDA II carries the highest risk of iron overload, with liver cirrhosis, diabetes and cardiac failure in later life.[226,227]

Inheritance and genetics

CDA II is also inherited as an autosomal recessive disorder,[208,221,228] but the gene or genes responsible have not yet been identified. Linkage analysis identified a putative locus on chromosome 20 in families from southern Italy,[229] but there is likely to be genetic heterogeneity.[230]

Laboratory findings

There is wide variation in the degree of anemia, both between different families and between siblings. The MCV is normal or slightly increased. The reticulocyte count is usually normal, or may be modestly raised. The blood film usually shows red cell anisocytosis, acanthocytes and basophilic stippling, and there may be occasional circulating binucleate normoblasts.

Unconjugated bilirubin is raised, and serum haptoglobin levels are low or undetectable. Impaired liver function tests may be secondary to cholelithiasis, or to hepatic iron loading. Serum ferritin levels increase with age, although with considerable individual variation. In a longitudinal study of 48 patients, the mean age at initiation of chelation therapy was 20 years (range 7 to 35 years).[222]

The characteristic feature of the red cells in CDA II, which gives the syndrome its acronym HEMPAS, is their lysis by acidified serum from some but not all normal individuals. The patient's own serum will not cause lysis, which helps to distinguish the syndrome from paroxysmal nocturnal hemoglobinuria. The test is also negative with sera from obligate heterozygotes.[231,232] It is thought that CDA II cells express an abnormal antigen to which approximately 40% of normal sera contain a complement-fixing IgM antibody, but the nature of this antigen has not been determined. CDA II red cells may also have abnormal complement activation control.[233]

CDA II red cells are strongly agglutinated by anti-i sera, even in adult life; I antigen is expressed normally.[221,232]

There are characteristic morphologic features of CDA II on bone marrow aspirate. There is erythroid hyperplasia, with binuclearity or multinuclearity affecting intermediate and late erythroblasts, the nuclei being equal in size and DNA content. Pseudo-Gaucher macrophages may be observed.[222]

Electron microscopy

Electron microscopy reveals a characteristic double membrane effect, caused by a linear structure running parallel to the plasma membrane, caused by residual endoplasmic reticulum.[234,235] Such changes are not unique to CDA type II, and may be seen to a lesser extent in other hemoglobinopathies.[236]

Pathogenesis

The underlying defect in CDA II is a failure of normal glycosylation of membrane proteins,[237] particularly band 3, the anion channel of the red cell. Polyacrylamide gel electrophoresis (PAGE) has shown that band 3 protein from CDA II red cells migrates faster than normal,[238,239] the reduction in molecular weight being the result of loss of glycosyl residues rather than an abnormal protein.[237] In CDA II there is a clustering of band 3 compared with the normal even distribution of the fully glycosylated protein.[240] Other membrane proteins, including band 4.5, and some plasma proteins, such as transferrin, are also underglycosylated. The primary molecular defect in CDA II is unknown.[241] There is no linkage with genes encoding common glycosylation enzymes.[242,243] Heterozygotes may also show evidence of abnormal glycosylation.[244]

Treatment

The management of CDA II depends upon the severity of anemia and the degree of iron overload. Splenectomy increases the hemoglobin in CDA II,[222,225] by reducing peripheral hemolysis.[191] However, splenectomy does not modulate the ineffective erythropoiesis of CDA II,[191] and consequently does not prevent iron loading.[222,225] The major indication for splenectomy is therefore to prevent transfusion dependence in severely anemic patients. Splenectomy has also been used to increase the hematocrit to a level that allows regular phlebotomy to facilitate the management of iron overload.

Ferritin levels should be monitored regularly, and iron chelation therapy or phlebotomy should be initiated in patients who demonstrate increasing ferritin levels.

Congenital dyserythropoietic anemia type III

CDA type III[245] is the rarest of the classified syndromes, although the striking bone marrow abnormalities meant that it was the first to be recognized, initially known as familial erythroid multinuclearity.[246] It is mainly inherited as an autosomal dominant disorder although there may be families with apparently recessive inheritance.[208] The abnormal gene has been located to 15q21-q25 in a Swedish family with dominant inheritance.[247]

Clinical features

Anemia is usually mild and is accompanied by slight icterus. Splenomegaly may occur but is absent in a substantial proportion of reported cases. The condition is usually discovered in young adult life unless there is a known family history. An increased incidence of monoclonal gammopathy[248] and retinal abnormalities, including angioid streaks and macular degeneration,[249] has been reported in a large Swedish kindred with CDA III.

Hematologic findings

There is mild macrocytic anemia with red cell anisocytosis and poikilocytosis. There may be evidence of intravascular hemolysis with hemosiderinuria and absent serum haptoglobin.[248] The acidified serum lysis test is negative[248] and there is variable expression of I and i antigens.[250,251]

The bone marrow shows erythroid hyperplasia with striking multinuclearity of the erythroblasts (up to 12 nuclei) in a single cell producing so-called "gigantoblasts".[195] The nuclei may be of the same or different maturity, with differing DNA content.[248,250,251] Similar appearances may occur in erythroleukemia, from which CDA type III should be differentiated.

Electron microscopy

Electron microscopy reveals nuclear clefts and autolytic areas within the cytoplasm with multiple nuclei within the cell.[252] There may be duplication of parts of the nuclear membrane.[248]

Management

The anemia in CDA III is usually mild, requiring no treatment.[245] Iron overload is unusual, despite the occurrence of ineffective erythropoiesis, probably as a consequence of intravascular hemolysis and hemosiderinuria.[248] Adult patients with CDA III should be screened for monoclonal gammopathy, and undergo regular ophthalmologic review to allow early detection and treatment[253] of neovascular changes in the retina.

Unclassified congenital dyserythropoietic anemias

A number of cases of CDA have been reported that do not fit the above classification.[193] In one family, a proband with mild anemia and multinucleated cells at all stages of erythroid differentiation had an affected child who died with hydrops fetalis.[254] There have been other reports of infants with hydrops fetalis and unusual types of CDA;[255,256] in most cases there was a history of previous neonatal deaths with hydrops or multiple abortions.[255] Possible explanations for such severe cases include double heterozygosity or homozygosity for autosomal dominant forms of CDA, new subtypes of CDA, or the coinheritance of other genetic modifiers of severity. Identification of the genes responsible for CDA II and CDA III will help to elucidate such cases, and facilitate further subclassification. The management of unclassified CDAs includes treatment of anemia, iron loading and gallstones, as for the main CDA types. In addition, bone marrow transplantation may be considered for severely affected children.[257,258]

Modifiers of severity in congenital dyserythropoietic anemia

Unbalanced globin chain synthesis with the formation of inclusion bodies containing precipitated globin chains may variably occur in the different types of CDA.[259–262] This provides a possible explanation for the finding that the coexistence of thalassemia trait may exacerbate the ineffective erythropoiesis of CDA II.[258] Gilbert syndrome has been identified as another potential genetic modifier of the severity of CDA II, the degree of hyperbilirubinemia being influenced by differences in the expression of uridine diphosphate glucuronosyl transferase.[263] It is not yet clear whether mutations associated with excess iron absorption in hereditary hemochromatosis influence the extent of iron loading in CDAs, as has been suggested in β-thalassemia trait.[264–266] Conversely, the severity of CDA may be ameliorated in other cases by as yet unidentified factors.[267]

Differential diagnosis of congenital dyserythropoietic anemia

It is important to make the diagnosis of CDA because of the risk of significant iron loading even in the presence of only mild anemia. CDA should be considered in any patient with evidence of a congenital anemia with raised bilirubin and reduced serum haptoglobin, especially in the presence of an inadequate reticulocytosis and abnormal red cell morphology on the blood film. Hereditary spherocytosis is the likeliest misdiagnosis in patients with CDA II,[225,268] based on clinical and laboratory similarities between the two disorders, including improvement in anemia after splenectomy. This carries the risk that evolving iron loading remains undetected until significant hemochromatosis has developed.[269,270]

The CDAs need to be distinguished from other congenital hemolytic anemias associated with ineffective erythropoiesis, notably β-thalassemia intermedia, especially if there is a reduced MCV, an uncommon finding in the CDAs.[193] Folate and vitamin B_{12} deficiency should be excluded in all age groups.

The mildness of the anemia in CDA may delay diagnosis until adolescence or adulthood when additional demands on hemopoiesis may produce symptomatic anemia, in which case the differential diagnosis will also include megaloblastic anemia, myelodysplasia and erythroleukemia (FAB M6).

> ### Key points
>
> **Differential diagnosis of chronic red cell aplasia in children**
>
> - Congenital red cell aplasia (Diamond–Blackfan anemia)
> - Chronic parvovirus B19 viremia
> - Immune-mediated pure red cell aplasia
> - Other congenital syndromes of bone marrow failure
>
> **Differential diagnosis of red cell aplasia in infancy**
>
> - Congenital red cell aplasia (Diamond–Blackfan anemia)
> - Early presentation of transient erythroblastopenia of childhood
> - Congenital parvovirus B19 infection
> - Alloimmune erythroid hypoplasia (maternal anti-Kell)
>
> **Practice point**
>
> Bone marrow transplant in Diamond–Blackfan anemia:
> - It is essential to exclude subclinical or mild DBA in sibling donors
>
> **Practice point**
>
> Iron loading in congenital dyserythropoietic anemias:
> - Iron overload caused by ineffective erythropoiesis can occur even in mild anemia
> - Splenectomy improves anemia in CDA II, but does not reduce iron loading

References

1. Josephs HW. Anaemia of infancy and early childhood. *Medicine* 1936; **15**: 307–451.
2. Diamond LK, Blackfan KD. Hypoplastic anaemia. *Am J Dis Child* 1938; **56**: 464–7.
3. Bresters D, Bruin MCA, Van Dijken PJ. Congenitale hypoplastische anemie in Nederland (1963–1989). *Tijdschrift Kindergeneeskunde* 1991; **59**: 203–10.
4. Ball SE, McGuckin CP, Jenkins G *et al.* Diamond–Blackfan anaemia in the U.K.: analysis of 80 cases from a 20-year birth cohort. *Br J Haematol* 1996; **94**: 645–53.
5. Willig TN, Niemeyer CM, Leblanc T *et al.* Identification of new prognosis factors from the clinical and epidemiologic analysis of a registry of 229 Diamond-Blackfan anemia patients. DBA group of Société d'Hematologie et d'Immunologie Pediatrique (SHIP), Gesellschaft für Padiatrische Onkologie und Hamatologie (GPOH), and the European Society for Pediatric Hematology and Immunology (ESPHI). *Pediatr Res* 1999; **46**: 553–61.
6. Vlachos A, Klein GW, Lipton JM. The Diamond Blackfan Anemia Registry: tool for investigating the epidemiology and biology of Diamond-Blackfan anemia. *J Pediatr Hematol Oncol* 2001; **23**: 377–82.
7. Van Hook JW, Gill P, Cyr D *et al.* Diamond–Blackfan anaemia as an unusual cause of nonimmune hydrops fetalis: A case report. *J Reprod Med Obstet Gynecol* 1995; **40**: 850–4.
8. Scimeca PG, Weinblatt ME, Slepowitz G, Harper RG, Kochen JA. Diamond–Blackfan syndrome: an unusual cause of hydrops fetalis. *Am J Pediatr Hematol Oncol* 1988; **10**: 241–3.
9. McLennan AC, Chitty LS, Rissik J, Maxwell DJ. Prenatal diagnosis of Blackfan–Diamond syndrome; case report and review of the literature. *Prenat Diagn* 1996; **16**: 349–53.
10. Rijhsinghani A, Wiechert RJ. Diamond–Blackfan anaemia in pregnancy. *Obstet Gynecol* 1994; **83** (suppl.): 827–9.
11. Balaban EP, Buchanan GR, Graham M, Frenkel EP. Diamond–Blackfan syndrome in adult patients. *Am J Med* 1985; **78**: 533–8.
12. Alter BP, Kumar M, Lockhart LL, Sprinz PG, Rowe TF. Pregnancy in bone marrow failure syndromes: Diamond-Blackfan anaemia and Shwachman-Diamond syndrome. *Br J Haematol* 1999; **107**: 49–54.
13. Alter, BP. Inherited bone marrow failure syndromes. In: Nathan DG, Orkin SH, Look AT, Ginsburg D (eds) *Nathan and Oski's Hematology of Infancy and Childhood*, 6th edn. Philadelphia: WB Saunders, 2003, pp. 280–365.
14. Gripp KW, McDonald-McGinn DM, La Rossa D *et al.* Bilateral microtia and cleft palate in cousins with Diamond-Blackfan anemia. *Am J Med Genet* 2001; **101**: 268–74.
15. Janov AJ, Leong T, Nathan DG *et al.* Diamond Blackfan anaemia. Natural history and sequelae of treatment. *Medicine* 1996; **75**: 77–8.

16. Alter BP. Childhood red cell aplasia. *Am J Pediatr Haematol Oncol* 1980; **2**: 121–39.

17. Cathie IAB. Erythrogenesis imperfecta. *Arch Dis Child* 1950; **25**: 313–24.

18. Aase JM, Smith DW. Congenital anaemia and triphalangeal thumbs: a new syndrome. *J Pediatr* 1969; **74**: 471–4.

19. Halperin DS, Freedman MH. Diamond–Blackfan anaemia: Etiology, pathophysiology, and treatment. *Am J Pediatr Hematol Oncol* 1989; **11**: 380–94.

20. Lanes R, Muller A, Palacios A. Multiple endocrine abnormalities in a child with Blackfan-Diamond anemia and hemochromatosis. Significant improvement of growth velocity and predicted adult height following growth hormone treatment despite liver damage. *J Pediatr Endocrinol Metab* 2000; **13**: 325–8.

21. Leblanc T, Gluckman E, Brauner R. Growth hormone deficiency caused by pituitary stalk interruption in Diamond-Blackfan anemia. *J Pediatr* 2003; **142**: 358.

22. Scott EG, Haider A, Hord J. Growth hormone therapy for short stature in Diamond Blackfan anemia. *Pediatr Blood Cancer* 2004; **43**: 542–4.

23. Santucci MA, Bagnara GP, Strippoli P *et al.* Long-term bone marrow cultures in Diamond-Blackfan anemia reveal a defect of both granulomacrophage and erythroid progenitors. *Exp Hematol* 1999; **27**: 9–18.

24. Casadevall N, Croisille L, Auffray I, Tchernia G, Coulombel L. Age related alterations in erythroid and granulopoietic progenitors in Diamond–Blackfan anaemia. *Br J Haematol* 1994; **87**: 369–75.

25. Giri N, Kang E, Tisdale JF *et al.* Clinical and laboratory evidence for a trilineage haematopoietic defect in patients with refractory Diamond-Blackfan anaemia. *Br J Haematol* 2000; **108**: 167–75.

26. Diamond LK, Wang WC, Alter BP. Congenital hypoplastic anaemia. *Adv Pediatr* 1976; **22**: 349–78.

27. Link MP, Alter BP. Fetal-like erythropoiesis during recovery from transient erythroblastopenia of childhood (TEC). *Pediatr Res* 1981; **15**: 1036–9.

28. Glader BE, Backer K. Elevated red cell adenosine deaminase activity: a marker of disordered erythropoiesis in Diamond–Blackfan anaemia and other haematologic diseases. *Br J Haematol* 1988; **68**: 165–8.

29. Whitehouse DB, Hopkinson DA, Evans DIK. Adenosine deaminase activity in Diamond–Blackfan syndrome. *Lancet* 1984; **ii**: 1398–9.

30. Filanovskaya LI, Nikitin DO, Togo AV, Blinov MN, Gavrilova LV. The activity of purine nucleotide degradation enzymes and lymphoid cell subpopulation in children with Diamond–Blackfan syndrome. *Gematologiia Transfuziologiia* 1993; **38**: 19–22.

31. Glader BE, Backer K, Diamond LK. Elevated erythrocyte adenosine deaminase activity in congenital hypoplastic anaemia. *N Engl J Med* 1983; **309**: 1486–90.

32. Whitehouse DB, Hopkinson DA, Pilz AJ, Arredondo FX. Adenosine deaminase activity in a series of 19 patients with the Diamond–Blackfan syndrome. *Adv Exp Med Biol* 1986; **195**: 85–92.

33. Willig TN, Perignon JL, Gustavsson P *et al.* High adenosine deaminase level among healthy probands of Diamond Blackfan anemia (DBA) cosegregates with the DBA gene region on chromosome 19q13. The DBA Working Group of Société d'Immunologie Pediatrique (SHIP). *Blood* 1998; **92**: 4422–7.

34. Orfali KA, Ohene-Abuakwa Y, Ball SE. Diamond Blackfan anaemia in the UK: clinical and genetic heterogeneity. *Br J Haematol* 2004; **125**: 243–52.

35. Gahr M, Scgroter W. The pattern of reactivated fetal erythropoiesis in bone marrow disorders of childhood. *Acta Paediatr Scand* 1982; **71**: 1013–18.

36. Van der Weyden MB, Harrison C, Hallam L, McVeigh D, Gan TE, Taaffe LM. Elevated red cell adenosine deaminase and haemolysis in a patient with a myelodysplastic syndrome. *Br J Haematol* 1989; **73**: 129–31.

37. Tani K, Fujii H, Takahashi K *et al.* Erythrocyte enzyme activities in myelodysplastic syndromes: elevated pyruvate kinase activity. *Am J Hematol* 1989; **30**: 97–103.

38. Hunter RE, Hakami N. The occurrence of congenital hypoplastic anaemia in half brothers. *J Pediatr* 1972; **81**: 346–8.

39. Gojic V, Van't Veer-Korthof ET, Bosch LJ, Puyn WH, Van Haeringen A. Congenital hypoplastic anaemia: another example of autosomal dominant transmission. *Am J Med Genet* 1994; **50**: 87–9.

40. Altman AC, Gross S. Severe congenital hypoplastic anaemia: transmission from a healthy female to opposite sex step-siblings. *Am J Pediatr Hematol Oncol* 1983; **5**: 99–101.

41. Lawton JWM, Aldrich JE, Turner TL. Congenital erythroid hypoplastic anaemia: autosomal dominant transmission. *Scand J Haematol* 1974; **13**: 276–80.

42. Gustavsson P, Skeppner G, Johansson B *et al.* Diamond-Blackfan anaemia in a girl with a de novo balanced reciprocal X;19 translocation. *J Med Genet* 1997; **34**: 779–82.

43. Gustavsson P, Willig TN, van Haeringen A *et al.* Diamond–Blackfan anaemia: genetic homogeneity for a gene on chromosome 19q13 restricted to 1.8 Mb. *Nat Genet* 1997; **16**: 368–71.

44. Gustavsson P, Garelli E, Draptchinskaia N *et al.* Identification of microdeletions spanning the Diamond-Blackfan anemia locus on 19q13 and evidence for genetic heterogeneity. *Am J Hum Genet* 1998; **63**: 1388–95.

45. Ramenghi U, Garelli E, Valtolina S *et al.* Diamond-Blackfan anaemia in the Italian population. *Br J Haematol* 1999; **104**: 841–8.

46. Draptchinskaia N, Gustavsson P, Andersson B *et al.* The gene encoding ribosomal protein S19 is mutated in Diamond-Blackfan anaemia. *Nat Genet* 1999; **21**: 169–75.

47. Willig TN, Draptchinskaia N, Dianzani I *et al.* Mutations in ribosomal protein S19 gene and diamond blackfan anemia: wide variations in phenotypic expression. *Blood* 1999; **94**: 4294–306.

48. Cmejla R, Blafkova J, Stopka T *et al.* Ribosomal protein S19 gene mutations in patients with diamond-blackfan anemia and identification of ribosomal protein S19 pseudogenes. *Blood Cells Mol Dis* 2000; **26**: 124–32.

49. Matsson H, Klar J, Draptchinskaia N *et al.* Truncating ribosomal protein S19 mutations and variable clinical expression in Diamond-Blackfan anemia. *Hum Genet* 1999; **105**: 496–500.

50. Ramenghi U, Campagnoli MF, Garelli E *et al.* Diamond-Blackfan anemia: report of seven further mutations in the RPS19 gene and evidence of mutation heterogeneity in the Italian population. *Blood Cells Mol Dis* 2000; **26**: 417–22.

51. Proust A, Da Costa L, Rince P *et al.* Ten novel Diamond-Blackfan anemia mutations and three polymorphisms within the rps19 gene. *Hematol J* 2003; **4**: 132–6.

52. Gazda H, Lipton JM, Willig TN *et al.* Evidence for linkage of familial Diamond-Blackfan anemia to chromosome 8p23.3-p22 and for non-19q non-8p disease. *Blood* 2001; **97**: 2145–50.

53. Freedman MH, Amato D, Saunders EF. Erythroid colony growth in congenital hypoplastic anaemia. *J Clin Invest* 1976; **57**: 673–7.

54. Freedman MH, Saunders EF. Diamond–Blackfan syndrome: evidence against cell-mediated erythropoietic suppression. *Blood* 1978; **51**: 1125–8.

55. Hoffman R, Zanjani ED, Vila J, Zaluky R, Lutton JD, Wasserman LR. Diamond–Blackfan syndrome: lymphocyte-mediated suppression of erythropoiesis. *Science* 1976; **193**: 899–900.

56. Steinberg MH, Colemen MF, Pennebaker JN. Diamond–Blackfan syndrome: evidence for T-cell mediated suppression of erythroid development and a serum blocking factor associated with remission. *Br J Haematol* 1979; **41**: 57–68.

57. Ershler WB, Ross J, Finlay JL, Shaidi NT. Bone marrow microenvironment defect in congenital hypoplastic anaemia. *N Engl J Med* 1980; **302**: 1321–7.

58. Bagnara GP, Zauli G, Vitale L *et al.* *In vitro* growth and regulation of bone marrow enriched CD34⁺ haematopoietic progenitors in Diamond–Blackfan anaemia. *Blood* 1991; **78**: 2203–10.

59. Tsai PH, Arkin S, Lipton JM. An intrinsic progenitor defect in Diamond-Blackfan anaemia. *Br J Haematol* 1989; **73**: 112–20.

60. Vlachos A, Federman N, Reyes-Haley C, Abramson J, Lipton JM. Hematopoietic stem cell transplantation for Diamond Blackfan anemia: a report from the Diamond Blackfan Anemia Registry. *Bone Marrow Transplant* 2001; **27**: 381–6.

61. Hamaguchi I, Ooka A, Brun A *et al.* Gene transfer improves erythroid development in ribosomal protein S19-deficient Diamond-Blackfan anemia. *Blood* 2002; **100**: 2724–31.

62. Hamaguchi I, Flygare J, Nishiura H *et al.* Proliferation deficiency of multipotent hematopoietic progenitors in ribosomal protein S19 (RPS19)-deficient Diamond-Blackfan anemia improves following RPS19 gene transfer. *Mol Ther* 2003; **7**: 613–22.

63. Gregory CJ, Eaves AC. Three stages of erythropoietic progenitor cell differentiation distinguished by a number of physical and biologic properties. *Blood* 1978; **51**: 527–37.

64. Nathan DG, Clarke BJ, Hillman DG, Alter BP, Housman DE. Erythroid precursors in congenital hypoplastic (Diamond-Blackfan) anemia. *J Clin Invest* 1978; **61**: 489–98.

65. Lipton JM, Kudisch M, Gross R, Nathan DG. Defective erythroid progenitor differentiation system in congenital hypoplastic (Diamond–Blackfan) anaemia. *Blood* 1986; **67**: 962–8.

66. Perdahl EB, Naprstek BL, Wallace WC, Lipton JM. Erythroid failure in Diamond–Blackfan anaemia is characterized by apoptosis. *Blood* 1994; **83**: 645–50.

67. Olivieri NF, Grunberger T, Ben-David Y *et al.* Diamond Blackfan anaemia: heterogeneous response of haematopoietic progenitor cells *in vitro* to the protein product of the Steel locus. *Blood* 1991; **78**: 2211–15.

68. Abkowitz JL, Sabo KM, Nakamoto B *et al.* Diamond–Blackfan anaemia: *in vitro* response of erythroid progenitors to the ligand for c-kit. *Blood* 1991; **78**: 2198–202.

69. Sieff CA, Yokoyama CT, Zsebo KM *et al.* The production of Steel factor mRNA in Diamond–Blackfan anaemia long-term cultures and interactions of Steel factor with erythropoietin and interleukin-3. *Br J Haematol* 1992; **82**: 640–7.

70. Alter BP, Knobloch ME, He L *et al.* Effect of stem cell factor on *in vitro* erythropoiesis in patients with bone marrow failure syndromes. *Blood* 1992; **80**: 3000–8.

71. McGuckin CP, Ball SE, Gordon-Smith EC. Diamond–Blackfan anaemia: Three patterns of *in vitro* response to haemopoietic growth factors. *Br J Haematol* 1995; **89**: 457–64.

72. Dunbar CE, Smith DA, Kimball J, Garrison L, Nienhuis AW, Young NS. Treatment of Diamond Blackfan anaemia with haematopoietic growth factors, granulocyte-macrophage colony stimulating factor and interleukin 3: sustained remissions following IL-3. *Br J Haematol* 1991; **79**: 316–21.

73. Gillio AP, Faulkner LB, Alter BP *et al.* Treatment of Diamond–Blackfan anaemia with recombinant human interleukin-3. *Blood* 1993; **82**: 744–51.

74. Olivieri NF, Feig SA, Valentino L, Berriman AM, Shore R, Freedman MH. Failure of recombinant human interleukin-3 therapy to induce erythropoiesis in patients with refractory Diamond–Blackfan anaemia. *Blood* 1994; **83**: 2444–50.

75. Ball SE, Tchernia G, Wranne L *et al.* Is there a role for interleukin-3 in Diamond–Blackfan anaemia? Results of a European multicentre study. *Br J Haematol* 1995; **91**: 313–18.

76. Fibach E, Manor D, Oppenheim A, Rachmilewitz EA. Proliferation and maturation of human erythroid progenitors in liquid culture. *Blood* 1989; **73**: 100–3.

77. Ohene-Abuakwa Y, Orfali KA, Marius C, Ball SE. Two-phase culture in Diamond Blackfan anemia: localization of erythroid defect. *Blood* 2005; **105**: 838–46.

78. Mauro VP, Edelman GM. The ribosome filter hypothesis. *Proc Natl Acad Sci USA* 2002; **99**: 12031–6.

79. Zimmermann RA. The double life of ribosomal proteins. *Cell* 2003; **115**: 130–2.

80. Gasser C. Aplastische anamia (chronische Erythroblastophtise) and Cortison. *Schweiz Med Wochenschr* 1951; **81**: 1241–2.

81. Krause PR, Klinman DM. Efficacy, immunogenicity, safety and use of live attenuated chickenpox vaccine. *J Pediatr* 1995; **127**: 518–25.

82. Ozsoylu S. High-dose intravenous corticosteroid treatment for patients with Diamond–Blackfan syndrome resistant or refractory to conventional treatment. *Am J Pediatr Hematol Oncol* 1988; **10**: 210–17.

83. Bernini JC, Carillo JM, Buchanan GR. High-dose intravenous methylprednisolone therapy for patients with Diamond–Blackfan anaemia refractory to conventional doses of prednisone. *J Pediatr* 1995; **127**: 654–9.

84. Buchanan GR. Oral megadose methylprednisolone therapy for refractory Diamond-Blackfan anemia. International Diamond-Blackfan Anemia Study Group. *J Pediatr Hematol Oncol* 2001; **23**: 353–6.

85. Wasser JS, Yolken R, Miller DR, Diamond L. Congenital hypoplastic anaemia (Diamond–Blackfan syndrome) terminating in acute myelogenous leukemia. *Blood* 1978; **51**: 991–5.

86. Glader BE, Flam MS, Dahl GV, Hyman CB. Haematologic malignancies in Diamond–Blackfan anaemia. *Pediatr Res* 1990; **27**: 142A.

87. Abkowitz JL, Schaison G, Boulad F *et al.* Response of Diamond-Blackfan anemia to metoclopramide: evidence for a role for prolactin in erythropoiesis. *Blood* 2002; **100**: 2687–91.

88. Splain J, Berman BW. Cyclosporin A treatment for Diamond–Blackfan anaemia. *Am J Hematol* 1992; **39**: 208–11.

89. Niemeyer CM, Baumgarten E, Holldack J *et al.* Treatment trial with recombinant human erythropoietin in children with congenital hypoplastic anaemia. *Contrib Nephrol* 1991; **88**: 276–81.

90. Fiorillo A, Poggi V, Migliorati R, Parasole R, Selleri C, Rotoli B. Unresponsiveness to erythropoietin therapy in a case of Blackfan Diamond anaemia. *Am J Hematol* 1991; **37**: 61.

91. Bejaoui M, Fitouri Z. Failure of immunosuppressive therapy and high-dose intravenous immunoglobulins in four transfusion-dependent, steroid-unresponsive Blackfan–Diamond anaemia patients. *Haematologica* 1993; **78**: 38–9.

92. August CS, King E, Gihens JH *et al.* Establishment of erythropoieis following bone marrow transplantation in a patient with congenital hypoplastic anaemia (Diamond–Blackfan syndrome). *Blood* 1976; **48**: 491–4.

93. Iriondo A, Garijo J, Baro J *et al.* Complete recovery of haemopoiesis following bone marrow transplant in a patient with unresponsive congenital hypoplastic anaemia (Blackfan–Diamond syndrome). *Blood* 1984; **64**: 348–51.

94. Wiktor-Jedrzejczak W, Szczylik C, Pojda Z *et al.* Success of bone marrow transplantation in congenital Diamond–Blackfan anaemia: a case report. *Eur J Haematol* 1987; **38**: 204–6.

95. Mugishima H, Gale RP, Rowlings PA *et al.* Bone marrow transplantation for Diamond–Blackfan anaemia. *Bone Marrow Transplant* 1995; **15**: 55–8.

96. Ohga S, Mugishima H, Ohara A *et al.* Diamond-Blackfan anemia in Japan: clinical outcomes of prednisolone therapy and hematopoietic stem cell transplantation. *Int J Hematol* 2004; **79**: 22–30.

97. Bonno M, Azuma E, Nakano T *et al.* Successful haematopoietic reconstitution by transplantation with umbilical cord blood cells in a patient with Diamond–Blackfan anaemia. *Blood* 1995; **86**: 938A.

98. Giardini C, Galimberti M, Lucarelli G. Bone marrow transplantation in thalassemia. *Ann Rev Med* 1995; **46**: 319–30.

99. Orfali KA, Wynn RF, Stevens RF, Chopra R, Ball SE. Failure of red cell production following allogeneic BMT for Diamond Blackfan anemia (DBA) illustrates the functional significance of high erythrocyte adenosine deaminase activity in the donor. *Blood* 1999; **94** (suppl. 1): 414a.

100. Zivny J, Jelinek J, Pospisilova D *et al.* Diamond blackfan anemia stem cells fail to repopulate erythropoiesis in NOD/SCID mice. *Blood Cells Mol Dis* 2003; **31**: 93–7.

101. van Dijken PJ, Verwijs W. Diamond-Blackfan anemia and malignancy. A case report and a review of the literature. *Cancer* 1995; **76**: 517–20.

102. Seip M. Malignant tumors in two patients with Diamond-Blackfan anemia treated with corticosteroids and androgens. *Pediatr Hematol Oncol* 1994; **11**: 423–6.

103. Turcotte R, Bard C, Marton D, Schurch W, Lafontaine E. Malignant fibrous histiocytoma in a patient with Blackfan-Diamond anemia. *Can Assoc Radiol J* 1994; **45**: 402–10.

104. Aquino VM, Buchanan GR. Osteogenic sarcoma in a child with transfusion-dependent Diamond-Blackfan anemia. *J Pediatr Hematol Oncol* 1996; **18**: 230–2.

105. Wranne L. Transient erythroblastopenia in infancy and childhood. *Scand J Haematol* 1970; **7**: 76–81.

106. Lovric VA. Anaemia and temporary erythroblastopenia in children. *Aust Ann Med* 1970; **1**: 34–9.

107. Kynaston JA, West NC, Reid MM. A regional experience of red cell aplasia. *Eur J Pediatr* 1993; **152**: 306–8.

108. Ware RE, Kinney TR. Transient erythroblastopenia in the first year of life. *Am J Hematol* 1991; **37**: 156–8.

109. Miller R, Berman B. Transient erythroblastopenia of childhood in infants < 6 months of age. *Am J Pediatr Hematol Oncol* 1994; **16**: 246–8.

110. Labotka RJ, Maurer MS, Honig GR. Transient erythroblastopenia of childhood: review of 17 cases including a pair of identical twins. *Am J Dis Child* 1981; **135**: 937–40.

111. Young RSR, Rannels DE, Hilmo A, Gerson JM, Goodrich D. Severe anaemia in childhood presenting as transient ischaemic attacks. *Stroke* 1983; **14**: 622–3.

112. Green N, Garvin J, Chutorian A. Transient erythroblastopenia of childhood presenting with papilledema. *Clin Ped* 1986; **25**: 278–9.

113. Michelson A, Marshall P. Transient neurological disorder associated with transient erythroblastopenia of childhood. *Am J Pediatr Hematol Oncol* 1987; **9**: 161–3.

114. Cherrick I, Karayalcin G, Landzowsky P. Transient erythroblastopenia of childhood: prospective study of fifty patients. *Am J Pediatr Hematol Oncol* 1994; **16**: 320–4.

115. Glader BE, Backer K. Comparative activity of erythrocyte adenosine deaminase and orotidine decarboxylase in Diamond-Blackfan anemia. *Am J Hematol* 1986; **23**: 135–9.

116. Hanada T, Koike K, Hirano C *et al.* Childhood transient erythroblastopenia complicated by thrombocytopenia and neutropenia. *Eur J Haematol* 1989; **42**: 77–80.

117. Wodzinski MA, Lilleyman JS. Transient erythroblastopenia of childhood due to human parvovirus B19 infection. *Br J Haematol* 1989; **73**: 127–31.

118. Wang WC, Mentzer WC. Differentiation of transient erythroblastopenia of childhood from congenital hypoplastic anaemia. *J Pediatr* 1976; **88**: 784–9.

119. Paglia D, Renner S, Valentine W, Nakatani M, Brockway R. The significance of distinctive enzyme profiles in transient erythroblastopenia of childhood and congenital hypoplastic anaemia. *Blood* 1991; **78**: 98A.

120. Karsten J, Anker AP, Odink RJ. Glycosylated haemoglobin and transient erythroblastopenia of childhood. *Lancet* 1996; **347**: 273.

121. Bhambhani K, Inoue S, Sanaik SA. Seasonal clustering of transient erythroblastopenia of childhood. *Am J Dis Child* 1988; **142**: 175–7.

122. Kubic PT, Warkentin PI, Levitt CJ, Coccia PF. Transient erythroblastopenia of childhood (TEC) occurring in clusters. *Pediatr Res* 1979; **13**: 435.

123. Elian JC, Frappaz D, Pozzetto B, Freycon F. Transient erythroblastopenia of childhood presenting with echovirus 11 infection. *Acta Paediatr* 1993; **82**: 492–4.

124. Freedman MH. Pure red cell aplasia in childhood and adolescence: pathogenesis and approaches to diagnosis. *Br J Haematol*. 1993; **85**: 246–53.

125. Koenig HM, Lightsey AL, Nelson DP, Diamond LK. Immune suppression of erythropoiesis in transient erythroblastopenia of childhood. *Blood* 1979; **54**: 742–6.

126. Dessypris EN, Krantz SB, Roloff JS, Lukens JN. Mode of

action of the IgG inhibitor of erythropoiesis in transient erythroblastopenia of childhood. *Blood* 1982; **59**: 114–23.

127. Freedman M, Saunders EF. Transient erythroblastopenia of childhood: varied pathogenesis. *Am J Hematol* 1983; **14**: 247–54.

128. Hanada T, Abe T, Takita H. T-cell-mediated inhibition of erythropoiesis in transient erythroblastopenia of childhood. *Br J Haematol* 1985; **59**: 391–2.

129. Freedman MH. "Recurrent" erythroblastopenia of childhood. *Am Dis Child* 1983; **137**: 458–60.

130. Anderson MJ, Higgins PG, Davis LR *et al*. Experimental parvoviral infection in humans. *J Infect Dis* 1985; **152**: 257–265.

131. Seip M. Transient erythroblastopenia in siblings. *Acta Paediatr Scand* 1982; **71**: 689–90.

132. Skeppner G, Forestier E, Henter JI, Wranne L. Transient red cell aplasia in siblings: a common environmental or a common hereditary factor? *Acta Paediatr* 1998; **87**: 43–7.

133. Gustavsson P, Klar J, Matsson H *et al*. Familial transient erythroblastopenia of childhood is associated with the chromosome 19q13.2 region but not caused by mutations in coding sequences of the ribosomal protein S19 (RPS19) gene. *Br J Haematol* 2002; **119**: 261–4.

134. Owren PA. Congenital haemolytic jaundice. The pathogenesis of the "haemolytic crisis". *Blood* 1948; **3**: 231–48.

135. Bell LM, Naides SJ, Stoffman P, Hodinka RL, Plotkin SA. Human parvovirus B19 infection among hospital staff members after contact with infected patients. *N Engl J Med* 1989; **321**: 485–91.

136. Cossart YE, Cant B, Field AM, Widdows D. Parvovirus-like particles in human sera. *Lancet* 1975; **i**: 72–7.

137. Pattison JR, Jones SE, Hodgson J *et al*. Parvovirus infections and hypoplastic crisis in sickle cell anaemia *Lancet* 1981; **i**: 664–5.

138. Serjeant GR, Topley JM, Mason K *et al*. Outbreak of aplastic crises in sickle cell anaemia associated with parvovirus-like agent. *Lancet* 1981; **ii**: 595–7.

139. Brownell AI, McSwiggan DA, Cubitt WD, Anderson MJ. Aplastic and hypoplastic episodes in sickle cell disease and thalassaemia intermedia. *J Clin Path* 1986; **39**: 121–4.

140. Harris JW. Parvovirus B19 for the haematologist. *Am J Hematol* 1992; **39**: 119–30.

141. Brown KE, Anderson SM, Young NS. Erythrocyte P antigen: cellular receptor for B19 parvovirus. *Science* 1993; **262**: 114–17.

142. Mortimer PP, Humphries RK, Moore JG *et al*. A human parvoviruslike virus inhibits haematopoietic colony formation *in vitro*. *Nature* 1983; **302**: 426–9.

143. Young NS, Mortimer PP, Moore JG, Humphries RK. Characterization of a virus that causes transient aplastic crisis. *J Clin Invest* 1984; **73**: 224–30.

144. Potter CG, Potter AC, Hatton CS *et al*. Variation of erythroid and myeloid precursors in the marrow and peripheral blood of volunteer subjects infected with human parvovirus (B19). *J Clin Invest* 1987; **79**: 1486–92.

145. Kudoh T, Yoto Y, Suzuki N *et al*. Human parvovirus B19-induced aplastic crisis in iron deficiency anemia. *Acta Paediatr Jpn* 1994; **36**: 448–9.

146. Tchernia G, Morinet F, Congard B, Croisille L. Diamond Blackfan anaemia: apparent relapse due to B19 parvovirus. *Eur J Pediatr* 1993; **152**: 209–10.

147. Kurtzman GJ, Ozawa K, Cohen B, Hanson G, Oseas R, Young NS. Chronic bone marrow failure due to persistent parvovirus B19 infection. *N Engl J Med* 1987; **317**: 287–94.

148. Frickhofen N, Young NS. Persistent parvovirus B19 infections in humans. *Microbial Pathogen* 1989; **7**: 319–27.

149. Kurtzman GJ, Cohen BJ, Field AM, Oseas R, Blaese RM, Young NS. Immune response to B19 parvovirus and an antibody defect in persistent viral infection. *J Clin Invest* 1989; **84**: 1114–23.

150. Nigro G, Gattinara GC, Mattia S, Caniglia M, Fridell E. Parvovirus B19-related pancytopenia in children with HIV infection. *Lancet* 1992; **340**: 145.

151. Gahr M, Pekrun A, Eiffert H. Persistence of parvovrius B19-DNA in blood of a child with severe combined immunodeficiency associated with pure red cell aplasia. *Eur J Pediatr* 1991; **150**: 470–2.

152. Kurtzman GJ, Cohen B, Meyers P, Amunullah A, Young NS. Persistent B19 parvovirus infection as a cause of severe chronic anaemia in children with acute lymphocytic leukaemia. *Lancet* 1988; **ii**: 1159–62.

153. Lefrere J-J, Mariotti M, Thauvin M. B19 parvovirus DNA in solvent/detergent-treated anti-haemophilia concentrates. *Lancet* 1994; **343**: 211–12.

154. Murray JC, Greisik MV, Leger F, McClain KL. B19 parvovirus-induced anaemia in a normal child. *Am J Ped Hematol Oncol* 1993; **15**: 420–3.

155. Salimans MM, Holsappel S, van de Rijke FM, Jiwa NM, Raap AK, Weiland HT. Rapid detection of human parvovirus B19 DNA by dot-hybridization and the polymerase chain reaction. *J Virol Methods* 1989; **23**: 19–28.

156. Kurtzman GK, Frickhofen N, Kimball J, Jenkins DW, Nienhuis AW, Young NS. Pure red cell aplasia of 10 years' duration due to persistent parvovirus B19 infection and its cure with immunoglobulin therapy. *N Engl J Med* 1989; **321**: 519–25.

157. Imamura N, Kuramoto A, Morimoto T, Ihara A. Pure red cell aplasia associated with acute lymphoblastic leukemia of pre-T-cell origin. *Med J Aust* 1986; **144**: 724.

158. Rubin RN, Walker BK, Ballas SK, Travis SF. Erythroid aplasia in juvenile rheumatoid arthritis. *Am J Dis Child* 1978; **132**: 760–2.

159. Schmid JR, Kiely JM, Harrison EG Jr *et al*. Thymoma associated with red cell agenesis: review of literature and report of cases. *Cancer* 1965; **18**: 216–30.

160. Clark DA, Dessypris EN, Krantz SB. Studies on pure red cell aplasia. XI. Results of immunosuppressive treatment of 37 patients. *Blood* 1984; **63**: 277–86.

161. Thompson DF, Gales MA. Drug-induced pure red cell aplasia. *Pharmacotherapy* 1996; **16**: 1002–8.

162. Hirai H. Two cases of erythroid hypoplasia caused by carbamazepine. *Jpn J Clin Haematol* 1977; **18**: 33–8.

163. Medberry CA, Pappas AA, Ackerman BH. Carbamazepine and erythroid arrest. *Drug Intell Clin Pharm* 1987; **21**: 439–42.

164. Dessypris EN, Redline S, Harris JW, Krantz SB. Diphenylhydantoin-induced pure red cell aplasia. *Blood* 1985; **65**: 789–94.

165. MacDougall LG. Pure red cell aplasia associated with sodium valproate therapy. *JAMA* 1982; **247**: 53–4.

166. Krantz SB, Kao V. Studies on red cell aplasia. I. Demonstration of a plasma inhibitor to heme synthesis and an antibody to erythroblastic nuclei. *Proc Natl Acad Sci USA* 1967; **58**: 493–500.

167. Nagasawa M, Okawa H, Yata J. A B cell line from a patient with pure red cell aplasia produces an immunoglobulin that

suppresses erythropoiesis. *Clin Immunol Immunopathol* 1991; **61**: 18–28.

168. Abkowitz JL, Kadin ME, Powell JS, Adamson JW. Pure red cell aplasia: lymphocyte inhibition of erythropoiesis. *Br J Haematol* 1986; **63**: 59–67.

169. Hanada T, Abe T, Nakamura H, Aoki Y. Pure red cell aplasia: relationship between inhibitory activity of T cells to CFU-E and erythropoiesis. *Br J Haematol* 1984; **58**: 107–13.

170. Corcione A, Pasino M, Claudio-Molinari AC, Acquila M, Marchese P, Mori PG. A paediatric case of pure red cell aplasia: successful treatment with anti-lymphocyte globulin and correlation with *in vitro* T cell-mediated inhibition of erythropoiesis. *Br J Haematol* 1991; **79**: 129–30.

171. Krantz SB. Pure red cell aplasia: biology and treatment. In: Feig SA, Freedman MH (eds) *Clinical Disorders and Experimental Models of Erythropoietic Failure*. Boca Raton, FL: CRC Press, 1993, pp. 85–124.

172. Casadevall N, Nataf J, Viron B *et al.* Pure red-cell aplasia and antierythropoietin antibodies in patients treated with recombinant erythropoietin. *N Engl J Med* 2002; **346**: 469–75.

173. Bennett CL, Luminari S, Nissenson AR *et al.* Pure red-cell aplasia and epoetin therapy. *N Engl J Med* 2004; **351**: 1403–8.

174. Locatelli F, Del Vecchio L. Pure red cell aplasia secondary to treatment with erythropoietin. *J Nephrol* 2003; **16**: 461–6.

175. Casadevall N, Cournoyer D, Marsh J *et al.* Recommendations on haematological criteria for the diagnosis of epoetin-induced pure red cell aplasia. *Eur J Haematol* 2004; **73**: 389–96.

176. Abkowitz JL, Powell JS, Nakamura JM, Kadin ME, Adamson JW. Pure red cell aplasia: response to therapy with antilymphocyte globulin. *Am J Hematol* 1986; **28**: 363–71.

177. Lacombe C, Casadevall N, Muller O, Varet B. Erythroid progenitors in adult chronic pure red cell aplasia: relationship of *in vitro* erythroid colonies to therapeutic response. *Blood* 1984; **64**: 71–7.

178. Charles RJ, Sabo KM, Kidd PG, Abkowitz JL. The pathophysiology of pure red cell aplasia: implications for therapy. *Blood* 1996; **87**: 4831–8.

179. Messner HA, Fauser AA, Curtis JE, Dotten D. Control of antibody-mediated pure red-cell aplasia by plasmapheresis. *N Engl J Med* 1981; **304**: 1334–8.

180. Public Health Laboratory Service Working Party on Fifth Disease. Prospective study of human parvovirus (B19) infection in pregnancy. *Br Med J* 1990; **33**: 1166–70.

181. Young NS. B19 parvovirus. *Baillière's Clin Haematol* 1995; **8**: 25–56.

182. Vaughan JL, Warwick R, Letsky E, Nicolini U, Rodeck CH, Fisk NM. Erythropoietic suppression in fetal anaemia because of Kell alloimmunization. *Am J Obstet Gynecol* 1994; **171**: 247–52.

183. Weiner CP, Widness JA. Decreased fetal erythropoiesis and haemolysis in Kell haemolytic anaemia. *Am J Obstet Gynecol* 1996; **174**: 547–51.

184. Manning M, Warwick R, Vaughan J, Roberts IAG. Inhibition of erythroid progenitor cell growth by anti-Kell: a mechanism for fetal anaemia in Kell-immunized pregnancies. *Br J Haematol* 1996; **93** (suppl. 1): 13.

185. Sahovic EA, Flick J, Graham CD, Stuart RK. Case report: isoimmune inhibition of erythropoiesis following ABO-incompatible bone marrow transplantation. *Am J Med Sci* 1991; **302**: 369–73.

186. Nilsson LR. Chronic pancytopenia with multiple congenital abnormalities (Fanconi's anaemia). *Acta Paediatr* 1960; **49**: 519–29.

187. Butturini A, Gale RP, Verlander PC, Adler-Brecher B, Gillio AP, Auerbach AD. Haematologic abnormalities in Fanconi anaemia: an International Fanconi Anaemia Registry study. *Blood* 1994; **84**: 1650–5.

188. German J, Schonberg S, Caskie S, Warburton D, Falk C, Ray JH. A test for Fanconi's anaemia. *Blood* 1987; **69**: 1637–41.

189. Boocock GR, Morrison JA, Popovic M *et al.* Mutations in SBDS are associated with Shwachman Diamond syndrome. *Nat Genet* 2003; **33**: 97–101.

190. Woloszynek JR, Rothbaum RJ, Rawls AS *et al.* Mutations of the SBDS gene are present in most patients with Shwachman-Diamond syndrome. *Blood* 2004; **104**: 3588–90.

191. Barosi G, Cazzola M, Stefanelli M, Ascari E. Studies of ineffective erythropoiesis and peripheral haemolysis in congenital dyserythropoietic anaemia type II. *Br J Haematol* 1979; **43**: 243–50.

192. Wickramasinghe SN. Congenital dyserythropoietic anemias. *Curr Opin Hematol* 2000; **7**: 71–8.

193. Heimpel H. Congenital dyserythropoietic anemias: epidemiology, clinical significance, and progress in understanding their pathogenesis. *Ann Hematol* 2004; **83**: 613–21.

194. Heimpel H, Wendt F. Congenital dyserythropoietic anemia with karyorrhexis and multinuclearity of erythroblasts. *Helv Med Acta* 1968; **34**: 103–15.

195. Wickramasinghe SN. Congenital dyserythropoietic anaemias: clinical features, haematological morphology and new biochemical data. *Blood Rev* 1998; **12**: 178–200.

196. Cazzola M, Barosi G, Bergamaschi G *et al.* Iron loading in congenital dyserythropoietic anaemias and congenital sideroblastic anaemias. *Br J Haematol* 1983; **54**: 649–54.

197. Cazzola M, Beguin Y, Bergamaschi G *et al.* Soluble transferrin receptor as a potential determinant of iron loading in congenital anaemias due to ineffective erythropoiesis. *Br J Haematol* 1999; **106**: 752–5.

198. Kostaridou S, Polychronopoulou S, Premetis E *et al.* Ineffective erythropoiesis underlies the clinical heterogeneity of congenital dyserythropoietic anemia type II (CDA II). *Pediatr Int* 2004; **46**: 274–9.

199. Tamary H, Shalev H, Luria D *et al.* Clinical features and studies of erythropoiesis in Israeli Bedouins with congenital dyserythropoietic anemia type I. *Blood* 1996; **87**: 1763–70.

200. Shalev H, Kapleushnik Y, Haeskelzon L *et al.* Clinical and laboratory manifestations of congenital dyserythropoietic anemia type I in young adults. *Eur J Haematol* 2002; **68**: 170–4.

201. Holmberg L, Jansson L, Rausing A, Henriksson P. Type I congenital dyserythropoietic anaemia with myelopoietic abnormalities and hand malformations. *Scand J Haematol* 1978; **21**: 72–9.

202. Brichard B, Vermylen C, Scheiff JM *et al.* Two cases of congenital dyserythropoietic anaemia type I associated with unusual skeletal abnormalities of the limbs. *Br J Haematol* 1994; **86**: 201–2.

203. Sabry MA, Zaki M, al Awadi SA, al Saleh Q, Mattar MS. Non-haematological traits associated with congenital dyserythropoietic anaemia type 1: a new entity emerging. *Clin Dysmorphol* 1997; **6**: 205–12.

204. Heimpel H, Wendt F, Klemm D, Schubothe H, Heilmeyer L. [Congenital dyserythropoietic anemia]. *Arch Klin Med* 1968; **215**: 174–94

205. Clauvel JP, Cosson A, Breton-Gorius J *et al.* [Congenital dyserythropoiesis (study of 6 cases).] *Nouv Rev Fr Hematol* 1972; **12**: 653–72.

206. Heimpel H, Forteza-Vila J, Queisser W, Spiertz E. Electron and light microscopic study of the erythroblasts of patients with congenital dyserythropoietic anemia. *Blood* 1971; **37**: 299–310.

207. Conde E, Mazo E, Baro J *et al.* Transmission and scanning electron microscopy study on congenital dyserythropoietic anemia type I. *Acta Haematol* 1983; **70**: 243–9.

208. Rossler J, Havers W. [Diagnosis and genetics of congenital dyserythropoietic anemias (CDA).] *Klin Padiatr* 2000; **212**: 153–8.

209. Dgany O, Avidan N, Delaunay J *et al.* Congenital dyserythropoietic anemia type I is caused by mutations in codanin-1. *Am J Hum Genet* 2002; **71**: 1467–74.

210. Lavabre-Bertrand T, Blanc P, Navarro R *et al.* alpha-Interferon therapy for congenital dyserythropoiesis type I. *Br J Haematol* 1995; **89**: 929–32.

211. Wickramasinghe SN. Response of CDA type I to alpha-interferon. *Eur J Haematol* 1997; **58**: 121–3.

212. Lavabre-Bertrand T, Ramos J, Delfour C *et al.* Long-term alpha interferon treatment is effective on anaemia and significantly reduces iron overload in congenital dyserythropoiesis type I. *Eur J Haematol* 2004; **73**: 380–3.

213. Parez N, Dommergues M, Zupan V *et al.* Severe congenital dyserythropoietic anaemia type I: prenatal management, transfusion support and alpha-interferon therapy. *Br J Haematol* 2000; **110**: 420–3.

214. Michaud AP, Bauman NM, Burke DK, Manaligod JM, Smith RJ. Spastic diplegia and other motor disturbances in infants receiving interferon-alpha. *Laryngoscope* 2004; **114**: 1231–6.

215. Dubois J, Hershon L, Carmant L *et al.* Toxicity profile of interferon alfa-2b in children: A prospective evaluation. *J Pediatr* 1999; **135**: 782–5.

216. Worle H, Maass E, Kohler B, Treuner J. Interferon alpha-2a therapy in haemangiomas of infancy: spastic diplegia as a severe complication. *Eur J Pediatr* 1999; **158**: 344.

217. Deb G, Jenkner A, Donfrancesco A. Spastic diplegia and interferon. *J Pediatr* 1999; **134**: 382.

218. Barlow CF, Priebe CJ, Mulliken JB *et al.* Spastic diplegia as a complication of interferon alfa-2a treatment of hemangiomas of infancy. *J Pediatr* 1998; **132**: 527–30.

219. Vesikari T, Nuutila A, Cantell K. Neurologic sequelae following interferon therapy of juvenile laryngeal papilloma. *Acta Paediatr Scand* 1988; **77**: 619–22.

220. Wickramasinghe SN, Hasan R, Smythe J. Reduced interferon-alpha production by Epstein-Barr virus transformed B-lymphoblastoid cell lines and lectin-stimulated lymphocytes in congenital dyserythropoietic anaemia type I. *Br J Haematol* 1997; **98**: 295–8.

221. Crookston JH, Crookston MC, Burnie KL *et al.* Hereditary erythroblastic multinuclearity associated with a positive acidified-serum test: a type of congenital dyserythropoietic anaemia. *Br J Haematol* 1969; **17**: 11–26.

222. Heimpel H, Anselstetter V, Chrobak L *et al.* Congenital dyserythropoietic anemia type II: epidemiology, clinical appearance, and prognosis based on long-term observation. *Blood* 2003; **102**: 4576–81.

223. Passi GR, Saran S. Neonatal hyperbilirubinemia due to hereditary spherocytosis. *Indian Pediatr* 2004; **41**: 199.

224. Tchernia G, Delhommeau F, Perrotta S *et al.* Recombinant erythropoietin therapy as an alternative to blood transfusions in infants with hereditary spherocytosis. *Hematol J* 2000; **1**: 146–52.

225. Iolascon A, Delaunay J, Wickramasinghe SN *et al.* Natural history of congenital dyserythropoietic anemia type II. *Blood* 2001; **98**: 1258–60.

226. Faruqui S, Abraham A, Berenfeld MR, Gabuzda TG. Normal serum ferritin levels in a patient with HEMPAS syndrome and iron overload. *Am J Clin Pathol* 1982; **78**: 97–101.

227. Halpern Z, Rahmani R, Levo Y. Severe hemochromatosis: the predominant clinical manifestation of congenital dyserythropoietic anemia type 2. *Acta Haematol* 1985; **74**: 178–80.

228. Verwilghen RL, Lewis SM, Dacie JV, Crookston JH, Crookston MC. Hempas: congenital dyserythropoietic anaemia (type II). *Q J Med* 1973; **42**: 257–78.

229. Gasparini P, Miraglia DG, Delaunay J *et al.* Localization of the congenital dyserythropoietic anemia II locus to chromosome 20q11.2 by genomewide search. *Am J Hum Genet* 1997; **61**: 1112–16.

230. Iolascon A, de Mattia D, Perrotta S *et al.* Genetic heterogeneity of congenital dyserythropoietic anemia type II. *Blood* 1998; **92**: 2593–4.

231. Enquist RW, Gockerman JP, Jenis EH, Warkel RL, Dillon DE. Type II congenital dyserythropoietic anemia. *Ann Intern Med* 1972; **77**: 371–6.

232. Erdmann H, Heimpel H, Buchta H. [Positive acid serum test and elevated agglutinability by Anti-i in patients with congenital dyserythropoietic anemia.] *Klin Wochenschr* 1970; **48**: 569–70.

233. Tomita A, Parker CJ. Aberrant regulation of complement by the erythrocytes of hereditary erythroblastic multinuclearity with a positive acidified serum lysis test (HEMPAS). *Blood* 1994; **83**: 250–9.

234. Alloisio N, Texier P, Denoroy L *et al.* The cisternae decorating the red blood cell membrane in congenital dyserythropoietic anemia (type II) originate from the endoplasmic reticulum. *Blood* 1996; **87**: 4433–9.

235. Fukuda MN, Klier G, Scartezzini P. Congenital dyserythropoietic anaemia type II (HEMPAS): characterization of aberrant intracellular organelles by immunogold electron microscopy. *Br J Haematol* 1987; **67**: 95–101.

236. Frisch B, Lewis SM, Sherman D, White JM, Gordon-Smith EC. The ultrastructure of erythropoiesis in two haemoglobinopathies. *Br J Haematol* 1974; **28**: 109–17.

237. Fukuda MN, Papayannopoulou T, Gordon-Smith EC, Rochant H, Testa U. Defect in glycosylation of erythrocyte membrane proteins in congenital dyserythropoietic anaemia type II (HEMPAS). *Br J Haematol* 1984; **56**: 55–68.

238. Anselstetter V, Horstmann HJ, Heimpel H. Congenital dyserythropoietic anaemia, types I and II: aberrant pattern of erythrocyte membrane proteins in CDA II, as revealed by two-dimensional polyacrylamide gel electrophoresis. *Br J Haematol* 1977; **35**: 209–15.

239. Baines AJ, Banga JP, Gratzer WB, Linch DC, Huehns ER. Red cell membrane protein anomalies in congenital dyserythropoietic anaemia, type II (HEMPAS). *Br J Haematol* 1982; **50**: 563–74.

240. Fukuda MN, Klier G, Yu J, Scartezzini P. Anomalous clustering of underglycosylated band 3 in erythrocytes and their precursor cells in congenital dyserythropoietic anemia type II. *Blood* 1986; **68**: 521–9.

241. Iolascon A, D'Agostaro G, Perrotta S *et al.* Congenital dyserythropoietic anemia type II: molecular basis and clinical aspects. *Haematologica* 1996; **81**: 543–59.

242. Iolascon A, Miraglia DG, Perrotta S *et al.* Exclusion of three candidate genes as determinants of congenital dyserythropoietic anemia type II (CDA-II). *Blood* 1997; **90**: 4197–200.

243. Lanzara C, Ficarella R, Totaro A *et al.* Congenital dyserythropoietic anemia type II: exclusion of seven candidate genes. *Blood Cells Mol Dis* 2003; **30**: 22–9.

244. Gockerman JP, Durocher JR, Conrad ME. The abnormal surface characteristics of the red blood cell membrane in congenital dyserythropoietic anaemia type II (HEMPAS). *Br J Haematol* 1975; **30**: 383–94.

245. Sandstrom H, Wahlin A. Congenital dyserythropoietic anemia type III. *Haematologica* 2000; **85**: 753–7.

246. Wolff JA, von Hofe FH. Familial erythroid multinuclearity. *Blood* 1951; **6**: 1274–83.

247. Lind L, Sandstrom H, Wahlin A *et al.* Localization of the gene for congenital dyserythropoietic anemia type III, CDAN3, to chromosome 15q21-q25. *Hum Mol Genet* 1995; **4**: 109–12.

248. Sandstrom H, Wahlin A, Eriksson M, Bergstrom I, Wickramasinghe SN. Intravascular haemolysis and increased prevalence of myeloma and monoclonal gammopathy in congenital dyserythropoietic anaemia, type III. *Eur J Haematol* 1994; **52**: 42–6.

249. Sandstrom H, Wahlin A, Eriksson M *et al.* Angioid streaks are part of a familial syndrome of dyserythropoietic anaemia (CDA III). *Br J Haematol* 1997; **98**: 845–9.

250. Wickramasinghe SN, Wahlin A, Anstee D *et al.* Observations on two members of the Swedish family with congenital dyserythropoietic anaemia, type III. *Eur J Haematol* 1993; **50**: 213–21.

251. Goudsmit R, Beckers D, De Bruijne JI *et al.* Congenital dyserythropoietic anaemia, type 3. *Br J Haematol* 1972; **23**: 97–105.

252. Bjorksten B, Holmgren G, Roos G, Stenling R. Congenital dyserythropoietic anaemia type III: an electron microscopic study. *Br J Haematol* 1978; **38**: 37–42.

253. Lim JI, Bressler NM, Marsh MJ, Bressler SB. Laser treatment of choroidal neovascularization in patients with angioid streaks. *Am J Ophthalmol* 1993; **116**: 414–23.

254. Roberts DJ, Nadel A, Lage J, Rutherford CJ. An unusual variant of congenital dyserythropoietic anaemia with mild maternal and lethal fetal disease. *Br J Haematol* 1993; **84**: 549–51.

255. Cantu-Rajnoldi A, Zanella A, Conter U *et al.* A severe transfusion-dependent congenital dyserythropoietic anaemia presenting as hydrops fetalis. *Br J Haematol* 1997; **96**: 530–3.

256. Carter C, Darbyshire PJ, Wickramasinghe SN. A congenital dyserythropoietic anaemia variant presenting as hydrops fetalis. *Br J Haematol* 1989; **72**: 289–90.

257. Ayas M, al Jefri A, Baothman A *et al.* Transfusion-dependent congenital dyserythropoietic anemia type I successfully treated with allogeneic stem cell transplantation. *Bone Marrow Transplant* 2002; **29**: 681–2.

258. Iolascon A, Sabato V, de Mattia D, Locatelli F. Bone marrow transplantation in a case of severe, type II congenital dyserythropoietic anemia (CDA II). *Bone Marrow Transplant* 2001; **27**: 213–15.

259. Wickramasinghe SN, Goudsmit R. Precipitation of beta-globin chains within the erythropoietic cells of a patient with congenital dyserythropoietic anemia, type III. *Br J Haematol* 1987; **65**: 250–1.

260. Wickramasinghe SN, Lee MJ, Furukawa T, Eguchi M, Reid CD. Composition of the intra-erythroblastic precipitates in thalassaemia and congenital dyserythropoietic anaemia (CDA): identification of a new type of CDA with intra-erythroblastic precipitates not reacting with monoclonal antibodies to alpha- and beta-globin chains. *Br J Haematol* 1996; **93**: 576–85.

261. Wickramasinghe SN, Pippard MJ. Studies of erythroblast function in congenital dyserythropoietic anaemia, type I: evidence of impaired DNA, RNA, and protein synthesis and unbalanced globin chain synthesis in ultrastructurally abnormal cells. *J Clin Pathol* 1986; **39**: 881–90.

262. Alloisio N, Jaccoud P, Dorleac E *et al.* Alterations of globin chain synthesis and of red cell membrane proteins in congenital dyserythropoietic anemia I and II. *Pediatr Res* 1982; **16**: 1016–21.

263. Perrotta S, del Giudice EM, Carbone R *et al.* Gilbert's syndrome accounts for the phenotypic variability of congenital dyserythropoietic anemia type II (CDA-II). *J Pediatr* 2000; **136**: 556–9.

264. Riva A, Mariani R, Bovo G *et al.* Type 3 hemochromatosis and beta-thalassemia trait. *Eur J Haematol* 2004; **72**: 370–4.

265. Melis MA, Cau M, Deidda F *et al.* H63D mutation in the HFE gene increases iron overload in beta-thalassemia carriers. *Haematologica* 2002; **87**: 242–5.

266. Ruiz-Arguelles GJ, Garces-Eisele J, Reyes-Nunez V *et al.* Heterozygosity for the H63D mutation in the hereditary hemochromatosis (HFE) gene may lead into severe iron overload in beta-thalassemia minor: observations in a thalassemic kindred. *Rev Invest Clin* 2001; **53**: 117–20.

267. Beauchamp-Nicoud A, Schischmanoff PO, Alloisio N *et al.* Suppression of CDA II expression in a homozygote. *Br J Haematol* 1999; **106**: 948–53.

268. Danise P, Amendola G, Nobili B *et al.* Flow-cytometric analysis of erythrocytes and reticulocytes in congenital dyserythropoietic anaemia type II (CDA II): value in differential diagnosis with hereditary spherocytosis. *Clin Lab Haematol* 2001; **23**: 7–13.

269. Hovinga JA, Solenthaler M, Dufour JF. Congenital dyserythropoietic anaemia type II (HEMPAS) and haemochromatosis: a report of two cases. *Eur J Gastroenterol Hepatol* 2003; **15**: 1141–7.

270. Greiner TC, Burns CP, Dick FR, Henry KM, Mahmood I. Congenital dyserythropoietic anemia type II diagnosed in a 69-year-old patient with iron overload. *Am J Clin Pathol* 1992; **98**: 522–5.

3

Inherited bone marrow failure syndromes

Yigal Dror

Introduction

Bone marrow failure can either be acquired throughout life (e.g., idiopathic aplastic anemia) or can occur as part of several inherited syndromes. Inherited marrow failure syndromes (IMFSs) are rare genetic diseases characterized by varying degrees of defective production of mature erythrocytes, granulocytes, and platelets in the bone marrow, leading to anemia, thrombocytopenia, and neutropenia. The designation "congenital" has a looser connotation and refers to conditions that manifest early in life, often at birth, regardless of causation. Thus, congenital marrow failure is not necessarily inherited, and may be due to acquired factors such as viruses and environmental toxins.

Although in all IMFSs the bone marrow is hypoproductive causing peripheral cytopenia, they constitute a heterogeneous group of disorders (Table 3.1), and are traditionally classified according to the lineage affected. In some IMFSs (e.g., Fanconi anemia) pancytopenia (two or more lineages affected) usually evolves. In others, one lineage is predominantly involved. Among the latter category are disorders with predominantly neutropenia (e.g., Kostmann neutropenia), anemia (e.g., Diamond–Blackfan anemia), or thrombocytopenia (e.g., thrombocytopenia absent radii).

A wide range of physical anomalies have been described in many IMFSs, with significant overlap among the various disorders. These include craniofacial, skeletal, cardiovascular, pulmonary, gastrointestinal, immunologic, renal, and neurologic anomalies as well as those of the skin, eyes, and ears.

All patterns of inheritance are associated with marrow failure disorders. Many IMFS cases are sporadic and could be either recessive or dominant traits with variable expression. Genes for many of the IMFSs have been identified and cloned, and can be used for diagnostic purposes (Table 3.1). A significant portion of the patients with IMFSs do not have known gene defects and cannot be accurately diagnosed by clinical and standard laboratory tests.[1]

Presentation with symptoms of marrow failure in IMFSs can be triggered or hastened by environmental exposures such as viruses, drugs, chemicals, or toxins. For example, there are reports of patients with IMFSs who developed hematologic symptoms following treatment with chloramphenicol,[2] or following a viral illness.[3]

The true incidence of the acquired vs inherited marrow failure syndromes is unknown. Older studies showed that about two-thirds of the patients with marrow failure had an acquired condition and one third inherited.[4] However, since most of these cases were diagnosed only on clinical findings, these figures are probably inaccurate. For example, recently a portion of patients with apparently "acquired" aplastic anemia or acute myeloblastic leukemia (AML) have been found to have IMFSs.[5]

Historically, the IMFSs were classified as "benign" hematology, which contrasted sharply with the malignant myeloid disorders. For example, patients with Kostmann syndrome often died early in life from complications of their disorders. However, in the current era of advanced supportive care and availability of recombinant cytokines and other therapeutics, patients with these conditions usually survive the early years of life and beyond. With the extended lifespan of patients, a new natural history for some of these disorders is evident. One of the most sobering observations is that most of these "benign" disorders confer an inordinately high predisposition to malignant transformation into myelodysplastic syndrome (MDS) and leukemia (particularly acute myeloblastic) as well as solid tumors.[6–11]

The true risk of cancer in the various IMFSs is unknown, but might be as high as 50% in certain IMFSs. Further, some patients with an apparently acquired MDS or AML are found to have a pre-existing marrow failure condition when investigated.[12] As the IMFSs are rare and no prospective studies with a consistent approach to diagnostic criteria for malignancy are available, there are major problems when trying to estimate the risk of malignancy based on the available data.

Table 3.1 Genes associated with inherited marrow failure syndromes.

Disorder	Gene	Protein	Gene locus	Inheritance	Reference
Fanconi anemia	FANCA	FANCA	16q24.3	AR	344
	FANCB	FANCB	Xp22.31	XLR	345
	FANCC	FANCC	9q22.3	AR	346, 347
	FANCD1/BRCA2	FANCD1/BRCA2	13q12.3	AR	39
	FANCD2	FANCD2	3p25.3	AR	348
	FANCE	FANCE	6p21.3	AR	349
	FANCF	FANCF	11p15	AR	350
	FANCG/XRCC9	FANCG	9p13	AR	351
	FANCI	(FANCI)	UK	AR	352
	FANCJ	(FANCJ)	UK	AR	352
	FANCL	FANCL/PHF9	2p16.1	AR	25
	UK	UK	UK	UK	
Shwachman–Diamond syndrome	SBDS	SBDS	7q11	AR	127
Dyskeratosis congenita	DKC1	Dyskerin	Xq28	XLR	156
	TERC	TERC	3q26	AD	157
Congenital amegakaryocytic thrombocytopenia	C-mpl	C-mpl	1p34	AR	180
Reticular dysgenesis	UK	UK	UK	UK	
Pearson syndrome	mDNA	Variable	mDNA	Maternal	194
Diamond–Blackfan anemia	RPS19	RPS19	19q13.3	AD	219
	UK	UK	8p	AD	
Congenital sideroblastic anemia	ALAS2	ALAS	Xp11.21	XL	251
	ABC7	ATP-binding cassette transporter 7	Xq13.1–q13.3	XL	252
	SLC19A2	Thiamine transporter 2	1q23.3	AR	253
Congenital dyserythropoietic anemia type I	CDAN1	Codanin I	15q15	AR	255
Congenital dyserythropoietic anemia type II	UK	UK	20q11.2	AR	
Congenital dyserythropoietic anemia type III	UK	UK	15q21–q25	AR	
Kostmann neutropenia	ELA2	Neutrophil elastase	19p13.3	AD	258
	GFI1	GFI1	1p22	AD	267
	WASP	WASP	Xp11.23–p11.22	XLR	268
Cyclic neutropenia	ELA2	Neutrophil elastase	19p13.3	AD	298
WHIM syndrome	CXCR4	CXCR4		AR	303
Nonsyndromic myelokathexis	UK	UK	UK	AR	
Glycogen storage diseases Ib	G6PT	G6PT	11q23	AR	306
Barth syndrome	Taz	Taffazins	Xq28	XL	307
Thrombocytopenia–absent radii	UK	UK	UK	AR	
Epstein/Fechtner/Sebastian/May–Hegglin/Alport syndrome	MYH9	Nonmuscle myosin heavy chain IIA	22q11–q13	AD	331
Mediterranean platelet disorder	GPIBA	GPIb	17pter–p12	AD	342
Montreal platelet disorder	UK	UK	UK	AD	
Familial autosomal dominant nonsyndromic thrombocytopenia	FLJ14813	Putative tyrosine kinase	10p11–12	AD	334
Thrombocytopenia with dyserythropoiesis	GATA1	GATA1	Xp11.23	XL	335
Thrombocytopenia with associated myeloid malignancies	CBFA2	CBFA2	21q22.1–22.2	AD	7
X-linked thrombocytopenia	WASP	WASP	Xp11.23	XL	
Thrombocytopenia with radioulnar dysostosis	HOXA11	HOXA11	7p15–p14.2	AD	340

AD, autosomal dominant; AR, autosomal recessive; XL, X-linked; XLR, X-linked recessive; UK, unknown.

Inherited marrow failure syndromes with predominantly pancytopenia

Fanconi anemia

This classical marrow failure disorder is typically inherited in an autosomal recessive manner with a heterozygote frequency of about 1 in 200, and occurs in all racial and ethnic groups. The original report by Professor Fanconi described pancytopenia combined with physical anomalies in three brothers.[13] A summary of the large body of published information on hundreds of patients with Fanconi anemia (FA) over the ensuing 80 years has underscored the clinical variability of the condition.[12,14] At presentation patients may have either a classic phenotype comprising physical anomalies and abnormal hematology, or typical physical anomalies but normal hematology, or normal physical features but abnormal hematology.

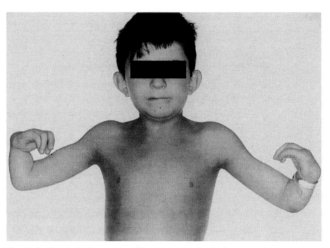

Fig. 3.1 Classical phenotype of Fanconi anemia. Patient has pigmentary changes around the neck, shoulders, and trunk, short stature, absent radii and thumbs bilaterally, microcephaly, and low-set ears.

Clinical manifestations

Hematologic features

A cardinal feature is the gradual onset of bone marrow failure involving one or more hematopoietic cell lineages. Thrombocytopenia usually develops initially, with the subsequent onset of granulocytopenia and anemia. Severe aplasia eventually develops in most cases but the full expression of pancytopenia is variable and occurs over a period of months to years. The development of aplastic anemia can be accelerated by intercurrent infections or by drugs such as chloramphenicol. Data from the International FA Registry showed that 86% of the patients developed hematologic abnormalities at a median of 7 years (range: birth to 31 years).[8] The actuarial risk of developing hematologic abnormalities increases with age, reaching 90–98% by 40 years.[14] Rosenberg and colleagues studied clinical risk factors for bone marrow failure in a cohort of 144 North American patients with FA.[15] They found that abnormal radii are the strongest predictor of early marrow failure. The cumulative incidence of marrow failure by age 10 years varied from 18% in the lowest risk group to 83% in the highest.[15]

Red blood cells are macrocytic with mean cell volumes often > 100 fL even before the onset of significant anemia. Erythropoiesis is characterized by increased fetal hemoglobin F and increased expression of i antigen, but not necessarily both features in individual cells. Increased hemoglobin F production is not clonal and has a heterogeneous distribution. Ferrokinetic studies indicate that most patients have an element of ineffective erythropoiesis as part of the marrow failure. Red blood cell lifespan may be slightly shortened but this is a minor component of the anemia.

In the early stages of the disease, the bone marrow can show erythroid hyperplasia, sometimes with dyserythropoiesis and even megaloblastic-appearing cells. As the disease progresses, the marrow becomes hypocellular and fatty, and shows a relative increase in lymphocytes, plasma cells, reticulum cells and mast cells. With full-blown marrow failure, the morphology on biopsy is identical to that seen in severe acquired aplastic anemia.

Nonhematologic manifestations

The presence of one or more characteristic congenital physical anomalies in the setting of bone marrow failure should strongly suggest a diagnosis of FA (Fig. 3.1). However, a portion of patients with FA may lack anomalies, and have been historically diagnosed with "Estren–Dameshek aplastic anemia".[16] With the introduction of clastogenic stress-induced chromosomal breakage analysis as a confirmatory test for FA, data from the International FA Registry showed that of 202 patients tested, 39% had aplastic anemia and anomalies, 30% had aplastic anemia without anomalies and 24% had anomalies only.[14] Seven percent had classical FA phenotype with negative chromosomal fragility testing.

The commonest physical anomaly is skin hyperpigmentation, a generalized brown melanin-like splattering, which is most prominent on the trunk, neck, and intertriginous areas and which becomes more obvious with age. Café-au-lait spots are common alone or combined with the generalized hyperpigmentation, and sometimes with vitiligo or hypopigmentation. The skin pigmentation should not be confused with hemosiderosis-induced bronzing in transfusion-dependent patients who have not been adequately chelated.

The majority of patients have short stature. Superimposed endocrinopathies might contribute to the growth defect. According to data from the International FA Registry, all 13 patients tested had abnormal spontaneous overnight growth hormone secretion; 21 of 48 (44%) patients tested had a subnormal response to growth hormone stimulation; 19 of

53 (36%) had overt or compensated hypothyroidism; 8 of 40 (25%) had impaired glucose tolerance; 28 of 39 (72%) had hyperinsulinemia.[17] Improvement in stature has been reported in patients with FA treated with growth hormone; however, it is unclear whether the use of growth hormone in this patient population increases the risk of malignancy.

Malformations involving the upper limbs are common, especially hypoplastic, supernumerary, bifid, or absent thumbs. Hypoplastic or absent radii in FA are always associated with hypoplastic or absent thumbs in contrast to the thrombocytopenia with thrombocytopenia absent radii syndrome, in which thumbs are always present. Less often, anomalies of the feet are seen, including toe syndactyly, short toes, a supernumerary toe, clubfoot, and flat feet. Congenital hip dislocation and leg abnormalities are occasionally seen.

Males often have gonadal and genitalia abnormalities, including an underdeveloped or micropenis, undescended, atrophic, or absent testes, hypospadias, phimosis, and an abnormal urethra. Female patients occasionally have malformations or atresia of the vagina, uterus, and ovary.

Many patients have a characteristic "facies" and unrelated patients can resemble each other almost as closely as siblings. The head and facial changes vary but commonly consist of microcephaly, small eyes, epicanthal folds, and abnormal shape, size, or positioning of the ears. About 10% of FA patients are mentally retarded. Renal anomalies occur but require imaging for documentation. Ectopic, pelvic, or horseshoe kidneys are often detected as well as duplicated, hypoplastic, dysplastic, or absent organs. Occasionally, hydronephrosis or hydroureter is present.

Cancer predisposition

The karyotype data, the defects in DNA repair, and the cellular damage that occur in FA patients translate into an enormous predisposition for malignancy. Two recent studies described the risk of malignancy in FA. Data from the International FA Registry study[14] demonstrated a crude rate of cancer of 23%; 179 patients developed 199 neoplasms. Of these neoplasms, 60% were hematologic and 40% were nonhematologic. The hematologic malignancies included AML (36%), MDS (31%), and acute lymphoblastic leukemia (3%). The authors suggested that the risk of hematologic and nonhematologic neoplasms increased with advancing age with a 33% and 28% cumulative incidence, respectively, by 40 years of age.

The second study is a survey of the literature from 1927 to 2001.[18] Two hundred patients (crude rate of 17%) had developed cancer at the median age of 16 years. In approximately 25% of patients with cancer, the malignancy preceded the diagnosis of FA. The author calculated that if the competing risks of aplastic anemia and leukemia could be removed, the estimated cumulative probability of development of a solid tumor is 76% by the age of 45 years.

The risk of advanced MDS/AML is higher for patients in whom a prior clonal marrow cytogenetic abnormality (MCA) had been detected.[8] Monosomy 7 or partial loss of 7q, rearrangements of 1p36 and 1q24–34, and rearrangements of 11q22–25 are the most frequently recurring cytogenetic changes. MCAs consisting of partial trisomies or tetrasomies of chromosome 3q conferred a high risk of transformation into advanced MDS or leukemia.[19]

Most of the solid tumors described in FA were squamous cell carcinomas involving the gastrointestinal tract at any site from the oropharynx to the anorectal-colonic area.[14,18] Less frequently, patients can develop carcinomas of the vulva, cervix, and breast or unusual combinations such as Wilms tumor with medulloblastoma, cancer of the vulva and tongue, hepatic carcinoma and cancer of the tongue, and hepatic carcinoma and esophageal carcinoma.[14,18]

Liver tumors, benign and malignant, as well as peliosis hepatis occur at increased frequency in FA.[14,18] The commonest tumors reported were adenomas and hepatocellular carcinoma. Since almost all patients were taking androgen therapy at the time the liver disease presented, androgens have been implicated as having a direct relationship in pathogenesis. Indeed, peliosis hepatis is reversible when androgens are stopped, and in three patients with tumors, discontinuation of androgens alone or coupled with hematopoietic stem cell transplantation (HSCT) effected a regression of the tumors.

Genetic aspects

FA has been reported in all ethnic groups, and is mostly inherited as an autosomal recessive condition. This was confirmed with the identification of the FA genes *A, C, D2/BRCA1, E, F, G, I, J,* and *L* (Table 3.1). Interestingly, it has long been known that the ratio of males to female diagnosed with the disorder is slightly more than one (1.06 to 1.2). This could be due to bias toward establishing the diagnosis more readily in males compared with females or due to prediagnosis early female death. However, the *FANCB* gene has recently been localized to Xp22.31, and it is thus inherited in an X-linked manner. Therefore, genetic counseling of families with FA should now depend on accurate genetic analysis.

A breakthrough in the search for the defective genes in FA evolved from the important observation that hybrid cells formed from FA and normal cells or from two unrelated FA patients resulted in correction of the abnormal chromosome fragility, a process known as complementation.[20,21] This enables classification of FA patients into various complementation groups and subsequently identification of the respective genes. Currently, at least 11 FA subgroups have been proposed and nine of the genes associated with these groups have already been identified (Table 3.1).

There can be discordance in clinical and hematologic findings among siblings, even in affected monozygotic twins.

However, a certain degree of correlation exists between genotype and phenotype. FA-A patients with homozygosity for null mutations tend to have an earlier onset of anemia and a higher incidence of leukemia than those with mutations producing an altered protein.[22] Also, FA-C patients with IVS4 + 4A > T or exon 14 mutations usually,[22,23] but not always,[24] have more somatic abnormalities, earlier onset of hematologic abnormalities, and poorer survival compared with patients with the *FANCC* exon 1 mutation and the non-FA-C population. FA-G patients had more severe cytopenia and a higher incidence of leukemia. FA-D, FA-E, and FA-F had higher frequencies of somatic abnormalities.

Pathogenesis

Protein complex

Solid data exist showing that the FA proteins interact in a common molecular pathway. The FA proteins FANCA, C, E, F, G, and L bind and form a complex, which is required for FANCD2 monoubiquitinylation. The ubiquitin ligase that performs this function might be FANCL.[25] After ubiquitination, FANCD2 can colocalize with FANCD1/BRCA2 and BRCA1 in "nuclear foci" following genotoxic stress.[25,26,29,30] Inactivating mutation of any one of the FA proteins in this pathway prevents the ultimate translocation of FANCD2 to the target nuclear foci. The precise functions of the FA proteins in the nucleus at a biochemical level are still unknown.

Mouse models

Knockout FA mouse models are available for *FANCC*, *FANCA*, and *FANCG*, but they do not completely mimic the human FA phenotype.[31,32] The mice do not exhibit developmental abnormalities or gross hematologic defects. However, their spleen cells have increased numbers of chromosomal aberrations in response to mitomycin C and diepoxybutane, the G_2–M progression of the cell cycle is abnormal,[33] hematopoietic progenitors are markedly sensitive to γ-interferon and have lower growth and differentiation potential in response to cytokines,[34] and both male and female mice have compromised gametogenesis and markedly impaired fertility.[31,32,35]

Chromosome breakage studies and abnormal DNA repair

A major finding in FA is abnormal chromosome fragility; this is seen readily in metaphase preparations of phytohemagglutinin-stimulated peripheral blood lymphocytes or cultured skin fibroblasts. The karyotype shows "spontaneously" occurring chromatid breaks, rearrangements, gaps, endoreduplications, and chromatid exchanges in cells from homozygous patients with FA. The abnormal chromosome pattern, number of breaks/cell, and variations in proportion of abnormal cells have no direct correlation with the hematologic or clinical course of individual patients.[23]

"Spontaneous" chromosomal breaks are occasionally absent in FA,[36] but are strikingly enhanced if clastogenic agents such as diepoxybutane or mitomycin C are added to the cultures.[36] Homozygous Fanconi cells are hypersensitive to many other oncogenic and mutagenic inducers, such as ionizing radiation, SV40 viral transformation, and alkylating and chemical agents including cyclophosphamide, nitrogen mustard, and platinum compounds. The increased chromosomal fragility is caused by a defect in DNA repair. Defects in mismatch repair, recombinational repair[37] and excision repair pathways[38] have been hypothesized. Mutations in any member of the FA protein complex reduce FANCD2 ubiquitinylation and its colocalization with BRCA1.[30] Some hypomorphic homozygous *BRCA2* (*FANCD1*) mutations prevent Rad51 localization in damage-induced nuclear foci,[39,40] which is required to protect cells and/or facilitate DNA repair.

Apoptosis

FA cells demonstrate G_2-phase cell cycle arrest.[41] This effect cannot be induced by DNA cross-linking agents. Several groups have shown that FA cells undergo accelerated apoptosis and are intolerant of oxidative stress.[42] FANCC enhances the function of GSTP1, which detoxifies byproducts of redox stress and xenobiotics, whereby it might protect cells from inducers of apoptosis.[43] FANCC associates with hsp70, upon exposure to either combinations of tumor necrosis factor (TNF) and interferon-γ (IFN-γ) or double-stranded RNA and IFN-γ. This interaction facilitates hsp70 binding to and inactivation of double-stranded RNA-dependent protein kinase, thereby protecting from apoptosis.[44] Mutations in the *FANCA*, *FANCC*, and *FANCG* genes markedly increase the amount of RNA-dependent protein kinase, leading to hypersensitivity of hematopoietic progenitor cells to growth inhibition by IFN-γ and TNF-α.[45]

The hematopoietic stem cell and progenitor phenotype

The frequency of erythroid colony-forming unit (CFU-E), erythroid burst-forming unit (BFU-E) and granulocyte-macrophage colony-forming unit (CFU-GM) cells is reduced in almost all patients after aplastic anemia becomes evident,[46,47] as well as in a few patients prior to the onset of aplastic anemia.[48] A defect in the response of early hematopoietic progenitors to specific cytokines has been proposed.[49] Because all hematopoietic cell lineages are affected in these studies, the basic defect either involves pluripotent hematopoietic stem cells and early progenitors or is due to faulty proliferative properties, or both.

Production of growth factors by the FA marrow stroma and the expression of their receptors on hematopoietic cells have not been systematically studied, and the results are variable.[50] Generation of the inhibitory cytokine TNF-α has been shown to be markedly heightened.[50]

Laboratory evaluation and diagnosis

About 75% of patients are between 3 and 14 years of age at the time of diagnosis with a mean age of about 8 years in males and 9 years in females.[12,14] It is noteworthy that 4% of the patients are diagnosed in the first year of life, and 10% after 15 years of age.

The diagnosis of FA is usually suspected after obtaining a medical, developmental, and family history, as well as conducting a physical examination. Low blood cell counts, red blood cell macrocytosis, high hemoglobin F, increased expression of the i antigen, and varying degrees of marrow hypoplasia are common findings, but are not specific for FA and can be seen in other IMFSs. In patients without physical anomalies, chromosomal breakage analysis using diepoxybutane or mitomycin C will specifically identify FA and lead to the correct diagnosis.

Since it was introduced in 1981[51] the chromosomal fragility test has become the gold standard for the diagnosis of FA. Fragile chromosomes can be readily seen in metaphase preparations of phytohemagglutinin-stimulated peripheral blood lymphocytes or cultured skin fibroblasts. "Spontaneous" chromosomal breaks are occasionally absent in true cases of homozygous FA, but become positive after the cells are treated with mitomycin C or diepoxybutane.[36] For definitive diagnostic purposes, the International FA Registry has defined FA as increased numbers of chromosome breaks/cell after exposure to diepoxybutane[36] with a mean of 8.96 (range 1.3–23.9) compared with normal controls of 0.06 (range 0–0.36). It must be noted that some patients with classical features of FA occasionally have a negative test. Whether this group represents a special subgroup of FA or a separate disorder has to be determined.

A new, rapid diagnostic test is Western blot of FANCD2 protein, which shows a slow band of monoubiquitinated isoforms in addition to a faster nonubiquitinated isoform. In most FA patients the defect lies upstream to this biochemical step, and thus only fast nonubiquitinated isoforms of FANCD2 are detected. Genetic testing for FA is complicated due to its association with multiple genes, and the inability to predict the location of the mutation in most cases. Complementation testing is done first followed by molecular analysis of the respective gene.

Prenatal diagnosis

Diagnostic testing can be performed on fetal amniotic fluid cells obtained at 16 weeks' gestation or on chorionic villus biopsy specimens at 9–12 weeks. A very high degree of prenatal diagnostic accuracy has been documented by looking at both spontaneous and diepoxybutane-induced breaks,[36] and genetic testing.[52]

Therapy and prognosis

Because of their clinical complexity, patients with FA should be supervised at a tertiary care center using a comprehensive and multidisciplinary approach. Due to early diagnosis and newer approaches to HSCT, the prognosis of patients with FA has been improved, and the median survival is currently 24 years of age.[14] Older female FA patients can be sexually active, become pregnant, and give birth to healthy children.[53]

Complications in FA include severe cytopenia (hemoglobin < 8 g/L, platelet counts < 20 × 10⁹/L, absolute neutrophil count < 0.5 × 10⁹/L), MDS with excess blasts (5–30%), and acute leukemia (blasts > 30%). If the patient is stable and has only minimal to moderate hematologic changes and no transfusion requirements, a period of observation is indicated. Blood counts may be monitored every 1–3 months and bone marrow aspirates and biopsies performed annually for morphology and cytogenetics to identify transformation into MDS/AML. Depending on the types of congenital anomalies, subspecialty consultations, for example, with cardiologists and orthopedic surgeons, can be arranged during this interval.

Hematopoietic stem cell transplantation

As most patients need hematopoietic stem cell transplantation (HSCT) at some stage of their disease, the author recommends HLA-typing for the whole family shortly after diagnosis. If no family member is a match, other options such as prenatal genetic diagnosis and *in vitro* fertilization for the selection of healthy donors for transplantation might be discussed with the family.

HSCT is currently the only curative therapy for the hematologic abnormalities of FA and the best donor source is an HLA-matched sibling. Initial efforts to transplant FA patients using standard preparative regimens were plagued by severe cytotoxicity and graft-versus-host disease (GVHD).[54] HSCT protocols for FA patients were subsequently dose-modified by Gluckman *et al.*[55] and others, and outcomes improved substantially.

In an analysis of 151 cases of FA patients from 42 institutions, who had HLA-identical sibling HSCT, the 2-year survival rate was 66%.[56] Factors associated with a favorable outcome were a younger patient age, higher pre-HSCT platelet count, use of antithymocyte globulin (ATG), use of low-dose cyclophosphamide (15–25 mg/kg) plus limited-field irradiation for pre-HSCT conditioning, and ciclosporine for GVHD prophylaxis. In a later European study, where all patients received low-dose cyclophosphamide and thoracoabdominal irradiation as transplant conditioning, the survival estimate was 74.4% at 54 months and 58.5% at 100 months.[57] Another report with a smaller number of patients showed an approximately 85% survival with a median follow-up of > 3 years.[58] This approach included cyclophosphamide, 20 mg/kg/day, thoracoabdominal irradiation 400 cGy and horse ATG. GVHD prophylaxis included posttransplant horse ATG, methylprednisolone, and ciclosporin.

Although there is still room for improving the overall survival rates of transplant in the matched sibling donor setting, the main challenges are currently in finding regimens with reduced long-term toxicity and eliminating a potential increase in the cancer risk above the inherent baseline rate. One such approach is eliminating irradiation. A conditioning regimen that omitted radiation and used a reduced dosage of cyclophosphamide showed 89% survival with a median follow-up of 285 days.[59] Fludarabine has increasingly been used as part of radiation-free conditioning regimens for FA since it was first used in this disease in 1997.[60,61] The results of these studies are encouraging; however, results of larger series are not yet available.

Results of HSCT with matched unrelated donors in FA have not been as good as with matched sibling donor HSCT, with a probability of 1-year survival of 34%[62] and 2-year survival of 29%.[56] Because of these dismal results, incorporating fludarabine in the preparatory regimens is of particular interest in this group of patients. Boulad et al.[63] analyzed 15 consecutive patients with FA with aplastic anemia, advanced MDS, or AML, who received granulocyte colony-stimulating factor (G-CSF) mobilized T-cell-depleted peripheral cell grafts from either partially mismatched related donors or unrelated donors (7–10 out of 10 HLA antigen match). Cytoreduction included total body irradiation (450 cGy), fludarabine (150 mg/m^2), and cyclophosphamide (40 mg/kg). Immuno-suppression included rabbit ATG and tacrolimus. All patients were fully engrafted. No patients required treatment for GVHD. With a median follow-up of 2.5 years, 13 of 15 patients were alive, and 11 of 15 were disease-free.

Wagner and colleagues[64] evaluated 98 unrelated donor transplants in FA for aplastic anemia (69%) or MDS/AML (31%). Fifty-four percent received cyclophosphamide and irradiation, and 46% received a fludarabine-containing preparative regimen. Twenty-two percent had a mismatch at a single locus. Seventy-one percent of grafts were T-cell depleted. Fludarabine-containing regimens resulted in significantly better engraftment rates, lower mortality, and better overall survival, and overcame the problem of diepoxybutane mosaicism in peripheral blood lymphocytes. Poor outcome was associated with receiving > 20 blood products prior to transplant. A European study also showed that delaying transplantation by the use of androgens was associated with poorer outcome posttransplantation.[65]

Cord blood cells are being used increasingly as a donor source. The first cord blood transplantation was performed in 1988 for a patient with FA using a matched sibling donor.[66] Cord cells from unrelated donors have been transplanted into FA patients.[58,67] A recent retrospective analysis of 72 patients with FA complicated by severe aplastic anemia or leukemia/MDS using HLA-identical or one to three HLA differences showed comparable overall survival (36%) to these authors' experience with the use of matched unrelated bone marrow transplant.[67] The main complications were non-engraftment and infections. Favorable factors were negative recipient cytomegalovirus (CMV) serology, nucleated cell dose of > 4.4 × 10^7/kg and use of fludarabine.

Transplant in FA with MDS or AML is associated with poorer outcome,[64] but is feasible. In these cases the preparative therapy was usually escalated, and included cyclophosphamide 40 mg/kg/day and total body irradiation 450 cGy with[64,68] or without fludarabine.[58] However, successful transplant in this setting using a fludarabine-containing regimen without the use of irradiation was also reported.[60]

Because of the increased risks associated with alternative donor marrow, the timing of the transplant when a matched sibling donor is not available is hotly debated. Traditionally only patients who failed androgen therapy were offered alternative donor transplant. However, a delay in the transplant and the use of androgen might expose the patients to more transfusions, infections, complications, and androgen-related toxicity, and may compromise the success of a subsequent HSCT.[64,65]

Preimplantation genetic diagnosis has recently been offered in combination with HLA typing in order to select a sibling embryo that is negative or heterozygous (but not homozygous) for the patient's FA gene mutations as well as HLA-matched to the patient. Many ethical issues are associated with this advanced procedure;[69] however, several successful transplants using this advanced technology have already been reported.[70,71]

Despite the clear-cut success in correcting the marrow failure of FA with HSCT, a subset of survivors will develop secondary cancers, particularly of the head and neck.[14,18] These malignancies reflect the ongoing genetic susceptibility of host nonhematopoietic tissue to cancer despite successful HSCT for marrow failure.

Hematopoietic growth factors

The potential for recombinant growth factor (cytokine) therapy for FA has not been fully explored but short-term data are encouraging.[72,73] An important multicenter clinical trial[72] examined the effect of prolonged administration of G-CSF in 12 FA patients with neutropenia. By week 8 of the study, all patients showed an increase in neutrophil counts. Some patients had clinically significant increase also in platelet counts and hemoglobin. In another study, patients without a matched sibling donor who did not have a MCA were given combination cytokine therapy consisting of G-CSF 5 µg/kg with erythropoietin 50 units/kg administered subcutaneously or intravenously three times a week.[58] Of 20 patients treated, all but 1 showed improved neutrophil numbers, 20% achieved a sustained rise in platelets, and 33% showed an increase in hemoglobin levels. However, more than half of the responders did not sustain the response after 1 year.

Since a marked predisposition to cancer is a feature of FA, the use of growth-promoting cytokines on a chronic basis for this disorder is a central issue. Development of new clones on G-CSF treatment was reported, and remains a significant concern.[72,73] However, appearance and disappearance of MCAs are common phenomena in FA patients and were not proven to be directly caused by G-CSF.[74]

Androgens

Androgen therapy has been used to treat FA for more than four decades. The overall response rate in the literature is about 50%,[12,18] heralded by reticulocytosis and a rise in hemoglobin within 1–2 months. If the other lineages respond, white cells increase next and finally platelets, but it may take many months to achieve the maximum response. When the response is deemed maximal, the androgens should be slowly tapered but not stopped entirely.

Oxymetholone is most frequently used at 2–5 mg/kg daily with preference for the lowest dose initially. Low-dose prednisone (5–10 mg orally every second day) is sometimes added to counter the androgen-induced growth acceleration. Danazol is another androgen that has recently been used in FA, but there are insufficient data to evaluate its efficacy and safety.

Almost all patients relapse when androgens are stopped. Many patients on long-term androgens eventually become refractory to therapy as marrow failure progresses. Potential side effects include masculinization, elevated hepatic enzymes, cholestasis, peliosis hepatis, and liver tumors. Those receiving androgens should be evaluated serially with liver chemistry profiles and ultrasonography and/or CT (computed tomography) scan of liver.

Gene therapy

The premise for gene therapy in FA is based on the presumption that corrected hematopoietic cells have a growth advantage. Strengthening this supposition are recent descriptions of rare patients with FA who had clinical improvement and spontaneous disappearance of cells with the FA phenotype due to intragenic mitotic recombination generating one allele with both FA mutations and one normal allele.[75]

Preclinical studies using retroviral vectors showed that the *FANCC* and *FANCA* genes can be successfully integrated into normal and FA cells.[76] This prompted a clinical trial in three FA-C patients[76,77] and four FA-A patients.[77] The patients underwent peripheral blood stem-cell harvesting. The CD34+ cell population was then infected with a retrovirus containing the wild-type copy of the respective FANC gene, followed by transfusion of these modified cells into the patient. These preliminary experiments failed to induce sufficient gene expression.[78] Lentivirus vectors have recently been studied for gene therapy in mice, and may be proven safe and useful for clinical gene therapy of FA hematopoietic cells.[79]

Shwachman–Diamond syndrome

Shwachman–Diamond syndrome (SDS) is an autosomal recessive multisystem disorder first described in the early 1960s by several groups.[80,81] The syndrome comprises a triad of bone marrow failure, pancreatic insufficiency and skeletal abnormalities.[82] In addition, the liver, kidneys, teeth, and immune system may also be affected.[9,10,82–85] SDS is also associated with a propensity for MDS and leukemia.[9,82,86–88] SDS is the third most common IMFS after Fanconi anemia and Diamond–Blackfan anemia. Although SDS is an autosomal recessive disorder, the ratio of males to females diagnosed with SDS is 1.7:1.[83]

Clinical manifestations

Hematologic features

Neutropenia is the most common hematologic abnormality, occurring in 88–100% of patients. It might be seen in the neonatal period,[82] and it can be either persistent or intermittent, fluctuating from severely low to normal levels. SDS neutrophils have defects in migration and chemotaxis in most patients.[84,86,89] The chemotactic defect might be due to abnormal distribution of concanavalin-A receptors or a cytoskeletal/microtubular abnormality,[89] and can be partially corrected *in vitro* and *in vivo*[90] by lithium.

Anemia with low reticulocytes occurs in up to 80% of the patients. The red blood cells are usually normochromic-normocytic, but can also be macrocytic. Fetal hemoglobin is elevated in 80% of patients.[91] The anemia is usually asymptomatic. Thrombocytopenia, with platelets less than 150×10^9/L, is seen in 24–88% of patients. Trilineage cytopenias occur in 10–65% of patients. Severe aplasia requiring transfusions has occasionally been reported.[82,92,93]

Bone marrow biopsy usually shows a hypoplastic specimen with increased fat deposition,[82,91] but marrows showing normal or even increased cellularity have also been observed.[83,86] Single-lineage hypoplasia is usually myeloid and occurs in 15–50% of patients.[9,83] Left-shifted granulopoiesis is a common finding.[82,83] Mild dysplastic changes in the erythroid, myeloid, and megakaryocytic precursors are commonly seen and may fluctuate; however, prominent multilineage dysplasia is less common, and if it occurs, may signify malignant myeloid transformation.

Multiple B- and T-cell defects have been reported in SDS.[94–98] In our series 7 of 14 patients had B-cell defects, 6 of 9 had at least one T-cell abnormality, and 5 of 6 had decreased percentages of circulating natural killer cells.[84]

Nonhematologic manifestations

Varying severity of pancreatic dysfunction due to abnormal acinar development and malabsorption is a hallmark of SDS.[83] Spontaneous improvement in pancreatic function occurs in up to 50% of the patients. Most patients with SDS have skeletal abnormalities including metaphyseal dysostosis, rib-cage abnormalities, which can lead to thoracic dystrophy and respiratory failure in the newborn period, delayed appearance of secondary ossification centers, clinodactyly, syndactyly, pes cavus, kyphosis, scoliosis, osteopenia, vertebral collapse, slipped femoral epiphysis, and supernumerary thumb or toe.[82,83,85,99–103]

Failure to thrive is common in SDS patients and is caused by various factors, including metaphyseal dysostosis, pancreatic insufficiency, feeding difficulties, and recurrent infections.[82,83] Mean birthweight is at the 25th percentile, but by age 1 year and later, over half of patients are below the 3rd percentile for height. When treated with pancreatic enzyme replacement, most patients continue to show a normal growth velocity, but remain consistently below the 3rd percentile for height and weight.[9]

Hepatomegaly or elevated serum liver enzymes are seen in 50–75% of patients, most often in young children, and tend to resolve with age. The liver disease is usually of little consequence. Delayed dentition of permanent teeth, dental dysplasia, increased risk of dental caries, and periodontal disease may also occur. Abnormalities of the kidneys, eyes, skin, testes, endocrine pancreas, heart, nervous system, and craniofacial structures have been reported.[82,83,104,105]

Cancer predisposition

A literature review identified 54 reported cases of SDS with marrow cytogenetic abnormalities (MCAs), MDS, or AML.[10] Of the 54 cases, 37 developed MCA/MDS at a median age of 8 years (range 2–42 years) and an additional 17 were diagnosed at the stage of overt leukemia at a median age of 14 years (range 1.5–37 years). Of the patients with MCA/MDS, 68% were males; of those with leukemia, 92% were males.

MCAs have been reported in 40 SDS patients in various stages of malignant myeloid transformation;[10] mostly i(7q) (44%) and del(12)(q12) (16%). i(7q) occurs rarely in other malignancies, and has not been reported in other IMFS. Among the patients with isolated i(7q), no progression into MDS with excess blasts or AML has been reported. However, 42% of the patients with non-i(7q) abnormalities of chromosome 7, particularly monosomy 7, either initially presented with advanced MDS/AML or progressed to them from earlier stages of MDS. Interestingly, MCAs in SDS can regress spontaneously.[88,106]

With regard to the cytological description of MDS, various morphologic types have been described. Nineteen SDS cases have been reported with cytogenetic abnormalities without prominent marrow dysplasia and without an increase in blasts.[86,87,103,106–111] Of these patients, four developed severe aplasia, and three developed more severe MDS/AML. Twelve reported SDS patients were diagnosed with MDS at the stage of refractory cytopenia with dysplasia,[86,95,107,109,112–116] eight of whom could be evaluated for disease progression: four developed AML. Only one case of refractory cytopenia with ring sideroblasts (without evidence of Pearson syndrome) in a patient with SDS, who eventually progressed to AML, was reported.[117] Six published SDS cases were diagnosed with MDS at the stage of refractory cytopenia with excess blasts.[86,108,119] Three of them progressed to AML.

Leukemia was reported in 26 SDS patients with a median age of 14 years (range 1.5–43 years).[82,86,104,113,117,120–125] Of these cases, nine were preceded by a documented MDS phase. Various types of AML have been described in SDS patients: AML-M0, M2, M4, M5, and M6. Acute lymphoblastic leukemia and juvenile myelomonocytic leukemia were rare. It is noteworthy that AML-M6 was particularly common in SDS, occurring in about 30% of cases with classifiable leukemia.

SDS-related leukemia carries a poor prognosis. Of the 26 reported cases of AML (as their initial presentation or after a period with MDS), 21 patients died either because of refractory disease or treatment-related toxicity.[10] Malignant myeloid transformation into MDS and AML in SDS patients while on G-CSF therapy has been reported,[11,107] but the causal relationship is unproven.

Genetic aspects

SBDS was identified originally by Lai and colleagues[126] in 2000. It has recently been found that about 90% of the families with clinical diagnosis of SDS were found to have mutations in *SBDS*, and 96% of the mutations are in exon 2.[127] The type of mutations include missense, nonsense, frameshift, and splice-site mutations as well as complex rearrangements comprising deletion/insertion.[127,128] Correlations are unlikely to exist between genotype and the phenotype in SDS, since patients with severe phenotype such as major skeletal abnormalities[100] or AML[129] have been found to have common mutations.

Pathogenesis

The function of the *SBDS* gene product is unknown. The mRNA is ubiquitously expressed.[127] The protein encoded by the *Saccharomyces cerevisiae* ortholog of *SBDS*, *YRL022c*, is essential for yeast survival. Indirect data from lower organisms suggested a role of the gene in RNA processing and ribosomal biogenesis.[130,131] Synthetic genetic arrays of *YHR087W*, a yeast homolog of the N-terminal domain of *SBDS*, suggested interactions with several genes involved in RNA and rRNA processing.[132] Austin and colleagues[133] have found that SBDS localizes to the nucleus, nucleolus, and cytoplasm of normal control fibroblasts, but it concentrates in the nucleolus during G_1 and G_2, and is diffusely distributed in the nucleus during S phase.

Bone marrow from patients with SDS is characterized by decreased frequency of CD34[+] progenitors,[91] which have a reduced ability to generate hematopoietic colonies of all lineages *in vitro*.[91,134,135] The stem cell defect comprises both the myeloid and lymphoid compartments,[84] and is likely to be related to accelerated apoptosis.[136] The increased tendency toward apoptosis was linked to hypersensitivity of marrow cells to Fas stimulation and increased Fas expression on marrow CD34[+], CD34[-]CD38[+], and CD34[-]CD38[-] cell populations.[136] In addition, SDS is characterized by an abnormal bone marrow stroma, which has decreased ability to support hematopoiesis from normal CD34[+] cells in long-term marrow stromal cultures.[91]

Compared with normal controls, mean telomere length of patients' marrow mononuclear cells at all ages tested was significantly shorter.[137] The data available on chromosomal instability in SDS are inconclusive. Increased frequencies of spontaneous chromosome aberrations in a patient's phytohemagglutinin-stimulated circulating lymphocytes was demonstrated by some groups,[138,139] but not by others.[140,141]

To study the relationship between *SBDS* and leukemia, we studied the association between *SBDS* gene mutations and *de novo* AML in children. Although we have found no *SBDS* mutations in 125 patients with *de novo* AML and in 4 patients with 7q abnormalities,[129] changes in expression levels or posttranslational modifications are still possible. We also analyzed two SDS cases who developed AML, and found that they had commonly occurring mutations: homozygosity for 258+2T→C or heterozygosity for 183–184TA→CT and 258+2T→C.[129] When SDS cases with early MDS were studied, various molecular and cellular parameters did not distinguish cases with acquired marrow cytogenetic abnormalities from the other SDS patients, including G-CSF receptor expression or *RAS* and *p53* mutation analysis.[88] However, SDS marrows demonstrated many characteristic MDS features, including defects in marrow stromal support of normal hematopoiesis, increased apoptosis mediated through the Fas pathway, high frequency of clonal marrow cytogenetic abnormalities, p53 protein overexpression and telomere shortening.[137,142,143] This raises the possibility that SDS has prominent pre-leukemic features from its inception.

Diagnosis

Clinical diagnosis is generally made in the first few years of life. The clinical diagnosis requires evidence of exocrine pancreatic dysfunction and characteristic hematologic abnormalities.[83,128,137] Low blood cell counts, red blood cell macrocytosis, high hemoglobin F, and varying degrees of marrow hypoplasia are usual findings. A cytogenetic finding of i(7q) is highly associated with SDS. Short stature, skeletal abnormalities, hepatomegaly, or biochemical abnormalities of the liver are supportive findings of the diagnosis. Attention should be given to ruling out:

- cystic fibrosis (most common cause of pancreatic insufficiency, with an abnormal sweat test);
- Pearson disease (pancreatic insufficiency and cytopenia, marrow ring sideroblasts, and vacuolated erythroid and myeloid precursors);
- cartilage hair hypoplasia (diarrhea, cytopenia, and metaphyseal chondrodysplasia, common in the Amish population); and
- other IMFSs.

Molecular diagnosis is now available. As the clinical diagnosis of SDS is usually difficult and patients may present at a stage when no clinical pancreatic insufficiency is evident it is probably advisable to test most or all suspected cases for mutations in the *SBDS* gene. It is noteworthy that about 10% of the SDS patients might be negative for mutations in *SBDS*.

Therapy and prognosis

As with Fanconi anemia, a multidisciplinary approach to the care of patients with SDS at a tertiary care center is recommended. Detection of asymptomatic MDS with excess blasts and AML with low blast count may prompt early treatment and improve prognosis. Therefore, in a stable patient with mild to moderate cytopenia, we routinely perform complete blood count and peripheral blood smear every 3–4 months as well as annual bone marrow testing to look for occult transformation. The frequency with which the screening tools should be applied is unknown, and probably depends on the severity of the bone marrow findings. The earliest reported ages of transformation were 1.5, 2, and 3 years, so if a screening program is planned it should probably start after diagnosis regardless of age.

Supportive care

In cases of fever and severe neutropenia, patients should be treated with intravenous antibiotics with broad-spectrum coverage until the infection clears up. G-CSF should be considered in such situations. G-CSF given for profound neutropenia has been effective in inducing a clinically beneficial neutrophil response.[107,144;145] Granulocyte–macrophage colony-stimulating factor (GM-CSF) was also shown to be effective in one patient[146] but not in others.[145] Despite low serum erythropoietin levels in one patient, administration of erythropoietin did not improve hemoglobin levels.[123] Thrombocytopenia and anemia may require respective chronic transfusions, sometimes with an iron chelation program.

Androgens

A few patients have received androgens plus steroids in the manner of treating patients with Fanconi anemia. Transient responses[93] and unsuccessful trials[92,123] have been reported. Because of the underlying liver abnormalities seen in SDS, the risk of androgen use might be even higher than it is in Fanconi anemia. Moreover, the worse outcome seen in Fanconi anemia patients who received androgens before HSCT is worrisome.[65]

Hematopoietic stem cell transplantation

The criteria for selecting patients for HSCT (related or alternative) should include severe cytopenia (hemoglobin < 8 g/L, absolute neutrophil count < 0.5×10^9/L, platelet count < 20×10^9/L), MDS with excess blasts and overt leukemia. In cases of frank leukemia, the patient may be started on chemotherapy to reduce tumor load before HSCT, but an effort to find a donor should be made at the time of diagnosis because of the high risk of therapy-related aplasia.

At present, HSCT provides the only curative option for the hematologic complications in SDS. Analysis of published case reports of SDS patients who underwent allogeneic HSCT suggested that complications are more common in SDS patients who receive chemotherapy or undergo HSCT than in patients with idiopathic blood dyscrasias.[10] The European Group for Blood and Marrow Transplantation has recently published results of HSCT using either matched-related sibling donor (23%) or unrelated donor or a family mismatched donor (77%) in 26 patients with SDS.[147] The conditioning regimen was based on busulfan (54%), total body irradiation (23%), fludarabine (15%), or other chemotherapy combinations (8%). GVHD prophylaxis comprised ciclosporin with or without methotrexate or T-cell depletion. Neutrophil and platelet engraftment were achieved in 81% and 65% of the patients. The incidence of grade III and IV acute GVHD was 24% and of chronic GVHD 29%. Overall survival was 64.5% with follow-up of 1.1 years. A trend toward a higher mortality rate was found in cases of AML/MDS versus severe aplastic anemia (56% vs 19%), but the difference was not significant. Results of a series of ten cases of SDS with severe aplastic anemia or MDS/AML from the French registry using unrelated (six cases) and related (four cases) donors, showed 5-year event-free survival rate of 60%.[148]

Complications are more common in SDS patients who receive chemotherapy or undergo HSCT than in patients with idiopathic blood dyscrasias. In a review of 36 patients with SDS who had been treated with chemotherapy alone[10] or with HSCT with or without irradiation, 83% died from complications related to the therapy, including prolonged severe aplasia, infections, cardiotoxicity, neurologic and renal complications, veno-occlusive disease, pulmonary disease, posttransplant graft failure, and GVHD.

Prognosis

On the basis of a literature review, Alter calculated the projected median survival of SDS patients as 35 years.[12] During infancy, morbidity and mortality are mostly related to malabsorption, infections, and thoracic dystrophy. Later in life the main causes of morbidity and mortality are hematologic or the treatment for the hematologic complications. Cytopenias tend to fluctuate in severity but never fully resolve. No remissions have been reported after symptomatic cytopenias or advanced malignant myeloid transformation.

Dyskeratosis congenita

Dyskeratosis congenita (DC) is characterized by ectodermal abnormalities,[149,150] bone marrow failure,[6] cancer predisposition,[6] and extreme telomere shortening.[151] With the recent advances in understanding the molecular basis of the disease, patients with hematologic abnormalities without dermatologic anomalies have been identified, which has changed dramatically the historical definition of the disease.[5]

Clinical features

Hematologic manifestations

The DC registry in Hammersmith, England, provides important data about the clinical features and genetic basis of DC.[6] About 50% of X-linked male patients with DC and 70% of autosomal recessive patients develop aplastic anemia, usually in the teenage years. The actuarial probability of marrow dysfunction in males is 94% by the age of 40 years.[6] Bone marrow dysfunction occurs less frequently in the autosomal dominant group. Some young patients can develop marrow failure prior to the clinical onset of the mucocutaneous manifestations. The initial hematologic change is usually thrombocytopenia, anemia, or both, followed by pancytopenia. The red cells are often macrocytic and the hemoglobin F can be elevated. Oddly, early bone marrow aspirations and biopsies may be hypercellular; however, with time all cellular elements decline.

Immunologic abnormalities, including reduced immunoglobulin levels, reduced T- and B-lymphocyte numbers, and reduced proliferation in response to mitogens, may occur in patients in DC. Severe combined immunodeficiency or abetagammaglobulinemia[152] can occur in patients carrying the *DKC1* gene mutation.

Nonhematologic manifestations

In most cases skin pigmentation and nail changes appear in the first 10 years of life, mucosal leukoplakia and excessive ocular tearing appear later, and by the mid-teens the serious complications of bone marrow failure and malignancy begin to develop. In some cases the marrow abnormalities may appear before the skin manifestations.

Cutaneous findings are the most consistent feature of the syndrome. Lacy reticulated skin pigmentation affecting the face, neck, chest, and arms is the most common finding (89%), and increases with age. There may also be a telangiectatic erythematous component. Nail dystrophy of the hands and feet is the next commonest finding (88%) (Fig. 3.2). It usually starts with longitudinal ridging, splitting, or pterygium formation, and may progress to complete nail loss. Leukoplakia

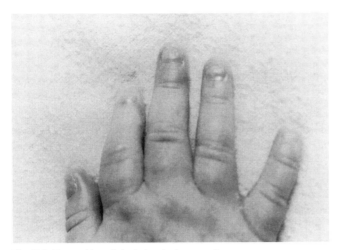

Fig. 3.2 Dystrophic nails in dyskeratosis congenita.

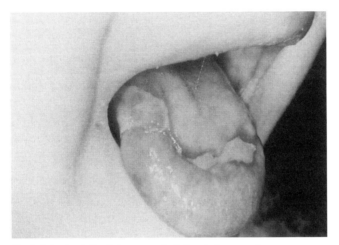

Fig. 3.3 Leukoplakia of the tongue in dyskeratosis congenita.

usually involves the oral mucosa, especially the tongue (78%) (Fig. 3.3) but can also be seen in the conjunctiva, anal, urethral, or genital mucosa. Hyperhidrosis of the palms and soles is common, and hair loss is sometimes seen. Eye abnormalities are observed in approximately 50% of cases.[6] Excessive tearing (epiphora) secondary to nasolacrimal duct obstruction is common. Other ophthalmologic manifestations include conjunctivitis, blepharitis, loss of eyelashes, strabismus, cataracts, and optic atrophy. Abnormalities of the teeth, particularly an increased rate of dental decay and early loss of teeth, are common. Skeletal abnormalities such as osteoporosis, avascular necrosis, abnormal bone trabeculation, scoliosis, and mandibular hypoplasia are seen in approximately 20% of cases.[6] Genitourinary abnormalities include hypoplastic testes, hypospadias, phimosis, urethral stenosis, and horseshoe kidney. Gastrointestinal findings, such as esophageal strictures, hepatomegaly, or cirrhosis, are seen in 10% of cases.[6,153]

The Hoyeraal–Hreidarsson syndrome is a severe variant of *DKC1*-associated DC, with cerebellar hypoplasia, microcephaly, growth retardation, immunodeficiency, and early-onset severe aplastic anemia.[152] A similar syndrome is Revesz syndrome, which is characterized by dystrophic nails, leukoplakia, aplastic anemia, cerebellar hypoplasia, growth retardation, microcephaly, and bilateral exudative retinopathy. The genetic defect has not yet been identified.[154]

Patients with DC are also prone to interstitial pulmonary disease with a restrictive defect as well as pulmonary vascular disease. This complication has been reported in patients after HSCT and in untransplanted patients.[6,155,175]

Cancer predisposition

Cancer develops in at least 10–15% of patients, usually in the third or fourth decades of life. The types of malignancies are similar to Fanconi anemia, although in DC solid tumors are more common than hematologic malignancies. All genetic subgroups can be affected with cancer.[12,19] Most of the cancers are squamous cell carcinoma or adenocarcinomas; the oropharynx and gastrointestinal tract are involved most frequently. Patients can develop multiple separate primary tumors. MDS and AML occur rarely.[6]

Genetic aspects

Approximately 85% of the 300 published cases of DC are male. The X-linked disease is caused by mutations in *DKC1* on chromosome Xq28.[156] Heterozygous mutations in the *TERC* gene are the cause for the autosomal dominant form of DC.[157] Familial cases with affected male and female siblings in one generation, and cases with known parental consanguinity fit an autosomal recessive inheritance pattern. The gene(s) for this group have not yet been identified.

The X-linked and autosomal recessive forms appear to have more physical anomalies and earlier onset of aplastic anemia. The X-linked disease is characterized by a higher incidence or severity of immune dysfunction. Clinically, the autosomal dominant group seems to be milder in its manifestations.[6]

Pathogenesis

The gene associated with the autosomal dominant DC, *TERC*, encodes for the RNA component of human telomerase, which is responsible for telomere maintenance.[151] DC cells are characterized by very short telomeres. In several acquired and inherited marrow failure syndromes, telomere length is reduced as a result of increased replicative stress. However, in DC there is also a telomerase defect, and the magnitude of this degenerative process is much more severe, so that patients develop aging-associated symptoms at an early stage.

The gene associated with the X-linked DC, *DKC1*, encodes for the protein dyskerin. Dyskerin is involved in pseudouridylation of nascent rRNA. In addition, dyskerin binds to *TERC*, facilitating telomere maintenance.

Clastogenic stress studies of DC cells are normal.[6,158] However, DC is a chromosome "instability" disorder of a different type than Fanconi anemia.[159] In some patients metaphase in peripheral blood cells, marrow cells, and fibroblasts in culture showed numerous spontaneous unbalanced chromosome rearrangements such as dicentrics, tricentrics, and translocations.

Clonogenic assays of marrow cells showed a marked reduction or absence of colony forming colonies of granulocytes, erythrocytes, monocytes and megakaryocytes (CFU-GEMM), BFU-E, CFU-E and CFU-GM progenitors.[46,160] Marrow stromal cells showed a normal ability to support growth of hematopoietic progenitors from normal marrow in three patients who were studied, but generation of progenitors from patient marrow cells inoculated onto normal stroma was reduced, suggesting that the defect in DC is of hematopoietic stem cell origin.[160]

Laboratory evaluation and diagnosis

The median age of diagnosis of the X-linked DC is 15 years (range 0.3–68 years), of the autosomal recessive form is 13 years (range 1.2–42 years), and of the autosomal dominant group is 25 years (range 7–58 years). Thrombocytopenia and anemia usually appear first, followed by pancytopenia. Severe cytopenia eventually develops in about 50% of the patients.

The diagnosis is frequently delayed, and some cases are accurately diagnosed many years after HSCT for apparently acquired aplastic anemia once the cutaneous manifestations become prominent. A detailed medical, developmental, and family history, along with a physical examination usually yield important diagnostic clues. Low blood cell counts, red blood cell macrocytosis, and high hemoglobin F are usual findings. Bone marrow cellularity can be normal or increased at the onset of cytopenia, but invariably decreases once the cytopenia deteriorates.

Mutation analysis of the *DKC1* and *TERC* genes can provide a molecular diagnosis for patients with the X-linked and autosomal dominant diseases. Selected patients with aplastic anemia who either have one or more DC-related nonhematologic manifestations or who do not respond to treatment with immunosuppressive therapy should be tested as well.[5]

Prenatal diagnosis
Prenatal diagnosis is now available to most patients with DC using molecular testing for *DKC1* and *TERC* of DNA from amniotic cells or chorionic villous cells.

Therapy and prognosis

The mean age of death is approximately 30 years.[12] The main causes of death relate to either bone marrow failure or malignancy.

Androgens
Androgens, usually combined with low-dose prednisone, can be expected to induce improved marrow function in about 40% of patients. If a response is seen and deemed to be maximal, the androgen dose can be slowly tapered but not usually stopped. As in Fanconi anemia, patients can become refractory to androgens as the aplastic anemia progresses.

Growth factors
Four patients were reported who responded to G-CSF therapy with significant increases in absolute neutrophil counts.[161,162] Similarly, GM-CSF therapy in two other patients resulted in improved neutrophil numbers.[163] A combination of G-CSF with erythropoietin was used in one case with DC and severe cytopenia, and improved counts of all cell lineages were observed.[164] Therefore, there appears to be potential benefit from cytokine therapy in selected patients with DC while waiting for HSCT or who are not eligible for transplant.

Hematopoietic stem cell transplantation
The only cure for patients who develop severe bone marrow complications is HSCT. To date, 25 patients with DC have reportedly undergone HSCT.[6,155,161,165–174] In most cases standard conditioning regimens were used.

Of the 19 reported cases of DC patients who were transplanted from a matched related donor (MRD), 11 survived more than 3 years. However, an additional 6 of these 19 died subsequently at 6–29 years posttransplant. Of the six reported cases of DC patients who were transplanted from a matched unrelated donor (MUD), three are alive after more than 3 years (including two patients from our institution who were initially reported to survive more than 1.5 years posttransplant).[161]

Short-term transplant-related toxicity is common in these populations, including sepsis, GVHD, and early death.[56,166,170] Vascular lesions and fibrosis involving various organs can occur in DC patients in both early and late periods after transplantation and carry a high mortality rate. Another striking complication for patients with DC after HSCT is bronchopulmonary disease. An inherent propensity for pulmonary disease[171] may explain the high incidence (up to 40%) of early and late fatal pulmonary complications after HSCT.[6,56,155,159,167]

Telomere shortening and chromosomal instability can explain hypersensitivity of DC patients to irradiation and chemotherapy.[60,172,173] The increased predisposition to posttransplant complications, especially pulmonary and vascular, the chromosomal instability, and the tendency to develop tumors highlight the need to avoid certain conditioning agents such as busulfan and irradiation. Reports of a reduced-intensity regimen incorporating fludarabine for

MRD[170] and MUD[161] HSCT in patients with DC have been published, showing decreased toxicity at short-term follow-up of 2–3 years. Longer follow-up is still needed to clarify whether long-term toxicity is also reduced by these regimens.

Congenital amegakaryocytic thrombocytopenia

In this section we refer to the syndrome of congenital amegakaryocytic thrombocytopenia (CAMT) as an autosomal recessive IMFS with predominantly pancytopenia, which usually presents in infancy with isolated thrombocytopenia due to reduced or absent marrow megakaryocytes, and frequently evolves into pancytopenia of varying degrees. In untreated cases, MDS with monosomy 7 and AML can develop at a later stage.[174] Nonhematologic manifestations occur in about a quarter of the patients.

Clinical features

Hematologic manifestations
Most patients present at birth or during the first year of life with a petechial rash, bruising, or bleeding. At presentation the platelets are typically moderately to severely reduced (with a median platelet count of $21 \times 10^9/L$,[174] but the hemoglobin levels and white blood cell counts are normal. Red cells may be macrocytic, and hemoglobin F can be increased. At diagnosis, bone marrow specimens show normal cellularity with markedly reduced or absent megakaryocytes. Aplastic anemia subsequently ensues in 39–75% of the patients at the age of 2–53 months.[174]

A second group of patients with CAMT present with moderate thrombocytopenia either early in infancy or later during childhood.[174] These patients are initially platelet transfusion-free, but tend to develop aplastic anemia during the first decade of life.

Nonhematologic manifestations
Roughly a quarter of patients have characteristic physical anomalies. Some affected sibships manifest both normal and abnormal physical findings in the same family. The most common manifestations in those with anomalies are neurologic and cardiac. Findings relating to cerebellar and cerebral atrophy are a recurrent theme, and developmental delay is a prominent feature in this group. Patients may also have microcephaly and an abnormal facies. Congenital heart disease with a variety of malformations can be detected, including atrial and ventricular septal defects, patent ductus arteriosus, tetralogy of Fallot, and coarctation of the aorta. Some of these can occur in combinations. Other anomalies include abnormal hips or feet, kidney malformations, eye anomalies, and cleft or high-arched palate.

Cancer predisposition

Patients with CAMT are prone to MDS/AML.[12,174] The typical course is the development of early thrombocytopenia, aplastic anemia, and then marrow cytogenetic abnormalities (usually monosomy 7), MDS and AML. The risk of malignant conversion is difficult to determine because of the rarity of the disease, paucity of published data, the possible patient heterogeneity, and the need for early HSCT due to the development of aplastic anemia. No solid tumors have yet been associated with the disease.

Genetic aspects

Mutations in the *MPL* (thrombopoietic receptor) gene are the cause of the disorder in most patients with CAMT, particularly,[178] but not exclusively,[179] in those without physical anomalies. Both alleles were mutated, confirming an autosomal recessive mode of inheritance.[178,180]

Pathogenesis

MPL mutations cause inactivation of the thrombopoietin receptor. The compensatory elevated levels of thrombopoietin[178,179] do not result in transmission of the receptor signals.[180,181] Thrombopoietin plays a critical role in the proliferation, survival, and differentiation of early and late megakaryocytes. This clearly explains the thrombocytopenia. However, thrombopoietin also promotes survival of hematopoietic stem cells; thus, it is possible that a defect in its receptor results in depletion of their pool. The number of colony forming units of megakaryocytes (CFU-Meg) progenitors might be normal initially, but declines as the disease progresses.[182,183]

Laboratory evaluation and diagnosis

The median age of diagnosis is 1.3 months (range 0–110 months) in the nonsyndromic cases and 2 days (range 0–18 months) in the syndromic cases.[12] The typical patient presents with isolated severe thrombocytopenia from birth. Once acquired diagnoses are excluded, IMFSs should be considered. In the first several months of life, red blood cell volume and hemoglobin F levels are difficult to interpret, but gradually can become abnormally high. If physical malformations, which are not characteristics of thrombocytopenia with absent radii syndrome, are observed, the diagnosis can be more readily suspected. The gold standard procedure for determining cellularity and marrow megakaryocyte pool is bone marrow biopsy. All patients with suspected CAMT should be offered *MPL* mutation analysis.

Therapy and prognosis

Without curative treatment, the mortality rate from thrombocytopenic bleeding, complications of aplastic anemia, or malignant myeloid transformation is close to 100%. For this reason, HLA typing of family members should be performed as soon as the diagnosis is confirmed to see if a matched related donor for HSCT exists. If not, a search for a matched unrelated donor should ensue as soon as the seriousness of the clinical picture dictates.

Platelet transfusions should be used as medically indicated and not just because of a low platelet count. Single donor platelets are preferred to minimize sensitization. All blood products should be irradiated and tested negative for CMV.

Corticosteroids have been used with no apparent efficacy. For aplastic anemia, androgens in combination with corticosteroids may induce a temporary partial response but the effect is short-lived. Based on the *in vitro* studies, several clinical trials have been conducted with interleukin-3 (IL-3), GM-CSF, and the fusion cytokine PIX321.[183] These cytokines may result in temporary hematologic improvement, but clearly are not curative. IL-3 and PIX321 are not available for clinical use. Other cytokines such as thrombopoietin and IL-11 are not licensed for children with IMFSs.

Hematopoietic stem cell transplantation

A review of publications from 1990 to 2000 yields five reports of a total of 15 CAMT patients who underwent HSCT.[184–188] Seven patients had received stem cells from a matched related donor using busulfan-based myeloablative regimens; all patients engrafted with minimal GVHD and had a good outcome. However, the outcome of eight patients who received unrelated or mismatched related donor transplants was inferior; five received total body irradiation-based conditioning. Initial graft failure occurred in three patients. Three patients died due to bronchiolitis obliterans with organizing pneumonia and infections. We have recently used a reduced-intensity transplantation regimen incorporating fludarabine 180 mg/m², ATG 160 mg/kg, and cyclophosphamide 120 mg/kg in a CAMT patient with aplastic anemia and acquired monosomy 7 who had no matched related donor. The patient had rapid and durable engraftment with minimal complications and is well 2 years posttransplantation.[189]

Other inherited marrow failure disorders with predominantly pancytopenia

Reticular dysgenesis is a congenital severe lymphohematopoietic stem cell disorder characterized by severe B- and T-cell immunodeficiency, thymic and lymph node aplasia, and cytopenia.[190] Neutropenia is the most common cytopenia, but anemia and thrombocytopenia can also occur. Bone marrow specimens are hypocellular with markedly reduced myeloid and lymphoid elements; erythroid and megakaryocytic series are usually normal. Clonogenic assays of hematopoietic progenitors consistently show reduced to absent colony growth, indicating that the underlying defect resides at the pluripotential lymphohematopoietic stem cell level.[191] The mode of inheritance is probably autosomal recessive, but an X-linked recessive mode is also possible in some cases. Similarly to other syndromes with severe combined immunodeficiency, the patients present with severe infections at birth or shortly thereafter. Neutrophil counts usually do not improve with administration of G-CSF,[191] and the patients often die within the first weeks of life unless they receive HSCT.[191]

Pearson disease is caused by deletional mutations in mitochondrial DNA,[192] and is associated with variable degrees of pancreatic dysfunction, pancytopenia, and metabolic acidosis.[193] Marrow aspirates show ring sideroblasts and vacuoles in myeloid and erythroid precursors. The cytopenia tends to improve with age.[194]

Pancytopenia due to hypoplastic bone marrow was also observed in Dubowitz syndrome,[195,196] Seckel syndrome,[197,198] and Schimke immuno-osseous dysplasia.[199]

Inherited marrow failure disorders with predominantly anemia

Diamond–Blackfan anemia

Diamond–Blackfan anemia (DBA) is an inherited form of pure red cell aplasia.[200] The syndrome is heterogeneous with respect to inheritance patterns, clinical and laboratory findings, and therapeutic outcome. About 80% of cases are apparently sporadic,[201] but the familial cases (20%) point to either autosomal dominant or autosomal recessive or X-linked recessive modes of inheritance. Using data from the European DBA registries,[202,203] the incidence of the disorder in Europe is 5–7 cases/million live births.

Clinical features

Hematologic manifestations

Anemia was once considered a universal component of the syndrome; however, studies of families with *RPS19* gene mutations have identified affected individuals without anemia.[204] Patients may present at birth with severe anemia and hydrops fetalis. In other cases the patient become symptomatic after birth and presents with pallor, weakness, cardiac failure, hepatosplenomegaly, and edema.

Median hemoglobin level at birth is 7 g/dL (range 2.6–14.8 g/dL). At presentation the median hemoglobin level is approximately 4 g/dL (range 1.7–9.1). The reticulocytes are decreased or absent. Macrocytosis is difficult to diagnose in the first 2 month of life. This might explain the observation that the mean corpuscular volume is abnormally high for age in 80% of the patients at presentation, and in apparently all patients afterward.[205] Peripheral blood smear is nondiagnostic. Most patients have normal platelet and neutrophil counts. Mild thrombocytopenia and neutropenia may occur in DBA, but severe thrombocytopenia and neutropenia are unusual findings.[206,209]

DBA erythrocytes manifest fetal erythroid characteristics, including[210] elevated levels of hemoglobin F, fetal amino acid profile of the hemoglobin F with high glycine to alanine ratio, and a high expression of the i antigen on the surface of red blood cells.

Studies of the red blood cell enzyme levels have shown an abnormal profile. For example, the activities of enolase, glyceraldehyde-3-phosphate dehydrogenase, phosphofructokinase, and glutathione peroxidase are increased;[211] in some cases the profile is similar to cord blood. The levels of several other enzymes resemble those in adult erythrocytes. For instance, carbonic anhydrase isoenzyme B activity is elevated and hexokinase has an adult type isoenzyme distribution.[210]

Glader and colleagues found elevated red blood cell adenosine deaminase levels in 90% of the patients, and in 17% of their parents.[212] As this abnormality is not found in red blood cells from normal cord blood samples, healthy children, or other marrow failure disorders, determination of the red blood cell adenosine deaminase level became a useful diagnostic test for DBA. Abnormalities involving pyrimidine enzymes in DBA erythrocytes have also been described, including elevated activities of orotate phosphoribosyl transferase[213] and orotidine monophosphate decarboxylase.[212,213]

Bone marrow biopsy and aspirate show a normocellular specimen in 90–95% of the patients. The myeloid to erythroid (mostly proerythroblasts) ratio is > 10:1. The myeloid and megakaryocytic lineages are usually unremarkable. In early stages of the disease, dyserythropoiesis changes might occur. Marrow cytogenetic abnormalities are extremely rare.

Nonhematologic manifestations

Obstetric complications such as miscarriages, stillbirth, pre-eclampsia, premature separation of the placenta and breech presentation have been reported in approximately 10% of the mothers of DBA patients. More than 10% of the patients have intrauterine growth retardation.

Physical anomalies have been reported in approximately 40% of the patients.[201,209] Short stature and failure to thrive are common. Craniofacial dysmorphisms include microcephaly, hypertelorism, microphthalmos, cataract, glaucoma, strabismus, microretrognathism, high-arched palate, cleft palate, and ear malformations. Some patients have characteristic facies consisting of snub nose, wide-set eyes, thick upper lip, and intelligent expression. Another characteristic facies consists of microcephaly, almond-shaped eyes, mild antimongoloid slant, and pointed chin. Neck anomalies

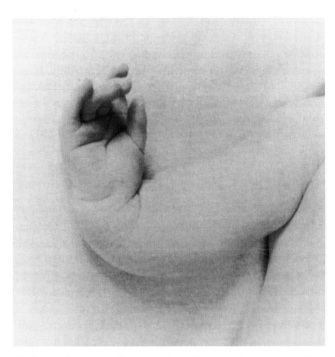

Fig. 3.4 Radial aplasia with preservation of the thumb in a newborn with TAR syndrome.

include pterygium coli, Klippel–Feil anomaly (fusion of the cervical vertebrae with fusion of the trapezius muscle), and Sprengel deformity (congenital elevation of the scapula). Thumb anomalies include bifid thumb (see Fig. 3.4), duplication, subluxation, hypoplasia, absence of thumb, and triphalangeal thumbs. The combination of hypoplastic anemia and a triphalangeal thumb is commonly referred to as Aase syndrome or Aase–Smith syndrome. Less commonly, patients may have weak or absent radial pulse along with flat thenar eminence. Urogenital anomalies include dysplastic kidneys, horseshoe kidneys, duplication of the ureters, renal tubular acidosis, and hypogonadism. Congenital heart disease includes ventricular septal defect and atrial septal defect. Other manifestations include congenital dislocation of the hip, achondroplasia, clubfoot, tracheoesophageal fistula, and mental retardation.

Cancer predisposition

Of the 354 patients registered in the DBA Registry of North America, 6 (1.7%) developed malignancies.[214] Reported malignancies in this registry and in the literature include MDS, AML, acute lymphoblastic leukemia, osteosarcoma, soft tissue sarcoma, Hodgkin lymphoma, non-Hodgkin lymphoma, gastric carcinoma, colon carcinoma, hepatocellular carcinoma, breast carcinoma, vaginal melanoma, and malignant fibrous histiocytoma. DBA is probably an additional genetic disease with inherent predisposition for cancer.

Genetic aspects

DBA affects both sexes equally, and has been reported in many ethnic groups including white people, black Africans, Arabs, East Indians, and Japanese. The study of a sporadic female case with DBA and a constitutional balanced reciprocal translocation 46,XX,t(X;19)(p21;q13),[215] as well as the identification of microdeletions at chromosome 19q13.2 in DBA patients,[216] linked the first DBA gene to the 19q13.2 locus. The breakpoint of the translocation t(X;19)(p21;q13) was found in *RPS19*.[217] The *RPS19* gene is 11 kb with six exons. Mutations in *RPS19* occur in approximately 25% of DBA patients, and include nonsense, frameshift, splice-site, missense, and deletional mutations.[217] A hotspot for missense mutations was identified between codons 52 and 62 of the *RPS19* gene.[204] The occurrence of mutations in one allele is congruent with the apparently autosomal dominant inheritance in this subgroup of patients. There seems to be no correlation between the *RPS19* genotype and phenotype. It is noteworthy that *RPS19* mutations were also found in some first-degree relatives presenting only with isolated high erythrocyte adenosine deaminase activity and/or macrocytosis.

A second DBA locus has been mapped to chromosome 8p22–p23 in about 35% of the cases,[218] but the candidate gene has not been identified yet. The linkage was found in families with vertical transmission of the disease, confirming an autosomal dominant inheritance in these families. About 40% of the patients neither carry *RPS19* mutations nor do they link to 8p22–p23.

Pathogenesis

DBA marrows are characterized by complete or nearly complete absence of erythroid precursors in 90% of the patients. The defect in DBA seems to be intrinsic to the hematopoietic stem cells and selectively limits their ability to differentiate into and expand the erythroid compartment. Clonogenic assays of marrow cells or CD34+ cells typically show absent BFU-E and CFU-E progenitors. Some patients show normal or even increased numbers of both progenitors or a block at the BFU-E stage.

Long-term bone marrow cultures showed normal stromal cell function in terms of its ability to support normal hematopoiesis.[219,220] However, DBA CD34+ cells had impaired ability to undergo granulocytic–monocytic differentiation in addition to their erythroid differentiation defect. These results underscore a stem cell defect in DBA rather than an isolated erythroid defect. This is in keeping with the clinical observation that in addition to anemia, patients can have neutropenia and thrombocytopenia.[206–208]

DBA erythroid progenitors demonstrate subnormal colony growth in response to erythropoietin.[221] The defect in colony growth can be partially corrected *in vitro* by the addition of combinations of factors, including glucocorticoids and erythropoietin,[222] stem cell factor and interleukin-3,[223] and stem cell factor and erythropoietin.[224]

RPS19 encodes for the ribosomal protein S19, which is associated with the ribosomal subunit 40S.[225] The exact role of *RPS19* in erythropoiesis is unclear. *RPS19* expression is highest at the earlier stages of erythropoiesis and decreases with differentiation.[226] Gene transfer of the wild-type *RPS19* into CD34+ cells from DBA patients with *RPS19* mutations improves erythroid colony growth,[227] proving the causative role of mutations in the gene in the pathogenesis of DBA.

In studies of CD34+ cells from DBA patients and CD34+ cells in which *RPS19* expression was reduced by approximately 50%, it has been shown that RPS19 promotes cell proliferation as well as differentiation into CFU-E progenitors.[228] Intermediate levels of RPS19 to approximately haploinsufficiency levels do not affect myeloid progenitors[223,228] or megakaryocytic progenitors.[223] It is likely that the genetic defects in the DBA gene(s) accelerates apoptosis of erythroid progenitor cells.[229,230]

The DBA defect does not reside in production of the major erythropoietic cytokines stem cell factor, interleukin-3, and erythropoietin; all are produced in normal or high levels in DBA patients. In addition, molecular analysis of the stem cell receptor gene and the stem cell factor gene found no mutations.

Laboratory evaluation and diagnosis

The median age of diagnosis is 2–3 months (range 0–64 years).[12] The typical patient presents with isolated anemia in the first year of life (90%). Presentation in the neonatal period requires exclusion of common causes of congenital anemia such as infections and hemolytic disorders. After the neonatal period, other causes of macrocytic anemia as well as transient erythroblastopenia of childhood have to be excluded before a diagnosis of DBA is made. Features of transient erythroblastopenia of childhood that can help distinguish it from DBA include: (i) onset usually at 1–4 years; (ii) preceding viral illness in more than half of the patients; (iii) normal red blood cell mean corpuscular volume while still in the reticulocytopenic phase; (iv) normal hemoglobin F and i antigen during the reticulocytopenic phase; (v) normal adenosine deaminase levels; and (vi) spontaneous recovery within 4–8 weeks. Another important differential diagnosis is parvovirus infection.

Once peripheral destruction, bleeding, and splenic sequestration are excluded, a primary marrow disorder should be considered. Bone marrow aspirate and biopsy should be done. If pure red cell aplasia is found, the most likely diagnosis in this age is DBA. If physical examination reveals characteristic DBA anomalies, particularly of the thumbs, the diagnosis is easily made. At any age, red blood cell volume and hemoglobin F levels should be ascertained and compared with the reference values based on age. Red blood cell adenosine deaminase level and clonogenic assays of marrow CD34[+] cells can be important diagnostic tools, though not available in most centers.

The diagnosis is based on the following characteristic features:

- anemia;
- presentation in the first 12 months of life;
- normochromic-macrocytic red blood cells;
- relative reticulocytopenia;
- normocellular marrow with selective, marked deficiency of erythroid precursors;
- increased serum erythropoietin in the anemic patients;
- normal white cell count;
- normal platelet counts;
- elevated hemoglobin F; and
- elevated red blood cell adenosine deaminase.

None of these diagnostic features occurs in 100% of the patients. Thus, all patients with suspected DBA should be offered genetic testing whenever possible. Unfortunately only the *RPS19* gene is available for testing, and thus, only 25% of the cases can be confirmed.

Treatment

Transfusions

Until a diagnosis of DBA is confirmed, the only treatment should be packed red cell transfusions. Complete correction of the hemoglobin by transfusions is not recommended as it might not be necessary and may prevent recovery of erythropoiesis in case the diagnosis is transient erythroblastopenia of childhood.

Most DBA patients are treated with a lifelong red blood cell transfusion program, either because they did not respond to prednisone or other medical treatment or they required high prednisone doses to maintain response. Approximately 15 mL/kg of leukocyte-depleted packed red blood cells on a monthly basis is usually required to allow normal activity and growth. After approximately 15 units of red blood cells, body iron stores should be carefully assessed. Liver biopsy[231] or superconducting quantum interference device (SQUID) susceptometer[232] are more accurate than serum ferritin, and routinely performed in large centers. Magnetic resonance imaging (MRI) of the liver has been explored,[233] but has not become a widely accepted method. The most common treatment of choice today for the treatment of iron overload is iron chelation with subcutaneous deferoxamine (desferrioxamine) infusion.

Hemoglobin levels before transfusions should be tailored to the individual patient and be maintained higher than 6–7 g/dL. Higher hemoglobin levels may be required to prevent symptoms and allow normal activity and optimal growth. Determination of pretransfusion hemoglobin levels is important also for detecting those rare patients who become transfusion independent either transiently or permanently.

Glucocorticoids

Oral prednisone or equivalent preparation is the mainstay of treatment for DBA.[221] Treatment with these drugs is usually begun once the diagnosis is confirmed. Some groups recommend waiting to administer glucocorticoids until the patient is approximately 1 year of age to minimize the adverse effect on growth. Approximately 65% of the patients respond to prednisone or prednisolone, and demonstrate reticulocytosis within 1–3 weeks followed by a rise in hemoglobin. The initial dose is usually 2 mg/kg daily, divided two to four times a day.[234] The prednisone trial may last for approximately 4 weeks as most patients will respond during this period. There are no known factors that can predict responsiveness to glucocorticoids. Once the hemoglobin level rises to 10 g/L or reaches a plateau of 7–9 g/L, the steroid dose can be slowly tapered to the minimal single dose on an alternate-day schedule or even once a week, which maintains the hemoglobin levels with an acceptable degree of side effects. The minimal effective dose varies, and might be as low as 0.05 mg/kg once a week. If the required glucocorticoid dose is too high (>0.5 mg/kg daily) or causes significant toxicity an alternative treatment should be sought. Growth curves and bone mineral density should be monitored periodically. Two-thirds of patients who initially respond to prednisone will continue the drug for life. The rest will either lose the response or require unacceptably high doses, which necessitates discontinuation of the drug.

Several groups studied the efficacy of high-dose methylprednisolone (30–100 mg/kg daily) for patients with DBA who failed conventional treatment of prednisone with either no response, partial response, or complete response.[235,236] However, relapses were common, and toxicity was significant.

Other medical treatment

Some patients who do not respond to prednisone can be treated successfully with ciclosporin.[237,238] Treatment with interleukin-3 induced rare sustained remissions in DBA patients.[239] However, it was removed from clinical use due to its unfavorable side effects. Erythropoietin levels are typically markedly elevated in DBA, and treatment trials have been unsuccessful.[240,241]

Hematopoietic stem cell transplantation

Although HSCT is the only known cure for the marrow failure in DBA, the indications for transplantation in DBA are unclear. The first factor in making a decision is the severity of the disease. Patients who either need no therapy or respond to relatively low doses of prednisone or respond to other medical therapies with minimal side effects are obviously not candidates for HSCT. Those who eventually need regular red blood cell transfusions and have personal or medical difficulties with iron chelation are potential candidates. Patients who are red blood cell transfusion-dependent but are properly chelated might have equal or better quality of life and equal or longer overall survival than transplanted patients. The second factor that has to be taken into account when consulting a patient or family about HSCT is that 10–15% of the patients may have spontaneous remission by their second decade of life. Third, the success of HSCT decreases when performed later in childhood or afterward.

The type of donor is critically important in DBA. Data from the European DBA Registry showed 11 of 13 (85%) successfully transplanted patients when performed with a matched sibling donor.[203] Data from the North American DBA Registry showed an overall survival of 88% with matched related donors compared with 14% when unrelated or mismatched related donors were used.[242]

Cord blood transplantation[243,244] and reduced toxicity regimens[245,246] have also been applied successfully in DBA, but represent a relatively small number of patients.

Long-term prognosis

The long-term outcome of DBA patients has still to be clarified. Based on literature review, Alter found that the projected median survival of DBA patients was 65 years.[12] Deaths are mainly due to the complications of iron overload and infections, and less commonly due to HSCT, leukemia, other cancer, or nonhematologic/oncologic complications.

Pregnancies of DBA females have been reported.[247,248] The pregnancy of a DBA mother might be complicated by worsening of the anemia, toxemia, labor arrest, fetal distress, intrauterine growth retardation, and preterm delivery.

Other inherited marrow failure syndromes with predominantly anemia

Congenital sideroblastic anemias are inherited or acquired disorders of mitochondrial iron utilization. Iron accumulation occurs in the mitochondria of red blood cell precursors. Perl's Prussian blue shows iron accumulation in a circular or ringed pattern around the nucleus in > 10% of cells. The genetic basis of the various forms of inherited sideroblastic anemias is summarized in Table 3.1. Treatment depends on the specific syndrome. Patients with X-linked sideroblastic anemia respond to pyridoxine. Patients with thiamine-responsive megaloblastic anemia respond to thiamine. In the other types of congenital sideroblastic anemia RBC transfusions are the mainstay of treatment. Hematopoietic stem cell transplantation is curative.[252] In Pearson syndrome the cytopenia improves with age and HSCT is not required.

Congenital dyserythropoietic anemias (CDAs) are inherited disorders with prominent morphologic dyserythropoiesis and ineffective erythropoiesis. Three main types of CDA exist, CDA I, II, and III, which differ in marrow morphology, serologic findings, and inheritance patterns (Table 3.1). The anemia in most patients is not severe and does not mandate chronic therapy. In cases with severe anemia splenectomy, a chronic RBC transfusion program or HSCT should be considered. Due to ineffective erythropoiesis and multiple transfusions, patients can develop iron overload necessitating iron chelation.

Inherited marrow failure disorders with predominantly neutropenia

Confusion and controversy prevail with regard to the terminology of childhood neutropenia. In the present chapter the term "congenital neutropenia" will be used for all cases of neutropenia, acquired or inherited, first noticed at birth or in the neonatal period. Congenital neutropenia can be mild, moderate, or severe. The term "chronic neutropenia" is reserved herein for a heterogeneous group of inherited or acquired disorders of myelopoiesis that last more than 6 months. Chronic neutropenia can be mild, moderate, or severe. Inherited bone marrow failure disorders with predominantly neutropenia are subtypes of chronic neutropenia. They can either be categorized as congenital neutropenia (such as Kostmann syndrome) or present later on in life (such as cyclic neutropenia).

Kostmann syndrome

Kostmann syndrome (KS) is a severe subtype of congenital neutropenia with onset in early childhood of profound neutropenia (absolute neutrophil count < 200/mL), recurrent life-threatening infections, and a maturation arrest of myeloid precursors at the promyelocyte-myelocyte stage of differentiation. KS was initially believed to be an autosomal recessive disorder, but with the clarification of the molecular basis of the disease it became evident that at least the majority of the cases (including the original families described by Dr Kostmann) are inherited in an autosomal dominant manner.

Clinical features

KS was first described in a large intermarried kinship in northern Sweden in 1956.[254] Subsequently, the disorder has been recognized widely, despite its rarity, and in various ethnic groups including Asians, American Indians, and black people.

About half the patients develop clinically impressive infections within the first month of life and 90% do so by 6 months. Skin abscesses are common but deep-seated tissue infections, septicemia, recurrent otitis media, pneumonia, advanced gingivostomatitis, and gut bacterial overgrowth also occurs.[254] Birth weights are generally unremarkable and physical examination is normal. Some patients with KS develop bone demineralization before and during G-CSF therapy.[255] The underlying pathogenesis is unclear but patients can develop bone pain and unusual fractures.

Neutropenia is profound in KS (usually < 200/µL but

often absolute). Compensatory monocytosis and sometimes eosinophilia is seen. At diagnosis, platelet numbers and hemoglobin values are normal. Humoral and cellular immunology is completely normal. Bone marrow specimens are usually normocellular. The striking classical finding is a maturation arrest at the promyelocyte-myelocyte stage of granulocytic differentiation. Cellular elements beyond are markedly reduced or totally absent. The other hematopoietic lineages are normal.

Genetic aspects

Most KS cases are inherited in an autosomal dominant fashion,[256] with the minority being sporadic or recessive.[257] More than 80% of the cases of KS are associated with mutations in one copy of the *ELA2* gene, which is the cause for almost all the autosomal dominant and the sporadic cases.[256] Although both healthy and affected family members have been reported to have the same *ELA2* genotype,[258] and although there is a lack of neutropenia in homozygous and heterozygous knockout mice,[259] it is now widely accepted that *ELA2* mutations are causative rather than just simply associated with KS.[260,262]

ELA2 encodes neutrophil elastase, a glycoprotein synthesized in the promyelocyte/myelocyte stages,[263] packed in the azurophilic cytoplasmic granules, and released in response to infection and inflammation.[264] Computerized modeling of neutrophil elastase showed that *ELA2* mutations in KS tend to cluster on the opposite face of the active site of the enzyme in contrast to cyclic neutropenia, where the mutations tend to cluster near the active site of the molecule.[256]

Mutations in the gene encoding the transcriptional repressor GFI1 were also identified in severe congenital neutropenia.[265] In addition, *WASP* gene mutations were described as a cause of severe congenital neutropenia in five related males from three generations.[266] In these cases the neutropenia was accompanied by monocytopenia and lymphocyte abnormalities.

Pathogenesis

The mechanisms for neutropenia in cases of mutations in *ELA2*, *GFI1*, or *WASP* are unknown. Neutrophil elastase normally localizes diffusely throughout the cytoplasm. *ELA2* mutations causing severe congenital neutropenia result in intracellular targeting of mutant neutrophil elastase to the nuclear and plasma membrane compartments.[267,268] The mutations are predicted to disrupt the AP3 protein recognition sequence, resulting in excessive membrane accumulation of elastase,[268] leading to premature apoptosis of differentiating (myeloblasts and promyelocytes) but not proliferating myeloid progenitor cells.[267,269] Data from clonogenic assays suggest that the defect is at the level of CFU-GM/CFU-G.[270,271] In case of GFI mutations, the mutated protein appears to cause overexpression of ELA2, and higher

neutrophil elastase levels in all subcellular compartments. *GFI1*-deficient mice also exhibit severe neutropenia.[272] In cases of *WASP* gene mutations, it has been suggested that the mutant protein is constitutively activated due to disruption of an autoinhibitory domain.[266]

Some patients with KS acquire G-CSF receptor mutations restricted to the myeloid lineage. These alterations are associated with the development of MDS/AML, and are not the cause of the neutropenia.[273]

Cancer predisposition

There is concern regarding the phenomenon of malignant myeloid transformation, which occurs in about 12.9% of the patients with KS, or an annual transformation rate of 2%.[219] Conversion to MDS/AML in the KS patients was associated with one or more cellular genetic abnormalities.[109] More than 90% of the patients develop clonal marrow cytogenetic abnormalities, mostly –7, or –7(q), but other abnormalities such as +21 or +8 have also been seen.[109,274,275] An activating *RAS* oncogene mutation, *K12D*, is acquired in approximately 50% of the patients with KS who develop malignant myeloid transformation.[109]

More than 80% of the patients who develop MDS/AML also acquire point nonsense G-CSF receptor mutations resulting in a truncated carboxy-terminal cytoplasmic domain of the receptor,[273,276] which leads to impaired ligand internalization, defective receptor downmodulation, enhanced proliferation in response to G-CSF,[277,278] diminished apoptosis,[279] and development of clonal marrow cytogenetic abnormalities.[278]

It is unclear whether G-CSF can be implicated in the malignant conversion of congenital neutropenic patients. On one hand, the crude number of MDS/AML among G-CSF-treated KS patients is 12.5%, or an annual transformation rate of 2%.[219] Furthermore, remission of AML after discontinuation of G-CSF was reported in a patient with KS on G-CSF.[280] On the other hand, leukemic transformation occurred in patients with KS also prior to the availability of G-CSF therapy.[281–285] With G-CSF therapy, most patients survive, which might thereby allow for the natural expression of leukemogenesis in this population. Also, MDS/AML has not been seen in patients with cyclic neutropenia who had been treated with G-CSF. Thus, it is still to be determined whether G-CSF hastens the appearance of leukemia in patients with an underlying genetic predisposition by giving growth advantage to the malignant clones.

Laboratory features and diagnosis

About half the patients present with infections within the first month of life. Complete blood counts and bone marrow testing in a neonate with severe infections are characteristic of KS. Later on in the first year of life, viruses are the most common cause of isolated neutropenia. An antecedent history of good health, the occurrence of a viral illness, active granulopoiesis up to the band stage in the bone marrow, demonstration of specific antibodies, and the transient nature of the neutropenia, distinguish this disorder from KS. The diagnosis can be supported by demonstrating specific antibodies on the patient granulocytes. Determination of immunoglobulin levels is an important part of the initial work-up of the neutropenic patients. Other IMFSs such as Shwachman–Diamond syndrome have to be ruled out. Genetic testing of the *ELA2* gene should be offered to all patients and families. If the test is negative a search for mutations in other genes such as *GFI1* or *WASP* can be considered.

Therapy and prognosis

Cytokines

Life-long treatment with G-CSF is currently the mainstay of management of patients with KS, and should be initiated as front-line treatment when the diagnosis is established.[274] Since the initial report of G-CSF treatment in KS in 1989,[286] hundreds of additional patients have been treated. The daily starting dose is 5 µg/kg subcutaneously, and this can be escalated by 5–10 µg/kg/day every 14 days until the desired neutrophil number is achieved. Neutrophils $> 0.5 \times 10^9$/L generally provide protection from infection, but target counts of about $1–2.5 \times 10^9$/L are clearly safer.

Complete response is defined by neutrophil counts of 1×10^9/L with doses up to 120 µg/kg/day. Ninety percent of patients show a complete response to G-CSF therapy, and infection-related events and antibiotic use are significantly decreased.[287] No response, as defined by absolute neutrophil counts of less than $0.5–1 \times 10^9$/L with doses of up to 120 µg/kg/day, is seen in less than 10% of the patients.

The vast majority of patients benefit substantially from G-CSF therapy with minimal adverse reactions, which include headache, general musculoskeletal pain, transient bone pain, and rash. These do not usually require discontinuation of G-CSF.[288] Osteopenia has been reported in KS patients who were treated with G-CSF for long periods. This complication might be related either to the treatment or to the underlying disorder,[289,290] and require periodic evaluation of the bone mineral density. The overall safety of long-term administration of G-CSF has been reviewed in detail by Freedman.[274]

The basis for the refractory state to G-CSF in the 10% of the patients with KS is unknown. In one case, a mutation in the extracellular domain of the G-CSF receptor was identified. Interestingly, small daily doses of oral prednisone administered to the patient with conventional doses of subcutaneous G-CSF resulted in complete neutrophil response and clinical improvement.[291] GM-CSF is not as effective as G-CSF, does not induce a consistent neutrophil response, and has more side effects. Prior to G-CSF, antibiotics were the mainstay of management for active infection and for prophylaxis.

Hematopoietic stem cell transplantation

Due to the extremely successful results with G-CSF in KS, HSCT is rarely offered to the patients. The current indications are either no response to G-CSF or malignant myeloid transformation with severe other lineage cytopenia or increased marrow blasts. Whether the accumulation of certain cytogenetic (e.g., monosomy 7) and molecular events (e.g., *G-CSFR* and *RAS* mutations) justifies transplant is unclear as a portion of these patients have stable disease for many years.

In the Severe Congenital Neutropenia International Registry database, 29 patients were transplanted; 18 due to MDS/AML[219] and 11 due to insufficient response to G-CSF.[292] Of the 11 patients who underwent HSCT due to a refractory disease, 8 had an HLA-matched sibling. Nine of the 11 patients survived without disease. Of the 18 transplanted patients who underwent HSCT for MDS/AML (mostly using mismatched related or unrelated donors), only 3 were cured.

Other inherited marrow failure syndromes with predominantly neutropenia

Cyclic neutropenia is an autosomal dominant disorder characterized by a regular, repetitive decrease in peripheral blood neutrophils at approximately 21-day intervals.[293] Patients usually present in infancy or childhood, and have a less severe infectious course compared with Kostmann syndrome. However, life-threatening infections such as *Clostridium* sp. sepsis, acute peritonitis, *Staphylococcus aureus* septicemia, mouth sores during the neutrophil nadir, and chronic gingivitis have been reported.[294,295] Diagnosis requires the demonstration of regular neutrophil cycles of 19–23 days, during which the neutrophil count typically fluctuates from normal/nearly normal for 16–19 days to moderately/severely low for 3–4 days. Daily treatment with G-CSF at doses of 1–5 µg/kg typically improves symptoms in most patients. Cyclic neutropenia is caused by heterozygous mutations in the *ELA2* gene, usually at the active site of neutrophil elastase,[257,296] without disrupting the enzymatic substrate cleavage by the active site.[257] The mutations seem to disturb a predicted transmembrane domain, leading to excessive granular accumulation of elastase and defective membrane localization of the enzyme.[268] The myeloid precursors are characterized by cycling increase in apoptosis.[269]

Myelokathexis is a rare autosomal dominant disorder with recurrent bacterial infections caused by reduced number and function of neutrophils.[297] Neutropenia is typically moderate to severe. Degenerative changes in the granulocytes are characteristic and include pyknotic nuclear lobes, fine chromatin filaments, and hypersegmentation.[297] Bone marrow specimens are usually hypercellular with granulocytic hyperplasia. The pathophysiology of myelokathexis has been attributed to a defective release of marrow cells into the peripheral blood.[297] Neutrophil precursors are characterized by depressed expression of Bcl-x and accelerated apoptosis.[298] G-CSF and GM-CSF ameliorate the neutropenia and lead to clinical improvement during episodes of bacterial infection.[297,299]

WHIM syndrome (warts, hypogammaglobulinemia, infections, and myelokathexis) is a subtype of myelokathexis,[300] caused by mutations in the chemokine receptor gene *CXCR4*.[301] The mutations result in enhanced chemotactic response of neutrophils in response to the CXCR4 ligand, CXCL12, which might account for the pathological retention of mature neutrophils in the bone marrow.[302]

Other disorders with isolated neutrophil production defects are glycogen storage disease type Ib,[303,304] and Barth syndrome.[305,306]

Inherited marrow failure disorders with predominantly thrombocytopenia

Thrombocytopenia with absent radii

The syndrome of thrombocytopenia with absent radii (TAR) was first described in 1929,[307] and subsequently defined in 1969.[308] The two features that are currently essential for the definition of the syndrome are hypomegakaryocytic thrombocytopenia and bilateral radial aplasia. This definition may change once the genetic basis is deciphered.

Clinical features

Hematologic manifestations
Most patients present with petechial rash or overt hemorrhage such as bloody diarrhea in the first week of life or later during the next 4 months. The diagnosis is usually made in the newborn period when thrombocytopenia is found in a patient with absent radii. Platelet counts at birth are usually between 15 and 30×10^9/L (range $7–92 \times 10^9$/L).[309,310]

Transient leukocytosis with a "left-shifted" granulocytic cell population is seen in the majority of patients, and is sometimes extreme ($>100 \times 10^9$/L). Anemia due to blood loss is sometimes present. Red cell size and hemoglobin F levels are normal.

Marrow specimens show normal to increased cellularity with decreased to absent megakaryocytes. The erythroid and myeloid lineages are normally represented. When a few megakaryocytes can be identified in biopsies, they are small, contain few nuclear segments, and show immature nongranular cytoplasm. If platelet counts increase spontaneously in patients after the first year of life, megakaryocytes increase in parallel and appear more mature morphologically. Platelet size is generally normal, with rare exception,[311] and function is unremarkable,[312] although some patients may show abnormal platelet aggregation and storage pool defects.[313]

Nonhematologic manifestations
Patients have radial aplasia (Fig. 3.4) with preservation of thumbs and fingers; this occurs bilaterally in almost all patients. Additional deformities in the upper extremity may be found and include radial club hands, hypoplasia of the carpals and phalanges, ulnae, humeri, and shoulder girdles, syndactyly, clinodactyly, and phocomelia. Characteristic findings also include a selective hypoplasia of the middle phalanx of the fifth finger and altered palmar contours. Malformations of the lower extremities are seen in about half of cases, and include hip dislocation, coxa valga, femoral torsion, tibial torsion, abnormal tibiofibular joints, small feet, valgus and varus foot deformities, syndactyly, clinodactyly, and phocomelia. Abnormal toe placement is commonly seen, especially the fifth toe overlapping the fourth. Other skeletal abnormalities include asymmetric first rib, cervical rib, cervical spinae bifida, fused cervical spine, and micrognathia.

One-third of patients have congenital heart defects. The most common are septal defects and tetralogy of Fallot. Facial hemangiomas are common, as well as redundant nuchal folds. Other abnormalities include dorsal pedal edema, hyperhidrosis, cows' milk intolerance, and kidney and genitourinary defects.[314]

Cancer predisposition

Of the 200 TAR patients reported in the literature, two developed AML[315,316] and one developed acute lymphoblastic leukemia.[317] Rare cases of solid tumors have also been reported. This literature might suggest a true, but low, predisposition to develop cancer.

Genetic aspects

The underlying genetic defect is unknown. Also, the inheritance of TAR syndrome has not been fully defined. However, family studies demonstrating occurrence of more than one sibling in the same families suggest that at least in some families the inheritance is autosomal recessive. Typically, parents of TAR patients are phenotypically normal, and females with TAR syndrome can conceive and give birth to hematologically and phenotypically normal offspring.

Pathogenesis

Thrombocytopenia in TAR syndrome is due to a defect in megakaryocytopoiesis/thrombocytopoiesis.[318,319] Marrow CFU-Meg progenitors are usually absent or reduced.[318,320,321] The few CFU-Meg colonies produced from these progenitors are small[322] or of abnormal morphology.[319] In differentiating liquid cultures, mature megakaryocytes (CD41+CD42+) demonstrated accelerated apoptosis, and earlier megakaryocytic precursors (CD34−CD41+CD42−) accumulated.[320]

Thrombopoietin levels in serum are consistently elevated in TAR syndrome.[323] Thrombopoietin-induced tyrosine phosphorylation of platelet proteins is absent or markedly decreased, but conflicting results have been published with regard to the expression of the thrombopoietin receptor.[320,323]

Laboratory evaluation and diagnosis

Almost all patients are diagnosed at the neonatal period or shortly after. The diagnosis can be missed if the patients do not bleed and a platelet count is not performed. The diagnosis is largely based on physical examination, skeletal survey, and blood counts. Extensive work-up to rule out acquired and other inherited causes of congenital thrombocytopenia is not always necessary, as most of the affected neonates are clinically well. Bone marrow examination is helpful to confirm hypo-megakaryopoiesis as the cause of the thrombocytopenia.

The main differential diagnosis of TAR syndrome is Fanconi anemia. In contrast to TAR syndrome, Fanconi anemia patients who lack their radii also have hypoplastic or absent thumbs. Fanconi anemia patients do not have skin hemangiomas, which are common in TAR patients, whereas TAR patients do not manifest skin pigmentation, as occurs in 65% of Fanconi anemia patients. Chromosome fragility testing is normal in TAR syndrome. Prenatal diagnosis has been demonstrated by quantitating platelet numbers obtained by fetoscopy or cordocentesis, and by ultrasound. In one confirmed case, a prenatal *in utero* platelet transfusion was given to effect a safe delivery.[324]

Therapy and prognosis

The thrombocytopenia is treated mostly with platelet transfusions, which should be used judiciously to avoid refractoriness and other transfusion reactions. Clinical bleeding and prophylaxis before surgical procedures are appropriate indications. Persistent platelet counts $< 10 \times 10^9/L$ may require preventive platelet transfusions on a regular basis. Whenever possible, single donor platelets should be considered to minimize the risk of alloimmunization. HLA partially matched donors for platelets may be required if patients become refractory to transfusions.

In exceptional situations, profound persistent life-threatening thrombocytopenia can be successfully treated by HSCT.[325] The role of thrombopoietic growth factors such as IL-11, IL-6, IL-3, and thrombopoietin in the management of TAR patients is unclear. Androgens, corticosteroids, and splenectomy are ineffective therapies for TAR syndrome.

The overall prognosis for survival and spontaneous remission is good, and patients rarely develop aplastic anemia or cancer. Deaths are usually due to intracranial or gastrointestinal bleeding. If patients survive the first year of life, platelet counts spontaneously increase inexplicably to levels that are hemostatically safe and which do not require platelet transfusional support. A minority of patients have sustained, profound thrombocytopenia. The actuarial survival reaches a plateau of 75% by the age of 4 years.[12]

Other inherited marrow failure syndromes with predominantly thrombocytopenia

The various syndromes with thrombocytopenia have been reviewed recently.[326,327] Clues for the specific diagnosis of the syndromes can be provided by a family history suggestive of an inherited pattern, age at diagnosis, and associated nonhematologic manifestations. A battery of tests, including bone marrow aspiration and biopsy, is usually required to establish a diagnosis. An algorithm to assist clinicians in the diagnosis of the inherited thrombocytopenia has been reported.[328]

MYH9-associated familial macrothrombocytopenia comprises an array of several syndromes (Alport, Fetchner, Ebstein, Sebastian, and May–Hegglin) that have classically been classified according to their nonhematologic manifestations.[326,327] *MYH9* encodes nonmuscle myosin heavy chain IIA, a cytoskeletal contractile protein.[329] The common features include autosomal dominant inheritance, large platelets, mild to moderate thrombocytopenia, normal numbers of megakaryocytes in the bone marrow, and variable platelet aggregation and secretion defects, which may rarely cause bleeding, requiring platelet transfusions.[330] Progression into aplastic anemia or leukemia has not thus far been reported.

Nonsyndromic thrombocytopenia associated with FLJ14813 gene mutations is characterized by an autosomal dominant inheritance, mild to moderate thrombocytopenia, normal platelet size and morphology, and mild bleeding tendency. Progression to leukemia is unlikely. Bone marrow specimens are of normal cellularity with normal to mildly reduced numbers of megakaryocytes, which can be small and have hypolobulated nuclei. Clonogenic assays show increased megakaryocytic progenitors.[331] FLJ14813 is a novel putative kinase.[332]

Familial thrombocytopenia with dyserythropoiesis is an X-linked disease with mild to severe bleeding tendency and mild to moderate dyserythropoiesis.[333,335] Platelets are normal to large size and the immune system is intact. Platelet counts are moderately to severely affected ($10–40 \times 10^9/L$), have variably low expression of GPIb, and their aggregation in response to ristocetin is reduced.[334] The anemia is variable in severity. Bone marrow biopsy specimens are hypercellular with dysplastic megakaryocytes having a peripheral nucleus and lack of nuclear segmentation or fragmentation as well as dysplastic erythroid precursors with mild megaloblastic changes with delayed nuclear maturation.[335] There are no reports of progression to severe aplastic anemia, MDS, or leukemia. The disorder is caused by missense mutations in GATA1,[333] a transcription factor important for both megakaryopoiesis and erythropoiesis. The treatment consists of platelet transfusion in case of bleeding, trauma, or preparation for surgery. Severe cases can be cured by allogeneic related or unrelated HSCT.[333]

Familial platelet disorder with associated myeloid malignancy is an autosomal dominant disease with a striking predisposition for hematologic malignancy.[336] The thrombocytopenia is mild to moderate, and platelets have normal size and morphology. The disorder is caused by mutations in the gene *CBFA2* (also called *AML1*).[7] Treatment of the thrombocytopenia is usually not required, but regular screening for leukemia is probably advisable and HSCT is potentially curative in the leukemic phase.

Thrombocytopenia associated with radioulnar synostosis is an autosomal dominant disorder with congenital thrombocytopenia, proximal radioulnar synostosis, clinodactyly, syndactyly, congenital hip dysplasia, and sensorineural deafness.[337] Patients are heterozygous for small deletional mutations in the *HOXA11* gene, which lead to truncation of the protein.[338] The thrombocytopenia can be severe and require platelet transfusions. The bone marrow shows absence of megakaryocytes. If the thrombocytopenia is severe or progresses to aplastic anemia, allogeneic HSCT can be curative.[337]

Thrombocytopenia is also part of Wiskott–Aldrich/XL-thrombocytopenia syndrome,[339] Mediterranean macrothrombocytopenia,[340] and Montreal platelet syndrome.[341]

Unclassifiable or poorly classified inherited marrow failure syndromes

Multiple cases of apparent IMFSs with or without anomalies have been reported. Further studies are needed to determine whether the cases are related to already categorized IMFSs or whether they constitute new syndromes. Because these disorders are rare, broad conclusions about management are difficult to formulate. For full-blown aplastic anemia with a hypocellular, fatty marrow, curative therapy with HSCT remains the first choice if a matched donor is identified. In familial cases, potential marrow donors must be thoroughly assessed clinically, hematologically, and by marrow morphology, clonogenic activity, and cytogenetics to ensure that latent or masked marrow dysfunction is not present. If a matched donor is not available, alternative options are androgens, growth factors and matched unrelated donor HSCT.

Acknowledgments

The author thanks Dr Melvin Freedman, the previous author of this chapter, Ms Roxanne Francis, and Ms LuAnn Brooker for their help in preparation of the chapter.

References

1. Steele JM, Klaassan R, Fernandez C *et al*. Disease progression in recently diagnosed patients with inherited marrow failure syndromes: A report from the Canadian Inherited Marrow Failure Registry (CIMFR). *Cancer and Blood* 2005; **44**: 538.
2. Vora AA, Kandoth WK, Athavale VB. Fanconi's anaemia. *Indian Pediatr* 1971; **8**: 40–2.
3. Jones R. Letter: Fanconi anemia: simultaneous onset of symptoms in two siblings. *J Pediatr* 1976; **88**: 152.
4. Windass B, Vowels MR, Hughes DO, White L. Aplastic anaemia in childhood: prognosis and approach to therapy. *Med J Aust* 1987; **146**: 15–19.
5. Vulliamy T, Marrone A, Dokal I, Mason PJ. Association between aplastic anaemia and mutations in telomerase RNA. *Lancet* 2002; **359**: 2168–70.
6. Dokal I. Dyskeratosis congenita in all its forms. *Br J Haematol* 2000; **110**: 768–79.
7. Song WJ, Sullivan MG, Legare RD *et al*. Haploinsufficiency of CBFA2 causes familial thrombocytopenia with propensity to develop acute myelogenous leukaemia. *Nat Genet* 1999; **23**: 166–75.
8. Butturini A, Gale RP, Verlander PC, Adler-Brecher B, Gillio AP, Auerbach AD. Hematologic abnormalities in Fanconi anemia: an International Fanconi Anemia Registry study. *Blood* 1994; **84**: 1650–5.
9. Mack DR, Forstner GG, Wilschanski M, Freedman MH, Durie PR. Shwachman syndrome: exocrine pancreatic dysfunction and variable phenotypic expression. *Gastroenterology* 1996; **111**: 1593–602.
10. Dror Y. Shwachman-Diamond syndrome. *Pediatr Blood Can* 2005; **45**(7): 892–901.
11. Freedman MH, Bonilla MA, Fier C *et al*. Myelodysplasia syndrome and acute myeloid leukemia in patients with congenital neutropenia receiving G-CSF therapy. *Blood* 2000; **96**: 429–36.
12. Alter BP. Inherited bone marrow failure syndromes. In: Nathan DG, Orkin SH, Ginsberg D, Look AT (eds) *Hematology of Infancy and Childhood*. Philadelphia: WB Saunders, 2003, pp. 280–365.
13. Fanconi G. Familiäre infantile perniziosaartige Anämie (perniziöses Blutbild und Konstitution). *Jahrbuch Kinder* 1927; **117**: 258.
14. Kutler DI, Singh B, Satagopan J *et al*. A 20-year perspective on the International Fanconi Anemia Registry (IFAR). *Blood* 2003; **101**: 1249–56.
15. Rosenberg PS, Huang Y, Alter BP. Individualized risks of first adverse events in patients with Fanconi anemia. *Blood* 2004; **104**: 350–5.
16. Estren S, Dameshek W. Familial hypoplastic anemia of childhood: Report of eight cases in two families with beneficial effect of splenectomy in one case. *Am J Dis Child* 1947; **73**: 671–87.
17. Wajnrajch MP, Gertner JM, Huma Z *et al*. Evaluation of growth and hormonal status in patients referred to the International Fanconi Anemia Registry. *Pediatrics* 2001; **107**: 744–54.
18. Alter BP. Cancer in Fanconi anemia, 1927–2001. *Cancer* 2003; **97**: 425–40.
19. Tonnies H, Huber S, Kuhl JS, Gerlach A, Ebell W, Neitzel H.

Clonal chromosomal aberrations in bone marrow cells of Fanconi anemia patients: gains of the chromosomal segment 3q26q29 as an adverse risk factor. *Blood* 2003; **101**: 3872–4.

20. Yoshida MC. Suppression of spontaneous and mitomycin C-induced chromosome aberrations in Fanconi's anemia by cell fusion with normal human fibroblasts. *Hum Genet* 1980; **55**: 223–6.

21. Duckworth-Rysiecki G, Cornish K, Clarke CA, Buchwald M. Identification of two complementation groups in Fanconi anemia. *Somat Cell Mol Genet* 1985; **11**: 35–41.

22. Faivre L, Guardiola P, Lewis C *et al.* Association of complementation group and mutation type with clinical outcome in Fanconi anemia. European Fanconi Anemia Research Group. *Blood* 2000; **96**: 4064–70.

23. Gillio AP, Verlander PC, Batish SD, Giampietro PF, Auerbach AD. Phenotypic consequences of mutations in the Fanconi anemia FAC gene: an International Fanconi Anemia Registry study. *Blood* 1997; **90**: 105–10.

24. Futaki M, Yamashita T, Yagasaki H *et al.* The IVS4 + 4 A to T mutation of the fanconi anemia gene FANCC is not associated with a severe phenotype in Japanese patients. *Blood* 2000; **95**: 1493–8.

25. Meetei AR, de Winter JP, Medhurst AL *et al.* A novel ubiquitin ligase is deficient in Fanconi anemia. *Nat Genet* 2003; **35**: 165–70.

26. Yamashita T, Kupfer GM, Naf D *et al.* The fanconi anemia pathway requires FAA phosphorylation and FAA/FAC nuclear accumulation. *Proc Natl Acad Sci USA* 1998; **95**: 13085–90.

27. Kupfer GM, Naf D, Suliman A, Pulsipher M, D'Andrea AD. The Fanconi anaemia proteins, FAA and FAC, interact to form a nuclear complex. *Nat Genet* 1997; **17**: 487–90.

28. Garcia-Higuera I, Kuang Y, Naf D, Wasik J, D'Andrea AD. Fanconi anemia proteins FANCA, FANCC, and FANCG/XRCC9 interact in a functional nuclear complex. *Mol Cell Biol* 1999; **19**: 4866–73.

29. Garcia-Higuera I, Kuang Y, Denham J, D'Andrea AD. The fanconi anemia proteins FANCA and FANCG stabilize each other and promote the nuclear accumulation of the Fanconi anemia complex. *Blood* 2000; **96**: 3224–30.

30. Garcia-Higuera I, Taniguchi T, Ganesan S *et al.* Interaction of the Fanconi anemia proteins and BRCA1 in a common pathway. *Mol Cell* 2001; **7**: 249–62.

31. Cheng NC, van de Vrugt HJ, van der Valk MA *et al.* Mice with a targeted disruption of the Fanconi anemia homolog Fanca. *Hum Mol Genet* 2000; **9**: 1805–11.

32. Koomen M, Cheng NC, van de Vrugt HJ *et al.* Reduced fertility and hypersensitivity to mitomycin C characterize Fancg/Xrcc9 null mice. *Hum Mol Genet* 2002; **11**: 273–81.

33. Rathbun RK, Faulkner GR, Ostroski MH *et al.* Inactivation of the Fanconi anemia group C gene augments interferon-gamma-induced apoptotic responses in hematopoietic cells. *Blood* 1997; **90**: 974–85.

34. Aube M, Lafrance M, Charbonneau C, Goulet I, Carreau M. Hematopoietic stem cells from fancc(–/–) mice have lower growth and differentiation potential in response to growth factors. *Stem Cells* 2002; **20**: 438–47.

35. Chen M, Tomkins DJ, Auerbach W *et al.* Inactivation of Fac in mice produces inducible chromosomal instability and reduced fertility reminiscent of Fanconi anaemia. *Nat Genet* 1996; **12**: 448–51.

36. Auerbach AD, Rogatko A, Schroeder-Kurth TM. International Fanconi Anemia Registry: relation of clinical symptoms to diepoxybutane sensitivity. *Blood* 1989; **73**: 391–6.

37. Papadopoulo D, Guillouf C, Mohrenweiser H, Moustacchi E. Hypomutability in Fanconi anemia cells is associated with increased deletion frequency at the HPRT locus. *Proc Natl Acad Sci USA* 1990; **87**: 8383–7.

38. Coppey J, Sala-Trepat M, Lopez B. Multiplicity reactivation and mutagenesis of trimethylpsoralen-damaged herpes virus in normal and Fanconi's anaemia cells. *Mutagenesis* 1989; **4**: 67–71.

39. Howlett NG, Taniguchi T, Olson S *et al.* Biallelic inactivation of BRCA2 in Fanconi anemia. *Science* 2002; **297**: 606–9.

40. Godthelp BC, Artwert F, Joenje H, Zdzienicka MZ. Impaired DNA damage-induced nuclear Rad51 foci formation uniquely characterizes Fanconi anemia group D1. *Oncogene* 2002; **21**: 5002–5.

41. Sabatier L, Dutrillaux B. Effect of caffeine in Fanconi anemia. I. Restoration of a normal duration of G2 phase. *Hum Genet* 1988; **79**: 242–4.

42. Rathbun RK, Christianson TA, Faulkner GR *et al.* Interferon-gamma-induced apoptotic responses of Fanconi anemia group C hematopoietic progenitor cells involve caspase 8-dependent activation of caspase 3 family members. *Blood* 2000; **96**: 4204–11.

43. Cumming RC, Lightfoot J, Beard K, Youssoufian H, O'Brien PJ, Buchwald M. Fanconi anemia group C protein prevents apoptosis in hematopoietic cells through redox regulation of GSTP1. *Nat Med* 2001; **7**: 814–20.

44. Pang Q, Keeble W, Christianson TA, Faulkner GR, Bagby GC. FANCC interacts with Hsp70 to protect hematopoietic cells from IFN-gamma/TNF-alpha-mediated cytotoxicity. *EMBO J* 2001; **20**: 4478–89.

45. Zhang X, Li J, Sejas DP, Rathbun KR, Bagby GC, Pang Q. The Fanconi anemia proteins functionally interact with the protein kinase regulated by RNA (PKR). *J Biol Chem* 2004; **279**: 43910–19.

46. Saunders EF, Freedman MH. Constitutional aplastic anaemia: defective haematopoietic stem cell growth in vitro. *Br J Haematol* 1978; **40**: 277–87.

47. Shihab-el-Deen A, Guevara C, Prchal JF. Bone marrow cultures in dysmyelopoietic syndrome: diagnostic and prognostic evaluation. *Acta Haematol* 1987; **78**: 17–22.

48. Daneshbod-Skibba G, Martin J, Shahidi NT. Myeloid and erythroid colony growth in non-anaemic patients with Fanconi's anaemia. *Br J Haematol* 1980; **44**: 33–8.

49. Bagnara GP, Strippoli P, Bonsi L *et al.* Effect of stem cell factor on colony growth from acquired and constitutional (Fanconi) aplastic anemia. *Blood* 1992; **80**: 382–7.

50. Rosselli F, Sanceau J, Gluckman E, Wietzerbin J, Moustacchi E. Abnormal lymphokine production: a novel feature of the genetic disease Fanconi anemia. II. In vitro and in vivo spontaneous overproduction of tumor necrosis factor alpha. *Blood* 1994; **83**: 1216–25.

51. Auerbach AD, Adler B, Chaganti RS. Prenatal and postnatal diagnosis and carrier detection of Fanconi anemia by a cytogenetic method. *Pediatrics* 1981; **67**: 128–35.

52. Levran O, Diotti R, Pujara K, Batish SD, Hanenberg H, Auerbach AD. Spectrum of sequence variations in the FANCA gene: an International Fanconi Anemia Registry (IFAR) study. *Hum Mutat* 2005; **25**: 142–9.

53. Alter BP, Frissora CL, Halperin DS *et al.* Fanconi's anaemia and pregnancy. *Br J Haematol* 1991; **77**: 410–18.

54. Gluckman E, Devergie A, Schaison G *et al.* Bone marrow transplantation in Fanconi anaemia. *Br J Haematol* 1980; **45**: 557–64.

55. Gluckman E, Devergie A, Dutreix J. Radiosensitivity in Fanconi anaemia: application to the conditioning regimen for bone marrow transplantation. *Br J Haematol* 1983; **54**: 431–40.

56. Gluckman E, Auerbach AD, Horowitz MM *et al.* Bone marrow transplantation for Fanconi anemia. *Blood* 1995; **86**: 2856–62.

57. Socie G, Devergie A, Girinski T *et al.* Transplantation for Fanconi's anaemia: long-term follow-up of fifty patients transplanted from a sibling donor after low-dose cyclophosphamide and thoraco-abdominal irradiation for conditioning. *Br J Haematol* 1998; **103**: 249–55.

58. Harris RE. Reduction of toxicity of marrow transplantation in children with Fanconi anemia. *J Pediatr Hematol Oncol* 1999; **21**: 175–6.

59. Flowers ME, Zanis J, Pasquini R *et al.* Marrow transplantation for Fanconi anaemia: conditioning with reduced doses of cyclophosphamide without radiation. *Br J Haematol* 1996; **92**: 699–706.

60. Kapelushnik J, Or R, Slavin S, Nagler A. A fludarabine-based protocol for bone marrow transplantation in Fanconi's anemia. *Bone Marrow Transplant* 1997; **20**: 1109–10.

61. Kurre P, Pulsipher M, Woolfrey A *et al.* Reduced toxicity and prompt engraftment after minimal conditioning of a patient with Fanconi anemia undergoing hematopoietic stem cell transplantation from an HLA-matched unrelated donor. *J Pediatr Hematol Oncol* 2003; **25**: 581–3.

62. MacMillan ML, Auerbach AD, Davies SM *et al.* Haematopoietic cell transplantation in patients with Fanconi anaemia using alternate donors: results of a total body irradiation dose escalation trial. *Br J Haematol* 2000; **109**: 121–9.

63. Boulad F, Auerbach AD, Kernan NA *et al.* Fludarabine (Flu) based cytoreductive regimen and T-cell depleted grafts from unrelated or mismatched related donors for the treatment of high risk patients with Fanconi anemia (FA). *Blood* 2004; **104**: 2152.

64. Wagner JE, Eapen M, Harris RE, MacMillan ML, Auerbach AD. Analysis of prognosis factors impacting engrafting and survival. *Blood* 2005; **104**: 824a.

65. Guardiola P, Pasquini R, Dokal I *et al.* Outcome of 69 allogeneic stem cell transplantations for Fanconi anemia using HLA-matched unrelated donors: a study on behalf of the European Group for Blood and Marrow Transplantation. *Blood* 2000; **95**: 422–9.

66. Gluckman E, Broxmeyer HA, Auerbach AD *et al.* Hematopoietic reconstitution in a patient with Fanconi's anemia by means of umbilical-cord blood from an HLA-identical sibling. *N Engl J Med* 1989; **321**: 1174–8.

67. Gluckman E, Vanderson R, Ionescu I *et al.* Results of unrelated cord blood transplants in Fanconi anemia. *Blood* 2004; **104**: 2145.

68. Boulad F, Gillio A, Small TN *et al.* Stem cell transplantation for the treatment of Fanconi anaemia using a fludarabine-based cytoreductive regimen and T-cell-depleted related HLA-mismatched peripheral blood stem cell grafts. *Br J Haematol* 2000; **111**: 1153–7.

69. Adams KE. Ethical considerations of applications of preimplantation genetic diagnosis in the United States. *Med Law* 2003; **22**: 489–94.

70. Verlinsky Y, Rechitsky S, Schoolcraft W, Strom C, Kuliev A. Preimplantation diagnosis for Fanconi anemia combined with HLA matching. *JAMA* 2001; **285**: 3130–3.

71. Bielorai B, Hughes MR, Auerbach AD *et al.* Successful umbilical cord blood transplantation for Fanconi anemia using preimplantation genetic diagnosis for HLA-matched donor. *Am J Hematol* 2004; **77**: 397–9.

72. Rackoff WR, Orazi A, Robinson CA *et al.* Prolonged administration of granulocyte colony-stimulating factor (filgrastim) to patients with Fanconi anemia: a pilot study. *Blood* 1996; **88**: 1588–93.

73. Scagni P, Saracco P, Timeus F *et al.* Use of recombinant granulocyte colony-stimulating factor in Fanconi's anemia. *Haematologica* 1998; **83**: 432–7.

74. Alter BP, Scalise A, McCombs J, Najfeld V. Clonal chromosomal abnormalities in Fanconi's anaemia: what do they really mean? *Br J Haematol* 1993; **85**: 627–30.

75. Gregory JJ Jr, Wagner JE, Verlander PC *et al.* Somatic mosaicism in Fanconi anemia: evidence of genotypic reversion in lymphohematopoietic stem cells. *Proc Natl Acad Sci USA* 2001; **98**: 2532–7.

76. Walsh CE, Grompe M, Vanin E *et al.* A functionally active retrovirus vector for gene therapy in Fanconi anemia group C. *Blood* 1994; **84**: 453–9.

77. Walsh C. Gene therapy for group A Fanconi anemia patients: Current update and future trials. *Fanconi Anemia Sc Lett* 2001; **30**: 9.

78. Liu JM, Kim S, Read EJ *et al.* Engraftment of hematopoietic progenitor cells transduced with the Fanconi anemia group C gene (FANCC). *Hum Gene Ther* 1999; **10**: 2337–46.

79. Yamada K, Ramezani A, Hawley RG *et al.* Phenotype correction of Fanconi anemia group A hematopoietic stem cells using lentiviral vector. *Mol Ther* 2003; **8**: 600–10.

80. Shwachman H, Diamond LK, Oski FA, Khaw K-T. The syndrome of pancreatic insufficiency and bone marrow dysfunction. *J Pediatr* 1964; **65**: 645–63.

81. Bodian M, Sheldon W, Lightwood R. Congenital hypoplasia of the exocrine pancreas. *Acta Paediatr* 1964; **53**: 282–93.

82. Aggett PJ, Cavanagh NP, Matthew DJ, Pincott JR, Sutcliffe J, Harries JT. Shwachman's syndrome. A review of 21 cases. *Arch Dis Child* 1980; **55**: 331–47.

83. Ginzberg H, Shin J, Ellis L *et al.* Shwachman syndrome: phenotypic manifestations of sibling sets and isolated cases in a large patient cohort are similar. *J Pediatr* 1999; **135**: 81–8.

84. Dror Y, Ginzberg H, Dalal I *et al.* Immune function in patients with Shwachman–Diamond syndrome. *Br J Haematol* 2001; **114**: 712–17.

85. Dror Y, Durie P, Marcon P, Freedman MH. Duplication of distal thumb phalanx in Shwachman–Diamond syndrome. *Am J Med Genet* 1998; **78**: 67–9.

86. Smith OP, Hann IM, Chessells JM, Reeves BR, Milla P. Haematological abnormalities in Shwachman–Diamond syndrome. *Br J Haematol* 1996; **94**: 279–84.

87. Dror Y, Squire J, Durie P, Freedman MH. Malignant myeloid transformation with isochromosome 7q in Shwachman–Diamond syndrome. *Leukemia* 1998; **12**: 1591–5.

88. Dror Y, Durie P, Ginzberg H *et al.* Clonal evolution in marrows of patients with Shwachman–Diamond syndrome: a prospective 5-year follow-up study. *Exp Hematol* 2002; **30**: 659–69.

89. Rothbaum RJ, Williams DA, Daugherty CC. Unusual surface distribution of concanavalin A reflects a cytoskeletal defect in neutrophils in Shwachman's syndrome. *Lancet* 1982; ii: 800–1.

90. Azzara A, Carulli G, Petrini M. Lithium effects on neutrophil motility in Shwachman–Diamond syndrome: evaluation by computer-assisted image analysis. *Br J Haematol* 2003; **123**: 369–70.

91. Dror Y, Freedman MH. Shwachman–Diamond syndrome: An inherited preleukemic bone marrow failure disorder with aberrant hematopoietic progenitors and faulty marrow microenvironment. *Blood* 1999; **94**: 3048–54.

92. Tsai PH, Sahdev I, Herry A, Lipton JM. Fatal cyclophosphamide-induced congestive heart failure in a 10-year-old boy with Shwachman–Diamond syndrome and severe bone marrow failure treated with allogeneic bone marrow transplantation. *Am J Pediatr Hematol Oncol* 1990; **12**: 472–6.

93. Barrios NJ, Kirkpatrick DV. Bone marrow transplant in Shwachman–Diamond syndrome. *Br J Haematol* 1991; **79**: 337–8.

94. Hudson E, Aldor T. Pancreatic insufficiency and neutropenia with associated immunoglobulin deficit. *Arch Intern Med* 1970; **125**: 314–16.

95. Aggett PJ, Harries JT, Harvey BA, Soothill JF. An inherited defect of neutrophil mobility in Shwachman syndrome. *J Pediatr* 1979; **94**: 391–4.

96. Sacchi F, Maggiore G, Marseglia G, Marconi M, Nespoli L, Siccardi AG. Association of neutrophil and complement defects in two twins with Shwachman syndrome. *Helv Paediatr Acta* 1982; **37**: 177–81.

97. Kornfeld SJ, Kratz J, Diamond F, Day NK, Good RA. Shwachman–Diamond syndrome associated with hypogammaglobulinemia and growth hormone deficiency. *J Allergy Clin Immunol* 1995; **96**: 247–50.

98. Maki M, Sorto A, Hallstrom O, Visakorpi JK. Hepatic dysfunction and dysgammaglobulinaemia in Shwachman–Diamond syndrome. *Arch Dis Child* 1978; **53**: 693–4.

99. Taybi H, Mitchell AD, Friedman GD. Metaphyseal dysostosis and the associated syndrome of pancreatic insufficiency and blood disorders. *Radiology* 1969; **93**: 563–71.

100. Makitie O, Ellis L, Durie PR *et al.* Skeletal phenotype in patients with Shwachman–Diamond syndrome and mutations in SBDS. *Clin Genet* 2004; **65**: 101–12.

101. Danks DM, Haslam R, Mayne V, Kaufmann HJ, Holtzapple PG. Metaphyseal chondrodysplasia, neutropenia, and pancreatic insufficiency presenting with respiratory distress in the neonatal period. *Arch Dis Child* 1976; **51**: 697–702.

102. Labrune M, Dommergues JP, Chaboche C, Benichou JJ. Shwachman's syndrome with neonatal thoracic manifestations. *Arch Fr Pediatr* 1984; **41**: 561–3.

103. Sokolic RA, Ferguson W, Mark HF. Discordant detection of monosomy 7 by GTG-banding and FISH in a patient with Shwachman–Diamond syndrome without evidence of myelodysplastic syndrome or acute myelogenous leukemia. *Cancer Genet Cytogenet* 1999; **115**: 106–13.

104. Savilahti E, Rapola J. Frequent myocardial lesions in Shwachman's syndrome. Eight fatal cases among 16 Finnish patients. *Acta Paediatr Scand* 1984; 73:642–651.

105. Dokal I, Rule S, Chen F, Potter M, Goldman J. Adult onset of acute myeloid leukaemia (M6) in patients with Shwachman–Diamond syndrome. *Br J Haematol* 1997; **99**: 171–3.

106. Smith A, Shaw PJ, Webster B *et al.* Intermittent 20q– and consistent i(7q) in a patient with Shwachman–Diamond syndrome. *Pediatr Hematol Oncol* 2002; **19**: 525–8.

107. Davies SM, Wagner JE, DeFor T *et al.* Unrelated donor bone marrow transplantation for children and adolescents with aplastic anaemia or myelodysplasia. *Br J Haematol* 1997; **96**: 749–56.

108. Passmore SJ, Hann IM, Stiller CA *et al.* Pediatric myelodysplasia: a study of 68 children and a new prognostic scoring system. *Blood* 1995; **85**: 1742–50.

109. Kalra R, Dale D, Freedman M *et al.* Monosomy 7 and activating RAS mutations accompany malignant transformation in patients with congenital neutropenia. *Blood* 1995; **86**: 4579–86.

110. Cunningham J, Sales M, Pearce A *et al.* Does isochromosome 7q mandate bone marrow transplant in children with Shwachman–Diamond syndrome? *Br J Haematol* 2002; **119**: 1062–9.

111. Raj AB, Bertolone SJ, Barch MJ, Hersh JH. Chromosome 20q deletion and progression to monosomy 7 in a patient with Shwachman–Diamond syndrome without MDS/AML. *J Pediatr Hematol Oncol* 2003; **25**: 508–9.

112. Faber J, Lauener R, Wick F *et al.* Shwachman–Diamond syndrome: early bone marrow transplantation in a high risk patient and new clues to pathogenesis. *Eur J Pediatr* 1999; **158**: 995–1000.

113. Arseniev L, Diedrich H, Link H. Allogeneic bone marrow transplantation in a patient with Shwachman–Diamond syndrome. *Ann Hematol* 1996; **72**: 83–4.

114. Woods WG, Roloff JS, Lukens JN, Krivit W. The occurrence of leukemia in patients with the Shwachman syndrome. *J Pediatr* 1981; **99**: 425–8.

115. Smith OP, Chan MY, Evans J, Veys P. Shwachman–Diamond syndrome and matched unrelated donor BMT. *Bone Marrow Transplant* 1995; **16**: 717–18.

116. Cesaro S, Guariso G, Calore E *et al.* Successful unrelated bone marrow transplantation for Shwachman–Diamond syndrome. *Bone Marrow Transplant* 2001; **27**: 97–9.

117. Huijgens PC, van der Veen EA, Meijer S, Muntinghe OG. Syndrome of Shwachman and leukaemia. *Scand J Haematol* 1977; **18**: 20–4.

118. Okcu F, Roberts WM, Chan KW. Bone marrow transplantation in Shwachman–Diamond syndrome: report of two cases and review of the literature. *Bone Marrow Transplant* 1998; **21**: 849–51.

119. Hsu JW, Vogelsang G, Jones RJ, Brodsky RA. Bone marrow transplantation in Shwachman–Diamond syndrome. *Bone Marrow Transplant* 2002; **30**: 255–8.

120. Caselitz J, Kloppel G, Delling G, Gruttner R, Holdhoff U, Stern M. Shwachman's syndrome and leukaemia. *Virchows Arch A Pathol Anat Histol* 1979; **385**: 109–16.

121. Gretillat F, Delepine N, Taillard F, Desbois JC, Misset JL.

Leukemic transformation of Shwachman's syndrome. *Presse Med* 1985; **14**: 45.

122. Strevens MJ, Lilleyman JS, Williams RB. Shwachman's syndrome and acute lymphoblastic leukaemia. *Br Med J* 1978; **2**: 18.

123. Seymour JF, Escudier SM. Acute leukemia complicating bone marrow hypoplasia in an adult with Shwachman's syndrome. *Leuk Lymphoma* 1993; **12**: 131–5.

124. Spirito FR, Crescenzi B, Matteucci C, Martelli MF, Mecucci C. Cytogenetic characterization of acute myeloid leukemia in Shwachman's syndrome. A case report. *Haematologica* 2000; **85**: 1207–10.

125. Lesesve JF, Dugue F, Gregoire MJ, Witz F, Dror Y. Shwachman–Diamond syndrome with late-onset neutropenia and fatal acute myeloid leukaemia without maturation: a case report. *Eur J Haematol* 2003; **71**: 393–5.

126. Lai CH, Chou CY, Ch'ang LY, Liu CS, Lin W. Identification of novel human genes evolutionarily conserved in *Caenorhabditis elegans* by comparative proteomics. *Genome Res* 2000; **10**: 703–13.

127. Boocock GR, Morrison JA, Popovic M *et al.* Mutations in SBDS are associated with Shwachman–Diamond syndrome. *Nat Genet* 2003; **33**: 97–101.

128. Woloszynek JR, Rothbaum RJ, Rawls AS *et al.* Mutations of the SBDS gene are present in most patients with Shwachman–Diamond syndrome. *Blood* 2004; **104**: 3588–90.

129. Majeed F, Jadko S, Freedman M, Dror Y. Mutation analysis of SBDS in pediatric acute myeloblastic leukemia. *Ped Blood and Cancer* 2005; **45**(7): 920–4.

130. Wu LF, Hughes TR, Davierwala AP, Robinson MD, Stoughton R, Altschuler SJ. Large-scale prediction of *Saccharomyces cerevisiae* gene function using overlapping transcriptional clusters. *Nat Genet* 2002; **31**: 255–65.

131. Koonin EV, Wolf YI, Aravind L. Prediction of the archaeal exosome and its connections with the proteasome and the translation and transcription machineries by a comparative-genomic approach. *Genome Res* 2001; **11**: 240–52.

132. Savchenko A, Krogan N, Cort JR *et al.* The Shwachman–Bodian–Diamond syndrome protein family is involved in RNA metabolism. *J Biol Chem* 2005; **280**: 19213–20.

133. Austin KM, Leary RJ, Shimamura A. The Shwachman–Diamond SBDS protein localizes to the nucleolus. *Blood* 2005; **106**: 1253–8.

134. Saunders EF, Gall G, Freedman MH. Granulopoiesis in Shwachman's syndrome (pancreatic insufficiency and bone marrow dysfunction). *Pediatrics* 1979; **64**: 515–19.

135. Suda T, Mizoguchi H, Miura Y *et al.* Hemopoietic colony-forming cells in Shwachman's syndrome. *Am J Pediatr Hematol Oncol* 1982; **4**: 129–33.

136. Dror Y, Freedman MH. Shwachman–Diamond syndrome marrow cells show abnormally increased apoptosis mediated through the Fas pathway. *Blood* 2001; **97**: 3011–16.

137. Thornley I, Dror Y, Sung L, Wynn RF, Freedman MH. Abnormal telomere shortening in leucocytes of children with Shwachman–Diamond syndrome. *Br J Haematol* 2002; **117**: 189–92.

138. Hershkovits BS, Dagan J, Freier S. Increased spontaneous chromosomal breakage in Shwachman syndrome. *J Pediatr Gastroenterol Nutr* 1999; **28**: 449–50.

139. Tada H, Ri T, Yoshida H, Ishimoto K, Kaneko M, Yamashiro Y *et al.* A case of Shwachman syndrome with increased spontaneous chromosome breakage. *Hum Genet* 1987; **77**: 289–91.

140. Fraccaro M, Scappaticci S, Arico M. Shwachman syndrome and chromosome breakage. *Hum Genet* 1988; **79**: 194.

141. Koiffmann CP, Gonzalez CH, Souza DH, Romani EG, Kim CA, Wajntal A. Is Shwachman syndrome (McKusick 26040) a chromosome breakage syndrome? *Hum Genet* 1991; **87**: 106–7.

142. Dror Y. P53 protein overexpression in Shwachman–Diamond syndrome. *Arch Pathol Lab Med* 2002; **126**: 1157–8.

143. Elghetany MT, Alter B. p53 protein overexpression in bone marrow biopsies of patients with Shwachman–Diamond syndrome has a prevalence similar to that of patients with refractory anemia. *Arch Pathol Lab Med* 2002; Apr, **126**(4): 452–5.

144. Grill J, Bernaudin F, Dresch C, Lemerle S, Reinert P. Treatment of neutropenia in Shwachman's syndrome with granulocyte growth factor (G-CSF). *Arch Fr Pediatr* 1993; **50**: 331–3.

145. van der Sande FM, Hillen HF. Correction of neutropenia following treatment with granulocyte colony-stimulating factor results in a decreased frequency of infections in Shwachman's syndrome. *Neth J Med* 1996; **48**: 92–5.

146. Vic PH, Nelken B, Mazingue F. Effect of recombinant human granulocyte and granulocyte and granulocyte-macrophage colony-stimulating factor in Shwachman's syndrome. *Int J Pediatr Hematol Oncol* 1996; **3**: 463–6.

147. Cesaro S, Oneto R, Messina C *et al.* Haematopoietic stem cell transplantation for Shwachman–Diamond disease: a study from the European Group for Blood and Marrow Transplantation. *Br J Haematol* 2005; **131**: 231–6.

148. Donadieu J, Michel G, Merlin E *et al.* Hematopoietic stem cell transplantation for Shwachman–Diamond syndrome: experience of the French neutropenia registry. *Bone Marrow Transplant* 2005; **36**(9): 787–92.

149. Zinnsser F. Atrophia cutis reticularis cum pigmentatione, dystrophia unguium et leukoplakia oris. *Ikonogr Dermatol (Hyoto)* 1906; **5**: 219–23.

150. Cole HN, Rauschkolb JC, Toomey J. Dyskeratosis congenita with pigmentation, dystrophia unguis and leukokeratosis oris. *Arch Dermatol Syphiligraph* 1920; **21**: 71–95.

151. Vulliamy TJ, Knight SW, Mason PJ, Dokal I. Very short telomeres in the peripheral blood of patients with X-linked and autosomal dyskeratosis congenita. *Blood Cells Mol Dis* 2001; **27**: 353–7.

152. Knight SW, Heiss NS, Vulliamy TJ *et al.* Unexplained aplastic anaemia, immunodeficiency, and cerebellar hypoplasia (Hoyeraal–Hreidarsson syndrome) due to mutations in the dyskeratosis congenita gene, DKC1. *Br J Haematol* 1999; **107**: 335–9.

153. Berezin S, Schwarz SM, Slim MS, Beneck D, Brudnicki AR, Medow MS. Gastrointestinal problems in a child with dyskeratosis congenita. *Am J Gastroenterol* 1996; **91**: 1271–2.

154. Revesz T, Fletcher S, al Gazali LI, DeBuse P. Bilateral retinopathy, aplastic anaemia, and central nervous system abnormalities: a new syndrome? *J Med Genet* 1992; **29**: 673–5.

155. Rocha V, Devergie A, Socie G *et al.* Unusual complications after bone marrow transplantation for dyskeratosis congenita. *Br J Haematol* 1998; **103**: 243–8.

156. Heiss NS, Knight SW, Vulliamy TJ *et al.* X-linked dyskeratosis congenita is caused by mutations in a highly conserved gene with putative nucleolar functions. *Nat Genet* 1998; **19**: 32–8.

157. Vulliamy T, Marrone A, Goldman F *et al.* The RNA component of telomerase mutated in autosomal dominated dyskeratosis congenita. *Nature* 2001; **413**: 432–5.

158. Pai GS, Yan Y, DeBauche DM, Stanley WS, Paul SR. Bleomycin hypersensitivity in dyskeratosis congenita fibroblasts, lymphocytes, and transformed lymphoblasts. *Cytogenet Cell Genet* 1989; **52**: 186–9.

159. Dokal I, Bungey J, Williamson P, Oscier D, Hows J, Luzzatto L. Dyskeratosis congenita fibroblasts are abnormal and have unbalanced chromosomal rearrangements. *Blood* 1992; **80**: 3090–6.

160. Marsh JC, Will AJ, Hows JM *et al.* "Stem cell" origin of the hematopoietic defect in dyskeratosis congenita. *Blood* 1992; **79**: 3138–44.

161. Dror Y, Freedman MH, Leaker M *et al.* Low-intensity hematopoietic stem-cell transplantation across human leucocyte antigen barriers in dyskeratosis congenita. *Bone Marrow Transplant* 2003; **31**: 847–50.

162. Oehler L, Reiter E, Friedl J *et al.* Effective stimulation of neutropoiesis with rh G-CSF in dyskeratosis congenita: a case report. *Ann Hematol* 1994; **69**: 325–7.

163. Russo CL, Glader BE, Israel RJ, Galasso F. Treatment of neutropenia associated with dyskeratosis congenita with granulocyte-macrophage colony-stimulating factor. *Lancet* 1990; **336**: 751–2.

164. Alter BP, Gardner FH, Hall RE. Treatment of dyskeratosis congenita with granulocyte colony-stimulating factor and erythropoietin. *Br J Haematol* 1997; **97**: 309–11.

165. Langston AA, Sanders JE, Deeg HJ *et al.* Allogeneic marrow transplantation for aplastic anaemia associated with dyskeratosis congenita. *Br J Haematol* 1996; **92**: 758–65.

166. Conter V, Johnson FL, Paoluccy P. Bone marrow transplantation for aplastic anemia associated with dyskeratosis congenita. *Am J Pediatr Hematol Oncol* 1988; **10**: 99–102.

167. Mahmoud HK, Schaefer UW, Schmidt CG, Becher R, Gotz GF, Richter HJ. Marrow transplantation for pancytopenia in dyskeratosis congenita. *Blut* 1985; **51**: 57–60.

168. Berthou C, Devergie A, D'Agay MFC *et al.* Late vascular complications after bone marrow transplantation for dyskeratosis congenita. *Br J Haematol* 1991; **79**: 335–6.

169. Yabe M, Yabe H, Hattori K *et al.* Fatal interstitial pulmonary disease in a patient with dyskeratosis congenita after allogeneic bone marrow transplantation. *Bone Marrow Transplant* 1997; **19**: 389–92.

170. Gungor T, Corbacioglu S, Storb R, Seger RA. Nonmyeloablative allogeneic hematopoietic stem cell transplantation for treatment of dyskeratosis congenita. *Bone Marrow Transplant* 2003; **31**: 407–10.

171. Treister N, Lehmann LE, Cherrick I, Guinan EC, Woo SB. Dyskeratosis congenita vs. chronic graft versus host disease: report of a case and a review of the literature. *Oral Surg Oral Med Oral Pathol Oral Radiol Endod* 2004; **98**: 566–71.

172. Ghavamzadeh A, Alimoghadam K, Nasseri P, Jahani M, Khodabandeh A, Ghahremani G. Correction of bone marrow failure in dyskeratosis congenita by bone marrow transplantation. *Bone Marrow Transplant* 1999; **23**: 299–301.

173. Lau YL, Ha SY, Chan CF, Lee AC, Liang RH, Yuen HL. Bone marrow transplant for dyskeratosis congenita. *Br J Haematol* 1999; **105**: 571.

174. Shaw PH, Haut PR, Olszewski M, Kletzel M. Hematopoietic stem-cell transplantation using unrelated cord-blood versus matched sibling marrow in pediatric bone marrow failure syndrome: one center's experience. *Pediatr Transplant* 1999; **3**: 315–21.

175. Paul SR, Perez-Atayde A, Williams DA. Interstitial pulmonary disease associated with dyskeratosis congenita. *Am J Pediatr Hematol Oncol* 1992; **14**: 89–92.

176. Ballmaier M, Germeshausen M, Schulze H *et al.* c-mpl mutations are the cause of congenital amegakaryocytic thrombocytopenia. *Blood* 2001; **97**: 139–46.

177. King S, Germeshausen M, Strauss G, Welte K, Ballmaier M. Congenital amegakaryocytic thrombocytopenia (CAMT): A detailed clinical analysis of 21 cases reveals different types of CAMT. *Blood* 2004; **104**: 740A.

178. van den Oudenrijn S, Bruin M, Folman CC *et al.* Mutations in the thrombopoietin receptor, Mpl, in children with congenital amegakaryocytic thrombocytopenia. *Br J Haematol* 2000; **110**: 441–8.

179. van den Oudenrijn S, Bruin M, Folman CC, Bussel J, de Haas M, dem Borne AE. Three parameters, plasma thrombopoietin levels, plasma glycocalicin levels and megakaryocyte culture, distinguish between different causes of congenital thrombocytopenia. *Br J Haematol* 2002; **117**: 390–8.

180. Muraoka K, Ishii E, Tsuji K *et al.* Defective response to thrombopoietin and impaired expression of c-mpl mRNA of bone marrow cells in congenital amegakaryocytic thrombocytopenia. *Br J Haematol* 1997; **96**: 287–92.

181. Ballmaier M, Germeshausen M, Krukemeier S, Welte K. Thrombopoietin is essential for the maintenance of normal hematopoiesis in humans: development of aplastic anemia in patients with congenital amegakaryocytic thrombocytopenia. *Ann N Y Acad Sci* 2003; **996**: 17–25.

182. Freedman MH, Estrov Z. Congenital amegakaryocytic thrombocytopenia: an intrinsic hematopoietic stem cell defect. *Am J Pediatr Hematol Oncol* 1990; **12**: 225–30.

183. Guinan EC, Lee YS, Lopez KD *et al.* Effects of interleukin-3 and granulocyte-macrophage colony-stimulating factor on thrombopoiesis in congenital amegakaryocytic thrombocytopenia. *Blood* 1993; **81**: 1691–8.

184. Henter JI, Winiarski J, Ljungman P, Ringden O, Ost A. Bone marrow transplantation in two children with congenital amegakaryocytic thrombocytopenia. *Bone Marrow Transplant* 1995; **15**: 799–801.

185. MacMillan ML, Davies SM, Wagner JE, Ramsay NK. Engraftment of unrelated donor stem cells in children with familial amegakaryocytic thrombocytopenia. *Bone Marrow Transplant* 1998; **21**: 735–7.

186. Lackner A, Basu O, Bierings M *et al.* Haematopoietic stem cell transplantation for amegakaryocytic thrombocytopenia. *Br J Haematol* 2000; **109**: 773–5.

187. Yesilipek A, Hazar V, Kupesiz A, Yegin O. Peripheral stem cell transplantation in a child with amegakaryocytic thrombocytopenia. *Bone Marrow Transplant* 2000; **26**: 571–2.

188. Kudo K, Kato K, Matsuyama T, Kojima S. Successful engraftment of unrelated donor stem cells in two children with congenital amegakaryocytic thrombocytopenia. *J Pediatr Hematol Oncol* 2002; **24**: 79–80.

189. Steele M, Hitzler JK, Doyle JJ, Yuille K, Dror Y. Germeshausch

M, Fernandez CV. Reduced-intensity hematopoietic stem-cell transplantation across human leukocyte antigen barriers in a patient with congenital amegakaryocytic thrombocytopenia and monosomy 7. *Pediatric Blood and Cancer* 2005; **45**(2): 212–16.

190. Gitlin D, Vawter G, Criag JM. Thymic alymphoplasia and congenital aleukocytosis. *Pediatrics* 1964; **33**: 184–92.

191. Roper M, Parmley RT, Crist WM, Kelly DR, Cooper MD. Severe congenital leukopenia (reticular dysgenesis). Immunologic and morphologic characterizations of leukocytes. *Am J Dis Child* 1985; **139**: 832–5.

192. Rotig A, Cormier V, Blanche S *et al*. Pearson's marrow-pancreas syndrome. A multisystem mitochondrial disorder in infancy. *J Clin Invest* 1990; **86**: 1601–8.

193. Pearson HA, Lobel JS, Kocoshis SA *et al*. A new syndrome of refractory sideroblastic anemia with vacuolization of marrow precursors and exocrine pancreatic dysfunction. *J Pediatr* 1979; **95**: 976–84.

194. Muraki K, Nishimura S, Goto Y, Nonaka I, Sakura N, Ueda K. The association between haematological manifestation and mtDNA deletions in Pearson syndrome. *J Inherit Metab Dis* 1997; **20**: 697–703.

195. Emami A, Vats TS, Schmike RN, Trueworthy RC. Bone marrow failure followed by acute myelocytic leukemia in a patient with Dubowitz syndrome. *Int J Pediatr Hematol Oncol* 1997; **4**: 187–91.

196. Walters TR, Desposito F. Aplastic anemia in Dubowitz syndrome. *J Pediatr* 1985; **106**: 622–3.

197. Upjohn C. Familial dwarfism associated with microcephaly, mental retardation and anaemia. *Proc R Soc Med* 1955; **48**: 334–5.

198. Butler MG, Hall BD, Maclean RN, Lozzio CB. Do some patients with Seckel syndrome have hematological problems and/or chromosome breakage? *Am J Med Genet* 1987; **27**: 645–9.

199. Boerkoel CF, O'Neill S, Andre JL *et al*. Manifestations and treatment of Schimke immuno-osseous dysplasia: 14 new cases and a review of the literature. *Eur J Pediatr* 2000; **159**: 1–7.

200. Diamond LK, Blackfan KD. Hypoplastic anemia. *Am J Dis Child* 1938; **56**: 464–7.

201. Halperin DS, Freedman MH. Diamond–Blackfan anemia: etiology, pathophysiology, and treatment. *Am J Pediatr Hematol Oncol* 1989; **11**: 380–94.

202. Ball SE, McGuckin CP, Jenkins G, Gordon-Smith EC. Diamond–Blackfan anaemia in the U.K.: analysis of 80 cases from a 20-year birth cohort. *Br J Haematol* 1996; **94**: 645–53.

203. Willig TN, Niemeyer CM, Leblanc T *et al*. Identification of new prognosis factors from the clinical and epidemiologic analysis of a registry of 229 Diamond–Blackfan anemia patients. DBA group of Société d'Hématologie et d'Immunologie Pédiatrique (SHIP), Gesellschaft für Padiatrische Onkologie und Hamatologie (GPOH), and the European Society for Pediatric Hematology and Immunology (ESPHI). *Pediatr Res* 1999; **46**: 553–61.

204. Willig TN, Draptchinskaia N, Dianzani I *et al*. Mutations in ribosomal protein S19 gene and diamond blackfan anemia: wide variations in phenotypic expression. *Blood* 1999; **94**: 4294–306.

205. Link MP, Alter BP. Fetal-like erythropoiesis during recovery from transient erythroblastopenia of childhood (TEC). *Pediatr Res* 1981; **15**: 1036–9.

206. Schofield KP, Evans DI. Diamond–Blackfan syndrome and neutropenia. *J Clin Pathol* 1991; **44**: 742–4.

207. Buchanan GR, Alter BP, Holtkamp CA, Walsh EG. Platelet number and function in Diamond–Blackfan anemia. *Pediatrics* 1981; **68**: 238–41.

208. Giri N, Kang E, Tisdale JF *et al*. Clinical and laboratory evidence for a trilineage haematopoietic defect in patients with refractory Diamond–Blackfan anaemia. *Br J Haematol* 2000; **108**: 167–75.

209. Vlachos A, Klein GW, Lipton JM. The Diamond Blackfan Anemia Registry: Tool for investigating the epidemiology and biology of Diamond–Blackfan anemia. *J Pediatr Hematol Oncol* 2001; **23**: 377–82.

210. Gahr M, Schroter W. The pattern of reactivated fetal erythropoiesis in bone marrow disorders of childhood. *Acta Paediatr Scand* 1982; **71**: 1013–18.

211. Wang WC, Mentzer WC. Differentiation of transient erythroblastopenia of childhood from congenital hypoplastic anemia. *J Pediatr* 1976; **88**: 784–9.

212. Glader BE, Backer K. Elevated red cell adenosine deaminase activity: a marker of disordered erythropoiesis in Diamond–Blackfan anaemia and other haematologic diseases. *Br J Haematol* 1988; **68**: 165–8.

213. Zielke HR, Ozand PT, Luddy RE, Zinkham WH, Schwartz AD, Sevdalian DA. Elevation of pyrimidine enzyme activities in the RBC of patients with congenital hypoplastic anaemia and their parents. *Br J Haematol* 1979; **42**: 381–90.

214. Lipton JM, Federman N, Khabbaze Y *et al*. Osteogenic sarcoma associated with Diamond–Blackfan anemia: a report from the Diamond–Blackfan Anemia Registry. *J Pediatr Hematol Oncol* 2001; **23**: 39–44.

215. Gustavsson P, Skeppner G, Johansson B *et al*. Diamond–Blackfan anaemia in a girl with a de novo balanced reciprocal X;19 translocation. *J Med Genet* 1997; **34**: 779–82.

216. Gustavsson P, Garelli E, Draptchinskaia N *et al*. Identification of microdeletions spanning the Diamond–Blackfan anemia locus on 19q13 and evidence for genetic heterogeneity. *Am J Hum Genet* 1998; **63**: 1388–95.

217. Draptchinskaia N, Gustavsson P, Andersson B *et al*. The gene encoding ribosomal protein S19 is mutated in Diamond–Blackfan anaemia. *Nat Genet* 1999; **21**: 169–75.

218. Gazda H, Lipton JM, Willig TN *et al*. Evidence for linkage of familial Diamond–Blackfan anemia to chromosome 8p23.3–p22 and for non-19q non-8p disease. *Blood* 2001; **97**: 2145–50.

219. Freedman M. Inherited forms of bone marrow failure. In: *Hofmann's Hematology: Basic Principles & Practice*, 4th edn. Hoffman R 2005 (Churchhill Livingstone).

220. Santucci MA, Bagnara GP, Strippoli P *et al*. Long-term bone marrow cultures in Diamond–Blackfan anemia reveal a defect of both granulomacrophage and erythroid progenitors. *Exp Hematol* 1999; **27**: 9–18.

221. Tsai PH, Arkin S, Lipton JM. An intrinsic progenitor defect in Diamond–Blackfan anaemia. *Br J Haematol* 1989; **73**: 112–20.

222. Chan HS, Saunders EF, Freedman MH. Diamond–Blackfan syndrome. I. Erythropoiesis in prednisone responsive and resistant disease. *Pediatr Res* 1982; **16**: 474–6.

223. Bagnara GP, Zauli G, Vitale L *et al*. In vitro growth and regulation of bone marrow enriched CD34+ hematopoietic progenitors in Diamond–Blackfan anemia. *Blood* 1991; **78**: 2203–10.

224. Olivieri NF, Grunberger T, Ben David Y *et al*.

Diamond–Blackfan anemia: heterogenous response of hematopoietic progenitor cells in vitro to the protein product of the steel locus. *Blood* 1991; **78**: 2211–15.

225. Da Costa L, Tchernia G, Gascard P *et al*. Nucleolar localization of RPS19 protein in normal cells and mislocalization due to mutations in the nucleolar localization signals in 2 Diamond–Blackfan anemia patients: potential insights into pathophysiology. *Blood* 2003; **101**: 5039–45.

226. Da Costa L, Narla G, Willig TN *et al*. Ribosomal protein S19 expression during erythroid differentiation. *Blood* 2003; **101**: 318–24.

227. Hamaguchi I, Ooka A, Brun A, Richter J, Dahl N, Karlsson S. Gene transfer improves erythroid development in ribosomal protein S19-deficient Diamond–Blackfan anemia. *Blood* 2002; **100**: 2724–31.

228. Miyake K, Flygare J, Kiefer T *et al*. Development of cellular models for ribosomal protein S19 (RPS19)-deficient diamond–blackfan anemia using inducible expression of siRNA against RPS19. *Mol Ther* 2005; **11**: 627–37.

229. Perdahl EB, Naprstek BL, Wallace WC, Lipton JM. Erythroid failure in Diamond–Blackfan anemia is characterized by apoptosis. *Blood* 1994; **83**: 645–50.

230. Flygare J, Kiefer T, Miyake K *et al*. Deficiency of ribosomal protein S19 in CD34+ cells generated by siRNA blocks erythroid development and mimics defects seen in Diamond–Blackfan anemia. *Blood* 2005; **105**: 4627–34.

231. Risdon RA, Barry M, Flynn DM. Transfusional iron overload: the relationship between tissue iron concentration and hepatic fibrosis in thalassaemia. *J Pathol* 1975; **116**: 83–95.

232. Sheth S. SQUID biosusceptometry in the measurement of hepatic iron. *Pediatr Radiol* 2003; **33**: 373–7.

233. Alustiza JM, Artetxe J, Castiella A *et al*. MR quantification of hepatic iron concentration. Gipuzkoa Hepatic Iron Concentration by MRI Study Group. *Radiology* 2004; **230**: 479–84.

234. Allen DM, Diamond LK. Congenital (erythroid) hypoplastic anemia: cortisone treated. *Am J Dis Child* 1961; **102**: 416–23.

235. Ozsoylu S. High-dose intravenous corticosteroid treatment for patients with Diamond–Blackfan syndrome resistant or refractory to conventional treatment. *Am J Pediatr Hematol Oncol* 1988; **10**: 217–23.

236. Buchanan GR. Oral megadose methylprednisolone therapy for refractory Diamond–Blackfan anemia. International Diamond–Blackfan Anemia Study Group. *J Pediatr Hematol Oncol* 2001; **23**: 353–6.

237. Bobey NA, Carcao M, Dror Y, Freedman MH, Dahl N, Woodman RC. Sustained cyclosporine-induced erythropoietic response in identical male twins with diamond–blackfan anemia. *J Pediatr Hematol Oncol* 2003; **25**: 914–18.

238. Alessandri AJ, Rogers PC, Wadsworth LD, Davis JH. Diamond–Blackfan anemia and cyclosporine therapy revisited. *J Pediatr Hematol Oncol* 2000; **22**: 176–9.

239. Ball SE, Tchernia G, Wranne L *et al*. Is there a role for interleukin-3 in Diamond–Blackfan anaemia? Results of a European multicentre study. *Br J Haematol* 1995; **91**: 313–18.

240. Niemeyer CM, Baumgarten E, Holldack J *et al*. Treatment trial with recombinant human erythropoietin in children with congenital hypoplastic anemia. *Contrib Nephrol* 1991; **88**: 276–80.

241. Fiorillo A, Poggi V, Migliorati R, Parasole R, Selleri C, Rotoli B. Unresponsiveness to erythropoietin therapy in a case of Blackfan Diamond anemia. *Am J Hematol* 1991; **37**: 65.

242. Vlachos A, Federman N, Reyes-Haley C, Abramson J, Lipton JM. Hematopoietic stem cell transplantation for Diamond Blackfan anemia: a report from the Diamond Blackfan Anemia Registry. *Bone Marrow Transplant* 2001; **27**: 381–6.

243. Bonno M, Azuma E, Nakano T *et al*. Successful hematopoietic reconstitution by transplantation of umbilical cord blood cells in a transfusion-dependent child with Diamond–Blackfan anemia. *Bone Marrow Transplant* 1997; **19**: 83–5.

244. Gluckman E, Rocha V, Boyer-Chammard A *et al*. Outcome of cord-blood transplantation from related and unrelated donors. Eurocord Transplant Group and the European Blood and Marrow Transplantation Group. *N Engl J Med* 1997; **337**: 373–81.

245. Gomez-Almaguer D, Ruiz-Arguelles GJ, Tarin-Arzaga LC *et al*. Reduced-intensity stem cell transplantation in children and adolescents: the Mexican experience. *Biol Blood Marrow Transplant* 2003; **9**: 157–61.

246. Ostronoff M, Florencio R, Campos G *et al*. Successful nonmyeloablative bone marrow transplantation in a corticosteroid-resistant infant with Diamond–Blackfan anemia. *Bone Marrow Transplant* 2004; **34**: 371–2.

247. Janov AJ, Leong T, Nathan DG, Guinan EC. Diamond–Blackfan anemia. Natural history and sequelae of treatment. *Medicine (Baltimore)* 1996; **75**: 77–8.

248. Alter BP, Kumar M, Lockhart LL, Sprinz PG, Rowe TF. Pregnancy in bone marrow failure syndromes: Diamond–Blackfan anaemia and Shwachman–Diamond syndrome. *Br J Haematol* 1999; **107**: 49–54.

249. Cotter PD, Baumann M, Bishop DF. Enzymatic defect in "X-linked" sideroblastic anemia: molecular evidence for erythroid delta-aminolevulinate synthase deficiency. *Proc Natl Acad Sci USA* 1992; **89**: 4028–32.

250. Allikmets R, Raskind WH, Hutchinson A, Schueck ND, Dean M, Koeller DM. Mutation of a putative mitochondrial iron transporter gene (ABC7) in X-linked sideroblastic anemia and ataxia (XLSA/A). *Hum Mol Genet* 1999; **8**: 743–9.

251. Fleming JC, Tartaglini E, Steinkamp MP, Schorderet DF, Cohen N, Neufeld EJ. The gene mutated in thiamine-responsive anaemia with diabetes and deafness (TRMA) encodes a functional thiamine transporter. *Nat Genet* 1999; **22**: 305–8.

252. Urban C, Binder B, Hauer C, Lanzer G. Congenital sideroblastic anemia successfully treated by allogeneic bone marrow transplantation. *Bone Marrow Transplant* 1992; **10**: 373–5.

253. Dgany O, Avidan N, Delaunay J *et al*. Congenital dyserythropoietic anemia type I is caused by mutations in codanin-1. *Am J Hum Genet* 2002; **71**: 1467–74.

254. Kostmann R. Infantile genetic agranulocytosis: A new recessive lethal disease in man. *Acta Paediatr Scand* 1956; **45** (suppl. 105): 1–368.

255. Dale DC, Cottle TE, Fier CJ *et al*. Severe chronic neutropenia: treatment and follow-up of patients in the Severe Chronic Neutropenia International Registry. *Am J Hematol* 2003; **72**: 82–93.

256. Dale DC, Person RE, Bolyard AA *et al*. Mutations in the gene encoding neutrophil elastase in congenital and cyclic neutropenia. *Blood* 2000; **96**: 2317–22.

257. Ancliff PJ, Gale RE, Liesner R, Hann IM, Linch DC. Mutations

in the ELA2 gene encoding neutrophil elastase are present in most patients with sporadic severe congenital neutropenia but only in some patients with the familial form of the disease. *Blood* 2001; **98**: 2645–50.

258. Germeshausen M, Schulze H, Ballmaier M, Zeidler C, Welte K. Mutations in the gene encoding neutrophil elastase (ELA2) are not sufficient to cause the phenotype of congenital neutropenia. *Br J Haematol* 2001; **115**: 222–4.

259. Belaaouaj A, McCarthy R, Baumann M *et al.* Mice lacking neutrophil elastase reveal impaired host defense against gram negative bacterial sepsis. *Nat Med* 1998; **4**: 615–18.

260. Ancliff PJ, Gale RE, Watts MJ *et al.* Paternal mosaicism proves the pathogenic nature of mutations in neutrophil elastase in severe congenital neutropenia. *Blood* 2002; **100**: 707–9.

261. Ancliff PJ. Congenital neutropenia. *Blood Rev* 2003; **17**: 209–16.

262. Horwitz M, Benson KF, Duan Z *et al.* Role of neutrophil elastase in bone marrow failure syndromes: molecular genetic revival of the chalone hypothesis. *Curr Opin Hematol* 2003; **10**: 49–54.

263. Fouret P, du Bois RM, Bernaudin JF, Takahashi H, Ferrans VJ, Crystal RG. Expression of the neutrophil elastase gene during human bone marrow cell differentiation. *J Exp Med* 1989; **169**: 833–45.

264. Cowland JB, Borregaard N. The individual regulation of granule protein mRNA levels during neutrophil maturation explains the heterogeneity of neutrophil granules. *J Leukoc Biol* 1999; **66**: 989–95.

265. Person RE, Li FQ, Duan Z *et al.* Mutations in proto-oncogene GFI1 cause human neutropenia and target ELA2. *Nat Genet* 2003; **34**: 308–12.

266. Devriendt K, Kim AS, Mathijs G *et al.* Constitutively activating mutation in WASP causes X-linked severe congenital neutropenia. *Nat Genet* 2001; **27**: 313–17.

267. Massullo P, Druhan LJ, Avalos BR. Aberrant processing and subcellular localization of the G185R neutrophil elastase mutant induces apoptosis of differentiating by not proliferating myeloid progenitor cells in severe congenital neutropenia. *Blood* 2003; **102**(11) Abstract 18.

268. Benson KF, Li FQ, Person RE, Albani D, Duan Z, Wechsler J. The genetic and cellular basis of hereditary neutropenia: Elastase or adaptin mutations disrupt their association and interfere with elastase's membrane and granule trafficking. *Nat Genet* 2003; **35**: 90–6.

269. Aprikyan AA, Kutyavin T, Stein S *et al.* Cellular and molecular abnormalities in severe congenital neutropenia predisposing to leukemia. *Exp Hematol* 2003; **31**: 372–81.

270. Amato D, Freedman MH, Saunders EF. Granulopoiesis in severe congenital neutropenia. *Blood* 1976; **47**: 531–8.

271. Komiyama A, Yamazaki M, Yoda S, Saitoh H, Morosawa H, Akabane T. Morphologic and functional heterogeneity of chronic neutropenia of childhood with normal neutrophil colony formation in vitro. *Am J Hematol* 1981; **11**: 175–82.

272. Karsunky H, Zeng H, Schmidt T *et al.* Inflammatory reactions and severe neutropenia in mice lacking the transcriptional repressor Gfi1. *Nat Genet* 2002; **30**: 295–300.

273. Dong F, Brynes RK, Tidow N, Welte K, Lowenberg B, Touw IP. Mutations in the gene for the granulocyte colony-stimulating-factor receptor in patients with acute myeloid leukemia preceded by severe congenital neutropenia. *N Engl J Med* 1995; **333**: 487–93.

274. Freedman MH. Safety of long-term administration of granulocyte colony-stimulating factor for severe chronic neutropenia. *Curr Opin Hematol* 1997; **4**: 217–24.

275. Weinblatt ME, Scimeca P, James-Herry A, Sahdev I, Kochen J. Transformation of congenital neutropenia into monosomy 7 and acute nonlymphoblastic leukemia in a child treated with granulocyte colony-stimulating factor. *J Pediatr* 1995; **126**: 263–5.

276. Dong F, Dale DC, Bonilla MA *et al.* Mutations in the granulocyte colony-stimulating factor receptor gene in patients with severe congenital neutropenia. *Leukemia* 1997; **11**: 120–5.

277. Ward AC, van Aesch YM, Schelen AM, Touw IP. Defective internalization and sustained activation of truncated granulocyte colony-stimulating factor receptor found in severe congenital neutropenia/acute myeloid leukemia. *Blood* 1999; **93**: 447–58.

278. Hermans MH, Antonissen C, Ward AC, Mayen AE, Ploemacher RE, Touw IP. Sustained receptor activation and hyperproliferation in response to granulocyte colony-stimulating factor (G-CSF) in mice with a severe congenital neutropenia/acute myeloid leukemia-derived mutation in the G-CSF receptor gene. *J Exp Med* 1999; **189**: 683–92.

279. Hunter MG, Avalos BR. Granulocyte colony-stimulating factor receptor mutations in severe congenital neutropenia transforming to acute myelogenous leukemia confer resistance to apoptosis and enhance cell survival. *Blood* 2000; **95**: 2132–7.

280. Jeha S, Chan KW, Aprikyan AG *et al.* Spontaneous remission of granulocyte colony-stimulating factor-associated leukemia in a child with severe congenital neutropenia. *Blood* 2000; **96**: 3647–9.

281. de Vries A, Peketh L, Joshua H. Leukaemia and agranulocytosis in a member of a family with hereditary leukopenia. *Acta Med Orient* 1958; **17**(1–2): 26–32.

282. Gilman PA, Jackson DP, Guild HG. Congenital agranulocytosis: prolonged survival and terminal acute leukemia. *Blood* 1970; **36**: 576–85.

283. Wong WY, Williams D, Slovak ML *et al.* Terminal acute myelogenous leukemia in a patient with congenital agranulocytosis. *Am J Hematol* 1993; **43**: 133–8.

284. Rosen RB, Kang SJ. Congenital agranulocytosis terminating in acute myelomonocytic leukemia. *J Pediatr* 1979; **94**: 406–8.

285. Miller RW. Childhood cancer and congenital defects. A study of U.S. death certificates during the period 1960–1966. *Pediatr Res* 1969; **3**: 389–97.

286. Bonilla MA, Gillio AP, Ruggeiro M *et al.* Effects of recombinant human granulocyte colony-stimulating factor on neutropenia in patients with congenital agranulocytosis. *N Engl J Med* 1989; **320**: 1574–80.

287. Dale DC, Bonilla MA, Davis MW *et al.* A randomized controlled phase III trial of recombinant human granulocyte colony-stimulating factor (filgrastim) for treatment of severe chronic neutropenia. *Blood* 1993; **81**: 2496–502.

288. Decoster G, Rich W, Brown SL. Safety profile of filgrastim (r-metHuG-CSF). In: Morstyn G, Dexter TM (eds) *Filgrastim (r-metHuG-CSF) in Clinical Practice*. New York: Marcel Dekker, 1994, p. 267.

289. Fewtrell MS, Kinsey SE, Williams DM, Bishop NJ. Bone mineralization and turnover in children with congenital neutropenia, and its relationship to treatment with recombinant human granulocyte-colony stimulating factor. *Br J Haematol* 1997; **97**: 734–6.

290. Yakisan E, Schirg E, Zeidler C et al. High incidence of significant bone loss in patients with severe congenital neutropenia (Kostmann's syndrome). J Pediatr 1997; **131**: 592–7.

291. Dror Y, Ward AC, Touw IP, Freedman MH. Combined corticosteroid/granulocyte colony-stimulating factor (G-CSF) therapy in the treatment of severe congenital neutropenia unresponsive to G-CSF: Activated glucocorticoid receptors synergize with G-CSF signals. Exp Hematol 2000; **28**: 1381–9.

292. Zeidler C, Welte K, Barak Y et al. Stem cell transplantation in patients with severe congenital neutropenia without evidence of leukemic transformation. Blood 2000; **95**: 1195–8.

293. Page AR, Good RA. Studies on cyclic neutropenia. Am J Dis Child 1957; **94**: 623.

294. Dale DC, Bolyard AA, Aprikyan A. Cyclic neutropenia. Semin Hematol 2002; **39**: 89–94.

295. Jonsson OG, Buchanan GR. Chronic neutropenia during childhood. A 13-year experience in a single institution. Am J Dis Child 1991; **145**: 232–5.

296. Horowitz M, Benson K, Person RE, Aprikyan AG, Dale DC. Mutations in ELA2, encoding neutrophil elastase, define a 21-day biological clock in cyclic haematopoiesis. Nat Genet 1999; **23**: 433–6.

297. Zuelzer WW. "Myelokathexis": a new form of chronic granulocytopenia. Report of a case. N Engl J Med 1964; **270**: 699–704.

298. Aprikyan AA, Liles WC, Park JR, Jonas M, Chi EY, Dale DC. Myelokathexis, a congenital disorder of severe neutropenia characterized by accelerated apoptosis and defective expression of bcl-x in neutrophil precursors. Blood 2000; **95**: 320–7.

299. Wetzler M, Talpaz M, Kellagher MJ, Gutterman JU, Kurzrock R. Myelokathexis: normalization of neutrophil counts and morphology by GM-CSF. JAMA 1992; **267**: 2179–80.

300. Gorlin RJ, Gelb B, Diaz GA, Lofsness KG, Pittelkow MR, Fenyk JR Jr. WHIM syndrome, an autosomal dominant disorder: clinical, hematological, and molecular studies. Am J Med Genet 2000; **91**: 368–76.

301. Hernandez PA, Gorlin RJ, Lukens JN et al. Mutations in the chemokine receptor gene CXCR4 are associated with WHIM syndrome, a combined immunodeficiency disease. Nat Genet 2003; **34**: 70–4.

302. Gulino AV, Moratto D, Sozzani S et al. Altered leukocyte response to CXCL12 in patients with warts, hypogamma-globulinemia, infections, myelokathexis (WHIM) syndrome. Blood 2004; **104**: 444–52.

303. Calderwood S, Kilpatrick L, Douglas SD et al. Recombinant human granulocyte colony-stimulating factor therapy for patients with neutropenia and/or neutrophil dysfunction secondary to glycogen storage disease type 1b. Blood 2001; **97**: 376–82.

304. Annabi B, Hiraiwa H, Mansfield BC et al. The gene for glycogen-storage disease type 1b maps to chromosome 11q23. Am J Hum Genet 1998; **62**: 400–5.

305. Bione S, D'Adamo P, Maestrini E, Gedeon AK, Bolhuis PA, Toniolo D. A novel X-linked gene, G4.5, is responsible for Barth syndrome. Nat Genet 1996; **12**: 385–9.

306. Kuijpers TW, Maianski NA, Tool AT et al. Neutrophils in Barth syndrome (BTHS) avidly bind annexin-V in the absence of apoptosis. Blood 2004; **103**: 3915–23.

307. Greenwald HM, Sherman I. Congenital essential thrombocytopenia. Am J Dis Child 1929; **38**: 1245–51.

308. Hall JG, Levin J, Kuhn JP, Ottenheimer EJ, van Berkum KA, McKusick VA. Thrombocytopenia with absent radius (TAR). Medicine (Baltimore) 1969; **48**: 411–39.

309. Hedberg VA, Lipton JM. Thrombocytopenia with absent radii. A review of 100 cases. Am J Pediatr Hematol Oncol 1988; **10**: 51–64.

310. Greenhalgh KL, Howell RT, Bottani A et al. Thrombocytopenia-absent radius syndrome: a clinical genetic study. J Med Genet 2002; **39**: 876–81.

311. Bessman JD, Harrison RL, Howard LC, Peterson D. The megakaryocyte abnormality in thrombocytopenia-absent radius syndrome. Blood 1983; **62** (suppl. 1): 143A.

312. Giuffre L, Cammarata M, Corsello G, Vitaliti SM. Two new cases of thrombocytopenia absent radius (TAR) syndrome: clinical, genetic and nosologic features. Klin Padiatr 1988; **200**: 10–14.

313. Day HJ, Holmsen H. Platelet adenine nucleotide "storage pool deficiency" in thrombocytopenic absent radii syndrome. JAMA 1972; **221**: 1053–4.

314. Hays RM, Bartoshesky LE, Feingold M. New features of thrombocytopenia and absent radius syndrome. Birth Defects Orig Artic Ser 1982; **18**(3B): 115–21.

215. Rao VS, Shenoi UD, Krishnamurthy PN. Acute myeloid leukemia in TAR syndrome. Indian J Pediatr 1997; **64**: 563–5.

316. Fadoo Z, Naqvi SM. Acute myeloid leukemia in a patient with thrombocytopenia with absent radii syndrome. J Pediatr Hematol Oncol 2002; **24**: 134–5.

317. Camitta BM, Rock A. Acute lymphoidic leukemia in a patient with thrombocytopenia/absent radii (Tar) syndrome. Am J Pediatr Hematol Oncol 1993; **15**: 335–7.

318. Homans AC, Cohen JL, Mazur EM. Defective megakaryocytopoiesis in the syndrome of thrombocytopenia with absent radii. Br J Haematol 1988; **70**: 205–10.

319. de Alarcon PA, Graeve JA, Levine RF, McDonald TP, Beal DW. Thrombocytopenia and absent radii syndrome: defective megakaryocytopoiesis–thrombocytopoiesis. Am J Pediatr Hematol Oncol 1991; **13**: 77–83.

320. Letestu R, Vitrat N, Masse A et al. Existence of a differentiation blockage at the stage of a megakaryocyte precursor in the thrombocytopenia and absent radii (TAR) syndrome. Blood 2000; **95**: 1633–41.

321. Kanz L, Kostielniak E, Welte K. Colony-stimulating activity (CSA) unique for the megakaryocytic hemopoietic cell lineage, present in the plasma of a patient with the syndrome of thrombocytopenia with absent radii (TAR). Blood 1989; **74** (suppl. 1): 247a.

322. al Jefri AH, Dror Y, Bussel JB, Freedman MH. Thrombocytopenia with absent radii: frequency of marrow megakaryocyte progenitors, proliferative characteristics, and megakaryocyte growth and development factor responsiveness. Pediatr Hematol Oncol 2000; **17**: 299–306.

323. Ballmaier M, Schulze H, Strauss G et al. Thrombopoietin in patients with congenital thrombocytopenia and absent radii: elevated serum levels, normal receptor expression, but defective reactivity to thrombopoietin. Blood 1997; **90**: 612–19.

324. Weinblatt M, Petrikovsky B, Bialer M, Kochen J, Harper R. Prenatal evaluation and in utero platelet transfusion for

thrombocytopenia absent radii syndrome. *Prenat Diagn* 1994; **14**: 892–6.

325. Brochstein JA, Shank B, Kernan NA, Terwilliger JW, O'Reilly RJ. Marrow transplantation for thrombocytopenia-absent radii syndrome. *J Pediatr* 1992; **121**: 587–9.

326. Drachman JG. Inherited thrombocytopenia: when a low platelet count does not mean ITP. *Blood* 2004; **103**: 390–8.

327. Geddis AE, Kaushansky K. Inherited thrombocytopenias: toward a molecular understanding of disorders of platelet production. *Curr Opin Pediatr* 2004; **16**: 15–22.

328. Balduini CL, Cattaneo M, Fabris F *et al.* Inherited thrombocytopenias: a proposed diagnostic algorithm from the Italian Gruppo di Studio delle Piastrine. *Haematologica* 2003; **88**: 582–92.

329. Seri M, Pecci A, Di Bari F *et al.* MYH9-related disease: May–Hegglin anomaly, Sebastian syndrome, Fechtner syndrome, and Epstein syndrome are not distinct entities but represent a variable expression of a single illness. *Medicine* 2003; **82**: 203–15.

330. Peterson LC, Rao KV, Crosson JT, White JG. Fechtner syndrome: a variant of Alport's syndrome with leukocyte inclusions and macrothrombocytopenia. *Blood* 1985; **65**: 397–406.

331. Drachman JG, Jarvik GP, Mehaffey MG. Autosomal dominant thrombocytopenia: incomplete megakaryocyte differentiation and linkage to human chromosome 10. *Blood* 2000; **96**: 118–25.

332. Gandhi MJ, Cummings CL, Drachman JG. FLJ14813 missense mutation: a candidate for autosomal dominant thrombocytopenia on human chromosome 10. *Hum Hered* 2003; **55**: 66–70.

333. Nichols KE, Crispino JD, Poncz M *et al.* Familial dyserythropoietic anaemia and thrombocytopenia due to an inherited mutation in GATA1. *Nat Genet* 2000; **24**: 266–270.

334. Freson K, Devriendt K, Matthijs G *et al.* Platelet characteristics in patients with X-linked macrothrombocytopenia because of a novel GATA1 mutation. *Blood* 2001; **98**: 85–92.

335. Mehaffey MG, Newton AL, Gandhi MJ, Crossley M, Drachman JG. X-linked thrombocytopenia caused by a novel mutation of GATA-1. *Blood* 2001; **98**: 2681–8.

336. Michaud J, Wu F, Osato M *et al.* In vitro analyses of known and novel RUNX1/AML1 mutations in dominant familial platelet disorder with predisposition to acute myelogenous leukemia: implications for mechanisms of pathogenesis. *Blood* 2002; **99**: 1364–72.

337. Thompson AA, Woodruff K, Feig SA, Nguyen LT, Schanen NC. Congenital thrombocytopenia and radio-ulnar synostosis: a new familial syndrome. *Br J Haematol* 2001; **113**: 866–70.

338. Thompson AA, Nguyen LT. Amegakaryocytic thrombocytopenia and radio-ulnar synostosis are associated with HOXA11 mutation. *Nat Genet* 2000; **26**: 397–8.

339. Jin Y, Mazza C, Christie JR *et al.* Mutations of the Wiskott–Aldrich Syndrome Protein (WASP): hotspots, effect on transcription, and translation and phenotype/genotype correlation. *Blood* 2004; **104**: 4010–19.

340. Savoia A, Balduini CL, Savino M *et al.* Autosomal dominant macrothrombocytopenia in Italy is most frequently a type of heterozygous Bernard–Soulier syndrome. *Blood* 2001; **97**: 1330–5.

341. Okita JR, Frojmovic MM, Kristopeit S, Wong T, Kunicki TJ. Montreal platelet syndrome: a defect in calcium-activated neutral proteinase (calpain). *Blood* 1989; **74**: 715–21.

342. Lo TF Jr, Rooimans MA, Bosnoyan-Collins L *et al.* Expression cloning of a cDNA for the major Fanconi anaemia gene, FAA. *Nat Genet* 1996; **14**: 320–3.

343. Meetei AR, Levitus M, Xue Y *et al.* X-linked inheritance of Fanconi anemia complementation group B. *Nat Genet* 2004; **36**: 1219–24.

344. Strathdee CA, Duncan AM, Buchwald M. Evidence for at least four Fanconi anaemia genes including FACC on chromosome 9. *Nat Genet* 1992; **1**: 196–8.

345. Strathdee CA, Gavish H, Shannon WR *et al.* Cloning of cDNAs for Fanconi's anaemia by functional complementation. *Nature* 1992; **356**: 763–7.

346. Timmers C, Taniguchi T, Hejna J *et al.* Positional cloning of a novel Fanconi anemia gene, FANCD2. *Mol Cell* 2001; **7**: 241–8.

347. de Winter JP, Leveille F, van Berkel CG *et al.* Isolation of a cDNA representing the Fanconi anemia complementation group E gene. *Am J Hum Genet* 2000; **67**: 1306–8.

348. de Winter JP, Rooimans MA, van Der WL *et al.* The Fanconi anaemia gene FANCF encodes a novel protein with homology to ROM. *Nat Genet* 2000; **24**: 15–16.

349. de Winter JP, Waisfisz Q, Rooimans MA *et al.* The Fanconi anaemia group G gene FANCG is identical with XRCC9. *Nat Genet* 1998; **20**: 281–3.

350. Levitus M, Rooimans MA, Steltenpool J *et al.* Heterogeneity in Fanconi anemia: evidence for 2 new genetic subtypes. *Blood* 2004; **103**: 2498–503.

4

Acquired aplastic anemia

Juliana Teo and Yigal Dror

Introduction

Acquired bone marrow failure or acquired aplastic anemia (AA) is characterized by pancytopenia with a hypocellular bone marrow in the absence of an inherited syndrome. The International Agranulocytosis and Aplastic Anemia Study[1] has defined aplastic anemia as hemoglobin $\leq$ 100 g/dL, platelet count $\leq 50 \times 10^9$/L, granulocytes $\leq 1.5 \times 10^9$/L, and a bone marrow biopsy demonstrating a decrease in cellularity and the absence of significant fibrosis or neoplastic infiltration.

Severe aplastic anemia (SAA) is diagnosed when there is less than 25% of normal bone marrow cellularity, determined by bone marrow biopsy, and at least two of the following peripheral blood findings: granulocytes $< 0.5 \times 10^9$/L, platelets $< 20 \times 10^9$/L, or absolute reticulocytes $\leq 40 \times 10^9$/L (<1% when corrected for hematocrit).[2]

Very severe AA is defined when the above criteria for SAA are met and the granulocyte count is $< 0.2 \times 10^9$/L. Moderate AA is defined when the criteria for SAA are not met. The category of disease severity is vital in dictating the urgency and choice of therapy, and is valuable in assessing prognosis. Due to the communality in referring to severe acquired aplastic anemia as SAA in the medical literature we will use herein these terms interchangeably.

Epidemiology

The incidence of AA in childhood (<15 years) is reported as 1–3 per million children per year.[1,3–5] The age of presentation peaks at 15–25 years and older than 60 years.[1,4] A high proportion of children (>70%) have severe disease at the time of presentation.[4,6] There is a slightly higher proportion of males. Most reports from Asia cite a two- to three-fold higher incidence of AA than that in the West, possibly due to environmental or genetic differences.[7,8] The strong inverse association between incidence of disease and socioeconomic standing in Thailand[8] supports an environmental etiology.

Etiology

Acquired AA can be classified into "idiopathic" and "secondary". Secondary AA can be attributed to a definable cause including:

- drugs and toxins;
- viral infections;
- hepatitis-associated AA, notably seronegative hepatitis;
- immune disorders, e.g., thymoma;
- paroxysmal nocturnal hemoglobinuria.

Seventy to eighty percent of the AA cases are idiopathic.[4,6,9] In a large prospective study by the French Cooperative Group,[4] the suspected etiology was recorded for 243 cases of AA in children and adults: 74% were idiopathic, 13% were associated with drugs, 5% with hepatitis, 5% with toxins, and the rest were categorized as miscellaneous including two cases that were pregnancy related. Of the drug exposures, only one was associated with chloramphenicol. Reduction in the use of chloramphenicol has not been accompanied by a parallel reduction in the incidence of AA,[10,11] and there is no evidence of its association with AA in Thailand.[8,12] The causative role of chloramphenicol in AA remains controversial.

Many case reports, case series, and large epidemiologic studies implicated a multitude of drugs in the etiology of AA, although the association might be circumstantial rather than causative.[4,8,12–14] Nevertheless, some studies have convincingly implicated certain medications. Kaufman et al.[15] incorporated data from several large-scale series studying the relationship of drugs in the etiology of AA. Comparisons were made between 454 patients with AA and 6458 controls. The strongest associations between AA and drugs were for penicillamine, gold, and carbamazepine. The other associated drugs include butazones, indometacin, diclofenac, sulfonamides, and furosemide. Chloramphenicol exposures were too few to provide an estimated risk. These studies, however, lacked accurate data about the drug exposure period and dose.

The French Cooperative Group studied 147 cases of AA compared with 287 hospitalized controls and 108 neighbors.[13] The results implicated gold salts, D-penicillamine, salicylates, and colchicine as risk factors for AA. However, the association between rheumatoid arthritis and AA confounded the ability to clearly link antiinflammatory agents with AA. Similarly, the use of non-phenicol antibiotics appeared to be linked to AA, but the history of a recent infectious episode confounded the interpretation of this result. The use of chloramphenicol and thiamphenicol was too limited to allow any conclusions.

Most of the patients in the above studies were adults. The incidence of drug-related AA in children was generally low, as the commonly implicated drugs are rarely used in childhood, with the exception of anticonvulsants (e.g., valproate and carbamezepine) and some nonsteroidal antiinflammatory drugs (NSAIDs, e.g., indometacin).

Exposure to environmental toxins, such as pesticides (e.g., DDT, chlordane, lindane),[8,16,17] paints,[18] and solvents[8] has often been implicated as a cause of AA, but not in all studies.[8] Prolonged exposure to benzene and its derivatives carries a particularly high risk of hematologic toxicities. Its metabolites have been implicated as a cause of aplasia,[19] DNA damage,[20] and apoptosis of hematopoietic cells.[21] A recent report demonstrated that chronic low-level exposure to benzene, at air levels considered safe by occupational guidelines, was also toxic to hematopoietic cells, particularly in susceptible individuals.[22]

A number of viruses have been implicated in the development of AA in a small portion of the patients. However, attributing causality to some viral agents may be difficult due to their ubiquitous nature. Implicated viruses include Ebstein–Barr virus,[23] cytomegalovirus,[24] human herpesvirus 6,[25] human immunodeficiency virus,[26] parvovirus B19,[27,28] hepatitis A[29] and B,[30] measles, mumps, rubella,[31] varicella, and flaviviruses.[32]

Hepatitis-associated AA occurs several weeks to several months after the onset of acute hepatitis of variable severity.[3,5,13,14,33] Most commonly, the hepatitis is seronegative for any known hepatitis viruses.[33–35] Preceding hepatitis is seen in 2–5% of patients with AA in studies from the West,[4,35] but is much higher in the East,[7] where it was implicated in up to 24% of the cases.[36] It appears to be more common in young males.[33] The hepatitis may follow a relatively benign course; however, the aplasia is associated with high mortality if untreated[37] or refractory.

The association between AA and fulminant liver failure following acute non-A, non-B, non-C hepatitis is well recognized. It appears to be more common in younger individuals, with a mean age of 10 years.[38] Aplastic anemia was reported in 28–33% of children and 5% of adults who underwent orthotopic liver transplantation for fulminant seronegative hepatitis.[39,40] In contrast, AA was reported in less than 1% of liver transplants for other reasons.[38,40] Although the cause of hepatitis and the associated AA is not known, there is evidence to support a T-cell immune-mediated mechanism against both systems.[33,41]

Paroxysmal nocturnal hemoglobinuria (PNH) is very uncommon in childhood, particularly before adolescence. It is characterized by episodic hemolysis, thrombosis, AA, and myelodysplastic syndrome (MDS). It is an acquired clonal disorder of hematopoietic stem cells due to an X-linked somatic mutation of the *PIGA* gene.[42] This results in abnormal biosynthesis of the cell membrane-anchoring phospholipid, glycosylphosphatidylinositol, and an absence of glycosylphosphatidylinositol-linked proteins, including the complement regulatory proteins, CD55 and CD59. Approximately 25% of adult patients with PNH present with or develop AA, and about 15% of adult patients with AA develop PNH in the recovery phase after immunosuppressive therapy (IST).[43–47] The pathophysiology of AA in PNH remains poorly understood. A small percentage of patients with PNH progress to leukemia.

Immunologic disorders are occasionally associated with acquired AA, albeit rarely. AA has been reported in patients with eosinophilic fasciitis,[48] thymoma,[49] Graves disease,[50] systemic lupus erythematosus,[51] rheumatoid arthritis,[13] Sjögren syndrome,[52] and transfusion-related graft-versus-host disease (GVHD).[53]

Inherited marrow failure syndromes have been estimated to represent approximately one-third of childhood AA, and are discussed in Chapter 3. Some of these patients may present with AA without characteristic physical anomalies, and even in their fifth and sixth decades. Recently, *TERC* and *TERT* mutations have been identified in some patients with apparently acquired AA,[54,55] suggesting that some of these patients may indeed have an inherited disorder. Advances in genetic and molecular diagnostic techniques may allow the diagnosis of these cases of seemingly "acquired" aplastic anemia. Differentiating inherited AA from the acquired forms is crucial since their therapy and prognoses differ.

Pathophysiology

Three main mechanisms have been implicated in the pathophysiology of acquired AA: an "autoimmune attack" on hematopoietic progenitor cells; inherent stem cell defects; and defects of the bone marrow stroma or microenvironment.

Cell-mediated autoimmunity was proposed as a major mechanism in the pathophysiology of idiopathic AA. The strongest evidence yet comes from the observed clinical response to IST. Also, there is an overrepresentation of HLA-DR2 in patients with AA as in autoimmune diseases.[56] *In vitro* hematopoietic colony formation was inhibited by patients' lymphocytes from both the circulation and bone marrow.[57] Predominance of CD8+ phenotype[58] or CD4+ cytotoxic cells[57] have been reported. *In vitro* and *in vivo* increases in inhibitory lymphokines have been demonstrated, including interferon-γ (IFN-γ), tumor necrosis factor-α (TNF-α), and interleukin-2 (IL-2),[58,59,60-62] reflecting a T-helper cell (Th1)-type response. These suppressive factors interfere with the mitotic cycle of hematopoietic precursors,[59] upregulate Fas receptors on CD34+ hematopoietic stem cells, and cause apoptosis.[63,64] The hematopoietic progenitor cells in patients who develop aplasia may have an enhanced sensitivity to these lymphokines, such as TNF-α.[65]

Many investigators have demonstrated oligoclonal expansion of specific T cells and skewed T-cell receptor Vβ repertoire in patients with AA.[57,59,66,67] The restricted T-cell clones can be cytotoxic to both autologous and allogeneic hematopoietic progenitor cells.[57] The size of the expanded T-cell clones correlates with disease activity, but they persist at low levels even after remission is achieved with IST.[59,66] Interestingly, there is molecular homology of these clones between patients, suggesting a limited number of antigens driving the immune response.[59] The detection of autoantibodies against hematopoietic antigens such as kinectin in some patients with AA[68] also suggests an immune mechanism.

Primary hematopoietic stem cell abnormalities have been demonstrated in acquired AA, including reduced numbers of CD34+ cells,[69] reduced multipotent and committed colony-forming cells, reduced long-term culture-initiating cells,[70,71] and a decrease in cobblestone area-forming cells.[72] The cure of AA following an infusion of hematopoietic stem cells implicates this deficiency. This is further supported by crossover experiments, in which patients' marrow cells that have been depleted of adherent cells grow poorly on normal stroma.[71,73] Also, bone marrow stroma has been shown to be of host origin, rather than donor, after hematopoietic stem cell transplantation (HSCT).[74] In addition, the observations of clonal evolution and persistence of stem cell deficiency and macrocytosis in some patients after recovery following IST further supports an underlying stem cell abnormality.

Several investigators have recently reported shortened telomere lengths in peripheral blood leukocytes from patients with AA compared with normal age-matched controls.[75,76] Telomere length improved after successful treatment with IST.[75,76] Like hemoglobin F, this might reflect "stress" hematopoiesis. However, telomere shortening might also be due to telomerase dysfunction.[54,55]

Abnormalities of the marrow stroma have been reported in a small proportion of the patients with AA. Approximately 50% of the patients have abnormal stromal cell proliferation[77] and do not form a confluent stromal layer in long-term cultures, or have morphologic differences from normal stroma.[71] Those patients with no stromal cell growth had a longer duration of aplasia.[77] Abnormal stromal secretion of hematopoietic growth factors has been found in patients with AA, including higher levels of macrophage inflammatory protein-1α and leukemia-inhibitory factor, a decrease in IL-1 receptor antagonist, and decreased IL-6 production in response to IL-1, TNF-α, and cytomegalovirus.[77,78] Despite these abnormalities in stromal morphology and in secretion of certain cytokines, the function of the aplastic stroma as measured by support of hematopoiesis from normal CD34+ cells was intact.[71,73] Also, patients with AA can be cured by HSCT despite preservation of their marrow stroma. This suggests a minor role of the marrow stroma in the pathogenesis of acquired AA.

Toxins, drugs, or their metabolites may be directly injurious by binding to macromolecules, triggering a hapten-directed immune response against stem or stromal cells. Similarly, viruses can directly infect stem cells, progenitor cells, or stromal cells leading to cytokine-mediated cell death by cytotoxic lymphocytes.[79] These mechanisms can lead either to stem cell loss through direct toxicity, microenvironmental failure, or to immune suppression of marrow elements by an activated immune system.[80] Individuals might be genetically more susceptible to toxins or viruses.

Clinical presentation

Children with AA usually present with symptoms related to their cytopenias. Thrombocytopenia causing increased bruising with or without mucosal bleeding is the most common initial presentation.[5] Pallor and fatigue are also common at presentation.[5] However, severe anemia of gradual onset is usually well compensated for by young children. Serious infections due to neutropenia are uncommon presenting symptoms. Apart from these presenting signs and symptoms, generally patients have been previously well with normal physical examinations and no dysmorphic features. Lymphadenopathy and hepatosplenomegaly are atypical. Most children have symptoms for less than 1 month, and > 80% for less than 3 months.[4,5]

Family history is often unremarkable; however, one study found an overrepresentation of bone marrow hypoplasia and hematologic malignancies in first-degree relatives.[5]

Natural history

In a series of 112 children with idiopathic AA, 71% met the criteria for SAA, 21% for moderate AA, and less than 5% for mild AA.[6] Two-thirds of patients with moderate disease progress to SAA at a median of 9.5 months (range 2–290 months) after diagnosis. The remaining patients persisted with moderate disease (21%), with a median of 32 months of follow-up, or underwent spontaneous complete resolution (12%), at a median of 7 months.[6]

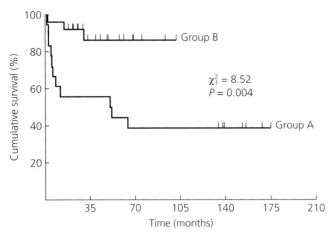

Fig. 4.1 Overall survival of all children receiving antithymocyte globulin. Three children in group A, and six in group B received a bone marrow transplant after failure of primary immunosuppressive therapy. Group A, 1973–1988 (n = 38); Group B, 1989–1996 (n = 37). Reproduced with permission from Ref. 83.

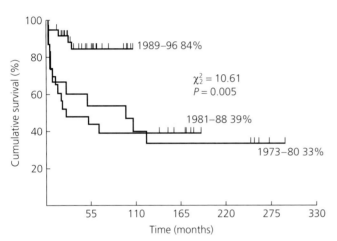

Fig. 4.2 Overall survival of children treated for aplastic anemia in three time periods. Group A, 1973–1988 (n = 38); Group B, 1989–1996 (n = 37). Reproduced with permission from Ref. 83.

Untreated SAA has a high mortality due to either infections or hemorrhagic events.[81] Supportive modalities, including transfusion and antibiotic therapy, have substantially improved survival. Accessibility to specific therapy, such as IST or HSCT, has dramatically changed the outlook for children diagnosed with AA. In this era of supportive and specific therapies, survival closely depends on the neutrophil count and duration of severe neutropenia. Causes of death include infections, bleeding and treatment-related complications. About one-third of the infections in AA are due to fungal infections.[5] A British study of acquired AA in childhood reported actuarial survival of 84% at 8 years for children treated between 1989 and 1996.[82] Figs 4.1–4.2.

Diagnosis and laboratory evaluation

Evaluation of the child with AA should include detailed family and developmental histories as well as careful physical examination to exclude other diagnoses and to screen for potential etiologies such as inherited bone marrow failure syndromes. A history of any previous hematologic derangements, drug exposure, and history that may suggest non-hematologic manifestations should be elucidated.

A complete blood count demonstrates pancytopenia and absolute reticulocytopenia. The peripheral blood smear commonly shows red blood cell macrocytosis. Levels of hemoglobin F and red cell mean corpuscular volume can be high in acquired AA, but less frequently and to a lesser degree compared with inherited bone marrow failure syndromes. The levels may remain elevated in patients who have clinically recovered.

Bone marrow examination is essential for confirmation of hypoplasia and to rule out other causes of pancytopenia. Bone marrow architecture can be determined and cellularity can be reliably graded according to severity by an adequate trephine biopsy of the bone marrow (Fig. 4.3). Prominent fibrosis is usually absent. Bone marrow aspirate usually shows empty particles and increased fat, reticulum, plasma, and mast cells, but is inadequate for accurate assessment of cellularity. Cellular morphology is usually normal. Bone marrow cytogenetics should be performed to rule out clonal disorder suggesting a hypoplastic MDS. Rarely, an acute leukemia presents initially with a period of hypoplastic anemia.[83] Clonogenic assays of marrow CD34+ cells might be helpful to distinguish between marrow underproduction versus peripheral destruction.

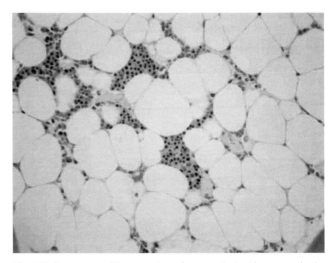

Fig. 4.3 Bone marrow biopsy specimen from a patient with severe aplastic anemia showing active hematopoiesis in less than 25% of the bone marrow space.

Careful attention to a possible underlying inherited marrow failure syndrome should be given, as a proportion of these patients will not have a dysmorphic appearance. Unfortunately, the only widely available screening test is the chromosome fragility test with mitomycin C or diepoxybutane to rule out Fanconi anemia (see Chapter 3). Rapid and cost-effective screening tests for other inherited bone marrow failure syndromes are greatly needed. A work-up for PNH is recommended, although this is a very uncommon finding in childhood AA. Deficiency of CD55 and CD59 on erythrocytes and leukocytes can be demonstrated by flow cytometry, which is currently the most sensitive test for detecting PNH clones.[84] Alternatively, a Ham acid serum test should be performed to look for evidence of PNH.

Measurement of serum vitamin B_{12} and red blood cell folate should also be undertaken to exclude dietary deficiency as a cause of pancytopenia and red blood cell macrocytosis. A limited immune work-up may implicate other etiologies and direct therapy differently. This might include quantitative immunoglobulins, direct antiglobulin test and antinuclear factor.

Viral serology, including cytomegalovirus, Epstein–Barr virus, parvovirus B19, hepatitis A, B, and C, human immunodeficiency virus, and herpes simplex virus type 6, is of value in diagnosis and for later management. Bone marrow may also be tested for viruses by culture or polymerase chain reaction (PCR) if aplasia is suspected to be due to a viral infection. A patient's cytomegalovirus (CMV) status has an impact on the choice of blood products used in supportive measures: a CMV-negative patient should ideally be offered CMV-negative blood products wherever possible.

Liver function tests, plasma electrolyte, urea, and creatinine determinations, and urinalysis are useful before specific therapy is administered. Extended red blood cell antigen phenotyping is recommended in addition to routine blood group and antibody screening. Provision of phenotypically matched red blood cells for transfusion would reduce sensitization, particularly in patients requiring long-term transfusion support. HLA-typing of the patient and the immediate family members is advisable at diagnosis, even when HSCT is not conducted as the first-line treatment, to facilitate the search for a suitable bone marrow donor in case treatment with IST is unsuccessful.

Treatment

Supportive care

Supportive modalities include chronic transfusion programs that treat and prevent major bleeding episodes and maintain hemoglobin, and antibiotics to treat infections. The provision of phenotypically matched red blood cell transfusions and single-donor platelet units would reduce alloimmunization,

particularly for the chronically transfused patients. Donation of blood products from members of the patient's family is not advisable, as HSCT using related donors might be warranted in the future. CMV-negative recipients should receive CMV-negative blood products wherever possible. We recommend filtering and irradiating all blood products.

Maintaining hemoglobin with transfusion of red blood cells allows for normal activities. Children better tolerate a greater degree of anemia than adults and can generally handle transfusion thresholds of between 60 and 70 g/L. Platelet transfusion support to treat and prevent life-threatening bleeding has probably resulted in the largest impact on the survival of patients with SAA. It has changed the leading cause of death from bleeding to infections. Reducing the transfusion threshold to 10×10^9/L in a stable patient has been found to be safe.[85] Other measures to prevent bleeding include avoidance of antiplatelet agents (e.g., NSAIDs) and avoidance of trauma.

The risk of serious bacterial and fungal infections correlates with the neutrophil count and duration of severe neutropenia. This risk is exacerbated during IST or HSCT. Prophylaxis for *Pneumocystis carinii* and fungal infections should be considered during IST. Neutropenic patients with fever should be treated aggressively with broad-spectrum antibiotics and with antifungal agents when clinically appropriate.

Hematopoietic stem cell transplantation (HSCT)

Matched sibling donor HSCT

The first successful HSCT in a patient with SAA was reported in 1970.[86] During the 1970s, HSCT was established as the best therapy for AA.[2] For children and young adults afflicted with SAA, early HSCT from an HLA-matched sibling donor is widely considered as the gold standard of care. Several trials reported overall survivals of 79–100% following matched sibling donor HSCT.[46,87–90] (Fig. 4.4) Cyclophosphamide (200 mg/kg over 4 days) is the most commonly used conditioning agent in HSCT for SAA. Various groups have used cyclophosphamide either alone or with limited-field irradiation or with low-dose total body irradiation.[91] Following the published excellent results from the Seattle group, there has been increasing enthusiasm for the use of cyclophosphamide with antithymocyte globulin (ATG) without irradiation,[88,89] showing superior survival outcomes, in the order of 80–90%,[46,89] in contrast to 55–67% when irradiation-based conditioning was used.[92] The need for conditioning therapy is borne out by the high incidence of graft failure seen with syngeneic HSCT. In a large report, 16 of 23 patients given syngeneic marrow without preparation failed to engraft.[93]

Failed engraftment in up to 32% was a significant problem in matched sibling HSCT for SAA in the 1970s.[94] Early transplantation with minimal pretransplant transfusion, the

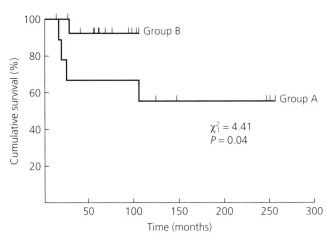

Fig. 4.4 Overall survival of all children receiving bone marrow transplantation. Group A, 1973–1988 (n = 38); Group B, 1989–1996 (n = 37). Reproduced with permission from Ref. 83.

addition of irradiation, and marrow nucleated cell dose > 3×10^8 cells/kg were all associated with a lower incidence of graft rejection.[87,91,94] Interestingly, the use of cyclosporin (cyclosporin) in the GVHD prophylactic regimens was associated with lower rates of graft failure.[91,94] Regimens incorporating cyclophosphamide and ATG in the preparation and cyclosporin with short-course methotrexate as GVHD prophylaxis reduced the engraftment failure rate to < 5%, even in heavily pretreated patients.[89]

Conditioning regimens incorporating thoraco-abdominal irradiation (TAI) are particularly associated with acute GVHD grades II–IV,[88,91] with a cumulative incidence of over 40% in a French study.[88] However, the use of cyclosporin with methotrexate, in particular when ATG was used in the conditioning regimen, reduced the incidence of acute GVHD to about 11%.[95] The incidence of chronic GVHD has not been influenced by cyclosporin, occurring in about 30% of patients.[87,89] Approximately one-fifth of patients who develop chronic GVHD die of associated complications.[87]

Long-term sequelae for growth and endocrine function have been minimal. Inclusion of irradiation in the preparatory regimen is a risk factor for reduced ultimate height.[96] The use of chemotherapeutic agents alone or with only low doses of radiation spares the thyroid gland. Secondary sexual characteristics develop at an appropriate age and the frequency of impairment to ovarian or testicular endocrine function is low. Many of these children have been able to have children.[87]

Secondary malignant tumors are of concern after successful HSCT. Although MDS and leukemia of donor origin can develop in up to 1% of the patients after HSCT for AA,[97–99] the more common problem is solid tumors, particularly epidermoid carcinomas. The reported incidences of secondary malignancies in AA are 3.5% at 10 years,[100] approximately 12% at 15 years,[88,100] and 13% at 20 years post-HSCT,[99]

respectively. Risk factors included treatment of GVHD with azathioprine and cyclosporin, the patient age, the use of irradiation, male sex, age at diagnosis, and the use of a radiation-based conditioning regimen.[88,99,100] The incidence of secondary solid tumors in patients transplanted without irradiation is generally lower than in those transplanted with irradiation: 1.4% at 10 years posttransplant according to the Seattle group.[101] Further, patients treated with TAI-based regimens who developed secondary solid malignancies did so within the radiation fields.[102]

The most common secondary solid tumors after HSCT for AA and for other indications are squamous-cell carcinomas of the head and neck, predominantly of the oropharynx, even if patients with Fanconi anemia or immunodeficiency are excluded.[88,99,101,103] Other types of secondary solid tumors in AA include brain tumors, papillary carcinoma of the thyroid, squamous-cell carcinoma of the skin, mammary carcinoma, gastric adenocarcinoma, and hepatocarcinoma. The outcome of patients with secondary tumors was poor as subsequent therapy is difficult.

Alternative donor HSCT

Matched sibling donors for HSCT are not available in the majority of cases with AA. Alternative HSCT generally requires a greater intensity of conditioning therapy to prevent graft failure and greater postinfusion immunosuppression to prevent GVHD.

The use of HLA-matched non-sibling family donors appears to give favorable outcomes,[104,105] although the reported cases are very few. The outcome of HSCT from mismatched family donors seems to depend on the degree of mismatch[104] and the preparatory regimens.[105] In the Seattle series[105] 12 of 16 patients with one-antigen mismatch donors, who were prepared with cyclophosphamide and TBI engrafted and 8 survived, compared with none among those transplanted with cyclophosphamide with or without ATG, but without TBI. Rare cases in which parental haploidentical hematopoietic stem cells have successfully been used for HSCT in SAA, have been reported.[106] The conditioning regimens included fludarabine, cyclophosphamide, and either total lymphoid irradiation (TLI) or busulfan, with high CD34[+] dose.

The outcome of HSCT from a matched unrelated donor for SAA is improving, but is inferior to that of matched sibling donors. In a multicenter North American report of 141 pretreated patients (median age 17.7 years), who received HSCT from unrelated donors for SAA, favorable outcomes were associated with age < 20 years (overall survival of 63%), HSCT within 3 years of diagnosis, and HLA-DRB1 matching (56% vs. 15% at 3 years).[107] Investigators in Japan have reported an overall survival of 69% at 5 years for those under 20 years. In addition to age, other unfavorable factors were transplantation more than 3 years after diagnosis, molecularly determined HLA-A or -B mismatch, and conditioning without ATG.[108] Encouraging results with novel conditioning regimens based on the use of Campath-1G have also been reported.[109]

The use of umbilical cord blood (UCB) as a source of stem cells for HSCT has been expanding.[110] Comparable outcomes were reported in a cohort of pediatric recipients of HSCT using unrelated donor UCB (predominantly 1–2 antigens; the rest were fully matched or 3-antigen mismatched) and unrelated donor (6/6 antigen matched) bone marrow transplanted for both hematologic malignancies and nonmalignant disorders.[110] Neutrophil recovery was significantly slower after UCB transplantation, but the probability of engraftment at day 45, the incidence of acute GVHD and 2-year survival (approximately 50%) were comparable between the groups. Chronic GVHD was less in UCB recipients although not statistically significant.

Immunosuppressive therapy

Autologous bone marrow reconstitution was noted, in the late 1960s and early 1970s, in a number of patients who received mismatched marrows.[86,111,112] This was also observed in some patients who were conditioned with cyclophosphamide and ATG but did not proceed with HSCT. These clinical observations combined with the extensive laboratory data discussed in the sections on Pathophysiology and Etiology above strongly suggested immune mechanisms in the pathogenesis of AA and led to the development of IST regimens in the treatment of AA.[113]

ATG with or without other agents or modalities, such as androgens, steroids and HSCT clearly emerged as more effective than supportive care alone.[114] Survival ranged from 30 to 70%, with responses typically occurring within the first 3–6 months following therapy. Equine ATG (e.g., Atgam; Pharmacia & Upjohn, Milton Keynes, UK) is more commonly used, and is usually administered at 100–160 mg/kg, in divided doses over 4–10 days. Rabbit ATG (e.g., Thymoglobuline; Imtix-Sangstat, Lyon, France) has also been shown to be effective, at doses of 2.5–3.5 mg/kg daily for 4–5 days.[115] Acute allergic reactions are common. Immune complex-mediated serum sickness typically manifests 10–14 days after initiation of therapy. These adverse effects have largely been ameliorated by the concurrent administration of prednisone, usually at 1–2 mg/kg/day, and premedication with antihistamines and acetaminophen (paracetamol).

Cyclosporin was shown to be effective.[116,118] The German group compared ATG and methylprednisolone versus ATG, methylprednisolone, and cyclosporin.[116] The response rate at 3 months was significantly higher in the group receiving cyclosporin (65 vs. 39%, $P < 0.03$), primarily because of an increased response rate in patients with severe disease.

The European Cooperative Group for Bone Marrow Transplantation (EBMT) compared ATG and methylprednisolone with or without oxymetholone.[119] Responses were significantly higher in the oxymethalone arm at 120 days (68% vs. 48%); however, the overall survival at 3 years did not reach statistical difference: 71% with androgens versus 65% without. Survival was influenced by the severity of the aplasia: the very severe group had a 43% 3-year survival compared with 78% for severe disease and 83% for moderate disease. This was particularly pronounced in females with severe aplasia.

Children treated with IST generally have better survival outcomes compared with adults;[118,120] but the reported survivals are variable and ranged from 54 to 100%.[22,46,121–124] This variability in outcomes may reflect the heterogeneity of treatment regimes, including administration of hematopoietic growth factors, inclusion of patients with clonal marrow cytogenetic abnormalities, and patients with inherited marrow failure syndromes. The EBMT SAA group recently reported a 5-year survival of 83% in 84 pediatric patients treated with IST.[46] Combination IST commonly used in most centers treating children with acquired AA consists of ATG, cyclosporin, and low- or intermediate-dose corticosteroids.[46,121,122] The authors use Atgam 40 mg/kg daily for 4 days, prednisone 0.5 mg/kg per dose twice daily for 14 days, and cyclosporin 6 mg/kg per dose twice daily to maintain blood levels of 150–200 µg/L.

Patients who failed to respond to the initial course of ATG treatment still have a substantial chance of response to repeated courses, using ATG from the same or an alternative animal source.[45,110] The EBMT SAA reported a 43% chance of response to a second treatment with ATG after the initial failure, and actuarial survivals at 13 years of 68.5% in those who responded after two courses versus 24.4% in those who did not receive a second course.[120] There was no significant increase in adverse effects following repeated ATG (of the same animal source)[120] and no significant difference in the risk of clonal disorders between patients receiving a single or multiple courses of ATG.[45]

A common problem in this treatment modality is recurrence of the aplasia in up to 35% of the patients at 5 years,[114] and a need for retreatment in 10–20%[111,112,114,121] within 4–37 months after withdrawal of cyclosporin. Patients treated with IST regain apparently normal hematopoiesis, but detailed studies revealed persistent defects in the number and function of hematopoietic progenitors.[70–73] IST reduces but does not eradicate the pathogenic T-cell clones, even in patients who respond.[57,66] Relapse was not associated with patient age, gender, interval between diagnosis and therapy, or absolute neutrophil count prior to treatment or 3 months posttherapy;[114] but it might be associated with rapid response to the original IST.[121] Approximately 50–70% of those who relapse respond to subsequent therapies,[111,114,121,125] with 60% still dependent on cyclosporin at 6–7 years.

There were promising results from an early pilot study of high-dose cyclophosphamide without HSCT in SAA.[147]

However, a prospective randomized study comparing ATG and cyclosporin with cyclophosphamide and cyclosporin had to be terminated prematurely due to an unacceptable incidence of invasive fungal infections and early deaths in the cyclophosphamide arm.[127] Follow-up of the survivors showed responses in 46% for the cyclophosphamide group compared with 75% in the ATG group, with no difference in relapse rate or clonal evolution.[128]

HSCT versus immunosuppressive therapy

There are no randomized trials comparing the two modalities. However, when compiling data from various studies, it appears that HSCT from an HLA-matched sibling generally gives superior long-term engraftment and survival (75–97%)[46,82,89,90,122,129] compared with IST (55–85%),[46,129,130] and is usually considered as the initial treatment of choice for children with SAA. Both the Seattle and Japanese experience demonstrated a considerable survival advantage of HSCT from an HLA-matched sibling over IST in children with AA.[44,90] Among 100 children in a Japanese study the overall survival was 97% in the HSCT group versus 55% in the IST group. In contrast, the data from the EBMT SAA group on a cohort of 227 children showed comparable overall survival at 5 years after treatment for both treatment modalities: 85% for HSCT from an HLA-matched sibling donor and 83% for IST.[46,129]

Successful HSCT is curative, results in a shorter duration of neutropenia and transfusion dependence in comparison with IST, and minimizes the risk of relapse and clonal evolution. The risks of HLA-matched sibling transplant versus the benefits are generally lower for patients younger than 40 years of age, although longer follow-up is necessary to evaluate morbidity associated with HSCT, particularly secondary malignancies.

For the majority of patients without a suitable HLA-matched sibling donor, IST remains the main treatment modality, and HSCT from an alternative donor is usually offered as a salvage therapy. Results of HSCT from alternative donors have generally been inferior to IST, and long-term survivals ranged up to 69%.[46,107,108] As outcomes improved with advances in donor selection, pretransplant conditioning incorporating high-dose cyclophosphamide, and GVHD prophylaxis, alternative donor HSCT may be offered at an earlier stage of the disease.

Androgens and growth factors

Androgens have no role as a single treatment agent for SAA,[9] unless other modalities are unavailable.[131] Androgen treatment can induce remission in 38% of children with nonsevere AA. The role of androgens as part of multiagent IST has been alluded to above. Bacigalupo *et al.*[119] demonstrated an increased rate of response in females with severe aplasia,

who received oxymethalone with the IST, although they were unable to demonstrate an improved survival.

Growth factors such as granulocyte colony-stimulating factor (G-CSF), granulocyte–macrophage colony-stimulating factor (GM-CSF) and interleukin-3 (IL-3) have been used as single agents in AA.[124,126,132–135] However, responses are rare and transient, and very high doses are sometimes necessary. Several studies have examined the impact of adding G-CSF to IST on response and long-term survival.[124,134] Although the use of G-CSF improves neutrophil counts in many patients, there was no significant difference in the rates of infectious episodes, overall hematologic response or survivals.[124,134]

Myelodysplastic syndrome

Several large studies have demonstrated an increased risk of MDS and/or leukemia in survivors of AA who had been treated with supportive care, androgens or IST.[43,45,47] Most commonly, patients are diagnosed at the stage of MDS and progress to leukemia, although occasionally patients present with overt leukemia. The actuarial risk of MDS/AML is 15% at 7 years post-IST.[44] MDS occurred at a median of 4.6 years (range 2.5–7.5) post-IST and AML at 5.0 years (range 2.8–7.6). The median age of these patients at the time of diagnosis of AA was 21 years (range 9–56).

Chromosomal aberrations can appear without morphologic signs of MDS/AML.[123] In one study, in 50% of the cases with marrow cytogenetic abnormalities after IST, the aberrant clone was present at diagnosis but detected retrospectively.[123] The group from the US National Institutes of Health[121] evaluated a large number of patients of all ages, with acquired AA whose bone marrow cytogenetics were normal at diagnosis.[136] The estimated rate of clonal evolution was 14% at 5 years and approximately 20% at 10 years.[136,137]

The relationship of G-CSF with MDS/AML in acquired AA is controversial.[137–139] In a prospective randomized study of IST with and without G-CSF in children with acquired AA, the risk of clonal evolution was proportional to the duration of G-CSF administration, particularly if it was longer than 180 days. Failure to respond to IST at 6 months was another risk factor in multivariate analysis. An earlier report also identified the duration and cumulative dose of G-CSF therapy as a risk factors in the development of MDS/AML in children with acquired AA.[140] These observations have not been borne out by other studies.[141–143] In these reports, there was no difference in the incidence of cytogenetic abnormalities between patients who received IST with or without G-CSF. Further studies are, therefore, required to investigate the safety of G-CSF in patients with AA.

A number of clonal marrow cytogenetic abnormalities have been reported at diagnosis of MDS/AML in patients with AA. The most common abnormalities are monosomy 7 (40–50%) and trisomy 8.[136,140,144] Patients with monosomy 7 and complex cytogenetics had higher rates of transformation to AML.[136]

As MDS/AML have also been reported in patients who received androgens or were treated with supportive care without IST,[47,145] it is likely that patients with AA have an inherent predisposition to malignant myeloid transformation, although the mechanism is unclear. MDS/AML secondary to AA are associated with poor survival.

Paroxysmal nocturnal hemoglobinuria

The incidence of PNH post-IST for AA is 8–22% at a median of 30 months (range 6–97 months),[45,47,136] or an actuarial risk of 13% at 7 years post-IST.[45] According to one study, 20% of PNH patients were less than 20 years old at the time of diagnosis with AA.[47] The hypothesis that PNH is a late complication of AA was refuted by demonstrating that PNH clones were always present at the time of diagnosis with AA, and no patient with normal glycosylphosphatidylinositol-linked proteins at diagnosis developed PNH after therapy.[84] Interestingly, PNH clones as determined by flow cytometry were not detected in patients who underwent HSCT or received ATG for renal transplantation, cancer patients on chemotherapy, large granular chronic lymphocytic leukemia, and normal controls.

PNH rarely presents in childhood. Twenty-six children were diagnosed with PNH between 1966 and 1991 at the Duke University Medical Centre.[146] More than 50% of them presented with AA, in contrast to adults (25%). All these children progressed to bone marrow failure during the course of their disease. In another study, none of the children who developed PNH post-AA progressed to MDS/AML, and at least one had spontaneous resolution of PNH.[47]

The cause of the high incidence of PNH in SAA patients treated with IST is unclear. The absence of PNH in patients with hypocellular marrow due to chemotherapy, irradiation, or inherited marrow failure syndromes suggests that PNH clonal expansion is not merely the result of hematopoietic failure.[84] Similarly, PNH clones are absent in patients with large granular chronic lymphocytic leukemia, whose cytopenias are thought to be due to natural killer-cell-mediated hematopoietic injury. Furthermore, their absence in patients who had received ATG for other reasons suggests that ATG-based therapy is not the cause of PNH.[84]

References

1. International Agranulocytosis and Aplastic Anemia Study. Incidence of aplastic anemia: the relevance of diagnostic criteria. *Blood* 1987; **70**: 1718–21.
2. Camitta BM, Thomas ED, Nathan DG *et al.* Severe aplastic anemia: a prospective study of the effect of early marrow transplantation on acute mortality. *Blood* 1976; **48**: 63–70.
3. Linet MS, McCaffrey LD, Morgan WF *et al.* Incidence of aplastic anemia in a three county area in South Carolina. *Cancer Res* 1986; **46**: 426–9.
4. Mary JY, Baumelou E, Guiguet M, The French Cooperative Group for Epidemiological Study of Aplastic Anemia. Epidemiology of aplastic anemia in France: a prospective multicentric study. *Blood* 1990; **75**: 1646–53.
5. Clausen N, Kreuger A, Salmi T, Storm-Mathisen I, Johannesson G. Severe aplastic anaemia in the Nordic countries: a population based study of incidence, presentation, course, and outcome. *Arch Dis Child* 1996; **74**: 319–22.
6. Howard SC, Naidu PE, Hu XJ *et al.* Natural history of moderate aplastic anemia in children. *Pediatr Blood Cancer* 2004; **43**: 545–51.
7. Young NS, Issaragrasil S, Chieh CW, Takaku F. Aplastic anaemia in the Orient. *Br J Haematol* 1986; **62**: 1–6.
8. Issaragrisil S. Epidemiology of aplastic anemia in Thailand. Thai Aplastic Anemia Study Group. *Int J Hematol* 1999; **70**: 137–40.
9. Camitta BM, Thomas ED, Nathan DG *et al.* A prospective study of androgens and bone marrow transplantation for treatment of severe aplastic anemia. *Blood* 1979; **53**: 504–14.
10. Mizuno S, Aoki K, Ohno Y, Sasaki R, Hamajima N. Time series analysis of age-sex specific death rates from aplastic anemia and the trend in production amount of chloramphenicol. *Nagoya J Med Sci* 1982; **44**: 103–15.
11. Bottiger LE, Furhoff AK, Holmberg L. Drug-induced blood dyscrasias. A ten-year material from the Swedish Adverse Drug Reaction Committee. *Acta Med Scand* 1979; **205**: 457–61.
12. Issaragrisil S, Kaufman DW, Anderson T *et al.* Low drug attributability of aplastic anemia in Thailand. The Aplastic Anemia Study Group. *Blood* 1997; **89**: 4034–9.
13. Baumelou E, Guiguet M, Mary JY. Epidemiology of aplastic anemia in France: a case-control study. I. Medical history and medication use. The French Cooperative Group for Epidemiological Study of Aplastic Anemia. *Blood* 1993; **81**: 1471–8.
14. The International Agranulocytosis and Aplastic Anemia Study. Risks of agranulocytosis and aplastic anemia. A first report of their relation to drug use with special reference to analgesics. *JAMA* 1986; **256**: 1749–57.
15. Kaufman DW, Kelly JP, Jurgelon JM *et al.* Drugs in the aetiology of agranulocytosis and aplastic anaemia. *Eur J Haematol Suppl* 1996; **60**: 23–30.
16. Roberts HJ. Pentachlorophenol-associated aplastic anemia, red cell aplasia, leukemia and other blood disorders. *J Fla Med Assoc* 1990; **77**: 86–90.
17. Rugman FP, Cosstick R. Aplastic anaemia associated with organochlorine pesticide: case reports and review of evidence. *J Clin Pathol* 1990; **43**: 98–101.
18. Guiguet M, Baumelou E, Mary JY. A case-control study of aplastic anaemia: occupational exposures. The French Cooperative Group for Epidemiological Study of Aplastic Anaemia. *Int J Epidemiol* 1995; **24**: 993–9.
19. Yardley-Jones A, Anderson D, Parke DV. The toxicity of benzene and its metabolism and molecular pathology in human risk assessment. *Br J Ind Med* 1991; **48**: 437–44.
20. Pellack-Walker P, Blumer JL. DNA damage in L5178YS cells following exposure to benzene metabolites. *Mol Pharmacol* 1986; **30**: 42–7.

21. Moran JL, Siegel D, Sun XM, Ross D. Induction of apoptosis by benzene metabolites in HL60 and CD34+ human bone marrow progenitor cells. *Mol Pharmacol* 1996; **50**: 610–15.

22. Lan Q, Zhang L, Li G *et al.* Hematotoxicity in workers exposed to low levels of benzene. *Science* 2004; **306**: 1774–6.

23. Baranski B, Armstrong G, Truman JT, Quinnan GV Jr, Straus SE, Young NS. Epstein–Barr virus in the bone marrow of patients with aplastic anemia. *Ann Intern Med* 1988; **109**: 695–704.

24. Sing GK, Ruscetti FW. The role of human cytomegalovirus in haematological diseases. *Baillière's Clin Haematol* 1995; **8**: 149–63.

25. Carrigan DR, Knox KK. Human herpesvirus 6 (HHV-6) isolation from bone marrow: HHV-6-associated bone marrow suppression in bone marrow transplant patients. *Blood* 1994; **84**: 3307–10.

26. Shah I, Murthy AK. Aplastic anemia in an HIV infected child. *Indian J Pediatr* 2005; **72**: 359–61.

27. Goto H, Ishida A, Fujii H *et al.* Successful bone marrow transplantation for severe aplastic anemia in a patient with persistent human parvovirus B19 infection. *Int J Hematol* 2004; **79**: 384–6.

28. Qian XH, Zhang GC, Jiao XY *et al.* Aplastic anaemia associated with parvovirus B19 infection. *Arch Dis Child* 2002; **87**: 436–7.

29. Domenech P, Palomeque A, Martinez-Gutierrez A, Vinolas N, Vela E, Jimenez R. Severe aplastic anaemia following hepatitis A. *Acta Haematol* 1986; **76**: 227–9.

30. McSweeney PA, Carter JM, Green GJ, Romeril KR. Fatal aplastic anemia associated with hepatitis B viral infection. *Am J Med* 1988; **85**: 255–6.

31. Kook H, Kim GM, Kim HJ, Kim CJ, Yoon WS, Hwang TJ. Rubella-associated aplastic anemia treated by syngeneic stem cell transplantations. *Am J Hematol* 2000; **64**: 303–5.

32. Nakao S, Lai CJ, Young NS. Dengue virus, a flavivirus, propagates in human bone marrow progenitors and hematopoietic cell lines. *Blood* 1989; **74**: 1235–40.

33. Brown KE, Tisdale J, Barrett AJ, Dunbar CE, Young NS. Hepatitis-associated aplastic anemia. *N Engl J Med* 1997; **336**: 1059–64.

34. Pol S, Thiers V, Driss F *et al.* Lack of evidence for a role of HCV in hepatitis-associated aplastic anaemia. *Br J Haematol* 1993; **85**: 808–10.

35. Hibbs JR, Frickhofen N, Rosenfeld SJ *et al.* Aplastic anemia and viral hepatitis. Non-A, non-B, non-C? *JAMA* 1992; **267**: 2051–4.

36. Liang DC, Lin KH, Lin DT, Yang CP, Hung KL, Lin KS. Post-hepatitic aplastic anaemia in children in Taiwan, a hepatitis prevalent area. *Br J Haematol* 1990; **74**: 487–91.

37. Hagler L, Pastore RA, Bergin JJ, Wrensch MR. Aplastic anemia following viral hepatitis: report of two fatal cases and literature review. *Medicine (Baltimore)* 1975; **54**: 139–64.

38. Itterbeek P, Vandenberghe P, Nevens F *et al.* Aplastic anemia after transplantation for non-A, non-B, non-C fulminant hepatic failure: case report and review of the literature. *Transpl Int* 2002; **15**: 117–23.

39. Cattral MS, Langnas AN, Markin RS *et al.* Aplastic anemia after liver transplantation for fulminant liver failure. *Hepatology* 1994; **20**: 813–18.

40. Tzakis AG, Arditi M, Whitington PF *et al.* Aplastic anemia complicating orthotopic liver transplantation for non-A, non-B hepatitis. *N Engl J Med* 1988; **319**: 393–6.

41. Lu J, Basu A, Melenhorst JJ, Young NS, Brown KE. Analysis of T-cell repertoire in hepatitis-associated aplastic anemia. *Blood* 2004; **103**: 4588–93.

42. Nishimura J, Murakami Y, Kinoshita T. Paroxysmal nocturnal hemoglobinuria: An acquired genetic disease. *Am J Hematol* 1999; **62**: 175–82.

43. De Planque MM, Bacigalupo A, Wursch A *et al.* Long-term follow-up of severe aplastic anaemia patients treated with antithymocyte globulin. Severe Aplastic Anaemia Working Party of the European Cooperative Group for Bone Marrow Transplantation (EBMT). *Br J Haematol* 1989; 73: 121–6.

44. Doney K, Leisenring W, Storb R, Appelbaum FR. Primary treatment of acquired aplastic anemia: outcomes with bone marrow transplantation and immunosuppressive therapy. Seattle Bone Marrow Transplant Team. *Ann Intern Med* 1997; **126**: 107–15.

45. Tichelli A, Gratwohl A, Nissen C, Signer E, Stebler GC, Speck B. Morphology in patients with severe aplastic anemia treated with antilymphocyte globulin. *Blood* 1992; **80**: 337–45.

46. Locasciulli A. Acquired aplastic anemia in children: incidence, prognosis and treatment options. *Paediatr Drugs* 2002; **4**: 761–6.

47. Najean Y, Haguenauer O. Long-term (5 to 20 years) evolution of nongrafted aplastic anemias. The Cooperative Group for the Study of Aplastic and Refractory Anemias. *Blood* 1990; **76**: 2222–8.

48. Kim SW, Rice L, Champlin R, Udden MM. Aplastic anemia in eosinophilic fasciitis: responses to immunosuppression and marrow transplantation. *Haematologia (Budapest)* 1997; **28**: 131–7.

49. Ritchie DS, Underhill C, Grigg AP. Aplastic anemia as a late complication of thymoma in remission. *Eur J Haematol* 2002; **68**: 389–91.

50. Das PK, Wherrett D, Dror Y. Remission of severe aplastic anemia induced by treatment for Graves' disease in a pediatric patient. *Pediatric Blood and Cancer* (in press).

51. Chute JP, Hoffmeister K, Cotelingam J, Davis TA, Frame JN, Jamieson T. Aplastic anemia as the sole presentation of systemic lupus erythematosus. *Am J Hematol* 1996; **51**: 237–9.

52. Quiquandon I, Morel P, Lai JL *et al.* Primary Sjogren's syndrome and aplastic anaemia. *Ann Rheum Dis* 1997; **56**: 438.

53. Anderson KC, Weinstein HJ. Transfusion-associated graft-versus-host disease. *N Engl J Med* 1990; **323**: 315–21.

54. Yamaguchi H, Calado RT, Ly H *et al.* Mutations in TERT, the gene for telomerase reverse transcriptase, in aplastic anemia. *N Engl J Med* 2005; **352**: 1413–24.

55. Vulliamy TJ, Walne A, Baskaradas A, Mason PJ, Marrone A, Dokal I. Mutations in the reverse transcriptase component of telomerase (TERT) in patients with bone marrow failure. *Blood Cells Mol Dis* 2005; **34**: 257–63.

56. Nimer SD, Ireland P, Meshkinpour A, Frane M. An increased HLA DR2 frequency is seen in aplastic anemia patients. *Blood* 1994; **84**: 923–7.

57. Nakao S, Takami A, Takamatsu H *et al.* Isolation of a T-cell clone showing HLA-DRB1*0405-restricted cytotoxicity for hematopoietic cells in a patient with aplastic anemia. *Blood* 1997; **89**: 3691–9.

58. Viale M, Merli A, Bacigalupo A. Analysis at the clonal level of T-cell phenotype and functions in severe aplastic anemia patients. *Blood* 1991; **78**: 1268–74.

59. Zeng W, Maciejewski JP, Chen G, Young NS. Limited heterogeneity of T cell receptor BV usage in aplastic anemia. *J Clin Invest* 2001; **108**: 765–73.

60. Hara T, Ando K, Tsurumi H, Moriwaki H. Excessive production of tumor necrosis factor-alpha by bone marrow T lymphocytes is essential in causing bone marrow failure in patients with aplastic anemia. *Eur J Haematol* 2004; **73**: 10–16.

61. Sloand E, Kim S, Maciejewski JP, Tisdale J, Follmann D, Young NS. Intracellular interferon-gamma in circulating and marrow T cells detected by flow cytometry and the response to immunosuppressive therapy in patients with aplastic anemia. *Blood* 2002; **100**: 1185–91.

62. Zeng W, Chen G, Kajigaya S *et al.* Gene expression profiling in CD34 cells to identify differences between aplastic anemia patients and healthy volunteers. *Blood* 2004; **103**: 325–32.

63. Philpott NJ, Scopes J, Marsh JC, Gordon-Smith EC, Gibson FM. Increased apoptosis in aplastic anemia bone marrow progenitor cells: possible pathophysiologic significance. *Exp Hematol* 1995; **23**: 1642–8.

64. Maciejewski J, Selleri C, Anderson S, Young NS. Fas antigen expression on CD34+ human marrow cells is induced by interferon gamma and tumor necrosis factor alpha and potentiates cytokine-mediated hematopoietic suppression in vitro. *Blood* 1995; **85**: 3183–90.

65. Kasahara S, Hara T, Itoh H *et al.* Hypoplastic myelodysplastic syndromes can be distinguished from acquired aplastic anaemia by bone marrow stem cell expression of the tumour necrosis factor receptor. *Br J Haematol* 2002; **118**: 181–8.

66. Risitano AM, Maciejewski JP, Green S, Plasilova M, Zeng W, Young NS. In-vivo dominant immune responses in aplastic anaemia: molecular tracking of putatively pathogenetic T-cell clones by TCR beta-CDR3 sequencing. *Lancet* 2004; **364**: 355–64.

67. Piao W, Grosse J, Czwalinna A, Ivanyi P, Ganser A, Franzke A. Antigen-recognition sites of micromanipulated T cells in patients with acquired aplastic anemia. *Exp Hematol* 2005; **33**: 804–10.

68. Hirano N, Butler MO, Bergwelt-Baildon MS *et al.* Autoantibodies frequently detected in patients with aplastic anemia. *Blood* 2003; **102**: 4567–75.

69. Scopes J, Daly S, Atkinson R, Ball SE, Gordon-Smith EC, Gibson FM. Aplastic anemia: evidence for dysfunctional bone marrow progenitor cells and the corrective effect of granulocyte colony-stimulating factor in vitro. *Blood* 1996; **87**: 3179–85.

70. Maciejewski JP, Selleri C, Sato T, Anderson S, Young NS. A severe and consistent deficit in marrow and circulating primitive hematopoietic cells (long-term culture-initiating cells) in acquired aplastic anemia. *Blood* 1996; **88**: 1983–91.

71. Marsh JC, Chang J, Testa NG, Hows JM, Dexter TM. The hematopoietic defect in aplastic anemia assessed by long-term marrow culture. *Blood* 1990; **76**: 1748–57.

72. Schrezenmeier H, Jenal M, Herrmann F, Heimpel H, Raghavachar A. Quantitative analysis of cobblestone area-forming cells in bone marrow of patients with aplastic anemia by limiting dilution assay. *Blood* 1996; **88**: 4474–80.

73. Novitzky N, Jacobs P. Immunosuppressive therapy in bone marrow aplasia: the stroma functions normally to support hematopoiesis. *Exp Hematol* 1995; **23**: 1472–7.

74. Scopes J, Ismail M, Marks KJ *et al.* Correction of stromal cell defect after bone marrow transplantation in aplastic anaemia. *Br J Haematol* 2001; **115**: 642–52.

75. Brummendorf TH, Rufer N, Holyoake TL *et al.* Telomere length dynamics in normal individuals and in patients with hematopoietic stem cell-associated disorders. *Ann NY Acad Sci* 2001; **938**: 293–303.

76. Ball SE, Gibson FM, Rizzo S, Tooze JA, Marsh JC, Gordon-Smith EC. Progressive telomere shortening in aplastic anemia. *Blood* 1998; **91**: 3582–92.

77. Holmberg LA, Seidel K, Leisenring W, Torok-Storb B. Aplastic anemia: analysis of stromal cell function in long-term marrow cultures. *Blood* 1994; **84**: 3685–90.

78. Dilloo D, Vohringer R, Josting A, Habersang K, Scheidt A, Burdach S. Bone marrow fibroblasts from children with aplastic anemia exhibit reduced interleukin-6 production in response to cytokines and viral challenge. *Pediatr Res* 1995; **38**: 716–21.

79. Frickhofen N, Liu JM, Young NS. Etiologic mechanisms of hematopoietic failure. *Am J Pediatr Hematol Oncol* 1990; **12**: 385–95.

80. Torok-Storb B. Etiological mechanisms in immune-mediated aplastic anemia. *Am J Pediatr Hematol Oncol* 1990; **12**: 396–401.

81. Davies SM, Walker DJ. Aplastic anaemia in the Northern Region 1971–1978 and follow-up of long term survivors. *Clin Lab Haematol* 1986; **8**: 307–13.

82. Pitcher LA, Hann IM, Evans JP, Veys P, Chessells JM, Webb DK. Improved prognosis for acquired aplastic anaemia. *Arch Dis Child* 1999; **80**: 158–62.

83. Liang R, Cheng G, Wat MS, Ha SY, Chan LC. Childhood acute lymphoblastic leukaemia presenting with relapsing hypoplastic anaemia: progression of the same abnormal clone. *Br J Haematol* 1993; **83**: 340–2.

84. Dunn DE, Tanawattanacharoen P, Boccuni P *et al.* Paroxysmal nocturnal hemoglobinuria cells in patients with bone marrow failure syndromes. *Ann Intern Med* 1999; **131**: 401–8.

85. Sagmeister M, Oec L, Gmur J. A restrictive platelet transfusion policy allowing long-term support of outpatients with severe aplastic anemia. *Blood* 1999; **93**: 3124–6.

86. Mathe G, Amiel JL, Schwarzenberg L *et al.* Bone marrow graft in man after conditioning by antilymphocytic serum. *Br Med J* 1970; **2**: 131–6.

87. Sanders JE, Storb R, Anasetti C *et al.* Marrow transplant experience for children with severe aplastic anemia. *Am J Pediatr Hematol Oncol* 1994; **16**: 43–9.

88. Ades L, Mary JY, Robin M *et al.* Long-term outcome after bone marrow transplantation for severe aplastic anemia. *Blood* 2004; **103**: 2490–7.

89. Storb R, Blume KG, O'Donnell MR *et al.* Cyclophosphamide and antithymocyte globulin to condition patients with aplastic anemia for allogeneic marrow transplantations: the experience in four centers. *Biol Blood Marrow Transplant* 2001; **7**: 39–44.

90. Kojima S, Horibe K, Inaba J *et al.* Long-term outcome of acquired aplastic anaemia in children: comparison between immunosuppressive therapy and bone marrow transplantation. *Br J Haematol* 2000; **111**: 321–8.

91. Gluckman E, Horowitz MM, Champlin RE *et al.* Bone marrow transplantation for severe aplastic anemia: influence of conditioning and graft-versus-host disease prophylaxis regimens on outcome. *Blood* 1992; **79**: 269–75.

92. Passweg JR, Socie G, Hinterberger W *et al.* Bone marrow transplantation for severe aplastic anemia: has outcome improved? *Blood* 1997; **90**: 858–64.

93. Hinterberger W, Rowlings PA, Hinterberger-Fischer M *et al.* Results of transplanting bone marrow from genetically identical twins into patients with aplastic anemia. *Ann Intern Med* 1997; **126**: 116–22.

94. McCann SR, Bacigalupo A, Gluckman E *et al.* Graft rejection and second bone marrow transplants for acquired aplastic anaemia: a report from the Aplastic Anaemia Working Party of the European Bone Marrow Transplant Group. *Bone Marrow Transplant* 1994; **13**: 233–7.

95. Storb R, Sanders JE, Pepe M *et al.* Graft-versus-host disease prophylaxis with methotrexate/cyclosporine in children with severe aplastic anemia treated with cyclophosphamide and HLA-identical marrow grafts. *Blood* 1991; **78**: 1144–5.

96. Cohen A, Duell T, Socie G *et al.* Nutritional status and growth after bone marrow transplantation (BMT) during childhood: EBMT Late-Effects Working Party retrospective data. European Group for Blood and Marrow Transplantation. *Bone Marrow Transplant* 1999; **23**: 1043–7.

97. Haltrich I, Muller J, Szabo J *et al.* Donor-cell myelodysplastic syndrome developing 13 years after marrow grafting for aplastic anemia. *Cancer Genet Cytogenet* 2003; **142**: 124–8.

98. Lawler M, Locasciulli A, Longoni D, Schiro R, McCann SR. Leukaemic transformation of donor cells in a patient receiving a second allogeneic bone marrow transplant for severe aplastic anaemia. *Bone Marrow Transplant* 2002; **29**: 453–6.

99. Deeg HJ, Socie G, Schoch G *et al.* Malignancies after marrow transplantation for aplastic anemia and fanconi anemia: a joint Seattle and Paris analysis of results in 700 patients. *Blood* 1996; **87**: 386–92.

100. Kolb HJ, Socie G, Duell T *et al.* Malignant neoplasms in long-term survivors of bone marrow transplantation. Late Effects Working Party of the European Cooperative Group for Blood and Marrow Transplantation and the European Late Effect Project Group. *Ann Intern Med* 1999; **131**: 738–44.

101. Witherspoon RP, Storb R, Pepe M, Longton G, Sullivan KM. Cumulative incidence of secondary solid malignant tumors in aplastic anemia patients given marrow grafts after conditioning with chemotherapy alone. *Blood* 1992; **79**: 289–91.

102. Pierga JY, Socie G, Gluckman E *et al.* Secondary solid malignant tumors occurring after bone marrow transplantation for severe aplastic anemia given thoraco-abdominal irradiation. *Radiother Oncol* 1994; **30**: 55–8.

103. Curtis RE, Rowlings PA, Deeg HJ *et al.* Solid cancers after bone marrow transplantation. *N Engl J Med* 1997; **336**: 897–904.

104. Bacigalupo A, Hows J, Gordon-Smith EC *et al.* Bone marrow transplantation for severe aplastic anemia from donors other than HLA identical siblings: a report of the BMT Working Party. *Bone Marrow Transplant* 1988; **3**: 531–5.

105. Wagner JL, Deeg HJ, Seidel K *et al.* Bone marrow transplantation for severe aplastic anemia from genotypically HLA-nonidentical relatives. An update of the Seattle experience. *Transplantation* 1996; **61**: 54–61.

106. Woodard P, Cunningham JM, Benaim E *et al.* Effective donor lymphohematopoietic reconstitution after haploidentical CD34+-selected hematopoietic stem cell transplantation in children with refractory severe aplastic anemia. *Bone Marrow Transplant* 2004; **33**: 411–18.

107. Deeg HJ, Seidel K, Casper J *et al.* Marrow transplantation from unrelated donors for patients with severe aplastic anemia who have failed immunosuppressive therapy. *Biol Blood Marrow Transplant* 1999; **5**: 243–52.

108. Kojima S, Matsuyama T, Kato S *et al.* Outcome of 154 patients with severe aplastic anemia who received transplants from unrelated donors: the Japan Marrow Donor Program. *Blood* 2002; **100**: 799–803.

109. Vassiliou GS, Webb DK, Pamphilon D, Knapper S, Veys PA. Improved outcome of alternative donor bone marrow transplantation in children with severe aplastic anaemia using a conditioning regimen containing low-dose total body irradiation, cyclophosphamide and Campath. *Br J Haematol* 2001; **114**: 701–5.

110. Barker JN, Davies SM, DeFor T, Ramsay NK, Weisdorf DJ, Wagner JE. Survival after transplantation of unrelated donor umbilical cord blood is comparable to that of human leukocyte antigen-matched unrelated donor bone marrow: results of a matched-pair analysis. *Blood* 2001; **97**: 2957–61.

111. Thomas ED, Storb R, Giblett ER *et al.* Recovery from aplastic anemia following attempted marrow transplantation. *Exp Hematol* 1976; **4**: 97–102.

112. Jeannet M, Speck B, Rubinstein A, Pelet B, Wyss M, Kummer H. Autologous marrow reconstitutions in severe aplastic anaemia after ALG pretreatment and HL-A semi-incompatible bone marrow cell transfusion. *Acta Haematol* 1976; **55**: 129–39.

113. Speck B, Gluckman E, Haak HL, van Rood JJ. Treatment of aplastic anaemia by antilymphocyte globulin with and without allogeneic bone–marrow infusions. *Lancet* 1977; **ii**: 1145–8.

114. Champlin R, Ho W, Gale RP. Antithymocyte globulin treatment in patients with aplastic anemia: a prospective randomized trial. *N Engl J Med* 1983; **308**: 113–18.

115. Di Bona E, Rodeghiero F, Bruno B *et al.* Rabbit antithymocyte globulin (r-ATG) plus cyclosporine and granulocyte colony stimulating factor is an effective treatment for aplastic anaemia patients unresponsive to a first course of intensive immunosuppressive therapy. Gruppo Italiano Trapianto di Midollo Osseo (GITMO). *Br J Haematol* 1999; **107**: 330–4.

116. Frickhofen N, Kaltwasser JP, Schrezenmeier H *et al.* Treatment of aplastic anemia with antilymphocyte globulin and methylprednisolone with or without cyclosporine. The German Aplastic Anemia Study Group. *N Engl J Med* 1991; **324**: 1297–304.

117. Doney K, Pepe M, Storb R *et al.* Immunosuppressive therapy of aplastic anemia: results of a prospective, randomized trial of antithymocyte globulin (ATG), methylprednisolone, and oxymetholone to ATG, very high-dose methylprednisolone, and oxymetholone. *Blood* 1992; **79**: 2566–71.

118. Rosenfeld S, Follmann D, Nunez O, Young NS. Antithymocyte globulin and cyclosporine for severe aplastic anemia: association between hematologic response and long-term outcome. *JAMA* 2003; **289**: 1130–5.

119. Bacigalupo A, Chaple M, Hows J *et al.* Treatment of aplastic anaemia (AA) with antilymphocyte globulin (ALG) and methylprednisolone (MPred) with or without androgens: a randomized trial from the EBMT SAA working party. *Br J Haematol* 1993; **83**: 145–51.

120. Locasciulli A, Bruno B, Rambaldi A *et al.* Treatment of severe aplastic anemia with antilymphocyte globulin, cyclosporine and two different granulocyte colony-stimulating factor regimens: a GITMO prospective randomized study. *Haematologica* 2004; **89**: 1054–61.

121. Gillio AP, Boulad F, Small TN *et al.* Comparison of long-term outcome of children with severe aplastic anemia treated with immunosuppression versus bone marrow transplantation. *Biol Blood Marrow Transplant* 1997; **3**: 18–24.

122. Fouladi M, Herman R, Rolland-Grinton M *et al.* Improved survival in severe acquired aplastic anemia of childhood. *Bone Marrow Transplant* 2000; **26**: 1149–56.

123. Fuhrer M, Burdach S, Ebell W *et al.* Relapse and clonal disease in children with aplastic anemia (AA) after immuno-suppressive therapy (IST): the SAA 94 experience. German/Austrian Pediatric Aplastic Anemia Working Group. *Klin Padiatr* 1998; **210**: 173–9.

124. Kojima S, Hibi S, Kosaka Y *et al.* Immunosuppressive therapy using antithymocyte globulin, cyclosporine, and danazol with or without human granulocyte colony-stimulating factor in children with acquired aplastic anemia. *Blood* 2000; **96**: 2049–54.

125. Schrezenmeier H, Marin P, Raghavachar A *et al.* Relapse of aplastic anaemia after immunosuppressive treatment: a report from the European Bone Marrow Transplantation Group SAA Working Party. *Br J Haematol* 1993; **85**: 371–7.

126. Guinan EC, Sieff CA, Oette DH, Nathan DG. A phase I/II trial of recombinant granulocyte-macrophage colony-stimulating factor for children with aplastic anemia. *Blood* 1990; **76**: 1077–82.

127. Tisdale JF, Dunn DE, Geller N *et al.* High-dose cyclophosphamide in severe aplastic anaemia: a randomised trial. *Lancet* 2000; **356**: 1554–9.

128. Tisdale JF, Maciejewski JP, Nunez O, Rosenfeld SJ, Young NS. Late complications following treatment for severe aplastic anemia (SAA) with high-dose cyclophosphamide (Cy): follow-up of a randomized trial. *Blood* 2002; **100**: 4668–70.

129. Bacigalupo A, Oneto R, Bruno B *et al.* Current results of bone marrow transplantation in patients with acquired severe aplastic anemia. Report of the European Group for Blood and Marrow transplantation. On behalf of the Working Party on Severe Aplastic Anemia of the European Group for Blood and Marrow Transplantation. *Acta Haematol* 2000; **103**: 19–25.

130. Halperin DS, Grisaru D, Freedman MH, Saunders EF. Severe acquired aplastic anemia in children: 11-year experience with bone marrow transplantation and immunosuppressive therapy. *Am J Pediatr Hematol Oncol* 1989; **11**: 304–9.

131. Marwaha RK, Bansal D, Trehan A, Varma N. Androgens in childhood acquired aplastic anaemia in Chandigarh, *Indian Trop Doct* 2004; **34**: 149–52.

132. Hord JD, Gay JC, Whitlock JA *et al.* Long-term granulocyte-macrophage colony-stimulating factor and immuno-suppression in the treatment of acquired severe aplastic anemia. *J Pediatr Hematol Oncol* 1995; **17**: 140–4.

133. Kojima S, Matsuyama T. Stimulation of granulopoiesis by high-dose recombinant human granulocyte colony-stimulating factor in children with aplastic anemia and very severe neutropenia. *Blood* 1994; **83**: 1474–8.

134. Gluckman E, Rokicka-Milewska R, Hann I *et al.* Results and follow-up of a phase III randomized study of recombinant human-granulocyte stimulating factor as support for immunosuppressive therapy in patients with severe aplastic anaemia. *Br J Haematol* 2002; **119**: 1075–82.

135. Ganser A, Lindemann A, Seipelt G *et al.* Effects of recombinant human interleukin-3 in aplastic anemia. *Blood* 1990; **76**: 1287–92.

136. Maciejewski JP, Risitano A, Sloand EM, Nunez O, Young NS. Distinct clinical outcomes for cytogenetic abnormalities evolving from aplastic anemia. *Blood* 2002; **99**: 3129–35.

137. Kojima S, Ohara A, Tsuchida M *et al.* Risk factors for evolution of acquired aplastic anemia into myelodysplastic syndrome and acute myeloid leukemia after immunosuppressive therapy in children. *Blood* 2002; **100**: 786–90.

138. Bessho M, Hotta T, Ohyashiki K *et al.* Multicenter prospective study of clonal complications in adult aplastic anemia patients following recombinant human granulocyte colony-stimulating factor (lenograstim) administration. *Int J Hematol* 2003; **77**: 152–8.

139. Kaito K, Kobayashi M, Katayama T *et al.* Long-term administration of G-CSF for aplastic anaemia is closely related to the early evolution of monosomy 7 MDS in adults. *Br J Haematol* 1998; **103**: 297–303.

140. Ohara A, Kojima S, Hamajima N *et al.* Myelodysplastic syndrome and acute myelogenous leukemia as a late clonal complication in children with acquired aplastic anemia. *Blood* 1997; **90**: 1009–13.

141. Schrezenmeier H, Hinterberger W, Hows J. Second immunosuppressive treatment of patients with aplastic anemia not responding to the first course of immunosuppression (IS): A report from the Working Party of Severe Aplastic Anemia for the EBMT. *Bone Marrow Transpl* 1995; **15** (suppl. 2): 65a.

142. Locasciulli A, Arcese W, Locatelli F, Di Bona E, Bacigalupo A. Treatment of aplastic anaemia with granulocyte-colony stimulating factor and risk of malignancy. Italian Aplastic Anaemia Study Group. *Lancet* 2001; **357**: 43–4.

143. Imashuku S, Hibi S, Bessho F *et al.* Detection of myelodysplastic syndrome/acute myeloid leukemia evolving from aplastic anemia in children, treated with recombinant human G-CSF. Pediatric AA Follow-up Study Group in Japan. *Haematologica* 2003; **88**: ECR31.

144. Maciejewski JP, Selleri C. Evolution of clonal cytogenetic abnormalities in aplastic anemia. *Leuk Lymphoma* 2004; **45**: 433–40.

145. Mir MA, Geary CG. Aplastic anaemia: an analysis of 174 patients. *Postgrad Med J* 1980; **56**: 322–9.

146. Ware RE, Hall SE, Rosse WF. Paroxysmal nocturnal hemoglobinuria with onset in childhood and adolescence. *N Engl J Med* 1991; **325**: 991–6.

147. Brodsky RA, Sensenbrenner LL, Jones RJ. Complete remission in severe aplastic anemia after high-dose cyclophosphamide without bone marrow transplantation. *Blood* 1996; **87**: 491–4.

Red Cell Disorders

5

Disorders of iron metabolism: iron deficiency, iron overload and the sideroblastic anemias

Andrew M. Will

The disorders of iron metabolism are of great importance in pediatric hematology. Iron deficiency anemia is arguably the commonest pediatric hematologic disorder and is certainly the most frequent cause of anemia in childhood. The problems of iron overload dominate the clinical course of all children receiving regular blood transfusions, and the sideroblastic anemias, although rare, need to be considered in the differential diagnosis of patients with anemias of uncertain origin.

Iron metabolism

Despite being one of the commonest substances in the natural world, iron is treated by the body as if it were a trace element. Iron is efficiently recycled and excretion is limited. In part, at least, this is because most naturally occurring iron is in the ferric (Fe^{3+}) form, which is highly insoluble and therefore relatively unavailable for absorption from the diet. Complex mechanisms to facilitate iron absorption have had to evolve.

Iron's importance in biochemistry lies in its ability to exist in two stable forms: the relatively inactive ferric (Fe^{3+}) and biochemically active ferrous (Fe^{2+}) state. This property makes it an ideal atom to be involved in electron transfer, which forms the basis of many enzyme-controlled biochemical reactions. Iron is therefore not just important as heme iron to carry oxygen but is also essential to the working of many of the body's enzyme systems (Table 5.1). Approximately half the enzymes of the Krebs cycle contain iron or require it as a cofactor. Therefore, although most of the iron metabolized each day is used to synthesize hemoglobin, chronic iron deficiency may produce a wide variety of effects other than anemia.

The potential reactivity of iron has led to the evolution of a group of specialized proteins to transport and store iron and regulate the iron-dependent synthetic pathways. Providing the ability of these proteins to contain ionic iron is maintained, iron can be safely stored and metabolized. In iron overload these systems become overwhelmed and the

Table 5.1 Iron-containing enzymes.

Cytochromes *a*, *b* and *c*
Succinate dehydrogenase
Cytochrome *c* oxidase
Cytochrome P450
Catalase
Myeloperoxidase
Tryptophan pyrrolase
Xanthine oxidase
NADH dehydrogenase
Ribonucleotide reductase

uncontrolled reactivity of ionic iron causes life-threatening tissue damage.

Humans appear to be unique in their inability to excrete excess iron.[1] Iron loss (about 1–1.5 mg/day) is achieved almost exclusively in the male by desquamation of skin and loss of mucosal cells from the gastrointestinal and urinary tracts.[2] In the female, iron is also lost through menstruation and during pregnancy. Iron loss by any of these means is relatively constant and cannot be altered in response to changes in body iron status. In the absence of a physiologic mechanism for the excretion of excess iron, iron balance is achieved by control of iron absorption.[3]

Iron absorption

Three factors are important in determining the amount of iron absorbed from the diet: total iron content of the diet, bioavailability of the iron in the diet, and control of iron absorption by the intestinal mucosal cells. Only the latter is responsive to body iron status and requirements.

Dietary iron content

Total iron content is probably the single most important dietary factor in determining the amount of iron absorbed

Table 5.2 Iron content of foodstuffs.

Foodstuff	Iron/100 g	Percent available for absorption
Rice flour	0.9	1
Bread	2.0	5
Wheat flour	2.3	5
Cod	0.9	10
Mackerel	1.0	10
Sardines in oil	1.5	10
Oysters	7.1	10
Beef sausages	2.4	
Chicken	3.0	>10
Pork chops	3.0	>10
Bacon (cooked)	3.3	
Beef (rump)	2.4	>10
(kidney)	6.5	
(liver)	12.1	

Table 5.3 Factors affecting iron absorption of nonheme iron from the gastrointestinal tract.

Increased absorption
Acids
   Vitamin C
   Hydrochloric acid
Solutes
   Sugars
   Amino acids (meats)

Decreased absorption
Alkalis
   Antacids
   Pancreatic secretions
   Hypochlorhydria
Precipitating agents (vegetables)
   Phytates
   Phosphates

from the gut. A mixed Western diet contains about 6 mg iron per 1000 kcal (4200 kJ).[4] An adult male will absorb about 10% of this (0.5–1 mg/day). In iron deficiency, the amount of iron absorbed can be increased to a maximum of 3.5 mg/day.[5] Large amounts of dietary iron do not block iron absorption but as the amount in the diet increases, the percentage absorbed decreases. Different foodstuffs contain different proportions of iron (Table 5.2); vegetarian diets are more likely to have an inadequate iron content than mixed diets.

Bioavailability of dietary iron

The bioavailability of dietary iron is also important in determining the amount of iron absorbed from the diet.[6] Dietary iron is in two forms: organic or heme iron derived from hemoglobin and myoglobin, and inorganic or nonheme iron. There is a different absorptive pathway by which iron can enter the gut mucosal cells for each of the two types of dietary iron.[3,7]

1 Heme iron is taken up directly by specialized receptors in the mucosal membrane[8] and passes unchanged into the cytoplasm where the porphyrin ring is cleaved and the iron released.[9] The heme iron pathway is relatively efficient and, unlike nonheme iron, absorption is little affected by the intraluminal factors discussed below. Although heme iron only accounts for about 10% of the total iron in a mixed diet, it accounts for up to 25% of the total iron absorbed.

2 Nonheme iron exists almost exclusively as insoluble ferric salts. To be absorbed the ferric salts must first be converted to the ferrous form and then bound to the intestinal iron transport protein, mucosal apotransferrin. Bound to apotransferrin, the nonheme iron can enter the gut mucosal cell. Within the cell, iron is cleaved from the mucosal transferrin and joins the same pool as heme-derived iron.

The uptake of nonheme iron by the gastrointestinal mucosal cells is affected by factors that enhance and inhibit absorption.[10,11]

• Foodstuffs vary in their ability to give up iron for absorption (see Table 5.2).[12] Rice, for example, is not only poor in total iron content but only 1–2% of this is available for absorption. Even relatively iron-rich vegetables such as spinach and wheat have only a small percentage of their total iron content available for absorption (1–2% and 5% respectively). In contrast, heme-rich animal-derived foodstuffs not only contain more iron per gram but a much higher percentage is available for absorption.

• Different foods can interact to either increase or decrease the absorption of iron from them (Table 5.3). Meat in the diet increases the absorption of even nonheme iron from the gut lumen. The addition of veal to a meal of maize can double the amount of iron absorbed from the cereal.[13] On the other hand, tannates in tea or coffee[14] and substances such as egg yolk have the opposite effect and reduce nonheme iron absorption.[15]

• Intraluminal factors influence the percentage of nonheme iron that can be reduced from the insoluble ferric to the soluble absorbable ferrous form.[16] Acids such as hydrochloric acid and vitamin C promote the production of ferrous iron, enhancing absorption, whereas antacids and hypochlorhydria reduce the amount of ferrous iron available from the diet. Phosphates and phytates, which are common in vegetables, also prevent the reduction of ferric to ferrous salts, thereby inhibiting iron absorption by forming insoluble complexes with iron salts.

The bioavailability of iron is clinically important. Vegans are at risk of iron deficiency even if their total dietary iron content appears satisfactory because the assimilation of iron from vegetable sources is inefficient. Moreover, the absorption of nonheme-derived iron is reduced by the absence of heme iron, and the increased intake of phytates and phosphates further reduces the availability of absorbable iron. In contrast, human milk has a low total iron content but the iron is in a form which is highly bioavailable[17] and which is also able to directly enhance the amount of iron absorbed from other foodstuffs in the early weaning diet.[18] Therefore, the vegan even with an apparently adequate total dietary iron content is at risk of iron deficiency but the breast-fed infant is less so.

Mucosal cell control

Gut mucosal cell control of iron absorption is not well defined but the amount of iron absorbed via the mucosa is responsive to body iron stores[19] and the erythropoietic activity of the bone marrow.[20] Increases in body iron lead to a reduction in iron absorbed from the gastrointestinal tract and when body iron stores are reduced, more iron is absorbed. Erythropoietic activity has the opposite effect: in conditions associated with high levels of erythropoietic activity, iron absorption is increased, but in disorders such as hypoplastic anemia where erythropoietic activity is reduced, iron absorption is reduced. The amount of dietary iron absorbed can be controlled at both phases of mucosal cell absorption.

1 *At the uptake of iron from the gut lumen into the mucosal cells.* For nonheme iron to be absorbed from the gut lumen across the brush border of the intestinal mucosal cells, iron must first be attached to the mucosal cell transport protein apo-transferrin.[21] The transferrin–iron complex produced is internalized by the small intestine, mainly in the duodenum and jejunum. Control of the uptake of dietary iron can be achieved during this phase of absorption because the amount of apo-transferrin secreted by the liver into the bile is inversely proportional to hepatic iron stores. Increased hepatic storage reduces the synthesis of apotransferrin by the liver, hence reducing gut mucosal cell iron uptake. A reduction in hepatic iron stores has the opposite effect.[22]

2 *During the transfer of iron to the portal blood.* Once inside the mucosal cells, the iron released from the transferrin–iron complex joins with heme-derived iron. Iron from this combined intracellular pool has two possible fates. It is either transferred to the portal blood for further metabolism within the body or combined with the mucosal cell storage protein apoferritin.[23] If the latter, the iron becomes trapped in the mucosal cell as storage ferritin. After 3–4 days the cell and any ferritin it contains are sloughed off into the intestinal lumen as the villus mucosal cell completes its lifespan. Control of absorption is achieved because the amount of apo-ferritin produced by the mucosal cells is dependent on body iron stores. When body iron stores are low, little is produced by the gut mucosal cells and a high percentage of the absorbed dietary iron can pass into the portal venous system. Conversely, when body iron stores are replete, the gut mucosal

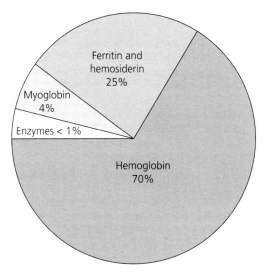

Fig. 5.1 Distribution of iron in man (adult male = 3.5–4.0 g).

cells produce more apoferritin, which traps absorbed dietary iron in the intestinal villus cells and this is later excreted in the feces.

Body iron distribution and turnover

The adult contains about 55 mg/kg of iron[4] and an adult male will have 3.5–4 g of iron in his body. The majority of that iron, about 70%, is carried in red blood cells as hemoglobin and most of the rest is stored as ferritin and hemosiderin, with approximately two-thirds within macrophages and one-third in hepatocytes. Small amounts of iron are present in myoglobin and traces in cellular enzymes (Fig. 5.1).

Although the distribution of iron in the body is fairly constant, the iron in the different compartments is continually being recycled. Each day about 25 mL of red blood cells need to be replaced. This represents a need for 25 mg of iron but only about 1 mg/day is absorbed from the diet. The other 24 mg required for red cell replacement alone needs to be recycled from senescent red cells and tissue stores. This daily iron cycle (Fig. 5.2) is reliant on plasma transferrin (TF), cell surface transferrin receptors (TFRs), and the storage protein ferritin. Intracellular control, in the erythroid cell at least, depends on the interaction of an iron-responsive binding protein (IRE-BP) with iron-responsive elements (IREs) present on the mRNA of TFR, ferritin and erythroid cell-specific δ-aminolevulinic acid synthetase (ALAS), the initial enzyme involved in the production of heme from glycine and succinyl-CoA in mitochondria (Fig. 5.3).

Transferrin

TF is the specialized plasma transport protein for iron.[24] It is a single polypeptide β-globulin of 679 amino acids with a molecular mass of 7957 kDa, and is mainly synthesized in the

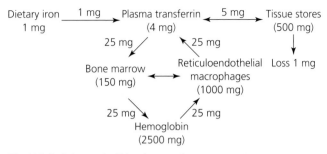

Fig. 5.2 Daily iron cycle. Values in parentheses represent average quantities of stored iron in a normal adult male. Other values represent average daily turnover in milligrams.

liver. Unusually for a transport protein, TF can be recycled after intracellular delivery of iron and it has a half-life of 8–10 days.[25] TF is produced from a single gene q21–qter on chromosome 32,[26] near the gene for its receptor.[27] Normally active structural variants have been described.

TF has two iron-binding sites, one at the N-terminal and one at the C-terminal domain.[28] It can therefore exist in four states: apotransferrin with no bound iron, as two different monoferric transferrins, and as diferric transferrins. At neutral pH, TF has a high affinity for binding ferric iron, and when fully iron saturated undergoes a conformational change that makes the diferric molecule more soluble and more resistant to enzymatic degradation. Diferric TF has about 3.5 times the affinity for TFR than either of the monoferric transferrins[29] and because of this the diferric form is

preferentially bound to cells for intracellular iron delivery. At neutral pH, apoferritin binds poorly to TFR.

Production of TF by the liver is inversely related to hepatocyte ferritin concentration, being increased when hepatic stores of iron are low and reduced when stores are increased.[30] Plasma TF concentration, usually measured as total iron-binding capacity (TIBC), is therefore a convenient assessment of iron stores.

Plasma TF is crucial for the daily iron cycle (see Fig. 5.2). At any one time, only about 4 mg of body iron is present bound to TF, yet every 24 hours > 30 mg of iron is transported throughout the body. Therefore, every day each molecule of TF carries several molecules of ferric iron between cells, and > 80% of this iron is transported to or reutilized in the bone marrow to make heme. The bulk of other daily iron turnover involves iron exchange with hepatocytes. There appears to be no alternative pathway for the iron to enter the red cell precursors. Congenital absence of TF is associated with severe iron deficiency anemia but uptake by nonerythropoietic tissues continues even in the absence of TF.[31]

Transferrin receptor

The TFR is a transmembrane glycoprotein that exists as a dimer of two subunits joined by a disulfide bond.[32] Each TFR can bind two TF molecules. At the neutral pH of the cell surface, TFR has an increased affinity for diferric TF compared with monoferric TF and this in turn is greater than the affinity of TFR for apotransferrin. Each TFR can therefore bind up to

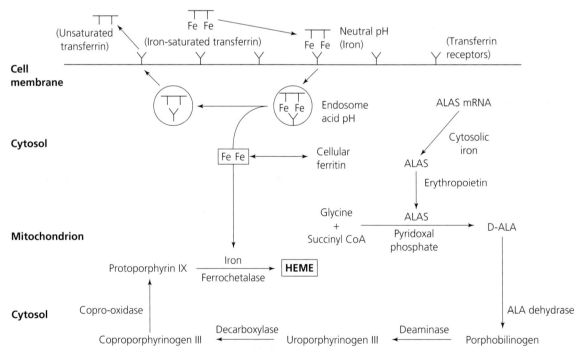

Fig. 5.3 Heme synthesis. Binding of iron-saturated transferrin to cell membrane transferrin receptors, endosome formation, release of iron into the cytosol, and the role of mitochondrial and cytosolic enzymes in the production of heme. ALAS, δ-aminolevulinic acid synthase.

four ferric ions and because the efficiency of TFR binding to TF is dependent on the degree of TF iron saturation, the plasma TF saturation (TIBC) directly affects the availability of iron for intracellular metabolism. In adults, a TIBC > 16% is needed to maintain normal erythropoiesis. Lower levels of about 7% are adequate to maintain red cell production in children.[33,34]

The number of TFRs present on a cell's surface reflects the ability of that cell to accept iron from circulating TF. TFRs are particularly numerous on cells that metabolize a large amount of iron, such as erythroid precursors, reticulocytes, and placental trophoblasts.[35]

Ferritin and hemosiderin

Iron can be stored as either ferritin or hemosiderin.[36] Ferritin is a water-soluble protein whose iron stores are relatively available for iron metabolism as and when required. In sudden hemorrhage, for example, iron loss can temporarily exceed supply. However, the extra blood cells required can be produced without interruption by using iron supplies mobilized from stored ferritin.

Hemosiderin in an insoluble protein–iron complex whose iron is less available, in the short term at least, for metabolic requirements. Unlike ferritin, hemosiderin is visible on light microscopy and stains deep blue with Perl's (Prussian Blue) reagent. It is found primarily in the Kupffer cells of the liver and the macrophages of the spleen and bone marrow. In iron overload, hemosiderin begins to be deposited in the parenchymal cells of the liver and other organs.

Ferritin is produced as a hollow spherical protein with 22–24 apoferritin subunits.[37] It has a molecular mass of 468 kDa. Six channels penetrate the spherical shell through which iron passes into the core. Up to about 4500 iron atoms can be contained in one ferritin molecule, mostly as ferric hydroxide with some ferric phosphate. Ferritin is usually about 50% saturated.

Two types of apoferritin subunit have been identified: L (light) and H (heavy).[38] In different tissues, different proportions of L and H chains are found in their respective ferritin molecules. Liver, a site of iron storage, contains ferritin consisting mainly of L chains but the heart, not normally a site of iron storage, has mainly H chains in its ferritin molecules. Ferritin with an excess of L chains may well be essential for long-term storage, whereas those mostly consisting of H chains may be more active in iron metabolism.[39]

Although different tissues may produce differing apoferritin spheres, all tissues need to be able to assemble the spheres quickly to protect themselves from the potential toxicity of free iron. As ferritin is produced, a small amount proportional to the intracellular ferritin concentration leaks into the plasma. Thus plasma ferritin concentration is related to cellular iron stores.[40]

Table 5.4 Sequence of detectable reduction in iron stores as iron deficiency anemia develops.

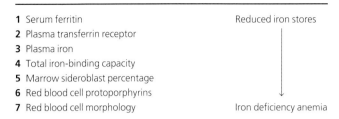

1 Serum ferritin	Reduced iron stores
2 Plasma transferrin receptor	
3 Plasma iron	
4 Total iron-binding capacity	
5 Marrow sideroblast percentage	
6 Red blood cell protoporphyrins	
7 Red blood cell morphology	Iron deficiency anemia

Assessment of body iron stores

Reduced iron stores

Detectable abnormalities occur in sequence as the magnitude of iron deficiency worsens (Table 5.4).[41] The eventual changes in red cell morphology are nonspecific and occur late. Of more importance, and usually the first indication of iron deficiency, are changes in red cell indices. Most modern automated instruments measure red blood cells, hemoglobin, and mean corpuscular volume (MCV) directly. The direct measurement of MCV has made this a sensitive parameter of red cell changes and it has overtaken the more traditional measurements of mean corpuscular hemoglobin concentration (MCHC) and mean corpuscular hemoglobin (MCH) as the primary indication of possible iron deficiency. Many modern blood counters produce two-dimensional red cell maps that can often demonstrate the presence of iron-deficient red cells.

No single confirmatory test is appropriate in all situations.
- Serum ferritin is a sensitive measurement of iron deficiency[40,41] but is an "acute-phase reactant" whose synthesis increases nonspecifically in response to inflammation, infection, or malignancy. Liver cell damage also raises the serum ferritin independently of body iron status.
- The increasing availability of radioimmunoassays of plasma TFR has provided a new method of diagnosing iron deficiency.[42] Plasma TFR concentration is proportional to marrow red cell turnover: erythroid hypoplasia (hypoplastic anemia, chronic renal failure) reduces and erythroid hyperplasia (chronic hemolytic anemia) increases plasma TFR. TFR levels are also increased in iron deficiency and, in the absence of other conditions causing erythroid hyperplasia, plasma TFR is a sensitive indicator of iron deficiency.[43] Unlike serum ferritin, plasma TFR is not affected by chronic inflammation or liver disease. Although available for a number of years, these methods have not been taken up by many hematology laboratories.
- Plasma iron and transferrin saturation (ratio of plasma iron to TIBC) provide a measure of current iron supply to the tissues. These tests are widely used but are strongly influenced by physiologic variation, concurrent inflammatory disease, and recent prior ingestion of iron.
- Free erythrocyte zinc protoporphyrin (ZPP) is a simple test

that can be performed on a drop of EDTA blood. This makes ZPP a convenient adjunct to MCV estimation and red cell mapping, as it is immediately available from the same blood sample that went through the blood count analyzer. In iron deficiency, protoporphyrin IX cannot combine with iron to form heme in the final step of heme synthesis. In the absence of iron, protoporphyrin combines with zinc to form ZPP, which is stable and persists throughout the lifespan of the red cell. Estimation of red cell ZPP provides an indication of iron supply to the red cell over a longer period than serum ferritin or plasma iron.[44] ZPP can therefore be used to confirm iron deficiency in a patient who has recently been started on iron supplements. ZPP may be affected by chronic inflammation but less so by acute infections of recent onset than the more traditional measurements of body iron.

• In difficult cases, bone marrow examination after staining with Perl's reagent will clarify the situation. In iron deficiency, neither the marrow macrophages nor erythroblasts contain iron. In the anemia of chronic disease there is plenty of iron present in the macrophages but none in the red cell precursors. Normally, about 20% of erythroblasts contain iron (sideroblasts).

Increased iron stores

In routine clinical practice, assessment of increased iron stores relies on repeated serum ferritin estimations and, if definitive diagnosis is required, on liver biopsy. However techniques developed using magnetic resonance imaging (MRI) are beginning to become increasingly used and in time are likely to have a major role in both the assessment and monitoring of the treatment of iron overload.

Plasma iron and TF saturation are poor indicators of reticuloendothelial iron overload. They are not reliably elevated by increased macrophage iron as occurs during the early stages of transfusion hemosiderosis. Serum ferritin, on the other hand, is elevated early even in macrophage iron deposition. As mentioned above, serum ferritin is influenced by several factors other than body iron status. Repeated measurements give a more reliable estimation of body iron stores than a single result.

Although marrow biopsy can give a subjective assessment of iron overload, liver biopsy provides much more useful information, including histologic assessment of the degree and distribution of hepatic iron stores and quantification of hepatic iron concentrations (fmol/g dry weight of liver tissue).[45] Liver biopsy is not to be undertaken lightly and is not practicable for regular assessment of body iron stores. Currently, repeat serum ferritin estimations have to be undertaken but noninvasive radiologic approaches are being developed and evaluated. Magnetic susceptometry using a superconducting quantum interference device (SQUID)[46] and dual-energy computed tomography[47] have both been developed but are not available for routine clinical use.

In the last few years, techniques using MRI have been developed.[48,49] These methods offer a repeatable and non-invasive quantitative assessment of body iron stores. Recent reports suggest that iron deposition among the internal organs is not uniform and that the oral chelator deferiprone may have the ability to preferentially remove cardiac iron compared with hepatic stores.[50] More work needs to be done but, if confirmed, the role of liver biopsy as the gold standard for estimating body iron stores will be called into question as it has always been assumed that liver iron levels reflect similar iron overload in the other internal organs.

Control of heme synthesis within the erythroblast (see Fig. 5.3)

In plasma, iron binds to apotransferrin to form monoferric and diferric TFs. At the neutral pH on the outside of the cell membrane, diferric TF binds preferentially to TFRs on the cell surface.[51] The iron-bearing TF–TFR complex rapidly clusters with other similar complexes and is internalized. Here, the clusters of iron–TF–TFR complexes coalesce with other similar clusters to form endosomes. Once within the cytosol, the pH within the endosome is lowered permitting release of iron into the cytosol. The apotransferrin–TFR complex remains tightly bound until it reaches the cell surface. Under the neutral pH conditions at the cell surface, the unsaturated apotransferrin is released to be recycled and bind with more iron. The TFRs remain at the cell surface ready to bind more diferric TF.[52]

Control of intracellular iron metabolism is mediated at the mRNA level by IRE-BP.[53] IRE-BP appears to be structurally identical to cytosolic aconitase, an iron–sulfur enzyme active in the Krebs cycle.[54] Evidence suggests that IRE-BP and cytosolic aconitase can reversibly convert from one form to another in response to alterations in intracellular iron availability.[55] This is mediated by changes in the molecular iron content of aconitase/IRE-BP internal iron–sulfur cluster.[56] Where intracellular iron is readily available, the aconitase enzymatic activity predominates, whereas low intracellular iron promotes the mRNA-binding activity of IRE-BP.

In the erythroid progenitors, IRE-BP acts by binding to IREs present on the mRNA of TFR, ferritin and ALAS, the first enzyme in the pathway for the formation of heme from glycine and succinyl-CoA. IRE-BP binding to the TFR IRE stabilizes TFR mRNA, reducing its cytoplasmic degradation and hence increasing the amount of cytoplasmic mRNA and the rate of TFR synthesis. More TFRs become available on the cell surface to bind diferric TF.[57] IRE-BP binding to ferritin and ALAS mRNA has the opposite effect of reducing translation of both ferritin and ALAS,[39,58] and thus reducing intracellular iron metabolism.

The effects of increased IRE-BP binding in the presence of low cytosolic iron and reduced IRE-BP binding in the presence of high cytosolic iron are summarized in Fig. 5.4. When

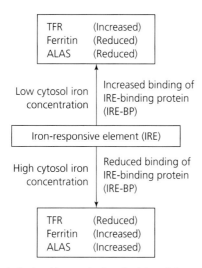

Fig. 5.4 Effect of cytosol iron content on the intracellular synthesis of transferrin receptors (TFR), ferritin, and δ-aminolevulinic acid synthase (ALAS) mediated via the iron-responsive element (IRE).

cytosolic iron is low, more TFRs are produced, which in turn increases the amount of iron-saturated TF taken into the cell. Storage and metabolism of iron by ferritin and ALAS are reduced, which again will tend to increase the iron content of the cytosol. The situation is reversed in the presence of high cytosolic iron levels. In consequence, iron uptake by erythroid cells has a positive effect, promoting ALAS activity. Increased ALAS activity increases protoporphyrin synthesis, thus coupling protoporphyrin production to iron availability within the erythroblast.[59] Under physiologic conditions, IRE-BP controls intracellular iron homeostasis.

Red cell cycle (Fig. 5.5)

Each day 25 mL of senescent red cells are destroyed. The globin chains are broken down into amino acids, which are then recycled to make more globin chains. The heme groups are split into iron and porphyrins. The porphyrins are metabolized and excreted as bilirubin. The iron is recycled

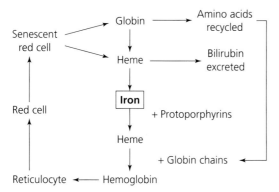

Fig. 5.5 Red cell cycle.

into the production of more red cell heme and combined with globin chains to form hemoglobin in erythroblasts and reticulocytes. Mature red blood cells survive 120 days on average before expressing red cell senescent antigen on their surface. This signals their imminent destruction and the initiation of the recycling process.

Iron deficiency

With the exception of the first few weeks of life, iron deficiency is by far the commonest cause of anemia in childhood. Depletion of iron stores, as indicated by a low serum ferritin without anemia, is even more frequent. Any child may develop iron deficiency but children from deprived inner-city backgrounds and from some ethnic minorities, notably Asian children, are particularly at risk, with the highest prevalence being seen in inner-city Asian toddlers. One UK study demonstrated iron deficiency in 39% of Asian infants.[60] Iron deficiency is not limited to Asian children and in the same study 20% of Afro-Caribbean and 16% of white inner-city toddlers were also iron deficient. In the vast majority of cases the deficiency of iron could have been prevented by simple dietary measures. In the USA, health education and public health programs introducing iron supplementation to the early weaning diet have significantly reduced the prevalence of iron deficiency in the pediatric population.[61] In the UK, similar approaches have been less successful.[62]

Etiology

In children, as in adults, iron balance is related to the ratio of iron absorbed from the diet to the amount lost from the tissues by desquamation and bleeding. However in children other factors are also important, namely the total amount of iron present at the time of birth and the increased demand for iron for growth, which is maximal in the first 6 months of life and during puberty.

In the adult, the approach to determining the cause of iron deficiency is dominated by the search for blood loss. In the child, especially under the age of 3 years, evaluation of the causes of iron deficiency requires an understanding of the developmental and dietary factors that affect total body iron stores.

Developmental factors

Fetus and neonate
The developing fetus is little affected by maternal iron stores. Only in extreme maternal iron deficiency is any degree of anemia seen in the fetus.[63] In general, the fetus acts as a parasite, receiving maternal iron at the expense of the mother. In the vast majority of cases, babies of iron-deficient mothers are born with normal hemoglobin concentrations. Infant serum

iron and TIBC are also usually normal in the presence of maternal iron deficiency.[64–66] At the same time as being able to sequester iron from the mother into the fetus, the placenta also acts as a barrier, excluding excess iron and preventing fetal iron overload. Consequently, maternal iron supplementation does not influence fetal iron status.[67]

A full-term infant at birth is iron replete, with an iron concentration of about 80 mg/kg body weight compared with 55 mg/kg body weight for an adult male;[68] 50 mg/kg is present as red blood cell iron, 25 mL/kg as storage iron, and 5 mg/kg as myoglobin.[69] The extra iron is needed to cope with the additional requirements of the accelerated rate of growth that takes place in the first few months of life. Iron stores at birth may be almost completely independent of maternal iron status but they are dependent on two other factors: birthweight and neonatal red cell mass.

Placental iron transport is insignificant until the third trimester when iron transport increases dramatically to as much as 4 mg/day. Infants born before 26 weeks' gestation have very low iron stores; in those born in the third trimester, iron stores are proportional to birthweight. A 1-kg preterm infant will have about 50 mg of total body iron compared with the 320 mg of a 4-kg full-term baby. The effect of this reduction is accentuated by the greater relative growth potential of the 1-kg preterm infant.

Red cell mass is determined by hemoglobin concentration and red cell volume. Although red cell volume is more or less uniform at 80–90 mL/kg, hemoglobin concentration at birth can vary from 13.5 to 21 g/dL in normal infants. The timing of umbilical cord clamping influences birth hemoglobin concentration (see also Chapter 9). At delivery, two-thirds of the red cells in the fetal circulation are in the infant and one-third in the placenta and cord. In the 3 min immediately following birth, uterine contractions will increase the amount of blood cells in the fetus to > 85%,[70] so early clamping of the cord can reduce the infant's iron content by between 15 and 30%.[71]

Infancy

During the first few weeks of life, erythropoiesis almost stops as the infant's red cell mass drops to a level appropriate for the oxygen-rich extrauterine environment.[72] Iron is stored until erythropoiesis resumes, usually when the infant's hemoglobin concentration has dropped to 11–12 g/dL.[73] In the normal term infant, the iron stored during this time is adequate to cope with the expected doubling of body weight that takes place in the first 5 months of life. After this time, iron absorption from the diet becomes critical to the maintenance of normal iron balance. It has been estimated that a term infant needs 100 mg of iron in the first year of life from the diet to maintain a hemoglobin level of 11 g/dL but a preterm infant may require two to four times as much.[74]

As stated above, newly born infants are iron replete. This is reflected by laboratory findings. Cord blood iron levels are high at 150–250 µg/dL, dropping to 130 µg/dL after 24 hours. Following resumption of erythropoiesis at 8 weeks, iron levels drop further to 80 µg/dL.[33] Serum ferritin is also raised at birth with levels between 100 and 200 µg/L; it then increases further over the first 8 weeks of life but then begins to drop following resumption of erythropoiesis.[37] At 1 year, the mean serum ferritin is usually 30 µg/L. Serum TF levels are proportional to gestational age. This is a developmental phenomenon and, at least in the preterm infant, is not related to iron status.[75]

Early childhood

During childhood total body iron increases in proportion to body weight. After 6 months of age, growth slows and the diet becomes more varied. As long as the diet has an adequate iron content, iron deficiency anemia is unusual. Even so, measured parameters of serum iron and TF saturation remain persistently low. TF saturations of 10% are not uncommon during early childhood but despite this erythropoiesis continues satisfactorily. Serum ferritin also remains low but levels < 10 µg/L indicate depletion of iron stores.

Puberty

At puberty, the secondary growth spurt increases iron requirements to allow for the increase in red cell and muscle mass. Another 80–90 mL of blood alone are required for every extra kilogram of lean body weight, equivalent to an extra 45 mg of iron; in addition to this is the iron required for new muscle myoglobin. This need for more iron is particularly marked in boys whose increase in lean body mass is on average double that seen in girls. In girls, however, as the growth spurt ends, menstruation begins and there is a need for extra iron to compensate for menstrual blood loss. Pregnancy can further increase the iron intake requirement of fertile females.

Dietary factors

The importance of dietary factors and the bioavailability of iron-containing foods has already been been discussed in the section on iron absorption (see p. 79).

These dietary factors are particularly important to the development of iron deficiency in early childhood. Human breast milk has a low total content of iron but, like heme iron, the iron present in breast milk is highly bioavailable and able to enhance the amount of iron absorbed from other foodstuffs in the early weaning diet.[18] Cows' milk, on the other hand, has a low total content of poorly bioavailable iron and its high phosphate content interferes with the absorption of iron from other foods. Cows' milk may also be associated with increased intestinal blood loss.[19] Thus, despite having an apparently low total iron intake, the breast-fed infant is relatively protected from iron deficiency in early childhood compared with the child with a high intake of cows' milk.

Table 5.5 Causes of iron deficiency in children.

Physiologic
Rapid growth (infancy and puberty)
Menarche
Pregnancy

Neonatal
Prematurity
Low birthweight
Blood loss (may be iatrogenic)
Erythropoietin therapy

Iron-poor diet
Excessive cows' milk
Vegetarian diet

Gastrointestinal
Hiatus hernia
Peptic ulceration/*Helicobacter pylori*
Esophageal varices
Meckel diverticulum
Celiac disease
Inflammatory bowel disease
Intestinal surgery
Polyposis coli
Milk-induced enteropathy
Parasitic worms
Atriovenous malformations
Hereditary hemorrhagic telangiectasia

Miscellaneous
Renal tract blood loss
Idiopathic pulmonary hemosiderosis
Bleeding diatheses

Table 5.6 Common causes of hypochromic microcytic anemia related to stage of childhood.

Neonatal period: iron deficiency unlikely

Rest of childhood: iron deficiency most common cause
Infancy and early childhood
    Dietary
    Prematurity
    Low birthweight

Later childhood
    Dietary
    Bleeding

Puberty
    Dietary
    Bleeding
    Increased demands: (i) menstruation; (ii) each 1 kg of weight gain
    = 80 mL blood and requires 45 mg of iron

A list of the causes of iron deficiency in childhood is given in Table 5.5. When considering the likely cause in a particular patient it is important to bear in mind the age of the child (Table 5.6). Under the age of 3 months, iron deficiency is rare and other causes of hypochromia and microcytosis should be sought. From 3 months to 3 years of age, poor diet often with excessive intake of cows' milk is the usual cause of a hypochromic, microcytic anemia. There may be history of premature birth or low birthweight. From 3 years of age to puberty, pure dietary iron deficiency becomes increasingly less likely and other etiologies, particularly gastrointestinal causes, should be considered. At puberty, the associated growth spurt in both sexes and onset of menstruation in girls make physiologic causes more common but other pathologies need to be excluded.

Diagnosis

The diagnosis of iron deficiency is usually straightforward. The patient is anemic with a low MCV. Some modern blood counters produce two-dimensional red cell maps that can aid the diagnosis by demonstrating the presence of iron-deficient red cells. In all cases confirmatory tests should be performed. There are a number of confirmatory tests available for diagnosing iron deficiency but as discussed above (see p. 85) no single one is appropriate in all situations. Most laboratories use the serum ferritin, although at times of rapid growth, particularly in early childhood and during puberty, a low serum ferritin may not reflect iron-deficient erythropoiesis. Furthermore, ferritin is an acute reactive protein and thus may be elevated during infections even in the presence of iron deficiency. ZPP levels are less affected by concomitant infection and are not affected by growth spurts and so may be a preferable method of diagnosing iron deficiency during childhood.

Usually one confirmatory test is adequate to confirm the diagnosis. In difficult cases, more investigations will be required and direct assessment of marrow iron stores may be needed. In others a trial of iron therapy may be useful. A dose of 3 mg/kg of elemental ferrous sulfate for 1 month should increase the hemoglobin of an iron-deficient subject by at least 1.0 g/dL in 4 weeks.[76] As long as the patient is compliant with iron therapy, failure to respond to a therapeutic trial excludes iron deficiency as the cause of anemia.

Differential diagnosis

The various causes of the hypochromic anemias are set out schematically in Fig. 5.6. Any process interfering with the formation or rate of production of hemoglobin will induce a reduction in mean red cell hemoglobin with resultant hypochromia of the red cells. The development of hypochromia is often associated with concomitant red cell microcytosis. A full clinical history, with particular reference to the age and racial origin of the child, birth history, any abnormal bleeding and, most importantly, a detailed assessment of

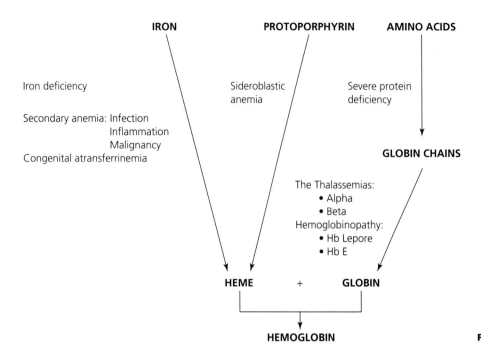

Fig. 5.6 Causes of the hypochromic anemias.

dietary intake, is essential to ensure the correct diagnosis of the cause of iron deficiency.

In most cases the differentiation between iron deficiency, secondary anemia, or a thalassemia trait is not difficult. However, it is not unusual for these conditions to coexist. Asian toddlers have a high incidence of iron deficiency but also commonly carry α- or β-thalassemia genes. In patients whose MCV improves but does not return to normal after an apparently adequate course of iron, thalassemia traits should be excluded.

In childhood, trivial viral infections are very common. These infections may falsely elevate iron and ferritin estimations and so can lead to diagnostic confusion. It is important to repeat any abnormal test results after the patient has recovered. Within a few weeks of recovery, any red cell abnormalities caused by infection should have returned to normal.

Although dietary iron deficiency is the predominant cause of iron deficiency anemia in children, abnormal blood loss must be considered in all patients. Worldwide, intestinal worm infections are the commonest cause of iron deficiency anemia due to blood loss. Hookworm infections with *Necator americanus* and *Ancylostoma duodenale* predominate but whipworm infection with *Trichuris trichiura* are also common. However, both these types of parasitic worms are mainly found in hot climates and are only likely to be seen in travellers to the tropics or in recently arrived immigrants. In the temperate regions of northern Europe, parasitic iron deficiency is uncommon and bleeding from a Meckel diverticulum, intestinal polyps, or peptic ulceration have to be considered as possible causes of iron deficiency secondary to intestinal hemorrhage.

Renal tract bleeding is usually obvious and is reported immediately by the patient or parent. However, pulmonary hemorrhage is sometimes less obvious, either because of chronic loss of iron into pulmonary macrophages (as seen in chronic pulmonary hemosiderosis) or because there is confusion as to whether the blood is coming from the upper airway or the gastrointestinal tract.

Although generally an idiopathic condition, *chronic pulmonary hemosiderosis* is occasionally associated with other disorders such as celiac disease and Goodpasture syndrome.[77,78] This rare condition affects predominantly children. It is characterized by repeated intraalveolar microhemorrhages, with the lost blood being taken up by pulmonary macrophages. The iron taken up by these macrophages is not recycled and over a period of time the patient becomes increasingly iron deficient. Pulmonary fibrosis develops and, if untreated, patients develop a severe restrictive lung defect with a significant degree of pulmonary arterial shunting. Chest radiography is often abnormal and diagnosis is made from the presence of iron-laden macrophages in bronchiolar lavage fluid. Limited successes with chloroquine,[79] cyclophosphamide,[80] and a combination of prednisolone and azathiaprine[81] have been reported but for most patients the outlook is poor.

Malabsorption syndromes need to be considered, especially in patients with symptoms suggestive of diarrhea, abdominal distension, and failure to thrive. This is in stark contrast to the toddler with excessive cows' milk intake, who is usually distinctly well-rounded.

Failure to respond to iron is usually due to failure to comply with therapy. However in some cases the diagnosis of iron deficiency will be incorrect. In addition to the common secondary anemias and thalassemia syndromes, there is a variety of inherited rare syndromes that may need to be considered such as congenital atransferrinemia or one of the sideroblastic anemias.

Inherited disorders of iron metabolism

Inherited disorders of iron metabolism are extremely rare. They are characterized by iron-deficient erythropoiesis with absent marrow iron stores despite the absorption of excessive quantities of iron into other tissues such as the heart and liver.

Congenital atransferrinemia[31]

Congenital absence of TF is an autosomal recessive disorder. Affected infants present at birth with a severe microcytic hypochromic anemia with a low serum iron and TIBC. Plasma TF is absent. The anemia does not respond to iron but transfusion with plasma can induce a reticulocyte response. Treatment is with blood transfusion and TF.[82]

Although bone marrow iron is absent, iron is absorbed from the gastrointestinal tract and deposited in the liver, pancreas, heart, and kidneys. One affected child died from the effects of myocardial hemosiderosis. Therefore, TF does not appear to be required for the release and transport of iron from the intestinal mucosal cells. However, the absence of TF prevents iron transport to the erythron.

Congenital microcytic hypochromic anemia with iron overload

Two sets of siblings have been described with a severe microcytic hypochromic anemia despite fully saturated TIBC and an increased serum iron.[83,84] Liver parenchymal cells contained excess iron and there was associated fibrosis. No iron was present in liver macrophages or the bone marrow, suggesting a functional defect of the transfer of iron to red cell precursors and macrophages.

Other syndromes

Three siblings have been described with a microcytic hypochromic anemia apparently due to an isolated abnormality of malabsorption and defective utilization of iron.[85] A single patient has also been described as having reduced iron incorporation into red cell precursors in the presence of a raised serum iron caused by an IgM autoantibody to TFR.[86]

Effects of iron deficiency

Anemia

Classically, there are four stages in the development of dietary iron deficiency.[76]
• Iron sufficiency: no anemia, red blood cells normal in number, microscopic appearance, size and biochemistry in the presence of adequate body iron stores.

• Iron deficiency: no anemia, red blood cells normal but iron stores are depleted with a low serum ferritin.
• Iron-deficient erythropoiesis: no anemia, iron stores depleted and abnormal red cells as demonstrated by a low MCV and abnormal biochemistry, i.e., raised ZPP.
• Iron-deficiency anemia: as above but with coexisting anemia.
However, as discussed above, during periods of rapid growth, children have reduced iron stores but with iron-sufficient erythropoiesis. So it is often difficult to assess a child with a low serum ferritin but a normal full blood count. Perhaps the best approach is to take a dietary history and give advice to improve dietary iron content if appropriate. It is also critical to evaluate the hemoglobin level found in the patient with the reference value for the child's age (see Chapter 37).

In most cases there is no difficulty in making the diagnosis. Dietary iron deficiency leads to a slow onset of anemia and the majority of toddlers present with a moderate to severe reduction of hemoglobin. Patients with abnormal bleeding will become symptomatic depending on the rate of blood loss. As for dietary-deficient toddlers, the peripheral blood changes are usually very obvious, with anemia, reduced MCV and MCH, and a raised red cell distribution width. The blood film is hypochromic and microcytic with pencil-shaped cells and occasional target red cells. Mild thrombocytosis of $500-700 \times 10^9$/L is often present. The etiology of the increase in platelets is unclear but the platelet count returns to normal with appropriate treatment of the iron deficiency.

The presence of symptoms depends on the degree of anemia and its rate of onset. Symptoms become more likely as the hemoglobin drops below 7 g/dL but many of the toddlers will have few if any symptoms despite often having much lower levels of hemoglobin than this. Children will often present with pallor, which has sometimes been missed by the usual carers and only noticed by a relative who has not seen the child for some time, reflecting the insidious onset of the anemia. Irritability is usual with excessive crying; less often there is a history of pica.

The clinical history is all-important in making the correct diagnosis as to the underlying cause of the iron deficiency. Physical signs other than pallor are unusual. The presence of abnormal bruising may suggest the presence of a bleeding diathesis, while telangiectasia of the mucous membranes of the mouth and lip or on the underside of the lower eyelid would point to a diagnosis of hereditary hemorrhagic telangiectasia. Nail abnormalities such as koilonychias are not often seen in children.

Growth and development

There is good evidence that iron deficiency, even in the absence of frank anemia, is associated with impaired testing of psychomotor function and reduced scholastic achievement.[87–91] Experiments in young rats have confirmed that iron deficiency during the early stages of development produces reversible changes in neurotransmitters and neural lipids and a permanent reduction in brain iron concentration.[92–98] Studies to determine whether treatment with iron can reverse the effects of iron deficiency in the developing human brain have produced variable results.[99,100] However there is no doubting the clinical transformation from an irritable listless child to a happy active toddler that is so often seen even in the first few weeks of iron therapy.

Growth is also affected. Even taking into account the poor overall nutrition prevalent in iron-deficient populations, treatment with iron has been shown to reverse the detrimental effects on growth.[101]

Although there remain gaps in our knowledge, iron deficiency must be taken very seriously especially in the first few years of life when neurodevelopment is as yet incomplete. Treatment needs to be effective, aggressively implemented, and followed up diligently to ensure compliance so that any avoidable neurologic damage might be prevented.

Management

Iron deficiency should be considered as a symptom and not as a specific disease entity *per se*. A thorough clinical history is an essential part of the assessment and management of the iron-deficient child. The extent of investigation required will depend on the age of the child and the patient's medical history. Where abnormal blood loss is suspected, technetium scanning for ectopic gastric mucosa in a Meckel diverticulum or endoscopy of the gastrointestinal tract may be an essential part of the patient's investigation. However, the majority of children with iron deficiency will be between 1 and 3 years of age with a generally poor diet and a history of excessive cows' milk intake. Some will have been born prematurely or with a low birthweight.

For all children the underlying cause needs to be found and treatment directed to this and not just to the prescription of iron, which will only temporarily improve the hemoglobin concentration. In most cases appropriate dietary advice will be necessary.

Prevention

Primary prevention, which aims to prevent the development of iron deficiency altogether, is an extremely important public health issue. Very many children are affected by iron deficiency and at a very early age before the nervous system has fully developed, at a time when it is potentially vulnerable to the effects of iron deficiency. Health education needs to be aimed at persuading mothers of young children of the benefits of breast-feeding in the first few months of life followed by appropriate weaning schedules. Infant formulary milk is already fortified with iron, as are many preprepared infant foods and cereals. In particular, mothers need to be

Table 5.7 Prevalence of iron deficiency anemia in UK toddlers.

Reference	Age (months)	Subject details	Reduction in Hb (percent < 11 g/dL)
60	15	Asian	39
		White	16
		Afro-Carribean	20
87	12–24	Mixed inner city	25 (<10.5 g/dL)
101	18	Inner city	26
102	12	Asian	26
		Non-Asian	12
103	18	Formula: iron fortified	2
		Cows' milk	33
104	15	Formula: iron fortified	0
		Formula: not iron fortified	9
	18	Formula: iron fortified	0
		Formula: not iron fortified	15
105	22	Asian	31
106	8–24	Asian	16
		White	9
107	18–29	National sample	12
	30–41		6
108	15	Formula: iron fortified	11
		Formula: not iron fortified	13
		Cows' milk	33

made aware of the dangers of excess cows' milk in the toddler diet, the primary cause of most early iron deficiency.

The evidence for a high incidence of iron deficiency in UK toddlers is incontrovertible (Table 5.7).[60,87,101–108] The impetus for systematic screening of young children in order to detect and treat iron deficiency early (i.e., secondary prevention) is increasing. Particularly as many clinical studies have demonstrated the potential reversibility of the neurologic effects of iron deficiency, there is increasing interest in screening for iron deficiency in early childhood. However, much work needs to be done to determine the best timing and most appropriate diagnostic methods.

Clinical management

1 Diagnosis: full blood count, blood film, confirmatory test of iron deficiency (i.e., ZPP).
2 Assessment of underlying cause: dietary history, birth history, presence of abnormal bleeding, family history, past medical/surgical history.
3 Investigation and treatment of any underlying cause found: dietary advice, scan for Meckel diverticulum, endoscopy.
4 Iron therapy.

Iron therapy

Oral iron

Elemental iron should be prescribed in a dose of 3 mg/kg up to a daily maximum of 180 mg, usually given as two divided doses. To avoid accidental iron overdosage, parents or guardians should be warned of the dangers of medicinal iron and all preparations should be kept in childproof containers and out of the reach of young children. The following preparations provide 3 mg of iron:

- 15 mg of ferrous sulfate;
- 9 mg of ferrous fumarate;
- 26 mg of ferrous gluconate;
- 9 mg of ferrous succinate;
- 17 mg of ferrous glycine sulfate;
- 21 mg of sodium iron edetate.

Note that adult preparations contain too much elemental iron and are unsuitable for young children.

Failure to respond to oral iron preparations is not uncommon and usually represents poor compliance. In most cases a change of preparation and impressing on the parent or carer the importance of adequate treatment, particularly with regard to neurodevelopmental problems, is all that is necessary to ensure an improved response. However, it is important to be aware that failure to respond or an incomplete response may be because the initial diagnosis of iron deficiency was incorrect or may indicate the coexistence of another abnormality such as a thalassemia trait.

All patients must be followed up until the blood count has returned to normal. After that time a further 3 months of treatment should be given to build up body iron stores. Ideally all patients should be checked again 6 months later to ensure that there has been no recurrence of the iron deficiency. Any recurrence needs to be investigated and the reason elucidated. In many cases the dietary advice given at diagnosis will not have been followed and needs to be reiterated. In others the possibility of underlying occult blood loss needs to be reconsidered.

Parenteral iron

Parenteral iron preparations are rarely indicated for the treatment of childhood iron deficiency and must only be considered if the diagnosis of iron deficiency is absolutely certain. The indications for parenteral iron preparations are:

- demonstrated intolerance to oral preparations;
- where there is a need to deliver iron rapidly to iron stores;
- in active inflammatory bowel disease where there is intolerance to oral iron;
- where there is demonstrated patient noncompliance with oral iron with a definite diagnosis of iron deficiency;
- where follow-up of the patient is impossible.

Contraindications for parenteral iron preparations include:

- anemias not due to iron deficiency;
- iron overload;
- history of hypersensitivity to parenteral iron preparations;
- history of severe allergy or anaphylactic reactions;
- clinical or biochemical evidence of liver damage;
- acute or chronic infection;
- neonates.

Only the intramuscular preparation containing iron, sorbitol, and citric acid (Jectofer) is licensed for use in children above 3 kg in weight. However some pediatricians are using the intravenous iron sucrose preparation Venofer, which has yet to be fully licensed for use in pediatrics.

The majority of children with iron deficiency are toddlers with inadequate diets. These children can be managed in the primary care setting in collaboration with the local hematology laboratory. However, all other children with iron deficiency need to be assessed in the hospital setting, where the full diagnostic facilities required are readily available. All cases without an obvious underlying cause for the iron deficiency and those who fail to respond as expected to therapy should be referred to a pediatric hematologist.

Sideroblastic anemias

The sideroblastic anemias are a heterogeneous group of disorders characterized by variable red cell hypochromia, anemia, and the presence of a significant number of ringed sideroblasts in the marrow. By definition, the ringed sideroblasts should total 10% or more of the nucleated red cell precursors.[109] Diagnostic ringed sideroblasts contain six or more siderotic granules arranged in a perinuclear collar around one-third or more of the erythroblast nucleus. These perinuclear granules consist of iron-laden mitochondria.[110]

All forms are characterized by failure to utilize iron properly during home synthesis in the mitochondria. Iron accumulates within the mitochondria and eventually adversely affects mitochondrial function. Premature erythroblast cell death follows, resulting in ineffective erythropoiesis.

The classification of the sideroblastic anemias is shown in Table 5.8. All forms of sideroblastic anemia are rare in childhood.[111] The congenital forms are occasionally encountered but the acquired forms are much less commonly seen in children than in adults.

Congenital sideroblastic anemias

Etiology

In most families affected by sideroblastic anemia, inheritance is X-linked and may be associated with the coinheritance of other X-linked traits such as glucose 6-phosphate dehydrogenase deficiency[112] or ataxia.[113] Female carriers may show minor changes with a variable population of circulating hypochromic red cells; the size of the hypochromic population in female carriers is probably dependent on random

Table 5.8 Classification of the sideroblastic anemias.

Congenital
Primary X-linked
Primary autosomal
Pearson syndrome
Stoddart variant
DIDMOAD or Wolfram syndrome
Syndromes of increased erythropoietic protoporphyrins

Acquired
Primary idiopathic also called refractory anemia with excess ringed sideroblasts (RARS; one of the myelodysplasias)

Secondary acquired
  Drugs: isoniazid, chloramphenicol
  Toxins: alcohol (chronic abuse), lead
  Copper deficiency
  Zinc excess
Diseases sometimes associated with an excess of ringed sideroblasts
  Hemolytic anemias
  Megaloblastic anemias
  Myeloid malignancies
  Autoimmune disorders

X-chromosome inactivation (lyonization). In some cases where lyonization is extreme, females are more severely affected.[114] In other families, females are affected because the sideroblastic anemia is inherited as an autosomal trait.[115,116]

Molecular basis (see Fig. 5.3)

The first step in the synthesis of heme from glycine and succinyl-CoA is catalyzed by ALAS in the presence of pyridoxal phosphate. Two types of ALAS exist in the body: one is a ubiquitous enzyme found in all tissues and is coded for by a gene on chromosome 3; the other is expressed by a gene on the X chromosome and is specific to erythroid cells.[117] This explains why most cases of inherited sideroblastic anemia are X-linked and why the synthesis of heme proteins other than hemoglobin is unaffected.

ALAS requires the presence of pyridoxal phosphate as a coenzyme to initiate mitochondrial heme production efficiently. In some cases of inherited X-linked sideroblastic anemia, mutant ALAS enzymes have been demonstrated.[118] Theoretically, pyridoxine in pharmacologic doses could act to improve the enzyme activity of a mutant ALAS in several ways and thereby improve the production of heme. It could stabilize the quaternary structure of mutant ALAS and thereby improve enzyme activity.[119] In other situations, pyridoxine might protect mutant ALAS from premature degradation by mitochondrial proteases.[119] Finally, the mutant enzyme might require a higher concentration of pyridoxal phosphate than is usually necessary to promote normal activity.[120]

In other families with sideroblastic anemia, defects of ferrochelatase and copro-oxidase have been described.[121,122] Copro-oxidase does not have pyridoxal phosphate as a cofactor, so these patients would not be expected to respond to pyridoxine therapy. In other patients, multiple or ill-defined enzyme deficiencies interfere with mitochondrial function and heme synthesis.[123] Some of these patients may respond to pyridoxine, others will not. Nevertheless, in all cases of inherited sideroblastic anemia a trial of pyridoxine therapy is indicated.[124]

Diagnosis

Most cases present in infancy or early childhood but less severe forms may pass unnoticed until adulthood. Some patients are discovered during routine testing of close relatives of a suspected patient. Others present late with the clinical effects of iron-overload liver disease, diabetes mellitus, or heart failure. Late presentation with iron over-load most often occurs in cases where anemia is mild or occasionally in female carriers. Examination is usually normal except for pallor but splenomegaly or hepatomegaly may be present.

Investigation reveals microcytosis with a variable degree of anemia. The microcytosis can be severe and an MCV of 50 fL can be seen in the more anemic patients. A novel form of macrocytic hereditary sideroblastic anemia was recently described.[125] The characteristic red cell dimorphism is most marked in cases with milder anemia and in female carriers. This can be detected by microscopic examination of the blood film or mechanically from erythrocyte volume distribution curves or red cell maps depending on the type of blood counter technology used. Serum iron and ferritin are elevated and TIBC reduced.

The dimorphic blood picture, raised serum iron, raised serum ferritin, and reduced TIBC may be confused with partially treated iron deficiency anemia, particularly as many patients will have already received iron, blood transfusions, or both. However, free erythrocyte porphyrins are normal and help to distinguish partially treated iron deficiency. Levels of protoporphyrin are reduced and coproporphyrin levels remain normal.

Other nonspecific abnormalities are often present, i.e., mild hyperbilirubinemia and reduced haptoglobins in the presence of a normal or only slightly increased reticulocytosis. Iron staining of peripheral blood will demonstrate circulating red cells that contain iron-laden mitochondrial remnants (Pappenheimer bodies). However, definitive diagnosis is most often made following microscopic examination of a bone marrow aspirate. Iron staining reveals the presence of large numbers of pathologic ringed sideroblasts. In inherited sideroblastic anemia, the ringed sideroblasts are predominantly seen in the late erythroblast population.

Table 5.9 Differentiation of hereditary from primary acquired sideroblastic anemia.

	Hereditary	Acquired
Red blood cell size	Microcytic	Macrocytic or normocytic
Ringed sideroblasts	Late erythroblasts	Early erythroblasts
Free red blood cell porphyrins	Normal	Increased
Red blood cell coproporphyrins	Normal	Increased
Marrow chromosomes	Normal	Abnormal in 60%
Relatives	Often abnormal	Normal

Differential diagnosis

Initial confusion with partially treated iron deficiency anemia will be clarified following iron staining of a bone marrow aspirate. It is important to consider performing a bone marrow aspirate in infants, especially males with unexplained iron deficiency anemia, or where investigation of microcytosis fails to elucidate a cause for the reduction in red cell size, particularly if the MCV has remained low despite iron therapy.

Once significant (>10%) numbers of ringed sideroblasts have been demonstrated, inherited sideroblastic anemia has to be differentiated from acquired disorders associated with the presence of excess ringed sideroblasts in the marrow (see Table 5.8). It is usually possible to differentiate inherited sideroblastic anemia from the primary acquired form on clinical grounds alone. In cases where there is uncertainty, laboratory findings will allow differentiation (Table 5.9). Red cell macrocytosis, raised red cell porphyrins, and the presence of marrow chromosomal abnormalities are particularly helpful. Investigation of close relatives is important as it helps to identify cases of inherited sideroblastic anemia and at the same time permits quantification of iron loading in asymptomatic siblings and carriers.

Other rare inherited disorders presenting in childhood can be associated with the presence of significant numbers of ringed sideroblasts in the marrow. Pearson *et al.*[126] have described a syndrome of refractory anemia presenting in early childhood as a severe transfusion-dependent normocytic or macrocytic anemia with reticulocytopenia. Neutropenia is usually present and a variable thrombocytopenia is common. Examination of the marrow reveals prominent degenerative cytoplasmic vacuolation in both erythroid and granulocytic precursors. Iron stores are markedly increased and ringed sideroblasts are prominent. The disease is not limited to the bone marrow; marked fibrosis of the exocrine pancreas was found at post-mortem examination of two children with the syndrome who died in the first 3 years of life, and three less severely affected children also showed *in vivo* evidence of abnormal pancreatic function. Pearson anemia probably represents a disorder of multiorgan cellular mitochondrial

dysfunction. A possible variant of Pearson anemia with early onset of severe pancytopenia and thyroid fibrosis has been described.[127]

Two children with DIDMOAD syndrome (Wolfram syndrome)[128] have been described as having a megaloblastic and sideroblastic anemia.[129] The patients were first cousins and both demonstrated a response to thiamine, with improvement in anemia and associated neutropenia and thrombocytopenia. Insulin requirements also reduced significantly following the introduction of thiamine therapy. The authors speculated that DIDMOAD syndrome might be a multisystem degenerative disorder caused by an inherited abnormality of thiamine metabolism.

Three reports have been published describing sideroblastic anemia in the presence of excess erythrocyte protoporphyrins.[130–132] These cases share some similarities with erythropoietic porphyria; two patients had skin photosensitivity and one developed liver disease with increased hepatic protoporphyrins.

Although primary acquired sideroblastic anemia is very unusual in childhood, secondary acquired cases do occur (see Table 5.8). A full drug history needs to be taken. Some drugs, like isoniazid, act as pyridoxine inhibitors; others like chloramphenicol may inhibit mitochondrial protein synthesis by interfering with ferrochelatase activity.

Lead toxicity is not uncommon in preschool children[133] and it can be associated with anemia and ringed sideroblasts in the marrow. Acute lead intoxication usually presents as lead encephalopathy with anemia as a late manifestation. However, chronic lead poisoning often coexists with iron deficiency and consequent microcytic anemia. Basophilic stippling, a precipitation of RNA and mitochondrial fragments, is often prominent on the blood film.[134] Lead binds to the red blood cell membrane and is absorbed into the red cell, interfering with several enzymes including ferrochelatase that are involved with heme synthesis.[135] Iron, heme intermediates, and ZPPs accumulate inside the red cells. An increase in free erythrocyte protoporphyrins is a useful screening test for lead poisoning and also helps to differentiate lead toxicity from sideroblastic anemia.[136] Diagnosis is confirmed by estimation of blood lead concentration. Treatment is based on the removal of the sources of lead ingestion and dual chelation therapy with dimercaprol (BAL) and calcium EDTA.[137]

Ringed sideroblasts may also be seen with abnormalities of other metals and occur in copper deficiency and zinc overload. Copper deficiency is only seen in malnourished premature babies[138] and in patients receiving long-term parenteral nutrition with inadequate copper supplementation.[139] Copper is absorbed almost exclusively during the last trimester and deficiency in a premature infant may be accentuated if the child is given copper-deficient feeds such as cows' milk at an early age. Early severe copper deficiency presents as a hypochromic anemia and neutropenia.

Examination of the marrow reveals ringed sideroblasts, vacuolation of erythroid and granulocytic precursors, and granulocytic maturation arrest. More chronic cases produce osteoporosis, depigmentation of the skin and hair, and central nervous system changes. The diagnosis is made by demonstrating a low serum copper and ceruloplasmin. The effects of copper deficiency are quickly reversed by daily treatment with 2–5 mg of copper sulfate orally or by the addition of 100–500 μg of copper to intravenous feeds. In excess, zinc interferes with copper absorption and can cause a secondary copper deficiency.[140] A high serum zinc is associated with low serum copper and ceruloplasmin levels. Discontinuation of zinc ingestion will reverse the changes over 2–3 months.

Other causes of secondary sideroblastic anemia are much commoner in adults than children. Ringed sideroblasts are only occasionally found in the marrows of children with myelodysplastic syndromes other than primary acquired sideroblastic anemia (refractory anemia with ringed sideroblasts). They can also rarely be seen in cases of acute myeloid leukemias. Careful examination of the marrow will distinguish these from primary inherited sideroblastic anemia. Significant numbers of ringed sideroblasts can sometimes be seen in juvenile rheumatoid arthritis,[141] and a single case of an antibody-mediated acquired sideroblastic anemia has been reported.[142]

Management

Between 25 and 50% of patients with hereditary sideroblastic anemia show some response to oral pyridoxine. A trial of pyridoxine 25–100 mg three times a day for 3 months is indicated in all patients. Response is variable and in many cases the MCV remains abnormal and residual microcytic hypochromic cells can be seen on the blood film. Responders should continue pyridoxine for life but because pyridoxine can produce a peripheral neuropathy, the dose should be titrated to the lowest daily dose that maintains response.[143] In one report, a patient who had not responded to oral pyridoxine responded to parenteral pyridoxal 5′-phosphate.[144] Folic acid supplements should also be given.

The majority of patients do not respond to pyridoxine and require regular blood transfusions that further increase iron overload. Strict adherence to chelation therapy with deferoxamine (desferrioxamine) is essential for long-term survival.

Mildly affected patients and even some female carriers may eventually develop symptoms of iron toxicity as a result of excess absorption from the diet.[145] These patients should be carefully monitored for excess iron deposition. If this is detected, most patients will tolerate therapeutic venesection to remove iron from the body.[146]

Splenectomy should be avoided, as it is associated with a high incidence of thromboembolism and persistent postoperative thrombocytosis.

Acquired sideroblastic anemias

Those occurring in childhood have been described above in the differential diagnosis of the inherited sideroblastic anemias.

Primary acquired idiopathic sideroblastic anemia/refractory anemia

Primary acquired idiopathic sideroblastic anemia is one of the myelodysplastic syndromes, refractory anemia with ringed sideroblasts (RARS).[147] RARS is usually a disease of the elderly and is seen only rarely in childhood. However, with the increasingly successful use of powerful chemotherapy and radiotherapy to treat pediatric malignancies, secondary forms of RARS may begin to be seen in pediatric practice.

In adults, RARS has a relatively benign course, with a 50-month median survival and about a 10% incidence of leukemic progression.[148] The more malignant forms are associated with marrow clonal chromosomal abnormalities other than trisomy 8, which has no adverse prognostic significance. However, monosomy 7 or partial deletion of the long arm of chromosome 7 in particular have a poor prognosis with an increased risk of leukemic transformation. Other factors associated with a poorer outcome are anemia requiring regular transfusions and hence early iron overload and the presence of associated neutropenia and/or thrombocytopenia. It is likely that the same factors are relevant to children as well.

In general, myelodysplasias occurring in children should be treated aggressively (see Chapter 4). If differentiation from inherited sideroblastic anemia is certain, and particularly in the presence of poor prognostic indicators, bone marrow transplantation should be considered early in the course of the disease. If a conservative approach is taken, patients must be closely monitored for iron overload and progression to more advanced types of myelodysplasia or frank leukemia.

Iron overload

Acute overdose

Accidental overdose is not uncommon, particularly in preschool children. A 1990 study of 339 cases found that 83.9% occurred in children under 6 years old.[149] This is because iron tablets look like sweets and are often available in the home because the child's mother is pregnant and has been prescribed iron supplements. Toxicity is directly related to the dose ingested. Doses > 60 mg/kg are likely to induce serious toxicity and ingestion of > 180 mg/kg may prove fatal.

Acute iron poisoning can be divided into four phases.

1 The patient experiences nausea and vomiting, abdominal

pain, and diarrhea due to irritation of the gastrointestinal tract. In some cases, ulceration can occur in the upper gastrointestinal tract during this phase with hematemesis and melena.

2 The patient appears to be well. Most recover at this stage but a minority progress to the third phase.

3 The patient develops iron encephalopathy, with fits and fluctuating conscious level, shock, metabolic acidosis, and acute renal tubular and hepatic necrosis.

4 Those that recover may go on to develop high intestinal obstruction with strictures, usually in the pyloric region. This fourth phase most often occurs in children 2–6 weeks after apparent recovery.

Treatment also depends on the amount of iron ingested. Where there is doubt about how many tablets, if any, have been taken, plain abdominal radiography may help to confirm significant overdose because iron tablets are radiopaque.

Serious toxicity occurs when the ability of TF and apoferritin to mop up the excess iron is exceeded. This is usually seen when serum iron is > 90 µmol/L and the TIBC is overwhelmed and toxic free iron oxy-radicals are generated. Guidelines suggest that when > 20 mg/kg has been ingested, gastric lavage should be performed.[150] If the patient is too young or cannot tolerate this procedure, an emetic should be administered. Patients who have taken > 40 mg/kg or an intentional overdose should be admitted for observation following lavage. In cases of significant overdose, deferoxamine should be given orally to prevent further absorption from the gastrointestinal tract and parenterally to remove iron already absorbed.

Chronic iron overload

The effects of chronic iron overload are most often seen in patients who have increased dietary iron absorption and/or are receiving regular blood transfusions. The extent of tissue damage is related to the total amount of iron absorbed, the speed of iron accumulation, and the distribution of iron in the body tissues. Iron stored in tissue macrophages appears to be relatively innocuous, whereas deposits in parenchymal cells are often associated with extensive tissue damage.

The mechanism producing cellular damage appears to be the same irrespective of the underlying cause of the iron overload. As tissue stores build up, the excess iron overwhelms the protective iron-binding proteins TF and ferritin. This allows increasing amounts of free non-TF-bound iron to exist as ionic iron in the plasma and tissues,[151] which promotes the production of free hydroxyl radicals. These oxy-radicals damage intracellular lipids, nucleic acids and proteins, disrupting intracellular organelles and breaking down intracellular lysosymes, which release hydrolytic enzymes into the cytosol and thereby cause further intracellular destruction. Cell death follows accompanied by pericellular necrosis and fibrosis.[152,153]

Table 5.10 Etiology of iron overload.

Increased gastrointestinal absorption
Hereditary hemochromatosis
Erythroid hyperplasia with ineffective erythropoiesis
    β-Thalassemia major
    β-Thalassemia intermedia
    Hemoglobin E/β-thalassemia
    Congenital dyserythropoietic anemias
    Pyruvate kinase deficiency
    Sideroblastic anemias
Atransferrinemias and other rare disorders of iron transport

Repeated red cell transfusions

Perinatal iron overload
Hereditary tyrosinemia (hypermethioninemia)
Zellweger syndrome (cerebrohepatorenal syndrome)
Neonatal hemochromatosis

Focal iron sequestration
Idiopathic hemochromatosis
Hallervorden–Spatz syndrome
Chronic hemoglobinuria

Etiology and distribution of abnormal iron deposition in the body

The clinical manifestations of iron overload differ according to the underlying disease process (Table 5.10).

In hereditary hemochromatosis, increased oral absorption causes a gradual increase in tissue iron and symptoms do not usually develop until middle age or later when total body iron stores have increased by 15–20 g.[154] Iron deposition is predominantly in parenchymal cells, initially in the liver but eventually affecting other organs.[155] In the rare cases presenting in childhood, the pattern of iron deposition is often more marked in the heart and thyroid.[156] In both the adult and pediatric forms, bone marrow macrophage iron deposition is unimpressive and may be absent.[157]

Excessive oral absorption of iron is also seen in the iron-loading anemias. These are the group of anemias associated with erythroid hyperplasia and ineffective erythropoiesis and include β-thalassemia major and intermedia, the congenital dyserythropoietic anemias, chronic hemolytic anemias, and some of the sideroblastic anemias. The iron distribution is similar to that seen in hereditary hemochromatosis and is predominantly in the parenchymal cells of the liver, spreading later to other organs. In some conditions such as β-thalassemia major, the increase in dietary iron absorption is of secondary importance to the iron deposition caused by the need for regular blood transfusions. In those conditions not requiring regular blood transfusions, increased oral iron absorption is the primary mechanism of iron overload. Although occurring more slowly than transfusion-related siderosis, this will eventually cause clinically significant tissue damage. Even patients with mild anemia can develop significant iron overload because the rate of iron deposition is not related to the severity of the underlying anemia.[145]

In transfusional iron overload, iron deposition occurs more quickly. Each unit of blood contains 200–250 mg of iron and most patients require > 200 mL/kg of blood annually, equivalent to about 200 mg/kg of iron each year.[158] Clinical symptoms usually appear when > 15 g of excess iron has been transfused. Initially, iron is stored in the marrow and reticuloendothelial macrophages, which have a storage capacity of about 10–15 g. When this storage capacity has been exceeded, parenchymal iron deposition occurs and tissue damage follows. Transfusional iron toxicity occurs relatively quickly. Iron-induced hepatic fibrosis has been detected in children under 3 years old.[159]

In the early stages of iron accumulation, histologic assessment of the pattern of iron deposition in the liver and bone marrow can help in differentiating the underlying cause. In advanced iron overload, however, the differences in tissue distribution disappear as iron deposition becomes more widespread.

Perinatal iron overload

Perinatal iron overload is rare and presumably occurs where the normal but poorly understood mechanisms for transferring iron from the maternal blood to the fetus via the trophoblast basement membrane and fetal endothelium fail to control entry of iron into the fetus.[160] Two distinct inherited disorders have been described. In hereditary tyrosinemia (hypermethioninemia), iron deposition is restricted to the liver, which is usually cirrhotic.[161] Pancreatic islet cell hyperplasia and renal abnormalities are also present. In Zellweger syndrome (cerebrohepatorenal syndrome), iron is deposited in the parenchymal cells of the liver, spleen, kidney, and lungs.[162]

The syndrome of neonatal hemochromatosis is less well defined and the underlying defect has not been identified.[163] In affected infants, iron is deposited in the parenchymal cells of the liver, heart, and endocrine organs but not in the bone marrow or spleen. Death usually occurs in the neonatal period from liver disease, which in some cases may precede widespread iron deposition.[164] The disorder may represent the common end stage of a group of disorders with different etiologies. In some cases an infective agent may be responsible; in others there is evidence of abnormal fetomaternal iron transport.

Focal iron overload

Focal sequestration of iron into the pulmonary alveolar macrophages occurs in idiopathic pulmonary hemosiderosis and in the basal ganglia of patients with the rare neurodegenerative disorder Hallervorden–Spatz syndrome.[165] In idiopathic pulmonary hemosiderosis, the iron sequestered in the

pulmonary macrophages is unavailable for iron metabolism and eventually iron deficiency anemia develops. The pathogenic role of the iron deposited in the central nervous system in Hallervorden–Spatz syndrome is uncertain. Renal hemosiderosis can occur in patients with chronic hemoglobinuria but is not associated *per se* with any renal dysfunction.

Clinical effects

Prior to the introduction of chelation therapy the clinical effects of iron overload presented in late childhood and the early teenage years in most regularly transfused patients. In hereditary hemochromatosis the slow rate of tissue iron overload usually delayed significant tissue damage until middle age or later. Generally, children developed normally during the first decade of life as long as adequate amounts of blood were transfused. In the second decade, patients often presented with growth failure and delayed or absent pubertal development. In the early teenage years, heart disease and abnormalities of liver function were commonly seen and a minority of patients developed hypothyroidism.[166] In the late teenage years, abnormalities of glucose tolerance and even diabetes mellitus occurred but the clinical picture was most often dominated by deteriorating heart disease that was frequently fatal before the age of 20.[167]

Iron chelation therapy has dramatically altered the clinical picture of iron overload. However, chelation regimens need to be strictly adhered to if they are to be effective, but unfortunately many patients fail to do so. In a study following variably chelated but regularly transfused thalassemic patients over a period of 21 years, the incidence of iron overload complications was still significant at 20 years of age; 30% had heart disease, 43% diabetes mellitus, 28% hypothyroidism, and 22% hypoparathyroidism. In patients older than 20, 60% had one or more iron-related, life-threatening complications.[168] The consequences of iron overload and the potential benefits of chelation therapy are shown in Table 5.11.

Heart

When total body iron is > 1 g/kg, significant amounts begin to be deposited in the myocardium and the conducting system of the heart.[158] In transfusional iron overload, the ECG changes of left ventricular hypertrophy and conduction defects may be detected by 10–12 years of age. Echocardiographic changes occur late in the disease process.[169] In inadequately chelated patients, cardiac disease is the commonest cause of death and may occur in the late teens.[167] Except in the rare childhood forms of hereditary hemochromatosis,[154] the cardiac effects of excessive iron deposition are only seen at a late stage of the illness in about 10–15% of the most seriously affected patients.

Liver

In hereditary hemochromatosis, iron is primarily deposited

Table 5.11 Complications of iron overload and the effect of chelation therapy.

Complication	Effect of chelation therapy	
	Protection	Reversibility of established disease
Liver	Yes	Yes
Heart	Yes	Yes
Endocrine		
Growth	Yes	Yes
Hypogonadism	Yes	No
Diabetes mellitus	Yes	No
Hypothyroidism	Yes	No
Hypoparathyroidism	Yes	No
Arthropathy	Unknown	
Infections	No (*Yersinia* seen with chelation therapy)	

in the parenchymal cells and so liver cell damage is initiated early and becomes clinically significant when the liver contains iron concentrations of about 5000 µg/g dry weight of liver.[170] However, because the development of iron overload in hemochromatosis is slow, liver disease usually takes decades to develop. In transfusional iron overload, iron is first deposited in the protective liver reticuloendothelial storage cells and about twice as much iron needs to be deposited in transfusional iron overload as in hereditary hemochromatosis before clinical problems develop.[171] Nevertheless, the rate of iron deposition in transfusional siderosis is so rapid that liver abnormalities can be detected within 2 years of initiating transfusion therapy.[172]

Hepatomegaly is detectable early followed by abnormal liver function tests. With further deposition parenchymal damage induces fibrosis, which may be present before 3 years of age.[159] Eventually, macronodular or mixed macronodular/micronodular cirrhosis develops. In adults with hemochromatosis the incidence of development of hepatoma in the cirrhotic liver is high.

In transfusional siderosis, liver disease was often multifactorial due to a high incidence of hepatitis B and C. Immunization of patients against hepatitis B and the introduction of effective screening tests for hepatitis B and C by the blood transfusion services have greatly reduced the incidence of viral hepatitis in these patients.

Endocrine system
Even well-transfused patients develop growth failure and hypogonadism in the second decade of life.[173] Poor pubertal growth in unchelated patients is probably caused by a combination of central hypogonadism[174] and reduced production

of insulin-like growth factor (IGF)-1.[175] Failure or delay of sexual development remains a problem for patients who do not fully comply with chelation regimens.

In one study a high incidence of abnormalities of glucose tolerance was demonstrated but frank diabetes mellitus only occurred in 6.5% of transfused unchelated thalassemics and usually not before 17 years of age. The incidence was higher in patients with a family history of diabetes.[176]

Hypothyroidism occurs in about 6% of unchelated thalassemics[166] and hypoparathyroidism in a similar number. Minor abnormalities of adrenal androgen secretion have also been described.

Joints
Arthropathy, particularly of large joints, is relatively common in older patients with hemochromatosis. It can also be seen at a younger age in a minority of patients with transfusional siderosis.[177]

Infections
The increased availability of iron may predispose to infection with a variety of bacteria and fungi, particularly *Yersinia enterocolitica* but also *Listeria monocytogenes*, *Escherichia coli*, *Vibrio vulnificus* and some *Candida* species.[178]

Management of iron overload

Iron chelation therapy

The introduction of effective iron chelation therapy has revolutionized the management of patients with iron overload disorders, and the problems of management of multiply transfused patients have shifted from detection and treatment of iron-induced organ damage to early detection and control of the unwanted effects of chelation. Modern pediatric practice is increasingly involved with the prevention rather than the management of iron overload (see Chapter 13 for details of iron chelation therapy).

Iron-loading anemias

Any condition associated with erythroid hyperplasia and ineffective erythropoiesis can be complicated by significant iron overload caused by increased gastrointestinal absorption. The degree of iron overload is not related to the degree of anemia and can occur even in those patients with little or no reduction in their hemoglobin concentration. The excess iron tends to be deposited in the parenchymal cells and so, as in hereditary hemochromatosis, tissue iron damage is initiated at an early stage of iron overload. Therefore, any patient with an iron-loading anemia needs to be monitored throughout life with intermittent estimations of serum ferritin. Any patient with a sustained significant rise in serum ferritin, especially if levels are continuing to increase, needs to be considered for treatment with therapeutic phlebotomy. Once significant iron overload has been confirmed, treatment should begin promptly as delay will only increase parenchymal tissue damage. For every 2 mL of blood venesected, approximately 1 mg of iron is removed from the body.

Despite being well tolerated by most patients with absent or mild anemia, phlebotomy should be initiated carefully. Between 5 and 10 mL/kg, up to a maximum of 500 mL, should be withdrawn per week, with the hemoglobin concentration and hematocrit checked prior to each venesection. As therapy continues there should be a progressive fall in serum ferritin. Eventually, serum iron and TIBC will return to normal when body iron stores become nearly depleted. Occasionally, serum iron may fall and the anemia become more severe in the presence of a persistently high serum ferritin. In this situation, suspending phlebotomy for a few weeks may allow iron to be mobilized from long-term iron stores, and then reintroduction of phlebotomy will be followed by further reductions in serum ferritin. When serum ferritin has become normal, weekly therapeutic phlebotomy should be discontinued. Thereafter, maintenance phlebotomy will be required every few weeks with the aim of keeping serum ferritin below 50 μg/L and TIBC normal.

A minority of patients cannot tolerate regular venesection, usually because of worsening anemia. They require regular transfusion to suppress erythropoiesis and hence reduce dietary iron absorption to normal and regular chelation therapy to remove the excess iron introduced by the transfused blood.

Patients on regular transfusion regimens

A regular transfusion regimen should not be introduced without proper consideration of the potential benefits for the patient and the risks involved. Iron chelation therapy is the crucial factor. Parents and patients must be educated about the effects of iron overload and the critical need for compliance with chelation. The physician in charge needs to have a comprehensive plan for the management of regular transfusion therapy and be able to carefully monitor the patient for the effects of iron overload and deferoxamine toxicity (see Chapter 13 for details of iron chelation therapy). The UK Thalassaemia Society has recently published the guideline document "Standards for the clinical care of children and adults with thalassemia in the UK: a full review of the necessary resources".[179] Although aimed at patients with β-thalassemia major, the basic principles are relevant to any child on long-term transfusion therapy.

Pretransfusion considerations (Table 5.12)
In all patients, the ultimate goal of transfusion therapy is to ensure normal growth and development and promote well-being.

Table 5.12 Preparations for the introduction of regular transfusion therapy.

State clinical aims

Plan regimen
    Type of red cells to be used
    Pretransfusion hemoglobin level
    Frequency of transfusion
    Logistics: who, when and where?
    Deferoxamine
        Initiation of therapy
        Initial dose
        Patient/parent training

Investigations
    Red cell antigen studies
    Baseline virology

Immunize against hepatitis B

In the hypoerythroblastic anemias, such as Diamond–Blackfan anemia, the only aim of therapy is to achieve the minimum hemoglobin concentration that ensures normal growth and development while preventing dyspnea and the other symptoms of clinical anemia. The appropriate level of pretransfusion hemoglobin will vary from patient to patient but in most at least 8 g/dL is necessary.

Those patients with anemias associated with erythroid hyperplasia and concomitant increase in iron absorption from the gastrointestinal tract also need regimens that promote normal growth and development. However, the regimen chosen for these patients must also adequately suppress marrow expansion and hypersplenism in order to prevent skeletal deformity and extramedullary hemopoiesis and at the same time reduce the excess absorption of dietary iron. In rare conditions such as pyruvate kinase deficiency, in which the oxygen dissociation curve is shifted to the right, relatively low levels of posttransfusion hemoglobin concentration may be adequate.[180] However, in the majority of patients, maintenance of a near-normal mean hemoglobin concentration is required.

Hypertransfusion regimens that aim for a trough hemoglobin of 9–10 g/dL are undoubtedly effective in preventing the physical effects of anemia and at the same time adequately suppress dietary iron absorption.[181] Supertransfusion regimens that aim for a higher pretransfusion hemoglobin of > 11 g/dL have been developed[182] but have not proven to be any more effective than hypertransfusion.[183]

Transfusions should aim to raise the patient's hemoglobin by about 4 g/dL and are given at 3 or 4 weekly intervals. Appropriately matched packed red cells with as long an expiry date as possible should be transfused. Attempts to improve the lifespan of transfused blood and hence increase the interval between transfusions by selecting out younger red cells from blood donations have been developed,[181] but in clinical practice these "neocytes" have been shown to prolong transfusion interval by only 13–16%.[184,185] Neocytes are about three times more expensive per unit and they increase donor exposure considerably. Leukocyte-depleted blood should be transfused to reduce the incidence of non-febrile transfusion reactions and to prevent the production of HLA antibodies, which is particularly important in patients who may at a later date be considered for bone marrow transplantation.

Logistic considerations are particularly important in pediatric patients. Children tolerate regular transfusion regimens better if they are treated in familiar surroundings by medical and nursing staff well known to them and who are skilled in the insertion of intravenous cannulae and the management of blood transfusions. Much of the pain associated with cannula insertion can be avoided by the use of topical anesthetic cream. Interference with schooling can be minimized with appropriate timing of outpatient appointments and by planning hospital visits well in advance. Schoolwork can be performed during hospitalization for transfusions.

The timing of the introduction of deferoxamine and the dose used is important. The side-effects of chelation therapy are most often seen when high doses are given before iron stores have significantly increased. A practical approach is to introduce deferoxamine when the serum ferritin is confirmed to be > 1000 μg/L. The serum ferritin should be maintained between 1000 and 2000 μg/L. The ratio of daily deferoxamine dose to serum ferritin should be assessed three to four times a year and should not exceed 0.025.

Prior to first transfusion, the patient's own red cell antigens should be identified, including full Rhesus genotype and Kell, Ss, Kidd, and Duffy types. It is not possible to transfuse fully matched red cells but units with the appropriate Rhesus and Kell type should be selected for routine use. If at a later date red cell antibodies develop, prior knowledge of the patient's own red cell antigens makes their identification much easier. Antibodies to these blood groups are particularly likely to complicate regular red cell transfusions in patients with sickle cell disease or β-thalassemia.[186]

Patients receiving regular blood transfusions need to be assessed at intervals to ensure that the aims of transfusion are being met and that the side-effects of iron overload or deferoxamine toxicity have not developed.

Hereditary hemochromatosis

The pediatrician is mainly involved with the screening of children for the possible inheritance of hemochromatosis rather than in treating established cases. However, hereditary hemochromatosis can in rare instances present in childhood, even in those as young as 2 years old.[157,187] Males and females are equally affected. The illness has a different clinical pattern in childhood from that seen in adults; the cardiac and gonadal consequences of iron overload predominate rather than the hepatic and pancreatic effects seen in adults.

Screening is best carried out using a combination of serum ferritin and TF saturation. If either or both of these are elevated, a confirmatory liver biopsy should be performed. Children presenting with idiopathic cardiomyopthy, hypogonadism, amenorrhea, diabetes mellitus, or arthritis should be tested to exclude hereditary hemochromatosis. Screening may need to be repeated at intervals in children at risk, as initial results may be normal in early childhood because the rate of iron overload occurs so slowly in most cases. Most often screening will be initiated following the diagnosis of hemochromatosis in an older relative. The gene for hereditary hemochromatosis has been mapped to the HLA class I region on chromosome 6,[188] and homozygotes and heterozygotes can be confidently diagnosed from HLA class I typing. Recently, a candidate gene, *HFE* (or HLA-H), has been identified and two FIFE mutations described.[189,190]

The treatment of iron overload in hereditary hemochromatosis is similar to that described above for the iron-loading anemias. The introduction of phlebotomy should not be delayed once diagnosis has been made. In cases where significant organ damage has occurred, iron chelation therapy may be required as well. When treatment is instituted at an early stage before significant organ damage has taken place, patients should have a normal life expectancy.[155]

References

1. Finch CA, Ragan HA, Dyer IA *et al.* Body iron loss in animals. *Proc Soc Exp Biol Med* 1986; **159**: 335.
2. Green R, Charlton R, Seftel H *et al.* Body iron excretion in man. *Am J Med* 1968; **45**: 336.
3. Finch CA, Huebers HA. Iron metabolism. *Clin Physiol Biochem* 1986; **4**: 5.
4. Committee on Iron Deficiency. Report of the American Medical Association Council on Foods and Nutrition. *JAMA* 1968; **203**: 407.
5. Finch CA, Cook JD, Labbe RF *et al.* Effect of blood donation on iron stores as evaluated by serum ferritin. *Blood* 1977; **50**: 441.
6. Cook JD, Lipschitz DA. Clinical measurements of iron absorption. *Clin Haematol* 1977; **6**: 567.
7. Turnbull AL, Cleton F, Finch CA. Iron absorption. IV. The absorption of hemoglobin iron. *J Clin Invest* 1962; **41**: 1898.
8. Finch CA, Huebers HA. Perspectives in iron metabolism. *N Engl J Med* 1982; **306**: 1520.
9. Weintraub LR, Weinstein MB, Huser HJ. Absorption of hemoglobin iron: the role of a heme-splitting substance in the intestinal mucosa. *J Clin Invest* 1968; **47**: 531.
10. Cook JD, Layrisse M, Martinez-Torres C *et al.* Food iron absorption measured by an extrinsic tag. *J Clin Invest* 1972; **51**: 805.
11. Hallberg L, Bjorn-Rasmussen E. Determination of iron absorption from whole diet: a new two-pool model using two radio-iron isotopes given as haem and and non-haem iron. *Scand J Haematol* 1972; **9**: 193.

12. Martinez-Torres C, Layrisse M. Nutritional factors in iron deficiency: food iron absorption. *Clin Haematol* 1973; **2**: 339.

13. Layrisse M, Martinez-Torres C, Roche M. The effect of interactions of various foods on iron absorption. *Am J Clin Nutr* 1968; **21**: 1175.

14. Disler PB, Lynch SR, Charlton RW *et al.* The effect of tea on iron absorption. *Gut* 1975; **16**: 193.

15. Callender ST, Marney SR, Warner GT. Eggs and iron absorption. *Br J Haematol* 1970; **19**: 657.

16. Crosby WH. Control of iron absorption by intestinal luminal factors. *Am J Clin Nutr* 1968; **21**: 1189.

17. McMillan JA, Oski FA, Lourie G *et al.* Iron absorption from human milk, simulated human milk and proprietary formulas. *Pediatrics* 1977; **60**: 896.

18. Saarinen UM, Siimes MA, Dallman PR. Iron absorption in infants: high bioavailability of breast milk iron is indicated by the extrinsic tag method of iron absorption and by the concentration of serum ferritin. *J Pediatr* 1977; **91**: 36.

19. Cook JD, Skikne BS. Intestinal regulation of body iron. *Blood Rev* 1987; **1**: 267.

20. Pootrakul P, Kitcharoen K, Yansukon P *et al.* The effect of erythroid hyperplasia on iron balance. *Blood* 1988; **71**: 1124.

21. Huebers HA, Huebers E, Csiba E *et al.* The significance of transferrin for intestinal iron absorption. *Blood* 1983; **61**: 283.

22. Idzerda RL, Huebers H, Finch CA, McKnight GS. Rat transferrin gene expression: tissue-specific regulation by iron deficiency. *Proc Natl Acad Sci USA* 1986; **83**: 3723.

23. Crosby WH. The control of iron balance by the intestinal mucosa. *Blood* 1963; **22**: 441.

24. Huebers HA, Finch CA. Transferrin: physiological behaviour and clinical implications. *Blood* 1984; **64**: 743.

25. Awai M, Brown EB. Clinical and experimental studies of the metabolism of I^{131}-labeled human transferrin. *J Lab Clin Med* 1963; **61**: 363.

26. Huerre C, Uzan G, Grzeschik K *et al.* The structural gene for transferrin (TF) maps to 3q21–qter. *Ann Genet* 1984; **27**: 5.

27. Rabin M, McClelland A, Kuhn L *et al.* Regional localisation of the human transferrin receptor gene to 3q26.2-qter. *Am J Hum Genet* 1985; **37**: 1112.

28. Bailey S, Evans RW, Garratt RC *et al.* Molecular structure of serum transferrin at 3.3-Å resolution. *Biochemistry* 1988; **27**: 5804.

29. Huebers J, Csiba E, Josephson B *et al.* Interaction of human diferric transferrin with reticulocytes. *Proc Natl Acad Sci USA* 1981; **78**: 621.

30. Morton AG, Tavill AS. The role of iron in the regulation of hepatic transferrin synthesis. *Br J Haematol* 1977; **36**: 383.

31. Goya N, Miyazaki S, Kodate S, Ushio B. A family of congenital atransferrinaemia. *Blood* 1972; **40**: 239.

32. McClelland A, Kuhn LC, Ruddle FH. The human transferrin receptor gene: genomic organisation and the complete primary structure of the receptor deduced from a cDNA sequence. *Cell* 1984; **39**: 267.

33. Saarinen UM, Siimes MA. Developmental changes in serum iron, total iron binding capacity, and transferrin saturation in infancy. *J Pediatr* 1977; **91**: 875.

34. Koeper MA, Dallman PR. Serum iron concentration and transferrin saturation in the diagnosis of iron deficiency in children: normal developmental changes. *J Pediatr* 1979; **91**: 870.

35. Iacopetta BJ, Morgan EH, Yeoh G. Transferrin receptors and iron uptake during erythroid cell development. *Biochim Biophys Acta* 1982; **687**: 204.

36. Aisen P, Listowski I. Iron transport and storage proteins. *Ann Rev Biochem* 1980; **49**: 357.

37. Worwood M. Ferritin in human tissues and serum. *Clin Haematol* 1982; **11**: 275.

38. Harrison PM, Andrews SC, Artymiuk PJ *et al.* Ferritin. In: Ponka P, Schulman HM, Woodworth RC (eds) *Iron Transport and Storage*. Boca Raton, FL: CRC Press, 1990, p. 81.

39. Munro H. The ferritin genes: their response to iron status. *Nutr Rev* 1993; **51**: 65.

40. Jacobs A, Worwood M. Ferritin in serum. Clinical and biochemical implications. *N Engl J Med* 1975; **292**: 951.

41. Herbert V. Anaemias. In: Paige DM (ed.) *Clinical Nutrition*, 2nd edn. St Louis: CV Mosby, 1988, p. 593.

42. Flowers CH, Skikne BS, Covell AM *et al.* The clinical measurement of serum transferrin receptor. *J Lab Clin Med* 1989; **114**: 368.

43. Skikne BS, Flowers CH, Cook JD. Serum transferrin receptor: a quantitative measure of tissue iron deficiency. *Blood* 1990; **75**: 1870.

44. Labbe RF, Reamer RL. Zinc protoporphyrin. *Semin Hematol* 1989; **26**: 40.

45. Brittenham GM, Danish EH, Harris JW. Assessment of bone marrow and body iron stores. *Semin Hematol* 1981; **18**: 194.

46. Brittenham GM, Farrell DE, Harris J *et al.* Magnetic susceptibility measurement of human iron stores. *N Engl J Med* 1982; **307**: 1671.

47. Leighton DM, Matthews R, de Campo M *et al.* Dual energy CT estimation of liver iron content in thalassaemic children. *Aust Radiol* 1988; **32**: 214.

48. Anderson LJ, Holden S, Davis B *et al.* Cardiovascular T2-star (T2*) magnetic resonance for the early diagnosis of myocardial iron overload. *Eur Heart J* 2001; **22**: 2171.

49. St Pierre TG, Clark PR, Cha-anusorn W *et al.* Non-invasive measurement and imaging of liver iron concentrations using proton magnetic resonance. *Blood* 2005; **105**: 855.

50. Anderson LJ, Wonke B, Prescott E *et al.* Comparisons of the effects of oral deferiprone and sub-cutaneous desferrioxamine on myocardial iron concentration and ventricular function in beta thalassemia major. *Lancet* 2002; **360**: 516.

51. Pippard MJ, Hoffbrand AV. Iron. In: Hoffbrand AV, Lewis SM (eds) *Postgraduate Haematology*, 3rd edn. London: Heinemann, 1989, pp. 82–97.

52. Irie S, Tavasolli M. Transferrin-mediated cellular iron uptake. *Am J Med Sci* 1987; **293**: 103.

53. Theil EC. The IRE (iron regulatory element) family: structures which regulate mRNA translation or stability. *Biofactors* 1993; **4**: 87.

54. Kennedy MC, Mende-Mueller L, Blondin GA *et al.* Purification and characterization of cytosolic aconitase from beef liver and its relationship to the iron responsive element binding protein. *Proc Natl Acad Sci USA* 1992; **89**: 11730.

55. Klausner RD, Rouault TA. A double life: cytosolic aconitase as a regulatory RNA binding protein. *Mol Biol Cell* 1993; **4**: 1.

56. Constable A, Quick S, Gray NK *et al.* Modulation of the RNA-binding activity of a regulatory protein by iron in-vitro:

switching between enzymatic and genetic function. *Proc Natl Acad Sci USA* 1992; **89**: 4554.

57. Leibold EA, Guo B. Iron-dependent regulation of ferritin and transferrin receptor expression by the iron-responsive element binding protein. *Annu Rev Nutr* 1992; **12**: 345.

58. Bhasker CR, Gurgeil G, Neupert B *et al.* The putative iron-responsive element in the human erythroid 5-aminolevulinate synthase mRNA mediates translational control. *J Biol Chem* 192; **268**: 12699.

59. May BK, Bhasker CR, Bawden MJ, Cox TC. Molecular regulation of 5-aminolevulinate synthase. Diseases related to heme synthesis. *Mol Biol Med* 1990; **7**: 405.

60. Marder E, Nicoll A, Polnay L, Shulman CE. Discovering anaemia at child health clinics. *Arch Dis Child* 1990; **65**: 892.

61. Dallman PR. Iron deficiency in the weanling. *Acta Paediatr Scand* 1986; **323** (suppl.): 59.

62. Childs F, Aukett MA, Darbyshire P *et al.* Does nutritional education work in preventing iron deficiency in the inner city? *Arch Dis Child* 1997; **76**: 144.

63. Singla PN, Chand S, Khanna S, Agarwal KN. Effect of maternal anaemia on the placenta and the newborn infant. *Acta Paediatr Scand* 1978; **67**: 645.

64. Lanzkowsky P. The influence of maternal iron-deficiency anaemia on the haemoglobin of the infant. *Arch Dis Child* 1961; **36**: 205.

65. Shott RJ, Andrews BF. Iron status of a medical high-risk populaton at delivery. *Am J Dis Child* 1972; **124**: 369.

66. Murray MJ, Murray AB, Murray NJ, Murray MB. The effect of iron status of Nigerian mothers on that of their infants at birth and 6 months, and on the concentration of iron in the breast milk. *Br J Nutr* 1978; **39**: 627.

67. Sturgeon P. Studies of iron requirements in infants. III. Influence of supplemental iron during normal pregnancy on mother and infant. B. The infant. *Br J Haematol* 1959; **5**: 45.

68. Rios E, Lipschitz DA, Cook JD, Smith NJ. Relationship of maternal and infant iron stores as assessed by determination of plasma ferritin. *Pediatrics* 1975; **55**: 694.

69. Widdowson EM, Spray CM. Chemical development *in utero*. *Arch Dis Child* 1951; **26**: 205.

70. Yao AC, Moinian M, Lind J. Distribution of blood between infant and placenta after birth. *Lancet* 1969; **ii**: 871.

71. Burman D. Iron requirements in infancy. *Br J Haematol* 1971; **19**: 657.

72. Finne PH, Halvorsen S. Regulation of erythropoiesis in the fetus and newborn. *Arch Dis Child* 1972; **47**: 683.

73. O'Brien RT, Pearson HA. Physiologic anemia of the newborn infant. *J Pediatr* 1971; **79**: 132.

74. Gorten MK. Iron metabolism in premature infants. III. Utilisation of iron as related to growth in infants with low birth weights. *Am J Clin Nutr* 1965; **17**: 322.

75. Galet S, Schulman HM, Bard H. The postnatal hypotransferrinemia of early preterm newborn infants. *Pediatr Res* 1976; **10**: 118.

76. Oski FA. Iron deficiency in infancy and childhood. *N Engl J Med* 1993; **329**: 190.

77. Bouros D, Panagou P, Rokkas T *et al.* Bronchoalveolar lavage findings in a young adult with idiopathic pulmonary hemosiderosis and celiac disease. *Eur Respir J* 1994; **7**: 1009.

78. van der Ent CK, Walencamp NJ, Donkerwolcke RA *et al.* Pulmonary haemosiderosis and immune complex glomerulonephritis. *Clin Nephrol* 1995; **43**: 339.

79. Bush A, Sheppard MN, Warner JO. Chloroquine in idiopathic pulmonary hemosiderosis. *Arch Dis Child* 1992; **67**: 625.

80. Colombo JL, Stolz SM. Treatment of life-threatening primary pulmonary hemosiderosis with cyclophosphamide. *Chest* 1992; **102**: 959.

81. Rossi GA, Balzano E, Battistini E *et al.* Long-term prednisolone and azathioprine treatment of a patient with idiopathic pulmonary hemosiderosis. *Pediatr Pulmonol* 1992; **13**: 176.

82. Schwick HG, Cap J, Goya N. Therapy of atransferrinaemia with transferrin. *J Clin Chem* 1978; **16**: 75.

83. Shahidi NT, Nathan DG, Diamond LK. Iron deficiency anaemia associated with an error of iron metabolism in two siblings. *J Clin Invest* 1964; **43**: 510.

84. Stavem P, Saltvedt E, Elgjo K, Rootwelt K. Congenital hypochromic microcytic anaemia with iron overload of the liver and hyperferraemia. *Scand J Haematol* 1973; **10**: 153.

85. Buchanan GR, Sheehan RG. Malabsorption and defective utilisation of iron in three siblings. *J Pediatr* 1981; **98**: 723.

86. Larrick JW, Human E. Acquired iron deficiency anemia caused by an antibody against the transferrin receptor. *N Engl J Med* 1984; **311**: 214.

87. Saarinen UM, Siimes MA. Serum ferritin in assessment of iron nutrition in healthy infants. *Acta Paediatr Scand* 1978; **67**: 741.

88. Parks YA, Wharton BA. Iron deficiency and the brain. *Acta Paediatr Scand* 1989; **361** (suppl.): 71.

89. de Andraca I, Castillo M, Walter T. Psychomotor development and behaviour in iron deficient anaemic infants. *Nutr Rev* 1997; **55**: 125.

90. Yager JY, Hartfield DS. Neurologic manifestations of iron deficiency in childhood. *Pediatr Neurol* 2002; **27**: 85.

91. Beard J. Iron deficiency alters brain development and functioning. *J Nutr* 2003; **133** (5 suppl. 1): 1468S.

92. Taylor EM, Crowe A, Morgan EH. Transferrin and iron intake by the brain: effects of altered iron status. *J Neurochem* 1991; **57**: 1584.

93. Dallman PR. Biochemical basis for the manifestations of iron deficiency. *Annu Rev Nutr* 1986; **6**: 13.

94. Larkin EC, Garratt BA, Rao GA. Relation of relative levels of nervonic to lignoceric acid in the brain of rat pups due to iron deficiency. *Nutr Rev* 1986; **6**: 309.

95. Ben-Shachar D, Ashkerrazi R, Youdim MBH. Long term consequences of early iron deficiency on dopaminergic neurotransmission. *Int J Dev Neurosci* 1986; **6**: 309.

96. Voorhess ML, Stuart MJ, Stockman JA, Oski FA. Iron deficiency anemia and increased urinary norepinephrine excretion. *J Pediatr* 1975; **86**: 542.

97. Symes AL, Missala K, Sourkes TL. Iron and riboflavin metabolism of a monoamine in the rat *in vivo*. *Science* 1971; **174**: 153.

98. Erikson KM, Jones BC, Hess EL *et al.* Iron deficiency decreases dopamine D_1 and D_2 receptors in rat brain. *Pharmacol Biochem Behav* 2001; **69**: 409.

99. Oski FA, Honig AS. The effects of therapy on the developmental scores of iron-deficient infants. *J Pediatr* 1978; **92**: 21.

100. Grantham-McGregor S, Ani C. A review of studies on the effect of iron deficiency on cognitive development in children. *J Nutr* 2001; **131**: 649S

101. Aukett MA, Parks YA, Scott PH *et al.* Treatment with iron increases weight gain and psychomotor development. *Arch Dis Child* 1986; **61**: 849.

102. Morton RE, Nysenbaum A, Price K. Iron status in the first year of life. *Pediatr Gastroenterol Nutr* 1988; **7**: 707.

103. Daly A, MacDonald A, Aukett A *et al.* Prevention of anaemia in inner city toddlers by an iron supplemented cows' milk formula. *Arch Dis Child* 1996; **75**: 9.

104. Stevens D, Nelson A. The effect of iron in formula milk after 6 months of age. *Arch Dis Child* 1995; **73**: 216.

105. Grindulis H, Scott PH, Belton NR, Wharton BA. Combined deficiency of iron and vitamin D in Asian toddlers. *Arch Dis Child* 1986; **61**: 843.

106. Mills AF. Surveillance for anaemia: risk factors in pattern of milk intake. *Arch Dis Child* 1990; **65**: 428.

107. Gregory JR, Collins DL, Davies PSW *et al. National Diet and Nutrition Survey: Children aged 1^1/$_2$ and 4^1/$_2$ years. Volume 1. Report of the Diet and Nutrition Survey.* London: HMSO, 1995.

108. Gill DG, Vincent S, Segal DS. Follow on formula in the prevention of iron deficiency: a multicentre study. *Acta Pediatrica* 1997; **86**: 683.

109. Bottomley S. Sideroblastic anaemia. *Clin Haematol* 1982; **11**: 389.

110. Cartwright GE, Deiss A. Sideroblasts, siderocytes and sideroblastic anemia. *N Engl J Med* 1975; **292**: 185.

111. MacGibbon BH, Mollen DL. Sideroblastic anaemia in man: observation on seventy cases. *Br J Haematol* 1965; **11**: 59.

112. Prasad AS, Tranchida L, Konno AT *et al.* Hereditary sideroblastic anaemia and glucose-6-phosphate dehydrogenase deficiency in a negro family. *J Clin Invest* 1968; **47**: 1415.

113. Pagon RA, Bird TD, Detter JC, Pierce I. Hereditary sideroblastic anaemia and ataxia: an X-linked recessive disorder. *J Med Genet* 1985; **22**: 267.

114. Weatherall DJ, Pembrey ME, Hall EG *et al.* Familial sideroblastic anaemia: problem of Xg and X chromosome inactivation. *Lancet* 1970; **ii**: 744.

115. Soslan G, Brodsky I. Hereditary sideroblastic anemia with associated platelet abnormalities. *Am J Hematol* 1989; **32**: 298.

116. van Waveran Hogervorst GD, van Roermund HPC, Snijders PJ. Hereditary sideroblastic anaemia and autosomal inheritance of erythrocyte dimorphism in a Dutch family. *Eur J Haematol* 1987; **38**: 405.

117. Bishop DF, Henderson AS, Astrin KH. Human delta-aminolevulinate synthase: assignment of the housekeeping gene to 3p21 and the erythroid-specific gene to X chromosome. *Genomics* 1990; **7**: 207.

118. Cox TC, Bottomley SS, Wiley JS *et al.* X-linked pyridoxine-responsive sideroblastic anemia due to a THR388-SER substitution in erythroid 5-aminolevulinate synthase. *N Engl J Med* 1994; **330**: 675.

119. Aoki Y, Muranaka S, Nakabayashi K, Ueda Y. Delta-aminolevulinic synthetase in erythroblasts of patients with pyridoxine-responsive anaemia. *J Clin Invest* 1979; **64**: 119.

120. Konopa L, Hoffbrand AV. Haem synthesis in sideroblastic anaemia. *Br J Haematol* 1979; **42**: 73.

121. Garby L. Chronic refractory hypochromic anaemia with disturbed haem-metabolism. *Br J Haematol* 1957; **3**: 55.

122. Stavem P, Romslo I, Rootwelt K, Emblem R. Ferrochelatase deficiency in the bone marrow in a syndrome of congenital hypochromic microcytic anaemia, hyperferraemia and iron over load of the liver. *Scand J Gastroenterol* 1985; **20** (suppl. 107): 73.

123. Aoki Y. Multiple enzymatic defects in mitochondria of haematological cells of patients with primary sideroblastic anaemia. *J Clin Invest* 1980; **66**: 43.

124. Raab SO. Pyridoxine responsive anaemia. *Blood* 1961; **18**: 285.

125. Tuckfield A, Ratnaike S, Hussein S, Metz J. A novel form of hereditary sideroblastic anaemia with macrocytosis. *Br J Haematol* 1997; **97**: 279.

126. Pearson HA, Lobel JS, Kocoshis SA *et al.* A new syndrome of refractory sideroblastic anemia with vacuolization of marrow precursors and exocrine pancreatic dysfunction. *J Pediatr* 1979; **95**: 976.

127. Stoddard RA, McCurnin DE, Shultenover SJ *et al.* Syndrome of refractory sideroblastic anemia with vacuolization of marrow precursors in the neonate. *J Pediatr* 1981; **99**: 259.

128. Anon. DIDMOAD (Wolfram) syndrome [editorial]. *Lancet* 1986; **i**: 1075.

129. Borgna-Pignalli C, Marradi P, Monetti N, Patrini C. Thiamine responsive anemia in DIDMOAD syndrome. *J Pediatr* 1989; **114**: 405.

130. Rothstein G, Lee R, Cartwright GE. Sideroblastic anaemia with dermal photosensitivity and greatly increased erythrocyte protoporphyrin. *N Engl J Med* 1969; **280**: 587.

131. Romslo I, Brun A, Sandberg S *et al.* Sideroblastic anaemia with markedly increased free erythrocyte porphyrin without dermal sensitivity. *Blood* 1982; **59**: 628.

132. Scott AJ, Ansford AJ, Webster BH, Stringer HCW. Erythropoietic protoporphyria with features of a sideroblastic anemia terminating in liver failure. *Am J Med* 1973; **54**: 251.

133. Lin-Fu JS. Vulnerability of children to lead exposure and toxicity. *N Engl J Med* 1973; **289**: 1289.

134. Paglia DE, Valentine WN, Dalgren JG *et al.* Effects of low-level lead exposure on pyrimidine-5-nucleotidase and other erythrocyte enzymes. Possible role of pyrimidine-5-nucleotidase in the pathogenesis of lead-induced anaemia. *J Clin Invest* 1975; **56**: 1164.

135. Goldberg A. Lead poisoning as a disorder of heme synthesis. *Semin Hematol* 1968; **5**: 424.

136. Piomelli S, Davidow B, Guinee VF *et al.* The FEP (free erythrocyte porphyrins) test: a screening micromethod for lead poisoning. *Pediatrics* 1973; **51**: 254.

137. Piomelli S, Rosen JF, Chisolm JJ, Graef JW. Management of childhood lead poisoning. *Pediatrics* 1984; **105**: 523.

138. Askenazi A, Levin S, Djaldetti M *et al.* The syndrome of neonatal copper deficiency. *Pediatrics* 1973; **52**: 525.

139. Zidar BL, Shadduck RK, Zeigler Z, Winklestein A. Observations on the anemia and neutropenia caused by copper deficiency. *Am J Hematol* 1977; **3**: 177.

140. Ramadurai J, Shapiro C, Kozloff M, Telfer M. Zinc abuse and sideroblastic anemia. *Am J Hematol* 1993; **42**: 227.

141. Harvey AR, Pippard MJ, Ansell BM. Microcytic anaemia in juvenile chronic arthritis. *Scand J Rheumatol* 1987; **16**: 53.

142. Ritchie AK, Hoffman R, Daimak N *et al.* Antibody-mediated sideroblastic anaemia: response to cytotoxic therapy. *Blood* 1979; **54**: 734.

143. Parry GJ, Bredesen DE. Sensory neuropathy with low-dose pyridoxine. *Neurology* 1985; **35**: 1466.

144. Mason DY, Emerson PM. Primary acquired sideroblastic anaemia: response to treatment with pyridoxal-5-phosphate. *Br Med J* 1973; **1**: 389.

145. Peto TEA, Pippard MJ, Weatherall DJ. Iron overload in mild sideroblastic anaemias. *Lancet* 1983; **i**: 375.

146. Weintraub LR, Conrad ME, Crosby WH. Iron loading anemia. Treatment with repeated phlebotomies and pyridoxine. *N Engl J Med* 1966; **275**: 169.

147. Bennett JM, Catovsky D, Daniel MT *et al.* Proposals for the classification of the myelodysplastic syndromes. *Br J Haematol* 1982; **51**: 189.

148. Third MIC Cooperative Study Group. Recommendations for a morphologic, immunological and cytogenetics (MIC) working classification of the primary and therapy-related myelodysplastic disorders. *Cancer Genet Cytogenet* 1988; **32**: 1.

149. Klein-Schwartz W, Odeka GM, Gorman RL *et al.* Assessment and management guidelines for acute iron ingestion. *Clin Pediatr* 1990; **29**: 316.

150. Hershko C, Peto TEA. Annotation: Non-transferrin plasma iron. *Br J Haematol* 1987; **66**: 149.

151. Halliwell B, Gutteridge JMC. Oxygen toxicity, oxygen radicals, transitional metals and disease. *Biochemistry* 1984; **219**: 1.

152. Slater TF. Free radical mechanisms in tissue injury. *Biochemistry* 1984; **222**: 1.

153. Niederau CR, Fisher R, Sonnenberg A *et al.* Survival and causes of death in cirrhotic and non-cirrhotic patients with primary hemochromatosis. *N Engl J Med* 1985; **313**: 1256.

154. Cartwright GE, Edwards CQ, Kravitz K *et al.* Hereditary hemochromatosis: phenotypic expression of the disease. *N Engl J Med* 1979; **301**: 175.

155. Haddy TB, Castro OL, Rana SR. Hereditary hemochromatosis in children, adolescents and young adults. *Am J Pediatr Hematol Oncol* 1988; **10**: 23.

156. Brink B, Disler P, Lynch S *et al.* Patterns of iron storage in dietary iron overload and idiopathic haemochromatosis. *J Lab Clin Med* 1977; **88**: 725.

157. Model B, Berdoukas V. *The Clinical Approach to Thalassaemia*. London: Grune & Stratton, 1984.

158. Iancu TC, Neustein HB. Ferritin in human liver cells of homozygous beta thalassaemia: ultrastructural observations. *Br J Haematol* 1977; **37**: 527.

159. Knisley AS, Grady RW, Kramer EE, Jones RL. Cytoferrin, maternal iron transport, and neonatal hemochromatosis. *Am J Pathol* 1989; **92**: 755.

160. Perry TL, Hardwick DF, Dixon G *et al.* Hypermethioninemia. *Pediatrics* 1965; **36**: 236.

161. Volpe JJ, Adams RD. Cerebro-hepato-renal syndrome of Zellweger. *Acta Neuropathol* 1972; **20**: 175.

162. Knisley AS, Harford JB, Klausner RD, Taylor SR. Neonatal hemochromatosis. *Am J Pathol* 1989; **134**: 439.

163. Hoogstraten J, Derek J de SA, Knisley AS. Fetal liver disease may precede extrahepatic siderosis in neonatal hemochromatosis. *Gastroenterology* 1990; **98**: 1699.

164. Dooling EC, Schoene WC, Richardson EP. Hallervorden–Spatz syndrome. *Arch Neurol* 1974; **30**: 70.

165. De Sanctis V, Pintor C, Aliquo MC. Prevalence of endocrine complications in patients with beta thalassaemia major: an Italian multicentre study. In: Pintor C, Muller EE, Loche S, New MI (eds) *Advances in Pediatric Endocrinology*. Berlin: Springer, 1992, pp. 127–33.

166. Zurlo MG, De Stephano P, Borgna-Pignatti C *et al.* Survival and causes of death in thalassaemia. *Lancet* 1989; **i**: 27.

167. Gabutti V, Piga A, Sachetti L *et al.* Quality of life and life expectancy in thalassaemic patients with complications. In: Buckner CD, Gale RP, Lucarelli G (eds) *Advances and Controversies in Thalassaemia Therapy: Bone Marrow Transplantation and Other Approaches*. New York: Liss, 1 989, pp. 35–41.

168. Ley TJ, Griffith P, Nienhuis AW. Transfusion haemosiderosis and chelation therapy. *Clin Haematol* 1982; **11**: 437.

169. Bassett ML, Halliday JW, Powell LW. Value of hepatic iron measurements in early haemochromatosis and determination of the critical iron level associated with fibrosis. *Hepatology (Am Soc Hematol Educ Program)* 1986; **6**: 24.

170. Risdon RA, Barry M, Flynn DM. Transfusional iron overload: the relationship between tissue iron concentration and hepatic fibrosis in thalassaemia. *J Pathol* 1975; **116**: 83.

171. Cohen AR. Management of iron overload in the pediatric patient. *Hematol Oncol Clin North Am* 1987; **1**: 521.

172. Borgna-Pignetti C, De Stephano P, Zonta L *et al.* Growth and sexual maturation in thalasssemia major. *J Pediatr* 1985; **106**: 150.

173. Kletzky OA, Costin G, Marrs RP *et al.* Gonadotrophin insufficiency in patients with thalassaemia major. *J Clin Endocrinol Metab* 1979; **48**: 901.

174. Herington AC, Wertha GA, Matthews RN, Gurger HG. Studies on the possible mechanism for deficiency of nonsuppressible insulin-like activity in thalassaemia major. *J Clin Endocrinol Metab* 1981; **12**: 293.

175. De Sanctis V, Zurlo MG, Senesi E *et al.* Insulin dependent diabetes in thalassaemia. *Arch Dis Child* 1988; **63**: 58.

176. Abbott DF, Gresham GA. Arthropathy in transfusional siderosis. *Br Med J* 1972; **1**: 1418.

177. Hershko C, Peto T, Wetherall DJ. Iron and infection. *Br Med J* 1987; **296**: 660.

178. UK Thalassaemia Society. Standards for the clinical care of children and adults with thalassaemia in the UK. Available at http://www.ukts.org/

179. Oski FA, Marshall BE, Delivoria-Papdopoulos M *et al.* Exercise with anemia: the role of the left-shifted or right-shifted oxygen hemoglobin equilibrium curve. *Ann Intern Med* 1971; **74**: 44.

180. Piomelli S, Danoff S, Becker M *et al.* Prevention of bone malformations and cardiomegaly in Cooley's anemia by early hypertransfusion regimen. *Ann NY Acad Sci* 1969; **165**: 427.

181. Propper RL, Button LN, Nathan DJ. New approaches to the transfusion management of thalassaemia. *Blood* 1980; **55**: 55.

182. Cazzola M, De Stefano P, Ponchio L *et al.* Relationship between transfusion regimen and suppression of erythropoiesis in beta thalassaemia major. *Br J Haematol* 1995; **89**: 473.

183. Cohen AR, Martin M, Schwartz E. A clinical trial of young red cell transfusions. *Pediatr Res* 1983; **17**: 231A.

184. Marcus RE, Wonke B, Bantock HM *et al*. A prospective trial of young red cells in 48 patients with transfusion dependent thalassaemia. *Br J Haematol* 1985; **60**: 153.

185. Coles SM, Klein HG, Holland PV. Alloimmunisation in two multitransfused populations. *Transfusion* 1981; **21**: 462.

186. Kaltwasser JP, Gottschalk R, Schalk KP *et al*. Non-invasive quantitation of liver iron-overload by magnetic resonance imaging. *Br J Haematol* 1990; **74**: 360.

187. Totaro A, Rommens JM, Grifa A *et al*. Hereditary hemochromatosis: generation of a transcription map within a refined and extended map of the HLA class 1 region. *Genomics* 1996; **31**: 319.

188. Feder JN, Gnirke A, Thomas W *et al*. A novel MHC class 1-like gene is mutated in patients with hereditary haemochromatosis. *Nat Genet* 1996; **13**: 399.

189. Bodmer JG, Parham P, Albert ED, Marsh SG on behalf of the WHO Nomenclature Committee for Factors of the HLA System. Putting a hold on HLA-H. *Nat Genet* 1997; **15**: 234.

6 Megaloblastic anemia and disorders of cobalamin and folate metabolism

Eric J. Werner

Megaloblastic anemia in childhood is most often due to either deficiency of vitamin B_{12} (cobalamin) or folate or to defects in their metabolism. It is the goal of this chapter to briefly discuss the metabolic pathways in which these vitamins play critical roles and the known defects in their absorption, transportation and metabolism. In addition, some defects in cobalamin metabolism that are not associated with megaloblastic anemia are also described here. For more complete discussion of cobalamin and folate metabolism, the reader is referred to recent reviews of various aspects of cobalamin and folate.[1,2] In this chapter, the terms "cobalamin" and "vitamin B_{12}" are used interchangeably.

Cobalamin (vitamin B_{12})

The cobalamins share the same structure: a planar corrin ring with a central cobalt atom, attached to a nucleotide structure, 5,6-dimethyl benziminazole, attached to ribose 3-phosphate (Fig. 6.1). The two main natural compounds have a methyl (CH_3) or a 5-deoxyadenosyl group attached to the cobalt atom. Cyanocobalamin was the form in which the vitamin was first isolated and this compound has been radioactively labeled with ^{57}Co or ^{58}Co for diagnostic uses. Hydroxocobalamin, which has the cobalt atom in the oxidized stable Co(III) state, is also used in therapy.

In nature, cobalamin is synthesized by microorganisms and is only present in foods of animal origin.[3] The steps of cobalamin absorption in the gastrointestinal tract are illustrated in Fig. 6.2. Cobalamin is released by enzymatic digestion from protein complexes in food in the acid pH of the stomach, where it it binds to R binder present in saliva and gastric juice. This binder is closely related to transcobalamin (TC) I present in plasma, and is similar to a binder in milk and other fluids. After release from R binder in the duodenum by pancreatic proteases, cobalamin binds to intrinsic factor (IF), a 45-kDa glycoprotein synthesized by gastric parietal cells. Cobalamin in bile is also attached to R binder and complexes with IF in the duodenum.[4] The IF–cobalamin complex

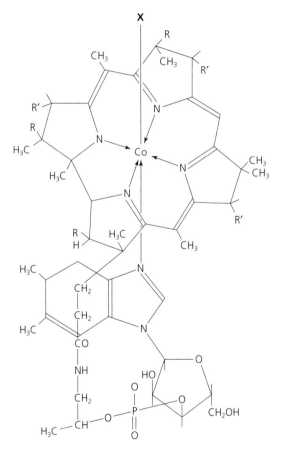

Fig. 6.1 Structure of cobalamin. A cobalt atom is at the center of a planar corrin ring. This is attached to a nucleotide, 5,6-dimethyl benziminazole ribose 3-phosphate. Attached to the cobalt atom at "X" may be a methyldeoxyadenosyl-, hydroxo- or cyano-moiety.

attaches to its receptor cubulin on the ileal brush border. The absorption of cobalamin by ileal receptors is limited to 1.5–2.5 μg from a single meal, although larger amounts have been documented.[5] A small fraction (<1%) of a large oral dose can be absorbed passively through the buccal, gastric and small intestinal mucosa.

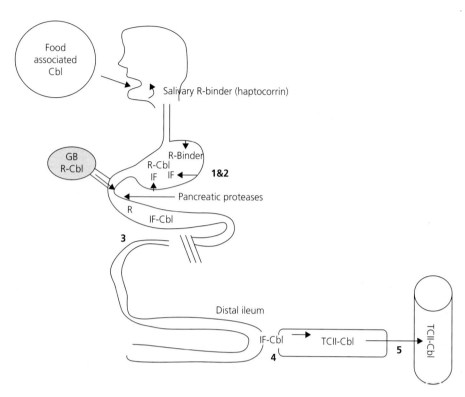

Fig. 6.2 Steps in cobalamin (Cbl) absorption. (1) Food-bound cobalamin is released from protein in stomach. (2) Cobalamin binds to R binder (haptocorrin) in the stomach. (3) Cobalamin is released from R binder in the proximal small intestine and binds to intrinsic factor (IF) produced by gastric parietal cells. (4) The IF–cobalamin complex is transported intracellularly through the cubulin receptor in the ileum. (5) Cobalamin is released into the plasma bound to transcobalamin II (TCII).

Within the enterocyte, the IF–cobalamin complex is digested, probably within lysosomes, and the cobalamin appears in portal blood attached to TCII, a 38-kDa polypeptide. The cobalamin–TCII complex has a rapid metabolic turnover with a half-life of about 6 min.[3]

In the plasma, cobalamin can bind to either TCI or TCII. TCI-bound cobalamin has a much slower turnover. The function of TCI and its bound cobalamin is unclear. Because 70–90% of cobalamin is bound to TCI, deficiency of TCII may be present with normal serum cobalamin levels.[6] The cobalamin bound to TCII is transported into various tissues where it is available for its metabolic function.

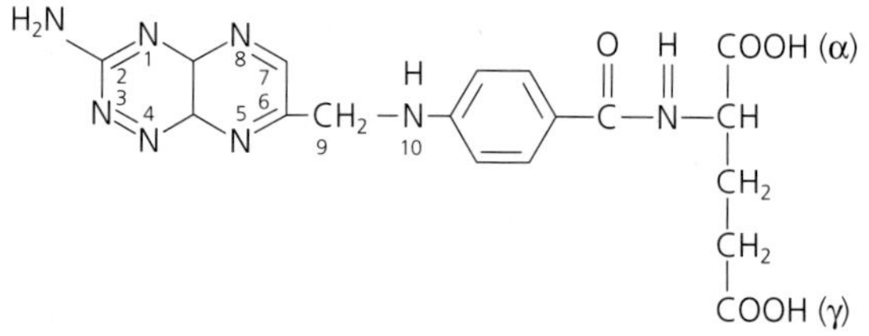

Folate

Folic acid (Fig. 6.3) is the parent compound of natural folates with the same vitamin activity, which are:

- reduced to tetrahydrofolate (THF) forms at positions 5, 6, 7 and 8;
- have single carbon units: methyl (CH_3-), formyl (CHO–), methylene ($CH_2=$), methenyl ($CH\equiv$) or formimino (CHNO–) attached to nitrogens N_5, N_{10} or both;
- have a chain of four to six glutamate moieties attached by γ-peptide bonds (polyglutamates). These are the active folate coenzymes whereas the monoglutamates are transport forms.

Folates are present in most foods, with especially high amounts in liver, leafy vegetables, fruits and yeast.[7] Cows' milk contains about 50–120 μg/L and human milk about 85 μg/L.[8]

Fig. 6.3 Structure of folic acid. Natural folates may contain a single carbon unit, i.e., methyl (CH_3-), methylene ($CH_2=$), methenyl ($CH\equiv$), formyl (CHO–), formimino (CHNO–), attached at the N_5 or N_{10} position. A chain of glutamic acid residues attached by peptide bond linkage are reduced to dihydro or tetrahydro forms at positions 7, 8 or 5, 6, 7, 8 in the pteridine portion respectively.

Beginning in 1998, the Food and Drug Administration (FDA) approved fortifying cereal-grain products with levels of folic acid at 140 μg per 100 g of cereal.[9] Cooking, especially in large volumes of water for prolonged periods, destroys folates, especially if vitamin C and other reducing agents that protect folates are first destroyed.[10] The first phase in the absorption of natural folates involves digestion of polyglutamates to monoglutamates. Absorption occurs in the small intestine via a saturable carrier process for relatively low intestinal concentrations of folate and by diffusion for high concentrations of folate or folic acid.[7] Folate is transported across cell membranes by one of at least two systems. Human reduced folate carrier-1, the gene for which has been localized to chromosome 21q22.3,[11] functions as a high-capacity low-

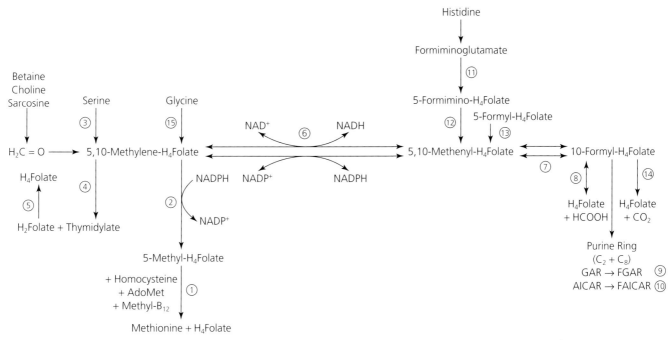

Fig. 6.4 Folate biochemical reactions: folate-mediated 1-carbon transfer reactions. 1, Methionine synthase; 2, methylene-tetrahydrofolate reductase; 3, serine hydroxymethyl-transferase; 4, thymidylate synthetase; 5, dihydrofolate reductase; 6, methylene-tetrahydrofolate dehydrogenase (either NADP or NAD dependent); 7, methenyl-tetrahydrofolate cyclohydrolase; 8, 10-formyl-tetrahydrofolate synthase; 9, GAR (5-phosphoribosylglycineamide transformylase; 10, AICAR (5-phosphoribosyl-5-aminoimidazole-4-carboxamide) transformase; 11, glutamate forminotransferase; 12, formimino-tetrahydrofolate cyclodeaminase; 13, 5,10-methenyl-tetrahydrofolate synthetase; 14, 10-formyl-tetrahydrofolate dehydrogenase; 15, glycine cleavage pathway; 16, folic acid is metabolized to tetrahydrofolate by dihydrofolate reductase. Reproduced with permission from Ref. 12.

affinity system.[12] In the second known system, folates bind to folate-binding proteins or folate receptors on the cell membrane and are internalized by a process called potocytosis.[13] Folate receptors are coded for by genes on chromosome 11q13.3–13.5.[12] Folic acid (pteroylglutamic acid) can be absorbed largely unchanged, especially when given in large, pharmacologic doses. It is converted to natural folates in the liver quite rapidly.[14] Bile contains about 100 µg/day[15] and interruption of the enterohepatic circulation leads to a fall in serum folate within 6 hours.[16] Total body folate stores in adults have been estimated to be 5–10 mg,[15] with some estimates as high as 12–28 mg,[8] which should be sufficient for about 1–4 months, especially if the enterohepatic circulation is intact.[8] Absence of dietary intake may lead to a fall in serum folate within 2–3 weeks.[15]

Folate in plasma is mostly either free or loosely and non-specifically bound to proteins such as albumin. Specific folate-binding proteins occur in small amounts in plasma. Their exact function is unclear.[15]

Cobalamin and folate metabolism

Cobalamin is known to have a role in two reactions in humans:

1 With a methyl group attached to the cobalt atom (methylcobalamin or MeCbl) it is a required cofactor for the enzyme methionine synthase in the conversion of homocysteine to methionine. This reaction requires 5-methyl-THF as a cofactor.

2 With 5′-deoxyadenosine attached to the cobalt atom (5′-deoxyadenosylcobalamin or AdoCbl) in the conversion of methylmalonyl-CoA to succinyl-CoA by the enzyme methylmalonyl-CoA mutase.

Folate takes part in intracellular biochemical reactions in its polyglutamate forms. As shown in Fig. 6.4, these coenzymes are involved in three amino acid interconversions: homocysteine to methionine, serine to glycine and forminino glutamic acid to glutamic acid; and in three reactions in DNA synthesis: formylation of the purines 5-phosphoribosyl-glycinamide (GAR) and 5-phosphoribosyl-5-aminoimidazole carboxamide (AICAR) and methylation of the pyrimidine deoxyuridine monophosphate (dUMP) to deoxythymidine monophosphate (dTMP, thymidylate). This last reaction is rate limiting for DNA synthesis. Thymidylate synthesis also causes oxidation of the folate coenzyme from the THF to dihydrofolate (DHF) state. The enzyme DHF reductase, inhibited by methotrexate for example, is required to return folate to the active THF state. Deficiency of folate reduces DNA replication by inhibiting thymidylate synthesis. The mechanism by which deficiency of cobalamin reduces DNA synthesis and causes megaloblastic anemia is also probably a result of reduced thymidylate synthesis. Plasma folate

(5-methyl-THF) entering cells is first "demethylated" to THF through the homocysteine–methionine reaction. Cobalamin deficiency reduces this reaction and so decreases cell THF concentration. Folate polyglutamate synthase, the intracellular enzyme needed to synthesize folate polyglutamates, requires THF (or formyl-THF) as substrate but cannot use methyl-THF as substrate.[12] Thus, cobalamin deficiency results in reduction in synthesis of all intracellular folate (polyglutamate) coenzymes. Total cell folate is reduced, plasma folate (methyl-THF) rises, and the intracellular folate reactions in DNA synthesis and amino acid conversion are impaired.

Inborn errors of vitamin B$_{12}$ transport and metabolism

Transport disorders

Intrinsic factor deficiency

This inherited form of pernicious anemia results from an absence of effective IF. Evidence of vitamin B$_{12}$ deficiency usually appears in early childhood after the first year of life, but may not appear until adolescence or adulthood. Patients typically show megaloblastic anemia, developmental delay and myelopathy.[17–20] They have normal gastric acid secretion and gastric cytology. In some cases, immunologically active but nonfunctional IF is produced, whereas in others none is found. An IF that is labile to destruction by acid and pepsin and with a low affinity for vitamin B$_{12}$ has also been reported.[21] Absorption of cobalamin is abnormal in children with IF deficiency, but is normalized when the vitamin is mixed with a source of normal IF. Inheritance is autosomal recessive and the gene for human IF has been localized to chromosome 11q13. Recently, a 4-bp deletion in the IF gene was described in a child with apparent congenital IF deficiency.[22]

Imerslund–Gräsbeck syndrome (defective vitamin B$_{12}$ transport by enterocytes)

Imerslund–Gräsbeck syndrome causes clinical manifestations of vitamin B$_{12}$ deficiency in childhood. Patients usually present within the first 2 years, although later presentation may occur.[23,24] Findings include pallor, weakness, anorexia, failure to thrive, recurrent infections and gastrointestinal symptoms.[20] Over 250 cases have been described and reports of patients predominate from Norway, Finland and the Middle East.[24] Patients with Imerslund–Gräsbeck syndrome have normal IF, no evidence of antibodies to IF, and normal intestinal morphology. They have a selective defect in vitamin B$_{12}$ absorption that is not corrected by treatment with IF. Proteinuria of the tubular type is a common feature and systemic vitamin B$_{12}$ corrects the anemia but not the proteinuria.[20]

Defects in two proteins have recently been described that account for Imerslund–Gräsbeck syndrome. Linkage studies from Finland documented a defect in the cubulin gene on chromosome 10. Cubulin appears to function as a receptor for IF on the ileal mucosa. Norwegian patients were subsequently found to have a defect in the AMN (amnionless) gene.[25] Recently, Fyfe et al.[26] have presented evidence that AMN complexes with cubulin and plays a critical role in its ability to bind and transport cobalamin. Deficiency or dysfunction of either protein appears to prevent absorption of cobalamin.

Transcobalamin (haptocorrin, R binder) deficiency

A deficiency or complete absence of TCI has been found in the plasma, saliva and leukocytes of very few individuals, but it is not clear if this deficiency is the cause of disease in any of these patients.[27–33] Zittoun et al.[32] described a boy with combined deficiency of R binder (TCI) and IF who had severe megaloblastic anemia and neurologic dysfunction. His father, who also had R-binder deficiency, was asymptomatic. TCI carries the majority of cobalamin in the plasma. However this percentage varies by location and with certain disease states.[34] Patients with severe deficiency of TCI may have a benign course.[29] Cobalamin levels are low, but TCII–vitamin B$_{12}$ (holotranscobalamin II) levels are normal, and the affected individuals may not be clinically cobalamin deficient. Carmel[33] found that of 567 samples referred for low cobalamin levels, three had undetectable TCI. Only one patient was available for study and she did not have abnormal neurologic findings, megaloblastic anemia or elevated levels of methylmalonic acid. Typically, individuals with TCI deficiency will have normal values for homocysteine and methylmalonic acid, will not show megaloblastic hematologic features and will have a normal Schilling test. Their plasma cobalamin levels should not respond to cobalamin supplementation. However, several patients with TCI deficiency have had neurologic sequelae, some of whom carried a diagnosis of multiple sclerosis.[6,29] The physiologic function of TCI is not known; roles as a scavenger of cobalamin analogs that may be toxic[35] or protectection of methylcobalamin from photolytic degradation have been proposed.[36]

Transcobalamin II deficiency

TCII deficiency is a rare autosomal recessive disorder.[20,37] Because TCI binds larger amounts of cobalamin in blood than TCII, serum cobalamin levels are often normal in TCII-deficient patients, but subnormal values have been reported.[34,38] Even though TCII in cord blood is of fetal origin,[39] infants with undetectable TCII in their plasma are usually born healthy but then demonstrate signs of cobalamin deficiency over the first several days of life. Usually, patients develop severe megaloblastic anemia in the first few months of life, but others present with pancytopenia or even isolated erythroid hypoplasia.[40] The presence of immature white cell precursors in an otherwise hypocellular marrow can result in the misdiagnosis of leukemia. Other symptoms include failure to thrive, weakness and diarrhea. Neurologic disease typically appears later, especially in untreated or undertreated patients.[41–44] The neurologic manifestations are more associated with diagnosis outside the neonatal period.[45] Severe immunologic deficiency with defective cellular and humoral immunity has been seen, as has defective granulocyte function. Long-term follow-up has documented persistence of neurologic deficits despite adequate therapy, although in some patients the neurologic damage may have occurred prior to diagnosis.[46] Laboratory findings should include macrocytic anemia, hyperhomocysteinemia and elevated levels of methylmalonic acid.[47]

The defect in TCII can be absent protein,[42,48] an inability to bind to cobalamin[49] or an inability to mediate cobalamin uptake into cells.[50] An abnormal Schilling test is usually found in TCII deficiency. This suggests that the TCII molecule may play a role in the IF-mediated transport of cobalamin across the ileal cell.

The TCII gene is located on chromosome 22.[51,52] The molecular basis of some of the variants has been defined. The first mutant alleles in TCII deficiency have included deletions[53] and nonsense mutations.[54] TCII is synthesized by amniocytes and prenatal diagnosis is possible even in the absence of known mutations in a family at risk.[55,56]

The mainstay of treatment for TCII deficiency has been high-dose cobalamin. Both oral treatment and systemic treatment have been used, although at least one patient redeveloped pancytopenia when transitioned to oral treatment,[46] and caution has been raised about using oral therapy.[57] Serum cobalamin levels must be kept very high (1000–10 000 pg/mL) in order to treat TCII-deficient patients successfully and this has been achieved with twice-weekly doses of hydroxocobalamin orally (500–1000 µg) or of systemic hydroxocobalamin (1000 µg) weekly or more often.[20,44,46]

Early and regular high-dose cobalamin therapy may lead to a favorable outcome.[58] Folate in the form of folic acid or folinic acid in milligram doses has been successful in reversing the hematologic findings in most patients. However, folate should not be given alone to patients with TCII deficiency as hematologic relapse and neurologic damage can occur when folate supplementation is given without cobalamin.[42,43]

Disorders of utilization

Methylmalonic acidurias

Disorders causing methylmalonic aciduria (MMA) are characterized by severe metabolic acidosis and the accumulation of large amounts of methylmalonic acid in blood, urine and cerebrospinal fluid (CSF). Patients with MMA have a defect in the nuclear-encoded mitochondrial matrix protein L-methylmalonyl-CoA mutase (mutase), which requires AdoCbl as a cofactor, and catalyzes the conversion of L-methylmalonyl-CoA to succinyl-CoA. The failure of this reaction to occur may be a result of a defect in the mutase enzyme itself or a defect in AdoCbl synthesis. The intracellular pathways and the potential defects are shown in Fig. 6.5. Defects that cause isolated abnormalities in mutase or AdoCbl will cause only MMA without homocysteinemia, while those that lead to abnormalities of both AdoCbl and MeCbl cause both MMA and homocysteinemia. Classification of the defects of cobalamin metabolism has been made largely on the basis of somatic cell complementation studies in cultured fibroblasts. The incidence of all forms of MMA determined by neonatal screening in Massachusetts is about 1 in 48 000.[59] Of 12 infants diagnosed in that state with MMA, three had mutase deficiency (two mild), six had defects in cobalamin synthesis (not further defined) and three were undefined. However, not all infants with elevated methylmalonic acid on newborn screen have disease, especially with mild elevations (<1400 µmol/mmol creatinine).[60]

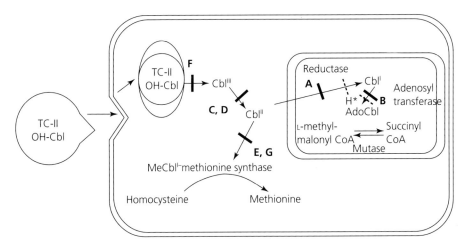

Fig. 6.5 Intracellular cobalamin metabolism and defects. Cbl[I], Cbl[II] and Cbl[III] refer to the oxidation state of the central cobalt atom of cobalamin. A–G refer to the sites of blocks that have been identified by complementation analysis. The site of block for CblH has not been identified. AdoCbl, adenosylcobalamin; MeCbl, methylcobalamin; TC, transcobalamin; OH-Cbl, hydroxocobalamin. The mitochondrial, lysosomal and cytoplasmic compartments are indicated. Modified from Ref. 198.

Deficiency of methylmalonyl-CoA mutase (mut^0, mut^-)

Mutations in the mutase apoenzyme result in MMA that is not responsive to cobalamin therapy.[20,37] Mature mutase purified from human liver is a dimer with a molecular weight of 150 000–160 000.[61] There are at least two types of mutase deficiency as defined in cultured fibroblasts from patients with MMA. Cell lines having no detectable mutase activity are designated mut^0; those with residual activity are called mut^-. Some cell lines synthesize no detectable protein, whereas others synthesize unstable proteins, and at least one has a mutation that interferes with transfer of the mutase to the mitochondria.[62,63] Variable levels of mRNA have been demonstrated in different mut^0 lines. Intragenic (interallelic) complementation has been seen between some mut lines.[64,65]

Patients with severe mutase deficiency rapidly become symptomatic with protein feeding. In a retrospective questionnaire study of patients with MMA, Matsui *et al.*[66] found lethargy (88%), recurrent vomiting (89%), failure to thrive (67%), dehydration (71%) and respiratory distress (50%) in patients with either mut^0 or mut^- defects. Of note, while the numbers were quite small (13 mut^0 and 5 mut^-), and not all patients were evaluated for each item, there were differences between these two disorders in the incidence of developmental delay (69% vs. 25%) and hepatomegaly (57% vs 0%). For normal children, urinary excretion of methylmalonic acid is < 0.04 mmol/24 hours and plasma concentrations are virtually undetectable. In contrast, in children with MMA, urinary excretion can exceed 2.1–49 mmol/24 hours and plasma concentrations range from 0.2 to 2.9 mmol/L (2.6–34 mg/dL).[62] Patients with MMA often have ketones and glycine in both blood and urine, hypoglycemia and hyperammonemia.[20,66] Matsui found leukopenia in about 60% and thrombocytopenia in 40% of patients with mutase deficiency. About half of the infants with mut^0 had anemia and methylmalonic acid has been shown to inhibit bone marrow stem cells in a concentration-dependent manner.[67] Interestingly, follow-up of children identified by newborn screening[59,60,68] has identified a number of individuals who excrete methylmalonic acid, have mutase deficiency by complementation analysis, and yet are clinically well and have never developed acidosis. Limited intellectual ability has been noted in several patients with mut^- disease; however, Varvogli *et al.*[69] described a 12 year old with the mut^- defect who scored in the 99th percentile on the National Acheivement Test and had a full-scale IQ of 129 on the Wechsler Intelligence Scale.

The cDNA for human mutase has been cloned and the gene localizes to chromosome 6p12–p21.2.[70] Over 50 mutations have been identified in human mutase,[70] including a large number near the carboxyl terminus which appear to alter AdoCbl binding to the enzyme.[65,71] A premature stop codon in the mitochondrial leader sequence has been described.[72] A common mutation (G717V) was found in five black patients who had a similar phenotype; of these, four were African-American and one was from Ghana.[73,74] In Japan, 6 of 16 patients studied shared one mutation (G425T),[75] while another mutation (N219Y) was identified in five unrelated Caucasian families from Turkey and France.[76]

Treatment consists of handling immediate issues such as hypoglycemia, acidosis and hyperammonemia and protein restriction using a formula deficient in valine, isoleucine, methionine and threonine, with the goal of limiting the amino acids that use the propionate pathway. While patients in the mut complementation class are not clinically responsive to vitamin B_{12}, a therapeutic trial of daily intramuscular hydroxocobalamin should be administered as soon as a diagnosis of MMA is considered until other cobalamin-responsive disorders have been excluded. Therapy with carnitine has been advocated.[77,78] Metronidazole may improve the clinical status of patients by reducing enteric propionate production by anaerobic bacteria.[79,80] A 7 year old with mut^- MMA and acute metabolic crisis and multiorgan dysfunction was found to have very low glutathione levels. Clinical and laboratory improvement were noted with ascorbate 2 g (120 mg/kg) daily.[81] Even with therapy, prognosis is guarded at best, with reports of brain infarctions and renal dysfunction as late complications.[82] Renal dysfunction was noted in two-thirds of patients with cobalamin-unresponsive MMA. In these patients the reduction of glomerular filtration rate correlated with age and the severity of the disease.[83]

Adenosylcobalamin deficiency (CblA, CblB, CblH)

Vitamin B_{12}-responsive MMA is caused by an intracellular deficiency in AdoCbl in both CblA and CblB. These two disorders are distinguished by complementation analysis. Recently, a gene called *MMAA* (for *m*ethyl*m*alonic *a*cidemia linked to the Cbl*A* complementation group) has been identified that is responsible for the CblA complementation group.[84] *MMAA* maps to chromosome 4q31.21. At least 22 mutations in *MMAA* have been identified.[85] The function of the protein product is not well understood, but appears to function within the mitochondria. In a single patient, fibroblasts behaved like those from CblA patients, but complementation was seen with CblA cells.[86] The defect in CblB lies in the cob(I)alamin adenosyltransferase enzyme, which participates in the final step in the synthesis of AdoCb1.[87] A gene for this protein (*MMAB*) has been mapped to chromosome 12q24 and several mutations have been identified from CblB patient cell lines.[88] Recently, a patient with clinical and biochemical features of CblA was found to have a new defect (CblH) by complementation analysis. The causative protein and/or gene product have not been identified.[89]

Most patients with CblA and CblB become sick early in the first year of life with symptoms that are similar to those seen in mutase deficiency.[66] The principal difference between defects in MMAA and MMAB as opposed to those in mutase is the clinical response to cobalamin treatment: 90% of CblA patients respond to vitamin B_{12}, with nearly 70% still well at up to 14 years of age. However, only 40% of patients with

CblB respond to therapy and only 30% show long-term survival. Therapy has been with systemic hydroxocobalamin or cyanocobalamin. Initial therapy also includes protein restriction avoiding proteins that utilize the proprionate pathway[20] Therapy with AdoCbl has not been successful, perhaps because of the inability of administered drug to get into the mitochondria.[90,91]

Both CblA and CblB are presumed to be inherited in an autosomal recessive manner. Roughly equal numbers of patients of both sexes have been reported, and obligate heterozygotes of CblB patients show decreased adenosyltransferase activity. Although prenatal therapy with vitamin B_{12} has had a good therapeutic result in a CblA patient, it is not certain whether therapy from birth would be equally effective.[92,93] In one patient, dosing of vitamin B_{12} to the mother was adjusted based on maternal methylmalonic acid levels.[94]

Combined deficiencies of adenosylcobalamin and methylcobalamin (CblC, CblD, CblF)

These three disorders result in failure of the cell to synthesize both MeCbl and AdoCbl.[62] Because these patients have a functional deficiency in both methionine synthase and mutase, homocystinuria, hypomethioninemia and MMA can develop. The metabolic defects occur after both endocytosis of TCII–vitamin B_{12} and hydrolysis of the TCII–vitamin B_{12} complex in the lysosome. In CblF disease, the defect appears to block the exit of vitamin B_{12} from the lysosome. In CblC and CblD disease, the defect is presumed to be in a cytosolic cob(III)alamin reductase or reductases.[95] Partial deficiencies of cyanocobalamin β-ligand transferase and microsomal cob(III)alamin reductase in CblC and CblD fibroblasts have been described.[96] When incubated with labeled cyanocobalamin, fibroblasts from CblC and CblD accumulate very little intracellular vitamin B_{12} and virtually no AdoCbl or MeCbl. In contrast, CblF fibroblasts accumulate excess vitamin B_{12} but it is all unmetabolized, nonprotein bound, and localized to lysosomes.[12,97] The definitive gene and protein abnormalities have not been identified.

Over 100 patients have been reported with CblC disease.[20,62] Most present in the first year of life, with a median age of onset of 1 month. Clinical features include poor feeding, failure to thrive, microcephaly, developmental delay and lethargy.[62,98,99] Most, but not all, have macrocytic megaloblastic anemia, and some have hypersegmented neutrophils and thrombocytopenia. Plasma homocysteine levels and urinary methylmalonic acid levels are increased while plasma methionine is decreased. There appears to be an early- and late-onset form of the disorder. Newborns may be difficult to recognize due to the nonspecific nature of their presenting symptoms and potential lack of laboratory features of metabolic disease.[100] Neurologic disorders such as poor cognitive function, dementia, delirium, myelopathy and tremor predominate in late-onset disease and hemato-

logic abnormalities may be absent.[62,101] An unusual pigmentary retinopathy with perimacular degeneration has been described,[98,102] as have cor pulmonale, hepatic failure and hemolytic–uremic syndrome.[62,103] It is likely that inheritance of CblC is autosomal recessive. Prenatal diagnosis has been successfully accomplished in CblC disease, using amniocytes, and the diagnosis has been ruled out using chorionic villus biopsy material and cells.[104,105]

Five patients with CblD have been reported. A pair of siblings presented at age 14 years and 1 year. The older child had neuromuscular and psychiatric disorders as well as mental retardation. He developed recurrent thrombosis in his late teens. The younger was clinically normal initially, but was developing academic problems by 13 years of age.[106] They did not have megaloblastic changes, but later abnormalities of the deoxyuridine suppression test that corrected with hydroxocobalamin were documented. This suggests the presence of a cobalamin-related defect in marrow DNA synthesis.[107] Recently, three additional patients were diagnosed with CblD by complementation group analysis. Two had significant neurologic problems, macrocytic red blood cells, elevated plasma homocysteine and low methionine levels. Neither had elevated urinary methylmalonic acid. The third patient was a premature infant who had several perinatal problems and a markedly elevated urinary methylmalonic acid but normal homocysteine. Early treatment with cobalamin was instituted. Because of the differing clinical picture associated with this complementation group result, the authors propose that mutations of different epitopes of the involved protein may lead to the disparate clinical presentations.[108]

Only five patients with CblF have been described so far. One died suddenly at 5 months of age despite a good clinical and biochemical response to cobalamin. Other findings in some patients have been small-for-gestational-age birthweight, growth retardation, stomatitis, dermatitis, hepatomegaly, hypoglycemia and arthritis.[20,109–111] Laboratory features may include megaloblastic anemia, thrombocytopenia, neutropenia, elevated homocysteine and decreased cobalamin absorption.[62] The defect is probably inherited as an autosomal recessive.[20]

Treatment of these disorders can be difficult, particularly in cases with early onset. Many patients with onset in the first month of life die.[62,99] Suggested therapy includes high-dose systemic hydroxocobalamin with a recommended dose of up to 1 mg daily,[20,62] although the need for daily therapy is unproven.[112] Two patients were recently documented to respond much more favorably to hydroxocobalamin than to cyanocobalamin.[113] Bartholomew *et al.*[112] found that systemic hydroxocobalamin was more effective than oral therapy and that betaine appeared to be helpful in combination with hydroxocobalamin in two patients. Neither folinic acid nor carnitine had any effect in these patients. The result of therapy with daily oral betaine and twice-weekly injections of hydroxocobalamin was reduced methylmalonic acid, normal serum methionine and homocysteine concentration, and resolution of lethargy, irritability and failure to thrive. However, complete reversal of the neurologic and retinal findings did not occur. Early diagnosis and treatment hopefully will improve outcome, but thus far surviving patients usually have moderate-to-severe developmental delay.[20] The patients with CblF disease responded to systemic therapy with hydroxocobalamin; the first patient responded to oral cobalamin.[62,109,111] The disease has been excluded in twins and in a single pregnancy by studies on amniocytes.[62]

Methylcobalamin deficiency (CblE, CblG)

Two groups of patients have been identified through complementation analysis with defects in methionine synthase activity but normal mutase activity, designated CblE and CblG. CblG is due to defects in methionine synthase while CblE is due to defects in the methionine synthase reductase enzyme that reduces cobalamin to its cob(I)alamin form necessary for function.[12] Clinically, patients with CblE and CblG present in the first few months of life with vomiting, poor feeding and lethargy.[12] Common findings include developmental delay, cerebral atrophy, feeding difficulty, seizures and megaloblastic anemia. Long-term neurologic damage is noted, but may be improved with early treatment. Although patients usually come to medical attention in the first 2 years of life, in one case the patient was diagnosed at age 21 years with findings resembling multiple sclerosis.[114] Other findings include electroencephalographic abnormalities, nystagmus, hypotonia, hypertonia, seizures, blindness and ataxia.[115] MMA is usually not present, but was transiently noted in one patient.[116] Both disorders are inherited in an autosomal recessive fashion. Visual abnormalities may be due to microvascular retinal damage.[117]

Following incubation in labeled cyanocobalamin, fibroblasts from both CblE and CblG patients show decreased intracellular levels of MeCbl in the presence of normal levels of AdoCbl.[118] The finding that in CblE extracts a relative deficiency in methionine synthetase activity can be seen when the assay is performed under suboptimal reducing conditions suggested that the defect was in a reducing system associated with the enzyme.[119,120] This has been confirmed with the identification of the methionine synthase reductase enzyme and its gene *MTRR*. This gene is localized to chromosome 5p15.2–15.3 and codes for a protein with 38% identity with human cytochrome P450 reductase.[121] Multiple defects in *MTRR* have been described in patients with CblE,[122] including one that appears to code for a less severe variant of the disorder.[123] CblG is due to defects in the methionine synthase enzyme. The gene for methionine synthase has been cloned and localized to chromosome 1q43.[124] Gene mutations that cause CblG have been identified.[124–126] Both CblE and CblG are inherited in an autosomal recessive pattern.

Systemic hydroxocobalamin, 1 mg administered at first daily and then decreased to once to three times weekly, has been recommended[12] and usually results in correction of the anemia and metabolic abnormalities. The neurologic changes are more reticent to treatment, but may improve gradually. A mother carrying an affected fetus was treated with twice-weekly hydroxocobalamin from the second trimester.[127] Long-term follow-up showed the child to be well at 14 years of age with a speech impediment.[12]

Inborn errors of folate metabolism and transport

Metabolic disorders

Methylenetetrahydrofolate reductase deficiency

Methylenetetrahydrofolate reductase (MTHFR) deficiency is the most common inborn error of folate metabolism and more than 40 cases are known.[12] The enzyme leads to the formation of 5-methyl-THF, a key component of the methionine synthase pathway for the conversion of homocysteine to methionine (see Fig. 6.4). Defects lead to neurologic manifestations similar to those of methionine synthase or cobalamin deficiency. Unlike cobalamin deficiency, megaloblastic anemia is rare in MTHFR deficiency.

The clinical manifestations of MTHFR deficiency are quite varied. Clinically asymptomatic but biochemically affected individuals have been reported.[128,129] In general, clinical severity is related to the proportion of methyl-THF in cells. In a review of 68 patients with MTHFR deficiency, 19% had clinical onset in the neonatal period, 49% between 3 months and 10 years of age and the remainder after age 10.[102] Neurologic abnormalities are the predominant finding, with developmental delay, hypotonia, lethargy, seizures and encephalopathy being frequently described.[102] Psychosis has also been described. Breathing disorders and microcephaly are often present along with motor and gait abnormalities.[102] The report of reversible psychiatric disturbances leads to speculation on the role of MTHFR deficiency in psychiatric disease.[130] Clinical manifestations of thrombotic disease, including stroke and retinal vein thrombosis, are also seen with MTHFR deficiency.[12,102,131,132] Thrombosis has been a prominent finding at autopsy in some patients.[20]

MTHFR-deficient patients have elevated urine homocysteine levels, although the amounts are less than seen in cystathionine synthase deficiency.[12] More than one determination of homocysteine excretion may be needed to eliminate the possibility of a false-negative value. Serum folate levels are generally but not always reduced while cobalamin levels are normal. Serum methionine levels are low or low-normal. Kanwar *et al.*[133] described the autopsy findings in a patient with MTHFR deficiency. The neurologic findings included perivascular demyelination and astrocytosis. Arterial vascular injury with intimal hyperplasia and extensive thrombosis was prominent. In the brain, the degree of demyelination was felt to be out of proportion to the vascular changes. Other post-mortem studies have also shown thrombosis and leukoencephalopathy.[134,135] There have been reports of patients with classic findings of subacute combined degeneration of the spinal cord similar to those described for vitamin B_{12} deficiency.[135,136]

The diagnosis of severe MTHFR deficiency has been made by direct measurement of enzyme activity in liver, leukocytes, cultured fibroblasts and lymphocytes. The specific activity of MTHFR in cultured fibroblasts is dependent on the stage of the culture cycle, being several fold higher in confluent cells than in cells in logarithmic growth. Therefore, it is important to compare activities of unknown samples and control cell lines in confluent cells. There is a rough correlation between residual enzyme activity and clinical severity.[137] In cultured fibroblasts, the proportion of total folate that is methyl-THF and the extent of labeled formate incorporated into methionine provide better correlations with clinical severity.[137,138] The gene for human MTHFR has been localized to chromosome 1p36.3. More than 30 mutations have been identified and there does not appear to be a predominant mutation in the families studied to date.[139] Prenatal diagnosis may be possible.[140–142] The inheritance appears to be autosomal recessive.[12]

The mechanism by which MTHFR and indeed cobalamin deficiency cause neuropathy is not well known. It may be due to undermethylation of proteins in the CNS caused by methionine deficiency, as betaine : homocysteine transferase, an alternative pathway for methionine production, is absent in the brain.[143] Since MTHFR is present in the mammalian brain and only methyl-THF can cross the blood–brain barrier, MTHFR deficiency may result in functionally low levels of folate in the brain.[20]

The prognosis is poor in severe MTHFR deficiency once there is evidence of neurologic involvement. Again, early recognition and treatment may improve the long-term neurologic outcome. Folic acid is given to maximize residual enzyme activity; and methyl-THF to replace the missing product of MTHFR.[12] Newborns should be given a trial of folic acid to assess responsiveness. Betaine appears to have improved the prognosis in patients both biochemically and developmentally.[102,144–146] Psychiatric symptoms also improved with betaine.[130] Other suggested agents include methionine to correct the deficiency of this amino acid; pyridoxine, which as a cofactor for cystathionine synthase may lower homocysteine levels; vitamin B_{12} because MeCbl is a cofactor for methionine synthetase; and carnitine, because of its requirement for adenosylmethionine.[12,102]

More than one case has been described in several families,

both affected males and females have been born to unaffected parents, and consanguinity has been reported, all features consistent with autosomal recessive inheritance.

Methylenetetrahydrofolate reductase polymorphisms

Two common polymorphisms have been identified in the MTHFR gene. The C677T (Ala to Val) transition when present in the homozygous form yields a thermolabile variant of MTHFR that has decreased activity at 37°C.[147] The 677T allele occurs with a higher frequency in whites compared with African-Americans or Africans. The frequency of this allele ranges from 0.17–0.19 in Asia to 0.27–0.36 in Western Europe.[148] Homozygous 677TT has about 30% of the activity of the wild-type enzyme[147] and individuals with this variant have about 22% and 24% higher homocysteine levels compared to persons with the 677CT and 677CC genotypes respectively.[149] Of note, the effect of the 677TT genotype on homocysteine levels may be more significant for people with relatively low folate levels.[149,150] Folate levels are reduced in children over 10 years of age with this genotype.[151] A second polymorphism has been described at position 1298 (A1298C) substituting a glutamine for alanine at that position. This mutation does decrease MTHFR activity but its effect on homocysteine levels is unclear.[152] These two mutations occur in linkage disequilibrium, with the combination of 677TT and 1298CC being extremely uncommon.[147]

While some studies have shown that hyperhomocysteinemia is a risk factor for both coronary artery disease and venous thromboembolism,[152] a recent metaanalysis revealed the correlation between MTHFR genotype and coronary artery disease to be weakly positive, with a 16% increase for those with the 677TT genotype.[153] Of interest, the increased risk was present in European but not North American populations, perhaps due to differences in folate status. While conflicting results have been obtained, it appears that no clear increased risk for venous thromboembolism can be assigned to the 677TT genotype.[154] In addition to risk of thrombotic disease, the 677TT genotype in the mother may increase the risk of neural tube defects in the newborn.

Several studies have documented a decreased rate of acute lymphoblastic leukemia in children and adults with the 677TT genotype.[155–157] Some studies have also shown a protective effect for the 1298C allele as well.[158] The story is less clear for non-Hodgkin lymphoma. Matsuo *et al.*[159] documented a decreased odds ratio for either the 677T or the 1298C alleles in adults with non-Hodgkin lymphoma. However, Skibola *et al.*[160] found an increased proportion of patients with subtypes of non-Hodgkin lymphoma to have the 677TT genotype and Stanulla *et al.*[161] found the representation of this genotype to be high in children with lymphoblastic lymphoma. Krajinovic *et al.*[158] found that the protective effect of the 677TT and 1298CC alleles was only present for Canadian children born before 1996, following which folate supplementation was recommended in Canada. Furthermore, one study documented decreased risk of childhood acute lymphoblastic leukemia if mothers received folate supplementation when pregnant.[162] The mechanism for the decreased risk of leukemia has not been proven, but it has been theorized that decreased MTHFR activity leads to increased levels of 5,10-methylenetetrahydrofolate available for purine and pyrimidine synthesis.[147]

Glutamate formiminotransferase deficiency

Histidine catabolism is associated with the transfer of a formimino group to THF, followed by the release of ammonia and the formation of 5,10-methenyltetrahydrofolate (see Fig. 6.4). The two steps in this reaction are carried out through a single bifunctional enzyme, formiminotransferase cyclodeaminase (FTCD) with two domains, glutamate formiminotransferase and formiminotetrahydrofolate cyclodeaminase.[163] Defects lead to build-up of formiminoglutamate (FIGLU). While rare, genetic defects in FTCD are the second most common genetic defect in folate metabolism, with more than 20 cases described.[12]

The clinical picture in patients with FTCD defects is quite inconsistent. Patients have been identified by elevation of FIGLU in the urine with or without histidine loading.[12] Some patients have had significant mental retardation, cortical atrophy, hypotonia, seizures and speech delay, while others do not appear to have significant neurologic problems.[12,164,165] Hematologic abnormalities including hypersegmented neutrophils and macrocytosis have also been described.[12,166] Decreased glutamate formiminotransferase activity in liver extracts (14–54% of control) and erythrocytes (35–37% of control) was seen in three patients,[165] although the ability to detect enzyme activity in erythrocytes is unclear.[12] Of note, three patients with malignancies were found to have increased urinary FIGLU and hydantoin proprionic acid (HPA) excretion that persisted after treatment.[12] This suggests that congenital FTCD deficiency may predispose to malignancy. In addition to elevated urinary excretion of FIGLU, serum folate levels are normal to increased and vitamin B_{12} levels are normal.[165,167]

As both males and females have been described, autosomal recessive inheritance is the probable means of transmission. The gene for FTCD has been cloned and maps to chromosome 21q22.3.[168] Gene abnormalities have been identified in patients with FTCD deficiency.[169] The gene is predominantly expressed in the liver with weak expression in the kidney. Of interest, FTCD appears to be the target antigen in type 2 autoimmune hepatitis.[170,171]

Treatment for this disorder is limited. Perry et al.[172] described two siblings who had massive urinary FIGLU excretion, speech delay and normal folate levels but whose FIGLU excretion decreased significantly with folate 5 mg

every 8 hours for 3 days or folinic acid 6 mg i.m. every 8 hours. However, others have not shown a response to folate treatment.[167,173] Methionine was not effective either clinically or biochemically in one patient.[167] As the relationship between clinical expression and FIGLU excretion is unclear, it is uncertain that reducing FIGLU excretion has clinical utility.

Transport disorders

Hereditary folate malabsorption

The process of folate absorption and transport is described above. Hereditary folate malabsorption (HFM) has also been called congenital malabsorption of folate; 18 patients have been described in the literature and the topic has been reviewed.[174] These children usually present in infancy with megaloblastic anemia, diarrhea, mouth ulcers, failure to thrive and usually progressive neurologic deterioration. Immunodeficiency is common and several infants had *Pneumocystis carinii* pneumonia either at diagnosis or shortly after treatment was initiated.[174,175] The neurologic disorders include mental retardation/developmental delay, seizures, intracranial calcifications and peripheral neuropathy.[174] The hematologic picture consists of megaloblastic anemia appearing in the first few months of life. The serum and red blood cell folate levels are low. Of significance, the folate level in the CSF is low, and lower than the serum level in folate-supplemented patients with HFM.[174] Excretion of FIGLU and orotic acid may be found in patients with HFM. All patients have a severe abnormality in the absorption of oral folic acid or reduced folates.

The defect in HFM remains to be identified. Malatack et al.[175] suggested that for HFM to occur defects must be present in both the high-capacity, pH-dependent active transport mechanism for folate and the low-capacity, pH-independent facilitated diffusion mechanism. Hence they propose that either there is a common component of both mechanisms or that the defects in the active transport system are more common than previously recognized. Even when blood folate levels are raised sufficiently to correct anemia, levels in the CSF remain low and the CSF/plasma folate ratio is reversed (normal > 3 : 1).[174–176]

The treatment of HFM requires maintaining adequate plasma and CSF folate levels. Folinic acid appears to be preferable to folic acid for obtaining adequate CSF levels, although the two may be used simultaneously.[176] Poncz and Cohen[177] reported that long-term folinic acid, initially 1.5 mg daily then decreased at age 6 years to five times weekly and then to three times weekly as a teenager, produced an excellent outcome in a single patient. Close monitoring of developmental functioning is important in addition to measurement of plasma and CSF folate concentrations. Many medications, such as anticonvulsants, antacids, histamine H_2 blockers and oral contraceptives, may further affect folate absorption and transport. This may be lead to changes in the adequacy of oral folinic acid treatment for patients with HFM.

There is a preponderance of females with HFM,[12] and the first reported male had atypical features,[178] including lack of mental retardation and correction of CSF folate levels in conjunction with correction of serum folate levels. Presumably affected siblings who died were noted in several of the families.[174] Consanguinity has been reported in several families, and the father of one patient has intermediate levels of folate absorption. These findings make autosomal recessive inheritance probable but unproven.

Cellular uptake defects

Although patients have been described with well-characterized abnormalities of folate uptake into cells, it is not clear that any of these represent primary defects. Branda *et al.*[179] reported an individual with severe aplastic anemia in whom folate treatment led to a dramatic recovery. There was an extensive family history of pancytopenia and leukemia. Studies revealed decreased uptake of 5-[14]CH$_3$-THF in lymphocytes and bone marrow cells, but normal uptake, polyglutamate formation and apparent function in thymidylate synthetase in mature erythrocytes and intestinal cells. This appeared to represent an inherited defect in folate cellular uptake in certain cells. In another family, the proband and three daughters had dyserythropoiesis without anemia.[180] There was abnormal methyl-THF uptake in red blood cells and bone marrow cells but not in lymphocytes. There was no clear correlation in the family between clinical findings and the disorder of cellular uptake.

Cerebral folate deficiency

5-Methyl-THF is actively transported into the CNS through binding to folate receptor protein 1 (FR1) attached to choroidal epithelial cells.[181] Wevers *et al.*[182] described an 18-year-old man with cerebellar symptoms, distal spinal muscular atrophy, pyramidal tract dysfunction and perceptive hearing loss who had severely low CSF but normal plasma and red blood cell folate levels. They suspected a defect in a folate-binding protein in the CSF leading to an isolated defect in the choroid plexus transport of folate. Subsequently, Ramaekers and Blau[181] reported 20 children who developed progressive neurologic findings beginning in infancy with deceleration of head growth, psychomotor retardation, cerebellar ataxia, spastic paraplegia, dyskinesia, visual disturbances and sensorineural hearing loss. Seven patients had seizures and seven had autistic features. CSF folate levels were low. The folate-binding affinity of FR1 was significantly reduced in four patients. Treatment with folinic acid 0.5–1 mg/kg daily or higher in some patients led to clinical improvement, especially in patients treated before 6 years of age.

Other inherited disorders associated with megaloblastic anemia

Thiamine-responsive megaloblastic anemia

Thiamine-responsive megaloblastic anemia, also known as Rogers syndrome, is a rare autosomal recessive disorder characterized by megaloblastic anemia, thrombocytopenia, diabetes mellitus, and sensorineural deafness.[183] The disorder is caused by abnormalities in the thiamine transporter protein THTR-1, encoded by the *SLC19A2* gene mapped to chromosome 1q23.2–23.3.[184,185] The THTR-1 protein has significant homology with the human reduced folate carrier protein.[185] Mutations in this gene have been reported in patients with thiamine-responsive megaloblastic anemia.[186–188] Other reported manifestations include retinitis pigmentosa, hypothyroidism, cardiac rhythm and structural abnormalities, optic nerve atrophy, and retinal dystrophy.[186,189,190] Villa *et al.*[191] reported an 18-year-old girl with thiamine-responsive megaloblastic anemia who suffered a stroke. The pathogenesis of the megaloblastic anemia appears to be related to decreased ribose formation.[192] Thiamine treatment improves the megaloblastic anemia and decreases insulin requirements.[183,193]

Hereditary orotic aciduria

Hereditary orotic aciduria is an autosomal recessive disease due to a defect in the last two enzyme activities of the pyrimidine *de novo* synthetic pathway: orotate phosphoribosyltransferase and orotidine-5′-monophosphate decarboxylase.[194] These two enzyme activities reside in a single bifunctional polypeptide, UMP synthase. The UMP synthase gene is localized to chromosome 3q13 and is approximately 15 kb in length.[194]

There have been 15 patients described with hereditary orotic aciduria and these patients have been recently reviewed.[194] Anemia is a consistent finding, with severe anisocytosis and macrocytosis. Hypochromia may be apparent. Leukopenia and neutropenia occur but thrombocytopenia has not been seen. Megaloblastic changes in the marrow are noted. Large amounts of orotic acid excreted in the urine may crystallize, causing urethral or ureteral obstruction. Orotic aciduria has also been noted in a patient with FTCD deficiency.[195] Malformations have been identified in several of these patients, including four individuals with congenital heart disease. Other abnormalities may include muscle weakness, strabismus, skeletal deformities and developmental delay, although these are not uniformly present. With treatment the prognosis is good, although the presence of malformations or immune deficiency may adversely affect prognosis. In addition, one patient had long-term neurologic degeneration.[194] The mainstay of treatment is uridine supplementation usually at a dose of 100–200 mg/kg daily, but dosing needs to be individualized.[194]

Acquired disorders of cobalamin metabolism (Table 6.1)

Nitrous oxide

It is well established that nitrous oxide (N_2O) is able to reversibly oxidize cobalamin from the cob(I) to cob(III) state. Because methionine synthase requires cobalamin in the fully reduced cob(I) state it is inactivated by nitrous oxide.[196] Myeloneuropathy has been reported in patients with vitamin B_{12} deficiency exposed to nitrous oxide.[197] Chronic nitrous oxide exposure has also resulted in myeloneuropathy.[198] Felmet *et al.*[199] described an 8-month-old infant who developed hypotonia, tremor and athetoid movements in association with macrocytic anemia 6 days after exposure to nitrous oxide. Three days later the infant had severe pancytopenia and megaloblastic changes in the bone marrow. Methylmalonic acid and homocysteine levels were markedly elevated. McNeely *et al.*[200] described an infant with a similar presentation 3 weeks after exposure to nitrous oxide anesthesia. Both infants had normal folate and very reduced cobalamin levels, responded well to cobalamin injections, and had evidence of maternal cobalamin deficiency. Selzer *et al.*[201] reported an infant with MTHFR deficiency who died after exposure to nitrous oxide anesthesia. Autopsy revealed asymmetric cerebral atrophy and severe demyelination. Transient elevated FIGLU excretion has been noted in some patients after nitrous oxide exposure.[202] While these case reports illustrate the potential for nitrous oxide to induce symptoms in at-risk individuals, the frequency of this problem appears to be very low.

Nutrition

Adult cobalamin stores are about 2000–3000 µg;[5] hence with a daily adult requirement of < 3 µg, it should take years for cobalamin deficiency to become symptomatic in the initially replete adult with an intact enterohepatic circulation. Adequate daily vitamin B_{12} intakes have been estimated to be 0.4 µg for infants < 6 months of age and 0.5–0.6 µg for those aged 6–12 months.[5] After infancy, the recommended dietary allowance (RDA) for cobalamin in children increases from 0.9 µg/day (1–3 years old) to 1.2 µg/day (4–8 years old) to 1.8 µg/day (9–13 years old) to 2.4 µg/day (14–18 years old). The RDA for pregnant women is 2.6 µg/day, with 2.8 µg/day during lactation. These figures assume normal absorption of this amount of the vitamin (approximately 50%) and an intact enterohepatic circulation.[5] The average American diet contains a mean of 4.6 µg/day (5.4 µg/day for males, 3.8 µg/day for females and 3.4 µg/day for adolescent females).[203] Vegan and macrobiotic diets contain little vitamin B_{12}. Holotranscobalamin II levels were reduced and homocysteine and methylmalonic acid levels were increased in a majority of nonsupplemented individuals who followed strict vegan or ovo-lacto diets,[204] although symptomatic changes or megaloblastic anemia appear to be uncommon in these people. Pregnant and lactating women have increased requirements for cobalamin.[5,205] Adolescents on vegetarian or macrobiotic diets may develop cobalamin deficiency with symptoms or cognitive changes.[206,207] There is a high incidence of cobalamin deficiency in developing countries such as Latin America.[208–210] It is unclear if this is entirely due to nutritional factors.[208]

Infants born to cobalamin-deficient mothers may become cobalamin deficient because of reduced placental transfer of cobalamin and, if breast-fed, because of cobalamin-deficient milk.[5,211,212] Several infants have been described who developed symptomatic cobalamin deficiency in infancy. Most were breast-fed infants of mothers who followed vegan diets.[213–217] These infants developed symptoms before the age of 18 months. Infants of mothers with pernicious anemia are rare because the disorder usually strikes after childbearing age and is associated with sterility.[218] Nevertheless, Lampkin *et al.*[219] reported an exclusively breast-fed 4-month-old infant who developed cobalamin deficiency. The mother had pernicious anemia and low levels of cobalamin in her milk. For older children, evidence of cobalamin deficiency has been noted in children and adolescents who follow vegetarianism without supplementation. Miller *et al.*[220] found that children fed a macrobiotic diet were more likely to have growth delay that correlated with elevations in methylmalonic acid.

Table 6.1 Acquired causes of cobalamin deficiency.

Nutritional
Maternal deficiency
Vegan

Malabsorption
Gastric
  Pernicious anemia
  Total or subtotal gastrectomy
Intestinal
  Stagnant loop syndrome
  Ileal resection
  Fish tapeworm
  Chronic tropical sprue

Malabsorption of cobalamin occurs in the following conditions but the deficiency is not usually sufficiently severe to cause megaloblastic anemia
  Gluten-induced enteropathy
  Cystic fibrosis and chronic pancreatitis
  Crohn disease uncomplicated by resection or stagnant loop
  Drugs: slow K, phenformin, metformin, cholestyramine

Malabsorption

Pernicious anemia

Pernicious anemia is an autoimmune disorder caused by antibodies against gastric parietal cells or intrinsic factor and is generally a disease of older adults. Pernicious anemia in children is quite rare, but has been reported in association with polyglandular autoimmune syndrome type I. Neufeld *et al.*[221] identified nine cases of pernicious anemia in 71 patients with this disorder. Typically, juvenile pernicious anemia presents in the first or second decade of life and is associated with other signs of endocrinopathy and atrophic gastritis.[222] As in adults, it may occur in any ethnic group and affects both sexes. Dahshan *et al.*[223] describe a case who presented at 17 years with prior history of diabetes mellitus at age 6, Graves disease at age 13 and schizophrenia at age 14. Many cases of polyglandular autoimmune syndrome type I are now classified as autoimmune polyendocrinopathy–candidiasis–ectodermal dystrophy (APECED). Features of APECED include candidiasis, alopecia, keratopathy, and multiple endocrine disorders including hypoparathyroidism, adrenal failure and insulin-dependent diabetes.[224] Multiple autoantibodies are described in this syndrome. Abnormalities of the *AIRE* gene, mapped to chromosome 21q22.3, may be responsible for this disorder.[225]

Other causes

Total or subtotal gastrectomy, intestinal stagnant loop syndrome and ileal resection may all cause severe cobalamin deficiency with megaloblastic anemia or neuropathy in children as in adults. Vitamin B_{12} deficiency has been seen in long-term follow-up of infants who had ileal resection for necrotizing enterocolitis.[226-228] In one report vitamin B_{12} absorption improved after several years.[229] Vitamin B_{12} deficiency has also been noted after neonatal subtotal gastrectomy.[230] Cobalamin absorption is decreased in children with cystic fibrosis,[231,232] perhaps due to impaired digestion of haptocorrins in the small intestine.[233] However, clinically significant cobalamin deficiency has been rarely reported in cystic fibrosis patients and one study found elevated cobalamin levels in these children.[234] The elevated levels may be due to liver disease and binding of cobalamin to TCI, and may not reflect the functional cobalamin status of these children. Supplemental cobalamin has been suggested for children with cystic fibrosis.[235] Other gastric illness such as infestation with *Diphyllobothrium latum* can deplete vitamin B_{12}.[236] *Helicobacter pylori* infection may play a role in cobalamin malabsorption.[208] A number of drugs, including proton pump inhibitors,[237] slow K, cholestyramine,[238] H_2 blockers,[196] and biguanides (metformin and phenformin),[239-241] have been reported to cause cobalamin malabsorption.

Food-cobalamin malabsorption

Food-cobalamin malabsorption has been described mainly in adults. It is manifested by an inability to absorb food-bound cobalamin with an intact ability to absorb free cobalamin. The Schilling test is normal. The disorder has been associated with atrophic gastritis, *Helicobacter* infection or partial gastrectomy.[196,242] The treatment is oral or systemic cobalamin supplementation.[243] It is likely that this disorder is due to an inability to remove cobalamin from R binders in food.

Folate deficiency (Table 6.2)

Nutrition

In the absence of clear data, the adequate folate intake for infants was estimated by determining the average intake of children fed predominantly human milk (~ 85 µg/L) and was found to be 65 µg/day or about 9.4 µg/kg daily for infants aged 0–6 months and 80 µg/day or about 8.8 µg/kg daily for those aged 7–12 months. The RDA for total folates in children increases from 150 µg/day (1–3 years old) to 200 µg/day (4–8 years old) to 300 µg/day (9–13 years old) to 400 µg/day (14–18 years old).[8] The RDA for pregnant women is

Table 6.2 Acquired causes of folate deficiency.

Nutritional
Inadequate poor-quality diet
Goats' milk
Special diets
Scurvy

Malabsorption
Gluten-induced enteropathy
Tropical sprue
Jejunal resection
Systemic infections

Increased requirements
Pregnancy, prematurity
Conditions with increased cell turnover
   Hemolytic anemias
   Widespread skin and other inflammatory diseases,
   e.g., tuberculosis, malaria
   Malignant diseases

Excess loss
Chronic dialysis

Drugs
Anticonvulsants, triamterene, sulfasalazine
Alcohol

Liver diseases

600 µg/day, with 500 µg/day during lactation.[8] Beginning in 1998, in the USA cereal-grain products have been fortified with 140 µg folic acid for every 100 g of cereal-grain.[9] This mandated folate supplementation of cereal-grain products has increased the American daily folate equivalent intake by about 200 µg to over 400 µg.[244]

Folate deficiency is common in children in underdeveloped countries. Villalpando *et al.*[245] found the incidence of severe folate deficiency to range from 2.8 to 13% for children < 4 years of age in Mexico, but was lower in those of higher socioeconomic status or higher vegetable intake.

Newborn infants have higher serum and red cell folate levels than adults but these fall in the first few weeks of life.[246,247] In premature infants the fall is steeper, folate reaches lower levels and folate deficiency with megaloblastic anemia may develop, especially if there are feeding difficulties, hemolytic disease, diarrhea or infection.[248] Goats' milk contains only 6 µg/L and infants fed only on this may develop clinically symptomatic deficiency.[249,250]

Pregnancy

Folate requirements are increased in pregnancy by about 200 µg/day to a total of 600 µg/day.[8] Folate is preferentially transferred to the fetus in a two-step process that involves placental folate-binding proteins.[20,251] Megaloblastic anemia may develop if the diet is inadequate and prophylactic folic acid is not given. Bone marrow examination showed that 25% or more of unsupplemented pregnant women had megaloblastic changes.[218] Folate deficiency can also lead to premature and low-birthweight infants.[218] Neonatal neural tube defects (spina bifida, meningocele, anencephaly) are associated with periconceptual folate deficiency.[252] In a randomized clinical trial, folate supplementation of 4 mg/day given to women with a previously affected child decreased the rate of neural tube defects by 72%.[253] In another trial, periconceptual folic acid supplementation of 400 µg/day decreased the rate of neural tube defects by 79% in a high-risk region.[254] Folic acid supplementation has also been shown in some studies to decrease the rate of cleft lip and palate,[255–257] and possibly conotruncal abnormalities.[258] Folate antagonists increase the rate of these deformities.[259] Similarly, the 677TT polymorphism in the MTHFR gene has been associated with increased neural tube defects.[260,261]

Malabsorption

Folate deficiency is very common in celiac disease (gluten-sensitive enteropathy).[262,263] The majority of patients with untreated celiac disease have anemia.[263] The anemia can be due to both iron and folate deficiency, hence a dimorphic picture may be seen. Anemia secondary to iron and folate deficiency may be present even in the absence of gastrointestinal symptoms.[264] Virtually all affected children have sub-

normal serum and red cell folate levels.[263] Malabsorption of cobalamin is frequent but cobalamin deficiency is generally not sufficiently severe to be the main cause of megaloblastic anemia.[263] While the presence of IgA anti-endomysial antibodies and transglutamase antibodies have a high sensitivity and specificity for celiac disease, the diagnosis is confirmed by endoscopy and biopsy. The intestinal lesion responds to withdrawal of gluten (glutamine-rich protein) from the diet. There is an increased risk of intestinal non-Hodgkin lymphoma as well as cancers of the mouth, pharynx and esophagus in adults.[265,266] Withdrawal of gluten also reduces the risk of subsequent development of cancer.[266]

Tropical sprue occurs in the local population and visitors to areas in the tropics where the condition is endemic. Generalized small intestinal malabsorption occurs. Folate and cobalamin deficiency are very common in tropical sprue.[267] In the chronic disease, cobalamin deficiency may become severe and cause megaloblastic anemia or neuropathy, even in the absence of gastrointestinal symptoms.[268] The cause of tropical sprue is likely to be an infection and antibiotic therapy is indicated. Therapy should also include folate and cobalamin (the latter especially for chronic cases).[268] Other acquired causes of folate malabsorption occasionally seen in childhood include inflammatory bowel disease[269,270] and gastric bypass.[271]

HIV infection[272] or systemic bacterial infections can cause folate deficiency.[273] Many medications are associated with folate deficiency and/or megaloblastic anemia. Phenytoin, carbamazepine, valproic acid and oral contraceptives may in some instances cause low folate levels.[274,275] Tobacco use has been associated with lower red blood cell folate levels.[274,276] Alcohol abuse is a common cause of folate deficiency for a number of reasons.[277,278]

Excess utilization

In a wide range of inflammatory and malignant diseases, folate requirements are increased (see Table 6.2). These include chronic hemolytic anemias, severe chronic infections and widespread skin diseases. Folate may also be lost by dialysis.[279] Conditions of increased folate need, e.g., sickle cell anemia, HIV infection, hepatitis and malaria, may increase the risk of the deficiency. In sickle cell disease, varying results have been seen. For instance, van der Dijs *et al.*[280] found elevated homocysteine levels in sickle cell patients that decreased by 50% with folate supplementation. In contrast, Rodriguez-Cortes *et al.*[281] found normal plasma homocysteine levels as well as serum and red cell folate values in unsupplemented sickle cell patients.

Antifolate drugs

Inhibitors of human dihydrofolate reductase (DHFR) include methotrexate, pyrimethamine and, to a much lesser degree, trimethoprim. Methotrexate causes megaloblastosis in humans whereas the main action of pyrimethamine is against malarial parasite DHFR. Trimethoprim acts against the bacterial enzyme and is at least 1000-fold less able than methotrexate to bind human DHFR.[282] Methotrexate is converted to polyglutamate forms in cells and this may result in prolonged inhibition of DNA synthesis. Alcohol, which may be the commonest cause of folate deficiency in the USA, has a variety of effects on folate metabolism, including decreased intestinal absorption and decreased hepatic storage as well as a direct effect on the bone marrow causing vacuolated normoblasts or megaloblasts.[282]

Tissue effects of cobalamin and folate deficiencies

The characteristic morphologic abnormalities of megaloblastic anemia are noted on the peripheral blood smear and bone marrow morphology. Anemia is usually but not always present and may be accompanied by neutropenia and thrombocytopenia. The mean cell volume is increased and erythrocyte morphology reveals macrocytosis and misshapen red blood cells. Neutrophil hypersegmentation, defined as > 5% of neutrophils with five clearly distinct lobes or the presence of any neutrophils with six clear lobes (Fig. 6.6). The bone marrow findings include dyserythropoiesis with less tightly condensed nuclear chromatin than appropriate for the degree of cytoplasmic maturation (nuclear–cytoplasmic dyssynchrony). There are giant bands and metamyelocytes. Of note, there is a relative decrease in late hematopoietic precursors due to ineffective hematopoeisis. This ineffective hematopoiesis also causes elevations in serum bilirubin and lactate dehydrogenase. The detailed mechanisms by which inhibition of DNA synthesis leads to the morphologic and biochemical features of megaloblastic anemia are unclear. One explanation has proposed that the intracellular

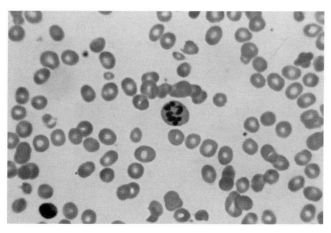

Fig. 6.6 Neutrophil hypersegmentation.

accumulation of uracil due to the inhibition of thymidylate synthetase leads to the formation of dUTP, which in turn is misincorporated into DNA. Excision of these uracil molecules can lead to breaks in the DNA.[143] Apoptosis appears to be increased in hematopoietic progenitors.[283]

As noted above, neuropathy due to cobalamin deficiency is seen in children with severe cobalamin deficiency as well as defects in cobalamin metabolism. Permanent mental retardation may result.[284,285] In older children and adults, features of a peripheral neuropathy mainly affecting the legs with, in severe cases, posterior column and pyramidal features are characteristic (subacute combined degeneration of the spinal cord). Paresthesiae, loss of sensation in the feet and unsteadiness in the dark are typical symptoms. Psychiatric and ophthalmic features may be present. The mechanism is not well understood, but may be related to undermethylation of myelin.[143] Neutrophil function defects have been described in cobalamin deficiency.[286,287]

The deficiencies affect epithelial surfaces. Glossitis, manifested as a painful, smooth, red tongue, may be a presenting feature.[288] Pathologically, squamous cells in the oral mucosa show nuclear and cytoplasmic enlargement.[289] Intestinal and other epithelial cells also show changes with folate or vitamin B_{12} deficiency.[290]

Serum bone alkaline phosphatase is reduced due to an effect on osteoblasts.[291] Reversible, diffuse hyperpigmentation due to hypermelanosis has been described in both children and adults with cobalamin defiency.[292–294]

Diagnosis

Measurement of serum cobalamin and serum and/or red cell folate are the most commonly used techniques. Both serum and red blood cell levels for folate and cobalamin can be measured by radiodilution, microbiological and chemiluminescence assays. Red blood cell assays are less affected by recent changes in diet or medications.[295] Typically, both serum and red blood cell folate levels will be reduced in folate deficiency and serum cobalamin levels are reduced in cobalamin deficiency. TCI levels exceed TCII levels in the plasma, although as previously noted the cobalamin attached to TCI is not in the metabolically active pool.[34] Elevations of TCI, as can occur in myelodysplastic syndrome or with oral contraceptive use, can cause normal serum cobalamin values in the presence of cobalamin deficiency. Similarly, deficiency of TCI can cause low serum cobalamin levels without disease.[33,296] Low red blood folate levels and normal to elevated serum folate levels are seen in cobalamin deficiency.[295] The mechanism for this "methylfolate trap" phenomenon is not clearly established.[143]

Metabolic assays may be helpful in diagnosing patients with mild deficiencies or who have false-positive results for serum folate or cobalamin. Serum methylmalonic acid is elevated in cobalamin but not folate deficiency and is sensitive for CblA, CblB, CblC, CblD and CblF.[196] It is also elevated in renal failure, thyroid disease, hemoconcentration, small bowel bacterial overgrowth and pregnancy.[196,297] Serum homocysteine is elevated in both folate and cobalamin deficiency.[196] Homocysteine is elevated in CblC, CblD, CblE, CblF and CblG, MTHFR deficiency and can also be elevated with the 677TT MTHFR polymorphism, especially when folate levels are suboptimal.[196] Homocysteine levels are less specific and are elevated in renal dysfunction, hypothyroidism, vitamin B_6 deficiency and with certain medications such as cholestyramine, carbamazepine and valproic acid.[196,297] Hence, patients with suspected cobalamin or folate deficiency and normal serum levels should be investigated with plasma or serum methylmalonic acid and homocysteine levels.[295] Recently, low levels of holotranscobalamin II have been shown to be another sensitive method for diagnosing cobalamin deficiency.[204] Holotranscobalamin II may be an early marker of cobalamin deficiency, with levels decreasing before there are other manifestations of the disorder.[298,299] The deoxyuridine suppression test is an indirect test of thymidylate synthesis. Deoxyuridine is added to bone marrow cells followed by exposure to ^{3}H-thymidine. In normal cells, deoxyuridine is rapidly converted to TTP and incorporated into DNA, suppressing the incorporation of ^{3}H-thymidine. In cells deficient in cobalamin or folate, there is a relative inability to convert deoxyuridine to thymidylate triphosphate, hence less suppression of ^{3}H-thymidine uptake into DNA. The test is corrected in cobalamin deficiency by cobalamin or 5-formyl-THF, but not by 5-methyl-THF. In folate deficiency, 5-formyl-THF and 5-methyl-THF both correct the test but cobalamin does not.[295] While the test is quite sensitive to early deficiency and can exclude other refractory macrocytic anemias such as myelodysplastic syndrome,[295] the test is only performed in specialized laboratories.

Tests of cobalamin absorption

The Schilling test is used to diagnose defects in cobalamin absorption. Fasting patients who are at least 3 days out from cobalamin exposure ingest a dose of ^{57}Co-labeled cobalamin. Thereafter, this labeled cobalamin is exceted into the urine, flushed by a large parenteral dose of unlabeled cobalamin. A 24-hour urine collection is analyzed for radioactivity. If subnormal amounts are excreted, a defect in cobalamin absorption is likely. The test can be repeated days later, administering exogenous IF with the ^{57}Co-labeled cobalamin. Correction of the defect confirms IF deficiency as occurs in congenital IF deficiency or pernicious anemia, but failure to correct with IF is not uncommon in patients with pernicious anemia.[295] In another modification of this test, ingested cobalamin is given with food such as eggs to investigate food-cobalamin malabsorption.[295]

Treatment

The treatment of disorders of cobalamin and folate metabolism and absorption has been previously discussed. Patients with severe anemia should be monitored closely for signs of heart failure. Transfusion should be given very slowly to avoid worsening the patient's cardiovascular status. In patients with severe anemia, close attention should be paid to electrolyte status to look for hypokalemia following initiation of treatment. High-dose folate may reverse the hematologic features of cobalamin deficiency, but the neurologic manifestations can progress. Hence, it is important to ensure that cobalamin deficiency is excluded before treating solely with folate.

Cobalamin deficiency is first treated by a series of intramuscular or subcutaneous injections of hydroxocobalamin (1000 µg in adults); usually six are given over a few weeks at intervals of a few days. Low doses of cobalamin (10 µg/day or 0.2 µg/kg daily subcutaneously for 2 days) may stimulate reticulocytosis and partially improve the metabolic state of the patient. Despite earlier reports of frequent mortality with treatment of severe cobalamin deficiency, Carmel[300] reported only a single death secondary to a coexisting disease in 219 patients with pernicious anemia of whom 101 had a hemoglobin ≤ 80 g/L. There is no comment on dosing of cobalamin treatment for these patients.[300] Maintenance is 1000 µg of hydroxocobalamin every 3 months. Vegans with cobalamin deficiency are also initially loaded with cobalamin and they may then be advised to eat food supplemented with cobalamin. Prophylactic cobalamin therapy is given to patients with an ileal resection or total gastrectomy.

Folate deficiency is initially corrected by giving folic acid 5 mg (100 µg/kg) daily for 4 months. The treatment is continued if the underlying condition causing folate deficiency cannot be reversed and daily folate dietary intake is not improved. Folinic acid (5-formyl-THF) is used to reverse the effect of methotrexate. Prophylactic folic acid is often given to children with severe hemolytic anemias, e.g., sickle cell anemia, thalassemia major and severe autoimmune hemolytic anemia, although as previously noted folate deficiency appears to be uncommon in patients with sickle cell disease. Periodic check of serum cobalamin levels may be advisable to avoid masking unsuspected cobalamin deficiency.[301] Folate (0.1 mg/day) and cobalamin (100 µg/month) supplementation to premature infants increased hemoglobin concentration in a randomized controlled trial.[302]

Other causes of megaloblastic and macrocytic anemia

Megaloblastic changes can be seen in the marrow in the

absence of disorders of cobalamin or folate. Drugs inhibiting synthesis of purine or pyrimidine DNA precursors at various points in DNA synthesis cause megaloblastic anemia. These drugs include hydroxycarbamide (hydroxyurea), mercaptopurine, 5-fluorouracil, cytosine arabinoside, zidovudine and others.[282] Erythropoiesis may also be megaloblastic in acute myeloid leukemia and myelodysplasia but the site of the presumed block in DNA synthesis is unknown. Congenital dyserythropoietic anemia types 1 and 3 have megaloblastic erythropoiesis.[303] These disorders are discussed elsewhere in this book.

Pappo *et al.*[304] reviewed the causes of macrocytosis in 146 children with a mean corpuscular volume > 90 fL; 35% were due to medications, principally anticonvulsants, zidovudine and immunosuppressive agents. Other causes were congenital heart disease (14%), Down syndrome (8%), reticulocytosis (8%) and marrow failure/myelodysplasia (4%). Neither cobalamin nor folate deficiency was identified, although extensive studies were not performed to rule them out. Macrocytic anemia has also been seen with hypothyroidism[305] and selenium deficiency.[306]

Acknowledgments

I would like to recognize the excellent work of Dr D.S. Rosenblatt and Dr A.V. Hoffbrand, who authored the chapter on this topic in the second edition of this book and which served as the backbone for this chapter.

References

1. Wickramasinghe SN. Morphology, biology and biochemistry of cobalamin- and folate-deficient bone marrow cells. *Baillières Clin Haematol* 1995; **8**: 441–59.

2. Banerjee R, Ragsdale SW. The many faces of vitamin B12: catalysis by cobalamin-dependent enzymes. *Annu Rev Biochem* 2003; **72**: 209–47.

3. Combs GF Jr. Vitamin B12. In: Combs GF Jr (ed.) *The Vitamins: Fundamental Aspects in Nutrition and Health*, 2nd edn. San Diego: Academic Press, 1998, pp. 403–20.

4. El Kholty S, Gueant JL, Bressler L *et al.* Portal and biliary phases of enterohepatic circulation of corrinoids in humans. *Gastroenterology* 1991; **101**: 1399–408.

5. Institute of Medicine. Vitamin B12. In: *Dietary Reference Intakes for Thiamin, Riboflavin, Niacin, Vitamin B6, Folate, Vitamin B12, Pantothenic Acid, Biotin, and Choline*. Washington, DC: National Academies Press, 1996, pp. 306–56.

6. Sigal SH, Hall CA, Antel JP. Plasma R binder deficiency and neurologic disease. *N Engl J Med* 1987; **317**: 1330–2.

7. Combs GF Jr. Folate. In: Combs GF Jr (ed.) *The Vitamins: Fundamental Aspects in Nutrition and Health*, 2nd edn. San Diego: Academic Press, 1998, pp. 377–401.

8. Institute of Medicine. Folate. In: *Dietary Reference Intakes for Thiamin, Riboflavin, Niacin, Vitamin B6, Folate, Vitamin B12, Pantothenic Acid, Biotin, and Choline*. Washington, DC: National Academies Press, 1998, pp. 196–305.

9. Rothenberg SP. Increasing the dietary intake of folate: pros and cons. *Semin Hematol* 1999; **36**: 65–74.

10. Seyoum E, Selhub J. Properties of food folates determined by stability and susceptibility to intestinal pteroylpolyglutamate hydrolase action. *J Nutr* 1998; **128**: 1956–60.

11. Sirotnak FM, Tolner B. Carrier-mediated membrane transport of folates in mammalian cells. *Annu Rev Nutr* 1999; **19**: 91–122.

12. Rosenblatt DS, Fenton WA. Inherited disorders of folate and cobalamin transport and metabolism. In: Scriver C, Baudet A, Sly W, Valle D (eds) *Metaboloic and Molecular Basis of Inherited Disease*, 8th edn. New York: McGraw-Hill, 2001, pp. 3897–933.

13. Brzezinska A, Winska P, Balinska M. Cellular aspects of folate and antifolate membrane transport. *Acta Biochim Pol* 2000; **47**: 735–49.

14. Pratt RF, Cooper BA. Folates in plasma and bile of man after feeding folic acid-³H and 5-formyltetrahydrofolate (folinic acid). *J Clin Invest* 1971; **50**: 455–62.

15. Herbert V. Folic acid. In: Shils ME, Olson JA, Shike M, Ross AC (eds) *Modern Nutrition in Health and Disease*, 9th edn. Baltimore: Williams & Wilkins, 1999, pp. 433–46.

16. Steinberg SE, Campbell CL, Hillman RS. Kinetics of the normal folate enterohepatic cycle. *J Clin Invest* 1979; **64**: 83–8.

17. Katz M, Mehlman CS, Allen RH. Isolation and characterization of an abnormal human intrinsic factor. *J Clin Invest* 1974; **53**: 1274–83.

18. Carmel R. Gastric juice in congenital pernicious anemia contains no immunoreactive intrinsic factor molecule: study of three kindreds with variable ages at presentation, including a patient first diagnosed in adulthood. *Am J Hum Genet* 1983; **35**: 67–77.

19. Remacha AF, Sambeat MA, Barcelo MJ, Mones J, Garcia-Die J, Gimferrer E. Congenital intrinsic factor deficiency in a Spanish patient. *Ann Hematol* 1992; **64**: 202–4.

20. Rosenblatt DS, Whitehead VM. Cobalamin and folate deficiency: acquired and hereditary disorders in children. *Semin Hematol* 1999; **36**: 19–34.

21. Yang YM, Ducos R, Rosenberg AJ *et al.* Cobalamin malabsorption in three siblings due to an abnormal intrinsic factor that is markedly susceptible to acid and proteolysis. *J Clin Invest* 1985; **76**: 2057–65.

22. Yassin F, Rothenberg SP, Rao S, Gordon MM, Alpers DH, Quadros EV. Identification of a 4-base deletion in the gene in inherited intrinsic factor deficiency. *Blood* 2004; **103**: 1515–17.

23. Rossler J, Breitenstein S, Havers W. Late onset of Imerslund–Grasbeck syndrome without proteinuria in four children of one family from the Lebanon. *Eur J Pediatr* 2003; **162**: 808–9.

24. Carmel R, Green R, Rosenblatt DS, Watkins D. Update on cobalamin, folate, and homocysteine. *Hematology (Am Soc Hematol Educ Program)* 2003; 62–81.

25. Tanner SM, Aminoff M, Wright FA *et al.* Amnionless, essential for mouse gastrulation, is mutated in recessive hereditary megaloblastic anemia. *Nat Genet* 2003; **33**: 426–9.

26. Fyfe JC, Madsen M, Hojrup P *et al.* The functional cobalamin (vitamin B12)-intrinsic factor receptor is a novel complex of cubilin and amnionless. *Blood* 2004; **103**: 1573–9.

27. Carmel R, Herbert V. Deficiency of vitamin B12-binding alpha globulin in two brothers. *Blood* 1969; **33**: 1–12.

28. Hall CA, Begley JA. Congenital deficiency of human R-type binding proteins of cobalamin. *Am J Hum Genet* 1977; **29**: 619–26.

29. Carmel R. R-binder deficiency. A clinically benign cause of cobalamin pseudodeficiency. *JAMA* 1983; **250**: 1886–90.

30. Carmel R. A new case of deficiency of the R binder for cobalamin, with observations on minor cobalamin-binding proteins in serum and saliva. *Blood* 1982; **59**: 152–6.

31. Jenks J, Begley J, Howard L. Cobalamin R binder deficiency in a woman with thalassemia. *Nutr Rev* 1983; **41**: 277–80.

32. Zittoun J, Leger J, Marquet J, Carmel R. Combined congenital deficiencies of intrinsic factor and R binder. *Blood* 1988; **72**: 940–3.

33. Carmel R. Mild transcobalamin I (haptocorrin) deficiency and low serum cobalamin concentrations. *Clin Chem* 2003; **49**: 1367–74.

34. Carmel R. The distribution of endogenous cobalamin among cobalamin-binding proteins in the blood in normal and abnormal states. *Am J Clin Nutr* 1985; **41**: 713–19.

35. Kolhouse JF, Kondo H, Allen NC, Podell E, Allen RH. Cobalamin analogues are present in human plasma and can mask cobalamin deficiency because current radioisotope dilution assays are not specific for true cobalamin. *N Engl J Med* 1978; **299**: 785–92.

36. Frisbie SM, Chance MR. Human cobalophilin: the structure of bound methylcobalamin and a functional role in protecting methylcobalamin from photolysis. *Biochemistry* 1993; **32**: 13886–92.

37. Linnell JC, Bhatt HR. Inherited errors of cobalamin metabolism and their management. *Baillières Clin Haematol* 1995; **8**: 567–601.

38. Carmel R, Ravindranath Y. Congenital transcobalamin II deficiency presenting atypically with a low serum cobalamin level: studies demonstrating the coexistence of a circulating transcobalamin I (R binder) complex. *Blood* 1984; **63**: 598–605.

39. Porck HJ, Frater-Schroder M, Frants RR, Kierat L, Eriksson AW. Genetic evidence for fetal origin of transcobalamin II in human cord blood. *Blood* 1983; **62**: 234–7.

40. Niebrugge DJ, Benjamin DR, Christie D, Scott CR. Hereditary transcobalamin II deficiency presenting as red cell hypoplasia. *J Pediatr* 1982; **101**: 732–5.

41. Meyers PA, Carmel R. Hereditary transcobalamin II deficiency with subnormal serum cobalamin levels. *Pediatrics* 1984; **74**: 866–71.

42. Burman JF, Mollin DL, Sourial NA, Sladden RA. Inherited lack of transcobalamin II in serum and megaloblastic anaemia: a further patient. *Br J Haematol* 1979; **43**: 27–38.

43. Thomas PK, Hoffbrand AV, Smith IS. Neurological involvement in hereditary transcobalamin II deficiency. *J Neurol Neurosurg Psychiatry* 1982; **45**: 74–7.

44. Zeitlin HC, Sheppard K, Baum JD, Bolton FG, Hall CA. Homozygous transcobalamin II deficiency maintained on oral hydroxocobalamin. *Blood* 1985; **66**: 1022–7.

45. Hall CA. The neurologic aspects of transcobalamin II deficiency. *Br J Haematol* 1992; **80**: 117–20.

46. Monagle PT, Tauro GP. Long-term follow up of patients with transcobalamin II deficiency. *Arch Dis Child* 1995; **72**: 237–8.

47. Barshop BA, Wolff J, Nyhan WL *et al.* Transcobalamin II deficiency presenting with methylmalonic aciduria and homocystinuria and abnormal absorption of cobalamin. *Am J Med Genet* 1990; **35**: 222–8.

48. Bibi H, Gelman-Kohan Z, Baumgartner ER, Rosenblatt DS. Transcobalamin II deficiency with methylmalonic aciduria in three sisters. *J Inherit Metab Dis* 1999; **22**: 765–72.

49. Qian L, Quadros EV, Regec A, Zittoun J, Rothenberg SP. Congenital transcobalamin II deficiency due to errors in RNA editing. *Blood Cells Mol Dis* 2002; **28**: 134–42; discussion 143–5.

50. Haurani FI, Hall CA, Rubin R. Megaloblastic anemia as a result of an abnormal transcobalamin II (Cardeza). *J Clin Invest* 1979; **64**: 1253–9.

51. Eiberg H, Moller N, Mohr J, Nielsen LS. Linkage of transcobalamin II (TC2) to the P blood group system and assignment to chromosome 22. *Clin Genet* 1986; **29**: 354–9.

52. Li N, Seetharam S, Seetharam B. Genomic structure of human transcobalamin II: comparison to human intrinsic factor and transcobalamin I. *Biochem Biophys Res Commun* 1995; **208**: 756–64.

53. Li N, Rosenblatt DS, Kamen BA, Seetharam S, Seetharam B. Identification of two mutant alleles of transcobalamin II in an affected family. *Hum Mol Genet* 1994; **3**: 1835–40.

54. Li N, Rosenblatt DS, Seetharam B. Nonsense mutations in human transcobalamin II deficiency. *Biochem Biophys Res Commun* 1994; **204**: 1111–18.

55. Rosenblatt DS, Hosack A, Matiaszuk N. Expression of transcobalamin II by amniocytes. *Prenat Diagn* 1987; **7**: 35–9.

56. Mayes JS, Say B, Marcus DL. Prenatal studies in a family with transcobalamin II deficiency. *Am J Hum Genet* 1987; **41**: 686–7.

57. Carmel R. Transcobalamin II deficiency and oral cobalamin therapy. *Blood* 1986; **67**: 1522–3.

58. Arlet JB, Varet B, Besson C. Favorable long-term outcome of a patient with transcobalamin II deficiency. *Ann Intern Med* 2002; **137**: 704–5.

59. Coulombe JT, Shih VE, Levy HL. Massachusetts Metabolic Disorders Screening Program. II. Methylmalonic aciduria. *Pediatrics* 1981; **67**: 26–31.

60. Sniderman LC, Lambert M, Giguere R *et al.* Outcome of individuals with low-moderate methylmalonic aciduria detected through a neonatal screening program. *J Pediatr* 1999; **134**: 675–80.

61. Fenton WA, Hack AM, Willard HR, Gertler A, Rosenberg LE. Purification and properties of methylmalonyl coenzyme A mutase from human liver. *Arch Biochem Biophys* 1982; **214**: 815–23.

62. Fenton W, Rosenberg L. Disorders of propionate and methylmalonate metabolism. In: Scriver C, Baudet A, Sly W, Valle D (eds) *Metaboloic and Molecular Basis of Inherited Disease*, 8th edn. New York: McGraw-Hill, 2001, pp. 2165–93.

63. Fenton WA, Hack AM, Kraus JP, Rosenberg LE. Immunochemical studies of fibroblasts from patients with methylmalonyl-CoA mutase apoenzyme deficiency: detection of a mutation interfering with mitochondrial import. *Proc Natl Acad Sci USA* 1987; **84**: 1421–4.

64. Raff ML, Crane AM, Jansen R, Ledley FD, Rosenblatt DS. Genetic characterization of a MUT locus mutation discriminating heterogeneity in mut0 and mut– methylmalonic aciduria by interallelic complementation. *J Clin Invest* 1991; **87**: 203–7.

65. Qureshi AA, Crane AM, Matiaszuk NV, Rezvani I, Ledley FD, Rosenblatt DS. Cloning and expression of mutations demonstrating intragenic complementation in mut0 methylmalonic aciduria. *J Clin Invest* 1994; **93**: 1812–19.

66. Matsui SM, Mahoney MJ, Rosenberg LE. The natural history of the inherited methylmalonic acidemias. *N Engl J Med* 1983; **308**: 857–61.

67. Inoue S, Krieger I, Sarnaik A, Ravindranath Y, Fracassa M, Ottenbreit MJ. Inhibition of bone marrow stem cell growth in vitro by methylmalonic acid: a mechanism for pancytopenia in a patient with methylmalonic acidemia. *Pediatr Res* 1981; **15**: 95–8.

68. Ledley FD, Levy HL, Shih VE, Benjamin R, Mahoney MJ. Benign methylmalonic aciduria. *N Engl J Med* 1984; **311**: 1015–18.

69. Varvogli L, Repetto GM, Waisbren SE, Levy HL. High cognitive outcome in an adolescent with mut– methylmalonic acidemia. *Am J Med Genet* 2000; **96**: 192–5.

70. Peters HL, Nefedov M, Lee LW et al. Molecular studies in mutase-deficient (MUT) methylmalonic aciduria: identification of five novel mutations. *Hum Mutat* 2002; **20**: 406.

71. Crane AM, Ledley FD. Clustering of mutations in methylmalonyl CoA mutase associated with mut– methylmalonic acidemia. *Am J Hum Genet* 1994; **55**: 42–50.

72. Ledley FD, Jansen R, Nham SU, Fenton WA, Rosenberg LE. Mutation eliminating mitochondrial leader sequence of methylmalonyl-CoA mutase causes mut0 methylmalonic acidemia. *Proc Natl Acad Sci USA* 1990; **87**: 3147–50.

73. Crane AM, Martin LS, Valle D, Ledley FD. Phenotype of disease in three patients with identical mutations in methylmalonyl CoA mutase. *Hum Genet* 1992; **89**: 259–64.

74. Adjalla CE, Hosack AR, Matiaszuk NV, Rosenblatt DS. A common mutation among blacks with mut– methylmalonic aciduria. *Hum Mutat* 1998; suppl. 1: S248–S250.

75. Ogasawara M, Matsubara Y, Mikami H, Narisawa K. Identification of two novel mutations in the methylmalonyl-CoA mutase gene with decreased levels of mutant mRNA in methylmalonic acidemia. *Hum Mol Genet* 1994; **3**: 867–72.

76. Acquaviva C, Benoist JF, Callebaut I et al. N219Y, a new frequent mutation among mut0 forms of methylmalonic acidemia in Caucasian patients. *Eur J Hum Genet* 2001; **9**: 577–82.

77. Roe CR, Hoppel CL, Stacey TE, Chalmers RA, Tracey BM, Millington DS. Metabolic response to carnitine in methylmalonic aciduria. An effective strategy for elimination of propionyl groups. *Arch Dis Child* 1983; **58**: 916–20.

78. Chalmers RA, Stacey TE, Tracey BM et al. L-Carnitine insufficiency in disorders of organic acid metabolism: response to L-carnitine by patients with methylmalonic aciduria and 3-hydroxy-3-methylglutaric aciduria. *J Inherit Metab Dis* 1984; **7** (suppl. 2): 109–10.

79. Thompson GN, Chalmers RA, Walter JH et al. The use of metronidazole in management of methylmalonic and propionic acidaemias. *Eur J Pediatr* 1990; **149**: 792–6.

80. Koletzko B, Bachmann C, Wendel U. Antibiotic therapy for improvement of metabolic control in methylmalonic aciduria. *J Pediatr* 1990; **117**: 99–101.

81. Treacy E, Arbour L, Chessex P et al. Glutathione deficiency as a complication of methylmalonic acidemia: response to high doses of ascorbate. *J Pediatr* 1996; **129**: 445–8.

82. Mahoney MJ, Bick D. Recent advances in the inherited methylmalonic acidemias. *Acta Paediatr Scand* 1987; **76**: 689–96.

83. Walter JH, Michalski A, Wilson WM, Leonard JV, Barratt TM, Dillon MJ. Chronic renal failure in methylmalonic acidaemia. *Eur J Pediatr* 1989; **148**: 344–8.

84. Dobson CM, Wai T, Leclerc D et al. Identification of the gene responsible for the cblA complementation group of vitamin B12-responsive methylmalonic acidemia based on analysis of prokaryotic gene arrangements. *Proc Natl Acad Sci USA* 2002; **99**: 15554–9.

85. Lerner-Ellis JP, Dobson CM, Wai T et al. Mutations in the MMAA gene in patients with the cblA disorder of vitamin B12 metabolism. *Hum Mutat* 2004; **24**: 509–16.

86. Cooper BA, Rosenblatt DS, Watkins D. Methylmalonic aciduria due to a new defect in adenosylcobalamin accumulation by cells. *Am J Hematol* 1990; **34**: 115–20.

87. Fenton WA, Rosenberg LE. The defect in the cbl B class of human methylmalonic acidemia: deficiency of cob(I)alamin adenosyltransferase activity in extracts of cultured fibroblasts. *Biochem Biophys Res Commun* 1981; **98**: 283–9.

88. Dobson CM, Wai T, Leclerc D et al. Identification of the gene responsible for the cblB complementation group of vitamin B12-dependent methylmalonic aciduria. *Hum Mol Genet* 2002; **11**: 3361–9.

89. Watkins D, Matiaszuk N, Rosenblatt DS. Complementation studies in the cblA class of inborn error of cobalamin metabolism: evidence for interallelic complementation and for a new complementation class (cblH). *J Med Genet* 2000; **37**: 510–13.

90. Batshaw ML, Thomas GH, Cohen SR, Matalon R, Mahoney MJ. Treatment of the cblB form of methylmalonic acidaemia with adenosylcobalamin. *J Inherit Metab Dis* 1984; **7**: 65–8.

91. Chalmers RA, Bain MD, Mistry J, Tracey BM, Weaver C. Enzymologic studies on patients with methylmalonic aciduria: basis for a clinical trial of deoxyadenosylcobalamin in a hydroxocobalamin-unresponsive patient. *Pediatr Res* 1991; **30**: 560–3.

92. van der Meer SB, Spaapen LJ, Fowler B, Jakobs C, Kleijer WJ, Wendel U. Prenatal treatment of a patient with vitamin B12-responsive methylmalonic acidemia. *J Pediatr* 1990; **117**: 923–6.

93. Ampola MG, Mahoney MJ, Nakamura E, Tanaka K. Prenatal therapy of a patient with vitamin-B12-responsive methylmalonic acidemia. *N Engl J Med* 1975; **293**: 313–17.

94. Evans MI, Duquette DA, Rinaldo P et al. Modulation of B12 dosage and response in fetal treatment of methylmalonic aciduria (MMA): titration of treatment dose to serum and urine MMA. *Fetal Diagn Ther* 1997; **12**: 21–3.

95. Mellman I, Willard HF, Youngdahl-Turner P, Rosenberg LE. Cobalamin coenzyme synthesis in normal and mutant human fibroblasts. Evidence for a processing enzyme activity deficient in cblC cells. *J Biol Chem* 1979; **254**: 11847–53.

96. Pezacka EH. Identification and characterization of two enzymes involved in the intracellular metabolism of cobalamin. Cyanocobalamin beta-ligand transferase and microsomal cob(III)alamin reductase. *Biochim Biophys Acta* 1993; **1157**: 167–77.

97. Vassiliadis A, Rosenblatt DS, Cooper BA, Bergeron JJ. Lysosomal cobalamin accumulation in fibroblasts from a patient with an inborn error of cobalamin metabolism

(cblF complementation group): visualization by electron microscope radioautography. *Exp Cell Res* 1991; **195**: 295–302.

98. Mitchell GA, Watkins D, Melancon SB *et al*. Clinical heterogeneity in cobalamin C variant of combined homocystinuria and methylmalonic aciduria. *J Pediatr* 1986; **108**: 410–15.

99. Rosenblatt DS, Aspler AL, Shevell MI, Pletcher BA, Fenton WA, Seashore MR. Clinical heterogeneity and prognosis in combined methylmalonic aciduria and homocystinuria (cblC). *J Inherit Metab Dis* 1997; **20**: 528–38.

100. Harding CO, Pillers DA, Steiner RD *et al*. Potential for misdiagnosis due to lack of metabolic derangement in combined methylmalonic aciduria/hyperhomocysteinemia (cblC) in the neonate. *J Perinatol* 2003; **23**: 384–6.

101. Roze E, Gervais D, Demeret S *et al*. Neuropsychiatric disturbances in presumed late-onset cobalamin C disease. *Arch Neurol* 2003; **60**: 1457–62.

102. Ogier de Baulny H, Gerard M, Saudubray JM, Zittoun J. Remethylation defects: guidelines for clinical diagnosis and treatment. *Eur J Pediatr* 1998; **157** (suppl. 2): S77–S83.

103. Russo P, Doyon J, Sonsino E, Ogier H, Saudubray JM. A congenital anomaly of vitamin B12 metabolism: a study of three cases. *Hum Pathol* 1992; **23**: 504–12.

104. Zammarchi E, Lippi A, Falorni S, Pasquini E, Cooper BA, Rosenblatt DS. cblC disease: case report and monitoring of a pregnancy at risk by chorionic villus sampling. *Clin Invest Med* 1990; **13**: 139–42.

105. Chadefaux-Vekemans B, Rolland MO, Lyonnet S, Rabier D, Divry P, Kamoun P. Prenatal diagnosis of combined methylmalonic aciduria and homocystinuria (cobalamin CblC or CblD mutant). *Prenat Diagn* 1994; **14**: 417–18.

106. Goodman SI, Moe PG, Hammond KB, Mudd SH, Uhlendorf BW. Homocystinuria with methylmalonic aciduria: two cases in a sibship. *Biochem Med* 1970; **4**: 500–15.

107. Carmel R, Goodman SI. Abnormal deoxyuridine suppression test in congenital methylmalonic aciduria–homocystinuria without megaloblastic anemia: divergent biochemical and morphological bone marrow manifestations of disordered cobalamin metabolism in man. *Blood* 1982; **59**: 306–11.

108. Suormala T, Baumgartner MR, Coelho D *et al*. The cblD defect causes either isolated or combined deficiency of methylcobalamin and adenosylcobalamin synthesis. *J Biol Chem* 2004; **279**: 42742–9.

109. Shih VE, Axel SM, Tewksbury JC, Watkins D, Cooper BA, Rosenblatt DS. Defective lysosomal release of vitamin B12 (cb1F): a hereditary cobalamin metabolic disorder associated with sudden death. *Am J Med Genet* 1989; **33**: 555–63.

110. Laframboise R, Cooper BA, Rosenblatt DS. Malabsorption of vitamin B12 from the intestine in a child with cblF disease: evidence for lysosomal-mediated absorption. *Blood* 1992; **80**: 291–2.

111. Rosenblatt DS, Laframboise R, Pichette J, Langevin P, Cooper BA, Costa T. New disorder of vitamin B12 metabolism (cobalamin F) presenting as methylmalonic aciduria. *Pediatrics* 1986; **78**: 51–4.

112. Bartholomew DW, Batshaw ML, Allen RH *et al*. Therapeutic approaches to cobalamin-C methylmalonic acidemia and homocystinuria. *J Pediatr* 1988; **112**: 32–9.

113. Andersson HC, Shapira E. Biochemical and clinical response to hydroxocobalamin versus cyanocobalamin treatment in patients with methylmalonic acidemia and homocystinuria (cblC). *J Pediatr* 1998; **132**: 121–4.

114. Carmel R, Watkins D, Goodman SI, Rosenblatt DS. Hereditary defect of cobalamin metabolism (cblG mutation) presenting as a neurologic disorder in adulthood. *N Engl J Med* 1988; **318**: 1738–41.

115. Watkins D, Rosenblatt DS. Functional methionine synthase deficiency (cblE and cblG): clinical and biochemical heterogeneity. *Am J Med Genet* 1989; **34**: 427–34.

116. Tuchman M, Kelly P, Watkins D, Rosenblatt DS. Vitamin B12-responsive megaloblastic anemia, homocystinuria, and transient methylmalonic aciduria in cb1E disease. *J Pediatr* 1988; **113**: 1052–6.

117. Poloschek CM, Fowler B, Unsold R, Lorenz B. Disturbed visual system function in methionine synthase deficiency. *Graefes Arch Clin Exp Ophthalmol* 2005; **243**: 497–500.

118. Watkins D, Rosenblatt DS. Genetic heterogeneity among patients with methylcobalamin deficiency. Definition of two complementation groups, cblE and cblG. *J Clin Invest* 1988; **81**: 1690–4.

119. Rosenblatt DS, Cooper BA, Pottier A, Lue-Shing H, Matiaszuk N, Grauer K. Altered vitamin B12 metabolism in fibroblasts from a patient with megaloblastic anemia and homocystinuria due to a new defect in methionine biosynthesis. *J Clin Invest* 1984; **74**: 2149–56.

120. Rosenblatt DS, Cooper BA. Selective deficiencies of methyl-B12 (cblE and cblG). *Clin Invest Med* 1989; **12**: 270–1.

121. Leclerc D, Wilson A, Dumas R *et al*. Cloning and mapping of a cDNA for methionine synthase reductase, a flavoprotein defective in patients with homocystinuria. *Proc Natl Acad Sci USA* 1998; **95**: 3059–64.

122. Wilson A, Leclerc D, Rosenblatt DS, Gravel RA. Molecular basis for methionine synthase reductase deficiency in patients belonging to the cblE complementation group of disorders in folate/cobalamin metabolism. *Hum Mol Genet* 1999; **8**: 2009–16.

123. Vilaseca MA, Vilarinho L, Zavadakova P *et al*. CblE type of homocystinuria: mild clinical phenotype in two patients homozygous for a novel mutation in the MTRR gene. *J Inherit Metab Dis* 2003; **26**: 361–9.

124. Leclerc D, Campeau E, Goyette P *et al*. Human methionine synthase: cDNA cloning and identification of mutations in patients of the cblG complementation group of folate/cobalamin disorders. *Hum Mol Genet* 1996; **5**: 1867–74.

125. Watkins D, Ru M, Hwang HY *et al*. Hyperhomocysteinemia due to methionine synthase deficiency, cblG: structure of the MTR gene, genotype diversity, and recognition of a common mutation, P1173L. *Am J Hum Genet* 2002; **71**: 143–53.

126. Gulati S, Baker P, Li YN *et al*. Defects in human methionine synthase in cblG patients. *Hum Mol Genet* 1996; **5**: 1859–65.

127. Rosenblatt DS, Cooper BA, Schmutz SM, Zaleski WA, Casey RE. Prenatal vitamin B12 therapy of a fetus with methylcobalamin deficiency (cobalamin E disease). *Lancet* 1985; **i**: 1127–9.

128. Marquet J, Chadefaux B, Bonnefont JP, Saudubray JM, Zittoun J. Methylenetetrahydrofolate reductase deficiency: prenatal diagnosis and family studies. *Prenat Diagn* 1994; **14**: 29–33.

129. Haworth JC, Dilling LA, Surtees RA *et al*. Symptomatic and

asymptomatic methylenetetrahydrofolate reductase deficiency in two adult brothers. *Am J Med Genet* 1993; **45**: 572–6.

130. Bonig H, Daublin G, Schwahn B, Wendel U. Psychotic symptoms in severe MTHFR deficiency and their successful treatment with betaine. *Eur J Pediatr* 2003; **162**: 200–1.

131. Baumgartner ER, Stokstad EL, Wick SH, Watson JE, Kusano G. Comparison of folic acid coenzyme distribution patterns in patients with methylenetetrahydrofolate reductase and methionine synthetase deficiencies. *Pediatr Res* 1985; **19**: 1288–92.

132. Loewenstein A, Goldstein M, Winder A, Lazar M, Eldor A. Retinal vein occlusion associated with methylenetetrahydrofolate reductase mutation. *Ophthalmology* 1999; **106**: 1817–20.

133. Kanwar YS, Manaligod JR, Wong PW. Morphologic studies in a patient with homocystinuria due to 5,10-methylenetetrahydrofolate reductase deficiency. *Pediatr Res* 1976; **10**: 598–609.

134. Wong PW, Justice P, Hruby M, Weiss EB, Diamond E. Folic acid nonresponsive homocystinuria due to methylenetetrahydrofolate reductase deficiency. *Pediatrics* 1977; **59**: 749–56.

135. Clayton PT, Smith I, Harding B, Hyland K, Leonard JV, Leeming RJ. Subacute combined degeneration of the cord, dementia and parkinsonism due to an inborn error of folate metabolism. *J Neurol Neurosurg Psychiatry* 1986; **49**: 920–7.

136. Beckman DR, Hoganson G, Berlow S, Gilbert EF. Pathological findings in 5,10-methylene tetrahydrofolate reductase deficiency. *Birth Defects* 1987; **23**: 47–64.

137. Rosenblatt DS, Cooper BA, Lue-Shing S *et al.* Folate distribution in cultured human cells. Studies on 5,10-CH2-H4PteGlu reductase deficiency. *J Clin Invest* 1979; **63**: 1019–25.

138. Boss GR, Erbe RW. Decreased rates of methionine synthesis by methylene tetrahydrofolate reductase-deficient fibroblasts and lymphoblasts. *J Clin Invest* 1981; **67**: 1659–64.

139. Tonetti C, Saudubray J-M, Echenne B, Landrieu P, Giraudier S, Zittoun J. Relations between molecular and biochemical abnormalities in 11 families from siblings affected with methylenetetrahydrofolate reductase deficiency. *Eur J Pediatr* 2003; **162**: 466–75.

140. Christensen E, Brandt NJ. Prenatal diagnosis of 5,10-methylenetetrahydrofolate reductase deficiency. *N Engl J Med* 1985; **313**: 50–1.

141. Wendel U, Claussen U, Diekmann E. Prenatal diagnosis for methylenetetrahydrofolate reductase deficiency. *J Pediatr* 1983; **102**: 938–40.

142. Zittoun J. Congenital errors of folate metabolism. *Baillères Clin Haematol* 1995; **8**: 603–16.

143. Wickramasinghe SN. The wide spectrum and unresolved issues of megaloblastic anemia. *Semin Hematol* 1999; **36**: 3–18.

144. Wendel U, Bremer HJ. Betaine in the treatment of homocystinuria due to 5,10-methylenetetrahydrofolate reductase deficiency. *Eur J Pediatr* 1984; **142**: 147–50.

145. Holme E, Kjellman B, Ronge E. Betaine for treatment of homocystinuria caused by methylenetetrahydrofolate reductase deficiency. *Arch Dis Child* 1989; **64**: 1061–4.

146. Ronge E, Kjellman B. Long term treatment with betaine in methylenetetrahydrofolate reductase deficiency. *Arch Dis Child* 1996; **74**: 239–41.

147. Frosst P, Blom HJ, Milos R *et al.* A candidate genetic risk factor for vascular disease: a common mutation in methylenetetrahydrofolate reductase. *Nat Genet* 1995; **10**: 111–13.

148. Robien K, Ulrich CM. 5,10-Methylenetetrahydrofolate reductase polymorphisms and leukemia risk: a HuGE minireview. *Am J Epidemiol* 2003; **157**: 571–82.

149. Brattstrom L, Wilcken DE, Ohrvik J, Brudin L. Common methylenetetrahydrofolate reductase gene mutation leads to hyperhomocysteinemia but not to vascular disease: the result of a meta-analysis. *Circulation* 1998; **98**: 2520–6.

150. Hanson NQ, Aras O, Yang F, Tsai MY. C677T and A1298C polymorphisms of the methylenetetrahydrofolate reductase gene: incidence and effect of combined genotypes on plasma fasting and post-methionine load homocysteine in vascular disease. *Clin Chem* 2001; **47**: 661–6.

151. Delvin EE, Rozen R, Merouani A, Genest J Jr, Lambert M. Influence of methylenetetrahydrofolate reductase genotype, age, vitamin B-12, and folate status on plasma homocysteine in children. *Am J Clin Nutr* 2000; **72**: 1469–73.

152. Key NS, McGlennen RC. Hyperhomocyst(e)inemia and thrombophilia. *Arch Pathol Lab Med* 2002; **126**: 1367–75.

153. Klerk M, Verhoef P, Clarke R, Blom HJ, Kok FJ, Schouten EG. MTHFR 677C→T polymorphism and risk of coronary heart disease: a meta-analysis. *JAMA* 2002; **288**: 2023–31.

154. Lee R, Frenkel EP. Hyperhomocysteinemia and thrombosis. *Hematol Oncol Clin North Am* 2003; **17**: 85–102.

155. Skibola CF, Smith MT, Kane E *et al.* Polymorphisms in the methylenetetrahydrofolate reductase gene are associated with susceptibility to acute leukemia in adults. *Proc Natl Acad Sci USA* 1999; **96**: 12810–15.

156. Wiemels JL, Smith RN, Taylor GM, Eden OB, Alexander FE, Greaves MF. Methylenetetrahydrofolate reductase (MTHFR) polymorphisms and risk of molecularly defined subtypes of childhood acute leukemia. *Proc Natl Acad Sci USA* 2001; **98**: 4004–9.

157. Franco RF, Simoes BP, Tone LG, Gabellini SM, Zago MA, Falcao RP. The methylenetetrahydrofolate reductase C677T gene polymorphism decreases the risk of childhood acute lymphocytic leukaemia. *Br J Haematol* 2001; **115**: 616–18.

158. Krajinovic M, Lamothe S, Labuda D *et al.* Role of MTHFR genetic polymorphisms in the susceptibility to childhood acute lymphoblastic leukemia. *Blood* 2004; **103**: 252–7.

159. Matsuo K, Hamajima N, Suzuki R *et al.* Methylenetetrahydrofolate reductase gene (MTHFR) polymorphisms and reduced risk of malignant lymphoma. *Am J Hematol* 2004; **77**: 351–7.

160. Skibola CF, Forrest MS, Coppede F *et al.* Polymorphisms and haplotypes in folate-metabolizing genes and risk of non-Hodgkin lymphoma. *Blood* 2004; **104**: 2155–62.

161. Stanulla M, Seidemann K, Schnakenberg E *et al.* Methylenetetrahydrofolate reductase (MTHFR) 677C→T polymorphism and risk of pediatric non-Hodgkin lymphoma in a German study population. *Blood* 2005; **105**: 906–7.

162. Thompson JR, Gerald PF, Willoughby ML, Armstrong BK. Maternal folate supplementation in pregnancy and protection against acute lymphoblastic leukaemia in childhood: a case-control study. *Lancet* 2001; **358**: 1935–40.

163. Mao Y, Vyas NK, Vyas MN *et al.* Structure of the bifunctional and Golgi-associated formiminotransferase cyclodeaminase octamer. *EMBO J* 2004; **23**: 2963–71.

164. Erbe RW. Genetic aspects of folate metabolism. *Adv Hum Genet* 1979; **9**: 293–354, 367–9.

165. Erbe RW. Inborn errors of folate metabolism (second of two parts). *N Engl J Med* 1975; **293**: 807–12.

166. Arakawa T. Congenital defects in folate utilization. *Am J Med* 1970; **48**: 594–8.

167. Duran M, Ketting D, de Bree PK *et al.* A case of formiminoglutamic aciduria. Clinical and biochemical studies. *Eur J Pediatr* 1981; **136**: 319–23.

168. Solans A, Estivill X, de la Luna S. Cloning and characterization of human FTCD on 21q22.3, a candidate gene for glutamate formiminotransferase deficiency. *Cytogenet Cell Genet* 2000; **88**: 43–9.

169. Hilton JF, Christensen KE, Watkins D *et al.* The molecular basis of glutamate formiminotransferase deficiency. *Hum Mutat* 2003; **22**: 67–73.

170. Lapierre P, Hajoui O, Homberg JC, Alvarez F. Formiminotransferase cyclodeaminase is an organ-specific autoantigen recognized by sera of patients with autoimmune hepatitis. *Gastroenterology* 1999; **116**: 643–9.

171. Muratori L, Sztul E, Muratori P *et al.* Distinct epitopes on formiminotransferase cyclodeaminase induce autoimmune liver cytosol antibody type 1. *Hepatology* 2001; **34**: 494–501.

172. Perry TL, Applegarth DA, Evans ME, Hansen S, Jellum E. Metabolic studies of a family with massive formiminoglutamic aciduria. *Pediatr Res* 1975; **9**: 117–22.

173. Niederwieser A, Matasovic A, Steinmann B, Baerlocher K, Kempken B. Hydantoin-5-propionic aciduria in folic acid nondependent formiminoglutamic aciduria observed in two siblings. *Pediatr Res* 1976; **10**: 215–19.

174. Geller J, Kronn D, Jayabose S, Sandoval C. Hereditary folate malabsorption: family report and review of the literature. *Medicine (Baltimore)* 2002; **81**: 51–68.

175. Malatack JJ, Moran MM, Moughan B. Isolated congenital malabsorption of folic acid in a male infant: insights into treatment and mechanism of defect. *Pediatrics* 1999; **104**: 1133–7.

176. Steinschneider M, Sherbany A, Pavlakis S, Emerson R, Lovelace R, De Vivo DC. Congenital folate malabsorption: reversible clinical and neurophysiologic abnormalities. *Neurology* 1990; **40**: 1315.

177. Poncz M, Cohen A. Long-term treatment of congenital folate malabsorption. *J Pediatr* 1996; **129**: 948.

178. Urbach J, Abrahamov A, Grossowicz N. Congenital isolated folic acid malabsorption. *Arch Dis Child* 1987; **62**: 78–80.

179. Branda RF, Moldow CF, MacArthur JR, Wintrobe MM, Anthony BK, Jacob HS. Folate-induced remission in aplastic anemia with familial defect of cellular folate uptake. *N Engl J Med* 1978; **298**: 469–75.

180. Howe RB, Branda RF, Douglas SD, Brunning RD. Hereditary dyserythropoiesis with abnormal membrane folate transport. *Blood* 1979; **54**: 1080–90.

181. Ramaekers VT, Blau N. Cerebral folate deficiency. *Dev Med Child Neurol* 2004; **46**: 843–51.

182. Wevers RA, Hansen SI, van Hellenberg Hubar JL, Holm J, Hoier-Madsen M, Jongen PJ. Folate deficiency in cerebrospinal fluid associated with a defect in folate binding protein in the central nervous system. *J Neurol Neurosurg Psychiatry* 1994; **57**: 223–6.

183. Ozdemir MA, Akcakus M, Kurtoglu S, Gunes T, Torun YA. TRMA syndrome (thiamine-responsive megaloblastic anemia): a case report and review of the literature. *Pediatr Diabetes* 2002; **3**: 205–9.

184. Neufeld EJ, Mandel H, Raz T *et al.* Localization of the gene for thiamine-responsive megaloblastic anemia syndrome, on the long arm of chromosome 1, by homozygosity mapping. *Am J Hum Genet* 1997; **61**: 1335–41.

185. Subramanian VS, Marchant JS, Parker I, Said HM. Cell biology of the human thiamine transporter-1 (hTHTR1). Intracellular trafficking and membrane targeting mechanisms. *J Biol Chem* 2003; **278**: 3976–84.

186. Lagarde WH, Underwood LE, Moats-Staats BM, Calikoglu AS. Novel mutation in the SLC19A2 gene in an African-American female with thiamine-responsive megaloblastic anemia syndrome. *Am J Med Genet* (Part A) 2004; **125**: 299–305.

187. Gritli S, Omar S, Tartaglini E *et al.* A novel mutation in the SLC19A2 gene in a Tunisian family with thiamine-responsive megaloblastic anaemia, diabetes and deafness syndrome. *Br J Haematol* 2001; **113**: 508–13.

188. Raz T, Labay V, Baron D *et al.* The spectrum of mutations, including four novel ones, in the thiamine-responsive megaloblastic anemia gene SLC19A2 of eight families. *Hum Mutat* 2000; **16**: 37–42.

189. Lorber A, Gazit AZ, Khoury A, Schwartz Y, Mandel H. Cardiac manifestations in thiamine-responsive megaloblastic anemia syndrome. *Pediatr Cardiol* 2003; **24**: 476–81.

190. Meire FM, Van Genderen MM, Lemmens K, Ens-Dokkum MH. Thiamine-responsive megaloblastic anemia syndrome (TRMA) with cone-rod dystrophy. *Ophthalmic Genet* 2000; **21**: 243–50.

191. Villa V, Rivellese A, Di Salle F, Iovine C, Poggi V, Capaldo B. Acute ischemic stroke in a young woman with the thiamine-responsive megaloblastic anemia syndrome. *J Clin Endocrinol Metab* 2000; **85**: 947–9.

192. Boros LG, Steinkamp MP, Fleming JC, Lee WN, Cascante M, Neufeld EJ. Defective RNA ribose synthesis in fibroblasts from patients with thiamine-responsive megaloblastic anemia (TRMA). *Blood* 2003; **102**: 3556–61.

193. Akinci A, Tezic T, Erturk G, Tarim O, Dalva K. Thiamine-responsive megaloblastic anemia with diabetes mellitus and sensorineural deafness. *Acta Paediatr Jpn* 1993; **35**: 262–6.

194. Webster DR, Becroft DMO, Gennup AHV, Van Kuilenburg ABP. Hereditary orotic aciduria and other disorders of pyrimidine metabolism. In: Scriver C, Baudet A, Sly W, Valle D (eds) *Metabolic and Molecular Basis of Inherited Disease*, 8th edn. New York: McGraw-Hill, 2001, pp. 2663–702.

195. Shin YS, Reiter S, Zelger O, Brunstler I, von Rucker A. Orotic aciduria, homocystinuria, formiminoglutamic aciduria and megaloblastosis associated with the formiminotransferase/cyclodeaminase deficiency. *Adv Exp Med Biol* 1986; **195**(A): 71–6.

196. Carmel R. Current concepts in cobalamin deficiency. *Annu Rev Med* 2000; **51**: 357–75.

197. Kinsella LJ, Green R. "Anesthesia paresthetica": nitrous oxide-induced cobalamin deficiency. *Neurology* 1995; **45**: 1608–10.

198. Pema PJ, Horak HA, Wyatt RH. Myelopathy caused by nitrous oxide toxicity. *AJNR Am J Neuroradiol* 1998; **19**: 894–6.

199. Felmet K, Robins B, Tilford D, Hayflick SJ. Acute neurologic decompensation in an infant with cobalamin deficiency exposed to nitrous oxide. *J Pediatr* 2000; **137**: 427–8.

200. McNeely JK, Buczulinski B, Rosner DR. Severe neurological impairment in an infant after nitrous oxide anesthesia. *Anesthesiology* 2000; **93**: 1549–50.

201. Selzer RR, Rosenblatt DS, Laxova R, Hogan K. Adverse effect of nitrous oxide in a child with 5,10-methylenetetrahydrofolate reductase deficiency. *N Engl J Med* 2003; **349**: 45–50.

202. Armstrong P, Rae PW, Gray WM, Spence AA. Nitrous oxide and formiminoglutamic acid: excretion in surgical patients and anaesthetists. *Br J Anaesth* 1991; **66**: 163–9.

203. Ervin RB, Wright JD, Wang CY, Kennedy-Stephenson J. Dietary intake of selected vitamins for the United States population: 1999–2000. Adv Data 2004; **339**: 1–4.

204. Herrmann W, Schorr H, Obeid R, Geisel J. Vitamin B-12 status, particularly holotranscobalamin II and methylmalonic acid concentrations, and hyperhomocysteinemia in vegetarians. *Am J Clin Nutr* 2003; **78**: 131–6.

205. Koebnick C, Hoffmann I, Dagnelie PC *et al*. Long-term ovo-lacto vegetarian diet impairs vitamin B-12 status in pregnant women. *J Nutr* 2004; **134**: 3319–26.

206. Ashkenazi S, Weitz R, Varsano I, Mimouni M. Vitamin B12 deficiency due to a strictly vegetarian diet in adolescence. *Clin Pediatr (Phila)* 1987; **26**: 662–3.

207. Louwman MW, van Dusseldorp M, van de Vijver FJ *et al*. Signs of impaired cognitive function in adolescents with marginal cobalamin status. *Am J Clin Nutr* 2000; **72**: 762–9.

208. Rogers LM, Boy E, Miller JW *et al*. Predictors of cobalamin deficiency in Guatemalan school children: diet, *Helicobacter pylori*, or bacterial overgrowth? *J Pediatr Gastroenterol Nutr* 2003; **36**: 27–36.

209. Diez-Ewald M, Torres-Guerra E, Layrisse M, Leets I, Vizcaino G, Arteaga-Vizcaino M. Prevalence of anemia, iron, folic acid and vitamin B12 deficiency in two Bari Indian communities from western Venezuela. *Invest Clin* 1997; **38**: 191–201.

210. Allen LH, Rosado JL, Casterline JE *et al*. Vitamin B-12 deficiency and malabsorption are highly prevalent in rural Mexican communities. *Am J Clin Nutr* 1995; **62**: 1013–19.

211. Jathar VS, Kamath SA, Parikh MN, Rege DV, Satoskar RS. Maternal milk and serum vitamin B12, folic acid, and protein levels in Indian subjects. *Arch Dis Child* 1970; **45**: 236–41.

212. Specker BL. Nutritional concerns of lactating women consuming vegetarian diets. *Am J Clin Nutr* 1994; **59** (5 suppl.): 1182S–1186S.

213. Renault F, Verstichel P, Ploussard JP, Costil J. Neuropathy in two cobalamin-deficient breast-fed infants of vegetarian mothers. *Muscle Nerve* 1999; **22**: 252–4.

214. Kuhne T, Bubl R, Baumgartner R. Maternal vegan diet causing a serious infantile neurological disorder due to vitamin B12 deficiency. *Eur J Pediatr* 1991; **150**: 205–8.

215. Weiss R, Fogelman Y, Bennett M. Severe vitamin B12 deficiency in an infant associated with a maternal deficiency and a strict vegetarian diet. *J Pediatr Hematol Oncol* 2004; **26**: 270–1.

216. Sklar R. Nutritional vitamin B12 deficiency in a breast-fed infant of a vegan-diet mother. *Clin Pediatr (Phila)* 1986; **25**: 219–21.

217. Higginbottom MC, Sweetman L, Nyhan WL. A syndrome of methylmalonic aciduria, homocystinuria, megaloblastic anemia and neurologic abnormalities in a vitamin B12-deficient breast-fed infant of a strict vegetarian. *N Engl J Med* 1978; **299**: 317–23.

218. Chanarin I. Folate and cobalamin. *Clin Haematol* 1985; **14**: 629–41.

219. Lampkin BC, Shore NA, Chadwick D. Megaloblastic anemia of infancy secondary to maternal pernicious anemia. *N Engl J Med* 1966; **274**: 1168–71.

220. Miller DR, Specker BL, Ho ML, Norman EJ. Vitamin B-12 status in a macrobiotic community. *Am J Clin Nutr* 1991; **53**: 524–9.

221. Neufeld M, Maclaren NK, Blizzard RM. Two types of autoimmune Addison's disease associated with different polyglandular autoimmune (PGA) syndromes. *Medicine (Baltimore)* 1981; **60**: 355–62.

222. McIntyre OR, Sullivan LW, Jeffries GH, Silver RH. Pernicious anemia in childhood. *N Engl J Med* 1965; **272**: 981–9.

223. Dahshan A, Poulick J, Tolia V. Special feature: pathological case of the month. Pernicious anemia and gastric atrophy in an adolescent female with multiorgan problems. *Arch Pediatr Adolesc Med* 2001; **155**: 609–10.

224. Ahonen P, Myllarniemi S, Sipila I, Perheentupa J. Clinical variation of autoimmune polyendocrinopathy–candidiasis–ectodermal dystrophy (APECED) in a series of 68 patients. *N Engl J Med* 1990; **322**: 1829–36.

225. Anon. An autoimmune disease, APECED, caused by mutations in a novel gene featuring two PHD-type zinc-finger domains. The Finnish-German APECED Consortium. Autoimmune Polyendocrinopathy–Candidiasis–Ectodermal Dystrophy. *Nat Genet* 1997; **17**: 399–403.

226. Davies BW, Abel G, Puntis JW *et al*. Limited ileal resection in infancy: the long-term consequences. *J Pediatr Surg* 1999; **34**: 583–7.

227. Skidmore MD, Shenker N, Kliegman RM, Shurin S, Allen RH. Biochemical evidence of asymptomatic vitamin B12 deficiency in children after ileal resection for necrotizing enterocolitis. *J Pediatr* 1989; **115**: 102–5.

228. Valman HB. Late vitamin B12 deficiency following resection of the ileum in the neonatal period. *Acta Paediatr Scand* 1972; **61**: 561–4.

229. Ooi BC, Barnes GL, Tauro GP. Normalization of vitamin B12 absorption after ileal resection in children. *J Paediatr Child Health* 1992; **28**: 168–71.

230. Quak SH, Joseph VT, Wong HB. Neonatal total gastrectomy. *Clin Pediatr (Phila)* 1984; **23**: 507–8.

231. Lindemans J, Neijens HJ, Kerrebijn KF, Abels J. Vitamin B12 absorption in cystic fibrosis. *Acta Paediatr Scand* 1984; **73**: 537–40.

232. Gueant JL, Champigneulle B, Gaucher P, Nicolas JP. Malabsorption of vitamin B12 in pancreatic insufficiency of the adult and of the child. *Pancreas* 1990; **5**: 559–67.

233. Monin B, Gueant JL, Vidailhet M, Michalski JC, Pasquet C, Nicolas JP. Excretion of cobalamin and haptocorrin in the meconium of cystic fibrosis, premature, and control neonates. *Am J Clin Nutr* 1987; **45**: 981–7.

234. Lindemans J, Abels J, Neijens HJ, Kerrebijn KF. Elevated serum vitamin B12 in cystic fibrosis. *Acta Paediatr Scand* 1984; **73**: 768–71.

235. Simpson RM, Lloyd DJ, Gvozdanovic D, Russell G. Vitamin B12 deficiency in cystic fibrosis. *Acta Paediatr Scand* 1985; **74**: 794–6.

236. Nyberg W, Grasbeck R, Saarni M, von Bornsdorff B. Serum vitamin B12 levels and incidence of tapeworm anemia in a population heavily infected with *Diphyllobothrium latum*. *Am J Clin Nutr* 1961; **9**: 606–12.

237. Howden CW. Vitamin B12 levels during prolonged treatment with proton pump inhibitors. *J Clin Gastroenterol* 2000; **30**: 29–33.

238. Andersen KJ, Schjonsby H. Intrinsic factor-mediated binding of cyanocobalamin to cholestyramine. *J Pharm Sci* 1978; **67**: 1626–7.

239. Filioussi K, Bonovas S, Katsaros T. Should we screen diabetic patients using biguanides for megaloblastic anaemia? *Aust Fam Physician* 2003; **32**: 383–4.

240. Andres E, Noel E, Goichot B. Metformin-associated vitamin B12 deficiency. *Arch Intern Med* 2002; **162**: 2251–2.

241. Gilligan MA. Metformin and vitamin B12 deficiency. *Arch Intern Med* 2002; **162**: 484–5.

242. Carmel R, Aurangzeb I, Qian D. Associations of food-cobalamin malabsorption with ethnic origin, age, *Helicobacter pylori* infection, and serum markers of gastritis. *Am J Gastroenterol* 2001; **96**: 63–70.

243. Andres E, Kurtz JE, Perrin AE *et al.* Oral cobalamin therapy for the treatment of patients with food-cobalamin malabsorption. *Am J Med* 2001; **111**: 126–9.

244. Bailey LB. Folate and vitamin B12 recommended intakes and status in the United States. *Nutr Rev* 2004; **62** (6 Pt 2): S14–S20; discussion S21.

245. Villalpando S, Montalvo-Velarde I, Zambrano N, Ramirez-Silva CI, Shamah-Levy T, Rivera JA. Vitamins A and C and folate status in Mexican children under 12 years and women 12–49 years: a probabilistic national survey. *Salud Publica Mex* 2003; **45** (suppl. 4): S508–S519.

246. Ek J. Plasma and red cell folate values in newborn infants and their mothers in relation to gestational age. *J Pediatr* 1980; **97**: 288–92.

247. Bjorke Monsen AL, Ueland PM, Vollset SE *et al.* Determinants of cobalamin status in newborns. *Pediatrics* 2001; **108**: 624–30.

248. Shojania AM. Folic acid and vitamin B12 deficiency in pregnancy and in the neonatal period. *Clin Perinatol* 1984; **11**: 433–59.

249. Parry TE. Goats' milk in infants and children. *Br Med J* 1984; **288**: 863–4.

250. Coleman R. Letter: A reminder: deficiency of folic acid in goat milk. *J Pediatr* 1976; **88**: 911.

251. Kamen BA, Caston JD. Purification of folate binding factor in normal umbilical cord serum. *Proc Natl Acad Sci USA* 1975; **72**: 4261–4.

252. Frenkel EP, Yardley DA. Clinical and laboratory features and sequelae of deficiency of folic acid (folate) and vitamin B12 (cobalamin) in pregnancy and gynecology. *Hematol Oncol Clin North Am* 2000; **14**: 1079–100, viii.

253. MRC Vitamin Study Research Group. Prevention of neural tube defects: results of the Medical Research Council Vitamin Study. *Lancet* 1991; **338**: 131–7.

254. Berry RJ, Li Z, Erickson JD *et al.* Prevention of neural-tube defects with folic acid in China. China–U.S. Collaborative Project for Neural Tube Defect Prevention. *N Engl J Med* 1999; **341**: 1485–90.

255. Shaw GM, Lammer EJ, Wasserman CR, O'Malley CD, Tolarova MM. Risks of orofacial clefts in children born to women using multivitamins containing folic acid periconceptionally. *Lancet* 1995; **346**: 393–6.

256. Itikala PR, Watkins ML, Mulinare J, Moore CA, Liu Y. Maternal multivitamin use and orofacial clefts in offspring. *Teratology* 2001; **63**: 79–86.

257. Loffredo LC, Souza JM, Freitas JA, Mossey PA. Oral clefts and vitamin supplementation. *Cleft Palate Craniofac J* 2001; **38**: 76–83.

258. Shaw GM, O'Malley CD, Wasserman CR, Tolarova MM, Lammer EJ. Maternal periconceptional use of multivitamins and reduced risk for conotruncal heart defects and limb deficiencies among offspring. *Am J Med Genet* 1995; **59**: 536–45.

259. Hernandez-Diaz S, Werler MM, Walker AM, Mitchell AA. Folic acid antagonists during pregnancy and the risk of birth defects. *N Engl J Med* 2000; **343**: 1608–14.

260. Botto LD, Yang Q. 5,10-Methylenetetrahydrofolate reductase gene variants and congenital anomalies: a HuGE review. *Am J Epidemiol* 2000; **151**: 862–77.

261. Kirke PN, Mills JL, Molloy AM *et al.* Impact of the MTHFR C677T polymorphism on risk of neural tube defects: case-control study. Br Med J 2004; **328**: 1535–6.

262. Farrell RJ, Kelly CP. Diagnosis of celiac sprue. *Am J Gastroenterol* 2001; **96**: 3237–46.

263. Hoffbrand AV. Anaemia in adult coeliac disease. *Clin Gastroenterol* 1974; **3**: 71–89.

264. Ciclitira PJ, Ellis HJ. Celiac disease. In: Yamada T (ed.) *Gastroenterology*. Philadelphia: Lippincott Williams & Wilkins, 2003, pp. 1580–98.

265. Askling J, Linet M, Gridley G, Haltersen TS, Ekstrom K, Ekbom A. Cancer incidence in a population-based cohort of individuals hospitalised with celiac disease or dermatitis herpetiformis. *Gastroenterology* 1992; **123**: 1428–35.

266. Holmes GK, Prior P, Lane MR, Pope D, Allan RN. Malignancy in coeliac disease: effect of a gluten free diet. *Gut* 1989; **30**: 333–8.

267. Lindenbaum J. Aspects of vitamin B12 and folate metabolism in malabsorption syndromes. *Am J Med* 1979; **67**: 1037–48.

268. Fantry GT, Fantry LE, James SP. Chronic infections of the small intestine. In: Yamada T (ed.) *Gastroenterology*. Philadelphia: Lippincott Williams & Wilkins, 2003, pp. 1561–79.

269. Papa A, De Stefano V, Danese S *et al.* Hyperhomocysteinemia and prevalence of polymorphisms of homocysteine metabolism-related enzymes in patients with inflammatory bowel disease. *Am J Gastroenterol* 2001; **96**: 2677–82.

270. Chowers Y, Sela BA, Holland R, Fidder H, Simoni FB, Bar-Meir S. Increased levels of homocysteine in patients with Crohn's disease are related to folate levels. *Am J Gastroenterol* 2000; **95**: 3498–502.

271. Strauss RS, Bradley LJ, Brolin RE. Gastric bypass surgery in adolescents with morbid obesity. *J Pediatr* 2001; **138**: 499–504.

272. Vilaseca MA, Sierra C, Colome C *et al.* Hyper-homocysteinaemia and folate deficiency in human immunodeficiency virus-infected children. *Eur J Clin Invest* 2001; **31**: 992–8.

273. Geerlings SE, Rommes JH, van Toorn DW, Bakker J. Acute folate deficiency in a critically ill patient. *Neth J Med* 1997; **51**: 36–8.

274. Lewis DP, Van Dyke DC, Stumbo PJ, Berg MJ. Drug and environmental factors associated with adverse pregnancy outcomes. Part I: Antiepileptic drugs, contraceptives, smoking, and folate. *Ann Pharmacother* 1998; **32**: 802–17.

275. Grace E, Emans SJ, Drum DE. Hematologic abnormalities in adolescents who take oral contraceptive pills. *J Pediatr* 1982; **101**: 771–4.

276. Mannino DM, Mulinare J, Ford ES, Schwartz J. Tobacco smoke exposure and decreased serum and red blood cell folate levels: data from the Third National Health and Nutrition Examination Survey. *Nicotine Tob Res* 2003; **5**: 357–62.

277. Lambie DG, Johnson RH. Drugs and folate metabolism. *Drugs* 1985; **30**: 145–55.

278. Weir DG, McGing PG, Scott JM. Folate metabolism, the enterohepatic circulation and alcohol. *Biochem Pharmacol* 1985; **34**: 1–7.

279. Teschner M, Kosch M, Schaefer RM. Folate metabolism in renal failure. *Nephrol Dial Transplant* 2002; **17** (suppl. 5): 24–7.

280. van der Dijs FP, Schnog JJ, Brouwer DA *et al.* Elevated homocysteine levels indicate suboptimal folate status in pediatric sickle cell patients. *Am J Hematol* 1998; **59**: 192–8.

281. Rodriguez-Cortes HM, Griener JC, Hyland K *et al.* Plasma homocysteine levels and folate status in children with sickle cell anemia. *J Pediatr Hematol Oncol* 1999; **21**: 219–23.

282. Scott JM, Weir DG. Drug-induced megaloblastic change. *Clin Haematol* 1980; **9**: 587–606.

283. Koury MJ, Price JO, Hicks GG. Apoptosis in megaloblastic anemia occurs during DNA synthesis by a p53-independent, nucleoside-reversible mechanism. *Blood* 2000; **96**: 3249–55.

284. Graham SM, Arvela OM, Wise GA. Long-term neurologic consequences of nutritional vitamin B12 deficiency in infants. *J Pediatr* 1992; **121**: 710–14.

285. Thomas PK, Hoffbrand AV. Hereditary transcobalamin II deficiency: a 22 year follow up. *J Neurol Neurosurg Psychiatry* 1997; **62**: 197.

286. Kaplan SS, Basford RE. Effect of vitamin B12 and folic acid deficiencies on neutrophil function. *Blood* 1976; **47**: 801–5.

287. Skacel PO, Chanarin I. Impaired chemiluminescence and bactericidal killing by neutrophils from patients with severe cobalamin deficiency. *Br J Haematol* 1983; **55**: 203–15.

288. Wray D. Common oral disease and oral manifestations of systemic disease. In: Shearman DJC, Finlayson N, Camilleri M, Carter D (eds) *Disease of the Gastrointestinal Tract and Liver*. New York: Churchill Livingstone, 1997, pp. 137–52.

289. DeMay R (ed.) *The Art and Science of Cytopathology*. Hong Kong: American Society of Clinical Pathology, 1996.

290. Odze RD, Goldman H. Systemic and miscellaneous disorders. In: Ming S-C, Goldman H (eds) *Pathology of the Gastrointestinal Tract*. Baltimore: Williams & Wilkins, 1998, pp. 399–429.

291. Carmel R, Lau KH, Baylink DJ, Saxena S, Singer FR. Cobalamin and osteoblast-specific proteins. *N Engl J Med* 1988; **319**: 70–5.

292. Mori K, Ando I, Kukita A. Generalized hyperpigmentation of the skin due to vitamin B12 deficiency. *J Dermatol* 2001; **28**: 282–5.

293. Simsek OP, Gonc N, Gumruk F, Cetin M. A child with vitamin B12 deficiency presenting with pancytopenia and hyperpigmentation. *J Pediatr Hematol Oncol* 2004; **26**: 834–6.

294. Sabatino D, Kosuri S, Remollino A, Shotter B. Cobalamin deficiency presenting with cutaneous hyperpigmentation: a report of two siblings. *Pediatr Hematol Oncol* 1998; **15**: 447–50.

295. Zittoun J, Zittoun R. Modern clinical testing strategies in cobalamin and folate deficiency. *Semin Hematol* 1999; **36**: 35–46.

296. Gardyn J, Mittelman M, Zlotnik J, Sela BA, Cohen AM. Oral contraceptives can cause falsely low vitamin B(12) levels. *Acta Haematol* 2000; **104**: 22–4.

297. Bjorke Monsen AL, Ueland PM. Homocysteine and methylmalonic acid in diagnosis and risk assessment from infancy to adolescence. *Am J Clin Nutr* 2003; **78**: 7–21.

298. Wickramasinghe SN, Fida S. Correlations between holo-transcobalamin II, holo-haptocorrin, and total B12 in serum samples from healthy subjects and patients. *J Clin Pathol* 1993; **46**: 537–9.

299. Herbert V, Fong W, Gulle V, Stopler T. Low holotranscobalamin II is the earliest serum marker for subnormal vitamin B12 (cobalamin) absorption in patients with AIDS. *Am J Hematol* 1990; **34**: 132–9.

300. Carmel R. Treatment of severe pernicious anemia: no association with sudden death. *Am J Clin Nutr* 1988; **48**: 1443–4.

301. Dhar M, Bellevue R, Carmel R. Pernicious anemia with neuropsychiatric dysfunction in a patient with sickle cell anemia treated with folate supplementation. *N Engl J Med* 2003; **348**: 2204–7.

302. Worthington-White DA, Behnke M, Gross S. Premature infants require additional folate and vitamin B-12 to reduce the severity of the anemia of prematurity. *Am J Clin Nutr* 1994; **60**: 930–5.

303. Foucar K. Anemias: erythrocyte maturation disorders. In: Foucar K (ed.) *Bone Marrow Pathology*, 2nd edn. Chicago: American Society of Clinical Pathologists, 1998, pp. 88–108.

304. Pappo AS, Fields BW, Buchanan GR. Etiology of red blood cell macrocytosis during childhood: impact of new diseases and therapies. *Pediatrics* 1992; **89**: 1063–7.

305. Chu JY, Monteleone JA, Peden VH, Graviss ER, Vernava AM. Anemia in children and adolescents with hypothyroidism. *Clin Pediatr (Phila)* 1981; **20**: 696–9.

306. Vinton NE, Dahlstrom KA, Strobel CT, Ament ME. Macrocytosis and pseudoalbinism: manifestations of selenium deficiency. *J Pediatr* 1987; **111**: 711–17.

7 Nonimmune neonatal anemias

Brenda E.S. Gibson and Christina Halsey

Anemia is the commonest hematologic abnormality in newborn babies and this chapter concentrates on the nonimmunologic causes of neonatal anemia. A careful history and examination combined with a few key investigations will help identify the cause of anemia in the majority of affected neonates.

Hematopoiesis in the neonatal period

Appreciation of the unique features of neonatal anemia requires an understanding of the many differences between fetal and adult hematopoiesis.

Erythropoiesis is switched off at birth
Although born with a hemoglobin (Hb) level significantly higher than that of the older child and adult, the rate of red cell production and hemoglobin synthesis in the neonate falls dramatically after birth.[1] At this time erythropoietin levels are virtually undetectable, which is thought to result from both the sudden increase in tissue oxygenation that occurs at birth and the switch from hepatic to renal erythropoietin production. Red cell production reaches a nadir at 2 weeks of age. Although bone marrow erythropoiesis gradually increases thereafter, there is a time lag before mature red cells appear in the circulation. Hence the hemoglobin is lowest at around 8 weeks of age and only attains more normal childhood values at 3–4 months of age.[2]

Neonatal red cells have a short half-life
The average lifespan of the red cells of the term and preterm neonate is 60–70 and 35–50 days respectively,[3] both considerably shorter than the 120-day lifespan of the adult red cell. The exact cause of the shortened red cell lifespan in neonates is unknown but probably reflects differing red cell membrane lipid composition in neonatal cells.

The major hemoglobin at birth is HbF ($\alpha_2\gamma_2$)
Fetal hemoglobin (HbF) comprises 70–80% of the total hemoglobin at birth. It remains static at this level until about 2 weeks of age when erythropoiesis recommences, and thereafter falls steadily to reach a level of less than 2% by the end of the first year of life. Although adult-type HbA ($\alpha_2\beta_2$) is produced in the embryo from 6–8 weeks gestation onwards, it remains at low levels until about 32 weeks' gestation. It gradually rises thereafter, reaching levels of 20–30% at birth and becomes the predominant hemoglobin by 3 months of age. This switch from fetal to adult hematopoiesis may be delayed in the sick premature infant. Small amounts of HbA$_2$ ($\alpha_2\delta_2$) and Hb Barts (γ^4 tetramers) are detectable in healthy neonates at birth. An understanding of the pattern of hemoglobin production, particularly when the switch from fetal to adult hematopoiesis occurs, explains the clinical manifestations of hemoglobinopathies in the neonatal period and in particular why α-chain abnormalities cause problems from early fetal life and why β-chain abnormalities may be difficult to diagnose in the neonatal period.

The neonatal red cell membrane is different from the adult red cell membrane
The neonatal red cell membrane shows many different properties to that of adult red cells. It has an altered lipid profile with increased total lipid content, increased mechanical fragility but relative resistance to osmotic lysis, and reduced expression of the blood group antigens A, B and I.

Neonatal red cell metabolism is different from adult red cell metabolism
There are many subtle differences between neonatal and adult red cell metabolism involving both the glycolytic and pentose phosphate pathways. This may increase the susceptibility of red cells to oxidant injury although the significance *in vivo* is unclear.

Hematologic values at birth

The diagnosis and treatment of neonatal anemia requires a knowledge of normal hemoglobin values for age and gestation and an awareness of factors that may produce artifactual results. Tables of age- and gestation-related reference values are given in Chapter 37. The following should be considered when assessing an infant with possible anemia.

Site of sampling

Blood samples collected by capillary sampling give consistently higher hemoglobin values than those collected simultaneously by the venous or arterial route. Studies have shown that capillary samples taken around the time of birth give an average hemoglobin value 2.3–3.5 g/dL higher than simultaneous venous samples.[4,5] The discrepancy is most marked in sick and premature infants and sample site differences should be taken into account when interpreting results, especially borderline results, in infants.

Quality of the sample

Neonatal sampling is difficult and samples may be small or partially clotted and collection tubes underfilled, all of which may produce false results. Capillary sampling from a good blood flow in a well-warmed extremity minimizes the recognized discrepancy between capillary and venous results. Because of the potential for artifactual error, a result suggesting a sudden or unexpected drop in hemoglobin should be repeated, if possible, before any other action is taken.

Timing of cord clamping at delivery

The average blood volume at birth in the healthy full-term infant is 86 mL/kg (range 69–107 mL/kg) and is higher in small-for-gestational-age and preterm infants.[6] The placental vessels contain approximately 150 mL of blood (range 50–200 mL). An increase in the hemoglobin concentration occurs uniformly in the first few hours after birth in all healthy newborns, because about one-quarter of the placental blood volume transfuses into the infant in the first 15 s after birth and 50% of the placental blood volume in the first minute. A delay in cord clamping allows more complete emptying of the placental vessels and can increase the infant's blood volume by 50–60%.[7] The rate of placental transfusion is increased in women who receive ergotamine derivatives at the onset of the third stage of labor and is decreased in placenta praevia, multiple pregnancies and after cesarean section. The advantages of late clamping of the umbilical cord may be greatest for premature infants in whom the red cell mass and total iron stores are decreased.[8] A hemoglobin concentration of less than 15 g/dL in the first week of life has been shown to be a significant predictor of severe refractory anemia of prematurity. The placental transfusion in preterm infants may also facilitate postnatal lung adaptation.[9]

Table 7.1 gives examples of how the variable management of the umbilical cord at birth can result in differences in blood volume, hematocrit and hemoglobin concentration; these can take up to 3 months to equalize.

Table 7.1 Effect of cord clamping on blood volume, hematocrit (Hct) and hemoglobin concentration (Hb).

	Early clamping	Late clamping
Blood volume at birth (mL/kg)	82	93
HCT (%) at 2 hours of age	0.47	0.63
HCT (%) at 24 hours of age	0.43	0.59
HCT (%) at 120 hours of age	0.44	0.59
Hb (g/dL) at 20–30 hours	15.6	19.3
Hb (g/dL) at 72–96 hours	18.1	19.7
Hb (g/dL) at 3 months	11.1	11.1

Gestational age

There is little variation in hemoglobin levels at birth between preterm and term infants but premature infants experience a more rapid and profound drop in hemoglobin postnatally (see below). The normal mean cell volume (MCV) is higher in preterm than term infants. The nucleated red cell and reticulocyte counts fall in inverse proportion to gestational age up until term, after which they rise again so that babies born after 40 weeks have higher reticulocyte counts than those born at term.[10] Red cell morphology also varies considerably with gestation, with increasing numbers of echinocytes (spiculated/burr like cells) seen with increasing prematurity. The gestational age is therefore very important when interpreting neonatal blood films.

Postnatal age

Postnatal age is also important in the interpretation of hematologic values. As already stated, erythropoiesis is effectively shut off at birth and this is followed by a steady decline in hemoglobin values to a nadir at around 8 weeks. This fall in hemoglobin is most marked in preterm infants. The reticulocyte count declines rapidly in nonanemic infants and is less than 1% by the end of the first week of life. Nucleated red blood cells also fall rapidly, usually disappearing from the circulation by 3 days of age, although small numbers may persist in premature infants until the end of the first week of life. The persistence of a reticulocytosis or of nucleated red cells can be a useful pointer to the cause of neonatal anemia (see Fig. 7.1).

Classification of neonatal anemia

There are three principal mechanisms that produce neonatal anemia:
- impaired red cell production;
- increased red cell destruction due to hemolysis;
- blood loss due to hemorrhage.

A stepwise approach to diagnosis should help identify the cause of the anemia and simplify management. However, in

Table 7.2 Hematologic causes of hydrops fetalis.

Impaired red cell production
Parvovirus B19 infection
Diamond–Blackfan anemia
Congenital dyserythropoietic anemias
Congenital leukemia

Increased red cell destruction
Immune hemolysis: Rh and Kell
α-Thalassemia major
Pyruvate kinase deficiency
Glucose phosphate isomerase deficiency
γβ-thalassemia
Rare unstable α-chain variants

Blood loss
Twin-to-twin transfusion syndrome
Fetomaternal hemorrhage

Table 7.3 Causes of anemia in the neonate.

Anemia secondary to blood loss
Concealed hemorrhage prior to birth or during delivery
  Fetomaternal
  Fetoplacental
  Twin-to-twin
Obstetric accidents, malformations of the cord or placenta
Internal hemorrhage
  Extracranial
  Intracranial
  Intraabdominal
  Pulmonary
Iatrogenic blood loss

Anemia as a result of a hemolytic process
Immune
  Alloimmune
  Autoimmune (passively acquired)
  Drug-induced
Infection
  Acquired (bacterial sepsis)
  Congenital: rubella, cytomegalovirus, etc.
Macroangiopathic and microangiopathic hemolytic anemias
Hereditary disorders of the red cell membrane
  Hereditary spherocytosis
  Hereditary elliptocytosis
  Other rare membrane disorders
Red cell enzyme deficiencies
  Glucose 6-phosphate dehydrogenase deficiency
  Pyruvate kinase deficiency
  Glucose phosphate isomerase deficiency
  Other rare enzyme deficiencies
Abnormal/unstable hemoglobins

Anemia due to impaired red cell production
Congenital red cell aplasia: Diamond–Blackfan anemia
Anemia of the preterm infant
Infection
  Bacterial sepsis
  Congenital infections
  Parvovirus B19 infection
Nutritional deficiencies
Congenital leukemia
Osteopetrosis

most cases, particularly anemias associated with prematurity and infection, the pathology may be multifactorial.

The timing of the onset of anemia can be helpful in identifying the likely cause.

• *Onset prior to birth.* Hydrops fetalis may be detected on antenatal ultrasound or be an unexpected finding at the time of birth. This condition has hematologic and nonhematologic causes but is characterized in the fetus and neonate by gross edema, ascites, pleural effusions, cardiac failure and profound anemia. The hematologic causes are listed in Table 7.2.

• *Onset in first 24 hours.* Severe anemia (hemoglobin < 8.0 g/dL) that presents around the time of birth is usually due to immune hemolysis or hemorrhage. Hydrops fetalis can result if either process has been chronic.

• *Onset after first 24 hours.* Anemia that becomes apparent after 24 hours is most often due to internal or external hemorrhage or nonimmune hemolytic disorders. Anemia due to impaired red cell production often manifests relatively late due to the boost in hemoglobin given to the baby by placental transfusion at birth, but if sufficiently severe, anemia due to impaired red cell production may lead to hydrops fetalis (see Table 7.2).

The causes of nonimmune neonatal anemia are listed in Table 7.3 and will be discussed in more detail; those which are immune-mediated are discussed in Chapter 8.

A diagnostic approach to neonatal anemia

The anemic fetus/neonate can present in one of four ways:
1 symptomatic anemia;
2 coincidental finding of a low hemoglobin;
3 hydrops fetalis detected before or at the time of birth;
4 jaundice/unconjugated hyperbilirubinemia.

The hematologic causes of hydrops fetalis are listed in Table 7.2. The presence of significant jaundice suggests a hemolytic process as a cause for the anemia.

The initial assessment of any anemic neonate should include the following.

Maternal history
• Preexisting medical conditions: bleeding disorders, hemoglobinopathies, red cell membrane defects, red cell enzymopathies.
• Antepartum conditions: drugs, maternal infection, trauma or vaginal bleeding.

- Helpful maternal investigations that may be available: full blood count during pregnancy, serologic tests, amniocentesis and ultrasound.

Birth history
- Method of delivery.
- Evidence of maternal hemorrhage.
- Fetal distress.
- Multiple pregnancies.
- Placental or umbilical cord pathology.

Family history
- Red cell membrane defects, hemoglobinopathies, red cell enzymopathies.
- Carrier status.
- History of consanguinity.

Neonatal history
- Gestation.
- Postnatal age at presentation of anemia.
- Ethnicity.
- Gender.

Examination
- Evidence of acute or chronic blood loss (see Table 7.4), organomegaly, congenital malformations and congenital infection.

Investigations
- Initial investigations: blood count, blood film, reticulocyte count and direct Coombs test.
- Subsequent investigations: dependent on results of initial assessment.

A diagnostic algorithm for the initial assessment and investigation of neonatal anemia is presented in Fig. 7.1.

Anemia secondary to blood loss

Bleeding can occur antenatally, during labor, or within the first few hours or days after birth. Neonates have a limited capacity to tolerate acute hemorrhage and prompt diagnosis and management are therefore essential for survival. The causes of blood loss can be considered in the following categories:
- concealed or occult hemorrhage prior to or during delivery;
- internal hemorrhage in the fetus or neonate;
- obstetric accidents;
- bleeding due to umbilical cord or placenta malformations;
- iatrogenic blood loss due to excessive sampling.

The clinical signs and symptoms of hemorrhage depend on the site, volume and rate of blood loss. It is usually relatively simple to distinguish acute from chronic blood loss on clinical grounds (Table 7.4). While life-threatening hemorrhage occurs in otherwise hematologically normal neonates, an

Table 7.4 Characteristics of acute and chronic blood loss in the neonate.

Acute blood loss
Pallor
Shallow tachypnea
Tachycardia
Poor peripheral perfusion
Hypotension
No organomegaly
Normochromic, macrocytic anemia (may have normal hemoglobin initially)
Reticulocytosis (may not be seen acutely)

Chronic blood loss
Pallor
Signs of cardiac failure
    Cardiac enlargement
    Tachypnea
    Hepatomegaly
    Ascites
Hypochromic, microcytic anemia
Reticulocytosis and nucleated red cells at birth

underlying bleeding diathesis should be considered in any infant presenting with unusual, unexplained or severe hemorrhage. It is important to remember that in acute blood loss the hemoglobin may initially be normal before falling rapidly in the subsequent few hours and therefore blood counts taken early may not reflect the degree of blood loss.

Concealed hemorrhage in the fetus prior to or during delivery

Occult hemorrhage can occur into the maternal circulation (fetomaternal), the placental circulation (fetoplacental) or, in the case of multiple pregnancies, into the fetus sharing the same placental blood supply (twin-to-twin).

Fetomaternal hemorrhage

Small numbers of fetal red cells (0.01 mL or more of blood) pass through the placental trophoblastic lining and enter the maternal circulation in more than 75% of normal pregnancies. Although this passage of red cells has been demonstrated from as early as 4–8 weeks' gestation, most significant spontaneous fetomaternal bleeding occurs in the third trimester or during labor and delivery. The risk in terms of both the frequency and magnitude of fetomaternal hemorrhage is increased by the use of invasive procedures during pregnancy and in a number of maternal conditions (Table 7.5).[11]

Clinical manifestations

Clinical manifestations vary with the size, rapidity and chronicity of the hemorrhage and the time at which the bleeding occurs with respect to delivery. In fetomaternal hemorrhage occurring at delivery, the volume of fetal blood

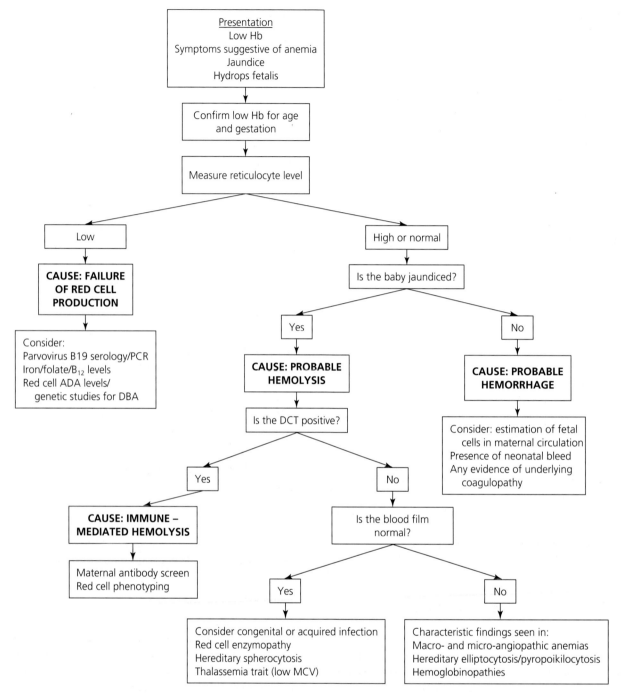

Fig. 7.1 A diagnostic algorithm for neonatal anemia. ADA, adenosine deaminase; DBA, Diamond–Blackfan anemia; DCT, direct Coombs test; MCV, mean cell volume; PCR, polymerase chain reaction.

detected in the maternal circulation is usually less than 0.5 mL but is greater than 15 mL in 0.3% of cases. Prior to delivery the acute loss of more than 20% of the fetal blood volume can lead to hydrops fetalis and stillbirth in the absence of intrauterine transfusion. Infants who survive will be clinically shocked, apneic and severely anemic. The same degree of blood loss over a more prolonged period of time may allow the fetus to compensate hemodynamically. Symptomatology is dependent on the degree of anemia: if mild it may go undetected, but if the hemoglobin is less than 12.0 g/dL the infant will usually display some signs of anemia such as pallor, tachypnea or poor feeding. Surviving infants with hemoglobin levels less than 4.0 g/dL at delivery have been reported.

Table 7.5 Conditions associated with increased risk and magnitude of fetomaternal hemorrhage.

Amniocentesis
Termination of pregnancy
Abdominal trauma
Chorioangioma or choriocarcinoma of placenta
Fetal blood sampling
Intrauterine transfusion
External cephalic version
Antepartum hemorrhage
Obstetric instrumentation
Manual removal of the placenta
Cesarean section
Pregnancy-induced hypertension

Laboratory diagnosis

The blood film is useful in distinguishing between acute and chronic blood loss. In acute blood loss, the red cells are normochromic and normocytic; in chronic blood loss, hypochromic and microcytic with anisopoikilocytosis. The reticulocyte count and nucleated red blood cell count are initially normal in acute blood loss but rise within the first few hours. A negative direct Coombs test and normal bilirubin will help distinguish anemia secondary to acute blood loss from that secondary to immune hemolysis.

A definitive diagnosis can only be made by demonstrating the presence of fetal red cells in the maternal circulation. The most widely used method is the Kleihauer–Betke technique of acid elution, although flow cytometer methods using fluorescent antibodies are increasingly employed.[12]

The Kleihauer test is based on the fact that at acid pH adult cells lose their hemoglobin whereas fetal hemoglobin resists elution and remains within erythrocytes. After appropriate staining, fetal cells appear pink and adult cells are seen as empty "ghosts". The ratio of fetal to adult cells can be determined by light microscopy. Evaluation of 6000 cells allows detection of bleeds greater than 0.4 mL. This technique is unreliable when maternal levels of fetal hemoglobin are increased as occurs in some hemoglobinopathies, in hereditary persistence of fetal hemoglobin, and in some normal women in whom pregnancy induces a rise in fetal hemoglobin, particularly in the first and second trimester.

Flow cytometric analysis permits the rapid, objective and reproducible evaluation of 50 000–100 000 red blood cells and is able to detect as little as 0.03 mL of fetal red cells in the maternal circulation.

If ABO incompatibility exists between maternal and fetal cells, the latter may be agglutinated and removed within hours from the maternal circulation by maternal antibody. It is therefore very important for an accurate assessment of the volume of fetomaternal hemorrhage that a maternal blood sample is taken as soon as a fetomaternal hemorrhage is suspected.

Fetoplacental hemorrhage

Rarely a transfusion of blood from the fetal circulation can accumulate within the placental tissue or retroplacentally rather than passing to the maternal circulation. If the infant is inadvertently held above the level of the placenta before the umbilical cord is cut at delivery, this can result in direct transfusion of blood from the fetus into the placenta.

Twin-to-twin transfusion

Approximately 70% of identical twin (monozygous) pregnancies share a placenta (monochorion). Vascular anastomoses within the placenta allow transfer of blood between the two fetuses. In about 15% of these monochorionic pregnancies the flow is sufficiently unbalanced to cause one fetus to become fluid overloaded with evidence of polyhydramnios and cardiac dysfunction, and the other to become anemic with evidence of poor renal function and oligohydramnios. This so-called twin-to-twin transfusion syndrome was previously diagnosed by a significant weight and hemoglobin discordance (>5 g/dL) at birth. Nowadays it is usually diagnosed antenatally by detection of markedly discrepant amniotic fluid volumes in the second trimester. Severe forms have a poor prognosis.[13] Several *in utero* interventions are employed to try to minimize the morbidity and mortality associated with this condition. A recent randomized trial showed some benefit for laser ablation of vascular anastomoses compared with serial removal of amniotic fluid from the polyhydramniotic twin.[14] However neither method was shown to be convincingly superior in all cases and further trials of intervention are indicated.

Obstetric accidents and malformations of the umbilical cord or placenta

Umbilical cord

In precipitous unattended or traumatic forceps deliveries, a normal umbilical cord can rupture and result in fetal hemorrhage. In normal deliveries, rupture can occur if the cord is abnormally short, entangled around the fetus or if it has vascular abnormalities such as venous tortuosity or an aneurysm.[15] Inflammation of the cord by meconium can weaken the vessels within it and predispose to rupture. If the hemorrhage is contained within the cord, a hematoma can form which can contain a large percentage of the fetal blood volume. In 1% of pregnancies there is a "velamentous" insertion of the cord into the edge of the placenta. This is more common in twin pregnancies and in pregnancies in which the placenta is low-lying (see below). In an estimated 1–2% of these pregnancies, fetal blood loss is significant and results in perinatal mortality of more than 60%.

Table 7.6 Classification of cranial bleeds in neonates.

	Clinical features	Risk factors	Timing	Outcome
Extracranial	*Subgaleal*: boggy swelling extending from orbital ridge to nape of neck (no limitation to spread) *Subaponeurotic/cephalhematoma*: swelling usually confined to one skull bone, i.e., does not cross sutures (extension limited by periosteal attachments)	Instrumental delivery, especially vacuum-assisted delivery, but 25% seen after normal vaginal delivery and 9% after cesarean section	Early: swelling apparent in first day of life	Can cause life-threatening hemorrhage. Once acute phase complete, recovery is usual. If large bleed, may see late hyperbilirubinemia, which is occasionally severe enough to require exchange transfusion
Intracranial (intraventricular, subarachnoid)	Diverse presentation from clinically asymptomatic to sudden collapse. Usually combination of bulging fontanelle, with neurologic signs: apnea, seizures, hypotonia. However, presentation may be with unexplained anemia alone	Prematurity, low birthweight, respiratory distress syndrome	Prenatal: very rare unless associated with hemorrhagic disorder such as NAIT 60% within first 24 hours 95% within first week	Depends on severity but can be associated with long-term neurologic sequelae

NAIT, neonatal alloimmune thrombocytopenia.

Placenta

Placenta previa and large placental abruptions can result in hemorrhage from both the fetal and maternal sides of the placenta and lead to neonatal anemia in surviving fetuses.[16] Fetal blood vessels in vasa previa are supported by the umbilical cord or placental tissues and traverse the amniotic sac in the lower segment of the uterus. If these vessels precede the presenting part during vaginal delivery they are at high risk of occlusion or laceration and this can result in life-threatening hemorrhage. The incidence of this condition is around 1 in 6000 pregnancies and is thought to be commoner with *in vitro* fertilization. The diagnosis is initially suspected on antenatal ultrasound and confirmed by Doppler studies. Hemorrhage is prevented by elective cesarean section before the onset of natural labor.

Massive fetal hemorrhage can be associated with accidental incision of the placenta at cesarean section; this complication is more likely if the placenta is anterior and low-lying.

Internal hemorrhage

Internal hemorrhage following a traumatic delivery is a well-recognized cause of neonatal anemia, although improvements in obstetric care and the increasing use of cesarean section for potentially difficult deliveries has resulted in a considerable decline in this complication. Nevertheless, all deliveries carry a risk of fetal hemorrhage, particularly if the fetus is large, small or abnormal, if the delivery is instrumental, or if antenatal care has been poor. A coincidental coagulopathy in the neonate, such as vitamin K deficiency or hemophilia, is likely to worsen the extent of any traumatic hemorrhage.

The clinical signs of anemia due to internal hemorrhage often present within 24–72 hours after birth, although with brisk hemorrhage their onset may be immediate, and are those of a shocked neonate with poor Apgar scores at delivery.

Cranial bleeds

Table 7.6 highlights the clinical features of extracranial and intracranial hemorrhage in neonates.[17-20] Severity of hemorrhage is variable but can be severe.

Intraabdominal hemorrhage

Breech deliveries of large-for-gestational-age infants are at particular risk of intraabdominal hemorrhage, although this complication has been described following normal deliveries. The hemorrhage can involve the adrenals, kidneys, liver and spleen or the retroperitoneal space. Retroperitoneal hemorrhage can present with bluish discoloration of the skin of the flank and sometimes a palpable mass and has been described following traumatic perforation or rupture of an umbilical artery by catheterization.

Rupture of the liver was previously reported in 1.2–9.6% of post-mortems carried out for investigation of stillbirth or neonatal death.[21] Despite improvements in obstetric care over the last few decades, small subcapsular hemorrhages probably occur more frequently after traumatic births than is clinically appreciated, particularly in low-birthweight infants. The severity depends on whether the hemorrhage is confined within the capsule of the liver (abdominal swelling and anemia but potential recovery) or whether the capsule ruptures. This complication usually presents 24–48 hours after delivery, with free blood in the peritoneal cavity and rapid onset of shock. Radiography of the abdomen reveals free fluid, and paracentesis confirms the presence of blood in the peritoneum.

The prognosis is typically poor but infants do survive with prompt resuscitation, blood transfusion and surgical repair.

Splenic rupture secondary to extreme splenic distension associated with severe hemolytic disease of the newborn is now an exceedingly rare event in countries with anti-D prophylactic programs, but splenic rupture can occur after apparently normal deliveries, most often in large-for-dates infants.[22]

Other sites

Pulmonary hemorrhage can occur in infants on ventilatory support, particularly in those born prematurely. Rarely, hemangiomas of the skin,[23] gastrointestinal tract[24] and thymus[25] can present with significant neonatal blood loss.

Iatrogenic blood loss

Despite the use of micromethods in modern neonatal practice, blood sampling losses in preterm babies is the commonest cause of neonatal anemia.[26] Blood sampling should be kept to a minimum and routine daily testing avoided if at all possible.

Anemia as a result of hemolysis

A hemolytic process is defined as a pathologic state that results in shortening of the normal red cell lifespan. Recognition of hemolysis, even if initially mild, is extremely important in the neonate as careful clinical monitoring and early intervention may prevent kernicterus and its sequelae. Neonatal hemolysis may be the first indication of an inherited red cell disorder, such as a red cell enzymopathy, a red cell membrane defect or a hemoglobinopathy, which will have consequences for the affected neonate throughout life. Neonatal anemia secondary to alloimmune hemolysis may have implications for future siblings.

In the neonate with hemolysis, hyperbilirubinemia may be a more prominent feature than anemia. The degree of anemia will depend on the rate of red cell destruction and the ability of the bone marrow to compensate by increasing red cell production. In addition, in some children, genetic variation in bilirubin conjugating mechanisms may lead to a disproportionately greater degree of hyperbilirubinemia than would be expected for the degree of red cell destruction (see discussion of G6PD deficiency below).

Laboratory results suggestive of hemolysis include:
1 the presence of persistently increased numbers of reticulocytes and/or nucleated red blood cells; although elevated at birth, these should normally be very low (<1%) by day 3 of life;
2 unconjugated hyperbilirubinemia especially in the first 48 hours after birth or an unusually high level;
3 a positive direct Coombs test (if immune in etiology);
4 characteristic red cell morphology (in some cases).
A Coombs test should be performed on any neonate suspected of a having hemolytic anemia. A positive Coombs test suggests immune-mediated hemolysis (discussed in Chapter 8).

The major causes of nonimmune hemolysis are (i) red cell membrane disorders, (ii) red cell enzymopathies, (iii) hemoglobinopathies, (iv) infections (both congenital and acquired) and (v) macroangiopathic and microangiopathic processes.

Red cell membrane disorders

These may be suspected by a positive family history or characteristic red cell morphology on a blood film. The commonest inherited red cell membrane defect is hereditary spherocytosis, which has an incidence of 1 in 5000 births. Hereditary pyropoikilocytosis is significant in that it may result in a severe transfusion-dependent anemia during the neonatal period. Red cell membrane disorders are discussed in more detail in Chapter 12.

Hereditary spherocytosis

This is a group of disorders caused by various mutations in proteins that comprise the red cell cytoskeleton. The cytoskeleton is responsible for the maintenance of red cell shape, deformability and elasticity, and hence patients with hereditary spherocytosis (HS) have fragile abnormally shaped cells that are particularly susceptible to extravascular hemolysis in the spleen. The inheritance pattern is usually autosomal dominant and most mutations are private, i.e., unique to each affected family. This explains the clinical heterogeneity and similar course within families.[27,28]

HS is commonly symptomatic in the neonatal period. In published series, 20–50% of affected individuals have a history of jaundice with or without anemia and mild splenomegaly in the newborn period.[29] Presentation is usually within the first 48 hours of life, but in 20% of neonates it is delayed beyond the first week. Severe anemia due to neonatal HS is rare, and the anemia is usually mild to moderate.

In the absence of a family history of HS the diagnosis is infrequently made in the neonatal period, when it is more difficult to confirm than later in childhood. The reticulocytosis and degree of splenomegaly can be variable and the number of spherocytes in the peripheral blood may not be significantly increased over the normal for this age group until the infant is 2–3 months of age. The haptoglobin level is an unreliable indicator of hemolysis in neonates. The osmotic fragility test, which is most commonly used to diagnose HS, is unreliable in the neonate, as the increased lipid content of the membrane of neonatal red cells renders them osmotically resistant. It is therefore important to perform an incubated osmotic fragility test and to include a control neonatal sample. It is often more practical to make a presumptive diagnosis of HS based on the blood film features and clinical findings and to defer formal testing until the baby is 6–12 months of age. Examination of parental blood films, one of which may show the typical morphologic features of HS, can be diagnostically rewarding.

Newer tests, such as the eosin-5-maleimide (EMA) binding dye test, have a higher predictive value but are not yet routinely available. Protein electrophoresis of the membrane proteins may be informative where there is diagnostic difficulty.

The main differential diagnosis is with ABO incompatibility, where spherocytosis is a striking feature, but spherocytes can also be seen in bacterial sepsis, hemolytic transfusion reactions and oxidative red cell injury. Morphologically, ABO incompatibility and HS may be indistinguishable. Maternal and infant blood groups and a Coombs test may be helpful, but if not, family studies may help differentiate HS from acquired conditions, as will the passage of time.

Management

The management is that of hyperbilirubinemia, which can usually be controlled with phototherapy, although kernicterus is a risk and exchange transfusion may be required. Hyperbilirubinemia may appear late and therefore babies born to parents with known HS should be carefully observed for jaundice during the first few days of life. Similarly it is important to monitor for the development of anemia, especially in those infants who do not mount an adequate reticulocyte response. Anemia may be more common in HS in the neonatal period than previously recognized. The hemoglobin is usually normal at birth but can drop precipitously during the first 5–30 days.[29] Transfusion is sometimes necessary but continued transfusion dependence is unusual. In these rare severe cases, erythropoietin may reduce or prevent the need for red cell transfusions.[30]

Supplementary dietary folic acid is recommended.[27] There is no evidence that children with HS who are symptomatic as neonates have a more severe form of the disease in later life.

Hereditary elliptocytosis and hereditary pyropoikilocytosis

These are a heterogeneous group of membrane disorders characterized by defective horizontal interactions between membrane proteins. There is some confusion with the nomenclature of these disorders, with "infantile poikilocytosis", "pyropoikilocytosis" and "pyknocytosis" all being used in the literature. There is no merit in this subclassification and all these disorders can be generically classified as hereditary pyropoikilocytosis (HPP). The diversity is not surprising as the genetic basis is complex, with hereditary elliptocytosis (HE) and HPP coexisting in the same families. HPP can be seen in homozygotes for HE mutations, in compound heterozygotes for two different HE mutations, or in individuals who inherit one HE mutation and a low expression spectrin allele such as α LELY.[28]

The commonest form of this condition, HE, is inherited in an autosomal dominant manner and other than the finding of 25–75% elliptocytes on the blood film, is generally a benign condition which does not cause any clinical symptoms.

In contrast, HPP results in a moderate to severe hemolytic anemia and jaundice and is morphologically characterized by marked red cell budding, fragmentation and variation in red cell shape (poikilocytosis). The blood film is very characteristic and HPP is one of the few causes of a low MCV (<70 fL) in neonates, the others being α-thalassemia and chronic iron deficiency. The correct diagnosis may be confirmed by examination of parental blood films when one or both may show features of classical HE.

The reason for the particularly severe phenotype seen in neonates is not well understood but may be related to the elevated free 2,3-diphosphoglycerate (2,3-DPG) levels in fetal cells, which may weaken spectrin–actin bonds leading to increased fragility.[31]

Management of HPP

In its milder forms, red cell fragmentation and subsequent hemolysis decline in the infant and the benign clinical picture of mild HE emerges by 6 months to 2 years of age. Supportive care with folic acid supplements and the judicious use of red cell transfusion is indicated. Investigations such as membrane protein analysis, osmotic fragility or EMA binding dye tests should be performed prior to transfusion.

In more severe cases, the red cell abnormalities do not improve with time and hemolysis persists with severe anemia, splenomegaly and early gallstone formation. Regular transfusion is necessary. Splenectomy is often effective at reducing or abolishing the transfusion requirement but is usually deferred until at least 3 years of age to reduce the risk of postsplenectomy sepsis.

Infantile pyknocytosis

This describes the association in early infancy of hemolytic anemia with unusual red cell morphology. The red cells are distorted, irregular and small with many projections. Spontaneous resolution is usual by 4–6 months of age. This disorder is probably heterogeneous and results from a number of different pathologies and has been described in association with HPP, glucose 6-phosphate dehydrogenase (G6PD) deficiency, and electrolyte disturbance. The term is therefore not useful and should probably be abandoned.[32]

Rare membrane defects

Dehydrated hereditary stomatocytosis is an inherited hemolytic anemia characterized by increased membrane permeability to sodium and potassium ions. It may be confused with HS. Although rare, it is associated with neonatal hepatitis and is a cause of perinatal ascites and therefore should be included in its differential diagnosis.[33]

Red cell enzyme deficiencies

Inherited disorders of red cell metabolism are an important cause of hemolytic anemia in early life (see also Chapter 9). Most enzymopathies have no distinct red cell morphology and their diagnosis depends on their inclusion in the differential diagnosis of hemolytic anemia in this age group. A family history and awareness of ethnicity may be helpful. Jaundice is again the prominent clinical finding but anemia can arise if the hemolysis is severe.

Glucose 6-phosphate dehydrogenase deficiency

This is the commonest of the red cell enzyme deficiencies. It is an X-linked disorder seen in individuals from the Mediterranean, Africa and Asia, and over 150 variants have been identified.[34] Female carriers are affected only if the normal gene on one X chromosome is inactivated by extreme lyonization.

G6PD is the first enzyme in the hexose-monophosphate shunt and is important in NADPH generation and in the regeneration of reduced glutathione, which protects the red cell from oxidative damage. Exposure to oxidant drugs, infection, acidosis or ingestion of fava beans can lead to denaturation of hemoglobin and extravascular hemolysis.

In global terms, G6PD deficiency is the commonest cause of severe neonatal jaundice. A family history or the ethnic origin may suggest the diagnosis. The onset of jaundice is often delayed until the second or third day of life and can be confused with "physiologic" jaundice, although the peak bilirubin is usually much higher. The degree of jaundice is often disproportionally high for the rate of hemolysis. Recent evidence suggests that decreased bilirubin conjugation and elimination play a major role in the pathogenesis of neonatal jaundice. There is an association between the degree of hyperbilirubinemia and the coinheritance of Gilbert syndrome due to a polymorphism in the promoter of the gene uridine diphosphate glucoronyltransferase (UGT1A).[35] Other genetic polymorphisms may also be involved.[36]

Although rare, massive acute hemolysis can occur, with or without obvious exposure to oxidant compounds, and may be fatal.[37]

The blood film is usually normal, although microspherocytes may be seen in severe cases. The diagnosis may be confirmed by enzyme assay but this may be within normal limits in the presence of a brisk reticulocytosis because reticulocytes have higher G6PD levels than mature red cells and in such circumstances the assay should be repeated when the acute hemolytic episode has subsided. Preterm infants have higher G6PD levels than term infants but this does not usually preclude the diagnosis.

Management

Early phototherapy is indicated and exchange transfusion may be necessary in severe cases. Parents and medical staff should be educated about avoidance of exposure to oxidant drugs and compounds. Maternal exposure to oxidant drugs may cause hemolysis in the neonate via transplacental transfer and has been reported for methylene blue and maternal ingestion of fava beans. Naphthalene, a major component of mothballs, is the most common domestic trigger for acute hemolysis. A list of drugs to be avoided can be found in the British National Formulary. Fat-soluble preparations of vitamin K (phytomenadione) are safe and all babies should receive vitamin K prophylaxis either intramuscularly or as an oral colloidal formulation. In contrast, water-soluble preparations of vitamin K (menadiol sodium phosphate) have been reported to cause severe hemolysis and are contraindicated. Folic acid supplements are not generally indicated except in severe variants associated with chronic hemolysis.

Pyruvate kinase deficiency

This is the second commonest red cell enzyme deficiency associated with neonatal hemolysis and the commonest red cell enzyme deficiency of the Embden–Meyerhof pathway. However, pyruvate kinase deficiency is relatively uncommon.[38] It is autosomal recessive in inheritance, and is primarily seen in northern Europeans, in whom there is wide variation in expression of the disorder although the severity remains fairly constant within a family. The block in the glycolytic pathway caused by pyruvate kinase deficiency results in an increase in 2,3-DPG levels. This improves oxygen delivery to the tissues and helps alleviate the clinical and biochemical effects of the anemia. However, in the neonate the hemolysis can be particularly severe, with jaundice developing within the first 24 hours of life associated with anemia, reticulocytosis and splenomegaly. Hydrops fetalis has been reported in severely affected families. Exchange transfusion is frequently required to avoid the risks of kernicterus. Infants who present at birth appear to have more severe hemolysis in later life. The blood film shows features of nonspherocytic hemolysis with a reticulocytosis and nucleated red blood cells. Irregularly contracted cells are seen in some but not all cases. Diagnosis can usually be made by direct enzyme assay or by demonstrating the carrier state in both parents. Although affected individuals usually have enzyme levels of about 5–40% of normal, there is not a good correlation between enzyme activity as measured *in vitro* and clinical severity and occasional patients with severe pyruvate kinase deficiency have completely normal enzyme activity when assayed by conventional methods. In these individuals, measurement of metabolic intermediates may demonstrate blockade at the pyruvate kinase step. Later, if multiple trans-fusions are required, splenectomy may lessen the transfusion requirement.

Glucose phosphate isomerase deficiency

This is the third commonest red cell enzymopathy and one-third of affected individuals develop symptoms in the neonatal period. Hydrops fetalis has been described.[39] Inheritance is autosomal recessive and the clinical mani-festations and morphologic features are similar to those of the other congenital nonspherocytic anemias.

Other enzymopathies

Other enzymopathies should be considered. Neonatal hemolysis may be the only presenting feature of conditions such as triose phosphate isomerase deficiency that have severe sequelae later in infancy and childhood. Clinical features and appropriate tests are discussed in Chapter 9.

Hemoglobinopathies (see also Chapters 10, 11 and 13)

As previously discussed, red blood cells contain approxim-ately 80% HbF ($\alpha_2\gamma_2$) and 20% HbA ($\alpha_2\beta_2$) at birth. There-fore hemoglobinopathies presenting in the neonatal period involve abnormalities of the α or γ chains. Abnormalities affecting γ-globin may be associated with severe clinical man-ifestations at birth which subside when the switch from fetal to adult hemoglobin occurs. The α-chain defects may behave differently in neonates compared with older infants and children, because in the neonatal period the α-chain is pre-dominantly paired with a γ-chain to form HbF, whereas in later infancy onwards it is paired with a β-chain to form HbA. Because β-globin synthesis is limited in the newborn, defects involving the β-globin gene rarely manifest in the first weeks of life.

Neonatal screening for hemoglobinopathies is now routinely performed in some countries and will lead to the increased detection of these disorders in the neonatal period, allowing early intervention.[40]

Globin-chain structural abnormalities

Most α-chain structural abnormalities have no clinical con-sequences in neonates or adults and most infants with these mutations are detected only by routine neonatal screening programs. Occasionally, an α-chain variant may be clinically significant in the neonate, but not in the adult. Hb Hasheron ($\alpha_2^{14Asp\rightarrow His}\beta_2$) can present as a transient hemolytic anemia in the newborn period because this α-chain variant is unstable when it associates with γ-globin but not β-globin chains. The hemolysis in the neonate resolves with transition from the fetal to the adult form of Hb Hasheron trait. Other rare α-

chain variants include Hb Taybe, which may be sufficiently unstable to cause hemolysis of a degree that can lead to hydrops fetalis.

Structural variants of the γ-chain also rarely cause clinical problems; if they do, these resolve as the γ to β switch occurs. HbF Poole is an unstable γ-chain variant that can be as-sociated with a significant hemolytic anemia in the neonatal period.

Neonatal sickle cell disease

Although β-chain abnormalities can be detected at birth using sensitive electrophoretic techniques, they do not usually cause clinical problems. The newborn with the commonest β-chain variant, sickle cell disease, is usually asymptomatic in the first few months of life due to the presence of HbF, which interferes with HbS polymerization within the red cell. However, hyperbilirubinemia may be more common in neonates with sickle cell disease than in the normal popula-tion and there has been a report of fatal sickling in a 5-day-old baby.[41] Despite the relative lack of symptoms in the majority of babies with sickle cell disease, it is important that they are started on penicillin prophylaxis and referred to a com-prehensive care provider early for parental education, support and other preventive measures including pneumococcal vac-cination. There is emerging evidence that such interventions reduce morbidity and mortality in this disease.[42,43]

Defective hemoglobin synthesis: the thalassemia syndromes (see also Chapter 13)

α-Thalassemias

A reduced rate of α-globin chain synthesis characterizes the α-thalassemias, which usually arise from a deletion of one or more of the four α-globin genes. In the presence of α-globin gene deletions, excess γ chains accumulate within the red cell and form a tetramer called Hb Barts (γ^4). The amount of Hb Barts is proportional to the number of affected α-globin genes. Clinical and laboratory features depend on the num-ber of genes deleted as described below.[44]

- Silent carrier α-thalassemia (α^+-thalassemia) occurs when one gene is deleted and is associated with a mild elevation of Hb Barts at birth (<2%) but no clinical manifestations.
- α-Thalassemia trait (α^0-thalassemia) occurs when two genes are deleted. The diagnosis is simpler in neonates than adults. It is the commonest cause of microcytic red cell indices (MCV < 95 fL), which are otherwise very rare in this age group. The diagnosis is confirmed by detection of an elevated level of Hb Barts of around 3–10% at birth, which disappears by 3 months of age after which the diagnosis is more difficult to make. This disorder is common in Southeast Asia, with an incidence of about 20% compared with 2–5% in African populations. In the latter, the α-thalassemia gene mutations are almost invariably on different chromosomes, i.e., the abnormal gene is always linked to a normal gene.

Consequently, offspring from two African α-thalassemia trait individuals will not inherit more than two α-thalassemia genes.[45] In Southeast Asians, the two gene mutations are usually on the same chromosome and if both parents pass on their affected chromosome, a four-gene deletion results (see below).

• If three α genes are deleted, HbH disease results. HbH consists of β[4] tetramers, is unstable, precipitates within the red cell and can be demonstrated by incubation of the blood with supravital oxidizing stains such as methylene blue. It can also be detected on hemoglobin electrophoresis or high-performance liquid chromatography (HPLC). HbH disease presents in the neonatal period with a significant microcytic, hemolytic anemia and a level of Hb Barts ranging from 20 to 40%. By 3 months of age, when the γ to β globin switch occurs, Hb Barts disappears and is replaced by HbH. Infants with HbH disease may require transfusion for severe anemia at birth but outwith this period the severity of the anemia is variable but often mild. The combination of two α gene deletions on one chromosome and a nondeletional α gene mutation on the other chromosome (e.g., Hb Constant Spring) may produce a particularly severe form of HbH disease that may be associated with hydrops fetalis.

• When all four α genes are deleted, no α-chain synthesis occurs, no HbF or HbA are produced and homozygous α-thalassemia results. This is a common cause of fetal death throughout Southeast Asia. These fetuses invariably become hydropic due to severe intrauterine anemia in the second or third trimester and are stillborn or die soon after birth. Those who survive to birth have a hemoglobin level of around 6–8 g/dL, with severe thalassemic changes on the peripheral blood film: microcytosis, hypochromia, poikilocytosis, target cells and nucleated red cells. The hemoglobin consists of approximately 80% Hb Barts, with the rest being the embryonic hemoglobin Hb Portland ($\zeta_2\gamma_2$). Hb Barts has an oxygen dissociation curve like myoglobin and is therefore unable to deliver oxygen to tissues. Intrauterine transfusions followed by a postdelivery transfusion program or hematopoietic stem cell transplantation have been reported to result in occasional survivors.[46] This disorder must be distinguished from other causes of hydrops fetalis due to severe anemia. In future, it is possible that *in utero* stem cell transplantation or gene therapy may be curative.

β-Thalassemias

Homozygous β-thalassemia does not cause symptoms in the newborn but during the γ to β globin switch, a microcytic anemia develops, nucleated red cells appear on the blood film and high levels of HbF persist. Any disorder that significantly alters the survival of fetal red cells, such as intrauterine blood loss or blood group incompatibility, can unmask β-thalassemia clinically at a younger age. Although generally asymptomatic, patients with β-thalassemia major can be detected by newborn screening by the presence of HbF alone on Hb electrophoresis or HPLC. This is not diagnostic and can be seen in patients with hereditary persistence of fetal hemoglobin (see Chapter 11) mutations or in premature neonates.[47]

γβ-Thalassemia

The β-globin cluster on chromosome 11 comprises closely linked genes that encode for embryonic (ε), fetal ($^G\gamma$ and $^A\gamma$) and adult (δ, β) globin chains. There are two γ genes on each chromosome termed $^G\gamma$ and $^A\gamma$ which differ in a single amino acid at position 136 (glycine and alanine respectively). Deletions of γ genes usually involve adjacent δ, β and sometimes ε genes also. Deletion of one γ gene is seen in $^G\gamma(^A\gamma\delta\beta)^0$-thalassemia. Homozygotes may have thalassemia intermedia and heterozygotes have a thalassemia trait-like picture with high HbF levels. $(\epsilon\gamma\delta\beta)^0$-Thalassemia involves deletion of both $^G\gamma$ and $^A\gamma$ on the same chromosome. Homozygous deletions have not been described, presumably because they would result in no fetal hemoglobin production and therefore be incompatible with *in utero* survival. Heterozygotes for $(\epsilon\gamma\delta\beta)^0$-thalassemia have a variable clinical phenotype but neonates may have a severe transfusion-dependent microcytic hemolytic anemia, and hydrops fetalis has been reported.[48] The disorder often improves with time, resembling β-thalassemia trait after 6 months of age when the switch to adult globin chain synthesis has been completed.

Infection

Both intrauterine and postnatally acquired infections can be associated with anemia in addition to other hematologic abnormalities in the neonatal period. The anemia may be multifactorial and due in part to marrow suppression and decrease in red cell production and in part to hemolysis. In severe bacterial sepsis, the hemolysis develops because of infection-induced small vessel damage and fibrin deposition, which can damage red cells and result in disseminated intravascular coagulation (see below).

Infections acquired by hematogenous spread *in utero* and associated with hemolysis include toxoplasmosis, cytomegalovirus, congenital syphilis and rubella (Table 7.7).[49] Herpes simplex infections are generally acquired from the cervix and vagina during delivery. The hemolytic process is thought to arise from direct injury to the red cell membrane or reticuloendothelial hyperplasia. Occasionally, antibody produced in response to infection can cross-react with antigen on the surface of the red cell producing a positive direct Coombs test leading to immune-mediated hemolysis.

Clinical suspicion of intrauterine infection in the neonate with hemolysis is often triggered by the associated findings of jaundice, chorioretinitis, pneumonitis, central nervous system abnormalities, growth retardation, skin lesions or hepatosplenomegaly. If the spleen is enlarged, hypersplenism can increase the rate of red cell destruction. Laboratory features include thrombocytopenia, leukocytosis with

Table 7.7 Congenital infections that may be complicated by anemia in the neonatal period.

Infection	Proportion of babies with any symptom of the infection	Laboratory features of the anemia
Cytomegalovirus	<10%	Hb 8.0–120 g/dL in first week Hb 5–10 g/dL at 3– weeks with reticulocytosis Blood film: poikilocytes, NRBCs
Herpes simplex	>90% have generalized disease	Mild microangiopathic changes
Rubella	>90% if infected in first trimester, less in second trimester	Mild anemia in 15–30% of infected infants Exaggerated postnatal decline in Hb
Toxoplasmosis	30–50%	Anemia in 40–50% of infected infants. Can be severe (Hb < 8.0 g/dL) and cause hydrops fetalis Reticulocytosis NRBCs on blood film
Syphilis	15% if mother untreated	>90% of infected infants are anemic. Can be severe (Hb < 8.0 g/dL). Reticulocytosis and NRBCs on blood film
Malaria	10% in endemic areas	Can be severe and life-threatening Reticulocytosis Parasitemia on blood film
Parvovirus	<10%	Reticulocytopenic anemia which can be mild to severe and cause hydrops fetalis Giant pronormoblasts in bone marrow with general erythroid hypoplasia

NRBCs, nucleated red blood cells.

immature forms (left shift), reticulocytosis and large numbers of nucleated red cells. Hyperbilirubinemia may be both conjugated and unconjugated due to the coexistence of hepatitis and hemolysis. The diagnosis is confirmed by serology or direct isolation of the infective agent from blood or an alternative site.

Although malaria remains a major health hazard in many parts of the world, vertical transmission appears to be rare, but when it does occur it can cause severe fetal infection and stillbirth.[50] All four species can produce congenital infection. The placenta is a preferential site for reproduction and growth of the malarial parasite, but also acts as a relative barrier to fetal infection. Maternal IgG crosses the placenta and provides additional protection to the fetus, which explains why congenital malaria is much commoner in infants born to nonimmune mothers. If the parasites are not eradicated, they may enter a latent phase that can delay presentation of malaria in the infected neonate for several weeks. Features of malaria in the newborn include fever, irritability, hepatosplenomegaly and jaundice as well as anemia, which is usually severe with associated reticulocytosis.

The diagnosis of congenital malaria requires a high index of clinical suspicion. The blood film should be carefully examined following suitable staining and blood should be sent for serologic testing to a reference laboratory that specializes in tropical diseases. If the diagnosis is suspected at birth, usually because the mother has been treated for malaria in pregnancy, the placental bed can be examined for the parasite and treatment instituted in the first days of life to prevent subsequent severe sequelae.

Parvovirus infection is discussed in the section on impaired red cell production.

Macroangiopathic and microangiopathic neonatal anemias

Macroangiopathic anemia

Severe cardiac defects, renal artery stenosis and large-vessel thrombi have been reported to cause hemolysis in the newborn by shear-related disruption to the red cell membrane and/or interaction of red cells with abnormal surfaces within the heart. The blood film may be very abnormal, with geometric red cell fragments. Thrombocytopenia and a coagulopathy may be present.

Disseminated intravascular coagulation

This is a common complication of neonatal infection, particularly bacterial infection. It can also be associated with severe birth asphyxia, respiratory distress syndrome, hypovolemia and hypothermia. A microangiopathic process results from red cell injury in partially occluded small blood vessels where red blood cells can be damaged by passage through fibrin strands or by trapping by damaged endothelium. There is accompanying thrombocytopenia and coagulopathy (see Chapter 29).

Hemangiomas

A microangiopathic hemolytic anemia can also occur in association with a giant hemangioma, i.e., Kasabach–Merritt syndrome. This can present at birth or during infancy. The predominant findings are of profound thrombocytopenia with anemia, hypofibrinogenemia and coagulopathy. Early recognition is important because the syndrome can be associated with considerable morbidity and mortality.[51]

Congenital thrombotic thrombocytopenic purpura

This is an inherited form of thrombotic thrombocytopenic purpura due to deficiency of von Willebrand cleaving protease (ADAMTS13). It can present in the neonatal period with thrombocytopenia, severe hyperbilirubinemia and a microangiopathic hemolytic anemia.[52]

Anemia secondary to impaired red cell production

With the exception of the physiologic anemia of prematurity, anemia secondary to impaired red cell production is relatively uncommon in the neonatal period. However, anemia due to inherited disorders associated with failure of red cell production, congenital infection and nutritional deficiencies or inborn errors of metabolism that affect absorption, transport or metabolism of hematinics can present in the neonatal period. Rarer causes of impaired red cell production at this age include congenital leukemia, Down syndrome with transient abnormal myelopoiesis, and osteopetrosis.

Inherited disorders of failure of red cell production

Inherited disorders of red cell production are all rare. Even in the neonatal period, failure of red cell production may be part of a pancytopenia, suggesting involvement of the stem cell, or a single cytopenia, suggesting involvement of committed erythroid progenitors. Some disorders typically present in the neonatal period and others more commonly outwith. Some disorders are associated with congenital abnormalities and others are not.

Diamond–Blackfan anemia

Diamond–Blackfan anemia is an uncommon inherited condition characterized by failure of erythropoiesis that results in a normochromic and usually macrocytic anemia with reticu-

locytopenia. The white cell and platelet counts are usually normal in infancy. The bone marrow shows an absence or a marked reduction in erythroid precursors. About 10% of patients are anemic at birth, 25% by 1 month of age and 90% by the end of the first year of life.[53] Infants presenting with hydrops fetalis have been reported.[54–56]

Approximately 10% of affected infants are of low birthweight (<2500 g).[53] Physical anomalies are seen in about 30% of patients and those evident in the neonatal period include microcephaly, cleft palate, flat thenar eminence, thumb deformities, web neck and eye anomalies.

The majority (75%) of cases are sporadic, but both autosomal dominant and autosomal recessive inheritance is described. Multiple genes for the disease probably exist but only the RPS 19 mutation has been identified to date. In patients without an identified mutation, the finding of elevated erythrocyte adenosine deaminase levels (measured before transfusion) helps support the diagnosis.

Steroid therapy should be instigated when the diagnosis is confirmed and the majority respond, at least initially. However, steroids started in early infancy have the potential to impair growth at the time when it is maximal and interfere later with routine infant immunizations.

Congenital dyserythropoietic anemia

Congenital dyserythropoietic anemia (CDA) is an uncommon inherited cause of anemia characterized by ineffective erythropoiesis and dysplastic morphology. The anemia is usually mild to moderate, but can be more severe and transfusion dependent. Very rarely it is severe enough to result in hydrops fetalis.[57,58]

CDA type 1 is characterized by macrocytic anemia, megaloblastic erythroid hyperplasia and nuclear chromatin bridging in bone marrow erythroid precursors with characteristic ultrastructural features on electron microscopy. In a retrospective review of 31 patients, about 50% had been investigated for anemia and early jaundice in the neonatal period, and had required blood transfusion during the first month of life.[59] Although the diagnosis of CDA type 1 is not usually made in the neonatal period, this study suggests that it should be considered in the differential diagnosis of neonatal anemia.

Hydrops fetalis has been reported secondary to profound anemia associated with atypical CDA characterized by peripheral blood, bone marrow and electron microscopy features resembling CDA type II, but with a negative acidified serum lysis test (Ham test).[57,58] These infants had remarkably similar hematologic findings of binuclear erythroblasts in the peripheral blood and erythroid hyperplasia with binuclear to multinuclear erythroblasts in the bone marrow. Fetal loss and consanguinity were common. Infants who survived were transfusion dependent and some received intrauterine transfusion.[57]

Pearson syndrome

Pearson syndrome, which is characterized by sideroblastic anemia and exocrine pancreatic dysfunction, results from a deletion of mitochondrial DNA. The anemia is usually macrocytic and presents before 1 month of age in 25% and by 6 months of age in 70% of affected individuals.[53] Hydrops fetalis has been reported.[60] Myeloid and erythroid precursors are vacuolated and sideroblasts, usually ring sideroblasts, are present in the bone marrow. Support with blood transfusion may be required.

Fanconi anemia

Fanconi anemia is characterized by increased chromosome breakage, progressive pancytopenia, predisposition to malignancy and an autosomal recessive pattern of inheritance. Associated congenital abnormalities include short stature (unhelpful diagnostically in the neonate), skin pigmentation, microophthalmia, genitourinary abnormalities and defects of the thumbs and radii. However some patients only have hematologic abnormalities and lack the congenital nonhematologic anomalies. Bone marrow failure generally starts during early school years, but hematologic presentation does occasionally occur in the neonatal period, and while this is most commonly with thrombocytopenia, there are reports of pancytopenia in this age group. Therefore Fanconi anemia should be considered as a cause of neonatal anemia and/or thrombocytopenia even in the absence of the typical congenital anomalies.[61]

Physiologic anemia of infancy/prematurity

The healthy term infant has a hemoglobin of around 16.5–18.5 g/dL; the level is influenced by a number of factors previously described, including the timing of cord clamping. The infant's hemoglobin remains reasonably stable during the first week of life and thereafter declines to reach a nadir of 10.5–12.5 g/dL by 8–10 weeks,[2] and this is referred to as the physiologic anemia of infancy. The hemoglobin concentration in the preterm infant is similar to that of the term infant at birth but the postnatal physiologic fall in hemoglobin, termed the physiologic anemia of prematurity, reaches its nadir earlier (4–8 weeks), is more profound (around 8 g/dL) and in both speed of onset and degree is directly related to the infant's gestation.

Pathophysiology of the anemia of infancy/prematurity

- Erythropoietin does not cross the placenta but is produced by the fetus. Levels rise with increasing gestation and are high in cord blood.[1] High erythropoietin levels are thought to be a physiologic response to low intrauterine oxygen tension and to be responsible for the infant's high hemoglobin at birth. The increase in oxygen tension after birth results in marked erythropoietin suppression, leading to almost undetectable levels and a subsequent fall in red cell production. The decline in hemoglobin production in the term infant reaches a nadir at 2 weeks of age, but in preterm infants may happen soon after birth, which is the reason that their hemoglobin nadir occurs earlier.

- Erythropoietin levels fall after birth and remain inappropriately low for the level of hemoglobin associated with the anemia of infancy and prematurity. This blunted response may partly be due to the fact that at this age the switch from liver to kidney as the site of erythropoietin production is incomplete and the liver may be less sensitive than the kidney to hypoxia. The number of erythroid progenitor cells have been shown to be relatively low for the degree of anemia, presumably secondary to a lack of erythropoietin drive, but burst forming unit-erythroid (BFU-E) colonies retain normal responsiveness to erythropoietin.[62,63]

- Pharmokinetic studies in animal models and preterm infants have shown that preterm infants require higher doses of recombinant human erythropoietin (r-HuEPO) because of more rapid clearance and greater volume of distribution; this may contribute to the preterm's low erythropoietin levels.

- Other factors that contribute to the severity of the anemia include rapid growth in the first few weeks of life with an increase in blood volume but no increase in red cell mass, shortened red cell survival in neonates, iatrogenic blood losses from blood sampling, and hematinic deficiencies.

Treatment of the anemia of prematurity

r-HuEPO is widely used in the management of preterm infants to reduce their transfusion requirements associated with the anemia of prematurity. However, there are many unanswered questions about r-HuEPO therapy in premature infants, including which preterms benefit, the optimal dose and scheduling of r-HuEPO, the optimal dose and route of iron and folate supplementation, and the appropriateness and safety of parenteral iron supplementation.[64]

The aim of r-HuEPO is to reduce both the number of infants who require any transfusion and the total number of transfusions required by those infants who cannot avoid transfusion because of their extreme prematurity. r-HuEPO has been shown to reduce the transfusion requirements of preterm infants weighing more than 1000–1250 g at birth,[65] although this is a group that less often requires transfusion and minimization of phlebotomy losses and stringent adherence to a transfusion policy is an attractive alternative.[66] The evidence for infants with a birthweight of less than 1000–1250 g is less convincing.

In a recent study, 172 preterm infants with a birthweight of 401–1000 g were randomized to receive r-HuEPO at a dose of 400 units/kg three times weekly or placebo supplemented with enteral and parenteral iron starting 4 days after birth.

There was no difference in the number of transfusions received by treated and control infants (4.3 ± 3.6 vs. 5.2 ± 4.2 respectively). Likewise, 118 infants with a birthweight of 1001–1250 g were similarly randomized and in this group there was no difference between treated and control infants in the number who received at least one transfusion (37% vs. 42% respectively). Hematocrits and reticulocyte counts were higher in treated infants and ferritin levels higher in controls. Therefore although r-HuEPO with iron supplementation stimulated erythropoiesis in infants weighing < 1250 g at birth, it did not impact on their transfusion requirements either by reducing the number of preterm infants who were exposed to allogeneic donor blood or the total number of transfusions required by preterm infants with a birthweight < 1000 g.[67]

Anemia during the first 2 weeks of life results predominantly from phlebotomy losses and the use of r-HuEPO during this period remains controversial. A multicentre, randomized, placebo-controlled trial investigated whether early administration reduced the total number of transfusions and in particular those required during the first 2 weeks of life; 114 preterms with a birthweight < 1250 g were randomized to receive r-HuEPO 1250 units/kg i.v. weekly or placebo from day 2 to day 14 of life. Subsequently, all patients received 750 units/kg s.c. weekly for an additional 6 weeks. All infants received oral iron 6 mg/kg daily and folic acid 2 mg daily. The early administration of r-HuEPO resulted in a higher hematocrit and reticulocyte count but this did not translate into a reduction in the total number of transfusions required during the first 2 weeks of life. A subgroup of the most severely ill infants (birthweight < 800 g and phlebotomy losses > 30 mL/kg) who received early r-HuEPO required fewer transfusions after the second week of treatment. Thrombocytosis (platelet count > 500×10^9/L) and neutropenia (neutrophil count < 1.0×10^9/L) were observed in 31% and 13% of infants respectively during treatment with r-HuEPO, but both were transient and unassociated with adverse events.[68]

Serum ferritin levels fall and red cells become hypochromic in infants who receive r-HuEPO. The optimal dose and route of iron supplementation to achieve the best response to r-HuEPO is not known or whether iron insufficiency limits the effectiveness of r-HuEPO. The American Academy of Pediatrics recommends a dose of 6 mg/kg daily,[69] but ferritin levels have fallen after even higher doses.[70] High oral doses may supply sufficient iron for erythropoiesis but storage iron may be depleted. Intravenous iron appears to maintain better serum ferritin concentrations and some have suggested that it be considered for patients with a low ferritin or those not established on enteral feeding.[71] Consideration should be given to the use of vitamin E with parenteral iron for its antioxidant properties. In a recent study, 42 preterm infants (<33 weeks and birthweight < 1500 g) received r-HuEPO 600 units/kg weekly and were randomized to receive oral ferrous lactate (12 mg/kg daily) or intravenous iron sucrose (6 mg/kg weekly). The hematocrit, reticulocyte count and number of transfusions were similar in both groups. Markedly higher ferritin levels ($P < 0.001$) were reported in the group receiving intravenous supplementation, the number of hypochromic cells was significantly greater ($P = 0.04$) in the group receiving oral supplementation, although present in both, and the mean daily weight gain greater ($P = 0.04$) in the group receiving intravenous supplementation.[71]

The aim of r-HuEPO is to reduce exposure to allogeneic blood. An alternative approach is to collect placental blood (PB), fractionate and store it in additive solutions in the same manner that would be applied to allogeneic donor blood. A recently reported study of 52 neonates showed no difference in efficacy and safety between autologous PB–RBC (red blood cell) transfusion and allogeneic RBC transfusion. All infants with a birthweight < 1000 g, but only 59% with a birthweight of 1000–2500 g and 58% of those infants who received surgery directly after delivery required allogeneic blood in addition to PB–RBCs. The mean hemoglobin increase after RBC transfusion of 10 mL/kg was 3 g/dL per kilogram of body weight following both allogeneic and PB–RBC blood; the posttransfusion fall in hemoglobin occurred faster in the PB–RBC group (0.32 vs. 0.24 g/dL daily; $P < 0.05$). The investigators concluded that preterm infants weighing less than 1000 g could not be supported by PB–RBC alone, but 40% of those with a birthweight of 1000–2500 g could be.[72]

In summary, r-HuEPO should be targeted at preterm infants for whom reducing phlebotomy losses and strict adherence to a transfusion policy cannot avert transfusion. Infants with a birthweight of less than 1000–1250 g are those with the greatest potential to benefit from r-HuEPO, because this is the group most likely to require transfusion. The evidence from controlled randomized trials is inconsistent but suggests that while r-HuEPO may reduce their total number of transfusions, it does not protect them from exposure to allogeneic donor blood. Neither does the use of autologous placental blood. Pedi-packs dedicated to one recipient continue to be important in reducing donor exposure. Further studies on the optimal dose and route of iron administration are required. r-HuEPO has the potential to reduce the risk of transfusion-related infection and appears safe but if iron supplementation is not optimal carries the risk of precipitating iron deficiency. Cost-effective use is important.

Infection

Congenital infection with cytomegalovirus, rubella, toxoplasmosis, herpes simplex and congenital syphilis often present with anemia but while this may be contributed to by marrow suppression, hemolysis generally plays a more important role. Adenovirus and particularly human parvovirus cause anemia by suppression of erythropoiesis.

Primary maternal infection with human parvovirus B19 during pregnancy can lead to intrauterine fetal infection resulting in profound anemia and nonimmune hydrops fetalis.[73] The virus infects bone marrow erythroid precursors and inhibits erythropoiesis. A retrospective review of consecutive cases of hydrops fetalis referred to a tertiary maternal fetal medicine center in the UK over a 30-month period implicated human parvovirus in 14.5% of those cases with a non-immune cause.[74] Most maternal infections with human parvovirus B19 cause no harm to the fetus and are associated with delivery of a healthy infant.[75] Fetal loss is highest when the infection occurs during the first 20 weeks of gestation.[76,77] The risk of transplacental transmission associated with primary maternal infection with human parvovirus B19 has variably been reported as 33–50%,[76,78] with a less than 5–9% risk of adverse outcome in the fetus.[76,79] Human parvovirus B19 virions can be demonstrated in the erythroid precursors of hydropic infants.

Diagnosis in the second trimester is by the ultrasound findings of a hydropic infant, the appropriate maternal serology and anemia on fetal blood sampling, if this is done prior to intrauterine transfusion, which has been used successfully to treat a number of infants with profound anemia and hydrops. Less severely affected infants who are delivered without transfusion will be anemic, reticulocytopenic and have giant pronormoblasts in their bone marrow which contain the viral particles. Viral DNA can be detected in the infant's serum and antibodies to human parvovirus B19 in maternal serum. The neonate generally requires only supportive care with red cell transfusions until the anemia resolves.

Transient pancytopenia secondary to bone marrow failure has been reported in a 5-day-old infant and attributed to echovirus type 11. Symptoms arose before 7 days of life, suggesting perinatal transmission. The infant was anemic (hemoglobin 7.1 g/dL), reticulocytopenic and had a hypocellular bone marrow. Echovirus type 11 was isolated from the infant's stool. The hemoglobin and neutrophil counts recovered but the infant received high-dose intravenous immunoglobulin for persistent thrombocytopenia.[80]

Virus-associated hemophagocytic syndrome has been reported in infants associated with Epstein–Barr virus, herpes simplex, cytomegalovirus and bacteria, and more recently following enteroviral infection.[81] The anemia is part of a pancytopenia and secondary to macrophage hemophagocytosis of red cells in the bone marrow. A previously affected sibling, a history of consanguinity and an early age at onset may suggest familial hemophagocytic lymphohistiocytosis, but both familial and sporadic forms can be associated with infection.

In infants born to mothers with HIV the perinatal prophylactic administration of zidovudine is associated with a rapidly reversible macrocytic anemia, thought secondary to marrow suppression. A placebo-controlled trial identified a significant reduction in hemoglobin concentration in newborns during the 6 weeks of treatment that normalized from 12 weeks of life onwards.[82]

Nutritional deficiencies

Hematinic deficiencies are rare in the neonatal period because the fetus is a successful parasite and unless maternal stores are extremely low will accumulate adequate stores by birth. However, the rapid growth which takes place in the neonatal period, particularly in the preterm infant, may deplete these.

Iron deficiency

Iron sufficiency is critical for rapidly developing fetal and neonatal tissue. Available iron is prioritized to hemoglobin synthesis in red cells when iron supply does not meet demands. Nonheme tissues such as skeletal muscle, heart and brain will become iron deficient before signs of iron deficiency anemia appear. Early iron deficiency appears to adversely affect cognitive development in infants, and the preterm infant may be at greater risk because of the relative immaturity and rapid growth rate of the preterm brain.[83]

Two-thirds of total body iron present in the term infant is acquired during the third trimester and the iron accumulated during fetal life is relatively independent of maternal iron stores. Iron stores are rarely depleted in the term infant before 6 months of age but this can occur earlier in the preterm infant who has a faster growth rate and less stored iron at birth. Multiple factors[83] can affect the infant's highly variable iron stores and preterm infants are more vulnerable:

- Antenatal and perinatal hemorrhage: fetomaternal hemorrhage, twin–twin transfusion, placenta previa or abruption, hemorrhage from the umbilical cord.
- Delayed clamping of the umbilical cord increases and early clamping decreases circulating hemoglobin and available iron.
- Gestational conditions: severe maternal iron deficiency, maternal hypertension with intrauterine growth retardation, maternal diabetes mellitus.
- Postnatal hemorrhage: phlebotomy losses, gastrointestinal blood loss.
- Erythropoietin without iron supplementation.

In addition to their lower iron stores and rapid growth rate with its attendant increase in blood volume and hemoglobin concentration, preterm infants are more likely to have significant phlebotomy losses and to receive r-HuEPO. r-HuEPO not only utilizes iron but if it reduces transfusion requirements, it deprives the preterm infant of a potential source of exogenous iron.

The early postnatal fall in hemoglobin concentration in the preterm infant is accompanied by an earlier (1–2 months of age) recovery of erythropoiesis. With the onset of erythropoiesis the serum ferritin level falls. Nontransfused infants who receive no iron supplementation have sufficient stores to sustain effective erythropoiesis only until they have doubled their birthweight.[84] Breast milk, cows' milk and unsupplemented formula are low in iron, although the iron in breast milk is more available. The American Academy of Pediatrics recommends iron supplementation at a dose of 2–4 mg/kg daily, up to 15 mg daily for preterm infants exclusively breast-fed, starting at 2 months of age, or when the birthweight doubles, and continued throughout the first year of life. Supplementation is not recommended for preterm infants receiving iron-fortified formula unless they are in negative iron balance or are receiving r-HuEPO. An incremented dose of iron of 6 mg/kg daily is recommended for those who receive exogenous erythropoietin or have pre-existing iron deficiency.[69] Even this dose may be inadequate to meet the iron needs of an optimal erythropoietin response.[71] Iron stores are depleted and red cells become hypochromic following r-HuEPO administration even with high-dose iron supplementation.[65,70,71] Early iron supplementation does not prevent or ameliorate physiologic anemia.

The main cause of iron loss in the preterm infant is through phlebotomy. Minimizing phlebotomy losses is important. Conservative transfusion practices with agreed transfusion thresholds are now common (see Table 7.8) and while these are to be supported, they may increase the risk of iron deficiency.

Indiscriminate iron supplementation should be avoided because of the poor antioxidant capabilities of preterm infants and the potential role of iron in several oxidant-related perinatal disorders. Preterm infants who are transfused may not need early iron supplementation. It may be important to maintain adequate vitamin E and ascorbic levels in the serum to prevent oxidative damage.

Inborn errors of iron metabolism

Iron metabolism is strictly regulated. There are relatively few genetic disorders that affect it and most are rare. Mutations in human genes regulating membrane iron transport causing simple iron deficiency have not yet been described.[85]

• *Congenital atransferrinemia.* This is a very rare autosomal recessive condition that usually presents in the first few months of life and is characterized by a virtual absence of transferrin, resulting in a severe hypochromic anemia and tissue iron overload.

• *Inherited sideroblastic anemia.* These anemias are characterized by a failure to utilize iron for heme synthesis. This results in hypochromic red cells, ineffective erythropoiesis with an increased demand for iron leading to increased iron absorption, ring sideroblasts in the bone marrow and tissue iron overload. The inheritance may be X-linked, associated with a mutation in the erythroid-specific 5-aminolevulinate synthase gene and be pyridoxine responsive or autosomal recessive and pyridoxine refractory. The latter has been described in the neonatal period.[86]

Vitamin B$_{12}$ deficiency

Vitamin B$_{12}$ deficiency with megaloblastic anemia has been reported in infants born to mothers with pernicious anemia.[87] The neonate's cobalamin level is directly related to maternal cobalamin levels and indirectly related to maternal metabolite levels of methylmalonic acid and homocysteine.[88,89] Infants of mothers with very low vitamin B$_{12}$ levels who are exclusively breast-fed are at particular risk.[90] If untreated these infants can develop neurologic problems as well as hematologic ones. Treatment is with vitamin B$_{12}$, which should be given intramuscularly if the cause is thought to be malabsorption.

Megaloblastosis associated with cobalamin C disease, a cobalamin-related metabolic disorder, has recently been reported in a 28-day-old infant.[91] The infant presented with failure to thrive, neurologic impairment, pancytopenia, megaloblastosis and hemolytic–uremic syndrome. The possibility of an underlying vitamin B$_{12}$ disorder was prompted by evidence of megaloblastic changes on the peripheral smear. Homocysteine and methylmalonic acid levels were elevated and the diagnosis confirmed by complementation studies using skin fibroblasts. Treatment was with parenteral hydroxocobalamin, carnitine and folinic acid.[91]

Folate deficiency

Folate deficiency is common in the preterm infant unless folate supplements are given. The preterm's rapid growth places it at particular risk of folate deficiency, which may be contributed to by additional factors such as infection, hemolysis, r-HuEPO administration and malabsorption secondary to diarrhea. Preterm infants routinely receive folate supplements. Rarely folate deficiency in the infant may be secondary to inherited disorders of absorption, transport and intracellular metabolism.

Management of neonatal anemia

This involves (i) identifying the cause of the anemia, (ii) preventive/prophylactic measures to lessen the anemia and/or hyperbilirubinemia and (iii) treatment which should only include red cell transfusion if absolutely indicated.

Diagnosis

The approach to diagnosis has been covered in the preceding sections and specific problems or issues related to diagnosis in the neonatal period highlighted.

Preventive/prophylactic measures

1 Routine blood sampling, the major cause of iatrogenic

blood loss, should be kept to a minimum and laboratory tests ordered judiciously.

2 Iron supplementation should adhere to the recommendation previously stated. Iron supplementation should be given to preterm infants who are exclusively breast-fed and those who receive r-HuEPO. Infants who are fed an iron-fortified formula should not receive supplemental iron unless they are in negative iron balance or are receiving r-HuEPO. Infants with chronic blood loss will also require iron supplements.

3 Preterm infants should receive folic acid supplements as should infants with hemolysis. Iron supplementation should be avoided in the latter group unless iron deficient because hemolysis increases gastrointestinal iron uptake and in this setting supplemental iron increases the risk of iron overload.

4 r-HuEPO is used for the treatment of anemia of prematurity as discussed previously. In addition, it may have a useful role in other areas such as the management of anemic babies born to Jehovah's Witnesses. R-HuEPO utilizes iron and reduces iron stores. High-dose iron supplementation should be given.

Transfusion

The decision to transfuse red cells to a neonate should not be taken lightly. There is increasing recognition of the potential hazards of transfusion, which are discussed in Chapter 33. The aim of transfusion is to ensure adequate tissue oxygenation and prevent clinically significant symptomatic anemia, but measuring these variables in neonates is difficult. Tissue oxygenation depends not only on the hemoglobin level but also on hemoglobin's ability to give up oxygen and on cardiopulmonary function. Therefore a transfusion trigger must take into account not just the hemoglobin level but the infant's clinical and physiologic state. A number of reviews and guidelines have attempted to identify transfusion thresholds but there is little evidence on which to base practice.[92,93] Table 7.8 lists possible transfusion thresholds based on consensus guidelines.[92]

Transfusion may hamper the diagnosis of certain inherited anemias, e.g., sickle cell disease, which would otherwise be identified by neonatal screening programs,[94] and diagnostic tests to identify the cause of the infant's anemia should be carried out before transfusion if at all possible.

Table 7.8 Suggested transfusion thresholds for anemic neonates.

Anemia in the first 24 hours of life	Hb 12 g/dL
Cumulative blood loss in 1 week in infant	
requiring intensive care	10% blood volume
Neonate receiving intensive care	Hb 12 g/dL
Acute blood loss	10% blood volume
Chronic oxygen dependency	Hb 11 g/dL
Late anemia, stable patient	Hb 7 g/dL

References

1. Finne PH, Halvorsen S. Regulation of erythropoiesis in the fetus and newborn. *Arch Dis Child* 1972; **47**: 683–7.
2. Matoth Y, Zaizov R, Varsano I. Postnatal changes in some red cell parameters. *Acta Paediatr Scand* 1971; **60**: 317–23.
3. Pearson HA. Life span of the fetal red blood cell. *J Pediatr* 1967; **70**: 166–71.
4. Thurlbeck SM, McIntosh N. Preterm blood counts vary with sampling site. *Arch Dis Child* 1987; **62**: 74–5.
5. Kayiran SM, Ozbek N, Turan M, Gurakan B. Significant differences between capillary and venous complete blood counts in the neonatal period. *Clin Lab Haematol* 2003; **25**: 9–16.
6. Maertzdorf WJ, Aldenhuyzen-Dorland W, Slaaf DW, Tangelder GJ, Blanco CE. Circulating blood volume in appropriate and small for gestational age full term and preterm polycythaemic infants. *Acta Paediatr Scand* 1991; **80**: 620–7.
7. Linderkamp O, Nelle M, Kraus M, Zilow EP. The effect of early and late cord-clamping on blood viscosity and other hemorheological parameters in full-term neonates. *Acta Paediatr Scand* 1992; **81**: 745–50.
8. Rabe H, Reynolds G, Diaz-Rossello J. Early versus delayed umbilical cord clamping in preterm infants. *Cochrane Database Syst Rev* 2004; (4): CD003248.
9. Wardrop CA, Holland BM. The roles and vital importance of placental blood to the newborn infant. *J Perinat Med* 1995; **23**: 139–43.
10. Hermansen MC. Nucleated red blood cells in the fetus and newborn. *Arch Dis Child* 2001; **84**: F211–F215.
11. Giacoia GP. Severe fetomaternal hemorrhage: a review. *Obstet Gynecol Surv* 1997; **52**: 372–80.
12. The estimation of fetomaternal haemorrhage. BCSH Blood Transfusion and Haematology Task Forces. *Transfus Med* 1999; **9**: 87–92.
13. Duncombe GJ, Dickinson JE, Evans SF. Perinatal characteristics and outcomes of pregnancies complicated by twin–twin transfusion syndrome. *Obstet Gynecol* 2003; **101**: 1190–6.
14. Senat MV, Deprest J, Boulvain M, Paupe A, Winer N, Ville Y. Endoscopic laser surgery versus serial amnioreduction for severe twin-to-twin transfusion syndrome. *N Engl J Med* 2004; **351**: 136–44.
15. Benirschke K. Obstetrically important lesions of the umbilical cord. *J Reprod Med* 1994; **39**: 262–72.
16. Bhide A, Thilaganathan B. Recent advances in the management of placenta previa. *Curr Opin Obstet Gynecol* 2004; **16**: 447–51.
17. Chadwick LM, Pemberton PJ, Kurinczuk JJ. Neonatal subgaleal haematoma: associated risk factors, complications and outcome. *J Paediatr Child Health* 1996; **32**: 228–32.
18. Ng PC, Siu YK, Lewindon PJ. Subaponeurotic haemorrhage in the 1990s: a 3-year surveillance. *Acta Paediatr Scand* 1995; **84**: 1065–9.
19. Pachman DJ. Massive hemorrhage in the scalp of the newborn infant: hemorrhagic caput succedaneum. *Pediatrics* 1962; **29**: 907–10.
20. Whitelaw A. Intraventricular haemorrhage and posthaemorrhagic hydrocephalus: pathogenesis, prevention and future interventions. *Semin Neonatol* 2001; **6**: 135–46.
21. Potter EL. Fetal and neonatal deaths: a statistical analysis of 2000 autopsies. *JAMA* 1940; **115**: 996–9.

22. Hui CM, Tsui KY. Splenic rupture in a newborn. *J Pediatr Surg* 2002; **37**: E3.

23. Svane S. Foetal exsanguination from hemangioendothelioma of the skin. *Acta Paediatr Scand* 1966; **55**: 536–9.

24. Golitz LE, Rudikoff J, O'Meara OP. Diffuse neonatal hemangiomatosis. *Pediatr Dermatol* 1986; **3**: 145–52.

25. Walsh SV, Cooke R, Mortimer G, Loftus BG. Massive thymic hemorrhage in a neonate: an entity revisited. *J Pediatr Surg* 1996; **31**: 1315–17.

26. Obladen M, Sachsenweger M, Stahnke M. Blood sampling in very low birth weight infants receiving different levels of intensive care. *Eur J Pediatr* 1988; **147**: 399–404.

27. Bolton-Maggs PH, Stevens RF, Dodd NJ, Lamont G, Tittensor P, King MJ. Guidelines for the diagnosis and management of hereditary spherocytosis. *Br J Haematol* 2004; **126**: 455–74.

28. Tse WT, Lux SE. Red blood cell membrane disorders. *Br J Haematol* 1999; **104**: 2–13.

29. Delhommeau F, Cynober T, Schischmanoff PO *et al*. Natural history of hereditary spherocytosis during the first year of life. *Blood* 2000; **95**: 393–7.

30. Tchernia G, Delhommeau F, Perrotta S *et al*. Recombinant erythropoietin therapy as an alternative to blood transfusions in infants with hereditary spherocytosis. *Hematol J* 2000; **1**: 146–52.

31. Mentzer WC Jr, Iarocci TA, Mohandas N *et al*. Modulation of erythrocyte membrane mechanical stability by 2,3-diphosphoglycerate in the neonatal poikilocytosis/elliptocytosis syndrome. *J Clin Invest* 1987; **79**: 943–9.

32. Dabbous IA, Bahlawan LE. Infantile pyknocytosis: a forgotten or a dead diagnosis? *J Pediatr Hematol Oncol* 2002; **24**: 507.

33. Rees DC, Portmann B, Ball C *et al*. Dehydrated hereditary stomatocytosis is associated with neonatal hepatitis. *Br J Haematol* 2004; **126**: 272–6.

34. Mehta A, Mason PJ, Vulliamy TJ. Glucose-6-phosphate dehydrogenase deficiency. *Baillières Best Pract Res Clin Haematol* 2000; **13**: 21–38.

35. Kaplan M, Renbaum P, Levy-Lahad E, Hammerman C, Lahad A, Beutler E. Gilbert syndrome and glucose-6-phosphate dehydrogenase deficiency: a dose-dependent genetic interaction crucial to neonatal hyperbilirubinemia. *Proc Natl Acad Sci USA* 1997; **94**: 12128–32.

36. Huang MJ, Kua KE, Teng HC, Tang KS, Weng HW, Huang CS. Risk factors for severe hyperbilirubinemia in neonates. *Pediatr Res* 2004; **56**: 682–9.

37. Dhillon AS, Darbyshire PJ, Williams MD, Bissenden JG. Massive acute haemolysis in neonates with glucose-6-phosphate dehydrogenase deficiency. *Arch Dis Child* 2003; **88**: F534–F536.

38. Zanella A, Bianchi P. Red cell pyruvate kinase deficiency: from genetics to clinical manifestations. *Baillières Best Pract Res Clin Haematol* 2000; **13**: 57–81.

39. Ravindranath Y, Paglia DE, Warrier I, Valentine W, Nakatani M, Brockway RA. Glucose phosphate isomerase deficiency as a cause of hydrops fetalis. *N Engl J Med* 1987; **316**: 258–61.

40. Henthorn JS, Almeida AM, Davies SC. Neonatal screening for sickle cell disorders. *Br J Haematol* 2004; **124**: 259–63.

41. Hegyi T, Delphin ES, Bank A, Polin RA, Blanc WA. Sickle cell anemia in the newborn. *Pediatrics* 1977; **60**: 213–16.

42. Bardakdjian-Michau J, Guilloud-Batailie M, Maier-Redelsperger M *et al*. Decreased morbidity in homozygous sickle cell disease detected at birth. *Hemoglobin* 2002; **26**: 211–17.

43. Vichinsky E, Hurst D, Earles A, Kleman K, Lubin B. Newborn screening for sickle cell disease: effect on mortality. *Pediatrics* 1988; **81**: 749–55.

44. Weatherall DJ. The thalassaemias. In: Stamatoyannopoulos G, Perlmutter R, Majerus PW, Varmus H (eds) *Molecular Basis of Blood Diseases*. Philadelphia: WB Saunders, 2000, pp. 183–226.

45. Dozy AM, Kan YW, Emberg SH *et al*. Alpha-globin gene organisation in blacks precludes the severe form of alpha-thalassaemia. *Nature* 1979; **280**: 605–7.

46. Thornley I, Lehmann L, Ferguson WS, Davis I, Forman EN, Guinan EC. Homozygous alpha-thalassemia treated with intrauterine transfusions and postnatal hematopoietic stem cell transplantation. *Bone Marrow Transplant* 2003; **32**: 341–2.

47. Heeney MM, Delgrosso K, Robinson R *et al*. Interpretation of fetal hemoglobin only on newborn screening for hemoglobinopathy. *J Pediatr Hematol Oncol* 2002; **24**: 499–502.

48. Kan YW, Forget BG, Nathan DG. Gamma-beta thalassemia: a cause of hemolytic disease of the newborn. *N Engl J Med* 1972; **286**: 129–34.

49. Klein JO, Remington JS. Current concepts of infections of the fetus and newborn infant. In: Remington JS, Klein JO (eds) *Infectious Diseases of the Fetus and Newborn Infant*. Philadelphia, WB Saunders, 2000, pp. 1–24.

50. Meerstadt PW. Congenital malaria. *Clin Exp Obstet Gynecol* 1986; **13**: 78–82.

51. Hall GW. Kasabach–Merritt syndrome: pathogenesis and management. *Br J Haematol* 2001; **112**: 851–62.

52. Schiff DE, Roberts WD, Willert J, Tsai HM. Thrombocytopenia and severe hyperbilirubinemia in the neonatal period secondary to congenital thrombotic thrombocytopenic purpura and ADAMTS13 deficiency. *J Pediatr Hematol Oncol* 2004; **26**: 535–8.

53. Alter BP. Inherited bone marrow failure syndromes. In: Nathan DG, Orkin SH, Look AT, Ginsburg D, (eds) *Nathan and Oski's Hematology of Infancy and Childhood* 6th edition. Philadelphia, PA: WB Saunders, 2003: pp. 280–365.

54. Saladi SM, Chattopadhyay T, Adiotomre PN. Nomimmune hydrops fetalis due to Diamond–Blackfan anemia. *Indian Pediatr* 2004; **41**: 187–8.

55. Dunbar AE III, Moore SL, Hinson RM. Fetal Diamond–Blackfan anemia associated with hydrops fetalis. *Am J Perinatol* 2003; **20**: 391–4.

56. Rogers BB, Bloom SL, Buchanan GR. Autosomal dominantly inherited Diamond–Blackfan anemia resulting in nonimmune hydrops. *Obstet Gynecol* 1997; **89**: 805–7.

57. Remacha AF, Badell I, Pujol-Moix N *et al*. Hydrops fetalis-associated congenital dyserythropoietic anemia treated with intrauterine transfusions and bone marrow transplantation. *Blood* 2002; **100**: 356–8.

58. Cantu-Rajnoldi A, Zanella A, Conter U *et al*. A severe transfusion-dependent congenital dyserythropoietic anaemia presenting as hydrops fetalis. *Br J Haematol* 1997; **96**: 530–3.

59. Shalev H, Kapelushnik J, Moser A, Dgany O, Krasnov T, Tamary H. A comprehensive study of the neonatal manifestations of congenital dyserythropoietic anemia type I. *J Pediatr Hematol Oncol* 2004; **26**: 746–8.

60. Oblender MG. Pearson syndrome presenting as non immune hydrops fetalis. *Clin Res* 1993; **41**: 803A.

61. Landmann E, Bluetters-Sawatzki R, Schindler D, Gortner L. Fanconi anemia in a neonate with pancytopenia. *J Pediatr* 2004; **145**: 125–7.

62. Emmerson AJ, Westwood NB, Rackham RA, Stern CM, Pearson TC. Erythropoietin responsive progenitors in anaemia of prematurity. *Arch Dis Child* 1991; **66** (7 special no.): 810–11.

63. Shannon KM, Naylor GS, Torkildson JC *et al.* Circulating erythroid progenitors in the anemia of prematurity. *N Engl J Med* 1987; **317**: 728–33.

64. Kling PJ, Winzerling JJ. Iron status and the treatment of the anemia of prematurity. *Clin Perinatol* 2002; **29**: 283–94.

65. Meyer MP, Meyer JH, Commerford A *et al.* Recombinant human erythropoietin in the treatment of the anemia of prematurity: results of a double-blind, placebo-controlled study. *Pediatrics* 1994; **93**: 918–23.

66. Avent M, Cory BJ, Galpin J *et al.* A comparison of high versus low dose recombinant human erythropoietin versus blood transfusion in the management of anaemia of prematurity in a developing country. *J Trop Pediatr* 2002; **48**: 227–33.

67. Ohls RK, Ehrenkranz RA, Wright LL *et al.* Effects of early erythropoietin therapy on the transfusion requirements of preterm infants below 1250 grams birth weight: a multicenter, randomized, controlled trial. *Pediatrics* 2001; **108**: 934–42.

68. Donato H, Vain N, Rendo P *et al.* Effect of early versus late administration of human recombinant erythropoietin on transfusion requirements in premature infants: results of a randomized, placebo-controlled, multicenter trial. *Pediatrics* 2000; **105**: 1066–72.

69. American Academy of Pediatrics. Nutritional needs of preterm infants. In: Kleinman RE (ed.) *Pediatric Nutrition Handbook*. Elk Grove Village, IL: American Academy of Pediatrics, 1998, pp. 55–87.

70. Bader D, Kugelman A, Maor-Rogin N *et al.* The role of high-dose oral iron supplementation during erythropoietin therapy for anemia of prematurity. *J Perinatol* 2001; **21**: 215–20.

71. Meyer MP, Haworth C, Meyer JH, Commerford A. A comparison of oral and intravenous iron supplementation in preterm infants receiving recombinant erythropoietin. *J Pediatr* 1996; **129**: 258–63.

72. Brune T, Garritsen H, Hentschel R, Louwen F, Harms E, Jorch G. Efficacy, recovery, and safety of RBCs from autologous placental blood: clinical experience in 52 newborns. *Transfusion* 2003; **43**: 1210–16.

73. Kinney JS, Anderson LJ, Farrar J *et al.* Risk of adverse outcomes of pregnancy after human parvovirus B19 infection. *J Infect Dis* 1988; **157**: 663–7.

74. Ismail KM, Martin WL, Ghosh S, Whittle MJ, Kilby MD. Etiology and outcome of hydrops fetalis. *J Matern Fetal Med* 2001; **10**: 175–81.

75. Koch WC. Fifth (human parvovirus) and sixth (herpesvirus 6) diseases. *Curr Opin Infect Dis* 2001; **14**: 343–56.

76. Public Health Laboratory Service Working Party on Fifth Disease. Prospective study of human parvovirus (B19) infection in pregnancy. *Br Med J* 1990; **300**: 1166–70.

77. Sohan K, Carroll S, Byrne D, Ashworth M, Soothill P. Parvovirus as a differential diagnosis of hydrops fetalis in the first trimester. *Fetal Diagn Ther* 2000; **15**: 234–6.

78. Koch WC, Harger JH, Barnstein B, Adler SP. Serologic and virologic evidence for frequent intrauterine transmission of human parvovirus B19 with a primary maternal infection during pregnancy. *Pediatr Infect Dis J* 1998; **17**: 489–94.

79. Brown KE. Human parvovirus B19 epidemiology and clinical manifestations. In: Anderson LJ, Young NS (eds) *Monographs in Virology: Human Parvovirus B19*. Basel: Karger, 1997, pp. 42–60.

80. Tarcan A, Ozbek N, Gurakan B. Bone marrow failure with concurrent enteroviral infection in a newborn. *Pediatr Infect Dis J* 2001; **20**: 719–21.

81. Barre V, Marret S, Mendel I, Lesesve JF, Fessard CI. Enterovirus-associated haemophagocytic syndrome in a neonate. *Acta Paediatr Scand* 1998; **87**: 469–71.

82. Le Chenadec J, Mayaux MJ, Guihenneuc-Jouyaux C, Blanche S. Perinatal antiretroviral treatment and hematopoiesis in HIV-uninfected infants. *AIDS* 2003; **17**: 2053–61.

83. Rao R, Georgieff MK. Neonatal iron nutrition. *Semin Neonatol* 2001; **6**: 425–35.

84. Ehrenkranz RA. Iron, folic acid and vitamin B12. In: Tsang RC, Luca A, Uauy R, Zlotkin S (eds) *Nutritional Needs of the Preterm Infant. Scientific Basis and Practical Guidelines*. New York: Williams & Wilkins, 1993, pp. 177–94.

85. Worwood M. Inborn errors of metabolism: iron. *Br Med Bull* 1999; **55**: 556–67.

86. Jardine PE, Cotter PD, Johnson SA *et al.* Pyridoxine-refractory congenital sideroblastic anaemia with evidence for autosomal inheritance: exclusion of linkage to ALAS2 at Xp11.21 by polymorphism analysis. *J Med Genet* 1994; **31**: 213–18.

87. Lampkin BC, Shore NA, Chadwick D. Megaloblastic anemia of infancy secondary to maternal pernicious anemia. *N Engl J Med* 1966; **274**: 1168–71.

88. Bjorke Monsen AL, Ueland PM, Vollset SE *et al.* Determinants of cobalamin status in newborns. *Pediatrics* 2001; **108**: 624–30.

89. Guerra-Shinohara EM, Paiva AA, Rondo PH, Yamasaki K, Terzi CA, D'Almeida V. Relationship between total homocysteine and folate levels in pregnant women and their newborn babies according to maternal serum levels of vitamin B12. *Br J Obstet Gynaecol* 2002; **109**: 784–91.

90. Johnson PR Jr, Roloff JS. Vitamin B12 deficiency in an infant strictly breast-fed by a mother with latent pernicious anemia. *J Pediatr* 1982; **100**: 917–19.

91. Kind T, Levy J, Lee M, Kaicker S, Nicholson JF, Kane SA. Cobalamin C disease presenting as hemolytic–uremic syndrome in the neonatal period. *J Pediatr Hematol Oncol* 2002; **24**: 327–9.

92. Gibson BE, Todd A, Roberts I *et al.* Transfusion guidelines for neonates and older children. *Br J Haematol* 2004; **124**: 433–53.

93. Murray NA, Roberts IA. Neonatal transfusion practice. *Arch Dis Child* 2004; **89**: F101–F107.

94. Reed W, Lane PA, Lorey F *et al.* Sickle-cell disease not identified by newborn screening because of prior transfusion. *J Pediatr* 2000; **136**: 248–50.

8 Immune hemolytic anemias

Bertil Glader

Introduction

Immune hemolytic anemias are a result of abnormal interactions between erythrocytes and the immune system. These occur after antibodies and/or complement components bind to red blood cell (RBC) surface antigens and thereby initiate RBC destruction via the mononuclear phagocytic system (extravascular hemolysis) or within the circulation (intravascular hemolysis).

Autoimmune hemolytic anemia (AIHA) is characterized by the production of antibodies directed against self RBC. AIHA is considered primary when hemolysis is present without other clinical problems; it is considered secondary when associated with immunologic abnormalities, infection, malignancy or administration of drugs.

Alloimmune hemolytic anemia follows exposure to RBC having nonself antigens. The resulting alloantibodies react with RBCs of the same antigenicity, but not with self RBCs. Allogeneic RBC exposure to fetal blood during pregnancy leads to hemolytic disease of the newborn. Similarly, allogeneic exposure during a blood transfusion can lead to acute or delayed hemolytic transfusion reactions.

Yet another type of immune-mediated hemolysis can occur as a result of an acquired intrinsic RBC defect that makes red cells susceptible to destruction by the normal immune system. Paroxysmal nocturnal hemoglobinuria (PNH) is an example of this type of hemolytic disorder.

This chapter reviews the mechanisms of immune hemolysis, the varied etiologies of AIHA in children, the causes and mechanisms of drug-induced immune hemolysis, the pathophysiology and clinical features of neonatal alloimmune hemolysis, and the biologic and clinical features of PNH.

Mechanisms of immune hemolysis

Factors known to determine the nature and severity of immunologically mediated RBC destruction include the following: specificity of red cell antigens; type and characteristics of anti-RBC antibodies; activation of serum complement proteins; and interaction with the mononuclear phagocytic (macrophage) system.[1]

Red blood cell antigens

The erythrocyte membrane contains structural and contractile proteins in conjunction with numerous enzymes and surface antigens. Glycophorin, an "intrinsic" membrane protein, carries the A-, B-, M- and N-specific blood group antigens, as well as receptors for viruses and other surface-reactive substances. The chemical composition of red blood antigens varies: ABO antigens are carbohydrate oligosaccharides, Rh antigens are proteins, MNS antigens are glycoproteins, and the P surface antigens are glycosphingolipids. Approximately 600 antigenic specificities have been recognized on RBCs, comprising almost 20 different blood group systems. The ABO and Rh antigens are the most important with regard to alloimmune hemolytic anemia.

ABO blood group

The ABO blood group is composed of two antigens, A and B. Two independent loci, ABO and H, are involved in determining the expression of ABO. The H gene locus, on chromosome 19, encodes a transferase that adds fucose to the terminal galactose of membrane oligosaccharides, and this structure is referred to as H substance. Group O individuals have the H antigenic determinant that is not detectable on A and B cell types. The genes for the ABO system, located on chromosome 9, encode transferases that add specific sugars to H substance, creating both A and B antigens. The ABH antigens occur frequently in other species, including bacterial flora of the gut; and this widespread occurrence probably accounts for the ubiquitous anti-A and anti-B reactivity of human sera (IgM isohemagglutinins), even in individuals never previously exposed to human blood groups through transfusion or pregnancy.

Rhesus system

The Rhesus (Rh) system is second only to the ABO blood group system in terms of clinical significance. Its importance lies in its antigenicity and the ease with which an Rh-negative person will form anti-Rh antibodies following transfusion with incompatible Rh-positive blood. In contrast to ABO antigens there are no naturally occurring antibodies to Rh antigens. Approximately 55% of incompatible blood transfusions that involve the D antigen result in the formation of anti-D, followed in frequency by Kell (approximately 20%). Whereas antibodies to ABO are predominantly of the IgM class, anti-Rh antibodies are IgG. Such antibodies can cross the placenta and thus cause significant morbidity and mortality, as in erythroblastosis fetalis (see below).

Unlike the ABO-H system, Rh blood types are restricted to the erythrocyte. This blood group is a complex system of several Rh antigens that are detected by specific antibodies. It is known that Rh blood group antigens are determined by at least two homologous but distinct membrane-associated proteins. Two of these membrane proteins have separate isoforms (C and c; E and e), which are detected by specific antibodies (anti-C and anti-c; anti-E and anti-e). The most important of the membrane Rh proteins is the D antigen. Rh-positive RBCs are those that possess this antigen. The symbol "d" (used to denote the absence of D, or Rh-negative) is not related to a specific antigen in that no anti-d serum has been identified. Rh proteins are encoded by two separate genes located on chromosome 1; they are designated Rh CcEe and Rh D.[2] The Rh CcEe gene encodes for both the C/c and E/e proteins. The Rh D gene encodes for the Rh D proteins. The Rh-negative phenotype results from deletion of the Rh D gene on both chromosomes. In most cases, the Rh-negative phenotype is also associated with Rh c and Rh e (i.e., Rh cde). The frequency of Rh negativity varies in different racial groups, ranging from a high of 30% in the Basque population to approximately 15% in Caucasians, lower in Africans (5%), and very low (<1%) in Asians. The Rh-positive phenotype may result from homozygosity (DD) or heterozygosity (Dd) for the D antigen; in Rh-positive Caucasians, approximately 44% are homozygous (DD) while 56% are heterozygous (Dd).

Immunoglobulins

All immunoglobulins have a common core structure consisting of two identical light chains (approximately 24 kDa) as well as two identical heavy chains (approximately 55 or 70 kDa). The antibody is constructed such that one light chain is attached to each heavy chain and the two heavy chains are attached to each other. The immunoglobulin heavy chains are of several types and their designation denotes the class of antibody: IgA, IgD, IgE, IgG and IgM. There are four IgG subclasses numbered according to decreasing serum concentration: IgG1 (9 mg/mL), IgG2 (3 mg/mL), IgG3 (1 mg/mL), IgG4 (0.5 mg/mL).

The ability of immunoglobulin to combine with antigen is dependent on a few amino acid residues at the end of each heavy chain, the Fab fragment, and each IgG molecule possesses two antigen-binding sites. The remainder of the antibody structure, called the Fc region because it can be crystallized, is responsible for other functions such as complement fixation and binding to Fc receptors on macrophages. The most common IgG encountered in AIHA reacts primarily at 37°C, although it may also have some reactivity at lower temperatures. A characteristic of IgG-mediated RBC destruction is the opsonization or clearance of autoantibodies via the macrophage Fc receptor located in the spleen.[3]

IgM has a pentameric structure with 10 antigen-binding sites and a molecular mass of approximately 900 kDa. IgM clearance of RBCs is characterized by efficient C1 fixation, complement binding and sequestration by the liver. Intravascular hemolysis may occur along with agglutination of RBCs secondary to the multiple binding sites on the IgM molecule. In AIHA, IgM molecules are usually temperature restricted, with optimum activity in the range 4–22°C. Thus, these molecules are termed cold reactive or cold agglutinins. The comparative features of IgG and IgM are listed in Table 8.1.

For an RBC antibody to cause agglutination, it must either overcome the net repulsive force (zeta potential) between RBCs or be structurally large enough to avoid this repellent force. IgM antibodies, because of their size, are capable of bridging this gap and causing agglutination. This is more of a problem for IgG antibodies but, depending on the density of RBC antigenic sites, this distance restriction may be overcome. For example, IgG anti-Rh antibodies do not agglutinate Rh-positive cells because there are at most 30 000 D sites per RBC. In contrast, IgG anti-A is effective at causing agglutination since there may be up to 1 000 000 A sites per RBC.

Table 8.1 General characteristics of antibodies.

	IgG	IgM
Geometric configuration	Monomer	Pentamer
Heavy chain isotype	γ	μ
Molecular mass (kDa)	150	900
Antigen-binding sites	2	10
Serum concentration (mg/dL)	1000–1500	85–205
Subclasses	IgG1, IgG2, IgG3, IgG4	None
Complement fixation	Occasionally	Yes
Fc-receptor binding	Yes	No
Agglutinates red blood cells	Rare	Yes
Crosses placenta	Yes	No

Complement system

The complement system comprises a series of plasma proteins that exist naturally in an inactive form. However, on stimulation by antigen–antibody complexes or bacterial polysaccharides they become activated, generating fragments capable of initiating and propagating immune effector functions. Two groups of proteins, the classical and alternate pathways, can trigger this proteolytic cascade.

The *classical pathway* is initiated by fixation of C1 to the Fc portion of the bound antibody (IgM or IgG) combined to a cell-surface antigen. This reaction requires two Fc complement receptor sites on an antibody molecule to be close together. Thus, the IgM molecule is efficient at C1-complement fixation when bound to the RBC membrane compared with the smaller, monomeric IgG antibody, which is a relatively poor activator of the classical complement pathway. The C1–antigen–antibody complex then initiates the activation of C4 and C2, respectively. The resultant C4b2b complex is known as C3 convertase because it catalyzes the cleavage of C3, resulting in fragments of C3a and C3b. The *alternate pathway*, which is of less significance in AIHA, leads to the same activation and cleavage of C3 but without an antigen–antibody binding requirement. Once C3b is generated, it possesses proteolytic activity that promotes cleavage of C5 into C5a and C5b. A common final effector sequence utilizing C5b though C9 leads to the generation of the membrane attack complex (MAC, C5b–9). This complex mediates cell lysis by creating pores in the antibody-coated cell membrane, increasing ionic permeability and thus causing osmotic lysis of the cell. C5 fixation is a relatively inefficient system in humans, and this inefficiency is partly explained by the existence of regulatory proteins that inactivate C3b before it can trigger C5 cleavage. These regulatory proteins have a central role in the pathophysiology of PNH-related hemolysis (see below).

Mononuclear phagocytic system

ABO-incompatible blood transfusion reactions are a consequence of circulating IgM antibodies that activate complement and thereby cause red cell lysis. This process is called intravascular hemolysis because immune-mediated destruction occurs within the circulation. In most immune hemolytic disorders, however, red cell destruction is primarily extravascular and RBCs are destroyed via phagocytosis by macrophages, particularly in the spleen and liver. This process involves binding of Fc receptors on macrophages to the Fc portion of IgG molecules attached to RBCs. Once bound, RBCs are phagocytosed and removed by macrophages. If not completely phagocytosed, partial removal of antibody–RBC membrane fragments results in a decrease in membrane surface area, and thereby spherocyte formation. These spherocytes have decreased deformability, become trapped in the reticuloendothelial system, and are subsequently removed by mononuclear phagocytes.

Immune reactions that result in C3b binding to RBCs also cause hemolysis by sequestration in the mononuclear phagocytic system. This occurs because reticuloendothelial macrophages have receptors for C3b as well as IgG. If complement components are present on RBCs, this can potentiate IgG-mediated extravascular hemolysis.

While the spleen is crucial in the clearance of IgG-sensitized cells, the Kupffer cells in the liver are capable of rapid sequestration and clearance of C3b-expressing cells sensitized by complement-binding IgM anti-RBC antibodies. Studies have shown that a greater number of IgG molecules per RBC are required for phagocytosis by the liver in a splenectomized animal.[4]

Antiglobulin test (Coombs test)

In 1945, Coombs[5] described a method to detect free (unbound) antibodies in serum, and this discovery later led to the demonstration and detection of RBCs coated *in vivo* with antibody and/or components of complement. This was a very important milestone in hematology. Prior to this there was no way to recognize antibody-coated RBCs, aside from those cases where there was visible agglutination (now known to be due to cold IgM antibodies). It was not possible to readily distinguish a common hereditary hemolytic disorder (hereditary spherocytosis) from an acquired hemolytic anaemia (AIHA) since both featured spherocytes in the peripheral blood smear. The ability to detect and characterize antibodies on RBCs has had a major impact on blood banking and on our ability to diagnose immune-mediated RBC destruction.

The antiglobulin test is used to generate visible agglutination of sensitized RBCs. The Coombs reagent for the antiglobulin test is produced by the injection of human globulin into a heterologous species, e.g., rabbit. The resultant serum antiglobulin is capable of overcoming the zeta potential to allow bridging of antibody-coated RBCs and thereby allows agglutination to occur. The direct antiglobulin test (DAT) entails mixing a subject's RBCs with polyspecific anti-human globulin that has both anti-IgG and anti-C3 activities (Fig. 8.1). If agglutination is seen with polyspecific reagents, the sample is next tested separately with specific reagents for anti-IgG or anti-C3. A positive DAT due to IgG is seen with warm autoantibodies that cause AIHA, hemolytic transfusion reactions, hemolytic disease of the newborn, some drug-induced antibodies, and following administration of various therapeutics including intravenous immunoglobulin and Rh immune globulin. A C3-positive DAT occurs with a cold IgG or IgM-mediated process, or it may occur with drug-related disorders. There is much overlap in antibody and C3 reactivity in the DAT, and sometimes both may be present. IgM autoantibodies generally detach from the RBC surface *in vivo*, so they are usually not detected in the DAT and are not present in an eluate made from a subject's RBCs.

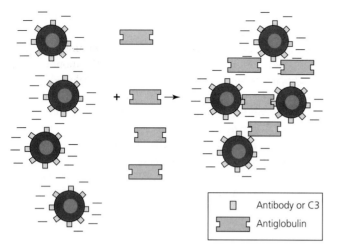

Fig. 8.1 The direct antiglobulin test entails mixing a subject's red blood cells (RBCs) with polyspecific anti-human globulin that has both anti-IgG and anti-C3 activities. The resultant serum antiglobulin is capable of overcoming the zeta potential to allow bridging of antibody-coated RBCs, and thereby allows macroscopically visible agglutination. If agglutination is seen with polyspecific reagents, the sample is next tested separately with specific reagents for anti-IgG or anti-C3.

Legend:
- Antibody or C3
- Antiglobulin

The indirect Coombs or antiglobulin test is a two-step process that identifies unbound (free) antibodies in the serum or in an eluate from RBCs that manifest positive DAT anti-IgG reactivity. This test is useful in blood-group compatibility testing and for cross-matching for transfusion. Patient serum is incubated with a panel of normal RBCs of known antigenicity. A similar approach can be used to study an eluate from RBCs known to be coated with an IgG antibody. Antiglobulin antibody is then added to the washed RBCs, and any agglutination that occurs indicates a reaction between antibody in the patient's serum or eluate and an antigen present on the RBC. By testing against a variety of RBCs with known antigenicity, the specificity of the involved antibody can be ascertained. Together with the DAT, results from serum and RBC eluate antibody studies help distinguish the different forms of AIHA.

Autoimmune hemolytic anemia: general considerations

AIHA is a result of antibodies produced against self RBC antigens. A working classification of AIHA relates to the thermal properties of the offending antibodies: warm AIHA vs. cold AIHA (Table 8.2). Cold AIHA can be further categorized into cold agglutinin disease and paroxysmal cold hemoglobinuria. Warm-reacting antibodies (usually IgG, usually polyclonal) react optimally at 37°C, whereas cold-reacting antibodies (IgG or IgM) react maximally at temperatures below 37°C. Each of the above types of AIHA exist as a primary disorder, with hemolysis being the only manifestation of disease. However, these different types of AIHA also can be associated with other underlying processes, with hemolysis being only one manifestation of the clinical condition.

The etiology of most RBC autoantibodies is not completely understood. One possibility is that autoimmune disease arises from the response to a foreign antigen when the foreign substance shows sufficient homology to a self antigen. In view of the association between AIHA and lymphoid neoplasms, as well as the concurrence with immunodeficiency syndromes and other autoimmune disorders, another possibility is that autoantibodies are a result of generalized immune system dysfunction. The immune system has several control mechanisms that regulate the balance between the need to tolerate self antigens and the need to respond appropriately to

Table 8.2 Characteristics of red cell antibodies in autoimmune hemolytic anemia (AIHA).

	Warm AIHA	Cold agglutinin disease	Paroxysmal cold hemoglobinuria
Immunoglobulin	IgG	IgM	IgG
Thermal reactivity	37°C	4°C	4°C
Fixes complement	Variable	Yes	Yes
Direct antiglobulin test			
4°C	–	–	IgG
37°C	IgG ± C3	C3	C3
Antigenic specificity	Rh	I/i	P
Site of red cell destruction	Extravascular	Extravascular Intravascular	Intravascular Extravascular
Therapy	Corticosteroids Anti-CD20 Splenectomy	Avoidance of cold Warm blood for transfusion	Avoidance of cold Warm blood for transfusion Corticosteroids

foreign antigens. Immune self-tolerance occurs centrally (in the thymus) via clonal deletion of developing lymphocyte precursors and peripherally with the elimination of leaky clones not eradicated by central tolerance. It is now known that peripheral tolerance is sustained by regulatory T cells via downregulation of both Th1 help for cell-mediated immunity and Th2 help for antibody production.[6] Regulatory T cells constitute 5–10% of CD4[+] T cells that are not Th1 or Th2; they express a unique transmembrane protein (CD25) on their surface. The antigens recognized by the T-cell receptor of these cells tend to be self peptides, and it is thought that these cells have a role in protecting against autoimmune disease. A mouse model of AIHA has been demonstrated to occur after repeated intraperitoneal injections of rat RBCs leading to the development of autoantibodies that also react with mouse RBCs. The end result is a hemolytic process similar to AIHA seen in humans.[7] Utilizing this mouse model, which produces AIHA in 30% of mice immunized to rat RBCs, it has been shown that anti-CD25 antibodies increase the development of AIHA to 90%, thus suggesting that CD25 may have a role in inducing this autoimmunity.[8]

This section focuses on the clinical and laboratory features of AIHA in children. Some of the clinical features of AIHA in children and adults are similar, but there are also significant differences. Several excellent overall reviews of AIHA are available.[9,10] Drug-induced immune hemolytic anemia is another category of hemolysis similar to AIHA and is considered separately in a later section.

Warm autoimmune hemolytic anemia

Children with AIHA are commonly seen in large pediatric medical centers. The incidence is somewhat less than that for immune thrombocytopenic purpura (ITP) but greater than that for aplastic anemia.[11] Warm autoantibodies are responsible for most cases of AIHA.[12,13] The peak incidence in children is in the first 4 years of life, often associated with viral illnesses, and is most commonly a primary disorder unrelated to any other disease process. In some children (as well as adults) warm AIHA can be associated with autoimmune conditions (systemic lupus erythematosus, rheumatoid arthritis) and immunodeficiency disorders (AIDS, hypogammaglobulinemia). Unique pediatric immune disorders associated with AIHA include Wiskott–Aldrich syndrome and autoimmune lymphoproliferative syndrome (ALPS).[14–16] In adults, but much less commonly in children, warm AIHA is secondary to lymphoid malignancies (chronic lymphocytic leukemia, lymphomas). In adults there is a female predilection for AIHA, presumably a reflection of the increased propensity for autoimmune disease in women. In children, however, no consistent difference of AIHA in boys and girls has been noted.[17–19] It is of interest that transient neonatal hemolysis due to passively acquired autoantibody can occur in infants born to mothers with AIHA.[20,21]

Clinical features

The clinical presentation and course of warm AIHA may be either mild, with symptoms attributable to a minor degree of anemia, or more complicated and severe. Children with AIHA frequently present with weakness, malaise, and fever. The symptoms may be of acute or insidious onset. Jaundice, pallor, edema, dark urine (hemoglobinuria), splenomegaly, and hepatomegaly often occur with severe hemolytic anemia. The child's presentation depends on not only the severity of the anemia but also the rapidity of onset of the hemolytic process. Additional physical findings may be present when the hemolytic process is secondary to an underlying disorder such as lupus or immunodeficiency. In cases of secondary disease, the symptoms of AIHA may precede recognition of the underlying illness by months to years but, ultimately, the signs and symptoms of the underlying disorder become manifest.

Laboratory features

Most children with AIHA are anemic at diagnosis, although the hemoglobin concentration varies considerably. It can be markedly decreased in patients with fulminant hemolysis or it may be normal in those with indolent disease. The mean corpuscular volume is usually elevated, reflecting reticulocytosis. Of note, however, reticulocytopenia can exist early in the disorder, presumably because anti-RBC antibodies also recognize an antigen present on RBC precursors, thereby resulting in intramedullary red cell destruction and "ineffective erythropoiesis".[22–24] Buchanan *et al.*[18] found that most children with moderate-to-severe anemia had inappropriately low reticulocyte counts, with 50% of patients having values of 5% or less. Bone marrow aspiration is seldom needed for diagnosis in children, but if done usually reveals normoblastic erythroid hyperplasia, even in those patients who are reticulocytopenic.[18] The peripheral blood smear manifests variable degrees of polychromatophilia, nucleated RBCs, erythrophagocytosis, and microspherocytes.

White blood cell counts may be low, normal, or elevated. Occasionally, the peripheral blood smear shows early white cell precursors (metamyelocytes, myelocytes, promyelocytes). Platelet counts are highly variable, varying from normal to elevated. Occasionally, patients may present with both immune thrombocytopenia and immune-mediated RBC hemolysis, as in Evans syndrome (see below).

Other laboratory findings include indirect hyperbilirubinemia and increased serum lactate dehydrogenase (LDH) activity as markers of increased RBC destruction. When intravascular hemolysis is severe, the released hemoglobin quickly depletes haptoglobin and produces hemoglobinemia. Because haptoglobin is an acute-phase reactant, its level may be normal or even increased if hemolysis is mild and there is adequate hepatic function. Significant hemoglobinemia that exceeds the renal reabsorptive capacity of hemoglobin leads to hemoglobinuria and the appearance of urinary hemosiderin.

A positive DAT establishes the diagnosis of AIHA. The factors that influence the risk of hemolysis are the presence of bound IgG1 and IgG3 antibodies,[25,26] the quantity of bound RBC autoantibodies and the resulting strength of the DAT.[27-29] The DAT is positive in over 95% of cases of warm AIHA, and it can be positive for IgG alone or IgG and C3.[12,13,30] Of note, the serologic pattern of the DAT at diagnosis does not help predict the clinical course in patients with warm AIHA. The vast majority of IgG autoantibodies are in the IgG1 subclass; the IgG3 subclass is the next most common, usually in combination with IgG1.[3,31] There is a small fraction of patients with a clinical picture that strongly suggests AIHA although the DAT is negative. It is thought that these DAT-negative cases may occur in patients with levels of IgG autoantibodies below the detectable threshold for the DAT or that there is an IgA autoantibody.[32-36] Warm autoantibodies are usually panagglutinins, which react with all cells on the diagnostic antibody panel and which presumably are directed at the Rh locus.[37] Other targeted antigens include membrane protein band 4.1, protein band 3, and glycophorin A.[38-41]

Treatment

Some children with warm antibody AIHA require no therapeutic intervention because of the mildness of the hemolytic process. Others, perhaps most, present emergently with severe hemolysis necessitating immediate medical management. In general, the goal of therapy is to reduce the hemolytic process to a clinically asymptomatic state with minimal medical side-effects. Close attention should always be paid to supportive care issues such as folic acid supplementation, hydration status, urine output, and cardiac status. Those cases associated with another related medical problem require that the underlying condition be managed in the hope of reducing autoantibody production. The mainstays of therapy for hemolytic anemia include steroids, RBC transfusions, and splenectomy. Other old and new pharmacologic approaches are also available. The therapies described in this section apply to warm AIHA. The similarities and differences in therapy for cold antibody AIHA are discussed in subsequent sections.

Steroids

Once anemia develops, glucocorticoids are the first line of therapy. More than three-quarters of all children with IgG autoantibodies show an initial response to high-dose steroids (prednisone 2–6 mg/kg daily). Glucocorticoids have two well-established mechanisms of action in the treatment of immune hemolysis. A rapid clinical response is attributed to the suppression of macrophage Fc and C3b receptors, with a resultant decrease in the rate of RBC phagocytosis. A reduction in hemolysis and a rise in hemoglobin level may be noticed within a few days. The second mechanism involves the suppression of antibody production and a fall in the level of circulating autoantibody. This effect will produce a delayed increase in the hemoglobin level over a period of several weeks. As hemolysis decreases (as monitored by both the hemoglobin and reticulocyte counts), doses of steroids should be tapered. If a relapse occurs, escalation to the initial therapeutic dose may be required. Risks and benefits of long-term steroid use must be weighed against changing to an alternative treatment modality. When administered in high doses or for prolonged periods, steroids have a number of well-known toxicities that include electrolyte imbalance, exacerbation of diabetes, increased appetite and weight gain, increased risk of infection, and adverse effects on growth.

Transfusions

RBC transfusions should be limited to cases of life-threatening anemia because the benefits are often transient as a result of antibody-mediated destruction of transfused cells. Donor RBCs are usually destroyed at the same rate as autologous RBCs.[42] Since warm autoantibodies in AIHA are usually panagglutinins, this invariably presents a problem when the transfusion service does the serologic work-up. An autoantibody reactive to all RBCs tested can mask an existing alloantibody by making all donor units appear cross-match incompatible, regardless of whether an alloantibody is present. The blood bank can attempt to find the least incompatible unit but the value of this in most cases is uncertain. In no case should a red cell transfusion be withheld in the presence of life-threatening anemia. Transfusions should be given slowly (5 mL/kg over 3–4 hours), especially in the setting of severe anemia. Also of concern is the risk of transfusion reaction due to the usual *in vitro* incompatibility of patient serum and donor RBCs, but in most cases this is more of a concern than a real problem.

Anti-CD20 (rituximab)

Rituximab is a chimeric human/mouse monoclonal antibody approved for the treatment of relapsed and refractory non-Hodgkin lymphoma. Since rituximab targets a pan-B-cell marker (CD20), any lymphoproliferative or immunologic disease where B cells play a pathogenic role may be amenable to treatment with this agent. Clinical studies now indicate that rituximab is effective in some patients, including children, with chronic ITP and chronic AIHA. Several reports indicate that children with refractory AIHA have durable remissions following a course of rituximab.[43-46] In one study of 15 children with refractory AIHA, 13 went into remission after two, three or four weekly doses of rituximab (375 mg/m^2 per dose).[45] Most importantly, 12 of these 13 children entering remission had not undergone splenectomy. Also, there were three relapses after several months remission, but all three of these children again remitted following a second course of rituximab.[45] These studies need further assessment but the data currently available suggest that rituximab should be added to the therapeutic armamentarium, and probably tried before splenectomy.

Splenectomy

For many years splenectomy has been the second line of treatment in patients who fail glucocorticoid therapy. However, this modality should now be considered a tertiary option, after a trial of anti-CD20 therapy (see above). Removal of the spleen theoretically has a twofold effect. First, it removes the primary site of extravascular hemolysis. Secondly, but probably less important, the spleen is also a site of antibody production. Studies indicate that splenectomy has a response rate of approximately 60–75%, but many of these patients require maintenance with lower doses of steroids, and some patients relapse months to years later. The procedure has a low morbidity and mortality rate. Due to the infection risk from encapsulated bacteria, patients should be vaccinated for pneumococcus and meningococcus, preferably before splenectomy is performed. Whenever possible, children should be over 5 years of age before splenectomy and the disease should be present for at least 6–12 months with no significant response to therapy. The decision to recommend splenectomy in patients with an underlying immunologic problem must be indiviualized for each affected patient, depending on the nature of the underlying disorder.

Other therapies

Some reports suggest that intravenous gammaglobulin is beneficial, while others show no benefit.[47–50] Most clinicians do not consider this a useful agent. Other therapies for AIHA run the gamut of those used in chronic ITP: danazol, vinca alkaloids, azathioprine, cyclophosphamide and others. In view of the greater rarity of AIHA as compared to ITP, insufficient evidence exists to be conclusive about the use of any of these. If azathioprine is used, it is necessary to continue the drug for 4–6 months before assessing that it is ineffective in decreasing autoantibody production. Plasmapheresis has shown a limited response in warm AIHA. A recent report also demonstrated effectiveness of hematopoietic stem cell tansplantation for refractory autoimmune cytopenias including AIHA.[51] Obviously this therapeutic modality should not be attempted until other interventions have failed.

Clinical course and prognosis

Many studies over the past several years allow for some generalizations about the clinical course in warm AIHA patients.[17–19,52,53] There appear to be two major groups of children with AIHA, a majority (50–70%) who have an acute course and a significant minority (30–50%) who have a more chronic course. The acute course is characterized by a sudden onset, often preceded by a viral infection, is seldom associated with underlying disorders, occurs in younger children (<4 years old), usually responds to steroids, and shows complete resolution within 3–4 months. In contrast, the chronic AIHA course is characterized by a more indolent onset, no prodromal infections, refractoriness to standard therapy, an ongoing need for other therapies such as splenectomy or other chemotherapy, frequent association with underlying medical conditions, and occurs in all ages but commonly in older children. Heisel and Ortega[19] observed an increased association of chronic AIHA with children over 12 years of age and, interestingly, also in children less than 2 years. This age distribution may reflect the early onset of congenital immune disorders in young children and the onset of autoimmune disorders in teenagers. It is intriguing that these patterns in acute and chronic AIHA are very similar to the acute and chronic pattern of ITP in children, and also parallel the major differences in childhood and adult ITP. In one study of 767 patients, 42.5% of the children had a transient acute clinical pattern of AIHA compared with only 4.5% of the adults. Also, adult AIHA is not associated with an infectious prodromal state, but there is a correlation with concurrent chronic illness. The adult mortality rate in one study was significantly higher (28.7%) than the corresponding pediatric rate (11%).[17] When mortality occurs in children with AIHA it almost always is seen in those with a chronic presentation. The cause of death is rarely from the anemia; more commonly it is a complication of therapy or the underlying medical condition. Some of the causes of death include postsplenectomy sepsis, infection in children with immunodeficiency disorders, renal failure in patients with systemic lupus erythematosus, bleeding in patients with associated thrombocytopenia (Wiscott–Aldrich syndrome, Evans syndrome), and complications from iron overload in massively transfused patients.

Evans syndrome

This disorder, first recognized over 50 years ago, is characterized by AIHA accompanied by immune thrombocytopenia. It results from the development of multiple autoantibodies targeting at least RBCs and platelets. In approximately 50% of cases, neutropenia also is present.[54] These autoantibodies are directed against specific antigens on erythrocytes and platelets and appear not to cross-react.[55,56] A variety of defects in cellular immunity have also been proposed, including decreased serum immunoglobulins, decreased T-helper (CD4) function and increased T-suppressor (CD8) cell function. Evans syndrome is a heterogeneous disorder and has been associated with many autoimmune conditions, collagen vascular disorders and malignancies.

An important recent observation is the association of Evans syndrome with ALPS.[57] The latter is a disorder of lymphocyte homeostasis, characterized by lymphoproliferation, autoimmune manifestations (AIHA, ITP), increased circulating double-negative T cells (CD3+CD4-CD8-), and impaired Fas-mediated apoptosis when studied *in vitro*.[14–16] In a study of 12 children with Evans syndrome, 7 (58%) were found to meet the diagnostic criteria for ALPS.[57] The significance of this finding is not entirely clear. It may turn out that many of the autoimmune cytopenias are variants of ALPS, and it seems reasonable to screen for double-negative T cells in children who have chronic single cytopenias such as AIHA or ITP.

If a patient has ITP and a positive DAT, even in the absence of hemolysis, Evans syndrome can be recognized at the time of identification of ITP. However, the converse is not true. The current lack of a diagnostic platelet antibody test does not allow distinction of "routine" AIHA from AIHA associated with Evans syndrome if the platelet count is normal.

The two major therapeutic regimens for autoimmune cytopenias, steroids and splenectomy, are generally not curative for Evans syndrome, and this has been a problem in long-term management of these patients. However, the drug rituximab, discussed previously for other cases of warm AIHA, has also induced sustained remissions in several patients with Evans syndrome.[45,58] This clinical observation needs to be followed, but the possibilities for successful therapy are encouraging. Also of interest, mycophenolate mofetil, a potent immunosuppressive drug used in organ transplantation, has reportedly helped the cytopenias in 12 of 13 patients with ALPS.[59] Obviously these therapeutic successes are of interest for all patients with chronic AIHA.

Cold agglutinin disease

Primary, or idiopathic, cold agglutinin disease is a chronic disease of adults over 50 years of age, associated with a monoclonal autoantibody, and characterized by chronic hemolysis and acrocyanosis when exposed to cold. This syndrome does not occur in children. However, secondary cold agglutinin disease is seen in both children and young adults, usually in association with acute infection. Cold agglutinins are IgM autoantibodies that cause clumping of erythrocytes at temperatures below 37°C, with maximal agglutination below 4°C. Clinical hemolysis in postinfectious cases is related to the normal immune response to infection. Symptoms appear 2–3 weeks after the infection starts (corresponding to the rising cold agglutinin titer) and resolve spontaneously 2–3 weeks later.

Cold agglutinins commonly are found in healthy children and adults (at titers of less than 1 : 32), but these low titers are of no clinical consequence.[60,61] In contrast, the autoantibodies in cold agglutinin hemolytic anemia are present in much higher titers (usually greater than 1 : 1000) and they also have a higher thermal amplitude, meaning that the *in vitro* temperature range at which agglutination occurs is increased. The normally occurring clinically insignificant cold agglutinins do not cause *in vitro* agglutination above 28°C, whereas

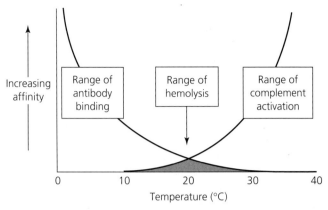

Fig. 8.2 Cold IgM autoantibodies are maximally reactive below 4°C while complement is maximally activated at 37°C. The area of overlap between these curves is the range of hemolysis. Modified with permission from Schubothe H. The cold hemagglutinin disease. *Semin Hematol* 1966; **3**: 27–47.

pathologic cold antibodies frequently continue to cause agglutination up to 37°C. Any hemagglutination seen at 37°C indicates a clinically significant cold autoantibody.

The pathophysiology of cold agglutinin disease is very temperature-dependent (Fig. 8.2). *In vivo*, pathologic cold IgM agglutinins bind erythrocytes in cooler peripheral areas of the microvasculature, such as the fingers, toes, ears, and nose. Upon return to warmer central areas of the circulation, bound IgM leads to activation of the complement pathway. In most cases C3b is deposited on the red cell membrane, but occasionally the entire complement cascade is activated to the membrane attack complex. At the same time, the higher temperatures cause dissociation of the IgM cold agglutinins, which thereby allows antibodies to bind to other RBCs in the colder peripheral circulation where the temperature may be 28–30°C. Since the complement cascade usually ends with C3b fixation, extravascular hemolysis by tissue macrophages is a major route of RBC destruction. However, when the complement cascade is completely activated, the end result is sometimes cell lysis with intravascular hemolysis.

Laboratory studies

In 1903, Landsteiner[62] noted that blood sometimes undergoes autoagglutination when chilled. It is now recognized that the presence of a cold agglutinin is often first suspected while performing a complete blood count in the clinical laboratory. RBC clumping artifactually increases the mean corpuscular volume and mean corpuscular hemoglobin concentration to very high levels, but these return to normal values after the blood is warmed.

The hemoglobin concentration in children with cold agglutinin disease is normal to mildly decreased. Reticulocyte count may be elevated. White blood cell and platelet counts are usually normal. The peripheral blood smear may show agglutination and polychromatophilia. Other laboratory findings reflecting red cell destruction include mildly elevated indirect serum bilirubin and LDH levels. Severe exacerbations can produce decreased haptoglobin, hemoglobinemia, and hemoglobinuria as markers of intravascular hemolysis.

Since cold agglutinins involve IgM autoantibodies and complement, the DAT is positive with polyspecific and anti-C3 reagents, but is negative with anti-IgG. Because the IgM autoantibodies dissociate from RBCs after C3 binding, they are not detected in the indirect antiglobulin test.

The IgM cold agglutinin is most frequently directed against the I/i erythrocyte membrane antigen group. The RBC surface densities of I/i are inversely proportional to one another. Neonatal RBCs almost exclusively express i antigen on their surface but, during infancy, antigen switching occurs and by 18 months of age I antigen is predominant. Antibody panels with adult RBCs will detect anti-I agglutinins while cord RBCs are needed to detect anti-i agglutinins. Secondary postinfectious cold agglutinins include anti-I associated with *Mycoplasma pneumoniae*, anti-i with Epstein–Barr virus (EBV), and both anti-I and anti-i with cytomegalovirus.[60,61] The majority of patients infected with *M. pneumoniae* transiently produce anti-I agglutinins, and in most cases these are not clinically significant. Similarly, the majority of anti-i cold antibodies secondary to infectious mononucleosis are benign, since up to 70% of affected patients have anti-i but less than 3% manifest any hemolysis.[63,64]

Treatment

Treatment of hemolysis associated with infection-related cold agglutinin disease is often not necessary. RBC transfusions are reserved for patients with significant hemolysis who are symptomatic. It should be noted that the presence of cold agglutinins often cause serologic difficulties during the blood bank work-up, and the blood bank may have to release least-incompatible RBC units that have a higher risk of containing an undetected alloantibody. The risk of further transfusion-related hemolysis can be reduced by using an in-line blood warmer at 37°C and by keeping the patient warm.[65]

Paroxysmal cold hemoglobinuria

In 1904, while describing an *in vitro* test to diagnose paroxysmal cold hemoglobinuria (PCH), Donath and Landsteiner first demonstrated the antibody which now carries their name.[66] The Donath–Landsteiner (DL) antibody is a biphasic, usually IgG, hemolysin that binds to erythrocytes at cooler temperatures, activates complement, and thereby causes hemolysis at warmer temperatures.[62] There are two clinical categories of PCH: a chronic form, which has been associated with late or congenital syphilis, and an acute transient form, found primarily in children. Chronic PCH is characterized

by intermittent episodes of hemolysis and hemoglobinuria occurring after cold exposure. Since the advent of antibiotic therapy, chronic PCH is now quite rare. Today, the vast majority of cases of Donath–Landsteiner hemolytic anemia occur transiently, and are found primarily in children recovering from upper respiratory infections.[67,68] The causative agent is often not identified. However several infectious agents have been implicated, including measles, mumps, EBV, cytomegalovirus, varicella zoster virus, adenovirus, influenza A, *M. pneumoniae*, *Haemophilus influenzae*, and *Escherichia coli*.

DL antibody-mediated AIHA was previously considered a rare event, but several reports investigating AIHA in children have found a relatively high incidence.[67,69,70] In a series of 42 children with AIHA, Sokol[69] found the DL antibody to have mediated 40% of cases. In another series of 68 children with AIHA, Gottsche *et al.*[70] found nearly one-third to be mediated by the DL antibody. In contrast, of 531 adults with AIHA, the DL antibody mediated none. All DL-mediated cases presented within 3 weeks of the onset of an apparent viral illness, most commonly an upper respiratory infection or enteritis. The vast majority of children diagnosed with DL-mediated AIHA have been aged 5 years or younger with no racial or gender predilection. Hemoglobinuria is the most common clinical finding, followed by jaundice and pallor. In the series reported by Sokol, hepatosplenomegaly was found in about 25% of cases.[69]

Laboratory features

Common laboratory findings include anemia with low hemoglobin levels (4–8 g/dL), and there is often reticulocytopenia early in the acute course, but this is followed by reticulocytosis. Leukopenia may also be seen early in the course but this is frequently followed by a marked leukocytosis $(10–80 \times 10^9/L)$. There are no changes in the platelet count. The peripheral blood smear may reveal normal RBC morphology, although polychromatophilia, spherocytosis, and nucleated red cells are commonly seen.[67,68] Erythrophagocytosis has also been noted, occurring much more frequently than in other cases of AIHA.[67,71] There is laboratory evidence for both intravascular and extravascular hemolysis as manifested by increased LDH, indirect bilirubinemia, decreased haptoglobin, hemoglobinemia, and hemoglobinuria.

In the acute transient form of PCH, the DL antibody is usually detectable only in the first several days after presentation.[70,71] The DL antibody binds to the erythrocyte at cold temperatures, and the binding site for this antibody is the P antigen of the erythrocyte membrane.[71] Once the DL antibody binds to the RBC, early complement components are fixed. The DL antibody has a weak binding affinity and releases at warmer temperatures; however, the early complement components remain fixed and, with warming, frequently activate the terminal complement sequence (through C8 and C9), thereby leading to intravascular hemolysis. Just as with cold aggutinin disease, cells with C3b complement coating alone are phagocytosed by the reticuloendothelial system. A small amount of weak-binding DL antibody may mediate severe RBC destruction by releasing from complement-bound cells and rebinding to new erythrocytes with the change in temperature between the peripheral and central circulation. Thus DL antibodies are very potent, and low titers can lead to severe hemolysis. However, since the period of antibody production is relatively brief, the disease usually resolves within a few weeks.[67,70]

As with cold agglutinin disease, the DAT is positive with polyspecific reagents and with anti-C3 reagents. However, with IgG-specific reagents, and at the standard temperature of 37°C, the DAT is usually negative. The indirect anti-globulin test is also negative. However, with cooling to 4°C, the DL antibody binds to the erythrocyte membrane, and the IgG DAT may become positive. Sometimes, it can be difficult to distinguish the DL antibody from a strong cold agglutinin that causes intravascular hemolysis.

The specific diagnosis of DL-mediated AIHA is confirmed by the DL antibody test. The direct DL test utilizes fresh blood from the patient to demonstrate hemolysis in auto-logous cells after incubation at 4°C followed by warming to 37°C. The indirect test utilizes the patient's serum in combination with washed group O erythrocytes, and fresh normal serum as a source of complement.[67] The cell suspensions are then incubated under three different conditions. One group of samples is incubated only at 0–4°C, a second group is incubated only at 37°C, while a third group is incubated first at 0–4°C for 30 min and then at 37°C for 60 min. The diagnosis of PCH is indicated when hemolysis is only observed in samples with patient's serum that have been incubated first at 0–4°C for 30 min and then at 37°C for 60 min.

Treatment

Since most cases of PCH are self-limited, treatment is usually symptomatic. As the DL antibody, like the cold agglutinin, binds at lower temperatures, keeping the patient warm is a mainstay of therapy. Similarly, warming of RBCs in a blood warmer prior to transfusion is important.[68] Transfusion with rare P-negative blood may be theoretically beneficial but this is not a realistic approach because of the rarity of this type of blood. High-dose intravenous immune globulin has not been shown to provide clear clinical benefit in DL antibody-mediated AIHA. Corticosteroids may depress antibody production and decrease complement receptor-mediated phagocytosis in the liver and spleen. However, since clinic-ally detectable production of the DL antibody is limited to a few days to weeks and, more importantly, because hemolysis is largely intravascular and mediated by terminal complement components, corticosteroids do not provide much clinical benefit. In cases of life-threatening PCH, plasmapheresis has proven to be helpful.[72]

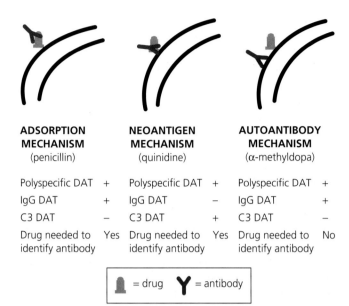

ADSORPTION MECHANISM (penicillin)		NEOANTIGEN MECHANISM (quinidine)		AUTOANTIBODY MECHANISM (α-methyldopa)	
Polyspecific DAT	+	Polyspecific DAT	+	Polyspecific DAT	+
IgG DAT	+	IgG DAT	−	IgG DAT	+
C3 DAT	−	C3 DAT	+	C3 DAT	−
Drug needed to identify antibody	Yes	Drug needed to identify antibody	Yes	Drug needed to identify antibody	No

🔋 = drug   Y = antibody

Fig. 8.3 Mechanisms of drug-induced immune hemolytic anemia, showing representative drugs and typical serologic studies. Note that drugs in the patient's serum or drug-treated red blood cells are needed to detect antibodies due to drug adsorption or neoantigen formation. DAT, direct antiglobulin test.

Drug-induced immune hemolytic anemia

For many years it has been known that drugs can cause immune hemolytic anemia. The majority of recognized cases were due to α-methyldopa and high-dose penicillin. Now-adays, the most common cause of drug-induced immune hemolytic anemia (DIIHA) is related to cephalosporins (see below).[1,73] DIIHA can result from three different types of interactions between drugs, antibodies, and RBC membrane components (Fig. 8.3).

1 *Drug adsorption mechanism.* This is seen with certain drugs, such as penicillin, that normally bind covalently to the RBC membrane. In itself, this causes no problems. However, at high doses of penicillin, antibody formation can occur, and the antibody combines with drug bound to the RBC membrane, and this can lead to red cell destruction. The IgG DAT test is positive if sufficient drug is present in the RBC membrane. In the absence of drug, the DAT is negative although antibody to drug may persist. Hemolysis occurs only when the drug is present in the blood.

2 *Neoantigen mechanism* (previously referred to as the immune complex mechanism). This occurs when the immune system perceives a drug–membrane interaction as foreign and produces antibody that binds to both the drug and components of the cell membrane. This mechanism is thought to explain quinidine-related immune hemolysis. The presence of drug or drug metabolites are necessary for antibody binding and RBC destruction. However, in contrast to the drug adsorption mechanism, the drug in the neoantigen mechanism is loosely bound and complement is also activated leading to C3 deposition. In contrast to the penicillin model, which requires high doses of drug to cause hemolysis, the neoantigen mechanism causes hemolysis with small doses of drug, and the degree of hemolysis can be quite severe. The DAT is positive for C3, but usually not IgG since the antibody is not bound to the cell.

3 *Autoantibody mechanism.* Antibody forms in response to drug, although the antibody also cross-reacts with the RBC membrane leading to DAT positivity. This type of drug-induced immune hemolysis is serologically indistinguishable from warm AIHA, and the diagnosis can only be confirmed if the patient responds to withdrawal of the drug. The DAT is positive in the absence of drug in the patient's blood sample. This type of hemolysis is seen with α-methyldopa. The DAT becomes positive in a significant fraction of patients taking α-methyldopa, but significant hemolysis occurs in only a few. These three mechanisms of DIIHA are not mutually exclusive. For example, cephalosporins are generally associated with immune hemolysis due to a drug adsorption mechanism or a neoantigen process, but they can also induce autoantibody formation.[74,75]

Over 100 different drugs have been implicated in DIIHA, although most cases are rare (Table 8.3). With the decreased use of intravenous penicillin and α-methyldopa, the incidence of drug-induced hemolysis associated with these agents has disappeared. Today, the majority of cases of DIIHA are due to second- and third-generation cephalosporins, especially cefotetan and ceftriaxone.[73,74,76,77] A report from the American Red Cross Blood Services in Los Angeles has indicated that of 119 cases of DIIHA studied over the past 26 years, 74 (83%) were due to cefotetan and 12 (10%) to ceftriaxone. Garraty[73] has summarized the published literature related to the clinical and laboratory features of DIIHA due to cefotetan and ceftriaxone.

• Cefotetan DIIHA most commonly occurs after a single dose of drug administered in conjunction with surgery. Previous exposure to drug is uncommon. Hemolysis occurs 1–13 days after receiving drug. Usually there is intravascular hemolysis with hemoglobinemia and hemoglobinuria. Hemoglobin levels are very low (mean 4.8 g/dL). Fatal hemolytic anemia and renal failure have occurred in 19% of patients. The DAT is always positive (anti-IgG 100%, anti-C3 86%) and almost all sera react with normal untreated RBCs in the presence of cefotetan.

• Ceftriaxone DIIHA is more acute and severe in children compared with adults. It occurs within a few minutes up to a mean of 6 days (children) or 9 days (adults). Fatal hemolytic anemia occurred in 6 of 9 children and 3 of 10 adults. There is usually a history of prior ceftriaxone exposure. The DAT is always positive (anti-IgG 75%, anti-C3 100%). Antibodies in sera are detected only in the presence of ceftriaxone (patient serum + drug + normal RBCs).

A positive DAT without clinical hemolysis is not an indica-

Table 8.3 Selected drugs reported to cause immune-mediated hemolytic anemia.

Amphotericin B
Ampicillin
Benzylpenicillin
Carbenicillin
Cefazolin
Cefotaxime
Cefotetan
Cefoxitin
Ceftazidime
Ceftriaxone
Cefalotin
Chlorpromazine
Cladribine
Erythromycin
Fludarabine
Furosemide
Hydralazine
Hydrochlorothiazide
Ibuprofen
Insulin
Interferon
Interleukin-2
Isoniazid
Mefloquine
Methadone
Methicillin
Methotrexate
Methyldopa
Paracetamol (acetaminophen)
Phenacetin
Phenytoin
Piperacillin
Probenecid
Procainamide
Quinidine
Ranitidine
Rifampicin
Sulfonamides
Sulindac
Tetracycline
Ticarcillin
Tolbutamide

Adapted with permission from Ref. 73.

tion for discontinuing any needed drug. In the presence of significant hemolysis, however, the suspected drug should be discontinued, particularly when other appropriate drugs are available. DIIHA usually resolves within a few days of stopping the drug. In severe cases, RBC transfusions may be given although the transfused red cells also may hemolyze at a similar rate.

Neonatal alloimmune hemolysis

Hemolysis due to alloimmune antibodies is seen with acute and delayed RBC transfusion reactions, following stem cell transplantation where there is an antigenic blood type difference between the donor and stem cell recipient, and during the neonatal period as a result of differences in maternal and fetal RBC antigens.[78] This section focuses on neonatal alloimmune hemolysis, the most common cause of hemolysis in newborn infants.

Neonatal alloimmune hemolysis is a consequence of maternal sensitization to fetal RBC antigens inherited from the father. Hemolysis occurs only in the fetus. The spectrum of clinical problems ranges from minimal hyperbilirubinemia to severe anemia with hydrops fetalis and/or kernicterus. Before effective prevention of Rh sensitization was available, hemolytic disease of the newborn was responsible for more than 10 000 deaths annually in the USA.[79] The incidence of alloimmune hemolysis nowadays is much less, but the majority of cases of serious alloimmune hemolysis are still due to Rh (D) incompatibility, although ABO maternal–fetal incompatibility is much more common. A much smaller fraction of neonatal hemolytic disease is due to sensitization to Kell, Duffy, Kidd, and other Rh antigens.

Rh hemolytic disease of the newborn

The role of Rh (D) antibody in classic erythroblastosis fetalis was first elucidated by Levine and Katzin in 1941.[80] The classification of Rh antibodies has been discussed above (see RBC antigens). The pathophysiology of alloimmune hemolysis resulting from Rh incompatibility includes the following: a Rh-negative mother, a Rh-positive fetus, leakage of fetal RBCs into the maternal circulation, and maternal sensitization to D antigen on fetal RBCs. The D antigen is the most immunogenic of the Rh antigens and there are no naturally occurring antibodies to Rh antigens. Immunization occurs almost exclusively during pregnancy. Small volumes of fetal RBCs enter the maternal circulation throughout gestation, although the major fetomaternal bleeding responsible for sensitization occurs during delivery.[81]

Rh hemolytic disease rarely ever occurrs during the first pregnancy. However, once sensitization occurs, reexposure to Rh (D) RBCs in subsequent pregnancies leads to an anamnestic response, with an increase in the maternal anti-D titer and an increased incidence of affected infants. In North America and Europe, significant hemolysis occurring in the first pregnancy is nowadays due to maternal exposure to Rh-positive RBCs from an earlier transfusion, fetal bleeding associated with a previous spontaneous or therapeutic abortion, ectopic pregnancy, or fetal bleeding associated with amniocentesis.

Prevention of Rh immunization in the mother

The major factor responsible for the reduced death rate has been development of Rh immune globulin to prevent maternal sensitization. Important early observations were that fetomaternal RBC transfer (and thereby sensitization) primarily occurred during delivery and that the frequency of Rh immune hemolytic disease was much lower in ABO-incompatible pregnancies (maternal RBC type O, fetal RBC type A or B). The apparent beneficial effect of ABO incompatibility was due to the fact that maternal anti-A and anti-B antibodies recognize the corresponding A and B fetal RBCs, leading to their destruction before sensitization could occur. As a result of these early observations, it became standard practice for unsensitized Rh-negative mothers to receive a single intramuscular dose of Rh immune globulin (300 µg) within 72 hours of delivering of a Rh-positive infant.[79] The anti-D immune globulin attaches to fetal Rh-positive RBCs in the maternal circulation, thereby leading to their rapid removal and preventing sensitization. The results of this therapy were remarkable, with the virtual elimination of Rh (D) sensitization as a major cause of hemolytic disease in newborns. However, because Rh immunoprophylaxis is not universally available, maternal sensitization still occurs in some developing countries due to failure to receive initial anti-D prophylaxis.

The current standard of practice is to administer a full dose of Rh immune globulin to all unsensitized Rh-negative women at 28 weeks' gestation, with an additional dose given at birth if the infant is Rh positive. Moreover, the dose of Rh immune globulin should be increased proportionally when there is evidence of larger than normal fetomaternal bleeding at delivery. All newborns should be screened using the rosette test to screen for fetal RBCs.[82] Positive results should be followed by a quantitative test such as the Kleihower–Betke stain.[83] In suspicious cases (e.g., placental abruption, neonatal anemia), the volume of fetal hemorrhage can be quantified using the Kleihauer–Betke procedure. Rh immune globulin also should be administered to unsensitized Rh-negative women after any event known to be associated with increased risk of fetomaternal hemorrhage (e.g., spontaneous or therapeutic abortion, amniocentesis, chorionic villus biopsy). The risk of anti-Rh sensitization ranges from 0.6 to 5.4% when nonsensitized Rh-negative women undergo amniocentesis.[84]

Prenatal management of the Rh-sensitized pregnancy

In utero, varying degrees of fetal hemolysis can occur, thereby leading to anemia, hepatosplenomegaly, and increased bilirubin formation. Bilirubin in the fetus is removed by the placenta into the maternal circulation, and thus hyperbilirubinemia is not a problem until after delivery. The major threat to the fetus is hydrops fetalis, and this can occur as early as 20–22 weeks' gestation. Hydrops fetalis is partly due to high-output cardiac failure secondary to severe anemia. Low colloid osmotic pressure resulting from hypoalbuminemia, a consequence of hepatic dysfunction, and a capillary leak syndrome secondary to tissue hypoxia also contribute to the edema of hydrops. The major focus of maternal and fetal prenatal management is to prevent severe anemia, hydrops and intrauterine death.

Maternal IgG anti-D titers should be determined at 12–16 weeks' gestation (first prenatal visit) and then at 28–32 weeks and 36 weeks in the completely asymptomatic case with no evident risk other than being Rh negative. Significant hemolytic disease may be indicated by the presence of measurable titers at the beginning of the pregnancy, a rapid rise in the titer, or a titer $\geq 1 : 64$. A history of a previously affected infant suggests a very high likelihood for similar or greater morbidity in association with subsequent Rh-positive pregnancies unless the fetus can be shown to be Rh negative.

Fetal assessment may be obtained through ultrasound, amniocentesis, and percutaneous umbilical blood sampling (PUBS). The development of high-resolution ultrasound has been a major advance that facilitates detection of early hydrops. Evaluation of skin and scalp edema, cardiac and pleural effusions as well as hepatosplenomegaly, ascites and placental thickening are used to assess the severity of the immune destructive process. Amniocentesis provides a means of evaluating hemolysis though spectrophotometric analysis of bilirubin content in amniotic fluid (ΔOD_{450}). Indications for amniocentesis include a maternal IgG anti-D titer of $\geq 1 : 16$ or ultrasonographic evidence of hydrops. Amniocentesis may be performed as early as 14–16 weeks' gestation. If testing or history indicate a high likelihood of fetal anemia with risk of death, ultrasound-guided PUBS can be performed to determine the fetal hemoglobin. Fetal hydrops does not occur until the hemoglobin concentration of the fetus decreases below 4 g/dL (or hematocrit below approximately 15%).

In the past, at-risk fetuses older than 32 weeks' gestation with evidence of mature lung function were delivered early. However, for those fetuses of less than 32 weeks' gestation with immature lung function, early delivery was not possible and fetal RBC transfusions were given. Initially, intrauterine RBC transfusions were administered through the peritoneal cavity, and this procedure ameliorated the anemia sufficiently to save many otherwise doomed fetuses.[85] However, the success rate with intrauterine RBC transfusions was much lower in some cases where hydrops was already present. This lack of response in some hydropic fetuses occurred because RBC absorption from the peritoneal cavity (complicated by ascites) was too slow to reverse the effects of severe anemia and hypoxia. Subsequently, the advent of ultrasound and PUBS has facilitated direct intravascular RBC transfusion to correct life-threatening anemia, with the reversal of established hydrops in most cases.[86,87] Both simple transfusions and exchange transfusions have been performed in

a number of fetuses.[88] Most perinatologists prefer simple RBC transfusion because of its shorter duration, aiming for a posttransfusion hematocrit no greater than 45% to avert circulatory overload.[89]

Diagnosis and management of Rh hemolytic disease in the neonate

Immediately following delivery of all infants born to a Rh-negative mother, blood should be evaluated for a direct Coombs test, ABO and Rh antigen screens, as well as hemoglobin concentration and reticulocyte count. If the Coombs test is positive, further evaluation is indicated to determine specific antibody identity and to prevent any delay in obtaining compatible blood should exchange or straight transfusion be necessary.

Mild hemolytic disease is most common, manifested by a positive DAT with minimal hemolysis, little or no anemia (cord blood hemoglobin > 14 g/dL), and minimal hyperbilirubinemia (cord blood bilirubin < 4 mg/dL). Aside from early phototherapy, these newborns generally require no therapy unless the postnatal rate of rise in bilirubin is greater than expected. Infants who do not become sufficiently jaundiced to require exchange transfusion are at risk of development of severe late anemia associated with a low reticulocyte count, usually at 3–6 weeks of age; thus, it is important to closely monitor hemoglobin levels after hospital discharge.

Moderate hemolytic disease is found in a smaller fraction of affected infants. This is characterized by hemolysis, moderate anemia (cord blood hemoglobin < 14 g/dL), and increased cord blood bilirubin levels (>4 mg/dL). The peripheral blood may reveal numerous nucleated RBCs, decreased numbers of platelets, and occasionally a leukemoid reaction with large numbers of immature granulocytes. The cause of thrombocytopenia is not understood, but it is unlikely to be an immune reaction because platelets lack Rh antigens. Similarly, the cause of the leukemoid reaction is not defined, although rarely it may be confused with congenital leukemia. Infants with Rh disease may also exhibit marked hepatosplenomegaly, a consequence of extramedullary hematopoiesis and sequestration of antibody-coated RBCs. The risk of development of bilirubin encephalopathy is high if these neonates do not receive treatment. Thus, early exchange transfusion with type-O Rh-negative fresh RBCs is usually necessary, in conjunction with intensive phototherapy. This approach has been responsible for the favorable outcome of most infants with moderate alloimmune hemolysis. It is common for newborns who receive an exchange transfusion to demonstrate a lower than normal hemoglobin concentration at the nadir of their "physiologic" anemia. In part this may be due to persistence of some anti-D antibody and destruction of the patient's own Rh (D)-positive RBCs. Therefore, follow-up of hemoglobin determinations for at least 2 months is important.

Table 8.4 Clinical and laboratory features of immune hemolysis due to Rh disease and ABO incompatibility.

	Rh disease	ABO incompatibility
Clinical features		
Frequency	Unusual	Common
Pallor	Marked	Minimal
Jaundice	Marked	Minimal to moderate
Hydrops	Common	Rare
Hepatosplenomegaly	Marked	Minimal
Laboratory features		
Blood type		
Mother	Rh (−)	O
Infant	Rh (+)	A or B
Anemia	Marked	Minimal
Direct Coombs test	Positive	Frequently negative
Indirect Coombs test	Positive	Usually positive
Hyperbilirubinemia	Marked	Variable
Red cell morphology	Nucleated cells	Spherocytes

ABO incompatibility

Hemolysis associated with ABO incompatibility is similar to Rh hemolytic disease in that maternal anti-A or anti-B antibodies enter the fetal circulation and react with A or B antigens on the erythrocyte surface (Table 8.4). In type A and B individuals, naturally occurring anti-B and anti-A isoantibodies are largely IgM molecules that do not cross the placenta. In contrast, the alloantibodies present in type O individuals are predominantly IgG molecules.[90] For this reason, ABO incompatibility is largely limited to type O mothers with type A or B fetuses. The presence of IgG anti-A or anti-B antibodies in type O mothers also explains why hemolysis caused by ABO incompatibility frequently occurs during the first pregnancy without prior "sensitization". ABO incompatibility is present in approximately 12% of pregnancies, although evidence of fetal RBC sensitization (i.e., positive DAT) is found in only 3% of births, and less than 1% of live births are associated with hemolysis.[81] The relative mildness of neonatal ABO hemolytic disease contrasts sharply with the findings in Rh incompatibility. In large part, this is because the A and B antigens are present in many tissues besides RBCs. Consequently, of the anti-A or anti-B antibodies that cross the placenta, only a small fraction actually bind to erythrocytes, the remainder being absorbed by other tissues.

Although hemolytic disease resulting from ABO incompatibility is milder than that resulting from Rh disease, severe hemolysis occasionally occurs, and hydrops fetalis has been reported. In these more severe cases it is essential to exclude other antibodies, as well as nonimmune causes of hemolysis such as glucose 6-phosphate dehydrogenase deficiency or hereditary spherocytosis (HS). In most cases, pallor and jaundice are minimal. Hepatosplenomegaly is uncommon. Laboratory features include minimal to moderate hyperbilirubinemia and, occasionally, some degree of anemia. The DAT is frequently negative, although the indirect antiglobulin test (neonatal serum plus adult A or B RBCs) is more commonly positive. This paradox is related to the fact that fetal RBCs, compared with adult erythrocytes, have less type-specific antigen on their surface.[91]

The peripheral blood smear in ABO incompatability is characterized by marked spherocytosis, and sometimes this can present a problem in distinguishing ABO incompatibility from HS. This is particularly true in those cases of ABO incompatability with a negative DAT. The osmotic fragility is abnormal in both and will not distinguish the two causes of spherocytosis. However, this is not an important clinical issue since the most important therapy for neonatal hemolysis should focus on controlling hyperbilirubinemia, and this is true for both HS and ABO incompatibility. Specific differentiation of ABO incompatability from HS can wait a few weeks to months; the former will disappear, while HS will persist.

Hemolysis in ABO incompatibility is usually mild, presenting with some degree of hyperbilirubinemia. Of major concern is that some infants with ABO incompatibility may be discharged home from medical establishments before significant clinical jaundice is evident. It is critical that infants with ABO incompatibility be monitored closely for evolving jaundice and hyperbilirubinemia in the first few days of life. In most cases hyperbilirubinemia is readily controlled by phototherapy.[92] When hyperbilirubinemia is more severe, exchange transfusion is necessary using group O Rh-compatible RBCs. Additional follow-up at 2–3 weeks of age to check for anemia in these infants is essential.

Minor blood group incompatibility

With the sharp decline of hemolytic disease due to Rh incompatibility, the proportion of cases caused by Rh c, Rh E, Kell, Duff, and Kidd incompatibility has increased from the previous estimate of 1–3% to as high as 20% (for Kell sensitization). The pathophysiology of these disorders is similar to that of Rh and ABO incompatibility. The infrequency of minor group incompatibility is primarily a reflection of the lower antigenicity of these RBC antigens. Diagnosis of minor group incompatibility is suggested by hemolytic anemia with a positive DAT in the absence of ABO or Rh incompatibility and with a negative maternal DAT. Definitive diagnosis requires identification of the specific antibody in neonatal serum or an eluate from neonatal RBCs. This is readily accomplished by testing maternal serum against a variety of known RBC antigens. With some antibodies such as Kell, antibody titer and amniocentesis findings may underestimate the severity of fetal hemolysis. Therefore, frequent ultrasound monitoring

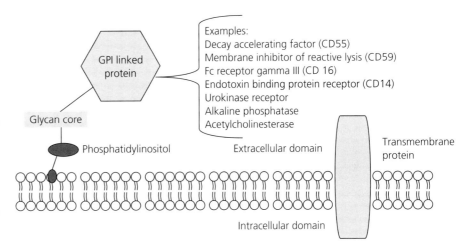

Fig. 8.4 The glycophosphatidilinositol (GPI) anchor for attachment of proteins to the cell membrane. The anchor is composed of a glycan core and phosphatidylinositol in the outer face of the lipid bilayer. This GPI structure covalently binds and anchors many proteins to the cell surface. In contrast to surface proteins that use the GPI anchor, transmembrane proteins span the entire bilayer and have extracellular, transmembrane, and intracellular domains. Some examples of GPI-linked proteins are shown.

may be necessary, with fetal blood sampling being done in worrisome cases. Fetal blood sampling is also useful in determining whether the fetus of a heterozygous father has inherited the offending RBC antigen. This identifies those fetuses that need further serial evaluations.

Paroxysmal nocturnal hemoglobinuria

PNH is a disorder characterized by intermittent episodes of intravascular hemolysis and hemoglobinuria. It is due to an acquired stem cell defect that renders RBCs susceptible to complement-mediated lysis.[93–96] In addition to hemolysis, venous thrombosis and bone marrow failure are features of this condition. PNH occurs primarily in adults, although occasionally it is recognized in children and adolescents.

In 1937, Thomas Hale Ham made the observation that red cells from patients with PNH were susceptible to lysis in an acidic environment, and this became the basis for the first laboratory test (Ham's test) to diagnose this disorder.[97,98] The reason for this complement sensitivity is that PNH red cells lack two membrane proteins that normally inhibit complement activation and thereby defend against the C5b–C9 MAC and resultant pore formation. One of these proteins is CD55 (decay-accelerating factor or DAF), which binds C3b and thereby prevents C5 cleavage and formation of the MAC. The other is CD59 (membrane inhibitor of reactive lysis or MIRL), which inhibits the insertion of C9 into the membrane.[99–101] Both of these proteins normally attach to the cell membrane via glycosylphosphatidylinositol (GPI), a cell membrane complex of a glycan core and phosphatidylinositol in the outer face of the lipid bilayer (Fig. 8.4). This GPI structure covalently binds and anchors many proteins to the cell surface.[102]

It is now known that PNH is due to an acquired mutation of the phosphatidylinositol glycan class A gene (*PIG-A*) in pluripotent hemopoietic stem cells. *PIG-A* encodes for a glycosyltransferase required for the synthesis of GPI.[103,104] The mutant stem cell has the capacity to form a hematopoietic clone of cells that are deficient in those proteins normally attached to the cell via the PGI anchor.[103,104] All marrow-derived cells (erythrocytes, granulocytes, platelets, and monocytes) are GPI deficient to varying degrees, thus supporting the concept that PNH is a clonal stem cell disorder. Study of glucose 6-phosphate dehydrogenase isozymes further supports the clonal basis of this condition.[105] Almost 200 different mutations in the *PIG-A* gene have been identified, some leading to complete inactivation of protein, other to partial inactivation. The abnormal PNH clone may be relatively small, affecting only a few percent of circulating erythrocytes and granulocytes or it may become dominant where almost all circulating cells are GPI deficient. Mature blood cells derived from this mutant hematopoietic clone can have a complete deficiency (type III) or partial deficiency (type II) of GPI proteins. In addition, patients with PNH have some cells with normal expression of GPI proteins (previously referred to as type I PNH cells).[106]

Clinical features

The classical hemolytic presentation of this disorder was first described more than 100 years ago, depicted as a paroxysmal hemolytic process that was often more frequent at night, associated with hemoglobinuria and abdominal and back pain. The reason why hemoglobinuria occurs in the morning is not known for sure. One consideration is that the pH is slightly lower during sleep, thereby facilitating complement activation and hemolysis. In practice, many patients have dark urine throughout the day whereas others never develop this symptom. In most cases hemolytic episodes occur every few weeks, although some patients have chronic unrelenting hemolysis with severe anemia. Occasionally, infection may trigger hemolysis, although often there is no identifiable reason. A common problem resulting from chronic intravascular hemolysis is iron deficiency, which occurs secondary to hemoglobinuria.

Another severe clinical complication of PNH is venous thrombosis; these thrombi occur in unusual locations, such as the hepatic, portal and mesenteric veins. The complications of venous thrombosis are often fatal, because the hypercoagulability observed in PNH is very difficult to treat even with aggressive anticoagulation. The cause of the hypercoagulable state in PNH is not well established. PNH platelets lack the GPI-linked complement regulatory proteins CD55 and CD59 and complement activation leads to platelet membrane vesiculation and the release of microparticles with procoagulant properties.[107] The levels of natural plasma anticoagulants (protein C, protein S, antithrombin III) are normal in PNH patients.[108]

Defective hematopoiesis is seen in many patients with PNH, either at presentation or during the course of the disease. The cause of this impaired hematopoiesis is not well understood, and it is not known whether GPI-linked surface proteins have a role in normal hematopoiesis. PNH can evolve into myelodysplasia or, less commonly, acute non-lymphoblastic leukemia.[109] However, a particularly interesting association exists between PNH and aplastic anemia in that one often evolves into the other.[110] The basis for this relationship between aplasia and PNH is not entirely clear. A commonly held view is that aplastic anemia is the result of an immunologic attack on hematopoietic stem cells.[111] Moreover, many patients with severe aplastic anemia have PNH cells at diagnosis, and the number of these cells often increases during the course of disease.[111,112] An interesting hypothesis that relates PNH and aplastic anemia is that the immunologic assault on stem cells may be mediated via GPI-anchored proteins. As a consequence, the PNH clone might be protected from immunologic destruction, thus giving them an apparent growth advantage over normal hematopoietic stem cells.[111,113]

Although primarily a disease of adults, PNH definitely occurs in children and adolescents, and the diagnosis should be considered for any child with unexplained cytopenia or thrombosis. In a report of 26 young patients with PNH, Ware et al.[114] noted the differences in clinical features compared with PNH in adults. Very few children had dark urine as a presenting symptom, and clinically obvious hemoglobinuria occurred in only 65% of children. Thrombosis occurred in approximately one-third of patients, and some died of this dreaded complication. All patients had laboratory evidence of defective or ineffective hematopoiesis, either at diagnosis or over the course of their disease. In a recent study of childhood PNH in the Netherlands, the vast majority presented with aplastic anemia or myelodysplasia.[115] No child presented with nocturnal hemoglobinuria.

Diagnosis

The original laboratory tests used to diagnose PNH were designed to show increased sensitivity of RBCs to complement lysis. However, both the acid hemolysis (Ham test) and the sugar-water test are now of historical interest only, having been replaced by flow cytometry detection of GPI-linked proteins. Peripheral blood erythrocytes and granulocytes can be analyzed by flow cytometry for surface expression of GPI-linked proteins such as CD16, CD48, CD55, or CD59.[116,117]

Treatment

Goals of therapy include pharmacologic methods of limiting hemolysis, red cell transfusions, treating and preventing iron deficiency or overload; the treatment and prevention of venous thrombosis; and attempts to replace abnormal stem cells through stem cell transplantation.

RBC transfusions are given to symptomatic anemic patients. Iron losses usually cannot be replenished simply from dietary sources and supplemental iron therapy is often necessary. There is a theoretical concern that iron supplementation in the iron-deficient patient can result in a burst of erythropoiesis and an increase in the number of PNH cells in the circulation, with subsequent exacerbation of hemolysis of the newly formed cells. This possible complication should be appreciated, but it should not prevent the patient from receiving iron therapy.

Therapy with oral corticosteroids (prednisone 1–2 mg/kg daily) can ameliorate hemolysis and is often recommended for 24–72 hours around the time of a hemolytic episode. A recent report suggested good results with eculizumab, a humanized monoclonal antibody that binds to C5, inhibiting its cleavage into C5a and C5b, thereby preventing the formation the C5b–9 complex. When given to transfusion-dependent PNH patients, hemolysis was decreased as manifested by a reduced serum LDH concentration, decreased transfusion requirements (with some patients becoming free of any transfusion need), and reduced hemoglobinuria in almost all patients.[118]

An ideal treatment for a disorder due to a stem cell mutation is the replacement of such progenitor cells with donor unaffected stem cells. Because stem cell transplantation can be curative therapy for PNH, it should be considered for selected patients if an HLA-matched donor is available.[119–121] Both related and unrelated matched donors have been used.

References

1. Petz LD, Garratty G. *Immune Hemolytic Anemias*, 2nd edn. Philadelphia: Churchill Livingstone, 2004.
2. Mouro I, Colin Y, Cherif-Zahar B, Cartron JP, Le Van Kim C. Molecular genetic basis of the human Rhesus blood group system. *Nat Genet* 1993; **5**: 62–5.
3. Engelfriet CP, Overbeeke MA, von dem Borne AE. Autoimmune hemolytic anemia. *Semin Hematol* 1992; **29**: 3–12.
4. Schreiber AD, Frank MM. Role of antibody and complement in the immune clearance and destruction of erythrocytes. II.

Molecular nature of IgG and IgM complement-fixing sites and effects of their interaction with serum. *J Clin Invest* 1972; **51**: 583–9.

5. Coombs. A new test for the detection of weak and "incomplete" Rh agglutinins. *Br J Exp Pathol* 1945; **26**: 255–66.

6. Sakaguchi S. Naturally arising CD4+ regulatory T cells for immunologic self-tolerance and negative control of immune responses. *Annu Rev Immunol* 2004; **22**: 531–62.

7. Playfair JH, Marshall-Clarke S. Induction of red cell autoantibodies in normal mice. *Nature New Biol* 1973; **243**: 213–14.

8. Mqadmi A, Zheng X, Yazdanbakhsh K. CD4+CD25+ regulatory T cells control induction of autoimmune hemolytic anemia. *Blood* 2005; **105**: 3746–8.

9. Dacie SJ. The immune haemolytic anaemias: a century of exciting progress in understanding. *Br J Haematol* 2001; **114**: 770–85.

10. Gehrs BC, Friedberg RC. Autoimmune hemolytic anemia. *Am J Hematol* 2002; **69**: 258–71.

11. Ware R. *Autoimmune Hemolytic Anemia*. Philadelphia: WB Saunders, 2003.

12. Sokol RJ, Hewitt S, Stamps BK. Autoimmune haemolysis: an 18-year study of 865 cases referred to a regional transfusion centre. *Br Med J* 1981; **282**: 2023–7.

13. Petz LD. Review: evaluation of patients with immune hemolysis. *Immunohematol* 2004; **20**: 167–76.

14. Drappa J, Vaishnaw AK, Sullivan KE, Chu JL, Elkon KB. Fas gene mutations in the Canale–Smith syndrome, an inherited lymphoproliferative disorder associated with autoimmunity. *N Engl J Med* 1996; **335**: 1643–9.

15. Sneller MC, Wang J, Dale JK *et al.* Clincial, immunologic, and genetic features of an autoimmune lymphoproliferative syndrome associated with abnormal lymphocyte apoptosis. *Blood* 1997; **89**: 1341–8.

16. Straus SE, Sneller M, Lenardo MJ, Puck JM, Strober W. An inherited disorder of lymphocyte apoptosis: the autoimmune lymphoproliferative syndrome. *Ann Intern Med* 1999; **130**: 591–601.

17. Habibi B, Homberg JC, Schaison G, Salmon C. Autoimmune hemolytic anemia in children. A review of 80 cases. *Am J Med* 1974; **56**: 61–9.

18. Buchanan GR, Boxer LA, Nathan DG. The acute and transient nature of idiopathic immune hemolytic anemia in childhood. *J Pediatr* 1976; **88**: 780–3.

19. Heisel MA, Ortega JA. Factors influencing prognosis in childhood autoimmune hemolytic anemia. *Am J Pediatr Hematol Oncol* 1983; **5**: 147–52.

20. Yam P, Wilkinson L, Petz LD, Garratty G. Studies on hemolytic anemia in pregnancy with evidence for autoimmunization in a patient with a negative direct antiglobulin (Coombs') test. *Am J Hematol* 1980; **8**: 23–9.

21. Burt RL, Prichard RW. Acquired hemolytic anemia in pregnancy: report of a case. *Obstet Gynecol* 1957; **10**: 444–50.

22. Conley CL, Lippman SM, Ness PM, Petz LD, Branch DR, Gallagher MT. Autoimmune hemolytic anemia with reticulocytopenia and erythroid marrow. *N Engl J Med* 1982; **306**: 281–6.

23. Greenberg J, Curtis-Cohen M, Gill FM, Cohen A. Prolonged reticulocytopenia in autoimmune hemolytic anemia of childhood. *J Pediatr* 1980; **97**: 784–6.

24. Liesveld JL, Rowe JM, Lichtman MA. Variability of the erythropoietic response in autoimmune hemolytic anemia: analysis of 109 cases. *Blood* 1987; **69**: 820–6.

25. Ravetch JV, Kinet JP. Fc receptors. *Annu Rev Immunol* 1991; **9**: 457–92.

26. LoBuglio AF, Cotran RS, Jandl JH. Red cells coated with immunoglobulin G: binding and sphering by mononuclear cells in man. *Science* 1967; **158**: 1582–5.

27. Garratty G, Nance SJ. Correlation between in vivo hemolysis and the amount of red cell-bound IgG measured by flow cytometry. *Transfusion* 1990; **30**: 617–21.

28. Lalezari P. Serologic profile in autoimmune hemolytic disease: pathophysiologic and clinical interpretations. *Semin Hematol* 1976; **13**: 291–310.

29. Dubarry M, Charron C, Habibi B, Bretagne Y, Lambin P. Quantitation of immunoglobulin classes and subclasses of autoantibodies bound to red cells in patients with and without hemolysis. *Transfusion* 1993; **33**: 466–71.

30. Chaplin H Jr. Clinical usefulness of specific antiglobulin reagents in autoimmune hemolytic anemias. *Prog Hematol* 1973; **8**: 25–49.

31. Garratty G. Factors affecting the pathogenicity of red cell auto and alloantibodies. *American Association of Blood Banks* 1989: 109.

32. Sokol RJ, Hewitt S, Booker DJ, Stamps R. Small quantities of erythrocyte bound immunoglobulins and autoimmune haemolysis. *J Clin Pathol* 1987; **40**: 254–7.

33. Schmitz N, Djibey I, Kretschmer V, Mahn I, Mueller-Eckhardt C. Assessment of red cell autoantibodies in autoimmune hemolytic anemia of warm type by a radioactive anti-IgG test. *Vox Sang* 1981; **41**: 224–30.

34. Sturgeon P, Smith LE, Chun HM, Hurvitz CH, Garratty G, Goldfinger D. Autoimmune hemolytic anemia associated exclusively with IgA of Rh specificity. *Transfusion* 1979; **19**: 324–8.

35. Reusser P, Osterwalder B, Burri H, Speck B. Autoimmune hemolytic anemia associated with IgA: diagnostic and therapeutic aspects in a case with long-term follow-up. *Acta Haematol* 1987; **77**: 53–6.

36. Salama A, Mueller-Eckhardt C. Autoimmune haemolytic anaemia in childhood associated with non-complement binding IgM autoantibodies. *Br J Haematol* 1987; **65**: 67–71.

37. Dacie JV, Cutbush M. Specificity of auto-antibodies in acquired haemolytic anaemia. *J Clin Pathol* 1954; **7**: 18–21.

38. Vos GH, Petz LD, Garratty G, Fudenberg HH. Autoantibodies in acquired hemolytic anemia with special reference to the LW system. *Blood* 1973; **42**: 445–53.

39. Wakui H, Imai H, Kobayashi R *et al.* Autoantibody against erythrocyte protein 4.1 in a patient with autoimmune hemolytic anemia. *Blood* 1988; **72**: 408–12.

40. Victoria EJ, Pierce SW, Branks MJ, Masouredis SP. IgG red blood cell autoantibodies in autoimmune hemolytic anemia bind to epitope on red blood cell membrane band 3 glycoprotein. *J Lab Clin Med* 1990; **115**: 74–88.

41. Leddy JP, Falany JL, Kissel GE, Passador ST, Rosenfeld SI. Erythrocyte membrane proteins reactive with human (warm-reacting) anti-red cell autoantibodies. *J Clin Invest* 1993; **91**: 1672–80.

42. Plapp FV, Beck ML. Transfusion support in the management of immune haemolytic disorders. *Clin Haematol* 1984; **13**: 167–83.

43. Ahrens. Treatment of refractory autoimmune haemolytic anaemia with anti-CD20 (rituximab). *Br J Haematol* 2001; **114**: 244–5.

44. Zecca M, De Stefano P, Nobili B, Locatelli F. Anti-CD20 monoclonal antibody for the treatment of severe, immune-mediated, pure red cell aplasia and hemolytic anemia. *Blood* 2001; **97**: 3995–7.

45. Zecca M, Nobili B, Ramenghi U *et al.* Rituximab for the treatment of refractory autoimmune hemolytic anemia in children. *Blood* 2003; **101**: 3857–61.

46. Quartier P, Brethon B, Philippet P, Landman-Parker J, Le Deist F, Fischer A. Treatment of childhood autoimmune haemolytic anaemia with rituximab. *Lancet* 2001; **358**: 1511–13.

47. Macintyre EA, Linch DC, Macey MG, Newland AC. Successful response to intravenous immunoglobulin in autoimmune haemolytic anaemia. *Br J Haematol* 1985; **60**: 387–8.

48. Flores G, Cunningham-Rundles C, Newland AC, Bussel JB. Efficacy of intravenous immunoglobulin in the treatment of autoimmune hemolytic anemia: results in 73 patients. *Am J Hematol* 1993; **44**: 237–42.

49. Bussel JB, Cunningham-Rundles C, Abraham C. Intravenous treatment of autoimmune hemolytic anemia with very high dose gammaglobulin. *Vox Sang* 1986; **51**: 264–9.

50. Salama A. IgG therapy in autoimmune haemolytic anaemia of warm type. *Blut* 1984; **48**: 391–2.

51. Passweg JR, Rabusin M, Musso M *et al.* Haematopoetic stem cell transplantation for refractory autoimmune cytopenia. *Br J Haematol* 2004; **125**: 749–55.

52. Zupanska B, Lawkowicz W, Gorska B *et al.* Autoimmune haemolytic anaemia in children. *Br J Haematol* 1976; **34**: 511–20.

53. Zuelzer WW, Mastrangelo R, Stulberg CS, Poulik MD, Page RH, Thompson RI. Autoimmune hemolytic anemia. Natural history and viral-immunologic interactions in childhood. *Am J Med* 1970; **49**: 80–93.

54. Evans RS, Takahashi K, Duane RT, Payne R, Liu C. Primary thrombocytopenic purpura and acquired hemolytic anemia: evidence for a common etiology. *AMA Arch Intern Med* 1951; **87**: 48–65.

55. Kakaiya RM, Sherman LA, Miller WV, Katz AJ. Nature of platelet antibody in Evans syndrome: a case report. *Ann Clin Lab Sci* 1981; **11**: 511–15.

56. Wang MY, McCutcheon E, Desforges JF. Fetomaternal hemorrhage from diagnostic transabdominal amniocentesis. *Am J Obstet Gynecol* 1967; **97**: 1123–8.

57. Teachey DT, Manno CS, Axsom KM *et al.* Unmasking Evans syndrome: T-cell phenotype and apoptotic response reveal autoimmune lymphoproliferative syndrome (ALPS). *Blood* 2005; **105**: 2443–8.

58. Mantadakis E, Danilatou V, Stiakaki E, Kalmanti M. Rituximab for refractory Evans syndrome and other immune-mediated hematologic diseases. *Am J Hematol* 2004; **77**: 303–10.

59. Koneti Rao V, Dugan F, Dale JK *et al.* Use of mycophenolate mofetil for chronic, refractory immune cytopenias in children with autoimmune lymphoproliferative syndrome. *Br J Haematol* 2005; **129**: 534–8.

60. Nydegger UE, Kazatchkine MD, Miescher PA. Immunopathologic and clinical features of hemolytic anemia due to cold agglutinins. *Semin Hematol* 1991; **28**: 66–77.

61. Roelcke D. Cold agglutination. *Transfus Med Rev* 1989; **3**: 140–66.

62. Landsteiner. Ueber Beziehungen zwischen dem Blutserum und den Korperzellen. *Munchen Med Wochenschr* 1903; **50**: 1812–14.

63. Jenkins WJ, Koster HG, Marsh WL, Carter RL. Infectious mononucleosis: an unsuspected source on anti-I. *Br J Haematol* 1965; **11**: 480–3.

64. Horwitz CA, Moulds J, Henle W *et al.* Cold agglutinins in infectious mononucleosis and heterophil-antibody-negative mononucleosis-like syndromes. *Blood* 1977; **50**: 195–202.

65. Rosenfield RE, Jagathambal. Transfusion therapy for autoimmune hemolytic anemia. *Semin Hematol* 1976; **13**: 311–21.

66. Donath. Uber paroxysmale haemoglobinurie. *Munchen Med Wochenschr* 1904; **51**: 1590–3.

67. Heddle NM. Acute paroxysmal cold hemoglobinuria. *Transfus Med Rev* 1989; **3**: 219–29.

68. Sokol RJ. Autoimmune haemolysis associated with Donath–Landsteiner antibodies. *Acta Haematol* 1982; **68**: 268–77.

69. Sokol RJ. Autoimmune hemolysis: a critical review. *Crit Rev Oncol Hematol* 1985; **4**: 125–54.

70. Gottsche B, Salama A, Mueller-Eckhardt C. Donath–Landsteiner autoimmune hemolytic anemia in children. A study of 22 cases. *Vox Sang* 1990; **58**: 281–6.

71. Wolach B, Heddle N, Barr RD, Zipursky A, Pai KR, Blajchman MA. Transient Donath–Landsteiner haemolytic anaemia. *Br J Haematol* 1981; **48**: 425–34.

72. Roy-Burman A, Glader BE. Resolution of severe Donath–Landsteiner autoimmune hemolytic anemia temporally associated with institution of plasmapheresis. *Crit Care Med* 2002; **30**: 931–4.

73. Garratty G. Review: drug-induced immune hemolytic anemia: the last decade. *Immunohematol* 2004; **20**: 138–46.

74. Arndt PA, Leger RM, Garratty G. Serology of antibodies to second- and third-generation cephalosporins associated with immune hemolytic anemia and/or positive direct antiglobulin tests. *Transfusion* 1999; **39**: 1239–46.

75. Shulman IA, Arndt PA, McGehee W, Garratty G. Cefotaxime-induced immune hemolytic anemia due to antibodies reacting in vitro by more than one mechanism. *Transfusion* 1990; **30**: 263–6.

76. Shammo JM, Calhoun B, Mauer AM, Hoffman PC, Baron JM, Baron BW. First two cases of immune hemolytic anemia associated with ceftizoxime. *Transfusion* 1999; **39**: 838–44.

77. Kakaiya R, Cseri J, Smith S, Silberman S, Rubinas TC, Hoffstadter A. A case of acute hemolysis after ceftriaxone: immune complex mechanism demonstrated by flow cytometry. *Arch Pathol Lab Med* 2004; **128**: 905–7.

78. Rowley SD. Hematopoietic stem cell transplantation between red cell incompatible donor–recipient pairs. *Bone Marrow Transplant* 2001; **28**: 315–21.

79. Freda VJ, Gorman JG, Pollack W, Bowe E. Prevention of Rh hemolytic disease: ten years' clinical experience with Rh immune globulin. *N Engl J Med* 1975; **292**: 1014–16.

80. Levine PK, Katzin EM. Isoimmunization in pregnancy: its

possible bearing on the etiology of erythroblastosis fetalis. *JAMA* 1941; **116**: 825.

81. Zipursky. Transplacental fetal hemorrhage after placental injury during delivery or amniocentesis. *Lancet* 1963; **ii**: 493.

82. Brecher M. *Technical Manual*, 14th edn. Bethesda, MD: American Association of Blood Banks, 2002.

83. Judd WJ. Practice guidelines for prenatal and perinatal immunohematology, revisited. *Transfusion* 2001; **41**: 1445–52.

84. Spinnato JA. Hemolytic disease of the fetus: a plea for restraint. *Obstet Gynecol* 1992; **80**: 873–7.

85. Liley. Intrauterine transfusion of fetus in hemolytic disease. *Br Med J* 1963; **2**: 1107.

86. Grannum PA, Copel JA, Moya FR *et al*. The reversal of hydrops fetalis by intravascular intrauterine transfusion in severe isoimmune fetal anemia. *Am J Obstet Gynecol* 1988; **158**: 914–19.

87. Rodeck CH, Nicolaides KH, Warsof SL, Fysh WJ, Gamsu HR, Kemp JR. The management of severe rhesus isoimmunization by fetoscopic intravascular transfusions. *Am J Obstet Gynecol* 1984; **150**: 769–74.

88. Grannum PA, Copel JA, Plaxe SC, Scioscia AL, Hobbins JC. In utero exchange transfusion by direct intravascular injection in severe erythroblastosis fetalis. *N Engl J Med* 1986; **314**: 1431–4.

89. Weiner CP, Williamson RA, Wenstrom KD, Sipes SL, Grant SS, Widness JA. Management of fetal hemolytic disease by cordocentesis. I. Prediction of fetal anemia. *Am J Obstet Gynecol* 1991; **165**: 546–53.

90. Abelson NM, Rawson AJ. Studies of blood group antibodies. V. Fractionation of examples of anti-B, anti-A,B, anti-P, anti-Jka, anti-Lea, anti-D, anti-CD, anti-K, anti-Fya, anti-s and anti-Good. *Transfusion* 1961; **1**: 116–23.

91. Voak D, Williams MA. An explanation of the failure of the direct antiglobulin test to detect erythrocyte sensitization in ABO haemolytic disease of the newborn and observations on pinocytosis of IgG anti-A antibodies by infant (cord) red cells. *Br J Haematol* 1971; **20**: 9–23.

92. Osborn LM, Lenarsky C, Oakes RC, Reiff MI. Phototherapy in full-term infants with hemolytic disease secondary to ABO incompatibility. *Pediatrics* 1984; **74**: 371–4.

93. Rotoli B, Luzzatto L. Paroxysmal nocturnal haemoglobinuria. *Baillières Clin Haematol* 1989; **2**: 113–38.

94. Rosse WF. Paroxysmal nocturnal hemoglobinuria: the biochemical defects and the clinical syndrome. *Blood Rev* 1989; **3**: 192–200.

95. Parker CJ. Historical aspects of paroxysmal nocturnal haemoglobinuria: "defining the disease". *Br J Haematol* 2002; **117**: 3–22.

96. Hillmen P, Lewis SM, Bessler M, Luzzatto L, Dacie JV. Natural history of paroxysmal nocturnal hemoglobinuria. *N Engl J Med* 1995; **333**: 1253–8.

97. Ham T. Chronic hemolytic anemia with paroxysmal nocturnal hemoglobinuria. A study of the mechanism of hemolysis in relation to acid–base equilibrium. *N Engl J Med* 1937; **217**: 915.

98. Ham T. Studies on the destruction of red blood cells. Chronic hemolytic anemia with paroxysmal nocturnal hemoglobinuria: an investigation of the mechanism of hemolysis with observations on five cases. *Arch Intern Med* 1939; **64**: 127.

99. Nicholson-Weller A, Burge J, Fearon DT, Weller PF, Austen KF. Isolation of a human erythrocyte membrane glycoprotein with decay-accelerating activity for C3 convertases of the complement system. *J Immunol* 1982; **129**: 184–9.

100. Fearon DT. Regulation of the amplification C3 convertase of human complement by an inhibitory protein isolated from human erythrocyte membrane. *Proc Natl Acad Sci USA* 1979; **76**: 5867–71.

101. Nicholson-Weller A, March JP, Rosenfeld SI, Austen KF. Affected erythrocytes of patients with paroxysmal nocturnal hemoglobinuria are deficient in the complement regulatory protein, decay accelerating factor. *Proc Natl Acad Sci USA* 1983; **80**: 5066–70.

102. Low MG, Saltiel AR. Structural and functional roles of glycosyl-phosphatidylinositol in membranes. *Science* 1988; **239**: 268–75.

103. Bessler M, Mason PJ, Hillmen P *et al*. Paroxysmal nocturnal haemoglobinuria (PNH) is caused by somatic mutations in the PIG-A gene. *EMBO J* 1994; **13**: 110–17.

104. Takeda J, Miyata T, Kawagoe K *et al*. Deficiency of the GPI anchor caused by a somatic mutation of the PIG-A gene in paroxysmal nocturnal hemoglobinuria. *Cell* 1993; **73**: 703–11.

105. Oni SB, Osunkoya BO, Luzzatto L. Paroxysmal nocturnal hemoglobinuria: evidence for monoclonal origin of abnormal red cells. *Blood* 1970; **36**: 145–52.

106. Rosse WF. Variations in the red cells in paroxysmal nocturnal haemoglobinuria. *Br J Haematol* 1973; **24**: 327–42.

107. Wiedmer T, Hall SE, Ortel TL, Kane WH, Rosse WF, Sims PJ. Complement-induced vesiculation and exposure of membrane prothrombinase sites in platelets of paroxysmal nocturnal hemoglobinuria. *Blood* 1993; **82**: 1192–6.

108. Griscelli-Bennaceur A, Gluckman E, Scrobohaci ML *et al*. Aplastic anemia and paroxysmal nocturnal hemoglobinuria: search for a pathogenetic link. *Blood* 1995; **85**: 1354–63.

109. Devine DV, Gluck WL, Rosse WF, Weinberg JB. Acute myeloblastic leukemia in paroxysmal nocturnal hemoglobinuria. Evidence of evolution from the abnormal paroxysmal nocturnal hemoglobinuria clone. *J Clin Invest* 1987; **79**: 314–17.

110. Lewis SM, Dacie JV. The aplastic anaemia–paroxysmal nocturnal haemoglobinuria syndrome. *Br J Haematol* 1967; **13**: 236–51.

111. Young NS. Acquired aplastic anemia. *Ann Intern Med* 2002; **136**: 534–46.

112. Mukhina GL, Buckley JT, Barber JP, Jones RJ, Brodsky RA. Multilineage glycosylphosphatidylinositol anchor-deficient haematopoiesis in untreated aplastic anaemia. *Br J Haematol* 2001; **115**: 476–82.

113. Chen G, Kirby M, Zeng W, Young NS, Maciejewski JP. Superior growth of glycophosphatidylinositol-anchored protein-deficient progenitor cells in vitro is due to the higher apoptotic rate of progenitors with normal phenotype in vivo. *Exp Hematol* 2002; **30**: 774–82.

114. Ware RE, Hall SE, Rosse WF. Paroxysmal nocturnal hemoglobinuria with onset in childhood and adolescence. *N Engl J Med* 1991; **325**: 991–6.

115. van den Heuvel-Eibrink MM, Bredius RG, te Winkel ML *et al*. Childhood paroxysmal nocturnal haemoglobinuria (PNH), a report of 11 cases in the Netherlands. *Br J Haematol* 2005; **128**: 571–7.

116. Hall SE, Rosse WF. The use of monoclonal antibodies and flow cytometry in the diagnosis of paroxysmal nocturnal hemoglobinuria. *Blood* 1996; **87**: 5332–40.

117. Schubert J, Schmidt RE. [Paroxysmal nocturnal hemoglobinuria. Diagnosis by fluorescence-activated cell analysis.] *Dtsch Med Wochenschr* 1992; **117**: 985–9.

118. Hillmen P, Hall C, Marsh JC *et al*. Effect of eculizumab on hemolysis and transfusion requirements in patients with paroxysmal nocturnal hemoglobinuria. *N Engl J Med* 2004; **350**: 552–9.

119. Lee JL, Lee JH, Lee JH *et al*. Allogeneic hematopoietic cell transplantation for paroxysmal nocturnal hemoglobinuria. *Eur J Haematol* 2003; **71**: 114–18.

120. Raiola AM, Van Lint MT, Lamparelli T *et al*. Bone marrow transplantation for paroxysmal nocturnal hemoglobinuria. *Haematologica* 2000; **85**: 59–62.

121. Saso R, Marsh J, Cevreska L *et al*. Bone marrow transplants for paroxysmal nocturnal haemoglobinuria. *Br J Haematol* 1999; **104**: 392–6.

9 Disorders of erythrocyte metabolism including porphyria

Disorders of erythrocyte metabolism

Lawrence Wolfe and Peter E. Manley

Red cell metabolism

Human erythrocytes are devoid of nuclei and cytoplasmic organelles in order to facilitate their deformability when passing through microcapillaries. Because they have no organelles, they are incapable of synthesizing proteins and lipids and have no capacity for oxidative phosphorylation, and have therefore developed a highly adapted metabolism.[1] Red cells rely completely on the catabolism of glucose (glycolysis) as an energy source to generate adenosine triphosphate (ATP). Red cell metabolic function includes generating compunds with the ability to protect red cell membranes and hemoglobin from oxidative damage, which maintains cell integrity and function. There are two major pathways involved in these important functions (Figs 9.1 and 9.2).

The Embden–Meyerhof pathway (Fig. 9.1) utilizes approximately 90% of available glucose and generates the ATP required for energy. The rate-limiting step is the conversion of glucose to glucose 6-phosphate (G6P) by hexokinase (HK). This pathway is also important in generating 2,3-diphosphoglycerate (2,3-DPG), which alters oxygen affinity, and nicotinamide adenine dinucleotide (NADH), which is used to restore methemoglobin to its functional state. Defects in the enzymes of this pathway are usually associated with chronic or congenital nonspherocytic hemolytic anemias.

The hexose monophosphate (HMP) shunt or pentose phosphate shunt (Fig. 9.2) utilizes approximately 10% of red cell glucose. The rate-limiting step in this pathway is the conversion of G6P to 6-phosphogluconate (6PG), which is catalyzed by glucose 6-phosphate dehydrogenase (G6PD). This pathway is the only way a red cell can produce nicotinamide adenine dinucleotide phosphate (NADPH). This then regenerates the pool of reduced glutathione (GSH). Reduced glutathione protects the red cell from oxidative damage from superoxide anions, methemoglobin, and hydrogen peroxide, which are formed during the reactions of hemoglobin with oxygen. These oxidants can also be formed when red cells are exposed to exogenous agents such as drugs or to oxygen products formed by granulocytes fighting infection. Therefore patients with defects in the HMP pathway tend to have acute hemolytic crises whenever an oxidant stress is applied.

In addition to these pathways the red cell has an additional mechanism to protect itself. Because the red cell relies mainly on ATP, it is critically important that the cell preserves its purine nucleotides. However pyrimidine nucleotides are toxic to red cells and must therefore be removed. The preservation and formation of the pool of nucleotides begins at the reticulocyte stage when ribosomal RNA is broken down. To successfully retain the purines needed and to remove the toxic pyrimidines the red cell has specific nucleotidases. The enzyme pyrimidine 5′-nucleotidase (P5′N) selectively dephosphorylates the pyrimidines CMP and UMP to cytidine and uridine, and this allows these molecules to passively diffuse from the red cell. Patients with defects in this enzyme have congenital nonspherocytic hemolytic anemias and basophilic stippling due to the excessive pyrimidines within the cell.

In the first half of the twentieth century, the initial attempts at classification were based on the autohemolysis test, in which saline-washed erythrocytes were incubated at 37°C and hemolysis was analyzed after 48 hours.[2] Autohemolysis was greater in all patients with congenital nonspherocytic hemolytic anemias. They were able to group the erythrocytes they tested into two types: type I, where hemolysis was

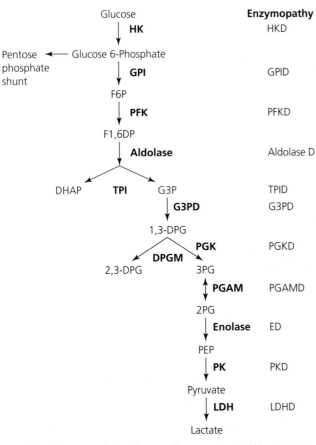

Fig. 9.1 Embden–Meyerhof pathway and known enzymopathies. Enzymes are bold; substrates are faint. 'D' added to the enzyme abbreviation in enzymopathy column indicates deficiency of that enzyme. HK, hexokinase; GPI, glucosephosphate isomerase; F6P, fructose 6-phosphate; PFK, phosphofructokinase; F1,6DP, fructose 1,6-diphosphate; DHAP, dihydroxyacetone phosphate; TPI, triosephosphate isomerase; G3P, glucose 3-phosphate; G3PD, glucose 3-phosphate dehydrogenase; 1,3-DPG, 1,3-diphosphoglycerate; DPGM, diphosphoglycerate mutase; 2,3-DPG, 2,3-diphosphoglycerate; PGK, phosphoglycerate kinase; 3PG, 3-phosphoglycerate; PGAM, phosphoglycerate mutase; 2PG, 2-phosphoglycerate; PEP, phosphoenolpyruvate; PK, pyruvate kinase; LDH, lactate dehydrogenase.

reduced if additional glucose was added; and type II, where hemolysis was unchanged or increased with the addition of glucose. It was noted that patients with type II erythrocytes contained low levels of ATP and high levels of 2,3-DPG.[3] It was felt that patients with these types of erythrocytes had an underlying defect in the glycolytic pathway and this was why glucose did not affect autohemolysis. This was confirmed when Valentine *et al.*[4] described the first cases of pyruvate kinase (PK) deficiency.

G6PD deficiency was first described when African-American soldiers developed an acute hemolytic crisis with hemoglobinuria after taking the antimalarial drug primaquine.[5]

Epidemiology

With the exception of PK and G6PD deficiency, the erythroenzymopathies are very uncommon (see Table 9.1 for prevalence).

Investigations when considering a diagnosis of red cell enzymopathy

Clinical findings

The most prominent clinical finding in a patient with a red cell enzymopathy is hemolysis. However, the hemolysis is not the same in all enzymopathies. The Embden–Meyerhof pathway is how the red cell generates the ATP needed for everyday survival and therefore patients with defects in this pathway will usually have constant chronic hemolysis. Patients with defects in the HMP shunt will usually have acute bouts of hemolysis when an oxidative stress is applied, and thus their disease appears episodic. In addition to hemolysis, these conditions can present with various syndromes, including splenomegaly, neurologic symptoms such as spasticity and hypotonia, and musculoskeletal symptoms such as

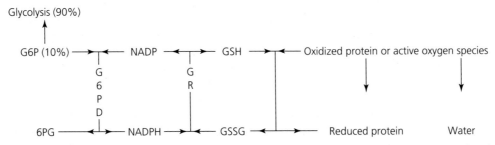

Fig. 9.2 Hexose monophosphate shunt. G6P (glucose 6-phosphate) is converted to 6PG (6-phosphogluconate) by G6PD (glucose 6-phosphate dehydrogenase) generating NADPH (nicotinamine adenine dinucleotide phosphate reduced), which regenerates GSH (glutathione) through interaction with GR (glutathione reductase) and GSSG (glutathione disulfide). Glutathione is then available for reducing active oxygen compounds or oxidized proteins especially hemoglobin.

Table 9.1 Prevalence of enzymopathies.

Type	Prevalence
Embden–Meyerhof pathway	
Hexokinase deficiency	22 cases described[6,7]
Glucosephosphate isomerase deficiency	60 cases described[8]
Phosphofructokinase deficiency	35 cases described[9]
Aldolase deficiency	5 cases described[10]
Triosephosphate isomerase deficiency	34 cases described[11]
Phosphoglycerate kinase deficiency	20 cases described[12]
Diphosphoglycerate mutase deficiency	20 cases described[13]
Phosphoglycerate mutase deficiency	5 cases described[14]
Enolase deficiency	3 cases described[15]
Pyruvate kinase deficiency	>400 cases described[16]
Lactose dehydrogenase deficiency	4 families described[17]
Hexose monophosphate shunt	
Glucose 6-phosphate dehydrogenase deficiency	400 million cases[18]
Glutathione synthetase	20 cases described[19]
Glutamylcysteine synthetase	3 cases described[20]
Glutathione reductase	3 cases described[21]
Erythrocyte nucleotide metabolism	
Pyrimidine-5′-nucleotidase deficiency	40 cases described[22]
Adenosine deaminase overexpression	14 cases[23–25]

easy fatiguability and severe muscle cramps. These patterns of presentation can help discriminate among the conditions. Although these symptoms are rare, the simultaneous appearance of muscle cramps with or without effort, myoglobinuria or rhabdomyolysis, and hemolytic anemia requires examination of red cell enzymes. Table 9.2 summarizes the symptoms of the red cell enzymopathies.

Erythrocyte morphology

In any hemolytic anemia, one of the first steps in the diagnostic process is examination of the peripheral blood smear. A large percentage of patients with hemolytic anemia can be detected by simple perusal of the smear. In addition, primary examination of the smear helps design the subsequent workup. In patients with defects of the Embden–Meyerhof pathway, most exhibit less active smears and little spherocytosis, often being termed "congenital nonspherocytic hemolytic anemia" or so-called "smear-negative" hemolysis (where there is no predominant morphology). This should lead the hematologist to specifically consider a small group of disorders including red cell metabolic defects and Wilson disease. The HMP shunt defects, when oxidative stress is present, may show "bite" and "blister" cell morphologies, but more characterisically the hematologist is asked to examine a smear after a bout of hemolysis or between attacks, and at these times it would appear normal. Patients with P5′N deficiency will have significant basophilic stippling of

their smears, reflecting the inability to clear pyrimidine nucleotides from the cytoplasm.

Patients with PK deficiency can have a high reticulocyte count, crenated burr cells, echinocytes, and dehydrated effete red cells, reflecting severe ATP depletion. Spherocytes are not elevated in patients with PK deficiency.

Laboratory information

Basic laboratory data

Patients who have any type of hemolytic anemia should have certain standard laboratory studies performed. These include (i) blood type and cross-match for red cell antibodies and to prepare the patient for transfusion if necessary, (ii) a complete blood count, (iii) blood smear and reticulocyte count, (iv) urinalysis to assess if hemolysis is intravascular, (v) serum lactate dehydrogenase (LDH), (vi) fractionated bilirubin and (vii) haptoglobin. Most patients with red cell enzymopathies will have a grossly normal osmotic fragility test.

Analysis of intermediate metabolites

When there is inhibition of a step in the glycolytic pathway, it can be helpful to examine the measurable intermediates proximal or distal to the deficient enzyme, such as 2,3-DPG and glutathione in HMP shunt defects. Red cell ATP can also be measured (Table 9.3). Analysis of these intermediates must be interpreted with caution because patients with anemia have increased levels of 2,3-DPG in order to improve oxygen delivery.[26] Another subtlety of evaluation involves the fact that hemolytic anemia leading to reticulocytosis will increase the population of young red cells, and their higher levels of ATP mask an overall depletion of ATP.

Triosephosphate isomerase (TPI) catalyzes the interconversion of dihydroxyacetone phosphate (DHAP) and glyceraldehyde 3-phosphate. If DHAP is not converted to glyceraldehyde 3-phosphate, it will spontaneously degrade to methylglyoxal.[27] These excessive intermediates can be measured when TPI deficiency is suspected. With the development of direct measurement for all enzymes of the glycolytic pathway, the analysis of intermediate metabolites is not obligatory but may be able to assist the investigator to target a specific enzyme. Patients with low levels of glutathione suggest deficiencies in either γ-glutamylcysteine or glutathione synthetase.[28,29]

Enzyme screening tests

Since these diseases are very rare, screening tests have been developed only for the more common disorders, such as G6PD deficiency. The fluorescent spot test is the oldest and most reliable screening test for G6PD.[30,31] It is based on the fluorescence of NADPH after G6P and NAD are added to a

Table 9.2 Clinical features associated with enzymopathies.

Enzyme	Inheritance	Hemolysis	Neurologic	Myopathy	Other
Embden–Meyerhof pathway					
Hexokinase deficiency	AR	+*			
Glucosephosphate isomerase deficiency	AR	+†	+ (rare)	+ (rare)	Fetal hydrops, splenomegaly, recurrent infection
Phosphofructokinase deficiency	AR	±‡		+	Myoglobinuria, myopathy, hyperuricemia
Aldolase deficiency	AR	+*	±	±	3 of 6 patients with rhabdomyolysis
Triosephosphate isomerase deficiency	AR	+*	+	+	Recurrent infection, sudden cardiac death, neonatal jaundice
Phosphoglycerate kinase deficiency	XL	+*	±	±	Myoglobinuria
Diphosphoglycerate mutase deficiency	AR	±			Erythrocytosis
Phosphoglycerate mutase deficiency	AR			+	Myoglobinuria
Enolase deficiency	AD	(+)†§			Spherocytosis
Pyruvate kinase deficiency	AR	+§			Iron overload
Lactose dehydrogenase deficiency	AR	+		+	
Hexose monophosphate shunt					
Glucose-6-phosphate dehydrogenase deficiency	XL	+†			Acidosis, 5-oxoprolinuria
Glutathione synthetase	AR	+*	+		Recurrent infection
γ-Glutamylcysteine synthetase	AR	+*	+		Favism, cataracts
Glutathione reductase	AR	+*			
Erthrocyte nucleotide metabolism					
Pyrimidine 5'-nucleotidase deficiency	AR	+‡			Basophilic stippling
Adenosine deaminase overexpression	AD	+*			
Adenylate kinase deficiency	AR	(+)			

* Nondiagnostic smear.

† Oxidant hemolysis morphology may appear.

‡ Stippling may be seen.

§ Active smear.

Parentheses indicate that link to enzyme deficiency is unproven.

AR, autosomal recessive; AD, autosomal dominant; XL, X-linked.

Table 9.3 Metabolic intermediates in red cell enzymopathies.

Defect	2,3-DPG levels	ATP levels	Comments
Proximal glycolysis: HK, GPI or PFK	Normal to low	Normal to low	Multiple variability within each defect
Distal glycolysis: PK or PGK	Elevated	Normal to low	Low ATP and 2,3-DPG more useful in PK deficiency PK deficiency also has high levels of 3-PG
Overproduction of ADA	Normal	Low	Due to rapid breakdown of adenosine

ADA, adenosine deaminase; 2,3-DPG, 2,3-diphosphoglycerate; GPI, glucosephosphate isomerase; HK, hexokinase; PFK, phosphofructokinase; 3-PG, 3-phosphoglycerate; PGK, phosphoglycerate kinase deficiency; PK, pyruvate kinase.

hemolysate of test cells. Recently, a new diagnostic kit has been described that detects patients with < 50% G6PD activity.[32,33] This test uses a formazan, WST-8, which is converted to an orange color detectable in the presence of G6PD and this is visible to the naked eye. New rapid microarray-based assays have also been developed to detect G6PD deficiency in specific populations.[34]

For PK, several screening tests have been developed but these may not detect some of the PK variants,[35] and they have not been extensively used.

The red cells of patients with P5'N deficiency exhibit a different spectral analysis and this can be used as a screening test for this disorder. Normal red blood cells have an absorption peak at 257 nm owing to the high percentage of adenosine compounds; patients with P5'N deficiency have a higher percentage of pyrimidine compounds, changing the absorption peak to 268 nm.[36]

Direct enzyme measurement and DNA measurement

Definitive diagnostic measurements are discussed with each specific disorder. All enzymes can be directly measured. Now that many mutations of the various enzymopathies have been discovered, DNA analysis can be performed to make the diagnosis. When direct enzyme measurement is employed there are a few pitfalls of which the investigator needs to be aware. In patients who have an episode of acute hemolysis, the most severely deficient red cells have usually been removed, especially in defects of the HMP shunt. When there is a reticulocytosis immediately following acute hemolysis or in patients who have recently been transfused, the enzyme levels can be read as abnormally high. Therefore correction for increased activity of enzymes and reticulocytes must be made. Some assays require leukocytes to be removed as they have higher levels of the enzyme.[37] The age of the patient being examined must also be taken into account when evaluating enzyme levels.[38]

Disorders of the Embden–Meyerhof pathway

Hexokinase deficiency

HK is the first enzyme of the pathway and plays an important role. HK phosphorylates glucose, forming G6P, using magnesium as a cofactor and ATP as a phosphate source. It provides the substrate for both the HMP shunt and anaerobic glycolysis necessary for red cell survival. HK deficiency is an autosomal recessive disease.

The enzyme

There are four major isozymes of mammalian HK.[39] The most prevalent isozyme involved in erythrocytes is HK-1. Recent studies have identified a specific erythroid isoform, HK-R.[40] The human HK-1 gene is located on chromosome 10q22,[41] which contains an erythroid cell-specific promoter.[42] HK activity initially declines rapidly. Specifically, HK-R activity, which is mainly expressed in reticulocytes, falls off quickly due to its short half-life (10 days). HK-1 becomes the predominant isoform as the erythrocyte ages because its half-life is much longer (66 days).[40] HK-1 is inhibited by its product G6P, which competitively inhibits ATP binding.[43] Mutations of the HK-1 gene have been reported and appear to decrease the enzyme's ability to undergo needed conformational changes during substrate binding.[44]

Clinical presentation

All patients with HK deficiency have hemolytic anemia.[45] The severity of the hemolysis is generally moderate. Severely affected individuals may have hyperbilirubinemia as a neonate. Patients may appear jaundiced or have splenomegaly. Development of gallstones may occur at an earlier age. Several affected patients have had congenital malformations or psychomotor retardation,[46] but it is not clear if these manifestations are directly caused by HK deficiency. Patients may also have severe tissue hypoxia because they are unable to decrease oxygen affinity and increase delivery to tissue by increasing the production of 2,3-DPG.

Diagnosis

Patients with HK deficiency may have a reduced level of 2,3-DPG, while ATP levels can be normal or reduced.[47,48] A moderate anemia with unremarkable red cell morphology is seen. The diagnosis of HK deficiency can be made by showing the enzyme to have aberrant kinetics, reduced stability, or altered electrophoretic mobility.[45] It is important to note that HK deficiency is an age-dependent enzyme with higher activity in reticulocytes than old erythrocytes. When interpreting the data it should include a comparison with other age-dependent enzymes such as PK or G6PD as an internal control and with HK levels in normal subjects with high reticulocyte counts. Otherwise the values can be interpreted as normal. Prenatal diagnosis of HK deficiency has been performed and described in a fetus with intrauterine growth retardation.[49]

Treatment

The treatment of patients with this disorder is to alleviate symptoms. It consists of transfusions and supplementation with folic acid; in severe cases (transfusion-dependent) splenectomy has abolished the need for transfusions.

Glucosephosphate isomerase deficiency

Glucosephosphate isomerase (GPI) catalyzes the isomerization of G6P to fructose 6-phosphate (F6P). Deficiency of this enzyme was first described in 1968,[50] and is the third most common cause of nonspherocytic hemolytic anemia after G6PD and PK deficiency. It is an autosomal recessive disease.

The enzyme

GPI is a dimeric enzyme with a molecular mass of 134 kDa. The gene encoding GPI is found on chromosome 19q13.1.[51] There are no isozymes for GPI, and thus in affected patients all tissues and cells are deficient in the enzyme. The majority of the gene defects (24 of the 29 found in this disorder) are point mutations.[52] More than 50% of patients affected with this disorder are compound heterozygotes. These mutations are very heterogeneous, with only 7 of the 29 mutations found in more than one family. GPI deficiency leads to a build-up of G6P, which is a potent inhibitor of HK. Deficiency of GPI affects not only anaerobic glycolysis but also the HMP shunt, leaving the patient susceptible to oxidative stress. The correlation between genotype and severity of disease has not been fully elucidated.

Sequencing of a protein called neuroleukin (NLK), which has neurotrophic and lymphokine properties, has shown that it is identical to GPI.[53,54] Deficiencies in NLK have been associated with motor neuron disease.[55]

Clinical presentation

Patients with GPI deficiency present with anemia, which varies from mild to severe. Patients also have variable degrees of jaundice, splenomegaly, and an increased risk of gallstones. As there are no isozymes of GPI, an affected patient has GPI deficiency in all tissues; thus GPI deficiency has also been associated with hydrops fetalis, neonatal death, and priapism.[56–58] The latter unusual symptom is theorized to be due to poor red cell deformability. Patients with GPI deficiency have had associated neurologic and white blood cell impairment. The homology with NLK has implicated GPI as the cause of these defects.[59,60] Hemolytic crises associated with GPI deficiency due to infection or exposure to oxidant drugs may occur. This may be due to the inability to recycle F6P through the HMP shunt.[50]

Diagnosis

A complete blood count shows a normochromic anemia with an increased reticulocyte count. Patients have decreased levels of ATP, 2,3-DPG, and GSH, due to decrease in HK secondary to high levels of G6P. GPI deficiency is mainly identified by the thermolability of the mutant in vitro. Enzyme activity can also be measured directly and is typically 10–40% of normal, with an increase in the G6P/F6P ratio.

Treatment

There is no specific therapy for GPI deficiency. Patients may require transfusions in acute situations or to maintain an adequate level of hemoglobin. In an acute hemolytic crisis, patients should be treated for any infection and have any offending oxidant agent removed, giving blood and fluid management to maintain adequate urine output. In patients who required chronic transfusion, splenectomy usually alleviated the need for continuation of transfusion therapy.[52]

Phosphofructokinase deficiency

Phosphofructokinase (PFK) catalyzes the principal rate-limiting step in glycolysis: the phosphorylation of F6P to fructose 1,6-diphosphate (FDP). Deficiency of this enzyme was first noted by Tauri et al.[61] It occurs as an autosomal recessive disease. It is also called glycogen storage disease VII or Tauri disease.

The enzyme

The heterogeneity of clinical syndromes associated with deficiency of PFK mirrors the complexity of its genetic control. PFK is a homotetrameric or heterotetrameric enzyme with three types of subunits: muscle (M), liver (L), and platelet (P) subunits are encoded by separate structural genes. The M subunit is isolated to chromosome 12q13,[62] the L subunit to chromosome 21q22,[63] and P subunit to chromosome 10p15.[64] Muscle PFK is composed entirely of M subunits, and liver PFK is made up entirely of L subunits. In red cells, both M and L subunits combine to form different tetramers, the relative proportions of which vary during development. This may explain the lower activity of PFK in neonatal red cells, the composition of which includes the relatively unstable L_4 isozyme that is not found in normal adult red cells. To date there have been 39 reports of unrelated families with PFK deficiency,[9] with multiple different mutations described in the PFK-M gene.[9,65] PFK-M deficiency appears to be more prevalent in people who are of Ashkenazi descent and have two typical mutations: one that alters a splice site or one which leads to nucleotide deletion in the PFK-M gene.[66,67]

Clinical findings

PFK deficiency can present with a variety of symptoms. It is characterized by myopathy or hemolysis. The majority of presenting symptoms relate to myopathy, including fatigue, muscle cramps, and exercise intolerance. The classic presentation has these symptoms exacerbated after a high-carbohydrate meal.[68] Patients can exhibit myoglobinuria secondary to rhabdomyolysis after exercise. Muscle weakness characteristically worsens during exercise because of the reliance of muscle cells on anaerobic glycolysis for energy generation. As red cell PFK is composed of both L and M subunits, red cells that have homotetrameric enzyme can be spared the full metabolic effects of M-subunit deficiency in classic PFK deficiency. Cases of PFK deficiency with isolated hemolysis and normal muscle enzyme activity have also been recognized.[69,70] When present, anemia is usually mild or moderate. In its most severe form, PFK deficiency may present at birth, cases having been described in infants deficient in all three isoforms. These patients suffer not only myopathy but also central nervous system dysfunction and cardiomyopathy, and can follow an inexorable course with death from respiratory failure in infancy.[71,72] Usually, the onset of symptoms is delayed until later childhood or even adult life. Increased purine generation in muscle and red cells may lead to hyperuricemia and arthropathy, which can be present even if no myopathy is present.[73]

Diagnosis

Patients may have a mild erythrocytosis due to reduced 2,3-DPG concentration, which occurs because the block is upstream from the formation of 2,3-DPG. Even in this situation the red cell lifespan is shortened. With the exception of prominent basophilic stippling seen in a few cases, red cell morphology is not helpful diagnostically. Patients can also have elevated serum creatine kinase and hyperuricemia. Reduced muscle PFK activity may be inferred from a failure of lactate production after anaerobic (ischemic) forearm exercise or by magnetic resonance spectroscopy.[74] The diagnosis of PFK deficiency can be confirmed by assay of red cell enzyme activity and intermediates. Typically, red cell PFK activity is about 50% of normal. Direct confirmation may be obtained by assay of enzyme activity on biopsied muscle tissue. Since muscle contains exclusively M_4 tetramers, the reduction in enzyme activity is correspondingly greater than in red cells.[75] In patients of Ashkenazi descent, genetic testing can be performed as 95% of these patients will have one of the two most common mutations.[76]

Treatment

Treatment is mainly through prevention. Avoidance of strenuous exercise can prevent episodes of muscle cramping, fatigue, and rhabdomyolysis. Anemia can be treated by red cell transfusions. There is one reported case in a patient with infantile PFK deficiency who showed some improvement in symptoms with a ketogenic diet; however this patient subsequently died.[77]

Aldolase deficiency

Aldolase is responsible for conversion of FDP to glyceraldehyde 3-phosphate and DHAP. The main enzyme that causes defects in erythrocyte glucose metabolism is aldolase A. Aldolase deficiency is an autosomal recessive disease.

The enzyme

Three tissue-specific isozymes, A, B and C, exist. Adolase C is found in brain. Aldolase B is expressed mainly in the liver, kidney, and intestine, where its main role is in exogenous fructose utilization, mutations in this enzyme causing fructose intolerance. Aldolase A is more ubiquitous and is the enzyme that drives the red cell glycolytic pathway.[78] Aldolase A is encoded on chromosome 16q22–24 and the

protein is a homotetramer.[79] Note that only six cases of hemolytic anemia due to inherited aldolase deficiency have been described.[80,81]

Clinical signs and symptoms

All patients with aldolase A deficiency have exhibited anemia, ranging from mild to severe; three of six patients had myopathy and one patient had mental retardation. In one case, myopathy characterized by exercise intolerance and rhabdomyolysis was a prominent manifestation.[82] Episodes of rhabdomyolysis were precipitated by fever. This was attributed to marked thermal instability of the mutant enzyme.

Diagnosis

All patients have a nonspherocytic hemolytic anemia. They can have hemoglobinuria and myoglobinuria. Patients with associated myopathy have elevated creatine kinase. Aldolase A enzyme activity can be measured and is low in patients with this disorder.

Treatment

In patients with severe anemia the treatment is red blood cell transfusion. One patient had resolution of transfusion requirements after splenectomy.[81] As with other shared enzymopathies with muscle involvement, strenuous exercise needs to be avoided.

Triosephosphate isomerase deficiency

TPI catalyzes with high efficiency the interconversion of the triosephosphates DHAP and glyceraldehyde 3-phosphate, the equilibrium favoring DHAP formation by a factor of 22 : 1. The clinical phenotype was first described by Schneider *et al.*[83] TPI deficiency is an autosomal recessive disease.

The enzyme

TPI is a homodimeric enzyme expressed in all cell types. It is encoded by a single gene on chromosome 12p13.[84,85] It is not only involved in glycolysis but is also an important enzyme in gluconeogenesis and triglyceride synthesis. To date, 14 mutations in the TPI gene have been identified.[11,86] The most common mutation found is a point mutation in codon 104 resulting in a substitution of Glu for Asp,[87] which creates a thermolabile unstable protein. The fact that TPI is a ubiquitous enzyme found in all cells is reflected in the multisystem nature of the clinical deficiency state. Patients with TPI deficiency have elevated levels of methylglyoxal, a degradation product of DHAP. This leads to increased glycation and nitrosation of proteins and may contribute to the pathogenesis of neurodegeneration.[27]

Clinical signs and symptoms

Patients who have TPI deficiency are either homozygotes or compound heterozygotes. Pure heterozygotes are clinically normal. TPI deficiency is the most severe disorder of the Embden–Meyerhof pathway. Patients with TPI deficiency usually present in the first year of life with nonspherocytic hemolytic anemia, which can result in neonatal jaundice. The degree of anemia in TPI deficiency is variable. Although severe anemia may be encountered, most patients require only occasional transfusions after the neonatal period. Patients also have an increased susceptibility to bacterial infections. This is most likely due to the deficiency of the leukocyte enzyme. The anemia may also worsen during periods of infection. Between 6 months and 2 years of age neuromuscular dysfunction becomes evident. The constellation of neurologic abnormalities observed in TPI deficiency includes motor delay or regression, spasticity, hypotonia, dystonic movements, opisthotonos, nystagmus, and optic atrophy.[87–89] These findings suggest that specific structures in the basal ganglia, brainstem, and spinal cord (anterior horn cells) are damaged in TPI deficiency.[89] Neuromuscular impairment is usually progressive, and most affected children fail to survive beyond 5 years of age. Rarely, the neurologic deficits may stabilize during childhood and there have been isolated cases in which there is no overt neurologic dysfunction.[90,91] Cognitive function is normal and correlates with the fact that there is little cortical damage in TPI deficiency. Patients have developmental delay more likely related to motor dysfunction than cognitive dysfunction. The cause of death in these patients is usually sudden and not well understood but cardiac arrhythmia has been invoked as a likely cause.

The mechanisms underlying the neuropathic effects of TPI deficiency are poorly delineated. Neuroimaging studies have failed to reveal extensive structural changes in the brain. Electrophysiologic studies show evidence of denervation myopathy in some cases. DHAP is an essential precursor in biosynthesis of ether glycerolipids (plasmalogens). Plasmalogen biosynthesis is impaired in peroxisomal disorders such as Zellweger syndrome and neonatal adrenoleukodystrophy, in which neurologic manifestations are prominent.[92] A kindred has been described in which only one of two affected siblings manifests neurologic dysfunction.[91] This was a family in which two Hungarian brothers were found, one with neurologic deficits and one without. As previously mentioned, patients with TPI deficiency have elevated levels of methylglyoxal, a degradation product of DHAP, which may lead to neurodegeneration. Interestingly, the one Hungarian brother with no neurologic deficits had lower levels of methylglyoxal than his brother with deficits.

Diagnosis

Morphologically, occasional spheroechinocytes may be visible on the blood film but there are no distinguishing features. TPI deficiency is diagnosed by assay of red cell enzyme activity in conjunction with metabolic intermediates. The biochemical hallmark of homozygous TPI deficiency is intracellular accumulation of DHAP. This is most marked (20–100 fold) in red cells which, unlike other tissues, lack the capacity to metabolize DHAP in the glycerol phosphate shuttle via α-glycerophosphate dehydrogenase. Recently, a sural nerve biopsy was performed in a patient with TPI deficiency confirming the peripheral neuropathy. However, because there is a dominant genetic defect among the many mutants described, DNA analysis of the many mutants described may be attempted on infants and family members suspected of TPI deficiency. As the disease can be devastating, DNA studies have been done prenatally as well.[86]

Treatment

Unfortunately there are no definitive treatments for TPI deficiency. Transfusion for anemia should be performed as needed clinically. Rapid treatment of infections should be initiated as patients can have worsening anemia and increased neurologic complications with infection. There have been recent studies looking at enzyme replacement as a treatment for TPI deficiency.[93,94]

Phosphoglycerate kinase deficiency

Phosphoglycerate kinase (PGK) is a key enzyme in the glycolytic pathway. It catalyzes the conversion of 1,3-diphosphoglycerate (1,3-DPG) to 3-phosphoglycerate (3-PG) with the concomitant generation of ATP. The deficiency is an X-linked inherited disease but, ironically, PGK deficiency was first recognized in a female with hemolytic anemia.[95]

The enzyme

PGK has two isozymes, PGK-1 and PGK-2. PGK-1 is the more abundant of the two and is expressed in all somatic cells. It is encoded by a single gene on the X chromosome (Xq13).[96] PGK-2 is encoded on chromosome 19 and is only expressed in late stages of spermatogenesis.[97] The PGK reaction can be bypassed by the Rapoport–Luebering shunt catalyzed by 2,3-diphosphoglyceromutase, forming 2,3-DPG. Only mutations in the PGK-1 gene have been found to cause the clinical symptoms seen in this enzyme deficiency. To date 16 mutants have been identified, including both missense and nonsense mutations.[9,98]

In hemizygous males, red cell PGK activity is usually less than 20% of normal. Enzyme levels in female heterozygotes vary not only because of lyonization, as in other X-linked disorders, but also because of the preferential survival of PGK-replete red cells that have the normal allele on their active X chromosome.

Clinical signs and symptoms

PGK deficiency is associated with nonspherocytic hemolytic anemia. Hemizygous males tend to have a more severe anemia than heterozygous females. The anemia may be exacerbated by an intercurrent infection. These patients may also suffer from neurologic dysfunction, including seizures, movement disorders, hemiplegia, aphasia, mental retardation, and behavioral disturbance including emotional lability. These are usually associated with severe enzyme deficiency in hemizygous males. Patients may also suffer from myopathy, including exercise intolerance, muscle cramps, rhabdomyolysis and myoglobinuria. Patients with myopathy do not usually have hemolytic anemia.[99]

While onset in the neonatal period with jaundice and seizures is reported, there may be latency in the appearance of neurologic manifestations with normal development in infancy.[100] The basis for the differing patterns of clinical expression in PGK deficiency is not understood since the same isozyme is expressed in all somatic cells.[101] Heterozygote females may manifest mild hemolysis but have normal neurologic function.

Diagnosis

The profile of red cell intermediates in affected males is consistent with a block in glycolysis at the PGK step. There will be a nonspherocytic hemolytic anemia on the blood smear if anemia is present. Reduction in the concentration of ATP is characteristic, as this step generates one molecule of ATP. Patients with defects in PGK will bypass this step via the Rapoport–Luebering shunt, thereby increasing levels of 2,3-DPG. Patients with myopathy can have an increase in myoglobinuria and creatine kinase. These patients may require a muscle biopsy to exclude glycogen storage diseases, which can present in a similar fashion (McArdle disease and Tauri disease). Enzyme levels of PGK-1 can be measured directly.

Treatment

Patients with severe hemolytic anemia require transfusions. In these patients, splenectomy has alleviated transfusions.[9] Patients with myopathy need to avoid strenuous exercise.

Phosphoglycerate mutase deficiency

Phosphoglycerate mutase catalyzes the reaction of 3-PG to 2-phosphoglycerate. This is a very rare disorder with only five cases reported.[14] There are two isozymes, a muscle isozyme, mapped to chromosome 7p13,[102] and a brain isozyme, mapped to chromosome 10q25.[103] It is an autosomal recessive disease and is caused by mutations in the muscle isozymes. Patients with this defect do not have hemolytic anemia. As the defect is in the muscle isoform, these patients exhibit exercise intolerance, muscle cramping, and rhabdomyolysis. These symptoms usually begin in childhood or adolescence. Diagnosis is by enzyme measurement, muscle biopsy, and elevated creatine kinase levels. There is no effective therapy for phosphoglycerate mutase deficiency. Patients with this disease need to avoid strenuous exercise.

Diphosphoglycerate mutase deficiency

Diphosphoglycerate mutase (DPGM) acts in the Rapoport–Luebering shunt to regulate the metabolism of 2,3-DPG. Its main catalytic function is the conversion of 1,3-DPG to 2,3-DPG. In addition, DPGM possesses phosphatase activity that is responsible for the conversion of 2,3-DPG to 3-PG and functions, albeit at low efficiency, as a monophosphoglycerate mutase. Human DPGM activity is confined to red cells. 2,3-DPG is the most abundant glycolytic intermediate and serves to lower the affinity of hemoglobin for oxygen, thereby shifting the oxygen dissociation curve to the right.

DPGM deficiency is an autosomal recessive illness, with only 20 cases described.[13] The phenotype of DPGM deficiency has been documented in most detail in a single kindred in which both homozygotes and heterozygotes exhibited erythrocytosis but no signs of hemolysis.[13,104]

Enolase deficiency

Enolase catalyzes the conversion of 2-phosphoglycerate to phosphoenolpyruvate (PEP). This enzyme is encoded by a gene located on chromosome 1q36.[105] This is also a very uncommon phenotype. Unlike the other deficiencies, enolase deficiency is an autosomal dominant disease. Patients with enolase deficiency do have spherocytic hemolytic anemia. Patients with this disorder may also be at increased risk for hemolysis after exposure to oxidant drugs. The pathogenesis for this deficiency is unknown and no mutations have been discovered. There is no therapy for this disorder but avoidance of oxidant drugs is suggested.

Pyruvate kinase deficiency

PK catalyzes the conversion of PEP to pyruvate and generates one ATP molecule. PK deficiency is the most frequent enzyme abnormality found in the Embden–Meyerhof pathway. It was first described in 1961 by Valentine *et al.*[4] PK deficiency is an autosomal recessive disease.

The enzyme

PK catalyzes the last reaction in the glycolytic pathway. It requires both magnesium and potassium for activity. The conversion of PEP to pyruvate is irreversible under physiologic conditions. Activity of the enzyme is increased in the presence of FDP.

The enzyme is a tetramer composed of four identical subunits. There are several isozymes present in mammalian tissue. The red cell (R) and liver (L) subunits are encoded by the PK-L/R gene found on chromosome 1q21.[106] These isoforms vary because of tissue-specific promoters, and because of this the R form is 31 amino acids longer than the L form.[107] The L form is also expressed in renal cortex and small intestine. The M isozyme is divided into two subsets, M1 and M2. Both are encoded on chromosome 15q22 by alternative mRNA splicing.[108,109] The M1 form is expressed in skeletal muscle, heart and brain. The M2 type is dominant during fetal life and is replaced in skeletal muscle, heart and brain by the M1 type. However, the M2 isoform remains the dominant form in leukocytes and platelets. In red blood cells, the M2 isoform is dominant in the progenitors but is eventually replaced by the R form.[110] This occurs in the normoblast and reticulocyte phase and is made up of L' tetramers (L_4') called PK-R1. Proteolysis converts the L' tetramer to a heterotetramer ($L_2'L_2$) called PK-R2, which is the main form in mature red cells.[111,112] In some cases of severe deficiency of the R subunit, reversion to synthesis of the M2 form may partially rescue the deficient phenotype.[113] This has been likened to the persistence of fetal hemoglobin in β-thalassemia. Persistence of the M2 isozyme in red cells may also account for the rare "high ATP" syndrome in which supraphysiologic PK activity leads to metabolic depletion of 2,3-DPG, with increased hemoglobin oxygen affinity and erythrocytosis.[114,115]

Patients with PK deficiency have mutations only in the PK-L/R gene. To date, 142 mutations have been described in PK deficiency.[116,117] The majority of them are missense, splicing, and stop codon mutations. Mutations of the enzyme are felt to potentially alter the affinity for PEP, alter the affinity for FDP, increase inhibition to ATP, or alter enzyme stability.[118] These mutations are spread throughout the coding region with no preference for the coding region.[119] Only two mutations have been found in the promoter region.[120] Most mutations have only been described once, but there are three mutations that are prevalent in different populations: 1468 C→T, 1529 G→A, and 1456 C→T. The 1456 C→T mutation is most common in southern Europe,[121] the 1468 C→T mutation is most common in Asia,[122] and the 1529 G→A mutation is most common in northern Europe and the USA.[123,124] This has prompted speculation as to whether deficiency of the liver enzyme may contribute to jaundice. Evidence of abnormal liver function in some cases of PK deficiency supports this possibility.

Pathophysiology of hemolytic anemia

The mechanism for hemolysis in PK deficiency is not well understood. It is felt that red blood cells become deficient in ATP, which leads to a cascade of events that begins with loss of cation homeostasis, with efflux of potassium and water leading to cellular dehydration and culminating in contraction and rigidity of erythroctyes, forming the characteristic crenated cells. These cells will then be removed in the reticuloendothelial system, particularly the spleen. This is not a full explanation as some patients with PK deficiency do not have low levels of ATP[125] and other disorders with ATP deficiency are not associated with hemolysis.[126] 2,3-DPG has been implicated in the hemolytic process. 2,3-DPG is an inhibitor of G6PD and may impair the HMP shunt. This may contribute to increased hemolysis in times of stress such as pregnancy or infection.[127] 2,3-DPG also inhibits the enzyme 5-phosphoribosyl-1-pyrophosphate. This mechanism is also not completely explanatory as patients with PK deficiency do not have severe hemolysis after exposure to oxidative agents as seen in G6PD deficiency and do not manifest the red cell changes on smear seen with classical oxidative hemolysis. 5-Phosphoribosyl-1-pyrophosphate is a critical enzyme in the purine salvage pathway that provides the red cell with adenine and thus this defect could diminish synthesis of NAD and NADPH, also leading to decreased red cell oxidant protection.[128] A high number of erythroid progenitors and reticulocytes are found in the spleen of PK-deficient patients, suggesting that there is ineffective erythropoiesis.[129] This is further substantiated by the paradoxical increase in the reticulocyte count in PK-deficient patients who undergo splenectomy.

Clinical presentation

Over 80% of cases present during childhood. The spectrum of clinical severity is wide.[130] However, it is important to note that the only gene affected in PK is the PK-L/R gene and the hepatic enzyme deficiency does not result in liver dysfunction. Therefore, the only clinical manifestations are limited to red blood cells. The clinical spectrum concerns chronic hemolytic anemia, which ranges from mild fully compensated anemia that remains undetected into later life to life-threatening anemia in the newborn period.[116] Anemia may also manifest *in utero*, causing nonimmune hydrops fetalis.[131,132] Neonatal jaundice is a common manifestation of PK deficiency and, if pronounced, may herald a severe course. Kernicterus, although rare, has been described. In severely affected cases, patients require chronic transfusion therapy. A particularly severe form of PK deficiency has been described in the Dutch Amish population in Pennsylvania.[133] As a result of the chronic hemolysis, other common clinical complications can result (Table 9.4).

An interesting aspect of PK deficiency is the ability of many of these patients to tolerate day-to-day life with hemoglobin levels as low as 6–7 g/dL. This is due to the fact that the PK defect is downstream from the production of 2,3-DPG. Patients can have high erythrocyte 2,3-DPG levels, which shifts the hemoglobin oxygen dissociation curve to the right, favoring oxygen delivery to the tissues.[134] Nonetheless, patients with severe anemia can have increased myocardial

Table 9.4 Clinical signs and symptoms in pyruvate kinase deficiency.

Hepatomegaly
Splenomegaly
Hyperbilirubinemia
Jaundice
Gallstones/cholecystitis
Iron overload causing liver damage
Skin ulcers
Aplastic crisis caused by infection

hypertrophy due to increased cardiac output secondary to the anemia.

Iron overload is also common in patients with PK deficiency and has been reported in more than half of nontransfusion-dependent patients.[135] The degree of iron overload can be exacerbated in patients who have undergone splenectomy or have defects in the *HFE* gene.

In severely affected children there may be growth delay and skeletal changes due to expanded erythropoiesis. Spinal cord compression due to extramedullary hematopoiesis has been described.[136] Exacerbation of hemolysis in PK deficiency may occur during intercurrent infection and, less consistently, in pregnancy[137] and during oral contraceptive use.[138] Quite often pregnancy is uncomplicated, with no adverse effects on maternal or fetal well-being.

Diagnosis

The presence of characteristic changes in red cell morphology, unusual among glycolytic disorders, may assist in the diagnosis of PK deficiency.[139] Typically, there is slight macrocytosis and poikilocytosis with ovalocytes and elliptocytes accompanied by polychromasia and occasional contracted crenated red cells (spheroechinocytes). The latter are accentuated after splenectomy. Patients with chronic hemolysis can have elevated LDH levels, low haptoglobin, and hyperbilirubinemia. Biochemically, PK deficiency is heterogeneous. Homozygotes typically exhibit < 25% and heterozygotes 40–60% residual enzyme activity. There is, however, considerable overlap and some PK-deficient variants are associated with normal or minimally reduced activity *in vitro*. Quantitative assays should be performed at high and low substrate concentrations in the presence or absence of the allosteric effector FDP in order to detect PK variants with abnormal kinetic properties. Accumulation of glycolytic intermediates preceding the PK step in glycolysis, particularly PEP, 2-phosphoglycerate, 3-PG, and 2,3-DPG,[140] but sometimes extending proximally due to feedback inhibition of other glycolytic enzymes by 2,3-DPG provides evidence of defective function *in vivo*. ATP formation is reduced but in the presence of marked reticulocytosis absolute levels may be normal. An increase in the ratio of 2,3-DPG to ATP has been found to be a more reliable predictor of PK deficiency.[141] The

majority of PK variants exhibit reduced stability and/or altered kinetic properties *in vitro*. The interpretation of kinetic studies in PK deficiency is complicated in compound heterozygotes by the varying proportion of tetramers formed by the two mutant subunits. As there are common mutations in patients with PK deficiency, DNA analysis can be performed for the diagnosis both prenatally and postnatally.[124,142]

Treatment

Therapy for PK deficiency is supportive. In fetal anemia with hydrops, intrauterine transfusions may need to be performed. In neonates with hyperbilirubinemia, exchange transfusion may be needed and then followed by chronic transfusions. As PK-deficient patients have high levels of 2,3-DPG, transfusions should be based on clinical symptoms and not the level of hemoglobin.

In severely affected patients who require prolonged transfusions, splenectomy can be performed. Delay until after the age of 5, if possible, is advisable. Splenectomy does not stop the hemolysis but removal of the spleen is accompanied by a rise in hemoglobin, which typically stabilizes at 1–3 g/dL higher than the level before splenectomy. There is a paradoxical rise in reticulocyte count that accompanies splenectomy, sometimes reaching 40–60%. It is important to note that there have been case reports of thrombosis in PK-deficient patients after splenectomy.[143,144]

Folic acid can be given to patients with PK deficiency as there is rapid cell turnover and there are no contraindications to do so. However, iron should be avoided in these patients as iron overload is a common problem in PK-deficient patients. It is important to monitor all patients with PK deficiency for signs and chemical levels suggestive of iron overload, especially if they have had a splenectomy or have a mutation of the *HFE* gene.

Bone marrow transplantation has been performed with success in one severely affected patient.[145] Gene transfer studies have been successful in animal models,[146,147] but a great deal of work remains before clinical trials are available.

Disorders of the hexose monophosphate shunt

Glucose 6-dehydrogenase deficiency

G6PD catalyzes the initial step in the HMP shunt. Though ubiquitously expressed by all cells, the pathophysiologic consequences of G6PD deficiency are confined almost exclusively to red blood cells, which lack the capacity to synthesize the enzyme and are inherently vulnerable to endogenous oxidative damage because of their role in oxygen transport. Through oxidation, G6PD converts G6P to 6PG and reduces NADP to NADPH in the process. This is the erythrocyte's only means of regenerating its supply of NADPH, which is crucial for maintaining glutathione levels and preventing oxidative damage to the red blood cell. G6PD deficiency is the most common human enzyme deficiency, with an estimated 400 million people affected. It was first described in the 1950s after a group of patients had a hemolytic crisis after taking the antimalarial drug primaquine.[5] It was quickly determined that patients with this deficiency do not have a chronic hemolytic process and are usually asymptomatic. As the metabolic role of G6PD has little to do with providing energy to the red blood cell, hemolysis only occurs when the red cell is under oxidative stress. G6PD deficiency is an X-linked disorder.

The enzyme

The gene for G6PD has been localized to the X chromosome (Xq28)[148] and has been cloned.[149,150] It comprises 13 exons encoding 515 amino acids and a GC-rich promoter. The active form of G6PD is a dimer that contains two binding sites for NADP and G6P.[151] The enzyme activity is the same in both males and females as one of the X chromosomes remains inactive. Hemizygous males carrying a defective variant gene express the deficiency, whereas most heterozygote women are clinically normal with a normal G6PD level in approximately 50% of their red cells. Those deficient cells in females are still susceptible to oxidative hemolysis.

Since the discovery of G6PD deficiency, over 300 variants of the gene have been reported.[152] The variants are almost all missense point mutations causing single amino acid substitutions.[153] There have been a few mutations described caused by small deletions.[154] Large deletions or frameshift mutations have not been identified and are thought to be incompatible with life.[152] Of the mutations, those that cause milder forms are not found in the C-terminal portion of the enzyme. There is a cluster of mutations that causes severe G6PD deficiency within exon 10, which encodes the amino acid sequence involved in the formation of the active dimer of the enzyme.[153]

G6PD variants have been classified by the World Heath Organization according to the level of residual enzyme activity and associated clinical manifestations (Table 9.5). The variants can also be divided into two forms, sporadic mutations and polymorphic mutations. Sporadic mutations are usually associated with more severe types of G6PD deficiency (class 1). Polymorphic mutations of G6PD have prevailed as they transfer a protective effect against malaria. These mutations tend to be less severe (class II or III) and do not outweigh the advantage of malaria protection; they have thus been transmitted throughout populations.[146,147,148]

Common G6PD variants include the following:
- *G6PD B.* This is considered the wild-type G6PD. It is found in most Caucasians, Asians and Blacks. In Black Africans there is another variant, G6PD A, which is found in 20–30% of this population. The A variant has an activity of approximately 90% of the wild type and people have normal phenotypes. The mutation in this variant is at nucleotide 376, which results in an Asn→Asp substitution.[155]
- *G6PD A⁻.* This is the most common variant, associated with mild to moderate hemolysis. It is found in 10–15% of African Blacks and African-Americans and has an enzyme activity of 10–15%. This variant has two mutations within the gene. The first mutation is the same one that results in the A variant. The second mutation occurs 95% of the time at nucleotide 202, resulting in a Val→Met substitution. There are less frequent mutations at nucleotide 680 or 968.[156]
- *G6PD Mediterranean variant.* This is the most common abnormal variant found in Caucasians. It is a single-base substitution at nucleotide 563 that causes a Ser→Phe substitution.[155] This causes a decrease in protein synthesis and therefore the enzyme's catalytic activity is much reduced, resulting in severe hemolysis (class II).[157]

Protection against malaria

There is a geographical correlation in the distribution of polymorphic variants of G6PD deficiency with areas known to be endemic for *Plasmodium falciparum* malaria. The mechanism for malaria resistance in G6PD deficiency is not known but there are multiple theories. One possibility is that after a deficient cell is infected with the parasite, there is an increase in oxidative stress in the cell and because of the deficient enzyme an increase in toxic oxidized species that impair the growth of the parasite.[156] Another possibility is that due to oxidative stress there is an increase in methemoglobin and Heinz body formation, causing membrane damage. In addition to the production of methemoglobin, ferriheme may be

Table 9.5 Classification of glucose 6-phosphate dehydrogenase variants.

Class	Enzyme activity (% of normal)	Examples	Clinical effects
I	Variable and rare (<10)	San Diego	CNSHA
II	<10	Mediterranean, Canton	AHA, NNJ
III	10–60	A⁻	AHA, NNJ
IV	100	A, B*	None
V	>100	Verona	None

* Wild type.
AHA, acute hemolytic anemia; CNSHA, chronic nonspherocytic hemolytic anemia; NNJ, neonatal jaundice.

released, which is also cytolytic. Both Heinz body formation and ferriheme can promote phagocytosis of the infected red cell by the reticuloendothelial system.[158,159]

Pathophysiology of hemolysis

Red cells deficient in G6PD cannot replete their glutathione reserves, which leaves them at risk from oxidative damage by other sulfhydryl-containing proteins as the glutathione diminishes. Oxidation of the sulfhydryl groups on hemoglobin leads to the formation of methemoglobin or sulfhemoglobin, which forms the insoluble Heinz bodies that attach to and damage the red cell membrane. There is also oxidation of membrane proteins, which causes the red cell to be less deformable and thus susceptible to phagocytosis in the spleen. Red blood cells can hemolyze intravascularly, especially in patients with very low levels of G6PD activity.

Clinical signs and symptoms

Acute hemolytic anemia

Under conditions of oxidative stress, acute hemolysis may occur abruptly in a child with G6PD deficiency who at other times is clinically well. Not all individuals, even those with the same G6PD variant, are equally susceptible. The most common trigger is infection followed by drugs or other exogenous oxidants. Table 9.6 lists common drugs associated with hemolysis. The release of peroxides generated during phagocytosis of bacteria may be important in triggering hemolysis during bacterial infection. Pneumonia, β-hemolytic streptococcal infection, viral hepatitis, *Escherichia coli* infection, and typhoid are particularly likely to precipitate hemolysis in children with G6PD deficiency.[160] More tenuously, diabetic ketoacidosis and hypoglycemia have been linked to acute hemolysis in G6PD-deficient subjects.[161]

The course and severity of acute hemolysis in G6PD deficiency is highly variable. Males are more frequently affected than females. The onset usually follows within 2–3 days of oxidative challenge. Constitutional symptoms, including irritability and lethargy, may herald overt hemolysis. Typically, these are followed by the development of fever sometimes accompanied by gastrointestinal symptoms. Hemoglobinuria ensues, the cardinal sign of intravascular hemolysis, with dark-red or brown urine often colloquially described as the color of Coca-Cola. This precedes or coincides with the onset of jaundice and is accompanied by signs of anemia with pallor, tachycardia and, if the hemolysis is severe, hypovolemic shock. The degree of anemia is variable but may be extremely severe. Other causes of intravascular hemolysis, such as *P. falciparum* malaria ("blackwater fever"), hemolytic transfusion reaction, autoimmune hemolysis, microangiopathy, paroxysmal cold hemoglobinuria, paroxysmal nocturnal hemoglobinuria, *Clostridium welchii* septicemia and

Table 9.6 Drugs associated with hemolysis in glucose 6-phosphate dehydrogenase deficiency.

Antimalarials
Primaquine
Pentaquine
Pamaquine

Sulfonamides and sulfones
Sulfanilamide
Sulfacetamide
Sulfapyridine
Sulfamethoxazole
Dapsone

Other antibacterial agents
Nitrofurantoin
Nalidixic acid
Chloramphenicol
Ciprofloxacin

Analgesic/antipyretic
Acetanilid
Acetylsalicylic acid (aspirin)

Miscellaneous
Probenecid
Dimercaprol
Vitamin K analogs
Naphthalene (mothballs)
Methylene blue
Ascorbic acid

babesiosis, should be considered in the differential diagnosis where appropriate.

Neonatal jaundice

Neonates born with G6PD deficiency are at increased risk for hyperbilirubinemia. The consequences can be serious and, if untreated, may have irreversible neurologic sequelae. In Africa and Southeast Asia, G6PD deficiency is a common cause of kernicterus.[162] Although early reports highlighted the prevalence of neonatal jaundice in Mediterranean and Southeast Asian infants, this complication affects all indigenous and immigrant populations in which G6PD deficiency occurs. Jaundice develops later than in Rhesus alloimmunization, typically on the second or third day of life, but can occur within the first day of life.[163] A hemolytic component may predominate when neonatal exposure occurs to oxidants,[164] for example drugs or naphthalene in the form of mothballs or in clothing. In the majority of cases, hyperbilirubinemia occurs in the absence of increased red cell breakdown or external exposure to oxidants. It is felt that the underlying mechanism of hyperbilirubinemia is primarily hepatic in origin.[165,166] Supporting this finding is that neonates with G6PD Mediterranean have a partial defect in bilirubin glucuronide conjugation similar to that seen in Gilbert disease.[167,168]

Favism

Hemolysis following ingestion of broad beans (*Vicia faba*), or favism, usually occurs within 1 day of ingestion of the beans. The highest incidence occurs in young boys. People who have hemolysis after ingestion of fava beans are always deficient in G6PD but not all variants are susceptible to this. The variant that is classically associated with favism is G6PD Mediterranean,[152] although it can occur in other variants including G6PD A⁻.[169] Variability in sensitivity to fava beans among individuals with G6PD deficiency and even in the same individual at different times suggests other factors, including perhaps absorption and metabolism of the toxic constituents. Maternal ingestion of fava beans[170] has been reported to cause hydrops fetalis *in utero* and to lead to hemolysis in breast-fed infants with G6PD deficiency.[171] Favism has even been attributed to inhalation of bean pollen.[172] The pyrimidine aglycones divicine and isouramil have been implicated as the toxic component of fava beans.[173,174] These chemicals deplete the red cell's glutathione stores and reduce the activity of catalase, both of which are important in reducing reactive oxidant species in the red cell.

Chronic nonspherocytic hemolytic anemia

In contrast to the episodic pattern of hemolysis associated with polymorphic G6PD variants, patients with class I G6PD deficiency have such low enzyme activity that they will have lifelong chronic hemolytic anemia. This will occur in the absence of oxidant stressors such as drug exposure and, to date, 90 variants have been classified as class I causing chronic nonspherocytic hemolytic anemia.[175] Such cases are usually sporadic and show no geographic or ethnic prediliction. All reported cases have been male. Neonatal jaundice, sometimes severe, is often the first manifestation. After infancy the clinical expression varies, from patients showing compensated hemolysis to those who become transfusion dependent. Most will have hemoglobin levels of 8–10 g/dL, with an elevated reticulocyte count. This reflects the heterogeneity of molecular defects among class I G6PD variants. Hemolysis in patients can be exacerbated by oxidative stress, particularly during intercurrent infection, and is occasionally accompanied by frank hemoglobinuria.

Even medications that are safe in patients with class II or III G6PD deficiency can cause hemolysis in class I patients. The spleen, though typically only moderately increased in size, may be sufficiently enlarged to cause hypersplenism. In the steady state, hemolysis is primarily extravascular, as evidenced by the absence of hemoglobinuria.

Diagnosis

The diagnosis of G6PD deficiency is usually recognized after an acute hemolytic crisis due to infection or after drug exposure. It is evidenced by the presence of characteristic poikilocytes, including "hemighosts" and "bite cells" on a blood smear. There may be marked reticulocytosis. Heinz bodies may be visualized by supravital staining with methyl violet. Since Heinz bodies are removed by the spleen and red cells containing them are rapidly destroyed, their appearance may be transient. Serum haptoglobin is absent. The urine may be described as the color of tea or Coca-Cola. These patients will have a negative Coombs test.

The fluorescent spot test is the oldest and most reliable screening test for G6PD.[30,31] It is based on the fluorescence of NADPH after G6P and NAD are added to a hemolysate of test cells. A new diagnostic kit to detect patients with < 50% G6PD activity has been described (see p. 174).[32,33] Other screening tests such as the methemoglobin reduction test measure the transfer of hydrogen ions from NADPH to an acceptor, in this case methemoglobin. The diagnosis of G6PD deficiency can also be confirmed by a quantitative assay of red cell activity, which measures by spectrophotometry the reduction of NADP to NADPH in the presence of G6P.[35]

A positive screening test should be confirmed by quantitative enzyme assay. Caution must be exercised in interpretation since false-negative results may occur. This rarely occurs in hemizygous Caucasian males but is more of an issue in heterozygous females and African-Americans (G6PD A⁻ enzyme activity is relatively well preserved in young red cells). This is especially true immediately after a hemolytic crisis and during the compensatory reticulocytosis. In practice, these limitations can usually be circumvented by assaying enzyme activity separately in old and young red cells fractionated by centrifugation, relating G6PD activity to that of another age-dependent enzyme (e.g., HK) performing a confirmatory test 2–3 months after the hemolytic crisis or by studying family members.

A specific problem arises in the diagnosis of chronic nonspherocytic hemolytic anemia in a G6PD-deficient child who originates from a population in which the prevalence of G6PD deficiency is high. In this situation, biochemical characterization of the G6PD variant is necessary. If this proves to be a common variant, an alternative explanation for chronic hemolysis must be sought. Genotypic diagnosis, which is feasible by rapid techniques for several polymorphic G6PD variants, is also useful in this context.

The diagnosis of G6PD deficiency in heterozygous females warrants special mention. Unbalanced mosaicism in favor of cells in which the active chromosome carries the wild-type G6PD allele may render the enzyme activity of a red cell lysate normal. In this situation (and after red cell transfusion), cytochemical staining with tetrazolium, which is capable of detecting minor populations of Gd⁻ red cells, may be helpful.[176] Somatic selection in favor of Gd⁺ red cells may also mask the heterozygous phenotype, particularly in the case of severely deficient variants.[177] If a common variant is suspected, genetic studies can be done on the family. New rapid microarray-based assays have also been developed to detect G6PD deficiency in specific populations.[34]

Treatment and prevention

Prevention plays an important role in reducing the risk of drug-induced hemolysis and favism in G6PD deficiency. In Sardinia, prospective neonatal screening combined with health education has resulted in a decline in the incidence of favism among children with G6PD deficiency.[178] In Singapore, screening has essentially eliminated kernicterus in the newborn.[179] Immunization against hepatitis A has been proposed, as this virus can cause significant hemolysis.[180] Once the diagnosis of G6PD deficiency has been made, parents should be counseled regarding avoidance of oxidants and the risk of hemolysis due to an infection. A list of drugs capable of causing hemolysis should be provided and screening of family members should be initiated. If it is necessary to give an individual with G6PD deficiency a drug that can cause hemolysis, such as primaquine for the treatment of *P. vivax* or *P. malariae* infection, dose reduction may reduce hemolysis to a tolerable level.[181,182]

Transfusion

Blood transfusion may be required and although no didactic rules apply, useful guidelines have been recommended by Luzzatto.[183] These advise immediate transfusion if the hemoglobin level is less than 7 g/dL or between 7 and 9 g/dL in the face of hemoglobinuria. At higher hemoglobin levels it may be justified to withhold transfusion, providing the child is kept under close observation and transfusion instigated if the hemoglobin falls below the threshold identified above. As G6PD deficiency is common in the population, blood donors can be G6PD deficient. Therefore, avoidance of transfusion with G6PD-deficient red cells is theoretically desirable, although in practice difficult to achieve. Recovery of hemoglobin to steady-state levels may take 3–6 weeks. This is quicker in the case of G6PD variants (e.g., A−) where enzyme activity is relatively well preserved in reticulocytes, making them less susceptible to destruction.

Neonatal jaundice

With respect to management, the degree of hyperbilirubinemia that triggers the need for phototherapy or exchange transfusion follows conventional criteria, adjusted for birthweight. A lower threshold may be applied in the face of rapid hemolysis. Prompt correction of hypoxia, acidosis, sepsis and other factors that exacerbate jaundice in the G6PD-deficient neonate is important. It is more important in neonates who require exchange transfusions to use blood from donors not deficient in G6PD.[152]

Chronic nonspherocytic hemolytic anemia

Individuals with type I G6PD deficiency will need more care throughout their lifetime. Patients usually have mild to moderate anemia and transfusion should be used only if the patient is symptomatic. Splenectomy has not had any significant benefit in these patients.[184] As with other chronic hemolytic anemias, patients may have increased iron absorption and they should be monitored for iron overload. They should also be evaluated for hereditary hemochromatosis as this puts them at even higher risk for iron overload. As a result of chronic hemolysis, they can also develop gallstones, causing cholecystitis, and prophylactic cholecystectomy can be considered. Care should still be taken to counsel these patients with regard to infection and oxidant medications as this can exacerbate hemolysis. Vitamin E can be given to these patients as an antioxidant, but its effect is controversial.[185,186] Folic acid can be given to these patients due to the rapid cell turnover.

Deficiencies of glutathione reductase, glutathione peroxidase, and glutathione synthesis

Glutathione, a tripeptide composed of glutamic acid, cysteine and glycine, is synthesized via sequential reactions catalyzed by γ-glutamylcysteine synthetase and glutathione synthetase. Glutathione is present in the red cell at millimolar concentrations, and in its reduced form (GSH) provides the main defense against oxidative damage. The conversion of harmful peroxides to water is catalyzed by glutathione peroxidase. Intracellular levels of GSH are maintained by both regeneration from oxidized glutathione, catalyzed by glutathione reductase, and *de novo* synthesis.

Of the two main enzymes of the HMP shunt, only deficiency of glutathione reductase has been reported to cause hemolysis, which has been reported in three siblings born of a consanguineous marriage.[21] Early cases of glutathione reductase deficiency have subsequently been shown to be due to inadequate synthesis of its cofactor, flavin-adenine dinucleotide, secondary to nutritional riboflavin deficiency.[187]

Of the enzymes involved in glutathione synthesis, hemolytic anemia due to γ-glutamylcysteine synthetase deficiency has been described, although it is very rare.[20] In one case, an affected patient developed progressive spinocerebellar ataxia.[188] Glutathione synthetase deficiency is the most common metabolic defect to cause GSH deficiency. Over 20 families with the condition have been reported.[19] Two phenotypes are recognized: when the enzyme deficiency is isolated to the red cell, there is mild hemolytic anemia, which may be exacerbated by oxidant stress; if all tissues are deficient in glutathione synthetase, this may result in a multisystem disorder characterized by hemolysis, metabolic acidosis, neurologic abnormalities, neutropenia, and susceptibility to bacterial infection. Acidosis is caused by the accumulation of 5-oxoproline, a metabolic product of γ-glutamylcysteine. Urinary excretion of 5-oxoproline is markedly elevated. Vitamin E has been used with clinical benefit in patients with recurrent infection,[189] but its overall efficacy is still under question.[190] As with G6PD deficiency, exposure to drugs with oxidative potential should be avoided.

Disorders of erythrocyte nucleotide metabolism

Pyrimidine 5'-nucleotidase deficiency

P5′N or uridine monophosphate hydrolase (UMPH) is involved in the removal of pyrimidines from the red blood cell, because ribosomal RNA is no longer needed for protein synthesis and the pyrimidines need to be removed from the cell. P5′N catalyzes the dephosphorylation of pyrimidine nucleoside monophosphates to their corresponding nucleosides. The nucleosides, uridine and cytidine, then diffuse across the red cell membrane. This allows the red cell to preserve phosphates and purines for ATP synthesis. P5′N deficiency is an autosomal recessive trait. It was initially described by Valentine et al.[191–193]

The enzyme

P5′N is a protein that exists as two isozymes, P5′N-1 and P5′N-2,[194] that have different substrate specificities and which are encoded by separate structural loci. P5′N-2 is localized to chromosome 17q23.2,[195] P5′N-1 to chromosome 7p15.[196] The predominant enzyme in the maturing red blood cell is P5′N-1 and is the more active of the two enzymes. It requires magnesium for activity. The associated defects causing hemolytic anemia are the result of a deficiency in P5′N-1 (UMPH-1). To date, 16 mutations have been described in the P5′N-1 gene.[196–199] They involve missense mutations, nonsense mutations, and large deletions causing decreased function of the enzyme. If the ribosomal RNAs remain and the pyrimidine nucleic acids cannot be removed, intracellular aggregates of RNA will accumulate within the cell. Approximately 40 cases have been reported.[200]

How intracellular accumulation of pyrimidines causes hemolysis is not known. Selective accumulation of CDP choline and CDP ethanolamine occurs in P5′N-1 deficiency and this may have an effect on structural aspects of the red cell membrane. Inhibition of glycolysis or adenine nucleotide salvage through competition of UTP and CTP with ATP has been postulated, as well as the fact that pyrimidines are strong chelators of magnesium that may inhibit other enzymes.[201]

Clinical signs and symptoms

Deficiency of P5′N is associated with hemolytic anemia of mild to moderate severity that may worsen during infection or pregnancy. The degree of anemia is variable, with hemoglobin levels ranging from 7.5 to 10 g/dL. The age of presentation ranges from infancy to adult life, but the majority of patients present at a younger age. They will have a reticulocytosis and also hyperbilirubinemia. Patients may have jaundice, pallor, and splenomegaly. A conspicuous feature of P5′N deficiency is basophilic stippling (ribonucleoprotein aggregates) due to impaired degradation of RNA, which may be visible in up to 5% of red cells. P5′N is also expressed in brain, kidney and spleen tissue.[202] Of note, mental retardation has been described in some P5′N-deficient individuals.[203]

It is also important to note that acquired P5′N deficiency is seen in lead poisoning[204] and underlies the mechanism of lead-induced hemolytic anemia.[205] P5′N is sensitive to inactivation by low concentrations of lead and exposed individuals show a dose-dependent depression of nucleotidase activity. Patients with severe acute lead toxicity have enzyme levels comparable to those found in homozygous deficiency states.

Diagnosis

A blood smear needs to be observed to look for basophilic stippling. Blood collected in EDTA must be examined fresh, since stippling is no longer discernible after 3 hours. P5′N is increased in young red cells.[206] When corrected for reticulocytosis, the enzyme activity in homozygous P5′N deficiency is generally about 5% of that in normal red cells. Normally, adenosine phosphates account for at least 97% of cellular nucleotides, causing ultraviolet absorption at 257 nm during spectral analysis. In P5′N deficiency, there is a much higher concentration of pyrimidine compounds and this shifts the ultraviolet absorption spectrum from the normal peak at 257 nm to 265–270 nm.[200] The diagnosis may be confirmed by measuring the enzyme levels directly.

Recently, patients with β-thalassemia and hemoglobin E have been shown to have low levels of P5′N deficiency and this can contribute to a marked increase in instability of these thalassemias.[207] Although the underlying mechanism is unknown, this suggests that the milieu of P5′N-deficient red cells may accentuate oxidative damage, a finding of potential importance in understanding the pathophysiology of HbE/β-thalassemia.

Treatment

Patients with P5′N deficiency are usually not transfusion dependent. However, in the presence of worsening anemia due to infection, especially with parvovirus B19, fever and pregnancy, patients may require intermittent red blood cell transfusion. Although patients with P5′N deficiency have splenomegaly, splenectomy has variable results and might be reserved to help those patients who are more severely affected.[208]

Adenosine deaminase overexpression

Adenosine deaminase (ADA) deaminates adenosine and 2′-deoxyadenosine to inosine and 2′-deoxyinosine respectively.

The ADA gene is localized to chromosome 20.[209] The mutations produce an increased expression, causing depletion of ATP. Clinically, overproduction of ADA is characterized by a well-compensated hemolytic anemia showing dominant inheritance. Red cell ADA levels are increased up to 100-fold, reflecting upregulation of transcription of the ADA gene. This phenomenon appears specific to red cells, since ADA levels in other cells are normal. Linkage studies indicate that the genetic defect responsible lies in *cis* rather than *trans* to the ADA gene,[210] but its identity remains obscure. Cases are very rare, with only 14 reported in the world's literature.

References

1. Beutler E. The red cell. In: *Hemolytic Anemia in Disorders of Red Cell Metabolism*. New York: Plenum, 1978, pp. 1–21.
2. Selwyn JG, Dacie JV. Autohemolysis and other changes resulting from the incubation *in vitro* of red cells from patients with congenital hemolytic anemia. *Blood* 1954; **9**: 414–38.
3. Robinson MA, Loder PB, De Gruchy GC. Red cell metabolism in non-spherocytic congenital haemolytic anemia. *Br J Haematol* 1961; **7**: 327–39.
4. Valentine WN, Tanaka KR, Miwa S *et al.* A specific erythrocyte glycolytic enzyme defect (pyruvate kinase) in three subjects with congenital non-spherocytic hemolytic anemia. *Trans Assoc Am Physicians* 1961; **74**: 100–10.
5. Carson PE, Flanagan CL, Ickes CE, Alving AS. Enzymatic deficiency in primaquine sensitive erythrocytes. *Science* 1956; **124**: 484–5.
6. Paglia DE, Shende A, Lanzkowsky P *et al.* Hexokinase "New Hyde Park": low activity erythrocyte isoenzyme in a Chinese kindred. *Am J Hematol* 1981; **10**: 107–17.
7. Bianchi M, Maganani M. Hexokinase mutations that produce nonspherocytic hemolytic anemia. *Blood Cells Mol Dis* 1995; **21**: 2–8.
8. Huppke P, Wünsch D, Pekrun A *et al.* Glucose phosphate isomerase deficiency: biochemical and molecular genetic studies on the enzyme variants of two patients with severe haemolytic anaemia. *Eur J Pediatr* 1997; **156**: 605–9.
9. Fujii H, Miwa S. Other erythrocyte enzyme deficiencies associated with non-haematological symptoms: phosphoglycerate kinase and phosphofructokinase deficiency. *Baillières Best Pract Res Clin Haematol* 2000; **13**: 141–8.
10. Yao DC, Tolan DR, Murray MF *et al.* Hemolytic anemia and severe rhabdomyolysis caused by compound heterozygous mutations of the gene for erythrocyte/muscle isozyme of aldolase, ALDOA$^{(Arg303X/Cys338Tyr)}$. *Blood* 2004; **103**: 2401–3.
11. Schneider AS. Triosephosphate isomerase deficiency: historical perspective and molecular aspects. *Baillières Best Pract Res Clin Haematol* 2000; **13**: 119–40.
12. MacMullin MF. The molecular basis of disorders of red cell enzymes. *J Clin Pathol* 1999; **52**: 241–4.
13. Rosa R, Prehu M-O, Beuzard Y, Rosa J. The first case of a complete deficiency of diphosphoglycerate mutase in human erythrocytes. *J Clin Invest* 1978; **62**: 907–15.
14. Tsujino S, Shanske S, Sakoda S *et al.* The molecular genetic basis of muscle phosphoglycerate mutase (PGAM) deficiency. *Am J Hum Genet* 1993; **52**: 472–7.
15. Lachant NA, Jennings MA, Tanaka KR. Partial erythrocyte enolase deficiency: a hereditary disorder with variable clinical expression. *Blood* 1986; **65**: A55.
16. Hirono A, Kanno H, Miwa S, Beutler E. Pyruvate kinase deficiency and other enzymopathies of the red cell. In: Scriver CR, Beaudet AL, Sly WS, Valle D (eds) *The Metabolic and Molecular Bases of Inherited Disease*, 8th edn. New York: McGraw-Hill, 2001, pp. 4637–64.
17. Sudo K, Maekawa M, Ikawa S *et al.* A missense mutation found in human lactate dehydrogenase-B (H) variant gene. *Biochem Biophys Res Commun* 1990; **168**: 672–6.
18. Beutler E. Glucose-6-dehydrogenase deficiency. *N Engl J Med* 1991; **324**: 169–74.
19. Hirono A, Iyori H, Sekine I *et al.* Three cases of hereditary nonspherocytic hemolytic anemia associated with red blood cell glutathione deficiency. *Blood* 1996; **87**: 2071–4.
20. Beutler E, Moroose R, Kramer L *et al.* Gamma-glutamylcysteine synthetase deficiency and hemolytic anemia. *Blood* 1990; **75**: 271–3.
21. Loos H, Roos D, Weening R, Houwerzill J. Familial deficiency of glutathione reductase in human blood cells. *Blood* 1976; **48**: 53–62.
22. Paglia DE, Valentine WN. Haemolytic anaemia associated with disorders of the purine and pyrimidine salvage pathways. *Clin Haematol* 1981; **10**: 81–98.
23. Valentine WN, Paglia DE *et al.* Herediatry hemolytic anemia with increased red cell adenosine deaminase (45 to 70-fold) and decreased adenosine triphosphate. *Science* 1977; **195**: 783–5.
24. Perignon JL, Hamet M *et al.* Biochemical study of a case of hemolytic anemia with increased (85-fold) cell adenosine deaminase. *Clin Chim Acta* 1982; **124**: 205–12.
25. Kanno H, Tani K *et al.* Adenosine deaminase (ADA) overproduction associated with congenital hemolytic anemia: case report and molecular analysis. *Jpn J Exp Med* 1988; **58**: 1–8.
26. Thomas HM III, Lefrak SS, Irwin RS *et al.* The oxyhemoglobin dissociation curve in health and disease. Role of 2,3-diphosphoglycerate. *Am J Med* 1974; **57**: 331–48.
27. Ahmed N, Battah, S, Karachalias N *et al.* Increased formation of methylgloxal and protein glycation, oxidation and nitrosation in triosephosphate isomerase deficiency. *Biochim Biophys Acta* 2003; **1639**: 121–32.
28. Boivin P, Galand C, Andre R, Debray J. Anémies hémolytiques congenitales avec deficit isole en glutathion reduit par deficit en glutathione synthetase. *Nouv Rev Fr Hematol* 1966; **6**: 859–66.
29. Konrad PN, Richards F II, Valentine WN, Paglia DE. Gammaglutamyl-cysteine synthetase deficiency. *N Engl J Med* 1972; **286**: 557–61.
30. Beutler E, Mitchell M. Special modifications of the fluorescent screening method for glucose-6-phosphate dehydrogenase deficiency. *Blood* 1968; **32**: 816–18.
31. Fairbanks VF, Beutler E. A simple method for detection of erythrocyte glucose-6-phosphate dehydrogenase (G-6-PD spot test) *Blood* 1962; **20**: 591.
32. Tantular IS, Kawamoto F. An improved, simple screening method for detection of glucose-6-phosphate dehydrogenase deficiency. *Trop Med Inter Health* 2003; **8**: 569–74.

33. Jalloh A, Tantular TS, Pusarawati S et al. Rapid epidemiologic assessment of glucose-6-phosphate dehydrogenase deficiency in malaria-endemic areas in Southeast Asia using a novel diagnostic kit. *Trop Med Inter Health* 2004; **9**: 615–23.

34. Bang-Ce Y, Hongquiong L, Zhensong L. Rapid detection of common Chinese glucose-6-phosphate dehydrogenase (G6PD) mutations by microarry-based assay. *Am J Hematol* 2004; **76**: 405–12.

35. Beutler E. *Red Cell Metabolism: A Manual of Biochemical Methods.* New York: Grune and Stratton, 1984.

36. International Committee for Standardization in Haematology. Recommended screening test for pyrimidine 5′-nucleotidase deficiency. *Clin Lab Haematol* 1989; **11**: 55–6.

37. Beutler E, Blume KG, Kaplan JC et al. International Committee for Standardization in Haematology: recommended methods for red cell enzyme analysis. *Br J Haematol* 1977; **35**: 331–40.

38. Konrad PN, Valentine WN, Paglia DE. Enzymatic activities and glutathione content of erythrocytes in the newborn: comparison with red cells of older normal subjects and those with comparable reticulocytosis. *Acta Haematol* 1972; **48**: 193–201.

39. Wilson JE. Hexokinase. *Rev Physiol Biochem Pharmacol* 1995; **126**: 65–198.

40. Murakami K, Blei, Tilton W et al. An isozyme of hexokinase specific for the human red blood cells (HK$_R$). *Blood* 1990; **75**: 770–5.

41. Shows TB, Eddy RL, Byers MG et al. Localization of the human hexokinase I gene (HK I) to chromosome 10q22. *Cytogenet Cell Genet* 1989; **51**: 1079a.

42. Murakami K, Blei F, Tilton W et al. Human HKR isozyme: organization of the hexokinase 1 gene, the erythroid-specific promoter, and transcription initiation site. *Mol Genet Metabol* 1999; **67**: 118–30.

43. Aleshin AE, Zeng C, Bourenkov GP, Bartunik HD, Fromm HJ, Honzatko RB. The mechanism of regulation of hexokinase: new insights from the crystal structure of recombinant human brain hexokinase complexed with glucose and glucose-6-phosphate. *Structure* 1998; **6**: 39–50.

44. Bianchi M, Crinelli R, Serafini G et al. Molecular bases of hexokinase deficiency. *Biochim Biophys Acta* 1997; **1360**: 211–21.

45. Kanno H. Hexokinase: gene structure and mutations. *Baillières Best Pract Res Clin Haematol* 2000; **13**: 83–8.

46. Gilsanz F, Meyer E, Paglia DE et al. Congenital hemolytic anemia due to hexokinase deficiency. *Am J Dis Child* 1978; **132**: 636–7.

47. Rijksen G, Akkerman JWN, Vandernwallbake AWL et al. Generalized hexokinase deficiency in the blood cells of a patient with nonspherocytic hemolytic anemia. *Blood* 1983; **61**: 12–18.

48. Newman P, Muir A, Parker AC. Non-spherocytic haemolytic anaemia in mother and son with hexokinase deficiency. *Br J Haematol* 1980; **46**: 537–47.

49. Kanno H, Ishikawa K, Fujii H et al. Severe hexokinase deficiency as a cause of hemolytic anemia, periventricular leucomalacia and intrauterine death of the fetus. *Blood* 1997; **80**: 8a.

50. Baughan MA, Valentine WN, Paglia DE et al. Hereditary hemolytic anemia associated with glucose phosphate isomerase (GPI) deficiency. A new enzyme defect of human erythrocytes. *Blood* 1968; **32**: 236–49.

51. McMorris FA, Chen TR, Ricciuti F et al. Chromosome assignments in man of the genes for two hexosephosphate isomerases. *Science* 1973; **179**: 1129–31.

52. Kugler W, Lakomek M. Glucose-6-phosphate isomerase deficiency. *Baillières Best Pract Res Clin Haematol* 2000; **13**: 89–101.

53. Chaput M, Claes V, Portetelle D et al. The neurotrophic factor neuroleukin is 90% homologous with phophohexose isomerase. *Nature* 1988; **332**: 454–5.

54. Faik P, Walker JIH, Redmill AAM, Morgan MJ. Mouse glucose-6-phosphate isomerase and neuroleukin have identical 3′ sequences. *Nature* 1988; **332**: 455–6.

55. Gurney ME, Belton AC, Cashman N, Antel JP. Inhibition of terminal axonal sprouting by serum from patients with amyotrophic lateral sclerosis. *N Engl J Med* 1984; **311**: 933–9.

56. Whitelaw AGL, Rogers PA, Hopkinson DA et al. Congenital haemolytic anaemia resulting from glucose phosphate isomerase deficiency: genetics, clinical picture, and prenatal diagnosis. *J Med Genet* 1979; **16**: 189–96.

57. Ravindranath Y, Paglia DE, Warrier I et al. Glucose phosphate isomerase deficiency as a cause of hydrops fetalis. *N Engl J Med* 1987; **316**: 258–61.

58. Goulding FJ. Priapism caused by glucose phosphate isomerase deficiency. *J Urol* 1976; **116**: 819–20.

59. Schroter W, Eber SW, Bardosi A et al. Generalized glucosephosphate isomerase (GPI) deficiency causing hemolytic anemia, neuromuscular symptoms and impairment of granulocytic function: a new syndrome due to a new stable GPI variant and diminished specific activity (GPI Homburg). *Eur J Pediatr* 1985; **144**: 301–5.

60. Kugler W, Breme K, Laspe P et al. Molecular basis of neurological dysfunction coupled with haemolytic anaemia in human glucose-6-phosphate isomerase (GPI) deficiency. *Hum Genet* 1997; **103**: 450–4.

61. Tauri S, Okuno G, Ikura Y et al. Phosphofructokinase deficiency in skeletal muscle: a new type of glycogenosis. *Biochem Biophys Res Commun* 1965; **19**: 517–23.

62. Howard T, Akots G, Bowden D. Physical and genetic mapping of the muscle phosphofructokinase gene (PFKM): reassignment to human chromosome 12q. *Genomics* 1996; **34**: 122–7.

63. Van Keuren M, Drabkin H, Hart I et al. Regional assignment of human liver-type 6-phosphofructokinase to chromosome 21q22.3 by using somatic cell hybrids and a monoclonal anti-L antibody. *Hum Genet* 1986; **74**: 34–40.

64. Morrison N, Simpson C, Fothergill-Gilmore L et al. Regional chromosomal assignment of the human platelet phosphofructokinase gene to 10p15. *Hum Genet* 1992; **89**: 105–6.

65. Raben N, Sherman JB. Mutations in muscle phosphofructokinase gene. *Hum Mutat* 1995; **6**: 1–6.

66. Sherman JB, Raben N, Nicastri C et al. Common mutations in the phosphofructokinase-M gene in Ashkenazi Jewish patients with glycogenesis VII and their population frequency. *Am J Hum Genet* 1994; **55**: 305–13.

67. Raben N, Sherman J, Miller F et al. A 5′ splice junction mutation leading to exon deletion in an Ashkenazic Jewish family with phosphofructokinase deficiency (Tarui disease). *J Biol Chem* 1993; **268**: 4963–7.

68. Haller RG, Lewis SF. Glucose-induced exertional fatigue in muscle phosphofructokinase deficiency. *N Engl J Med* 1991; **324**: 364–9.

69. Miwa S, Sato T, Murao H *et al*. A new type of phosphofructokinase deficiency: hereditary nonspherocytic hemolytic anemia. *Acta Haematol Jpn* 1972; **35**: 113–18.

70. Waterbury L, Frenkel EP. Hereditary nonspherocytic hemolysis with erythrocyte phosphofructokinase deficiency. *Blood* 1972; **39**: 415–25.

71. Amit R, Bashan N, Abarbanel JM *et al*. Fatal familial infantile glycogen storage disease: multisystem phosphofructokinase deficiency. *Muscle Nerve* 1992; **15**: 455–8.

72. Servidei S, Bonilla E, Diedrich RG *et al*. Fatal infantile form of phosphofructokinase deficiency. *Neurology* 1986; **36**: 1465–70.

73. Mineo I, Kono N, Hara N *et al*. Myogenic hyperuricemia. A common pathophysiologic feature of glycogenosis types III, V, and VII. *N Engl J Med* 1987; **317**: 75–80.

74. Duboc D, Jehenson P, Dinh ST *et al*. Phosphorus NMR spectroscopy study of muscular enzyme deficiencies involving glycogenolysis and glycolysis. *Neurology* 1987; **37**: 663–71.

75. Layzer RB, Rasmussen J. The molecular basis of muscle phosphofructokinase deficiency. *Arch Neurol* 1974; **31**: 411–17.

76. Raben N, Sherman JB, Adams E, *et al*. Various classes of mutations in patients with phosphofructokinase deficiency (Tarui's disease). *Muscle Nerve* 1995; **3**: S35–S38.

77. Swoboda KJ, Specht L, Jones HR *et al*. Infantile phosphofructokinase deficiency with arthrogryposis: clinical benefit of a ketogenic diet. *J Pediatr* 1997; **131**: 932–4.

78. Salvatore F, Izzo P, Paolella G. Aldolase gene and protein families: structure, expression and pathophysiology. In: Blasi F (ed.) *Horizons in Biochemistry and Biophysics*, vol. 8. Chichester: John Wiley & Sons, 1986, pp. 611–65.

79. Kikuta A, Yoshida MC, Sakakibara M *et al*. Molecular gene mapping for the structural gene for human aldolase A (ALDOA) to chromosome 22 [abstract]. *Cytogenet Cell Genet* 1985; **40**: 674.

80. Esposito G, Vitagliano L, Costanzo P. Human aldolase A natural mutants: relationship between flexibility of the C-terminal region and enzyme function. *Biochem J* 2004; **380**: 51–6.

81. Yao DC, Tolan DR, Murray MF *et al*. Hemolytic anemia and severe rhabdomyolysis caused by compound heterozygous mutations of the gene for erythrocyte/muscle isozyme of aldolase, ALDOA(Arg303X/Cys338Tyr). *Blood* 2004; **103**: 2401–3.

82. Kreuder J, Borkhardt A, Repp R *et al*. Inherited metabolic myopathy and hemolysis due to a mutation in aldolase A. *N Engl J Med* 1996; **334**: 1100–4.

83. Schneider AS, Valentine WN, Hattori M, Heins HL. Hereditary hemolytic anemia with triosephosphate isomerase deficiency. *N Engl J Med* 1965; **272**: 229–35.

84. Jongsma AP, Los WR, Hagemeijer A. Evidence for synteny between the human loci for triose phosphate isomerase, lactate dehydrogenase-B, and peptidase-B and the regional mapping of these loci on chromosome 12. *Cytogenet Cell Genet* 1974; **13**: 106–7.

85. Rethore MO, Kaplan JC, Junien C *et al*. 12pter to 12p12.2: possible assignment of human triose phosphate isomerase. *Hum Genet* 1977; **36**: 235–7.

86. Wilmshurst JM, Wise GA, Pollard JD, Ouvrier RA. Chronic axonal neuropathy with triosephosphate isomerase deficiency. *Pediatr Neurol* 2004; **30**: 146–8.

87. Schneider A, Westwood B, Yim C *et al*. Triosephosphate isomerase deficiency: repetitive occurrence of point mutation in amino acid 104 in multiple apparently unrelated families. *Am J Hematol* 1995; **50**: 263–8.

88. Valentine WN, Schneider AS, Baughan MA *et al*. Hereditary hemolytic anemia with triosephosphate isomerase deficiency. *Am J Med* 1966; **41**: 27–41.

89. Poll-The BW, Aicardi J, Girot R, Rosa R. Neurological findings in triosephosphate isomerase deficiency. *Ann Neurol* 1985; **17**: 439–43.

90. Harris SR, Paglia DE, Jaffe ER, Valentine WN, Klein RL. Triosephosphate isomerase deficiency in an adult [abstract]. *Clin Res* 1970; **18**: 529.

91. Hollan S, Fujii H, Hirono A *et al*. Hereditary triosephosphate isomerase (TPI) deficiency: two severely affected brothers, one with and one without neurological symptoms. *Hum Genet* 1993; **92**: 486–90.

92. Lazarow PB, Moser HW. Disorders of peroxisome biogenesis. In: Scriver CH, Beaudet AI, Sly WS, Valle D (eds) *The Metabolic and Molecular Bases of Inherited Disease*, vol. 2. New York: McGraw Hill, 1995, pp. 2287–324.

93. Ationu A, Humphries A, Wild B *et al*. Towards enzyme-replacement treatment in triosephosphate isomerase deficiency. *Lancet* 1999; **353**: 1155–6.

94. Ationu A, Humphries A, Lalloz MR *et al*. Reversal of metabolic block in glycolysis by enzyme replacement in triosephosphate isomerase-deficient cells. *Blood* 1999; **94**: 3193–8.

95. Kraus AP, Langston MF Jr, Lynch BL. Red cell phosphoglycerate kinase deficiency: a new cause of non-spherocytic hemolytic anemia. *Biochem Biophys Res Commun* 1968; **30**: 173–7.

96. Willard HF, Goss SJ, Holmes MT, Munroe DL. Regional localization of the phosphoglycerate kinase gene and pseudogene on the human X chromosome and assignment of a related DNA sequence to chromosome 19. *Hum Genet* 1985; **71**: 138–43.

97. Gartler SM, Riley DE, Lebo RV *et al*. Mapping of human autosomal phosphoglycerate kinase sequence to chromosome 19. *Somat Cell Mol Genet* 1986; **12**: 395–401.

98. Hamano T, Mutoh T, Sugie H *et al*. Phosphoglycerate kinase deficiency: an adult myopathic form with a novel mutation. *Neurology* 2000; **54**: 1188–90.

99. Rosa R, George C, Fardeau M *et al*. A new case of phosphoglycerate kinase deficiency: PGK Creteil associated with rhabdomyolysis and lacking hemolytic anemia. *Blood* 1982; **60**: 84–91.

100. Konrad PNJ, McCarthy DJ, Mauer AM *et al*. Erythrocyte and leukocyte phosphoglycerate kinase deficiency with neurologic disease. *J Pediatr* 1973; **82**: 456–60.

101. Beutler E. Electrophoresis of phosphoglycerate kinase. *Biochem Genet* 1969; **3**: 189–95.

102. Edwards Y, Sakoda S, Schon E *et al*. The gene for human muscle-specific phosphoglycerate mutase, PGAMM, mapped to chromosome 7 by polymerase chain reaction. *Genomics* 1989; **5**: 948–51.

103. Junien C, Despoisse S, Turleau C *et al*. Assignment of

phosphoglycerate mutase (PGAMA) to human chromosome 10: regional mapping of GOT1 and PGAMA sub-bands 10q26.1 (or q25.3). *Ann Genet* 1982; **25**: 25–7.

104. Lemarchandel V, Joulin V, Valentin C *et al.* Compound heterozygosity in a complete erythrocyte bisphosphoglycerate mutase deficiency. *Blood* 1992; **80**: 2643–9.

105. Giallongo A, Feo S, Moore R *et al.* Molecular cloning and nucleotide sequence of a full-length cDNA for human alpha enolase. *Proc Natl Acad Sci USA* 1986; **83**: 6741–5.

106. Satoh H, Tani K, Yoshida MC *et al.* The human liver-type pyruvate kinase (PKL) gene is on chromosome 1 at band q21. *Cytogenet Cell Genet* 1988; **47**: 132–3.

107. Noguchi T, Yamada K, Inoue H *et al.* The L- and R-type isozymes of rat pyruvate kinase are produced from a single gene by use of different promoters. *J Biol Chem* 1987; **262**: 14366–71.

108. Noguchi T, Inoue H, Tanaka T. The M1- and M2-type isozymes of rat pyruvate kinase are produced from the same gene by alternative RNA splicing. *J Biol Chem* 1986; **261**: 13807–12.

109. Tani K, Yoshida MC, Satoh H *et al.* Human M_2-type pyruvate kinase: cDNA cloning, chromosomal assignment and expression in hepatoma. *Gene* 1988; **73**: 509–16.

110. Takegawa S, Fujii H, Miwa S. Change of pyruvate kinase isozymes from M_2- to L-type during development of the red cell. *Br J Haematol* 1983; **54**: 467–74.

111. Marie J, Simon M-P, Dreyfus J-C, Kahn A. One gene, but two messenger RNAs encode liver L and red cell L' pyruvate kinase subunits. *Nature* 1981; **292**: 70–2.

112. Kahn A, Marie J, Garreau H, Sprengers ED. The genetic system of the L-type pyruvate kinase forms in man. Subunit structure, interrelation and kinetic characteristics of the pyruvate kinase enzymes from erythrocytes and liver. *Biochim Biophys Acta* 1978; **523**: 59–74.

113. Takegawa S, Miwa S. Change of pyruvate kinase (PK) isozymes in classical type PK deficiency and other PK deficiency cases during red cell maturation. *Am J Hematol* 1984; **16**: 53–8.

114. Max-Audit I, Rosa R, Marie J. Pyruvate kinase hyperactivity genetically determined: metabolic consequenes and molecular characterization. *Blood* 1980; **56**: 902–9.

115. Staal GEJ, Vansen G, Roos D. Pyruvate kinase and the "high ATP syndrome". *J Clin Invest* 1984; **74**: 231–5.

116. Zanella A, Bianchi P. Red cell pyruvate kinase deficiency: from genetics to clinical manifestations. *Baillèeres Best Pract Res Clin Haematol* 2000; **13**: 57–81.

117. Zanella A, Bianchi P, Fermo E *et al.* Molecular characterization of the PK-LR gene in sixteen pyruvate kinase-deficient patients. *Br J Haematol* 2001; **113**: 43–8.

118. Wang C, Chiarelli LR, Bianchi P. Human erythrocyte pyruvate kinase: characterization of the recombinant enzyme and a mutant form (R510Q) causing nonspherocytic hemolytic anemia. *Blood* 2001; **98**: 3113–20.

119. Muirhead H, Clayden DA, Barford D *et al.* The structure of cat muscle pyruvate kinase. *EMBO J* 1986; **5**: 475–81.

120. Van Solinge WW, van Wijk HA, Kraaijenhagen RJ *et al.* Novel mutations in the human red cell type pyruvate kinase gene: two promoter mutations in cis, a splice site mutation, a nonsense and three missense mutations [abstract]. *Blood* 1997; **90** (suppl. 1): 1197.

121. Zanella A, Bianchi P, Baronciani L *et al.* Molecular characterization of PK-LR gene in pyruvate kinase-deficient Italian patients. *Blood* 1997; **89**: 3847–52.

122. Kanno H, Fujii H, Miwa S. Molecular heterogeneity of pyruvate kinase deficiency identified by single strand conformational polymorphism (SSCP) analysis [abstract]. *Blood* 1994; **84** (suppl. 1): 13a.

123. Baronciani L, Beutler E. Molecular study of pyruvate kinase deficient patients with hereditary nonspherocytic hemolytic anemia. *J Clin Invest* 1995; **95**: 1702–9.

124. Baronciani L, Beutler E. Analysis of pyruvate kinase-deficiency mutations that produce nonspherocytic hemolytic anemia. *Proc Natl Acad Sci USA* 1993; **90**: 4324–7.

125. Valentine WN, Paglia DE. The primary cause of hemolysis in enzymopathies of anaerobic glycolysis: a viewpoint. *Blood Cells* 1980; **6**: 819–21.

126. Beutler E. The primary cause of hemolysis in enzymopathies of anaerobic glycolysis: "A viewpoint". A commentary. *Blood Cells* 1980; **6**: 827.

127. Tomoda A, Lachant NA, Noble NA, Tanaka KR. Inhibition of the pentose phosphate shunt by 2,3-diphosphoglycerate in erythrocyte pyruvate kinase deficiency. *Br J Haematol* 1983; **54**: 475–84.

128. Zerez CR, Tanaka KR. Impaired nicotinamide adenine dinucleotide synthesis in pyruvate kinase-deficient human erythrocytes: a mechanism for decreased total NAD content and a possible secondary cause of hemolysis. *Blood* 1987; **69**: 999–1005.

129. Aizawa S, Kohdera U, Hiramoto M *et al.* Ineffective erythropoiesis in the spleen of a patient with pyruvate kinase deficiency. *Am J Hematol* 2003; **74**: 68–72.

130. Tanaka KR, Paglia DE. Pyruvate kinase deficiency. *Semin Hematol* 1971; **8**: 367–95.

131. Hennekam RCM, Beemer FA, Cats BP *et al.* Hydrops fetalis associated with red cell pyruvate kinase deficiency. *Genet Couns* 1990; **1**: 75–7.

132. Ferreira P, Morais L, Costa R *et al.* Hydrops fetalis associated with erythrocyte pyruvate kinase deficiency. *Eur J Pediatr* 2000; **159**: 481–2.

133. Bowman HS, McKusick VA, Dronamraju KR. Pyruvate kinase deficient hemolytic anemia in an Amish isolate. *Am J Hum Genet* 1965; **17**: 1–8.

134. Delivoria-Papadopoulos M, Oski FA, Gottlieb AJ. Oxygen-hemoglobin dissociation curves: effect of inherited enzyme defects of the red cell. *Science* 1969; **165**: 601–2.

135. Zanella A, Berzuini A, Colombo MB *et al.* Iron status in red cell pyruvate kinase deficiency: study of Italian cases. *Br J Haematol* 1993; **83**: 485–90.

136. Rutgers MJ, van der Lugt PJ, van Turnhout JM. Spinal cord compression by extramedullary hemopoietic tissue in pyruvatekinase-deficiency-caused hemolytic anemia. *Neurology* 1979; **29**: 510–13.

137. Fanning J, Hinkle RS. Pyruvate kinase deficiency hemolytic anemia: two successful pregnancy outcomes. *Am J Obstet Gynecol* 1985; **153**: 313–14.

138. Kendall AG, Charlow GF. Red cell pyruvate kinase deficiency: adverse effect of oral contraceptives. *Acta Haematol* 1977; **57**: 116–20.

139. Dacie J. *The Haemolytic Anaemias, Vol. I. The Hereditary*

Haemolytic Anaemias, 3rd edn. Edinburgh: Churchill Livingstone, 1985.
140. Lestas AN, Kay LA, Bellingham AJ. Red cell 3-phosphoglycerate level as a diagnostic aid in pyruvate kinase deficiency. *Br J Haematol* 1987; **67**: 485–8.
141. Buc HA, Leroux JP, Garreau H *et al.* Metabolic regulation in enzyme deficient red cells. *Enzyme* 1974; **18**: 19–36.
142. Baronciani L, Beutler E. Prenatal diagnosis of pyruvate kinase deficiency. *Blood* 1994; **84**: 2354–6.
143. Bertrand P, Feremans WW, Barroy JP *et al.* Complications vasculaire dans un cas d'anemie hemolytique par deficit en pyruvate kinase. *Acta Chir Belg* 1982; **82**: 533–7.
144. Chou R, DeLoughery TG. Recurrent thromboembolic disease following splenectomy for pyruvate kinase deficiency. *Am J Hematol* 2001; **67**: 197–9.
145. Tanphaichitr VS, Suvatte V, Issaragrisil S *et al.* Successful bone marrow transplantation in a child with red blood cell pyruvate kinase deficiency. *Bone Marrow Transplant* 2000; **26**: 689–90.
146. Tani K, Yoshikubo T, Ikebuchi K *et al.* Retrovirus-mediated gene transfer of human pyruvate kinase (PK) cDNA into murine hematopoietic cells: implications for gene therapy of human PK deficiency. *Blood* 1994; **83**: 2305–10.
147. Richard RE, Weinreich M, Chang KH *et al.* Modulating erythrocyte chimerism in a mouse model of pyruvate kinase deficiency. *Blood* 2004; **103**: 4432–9.
148. Kirkman HN, Hendrickson EM. Sex-linked electrophoretic difference in glucose-6-phosphate dehydrogenase. *Am J Hum Genet* 1963; **15**: 241–58.
149. Martini G, Toniolo D, Vulliamy T *et al.* Structural analysis of the X-linked gene encoding human glucose 6-phosphate dehydrogenase. *EMBO J* 1986; **5**: 1849–55.
150. Takizawa T, Huang IY, Ikuta T, Yoshida A. Human glucose-6-phosphate dehydrogenase: primary structure and cDNA cloning. *Proc Natl Acad Sci USA* 1986; **83**: 4157–61.
151. Mason, PJ. New insights into G6PD deficiency. *Br J Haematol* 1996; **94**: 585–91.
152. Beutler E. G6PD deficiency. *Blood* 1994; **84**: 3613–36.
153. Mehta A, Mason PJ, Vulliamy TJ. Glucose-6-phosphate dehydrogenase deficiency. *Baillèeres Best Pract Res Clin Haematol* 2000; **13**: 21–38.
154. Hirono A, Fujii H, Miwa S. Identification of two novel deletion mutations in glucose-6-phosphate dehydrogenase gene causing hemolytic anemia. *Blood* 1995; **85**: 1118–21.
155. Vulliamy TJ, D'Urso M, Battistuzzi G *et al.* Diverse point mutations in the human glucose-6-phosphate dehydrogenase gene cause enzyme deficiency and mild or severe hemolytic anemia. *Proc Natl Acad Sci USA* 1988; **85**: 5171–5.
156. Ruwende C, Hill A. Glucose-6-phosphate dehydrogenase deficiency and malaria. *J Mol Med* 1998; **76**: 581–8.
157. Piomelli S, Corash LM, Davenport DD *et al.* In vivo lability of glucose-6-phosphate dehydrogenase in GdA$^-$ and GdMediterranean deficiency. *J Clin Invest* 1968; **47**: 940–8.
158. Giribaldi G, Ulliers D, Mannu F *et al.* Growth of *Plasmodium falciparum* induces stage-dependent haemichrome formation, oxidative aggregation of band 3, membrane deposition of complement and antibodies, and phagocytosis of parasitized erythrocytes. *Br J Haematol* 2001; **113**: 492–9.
159. Janney SK, Joist JJ, Fitch CD. Excess release of ferriheme in G6PD-deficient erythrocytes: possible cause of hemolysis and resistance to malaria. *Blood* 1986; **67**: 331–3.
160. Choremis C, Kattamis CA, Kyriazakou M, Gavrillidou E. Viral hepatitis in G6PD deficiency. *Lancet* 1966; **i**: 269–70.
161. Gellady A, Greenwood RD. G-6-PD hemolytic anemia complicating diabetic ketoacidosis. *J Pediatr* 1972; **80**: 1037–8.
162. Luzzatto L, Mehta A. Glucose 6-phosphate dehydrogenase deficiency. In: Scriver CH, Beaudet AL, Sly WS, Valle D (eds) *The Metabolic and Molecular Bases of Inherited Disease*, vol. 3. New York: McGraw Hill, 1995, pp. 3367–98.
163. Kaplan M, Algur N, Hammerman C. Onset of jaundice in glucose-6-phosphate dehydrogenase-deficient neonates. *Pediatrics* 2001; **108**: 956–9.
164. Owa JA. Relationship between exposure to iatrogenic agents, glucose-6-phosphate dehydrogenase deficiency and neonatal jaundice in Nigeria. *Acta Paediatr Scand* 1989; **78**: 848–52.
165. Meloni T, Costa S, Cutillo S. Haptoglobin, hemopexin, hemoglobin and hematocrit in newborns with erythrocyte glucose-6-phosphate dehydrogenase deficiency. *Acta Haematol* 1975; **54**: 284–8.
166. Kaplan M, Vreman HJ, Hammerman C *et al.* Contribution of haemolysis to jaundice in Sephardic Jewish glucose-6-phosphate dehydrogenase deficient neonates. *Br J Haematol* 1996; **93**: 822–7.
167. Kaplan M, Rubaltelli FF, Hammerman C *et al.* Conjugated bilirubin in neonates with glucose-6-phosphate dehydrogenase deficiency. *J Pediatr* 1996; **128**: 695–7.
168. Kaplan M, Renbaum P, Levy Lahad E *et al.* Gilbert syndrome and glucose-6-phosphate dehydrogenase deficiency. A dose-dependent genetic interaction crucial to neonatal hyperbilirubinemia. *Proc Natl Acad Sci USA* 1997; **94**: 12128–32.
169. Galiano S, Gaetani GF, Barabino A *et al.* Favism in the African type of glucose-6-phosphate dehydrogenase deficiency (A–). *Br Med J* 1990; **300**: 236.
170. Kattamis CA, Kyriazakou M, Chaidas S. Favism. Clinical and biochemical data. *J Med Genet* 1969; **6**: 34–41.
171. Mentzer WC Jr, Collier E. Hydrops fetalis associated with erythrocyte G-6-PD deficiency and maternal ingestion of fava beans and ascorbic acid. *J Pediatr* 1975; **86**: 565–7.
172. Dacie J. Hereditary enzyme-deficiency haemolytic anaemias III: deficiency of glucose-6-phosphate dehydrogenase. In: *The Haemolytic Anaemias, Vol. 1. The Hereditary Haemolytic Anaemias*, 3rd edn. Edinburgh: Churchill Livingstone, 1985, pp. 364–418.
173. Chevion M, Navok T, Glaser G, Mager J. The chemistry of favism-inducing compounds. The properties of isouramil and divicine and their reaction with glutathione. *Eur J Biochem* 1982; **127**: 405–9.
174. Gaetani GF, Rolfo M, Arena S *et al.* Active involvement of catalase during hemolytic crises of favism. *Blood* 1996; **88**: 1084–8.
175. Beutler E. The genetics of glucose-6-phosphate dehydrogenase deficiency. *Semin Hematol* 1990; **27**: 137–64.
176. Van Noorden CJF, Vogels IMC. A sensitive cytochemical staining method for glucose-6-phosphate dehydrogenase activity in individual erythrocytes. II. Further improvements of the staining procedure and some observations with glucose-6-phosphate dehydrogenase deficiency. *Br J Haematol* 1985; **60**: 57–63.
177. Filosa S, Giacometti N, Cai WW *et al.* Somatic cell selection is a

major determinant of the blood cell phenotype in heterozygotes for glucose 6-phosphate dehydrogenase mutations causing severe enzyme deficiency. *Am J Hum Genet* 1996; **59**: 887–95.

178. Meloni T, Forteleoni G, Meloni GF. Marked decline of favism after neonatal glucose-6-phosphate dehydrogenase screening and health education. The northern Sardinian experience. *Acta Haematol* 1992; **87**: 29–31.

179. Tay JS. Medical genetics in Singapore. *Southeast Asian J Trop Med Public Health* 1995; suppl. 1: 19–25.

180. Chau TN, Lai ST, Lai JY, Yuen H. Haemolysis complicating acute viral hepatitis in patients with normal or deficient glucose-6-phosphate dehydrogenase activity. *Scand J Infect Dis* 1997; **29**: 551–3.

181. Brewer GJ, Zarafonetis CJ. The haemolytic effect of various regimens of primaquine with chloroquine in American Negroes with G6PD deficiency and the lack of an effect of various antimalarial suppressive agents on erythrocyte metabolism. *Bull World Health Organ* 1967; **36**: 303–8.

182. Buchachart K, Krudsood S, Singhasivanon P *et al*. Effect of primaquine standard dose (15 mg/day for 14 days) in the treatment of vivax malaria patients in Thailand. *Southeast Asian J Trop Med Public Health* 2001; **32**: 720–6.

183. Luzzatto L. Glucose-6-phosphate dehydrogenase deficiency and hemolytic anemia. In: Nathan DG, Orkin SH (eds) *Nathan and Oski's Hematology of Infancy and Childhood*. Philadelphia: WB Saunders, 1998, pp. 704–26.

184. Beutler E, Mathai CK, Smith JE. Biochemical variants of glucose-6-phosphate dehydrogenase giving rise to congenital nonspherocytic hemolytic disease. *Blood* 1968; **31**: 131–50.

185. Corash L, Spielberg S, Bartsocas C *et al*. Reduced chronic hemolysis during high-dose vitamin E administration in Mediterranean-type glucose-6-phosphate dehydrogenase deficiency. *N Engl J Med* 1980; **303**: 416.

186. Johnson GJ, Vatassery GT, Finkel B, Allen DW. High-dose vitamin E does not decrease the rate of chronic hemolysis in glucose-6-phosphate dehydrogenase deficiency. *N Engl J Med* 1983; **308**: 1014–17.

187. Beutler E. Effect of flavin compounds on glutathione reductase activity: *in vivo* and *in vitro* studies. *J Clin Invest* 1969; **48**: 1957–66.

188. Konrad PN, Richards F II, Valentine WN, Paglia DE. Gammaglutamyl-cysteine synthetase deficiency. *N Engl J Med* 1972; **286**: 557–61.

189. Boxer LA, Oliver JM, Spielberg SP. Protection of granulocytes by vitamin E in glutathione synthetase deficiency. *N Engl J Med* 1979; **301**: 901–5.

190. Prchal JT, Crist WM, Roper M, Wellner VP. Hemolytic anemia, recurrent metabolic acidosis, and incomplete albinism associated with glutathione synthetase deficiency. *Blood* 1983; **62**: 754–7.

191. Valentine WN, Anderson HM, Paglia DE *et al*. Studies on human erythrocyte nucleotide metabolism. II. Nonspherocytic hemolytic anemia, high red cell ATP, and ribosephosphate pyrophosphokinase (RPK, E.C.2.7.6.1) deficiency. *Blood* 1972; **39**: 674–84.

192. Valentine WN, Bennett JM, Krivit W *et al*. Nonspherocytic haemolytic anaemia with increased red cell adenine nucleotides, glutathione and basophilic stippling and ribosephosphate pyrophosphokinase (RPK) deficiency: studies on two new kindreds. *Br J Haematol* 1973; **24**: 157–67.

193. Valentine WN, Fink K, Paglia DE *et al*. Hereditary hemolytic anemia with human erythrocyte pyrimidine 5′-nucleotidase deficiency. *J Clin Invest* 1974; **54**: 866–79.

194. Hirono A, Fujii H, Natori H *et al*. Chromatographic analysis of human erythrocyte pyrimidine 5′ nucleotidase from five patients with pyrimidine 5′ nucleotidase deficiency. *Br J Haematol* 1987; **65**: 35–41.

195. Wilson DE, Swallow DM, Povey S. Assignment of the human gene for uridine 5′-monophosphate phosphohydrolase (UMPH2) to the long arm of chromosome 17. *Ann Hum Genet* 1986; **50**: 223–7.

196. Marinaki AM, Escuredo E, Duley JA *et al*. Genetic basis of hemolytic anemia caused by pyrimidine 5′ nucleotidase deficiency. *Blood* 2001; **97**: 3327–32.

197. Kanno H, Takizawa T, Miwa S, Fujii H. Molecular basis of Japanese variants of pyrimidine 5′-nucleotidase deficiency. *Br J Haematol* 2004; **126**: 265–71.

198. Balta G, Gumruk F, Skarsu N *et al*. Molecular characterization of Turkish patients with pyrimidine 5′ nucleotidase-I deficiency. *Blood* 2003; **102**: 1900–3.

199. Bianchi P, Fermo E, Alfinito F *et al*. Molecular characterization of six unrelated Italian patients affected by pyrimidine 5′-nucleotidase deficiency. *Br J Haematol* 2003; **122**: 847–51.

200. Vives i Corrons JL. Chronic non-spherocytic haemolytic anaemia due to congenital pyrimidine 5′ nucleotidase deficiency: 25 years later. *Baillières Best Pract Res Clin Haematol* 2000; **13**: 103–18.

201. Rees DC, Duley JA, Marinaki AM. Pyrimidine 5′ nucleotidase deficiency. *Br J Haematol* 2003; **120**: 375–83.

202. Beutler E, West C. Tissue distribution of pyrimidine-5′-nucleotidase. *Biochem Med* 1982; **27**: 334–41.

203. Beutler E, Baranko PV, Feagler J *et al*. Hemolytic anemia due to pyrimidine-5′-nucleotidase deficiency: report of eight cases in six families. *Blood* 1980; **56**: 251–5.

204. Paglia DE, Valentine WN, Dahlgren JG. Effects of low-level lead exposure on pyrimidine 5′-nucleotidase and other erythrocyte enzymes. *J Clin Invest* 1975; **56**: 1164–9.

205. Valentine WN, Paglia DE, Fink K, Madokoro G. Lead poisoning. Association with hemolytic anemia, basophilic stippling, erythrocyte pyrimidine 5′-nucleotidase deficiency and intraerythrocyte accumulation of pyrimidines. *J Clin Invest* 1976; **58**: 926–32.

206. Beutler E, Hartman G. Age-related red cell enzymes in children with transient erythroblastoma of childhood and with hemolytic anemia. *Pediatr Res* 1985; **19**: 44–7.

207. Vives i Corrons JL, Pujades MA, Aguilar i Bascompte JL *et al*. Pyrimidine 5′nucleotidase and several other red cell enzyme activities in beta-thalassaemia trait. *Br J Haematol* 1984; **56**: 483–94.

208. McMahon JN, Lieberman JE, Gordon-Smith EC, Egan EL. Hereditary haemolytic anaemia due to red cell pyrimidine 5′-nucleotidase deficiency in two Irish families with a note on the benefit of splenectomy. *Clin Lab Haematol* 1981; **3**: 27–34.

209. Wiginton DA, Kaplan DJ, States JC. Complete sequence and structure of the gene for human adenosine deaminase. *Biochemistry* 1986; **25**: 8234–44.

210. Chen FH, Tartaglia AP, Mitchell BS. Hereditary overexpression of adenosine deaminase in erythrocytes: evidence for a cis-acting mutation. *Am J Hum Genet* 1993; **53**: 889–93.

Porphyria

Lawrence Wolfe and Peter E. Manley

Porphyrias are a group of metabolic disorders caused by genetic or acquired deficiencies in the enzymes of the heme biosynthetic pathway.[1] They were first classified by Gunther in 1911. The causative effect was discovered by Meyer-Betz in 1912 who actually injected himself with hematoporphyrin and developed skin photosensitivity.[2] Porphyrias can be divided into two distinct groups based on their clinical characteristics: the first group causes neuroviscerals crises and is associated with overproduction of δ-aminolevulinic acid (ALA) or porphobilinogen (PBG);[3] the second group is associated with skin lesions due to photosensitization by porphyrins. Each type of porphyria has a characteristic pattern of overproduction of heme precursors. The particular precursor or substrate that is elevated allows determination of the specific enzyme deficiency in the biosynthetic pathway. With specific diagnosis, a comprehensive treatment plan can be developed.

Our first goal is to offer an approach to the clinical appreciation of the porphyrias, their work-up and their diagnosis. Each individual disease is then considered further, including a more detailed discussion of therapeutic approaches.

Epidemiology

Porphyrias are uncommon in the pediatric population and patients rarely present with hematologic complications. Those that do present with hemolytic or hypoproliferative anemia (congenital erythropoietic porphyria, hepatoerythropoietic porphyria, and erythropoietic porphyria) also have concomitant photodermatitis, pointing toward porphyria as

Table 9.7 Prevalence of the porphyrias.

Type	Prevalence
Acute intermittent porphyria	1 in 50 000[1]
δ-Aminolevulinic acid dehydratase deficiency porphyria	5 reported cases[4]
Congenital erythropoietic porphyria	150 reported cases[5]
Erythropoietic protoporphyria	1 in 75 000–200 000[6]
Hepatoerythropoietic protoporphyria	30 reported cases[7–9]
Hereditary coproporphyria	1 in 500 000[10]
Porphyria cutanea tarda	1 in 10 000[11]
Variegate porphyria	3 in 1000 in South Africa[12]
	1 in 100 000[13,14]

the diagnosis. However, because this is a problem with heme synthesis, the pediatric hematologist may be called upon to evaluate a patient with suspected porphyria, even in the absence of hematologic issues, to make the diagnosis by ordering the appropriate tests, interpret the test results, and manage the therapy of these patients. Table 9.7 lists the prevalence of the porphyrias among reported populations.

Classification

Table 9.8 shows the classifications of the porphyrias along with their corresponding clinical symptoms. It can be clearly seen from the age of presentation column in this table that δ-aminolevulinic acid dehydratase (ALAD) deficiency porphyria, congenital erythropoietic porphyria, erythropoietic porphyria, variegate porphyria, and hepatoerythropoietic porphyria may present in the pediatric age range while the more common acute intermittent porphyria and porphyria cutanea tarda usually appear later.

An additional challenge is the diagnosis of latent disease in offspring of affected adults. Prior to the biochemical classification of the porphyrias, they were predominantly identified by which tissues appeared to produce the toxic porphyrin metabolite (hepatic vs. erythroid) or what symptoms were produced (acute and neuroviscerals vs. cutaneous). Ironically, major hematologic problems do not appear in the general classification scheme of these diseases. Significant hemolytic anemia occurs rarely and total heme deficiency or attendant hypoproliferative anemia is uncommon as well (Table 9.9). We will use clinical classifications in discussion of diagnosis and move toward biochemical classification in discussing therapy, which requires more understanding of pathophysiology. This is because treatment relates to preventing metabolite build-up, shutting down overproduction, or protecting against the effects of created toxic metabolites.

Clinical signs and symptoms when considering a diagnosis of porphyria

Heme intermediates are all toxic when produced in excessive amounts. These disturbances can present clinically in two ways. The hepatic porphyrias present with neuroviscerals complications and the cutaneous porphyrias present predominantly with skin findings due to photosensitization.

Table 9.8 Characteristics of the porphyrias.

Disorder	Neurovisceral crises	Skin lesion	Age at presentation	Inheritance
Acute porphyrias				
ALAD deficiency porphyria	+	−	Any age	AR
Acute intermittent porphyria	+	−	Second to third decade	AD
Hereditary coproporphyria	+	+*	Fifth decade	AD
Variegate porphyria	+[†]	+[†]	Before puberty	AD
Cutaneous porphyrias				
Congenital erythropoietic porphyria	−	+	Before age 1	AR
Erythropoietic protoporphyria	−	+	Childhood before age 4	AD[‡]
Hepatoerythropoietic protoporphyria	−	+	Early childhood	AR
Porphyria cutanea tarda	−	+	20–80 years	Variable[§]

* Some patients can experience chronic neuropathy without acute crises.
† Patients may present with skin lesions, neurovisceral attacks, or both.
‡ Related to coinheritance of both a ferrochelatase gene mutation and weak normal allele.[15]
§ Dominant in familial porphyria cutanea tarda but disease can also be acquired.
ALAD, δ-aminolevulinic acid dehydratase; AR, autosomal recessive; AD, autosomal dominant.

Table 9.9 Presentation of single and mixed manifestations of porphyria.

Neurovisceral	Photosensitivity	Hematologic
ALAD deficiency porphyria	Porphyria cutanea tarda	**Congenital erythropoietic porphyria**
Acute intermittent porphyria	**Congenital erythropoietic porphyria**	**Hepatoerythropoietic porphyria**
Hereditary coproporphyria	**Hepatoerythropoietic porphyria**	**Erythropoietic protoporphyria**
Variegate porphyria	**Erythropoietic protoporphyria**	
	Hereditary coproporphyria	
	Variegate porphyria	

Porphyrias in italic share neurovisceral and photosensitivity symptoms. Porphyrias in bold share photosensitivity and hematologic symptoms (usually hemolytic anemia or hypoproliferative anemia). Note that hematologic symptoms may not be prominent and these porphyrias usually present to the physician because of severe photosensitivity.
ALAD, aminolevulinic acid dehydratase.

Tables 9.10 and 9.11 list common signs and symptoms seen in patients with acute hepatic/neurovisceral porphyrias and the cutaneous porphyrias respectively. In the case of cutaneous porphyria, the pathogenesis is well understood and can readily be reproduced experimentally. In contrast, the mechanism of neurologic manifestations remains uncertain.

Neurovisceral manifestations

As with all hepatic porphyrias, the initial sign of an acute attack is abdominal pain, which often radiates to the back, thighs or buttocks. This can be accompanied by diarrhea, anorexia, constipation, vomiting, and abdominal distension. There may be some guarding but no true peritoneal findings. Central nervous system (CNS) symptoms include mental confusion, neuropathy, and seizures. Psychiatric symptoms include anxiety, depression, phobias, and psychosis. These psychiatric manifestations can appear simultaneously or exclusively and can potentially be the sole feature of the disease.

More intense attacks include seizures, which may be provoked by hyponatremia, caused by inappropriate secretion of vasopressin, or by direct metabolic affects on the CNS.[18] These severe attacks may progress within days to a predominantly motor neuropathy, which may remain peripheral or become generalized with respiratory paralysis. Moderate tachycardia and hypertension are common; patients with fluctuating blood pressure and/or arrhythmias are at particular risk for cardiac arrest.[16]

These manifestations flare and then settle as the stimulus to heme production fades or is halted medically. The neuropathy will reverse slowly as axons grow back from the periphery. Long-term complications include physical disability, hypertension, chronic renal failure, and an increased risk of hepatocellular carcinoma.[16]

Table 9.10 Signs and symptoms of the acute hepatic/neurovisceral porphyrias.

Abdominal pain
Vomiting
Constipation
Muscle weakness
Polyneuropathy
Bulbar neuropathy causing respiratory paralysis
Head, neck and chest pain
Psychiatric symptoms
Tachycardia
Seizures
Fever
Diarrhea

Table 9.11 Signs and symptoms of cutaneous porphyrias.

Light-induced skin lesions causing:
  Pruritis
  Burning
  Edema
  Erythema
  Waxy thickening of the skin
  Purpura
  Blistering
  Scarring
  Hyperpigmentation
  Hypertrichosis
Hemolytic anemia
Splenomegaly
Keratoconjunctivitis

Diagnosis of acute hepatic porphyria

As porphyria is not a common illness, there are many factors that need to be considered when determining if further work-up should commence. Pure neurovisceral porphyrias (acute intermittent porphyria and ALAD porphyria) are difficult to diagnose, as symptoms may fall into the background of mistaken psychiatric or neurologic diagnosis. Moreover, the requirement in neurovisceral or hepatic porphyria for an inciting event to occur that triggers heme synthesis in order for the disease to manifest can be an additional confounding factor. Because of these issues there should be a complete family history, looking at both medical and psychiatric history, as the majority of hepatic porphyrias are autosomal dominant in nature. A detailed description of the attacks, especially considering behaviors or events prior to the attack, is critical. The clinician is basically looking for characteristics that may stimulate the production of ALA (see later). This stimulation can be due to hormonal shifts in either gender, but premenstrual attacks may be the first sign of disease in women. The induction of even a brief starvation state from stress or planned dieting also begins the process of ALA synthesis. Smoking or medications that induce hepatic cytochrome P450 enzymes can precipitate an attack. In those rare conditions where photosensitivity and neurovisceral disease appear simultaneously (hereditary coproporphyria and variegate porphyria), suspicion of porphyria and the ensuing investigation are much clearer. If after this the suspicion for hepatic porphyria is high, the investigation should proceed.

Pathogenesis of neurovisceral disease

Acute attacks of porphyria are always associated with induction of hepatic ALA synthase (ALAS1) activity and a marked increase in production of ALA over the basal level for that patient. These changes are often provoked by drugs, particularly those that induce cytochrome P450 proteins. Associated histopathologic lesions include axonal degeneration and chromatolysis, particularly of the anterior horn cells of the spinal cord and brainstem nuclei, with some secondary demyelination.

Numerous hypotheses have attempted to relate signs and symptoms to neuronal dysfunction. Attention has focused on several putative mechanisms of this dysfunction that are not mutually exclusive.
• Neurotoxicity is due to the effects of ALA and not PBG. This is supported by the fact that in ALAD deficiency porphyria, PBG levels are normal but similar symptoms are seen. Therefore it is felt that ALA is the main toxic intermediate.
• ALA is a γ-aminobutyric acid (GABA), glutamate, and aspartate analog and can bind to GABA receptors; this is thought to be neurotoxic. In addition, ALA can inhibit GABA binding to synaptic membranes.[17,18]
• Neuronal heme deficiency.[18]
• Decreased plasma melatonin levels,[19] which enhance ALA-mediated lipid peroxidation.[20,21]
Clearly, there is still mystery and confusion about pathophysiology. For instance, neurovisceral attacks are *always* associated with overproduction of ALA. However, there is no clear dose–response relationship between ALA concentration and neuronal dysfunction. For example, asymptomatic patients often excrete excess ALA.

Various effects of ALA on neuronal function have been demonstrated in animal experiments and *in vitro* preparations but their physiologic relevance is uncertain. Administration of ALA to normal subjects has no discernible effect on plasma concentrations, similar to patients during acute attacks.[22] The blood–brain barrier is relatively impermeable to ALA; concentrations in cerebrospinal fluid (usually < 12 nmol/L) are about 10-fold lower than in plasma.[23] Decreased tryptophan deoxygenase activity in the liver leads to increased delivery of tryptophan to the brain and formation of serotonin (or 5-hydroxytryptamine, 5-HT). Plasma 5-HT concentrations are increased in acute porphyria[24] and serotonergic effects may underlie some clinical symptoms, particularly those ascribed to the autonomic nervous system.[18] A recent study looking at patients who were homozygous dominant for acute intermittent porphyria has provided new insight into the neurotoxicity of the acute porphyria.[25] The homozygous dominant patients had white matter changes in areas susceptible to excitotoxic agents. These patients did not have mitochondrial dysfunction and if neuronal heme deficiency was important, it would be expected that there would also be changes in the gray matter, where neurons reside. This lends credence to the toxicity of ALA through either a direct effect or increased binding to GABA receptors.

Cutaneous manifestations

After excluding drug-induced causes, direct sun-related rashes (e.g., polymorphous light eruption), and systemic lupus, porphyria should be considered as a potentially important diagnostic consideration.

Diagnosis of cutaneous porphyria

As with the hepatic porphyrias, the cutaneous porphyrias are very uncommon. However, the clinical presentation may make it easier to proceed with a work-up for cutaneous porphyria. Patients with cutaneous porphyria present clinically in one of two ways, dictated primarily by the partitioning of specific porphyrin metabolites into the skin.

In erythropoietic protoporphyria (EPP), because of the ability of the lipophilic protoporphyrins to penetrate into the upper dermal layers, one sees immediate pain on skin exposure to natural and even artificial light and waxy thickening of the skin without skin fragility. When photosensitivity appears with evidence of hemolytic anemia and/or liver disease, EPP must be considered. EPP should be suspected when there is a history of a child complaining of skin pain when immediately exposed to the sun. When this is coupled with anemia or signs of liver disease, investigations for EPP should be initiated.

All other cutaneous porphyrias may lead to skin fragility and subepidermal bullae, often associated with hypertrichosis and patchy pigmentation due to the accumulation of water-soluble uroporphyrinogens and coproporphyrins. The most common type of cutaneous porphyria is porphyria cutanea tarda (PCT). PCT is most often acquired and if a patient presents with skin findings that suggest cutaneous porphyria, PCT should be considered early on and a search for an underlying cause should be initiated. Because these illnesses often depend on adult behaviors (Table 9.12), PCT is rarely encountered in childhood. Cases of severe photodermatitis in childhood raise the possibility of the rare illness congenital erythropoietic porphyria (CEP). This is a very uncommon disorder and the patient usually has very distinctive findings such as pink urine (which will stain the diaper),

Table 9.12 Diseases associated with sporadic porphyria cutanea tarda.[26]

Alcoholism
Hemochromatosis
β-Thalassemia
Diabetes mellitus
Hepatitis C infection
Cytomegalovirus infection
HIV infection
Systemic lupus erythematosus
Renal failure/dialysis
Hepatocellular carcinoma
Hematologic malignancy

brown/red discoloration of the teeth, and phototoxic burning on light exposure.

Pathogenesis of cutaneous manifestations

Despite clinical differences in the expression of photosensitivity, the histopathologic changes in light-exposed skin are qualitatively similar in all porphyrias. The characteristic finding is the presence of amorphous, hyaline, PAS-positive material in and around the walls of small blood vessels in the dermis and, often, also at the dermoepidermal junction.[27,28] This material is derived from the walls and contents of blood vessels and represents the cumulative reparative response to repeated cycles of endothelial cell injury with local leakage of vascular contents.[29] Bullae are formed by a split in the lamina lucida of the basement membrane;[30] dermal papillae, stiffened by hyaline deposits, project into the floor and there is no surrounding inflammatory infiltrate.

These changes are provoked by the oxygen-dependent action of light at wavelengths around 400 nm on porphyrins in the dermis. Light at this wavelength penetrates the deeper layers of the dermis and passes through window glass. This energy is strongly absorbed by porphyrins (Soret absorption peak), generating an excited state that either returns rapidly to the ground state with emission of red light (fluorescence) or undergoes intersystem crossing to the longer-lived triplet state. Triplet-state porphyrins react with molecular oxygen by transferring energy to form singlet oxygen species or, less efficiently, by electron transfer to form a superoxide anion. They may also directly initiate other free radical reactions.

Oxygen free radicals are the most important mediators of photodamage to the skin. Since they are short-lived, the site of photodamage is determined largely by the distribution of porphyrins within the cell. Protoporphyrin has particular affinity for membrane lipids, both the endothelial cells and epithelial cells, while more water-soluble porphyrins preferentially accumulate in the lower dermis and cells of the basement membrane zone. These differences in distribution may explain the clinical differences between EPP and the other cutaneous porphyrias (CEP, PCT). Porphyrin-catalyzed photodynamic reactions damage proteins, lipids and DNA,[31] and may activate complement, especially in endothelial cells in EPP,[32] degranulate mast cells,[33] and enhance degradation of dermal components by metalloproteinases.[34]

Diagnosing porphyria and attending to family members

When a diagnosis of porphyria is suspected, the appropriate laboratory markers need to be collected and correctly interpreted (Table 9.13). Once the history, physical examination, and screening laboratory tests have revealed which porphyria(s) might be possible (see Table 9.9), scrutiny of Tables 9.13 and 9.14 and the sections on diagnosis above will provide clarification of the porphyria(s) under consideration. This will ensure that stool and urine porphyrins are measured (there is a tendency to forget their importance) as well as blood enzymes and porphyrins when appropriate.

Identification of asymptomatic affected individuals is an essential part of the management of families with acute intermittent porphyria (AIP), hereditary coproporphyria (HCP) or variegate porphyria (VP). Detection of latent porphyria during childhood before there is any real risk of acute porphyria should be the goal of the physician encountering signs or symptoms of porphyria in any member of a family (Table 9.14).

There are issues to consider in the laboratory analysis of the porphyrias. Metabolite measurements are normal before puberty, with the possible exception of the fecal coproporphyrin isomer ratio in some children with latent HCP.[35]

Assay of PBG deaminase activity in erythrocytes is currently the most widely used method for detection of latent AIP. Enzyme activity decreases markedly as erythrocytes age and is dependent on the age distribution of the circulating cells. Its use should be restricted to hematologically normal individuals over the age of 8 months. Enzyme methods for the detection of latent HCP and VP require nucleated cells and are technically more complex than the PBG deaminase assay (Table 9.13).

New mutations for the porphyrias are being discovered frequently. However, there is no single test for all these DNA variations. Therefore, DNA testing is not suitable for screening for porphyrias, except within families. For these reasons, DNA testing is most meaningful only after standard testing for porphyria has confirmed a diagnosis.

Heme biosynthesis and pathway (Fig. 9.3)

Daily heme synthesis in normal adults is about 7 μmol/kg. The majority is produced within the bone marrow and used for hemoglobin formation. The remainder of the synthesis occurs in the liver. Approximately half is incorporated into the hemeproteins of the cytochrome P450 enzymes. Heme is also incorporated into heme proteins, the mitochondrial and microsomal cytochromes involved in the electron and oxygen transport chain.[38] Heme synthesis starts in the mitochondria. The intermediate steps take place in the cytosol and the products of synthesis then reenter the mitochondria for the final two steps in the process.

Table 9.13 Laboratory measurements for the porphyrias.

Porphyria	Enzyme	Urine	Stool	Plasma	RBC
ALAD deficiency	ALAD	ALA+++	–	–	
AIP	PBGD	*ALA+++/PBG+++ †ALA+/PBG+	– –	– –	
CEP	UROS	URO I++ COPRO I+	URO I+	URO I+ COPRO ++	URO I+
PCT/HEP	UROD	*URO I+++ †URO I+	*ISOCOPRO++ †ISOCOPRO+	Fluorescence 620 nm	
HCP	CPO	†ALA/PBG++/COPROIII++ †COPRO III+	*COPRO III++++ †COPRO III+++	COPRO III+	
VP	PPO	*ALA/PBG++/URO/COPROIII++ †COPRO III+	*COPROIII/PP++ †COPROIII/PP++	Fluorescence 625 nm	
EPP	Ferrochelatase	Normal	PP+	Fluorescence 630 nm	Free PP+

* During acute attack.

† During remission.

ALA, aminolevulinic acid; ALAD, aminolevulinic acid dehydratase; AIP, acute intermittent porphyria; CEP, congenital erythropoietic porphyria; COPRO, corproporphyrin; CPO, coproporphyrinogen III oxidase; EPP, erythropoietic protoporphyria; HCP, hereditary coproporphyria; ISOCOPRO, isocoproporphyrin; PBG, porphobilinogen; PBGD, porphobilinogen deaminase; PCT, porphyria cutanea tarda; PP, protoporphyrin; PPO, protoporphyrinogen oxidase; URO, uroporphyrin; UROD, uroporphyrinogen III decarboxylase; UROS, uroporphyrinogen III synthase; VP, variegate porphyria.

Table 9.14 Identification of latent acute autosomal dominant porphyrias.[35–37]

Disease	Test	Limitations	Sensitivity	Specificity
AIP	Urinary PBG Erythrocyte PBGD	Normal before puberty Not before age of 8 months	Low Overlap between AIP and normal ranges contains 10–20% of asymptomatic relatives	High
HCP	Fecal coproporphyrin (isomer III/I ratio)	Sensitivity in children not established	High*	High*
	CPO	Requires fresh lymphocytes or cell culture; technically complex	ND	ND
VP	Fecal porphyrins; copro isomer ratio	Normal before puberty	36% at age 15 or over	
	Fluorescence emission spectroscopy of plasma	Normal before puberty	86% at age 15 or over	100%†
	PPO	Requires fresh lymphocytes or cell culture; technically complex	ND	ND

* For adults.

† When erythrocyte free protoporphyrin concentration is normal.

AIP, acute intermittent porphyria; CPO, coproporphyrinogen oxidase; HCP, hereditary coproporphyria; ND, not determined (overlap between activities for affected and unaffected individuals small); PBG, porphobilinogen; PBGD, porphobilinogen deaminase; PPO, protoporphyrinogen oxidase; VP, variegate porphyria.

Regulation of heme is through the first enzyme in the pathway, ALAS. There are two forms of ALAS. ALAS1 is produced in the liver and other tissues; the gene that codes for this enzyme is found on chromosome 3 (3p21.1). The ALAS2 isozyme is specifically found in the erythroid line and is encoded on the X chromosome (Xp11.21).[39] This enzyme catalyzes the reaction of glycine and succinyl-CoA to form ALA. Deficiencies in the ALAS1 enzyme have not been described. Defects in ALAS2 do not cause porphyria but are responsible for X-linked sideroblastic anemia.[40]

Regulation of heme synthesis in the liver is through ALAS1. The activity of ALAS is substantially lower than the subsequent enzymes, with the exception of PBG deaminase in nonerythroid cells. In the liver ALAS1 levels are rapidly turned over in response to metabolic needs. ALAS1 is under positive control by porphyrinogenic chemicals and under negative control by heme.[41] Its levels can be increased by drugs that increase hepatic cytochrome P450, a rapidly metabolized heme protein,[42] or by induction of heme oxygenase, which will degrade heme.[43] When there is excess heme in the cellular heme pool, this will inhibit ALAS1 via negative feedback regulation. This can also be accomplished by giving exogenous heme or by inhibiting heme oxygenase, methods relied upon for treatment of severe acute attacks.[44,45] The regulation of ALAS1 occurs at several levels, by destabilization of ALAS1 mRNA by heme or by decreasing the rate of entry of the enzyme into the mitochondria.[42]

ALAS2 is not under the direct control of heme production. Rather it is under the control of the iron supply. However, heme does play an important role in providing iron in heme synthesis. In higher concentrations heme inhibits the acquisition of iron from transferrin and diminishes the availability of iron. Within the mRNA of ALAS2 there is an iron-responsive element (IRE). In the absence of iron, iron regulatory proteins bind to the IRE on mRNA, blocking translation of the enzyme.[46,47]

Acute hepatic porphyrias

ALAD and ALAD deficiency porphyria

ALAD is the enzyme involved in the second step of heme synthesis; it is also known as porphobilinogen synthase. It catalyzes the formation of PBG from two ALA molecules. Its deficiency is the least common of all the porphyrias. It was initially described by Doss *et al.*[48] There have been only five reported cases of this disease in the literature.[4] It is an autosomal recessive disorder.

The enzyme

Human ALAD is encoded by a single 13-kb gene on chromosome 9 (9q34) that contains 13 exons.[49] The enzyme is an octamer with identical 35-kDa subunits. It contains eight Zn^{2+} atoms, of which four are needed for catalytic activity. The zinc atoms allow the interaction with the octameric enzyme and the first ALA molecule.[50] ALAD is inhibited by compounds of clinical importance. Heavy metals, especially lead, act as potent inhibitors of the enzyme by displacing zinc, which is essential for catalytic activity;[51] the intermediate succinylacetone, which is formed in hereditary tyrosinemia, is also a potent inhibitor of ALAD.[52,53]

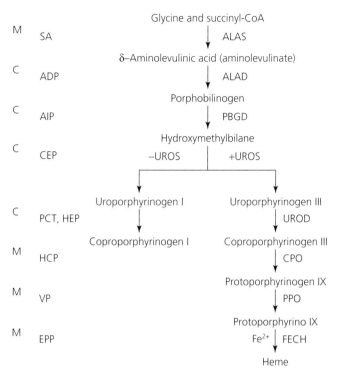

Glycine and succinyl-CoA

M SA   ALAS

δ–Aminolevulinic acid (aminolevulinate)

C ADP   ALAD

Porphobilinogen

C AIP   PBGD

Hydroxymethylbilane

C CEP   −UROS   +UROS

Uroporphyrinogen I   Uroporphyrinogen III

C PCT, HEP   UROD

Coproporphyrinogen I   Coproporphyrinogen III

M HCP   CPO

Protoporphyrinogen IX

M VP   PPO

Protoporphyrino IX

M EPP Fe^{2+} FECH

Heme

Fig. 9.3 Heme synthesis. M, reactions that occur in mitochondria; C, reactions that occur in cytosol. ALAS, δ-aminolevulinic acid synthetase; ALAD, δ-aminolevulinic acid dehyratase; PBGD, porphobilinogen deaminase; UROS, uroporphyrinogen III synthase; UROD, uroporphyrinogen III decarboxylase; CPO, coproporphyrinogen III oxidase; PPO, protoporphyrinogen oxidase; FECH, ferrochelatase; SA, X-linked sideroblastic anemia; ADP, δ-aminolevulinic acid dehydratase deficiency porphyria; AIP, acute intermittent porphyria; CEP, congenital erythropoietic porphyria; PCT, porphyria cutanea tarda; HEP, hepatoerythropoietic porphyria; HCP, hereditary coproporphyria; VP, variegate porphyria; EPP, erythropoietic protoporphyria.

All the mutations have been identified. With the exception of one patient, all the patients were compound heterozygotes.[54–57] The patient who only had one mutant allele was asymptomatic and was identified through newborn screening for tyrosinemia.[58] Three patients were diagnosed with this disease at an early age and all their mutations were early stop codons, mutations in the substrate-binding site, or mutations in the zinc-binding site. One patient, an elderly man, did not develop any symptoms until he developed a myeloproliferative syndrome. He had two mutations: one of these did not affect the folding of the enzyme and thus the enzyme could function properly. When he developed his myeloproliferative syndrome with polycythemia, a preference occurred for one erythroid clone. It was found that this erythrocyte clone carried the nonfunctional ALAD allele.[4]

Clinical presentation

The age at presentation can be variable. Disease has been seen in a newborn, a teenager and the elderly man described above, who developed the symptoms after he was diagnosed with a myeloproliferative disorder.[48,59,60] Clinical symptoms have included colicky abdominal pain and polyneuropathy. The affected infant had generalized hypotonia and respiratory insufficiency. His treatment eventually required liver transplantation.[59] There were no significant hematologic abnormalities in these patients, although myeloproliferative disorders may occur.

Diagnosis

Conditions where ALAD are suppressed need to be excluded, as this type of porphyria is very uncommon. These include lead poisoning, zinc deficiency, chronic renal insufficiency,[61] and diabetes mellitus.[62] Symptoms similar to ALAD porphyria can present in patients with these medical problems, with elevation of urine ALA. ALA is excreted exclusively in the urine and normal excretion is less than 7 mg in 24 hours. In a patient with ALAD porphyria, ALA excretion will be three to ten times higher. This disease can be distinguished from AIP in that PBG excretion will be normal to only slightly above normal in the latter disease. Total porphyrin levels will also be elevated in a nonspecific fashion in ALAD porphyria. In addition, erythrocytes and lymphocytes can be assayed for ALAD activity, which is less than 5% of normal levels.

PBG deaminase and acute intermittent porphyria

PBG deaminase (PBGD) is the third enzyme in the synthesis of heme. It is responsible for the conversion of PBG into hydroxymethylbilane. AIP is due to a decrease in the production of this enzyme. This porphyria is an autosomal dominant disorder. Patients who inherit this disease will have levels 50% of normal. Approximately 90% of patients will have no clinical symptoms throughout their entire life. AIP is the most common type of acute hepatic porphyria.

The enzyme

PBGD (hydroxymethylbilane synthase) catalyzes the head-to-tail polymerization of four PBG molecules to form the linear tetrapyrrole, hydroxymethylbilane (pre-uroporphyrinogen). The discovery by ^{13}C NMR spectroscopy of the extremely unstable product of this reaction initiated a series of investigations that have produced an almost complete picture of the mechanism of this fascinating and unique enzyme.[63–65] The structure of the enzyme from *Escherichia coli* has been determined by X-ray crystallography at 0.176 nm resolution.[63] It contains three domains of similar size with a deep catalytic cleft between domains 1 and 2. The shape of these two domains resembles transferrin and the periplasmic binding proteins, proteins that undergo marked conformational change on interaction with their ligands.

PBGD first binds to two molecules of PBG. This forms a dipyrrolmethane cofactor that allows for the binding sites for subsequent PBG molecules to form a linear tetrapyr-role, hydroxymethylbilane (HMB).[66] HMB is a very un-stable molecule and a short intermediate to the next step. Uroporphyrinogen III cosynthase needs to be present to quickly convert HMB to uroporphyrinogen III that can then continue to form heme. If this enzyme is not present, HMB will spontaneously convert to uroporphyrinogen I, which cannot go on to form heme molecules.

Human PBGD exists in two forms: a 40-kDa erythroid isozyme and a housekeeping (or ubiquitous) isozyme that contains an additional 17 amino acids at its NH_2-terminus and which is expressed in all tissues. Both are encoded by a single 10-kb gene on chromosome 11 (11q24.1–24.2) contain-ing 15 exons.[67] Tissue-specific expression is determined by separate erythroid and ubiquitous promoters 5' to exons 2 and 1, with translation initiation codons in exons 3 and 1, respectively.[68] More than 100 mutations that cause AIP have been identified in the PBGD gene.[69] AIP can be divided into three groups.[70]

• *Type 1 mutations*: PBGD activity is decreased by 50% in all tissues. The mutations are usually single-base substitutions or deletions. This will lead to single amino acid changes or truncated proteins.

• *Type 2 mutations* occur in less than 5% of patients with AIP. These are characterized by decreased PBGD activity in non-erythroid cells (50% of normal) but normal erythroid PBGD activity. The defect in this mutation is due to a single-base substitution in the 5' splice donor site of intron 1. Since ery-throid PBGD uses a promoter downstream of the mutation site, its production is not compromised.[71]

• *Type 3 mutations*: PBGD activity is 50% of normal in all tissues. These lesions are CRIM positive. Mutations occur mostly in exons 10 and 12, which are felt to be the regions essential for catalytic activity and substrate binding.[64]

Clinical presentation

Patients with this disease usually present after puberty, although there have been a few cases of symptoms at a younger age.[72,73] This disease is more common in women than men. As mentioned previously in the discussion of neurovisceral presentations, the initial sign of an acute attack is abdominal pain, which often radiates to the back, thighs or buttocks. Urinary retention, incontinence and dysuria can also occur. Cardiac and autonomic symptoms also appear and patients can succumb to blood pressure extremes or arrhythmias. In addition, hypertension may become sus-tained between the acute exacerbations of AIP. CNS symp-toms include mental confusion and seizures. Seizures can be the result of hyponatremia, a result in some patients of inappropriate secretion of vasopressin, or possibly a result of metabolic effects on the CNS.[18] Peripheral neuropathy is a common feature of AIP. This usually begins in the lower extremities but can also involve the upper extremities. In severe attacks, bulbar involvement can appear, leading to irreversible CNS damage or death. Psychiatric complaints are prevalent in AIP. In addition to formal psychiatric diagnoses, patients can also enter an altered state of consciousness rang-ing from somnolence to true coma. Psychiatric symptoms may represent the sole feature of the disease.[74] There is little evidence that acute porphyria causes long-term psychiatric illness, apart from generalized anxiety.[75] See Table 9.15 for a comprehensive analysis of symptom frequency in this complex illness.

Most patients have only one severe attack; a minority suffer from repeated attacks over several years. Regular premenstrual

Table 9.15 Signs that occur in attacks of acute intermittent porphyria.*

Symptom/sign	Goldberg (1959) ($n = 50$)	Stein & Tschudy (1970) ($n = 46$)	Mustajoki & Nordmann (1993) ($n = 51$)	Hift (1986–95) ($n = 92$)
Abdominal pain	94	95	96	98
Nonabdominal pain	52	50	25	
Vomiting	88	43	84	85
Constipation	84	48	78	28
Psychologic symptoms	58	40	19	2
Convulsions	16	20		5
Muscle weakness	68	60	8	7
Sensory loss	38	26		2
Hypertension (diastolic blood pressure > 85 mmHg)	54	36	57	68
Tachycardia (>80/min)	64	80	79	57
Hyponatremia (<135 nmol/L)			32	39

* All values are percentages.
Reprinted with permission from Ref. 16.

attacks may occur in young women and may be initiated by the return of menstruation after pregnancy. The prognosis for most patients is good; few attacks now end fatally, particularly if the diagnosis is made early.[76,77] The neuropathy reverses slowly as axons grow back from the periphery. Long-term complications in patients with AIP include physical disability, chronic renal failure, and an increased risk of hepatocellular carcinoma.[16] The risk of hepatocellular carcinoma is thought to be due to increased reactive oxygen species that initiate DNA strand breaks.[78]

Precipitating factors

Precipitating factors responsible for attacks in AIP are those events that cause an increase in ALAS1 (see previous discussion). With the upregulation of ALAS1 and the limiting levels of PBGD, an increase in both ALA and PBG occurs, precipitating an attack. In adults, most attacks are provoked by drugs, particularly those that induce cytochrome P450 (Table 9.16), and menstruation.[16,76,79,80] Exogenous estrogens and progesterones can also precipitate attacks, although the exact mechanism is not known.[81,82] Other precipitants include alcohol, smoking, calorie restriction, infection and stress. Caloric restriction, most notably lack of carbohydrate, increases heme oxygenase, which also increases ALAS1 due to decrease in hepatic heme concentrations.[83] Of note, patients with AIP who developed type II diabetes have been reported to have a *decrease* in their acute attacks. This may be due to increase in glucose levels and higher amounts of carbohydrate.[84] In the past, general surgery has been hazardous but the dangers seem largely to be related to use of inappropriate drugs and anesthetic agents. Provided the diagnosis of porphyria is known in advance and the patient is managed accordingly, surgery need not be discouraged.[16]

Diagnosis

The diagnosis of AIP can be established by finding elevated PBG or ALA in the urine. Total urine porphyrins will be elevated. One method for measuring PBG in urine is ion-exchange chromatography followed by reaction with Ehrlich's aldehyde reagent (*p*-aminodimethylbenzaldehyde in HCl) to produce a red product.[85,86] There are rapid tests designed to detect PBG in the urine, such as the Watson–Schwartz test and the Hoesch test.[87] Screening tests, such as the Watson–Schwartz test, are less sensitive and less specific.[85,86] Newer techniques have improved the detection by measuring PBG in its native form, improving the sensitivity of the diagnosis.[88] Positive screening tests should always be confirmed by a specific, quantitative method. In AIP, PBG and ALA urine excretion usually remains increased for many weeks after the onset of an acute attack. Erythrocyte PBGD activity may be measured to determine the patient's type of PBGD deficiency. Type II AIP patients should have normal

Table 9.16 Drug safety in neurovisceral/hepatic porphyria.*

Safe
Acetaminophen (paracetamol)
Aspirin
Atropine
Bromides
Cimetidine
Chloral hydrate
Estrogens[†‡]
Glucocorticoids
Insulin
Narcotic analgesics
Penicillin and derivatives
Phenothiazines
Ranitidine[†§]
Serotonin reuptake inhibitors (antidepressants)
Streptomycin

Unsafe
Alcohol
Antiepilepsy drugs: phenytoin[†]
Barbiturates[†]
Birth control pills
Calcium channel blockers:[¶] nifedipine
Carbamazepine[†]
Carisoprodol[†]
Clonazepam
Danazol[†]
Diclofenac[†]
Diones: trimethadione, paramethadione
Ergots
Ethchlorvynol[†]
Felbamate
Glutethimide[†]
Griseofulvin[†]
Mephenytoin
Meprobamate[†]
Methyprylon
Metoclopramide[†]
Pimidone[†]
Progesterone:[†] progestins/synthetic
Pyrazinamide[†]
Pyrazolones: aminopyrine, antipyrine
Rifampin
Sedatives
Succinimides: ethosuximide, methsuximide
Sulfonamide antibiotics[†]
Tranquilizers
Valproic acid[†]

* Excerpted from www.porphyriafoundation.com
† Porphyria is listed as a contraindication, warning, precaution, or adverse effect in 1994 US labeling for these drugs.
‡ There is little evidence that estrogens alone are harmful in acute porphyrias. They have been implicated as harmful based mostly on experience with estrogen–progestin combinations and because they can exacerbate porphyria cutanea tarda. Some patients with acute intermittent porphyria, hereditary coproporphyria, variegate porphyria and aminolevulinic acid dehydratase deficiency porphyria may tolerate a low-dose estrogen patch.
§ Although porphyria is listed as a precaution in US labeling for this drug, it is regarded as safe by other sources.
¶ There is strong evidence in laboratory studies and some clinical evidence that these agents may be harmful.
The text of this table was prepared by Karl E. Anderson and Douglas E. Goeger of Texas Medical Branch at Galveston.

erythrocyte PBGD levels. Type I and type III patients (representing the vast majority of defects) will have 50% or less of normal PBGD activity. If there is any confusion about the presence of additional hematologic or cutaneous disease in a patient thought to have AIP with normal red cell PBGD activity (type II), fecal porphyrins should be evaluated (see below).

Hereditary coproporphyria and coproporphyrinogen oxidase

HCP occurs when there is a defect in the enzyme coproporphyrinogen oxidase (CPO). CPO is involved in the sixth step of heme synthesis. It converts coproporphyrinogen III to protoporphyrinogen IX. This is an autosomal dominant hepatic porphyria. Patients who inherit this disorder will have enzyme activity 50% of normal. Symptoms of this disease are similar to AIP but a subset of patients will have cutaneous photosensitivity.

The enzyme

CPO is a mitochondrial enzyme and it is at this step in heme synthesis that the process reenters the mitochondria for completion to form heme. CPO is involved in the sequential hydrogenation and decarboxylation of the 2- and 4-propionate side-chains of coproporphyrinogen III to protoporphyrinogen IX, with formation of the tricarboxylic intermediate, harderoporphyrinogen. Coproporphyrinogen I is not metabolized so it is at this stage that the pathway becomes specific for the asymmetric series III isomers. Human CPO is encoded by a single 14-kb gene on chromosome 3 (3q12) that contains seven exons.[89] Human CPO is a metal-free 74-kDa homodimer situated in the mitochondrial intermembrane space, possibly loosely attached to the outer surface of the inner membrane.[90,91] It is synthesized as a precursor with a 110 amino acid presequence that directs it to the intermembrane space.[89] For mammalian CPOs to function, they have an absolute requirement for molecular oxygen; no cofactors have been identified as a requirement for function. In erythroid cells CPO transcripts increase during cell differentiation. Functional analysis of the promoter has demonstrated that the synergistic action of an Sp-1 like element, a GATA site, and a novel regulatory element (CPO promoter regulatory element) that interacts with a leucine zipper-like structure, K1p1, are perquisites for activity in erythroid cells.[92] Conversely, in nonerythroid cells the GATA site is not required, indicating that regulation of CPO is tissue-specific.[93]

Multiple different mutations have been described in the CPO gene.[94–97] There are two mutations that result in elevated levels of the intermediate porphyrin harderoporphyrinogen. These involve exon 6, which implies that this region is important for the decarboxylation in the conversion of harderophorphyrinogen to protoporphyrinogen.[98]

Patients with this defect are said to have harderoporphyria. It is also important to note that the clinical severity of HCP does not correlate with inactivation of the CPO mutation.[98]

Clinical presentation

Symptoms in HCP rarely present before puberty. There have been some cases of homozygous HCP that presented before puberty with neurovisceral symptoms, hemolytic anemia and jaundice. The patients who presented with hemolytic anemia had the subset condition harderoporphyria.[99,100] As HCP is a hepatic porphyria, it presents in a similar fashion to that of AIP. The common presentation is again with abdominal pain, vomiting, neuropathy, and psychiatric symptoms. However, up to 30% of patients may present with skin lesions. The skin lesions are very similar to those seen in PCT.

HCP is exacerbated by many of the same factors that precipitate attacks in AIP, such as medications, stress, fasting, and alcohol consumption. These patients, as in AIP, are also at increased risk for hepatocellular carcinoma.

Laboratory diagnosis

Patients with HCP will have elevated levels of ALA, PBG, and coproporphyrin (predominantly in the type III form) in the urine. These patients differ from patients with AIP in that ALA and PBG levels drop quickly. In the quiescent state, affected patients will excrete predominantly coproporphyrin III in their feces and the ratio of this to coproporphyrin I will be elevated. The enzyme can be directly measured in mononuclear cells but this should not be used as the sole diagnostic tool for this disease.[101] Patients with harderoporphyria will have harderoporphyrin in their feces as well as coproporphyrin. As HCP can have both cutaneous and neurovisceral findings, it is important that it not be confused with AIP or PCT. Therefore, fecal porphyrin analysis is critical when this diagnosis is considered. Only HCP will have elevated levels of coproporphyrin.

Variegate porphyria and protoporphyrinogen oxidase

VP is an autosomal dominant hepatic porphyria. It occurs when there is a defect in the enzyme protoporphyrinogen oxidase (PPO). Enzyme levels are less than 50% of normal. PPO is the seventh step in the formation of heme. It converts protoporphyrinogen IX to protoporphyrin IX. The term "variegate" was applied because VP can present with neurovisceral symptoms or cutaneous symptoms or both.

The enzyme

Human PPO is encoded by a gene on chromosome 1 (1q21–23) that contains 13 introns spread over 5.5 kb.[102–104]

PPO is a flavoprotein with an absolute requirement for molecular oxygen.[105] This enzyme catalyzes the removal of six hydrogen atoms from the porphyrinogen nucleus. The enzyme is associated with the inner mitochondrial membrane but no transmembrane-spanning region has been identified.[106] Unlike the other mitochondrial enzymes of heme synthesis, PPO is not synthesized with a presequence to target import into the mitochondria.[104]

More than 100 disease-specific mutations of the PPO gene have been identified.[107] However, there is less allelic heterogeneity as an estimated 20 000 descendants of a South African individual have been demonstrated to have inherited the same PPO mutation.[108] There is even less heterogeneity in Finnish and Swedish populations.[14,109]

Clinical presentation

As with all hepatic porphyrias, neurovisceral attacks are common, leading to abdominal pain, nausea, vomiting, tachycardia, hypertension, neuropathy, back pain, and psychiatric symptoms. However, in comparison with AIP, attacks of VP are generally milder and recurrent attacks less frequent.[110]

Although VP is classified as a hepatic porphyria, cutaneous photosensitivity is common. Lesions are very similar to those seen in PCT and HCP. These include vesicles, bullae, erosions, hyperpigmentation and hypertrichosis of sun-exposed areas. Skin findings are less prevalent in the northern countries where sun exposure is less intense.

VP is exacerbated by many of the same factors that precipitate attacks in AIP, such as medications, stress, fasting, and alcohol consumption. These patients, as in AIP, are also at increased risk for hepatocellular carcinoma.

Of specific importance to the pediatrician, 12 unrelated patients with homozygous VP have been described.[111,112] Except for one patient, all have developed skin fragility, subepidermal bullae and hypertrichosis before the age of 2 years. Other clinical manifestations include growth retardation, clinodactyly and flexion deformities of the fingers, mental retardation, convulsions, and nystagmus.

Laboratory diagnosis

Patients experiencing an acute attack of VP will have elevated urinary ALA, PBG and uroporphyrin. Patients will also have increased fecal protoporphyrin and coproporphyrin III. Fecal X-porphyrins are ether/acetic acid-soluble porphyrins extracted from feces. X-porphyrins are significantly elevated in VP. However, the most effective way to diagnose VP is by measurement of plasma porphyrin levels. Plasma porphyrins are especially increased in patients with cutaneous findings. In VP, dicarboxylporphyrin is bound tightly to plasma proteins. In order to distinguish VP from the other porphyrias, plasma emission scanning can be done. Plasma porphyrins have an emission maximum at 626 nm, unlike any other porphyria.[113,114]

Treatment of hepatic porphyrias

Acute attack

In a patient with acute hepatic porphyria exacerbation, the cause of the attack needs to be quickly identified. All medications that could potentially cause an increase in cytochrome production and thus increase ALAS synthesis need to be stopped. If the attack was brought on by infection, the infection needs treatment. Carbohydrate loading is the next approach to treatment. The patient should receive high doses of glucose because it is effective at inhibiting ALAS production. An adequate dose is 300–400 g daily. In sick patients this can be administered via nasogastric tube or intravenously through central venous lines. In patients with initial severe neurologic involvement or in those who have not responded to carbohydrate loading over 1–2 days, heme preparations are the next choice. They consistently reduce ALAS formation, but have side-effects that reserve them for severe disease or when patients fail to respond to glucose treatment. Hemin (Panhematin; Abbot) should be given during an acute attack. This is the most effective agent for reducing acute neurovisceral attacks.[44] The recommended dose for treatment is 3–4 mg/kg once a day for at least 4 days. The side-effects of hemin are phlebitis and coagulopathy. Although acute hemorrhage has not been seen with the use of hemin, concurrent anticoagulant therapy should not be used. To decrease the risk of phlebitis, patients will sometimes require the placement of a central venous catheter. Heme arginate preparations (Normosang; Orphan Europe, Paris) are available outside the USA and significantly reduce the risk of adverse events.

Cimetidine has also been shown to suppress ALAS and can be used as an alternative if standard modalities are not available. Doses of 800 mg/day in adults have had a positive effect during acute attacks.[115] Heme oxygenase inhibitors can also be used. However, these drugs (e.g., tin protoporphyrin) have toxic side-effects and zinc mesoporphyrin is not widely available.[116,117] Patients may also require antiemetics, pain control, antihypertensive agents, and close monitoring of electrolytes. If patients have bulbar dysfunction that leads to respiratory difficulty, mechanical ventilation may be required. Currently, recombinant PBGD is being studied in the treatment of acute attacks of AIP.

Prevention

As this disease has many triggers, the best way to avoid an acute attack is to avoid those factors known to exacerbate hepatic porphyrias. A list of potentially safe and unsafe agents can be found at the American Porphyria Foundation website (www.porphyriafoundation.com) (see also Table 9.16). For women whose acute exacerbations occur during menstruation, suppression of ovulation with LHRH analogs can reduce the number of attacks.[118] Care needs to be taken to treat infections and monitor these patients when they have any surgical procedures. Patients need to avoid episodes of starvation or reduced caloric intake, which can also exacerbate this disease. In patients with frequent recurrent attacks, weekly administration of hemin may help control the disease.[119,120] Liver transplantation has been successful in two patients, one with AIP and one with VP who failed all other treatments.[121,122] New research into gene therapy has looked into transferring the enzyme PBGD via viral vectors into hepatocytes. This approach is still in its very early stages.[123,124]

Photocutaneous porphyrias

Congenital erythropoietic porphyria and uroporphyrinogen III synthase

CEP is an autosomal recessive disease that is due to a deficiency of the enzyme uroporphyrinogen III synthase (UROS). It is also called Gunther disease. UROS is the fourth step in the formation of heme. It converts HMB to uroporphyrinogen III. Enzyme levels of UROS in this disorder are markedly deficient but not absent and are usually less than 1%.

The enzyme

The human UROS gene on chromosome 10 (10q25.2–26.3) covers 45 kb and contains nine exons that encode a 29-kDa protein.[125] UROS catalyzes both cyclization and reversal of the orientation of ring D of HMB to give the uroporphyrinogen III isomer, which is the common precursor of all tetrapyrrolic pigments. In the absence of UROS, HMB rapidly cyclizes to the symmetrical hexahydroporphyrin, uroporphyrinogen I, and this molecule has no physiologic function. This molecule is then converted to coproporphyrinogen I and cannot be metabolized further. Several mechanisms for this unique reaction have been suggested; current evidence favors the formation of a spiro-intermediate, an unusual molecular configuration that would yield the products seen in the normal patient.[126] In addition, like ALAS there are two forms of this enzyme, an erythroid-specific and a housekeeping form.[127]

To date, 36 mutations in the UROS gene that cause CEP in homozygotes or compound heterozygotes have been characterized.[128] The majority of patients with CEP are compound heterozygotes for the UROS mutations. The most common mutation (C73R) represents about 35% of mutant alleles, followed by L4F and T228M mutations representing 7% and 6% respectively. There is a correlation between the genotype and

phenotype of patients with CEP. Those patients homozygous for the C73R mutation have a UROS activity of < 2% and have particularly severe disease. Patients who have mutations that express some residual activity have milder forms of the disease. Some of these have been identified in patients with only mild cutaneous symptoms.[129]

Clinical features

The age at onset and clinical severity of CEP are highly variable. It can range from nonimmune hydrops fetalis *in utero* due to severe hemolytic anemia to milder later-onset forms in which patients only develop cutaneous lesions. There are a number of factors that cause this phenotypic variability, including the amount of UROS activity,[129] the degree of hemolysis and subsequent stimulation of erythropoiesis, and the amount of exposure to ultraviolet (UV) light. Most patients have the severe infantile-onset form.[130]

Cutaneous involvement

Common early signs are blisters and erosions on light-exposed skin, especially on the hands and face. The severe and persistent skin lesions resemble those of other bullous porphyrias: subepidermal bullae, skin fragility with erosions and vesicles, which contain serous fluid and are prone to rupture and infection. The serous fluid will fluoresce due to the high content of porphyrin. Milia, hypertrichosis (particularly of the face), and patchy pigmentation are all common.[131] Repetitive cycles of symptomatic episodes lead to photomutilation, with erosion and resorption of the terminal phalanges, contractures, destruction of the ears, nose and eyelids, and scarring alopecia. Corneal scarring may lead to blindness.

Hematologic involvement

Clinical manifestations are not confined to the skin. Hemolytic anemia and splenomegaly are common. On a peripheral smear, anisocytosis, poikilocytosis, polychromasia, basophilic stippling, reticulocytes, and nucleated red blood cells can be seen. Neonates can have hyperbilirubinemia due to anemia and if CEP is not recognized, treatment using phototherapy can be quite harmful. Splenomegaly will usually develop because of the increased turnover of damaged red blood cells. Hypersplenism causing anemia, thrombocytopenia and leukopenia eventually occurs. This may result in purpura, bruising and hemorrhagic blisters. Hydrops fetalis, extensive bruising and hepatosplenomegaly may be present at birth due to severe hemolytic anemia.

Additional clinical features

Pink or red staining of diapers or pink/red-brown amniotic fluid due to increased urinary porphyrins may be the first sign of disease. Porphyrin from CEP can be deposited in the bones and teeth. This causes the teeth to appear reddish-brown in natural light (erythrodontia). The teeth will also fluoresce when exposed to long-wavelength UV light. Porphyrin deposition in the bones will cause bone loss due to demineralization.[132] Bone loss may also occur secondary to erythroid marrow expansion to compensate for ineffective erythropoiesis.[133] Other skeletal changes include bone resorption from photomutilation and decreased bone density with pathologic fractures. Vitamin D metabolism may be impaired because of the avoidance of sunlight.

Diagnosis

Investigations for CEP should be initiated in patients with pink- or red-stained diapers and skin photosensitivity. In patients with CEP, urine porphyrins, uroporphyrinogen I and coproporphyrinogen I are significantly elevated. Fecal and plasma coproporphyrinogen I levels are also increased. A Wood's light will demonstrate fluorescence of teeth. Assays for UROS enzyme activity have been developed as well as detection of the gene mutations, which can help with genotype/phenotype correlations.[134] If a family has already had an infant with CEP, prenatal testing can be performed to detect if the fetus has the disease and then the necessary precautions can be taken to prevent the harmful effects of phototherapy for neonatal hyperbilirubinemia. Prenatal detection can be performed by direct observation of UROS gene mutations or measurement of UROS activity in cultured amniotic cells.[135,136]

Treatment

Treatment of these patients involves multiple interventions. The first is sun protection or sun avoidance. If a patient needs to go out in the sun, adequate coverage of skin is needed; sunscreens and β-carotene have been beneficial in protecting the skin.[137] If any of the patient's bullae or vesicles become infected, rapid treatment should be initiated to prevent scarring.

Patients with severe hemolytic anemia will require blood transfusions. Blood transfusions have multiple benefits: they suppress erythropoiesis, decreasing the amount of porphyrins and thus photosensitivity. If a patient develops hypersplenism, splenectomy may alleviate the thrombocytopenia and reduce the number of transfusions.[137] To achieve the desired benefit from transfusion therapy, the patient's hematocrit should be kept above 32% and deferoxamine should be administered appropriately to avoid iron overload.[131] Other therapies that have been useful include hydroxycarbamide to reduce porphyrin synthesis and oral charcoal to increase the fecal loss of porphyrins.[138,139] These therapies are more effective in patients with milder forms of the disease.

Hematopoietic stem cell transplant (HSCT) has been used and can be curative in patients with CEP. Ten patients have undergone HSCT, with nine surviving with a significant reduction in symptoms and signs of their disease.[140] Future directions include using gene therapy to introduce UROS activity into the hematopoietic stem cells of patients with CEP. This approach would avoid the toxicities associated with allogeneic HSCT.

Porphyria cutanea tarda, hepatoerythropoietic porphyria and uroporphyrinogen decarboxylase

PCT is the most common type of porphyria, with onset usually in adulthood. It is due to a defect in the enzyme uroporphyrinogen decarboxylase (UROD). There are three different forms of PCT.

• Type I represents approximately 80% and is known as the sporadic form. In these patients, levels of UROD are decreased only in the liver and not in red blood cells. Levels of UROD are only low during acute attacks and return to more normal levels once treatment is initiated.[141] This is most common in male patients and is the result of certain disease associations (see Table 9.12).

• Type II represents approximately 20% of patients. This is the autosomal dominant form of PCT and shows a 50% reduction of UROD activity. Activation of PCT in these patients occurs more readily if they contract any of the disorders listed in Table 9.12 as they already have a 50% reduction in the enzyme.

• Type III resembles type I in that no mutation is detected but disease occurs in more than one family member, suggesting there is an inherited predisposition. Patients with type III disease can have onset of disease at an earlier age than patients with type I or type II.

Patients with hepatoerythropoietic porphyria (HEP) are homozygous or compound heterozygous for UROD deficiency and this porphyria is very uncommon.

The enzyme

The cytosolic enzyme UROD is the fifth step in heme formation. It catalyzes the decarboxylation of uroporphyrinogens I and III to the corresponding coproporphyrinogens.[142] The enzyme decarboxylates all four isomers but the type III isomer is decarboxylated the fastest. Human UROD is an 82-kDa homodimer[143] encoded by a gene on chromosome 1 (1p34) that contains 10 exons spread over 3 kb.[7] With uroporphyrinogen III as a substrate and under physiologic conditions, the acetic acid substituents are decarboxylated in a clockwise order around the porphyrinogen macrocycle, starting at ring D, with the formation of 7-, 6- and 5-carboxyl intermediates. The affinity of the enzyme for substrate decreases with the removal of each carboxyl group from the substrate. All URODs are inhibited by sulfhydryl group-containing reagents, including heavy metals. Evidence from study of natural mutants and from site-directed mutagenesis experiments is consistent with the hypothesis that each side-chain is decarboxylated at the same catalytic site,[142,144] but the mechanism by which the substrate rotates remains obscure.

Patients with the sporadic forms of PCT do not have any evidence of UROD mutations.[141] In the familial form of PCT, over 45 different mutations have been reported.[107] Patients with HEP, although they have mutations in both UROD alleles, still have some residual UROD activity. However, most mutations found in HEP are not found in familial PCT. Thus, the mutations in familial PCT appear to be more critical to enzyme activity than those found in HEP.[145]

Pathogenesis

To cause the symptoms of PCT, approximately 75% of the enzyme needs to be inhibited.[141] Abnormal iron metabolism appears to be a major precipitating factor in PCT. This is most likely due to the production of oxygen free radicals produced by reactive intracellular iron. Patients with PCT typically have higher levels of iron compared with control populations. Not surprisingly, patients with PCT commonly have mutations in the *HFE* gene that is associated with hemochromatosis.[146–148] Polyhalogenated hydrocarbons such as hexacholorbenzene inhibit UROD and can cause PCT. This is sometimes referred to as toxic porphyria. Estrogen-containing contraceptives can precipitate PCT in women.[149]

Clinical features

Patients with PCT can have blisters and erosions on light-exposed skin especially on the hands and face. These subepidermal bullae, which contain serous fluid, then denude and become crusted. These heal slowly and are prone to infections. Facial hypertrichosis and hyperpigmentation are common. Cutaneous thickening of the skin with scarring and calcification can be seen and is sometime termed "pseudoscleroderma".[150] Milia may also develop within the areas of bullae. Patients may also develop onycholysis. In patients with HEP, the skin findings are similar to those found in CEP.

Patients with PCT almost always have liver dysfunction, even in cases not associated with hepatitis C. Porphyrin levels within the liver and needle-like inclusions have been found in the cytoplasm of hepatocytes. It is thought that these may be composed of uroporphyrin and may cause liver damage in PCT.[107]

Diagnosis

When an apparently "acquired" porphyria is discovered, PCT should be considered and an analysis of underlying causes initiated (see Table 9.12). Patients with evidence of PCT will have increased uroporphyrin I. In the feces, isocoproporphyrin (coproporphyrin I) is dominant. However, concentrations of coproporphyrin and X-porphyrin may also be elevated. Uroporphyrin and 7-carboxyporphyrin are elevated in the liver. Plasma porphyrins will fluoresce at 620 nm. Sporadic and familial (type II) PCT can be distinguished by

measuring erythrocyte UROD activity.[151] In children, measurement of erythrocyte UROD activity and protoporphyrin concentration is required to distinguish HEP from type II PCT.

Treatment

When patients are diagnosed with PCT, an underlying cause for this disease needs to be evaluated. Infectious diseases should be investigated and treated, precipitating factors should be removed, evaluation for hepatitis C and hepatocellular carcinoma should be initiated, and testing for hemochromatosis accomplished.

The most effective treatments for PCT are low-dose chloroquine and phlebotomy. Phlebotomy was introduced in 1961 and remains the standard of care. It can induce remissions in most patients. There are many different protocols for phlebotomy in patients with PCT.[152] These may be similar to those used in hereditary hemochromatosis, commonly removing 300–450 mL of blood every 1–2 weeks and continuing until the ferritin level is at the lower limit of normal. Urinary porphyrin levels are monitored every 3 months during this time. Care must be taken to keep the hemoglobin above 10 g/dL.

When phlebotomy is contraindicated or when there is not marked iron overload, low-dose chloroquine is the most effective alternative (200–250 mg once to twice a week or hydroxychloroquine 100 mg twice a week). The mechanism of effect is not well understood. It is important for patients when beginning this treatment to know that normal doses of chloroquine (200 mg/day) can cause a hepatitis-like syndrome from the initial release of stored porphyrins in the liver. In this case, urinary porphyrins will significantly increase. In severe cases, both treatment modalities can be used. Urinary porphyrins should be monitored. In preliminary studies thalidomide appears to have some efficacy in treating PCT.[153]

Patients with end-stage renal disease can have severe forms of PCT. Porphyrins in this patient population are not easily dialyzable. In these patients the treatment of choice has become erythropoietin. This can correct anemia, mobilize iron and raise the hemoglobin enough to enable phlebotomy to decrease iron levels.[154,155]

Erythropoietic protoporphyria and ferrochelatase

EPP is an autosomal dominant disease due to a deficiency in the enzyme ferochelatase (FECH). FECH is the last step in heme formation. It catalyzes the insertion of iron into protoporphyrin IX.

The enzyme

Human FECH is encoded by a single 45-kb gene on chromosome 18 (18q21.3) that contains 11 exons. The gene contains two polyadenylation sites, the upstream site producing a 2.2-kb transcript that may be used preferentially in erythroid cells.[80,156] Newly synthesized FECH contains a sequence that directs transport into the mitochondrion and is then cleaved to form the mature 40-kDa protein. FECH functions *in vitro* as a monomer,[157] but radiation inactivation experiments suggest that it may be present in the mitochondrial membrane as a dimer.[158] Mammalian but not bacterial FECH has a carboxy-terminal extension that contains a [2Fe–2S] cluster.[159] Removal of this extension inactivates the enzyme, an unexpected finding in view of the similarity of the remaining sequence with those of active bacterial enzymes.[160] In addition to protoporphyrin IX and Fe^{2+}, other dicarboxylic porphyrins (mesoporphyrin, deuteroporphyrin) and metals (Zn^{2+}, Co^{2+}) serve as substrates. Mechanistic studies using *N*-alkylporphyrins as inhibitors suggest that the porphyrin ring becomes distorted during the reaction in order to facilitate Fe^{2+} insertion. The residues that bind Fe^{2+} have not been unequivocally identified. More recent site-directed mutagenesis experiments implicate histidine residues, particularly H263 in the human enzyme.[157]

Over 70 mutations of the FECH gene have been identified.[161] Most patients who inherit a mutant allele are asymptomatic. For protoporphyrin to accumulate to the level that will cause clinical symptoms, enzyme activity must be below 35%.[162] In most patients this is due to inheritance of a wild-type allele that has low expression of FECH in addition to a mutated allele (IVS3-48C allele).[15,163]

Autosomal recessive EPP, unlike homozygous variants of the other autosomal dominant porphyrias, is not phenotypically distinct. Prevalence in UK patients with EPP is 3% and those patients who have autosomal recessive disease have a higher risk of liver disease.[161]

Clinical presentation

EPP usually presents in early childhood. It is characterized by skin pain with erythema, itching and edema that develops rapidly on sun exposure. The pain after sun exposure can sometimes last for several days. Some patients initially manifest their illness as solar urticaria. These lesions occur mainly on the face and hands. If sun exposure is not avoided, chronic lesions develop with waxy thickening of the skin and scarring. Photosensitivity is worse during the summer months and may be exacerbated by heat exposure or temperature gradients.[164] In approximately 25% of patients with EPP, anemia can be found. This can be due to disturbed erythropoiesis or hemolysis.[165]

Liver disease is the most prevalent additional manifestation observed in this cutaneous porphyria. Protoporphyrin is lipophilic and is excreted in bile and enters the enterohepatic circulation; excess protoporphyrin will be taken up by hepatocytes and can exacerbate hepatotoxicity and biliary cholestasis. Patients can suffer from biliary stones causing obstruction and elevated liver enzymes, and a minority of patients will develop severe liver disease and failure.

Diagnosis

Patients will have increased free protoporphyrin in the feces and the plasma, with plasma fluorescence at 630 nm. Urinary porphyrin levels should be normal. There are also changes in the pattern of porphyrin levels that can be indicative of liver disease. Patients will have an increase in erythrocyte and plasma protoporphyrin and a decrease in stool protoporphyrin. There is also an increase in coproporphyrin I levels in the urine.[164]

Treatment

In patients with EPP, skin protection is very important as sun exposure can be debilitating. Sun avoidance, even through windows, is very important. Protective clothing and sunscreens should be used routinely. Care should be taken in patients with EPP undergoing surgery as prolonged exposure of internal organs to artificial light can severely burn internal organs and exacerbate anemia. β-Carotene has been used since 1970 to successfully diminish photosensitivity.[166] Doses range from 30 to 180 mg/day depending on the size of the patient. Other therapies, such as oral cysteine, phototherapy with narrow-band UVB (TL01 therapy), and cholestyramine to increase protoporphyrin excretion, have been used.[26] In patients with fulminant liver failure, liver transplantation is required.[167] Transfusion and exchange transfusion may decrease serum protoporphyrin levels.[168] Although these procedures may be valuable for acute toxicity,[169] they may not significantly reduce chronic liver toxicity or prevent progression to hepatic failure. The only way to induce remission in this disease is through HSCT.[167,170,171,172] Gene therapy attempting to express the FECH gene in hematopoietic stem cells is under investigation. Some animal models have shown success using this approach.[170]

References

1. Anderson KE, Sassa S, Bishop DF, Desnick RJ. The porphyrias. In: Scriver CR, Beaudet AL, Sly WS, Valle D (eds) *The Metabolic and Molecular Bases of Inherited Disease*, 8th edn. New York: McGraw-Hill, 2001, vol. 1, pp. 2991–3062.
2. Elder GH. The cutaneous porphyrias. In: Hawk JLM (ed.) *Photodermatology*. London: Arnold, 1999, pp. 171–97.
3. Elder GH. Hepatic porphyrias in children. *J Inherited Metab Dis* 1997; **20**: 237–46.
4. Maruno M, Furuyama K, Akagi R *et al*. Highly heterogeneous nature of δ aminolevulinate dehydratase (ALAD) deficiencies in ALAD porphyria. *Blood* 2001; **97**: 2972–8.
5. Desnick RJ, Astrin KH. Congenital erythropoietic porphyria:

advances in pathogenesis and treatment. *Br J Haematol* 2002; **117**: 779–95.

6. Todd DJ. Erythropoietic porphyria. *Br J Dermatol* 1994; **131**: 751–66.

7. Moran Jimenez MJ, Ged C, Romana M *et al.* Uroporphyrinogen decarboxylase: complete gene sequence and molecular study of three families with hepatoerythropoietic porphyria. *Am J Hum Genet* 1996; **58**: 712–21.

8. Hift R, Meissner PN, Todd G. Hepatoerythropoietic porphyria precipitated by viral hepatitis. *Gut* 1993; **34**: 1632–4.

9. Parsons JL, Sahn EE, Holden KR *et al.* Neurologic disease in a child with hepatoerythropoietic porphyria. *Pediatr Dermatol* 1994; **11**: 216–21.

10. With TK. Hereditary coproporphyria and variegate porphyria in Denmark. *Dan Med Bull* 1983; **30**: 106.

11. Elder GH. Porphyria cutanea tarda. *Semin Liver Dis* 1998; **18**: 67–75.

12. Kirsch RE, Meissner PN, Hift RJ. Variegate porphyria. *Semin Liver Dis* 1998; **181**: 33–41.

13. Fraunberg M, Timonen K, Mustajoki P, Kauppinen R. Clinical and biochemical characteristics and genotype–phenotype correlation in Finnish variegate porphyria patients. *Eur J Hum Genet* 2002; **10**: 649–57.

14. Wiman A, Harper P, Floderus Y. Nine novel mutations in the protoporphyrinogen oxidase gene in Swedish families with variegate porphyria. *Clin Genet* 2003; **64**: 122–30.

15. Gouya L, Puy H, Robreau AM *et al.* The penetrance of dominant erythropoietic protoporphyria is modulated by the expression of wildtype FECH. *Nat Genet* 2002; **30**: 27–8.

16. Meyer UA, Schuurmans MM, Pindberg RLP. Acute porphyrias: Pathogenesis of neurological manifestations. *Semin Liver Dis* 1998; **18**: 43–52.

17. Brennan MJ, Cantrill RC, Kramer S. Effect of delta-aminolaevulinic acid on GABA receptor binding in synaptic plasma membranes. *Int J Biochem* 1980; **12**: 833–5.

18. Mayer UA, Schuurmans MM, Pindberg RLP. Acute porphyrias: pathogenesis of neurological manifestations. *Semin Liver Dis* 1998; **18**: 43–52.

19. Puy H, Deybach JC, Bogdan A *et al.* Increased delta-aminolevulinic acid and decreased pineal melatonin production. A common event in acute porphyria studies in the rat. *J Clin Invest* 1996; **97**: 104–10.

20. Princ FG, Juknat AA, Maxit AG *et al.* Melatonin's antioxidant protection against delta-aminolevulinic acid- induced oxidative damage in rat cerebellum. *J Pineal Res* 1997; **23**: 40–6.

21. Carneiro RC, Reiter RJ. Delta-aminolevulinic acid-induced lipid peroxidation in rat kidney and liver is attenuated by melatonin: an in vitro and in vivo study. *J Pineal Res* 1998; **24**: 131–6.

22. Mustajoki P, Himberg JJ, Tokola O *et al.* Rapid normalization of antipyrine oxidation by heme in variegate porphyria. *Clin Pharmacol Ther* 1992; **51**: 320–4.

23. Gorchein A, Webber R. δ-Aminolevulinic acid in plasma, cerebrospinal fluid, saliva and erythrocytes: studies in normal, uraemic and porphyric subjects. *Clin Sci* 1987; **72**: 103–12.

24. Puy H, Deybach J-C, Baudry P *et al.* Decreased nocturnal plasma melatonin levels in patients with recurrent acute intermittent porphyria attacks. *Life Sci* 1993; **53**: 621–7.

25. Solis C, Marinez-Bermejo A, Naidich TP *et al.* Acute intermittent porphyria: studies of the severe homozygous dominant disease provides insights into the neurologic attacks in acute porphyria. *Arch Neurol* 2004; **61**: 1764–70.

26. Murphy GM for the British photodermatology group. The cutaneous porphyrias: a review. *Br J Dermatol* 1999; **140**: 573–81.

27. Wolff K, Hönigsmann H, Rauschmeier W *et al.* Microscopic and fine structural aspects of porphyrias. *Acta Derm Venereol* 1982; **100** (suppl.): 17–28.

28. Epstein JH, Tuffanelli DL, Epstein WL. Cutaneous changes in the porphyrias: a microscopic study. *Arch Dermatol* 1973; **107**: 689–98.

29. Wick G, Hönigsmann H, Timpl R. Immunofluorescence demonstration of type IV collagen and a noncollagenous glycoprotein in thickened vascular basal membranes in protoporphyria. *J Invest Dermatol* 1979; **73**: 335–8.

30. Dabski C, Beutner EH. Studies of laminin and type IV collagen in blisters of porphyria cutanea tarda and drug-induced pseudoporphyria. *J Am Acad Dermatol* 1991; **25**: 28–32.

31. Spikes JD. Photobiology of porphyrins. In: Doiron DR, Gomer CF (eds) *Porphyrin Localization and Treatment of Tumors*. New York: Liss, 1984, pp. 19–39.

32. Lim HW, Poh-Fitzpatrick MB, Gigh I. Activation of the complement system in patients with porphyrias after irradiation *in vivo. J Clin Invest* 1984; **74**: 1961–5.

33. Glover RA, Bailey CS, Barrett KE *et al.* Histamine release from rodent and human mast cells induced by protoporphyrin and ultraviolet light: studies of the mechanism of mast-cell activation in erythropoietic protoporphyria. *Br J Dermatol* 1996; **134**: 880–5.

34. Herrmann G, Wlaschek M, Bolsen K *et al.* Photosensitization of uroporphyrin augments the ultraviolet A-induced synthesis of matrix metalloproteinases in human dermal fibroblasts. *J Invest Dermatol* 1996; **107**: 398–403.

35. Blake D, McManus J, Cronin V *et al.* Fecal coproporphyrin isomers in hereditary coproporphyria. *Clin Chem* 1992; **38**: 96–100.

36. Nordmann Y, Deybach JC. Human hereditary porphyrias. In: Dailey HA (ed.) *Biosynthesis of Heme and Chlorophylls*. New York: McGraw-Hill, 1990, pp. 491–542.

37. Long C, Smyth SJ, Woolf J *et al.* Detection of latent variegate porphyria by fluorescence emission spectroscopy of plasma. *Br J Dermatol* 1993; **129**: 9–13.

38. Mauzerall DC. Evolution of porphyrins. *Clin Dermatol* 1998; **16**: 195–201.

39. Bishop DF, Henderson AS, Astrin KH. Human delta-aminolevulinate synthase: assignment of the housekeeping gene 3p21 and the erythroid-specific gene to the X chromosome. *Genomics* 1990; **7**: 207–14.

40. May A, Bishop DF. The molecular biology and pyridoxine responsiveness of X-linked sideroblastic anaemia. *Haematologica* 1998; **83**: 56–70.

41. Granick S, Sassa S. Delta-aminolevulinic acid synthetase and the control of heme and chlorophyll synthesis. In: Vogel HJ (ed.) *Metabolic Regulation*. New York: Academic Press, 1971, p. 71.

42. May BK, Dogra SC, Sadlon TJ *et al.* Molecular regulation of haem biosynthesis in higher vertebrates. *Prog Nucl Acids Res Mol Biol* 1995; **51**: 1–51.

43. Tenhunen R, Marver HS, Schmid R. Microsomal heme oxygenase. *J Biol Chem* 1969; **244**: 6388–94.

44. Mustajoki P, Tenhunen R, Pierach C, Volin L. Heme in the treatment of porphyrias and hematological disorders. *Semin Hematol* 1989; **26**: 1–9.

45. Kappas A, Simionatto CS, Drummond GS, Sassa S, Anderson KE. The liver excretes large amounts of heme into bile when heme oxygenase is inhibited competitively by Sn-protoporphyrin. *Proc Natl Acad Sci USA* 1985; **82**: 896–900.

46. Ponka P. Tissue-specific regulation of iron metabolism and heme synthesis: distinct control mechanism in erythroid cells. *Blood* 1997; **89**: 1–25.

47. Ponka P. Cell biology of heme. *Am J Med Sci* 1999; **318**: 241–56.

48. Doss M, von Tiepermann R, Schneider J, Schmid H. New type of hepatic porphyria with porphobilinogen synthase defect and intermittent acute clinical manifestations. *Klin Wochenschr* 1979; **57**: 1123–7.

49. Potluri VR, Astrin KH, Wetmur JG *et al*. Human delta-aminolevulinate dehydratase: chromosomal localization to 9q34 by in situ hybridization. *Hum Genet* 1987; **76**: 236–9.

50. Kaya AH, Plewinska M, Wong DM, Desnick RJ, Wetmur JG. Human δ-aminolevulinate dehydratase (ALAD) gene: structure and alternative splicing of the erythroid and housekeeping mRNAs. *Genomics* 1994; **19**: 242–8.

51. Granick JL, Sassa S, Kappas A. Some biochemical and clinical aspects of lead intoxication. In: Bodansky O, Latner AL (eds) *Advances in Clinical Chemistry*. New York: Academic Press, 1978, p. 287.

52. Sassa S, Kappas A. Hereditary tyrosinemia and the heme biosynthetic pathway. Profound inhibition of delta-aminolevulinic acid dehydratase activity by succinylacetone. *J Clin Invest* 1983; **71**: 625–34.

53. Lindblad B, Lindstedt S, Steen G. On the enzymic defects in hereditary tyrosinemia. *Proc Natl Acad Sci USA* 1977; **74**: 4641–5.

54. Ishida N, Fujita H, Noguchi T *et al*. Message amplification phenotyping of an inherited delta-aminolevulinate dehydratase deficiency in a family with acute hepatic porphyria. *Biochem Biophys Res Commun* 1990; **172**: 237–42.

55. Plewinska M, Thunell S, Holmberg L *et al*. Delta-aminolevulinate dehydratase deficient porphyria: identification of the molecular lesions in a severely affected homozygote. *Am J Hum Genet* 1991; **49**: 167–74.

56. Akagi R, Shimizu R, Furuyama K *et al*. Novel molecular defects of the delta-aminolevulinate dehydratase gene in a patient with inherited acute hepatic porphyria. *Hepatology* 2000; **31**: 704–8.

57. Akagi R, Nishitani C, Harigae H *et al*. Molecular analysis of delta-aminolevulinate dehydratase deficiency in a patient with an unusual late-onset porphyria. *Blood* 2000; **96**: 3618–23.

58. Akagi R, Yasui Y, Harper P, Sassa S. A novel mutation of delta-aminolaevulinate dehydratase in a healthy child with 12% erythrocyte enzyme activity. *Br J Haematol* 1999; **106**: 931–7.

59. Thunell S, Holmberg L, Lundgren J. Aminolevulinate dehydratase porphyria in infancy: a clinical and biochemical study. *J Clin Chem Clin Biochem* 1987; **25**: 5–14.

60. Hassoun A, Verstraeten L, Mercelis R, Martin J-J. Biochemical diagnosis of a hereditary aminolaevulinate dehydratase deficiency in a 63-year-old man. *J Clin Chem Clin Biochem* 1989; **27**: 781–6.

61. Guolo M, Stella AM, Melito V *et al*. Altered 5-aminolevulinic acid metabolism leading to pseudoporphyria in hemodialysed patients. *Int J Biochem Cell Biol* 1996; **28**: 311–17.

62. Fernandez-Cuartero B, Rebollar JL, Batlle A, Enriquez de Salamanca R. Delta-aminolevulinate dehydratase (ALA-D) activity in human and experimental diabetes mellitus. *Int J Biochem Cell Biol* 1999; **31**: 479–88.

63. Louie GV, Brownlie PD, Lambert R *et al*. The three-dimensional structures of mutants of porphobilinogen deaminase: a flexible multidomain polymerase with a single catalytic site. *Nature* 1992; **359**: 33–9.

64. Brownlie PD, Lambert R, Louie GV *et al*. The three-dimensional structures of mutants of porphobilinogen deaminase: toward an understanding of the structural basis of acute intermittent porphyria. *Protein Sci* 1994; **3**: 1644–50.

65. Jordan PM. Porphobilinogen deaminase: mechanism of action and role in the biosynthesis of uroporphyrinogen III. In: *The Biosynthesis of the Tetrapyrrole Pigments*. Ciba Foundation Symposium 180. Chichester: John Wiley & Sons, 1994, pp. 70–96.

66. Jordan PM, Warren MJ. Evidence for a dipyrromethane cofactor at the catalytic site of *E. coli* porphobilinogen deaminase. *FEBS Lett* 1987; **225**: 87–92.

67. Yoo HW, Warner CA, Chen CH, Desnick RJ. Hydroxymethylbilane synthase: complete genomic sequence and amplifiable polymorphisms in the human gene. *Genomics* 1993; **15**: 21–7.

68. Chretien S, Dubart A, Beaupain D *et al*. Alternative transcription and splicing of the human porphobilinogen deaminase gene result either in tissue-specific or in housekeeping expression. *Proc Natl Acad Sci USA* 1988; **85**: 6–10.

69. Puy H, Deyback JC, Lamoril J *et al*. Molecular diagnosis of PBG deaminase gene defects in acute intermittent porphyria. *Am J Hum Genet* 1997; **60**: 1373–83.

70. Sassa S, Kappas A. Molecular aspects of the inherited porphyrias. *J Intern Med* 2000; **247**: 169–78.

71. Puy H, Gross U, Deybach JC *et al*. Exon 1 donor splice site mutations in the porphobilinogen deaminase gene in the non-erythroid variant form of acute intermittent porphyria. *Hum Genet* 1998; **103**: 570–5.

72. Barclay N. Acute intermittent porphyria in childhood: a neglected diagnosis? *Arch Dis Child* 1974; **49**: 404–5.

73. Beauvais P, Klein M-L, Denave L *et al*. Porphyrie ague intermittente a l'age de quatre mois. *Arch Fr Pediatr* 1976; **33**: 987–92.

74. Burgovne K, Swartz R, Ananth J. Porphyria: reexamination of psychiatric implications. *Psychother Psychosom* 1995; **64**: 121.

75. Crimlisk HL. The little imitator – porphyria: a neuropsychiatric disorder. *J Neurol Neurosurg Psychiatry* 1997; **62**: 319–28.

76. Kauppinen R, Mustajoki P. Prognosis of acute porphyria: occurrence of acute attacks, precipitating factors and associated diseases. *Medicine* 1992; **71**: 1–13.

77. Jeans JB, Savik K, Gross CR *et al*. Mortality in patients with acute intermittent porphyria requiring hospitalization: a United States case series. *Am J Med Genet* 1996; **65**: 269–73.

78. Onuki J, Teixeira PC, Medeiros MH *et al*. Is 5-aminolevulinic acid involved in the hepatocellular carcinogenesis of acute intermittent porphyria? *Cell Mol Biol* 2002; **48**: 17–26.

79. Moore MR, McColl KEL, Rimington C, Goldberg A. *Disorders of Porphyrin Metabolism.* New York: Plenum, 1987.

80. Anderson K. The porphyrias. In: Zakim D, Boyer TD (eds) *Hepatology: A Textbook of Liver Disease.* Philadelphia: WB Saunders, 1995, pp. 417–63.

81. Andersson C, Innala E, Backstrom T. Acute intermittent porphyria in women: clinical expression, use and experience of exogenous sex hormones. A population-based study in northern Sweden. *J Intern Med* 2003; **254**: 176–83.

82. Levit EJ, Nodine JH, Perloff WH. Progesterone-induced porphyria: case report. *Am J Med* 1957; **22**: 831.

83. Rodgers PA, Stevenson DK. Developmental biology of heme oxygenase. *Clin Perinatol* 1990; **17**: 275–91.

84. Andersson C, Bylesjo I, Lithner F. Effects of diabetes mellitus on patients with acute intermittent porphyria. *J Intern Med* 1999; **245**: 193–7.

85. Bonkovsky H, Barnard G. Diagnosis of porphyric syndromes: a practical approach in the era of molecular biology. *Semin Liver Dis* 1998; **18**: 57–65.

86. Elder GH, Smith SG, Smyth SJ. Laboratory investigation of the porphyrias. *Ann Clin Biochem* 1990; **27**: 395–412.

87. Lamon J, With TK, Redeker AG. The Hoesch test: bedside screening for urinary porphobilinogen in patients with suspected porphyria. *Clin Chem* 1974; **20**: 1438–40.

88. Ford RE, Magera MJ, Kloke KM, Chezick PA, Fauq A, McConnell JP. Quantitative measurement of porphobilinogen in urine by stable-isotope dilution liquid chromatography-tandem mass spectrometry. *Clin Chem* 2001; **47**: 1627–32.

89. Belfau-Larue M-H, Martasek P, Grandchamp B. Coproporphyrinogen oxidase: gene organisation and description of a mutation leading to exon 6 skipping. *Hum Mol Genet* 1994; **3**: 1325–30.

90. Medlock AE, Dailey HA. Human coproporphyrinogen oxidase is not a metalloprotein. *J Biol Chem* 1996; **271**: 32507–10.

91. Dailey HA. Conversion of coproporphyrinogen to protoheme in higher eukaryotes and bacteria: terminal three enzymes. In: Dailey HA (ed.) *Biosynthesis of Heme and Chlorophylls.* New York: McGraw-Hill, 1990, p. 123.

92. Takahashi S, Taketani S, Akasaka JE *et al.* Differential regulation of coproporphyrinogen oxidase gene between erythroid and nonerythroid cells. *Blood* 1998; **92**: 3436–44.

93. Takahashi S, Furuyama K, Kobayashi A *et al.* Cloning of a coproporphyrinogen oxidase promoter regulatory element binding protein. *Biochem Biophys Res Commun* 2000; **273**: 596–602.

94. Martasek P, Nordmann Y, Grandchamp B. Homozygous hereditary coproporphyria caused by an arginine to tryptophane substitution in coproporphyrinogen oxidase and common intragenic polymorphisms. *Hum Mol Genet* 1994; **3**: 477–80.

95. Lamoril J, Deybach JC, Puy H *et al.* Three novel mutations in the coproporphyrinogen oxidase gene. *Hum Mutat* 1997; **9**: 78–80.

96. Schreiber WE, Zhang X, Senz J, Jamani A. Hereditary coproporphyria: exon screening by heteroduplex analysis detects three novel mutations in the coproporphyrinogen oxidase gene. *Hum Mutat* 1997; **10**: 196–200.

97. Gross U, Puy H, Kuhnel A *et al.* Molecular, immunological, enzymatic and biochemical studies of coproporphyrinogen oxidase deficiency in a family with hereditary coproporphyria. *Cell Mol Biol* 2002; **48**: 49–55.

98. Lamoril J, Puy H, Whatley SD *et al.* Characterization of mutations in the CPO gene in British patients demonstrates absence of genotype–phenotype correlation and identifies relationship between hereditary coproporphyria and harderoporphyria. *Am J Hum Genet* 2001; **68**: 1130–8.

99. Kuhnel A, Gross U, Doss MO. Hereditary coproporphyria in Germany: clinical–biochemical studies in 53 patients. *Clin Biochem* 2000; **33**: 465–73.

100. Lamoril J, Puy H, Gouya L *et al.* Neonatal hemolytic anemia due to inherited harderoporphyria: clinical characteristics and molecular basis. *Blood* 1998; **91**: 1453–7.

101. Gross U, Gerlack R, Kuhnel A *et al.* A description of an HPLC assay of coproporphyrinogen III oxidase activity in mononuclear cells. *J Inherited Metab Dis* 2003; **26**: 565–70.

102. Taketani S, Inazawa J, Abe T *et al.* The human protoporphyrinogen oxidase gene (PPOX): organization and location to chromosome 1. *Genomics* 1995; **29**: 698–703.

103. Roberts AG, Whatley SD, Daniels J *et al.* Partial characterization and assignment of the gene for protoporphyrinogen oxidase and variegate porphyria to human chromosome 1q23. *Hum Mol Genet* 1995; **4**: 2387–90.

104. Puy H, Robréau A-M, Rosipal R, Nordmann, Y, Deybach J-C. Protoporphyrinogen oxidase: complete genomic sequence and polymorphisms in the human gene. *Biochem Biophys Res Commun* 1996; **226**: 227–30.

105. Dailey TA, Dailey HA. Expression, purification and characteristics of mammalian protoporphyrinogen oxidase. *Methods Enzymol* 1997; **281**: 340–9.

106. Deybach JC, da Silva V, Grandchamp B, Nordmann Y. The mitochondrial location of protoporphyrinogen oxidase. *Eur J Biochem* 1985; **149**: 431–5.

107. Nordmann Y, Puy H. Human hereditary hepatic porphyrias. *Clin Chim Acta* 2002; **325**: 17–37.

108. Meissner PN, Dailey TA, Hift RJ *et al.* A R59W mutation in human protoporphyrinogen oxidase results in decreased enzyme activity and is prevalent in South Africans with variegate porphyria. *Nat Genet* 1996; **13**: 95–7.

109. von und zu Fraunberg M, Timonen K, Mustajoki P *et al.* Clinical and biochemical characteristics and genotype–phenotype correlation in Finnish variegate porphyria patients. *Eur J Hum Genet* 2002; **10**: 649–57.

110. Kirsch RE, Meissner PN, Hift RJ. Variegate porphyria. *Semin Liver Dis* 1998; **18**: 33–41.

111. Hift R, Meissner PN, Todd G *et al.* Homozygous variegate porphyria: an evolving clinical syndrome. *Postgrad Med J* 1993; **69**: 781–6.

112. Roberts AG, Whatley SD, Dailey TA *et al.* Molecular characterization of homozygous variegate porphyria. *J Inherited Metab Dis* 1996; **19** (suppl. 1): 17.

113. Poh-Fitzpatrick MB. A plasma porphyrin fluorescence marker for variegate porphyria. *Arch Dermatol* 1980; **116**: 543–7.

114. Longas MO, Poh-Fitzpatrick MB. A tightly bound protein–porphyrin complex isolated from the plasma of a patient with variegate porphyria. *Clin Chim Acta* 1982; **118**: 219–28.

115. Rogers, PD. Cimetidine in the treatment of acute intermittent porphyria. *Ann Pharmacother* 1997; **31**: 365–7.

116. Bonkovsky HL. Advances in understanding and treating

"the little imitator", acute porphyria. *Gastroenterology* 1993; **105**: 590–4.

117. Dover SB, Moore MR, Fitzsimmons EJ *et al.* Tin protoporphyrin prolongs the biochemical remission produced by heme arginate in acute hepatic porphyria. *Gastroenterology* 1993; **105**: 500–6.

118. Anderson KE, Spitz IM, Bardin CW, Kappas A. A gonadotropin releasing hormone analogue prevents cyclical attacks of porphyria. *Arch Intern Med* 1990; **150**: 1469–74.

119. Tenhunen R, Mustajoki P. Acute porphyria: treatment with heme. *Semin Liver Dis* 1998; **18**: 53–5.

120. Elder GH, Hift RJ. Treatment of acute porphyria. *Hosp Med* 2001; **62**: 422–5.

121. Soonawalla ZF, Orug T, Badminton MN *et al.* Liver transplantation as a cure for acute intermittent porphyria. *Lancet* 2004; **363**: 705–6.

122. Stojeba N, Meyer C, Jeanpierre C *et al.* Recovery from a variegate porphyria by a liver transplantation. *Liver Transplant* 2004; **10**: 935–8.

123. Johansson A, Moller C, Harper P. Correction of the biochemical defect in porphobilinogen deaminase deficient cells by non-viral gene delivery. *Mol Cell Biochem* 2003; **250**: 65–71.

124. Johansson A, Nowak G, Moller C, Harper P. Non-viral delivery of the porphobilinogen deaminase cDNA into a mouse model of acute intermittent porphyria. *Mol Genet Metab* 2004; **82**: 20–6.

125. Tsai SF, Bishop DF, Desnick RJ. Human uroporphyrinogen III synthase: molecular cloning, nucleotide sequence, and expression of a full-length cDNA. *Proc Natl Acad Sci USA* 1988; **85**: 7049.

126. Shoolingin-Jordan PM. Porphobilinogen deaminase and uroporphyrinogen III synthase. *J Bioenerg Biomembr* 1995; **27**: 181–96.

127. Aizencang G, Solis C, Bishop DF, Warner C, Desnick RJ. Human uroporphyrinogen-III synthase: genomic organization, alternative promoters, and erythroid-specific expression. *Genomics* 2000; **70**: 223–31.

128. Desnick RJ, Astrin KH. Congenital erythropoietic porphyria: advances in pathogenesis and treatment. *Br J Haematol* 2002; **117**: 779–95.

129. Warner CA, Poh-Fitzpatrick MB, Zaider EF *et al.* Congenital erythropoietic porphyria. A mild variant with low uroporphyrin I levels due to a missense mutation (A66V) encoding residual uroporphyrinogen III synthase activity. *Arch Dermatol* 1992; **128**: 1243–8.

130. Fritsch C, Bolsen K, Ruzicka T, Günter G. Congenital erythropoietic porphyria. *J Am Acad Dermatol* 1997; **36**: 594–610.

131. Poh-Fitzpatrick MB. The erythropoietic porphyrias. *Dermatol Clin* 1986; **4**: 291–8.

132. Piomelli S, Poh-Fitzpatrick MB, Seaman C *et al.* Complete suppression of the symptoms of congenital erythropoietic porphyria by long-term treatment with high-level transfusions. *N Engl J Med* 1986; **314**: 1029–31.

133. Laorr A, Greenspan A. Severe osteopenia in congenital erythropoietic porphyria. *Can Assoc Radiol J* 1994; **45**: 307–9.

134. Shoolingin-Jordan PM, Leadbeater R. Coupled assay for uroporphyrinogen III synthase. *Methods Enzymol* 1997; **281**: 327–36.

135. Deybach JC, Grandchamp B, Grelier M *et al.* Prenatal exclusion of congenital erythropoietic porphyria (Gunther's disease) in a fetus at risk. *Hum Genet* 1980; **53**: 217–21.

136. Ged C, Moreau-Gaudry F, Taine L *et al.* Prenatal diagnosis in congenital erythropoietic porphyria by metabolic measurement and DNA mutation analysis. *Prenat Diagn* 1996; **16**: 83–6.

137. Mathews-Roth MM, Pathak MA, Fitzpatrick TB *et al.* Beta carotene therapy for erythropoietic protoporphyria and other photosensitivity diseases. *Arch Dermatol* 1977; **113**: 1229–32.

138. Guarini L, Piomelli S, Poh Fitzpatrick MB. Hydroxyurea in congenital erythropoietic porphyria [letter]. *N Engl J Med* 1994; **330**: 1091–2.

139. Tishler PV, Winston SH. Rapid improvement in the chemical pathology of congenital erythropoietic porphyria with treatment with superactivated charcoal. *Methods Find Exp Clin Pharmacol* 1990; **12**: 645–8.

140. Dupuis-Girod S, Akkari V, Ged C *et al.* Successful match-unrelated donor bone marrow transplantation for congenital erythropoietic porphyria (Gunther disease). *Eur J Pediatr* 2005; **164**: 104–7.

141. Elder GH, Urquhart AJ, De Salamanca RE *et al.* Immunoreactive uroporphyrinogen decarboxylase in the liver in porphyria cutanea tarda. *Lancet* 1985; **ii**: 229–33.

142. Elder GH, Roberts AG. Uroporphyrinogen decarboxylase. *J Bioenerg Biomembr* 1995; **27**: 207–14.

143. Phillips JD, Whitby FG, Kushner JP, Hill CP. Characterization and crystallization of human uroporphyrinogen decarboxylase. *Protein Sci* 1997; **6**: 1343–6.

144. Wyckoff EE, Phillips JD, Sowa AM, Franklin MR, Kushner JK. Mutational analysis of human uroporphyrinogen decarboxylase. *Biochim Biophys Acta* 1996; **1298**: 294–304.

145. Roberts AG, Elder GH, De Salamanca RE *et al.* A mutation (G281E) of the human uroporphyrinogen decarboxylase gene causes both hepatoerythropoietic porphyria and overt familial porphyria cutanea tarda: biochemical and genetic studies on Spanish patients. *J Invest Dermatol* 1995; **104**: 500–2.

146. Roberts AG, Whatley SD, Morgan RR *et al.* Increased frequency of the haemochromatosis Cys282Tyr mutation in sporadic porphyria cutanea tarda. *Lancet* 1997; **349**: 321–3.

147. Sampietro M, Piperno A, Lupica L *et al.* High prevalence of the His63Asp HFE mutation in Italian patients with porphyria cutanea tarda. *Hepatology* 1998; **27**: 181–4.

148. Lamoril J, Andant C, Gouya L *et al.* Hemochromatosis (HFE) and transferrin receptor-1 (TFRC1) genes in sporadic porphyria cutanea tarda (sPCT). *Cell Mol Biol* 2002; **48**: 33–41.

149. Bulaj ZJ, Phillips JD, Ajioka RS *et al.* Hemochromatosis genes and other factors contributing to the pathogenesis of porphyria cutanea tarda. *Blood* 2000; **95**: 1565–71.

150. Grossman ME, Poh-Fitzpatrick MB. Porphyria cutanea tarda. Diagnosis and management. *Med Clin North Am* 1980; **64**: 807–27.

151. Held JL, Sassa S, Kappas A *et al.* Erythrocyte uroporphyrinogen decarboxylase activity in porphyria cutanea tarda: a study of 40 consecutive patients. *J Invest Dermatol* 1989; **93**: 332–4.

152. Badminton MN, Elder GH. Management of acute and cutaneous porphyrias. *Int J Clin Pract* 2002; **56**: 272–8.

153. Monastirli A, Georgiou S, Bolsen K *et al.* Treatment of porphyria cutanea tarda with oral thalidomide. *Skin Pharmacol Appl Skin Physiol* 1999; **12**: 305–11.

154. Anderson KE, Goeger DE, Carson RW *et al.* Erythropoietin for the treatment of porphyria cutanea tarda in a patient on long-term hemodialysis *N Engl J Med* 1990; **322**: 315–17. Erratum in *N Engl J Med* 1990; **322**: 1616.

155. Peces R, Salamanca R, Fontanellas A *et al.* Successful treatment of haemodialysis-related porphyria cutanea tarda with erythropoietin. *Nephrol Dial Transplant* 1994; **9**: 433–5.

156. Taketani S, Inazawa J, Nakahashi Y, Abe T, Tokunaga R. Structure of the human ferrochelatase gene. Exon/intron gene organization and location of the gene to chromosome 18. *Eur J Biochem* 1992; **205**: 217–22.

157. Ferreira GC, Ricardo F, Lloyd SG, Moura I, Moura JJG, Huynh BH. Structure and function of ferrochelatase. *J Bioenerg Biomembr* 1995; **27**: 221–30.

158. Straka JG, Bloomer JR, Kempner ES. The functional size of ferrochelatase determined *in situ* by radiation inactivation. *J Biol Chem* 1991; **266**: 24637–41.

159. Franco R, Moura JJG, Moura I *et al.* Characterization of the iron-binding site in mammalian ferrochelatase by kinetic and Mössbauer methods. *J Biol Chem* 1995; **270**: 26352–7.

160. Schneider-Yin X, Gouya L, Dorsey M *et al.* Mutations in the iron-sulfur cluster ligand of the human ferrochelatase lead to erythropoietic protoporphyria. *Blood* 2000; **96**: 1545–9.

161. Whatley SD, Mason NG, Khan M *et al.* Autosomal recessive erythropoietic protoporphyria in the United Kingdom: prevalence and relationship to liver disease. *J Med Genet* 2004; **41**: e105.

162. Rossi E, Costin KA, Garcia-Webb P. Ferrochelatase activity in human lymphocytes, as quantified by a new high-performance liquid-chromatographic method. *Clin Chem* 1988; **34**: 2481–5.

163. Gouya L, Puy H, Lamoril J *et al.* Inheritance in erythropoietic protoporphyria: a common wild-type ferrochelatase allelic variant with low expression accounts for clinical manifestation *Blood* 1999; **93**: 2105–10.

164. Lecha M. Erythropoietic protoporphyria. *Photodermatol Photoimmunol Photomed* 2003; **19**: 142–6.

165. Mathews-Roth MM. Anemia in erythropoietic protoporphyria [letter]. *JAMA* 1974; **230**: 824.

166. Mathews-Roth MM, Pathak MA, Fitzpatrick TB *et al.* Beta-carotene as a photoprotective agent in erythropoietic protoporphyria. *N Engl J Med* 1970; **282**: 1231–4.

167. Meerman L, Haagsma EB, Gouw AS *et al.* Long-term follow-up after liver transplantation for erythropoietic protoporphyria. *Eur J Gastroenterol Hepatol* 1999; **11**: 431–8.

168. Eichbaum QG, Dzik WH *et al.* Red blood cell exchange transfusion in two patients with advanced erthropoetic protoporphyria. *Transfusion* 2005; **45**: 208–13.

169. Van Wijk HV, van Hattum J *et al.* Blood transfusion therapy for acute cholestasis in protoporphyria. *Dig Dis Sci* 1988; **33**: 1621–5.

170. Pratschke J, Steinmuller T *et al.* Orthoptic liver transplantation for hepatic associated metabolic disorders. *Clinical Transplantation* 1998; **12**: 228–32.

171. Poh-Fitzpatrick MB, Wang X, Anderson KE *et al.* Erthopoietic protoporphyria: altered phenotype after bone marrow transplantation for myelogenous leukemia in a patient heteroallelic for ferrochelatase gene mutations. *J Am Dermatol* 2002; **46**: 861–6.

172. Fontanellas A, Mazurier F, Landry M *et al.* Reversion of hepatobiliary alterations by bone marrow transplantation in a murine model of erythropoietic protoporphyria. *Hepatology* 2000; **32**: 73–81.

10 Sickle cell disease

Corrina McMahon

Introduction

The first recorded description of sickle cell crisis was by Africanus Horton who noted the association of bone pains and cold weather.[1] The first medical description of sickle cell disease was published in 1910. It described thin sickle-shaped red cells occurring in a Caribbean student who was hospitalized with back and muscle pain and suggested that the illness might be related to the abnormally shaped cells.[2] In 1949 Pauling and Itano described sickle cell anemia as the first molecular disease when they found that hemoglobin from a patient with sickle cell anemia (HbS) differed in electrophoretic mobility from normal hemoglobin (HbA) and that hemoglobin from a subject with sickle cell trait was a mixture of HbS and HbA.[3] Some years later Ingram described the valine for glutamine substitution of normal hemoglobin that produces HbS.[4]

Sickle cell disease (SCD) is a generic term for a group of disorders that includes homozygous sickle cell anemia (HbSS), sickle cell hemoglobin C disease (HbSC), sickle cell thalassemia disease (S/thal) and other compound heterozygous conditions. They are all characterized by the presence of the mutated β-globin gene, β^S-globin, and all cause clinical disease.[5] Homozygous HbSS and compound heterozygosity for β^0-thalassemia have the most severe phenotype. Compound heterozygosity with HbC, and β^+-thalassemia have a less severe phenotype and an increased life expectancy. Sickle cell trait (HbAS) is the carrier state and is not classified as a sickle cell disease.

Epidemiology

The β^S-globin gene mutation has arisen independently several times and at least five mutations, four in Africa and one in India, have been selected and expanded.[6] The three major African genotypes are localized exclusively to one major geographical area: Benin to central west Africa, Senegal to the African west coast and Bantu (Central African Republic) to central Africa. The Arab–Indian mutation probably originated in the Indus valley and extended to Saudi Arabia, Bahrain, Kuwait and Oman.[7] The African and Arab slave trades have been responsible for genetic dissemination throughout Europe and America and more recently war and economic migration has brought the gene to countries where it was formerly unknown. In many cases there is now a considerable admixture of the African genotypes in America and Europe.

The prevalence of sickle cell trait in western, central and eastern Africa is 5–40% but is less common in northern and southern Africa.[8] It occurs in 8% of the African-American population and SCD affects about 1 in 600 African-Americans.[9] In the UK, it is estimated that about 3000 babies (0.47%) are born each year with sickle cell trait and 0.28 per 1000 conceptions are affected by SCD.[10]

The median life expectancy for those with homozygous SCD (HbSS) in the USA was reported at 42 years for males and 48 years for females in 1994, whereas those with HbSC had a median life expectancy of 60 and 68 years respectively. The study found that 33% of deaths occurred during an acute crisis; the other major cause of death was acute organ failure.[11] Factors that predict adverse outcome are dactylitis, severe anemia (hemoglobin < 7 g/dL), and leukocytosis within the first 2 years of life.[12] A 2004 study clearly demonstrates the influence of aggressive management strategies in childhood. It reports a death rate of 0.4 per 100 patient-years and a sickle-related survival rate of 93.6% by 18 years of age. The mean age of death in this study was 5.6 years and the most common cause of death was infection.[13] The most common portal of entry for infection is the upper respiratory tract and death commonly occurs within the first 24 hours following an acute presentation.[14] The situation in Africa is quite different. In 1989 the death rate was estimated to be 50% before the age of 1 year in Nigeria,[15] and in Kenya some years later it was noted that 77% of those with SCD were aged less than 15 years, suggesting that most died in their teenage years.[16]

Pathophysiology

SCD is caused by a single point mutation at codon 6 of the β-globin gene that results in a valine → glutamine substitution. The resultant mutant hemoglobin (HbS) polymerizes when deoxygenated (Table 10.1) because valine can dock with complementary sites on adjacent globin chains. Polymerization depends on intracellular HbS concentration, the degree of cell deoxygenation, pH and the intracellular concentration of fetal hemoglobin (HbF). The polymers form bundles that distort the red cell into the classic sickled or crescent shape and interfere with red cell membrane structure and deformability.[7] Some coinherited or acquired conditions, e.g., hereditary persistence of HbF and α-thalassemia, can reduce HbS polymerization and reduce sickling (Table 10.2).

Damage to the red cell membrane produces a series of abnormal sodium, potassium and calcium fluxes that lead to red cell dehydration (Table 10.3).[7,17] Red cell dehydration increases the intracellular HbS concentration and promotes sickling.

Vasoocclusion, the key feature of SCD, is the end result of a series of red cell, endothelial, monocyte and platelet interactions (Table 10.3). A proposed unified schema is that the endothelium is activated by cytokines released by infection, inflammation or directly by migrating leukocytes.[18] The red cell adheres to the endothelium through a series of mechanisms, either directly via exposed red cell membrane phosphatidylserine or sulfated glycans, or by using soluble adhesion molecules (e.g., integrins and thrombospondin and/or high-molecular-weight von Willebrand factor) as a bridge.[18,19,21] Adherent leukocytes and red cells narrow

Table 10.1 Factors contributing to sickle cell crisis.

Deoxygenation
Dehydration
Infection
Pyrexia
Change in temperature
Acidosis
Exercise
Menstruation (some women only)

Table 10.2 Disease modifiers.

Coinheritance of hereditary persistence of fetal hemoglobin
Coinheritance of any other disorder of β-globin giving rise to increased HbF levels
Saudi-Arabian/Indian and Senegal phenotypes (increased HbF)
Coinheritance of α-thalassemic trait
Iron deficiency

Table 10.3 Factors contributing to sickle cell crisis.

HbS polymerization

An increase in red cell dehydration[7,17]
Increased cation (sodium, potassium, magnesium and calcium) membrane permeability
Calcium ion entry activates the Gardos channels
Activation of the Gardos channels (calcium-sensitive K^+-efflux channels) triggers the loss of potassium and water and leads to red cell dehydration
K/Cl cotransporter mechanism is activated by lower pH and deoxygenation contributing to intracellular dehydration

Disruption of the red cell bilayer and exposure of phosphatidylserine[7]

Upregulation of endothelial adhesion molecules[18]
Leukocyte activation and adherence to the endothelium
Adherence of the red cell to the endothelium

Nitric oxide depletion by free heme[21]
Reduction of nitric oxide
Loss of nitric oxide-associated vasodilatation
Upregulation of adhesion molecules

the diameter of the blood vessel, slowing blood flow and trapping dense sickled cells. The increase in blood transit time also increases red cell sickling and, finally, blood vessel occlusion occurs. This produces ischemia and finally necrosis, which causes cytokine release and perpetuates the sickle event.[7,19,20]

Sickle cell trait

Sickle cell trait is a benign condition produced when a gene containing the HbS mutation is inherited along with a normal β-globin gene, and is described as HbAS. The individual with HbAS is considered to be a carrier of the sickle cell genetic mutation. Two HbAS partners have a 25% risk of having a child with HbSS and this risk remains the same for each pregnancy. The diagnosis of HbAS is made when the quantity of HbA exceeds that of HbS on hemoglobin testing. Individuals with sickle cell trait can suffer an excessive incidence of hematuria and a urine-concentrating defect. This is probably caused by microvascular injury in the vasa recta of the renal medulla, which has a hypoxic acidotic environment conducive to sickling even in the presence of HbA. Nevertheless, HbAS should only be considered as the cause of hematuria when other possibilities have been excluded. There are reports that individuals with sickle cell trait can develop sickle cell crisis and there is an increased incidence of sudden death in some individuals with HbAS. This is probably related to heat exhaustion brought on by rigorous exercise in hot weather. A liberal fluid intake, gradual acclimatization and the avoidance of overexertion is suggested for individuals with sickle cell trait in hot climates.[22]

Laboratory features

HbF is the predominant hemoglobin at birth, comprising about 80% of all detectable hemoglobins. HbA usually comprises 20% of all hemoglobins and HbA_2 is normally not detectable to any major extent. By 6 months of age, HbA has become the major hemoglobin and HbF has fallen to about 5–10%, while HbA_2 has reached adult levels but may continue to rise for 1–2 years.

Individuals with HbSS, HbSC, HbS/β^0-thalassemia do not produce HbA. Individuals with HbS/β^+-thalassemia produce some HbA, usually 3–20%. HbA_2 is elevated in those with an associated β^+ or β^0 thalassemia. HbF may continue to be present at higher than expected levels in those with HbSS.[23]

Blood count

The blood count in sickle disease is normal for the first 2 months. The blood count in those with HbSS and HbS/β^0-thalassemia will usually demonstrate a moderate anemia by 6–12 months and a reticulocytosis because of hemolysis. A sustained reticulocytosis above 25% is unusual and suggests recovery from an acute event, hypersplenism or, occasionally, a superimposed autoimmune anemia. Individuals with HbSC or HbS/β^+-thalassemia may be normal or have mild anemia. Individuals with higher HbF levels tend to have higher hemoglobin levels.[23]

Blood film

The red cells in HbSS vary in size and shape. There is increased polychromasia, red cell fragments, and a variable number of hypochromic or target cells. The characteristic dense sickled cells occur in variable amounts. They are not usually present for the first few months of life because of the high HbF level. The number of sickled cells is variable and ranges from only an occasional finding to 30–40% of all red cells.[24] Some investigators report an increased number of sickled cells during a sickle crisis but this has not been confirmed by all.[25] In addition to the classical sickled cell there are other cells, often called 'boat-shaped' that are elongated and pointed at one or both ends. Howell–Jolly bodies are usually found by 1 year of age and represent evidence of hyposplenism. The presence of many target cells and hypochromia may indicate coexistent α-thalassemia trait. Those individuals who are taking hydroxycarbamide therapy often exhibit a macrocytosis.

The peripheral blood of individuals with HbSC shows less polychromasia and Howell–Jolly bodies are usually not seen. Target cells are a common feature. Sickled cells are not often seen but 'boat cells' are common. The characteristic feature is the presence of SC poikilocytes. These are misshapen cells that contain irregularly shaped crystals that jut out at various angles or they may appear similar to sickle cells but on closer inspection have a straight-sided crystal present.[24]

Individuals with HbS/β^+-thalassemia have only occasional boat-shaped cells and no sickle cells. They have more thalassemic features, including hypochromic microcytic cells, sometimes with basophilic stippling, and frequent target cells.

Other investigations

Patients with HbSS and HbS/β^0-thalassemia will have evidence of hemolysis such as elevated lactate dehydrogenase and bilirubin levels and low haptoglobin levels.

Sickle solubility test

This is a simple, quick test to detect the presence of HbS. A sample of the patient's red cells is mixed with a deoxygenating substance. If the solution becomes turbid, the presence of HbS is suggested, although this needs to be confirmed by more definitive testing. A positive solubility test does not distinguish HbAS, HbSC, HbSS or HbS/$\beta^{+/0}$-thalassemia. It may give a false-negative result in children less than 6 months of age and is not recommended in this age group. It may also be negative in extreme anemia or following blood transfusion. False-positive results can occur in those with elevated white cell counts and with hyperproteinemic or hyperlipidemic states because of plasma turbidity, and for this reason the use of plasma-free red cells is recommended.

Definitive testing (Table 10.4)

Hemoglobin electrophoresis relies on the fact that different hemoglobins will separate from each other when exposed to a charge gradient and can be visualized using a staining process. Acid and alkaline medium is used to further characterize the hemoglobins, which have differing mobilities in different media. Hemoglobin electrophoresis is difficult to interpret and may be imprecise in the neonate.

High-performance liquid chromatography (HPLC) has now superseded hemoglobin electrophoresis as the first-line test for variant hemoglobins. This technology involves the capture of positively charged hemoglobin molecules onto a negatively charged solid column, followed by their elution into a liquid phase and capture at a rate that depends on

Table 10.4 Methodologies used for hemoglobin identification.

Hemoglobin electrophoresis
High-performance liquid chromatography
Isoelectric focusing
Mass spectrometry
DNA testing

their charge. Some hemoglobins (e.g., HbF) will elute quite quickly, whereas others (e.g., HbS and HbC) take some minutes. The speed of elution and the quantity of hemoglobin present is calculated using a computerized program.

Isoelectric focusing is often used as a confirmatory test if a hemoglobin variant is detected on HPLC. It gives a pattern similar to that of conventional hemoglobin electrophoresis but allows better separation and definition of hemoglobin variants. It relies on the fact that the net charge of a protein or hemoglobin depends on the pH in the surrounding solution. Various hemoglobins are separated on the gel according to the point where they have no net charge (isoelectric point).

All variant hemoglobins should be characterized using two different methodologies. Sometimes it proves impossible to definitively identify a mutant hemoglobin using any of the above techniques. DNA analysis can be useful to identify the mutant hemoglobin by determining the type of mutation and the gene it affects (e.g., α- or β-globin genes).

Neonatal screening

Early diagnosis facilitates parental education and the introduction of preventive vaccination and antibiotic programs. Universal neonatal screening is now undertaken in many American states and in the UK. It is performed using a blood spot technique from a heel-prick, often when blood is taken for inherited metabolic disease screening. Blood can be taken by direct venipuncture or by umbilical cord blood sampling. The latter may give inaccurate results if contaminated by maternal blood and is least favored.

Surgery and sickle cell disease

Patients with SCD may require surgery because of the complications associated with this disease, e.g., gallstones and avascular necrosis of the femoral head, or for completely unrelated complaints. Surgery and general anesthesia in SCD are not without complications. Early reviews reported a perioperative mortality rate of 10% and a postoperative complication rate of up to 50%.[26] This was due, at least in part, to anemia, an increased tendency for red cells to sickle because of hypoxia and hypoperfusion, and because of the complications of SCD such as renal impairment and pulmonary disease. The cooperative study of surgery and anesthesia issued its findings in 1995 for the period 1978–88, during which 1079 surgical procedures were performed on 717 patients. Cholecystectomy and splenectomy accounted for 24% of all surgery; 93% of the patients had preoperative blood transfusion. The overall mortality rate within 30 days of surgery was 1.1% but no death was reported in patients under the age of 14 years. Sickle complications were more likely to occur with regional than with general anesthesia.[27] A more recent study

of laparoscopic versus open splenectomy or cholecystectomy in children found that acute chest syndrome (ACS) occurred in 20% of cases. Importantly, laparoscopic surgery did not reduce the incidence of complications and was associated with a longer operating time.[28] Another study found that a history of pulmonary disease identified patients at risk for sickle-related events following adenotonsillectomy.[29]

It was accepted for many years that blood transfusion was a necessary prerequisite for all but the most minor of surgical or anesthetic procedures. The aim was to reduce the percentage of sickle hemoglobin to 30% in order to reduce the ability to sickle and to correct anemia.[26] Blood transfusion could be administered by two methods: exchange transfusion or by giving a number of transfusions over a period of weeks. Some centers adopted a more conservative approach and transfused to correct anemia without aiming to reduce the HbS level. In 1988 a multicenter study was commenced to address the question of perioperative care and to attempt to define whether aggressively transfusing to achieve an HbS level under 30% or simple 'top-up' transfusion was the best transfusion policy. The necessity of administering blood was not addressed. The results demonstrated that chest syndrome developed in 10% of patients and resulted in two deaths (0.33%), but the frequency of serious complications was similar in both transfusion groups (30%) and the incidence of transfusion-related complications was greater in the group aggressively transfused to HbS < 30%. It was concluded that simple transfusion to a hemoglobin level of 10 g/dL was as effective as aggressive transfusion.[26] In the case of HbSC, a study of outcomes demonstrated that individuals undergoing abdominal surgery without transfusion had a sickle-related complication rate of 35%, whereas those who received transfusion preoperatively had no sickle-related complications. This prompted the recommendation that individuals with HbSC undergoing abdominal surgery should receive blood transfusion but that transfusion was not necessary for simple procedures such as myringotomy.[30] New understanding of the pathophysiology of SCD and newer anesthetic techniques suggests that blood transfusion may not always be necessary. A randomized controlled trial comparing 'top-up' transfusion to no transfusion is long overdue.

Irrespective of the decision to transfuse or not, there are some simple precautions that are applicable to every child undergoing surgery.

• Ensure that the child is well hydrated for a minimum of 8 hours prior to surgery. Intravenous hydration should continue during and following surgery.

• Ensure that he/she remains adequately oxygenated during and following the procedure using supplemental oxygen. Some centers have used positive airway pressure for those undergoing abdominal surgery but most children find this unacceptable when fully awake.

• Ensure that the surrounding ambient temperature is adequate at all times.

• Intraoperative monitoring should include temperature, blood pressure, electrocardiographic features and oxygen levels. Postoperatively, blood pressure and oxygen levels (with pulse oximetry) should continue to be monitored.

• Incentive spirometry and physiotherapy should be undertaken once the child is awake.

Some surgical procedures require the use of a tourniquet. Logically, this should create a static reservoir of sickled red cells, because of the hypoxic and acidotic conditions, which can be released back into the system when the tourniquet is removed.[22,23] Some have advocated prior exchange transfusion to reduce the potential risk.[23] In practice the use of a tourniquet does not appear to cause problems.[31,32]

Specific problems in children with sickle cell disease (Table 10.5)

Growth and development

Studies of individuals with HbSS and HbS/β^0-thalassemia in the USA, Jamaica, Italy and Nigeria suggest that growth delay is common and most evident in the adolescent

Table 10.5 Types of sickle events.

Hyposplenism/infection

Anemia
Hemolytic
Aplastic
Anemia of chronic disease (e.g., renal failure)

Vasoocclusive
Bone
Abdominal
  Splenic sequestration
  Bowel infarction
  Hepatic sequestration
  Hepatic infarction
  Gallstones
Chest
  Acute chest syndrome
  Chronic lung disease/pulmonary hypertension
Heart
Eye
Kidney
  Renal concentrating defect/enuresis
  Proteinuria
  Acute renal failure
  Chronic renal failure
Priapism
Leg ulcers
Cerebral
  Stroke
  Silent infarction
  Neurocognitive disorders

years.[33–36] It is suggested that weight deficit tends to be greater than height deficit.[33] The Jamaican cohort study found that differences in weight between infants with HbSS and HbAA had emerged by the first year of life and reached significance in girls at 12 months and boys by 21 months.[37] There is a 1–2 year delay in sexual development and bone age may be delayed by as much as 4 years.[23,34] Most individuals will attain their expected height centile by adulthood but weight may remain below the appropriate growth centile.[22] Specific height and weight growth reference curves have been derived for children with SCD aged 0–18 years in order to identify coincidental growth problems.[38] No specific endocrine abnormality has been identified in individuals with SCD.

Children with SCD have increased resting energy expenditure, possibly due to anemia and increased cardiac output and this may contribute to poor growth.[39] It has also been suggested that these children may have increased protein requirements and are at risk of protein-energy malnutrition. They have marked reductions in fat-free mass and reduced body fat, indicating reduced energy stores.[40] Interventional studies will be necessary to determine if increased nutritional support can increase body habitus in those with SCD.

Plasma zinc levels are low in adults with symptomatic SCD and urinary loss of zinc is increased. Zinc deficiency reduces helper T cells and cell-mediated immunity. Zinc supplementation has been reported to improve sexual development and growth.[41] It has also reduced the number of bacterial infections, hospitalizations and vasoocclusive episodes.[42] Nevertheless, routine zinc supplementation has not gained popularity.

Contraception and pregnancy

There is no evidence to suggest that there is an increased risk of infertility in females with SCD. Oral contraceptive agents can be recommended when requested and there is no evidence that they are more hazardous to women with SCD.[43] Depot progestogens are a useful alternative for those who cannot take oral preparations. Intrauterine contraceptive devices have an increased risk of uterine and tubal infection and should be used with caution.[44]

The risk of spontaneous miscarriage was reported to be as high as 25% in the past but now appears to be similar to that of the normal population.[43–45] The incidence of intrauterine growth restriction may be as high as 21% and may be explained by maternal anemia and placental insufficiency from vascular occlusion and fibrosis.[44,46] Perinatal mortality rates are increased and range between 1 and 8% in the USA and UK, whereas in Africa they are as high as 12–19%. Hypertension and preeclampsia may complicate up to one-third of all pregnancies and an increase in maternal mortality rates for women with SCD is reported.[44] There is an increased rate of urinary tract infection; urine analysis should be undertaken at least monthly and positive results treated aggressively. Anemia may be exacerbated and a drop in hemoglobin of more than 20% may necessitate simple 'top-up' transfusion.[43] ACS, painful crises and cerebrovascular events have all been reported but the incidence does not appear higher than in the nonpregnant state. There is no proof that prophylactic blood transfusion alters pregnancy outcome and it should be reserved for those patients with a prior history of perinatal mortality, and those with preeclampsia, ACS, new neurologic event, severe anemia and twin pregnancy.[43]

Infection

The rate of pneumococcal infection is 30–100 times that of normal children and it has been one of the commonest causes of death in children under 5 years of age.[47] All children with SCD have splenic dysfunction, irrespective of spleen size, and complete dysfunction has developed in most children with HbSS by 2 years of age.[47] This causes increased susceptibility to encapsulated organisms such as *Streptococcus pneumoniae* (pneumococcus), *Haemophilus influenzae*, and *Neisseria meningitidis*. The National Institutes of Health (NIH) cooperative study of SCD found that 66% of infections in children under 6 years old were due to pneumococcus, whereas 50% of infections in children over 6 years old were caused by Gram-negative organisms. *Escherichia coli* was responsible for 73% of urinary tract infections and *Salmonella* species caused 77% of cases of osteomyelitis.[48,49] A Jamaican study confirmed these findings and suggested that *H. influenzae* was also predominantly found in children less than 5 years of age, whereas *E. coli* and *Klebsiella* species predominated in children over 10 years of age. In this study, *E. coli* was found almost exclusively in girls.[50] *Mycoplasma* species may be responsible for up to 16% of ACS cases and *Chlamydia pneumoniae* has also been implicated as a causative agent in others.[47]

Other types of immunologic dysfunction have been noted in children with SCD. There are decreased opsonin levels, which normally promote phagocytosis.[23,47] The alternative pathway of complement activation is also found to be defective by some investigators[51] though not by others.[52,53] Abnormal neutrophil kinetics have been noted, with a decrease in marginating pool numbers in favor of increased numbers in the circulating pool, reducing the half-life of the neutrophil.[54] It is also suggested that cellular immunity, T-helper cell function and interleukin-2 production is adversely affected by zinc deficiency, common in SCD, and that zinc supplementation reduces the incidence of infection.[42]

Management of infection

Prophylaxis (Table 10.6)

Penicillin prophylaxis should be commenced in the newborn period and continued for at least 5 years. The PROPS II study of 400 children aged 5 years randomized to receive penicillin

Table 10.6 Proposed management strategies.

Early intervention

Penicillin
Folic acid
Vaccination
Fluids
Rest
Nutrition

Management of acute events

General measures
Assessment
Blood tests (full blood count, reticulocyte count, biochemistry, cultures)
Chest radiography
Hydration (5% dextrose or 2.5% dextrose + 0.45% saline)
Oxygen (if saturation < 95%)

Specific measures
Antibiotics
Transfusion
　Simple 'top-up' transfusion
　Exchange transfusion
Pain management

Preventive strategies

Central nervous system
Transcranial Doppler ultrasonography
MRI
Psychometric testing

Heart/lungs
Echocardiography plus tricuspid jet velocity
Sleep studies for nocturnal hypoxia

Kidneys
Early morning urine for urine osmolality

Bones
MRI
Surgical intervention

Nutritional
High energy

Eyes
Ophthalmology review

MRI, magnetic resonance imaging.

or placebo demonstrated no significant difference after 3 years follow-up provided that there was no history of prior pneumococcal infection or splenectomy.[55] Nevertheless, some clinicians continue penicillin prophylaxis beyond the age of 5 years. An alternative (but unproved) approach for children over 5 years old would be to commence penicillin at the onset of fever, theoretically providing some treatment while the child is on the way to the doctor.[56] The British Committee for Standards in Haematology (BCSH) guidelines for those with a hyposplenic state suggest that penicillin prophylaxis should continue for life. Those with penicillin allergy should receive erythromycin twice daily.[57]

Pneumococcal vaccination should be administered from 2 months of age. The pentavalent conjugated pneumococcal vaccine (CPV) Prevenar is suitable for children under 2 years. The polyvalent (23-valent) polysaccharide pneumococcal vaccine (PPV) Pneumovax is recommended at 24 months of age. There is no consensus as to whether a further PPV booster should be given and, if so, when and for how long, but a recent study suggested that PPV was 80% effective within 3 years of vaccination and that children with SCD of all ages may benefit from PPV boosted with CPV.[58] Another study demonstrated higher IgG pneumococcal antibody concentrations when CPV and PPV were given as a combination 2 months apart.[59] The BCSH guidelines are quite clear and recommend 5-yearly PPV boosters for life.[57]

Hepatitis B vaccination is now a routine practice in many centers and may be commenced at 2 months of age. Influenza should be administered yearly as viral influenza can cause severe morbidity in individuals with SCD.

Acute management

Most antibiotic therapy is commenced empirically before culture reports are available. Empiric antibiotic cover should aim to treat pneumococcal and *H. influenzae* infections. A child with chest infiltrates should, in addition, receive antibiotics that will treat *Mycoplasma* and *Chlamydia* species. Urinary tract infections should be treated with antibiotics that cover Gram-negative organisms. Treatment of osteomyelitis and septic arthritis requires antibiotics specific for *Salmonella* and *Staphylococcus aureus*. If a child has recently returned from Africa and has fever and diarrhea, typhoid fever should be considered.

Parents and clinicians should be aware that a temperature over 38.5°C in a child with SCD should be treated as an emergency. The child should have a full blood profile, cultures (blood, urine and throat), oxygen saturations and possibly chest radiography performed (see Table 10.6). Other investigations, such as lumbar puncture, should be performed if there is evidence of meningitis. Periosteal or joint aspiration should be undertaken if there is evidence of osteomyelitis or septic arthritis.[60]

Anemia

The first four cases of SCD reported in the literature described anemia and jaundice, consistent features of HbSS. Homozygous SCD is a hemolytic disease. The mean red cell survival time is about 12 days. The rate of hemolysis is determined by the degree of HbS polymerization, the number of irreversibly sickled cells, gender and the presence of α^+-thalassemia.[61] Vigorous exercise also increases the hemolytic rate.[62] The usual hemoglobin level for those with HbSS is 6–9 g/dL.[23] The individuals are usually asymptomatic at these levels because of a right-shift in the oxygen dissociation curve due to HbS that enhances oxygen delivery to the tissues.[22]

When patients are well, the hemoglobin deviates very little and a falling hemoglobin may signify the early onset of renal failure.[23]

An acute precipitous drop in hemoglobin can occur in SCD and lead to cardiac failure and death. There are three main reasons for this: acute splenic sequestration (discussed later in this chapter), hyperhemolysis or parvovirus B19 infection.

Hyperhemolysis

Accelerated hemolysis can occur in association with an acute sickle event, most commonly due to infection and ACS.[56] It is associated with an increased reticulocyte count above baseline values. Malaria can cause severe life-threatening hemolysis and should be considered if there is a history of travel to malaria zones. A sudden unexpected fall in hemoglobin in an individual who has recently received a red cell transfusion should raise the possibility of a hemolytic transfusion reaction and appropriate investigations are required. Glucose 6-phosphate dehydrogenase deficiency often occurs in children with SCD but there is little evidence that it contributes to anemia.

Parvovirus B19

This infectious agent causes profound anemia because of a direct cytotoxic effect on the erythroid precursors, although occasionally other progenitors are also affected. The normal lifespan of a red cell in SCD is much shortened as previously described and any cessation in erythropoiesis will have a marked effect. The patient may have signs of fever, upper respiratory tract infection and/or gastrointestinal symptoms. The reticulocytopenia begins 5 days after exposure and can last 7–10 days. Exacerbation of the anemia occurs shortly after the onset of reticulocytopenia. In the recovery phase patients may be thought to have a hyperhemolytic event because of the association of anemia with a massive reticulocytosis. The diagnosis can be made by measuring parvoviral IgM levels, which will be positive, or by identification of the virus using polymerase chain reaction. There is no recorded case of parvoviral reinfection and protective immunity appears lifelong.[56,63]

Vasoocclusive events

Most patients with homozygous SCD will experience a painful vasoocclusive event at some point in their life. The degree of severity of disease varies from patient to patient and is only partially explained by HbF levels and other known disease modifiers (see Table 10.2). Vasoocclusive episodes account for over 90% of all emergency hospital admissions and will most likely result in the patient's death either because of acute organ failure or chronic organ damage.[11,64] Factors that may precipitate sickling and vasoocclusion include

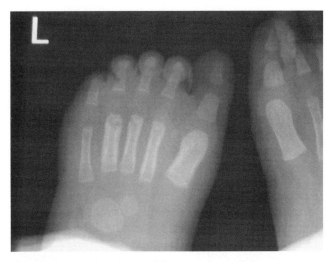

Fig. 10.1 Periosteal reaction, medullary expansion and inflammation in first to fourth metatarsal bones and focal lucency at the head of the third and fourth metatarsal bones in a boy aged 14 months with recurrent dactylitis.

hypoxia, dehydration and cold weather (see Table 10.1).[5] The following sections detail the organ systems involved either acutely or chronically and give some suggested management strategies.

Bone and joints

Acute problems

Dactylitis (hand–foot syndrome)

Dactylitis is caused by vasoocclusion and necrosis affecting the bone marrow and inner third of the cortex of the small bones of the hands or feet.[23] It occurs most frequently in children aged 6 months to 2 years old. It presents as an acute painful swelling of the dorsum of the hands or feet and extends into the fingers and toes. It is usually associated with fever. It can take at least 1 week to resolve and tends to recur. Radiologic bone abnormalities may take 2 weeks to appear and include periosteal reaction, translucency or opacity of the diaphysis, and occasional bone loss (Fig. 10.1).[65] Recurrent events can lead to bone deformity or early fusion of the epiphysis resulting in shortened digits. It is suggested that an episode of dactylitis in the first 2 years of life may predict severe manifestations of SCD in later life.[12] Infection should be considered if the symptoms and signs do not resolve with conservative management.

Bones and joints

The common sites of infarction are the spine, pelvis and long bones. Affected vertebrae may exhibit a 'codfish' appearance due to collapse of the endplates. The commonest long bones affected are the humerus, tibia and femur.[66] The distal segment between the diaphysis and metaphysis is most often involved in children less than 10 years old and there may be local tenderness, warmth and swelling with impaired movement of the adjacent joint.[23,56] Often the pain is more diffuse and nonspecific and is due to bone marrow infarction and necrosis. The child is often pyrexial and a leukocytosis is usually present, probably due to the underlying inflammatory response. The pain may last several days.

Management

Warmth, hydration and adequate pain relief are the cornerstones of management. Small children may require only nonsteroidal antiinflammatory drugs (NSAIDs) whereas older children may also require opiate analgesia (see section on pain management). If the pyrexia persists, particularly if it is associated with fluctuant swelling, osteomyelitis or septic arthritis should be considered.

Chronic bone disease

Osteonecrosis or avascular necrosis (AVN) is painful and disabling. It can occur with all types of SCD but is most common in those with HbSS/α-thalassemia. The incidence is 2.5 per 100 patient-years for hip and shoulder joints, and AVN of the femoral head has been described in children as young as 5 years of age. The median age of diagnosis among African-Americans is 28–36 years,[67] among Jamaicans the median age of onset is 20 years,[68] while among Nigerians the mean age of onset is 13.7 years.[69] Of those with shoulder disease, 75% will also have hip disease.[69,70] Shoulder disease can be asymptomatic but hip disease may present acutely with symptoms suggestive of septic arthritis or may have a more insidious course with pain and limitation of movement. The course from early disease to collapse of the femoral head can be as short as 2 years. The cause of AVN is unclear but may be due, in part, to microinfarction of the cancellous bone.[22] Plain bone radiographs are normal in early disease but magnetic resonance imaging (MRI) may show bone and bone marrow necrosis. Some evidence suggests that core decompression early in the course of the disease may halt the progression of necrosis at least in the short term and relieve pain and loss of function.[71,72] Ultimately, joint replacement is usually needed but because these have a limited lifespan and will need to be revised, their use in teenagers and young adults should be postponed if possible. This makes MRI surveillance and early intervention with core decompression an attractive option.

Abdomen

Acute splenic sequestration

Acute splenic sequestration is a major cause of mortality in children with SCD. The mortality rate for a first event was 12% in a Jamaican series and 20% for those with recurrent disease.[73] It is caused by intrasplenic trapping of red cells and is defined as a hemoglobin decrease of at least 2 g/dL associated with a markedly elevated reticulocyte count and acutely enlarging spleen.[56] The attacks are often associated with viral or bacterial infection. Recurrent splenic sequestration is common and occurs in at least 50% of those who survive the first episode.[73] Sequestration can occur in children as young as 5 weeks but is seen most often in children between the ages of 3 months and 5 years. We have noticed splenic sequestration occurring in children as old as 10 years who are receiving disease-modifying therapy such as chronic blood transfusion or hydroxycarbamide, possibly because these treatment modalities delay splenic fibrosis. It is also reported in older children and adults with HbSC and HbSS/β+-thalassemia.[74,75]

Management

Early diagnosis is important and parental instruction in abdominal examination and the detection of splenomegaly has become one of the cornerstones of management.[76] The treatment of splenic sequestration is directed towards the correction of hypovolemia with blood transfusion. The aim of transfusion is to raise the hemoglobin to 7 g/dL; however, as some of the red cells sequestered in the spleen will be released as the spleen regresses, the final hemoglobin will often be higher than predicted on the basis of the volume of red cells administered.[77]

Recurrence may be prevented by splenectomy or perhaps by chronic transfusion. We have not found chronic transfusion to be effective even when the HbS level is less than 20%. Kinney *et al*.[78] have reported similar findings in patients receiving blood transfusion whose HbS was less than 30%. A study by Wright *et al*.[79] found that mortality or bacteremic episodes did not differ between children post splenectomy and a control group and recommended that splenectomy should not be deferred due to concerns about infection risk. However, the recommendations of the NIH are that patients who have life-threatening splenic sequestration requiring transfusion should have a splenectomy shortly after the event or be placed on a chronic transfusion program. Further recommendations are that children less than 2 years who have had a severe episode should be placed on chronic transfusion to keep the HbS below 30% until splenectomy can be considered over the age of 2 years.[56]

Abdominal painful crisis

This is a term used to describe any complication in which abdominal pain is prominent and not caused by any other obvious intraabdominal pathology.[23] It usually affects younger children. The pain may be mild and transient to severe and generalized, sometimes with features of intestinal obstruction. Radiologic investigation has, in some cases, found a localized nonfunctioning segment of bowel that recovers function after 3–4 days of conservative management,[23] but often there is no discernible cause.

Hepatic sequestration

This is a rare condition in children and is analogous to splenic sequestration. It is recognized by rapid hepatic enlargement in association with a falling hemoglobin and rising reticulocyte count. The bilirubin level increases and alkaline phosphatase may also be elevated. The transaminases may be normal. Exchange transfusion is recommended because of the risk of hyperviscosity with simple transfusion.[80]

Acute hepatic necrosis

Acute hepatic necrosis and failure can occur in the absence of viral liver disease and in association with other sickle cell-related vasoocclusive events. Exchange transfusion can bring about a rapid improvement in clinical and biochemical parameters.[81]

Gallstones

There is an increased incidence of gallstones in individuals with SCD. They may develop before the age of 4 years and have been reported in 17–33% of patients aged between 2 and 18 years and in over 50% of the adult population.[82] Coexistent α-thalassemia decreases the chance of developing gallstones, possibly because it reduces the rate of hemolysis.[83] Fever, nausea, vomiting and abdominal pain are nonspecific features of cholecystitis and careful evaluation is necessary to exclude other potential causes, as gallstones are not always symptomatic. Laparoscopic cholecystectomy is the treatment of choice for symptomatic gallstones.[56]

Renal manifestations

The environment of the renal medulla is hypoxic, acidotic and hypertonic, all of which promote HbS polymerization. This makes the medulla particularly susceptible to injury.[84]

Hyposthenuria, an inability to concentrate urine properly, is the commonest renal abnormality. It may present with enuresis, often at night. It also makes individuals with SCD more susceptible to dehydration than normal individuals.[85] Other abnormalities frequently found include impaired renal acidification, decreased potassium secretion and hematuria.[86] Hematuria occurs most often in males and is usually unilateral, arising from the left kidney in 80% of cases.

Proteinuria is an early manifestation of sickle nephropathy and affects at least 6% of children with SCD. It is associated with lower hemoglobin concentrations, higher mean corpuscular volume and higher white cell counts.[87] The nephrotic syndrome is estimated to occur in 4% of patients with SCD and renal failure seems virtually inevitable once nephrotic syndrome intervenes.[88] Angiotensin-converting enzyme (ACE) inhibitors decrease urinary protein excretion and may delay the onset of nephropathy.[89]

Renal failure

Acute renal failure has been reported in 10.3% of patients hospitalized with SCD.[90] It can arise as a result of dehydration during a sickle cell crisis or secondary to rhabdomyolysis, sepsis and drug nephrotoxicity. Rhabdomyolysis is a common finding in patients who develop multiorgan failure syndrome (i.e., renal, pulmonary and hepatic failure) during a painful vasoocclusive episode but it may respond dramatically to aggressive red cell exchange.[91]

The overall prevalence of chronic renal failure in SCD is about 4.5% and is age related. Predictors of chronic renal failure include hypertension, proteinuria, hematuria, increasingly severe anemia, nephrotic syndrome and inheritance of the Bantu phenotype.[92] Factors that may slow disease progression include avoidance of NSAIDs, use of ACE inhibitors and control of hypertension. Renal transplantation is an appropriate form of renal replacement in those with end-stage renal disease. Patient and graft survival results are comparable to those obtained in other groups of patients.[93] However, recurrence of hyposthenuria and nephropathy after transplant has been described.

Priapism

Priapism is a sustained, painful, involuntary erection and is a well-recognized complication of SCD. It is due to vasoocclusive obstruction to venous drainage of the penis. It is classified as 'prolonged' if it lasts more than 3 hours and 'stuttering' if it lasts more than a few minutes but less than 3 hours and resolves spontaneously. Stuttering priapism may recur and become prolonged. Prolonged priapism is a urologic emergency. Recurrent prolonged episodes ultimately lead to fibrosis and impotence. It may affect more than 30% of males with SCD. Recently, polymorphisms in a gene (*KLOTHO*) that regulates endothelial growth factor expression and endothelial nitric oxide release has been implicated in the etiology of priapism.[94] The mean age at the time of the initial episode has been reported as 12 years and the probability of experiencing priapism by the age of 20 years was 89%.[95]

Management

The patient should attempt to urinate as soon as the priapism begins and take extra fluids and analgesia. If the priapism lasts longer than 2 hours, the patient should be encouraged to seek medical attention. Conservative management includes analgesia, hydration, anxiolytic therapy and possibly exchange blood transfusion. This is usually effective in young children and should be tried first. If the penile shaft fails to soften, then aspiration and irrigation of the cavernosa may be successful. Early surgical intervention is necessary in adults as medical treatment is less successful.[5] Shunting may be necessary to prevent recurrent episodes. Recently, an oral α-adrenergic agent, etilefrine, has been found effective in preventing recurrence.[96,97] There is anecdotal evidence that hydroxycarbamide may prevent priapism but further studies are needed.[98]

Leg ulcers

Between 10 and 20% of individuals with SCD will develop painful indolent leg ulcers usually over the lateral or medial malleolus. Occasionally they are found on the dorsum of the foot or over the tibia. They can be single or multiple. Some will heal quickly whereas others may be present for years.

There is no definitive treatment for leg ulcers. The area should be kept clean and infection treated promptly. A variety of dressings have been tried and no single one has shown superiority. Intravenous arginine butyrate has produced rapid healing of ulcers,[99] but a role for hydroxycarbamide seems unclear because it is implicated in ulcer formation in patients with myeloproliferative disease.[100]

Pulmonary manifestations

Acute chest syndrome

ACS is the second most common cause of hospitalization in patients with SCD and is responsible for 25% of deaths.[101] The incidence ranges from 24.5 events per 100 patient-years in young children to 8.8 events per 100 patient-years in older adults. Fever, cough, chest pain and pulmonary infiltrates on chest radiography are the common presenting features and the condition may rapidly progress to life-threatening respiratory insufficiency and total 'white out' on chest radiographs (Fig. 10.2).[21] The most common etiologic factors are infection, pulmonary fat embolism or pulmonary infarction but it may be multifactorial. The commonest infective organisms isolated in children are virus, *Mycoplasma pneumoniae* and *Chlamydia pneumoniae*. Pulmonary infarction is the sole cause of ACS in 20% of cases but is a major factor in all events.[101] Factors influencing the frequency of ACS include the degree of anemia, low HbF levels, high steady-state white

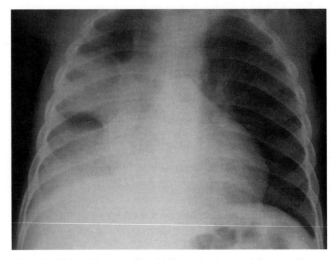

Fig. 10.2 Right midzone and basal infiltrate in a boy aged 5 years with acute chest syndrome.

cell count, younger age group, seasonal variation (especially in the young) and bronchoreactive lung disease. Higher hemoglobin levels and winter season increases the frequency of episodes. Bronchoreactive lung disease is common in individuals with SCD and is present in 43% of children during the steady state. It often worsens during ACS and may contribute to progressive lung injury.[101,103] Hemoglobin levels may drop by at least 1 g/dL during the event and the white cell counts double. A platelet count of less than $200 \times 10^9/L$ is a strong predictor of morbidity and mortality.[101] The patient may become more unstable during the first few days following admission; 15% of all patients require intubation and the average mortality rate is 3%, rising to 9% in those over 18 years of age.

Management

Supplemental oxygen should be administered to those whose oxygen saturation is less than 95%. Hydration is important but overhydration can worsen the condition. Adequate pain relief should be administered but oversedation avoided. Incentive spirometry has been shown to be beneficial in the prevention and management of ACS. Airways hyperreactivity is treated with bronchodilators. Intravenous broad-spectrum antibiotics including a macrolide or quinolone should be administered. Top-up blood transfusion, to achieve a final hemoglobin of 10 g/dL, has been shown to be effective in children with ACS and should be administered if there is evidence of hypoxemia.[56,104] In severe cases exchange transfusion may be necessary. Mechanical ventilation may be necessary for those with life-threatening respiratory failure and use of extracorporeal membrane oxygenation may be beneficial.[105] Dexamethasone and inhaled nitric oxide also show promise but further study is necessary to determine their role.[106,107]

Chronic pulmonary disease

Chronic pulmonary disease is a disease of adults with SCD and affects up to 32% of patients.[108] The true incidence is unknown as the early stages of disease are asymptomatic. The etiology is multifactorial and includes lung damage from ACS, chronic oxygen desaturation or sleep hypoventilation, repeated episodes of thromboembolism, and hemolytic anemia-associated pulmonary hypertension due to reduced nitric oxide/arginine levels.[56,101,109] Survival for those with symptomatic sickle cell-related pulmonary hypertension appears to be shorter than for those with primary pulmonary hypertension, with reports suggesting a 2-year mortality of 50% compared with a 2.8-year median survival for those with primary pulmonary hypertension.[110] The HbF level, white cell or platelet count and the use of hydroxycarbamide appears unrelated to the development of pulmonary hypertension.[108] A recent study of infants aged 3–30 months found evidence of early abnormal lung function in those with HbSS

that had a possible relationship to airways reactivity.[111] This suggests that the injury which culminates in later pulmonary damage may begin at a very early age and may require early intervention if progression is to be halted. The HUG-Infant trial may give some information on the role of hydroxycarbamide as an early intervention strategy. The use of arginine supplementation may also be of benefit.[112]

Cerebrovascular disease

Stroke

Children with SCD have a 200-fold increased risk of stroke, with a prevalence rate of 11%.[113,114] The incidence of ischemic stroke is highest in children aged 1–9 years, whereas intracranial hemorrhage is most common in adults. Cerebral infarction may occur as a result of fibrous proliferation of the intima affecting the distal internal carotid, proximal middle cerebral artery and the proximal anterior cerebral artery. This leads to vasoocclusion and the development of collaterals.[115] Patients with a history of stroke typically have infarcts in the cortex and deep white matter. The patterns of infarction include wedge-shaped lesions of large-vessel territories, border zone infarctions particularly of the middle cerebral artery territory, and small punctate lesions of the deep white matter.[116] High white cell count, low hemoglobin levels, and recent episodes of ACS have all been associated with high risk of infarction.[115] Specific HLA types (DPB1*0401, A*0102, A*2612) may also be associated with small- and large-vessel stroke but further evaluation is required to confirm this preliminary finding.[113]

Management

The child should undergo evaluation with computed tomography or MRI to determine the cause of the neurologic deficit. Intravenous hydration should be given. Exchange blood transfusion should be undertaken as soon as possible, aiming to reduce HbS to less than 30%. This usually requires a one-volume exchange. A chronic transfusion program should be instituted to maintain HbS less than 30% as studies have shown that untransfused patients have a stroke recurrence rate as high as 70% whereas it is about 10% in a transfused group of patients.[22] The duration of a chronic transfusion program is unclear as strokes have recurred when transfusions have stopped even after 5–12 years of therapy.[117] Recently, it has been suggested that hydroxycarbamide overlapping blood transfusion for some months and then continued alone may be an alternative to blood transfusion for long-term stroke prevention.[118,119]

Prevention

Transcranial Doppler ultrasonography (TCD) measures blood flow through intracranial blood vessels. Blood flow velocity is higher through stenotic vessels. The STOP study screened patients with HbSS and HbS/β⁰-thalassemia, aged 2–16 years, using TCD. Time-averaged mean velocities were measured in the middle cerebral, distal internal carotid and anterior cerebral arteries. Flow rates of 200 cm/s were considered abnormal. Those with abnormal flow were randomized to a blood transfusion group, aiming to keep HbS below 30%, or an observation group. After 24 months, 10 cerebral infarctions had occurred in the observation group compared with only one in the transfusion group and the study was closed.[119] This has led to the recommendation that all children aged 2–16 years be screened by TCD and chronic transfusion strongly considered if abnormal.[56]

Silent infarction

MRI has identified silent infarcts in at least 17% of children who have not had a clinical stroke.[121] These children perform poorly on psychometric testing and are educationally disadvantaged.[122] A multivariate analysis identified low pain event rate, leukocyte count above 11.8×10^9/L, the Senegal sickle haplotype and a previous history of seizures as risk factors for silent infarction.[121] Silent infarcts are prominent in children under 4 years, with a possible incidence of 11%.[123] Those children with abnormal TCD and MRI seem at increased risk of stroke or new silent infarction and chronic transfusion appears to reduce this risk.[124] However, the relationship between abnormal TCD and silent infarction is not clear. Wang et al.[123] demonstrated that of the 17 patients they identified as having silent infarction, only four had abnormal TCD and one had a conditional result.[123] Further study is required to confirm the preliminary data that blood transfusion has a role in the management of silent infarction, particularly in those with normal TCD. Recently it has been suggested that nocturnal hypoxemia may also have a role in the development of cerebral events and it is suggested that screening for, and management of, this problem may be an effective alternative to prophylactic blood transfusion.[125]

Eye disease

Sickle cell vasoocclusion can affect the vascular bed within the eye, often with devastating consequences. There are two main types of eye disease described in SCD: nonproliferative and proliferative disease.

Nonproliferative disease

Conjunctival vascular occlusions are more marked in HbSS and HbS/β⁰-thalassemia and consist of saccular or multiple short comma-shaped capillary segments often packed with red cells.[23] Iris atrophy can occur as part of a more generalized anterior segment ischemia or as an isolated finding with papillary irregularity and white patches on the iris. Other findings include retinal pigmentary changes, abnormalities of the retinal vasculature, macula, choroids and optic disk.

They are apparent by ophthalmoscopy but rarely have visual sequelae.[56]

Proliferative disease

This is more common in those individuals with HbSC disease and affects 5–10% of all those with SCD. It involves the growth of abnormal vascular fronds, most likely due to peripheral retinal arteriolar occlusions and ischemia stimulating angiogenesis.[56] They can vary from small vessel loops to large complex lesions occupying a large segment of the retinal periphery.[23] It can occur as early as 8 years of age and affects males more frequently than females.[23] Sudden blindness may occur because of vitreous hemorrhage and from mechanical traction created by chronic enlarging fibrovascular retinal membranes.[56]

Management

All children with sickle cell hemoglobinopathies should have yearly dilated eye examination carried out by an ophthalmologist experienced in retinal disease. Any individual who experiences a change in vision should have an immediate ophthalmologic consultation. Treatment is usually reserved for those with proliferative retinopathy and consists of laser photocoagulation or cryotherapy to induce regression of the neovascular tissue. Surgery is required for retinal detachment or nonresolving vitreous hemorrhage.[56]

General management strategies (Table 10.6)

The management of acute sickle events includes rapid assessment that should include blood pressure and pulse oximetry measurements. Blood testing is usually required as many children appear well even if they have increasing anemia. Blood testing should include full blood count, reticulocyte estimation and blood film. Blood chemistry measurement of urea, sodium, potassium, creatinine and bilirubin may be useful. Blood, urine and throat cultures are required if the child has a fever and chest radiography can be useful as early chest syndrome may have few clinical signs. Intravenous hydration is often required but 0.9% 'normal' saline is best avoided because of the large salt load. Dextrose 5% or dextrose 2.5% + 0.45% saline are preferred options. Broad-spectrum antibiotics are commenced in ill pyrexial children. Macrolide antibiotics are added for those with chest signs and other specific antibiotics should be considered depending on the clinical presentation.

Blood transfusion can be life-saving. It should be considered if the hemoglobin level falls below 6 g/dL. Simple 'top-up' transfusion restores blood volume in acute splenic sequestration and improves oxygenation in ACS with evidence of hypoxemia. Exchange transfusion is of benefit in severe chest crisis, stroke or transient ischemic episode, and acute hepatic sequestration or hepatic necrosis. Exchange transfusion should be considered for prolonged unresolving priapism in children. The blood given should be fully ABO, Rhesus and Kell matched as a minimum requirement. All children with SCD should have extended red cell phenotyping undertaken when they are older than 6 months of age. Administration of phenotypically matched red cells will reduce the incidence of alloimmunization.

Pain management

Recurrent episodes of acute severe pain are the hallmarks of SCD. Different individuals have different mechanisms for dealing with pain and pain perception depends on a series of poorly understood interactions between physical and psychologic factors. A formal pain assessment should be made using one of the pain assessment tools appropriate to the patient's age and cognitive abilities, e.g., Wong-Baker Faces Pain Rating Scale. Initial management should be aimed at providing rapid and adequate pain control, which should be maintained using parenteral or oral analgesia. Provision for extra bolus analgesia should be made for breakthrough pain. Analgesia is administered using a 'step-up analgesic ladder' template, starting with paracetamol (acetaminophen) and NSAIDs (if not contraindicated by liver or renal disease) for mild pain, moving on to a mild opioid in addition to NSAIDs and paracetamol, and finally for severe pain a strong opioid is given with NSAIDs.[126] Antiemetic medication and laxatives should be prescribed with opioids. Adjunctive therapy, including massage, distraction and anxiolytic medication, may be beneficial. Pain score, blood pressure, pulse, respiratory rate, oxygen saturation and level of consciousness should be monitored regularly.

Long-term surveillance strategies

It has been suggested that many of the individuals who develop multiorgan failure had, for most of their lives, been considered to have mild SCD.[11] The surveillance regimen suggested here is designed to allow early identification of organ dysfunction. The specific pathophysiology in many cases remains unclear but it is hoped that early therapeutic intervention can halt disease progression. Controlled clinical trials are required in many cases to determine the most appropriate treatment modalities.

Long-term therapeutic options

Blood transfusion

Acute indications for blood transfusion are discussed above. The role of chronic blood transfusion is to suppress endogenous red cell production and reduce HbS to less than 30%. Red cells that are leukocyte depleted and phenotypically matched for Rhesus, Kell and Duffy antigens are usually administered every 3–4 weeks. Indications for chronic transfusion therapy include:

- primary stroke prevention in those with abnormal TCD;
- secondary stroke prevention;
- anemia associated with chronic renal failure;
- severe debilitating pain;
- complicated pregnancy (twin or previous fetal loss).

Possible indications for chronic transfusion therapy include:

- silent infarction;
- splenic sequestration while awaiting surgery;
- priapism;
- pulmonary hypertension.

Blood transfusion is not without complication and the benefits of transfusion must be weighed against these complications. Acute transfusion reactions may occur. Alloimmunization can occur in 30% of patients and antibodies to K, E, C and Jkb accounted for 82% of alloantibodies in one study.[127] Delayed hemolysis can occur 6–10 days following transfusion and can mimic or precipitate an acute sickle event. The direct Coombs test is usually negative but hemoglobinuria is a frequent finding.[128] The risks of viral transmission have diminished with improved blood banking procedures, although there is a new and as yet poorly defined risk of prion transmission. Iron overload is a definite risk with prolonged transfusion therapy. Iron stores must be monitored, usually by measuring serum ferritin, and iron chelation instituted once ferritin levels exceed 1000 ng/mL.[56]

Hydroxycarbamide

Hydroxycarbamide is a ribonucleotide inhibitor that impedes DNA synthesis by preventing the formation of deoxyribonucleotides. All the mechanisms of action in SCD have not been fully elucidated but some properties have been noted. It increases HbF levels and reduces neutrophils, monocytes and reticulocytes.[129] It improves red cell hydration and deformability[126] and reduces red cell endothelial adherence.[131] It may also generate nitric oxide, a potent vasodilator.[22]

Initial studies of hydroxycarbamide in adults suggested that it reduced the frequency of painful crises, ACS, blood transfusions and hospitalizations.[129] A recently published 9-year follow-up study of the original group now confirms a 40% reduction in mortality.[132] Similar studies in children confirmed its efficacy and lack of life-threatening events,[133,134] and a 9-year follow-up study has shown sustained HbF levels without effects on growth or increased numbers of acquired DNA mutations.[135] One of the unanswered questions is whether hydroxycarbamide given prior to the onset of chronic organ dysfunction could prevent damage. Preliminary data suggested benefits even in young children and now that the cooperative study of hydroxycarbamide in infants (HUG-Infants) has commenced, its findings will be eagerly awaited.[136] Hydroxycarbamide is potentially mutagenic and carcinogenic and both cancer and leukemia have been reported in patients receiving the drug. It remains unclear if the incidence of cancer is higher in this group than in the general population.[137]

Hematopoietic cell transplantation

Stem cell transplantation is the only current therapy that has the potential to cure SCD. There have been about 200 transplants from HLA-identical siblings worldwide and there is an 85% survival, free of SCD, with a follow-up in some cases of 11 years. There is a 5% transplant-related mortality and 5% of patients experience chronic graft-versus-host disease. Neurologic complications such as seizures can occur during transplant and may in part be related to hypertension. The current indications for stem cell transplant are:[56]

- availability of a fully HLA-matched sibling donor;
- patient age < 16 years with HbSS or HbS/β^0-thalassemia;
- previous stroke;
- abnormal MRI or neuropsychologic function;
- recurrent chest syndrome or stage I/II sickle lung disease;
- recurrent vasoocclusive episodes;
- sickle nephropathy;
- AVN of multiple joints.

Volunteer unrelated transplants, umbilical cord blood and nonmyeloablative transplants are the subject of clinical trial. Currently, there are no comparative studies of blood transfusion, hydroxycarbamide or stem cell transplantation that would permit recommendation of one intervention over the others.

The Future

Drug therapies that specifically target one aspect of the sickle pathologic process are being developed (Table 10.7). Drugs

Table 10.7 Experimental therapies for the management of sickle cell disease.

Agents to increase HbF
 Butyrate
 Decitabine
Nitric oxide promoters
 Nitric oxide
 Arginine
 Citrulline
Red cell membrane channel blockers
 Magnesium
 Arginine
 Clotrimazole derivatives
Endothelial interactions/decreased activation
 Antiadhesion molecules
 Sulfasalazine
Combinations

such as arginine that increase the availability of nitric oxide are undergoing phase I studies and have shown some benefit in pulmonary hypertension.[138] Agents such as decitabine, which act by hypomethylation of the γ-globin genes, produce a rise in HbF levels and have shown effect even in individuals previously resistant to hydroxycarbamide.[139] Short-chain fatty acids and their derivatives enhance γ-globin gene expression and can induce significant HbF increase.[137] Clotrimazole derivatives and magnesium inhibit erythrocyte membrane electrolyte fluxes and can prevent red cell dehydration, thus reducing HbS concentration and polymerization. Antibodies targeting endothelial adhesion mechanisms have been developed in rat models and are now awaiting further development. Alternatives to sibling transplantation are being actively pursued as few patients have fully matched sibling donors and advances in this area can be expected. Gene therapy is still at the developmental stage and is moving slowly. It is unlikely that any major advance will be seen in the near future. Our knowledge of the mechanisms underlying the sickling process has grown enormously over the past 10 years; however, one suspects there is much left to understand, particularly in the area of vascular biology about this complex disease.

References

1. Africanus Horton JB. *The Diseases of Tropical Climates and their Treatment*. London: Churchill, 1874.
2. Herrick JB. Peculiar elongated and sickled red blood corpuscles in a case of severe anaemia. *Arch Intern Med* 1910; **6**: 517–21.
3. Pauling L, Itano HA, Singer SJ, Wells IC. Sickle cell anaemia, a molecular disease. *Science* 1949; **10**: 543–8.
4. Ingram VM. Gene mutations in human haemoglobin: the chemical difference between normal and sickle haemoglobin. *Nature* 1957; **180**: 326–8.
5. Okpala I. The management of crisis in sickle cell disease. *Eur J Haematol* 1998; **60**: 1–6.
6. Ohene-Frempong K. Sickle cell disease in the United States of America and Africa. *Hematology (Am Soc Hematol Educ Program)* 1999: 64–72.
7. Stuart MJ, Nagel RL. Sickle cell disease. *Lancet* 2004; **364**: 1343–60.
8. Diallo D, Tchernia G. Sickle cell disease in Africa. *Curr Opin Hematol* 2002; **9**: 111–16.
9. Fixler J, Styles L. Sickle cell disease. *Pediatr Clin North Am* 2002; **49**: 1193–210.
10. Hickman M, Modell B, Greengross P *et al.* Mapping the prevalence of sickle cell and beta thalassaemia in England: estimating and validating ethnic-specific rates. *Br J Haematol* 1999; **104**: 860–7.
11. Platt OS, Brambilla DJ, Rosse WF *et al.* Mortality in sickle cell disease. Life expectancy and risk factors for early death. *N Engl J Med* 1994; **330**: 1639–44.
12. Miller ST, Sleeper LA, Pegelow CH *et al.* Prediction of adverse outcomes in children with sickle cell disease. *N Engl J Med* 2000; **342**: 83–9.

13. Quinn CT, Rogers ZR, Buchanan GR. Survival of children with sickle cell disease. *Blood* 2004; **103**: 4023–7.

14. Manci EA, Culberson DE, Yang YM *et al*. Causes of death in sickle cell disease: an autopsy study. *Br J Haematol* 2003; **123**: 359–65.

15. Fleming AF. The presentation, management and prevention of crisis in sickle cell disease in Africa. *Blood Rev* 1989; **3**: 18–28.

16. Aluoch JR, Aluoch LHM. Survey of sickle cell disease in Kenya. *Trop Geogr Med* 1993; **45**: 18–21.

17. Bookchin RM, Lew VL. Sickle red cell dehydration: mechanisms and interventions *Curr Opin Hematol* 2002; **9**: 107–10.

18. Kaul DK, Tsai HM, Liu XD, Nakada MT, Nagel RL, Coller BS. Monoclonal antibodies to aVb3 (7E3 and LM609) inhibit sickle red blood cell endothelium interactions induced by platelet-activating factor. *Blood* 2000; **95**: 368–74.

19. Frennette PS. Sickle cell vaso-occlusion: multistep and multicellular paradigm *Curr Opin Hematol* 2002; **9**: 101–6.

20. Barabino GA, Liu XD, Ewenstein BM, Kaul DK. Anionic polysaccharides inhibit adhesion of sickle erythrocytes to the vascular endothelium and result in improved hemodynamic behaviour. *Blood* 1999; **93**: 1422–9.

21. Stuart MJ, Setty BN. Sickle cell acute chest syndrome: pathogenesis and rationale for treatment. *Blood* 1999; **94**: 1555–60.

22. Ohene-Frempong K, Steinberg MH. Clinical aspects of sickle cell anemia in adults and children. In: Steinberg MH, Forget BG, Higgs DR, Nagel RL (eds) *Disorders of Haemoglobin*. Cambridge: Cambridge University Press, 2001, pp. 611–70.

23. Serjeant GR, Serjeant BE. *Sickle Cell Disease*, 3rd edn. Oxford: Oxford University Press, 2001.

24. Bain BJ. *Haemoglobinopathy Diagnosis*. Oxford: Blackwell Science, 2001.

25. Bunn HF. Sickle hemoglobin and other haemoglobin mutants. In: Stamatoyannopoulos G, Nienhuis AW, Majerus PW, Varmus H (eds) *The Molecular Basis of Blood Diseases*, 2nd edn. Philadelphia: WB Saunders, 1994, pp. 207–56.

26. Vichinsky EP, Haberkern CM, Neumayr L *et al*. A comparison of conservative and aggressive transfusion regimens in the perioperative management of sickle cell disease. *N Engl J Med* 1995; **333**: 206–14.

27. Koshy M, Weiner SJ, Miller ST *et al*. Surgery and anesthesia in sickle cell disease. Cooperative study of sickle cell diseases. *Blood* 1995; **86**: 3676–84.

28. Wales PW, Carver E, Crawford MW, Kim PC. Acute chest syndrome after abdominal surgery in children with sickle cell disease: is laparoscopic approach better? *J Pediatr Surg* 2001; **36**: 718–21.

29. Waldron P, Pegelow C, Neumayr L *et al*. Tonsillectomy, adenoidectomy, and myringotomy in sickle cell disease: perioperative morbidity. Preoperative Transfusion in Sickle Cell Disease Study Group. *J Pediatr Hematol Oncol* 1999; **21**: 129–35.

30. Neumayr L, Koshy M, Haberkern C *et al*. Surgery in patients with haemoglobin SC disease. Preoperative Transfusion in Sickle Cell Disease Study Group. *Am J Hematol* 1998; **57**: 101–8.

31. Adu-Gyamfi Y, Sankarankutty M, Marwa S. Use of a tourniquet in patients with sickle cell disease. *Can J Anaesth* 1993; **40**: 24–7.

32. Vipond AJ, Caldicott LD. Major vascular surgery in a patient with sickle cell disease. *Anaesthesia* 1998; **53**: 1204–6.

33. Platt OS, Rosenstock W, Espeland MA. Influence of sickle haemoglobinopathies on growth and development. *N Engl J Med* 1984; **311**: 7–12.

34. Singhal A, Thomas P, Cook R *et al*. Delayed adolescent growth in homozygous sickle cell Disease. *Arch Dis Child* 1994; **71**: 404–8.

35. Caruso-Nicoletti M, Mancuso M, Spadaro G *et al*. Growth and development in white patients with sickle cell diseases. *Am J Pediatr Hematol Oncol* 1992; **14**: 285–8.

36. Modebe O, Ifenu SA. Growth retardation in homozygous sickle cell disease: role of calorie intake and possible gender related differences. *Am J Hematol* 1993; **44**: 149–54.

37. Stevens MCG, Maude GH, Cupidore L, Jackson H, Hayes RJ, Serjeant GR. Prepubertal growth and skeletal maturation in sickle cell disease. *Pediatrics* 1986; **78**: 124–32.

38. Thomas PW, Singhal A, Hemmings-Kelly M, Sergeant GR. Height and weight reference curves for homozygous sickle cell disease. *Arch Dis Child* 2000; **82**: 204–8.

39. Barden EM, Zemel BBS, Kawchak DA, Goran MI, Ohene-Frempong K, Stallings VA. Total and resting energy expenditure in children with sickle cell disease. *J Pediatr* 2000; **136**: 73–9.

40. Barden EM, Kawchak DA, Ohene-Frempong K, Stallings VA, Zemel BS. Body composition in children with sickle cell disease. *Am J Clin Nutr* 2002; **76**: 218–25.

41. Leonard MB, Zemel BS, Kawchak DA, Ohene-Frempong K, Stallings VA. Plasma zinc status, growth and maturation in children with sickle cell disease. *J Pediatr* 1998; **132**: 467–71.

42. Prasad AS, Beck FWJ, Kaplan J *et al*. Effect of zinc supplementation on incidence of infections and hospital admissions in sickle cell diseases (SCD). *Am J Hematol* 1999; **61**: 194–202.

43. Kosey M. Sickle cell disease and pregnancy. *Blood Rev* 1995; **9**: 157–64.

44. Khare M, Bewley W, Okpala I. Management of pregnancy in sickle cell disease. In: *Practical Management of Haemoglobino-pathies*. Oxford: Blackwell Publishing, 2004, pp. 107–19.

45. Rahimy MC, Gangbo A, Adjou R *et al*. Effect of active prenatal management on pregnancy outcome in sickle cell disease in an African setting. *Blood* 2000; **96**: 1685–9.

46. Anyaegbunam A, Mikhail M, Axioitis C, Morel ML, Merkatz IR. Placental histology and placental/fetal weight ratios in pregnant women with sickle cell disease: relationship to pregnancy outcome. *J Assoc Acad Minor Phys* 1994; **5**: 123–5.

47. Overturf GD. Infections and immunizations of children with sickle cell disease. *Adv Pediatr Infect Dis* 1999; **14**: 191–218.

48. Zarkowsky HS, Gallagher D, Gill FM *et al*. Bacteraemia in sickle haemoglobinopathies. *J Pediatr* 1986; **109**: 579–85.

49. Sadat-Ali M. The status of acute osteomyelitis in sickle cell disease. A 15-year review. *Int Surg* 1998; **83**: 84–7.

50. Magnus SA, Hambleton IR, Moosdeen F, Sergeant GR. Recurrent infections in homozygous sickle cell disease. *Arch Dis Child* 1999; **80**: 537–41.

51. Hand W, King NL. Serum opsonization of salmonella in sickle cell anaemia. *Am J Med* 1978; **64**: 388–95.

52. Bjornson AB, Gaston MH, Zellner CL. Decreased opsonization for *Streptococcus pneumoniae* in sickle cell disease: studies on

selected complement components and immunoglobulins. *J Pediatr* 1977; **91**: 371–8.

53. Field R, Strunk R, Overturf G. Opsonization of salmonella lipopolysaccaride in sickle cell disease. *Pediatr Res* 1981; **15**: 167–211.

54. Boggs DR, Hyde F, Stodes C. An unusual pattern of neutrophil kinetics in sickle cell anemia. *Blood* 1973; **41**: 59–65.

55. Falletta JM, Woods GM, Verter JI *et al*. Discontinuing penicillin prophylaxis in children with sickle cell disease. Prophylactic Penicillin Study II. *J Pediatr* 1995; **127**: 685–90.

56. US Department of Health and Human Services. *The Management of Sickle Cell Disease*, 4th edn. NIH, Bethesda, Maryland, USA: National Institutes of Health, 2002.

57. BSCH guidelines for the prevention and treatment of infection in patients with absent or dysfunctional spleens. *Br Med J* 1996; **312**: 430–4.

58. Adamkiewitz TV, Sarnaik S, Buchanan GR *et al*. Invasive pneumococcal infections in children with sickle cell disease in the era of penicillin prophylaxis, antibiotic resistance and 23-valent pneumococcal polysaccharide vaccination. *J Pediatr* 2003; **143**: 438–44.

59. Vernacchio L, Neufeld EJ, MacDonald K *et al*. Combined schedule of 7-valent pneumococcal conjugate vaccine followed by 23-valent pneumococcal vaccine in children and adults with sickle cell disease. *J Pediatr* 1998; **133**: 275–8.

60. Booz MM, Hariharan V, Aradi AJ, Malki AA. The value of ultrasound and aspiration in differentiating vaso-occlusive crisis and osteomyelitis in sickle cell disease patients. *Clin Radiol* 1999; **54**: 636–9.

61. Serjeant GR, Serjeant BE, Stephens S *et al*. Determinants of haemoglobin level in steady state homozygous sickle cell disease. *Br J Haematol* 1996; **92**: 143–9.

62. Platt OS Exercise-induced hemolysis in sickle cell anemia: shear sensitivity and erythrocyte dehydration. *Blood* 1982; **59**: 1055–60.

63. Serjeant GR, Serjeant BE, Thomas PW *et al*. Human parvovirus infection in homozygous sickle cell disease. *Lancet* 1993; **341**: 1237–40.

64. Brozovic M, Davies SC, Brownell AI. Acute admissions of patients with sickle cell disease who live in Britain. *Br Med J* 1987; **294**: 1206–8.

65. Burko H, Watson J, Robinson M. Unusual bone changes in sickle cell disease in childhood. *Radiology* 1963; **80**: 957–62.

66. Keeley K, Buchanan GR. Acute infarction of the long bones in children with sickle cell anemia. *J Pediatr* 1982; **101**: 170–5.

67. Milner PF, Kraus AP, Sebes JI *et al*. Sickle cell disease as a cause of osteonecrosis of the femoral head. *N Engl J Med* 1991; **325**: 1476–81.

68. Lee REJ, Golding JSR, Serjeant GR. The radiological features of avascular necrosis of the femoral head in homozygous sickle cell disease. *Clin Radiol* 1981; **32**: 205–14.

69. Ebong WW. Avascular necrosis of the femoral head associated with haemoglobinopathy. *Trop Geogr Med* 1977; **29**: 19–23.

70. Milner PF, Kraus AP, Sebes JI *et al*. Osteonecrosis of the humeral head in sickle cell disease. *Clin Orthop* 1993; **289**: 136–43.

71. Mont MA, Carbone JJ, Fairbank AC. Core decompression versus non-operative management for osteonecrosis of the hip. *Clin Orthop Relat Res* 1996; **324**: 169–78.

72. Styles LA, Vichinsky EP. Core compression in avascular necrosis of the hip in sickle cell disease. *Am J Hematol* 1996; **52**: 103–7.

73. Topley JM, Rogers DW, Stevens MCG *et al*. Acute splenic sequestration and hypersplenism in the first 5 years in homozygous sickle cell disease. *Arch Dis Child* 1981; **56**: 765–9.

74. Aquino VM, Norvell JM, Buchanan GR. Acute splenic complications in children with sickle cell–hemoglobin C disease. *J Pediatr* 1997; **130**: 961–5.

75. Orringer EP, Fowler VG Jr, Owens CM *et al*. Case report: splenic infarction and acute splenic sequestration in adults with haemoglobin SC disease. *Am J Med Sci* 1991; **302**: 374–9.

76. Powell RW, Levine GL, Yang YM, Mankad VN. Acute splenic sequestration crisis in sickle cell disease: early detection and treatment. *J Pediatr Surg* 1992; **27**: 215–19.

77. Casey JR, Kinney TR, Ware RE. Acute splenic sequestration in the absence of palpable splenomegaly. *Am J Pediatr Hematol Oncol* 1994; **16**: 181–2.

78. Kinney TR, Ware RE, Schultz WH *et al*. Long-term management of splenic sequestration in children with sickle cell disease. *J Pediatr* 1990; **117**: 194–9.

79. Wright JG, Hambleton IR, Thomas PW *et al*. Post splenectomy course in homozygous sickle cell disease. *J Pediatr* 1999; **134**: 304–9.

80. Lee ESH, Chu PCM. Reverse sequestration in a case of sickle cell crisis. *Postgrad Med J* 1996; **72**: 487–8.

81. Stephan JL, Merpit-Gonon E, Richard O, Raynaud-Ravni C, Freycon F. Fulminant liver failure in a 12-year-old girl with sickle cell anaemia: favourable outcome after exchange transfusions *Eur J Pediatr* 1995; **154**: 469–71.

82. Walker TM, Hambleton IR, Serjeant GR. Gallstones in sickle cell disease: observation from the Jamaican cohort study. *J Pediatr* 2000; **136**: 80–5.

83. Haider MZ, Ashebu S, Aduh P, Adekile AD. Influence of alpha-thalassaemia on cholelithiasis in SS patients with elevated HbF. *Acta Haematol* 1998; **100**: 147–50.

84. Statius van Eps LW, Pinedo-Veels C, deVries CH *et al*. Nature of the concentrating defect in sickle cell nephropathy. Microradioangiographic studies. *Lancet* 1970; **i**: 450–2.

85. Allon M. Renal abnormalities in sickle cell disease. *Arch Intern Med* 1990; **150**: 501–4.

86. Pham PT, Pham PC, Wilkinson AH, Lew SQ. Renal abnormalities in sickle cell disease. *Kidney Int* 2000; **57**: 1–8.

87. Wigfall DR, Ware RE, Burchinal MR, Kinney TR, Foreman JW. Prevalence and clinical correlates of glomerulopathy in children with sickle cell disease. *J Pediatr* 2000; **136**: 749–53.

88. Bakir AA, Hathiwala SC, Ainis H *et al*. Prognosis of the nephrotic syndrome in sickle cell glomerulonephropathy: a retrospective study. *Am J Nephrol* 1987; **7**: 110–15.

89. Falk RJ, Scheinman J, Phillips G *et al*. Prevalence and pathologic features of sickle cell nephropathy and response to inhibition of angiotensin-converting enzyme. *N Engl J Med* 1992; **326**: 910–15.

90. Sklar AH, Perez JC, Harp RJ, Caruana RJ. Acute renal failure in sickle cell anemia. *Int J Artif Organs* 1990; **13**: 347–51.

91. Hassell KL, Eckman JR, Lane PA. Acute multiorgan failure syndrome: a potentially catastrophic complication off severe sickle cell pain episodes. *Am J Med* 1994; **96**: 155–62.

92. Powars DR, Elliott-Mils DD, Chan L *et al*. Chronic renal failure

in sickle cell disease: risk factors, clinical course, and mortality. *Ann Intern Med* 1991; **115**: 614–20.

93. Warady BA, Sullivan EK. Renal transplantation in children with SCD: a report of the North American Pediatric Renal Transplant Cooperative study (NAPRTCS). *Pediatr Transplant* 1998; **2**: 130–3.

94. Nolan VG, Baldwin C, Ma Q *et al*. Association of single nucleotide polymorphisms in klotho with priapism in sickle cell anaemia. *Br J Haematol* 2005; **128**: 266–72.

95. Mantadakis E, Cavender JD, Rogers ZR, Ewalt DH, Buchanan GR. Prevalence of priapism in children and adolescents with sickle cell anemia. *J Pediatr Hematol Oncol* 1999; **21**: 518–22.

96. Virag R, Bachir D, Lee H, Galacteros F. Preventive treatment of priapism in sickle cell disease with oral and self intracavernous injection of etilefrine. *Urology* 1996; **47**: 777–81.

97. Davies SC, Roberts-Harewood M. Blood transfusion in sickle cell disease. *Blood Rev* 1997; **11**: 57–71.

98. Saad ST, Lajolo C, Gilli S *et al*. Follow-up of sickle cell disease patients with priapism treated with hydroxyurea. *Am J Hematol* 2004; **77**: 45–9.

99. Sher GD, Olivieri NF. Rapid healing of chronic leg ulcers during arginine butyrate therapy in patients with sickle cell disease and thalassaemia. *Blood* 1994; **84**: 2378–80.

100. Best PJ, Daoud MS, Pittelkow MR *et al*. Hydroxyurea-induced leg ulceration in 14 patients. *Ann Intern Med* 1998; **128**: 29–32.

101. Vichinsky E. Understanding the pathophysiology and treatment of pulmonary injury in sickle cell disease. *Hematology (Am Soc Hematol Educ Program)* 2002; 16–22.

102. Vichinsky EP, Neumayr LD, Earles AN *et al*. Causes and outcomes of acute chest syndrome in sickle cell disease. National Acute Chest Syndrome Study Group. *N Engl J Med* 2000; **342**: 1855–65.

103. Castro O, Brambilla DJ, Thorington B *et al*. The acute chest syndrome in sickle cell disease: incidence and risk factors. The cooperative study of sickle cell disease. *Blood* 1994; **84**: 643–9.

104. Emre U, Miller ST, Gutierez M, Steiner P, Rao SP, Rao M. Effect of transfusion in acute chest syndrome of sickle cell disease. *J Pediatr* 1995; **127**: 901–4.

105. Pelidis MA, Kato GJ, Resar LM *et al*. Successful treatment of life threatening acute chest syndrome in sickle cell disease with venovenous extracorporeal membrane oxygenation. *J Pediatr Hematol Oncol* 1997; **19**: 459–61.

106. Bernini JC, Rogers ZR, Sandler ES *et al*. Beneficial effect of intravenous dexamethasone in children with mild to moderately severe acute chest syndrome complicating sickle cell disease. *Blood* 1998; **92**: 3082–9.

107. Sullivan KJ, Goodwin SR, Evangelist J *et al*. Nitric oxide successfully used to treat acute chest syndrome of sickle cell disease in a young adolescent. *Crit Care Med* 1999; **27**: 2563–8.

108. Gladwin MT, Sachdev V, Jison ML *et al*. Pulmonary hypertension as a risk factor for death in patients with sickle cell disease. *N Engl J Med* 2004; **350**: 886–95.

109. Jison ML, Gladwin MT. Hemolytic anaemia-associated pulmonary hypertension of sickle cell disease and the nitric oxide/arginine pathway. *Am J Respir Crit Care Med* 2003; **168**: 3–4.

110. Castro O, Hoque M, Brown BD. Pulmonary hypertension in sickle cell disease: cardiac catherization results and survival. *Blood* 2003; **101**: 1257–61.

111. Koumbourlis AC, Hurlet-Jensen A, Bye MR. Lung function in infants with sickle cell disease. *Pediatr Pulmonol* 1997; **24**: 277–81.

112. Morris CR, Morris SM Jr, Hagar W *et al*. Arginine therapy: a new treatment for pulmonary hypertension in sickle cell disease? *Am J Respir Crit Care Med* 2003; **168**: 63–9.

113. Hoppe C, Klitz W, Noble J, Vigil L, Vichinsky E, Styles L. Distinct HLA associations by stroke subtype in children with sickle cell disease. *Blood* 2003; **101**: 2865–9.

114. Pegelow CH, Macklin EA, Moser FG *et al*. Longitudinal changes in brain magnetic resonance imaging findings in children with sickle cell disease. *Blood* 2002; **99**: 3014–18.

115. Abboud MR, Cure J, Granger S *et al*. Magnetic resonance angiography in children with sickle cell disease and abnormal transcranial Doppler ultrasonography findings enrolled in the STOP study. *Blood* 2004; **103**: 2822–6.

116. Adams RJ. Stroke prevention and treatment in sickle cell disease. *Arch Neurol* 2001; **58**: 565–8.

117. Wang WC, Kovnar EH, Tonkin IL *et al*. High risk of recurrent stroke after discontinuance of five to twelve years of transfusion therapy in patients with sickle cell disease. *J Pediatr* 1991; **118**: 377–82.

118. Ware RE, Zimmermann SA, Schultz WH. Hydroxyurea as an alternative to blood transfusion for the prevention of recurrent stroke in children with sickle cell disease. *Blood* 1999; **94**: 3022–6.

119. Ware RE, Zimmermann SA, Sylvestre PB *et al*. Prevention of secondary stroke and resolution of transfusional iron overload in children with sickle cell anemia using hydroxyurea and phlebotomy. *J Pediatr* 2004; **145**: 346–52.

120. Adams R, McKie V, Hsu L *et al*. Prevention of first stroke by transfusion in children with sickle cell disease and abnormal results of transcranial Doppler ultrasonography. *N Engl Med* 1998; **339**: 5–11.

121. Kinney TR, Sleeper LA, Wang WC *et al*. Silent cerebral infarcts in sickle cell anemia: a risk factor analysis. *Pediatrics* 1999; **103**: 640–5.

122. Armstrong FD, Thompson RJ Jr, Wang WC *et al*. Cognitive functioning and brain MRI in children with SCD. *Pediatrics* 1996; **97**: 864–70.

123. Wang WC, Langston JW, Steen RG *et al*. Abnormalities of the central nervous system in very young children with sickle cell anemia. *J Pediatr* 1998; **132**: 994–8.

124. Pegelow CH, Wang W, Granger S *et al*. Silent infarcts in children with sickle cell anaemia and abnormal cerebral artery velocity. *Arch Neurol* 2001; **58**: 2017–21.

125. Kirkham FJ, Hewes DK, Prengler M *et al*. Nocturnal hypoxaemia and central-nervous-system events in sickle-cell disease. *Lancet* 2001; **357**: 1656–9.

126. Rees DC, Olujohungbe AD, Parker NE *et al*. Guidelines for the management of the acute painful crisis in sickle cell disease. *Br J Haematol* 2003; **120**: 744–52.

127. Vichinsky EP, Earles A, Johnson RA *et al*. Alloimmunisation in sickle cell anemia and transfusion of racially unmatched blood. *N Engl J Med* 1990; **322**: 1617–21.

128. Talano JA, Hillery CA, Gottschall JL, Baylerian DM, Scott JP. Delayed hemolytic transfusion reaction/hyperhemolysis syndrome in children with sickle cell disease. *Pediatrics* 2003; **111**: 661–5.

129. Charache S, Terrin ML, Moore RD *et al*. Hydroxyurea and sickle cell anemia: clinical utility of a myelosuppressive 'switching' agent. *Medicine (Baltimore)* 1996; **75**: 300–26.

130. Ballas SK, Dover GJ, Charache S. Effect of hydroxyurea on the rheological properties of sickle erythrocytes in vivo. *Am J Hematol* 1991; **32**: 104–11.

131. Adragna NC, Fonseca P, Lauf PK. Hydroxyurea affects cell morphology, cation transport and red cell adhesion in cultured vascular endothelial cells. *Blood* 1994; **83**: 553–60.

132. Steinberg MH, Barton F, Castro O *et al*. Effects of hydroxyurea on mortality and morbidity in adult sickle cell anemia: risks and benefits up to 9 years of treatment. *JAMA* 2003; **289**: 1645–51.

133. Kinney TR, Helms RW, O'Branski EE *et al*. Safety of hydroxyurea in children with sickle cell anemia: results of the HUG-KIDS study, a phase I/II trial. *Blood* 1999; **94**: 1550–4.

134. Ferster A, Tahriri P, Vermylen C, Sturbois G, Corazza F. Five years of experience with hydroxyurea in children and young adults with sickle cell disease. *Blood* 2001; **97**: 3628–32.

135. Zimmerman SA, Schultz WH, Davis JS *et al*. Sustained long-term haematologic efficacy of hydroxyurea at maximum tolerated dose in children with sickle cell disease. *Blood* 2004; **103**: 2039–45.

136. Wang WC, Wynn LW, Rogers ZR, Scott JP, Lane PA, Ware RE. A 2 year pilot trail of hydroxyurea in very young children with sickle cell anemia. *J Pediatr* 2001; **139**: 790–6.

137. Buchanan GR, De Baun MR, Quill CT and Steinberg MH. Sickle cell disease. *Hematology (Am Soc Hematol Educ Program)* 2004; 35–47.

138. Morris CR, Kuypers FA, Larkin S *et al*. Arginine therapy: a novel strategy to induce nitric oxide production in sickle cell disease. *Br J Haematol* 2000; **111**: 498–500.

139. Saunthararajah Y, Hillery CA, Lavelle D *et al*. Effects of 5-aza-2'-deoxycytidine on fetal haemoglobin levels, red cell adhesion and hematopoietic differentiation in patients with sickle cell disease. *Blood* 2003; **102**: 3865–70.

11 Hemoglobin variants and the rarer hemoglobin disorders

Andreas E. Kulozik

Introduction

Hemoglobin is a tetrameric protein complex consisting of two pairs of globin chains with a combined molecular mass of 64 400 Da. One type of globin chain is coded at the tip of the short arm of chromosome 16 where the α-globin gene cluster containing the embryonic ζ and the adult α2 and α1 genes is located.[1] The other type is coded on the short arm of chromosome 11 (11p14) by the β-globin gene cluster containing the embryonic ε, fetal $^G\gamma$ and $^A\gamma$, and adult δ and β genes.[1] Each of the four subunits is covalently bound to the ferroprotoporphyrin heme as a ligand. The structure and function of hemoglobin enable it to be soluble and stable in the erythrocyte, and to allow uptake, transport and release of large quantities of oxygen under physiologic conditions.

As of January 2005, 896 functionally relevant and functionally silent hemoglobin variants have been described and deposited in the hemoglobin variant database.[2] This chapter reviews aspects of normal hemoglobin structure and function and describes the less common pathologic hemoglobin anomalies.

Hemoglobin structure

Primary structure

The globin chains are coded in the α- and β-gene cluster (Fig. 11.1) and contain 141 and 146 amino acids respectively.[3] The strong evolutionary and functional kinship of these proteins is reflected by the high degree of sequence homology. The α- and ζ-chains show identity at 84 of 141 residues (60%). The homology of the ε, γ, δ and β genes is even more striking, with an identity of 94 of 146 residues (64%). The heme is bound covalently between the iron and the proximal F8 His

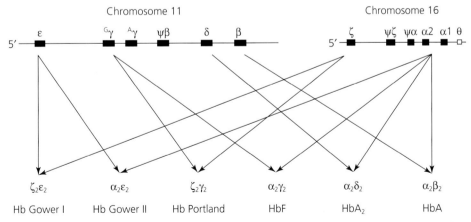

Fig. 11.1 The α- and β-globin gene clusters on chromosomes 11 and 16. The β-globin gene cluster contains the embryonic ε-, fetal γ-, and adult δ- and β-globin genes. In addition, there is a nonexpressed pseudogene (ψβ) with significant sequence homology to the β gene. The α-globin gene cluster contains the embryonic ζ- and adult α-globin genes. In addition, there are various pseudogenes (ψζ, ψα1, θ). Different hemoglobins are produced in the course of ontogeny; all contain two α- or ζ-chains and two β- or β-like chains (embryonic stage: Hb Gower I, Hb Gower II, Hb Portland; fetal stage: HbF; postnatal and adult stage: HbA₂, HbA).

at position 87 in the α-chain and at position 92 in the β-chain. The functionally important residues, such as those at the α–β interfaces or at the heme-binding sites, are especially highly conserved.

Secondary structure

The globin chains are wound up into segments of α-helices that are interrupted by non-helical configurations where the polypeptide chains bend.[3] The helices, with 3.6 amino acids per turn, are stabilized by H-bonds between the carbonyl and amino groups of residues four positions apart. The β-chain consists of eight helical segments (designated A–H). The α-chain is similar, although the D helix has been deleted in the course of evolution by a functionally neutral mutation.[4] The residues can be assigned to their position in the helices and the degree of homology between globin chains is particularly striking when the alignment is oriented at the secondary structure. For example, the heme-binding histidines at positions 87 in the α-chain and 92 in the β-chain are at position 8 in the F helix (F8) in both globin chains. Homologous positions in the globins are therefore best represented by the helical designation rather than by their numerical position in the primary structure.

Tertiary and quaternary structure

Much of the information available about the three-dimensional structure and the function of hemoglobin has been obtained by X-ray crystallography.[5–10] Tertiary structure refers to the steric relationship of residues within the individual globin chain, whereas quaternary structure refers to subunit interactions. Both determine the functionally important three-dimensional structure of the entire tetrameric protein –heme complex and are therefore dealt with together.

The helices of the individual globin chains form a compact spherical structure (Fig. 11.2). The residues facing outward are mainly polar, whereas those facing inwards are mainly non-polar. This distribution is responsible for both the excellent solubility of hemoglobin and its high degree of stability by blocking the influx of water into the central part of the complex.

Near to the surface, the heme molecule is suspended between the proximal and distal histidines at position F8 and E7. The six electrons in the outermost orbital of the ferrous iron (Fe^{2+}) coordinate with the four nitrogens of the pyrrole molecule, the imidazole nitrogen of His F8 and the oxygen. Additionally, there are multiple contacts to mainly non-polar residues of the heme pocket between the E and F helices, but also to residues of the C, G and H helices. The porphyrin ring is held in this pocket by 60 hydrophobic bonds, conferring a high degree of stability. The functional importance of these contact points is highlighted by their strong evolutionary conservation and by the effect of amino acid substitutions that result in unstable hemoglobin variants.

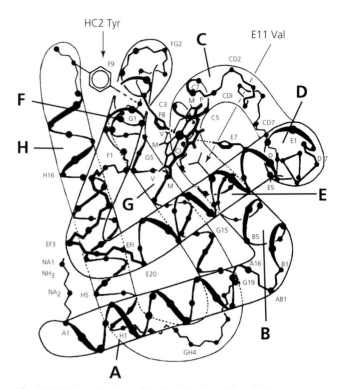

Fig. 11.2 Tertiary structure of the β-globin chain. The α-helices are designated A–F from the N- to the C-terminal. Modified with permission from Ref. 84.

The four subunits are assembled to form an ellipsoid measuring $6.4 \times 5.5 \times 5.0$ nm. In the center of the tetrameric complex runs a twofold, dyad axis of symmetry, which means that any part of the molecule will superimpose on an identical counterpart if rotated by 180° around this axis (Fig. 11.3).[11] The α and β chains have two interfaces between each other, one between the α_1 (α_2) and β_1 (β_2) and the other between the α_1 (α_2) and β_2 (β_1) chains. The $\alpha_1\beta_1$ ($\alpha_2\beta_2$) contact is established by about 40 van der Waals and H-bonds involving 16 α-chain and 17 β-chain residues.[3] The characteristic of the $\alpha_1\beta_2$ contact is that there are two possible conformations that are assumed while oxygenated or deoxygenated. The deoxy form is tight (T-form) with about 40 van der Waals and H-bonds,[3] whereas the oxy form is relaxed by about 0.7 nm and established by only 22 van der Waals and H-bonds (R-form). Consequently, oxyhemoglobin is less stable than deoxyhemoglobin. This allosteric movement at the $\alpha_1\beta_2$ interface is also paramount to the cooperative effect of oxygen binding. Calculations of conformational energies and direct structural analyses suggest that oxygen binding to the T-form puts an increased strain on the $\alpha_1\beta_2$ ($\alpha_2\beta_1$) interface that can be relieved by the conformational change to the R-form, which can then more readily accept more oxygen at the other hemes in the complex. Mechanistically, the transition from the T-form to the R-form requires oxygen binding according to a "symmetry rule," i.e., whenever oxygen binding creates a

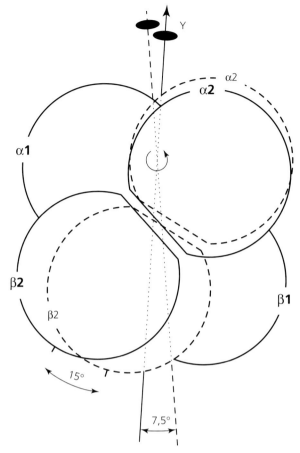

Fig. 11.3 Quaternary structure of hemoglobin in the T (solid line) and R (dotted line) quaternary conformations. The α_1/β_1 contact remains unchanged, whereas the α_1/β_2 contact rotates by about 15° when the allosteric switch occurs. Modified with permission from Ref. 11.

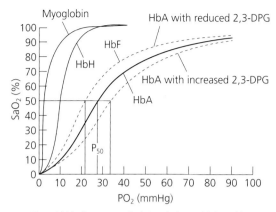

Fig. 11.4 Sigmoid binding curve of HbF and HbA at high and low 2,3-diphosphoglycerate (2,3-DPG) concentrations. The hyperbolic binding curves of myoglobin and HbH, which do not show a cooperative effect on oxygen binding, are shown for comparison. Modified with permission from Ref. 84.

4 mol of O_2; as 1 mol of a gas at standard temperature and pressure is 22.4 L, 1 g of hemoglobin can bind 1.39 mL of O_2. At a hemoglobin concentration of 15 g/dL, 100 mL of blood can thus transport ~ 20 mL of O_2.

The basic mechanism is the cooperative effect of the subunits, which is structurally based on the allosterism of the R-form and T-form. This means that binding of oxygen induces allosteric changes in particular at the the $\alpha_1\beta_2$ contact that facilitate the uptake of further oxygen molecules (homotropism). This cooperative effect is modified by the influence of other molecules, such as 2,3-DPG, H^+, Cl^- and CO_2 (heterotropism). The physiologic corollary of this cooperative effect is the sigmoid binding curve of hemoglobin, i.e., oxygen is rapidly loaded and unloaded at physiologic oxygen tensions (Fig. 11.4).

Homotropic interactions of oxygen binding

A powerful model of oxygen binding was proposed by Monod *et al.*[14] which was later modified.[12] According to this model, the R-form and the T-form are in equilibrium and differ in their oxygen affinity. The binding of the ligand to the individual subunit causes the tertiary structure to relax. When one subunit of each $\alpha_1\beta_1$ and $\alpha_2\beta_2$ dimer is oxygenated, the quaternary switch to the R conformation occurs, facilitating oxygen loading of the remaining two subunits. This basic shift of the equilibrium induced by the ligand itself is modified heterotropically by CO_2, 2,3-DPG and chloride as detailed below.

Heterotropic interactions of oxygen binding

Bohr effect

Bohr, Hasselbalch and Krogh showed in 1904 that oxygen

tetramer with at least one ligated subunit on each dimeric half-molecule ($\alpha_1\beta_1$ or $\alpha_2\beta_2$), quaternary switching occurs.[12]

The T-form is further stabilized by chloride and 2,3-diphosphoglycerate (2,3-DPG), which confer intra- and inter-subunit salt bonds. Cl^- establishes two bonds between the N-terminal Val of α_2 to α_2 131 Ser and α_1 141 Arg and also neutralizes repulsive forces of positively charged residues in the central cavity.[13] 2,3-DPG is a polyanion that associates with the positive charges of the N-terminal amino groups of Lys 82 and of the histidines 2 and 143 of the β-chains. When 2,3-DPG is lost during oxygenation, Cl^- and H^+ ions are ejected from the central cavity.

Hemoglobin function

The chief function of hemoglobin is to take up oxygen in the lungs and transport it to the peripheral tissues, where it is unloaded in exchange for CO_2. The quantities of oxygen transported are enormous: 1 mol of hemoglobin can bind affinity is reduced by CO_2. The major mechanism of the Bohr effect is the formation of carbonic acid from CO_2 and H_2O, catalyzed by carbonic anhydrase ($CO_2 + H_2O \leftrightarrow H_2CO_3$); carbonic acid readily dissociates into HCO_3^- and H^+. HCO_3^- is rapidly exported into the plasma in exchange for Cl^-, thus decreasing intracellular pH. The protons stabilize the T-form by forming H-bonds, predominantly at β 146 His but also at β 94 Asp, α 122 His and the N-terminal amino groups.[15–18] On oxygenation these protons are extruded, breaking the salt bonds and changing the pK_a, from 8.0 in deoxyhemoglobin to 7.1 in oxyhemoglobin.[8,19–21] The Bohr effect therefore facilitates gas exchange, because oxygen affinity is decreased and oxygen unloaded at high concentrations of CO_2, i.e., in the peripheral tissues. Conversely, when CO_2 is exhaled in the lungs and intracellular pH rises, oxygen affinity is increased, which favors oxygen uptake.

A smaller portion of the CO_2 is directly bound to reactive amino groups to form carbamino complexes that also stabilize the T-form. However, in comparison to the Bohr effect, carbamino formation is probably of much less significance in terms of controlling allosterism and cooperative oxygen binding.[22]

Interaction with chloride

Chloride is transported into the red cell when bicarbonate is exported during protonation and deoxygenation (see above). Chloride reinforces the stabilization of the T-form by neutralizing electrostatic repulsion by an excess of positive charges in the central cavity of the molecule.[13,23,24] Additionally, Cl binding at the N-terminus of the α-chains appears to stabilize protonation and the T-form, thus modulating allosterism. Upon oxygenation, chloride is released together with the protons that are required for the reverse carbonic anhydrase reaction. The efficiency of the Bohr effect is reduced to about half in a chloride-depleted system, demonstrating the physiologic importance of the chloride interaction.[25] Clinically, the importance of the interaction of chloride with positively charged residues is demonstrated by the variants with altered oxygen affinity and additional or missing positive charges in the central cavity of the molecule.[13]

Interaction with 2,3-DPG

2,3-DPG is a polyanion with a high affinity for positively charged residues in the hemoglobin complex. It is a potent modifier of oxygen affinity[26,27] and forms H-bonds with the N-terminal amino groups, the imidazole of β 143 His, and the amino groups of β 82 Lys in the T-conformation. In the R-conformation, these interactions are much weaker.[28,29] 2,3-DPG thus stabilizes deoxyhemoglobin and reduces oxygen affinity. The higher oxygen affinity of HbF in comparison to HbA is due to a sequence difference between the γ and

β chains: β 143 His corresponds to γ 143 Ser, which is an uncharged amino acid that does not bind to 2,3-DPG.

The concentration of intracellular 2,3-DPG can be upregulated in conditions of chronic hypoxia, thus reducing oxygen affinity and increasing oxygen availability in peripheral tissues. This is also one of the compensatory mechanisms of chronic anemia.

Hemoglobin variants

Adult hemoglobins

HbA

After completion of the fetal to adult switch (see below), HbA ($\alpha_2\beta_2$) is the predominant hemoglobin. HbA is posttranslationally glycosylated at the N-terminal valine and at internal lysine residues. This is a two-step reaction, first quickly and reversibly transforming the Hb–NH_2 group to an aldimine and then slowly and irreversibly to a ketoamine. The posttranslational modifications can be identified as fast-eluting fractions (HbA$_{Ia–c}$) on column chromatography (Fig. 11.5). One of these fractions (HbA$_{Ic}$) can be readily quantified and is a useful marker for the long-term metabolic control of patients with diabetes mellitus. In rare cases of substitutions of the N-terminal Val residue, HbA can be acetylated, in this respect resembling HbF. In cation exchange chromatography, these variants may be mistakenly identified as raised HbA$_{Ic}$.[30–32]

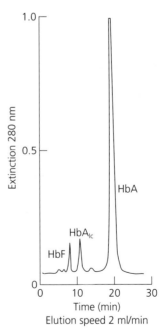

Fig. 11.5 Quantitation of HbF and HbA$_{Ic}$ by fast protein liquid chromatography (Mono S® HR 5/5, Pharmacia). Modified with permission from Ref. 84.

HbA$_2$

About 2.5% of adult hemoglobin is HbA$_2$ ($\beta_2\delta_2$). Functionally, HbA$_2$ is identical to HbA, although due to its low level of expression it is physiologically irrelevant and total lack of its synthesis has no clinical effect.

The δ-chain is highly homologous to the β-chain and differs by only 10 amino acids. Because of the difference in charge, HbA$_2$ can be easily separated from HbA by electrophoresis or chromatography. The δ-globin gene is located immediately 5' of the β-globin gene (see Fig. 11.1) and switched on roughly in parallel to the β gene. The much lower level of δ-globin expression results from the following.

1 Reduced transcriptional activity of the δ-globin gene, which is caused by the relative inefficiency of its promoter[33] and probably by the lack of, or a less efficiently functioning, enhancer in the second intron.[34]

2 Reduced δ-globin mRNA stability.[35]

3 A lesser affinity of δ-globin chains for α-globin chains.[36] This characteristic is exploited for the diagnosis of heterozygous β-thalassemia. When β-globin chains are present in low concentrations, δ-globin chains are able to form tetramers with α-chains and HbA$_2$ levels thus increase. Conversely, in α-thalassemia, HbA$_2$ may be decreased.

Fetal hemoglobin

Structure and function

Structurally and functionally, fetal hemoglobin (HbF; $\alpha_2\gamma_2$) is similar to HbA. However, there are some significant differences. The amino acid sequence of the γ-chain differs from the β-chain at 39 residues; 22 of these occur at the external surface, explaining the different electrophoretic/chromatographic behavior and the increased solubility of HbF. Four substitutions are located at the $\alpha_1\beta_1$ ($\alpha_1\gamma_1$) interface, which results in the increased stability of HbF. The $\alpha_1\beta_2$ ($\alpha_1\gamma_2$) contacts are identical in both HbA and HbF, which is reflected by similar cooperative effects of oxygen binding in both hemoglobins. The substitution β 143 His $\rightarrow$ γ 143 Ser causes a diminished interaction of HbF with 2,3-DPG, thus increasing oxygen affinity of fetal red cells.[37] The diagnostically important increased resistance of HbF to alkali (see below) can be explained by the β 112 Cys $\rightarrow$ γ 112 Thr and β 130 Tyr $\rightarrow$ γ 130 Trp substitutions.[38]

HbF is structurally heterogeneous. The γ-globin chains are coded for by two closely linked genes that are located between the ϵ and the δ genes within the β-globin gene cluster (see Fig. 11.1). The amino acid sequence that is coded for by the more 5' gene differs from that of the 3' gene at position 136, where the 5' gene codes for a glycine ($^G\gamma$) and the 3' gene for an alanine ($^A\gamma$) residue.[39] During fetal life, about 75% of the HbF contains $^G\gamma$ chains, whereas the small amounts of HbF present in adult life contain predominantly $^A\gamma$ chains.[40]

In addition to these allelic differences, the $^A\gamma$ gene contains a common polymorphism coding for either Ile ($^A\gamma^I$) or Thr ($^A\gamma^T$) at position 75.[41] The major posttranslational modification of HbF is by acetylation at the N-terminal Gly, which results in a more negatively charged component (HbF$_1$).

Diagnostic and therapeutic relevance

Following the fetal to adult hemoglobin switch during the first 6 months of life there are only trace amounts of HbF in the peripheral blood.[42] The discovery of a method to differentiate fetal from adult red cells by acid HbA elution[43] and the identification of fetal red cells in the maternal circulation post partum was part of the logical foundation for anti-D prophylaxis in Rh-negative mothers (see Chapter 10). Practically, this method is useful for the estimation of fetomaternal blood transfusion.[44]

Increased HbF levels occur in both hemoglobin disorders and acquired hematopoietic diseases. In sickle cell disease (see Chapter 11), HbF is raised as a result of selective survival of F cells. In patients from Saudi Arabia and India, HbF synthesis is increased and associated with a milder clinical phenotype.[45,46] The sickle cell mutation in Asia occurred on a different genetic background from that in African patients.[47] There is probably more than one genetic factor responsible for the raised HbF levels, which are both probably linked and not linked to the β-globin gene cluster.[48–51] The clinical benefit of hydroxycarbamide in the treatment of sickle cell disease is related to an increase of HbF, although HbF-independent factors probably play an additional important role.[52]

In patients with homozygous β-thalassemia, the increase of the relative HbF is pathognomonic (see Chapter 15). While HbF synthesis per cell is not increased in most patients, in absolute terms F cells are produced in larger numbers than normal by the greatly expanded bone marrow. These cells subsequently survive selectively because the imbalance between α-chain and non-α-chain synthesis is less marked in F cells than in cells not expressing γ-globin.[53] If genetic determinants that increase globin gene expression per cell are present, such as point mutations of the γ-globin gene promoters or deletions of the β-globin gene cluster,[54] the clinical and hematologic manifestations of homozygous β-thalassemia can be considerably ameliorated and adult individuals with hereditary persistence of HbF and 100% HbF can be perfectly healthy (see Chapter 15). Pharmacologic attempts to reactivate HbF synthesis have been promising but have not been shown to be applicable to most patients in large-scale trials.[55–57]

There are a multitude of acquired conditions associated with an increase of HbF. This is invariably so in, and is a diagnostic feature of, juvenile chronic myeloid leukemia, Fanconi anemia and erythroleukemia.[58–62] Raised HbF levels can be commonly seen, but are not of specific diagnostic value, in other myeloproliferative disorders and during the

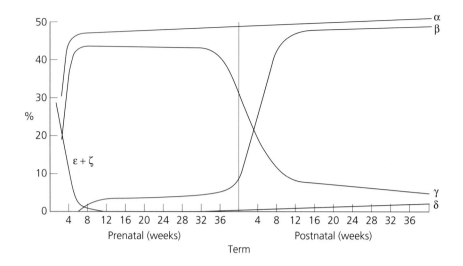

Fig. 11.6 Developmental changes in globin synthesis.

hematologic recovery following bone marrow transplantation or intensive chemotherapy.[63]

Embryonic hemoglobins

During weeks 2–14 of embryonic life the yolk sac produces three different hemoglobins: $\zeta_2\varepsilon_2$ (Hb Gower I), $\alpha_2\varepsilon_2$ (Hb Gower II), and $\zeta_2\gamma_2$ (Hb Portland).[64–66] The ε-chains are homologous to the β and γ chains and are coded for by a single gene at the 5′ end of the β-globin gene cluster (see Fig. 11.1). The ζ-chain is homologous to the α-chain and is coded for by a single gene at the 5′ end of the α-globin gene cluster (see Fig. 11.1). All three embryonic hemoglobins show allosterism, a cooperative effect on oxygen binding, and sensitivity to 2,3-DPG, but they exhibit a higher oxygen affinity than HbA and a decreased Bohr effect.[67] Under normal conditions these hemoglobins are not detectable during fetal or postnatal life. However, in deletional α^0-thalassemia, embryonic hemoglobins can be found at later stages of development.[68–70]

Developmental changes

The individual globin genes are activated to high levels of expression selectively in erythroid cells and programmed to be predominantly expressed at specific developmental stages. In both clusters on chromosomes 11 and 16 the globin genes are arranged in the order of their expression during development (see Fig. 11.1). About 14 days following conception, Hb Gower I and II, Hb Portland, and a little later HbF, begin to be synthesized in the yolk sac. By about 8 weeks the embryonic genes are silenced and HbF becomes the predominant hemoglobin and is synthesized in the fetal liver and spleen, and increasingly also in the bone marrow. HbA is made in small amounts during this period. At around birth, γ-globin chain and HbF synthesis are substituted by β-globin

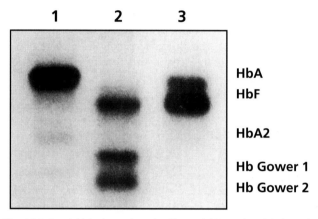

Fig. 11.7 Starch bloc electrophoresis of hemoglobins at the adult (lane 1), embryonic (lane 2), and fetal (lane 3) stages of development.

chain and HbA synthesis. Postnatally, the bone marrow becomes the only site of normal erythropoiesis (Figs 11.6 and 11.7).[71]

In the α-globin gene cluster there is a genetic embryonic (ζ) to fetal/adult (α) switch, whereas the β-globin gene cluster performs an embryonic (ε) to fetal (γ) and a fetal to adult (β) switch in gene expression. These switches are important paradigms of ontogenetic gene regulation and have therefore been the subject of intense study by biologists. The motivation for the medical sciences to study the fetal to adult hemoglobin switch results from the interest in reactivating γ-globin gene expression as a therapeutic option for the hemoglobinopathies.

The mechanisms responsible for the developmental specificity of hemoglobin synthesis are dependent on specific sequences within both the promoters and remote regulatory sequences.[72–75] These DNA sequences interact with erythroid-specific and ubiquitous transcription factors, which results in the activation or silencing of the individual genes.

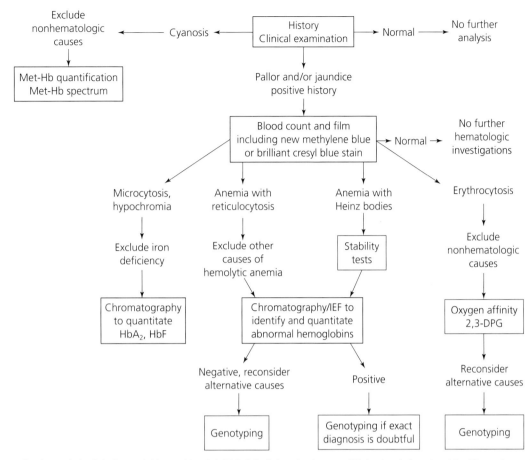

Fig. 11.8 Strategy for the analysis of the hemoglobinopathies. 2,3-DPG, 2,3-diphosphoglycerate; IEF, isoelectric focusing; Met-Hb, methemoglobin.

Experiments in transgenic mice and the analysis of naturally occurring mutants suggest that the individual genes can be either autonomously regulated or require competition with other genes of the cluster.[54,76–81]

Methods of hemoglobin identification

The practical approach to hemoglobin analysis is summarized in Fig. 11.8. The laboratory hematologist needs to be informed about relevant clinical details, in particular any recent erythrocyte transfusions, results of routine hematology, and iron status. The blood needs to be anticoagulated with EDTA or citrate and, except for the analysis of highly unstable variants or HbH in the diagnosis of α-thalassemia, can be stored for a few days. Generally, a blood volume of 5 mL is sufficient to perform all necessary analyses.

Routine hematology

This should include a complete blood count, including erythrocyte indices and reticulocytes, and careful examination of a blood film.

Cytologic tests

These tests are valuable, simple, and reproducible but are relatively labor-intensive as they are not automated.

HbF cells (Kleihauer technique)

This technique is based on the acid elution of HbA but not HbF from single cells.[43] The thin film is fixed and dried in 80% ethanol and then incubated for 5 min in a citrate-phosphate buffer at pH 3.2 and 37°C. The slide is then rinsed and stained with hematoxylin and eosin. HbA cells appear as empty ghosts, whereas HbF cells are stained (Fig. 11.9). If HbF cells are not present, there is no need to quantitate HbF by more sensitive techniques such as alkali denaturation or chromatography.

Inclusion bodies

HbH cells and Heinz bodies that reflect denatured hemoglobin can be identified by incubation for 30 min at room temperature of a drop of blood with a drop of brilliant cresyl blue or new methylene blue.[82] Microscopically, Heinz bodies are coarse and rather plump and located peripherally against the membrane, whereas HbH inclusions are smaller

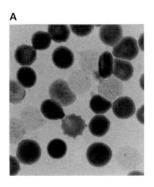
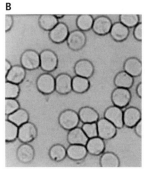
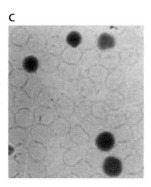

Fig. 11.9 Kleihauer technique. Acid elution of HbA and demonstration of HbF in single red cells: (A) cord blood; (B) normal adult blood; (C) maternal blood after fetomaternal transfusion. Modified with permission from Ref. 84.

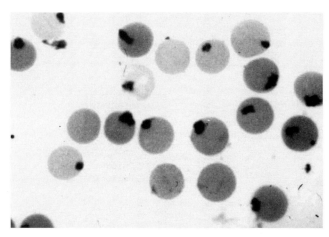

Fig. 11.10 Heinz bodies in a brilliant cresyl blue-stained film of a patient with Hb Köln.

and more evenly distributed within the cell. The Kleihauer technique (see above) is also useful for the demonstration of inclusion bodies (Fig. 11.10).

Sickle test

This test was used to demonstrate HbS in blood films and is now dispensable, because hemoglobin electrophoresis or chromatography are more useful quantitative methods and can distinguish heterozygotes, homozygotes, and compound heterozygotes.[82]

Denaturation tests

HbF

Denaturation by alkali is the classic technique for determining HbF quantitatively.[83] In principle, this is based on the increased stability of HbF over HbA in the presence of alkali due to the amino acid substitutions at positions 112 (β Cys $\rightarrow$ γ Thr) and 130 (β Tyr $\rightarrow$ γ Trp). The detailed protocol of alkali denaturation of a cyanmethemoglobin solution has to be followed accurately with respect to the concentrations of hemoglobin solution, NaOH, and ammonium sulfate, as well as to the timing and temperature. The method is reliable for

low HbF concentrations. At higher concentrations (>20%) the alkali denaturation method tends to underestimate, because some of the HbF is coprecipitated with the HbA.

Unstable variants

If an unstable variant cannot be specifically identified by electrophoretic, chromatographic, or isoelectric focusing techniques, its presence may be demonstrated as Heinz bodies or by an increased denaturation by heat or isopropanol.[82] For the heat denaturation test a buffered cyanmethemoglobin solution is incubated at 69.5°C for 6 min, which results in the precipitation of unstable variants. For the isopropanol test the hemolysate is incubated with 17% buffered isopropanol at 37°C, which also results in the precipitation of unstable hemoglobins. If the specific identification of the variant is not possible by standard techniques, DNA analysis is probably the most economic diagnostic procedure to be employed next.

Solubility test

This method is still used by some laboratories to discriminate HbS from other rarer variants with the same electrophoretic behavior. However, DNA analysis is now the more efficient method to identify the variant.

Spectral analysis

This is a method to identify HbM anomalies that show a characteristic methemoglobin spectrum at 450–650 nm (Fig. 11.11). The hemolysate is transformed completely into methemoglobin by potassium ferricyanide and the absorption compared to a normal control with an identical concentration and pH.[84]

Oxygen affinity

The oxygen dissociation curve can be measured by using commercially available tonometers. In principle, red cells are deoxygenated and suspended at a low concentration at a defined temperature and pH. Oxygen at known P_{O_2} is then added stepwise and the amount of oxyhemoglobin measured by spectrometry (see Fig. 11.4).

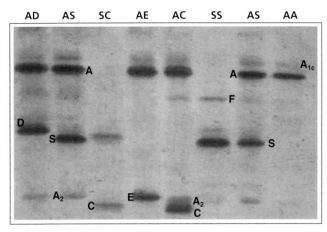

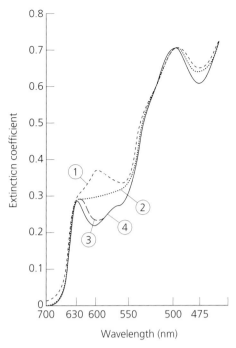

Fig. 11.11 Methemoglobin spectrum of HbM Saskatoon (curve 1), HbM Boston (curve 2), and HbM Milwaukee (curve 3) in comparison to normal methemoglobin (curve 4). Modified with permission from Ref. 84.

Fig. 11.12 Immobilized pH gradient of common hemoglobin variants. Kindly provided by Dr P. Sinha.

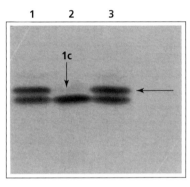

Fig. 11.13 Immobilized pH gradient of Hb Okayama (arrow) (lanes 1 and 3) and a normal control with HbA_{1c} in the same position (lane 2). Kindly provided by Dr P. Sinha.

Hemoglobin electrophoresis

The identification of hemoglobin variants by electrophoretic techniques depends on the introduction of a charge difference by the amino acid substitution. Commonly used routine methods are alkaline cellulose acetate and acid agar-gel electrophoresis of hemolysates.[82] Although the commoner variants are detected with these methods, 45 of all pathologic hemoglobin variants are not associated with a charge difference and are therefore electrophoretically silent. Furthermore, electrophoretic methods are generally unreliable for the quantitation of hemoglobin variants. An exception is the technically difficult and laborious starch bloc electrophoresis that results in particularly sharp bands that allow reproducible quantitative measurements (see Fig. 11.7).[84]

Isoelectric focusing

A pH gradient is generated in a polyacrylamide gel, separating the loaded hemoglobins according to their pK_a. In contrast to hemoglobin electrophoresis, this method does not rely on the charge and many variants not detectable by electrophoretic methods can be identified by isoelectric focusing.[85] The technical effort associated with isoelectric focusing can be much reduced by using immobilized pH gradients in polyacrylamide gels, which can be used to detect common (Fig. 11.12) and rare (Fig. 11.13) variants with a high degree of sensitivity and specificity.[86]

Chromatography

With these methods, hemoglobin variants can be reliably identified and quantitated. Recently, in larger laboratories, high-performance liquid chromatography and fast protein liquid chromatography techniques have largely superseded the formerly used DEAF-Sephadex chromatography (see Fig. 11.5). Apart from their high degree of accuracy and reproducibility, chromatographic methods can also be used to prepare samples for further biochemical and biophysical analysis.

Mass spectrometry

This method has recently been introduced to accurately determine the molecular weight of globin chains. The likely amino acid substitution can thus be predicted without protein sequencing. This method complements DNA sequencing in that it detects posttranslational modifications.[87] However, the immense cost of the equipment and the special expertise required limit this technique to specialized laboratories.

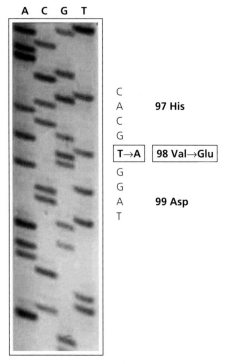

A C G T

C
A   97 His
C
G

T→A   98 Val→Glu

G
G
A   99 Asp
T

Fig. 11.14 Characterization of an unstable variant by DNA sequence analysis. The G*T*G→G*A*G mutation in codon 98 can be demonstrated directly and the Val→Glu amino acid substitution of Hb Mainz deduced according to the genetic code.

DNA analysis

The invention of the polymerase chain reaction (PCR)[88,89] caused a revolution in clinically applied molecular biology. PCR-amplified DNA can also be subjected to various diagnostic procedures such as allele-specific oligonucleotide hybridization, restriction enzyme analysis,[90,91] or automated direct sequencing.[92] The structure of variant hemoglobins and the amino acid substitution can thus be indirectly determined (Fig. 11.14), although posttranslational modifications detectable by biochemical analysis do, of course, remain unidentified.[87,93–96] Molecular genetic techniques are particularly useful in prenatal diagnosis.[97]

Rare hemoglobin disorders

Unstable variants (congenital Heinz body hemolytic anemia)

Hemoglobin is a highly organized complex whose function and stability is dependent on the subtle arrangement of the various structural features described above. Many mutations thus lead to some degree of instability that can be recognized by *in vitro* testing but do not result in significant clinical consequences. The clinical definition of unstable hemoglobinopathies therefore refers to congenital Heinz-body hemolytic anemia (CHBA) only.[98,99] A continuously updated list of the variants can be found in the globin database.[2]

Pathogenesis

The common pathway for unstable hemoglobin denaturation is the relaxation of the strict steric organization, which then favors the R configuration and thus the oxygenated state. In oxyhemoglobin, ferrous iron is more likely to be oxidized to the ferric form (Hb Fe^{2+} + O_2 → Hb Fe^{3+} + O_2^-). Both the superoxide anion and hydrogen peroxide can induce the generation of more methemoglobin. As ferriheme has a lower affinity for globin, this in itself may lead to heme loss and rapid denaturation.[100,101] Additionally, the distortion of the quaternary configuration allows the E7 histidine directly but reversibly to bind to the oxidized heme (reversible hemichrome). If on further distortion other residues bind to the oxidized heme, this is irreversible and results in denaturation and finally precipitation as a Heinz body. These become attached to the inner surface of the red cell membrane and cause trapping in the spleen where the inclusions are removed or hemolysis occurs. In addition to this rather mechanical view of splenic hemolysis, autologous antibodies have been reported to bind to modified membrane constituents.[102,103]

Many unstable variants can be detected electrophoretically (see Fig. 11.15). However, if instability is severe in the so-called hyperunstable hemoglobins, protein-based analytical techniques are not sufficient (see below). In some such variants the clinical features are remarkably mild.[104] In others, there is marked ineffective erythropoiesis with low reticulocyte counts for the degree of anemia and unbalanced synthesis of α-globin/non-α-globin chains, suggesting that an early step of complex formation such as dimerization may be affected.[105–110]

There are five different and not mutually exclusive molecular mechanisms destabilizing the three-dimensional structure of the complex. In some variants the mechanism for instability cannot be predicted from the amino acid substitution and X-ray crystallography data are not available.

Destabilization of the globin–heme interaction

Heme is bound to the heme pocket at the surface of the complex where nonpolar residues in the CD, E, F, and FG regions interact hydrophobically with the porphyrin ring. Many of the clinically relevant unstable variants, including the most common Hb Köln (β 98 [FG5] Val → Met), affect these residues resulting in a weaker globin to heme link.[111,112]

If the F8 histidine is substituted in Hb Istanbul (β 92 His → Gln),[113] Hb Mozhaisk (β 92 His → Arg),[114] and Hb Newcastle (β 92 His → Pro),[115] heme cannot be bound to globin, which results in instability.

The E7 histidine binds directly to molecular oxygen and, together with E11 Val, produces a steric configuration that prevents access of larger molecules to the heme pocket. If E7 His is substituted by Arg in Hb Zürich (β 63 His → Arg), a molecular gap is opened that allows oxidant substances, such as sulfonamide drugs, to attack the ferrous iron, resulting in methemoglobin formation that triggers denaturation. In Hb Zürich, ferrous iron oxidation can be inhibited by CO (e.g., in smokers) resulting in a decrease of Heinz bodies.

A substitution of E11 Val was the first unstable hemoglobin to be characterized at the molecular level.[116] This rare variant has been described in four families from the UK, Japan, and Russia, and results in considerable anemia (Hb 5–8 g/dL) with regular transfusion requirements.[87] In the initial protein analysis, E11 Val was found to be substituted by Asp and was designated Hb Bristol. Subsequent DNA analysis showed a GTG→ATG mutation of codon 67, thus replacing the codon of Val with Met, not Asp. Met has therefore been posttranslationally modified to Asp. Posttranslational modifications have also been observed in Hb Redondo (β 92 His → Asn → Asp), Hb La Roche-sur-Yon (β 81 Leu → His → β 80 Asn → Asp), and Hb Atlanta-Coventry (β 75 Leu → Pro → β 141 Leu deleted).[87,93–96]

Disruption of secondary structure

The predominant secondary structure of globin chains is the α-helix, which is crucial for the tight assembly of the tertiary and quaternary structure. Any substitution that inhibits α-helix formation is therefore likely to be associated with clinical manifestations. Proline cannot participate in helix formation and variants introducing this residue are almost always unstable. An exception is the stable variant Hb Singapore (α 141 Arg → Pro) where the proline is located at the C-terminal end of the chain, which does not participate in helix formation.[117]

Substitutions at the hydrophobic core

The interior of the complex is highly hydrophobic. A common mechanism of destabilization is a substitution of a charged for an uncharged amino acid, thus allowing water to enter into the tightly fitting core.[118] Similarly, the tight steric fit may be disturbed by the replacement of one hydrophobic residue with another. Finally, if the strong $\alpha_1\beta_1$ interface is relaxed, the internal SH groups may become highly reactive as is the case in Hb Tacoma and Hb Philly.[119,120]

Amino acid deletions

Deletions of amino acids can have a serious effect on the conformation of the entire complex, which may be so severe that a thalassemic phenotype develops.

Elongation of a subunit

These variants are caused by DNA insertions, by mutations of the translation termination codon (Ter), or by a frameshift in the third exon putting Ter out of frame. If translation is continued into the 3′ untranslated region (UTR) of the α-globin gene, the mRNA becomes unstable and this is associated with a thalassemic phenotype.[121,122]

Genetics

Unstable hemoglobins are inherited as an autosomal dominant trait with CHBA in the heterozygote. As the clinical consequences are part of the definition of unstable hemoglobinopathies, it is not surprising that β variants are more common than α variants. Each of the two β-globin alleles directs 50% of the total β-globin chain synthesis, whereas there are two α_2 globin and two α_1-globin alleles of which α_2 is expressed at about twice the level of α_1.[123,124] Each α_2 allele thus accounts for about 30–35% and each α_1 allele for about 15–20% of the total α-chain synthesis. The α_1 variants are therefore mildly expressed phenotypically even when present homozygously.[125] Also, analogous amino acid substitutions lead to clinically milder presentations in the α-globin than in the β-globin chains. Thus, α-chain variants are less likely to be identified than β-chain variants (e.g., Hb Iwata α F8 His → Arg, no anemia, 5% abnormal hemoglobin[126] vs. Hb Mozhaisk β F8 His → Arg, Hb 7 g/dL, 32% abnormal hemoglobin and CHBA).[114]

Variants of the γ-chain are rare. In HbF Poole (^{G}γ 130 Trp → Gly) there is neonatal (and presumably fetal) hemolytic anemia that disappears with the fetal to adult hemoglobin switch after the first few months of life.[127] More severe γ-chain variants are not known, probably due to the duplication of the γ genes and to the negative selection bias presumably operating in fetal hemoglobinopathies.

No selective pressure seems to have favored unstable hemoglobins in the course of evolution. Therefore, these variants are generally rare and have often been described in single families only. Spontaneous mutations are not uncommon.

There are single reports of patients who are compound heterozygotes for an unstable variant and a thalassemic mutation. The clinical picture of these cases depends on the degree of instability of the abnormal variant; some are mildly affected,[128,129] whereas others exhibit severe hemolytic disease.[130] Homozygotes are also exceedingly rare. A patient with homozygous Hb Bushwick (β74 (E18) Gly → Val) was reported to suffer from chronic anemia caused by a combination of hemolysis and ineffective erythropoiesis that was severely exacerbated at times of infection.[131]

Clinical features

The age at presentation and the severity of CHBA depends on the degree of instability and on the type of chain affected. For the reasons discussed above, β-chain variants tend to be more severe than α-chain variants. In severe CHBA, patients may become symptomatic in early childhood. They present either with chronic anemia, a hemolytic crisis associated with fever and/or oxidant stress of sulfonamide medication, or with an aplastic crisis usually following parvovirus infection.[132] The urine is often dark due to the presence of bilirubin degradation products (mesobilifuscinuria). Pigment gallstones are also common and may cause colic. Milder unstable variants may not be associated with any clinical symptoms and may only be detected fortuitously.

The findings on clinical examination depend on the severity of the hemolysis. Jaundice and splenomegaly are common. In some, this may be associated with hypersplenism. Cyanosis may be noted in those with a significant methemoglobin concentration (e.g., Hb Freiburg).[133] Occasionally, leg ulcers have been described.[134,135]

The hyperunstable and thalassemic variants can be mild but often cause severe anemia and may present as thalassemia intermedia or even thalassemia major (see below). They differ from other types of CHBA in that Heinz bodies are not necessarily seen, the abnormal hemoglobin cannot be identified by hemoglobin analysis, and the α/non-α ratio is often unbalanced. Ineffective erythropoiesis may be suggested by low reticulocyte counts for the degree of anemia and the degree of plasma transferrin receptor elevation, and by inclusion bodies in the erythroblasts in the bone marrow (Table 11.1).

Laboratory diagnosis

Routine hematology shows signs of hemolytic anemia with reticulocytosis, indirect hyperbilirubinemia, and decreased haptoglobin. Blood films stained with new methylene blue or brilliant cresyl blue show Heinz bodies (see Fig. 11.10). Hemoglobin analysis often demonstrates characteristic findings, allowing the identification of the abnormal variant (Fig. 11.15). Otherwise, DNA analysis will establish the definite diagnosis (see Fig. 11.14).

Treatment

Most patients with CHBA do not require specific treatment. If severe hemolysis is present, folic acid should be supplemented, oxidant drugs avoided, and increased awareness exercised at times of pyrexia. Paracetamol (acetaminophen) or acetylsalicylic acid are generally safe. Sulfonamides should be avoided.

Splenectomy

This is clearly indicated in cases with hypersplenism but has been tried in other patients with varied success. Generally, caution is adequate because of the danger of postsplenectomy septicemia, particularly in young children, and because of postsplenectomy thromboembolism.[136–138] Penicillin prophylaxis is mandatory and vaccination against *Streptococcus pneumoniae* and *Neisseria meningitidis* is indicated and should ideally be performed 3 months before the operation.[139,140] The duration of penicillin prophylaxis is controversial and

recommendations are often based on anecdotal reports. Controlled studies are difficult because of the rarity of this complication and the uncertain long-term compliance of patients. However, there are numerous reports of postsplenectomy septicemia occurring many years after the operation and the risk probably depends on the underlying disorder. There are also reports of postsplenectomy pulmonary embolism following the development of polycythemia and pulmonary hypertension in unstable hemoglobinopathies.[141,142] Priapism following splenectomy in a patient with the hyperunstable Hb Olmsted (β 141 [H19] Leu $\rightarrow$ Arg) has been reported,[143] which is also a well-recognized complication of splenectomy in thalassemia intermedia.[144–146]

Cholecystectomy

Gallstones are often asymptomatic and do not generally require treatment. However, in patients with colic or stones in the bile duct, surgical treatment may be warranted.

Hydroxycarbamide

This drug has a definite place in the therapy of adults and children with sickle cell disease[52,147–150] and possibly in thalassemia intermedia.[51,152] There has also been a report of two adult patients with severe CHBA who benefited from hydroxycarbamide treatment.[153]

Thalassemic variants

In these variants there is, in addition to the structural abnormality, a net decrease in globin chain synthesis, which may be caused by reduced transcriptional activity, a decrease in mRNA processing efficiency or mRNA stability, or increased posttranslational degradation (see Table 11.1). There are clinical and hematologic characteristics of thalassemia (Fig. 11.16), such as hypochromia, microcytosis, splenomegaly, and anemia due to ineffective erythropoiesis and dyserythropoiesis in the β-chain variants or signs of hemolysis in the α-chain variants.

Pathogenesis and clinical features

The paradigm of this type of hemoglobin variant is Hb Lepore, which contains a $\delta\beta$ fusion chain. This is coded for by a $\delta\beta$-globin fusion gene that is the result of an unequal crossover event between the highly homologous δ- and β-globin genes. The cross-over has occurred at three different points: Hb Lepore Boston ($\delta87\beta116$),[154,155] Hb Hollandia ($\delta22\beta50$),[156] and Hb Baltimore ($\delta50\beta86$).[157,158] These variants do not differ in their pathogenetic or clinical effect. The transcriptional activity of these fusion genes is controlled by the δ-globin gene promoter containing only a single CACCC-box and is thus much reduced compared with the β-globin gene that contains this regulatory element in duplicate. Heterozygotes

Table 11.1 Thalassemic hemoglobin variants.

Reference	Variant type and name	Mutation	Mechanism
Reduced transcriptional activity			
154–161	Hb Lepore Boston	δβ-globin gene fusion	Transcriptional control by 5-globin gene promoter
	Hb Lepore Hollandia		
	Hb Lepore Baltimore		
Impaired mRNA processing efficiency			
162	HbE	β 26 Glu → Lys	Activation of a cryptic splice site
163	Hb Knossos	β 27 Ala → Ser	Activation of a cryptic splice site
169	Hb Monroe	β 30 Arg › Thr	Mutation of the splice donor consensus sequence
Reduced mRNA stability			
121, 122, 170, 171	Hb Constant Spring	α 142 Ter → Gln	Associated with translational readthrough into the 5′-UTR
172	Hb Icaria	α 142 Ter → Lys	See Hb Constant Spring
173	Hb Koya Dora	α 142 Ter → Ser	See Hb Constant Spring
174	Hb Seal Rock	α 142 Ter → Glu	See Hb Constant Spring
Reduced posttranslational stability			
178	Hb Suan Dok	α 109 Leu → Arg	Hyperunstable
179	Hb Quong Sze	α 125 Leu → Pro	Hyperunstable
180	Hb Toyama	α 136 Leu → Arg	Hyperunstable
110	Hb Chesterfield	β 28 Leu → Arg	Hyperunstable
104	No name	β 30–31 + Arg	Hyperunstable
181	Hb Korea	β 33–34 Val-Val → 0–0	Hyperunstable
177	Hb Dresden	β 33–35 Val-Val-Tyr → 0–0-Asp	Hyperunstable
182	Hb Cagliari	β 60 Val → Glu	Hyperunstable
183	Hb Agnana	β 94 + TG	Hyperunstable
107	Hb Terre Haute	β 106 Leu → Arg	Hyperunstable
108	Hb Manhattan	β 109 ΔG	Extended hyperunstable β chain of 156 amino acids
184	Hb Showa-Yakushiji	β 110 Leu → Pro	Hyperunstable
185, 186	Hb Brescia/Durham-NC	β 114 Leu → Pro	Hyperunstable
187	Hb Geneva	β 114 ACT, +G	Hyperunstable
188	FS 123 AA (β chain Makabe)	β 123 ACC → -CC	Extended hyperunstable one chain of 156 amino acids
189	FS 124 AA	β 124 CCA → CC-	Extended unstable F3 chain of 156 amino acids
189	No name	β 124–125 + Pro	?
190	Hb Vercelli	β 126 GTG → G-G	Extended unstable F3 chain of 156 amino acids
191	Hb Neapolis	β 126 Val → Gly	Hyperunstable
108	Hb Houston	β 127 Ala → Pro	Hyperunstable
192, 193	F1-chain Gunma	β 127–128 Gln-Ala → Pro	Hyperunstable, shortened by one residue
105	No name	β 128–135 rearrangement (4 bp 128/129 deleted, 11 by 132–135 deleted, CCACA inserted)	Hyperunstable
194	No name	β 134–137 Val-Ala-Gly-Val → Gly-Arg	Hyperunstable, shortened by two residues
Premature translational termination			
195	NS 121	β 121 Glu → Ter	Premature termination of translation
196	NS 127	β 127 Gln → Ter	Premature termination of translation

for the Hb Lepore anomaly are hypochromic, with about 7–15% of the variant and 2–3% HbF. Compound heterozygotes with a $β^0$ or a severe $β^+$ allele on the other chromosome are usually transfusion dependent, as are the rare cases of homozygotes.[159–161]

The commonest thalassemic hemoglobin variant is HbE (β 26 Glu → Lys), which reaches extraordinarily high gene frequencies in Southeast Asia. Both the $β^E$ mutation and the much rarer variant Hb Knossos (β 27 Ala → Ser) cause activation of a cryptic splice site in exon 1 of the β-globin gene and thus defective mRNA processing. In addition, HbE is mildly unstable, which contributes to the reduced

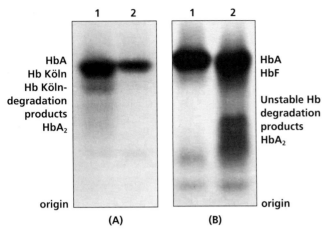

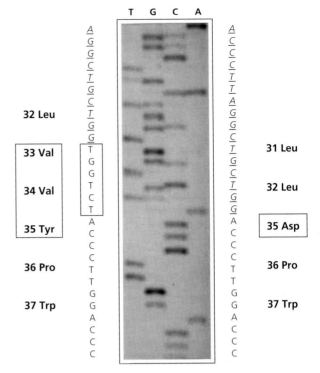

Fig. 11.15 Characterization of unstable variants by starch bloc electrophoresis. Hemolysate of a patient with Hb Köln (A, lane 1) and another with an unidentified unstable hemoglobin (B, lane 2) is compared to a normal control (A, lane 2 and B, lane 1). Modified with permission from Ref. 84.

Fig. 11.17 Sequence analysis of the β-globin gene in Hb Dresden. The TGGTCT deletion of a hexanucleotide within codons 33–35 can be readily identified and the structure of the abnormal globin deduced.

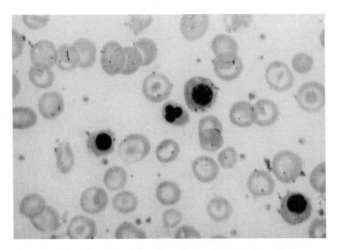

Fig. 11.16 Peripheral blood film of a splenectomized patient with the highly unstable and thalassemic variant Hb Dresden (β 33–35 Val-Val-Tyr → 0–0-Asp) showing marked hypochromia, target cells, and dysplastic normoblasts. Hemoglobin electrophoresis and immobilized pH gradient showed high levels of HbF. The abnormal hemoglobin could not be identified by these methods.

availability of these globin chains. HbE causes hemolysis in the homozygote and thalassemia intermedia or major when in compound with a β⁰-thalassemia mutation. Hb Knossos/β⁰-thalassemia compound heterozygotes have been described as exhibiting the phenotype of thalassemia intermedia or major.[162–168]

Another example of a variant with impaired splice efficiency is Hb Monroe (β 30 Arg → Thr). The G → C mutation affects the last nucleotide of the first exon, which is part of the consensus sequence of the splice donor site surrounding the invariant GT dinucleotide.[169] Hb Monroe is a severe

β⁺-thalassemia mutation with < 1% residual activity. mRNA stability and globin chain synthesis and stability are reduced in termination codon mutations that cause ribosomal readthrough into the 3′-UTR and an elongation of the α-globin chain (Hb Constant Spring, Hb Icaria, Hb Koya Dora, Hb Seal Rock). Clinically, these defects are typical thalassemia mutations and the variants are detectable in small amounts.[121,122,170–174]

Finally, a thalassemic phenotype of hemoglobin variants may be caused posttranslationally. In some of these variants the globin chains are markedly unstable and degraded before they can be incorporated into the tetramer. Others cause hyperinstability of the complete hemoglobin molecule. In either case, protein-based analytical techniques are unlikely to be informative and DNA analysis has to be employed (Fig. 11.17). A special type of abnormality that may be classified with this group of variants is characterized by premature translational stop codons in the third β-globin exon, which results in the synthesis of C-terminally truncated and nonfunctional globin chains. In all these mutations, the erythropoietic precursor in the bone marrow has to degrade α- and β-globin chains, which overloads the proteolytic capacity of the system and causes ineffective erythropoiesis.[105,175,176] The clinical hallmark of these abnormalities is the dominant mode of inheritance of the thalassemic phenotype, which may be mild or severe with chronic transfusion requirements.

Genetics

In these variants typical features of thalassemia are seen in the heterozygote. If expressed in sufficient amounts, the diagnosis may be made by hemoglobin analysis. Otherwise, DNA analysis will identify the gene mutation, enabling the deduction of the amino acid substitution in most cases.

Treatment

Treatment guidelines for thalassemia intermedia and major are described in Chapter 15.

Variants with increased oxygen affinity

In these variants the equilibrium between the R-quaternary and T-quaternary conformation is disturbed and the R form is more readily assumed. The sigmoid oxygen binding curve is shifted to the left, i.e., oxygen uptake in the lungs is facilitated and oxygen release in the peripheral tissues impeded. Many variants with altered oxygen affinity are also unstable to some degree. In contrast to CHBA, the clinical hallmark of variants with altered oxygen affinity is erythrocytosis/polycythemia but not hemolysis. A continuously updated list of the variants can be found in the globin database.[2]

Pathogenesis

The more the oxygen binding curve is shifted to the left, the more difficult it is for the tetramer to change its quaternary conformation. Generally, this loss of allosterism results in loss of the cooperative and Bohr effects. These variants thus resemble other hemoproteins such as myoglobin, and with an increasing degree of oxygen affinity tend not to function as oxygen carriers. Although there is no hypoxemia, oxygen availability is decreased. This results in erythropoietin production and erythrocytosis as a compensatory mechanism. Most patients with high-affinity variants show normal exercise tolerance, although blood loss or venesection to a numerically normal hemoglobin may result in clinically relevant hypoxia.[197–200]

Many high-affinity variants have substitutions at the $\alpha_1\beta_2$ interface, where most of the allosteric changes occur. The C-terminal ends of the subunits are also important sites for high-affinity variants because they greatly contribute to the stabilization of the T-conformation forming salt bonds (α 141 Arg, β 146 His) and to the anchoring of the loose end in a pouch between the F and H helices (α 140 Tyr, β 145 Tyr). In addition, 2,3-DPG binding can be affected by changes of β 143 His or β 82 Lys.[15,201–212]

Genetics

High-affinity traits are autosomal dominant, with α variants usually less apparent than β variants for the reasons discussed

above. Homozygotes or compound heterozygotes with β-thalassemia mutations are rare and expected to be viable only in variants with a moderate increase in oxygen affinity and preserved functional properties. For example, the high-affinity variant Hb Headington (β 72 [E16] Ser $\rightarrow$ Arg) exhibits a moderate decrease in cooperativity and a normal Bohr effect. In compound with $\delta\beta^0$-thalassemia, a 62-year-old male has been reported to have erythrocytosis but no symptoms related to this abnormality.[213] Rather more severely, a patient with thalassemia intermedia has been reported to be compound heterozygous for $\delta\beta^0$-thalassemia and Hb Crete (β 129 [H7] Ala $\rightarrow$ Pro), which is an unstable variant with high oxygen affinity but normal Bohr effect.[214]

Clinical features

Most patients are asymptomatic but may present with a violaceous complexion or peripheral cyanosis. Splenomegaly occurs in some patients but is not common. Most commonly, high-affinity variants are detected on a routine blood count showing erythrocytosis. Hyperviscosity-related symptoms do not usually occur, although there are anecdotal reports of exceptions.[215] In theory, oxygen delivery to the fetus will be affected if the mother's blood contains a high-affinity hemoglobin. In practice, however, this is not the case and for mothers with an exclusive or predominant occurrence of HbF, fetal outcome is normal.[216–218]

Laboratory diagnosis

The blood count shows erythrocytosis to be the commonest abnormality. The hemoglobin ranges between 17 and 22 g/dL. In some patients, leukocytosis has been reported and polycythemia vera must be carefully excluded in these cases.

Only about 50% of all high-affinity variants are detectable electrophoretically. The diagnosis can be established by measuring the oxygen dissociation curve of the hemolysate[219] and by DNA analysis.

Treatment

Variants with high oxygen affinity cause benign changes in the hematologic parameters. Erythrocytosis is the mode of compensation for decreased oxygen availability. Phlebotomy should therefore not generally be performed but exceptions may be the rare cases with symptoms related to hyperviscosity. It is important to establish the correct diagnosis in order to avoid inappropriate therapy.[220]

Variants with decreased oxygen affinity

Pathogenesis

In these rare variants the T-conformation is stabilized, thus impeding oxygen uptake and facilitating oxygen unloading. This right shift of the oxygen binding curve leads to good oxygen availability to the peripheral tissues but a less active hematopoietic stimulus, and slight anemia is a possible feature.

Clinical features

Heterozygous individuals are healthy but may have slight anemia without functional consequences. Cyanosis due to incomplete oxygen loading is a feature of some low-affinity variants such as Hb Kansas (β 102 Asn → Thr), Hb Beth Israel (β 102 Asn → Ser) and Hb St Mande (β 102 Asn → Tyr). However, exercise tolerance is not affected, because of the facilitated oxygen delivery.[221–224] As there are no functionally significant clinical symptoms, treatment is not required.

HbM anomalies

The HbM anomalies are rare variants that occur throughout the world. They are characterized by amino acid substitutions of the heme iron-binding region that cause permanent and virtually complete oxidation of the heme iron to the ferric (Fe^{3+}) form. HbM variants are therefore unable to carry oxygen and have a typical methemoglobin absorption spectrum. Instability is not a prominent feature of the M hemoglobins, which also differentiates M hemoglobins from the unstable variants with a high rate of spontaneous oxidation, such as Hb Freiburg, Hb Tübingen, and Hb St Louis. Heterozygotes are cyanotic without any other clinical symptoms.

Pathogenesis

Normal hemoglobin is slowly oxidized to methemoglobin at a calculated rate of 3% daily. There are five known adult and two fetal HbM variants (Table 11.2). Six of these are His → Tyr substitutions of the proximal (F8) or the distal (E7) heme-binding site. Tyr forms a covalent bond with ferric iron which is thus stabilized.[225] In HbM Milwaukee, the hydrophobic Val at position β 67 is substituted by the polar Glu, which binds covalently to the ferric heme iron exactly one helical winding carboxy-terminal of His E7.[226] Methemoglobin formation stabilizes the R-quaternary conformation, which

obliterates hemoglobin function both directly by blocking oxygen loading of the affected subunits and indirectly by increasing oxygen affinity of the normal subunits, thus impeding oxygen delivery.[227,228]

Normally, methemoglobin is efficiently reduced to ferrohemoglobin by the NADH-dependent cytochrome b_5 reductase and to a much lesser extent by the NADPH-dependent flavin reductase.[229–234] The normal methemoglobin concentration is < 1%. Three of the five known adult M hemoglobins cannot be enzymatically reduced and the other two are oxidized too fast for the enzyme to be effective.[235] Clinical tolerance of methemoglobin depends on the acuteness of its formation, very much analogous to the tolerance of anemia. In chronic cases, such as those with M hemoglobins or those with cytochrome b_5 reductase deficiency,[236] methemoglobin concentrations of up to 40% are well tolerated. In contrast, when methemoglobinemia develops suddenly following intoxication with oxidant drugs or chemicals, symptoms of hypoxia may start at levels of 20%.[237] Toxic methemoglobinemia is most likely to occur in infants, whose cytochrome b_5 reductase is only about half as active as that of adults.[238]

Genetics and clinical features

M hemoglobins are inherited in an autosomal dominant fashion, although spontaneous mutations are common. Heterozygotes are cyanotic without impairment of physical abilities. The lower levels of α HbM than β HbM can be explained by the presence of four α-globin but only two β-globin genes in the genome (see above). Homozygotes have not yet been described. Newborns with HbFM variants present with transient cyanosis that disappears with the fetal to adult hemoglobin switch.

Laboratory diagnosis

In alkaline hemoglobin electrophoresis, M hemoglobins may be detected as a grayish-green band that migrates slightly more slowly than HbA. At pH 7.0, HbM can be separated from normal methemoglobin following ferricyanide oxidation. The absorption spectrum of HbM at pH 6.8–7.0 is characteristically changed in comparison to normal

Table 11.2 HbM anomalies.

	Structure	Hb (g/dL)	Variant (%)	Hematology
HbM Boston[225]	α58 (E7) His → Tyr	15	25–32	Cyanosis
HbM Iwate[239]	α87 (F8) His → Tyr	17	20–27	Cyanosis
HbM Saskatoon[240]	β63 (E7) His → Tyr	13–16	35–40	Cyanosis and some degree of hemolysis
HbM Hyde Park[241]	β92 (F8) His → Tyr	10–12.5	25–40	Cyanosis and some degree of hemolysis
HbM Milwaukee[242]	β67 (E11) Val → Glu	14–15	26–40	Cyanosis
HbFM Osaka[243]	γ63 (E7) His → Tyr			Cyanosis of the newborn
HbFM Fort Ripley[244,245]	γ92 (F8) His → Tyr			Cyanosis of the newborn

Table 11.3 Differential diagnosis of cyanosis.

Inadequate oxygenation
Pulmonary disease
Cardiac disease with right-to-left shunting
Congestive heart failure and shock
Hemoglobin variants with decreased oxygen affinity

Methemoglobinemia
Inherited
   Cytochrome b_5 reductase deficiency
   M hemoglobins
   Unstable hemoglobins with a high rate of spontaneous oxidation
    (Hb Freiburg, Hb Tübingen, Hb St Louis)
Acquired
   Drugs
   Toxins
   Cows' milk protein intolerance
   Helicobacter pylori infection in infancy

Sulfhemoglobinemia
Acquired: toxins, drugs

---

methemoglobin, although DNA analysis is probably the most efficient method to confirm the diagnosis.

Treatment

The most important treatment is to establish the diagnosis (Table 11.3) and to reassure the patient and parents of the normal physical prognosis. Unnecessary and possibly dangerous diagnostic procedures to exclude heart and lung disease must be avoided. Redox agents such as methylene blue or ascorbic acid have no effect.

Cyanosis occurs at levels of normal deoxyhemoglobin > 5 g/dL. It follows that acquired conditions that result in inadequate oxygenation are the commonest causes of cyanosis. In severe polycythemia, cyanosis may occur in the absence of hypoxemia. Methemoglobinemia or sulfhemoglobinemia are rare causes of cyanosis (>1.5 g/dL methemoglobin; >0.5 g/dL sulfhemoglobin) and may be inherited or acquired.

References

1. Weatherall DJ, Clegg JB. *The Thalassaemia Syndromes*. Oxford: Blackwell Scientific Publications, 1981.
2. Hardison RC, Chui DHK, Riemer C *et al.* Databases of human hemoglobin variants and other resources at the Globin Gene Server. http://globin.cse.psu.edu/hbvar/menu.html
3. Bunn HF, Forget BG. *Hemoglobin: Molecular, Genetic and Clinical Aspects*. Philadelphia: WB Saunders, 1986.
4. Komiyama NH, Shih DT, Looker D, Tame J, Nagai K. Was the loss of the D helix in α globin a functionally neutral mutation? *Nature* 1991; **352**: 349–51.
5. Perutz MF, Lehmann H. Molecular pathology of human haemoglobin. *Nature* 1968; **219**: 902–9.
6. Perutz MF, Muirhead H, Cox JM, Goaman LC. Three-dimensional Fourier synthesis of horse oxyhaemoglobin at 2.8 Å resolution: the atomic model. *Nature* 1968; **219**: 131–9.
7. Perutz MF, Miurhead H, Cox JM *et al.* Three-dimensional Fourier synthesis of horse oxyhaemoglobin at 2.8 Å resolution: (1) X-ray analysis. *Nature* 1968; **219**: 29–32.
8. Fermi G, Perutz MF, Shaanan B, Fourme R. The crystal structure of human deoxyhaemoglobin at 1.74 Å resolution. *J Mol Biol* 1984; **175**: 159–74.
9. Liddington R, Derewenda Z, Dodson E, Hubbard R, Dodson G. High resolution crystal structures and comparisons of T-state deoxyhaemoglobin and two liganded T-state haemoglobins: T(α-oxy)haemoglobin and T(met)haemoglobin. *J Mol Biol* 1992; **228**: 551–79.
10. Paoli M, Liddington R, Tame J, Wilkinson A, Dodson G. Crystal structure of T state haemoglobin with oxygen bound at all four haems. *J Mol Biol* 1996; **256**: 775–92.
11. Fermi G, Perutz M. Hemoglobin and myoglobin. In: Philipps DC, Richards FM (eds) *Atlas of Molecular Structures in Biology*. Oxford: Clarendon Press, 1981.
12. Ackers GK, Doyle ML, Myers D, Daugherty MA. Molecular code for cooperativity in hemoglobin. *Science* 1992; **255**: 54–63.
13. Perutz MF, Shih DT, Williamson D. The chloride effect in human haemoglobin. A new kind of allosteric mechanism. *J Mol Biol* 1994; **239**: 555–60.
14. Monod J, Wyman J, Changeux JP. On the nature of allosteric transitions: a plausible model. *J Mol Biol* 1965; **12**: 88–95.
15. Perutz MF. Stereochemistry of cooperative effects in haemoglobin. *Nature* 1970; **228**: 726–39.
16. Perutz MF, Kilmartin JV, Nishikura K, Fogg JH, Butler PJ, Rollema HS. Identification of residues contributing to the Bohr effect of human haemoglobin. *J Mol Biol* 1980; **138**: 649–68.
17. Kilmartin JV, Fogg JH, Perutz MF. Role of C-terminal histidine in the alkaline Bohr effect of human hemoglobin. *Biochemistry* 1980; **19**: 3189–93.
18. Nishikura K. Identification of histidine-122α in human haemoglobin as one of the unknown alkaline Bohr groups by hydrogen-tritium exchange. *Biochem J* 1978; **173**: 651–7.
19. Shih DT, Luisi BF, Miyazaki G, Perutz MF, Nagai K. A mutagenic study of the allosteric linkage of His (HC3) 146β in haemoglobin. *J Mol Biol* 1993; **230**: 1291–6.
20. Perutz MF, Muirhead H, Mazzarella L, Crowther RA, Greer J, Kilmartin JV. Identification of residues responsible for the alkaline Bohr effect in haemoglobin. *Nature* 1969; **222**: 1240–3.
21. Kilmartin JV, Breen JJ, Roberts GC, Ho C. Direct measurement of the pK values of an alkaline Bohr group in human hemoglobin. *Proc Natl Acad Sci USA* 1973; **70**: 1246–9.
22. Bauer C, Schroder E. Carbamino compounds of haemoglobin in human adult and foetal blood. *J Physiol* 1972; **227**: 457–71.
23. Kelly RM, Hui HL, Noble RW. Chloride acts as a novel negative heterotropic effector of hemoglobin Rothschild (β 37 Trp → Arg) in solution. *Biochemistry* 1994; **33**: 4363–7.
24. Bonaventura C, Arumugam M, Cashon R, Bonaventura J, Moo Penn WF. Chloride masks effects of opposing positive charges in Hb A and Hb Hinsdale (β 139 Asn → Lys) that can modulate cooperativity as well as oxygen affinity. *J Mol Biol* 1994; **239**: 561–8.

25. Rollema HS, de Bruin SH, Janssen LH, van Os GA. The effect of potassium chloride on the Bohr effect of human hemoglobin. *J Biol Chem* 1975; **250**: 1333–9.

26. Chanutin A, Curnish RR. Effect of organic and inorganic phosphates on the oxygen equilibrium of human erythrocytes. *Arch Biochem Biophys* 1967; **121**: 96–102.

27. Benesch R, Benesch RE. The effect of organic phosphates from the human erythrocyte on the allosteric properties of hemoglobin. *Biochem Biophys Res Commun* 1967; **26**: 162–7.

28. Gupta RK, Benovic JL, Rose ZB. Location of the allosteric site for 2,3-bisphosphoglycerate on human oxy- and deoxyhemoglobin as observed by magnetic resonance spectroscopy. *J Biol Chem* 1979; **254**: 8250–5.

29. Arnone A. X-ray diffraction study of binding of 2,3-diphosphoglycerate to human deoxyhaemoglobin. *Nature* 1972; **237**: 146–9.

30. Boissel JP, Kasper TJ, Shah SC, Malone JI, Bunn HF. Aminoterminal processing of proteins: hemoglobin South Florida, a variant with retention of initiator methionine and N α-acetylation. *Proc Natl Acad Sci USA* 1985; **82**: 8448–52.

31. Vasseur C, Blouquit Y, Kister J *et al.* Hemoglobin Thionville. An α-chain variant with a substitution of a glutamate for valine at NA-1 and having an acetylated methionine NH2 terminus. *J Biol Chem* 1992; **267**: 12682–91.

32. Boissel JP, Kasper TJ, Bunn HF. Cotranslational amino-terminal processing of cytosolic proteins. Cell-free expression of site-directed mutants of human hemoglobin. *J Biol Chem* 1988; **263**: 8443–9.

33. Humphries RK, Ley T, Turner P, Moulton AD, Nienhuis AW. Differences in human α-, β- and δ-globin gene expression in monkey kidney cells. *Cell* 1982; **30**: 173–83.

34. LaFlamme S, Acuto S, Markowitz D, Vick L, Landschultz W, Bank A. Expression of chimeric human β- and δ-globin genes during erythroid differentiation. *J Biol Chem* 1987; **262**: 4819–26.

35. Ross J, Pizarro A. Human β and δ globin messenger RNAs turn over at different rates. *J Mol Biol* 1983; **167**: 607–17.

36. Bunn HF, Forget BG. *Hemoglobin: Molecular, Genetic and Clinical Aspects*. Philadelphia: WB Saunders, 1986, pp. 417–21.

37. Frier JA, Perutz MF. Structure of human foetal deoxyhaemoglobin. *J Mol Biol* 1977; **112**: 97–112.

38. Perutz MF. Mechanism of denaturation of haemoglobin by alkali. *Nature* 1974; **247**: 341–4.

39. Schroeder WA, Huisman TH, Shelton JR *et al.* Evidence for multiple structural genes for the γ chain of human fetal hemoglobin. *Proc Natl Acad Sci USA* 1968; **60**: 537–44.

40. Schroeder WA. The synthesis and chemical heterogeneity of human fetal hemoglobin: overview and present concepts. *Hemoglobin* 1980; **4**: 431–46.

41. Ricco G, Mazza U, Turi RM *et al.* Significance of a new type of human fetal hemoglobin carrying a replacement isoleucine replaced by threonine at position 75 (E19) of the γ chain. *Hum Genet* 1976; **32**: 305–13.

42. Bard H. The postnatal decline of hemoglobin F synthesis in normal full-term infants. *J Clin Invest* 1975; **55**: 395–8.

43. Kleihauer E, Braun HKB. Demonstration von fetalem Hämoglobin in den Erythrocyten eines Blutausstrichs. *Klin Wochenschr* 1957, **35**: 637–8.

44. Kleihauer E, Hötzel U, Betke K. Die materno-fetale Transfusion. *Monatsschr Kinderheilkd* 1967; **115**: 145–6.

45. Kar BC, Satapathy RK, Kulozik AE *et al.* Sickle cell disease in Orissa State, India. *Lancet* 1986; **ii**: 1198–201.

46. Padmos MA, Roberts GT, Sackey K *et al.* Two different forms of homozygous sickle cell disease occur in Saudi Arabia. *Br J Haematol* 1991; **79**: 93–8.

47. Kulozik AE, Wainscoat JS, Serjeant GR *et al.* Geographical survey of βˢ-globin gene haplotypes: evidence for an independent Asian origin of the sickle-cell mutation. *Am J Hum Genet* 1986; **39**: 239–44.

48. Kulozik AE, Kar BC, Satapathy RK, Serjeant BE, Serjeant GR, Weatherall DJ. Fetal hemoglobin levels and βˢ-globin haplotypes in an Indian population with sickle cell disease. *Blood* 1987; **69**: 1742–6.

49. Thein SL, Sampietro M, Rohde K *et al.* Detection of a major gene for heterocellular hereditary persistence of fetal hemoglobin after accounting for genetic modifiers. *Am J Hum Genet* 1994; **54**: 214–28.

50. Chang YC, Smith KD, Moore RD, Serjeant GR, Dover GJ. An analysis of fetal hemoglobin variation in sickle cell disease: the relative contributions of the X-linked factor, β-globin haplotypes, α-globin gene number, gender, and age. *Blood* 1995; **85**: 1111–17.

51. Craig JE, Rochette J, Fisher CA *et al.* Dissecting the loci controlling fetal hemoglobin production on chromosomes 11p and 6q by the regressive approach. *Nat Genet* 1996; **12**: 58–64.

52. Charache S, Terrin ML, Moore RD *et al.* Effect of hydroxyurea on the frequency of painful crises in sickle cell anemia. Investigators of the Multicenter Study of Hydroxyurea in Sickle Cell Anemia. *N Engl J Med* 1995; **332**: 1317–22.

53. Weatherall DJ, Clegg JB, Wood WG. A model for the persistence or reactivation of fetal hemoglobin production. *Lancet* 1976; **ii**: 660–3.

54. Wood WG. Increased HbF in adult life. *Baillière's Clin Haematol* 1993; **6**: 177–213.

55. Perrine SP, Ginder GD, Faller DV *et al.* A short-term trial of butyrate to stimulate fetal-globin-gene expression in the β-globin disorders. *N Engl J Med* 1993; **328**: 81–6.

56. Sher GD, Ginder GD, Little J, Yang S, Dover GJ, Olivieri NF. Extended therapy with intravenous arginine butyrate in patients with β-hemoglobinopathies. *N Engl J Med* 1995; **332**: 1606–10.

57. Reich S, C. Bührer B, Vetter D *et al.* Oral isobutyramide reduces transfusion requirements in some patients with homozygous β-thalassemia. *Blood* 2000; **96**: 3357–63.

58. Weatherall DJ, Brown MJ. Juvenile chronic myeloid leukaemia. *Lancet* 1970; **i**: 526.

59. Maurer HS, Vida LN, Honig GR. Similarities of the erythrocytes in juvenile chronic myelogenous leukemia to fetal erythrocytes. *Blood* 1972; **39**: 778–84.

60. Pagnier J, Lopez M, Mathiot C *et al.* An unusual case of leukemia with high fetal hemoglobin: demonstration of abnormal hemoglobin synthesis localized in a red cell clone. *Blood* 1977; **50**: 249–58.

61. Krauss JS, Rodriguez AR, Milner PF. Erythroleukemia with high fetal hemoglobin after therapy for ovarian carcinoma. *Am J Clin Pathol* 1981; **76**: 721–2.

62. Miniero R, David O, Saglio G, Paschero C, Nicola P. The Hbf in Fanconi's anemia. [Authors' transl.] *Pediatr Med Chir* 1981; **3**: 167–70.

63. Alter BP, Rappeport JM, Huisman TH, Schroeder WA, Nathan DG. Fetal erythropoiesis following bone marrow transplantation. *Blood* 1976; **48**: 843–53.

64. Huehns ER, Flynn FV, Butler EA, Beaven GH. Two new haemoglobin variants in a young human embryo. *Nature* 1961; **189**: 1877–9.

65. Capp GL, Rigas DA, Jones RT. Evidence for a new haemoglobin chain (C-chain). *Nature* 1970; **228**: 278–80.

66. Capp GL, Rigas DA, Jones RT. Hemoglobin Portland 1: a new human hemoglobin unique in structure. *Science* 1967; **157**: 65–6.

67. Hofmann O, Mould R, Brittain T. Allosteric modulation of oxygen binding to the three human embryonic haemoglobins. *Biochem J* 1995; **306**: 367–70.

68. Todd D, Lai MC, Beaven GH, Huehns ER. The abnormal haemoglobins in homozygous α-thalassaemia. *Br J Haematol* 1970; **19**: 27–31.

69. Chui DH, Wong SC, Chung SW, Patterson M, Bhargava S, Poon MC. Embryonic α-globin chains in adults: a marker for α-thalassemia1 haplotype due to a greater than 17.5-kb deletion. *N Engl J Med* 1986; **314**: 76–9.

70. Chung SW, Wong SC, Clarke BJ, Patterson M, Walker WH, Chui DH. Human embryonic ζ-globin chains in adult patients with α-thalassemias. *Proc Natl Acad Sci USA* 1984; **81**: 6188–91.

71. Weatherall DJ, Clegg JB. *The Thalassaemia Syndromes*. Oxford: Blackwell Scientific, 1981, pp. 58–70.

72. Grosveld F, van Assendelft GB, Greaves DR, Kollias G. Position-independent, high-level expression of the human β-globin gene in transgenic mice. *Cell* 1987; **51**: 975–85.

73. Tuan D, Solomon W, Li Q, London IM. The "R-like-globin" gene domain in human erythroid cells. *Proc Natl Acad Sci USA* 1985; **82**: 6384–8.

74. Sharpe JA, Chan Thomas PS, Lida J, Ayyub H, Wood WG, Higgs DR. Analysis of the human α globin upstream regulatory element (HS-40) in transgenic mice. *EMBO J* 1992; **11**: 4565–72.

75. Vyas P, Vickers MA, Simmons DL, Ayyub H, Craddock CF, Higgs DR. Cis-acting sequences regulating expression of the human α-globin cluster lie within constitutively open chromatin. *Cell* 1992; **69**: 781–93.

76. Amrolia PJ, Cunningham JM, Ney P, Nienhuis AW, Jane SM. Identification of two novel regulatory elements within the 5'-untranslated region of the human A γ-globin gene. *J Biol Chem* 1995; **270**: 12892–8.

77. Jane SM, Ney PA, Vanin EF, Gumucio DL, Nienhuis AW. Identification of a stage selector element in the human γ-globin gene promoter that fosters preferential interaction with the 5' HS2 enhancer when in competition with the β-promoter. *EMBO J* 1992; **11**: 2961–9.

78. Raich N, Enver T, Nakamoto B, Josephson B, Papayannopoulou T, Stamatoyannopoulos G. Autonomous developmental control of human embryonic globin gene switching in transgenic mice. *Science* 1990; **250**: 1147–9.

79. Raich N, Clegg CH, Grofti J, Romeo PH, Stamatoyannopoulos G. GATA1 and YY1 are developmental repressors of the human ε-globin gene. *EMBO J* 1995; **14**: 801–9.

80. Orkin SH. Globin gene regulation and switching: circa 1990. *Cell* 1990; **63**: 665–72.

81. Stamatoyannopoulos G. Control of globin gene expression during development and erythroid differentiation. *Exp Hematol* 2005, **33**: 259–71.

82. Dacie JV, Lewis SM. *Practical Haematology*. Edinburgh: Churchill Livingstone, 1984, pp. 179–99.

83. Betke K, Marti HR, Schlicht I. Estimation of small percentages of foetal hemoglobin. *Nature* 1959; **184**: 1877–8.

84. Kleihauer E, Kohne E, Kulozik AE. *Anomale Hämoglobine and Thalassämiesyndrome*. Landsberg: Ecomed, 1996, pp. 57–67.

85. Monte M, Beuzard Y, Rosa J. Mapping of several abnormal hemoglobins by horizontal polyacrylamide gel isoelectric focusing. *Am J Clin Pathol* 1976; **66**: 753–9.

86. Sinha P, Galacteros F, Righetti PG, Kohlmeier M, Kottgen E. Analysis of hemoglobin variants using immobilized pH gradients. *Eur J Clin Chem Clin Biochem* 1993; **31**: 91–6.

87. Rees DC, Rochette J, Schofield C *et al*. A novel silent posttranslational mechanism converts methionine to aspartate in hemoglobin Bristol (β 67 [E11] Val-Met → Asp). *Blood* 1996; **88**: 341–8.

88. Mullis KB, Faloona FA. Specific synthesis of DNA *in vitro* via a polymerase-catalyzed chain reaction. *Methods Enzymol* 1987; **155**: 335–50.

89. Mullis K, Faloona F, Scharf S, Saiki R, Horn G, Erlich H. Specific enzymatic amplification of DNA *in vitro*: the polymerase chain reaction. *Cold Spring Harb Symp Quant Biol* 1986; **51**: 263–73.

90. Chehab FF, Doherty M, Cai SP, Kan YW, Cooper S, Rubin EM. Detection of sickle cell anemia and thalassaemias. *Nature* 1987; **329**: 293–4. Published erratum appears in *Nature* 1987; **329**: 678.

91. Kulozik AE, Lyons J, Kohne E, Bartram CR, Kleihauer E. Rapid and non-radioactive prenatal diagnosis of β thalassaemia and sickle cell disease: application of the polymerase chain reaction (PCR). *Br J Haematol* 1988; **70**: 455–8.

92. Thein SL, Hinton J. A simple and rapid method of direct sequencing using Dynabeads. *Br J Haematol* 1991; **79**: 113–15.

93. George PM, Myles T, Williamson D, Higuchi R, Symmans WA, Brennan SO. A family with haemolytic anaemia and three β-globins: the deletion in haemoglobin Atlanta-Coventry (β 75 Leu → Pro, 141 Leu deleted) is not present at the nucleotide level. *Br J Haematol* 1992; **81**: 93–8.

94. Wajcman H, Vasseur C, Blouquit Y *et al*. Hemoglobin Redondo [β 92 (F8) His → Asn]: an unstable hemoglobin variant associated with heme loss which occurs in two forms. *Am J Hematol* 1991; **38**: 194–200.

95. Brennan SO, Shaw J, Allen J, George PM. β 141 Leu is not deleted in the unstable haemoglobin Atlanta-Coventry but is replaced by a novel amino acid of mass 129 daltons. *Br J Haematol* 1992; **81**: 99–103.

96. Wajcman H, Kister J, Vasseur C *et al*. Structure of the EF corner favors deamidation of asparaginyl residues in hemoglobin: the example of Hb La Roche-sur-Yon [β 81 (EF5) Leu → His]. *Biochim Biophys Acta* 1992; **1138**: 127–32.

97. Old JM, Fitches A, Heath C *et al*. First-trimester fetal diagnosis for hemoglobinopathies: report on 200 cases. *Lancet* 1986; **ii**: 763–7.

98. Rieder RF. Human hemoglobin stability and instability: molecular mechanisms and some clinical correlations. *Semin Hematol* 1974; **11**: 423–40.

99. Williamson D. The unstable hemoglobins. *Blood Rev* 1993; **7**: 146–63.

100. Jacob H, Winterhalter K. Unstable hemoglobins: the role of heme loss in Heinz body formation. *Proc Natl Acad Sci USA* 1970; **65**: 697–701.

101. Jacob HS, Winterhalter KH. The role of hemoglobin heme loss in Heinz body formation: studies with a partially heme-deficient hemoglobin and with genetically unstable hemoglobins. *J Clin Invest* 1970; **49**: 2008–16.

102. Low PS, Waugh SM, Zinke K, Drenckhahn D. The role of hemoglobin denaturation and band 3 clustering in red blood cell aging. *Science* 1985; **227**: 531–3.

103. Waugh SM, Willardson BM, Kannan R *et al.* Heinz bodies induce clustering of band 3, glycophorin, and ankyrin in sickle cell erythrocytes. The role of hemoglobin denaturation and band 3 clustering in red blood cell aging. *J Clin Invest* 1986; **78**: 1155–60.

104. Arjona SN, Eloy Garcia JM, Gu LH, Smetanina NS, Huisman TH. The dominant β-thalassaemia in a Spanish family is due to a frameshift that introduces an extra CGG codon (= arginine) at the 5′ end of the second exon. *Br J Haematol* 1996; **93**: 841–4.

105. Thein SL, Hesketh C, Taylor P *et al.* Molecular basis for dominantly inherited inclusion body β-thalassemia. *Proc Natl Acad Sci USA* 1990; **87**: 3924–8.

106. Girodon E, Ghanem N, Vidaud M *et al.* Rapid molecular characterization of mutations leading to unstable hemoglobin β-chain variants. *Ann Hematol* 1992; **65**: 188–92.

107. Coleman MB, Steinberg MH, Adams JGD. Hemoglobin Terre Haute arginine β 106. A posthumous correction to the original structure of hemoglobin Indianapolis. *J Biol Chem* 1991; **266**: 5798–800.

108. Kazazian HH Jr, Dowling CE, Hurwitz RL, Coleman M, Stopeck A, Adams JGD. Dominant thalassemia-like phenotypes associated with mutations in exon 3 of the β-globin gene. *Blood* 1992; **79**: 3014–18.

109. Thein SL, Wood WG, Wickramasinghe SN, Galvin MC. β-Thalassemia unlinked to the β-globin gene in an English family. *Blood* 1993; **82**: 961–7.

110. Thein SL, Best S, Sharpe J, Paul B, Clark DJ, Brown MJ. Hemoglobin Chesterfield (β 28 Leu → Arg) produces the phenotype of inclusion body b thalassemia [letter]. *Blood* 1991; **77**: 2791–3.

111. Jones RV, Grimes AJ, Carrell RW, Lehmann H. Koln haemoglobinopathy. Further data and a comparison with other hereditary Heinz body anemias. *Br J Haematol* 1967; **13**: 394–408.

112. Carrell RW, Lehmann H, Hutchison HE. Haemoglobin Koln (β-98 valine → methionine): an unstable protein causing inclusion-body anaemia. *Nature* 1966; **210**: 915–16.

113. Aksoy M, Erdem S, Efremov GD *et al.* Hemoglobin Istanbul: substitution of glutamine for histidine in a proximal histidine (F8(92)). *J Clin Invest* 1972; **51**: 2380–7.

114. Spivak VA, Molchanova TP, Postnikov YuV, Aseeva EA, Lutsenko IN, Tokarev YuN. A new abnormal hemoglobin: Hb Mozhaisk β 92 (F8) His leads to Arg. *Hemoglobin* 1982; **6**: 169–81.

115. Finney R, Casey R, Lehmann H, Walker W. Hb Newcastle: β92 (F8) His replaced by Pro. *FEBS Lett* 1975; **60**: 435–8.

116. Steadman JH, Yates A, Huehns ER. Idiopathic Heinz body anaemia: Hb-Bristol (β 67 (E11) Val to Asp). *Br J Haematol* 1970; **18**: 435–46.

117. Clegg JB, Weatherall DJ, Boon WH, Mustafa D. Two new haemoglobin variants involving proline substitutions. *Nature* 1969; **222**: 379–80.

118. Perutz MF, Kendrew JC, Watson HC. Structure and function of haemoglobin. II. Some relations between polypeptide chain configuration and amino acid sequence. *J Mol Biol* 1965; **13**: 669–78.

119. Brimhall B, Jones RT, Baur EW, Motulsky AG. Structural characterization of hemoglobin Tacoma. *Biochemistry* 1969; **8**: 2125–9.

120. Rieder RF, Oski FA, Clegg JB. Hemoglobin Philly (β 35 tyrosine phenylalanine): studies in the molecular pathology of hemoglobin. *J Clin Invest* 1969; **48**: 1627–42.

121. Weiss IM, Liebhaber SA. Erythroid cell-specific determinants of α-globin mRNA stability. *Mol Cell Biol* 1994; **14**: 8123–32.

122. Weiss IM, Liebhaber SA. Erythroid cell-specific mRNA stability elements in the α 2-globin 3′ nontranslated region. *Mol Cell Biol* 1995; **15**: 2457–65.

123. Liebhaber SA, Kan YW. Differentiation of the mRNA transcripts originating from the α1- and α2-globin loci in normals and α-thalassemics. *J Clin Invest* 1981; **68**: 439–46.

124. Liebhaber SA, Cash FE, Ballas SK. Human α-globin gene expression. The dominant role of the α2-locus in mRNA and protein synthesis. *J Biol Chem* 1986; **261**: 15327–33.

125. Darbellay R, Mach Pascual S, Rose K, Graf J, Beris P. Haemoglobin Tunis-Bizerte: a new α1 globin 129 Leu → Pro unstable variant with thalassaemic phenotype. *Br J Haematol* 1995; **90**: 71–6.

126. Ohba Y, Miyaji T, Hattori Y, Fuyuno K, Matsuoka M. Unstable hemoglobins in Japan. *Hemoglobin* 1980; **4**: 307–12.

127. Lee Potter JP, Deacon Smith RA, Simpkiss MJ, Kamuzora H, Lehmann H. A new cause of haemolytic anemia in the newborn. A description of an unstable fetal hemoglobin: F Poole, α2-G-γ2 130 tryptophan yields glycine. *J Clin Pathol* 1975; **28**: 317–20.

128. Galacteros F, Loukopoulos D, Fessas P *et al.* Hemoglobin Koln occurring in association with a β zero thalassemia: hematologic and functional consequences. *Blood* 1989; **74**: 496–500.

129. Vassilopoulos G, Papassotiriou I, Voskaridou E *et al.* Hb Arta [β45 (CD4) Phe → Cys]: a new unstable haemoglobin with reduced oxygen affinity in trans with β-thalassaemia. *Br J Haematol* 1995; **91**: 595–601.

130. Curuk MA, Dimovski AJ, Baysal E *et al.* Hb Adana or a 2 (59) (E8) Gly → Asp β2, a severely unstable α1-globin variant, observed in combination with the -(α)20.5 Kb α-thal-1 deletion in two Turkish patients. *Am J Hematol* 1993; **44**: 270–5.

131. Srivastava P, Kaeda JS, Roper D, Vulliamy TJ, Buckley M, Luzzatto L. Severe hemolytic anemia associated with the homozygous state for an unstable hemoglobin variant (Hb Bushwick). *Blood* 1995; **86**: 1977–82.

132. Serjeant GR, Serjeant BE, Thomas PW, Anderson MJ, Patou G, Pattison JR. Human parvovirus infection in homozygous sickle cell disease. *Lancet* 1993; **341**: 1237–40.

133. Jones RT, Brimhall B, Huisman TH, Kleihauer E, Betke K. Hemoglobin Freiburg: abnormal hemoglobin due to deletion of a single amino acid residue. *Science* 1966; **154**: 1024–7.

134. Jackson JM, Yates A, Huehns ER. Haemoglobin Perth: β-32 (B14) Leu leads to Pro, an unstable haemoglobin causing haemolysis. *Br J Haematol* 1973; **25**: 607–10.

135. Dianzam I, Ramus S, Cotton RG, Camaschella C. A spontaneous mutation causing unstable Hb Hammersmith: detection of the β42 TTT–TCT change by CCM and direct sequencing. *Br J Haematol* 1991; **79**: 127–9.

136. Linet MS, Nyren O, Gridley G *et al.* Causes of death among patients surviving at least one year following splenectomy. *Am J Surg* 1996; **172**: 320–3.

137. Lehne G, Hannisdal E, Langholm R, Nome O. A 10-year experience with splenectomy in patients with malignant non-Hodgkin's lymphoma at the Norwegian Radium Hospital. *Cancer* 1994; **74**: 933–9.

138. Cullingford GL, Watkins DN, Watts AD, Mallon DF. Severe late postsplenectomy infection. *Br J Surg* 1991; **78**: 716–21.

139. Lane PA. The spleen in children. *Curr Opin Pediatr* 1995; **7**: 36–41.

140. Reid MM. Splenectomy, sepsis, immunisation, and guidelines. *Lancet* 1994; **344**: 970–1.

141. Egan EL, Fairbanks VF. Postsplenectomy erythrocytosis in hemoglobin Koln disease. *N Engl J Med* 1973; **288**: 929–31.

142. Beutler E, Lang A, Lehmann H. Hemoglobin Duarte: (α2 β2 δ2 (E6) Ala leads to Pro): a new unstable hemoglobin with increased oxygen affinity. *Blood* 1974; **43**: 527–35.

143. Thuret I, Bardakdjian J, Badens C *et al.* Priapism following splenectomy in an unstable hemoglobin: hemoglobin Olmsted β141 (H19) Leu → Arg. *Am J Hematol* 1996; **51**: 133–6.

144. Rao KR, Patel AR. Priapism and thalassaemia intermedia [letter]. *Br J Surg* 1986; **73**: 1048.

145. Jackson N, Franklin IM, Hughes MA. Recurrent priapism following splenectomy for thalassaemia intermedia. *Br J Surg* 1986; **73**: 678.

146. Macchia P, Massei F, Nardi M, Favre C, Brunori E, Barba V. Thalassaemia intermedia and recurrent priapism following splenectomy [letter]. *Haematologica* 1990; **75**: 486–7.

147. Jayabose S, Tugal O, Sandoval C *et al.* Clinical and hematologic effects of hydroxyurea in children with sickle cell anemia. *J Pediatr* 1996; **129**: 559–65.

148. Scott JP, Hillery CA, Brown ER, Misiewicz V, Labotka RJ. Hydroxyurea therapy in children severely affected with sickle cell disease. *J Pediatr* 1996; **128**: 820–8.

149. Ferster A, Vermylen C, Cornu G *et al.* Hydroxyurea for treatment of severe sickle cell anemia: a pediatric clinical trial. *Blood* 1996; **88**: 1960–4.

150. Claster S, Vichinsky E. First report of reversal of organ dysfunction in sickle cell anemia by the use of hydroxyurea: splenic regeneration. *Blood* 1996; **88**: 1951–3.

151. Zeng YT, Huang SZ, Ren ZR *et al.* Hydroxyurea therapy in β-thalassaemia intermedia: improvement in haematological parameters due to enhanced β-globin synthesis. *Br J Haematol* 1995; **90**: 557–63.

152. Haljar FM, Pearson HA. Pharmacologic treatment of thalassemia intermedia with hydroxyurea. *J Pediatr* 1994; **125**: 490–2.

153. Rose C, Bauters F, Galacteros F. Hydroxyurea therapy in highly unstable hemoglobin carriers [letter]. *Blood* 1996; **88**: 2807–8.

154. Baird M, Schreiner H, Driscoll C, Bank A. Localization of the site of recombination in formation of the Lepore Boston globin gene. *J Clin Invest* 1981; **68**: 560–4.

155. Mavilio F, Giampaolo A, Care A, Sposi NM, Marinucci M. The δ β crossover region in Lepore boston hemoglobinopathy is restricted to a 59 base pairs region around the 5′ splice junction of the large globin gene intervening sequence. *Blood* 1983; **62**: 230–3.

156. McDonald MJ, Noble RW, Sharma VS, Ranney HM, Crookston JH, Schwarz JM. A comparison of the functional properties of two lepore haemoglobins with those of haemoglobin A1. *J Mol Biol* 1975; **94**: 305–10.

157. Metzenberg AB, Wurzer G, Huisman TH, Smithies O. Homology requirements for unequal crossing over in humans. *Genetics* 1991; **128**: 143–61.

158. Ostertag W, Smith EW. Hemoglobin-Lepore-Baltimore, a third type of a δ, β crossover (δ 50, β 86). *Eur J Biochem* 1969; **10**: 371–6.

159. Camaschella C, Serra A, Bertero MT *et al.* Molecular characterization of Italian chromosomes carrying the Lepore Boston gene. *Acta Haematol* 1989; **81**: 136–9.

160. Efremov DG, Efremov GD, Zisovski N *et al.* Variation in clinical severity among patients with Hb Lepore-Boston-β-thalassaemia is related to the type of β-thalassaemia. *Br J Haematol* 1988; **68**: 351–5.

161. Quattrin N, Luzzatto L, Quattrin S Jr. New clinical and biochemical findings from 235 patients with hemoglobin Lepore. *Ann NY Acad Sci* 1980; **344**: 364–74.

162. Orkin SH, Kazazian HH Jr, Antonarakis SE, Ostrer H, Goff SC, Sexton JP. Abnormal RNA processing due to the exon mutation of β E-globin gene. *Nature* 1982; **300**: 768–9.

163. Orkin SH, Antonarakis SE, Loukopoulos D. Abnormal processing of β Knossos RNA. *Blood* 1984; **64**: 311–13.

164. Wong SC, Ali MA. Hemoglobin E diseases: hematological, analytical, and biosynthetic studies in homozygotes and double heterozygotes for α-thalassemia. *Am J Hematol* 1982; **13**: 15–21.

165. Fairbanks VF, Oliveros R, Brandabur JH, Willis RR, Fiester RE. Homozygous hemoglobin E mimics β-thalassemia minor without anemia or hemolysis: hematologic, functional, and biosynthetic studies of first North American cases. *Am J Hematol* 1980; **8**: 109–21.

166. Arous N, Galacteros F, Fessas P *et al.* Structural study of hemoglobin Knossos, β27 (B9) Ala leads to Ser. A new abnormal hemoglobin present as a silent β-thalassemia. *FEBS Lett* 1982; **147**: 247–50.

167. Fessas P, Loukopoulos D, Loutradi Anagnostou A, Komis G. "Silent" β-thalassaemia caused by a "silent" β-chain mutant: the pathogenesis of a syndrome of thalassaemia intermedia. *Br J Haematol* 1982; **51**: 577–83.

168. Vetter B, Schwarz C, Kohne E, Kulozik AE. β-Thalassemia in the immigrant and non-immigrant German populations. *Br J Haematol* 1997; **97**: 266–77.

169. Vidaud M, Gattoni R, Stevenin J *et al.* A 5′ splice-region G-C mutation in exon 1 of the human β-globin gene inhibits pre-mRNA splicing: a mechanism for β⁺-thalassaemia. *Proc Natl Acad Sci USA* 1989; **86**: 1041–5.

170. Milner PF, Clegg JB, Weatherall DJ. Haemoglobin-H disease due to a unique haemoglobin variant with an elongated α-chain. *Lancet* 1971; **i**: 729–32.

171. Clegg JB, Weatherall DJ, Milner PF. Hemoglobin Constant Spring: a chain termination mutant? *Nature* 1971; **234**: 337–40.

172. Clegg JB, Weatherall DJ, Contopolou Griva I, Caroutsos K, Poungouras P, Tsevrenis H. Hemoglobin Icaria, a new

chain-termination mutant which causes a thalassaemia. *Nature* 1974; **251**: 245–7.

173. De Jong WW, Meera Khan P, Bernini LF. Hemoglobin Koya Dora: high frequency of a chain termination mutant. *Am J Hum Genet* 1975; **27**: 81–90.

174. Merritt D, Jones RT, Head C *et al.* Hemoglobin Seal Rock [(α2) 142 Term-Glu, codon 142 TAA-GAA] an extended α chain variant associated with anemia, microcytosis and α-thalassaemia-2 (–3.7 kb). *Hemoglobin* 1997; **21**: 331–44.

175. Hanash SM, Rucknagel DL. Proteolytic activity in erythrocyte precursors. *Proc Natl Acad Sci USA* 1978; **75**: 3427–31.

176. Holbrook J, Neu-Yilik G, Hentze MW, Kulozik AE. Nonsense mediated decay approaches the clinic. *Nat Genet* 2004; **36**: 801–9.

177. Vetter B, Neu-Yilik G, Kohne E *et al.* Dominant β-thalassaemia: a highly unstable haemoglobin is caused by a novel 6 bp deletion of the β-globin gene. *Br J Haematol* 2000; **108**: 176–81.

178. Weiss I, Cash FE, Coleman MB *et al.* Molecular basis for α-thalassaemia associated with the structural mutant hemoglobin Suan-Dok (α2 109 Leu → Arg). *Blood* 1990; **76**: 2630–6. Published erratum appears in *Blood* 1991; **77**: 1404.

179. Goossens M, Lee KY, Liebhaber SA, Kan YW. Globin structural mutant α 125 Leu leads to Pro is a novel cause of α-thalassaemia. *Nature* 1982; **296**: 864–5.

180. Ohba Y, Yamamoto K, Hattori Y, Kawata R, Miyaji T. Hyperunstable hemoglobin Toyama [α2 136 (H19) Leu → Arg β2]: detection and identification by *in vitro* biosynthesis with radioactive amino acids. *Hemoglobin* 1987; **11**: 539–56.

181. Park SS, Barnetson R, Kim SW, Weatherall DJ, Thein SL. A spontaneous deletion of β 33/34 Val in exon 2 of the β globin gene (Hb Korea) produces the phenotype of dominant β thalassaemia. *Br J Haematol* 1991; **78**: 581–2.

182. Podda A, Galanello R, Maccioni L *et al.* Hemoglobin Cagliari (β 60 [E4] Val → Glu): a novel unstable thalassemic hemoglobinopathy. *Blood* 1991; **77**: 371–5.

183. Ristaldi MS, Pirastu M, Murru S *et al.* A spontaneous mutation produced a novel elongated β-globin chain structural variant (Hb Agnana) with a thalassemia-like phenotype [letter]. *Blood* 1990; **75**: 1378–9.

184. Kobayashi Y, Fukumaki Y, Komatsu N, Ohba Y, Miyaji T, Miura Y. A novel globin structural mutant, Showa-Yakushiji (β110 Leu → Pro) causing a β-thalassaemia phenotype. *Blood* 1987; **70**: 1688–91.

185. Murru S, Poddie D, Sciarratta GV *et al.* A novel β-globin structural mutant, Hb Brescia (β114 Leu → Pro), causing a severe β-thalassaemia intermedia phenotype. *Hum Mutat* 1992; **1**: 124–8.

186. de Castro CM, Devlin B, Fleenor DE, Lee ME, Kaufman RE. A novel β-globin mutation, β Durham-NC [β114 Leu → Pro], produces a dominant thalassemia-like phenotype. *Blood* 1994; **83**: 1109–16.

187. Beris P, Miescher PA, Diaz Chico JC *et al.* Inclusion body β-thalassaemia trait in a Swiss family is caused by an abnormal hemoglobin (Geneva) with an altered and extended β chain carboxy-terminus due to a modification in codon β114. *Blood* 1988; **72**: 801–5.

188. Fucharoen S, Kobayashi Y, Fucharoen G *et al.* A single nucleotide deletion in codon 123 of the β-globin gene causes an inclusion body β-thalassaemia trait: a novel elongated globin chain β Makabe. *Br J Haematol* 1990; **75**: 393–9.

189. Curuk MA, Molchanova TP, Postnikov YuV *et al.* β-Thalassemia alleles and unstable hemoglobin types among Russian pediatric patients. *Am J Hematol* 1994; **46**: 329–32.

190. Murru S, Loudianos G, Deiana M *et al.* Molecular characterization of β-thalassemia intermedia in patients of Italian descent and identification of three novel β-thalassemia mutations. *Blood* 1991; **77**: 1342–7.

191. Pagano L, Lacerra G, Camardella L *et al.* Hemoglobin Neapolis, β126 (H4) Val → Gly: a novel β-chain variant associated with a mild β-thalassemia phenotype and displaying anomalous stability features. *Blood* 1991; **78**: 3070–5.

192. Hattori Y, Yamane A, Yamashiro Y *et al.* Characterization of β-thalassemia mutations among the Japanese. *Hemoglobin* 1989; **13**: 657–70.

193. Fucharoen S, Fucharoen G, Fukumaki Y *et al.* Three-base deletion in exon 3 of the β-globin gene produced a novel variant (β Gunma) with a thalassemia-like phenotype [letter]. *Blood* 1990; **76**: 1894–6.

194. Oner R, Oner C, Wilson JB, Tamagnini GP, Ribeiro LM, Huisman TH. Dominant β-thalassaemia trait in a Portuguese family is caused by a deletion of (G)TGGCTGGTGT(G) and an insertion of (G)GCAG(G) in codons 134, 135, 136 and 137 of the β-globin gene. *Br J Haematol* 1991; **79**: 306–10.

195. Fei YJ, Stoming TA, Kutlar A, Huisman TH, Stamatoyannopoulos G. One form of inclusion body β-thalassemia is due to a GAA–TAA mutation at codon 121 of the β chain [letter]. *Blood* 1989; **73**: 1075–7.

196. Hall GW, Franklin IM, Sura T, Thein SL. A novel mutation (nonsense β127) in exon 3 of the β globin gene produces a variable thalassaemic phenotype. *Br J Haematol* 1991; **79**: 342–4.

197. Butler WM, Spratling L, Kark JA, Schoomaker EB. Hemoglobin Osler: report of a new family with exercise studies before and after phlebotomy. *Am J Hematol* 1982; **13**: 293–301.

198. Winslow RM, Butler WM, Kark JA, Klein HG, Moo Penn W. The effect of bloodletting on exercise performance in a subject with a high-affinity hemoglobin variant. *Blood* 1983; **62**: 1159–64.

199. Wranne B, Berlin G, Jorfeldt L, Lund N. Tissue oxygenation and muscular substrate turnover in two subjects with high hemoglobin oxygen affinity. *J Clin Invest* 1983; **72**: 1376–84.

200. Wranne B, Jorfeldt L, Berlin G *et al.* Effect of haemodilution on maximal oxygen consumption, blood lactate response to exercise and cerebral blood flow in subjects with a high-affinity haemoglobin. *Eur J Haematol* 1991; **47**: 268–76.

201. Mavilio F, Marinucci M, Tentori L, Fontanarosa PP, Rossi U, Biagiotti S. Hemoglobin Legnano (α2 141 (HC3) Arg replaced by Leu β2): a new abnormal human hemoglobin with high oxygen affinity. *Hemoglobin* 1978; **2**: 249–59.

202. Shimasaki S. A new hemoglobin variant, hemoglobin Nunobiki [α141 (HC3) Arg → Cys]. Notable influence of the carboxy-terminal cysteine upon various physico-chemical characteristics of hemoglobin. *J Clin Invest* 1985; **75**: 695–701.

203. Kosugi H, Weinstein AS, Kikugawa K, Asakura T, Schroeder WA. Characterization and properties of Hb York (β146 His leads to Pro). *Hemoglobin* 1983; **7**: 205–26.

204. Schneider RG, Bremner JE, Brimhall B, Jones RT, Shih TB. Hemoglobin Cowtown (β146 HC3 His → Leu): a mutant with high oxygen affinity and erythrocytosis. *Am J Clin Pathol* 1979; **72**: 1028–32.

205. Shih T, Jones RT, Bonaventura J, Bonaventura C, Schneider RG. Involvement of His HC3 (146) β in the Bohr effect of human hemoglobin. Studies of native and N-ethylmaleimide-treated hemoglobin A and hemoglobin Cowtown (#146 His replaced by Leu). *J Biol Chem* 1984; **259**: 967–74.

206. Nagel RL, Gibson QH, Hamilton HB. Ligand kinetics in hemoglobin Hiroshima. *J Clin Invest* 1971; **50**: 1772–5.

207. Bonaventura C, Bonaventura J, Amiconi G, Tentori L, Brunori M, Antonini E. Hemoglobin Abruzzo (β143 (H21) His replaced by Arg). Consequences of altering the 2,3-diphosphoglycerate binding site. *J Biol Chem* 1975; **250**: 6273–7.

208. Perutz MF. Stereochemical interpretation of high oxygen affinity of haemoglobin Little Rock (α2 β2 143 His leads to Gln). *Nature New Biol* 1973; **243**: 180.

209. Jensen M, Oski FA, Nathan DG, Bunn HF. Hemoglobin Syracuse (α2 β2–143(H21) His leads to Pro), a new high-affinity variant detected by special electrophoretic methods. Observations on the autooxidation of normal and variant hemoglobins. *J Clin Invest* 1975; **55**: 469–77.

210. Bonaventura J, Bonaventura C, Sullivan B *et al.* Hemoglobin Providence. Functional consequences of two alterations of the 2,3-diphosphoglycerate binding site at position β82. *J Biol Chem* 1976; **251**: 7563–71.

211. Sugihara J, Imamura T, Nagafuchi S, Bonaventura J, Bonaventura C, Cashon R. Hemoglobin Rahere, a human hemoglobin variant with amino acid substitution at the 2,3-diphosphoglycerate binding site. Functional consequences of the alteration and effects of bezafibrate on the oxygen bindings. *J Clin Invest* 1985; **76**: 1169–73.

212. Ikkala E, Koskela J, Pikkarainen P *et al.* Hb Helsinki: a variant with a high oxygen affinity and a substitution at a 2,3-DPG binding site (β82[EF6] Lys replaced by Met). *Acta Haematol* 1976; **56**: 257–75.

213. Rochette J, Barnetson R, Kiger L *et al.* Association of a novel high oxygen affinity haemoglobin variant with δ β thalassaemia. *Br J Haematol* 1994; **86**: 118–24.

214. Maniatis A, Bousios T, Nagel RL *et al.* Hemoglobin Crete (β129 ala leads to pro): a new high-affinity variant interacting with β⁰- and δβ⁰-thalassemia. *Blood* 1979; **54**: 54–63.

215. Charache S, Weatherall DJ, Clegg JB. Polycythemia associated with a hemoglobinopathy. *J Clin Invest* 1966; **45**: 813–22.

216. Charache S, Catalano P, Burns S *et al.* Pregnancy in carriers of high-affinity hemoglobins. *Blood* 1985; **65**: 713–18.

217. Kulozik AE, Bellan Koch A, Kohne E, Kleihauer E. A deletion/inversion rearrangement of the β-globin gene cluster in a Turkish family with δβ⁰-thalassaemia intermedia. *Blood* 1992; **79**: 2455–9.

218. Kaeda JS, Prasad K, Howard RJ, Mehta A, Vulliamy T, Luzzatto L. Management of pregnancy when maternal blood has a very high level of fetal haemoglobin. *Br J Haematol* 1994; **88**: 432–4.

219. Lichtman MA, Murphy MS, Adamson JW. Detection of mutant hemoglobins with altered affinity for oxygen. A simplified technique. *Ann Intern Med* 1976; **84**: 517–20.

220. Bagby GC Jr, Richert Boe K, Koler RD. 32P and acute leukemia: development of leukemia in a patient with hemoglobin Yakima. *Blood* 1978; **52**: 350–4.

221. Bunn HF. Subunit dissociation of certain abnormal human hemoglobins. *J Clin Invest* 1969; **48**: 126–38.

222. Gibson QH, Riggs A, Imamura T. Kinetic and equilibrium properties of hemoglobin Kansas. *J Biol Chem* 1973; **248**: 5976–86.

223. Nagel RL, Lynfield J, Johnson J, Landau L, Bookchin RM, Harris MB. Hemoglobin Beth Israel. A mutant causing clinically apparent cyanosis. *N Engl J Med* 1976; **295**: 125–30.

224. Arous N, Braconnier F, Thillet J *et al.* Hemoglobin Saint Mande β 102 (G4) Asn replaced by Tyr: a new low oxygen affinity variant. *FEBS Lett* 1981; **126**: 114–16.

225. Pulsinelli PD, Perutz MF, Nagel RL. Structure of hemoglobin M Boston, a variant with a five-coordinated ferric heme. *Proc Natl Acad Sci USA* 1973; **70**: 3870–4.

226. Perutz MF, Pulsinelli PD, Ranney HM. Structure and subunit interaction of haemoglobin M Milwaukee. *Nature New Biol* 1972; **237**: 259–63.

227. Nagai M, Takama S, Yoneyama Y. Reduction and spectroscopic properties of haemoglobins M. *Acta Haematol* 1987; **78**: 95–8.

228. Nagai M, Yoneyama Y, Kitagawa T. Characteristics in tyrosine coordinations of four hemoglobins M probed by resonance Raman spectroscopy. *Biochemistry* 1989; **28**: 2418–22.

229. Passon PG, Reed DW, Hultquist DE. Soluble cytochrome β 5 from human erythrocytes. *Biochim Biophys Acta* 1972; **275**: 51–61.

230. Kuma F, Ishizawa S, Hirayama K, Nakajima H. Studies on methemoglobin reductase. I. Comparative studies of diaphorases from normal and methemoglobinemic erythrocytes. *J Biol Chem* 1972; **247**: 550–5.

231. Kuma F, Inomata H. Studies on methemoglobin reductase. II. The purification and molecular properties of reduced nicotinamide adenine dinucleotide-dependent methemoglobin reductase. *J Biol Chem* 1972; **247**: 556–60.

232. Choury D, Leroux A, Kaplan JC. Membrane-bound cytochrome b5 reductase (methemoglobin reductase) in human erythrocytes. Study in normal and methemoglobinemic subjects. *J Clin Invest* 1981; **67**: 149–55.

233. Yubisui T, Matsuki T, Tanishima K, Takeshita M, Yoneyama Y. NADPH-flavin reductase in human erythrocytes and the reduction of methemoglobin through flavin by the enzyme. *Biochem Biophys Res Commun* 1977; **76**: 174–82.

234. Tomoda A, Yubisui T, Tsuji A, Yoneyama Y. Changes in intermediate haemoglobins during methaemoglobin reduction by NADPH-flavin reductase. *Biochem J* 1979; **179**: 227–31.

235. Nagai M, Yubisui T, Yoneyama Y. Enzymatic reduction of hemoglobins M Milwaukee-1 and M Saskatoon by NADH-cytochrome b5 reductase and NADPH-flavin reductase purified from human erythrocytes. *J Biol Chem* 1980; **255**: 4599–602.

236. Jaffe ER, Hsieh HS. DPNH-methemoglobin reductase deficiency and hereditary methemoglobinemia. *Semin Hematol* 1971; **8**: 417–37.

237. Mansouri A, Lurie AA. Concise review: methemoglobinemia. *Am J Hematol* 1993; **42**: 7–12.

238. Bartos HR, Desforges JF. Erythrocyte DPNH dependent diaphorase levels in infants. *Pediatrics* 1966; **37**: 991–3.

239. Sick H, Gersonde K. Co-binding studies on Hb M Iwate. Allostery of a T state hemoglobin. *Biochim Biophys Acta* 1979; **581**: 34–43.

240. Nagai M, Kitagawa T, Yoneyama Y. Molecular pathology of hemoglobin M Saskatoon disease. *Biomed Biochim Acta* 1990; **49**: 5317–22.

241. Ranney HM, Nagel RL, Heller P, Udem L. Oxygen equilibrium of hemoglobin M-Hyde Park. *Biochim Biophys Acta* 1968; **160**: 112–15.

242. Udem L, Ranney HM, Bunn HF, Pisciotta A. Some observations on the properties of haemoglobin M Milwaukee-1. *J Mol Biol* 1970; **48**: 489–98.

243. Hayashi A, Fujita T, Fujimura M, Titani K. A new abnormal fetal hemoglobin, Hb FM-Osaka (α2 72 63 His replaced by Tyr). *Hemoglobin* 1980; **4**: 447–8.

244. Glader BE. Hemoglobin FM-Fort Ripley: another lesson from the neonate. *Pediatrics* 1989; **83**: 792–3.

245. Hain RD, Chitayat D, Cooper R *et al*. Hb FM-Fort Ripley: confirmation of autosomal dominant inheritance and diagnosis by PCR and direct nucleotide sequencing. *Hum Mutat* 1994; **3**: 239–42.

12 Red cell membrane abnormalities

Patrick G. Gallagher

The erythrocyte membrane provides a protective layer between hemoglobin and other intracellular components and the extracellular environment. It facilitates the transport of cations, anions, urea, water, and other small molecules in and out of the cell, but denies entry to larger molecules, particularly if they are charged. It is a sturdy yet flexible container, consisting of a lipid bilayer studded with numerous integral proteins and an underlying proteinaceous membrane skeleton. With only a limited capacity for repair or self-renewal, it lasts the entire 120-day lifespan of the normal red cell. This chapter summarizes the structure and functions of the normal red cell membrane and reviews the major red cell membrane abnormalities that cause human disease.

Membrane lipids

Components

Lipids comprise about 50% of the weight of the erythrocyte membrane. The average human red cell contains about 455 million lipid molecules, all found within the lipid bilayer of the plasma membrane. Phospholipids and unesterified cholesterol, present in nearly equimolar concentrations, predominate, but there are small amounts of glycolipids, primarily globoside, the parvovirus receptor.[1-4] The major phospholipids are phosphatidylcholine, phosphatidylethanolamine, sphingomyelin, and phosphatidylserine. Small quantities of phosphatidic acid, phosphatidylinositol and lysophosphatidylcholine are also found. The typical phospholipids, with the exception of sphingomyelin and lysophosphatidylcholine, are composed of a glycerol backbone with two medium-chain fatty acids attached via an ester or vinyl linkage. The composition of fatty acids partially determines the properties of the various phospholipids and can affect membrane properties.[5] A family of red cell enzymes with specificity for each phospholipid class is thought to maintain the precise fatty acyl composition characteristic of that class.[6] Lysophospholipids, the precursors of phospholipids, have a single fatty acid attached to the first position of the glycerol backbone.

Phosphoinositides are phospholipids with a phosphoinositol-containing polar head group, which may be mono-phosphorylated (phosphatidylinositol-4-monophosphate) or bi-phosphorylated (phosphatidylinositol-4,5-bisphosphate).[7] Although representing only 2–5% of membrane phospholipids, phosphoinositides have considerable biologic activity and are involved in maintaining red cell shape and deformability.[8] Some membrane proteins, including proteins involved in complement regulation, are anchored to the red cell membrane through a phosphoinositol lipid domain.[9] This allows these proteins to move laterally in the membrane, preventing complement-mediated membrane damage. Phosphoinositol-anchored proteins are lost through the release of lipid-enriched vesicles from the cell during the membrane remodeling that accompanies reticulocyte maturation or cell aging. This process of vesiculation and loss of complement regulatory proteins is accelerated in sickle cell anemia by repeated cycles of sickling, making these cells sensitive to complement-mediated lysis.[10]

Organization and dynamics

Under physiologic conditions, the lipid bilayer is in a liquid state allowing both the transmembrane proteins and the cell surface molecules to move in the plane of the membrane. Bilayer fluidity is influenced by several factors, including temperature, which determines the phase transition between a liquid and gel state, the content of free cholesterol (the rigid sterol ring of which decreases lipid bilayer fluidity), and the length and the degree of unsaturation of phospholipid fatty acids. The saturated fatty acids have a relatively rigid backbone, resisting motion, while unsaturated fatty acids have relatively unrestricted movements, thereby increasing the fluidity of the lipid bilayer.

Phospholipids are asymmetrically distributed throughout

the membrane. Phosphatidylserine and phosphatidylethanolamine are primarily in the inner leaflet, while sphingomyelin and phosphatidylcholine are concentrated in the outer half of the bilayer. This asymmetric distribution of phospholipids is a dynamic system involving a constant exchange ("flip-flop") between the phospholipids of the two bilayer leaflets.[11,12] In pathologic states, outward exposure of phosphatidylserine, such as occurs in sickle cell disease, β-thalassemia, diabetes and other disorders, leads to activation of blood clotting via conversion of prothrombin to thrombin and red cell attachment to macrophages of the reticuloendothelial system, marking them for destruction.[13–17] Factors maintaining normal phospholipid asymmetry include a "flippase" or aminophospholipid translocase, which is responsible for magnesium ATP-dependent translocation of phosphatidylserine and phosphatidylethanolamine from the outer leaflet to the inner one; a "floppase" or phospholipid translocase, which moves phospholipids from the outer leaflet to the inner one; and a calcium-dependent phospholipid "scramblase", which facilitates bidirectional movements of phospholipids in the bilayer.[18–21]

Changes in the asymmetric distribution of phospholipids have profound effects on red cell shape and other properties. Increasing flip-flop rates perturb phospholipid asymmetry. Examples include an increase in cytosolic calcium, which induces phospholipid scrambling, oxidative cross-linking of membrane proteins, or, in deoxygenated sickled red cells, uncoupling of the lipid bilayer from the underlying skeleton at the tips of the sickle cell spicules.

Glycolipids and cholesterol are intercalated between membrane phospholipids with their long axes perpendicular to the bilayer plane.[22] Cholesterol molecules are distributed evenly across the bilayer but glycolipids are localized to the outer leaflet where they contribute to the structure of the blood group antigens. The shape of the lipid bilayer is responsive to slight variations in the surface area of either the inner or outer leaflet, termed the "bilayer couple effect". This effect predicts that erythrocyte membrane shape changes are the result of expansion of one lipid leaflet compared with the other and that commensurate alteration of the unperturbed leaflet can compensate for such expansion, restoring the normal biconcave shape.[23] Increasing the surface area of the inner leaflet produces a stomatocytic change in shape whereas increasing that of the outer leaflet transforms the cell into an echinocyte.

There is an increasing realization that lipids exist in different domains within each of the bilayer leaflets.[24,25] Large lipid-rich macroscopic domains have been observed in the membrane. Lipids have also been found in protein-bound microscopic domains. Recently, the presence of lipid-associated domains associated with the detergent-resistant fraction of the membrane, termed "lipid rafts" by some, has been described.[26] The precise functions of these specific domains have yet to be elucidated. It has been suggested that lipid rafts play a role in facilitating malarial invasion of the erythrocyte.[27–29]

Lipid renewal pathways

Mature erythrocytes are unable to synthesize fatty acids, phospholipids, or cholesterol and thus exchange pathways are the mechanism of lipid modification of red blood cells. In the circulation, erythrocyte cholesterol is rapidly exchanged with unesterified cholesterol from plasma lipoproteins.[30] The outer bilayer phospholipids, phosphatidylcholine and sphingomyelin, are slowly exchanged with plasma lipids. Phosphatidylserine and phosphatidylethanolamine, located in the inner bilayer, do not participate in lipid exchange. Another potential lipid renewal pathway is fatty acid acylation. This is an ATP-dependent process in which fatty acids combine with lysophosphatides to remake the native phospholipids, renewing damaged or lost fatty acid side-chains. The composition of red cell phospholipids is quite distinct from that of plasma phospholipids, suggesting that specific pathways exist in red cells to remodel phospholipids to optimize their function. Dietary changes have only a minimal effect on the composition of red cell membrane phospholipids.[31] In contrast, it is likely that oxidant damage, particularly to unsaturated fatty acid groups, can alter membrane structure and function. Removal of oxidized fatty acids and replacement by normal fatty acids appears to be essential for red cell survival.

Membrane proteins

The red cell membrane contains about a dozen major proteins and hundreds of minor ones. The major proteins of the red cell membrane (Fig. 12.1 and Table 12.1) and their disorders have been intensively studied. Membrane proteins may be classified as either integral, i.e., penetrating or crossing the lipid bilayer and interacting with the hydrophobic lipid core, or peripheral, i.e., interacting with integral proteins or lipids at the membrane surface but not penetrating into the bilayer core.

Components

The integral membrane proteins include glycophorins A, B, C, and D, which possess membrane receptors and antigens, and transport proteins such as band 3, the erythrocyte anion exchanger.[32–34] The glycophorins, which provide most of the negative surface charge red cells require to avoid sticking to each other and to the vascular wall, carry receptors for *Plasmodium falciparum* and various viruses and bacteria, and serve as conduits for transmembrane signaling.[35] Band 3, the major integral protein of the red cell, serves many functions, including as a chloride–bicarbonate exchanger, a binding site for a variety of enzymes and cytoplasmic membrane

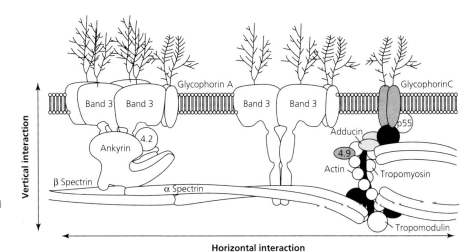

Fig. 12.1 Erythrocyte Membrane. A model of the major proteins of the erythrocyte membrane is shown: α and β spectrin, ankyrin, band 3 (the anion exchanger), 4.1 (protein 4.1) and 4.2 (protein 4.2), actin and glycophorin. Reproduced with permission from Tse WT, Lux SE Red blood cell membrane disorders. *Br J Haematol* 1999; **104**: 2.

Table 12.1 Major human erythrocyte membrane proteins.

SDS gel band*	Protein	Molecular weight × 10³ (gel/calculated)	Approximate proportion (weight %)	Monomer copies per cell (×10³)	Chromosome location	Gene	Associated diseases
1	α-Spectrin	240/281	14	242 ± 20	1q22–q23	SPTA1	HE, HPP, HS
2	β-Spectrin	220/246	13	242 ± 20	14q23–q24.2	SPTB	HE, HPP, HS, HAc
2.1	Ankyrin	210/206	6	124 ± 11	8p11.2	ANK1	HS
2.9†	α-Adducin	103/81	<1	≈ 30	4p16.3	ADDA	–
	β-Adducin	97/80	<1	≈ 30	2p13–p14	ADDB	–
3‡	AE1	90–100/102	29	≈ 1200	17q12–q21	EPB3	HS, SAO, HA
4.1	Protein 4.1	80 + 78/66§	5	≈ 200	1p33–p34.2	EL1	HE
4.2	Pallidin	72/77	5	≈ 250	15q15–q21	ELB42	HS
4.9†	Dematin	48 + 52/43 + 46	1	≈ 140	8p21.1	–	–
	p55	55/53		≈ 80	Xq28	MPP1	–
5	β-Actin	43/42	6	≈ 500	7pter–q22	ACTB	–
	Tropomodulin	43/41		≈ 30	9q22	TMOD	–
6	G3PD	35/36	5	≈ 500	12q13	GAPD	–
7	Stomatin	31/32	4	–	9q33–q34	EPB72	HSt
	Tropomyosin	27 + 29/28		≈ 70	1q31	TPM3	–
8	Protein 8	23/–	1–2	≈ 200	–	–	–
PAS-1¶	Glycophorin A	36/14	1.6	≈ 1000	4q31	GYPA	–
PAS-2¶	Glycophorin C	32/14	0.1	≈ 200 (C + D)	2q14–q21	GYPC	HE
PAS-3¶	Glycophorin B	20/8	0.2	≈ 200	4q31	GYPB	None
	Glycophorin D	23/11	0.02	≈ 200 (C + D)	2q14–q21	GYPD	HE
	Glycophorin E**	–/–	–	–	4q31	GYPE	–

* Numbering system of bands 1–8 refer to Coomassie blue-stained gels; PAS-1 to PAS-3 refer to periodic acid–Schiff-stained gels.

† The α and β adducins lie in the upper part of SDS gel band 3. Band 4.9 contains both dematin and p55; band 5 contains β-actin and tropomodulin; band 7 contains stomatin and tropomyosin.

‡ The protein runs as a broad band on SDS gels due to heterogeneous glycosylation.

§ Protein 4.1 is a doublet (4.1a and 4.1b) on SDS gels. Protein 4.1a is derived from 4.1b by slow deamidation. Its proportion is a measure of red blood cell age.

¶ The glycophorins (GpA–GpD) are visible only on PAS-stained gels.

** Glycophorin E mRNA has been identified but it is not certain that the mRNA is translated.

HE, hereditary elliptocytosis; HS, hereditary spherocytosis; HPP, hereditary pyropoikilocytosis; HAc, hereditary acanthocytosis; HSt, hereditary stomatocytosis; SAO, Southeast Asian ovalocytosis; AE1, anion exchange protein 1 (erythroid anion exchange protein); G3PD, glyceraldehyde 3-phosphate dehydrogenase. Reprinted with permission from Ref. 178.

components, and a participant in regulation of red cell deformability, intermediary metabolism, senescence, and shape.[36,37] Other integral proteins include the Rh proteins, Kell and Duffy antigens, glucose, urea and amino acid transporters, Na^+/K^+-ATPase, Ca^{2+}-ATPase, Mg^{2+}-ATPase, various kinases and phosphatases, acetylcholinesterase, decay accelerating factor, complement proteins, and receptors for transferrin, insulin, insulin-like growth factors, thyroid hormone, parathyroid hormone, β-adrenergic agonists, cholinergic agents, diphtheria toxin, ceruloplasmin and opiates.

Peripheral membrane proteins include the structural proteins of the spectrin-based erythrocyte membrane skeleton and enzymes such as glyceraldehyde 3-phosphate dehydrogenase. The membrane skeleton is composed of an intricately interwoven meshwork of proteins and is largely responsible for the biconcave disk shape of the red cell.[38–40] It comprises approximately half the membrane protein mass and is primarily composed of spectrin. Spectrin is composed of two subunits, α and β spectrin, encoded by separate genes, that both contain 106 amino acid α-helical "spectrin repeats" composed of triple helices connected by short connecting regions. The α- and β-spectrin chains intertwine in an antiparallel manner to form 100-nm long heterodimers, which self-associate head to head to form tetramers and oligomers. These higher-order molecules provide significant flexibility and structural support for the lipid bilayer, helping maintain cellular shape. Disruption of spectrin self-association leads to membrane instability, altered membrane deformability and mechanical properties, and abnormal erythrocyte shape.

The primary linkage of spectrin to the erythrocyte membrane is mediated by the binding of spectrin to ankyrin, which in turn binds to band 3.[41] Protein 4.2 binds to band 3 and probably binds to ankyrin, possibly promoting their interaction.[42] Disruption of the spectrin–ankyrin–band 3 linkage or the band 3–protein 4.2 interaction leads to membrane loss and the phenotype of spherocytosis.

A second linkage of spectrin to the plasma membrane is mediated by its association with a multiprotein "junctional complex" that includes spectrin, protein 4.1, and actin.[43] Protein 4.1, a protein with numerous erythroid and nonerythroid isoforms,[44] interacts with spectrin and actin as well as proteins in the overlying lipid bilayer, including band 3, glycophorin C, p55, calmodulin, CD44, pIC1n, CASK, mature parasite-infected antigen, and phosphatidylserine. Other important peripheral membrane proteins include p55 (which interacts with protein 4.1 and glycophorin C), the β subtype of actin, adducin, a heteromer of structurally related proteins, α-adducin, β-adducin or γ-adducin, which plays a role in the early assembly of the spectrin/actin complex by capping the ends of fast-growing actin filaments and by recruiting spectrin to the ends of actin filaments, dematin, tropomyosin, and tropomodulin. Disruption of the protein–protein interactions of the junctional complex also leads to membrane defects and inherited hemolytic anemia.

Membrane synthesis

Membrane proteins are synthesized early in the differentiation of erythroid progenitor cells. Events controlling membrane synthesis and assembly are poorly understood. There is considerable *in vitro* evidence suggesting that spectrin and ankyrin are assembled onto the membrane in only small amounts until band 3 is synthesized and introduced into the bilayer, providing an attachment site for ankyrin, spectrin, and the other skeletal proteins in sequence.[45] These data suggested a pivotal role for band 3 in membrane assembly. However, creation of a band 3 knockout mouse has led to reexamination of the role of band 3 in membrane protein assembly, because nearly normal amounts of skeletal proteins are present in the erythrocyte membranes of these mice despite the total absence of band 3.[46] Further studies have shown that protein 4.2 can assemble on the membrane in the absence of band 3. There is asymmetric synthesis of α and β spectrin, the former exceeding the latter by several fold. Proteins not incorporated into the membrane are rapidly degraded and lost. Similarly, large excesses of protein 4.1 are generated relative to the amount actually incorporated into the membrane skeleton. Overall, membrane protein biosynthesis and incorporation can be viewed as a somewhat inefficient process.

Membrane deformability

The normal red cell has a biconcave disk shape in the resting state, but in circulation it assumes elliptical, parachute-like, or other shapes in response to circulatory shear forces. Its ability to deform is determined by the surface area–volume ratio, cytoplasmic viscosity, and membrane material properties.[47] A decrease in the surface area–volume ratio, as is seen in spherocytes, reduces deformability and may impede passage of the red cell through constricted areas of the microcirculation, as found in the spleen. Changes in cytoplasmic viscosity are usually the result of osmotic movement of water into or out of the red cell. Movement of water into the cell decreases cytoplasmic viscosity but causes an increase in cell volume without affecting surface area, thus adversely affecting deformability. Movement of water out of the cell increases cytoplasmic viscosity and consequently decreases deformability. Optimal deformability is noted at physiologic plasma osmolarity (290 mosmol). Membrane material properties are complex, as the membrane behaves as a solid, semisolid or liquid depending on the duration and strength of the deforming force exerted. The force required to increase surface area is primarily determined by the lipid bilayer, whereas most other behaviors such as elasticity, elastic recoil, and yield shear stress are determined by the intrinsic and cytoskeletal protein network.[48] Many of the proteins of the red cell membrane are subject to posttranslational modification by phosphorylation, glycosylation, myristylation, fatty acid acylation, sulfhydryl-mediated oxidation, calmodulin, calpain-mediated proteolysis, and other processes that affect membrane properties in various ways.

Membrane transport

Water, urea, glucose, anions, and many other molecules move across the red cell membrane. This discussion is limited to cations, as disorders of cation transport are those most frequently associated with various human red cell disorders.[49,50] The normal red cell has an internal cation content quite different from that of the surrounding plasma.[51] The red cell K^+ concentration is high (~140 mmol/L cell water) compared with plasma K^+ concentrations of 4–5 mmol/L, whereas the red cell Na^+ concentration is low (~10 mmol/L cell water) compared with the plasma Na^+ concentration of about 140 mmol/L.[52] These concentration gradients lead to a small passive movement across the lipid bilayer of Na^+ into and K^+ out of the cell. Cation homeostasis is maintained by the active transport of Na^+ out of and K^+ into the cell with a 3 : 2 stoichiometry that exactly equals the normal passive movement of these cations. The Na^+/K^+-ATPase pump responsible for active transport couples the hydrolysis of ATP to the movement of Na^+ and K^+. The pump is a multimer composed of a catalytic α subunit and smaller β and γ subunits. Two other cation transport pathways are of importance, the Gardos channel and K/Cl cotransport. The Gardos channel is activated by increased intracellular Ca^{2+}, usually the result of ATP depletion, and promotes loss of intracellular K^+ and ultimately cell dehydration.[53] The volume-activated K/Cl cotransport pathway, also leads to cell dehydration secondary to the loss of K^+.[54] Both these pathways have been targeted to prevent cellular dehydration and sickling in sickle cell disease.[49,55] Finally, mechanical stretching of the membrane may lead to cation loss, a process likely to be of importance in the cellular dehydration that follows sickling deformation of hemoglobin SS red cells. The molecular basis of this pathway is unknown.

Fetal and neonatal red cell membranes

The membranes of fetal and neonatal erythrocytes differ from those of adult cells.[56] Increased myosin, cholesterol, and lipid phosphorus, and decreased aquaporin have been observed,[56–58] but the functional significance of these observations is unknown. Increased potassium loss, reduced chloride/bicarbonate exchange, and decreased water transport are other features of neonatal red cells.[59] The blood group antigen systems of neonatal cells are not fully developed and there are expression differences in the Ii antigen of band 3. There is significant variation in size and shape of neonatal cells. Thus irregularly shaped cells such as poikilocytes, acanthocytes, and burr cells are much more common on peripheral blood smears from neonates than on those from adults. There is a striking loss of surface area as neonatal red cells age[57] and this, along with cation loss and dehydration, creates a subpopulation of dense, poorly deformable, older cells destined for early destruction, contributing to the shortened life of the neonatal erythrocyte.[60] The neonatal erythrocyte exhibits decreased deformability, reflected in increased osmotic resistance, which normalizes by 4–6 weeks of age. The practical correlate of this observation is that osmotic fragility curves generated from control neonatal erythrocytes should be used when testing a neonate for hereditary spherocytosis (HS) (see below). The performance of osmotic fragility testing need only be delayed in cases when there is potential for confusion between HS and spherocytosis from other causes, e.g., ABO incompatibility.

Hereditary spherocytosis

The hallmark of this group of heterogeneous disorders is the presence of spherocytes on the peripheral blood smear.[61,62] Hemolysis is commonly accompanied by anemia of variable severity. Inheritance is autosomal dominant in two-thirds to three-quarters of patients. In the remainder, inheritance is autosomal recessive or due to a *de novo* mutation.[63–66] The incidence of HS is about 1 in 2500–4000 in northern European populations, but this is likely to be an underestimate as mild cases are often not diagnosed.[67] In other parts of the world, the disease is thought to be less common, although comprehensive population survey data are unavailable.

Clinical features

Anemia in HS may be absent, mild, moderate, or severe to the point of threatening life.[63] Patients with "typical" HS suffer from mild to moderate anemia.

• *Mildly affected individuals* exhibit no anemia, have modest reticulocytosis, and may not be detected until adolescence or adult life. They maintain normal hemoglobin levels in the face of accelerated erythrocyte destruction by virtue of an erythropoietin-driven increase in erythropoiesis.[68]

• *Moderately affected individuals* are more anemic, have higher reticulocyte counts and elevated serum bilirubin levels, may require occasional transfusions, and are usually detected in infancy or childhood. As noted in the earliest descriptions of HS, mild intermittent jaundice may be the only symptom of the disease. Splenomegaly develops in most patients, with the spleen occasionally reaching large dimensions.

• *Severely affected individuals* have marked hemolysis, anemia, hyperbilirubinemia, splenomegaly, and typically require regular red cell transfusions, particularly during infancy and early childhood.[63] Some of these infants present in the first few months of life with severe life-threatening hemolysis.[69] In the most severe cases, there is prenatal onset; hydrops fetalis and *in utero* demise may occur.[70] As in other chronic hemolytic anemias, exacerbations of anemia may be aplastic, hemolytic, or megaloblastic in origin.

• *Aplastic crisis* may occur as a result of transient marrow suppression by parvovirus B19 or other viral infections. Parvovirus B19 selectively infects erythroid precursors and inhibits their growth. The ensuing anemia, often severe, may be the first manifestation of HS. Multiple family members with undiagnosed HS who are infected with parvovirus have developed aplastic crises at the same time, leading to descriptions of "outbreaks" of HS. Infection with parvovirus is a particular danger to susceptible pregnant women because it can infect the fetus, leading to fetal anemia, hydrops fetalis, and fetal demise.

• *Increased hemolysis* may accompany viral illnesses, probably as a consequence of concomitant splenomegaly associated with the illness (the crucial role of the spleen in spherocyte destruction is discussed below).

• *Megaloblastic anemia* may be superimposed on the chronic hemolytic anemia of HS due to an unmet increased demand for folate to support erythropoiesis. This typically occurs in patients with increased folate demands, i.e., those recovering from an aplastic crisis, pregnant women, and the elderly. Megaloblastic crisis in pregnancy has been reported as the first manifestation of HS.

When detected in the neonatal period, HS is frequently accompanied by jaundice, requiring treatment with phototherapy or exchange transfusion.[63] This is thought to be due to coinheritance of Gilbert syndrome. In the neonatal period, spherocytosis on the peripheral blood smear and reticulocytosis are often minimal or even absent.[71]

Complications

A common complication is the formation of bilirubinate gallstones, found in at least half of adult patients with HS. Gallstones have been detected in infancy, but they are most likely to be found in older children and young adults.[72] The coinheritance of Gilbert syndrome markedly increases the risk for gallstones.[73,74] Because of their high incidence, HS patients should be periodically examined by ultrasound for the presence of gallstones, beginning early in childhood.

Rare complications or associations include leg ulcers and/or dermatitis that heal after splenectomy, gout, extramedullary hematopoietic tumors,[75,76] spinocerebellar degenerative syndromes, hypertrophic cardiomyopathy, and movement disorder with myopathy. A number of cases of HS and hematologic malignancy, including myeloproliferative disorders and leukemia, have been reported. It has been suggested that persistent hematopoietic stress predisposes to the development of these disorders.

Laboratory diagnosis

Many cases of HS are initially suspected because spherocytes are found on the peripheral blood smear in a patient with a family history of HS (Fig. 12.2). Spherocytes are a feature of many hemolytic anemias, so their identification on the peripheral blood smear alone is not sufficient to establish a diagnosis of HS (see below). Typical HS patients have obvious spherocytes lacking central pallor on peripheral blood smear. Less commonly, only a few spherocytes are present or, in severe cases, there are numerous small dense spherocytes and bizarre erythrocyte morphology with anisocytosis and poikilocytosis. Molecular studies have shown that specific morphologic findings are associated with certain membrane protein defects, such as "pincered" erythrocytes (band 3), spherocytic acanthocytes (β spectrin), or spherostomatocytes (protein 4.2) (Fig. 12.2).

Routine blood counts in HS reveal anemia and reticulocytosis to varying degrees, with most patients exhibiting mild to moderate anemia. Despite the increased percentage of reticulocytes with a larger volume than mature red cells, mean corpuscular volume (MCV) is normal or slightly low. The most helpful red cell index is mean corpuscular hemoglobin concentration (MCHC), which is usually elevated, reflecting red cell dehydration.[77] When combined with elevated red cell distribution width (RDW, > 14), an elevated MCHC (>35 g/dL) suggests the diagnosis of HS. In unsplenectomized children, MCHC > 35 g/dL and RDW > 14 has a sensitivity of 63% and specificity of 100% for the diagnosis of HS.[78] Measurement of MCV by light scatter analysis provides a histogram of MCHCs that has been claimed to identify nearly all patients with HS.

The reduced surface area–volume ratio characteristic of spherocytes increases their susceptibility to osmotic lysis in hypotonic solutions. This is the basis of the osmotic fragility test, in which red cells are suspended in buffered salt solutions of decreasing tonicity and the degree of hemolysis determined (Fig. 12.3). Incubation of blood specimens for 24 hours in the absence of metabolic substrate accentuates the osmotic fragility of spherocytes and makes easier the distinction of this disease from others. Surprisingly, even after incubation, up to 15% of samples have normal osmotic fragility.[77] The finding of increased osmotic fragility is not unique to HS and is also present in other conditions associated with spherocytosis. In nonsplenectomized HS subjects, a "tail" of the osmotic fragility curve may be present, indicating a subpopulation of particularly fragile red cells conditioned by splenic stasis. This subpopulation of cells disappears after splenectomy. The relative contributions of cell dehydration and surface area deficiency can be accurately determined by osmotic gradient ektacytometry, available only in specialized laboratories.[77]

Other tests used in the diagnosis of HS are not widely used (e.g., glycerol lysis test, pink test, hypertonic cryohemolysis, and skeleton gelation test). The former two tests, which employ glycerol to retard the osmotic swelling of red cells, are preferred in some laboratories because they are easy to

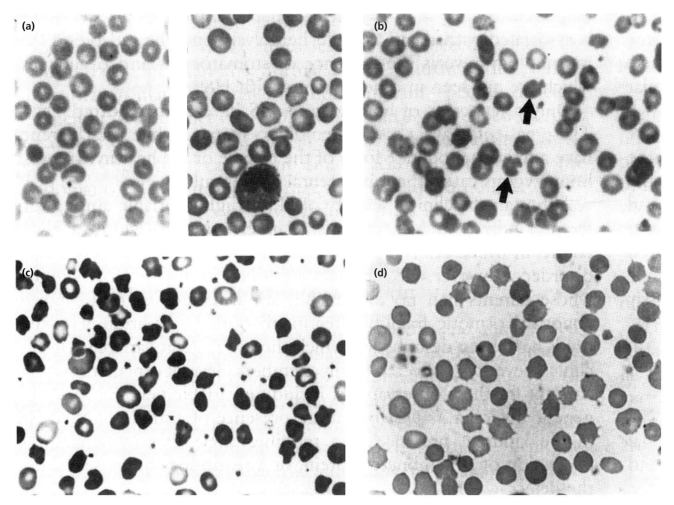

Fig. 12.2 Peripheral blood smears in hereditary spherocytosis (HS). (a) Two blood smears of typical moderately severe HS with a mild deficiency of red cell spectrin and ankyrin. Although many cells have spheroidal shape, some retain a central concavity. (b) HS with pincered red cells (arrows), as typically seen in HS associated with band 3 deficiency. Occasional spiculated red cells are also present. (c) Severe atypical HS due to severe combined spectrin and ankyrin deficiency. In addition to spherocytes, many cells have irregular contour. (d) HS with isolated spectrin deficiency due to a β-spectrin mutation. Some of the spherocytes have prominent surface projections resembling spheroacanthocytes. Reproduced with permission from Gallagher PG, Jarolim P. Red cell membrane disorders. In: Hoffman R, Benz EJ Jr, Shattil SJ *et al.* (eds) *Hematology: Basis Principles and Practice*, 4th edn. Philadelphia: WB Saunders, 2005, pp. 669–91.

perform and can be adapted to microsamples. Flow cytometric analysis of eosin-5-maleimide binding to erythrocytes, which reflects relative amounts of Rh-related integral membrane proteins and band 3, has recently been explored as a screening test for HS diagnosis.[79] Specialized testing, such as membrane protein quantitation, ektacytometry, and genetic analyses, are available for studying difficult cases or when additional information is desired.

Other laboratory manifestations in HS are markers of ongoing hemolysis. Reticulocytosis, increased bilirubin, increased lactate dehydrogenase, increased urinary and fecal urobilinogen, and decreased haptoglobin reflect increased erythrocyte production or destruction.

Differential diagnosis

Acquired immune hemolytic disease is the condition that most closely resembles HS. It can be ruled out by the absence of a family history of hemolytic anemia, the presence of a positive direct antiglobulin test or other manifestations of autoimmune disease, and a relative lack of exacerbation of hemolysis in the incubated osmotic fragility test. In the neonate, some cases of ABO incompatibility may be excluded by mother/infant blood group typing, and by a negative antiglobulin test of newborn red cells. Other diseases in which spherocytes may be seen, such as unstable hemoglobinopathies, glucose 6-phosphate dehydrogenase (G6PD) deficiency, microangiopathic hemolytic anemia, or clostridial sepsis, is distinguished from HS by differences in clinical course, red cell morphology, and clinical laboratory tests specific for each disease. The mechanism of spherocyte production is usually loss of membrane surface area in excess of loss of cell volume. Membrane loss may be secondary to oxidant injury, as in G6PD deficiency or hemoglobin H disease.

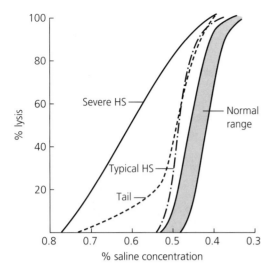

Fig. 12.3 Osmotic fragility curves in hereditary spherocytosis (HS). The shaded area is the normal range. Results representative of both typical and severe HS are shown. A "tail", representing very fragile erythrocytes that have been conditioned by the spleen, is common in many HS patients prior to splenectomy. Reproduced with permission from Dacie J. Hereditary spherocytosis. In: *The Haemolytic Anaemias*. Edinburgh: Churchill Livingstone, 1985, pp. 134–215.

In immune hemolytic anemia, interaction of membrane–antibody complexes with the reticuloendothelial system leads to membrane loss through phagocytosis. Venoms may contain phospholipases or other membrane-active enzymes that induce spherocyte formation. Various types of mechanical hemolytic anemia may generate spherocytes in the process of erythrocyte fragmentation. With the exception of autoimmune hemolytic anemia, spherocytes are rarely the sole or dominant morphologic abnormality noted in these conditions. Macrospherocytes may be seen when red cell water content is increased and the cell swells, as is the case in hereditary hydrocytosis.

Pathophysiology

The molecular basis of HS is heterogeneous and thus it is likely that the loss of membrane surface area is a consequence of several molecular mechanisms whose common denominator is a weakening of protein–protein interactions that link the membrane skeleton to the lipid bilayer, leading to microvesiculation, loss of membrane surface area, decreased surface area–volume ratio, and spherocytosis (Fig. 12.4). Defects of spectrin, ankyrin, or protein 4.2 lead to reduced density of the membrane skeleton, causing destabilization of the lipid bilayer with the resultant loss of band 3-containing microvesicles. Abnormalities of band 3 result in band 3 deficiency, leading to loss of the lipid-stabilizing effect of band 3 and releasing band 3-free microvesicles from the membrane. Both pathways ultimately result in the loss of membrane material with a reduction in membrane surface area. The ensuing decrease in membrane surface area with formation of spherocytes is paralleled by a decrease in erythrocyte deformability that predisposes the cells to splenic entrapment and conditioning.

The spleen plays a secondary, but important, role in the pathobiology of HS. Splenic destruction of abnormal erythrocytes with decreased deformability is the primary cause of hemolysis experienced by patients with HS.[80] Reticulocytes are not spherocytic, indicating that the spherocytic change in shape appears after reticulocyte maturation in the circulation.

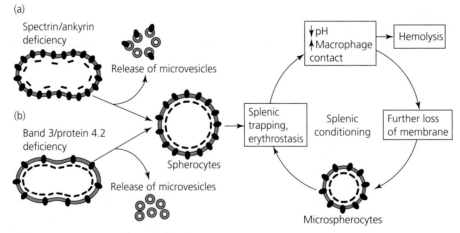

Fig. 12.4 Pathophysiology of hereditary spherocytosis. The primary defect in hereditary spherocytosis is a deficiency of membrane surface area. Decreased surface area may produced by two different mechanisms. (a) Defects of spectrin or ankyrin lead to reduced density of the membrane skeleton, destabilizing the overlying lipid bilayer and releasing band 3-containing microvesicles. (b) Defects of band 3 or protein 4.2 lead to band 3 deficiency and loss of its lipid-stabilizing effect. This results in the loss of band 3-free microvesicles. Both pathways result in membrane loss, decreased surface area, and formation of spherocytes with decreased deformability. These deformed erythrocytes become trapped in the hostile environment of the spleen where splenic conditioning inflicts further membrane damage, amplifying the cycle of red cell membrane injury. Reproduced with permission from Gallagher PG, Jarolim P. Red cell membrane disorders. In: Hoffman R, Benz EJ Jr, Shattil SJ *et al.* (eds) *Hematology: Basis Principles and Practice*, 3th edn. Philadelphia: WB Saunders, 2000, pp. 576–610.

Repeated passages through the splenic cords, a process termed "splenic conditioning", promotes membrane loss leading to a reduction in surface area–volume ratio and a progressively more spheroid red cell. Reflecting this process, red cells obtained from the splenic vein have greater osmotic fragility than those obtained from the splenic artery. The more spheroidal the red cell, the greater the likelihood that its lack of deformability will prevent its passage through the narrow fenestrations of the splenic cords. Some of these conditioned red cells reenter the systemic circulation, as revealed by the "tail" of the osmotic fragility curve (see Fig. 12.3), indicating the presence of a subpopulation of cells with markedly reduced surface area. After splenectomy, this red cell population disappears.

Detained in the fenestrations of the splenic sinuses, the red cell is subjected to an acidotic, metabolically unfavorable environment where oxidants are prevalent and phagocytic reticuloendothelial cells are ubiquitous. Secondary lesions, such as 2,3-diphosphoglycerate (2,3-DPG) depletion, occur in this setting. Nondeformable spherocytes accumulate in the red pulp, which becomes grossly enlarged. The central importance of the spleen in the production and destruction of spherocytes is most clearly seen when the spleen is removed surgically, for this procedure virtually eliminates hemolysis and anemia in moderately severe cases and eliminates the need for transfusion and partially corrects the anemia in severe cases.

Molecular genetics

HS is the clinical consequence of mutations in the genes encoding ankyrin, band 3, α and β spectrin, or protein 4.2.[81–83] The molecular basis of HS is heterogeneous and is frequently classified based on findings after quantitation of membrane proteins from HS patients. These abnormalities are combined deficiency of spectrin and ankyrin, isolated deficiency of spectrin, deficiency of band 3, and deficiency of protein 4.2[84]

Combined deficiency of spectrin and ankyrin

Combined spectrin and ankyrin deficiency is the most common abnormality of the erythrocyte membrane in approximately half to two-thirds of typical HS patients. Ankyrin is the primary binding site on the membrane for the spectrin-based membrane skeleton. Thus ankyrin deficiency leads to a proportional decrease in spectrin assembly on the membrane despite normal spectrin synthesis. Most ankyrin defects are private point mutations in the coding region of the ankyrin gene associated with decreased mRNA accumulation, i.e., deletion, frameshift, or nonsense mutations.[83,85] In some cases, mutations of the ankyrin promoter leading to decreased ankyrin expression have been found.[86] Approximately 15–20% of ankyrin gene mutations reported are *de novo* mutations.[66,87]

A few patients with atypical HS associated with karyotypic abnormalities involving deletions or translocations of the ankyrin gene locus on chromosome 8p have been described. Ankyrin deletions may be part of a contiguous gene syndrome, with manifestations of spherocytosis, mental retardation, typical facies, and hypogonadism.[88]

Isolated spectrin deficiency

The reported mutations of isolated spectrin deficiency include defects of both α and β spectrin. Since α spectrin is synthesized in excess and β-spectrin synthesis is rate limiting for membrane assembly of spectrin tetramer, it is not surprising that mutation of a single β-spectrin allele is sufficient to cause spherocytosis while both α-spectrin alleles must be affected for the same to occur.

Mutations of the β-spectrin gene have been identified in a number of patients with dominantly inherited HS associated with spectrin deficiency.[89,90] With rare exceptions, these mutations are private and are associated with decreased β-spectrin mRNA accumulation. β-Spectrin[Kissimmee], a point mutation located in the highly conserved region of β spectrin involved in the interaction with protein 4.1, is dysfunctional in its *in vitro* binding to protein 4.1 and thereby the linkage of spectrin to actin.[91]

In recessive HS associated with isolated spectrin deficiency, the defect involves α spectrin.[62,92,93] In normal erythroid cells, α spectrin is synthesized in large excess of β spectrin. Thus, subjects with one normal and one defective α-spectrin allele are expected to be asymptomatic, because α-spectrin production remains in excess of β-spectrin synthesis, allowing normal amounts of spectrin heterodimers to be assembled on the membrane. Patients who are homozygotes or compound heterozygotes for α-spectrin defects may suffer from severe HS.[94,95]

Deficiency of band 3

Deficiency of band 3 is found in a subset of HS patients who present with a phenotype of mild to moderate dominantly inherited HS with mushroom-shaped or "pincered" red cells. Most, if not all, of these patients also have concomitant protein 4.2 deficiency, and a reduction in red cell anion transport proportional to the band 3 deficiency. More than 50 different band 3 mutations associated with HS have been reported.[82] These mutations are spread throughout band 3 in both the cytoplasmic domain and the membrane-spanning domains. Many of these are frameshift or nonsense mutations associated with complete or near-complete absence of mutant allele mRNA in reticulocytes.[96,97] A number of band 3 missense mutations clustered in the membrane-spanning domain that replace highly conserved arginines have been described.[98] In these HS cases, the mutant band 3 most likely does not fold and insert into the endoplasmic reticulum and ultimately into the erythrocyte membrane after synthesis. Finally, alleles have been identified that influence band 3 expression and that, when inherited in *trans* to a band 3 mutation, aggravate band 3 deficiency and worsen the clinical severity of disease.[99]

Deficiency of protein 4.2

HS associated with isolated protein 4.2 deficiency is an autosomal recessive condition that is usually found in individuals of Japanese ancestry.[100] In these cases, an almost total absence of protein 4.2 from the erythrocyte membranes of homozygous patients is detected. Protein 4.2-deficient erythrocytes may also have a decreased content of ankyrin and band 3. Protein 4.2 deficiency also occurs in association with band 3 mutations, probably as a result of abnormal binding of protein 4.2 to the cytoplasmic domain of band 3.[101]

Treatment

Splenectomy cures or markedly improves the anemia in most patients with HS.[63,77,92] Even patients with severe HS exhibit significant clinical improvement, with the degree of spectrin deficiency in HS erythrocytes correlating with the response to splenectomy (Fig. 12.5). After splenectomy, erythrocyte lifespan normalizes, transfusion requirements are decreased or eliminated, and the risk of cholelithiasis is reduced. Reticulocyte counts fall to normal or near normal, spherocytosis and altered osmotic fragility persist, but the "tail" of the osmotic fragility curve, created by conditioning of a subpopulation of spherocytes by the spleen, disappears.

Laparoscopic splenectomy is now the surgical method of choice, resulting in less postoperative discomfort, quicker recovery time, shorter hospitalization, and decreased costs.[102,103] Even huge spleens can be removed laparoscopically.

The benefits of splenectomy must be balanced against the immediate and long-term risks of the procedure. Operative complications of splenectomy include local infection, bleeding, and pancreatitis. The most feared long-term complication of splenectomy is overwhelming sepsis, often fatal, with encapsulated bacteria, especially *Streptococcus pneumoniae*.[104] One review of 850 postsplenectomy HS cases comprising mostly infants and children found that 30 (3.52%) developed sepsis and 19 (2.23%) died of infection.[105] Another report of 226 splenectomized HS patients estimated the mortality from overwhelming sepsis to be 0.73 per 1000 years. The mortality rates for the 35 children who underwent splenectomy prior to 6 years of age and for the 191 individuals who were older than 6 at the time of splenectomy were 1.12 per 1000 and 0.66 per 1000 years of life after splenectomy, respectively, both far exceeding the rates in the general population.[104] These rates may overestimate the current risk of sepsis, since most of the participants underwent splenectomy prior to the introduction of the pneumococcal vaccine.

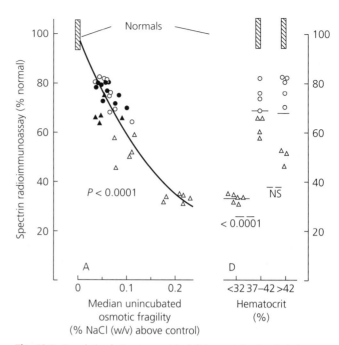

Fig. 12.5 Correlation between spectrin deficiency and unincubated osmotic fragility in hereditary spherocytosis (HS). Spectrin content, as measured by radioimmunoassay, is shown on the vertical axis and osmotic fragility, as measured by NaCl concentration producing 50% hemolysis of erythrocytes, is shown on the horizontal axis. Circles represent patients with typical autosomal dominant HS; triangles represent patients with atypical nondominant spherocytosis. Open symbols represent patients who have undergone splenectomy. The right panel shows the hematocrit of each patient at least 4 months post splenectomy. Reproduced with permission from Ref. 92.

The introduction of pneumococcal, *Haemophilus influenzae*, and meningococcal vaccines and the promotion of early antibiotic therapy for febrile children who have had a splenectomy have led to decreases in the incidence of overwhelming postsplenectomy infection.[106] Some recommend daily oral penicillin prophylaxis, although data to support this are lacking. Others advise having antibiotics available at home for immediate treatment of any significant fever. The emerging risk of penicillin-resistant pneumococcal infections requires vigilance and prompt selection of appropriate antibiotics in ill patients with suspected pneumococcal infection.

In the past, splenectomy was considered "routine" in HS patients. However, the risk of overwhelming postsplenectomy infection, the emergence of penicillin-resistant pneumococci, and growing recognition of increased risk of cardiovascular disease, particularly thrombosis and pulmonary hypertension, have led to reevaluation of the role of splenectomy in HS.[107,108] Recent HS management guidelines recognize these important considerations and recommend detailed discussion between health-care providers, patient, and family when splenectomy is considered.[109] For instance, splenectomy may pose special risks for individuals living in geographic regions where parasitic diseases such as

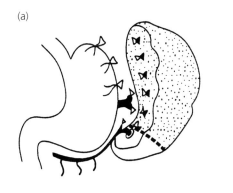
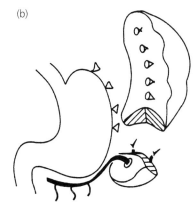

Fig. 12.6 Surgical technique used for partial (about 80%) splenectomy. (a) All vascular pedicles supplying the spleen are divided except those arising from the left gastroepiploic vessels. (b) The upper pole of the spleen is removed at the boundary between the well-perfused and poorly perfused tissue. Reproduced with permission from Tchernia G, Gauthier F, Mielot F *et al.* Initial assessment of the beneficial effect of partial splenectomy in hereditary spherocytosis. *Blood* 1993; **81**: 2014.

malaria or babesiosis occur. One approach is to splenectomize patients with severe hemolytic anemia and those suffering from significant signs or symptoms of anemia, including growth failure, skeletal changes, leg ulcers, and extramedullary hematopoietic tumors. Routine use of splenectomy in patients with moderate HS and compensated asymptomatic anemia is controversial. Patients with mild HS and compensated hemolysis can be followed carefully and referred for splenectomy if clinically indicated.

The higher risk of overwhelming sepsis in young children who undergo splenectomy makes it important to defer the operation until at least 6 years of age in all but the most severely affected patients. Recently, partial splenectomy via open laparotomy has been advocated for infants and young children with severe hemolysis and transfusion-dependent anemia (Fig. 12.6).[110–113] The goals of this procedure are to preserve the immunologic functions of the spleen while reducing the degree of splenic entrapment and destruction of spherocytic red cells and palliating hemolysis and anemia. Long-term data for this procedure are lacking. Rapid regrowth of the spleen may limit its effectiveness. In many cases, complete splenectomy is required, but hopefully at a time when the patients are considerably older and the risk of sepsis is less.

Supportive care with daily oral folic acid is warranted.

Hereditary elliptocytosis

The elliptocytosis syndromes are a heterogeneous group of hereditary erythrocyte disorders that have in common the presence of elongated, oval or elliptical cigar-shaped red cells on peripheral blood smear.[114] Inheritance is usually autosomal dominant. The incidence of elliptocytosis in the USA is not greater than 1 in 2000–4000,[115] but in malarial regions of Africa it may reach 1.6% of the population[116] and in malarial areas of Southeast Asia 30% or higher.

Clinical syndromes

Elliptocytic red cell morphology is the common denominator

in all but the clinically silent forms of this group of patients (Fig. 12.7). Hemolytic anemia ranges from absent to life-threatening. Severe hemolysis is usually a consequence of homozygosity or compound heterozygosity for spectrin self-association site mutations. The clinical features generally fall into one of the following categories as defined by Palek and Jarolim.[117]

Silent carrier

These individuals are clinically and hematologically normal, but usually have subtle defects in membrane skeletal properties that can be detected in the laboratory. The responsible mutation is most commonly the low-expression spectrin variant, α spectrin^{LELY} (see below), but occasionally one of the structural spectrin mutations usually associated with common hereditary elliptocytosis (HE) may be clinically silent. Silent carriers are usually only detected during analysis of pedigrees containing individuals with more clinically obvious forms of elliptocytosis.

Common hereditary elliptocytosis

This is the most frequent type of HE. Most patients are asymptomatic and come to medical attention only because of the presence of elliptocytes on the peripheral blood smear (Fig. 12.7). Transient hemolytic anemia with more striking morphologic abnormalities (schistocytes, fragments, budding forms, and microcytes) (Fig. 12.7) may be encountered during the neonatal period and infancy, but they usually evolve into typical asymptomatic HE throughout childhood. Episodic hemolysis and morphologic changes like those seen in transient neonatal poikilocytosis may also occur during acute or chronic illnesses characterized by reticuloendothelial hyperplasia,[118,119] vitamin B_{12} deficiency,[120–122] or altered microvasculature.[123] Rarely, common HE is associated with lifelong hemolysis. This usually implies the inheritance of an unusually severe spectrin mutation or coinheritance of a low-expression mutation that increases the relative amount of the mutant α-spectrin polypeptide. Homozygous or compound

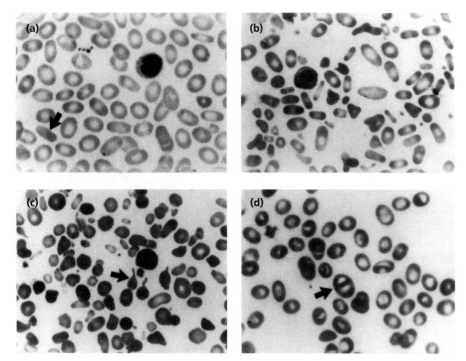

Fig. 12.7 Peripheral blood smears from subjects with various forms of hereditary elliptocytosis (HE). (a) Simple heterozygote with mild common HE associated with an elliptogenic spectrin mutation. Note predominant elliptocytosis with some rod-shaped cells (arrow) and virtual absence of poikilocytes. (b) "Homozygous" common HE due to doubly heterozygous state for two α-spectrin mutations. Both parents have mild HE. There are many elliptocytes as well as numerous fragments and poikilocytes. (c) Hereditary pyropoikilocytosis: the patient is a double heterozygote for mutant α spectrin and a defect characterized by reduced synthesis of this protein. Note prominent microspherocytosis, micropoikilocytosis, and fragmentation. Only a few elliptocytes are present. Some poikilocytes are in the process of budding (arrow). (d) Southeast Asian (Melanesian) ovalocytosis. The majority of cells are oval, some of them containing either a longitudinal slit or a transverse ridge (arrow). Reproduced with permission from Ref. 117.

heterozygous HE is also often associated with chronic hemolysis, which ranges from moderate to life-threatening and may be accompanied by splenomegaly and other findings of chronic hemolysis.

Hereditary pyropoikilocytosis

Hereditary pyropoikilocytosis (HPP) is the most severe of the elliptocytosis syndromes.[120,124] The hallmark of this disorder is that the red cells resemble those seen in burn patients and, indeed, are susceptible to budding and fragmentation on heating to 46°C, whereas normal red cells are unaffected at temperatures below 50°C.[117] It is now established that HPP represents a subtype of common HE, as evidenced by the coexistence of HE and HPP in the same family and by the presence of the same molecular defect of spectrin. Unlike patients with HE, HPP erythrocytes are also partially deficient in spectrin. In some HPP probands, one HE parent has a structural mutation of α-spectrin while the other parent is fully asymptomatic and has no detectable biochemical abnormality. The asymptomatic parent carries a silent "thalassemia-like" defect of spectrin synthesis, enhancing the relative expression of the spectrin mutant and leading to a superimposed spectrin deficiency in the HPP proband. Other HPP probands have inherited two structural mutations of spectrin from HE parents in a homozygous or compound heterozygous manner. The thermal instability of spectrin originally reported as diagnostic of HPP is not unique for this disorder; it is also found in the erythrocytes of some HE patients.

Hemolytic anemia usually first appears in the neonatal period and resembles the transient neonatal hemolysis described above in common HE infants. However, in HPP the morphologic abnormalities of the red cells (poikilocytes, spherocytes, fragmentation, and extreme microcytosis) (Fig. 12.7) and the hemolytic anemia is lifelong rather than transient. An abundance of microspherocytes and, often, a paucity of elliptocytes on the peripheral blood smear are features that distinguish HPP from the hemolytic forms of common HE. HPP patients develop splenomegaly, may require transfusions for episodes of anemia, and often require splenectomy. HPP is seen predominantly in black subjects, but it has also been diagnosed in Arabs and Caucasians.

Spherocytic elliptocytosis

Typically seen only in Caucasians, this is a dominantly inherited disorder producing mild-to-moderate hemolysis, splenomegaly, and red cells that range from spherocytes to elliptocytes. The elliptocytes are often few in number and fragmentation, budding and extreme microcytosis are absent, distinguishing spherocytic elliptocytosis from HPP and the other hemolytic forms of common HE.

Southeast Asian ovalocytosis

Common in New Guinea and other malaria-ridden regions of Southeast Asia, Southeast Asian ovalocytosis is a dominant asymptomatic condition that is thought to confer protection against *P. falciparum* infection.[125,126] The red cells are often described as stomatocytic elliptocytes and have a unique appearance on the peripheral blood smear (Fig. 12.7).

Heterozygotes are not anemic. The homozygous state has never been seen and is thought to be lethal *in utero*.[127]

Diagnosis

A careful inspection of the peripheral blood smear is the first step in identifying the various clinical forms of elliptocytosis. Red cell indices are normal in common HE, whereas profound microcytosis and and increased MCHC are features of HPP. Hematologic evaluation of the parents and siblings is usually helpful in defining the pattern of inheritance. Osmotic fragility is increased in HPP and homozygous common HE but normal in the less severe subtypes.[117]

Specialized testing, such as membrane protein quantitation, tryptic digestion of spectrin, spectrin self-association studies, ektacytometry, and genetic analyses, are available for studying difficult cases or when additional information is desired. Prenatal diagnosis has been accomplished by direct examination of fetal red cells and membrane proteins. If the specific mutation(s) present in the family is known, prenatal diagnosis by analysis of fetal DNA is also feasible.

Pathophysiology

Weakening of membrane skeleton protein interactions by mutations altering protein structure, function, or amount leads to diminished membrane mechanical stability and ultimately, in severe cases, to hemolysis. The α- and β-spectrin mutations near the αβ-spectrin heterodimer self-association region impair spectrin tetramer formation, while protein 4.1 or glycophorin deficiency affects spectrin–actin–protein 4.1 junctional complex formation and membrane attachment.

Elliptocytes form as the red cell matures, since immature red cells in the HE syndromes do not exhibit any morphologic abnormalities.[117] Acquisition of the elliptocytic shape is thought to be the result of the repeated episodes of elliptocytic deformation that all red cells experience during each circulatory cycle. Whereas normal red cells regain a discocytic configuration by a process of elastic recoil, HE red cells become locked into the elliptocytic configuration by disruption of the normally abundant interconnections between the membrane proteins.

The elliptocytic shape *per se* does not necessarily shorten the lifespan of the red cell. For example, Southeast Asian ovalocytes, despite being rigid cells with a membrane mechanical stability greater than normal, have a normal lifespan.[117] Although mechanical fragility is impaired, leading to fragmentation and microcytosis, intravascular hemolysis appears to play little role in red cell destruction since hemoglobinuria, hemoglobinemia, or hemosiderinuria are not features of hemolytic elliptocytosis. In fact, considerable hemolysis must occur within the spleen, since splenectomy usually reduces the hemolytic rate.

Alterations in the microcirculation or transient developmental factors present during fetal and early postnatal life can generate poikilocytosis and hemolysis in individuals with common HE. Transient neonatal poikilocytosis and hemolysis is thought to occur as a consequence of the high concentrations of fetal hemoglobin in neonatal red cells. Because fetal hemoglobin does not bind 2,3-DPG, large amounts of free 2,3-DPG are available in the neonatal red cell to interact with and destabilize the membrane skeleton.[128] In normal neonatal red cells this does not appear to have a discernible effect on red cell shape or survival, but in red cells whose membrane skeleton is weakened by an inherited defect, the sum of the effects of 2,3-DPG and the inherited defect is sufficient to decrease mechanical stability, producing poikilocytosis and hemolytic anemia. As fetal hemoglobin levels decline over the first few months of life, the contribution of 2,3-DPG to the hemolytic process wanes, hemolysis disappears, and poikilocytes are replaced by the elliptocytes characteristic of common HE.

Molecular genetics

The variable clinical severity of HE is a consequence of mutations in α or β spectrin, protein 4.1, glycophorin C, or band 3. These mutations lead to quantitative or qualitative defects in the mutant protein.[81,114]

Spectrin mutations

The most common defects in HE are mutations of α or β spectrin.[129,130] The side-to-side, antiparallel self-association of these proteins into a flexible rod-like αβ heterodimer forms the building block of the spectrin tetramer.[33,131] Spectrin heterodimers associate head to head to form spectrin tetramers, the major structural subunits of the membrane skeleton. Spectrin tetramers are interconnected into a two-dimensional lattice through binding, at their distal ends, to actin oligomers with the aid of protein 4.1 at the junctional complex.[132] Spectrin dimer–tetramer interconversion is governed by a simple thermodynamic equilibrium that under physiologic conditions strongly favors spectrin tetramers.[133,134] The contact site between the α- and β-spectrin chains of the opposed heterodimers is an atypical triple helical repeat in which one helix is contributed by the NH$_2$-terminus of α spectrin and two helices are contributed by the COOH-terminus of β-spectrin.

Most α-spectrin defects are at, or near, the NH$_2$-terminus of α spectrin involved in heterodimer self-association site, impairing self-association of spectrin into tetramers (Fig. 12.8).[129,135] Most α-spectrin mutations are point mutations.[130] These mutations create abnormal proteolytic cleavage sites that typically reside in the third helix of a repetitive segment and give rise to abnormal tryptic peptides on two-dimensional tryptic peptide maps of spectrin.

Elliptocytogenic β-spectrin mutations are COOH-terminal point mutations or truncations that disrupt the formation

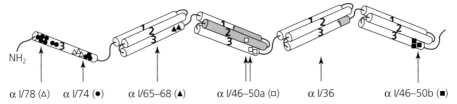

α I/78 ($\triangle$) α I/74 ($\bullet$) α I/65–68 ($\blacktriangle$) α I/46–50a ($\square$) α I/36 α I/46–50b ($\blacksquare$)

Fig. 12.8 A model of the spectrin self-association site: a triple helical model of the spectrin repeats that constitute the spectrin self-association site. The symbols denote positions of various genetic defects identified in patients with hereditary elliptocytosis or hereditary pyropoikilocytosis. Limited tryptic digestion of spectrin followed by two-dimensional gel electrophoresis identifies abnormal cleavage sites in spectrin associated with different mutations. These cleavage sites are denoted by arrows. Reproduced with permission from Gallagher PG, Tse WT, Forget BG. Clinical and molecular aspects of disorders of the erythrocyte membrane skeleton. *Semin Perinatol* 1990; **14**: 351.

of the combined β triple-helical repetitive segment and consequently the self-association of spectrin heterodimers to tetramers (Fig. 12.8).[129,130] All these mutations open a proteolytic cleavage site residing in the third helix of the combined repetitive segment, which gives rise to a 74-kDa αI peptide on tryptic peptide mapping of erythrocyte spectrin.

Although most spectrin mutations reside in the vicinity of the $\alpha\beta$-spectrin self-association site, a few mutations residing in the αII domain have been described. These mutations are asymptomatic in the simple heterozygous state but cause hemolytic anemia, which may be severe, in homozygous patients.[136–138]

The large number of α-spectrin mutations has allowed correlations to be established between clinical severity and the nature of the mutation. Mutations near the site of dimer–dimer self-association at the NH$_2$-terminus of α spectrin are the most likely to interfere with tetramer formation and lead to clinical symptoms. Another important determinant of clinical severity is the amount of mutant spectrin polypeptides present. In general, the greater the percentage of mutant spectrin, the more severe the clinical course. Variation in the amount of mutant spectrin found in members of a given pedigree is sometimes due to homozygous or heterozygous inheritance of the structural mutation, but more often it is due to the presence or absence of a low-expression α-spectrin mutation inherited in *trans* to a single mutant α-spectrin allele.

The commonest example of a low-expression allele is α-spectrin^{LELY}, which is present in 20–30% of α-spectrin alleles in the normal population.[139,140] The primary mutation, which is in intron 45, leads to variable splicing and loss of exon 46 in about half of the mRNA synthesized. α-Spectrin polypeptides lacking exon 46 sequences do not participate as avidly as do normal α-spectrin polypeptides in dimer and tetramer assembly and are therefore vulnerable to loss by proteolysis.[141] The ultimate effect of such a mutation is to reduce the quantity of α spectrin available for assembly into the membrane. Since more α than β spectrin is normally synthesized, a moderate reduction in α spectrin need not alter the number of $\alpha\beta$-spectrin dimers finally assembled into the membrane. It will, however have the effect of increasing the fraction

of α spectrin to the non-spectrin^{LELY} allele. If this allele bears a mutation that is associated with elliptocytosis, the greater quantity of the mutant spectrin in the membrane will usually be associated with greater clinical severity. In contrast, if the α-spectrin^{LELY} mutation is inherited in *cis* with an elliptocytic mutation, there will be a reduced quantity of the mutant spectrin in the membrane and a milder clinical picture.

Protein 4.1 mutations

Protein 4.1 mutations are a much less common cause of elliptocytosis than spectrin mutations. Protein 4.1 has several domains involved in protein–protein interactions, including a spectrin-binding domain where 4.1 binds to the distal end of the spectrin $\alpha\beta$ heterodimer, markedly increasing the binding of spectrin to oligomeric actin, and an NH$_2$-terminal domain, where 4.1 interacts with glycophorin C, phosphatidylinositol, and phosphatidylserine, facilitating the attachment of the distal end of spectrin to the membrane.[33,132] Studies of 4.1 mRNA from normal erythroid cells have revealed 4.1 isoforms resulting from complex tissue- and developmental stage-specific patterns of alternate mRNA splicing.[142–147] Alternate translation initiation sites are present in the protein 4.1 mRNA. When an upstream AUG is utilized, isoforms greater than 80 kDa are synthesized. During erythropoiesis, this upstream AUG is spliced out and a downstream AUG is utilized, leading to the production of the 80-kDa mature erythroid protein 4.1 isoform.[143]

Partial protein 4.1 deficiency is associated with mild dominant HE, while complete deficiency (a homozygous state) leads to severe hemolytic HE.[148,149] Homozygous 4.1(–) erythrocytes fragment more rapidly than normal at moderate shear stresses, an indication of their intrinsic instability.[121] Homozygous protein 4.1(–) erythrocytes also lack p55 and have only 30% of the normal content of glycophorin C. Electron microscopic studies of homozygous 4.1(–) erythrocyte membranes revealed a markedly disrupted skeletal network with disruption of the intramembrane particles, suggesting that protein 4.1 plays an important role in maintenance of not only the skeletal network but also the integral proteins of the membrane structure.[150]

Mutations associated with 4.1 deficiency have included a deletion that includes the exon encoding the erythroid transcription start site and mutations of the transcription initiation codon.[114] Qualitative defects of protein 4.1 include deletions and duplications of the exons encoding the spectrin-binding domain, leading to either truncated or elongated forms of protein 4.1.

Glycophorin C deficiency

Glycophorin C deficiency with elliptocytosis, the Leach phenotype,[151,152] is usually due to a large deletion of genomic DNA (~7 kb) that removes exons 3 and 4 from the GPC/GPD locus. In contrast to other forms of HE, which are dominantly inherited, heterozygous carriers are asymptomatic, with normal red blood cell morphology; homozygous subjects have no anemia and only mild elliptocytosis apparent on the peripheral blood film.[153] Glycophorin C-deficient subjects are also partially deficient in protein 4.1 and lack p55, presumably because these proteins form a complex and recruit or stabilize each other on the membrane.[154] It has been speculated that the protein 4.1 deficiency in Leach erythrocytes is the cause of the elliptocytic shape. In contrast, subjects deficient in glycophorin A, the major transmembrane glycoprotein, are asymptomatic.

Resistance to malaria

As is the case with other erythrocyte variants such as hemoglobinopathies, enzymopathies, and blood group antigens, alterations in red cell membrane structure that lead to elliptocytosis may provide resistance against malaria. This property has been attributed to diminished invasion, poor intraerythrocytic growth, or diminished cytoadherence of infected erythrocytes.[155] A high prevalence of HE in regions where malaria has been or is endemic, such as the approximately 1.6% incidence of common HE in inhabitants of Benin in West Africa, suggests positive evolutionary selection.[116,156] Convincing data are available for heterozygous Southeast Asian ovalocytosis, which in one study was found in approximately 15% of inhabitants of the Madang area of Papua New Guinea but in only 9% of those who had uncomplicated *P. falciparum* malaria, and in none of those with potentially life-threatening cerebral malaria.[157]

Treatment

Most cases of HE require no specific therapy. Supportive care measures such as supplemental folic acid or occasional red cell transfusions for episodes of anemia (usually related to infection) may be helpful. When hemolysis is severe, splenectomy may eliminate the need for regular red cell transfusions and improve the anemia. As in HS, the increased risk of bacterial infection following splenectomy in infancy or early childhood is a reason to wait until later childhood or adolescence before considering surgery.

Echinocytes and acanthocytes

Echinocytes and acanthocytes are types of spiculated red blood cells. Echinocytes have serrated edges over the entire surface of the cell and often appear crenated in a blood smear. Acanthocytes have only a few spicules of varying size that project from the cell surface at irregular intervals. They appear contracted and dense on stained peripheral blood smears. Wet preparations or scanning electron micrographs can be used to distinguish the two types of cells. Echinocytes can be produced *in vitro* by washing red cells in saline, by interactions between glass and red cells, and by insertion of amphipathic compounds that localize to the exterior leaflet of the lipid bilayer. High pH, ATP depletion, and Ca^{2+} accumulation can also cause echinocytosis. Echinocytes are seen in neonates and in patients with uremia, those who have defects in glycolytic metabolism, after splenectomy, and in some patients with microangiopathic hemolytic anemia. Acanthocytosis and echinocytes may be found in patients with liver damage, abetalipoproteinemia, unusual neurologic symptoms, anorexia nervosa, McLeod and In(Lu) blood groups, myelodysplasia, and hypothyroidism.

Abetalipoproteinemia

Progressive ataxia, atypical retinitis pigmentosa, a celiac syndrome, and acanthocytosis are the primary manifestations of abetalipoproteinemia.[158] Absorption of lipids through the intestine is defective, serum cholesterol levels are extremely low, and serum β lipoprotein is absent in this hereditary disease. The disease is due to failure to synthesize or secrete lipoprotein-containing products of the apolipoprotein B gene, the B apoproteins B100 and B48, or to defects in the microsomal triglyceride transfer protein, required for secretion of apoprotein B-containing lipoproteins.[159–161] A wide spectrum of clinical manifestations may be observed depending on the extent to which apolipoprotein B-mediated metabolic processes are affected. All patients have some degree of neurologic impairment and acanthocytes. The acanthocytic shape is not present in young erythrocytes but accumulates with cell aging. In severe cases, up to 50–90% of the erythrocytes are acanthocytes. Despite the profound morphologic abnormality, anemia may be absent or manifest as a very mild normocytic anemia with normal or slightly elevated reticulocyte counts.

In the abetalipoproteinemic acanthocytic erythrocyte, the outer leaflet of the red cell membrane is markedly enriched in sphingomyelin, mirroring the altered plasma lipid profile of these patients presumably due to lipid exchange. In contrast to the spur cell anemia of liver disease (see below), erythrocyte membrane cholesterol is normal or slightly increased. The molecular basis of the acanthocytic shape is unknown but is presumed to be due to an increase in surface area of the outer leaflet of the lipid bilayer relative to the inner leaflet.

Patients may become deficient in vitamin E due to fat malabsorption, rendering their acanthocytic red cells susceptible to hemolysis following *in vitro* incubation in dilute solutions of hydrogen peroxide. Whether vitamin E deficiency influences the various clinical manifestations of this disease is not known. However, children who have chronic liver disease and develop vitamin E deficiency have been reported to develop acanthocytosis as well as neurologic dysfunction. Retinal and neuromuscular abnormalities may be stabilized by the administration of vitamin E.

Chorea-acanthocytosis

This syndrome is characterized by acanthocytes, normolipoproteinemia, and progressive neurologic disease beginning in adolescence or adult life.[162] The neurologic manifestations are varied and include limb chorea, progressive orofacial dyskinesia, tongue-biting, muscle wasting, and hypotonia. The relationship between the red cell changes and neurologic manifestations is unclear. Recent cloning of the chorein gene and identification of mutations in affected patients have not significantly extended our understanding of the pathophysiology of this disorder.[2,163,164] Chorein does not belong to any known gene family.

Other neuroacanthocytosis syndromes

Neurocanthocytosis is the term applied to a group of disorders with great phenotypic and genetic heterogeneity.[165,166] In addition to the chorea-acanthocytosis syndrome described above and the X-linked McLeod syndrome described below, acanthocytosis is found in other neurodegenerative disorders including Huntington disease-like 2 and pantothenate kinase-associated neurodegeneration, formerly known as Hallervorden–Spatz syndrome and its allelic variant HARP syndrome (*h*ypobetalipoproteinemia, *a*canthocytosis, *r*etinitis pigmentosa, *p*allidal degeneration).[167–172] Variants of all these disorders have been found, including syndromes with chorea-acanthocytosis and myopathy and with chorea-acanthocytosis, spherocytosis and hemolysis. The etiology of the acanthocytic phenotype in these disorders is unknown. Further investigation of the precise defect in the red cell may provide insights into the pathophysiologic processes affecting the brain.

Miscellaneous disorders

A variety of additional disorders are associated with either acanthocytes or echinocytes.

Anorexia nervosa

Patients with anorexia nervosa may have acanthocytes on peripheral smear.[173] The mechanisms responsible have not been defined and considerable variation in the number of acanthocytes exists between patients. Anemia is rare and is usually hypoplastic and not hemolytic. It is accompanied by other cytopenias, attributed to malnutrition and starvation.

Liver disease

Patients with liver disease may develop either target cells or spur cells. Those with target cells have a reversible disorder primarily related to the increased unesterified cholesterol content of the plasma associated with lecithin-cholesterol acyltransferase (LCAT) inhibition (see below) and do not have hemolysis. In contrast, patients with advanced hepatocellular disease have 20–30% acanthocytes in their peripheral blood and moderate-to-severe hemolysis. Echinocytes and target cells may also be present. In contrast to target cells, where there is a proportionate increase in red cell cholesterol and phospholipid, in spur cells or acanthocytes associated with hepatocellular liver disease there is not only an increase in both cholesterol and phospholipid but a dramatic increase in the ratio of cholesterol to phospholipid. The precise impact of this imbalance of lipids on membrane properties and the profound hemolysis associated with this condition has not been determined. In addition to these quantitative lipid abnormalities, a defect in the remodeling of membrane phospholipids is present. To add additional complexity to the picture, some patients with advanced hepatocellular liver disease, particularly children, develop spur cells but do not have abnormalities in membrane lipids.

Vitamin E deficiency

Echinocytes and occasional acanthocytes are a feature of vitamin E deficiency. Previously noted in premature infants due to feeding of formulas with inadequate vitamin E content and very high polyunsaturated fatty acids, this condition is now limited to patients who have fat malabsorption, often related to liver disease, abetalipoproteinemia, or cystic fibrosis.[174] Parenteral administration of vitamin E will correct the deficiency in patients with impaired gastrointestinal absorption of this vitamin.

Blood group abnormalities

Acanthocytes have been associated with certain abnormalities of the blood group systems. In McLeod syndrome, an X-linked inherited anomaly of the Kell blood group system, red cells, leukocytes, or both cell types react poorly with Kell antisera but behave normally in other blood group reactions. Affected cells lack XK, a membrane protein that is linked to

Kell, a zinc endopeptidase that carries the Kell antigens.[175–177] Males have variable acanthocytosis (8–85%) and mild compensated hemolysis. Females have only occasional acanthocytes and very mild or no hemolysis. Some patients with McLeod syndrome develop a neuropathy or myopathy. Psychiatric symptoms, seizures, and peripheral neuropathy with muscle denervation have also been reported. The XK gene is less than 500 kb from the chronic granulomatous disease (CGD) locus. Thus some males with chromosomal deletions involving this region have both McLeod syndrome and CGD. It is important to identify these patients because if they are transfused, they may develop antibodies compatible only with McLeod red cells.

The commonest cause of the null Lutheran phenotype Lu(a–b–) is the presence of an inhibitor called In(Lu) that partially suppresses expression of Lu_a and Lu_b, rendering these antigens undetectable by standard agglutination tests. About 1 in 5000 individuals inherits this dominantly acting inhibitor. Patients with this inhibitor have normal, poikilocytic, or acanthocytic red cells but no hemolysis.

Uremia

Echinocytes are found in the blood smear of patients who develop uremia and hemolysis. These are secondary to an extra corpuscular factor that appears to affect red cell metabolism and results in elevated levels of intracellular calcium, a factor known to induce echinocytosis. Red cells from patients with uremia survive normally when infused into nonuremic recipients.

Other disorders

Approximately 50% of patients with hypothyroidism have a small number (0.5–2%) of acanthocytes on peripheral blood smears. Due to the high incidence of hypothyroidism relative to other disorders causing acanthocytosis, it has been suggested that thyroid testing be considered in patients with acanthocytosis.[178]

Target cells

Target cells are red cells that have an increased surface area–volume ratio. The redundant membrane creates what appears to be a hyperchromic bull's-eye in the center of the red cell when viewed on a stained peripheral blood smear. Target cells are generated either by increasing the membrane lipid content and thus the surface area or by decreasing cell volume. The latter is the consequence of decreased hemoglobin synthesis (thalassemia or iron deficiency), the presence of certain structural mutations of hemoglobin (S, C, D, E), or of primary disorders of cell hydration. Generally, an increase in membrane surface area does not affect red cell survival, while reduced volume from cellular dehydration or reduced hemoglobin synthesis often may.

Target cells are often seen in the peripheral blood smear of patients who have obstructive liver disease, reflecting a balanced increase in phospholipids and cholesterol.[179,180] Unesterified cholesterol in the plasma increases in concentration as a result of the inhibition of LCAT by bile salts. The central role of abnormal plasma lipids in the formation of target cells can be shown *in vitro* by incubation of normal red cells in plasma from patients with obstructive liver disease or, conversely, by incubating target cells in normal plasma. In the former situation, target cells are formed and in the latter they disappear. This is the basis for the observation that in patients with HS who develop temporary obstructive jaundice as a result of gallstones, the hemolytic process improves and osmotic fragility may become normal. In this setting, the increase in membrane surface area normalizes the previously abnormal surface area–volume ratio of spherocytes.

Target cells are also seen in hereditary LCAT deficiency, a rare disease due to a mutation in the LCAT gene.[181,182] Plasma unesterified cholesterol and phospholipid concentrations are increased. The disorder, which exhibits an autosomal recessive mode of inheritance, is characterized by anemia, corneal opacities, hyperlipemia, proteinuria, chronic nephritis, and premature atherosclerosis. A moderate normochromic normocytic anemia accompanied by prominent target cell formation and decreased red cell osmotic fragility is noted. Serum and red cell lipids are improved *in vivo* when LCAT is provided by infusions of normal plasma.

In the first few weeks following splenectomy, target cells appear, reaching levels of 2–10%. Like other target cells, membrane lipids are increased, osmotic fragility is decreased, and the mean surface area–volume ratio is increased.[117,183] The spleen normally removes excess membrane from red cells, a process called splenic conditioning. The exact mechanism responsible is not defined, although the reduction in red cell lipid content suggests that lipases may be involved. After splenectomy, red cells may eventually lose their excess lipid by conditioning in nonsplenic sites, gradually leading to the disappearance of target cells.

Disorders of hydration and cation transport

The hereditary stomatocytosis syndromes are a group of inherited disorders characterized by erythrocytes with a mouth-shaped (stoma) area of central pallor on peripheral blood smear (Fig. 12.9).[184–186] Stomatocytosis is associated with abnormalities in red cell hydration and cation transport that lead to changes in red cell volume, which may be either increased (hydrocytosis) or decreased (xerocytosis), or in some cases near normal. The pathobiology of the stomatocytic shape is poorly understood and the molecular basis

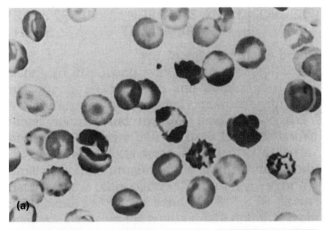

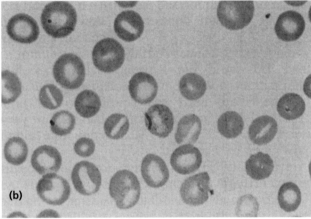

Fig. 12.9 Red cell morphology in disorders of cell hydration: (a) hereditary xerocytosis; (b) hereditary hydrocytosis. Reproduced with permission from Ref. 184.

of this group of disorders is unknown. Primary disorders of cellular metabolism or hemoglobinopathies may produce a secondary abnormality of cell hydration that contributes to the hemolytic process. This section focuses on the primary disorders of cell hydration.

Xerocytosis

Clinical features

The dehydrated stomatocytosis syndromes, also known as xerocytosis or dessicytosis, are characterized by contracted and spiculated red cells, variable numbers of stomatocytes, and target cells on peripheral blood smear.[185] Little or no anemia is usually found, although red cell lifespan may be considerably shortened.[187] Splenomegaly and other markers of chronic hemolysis are uncommon. Inheritance has usually been autosomal dominant. A clinical syndrome of xerocytosis, perinatal ascites, nonimmune hydrops fetalis, and pseudohyperkalemia has been described in several kindreds.[188, 189]

Laboratory findings

The hallmark of xerocytosis is red cell dehydration, which is most easily detected by examination of the red cell indices (high MCHC) or the osmotic fragility curve (increased osmotic resistance). These tests serve to separate xerocytosis from spherocytosis, where the MCHC may be elevated but osmotic fragility is usually increased. A simple test may reveal resistance of xerocytes to heat-induced budding and fragmentation.[190] Target cells and occasional bizarre red cells where the hemoglobin is puddled at each pole are seen on the peripheral blood smear (Fig. 12.9).[191] The reticulocyte count is often increased to a level higher than that expected for the degree of anemia. Ultimately, the diagnosis of xerocytosis depends on recognizing the abnormalities listed above and eliminating from consideration other diseases such as hemoglobinopathies or pyruvate kinase deficiency that may produce similar abnormalities.

Pathophysiology

The basic red cell abnormality in xerocytosis is passive loss of intracellular K^+ in excess of accumulation of intracellular Na^+, leading to a gradual decline in total intracellular cations and an obligate loss of cell water to maintain osmotic balance. Active transport of cations via the Na^+/K^+-ATPase pump does not restore cation homeostasis but rather exaggerates the defect, since the fixed stoichiometry of the pump (3 Na^+ out, 2 K^+ in) leads to a further net loss of cations from the cell.[192] A primary pathway for cellular dehydration in hemoglobinopathies (HbSS and HbSC disease) is volume-dependent KCl cotransport. This pathway has not been characterized extensively in xerocytes, but in one family there was evidence that it was abnormal.[193] The dehydrated xerocyte is rigid due to its increased cytoplasmic viscosity[194] and perhaps also to intrinsic membrane rigidity induced by complexing of globin to spectrin.[195] The rigidity of the xerocyte may contribute to its shortened lifespan by increasing its sensitivity to shear-induced hemolysis in the circulation.[196] Xerocytes resemble HS erythrocytes in their proclivity to vesiculation and loss of membrane surface area after metabolic depletion in vitro.[197] Like other dehydrated red cells, xerocytes are susceptible to injury by exogenous oxidants, a susceptibility that can be prevented by prior rehydration of the cells.[195,198]

The primary molecular event responsible for xerocytosis is unknown. The gene for xerocytosis has been mapped to 16q23–q24.[199] Isolated pseudohyperkalemia is allelic to xerocytosis and also shows linkage to this region.[199]

Treatment

No specific treatment is available or usually required. Splenectomy is of little or no benefit, and in some cases may be deleterious, predisposing to life-threatening thrombotic episodes (see below).

Hydrocytosis (stomatocytosis)

Clinical features

Mild-to-moderate lifelong hemolytic anemia, often accompanied by splenomegaly, jaundice, and other complications of hemolysis, are seen in hydrocytosis.[184,200] Some affected individuals develop evidence of iron overload, even in the absence of blood transfusions.[201] Hydrocytosis is a rare disorder but in informative pedigrees, inheritance has been autosomal dominant.[4,202–206]

Laboratory findings

As implied by the name, cell water is increased in hydrocytes, causing them to swell and appear on the peripheral blood smear as stomatocytes (Fig. 12.9). The swollen waterlogged cells can also be recognized by the unusually high MCV (often > 120 fL) and low MCHC seen in this condition. The osmotic fragility of hydrocytes is increased. Unlike normal red cells, hydrocytes are low in K^+ and high in Na^+. The total monovalent cation content (Na^+ and K^+) of hydrocytes is greater than that of normal red cells. Increased osmotic fragility is found in both hydrocytosis and HS, but the two disorders are easily distinguished on the basis of their morphology, red cell indices, and red cell monovalent cation content.

Pathophysiology

Like xerocytosis, hydrocytosis is caused by an abnormality in passive monovalent cation flux. The dominant abnormality is increased passive influx of Na^+, which is not matched by an equivalent outflow of K^+. Active cation transport by the Na^+/K^+-ATPase pump, although greatly increased, is unable to prevent the accumulation of intracellular Na^+ and the resulting increase in monovalent cation content causes osmotic movement of water into the cell, cell swelling, and transformation from diskocyte to stomatocyte morphology. Metabolic depletion, by preventing ATP generation for the Na^+/K^+-ATPase pump, inhibits active transport of Na^+ out of the cell and accelerates water accumulation and cell swelling. The favorable effect of splenectomy on the rate of hemolysis is most likely due to removal of the organ where metabolic depletion of red cells is most likely to occur.

The molecular basis for hydrocytosis is not known. Red cells from many patients lack or are deficient in stomatin, an integral membrane protein also present in lipid rafts. The precise function of stomatin is unknown but it has been hypothesized to be involved in lipid rafts of the plasma membrane and a multimeric signaling complex of the actin cytoskeleton, mechanosensation, nociception, and a membrane-bound proteolytic process. Mutations have not been found in stomatin cDNA from patients with hydrocytosis and the stomatin mRNA content of reticulocytes is normal.[207] A stomatin knockout mouse had no erythroid phenotype.[208] A homozygous stomatin mutation has been described in a child with severe multisystem disease with a dyserythropoietic, sideroblastic erythroid, not hydrocytosis, phenotype.[209]

Cryohydrocytosis, another condition associated with abnormal cation transport and overhydrated red cells, is distinguished from hydrocytosis by the profound increase in cation permeability that occurs *in vitro* at low temperature (4°C).[210] A similar susceptibility to cold-induced cation permeability in which K^+ loss predominates and xerocytes instead of hydrocytes are present has also been described.

Treatment

Splenectomy may decrease the hemolytic rate[6,211] but is to be avoided if possible because of an unusually high risk of serious thrombotic complications and chronic pulmonary hypertension after splenectomy.[200] This has been attributed to increased erythrocyte–endothelial cell adhesion due to erythrocyte phosphatidylserine exposure.[212,213] Fortunately, the majority of patients are able to maintain an adequate hemoglobin level, so that splenectomy is not required.

Other disorders with stomatocytosis

Hydrocytosis and xerocytosis represent the extremes of a spectrum of red cell permeability defects. Patients with features of both conditions have been reported, with variability in the severity of permeability defects, stomatin deficiency, hemolysis, anemia, and numbers of stomatocytes.[185,186,210,214] These patients have been categorized as "intermediate" syndromes. These observations suggest that hereditary stomatocytosis is a complex collection of syndromes caused by various molecular defects. As detailed below, in some cases these defects have been elucidated.

Rh deficiency syndrome

Stomatocytosis is also present on peripheral blood smears of patients with Rh deficiency syndrome. Erythrocytes from these rare individuals have either absent (Rh_{null}) or markedly reduced (Rh_{mod}) Rh antigen expression. There is mild to moderate hemolytic anemia. Rh proteins are part of a multiprotein complex that includes two Rh proteins and two Rh-associated glycoproteins (RhAG).[215] Other proteins that associate with this complex include CD47, LW, glycophorin B, and protein 4.2.[216,217] The Rh–RhAG complex interacts with ankyrin to link the membrane skeleton to the lipid bilayer.

Rh_{null} erythrocytes have increased osmotic fragility, reflecting dehydration and reduced membrane surface area. K^+

transport and Na^+/K^+ pump activity are increased, possibly because of reticulocytosis. Phospholipid asymmetry is also altered. Though the clinical syndromes are the same, the genetic basis of the Rh deficiency syndrome is heterogeneous, and at least two groups have been defined. The "amorph" type is due to defects involving the *RH30* locus encoding the RhD and RhE polypeptides.[218,219] The "regulatory" type of Rh_{null} and Rh_{mod} phenotypes results from suppressor or "modifier" mutations at the *RH50* locus. When one chain of the Rh–RhAG complex is absent, the complex is either not transported to the membrane or is assembled at the membrane.

Familial deficiency of high-density lipoproteins

Familial deficiency of high-density lipoproteins leads to accumulation of cholesteryl esters in many tissues. Hematologic manifestations include a moderately hemolytic anemia with stomatocytosis. Erythrocyte membranes have low free cholesterol content, leading to a decreased cholesterol/phospholipid ratio and a relative increase in phosphatidylcholine.

Sitosterolemia

Sitosterolemia is a recessively inherited condition associated with early-onset xanthomatosis, atherosclerosis, and elevated plasma levels of plant sterols. Defects in the ABCG5 or ABCG8 cotransporters lead to increased intestinal absorption and decreased biliary elimination of all sterols, particularly plant sterols. Hematologically, the patients present with macrothrombocytopenia and a stomatocytic hemolytic anemia.[218,219]

Acquired stomatocytosis

Stomatocytes have been found in several acquired conditions, including neoplasms, cardiovascular and hepatobiliary disease, alcoholism, and therapy with drugs, some of which are known to be stomatocytogenic *in vitro*. Sometimes, the percentage of stomatocytes on the peripheral blood smear may approach 100%. However, the clinical significance of these findings is unclear.

References

1. Op den Kamp JA. Lipid asymmetry in membranes. *Annu Rev Biochem* 1979; **48**: 47–71.
2. Dobson-Stone C, Danek A, Rampoldi L *et al*. Mutational spectrum of the CHAC gene in patients with chorea-acanthocytosis. *Eur J Hum Genet* 2002; **10**: 773–81.
3. Sweeley CC, Dawson G. Lipids of the erythrocyte membrane In: Jamieson GA, Greenwalt TJ (eds) *Red Cell Membrane Structure and Function*. Philadelphia: JB Lippincott, 1969, pp. 172–227.
4. Van Deenen LL, DeGier J. Lipids of the red blood cell membranes. In: Surgenor DM (ed.) *The Red Blood Cell*. New York: Academic Press, 1974, p. 148.
5. Bevers EM, Comfurius P, Dekkers DW *et al*. Transmembrane phospholipid distribution in blood cells: control mechanisms and pathophysiological significance. *Biol Chem* 1998; **379**: 973–86.
6. Lubin BH, Kuypers FA. Phospholipid repair in human erythrocytes. In: Davies KJ (ed.) *Oxidative Damage and Repair: Chemical, Biological, and Medical Aspects*. New York: Pergamon Press, 1991, pp. 557–64.
7. Berridge MJ. Inositol trisphosphate and calcium signalling. *Nature* 1993; **361**: 315–25.
8. Hogan A, Yakubchyk Y, Chabot J *et al*. The phosphoinositol 3,4-bisphosphate-binding protein TAPP1 interacts with syntrophins and regulates actin cytoskeletal organization. *J Biol Chem* 2004; **279**: 53717–24.
9. Devaux PF, Morris R. Transmembrane asymmetry and lateral domains in biological membranes. *Traffic* 2004; **5**: 241–6.
10. Test ST, Woolworth VS. Defective regulation of complement by the sickle erythrocyte: evidence for a defect in control of membrane attack complex formation. *Blood* 1994; **83**: 842–52.
11. Balasubramanian K, Schroit AJ. Aminophospholipid asymmetry: a matter of life and death. *Annu Rev Physiol* 2003; **65**: 701–34.
12. Devaux PF. Lipid transmembrane asymmetry and flip-flop in biological membranes and in lipid bilayers. *Curr Opin Struct Biol* 1993; **3**: 489–94.
13. Borisenko GG *et al*. Macrophage recognition of externalized phosphatidylserine and phagocytosis of apoptotic Jurkat cells: existence of a threshold. *Arch Biochem Biophys* 2003; **413**: 41–52.
14. Eldor A, Rachmilewitz EA. The hypercoagulable state in thalassemia. *Blood* 2002; **99**: 36–43.
15. Kuypers FA, de Jong K. The role of phosphatidylserine in recognition and removal of erythrocytes. *Cell Mol Biol* 2004; **50**: 147–58.
16. Williamson P, Schlegel RA. Transbilayer phospholipid movement and the clearance of apoptotic cells. *Biochim Biophys Acta* 2002; **1585**: 53–63.
17. Yasin Z, Witting S, Palascak MB *et al*. Phosphatidylserine externalization in sickle red blood cells: associations with cell age, density, and hemoglobin F. *Blood* 2003; **102**: 365–70.
18. Daleke DL. Regulation of transbilayer plasma membrane phospholipid asymmetry. *J Lipid Res* 203; **44**: 233–42.
19. Daleke DL, Lyles JV. Identification and purification of aminophospholipid flippases. *Biochim Biophys Acta* 2000; **1486**: 108–27.
20. Sims PJ, Wiedmer T. Unraveling the mysteries of phospholipid scrambling. *Thromb Haemost* 2001; **86**: 266–75.
21. Zhou Q, Zhao J, Stout JG *et al*. Molecular cloning of human plasma membrane phospholipid scramblase. A protein mediating transbilayer movement of plasma membrane phospholipids. *J Biol Chem* 1997; **272**: 18240–4.
22. Ohvo-Rekila H, Ramstedt B, Leppimaki P *et al*. Cholesterol interactions with phospholipids in membranes. *Prog Lipid Res* 2002; **41**: 66–97.
23. Sheetz MP, Singer SJ. Biological membranes as bilayer couples. A molecular mechanism of drug–erythrocyte interactions. *Proc Natl Acad Sci USA* 1974; **71**: 4457–61.
24. Holthuis JC, van Meer G, Huitema K. Lipid microdomains,

lipid translocation and the organization of intracellular membrane transport. *Mol Membr Biol* 2003; **20**: 231–41.

25. Koumanov KS, Wolf C, Quinn PJ. Lipid composition of membrane domains. *Subcell Biochem* 2004; **37**: 153–63.

26. Salzer U, Prohaska R. Stomatin, flotillin-1, and flotillin-2 are major integral proteins of erythrocyte lipid rafts. *Blood* 2001; **97**: 1141–3.

27. Hiller NL, Akompong T, Marrow JS *et al.* Identification of a stomatin orthologue in vacuoles induced in human erythrocytes by malaria parasites. A role for microbial raft proteins in apicomplexan vacuole biogenesis. *J Biol Chem* 2003; **278**: 48413–21.

28. Murphy SC, Samuel BU, Harrison T, Speicher KD *et al.* Erythrocyte detergent-resistant membrane proteins: their characterization and selective uptake during malarial infection. *Blood* 2004; **103**: 1920–8.

29. Samuel BU, Mohandas N, Harrison T *et al.* The role of cholesterol and glycosylphosphatidylinositol-anchored proteins of erythrocyte rafts in regulating raft protein content and malarial infection. *J Biol Chem* 2001; **276**: 29319–29.

30. Shohet SB, Nathan DG, Karnovsky ML. Stages in the incorporation of fatty acids into red blood cells. *J Clin Invest* 1968; **47**: 1096–108.

31. Farquhar JW, Ahrens EH Jr. Effects of dietary fats on human erythrocyte fatty acid patterns. *J Clin Invest* 1963; **42**: 675–85.

32. Alper SL, Darman RB, Chernova MN *et al.* The AE gene family of Cl/HCO_3^- exchangers. *J Nephrol* 2002; **15** (suppl. 5): S41–S53.

33. Morrow JS, Rimm DL, Kennedy SP *et al.* Of membrane stability and mosaics: the spectrin cytoskeleton. In: Hoffman J, Jamieson J (eds) *Handbook of Physiology.* London: Oxford, University Press, 1997, pp. 485–540.

34. Tanner MJ. Band 3 anion exchanger and its involvement in erythrocyte and kidney disorders. *Curr Opin Hematol* 2002; **9**: 133–9.

35. Cartron JP, Le Van Kim C, Colin Y. Glycophorin C and related glycoproteins: structure, function, and regulation. *Semin Hematol* 1993; **30**: 152–68.

36. Bruce LJ, Beckmann R, Ribeiro ML *et al.* A band 3–based macrocomplex of integral and peripheral proteins in the RBC membrane. *Blood* 2003; **101**: 4180–8.

37. Kanki T, Young MT, Sakaguchi M *et al.* The N-terminal region of the transmembrane domain of human erythrocyte band 3. Residues critical for membrane insertion and transport activity. *J Biol Chem* 2003; **278**: 5564–73.

38. Dias BG *et al.* Differential regulation of brain derived neurotrophic factor transcripts by antidepressant treatments in the adult rat brain. *Neuropharmacology* 2003; **45**: 553–63.

39. Discher DE. New insights into erythrocyte membrane organization and microelasticity. *Curr Opin Hematol* 2000; **7**: 117–22.

40. Discher DE, Carl P. New insights into red cell network structure, elasticity, and spectrin unfolding: a current review. *Cell Mol Biol Lett* 2001; **6**: 593–606.

41. Mohler PJ, Bennett V. Defects in ankyrin-based cellular pathways in metazoan physiology. *Front Biosci* 2005; **10**: 2832–40.

42. Cohen CM, Dotimas E, Korsgren C. Human erythrocyte membrane protein band 4.2 (pallidin). *Semin Hematol* 1993; **30**: 119–37.

43. Gilligan DM, Bennett V. The junctional complex of the membrane skeleton. *Semin Hematol* 1993; **30**: 74–83.

44. Conboy JG. Structure, function, and molecular genetics of erythroid membrane skeletal protein 4.1 in normal and abnormal red blood cells. *Semin Hematol* 1993; **30**: 58–73.

45. Hanspal M, Palek J. Biogenesis of normal and abnormal red blood cell membrane skeleton. *Semin Hematol* 1992; **29**: 305–19.

46. Peters LL, Shivdasani RA, Liu SC *et al.* Anion exchanger 1 (band 3) is required to prevent erythrocyte membrane surface loss but not to form the membrane skeleton. *Cell* 1996; **86**: 917–27.

47. Lee JC, Discher DE. Deformation-enhanced fluctuations in the red cell skeleton with theoretical relations to elasticity, connectivity, and spectrin unfolding. *Biophys J* 2001; **81**: 3178–92.

48. Mohandas N, Chasis JA. Red blood cell deformability, membrane material properties and shape: regulation by transmembrane, skeletal and cytosolic proteins and lipids. *Semin Hematol* 1993; **30**: 171–92.

49. Bookchin RM, Lew VL. Sickle red cell dehydration: mechanisms and interventions. *Curr Opin Hematol* 2002; **9**: 107–10.

50. Ellory JC, Gibson JS, Stewart GW. Pathophysiology of abnormal cell volume in human red cells. *Contrib Nephrol* 1998; **123**: 220–39.

51. Brugnara C. Erythrocyte membrane transport physiology. *Curr Opin Hematol* 1997; **4**: 122–7.

52. Jorgensen PL, Hakansson KO, Karlish SJ. Structure and mechanism of Na,K-ATPase: functional sites and their interactions. *Annu Rev Physiol* 2003; **65**: 817–49.

53. Maher AD, Kuchel PW. The Gardos channel: a review of the Ca^{2+}-activated K^+ channel in human erythrocytes. *Int J Biochem Cell Biol* 2003; **35**: 1182–97.

54. Adragna NC, Fulvio MD, Lauf PK. Regulation of K-Cl cotransport: from function to genes. *J Membr Biol* 2004; **201**: 109–37.

55. Brugnara C. Sickle cell disease: from membrane pathophysiology to novel therapies for prevention of erythrocyte dehydration. *J Pediatr Hematol Oncol* 2003; **25**: 927–33.

56. Matovcik LM, Mentzer WC. The membrane of the human neonatal red cell. *Clin Haematol* 1985; **14**: 203–21.

57. Matovcik LM, Chiu D, Lubin B *et al.* The aging process of human neonatal erythrocytes. *Pediatr Res* 1986; **20**: 1091–6.

58. Matovcik LM, Groschel-Stewart U, Schrier SL. Myosin in adult and neonatal human erythrocyte membranes. *Blood* 1986; **67**: 1668–74.

59. Agre P, Smith BL, Baumgarten R *et al.* Human red cell Aquaporin CHIP. II. Expression during normal fetal development and in a novel form of congenital dyserythropoietic anemia. *J Clin Invest* 1994; **94**: 1050–8.

60. Lane PA, Galili U, Iarocci TA *et al.* Cellular dehydration and immunoglobulin binding in senescent neonatal erythrocytes. *Pediatr Res* 1988; **23**: 288–92.

61. Eber S, Lux SE. Hereditary spherocytosis: defects in proteins that connect the membrane skeleton to the lipid bilayer. *Semin Hematol* 2004; **41**: 118–41.

62. Tse WT, Gallagher PG, Jenkins PB *et al.* Amino-acid

substitution in alpha-spectrin commonly coinherited with nondominant hereditary spherocytosis. *Am J Hematol* 1997; **54**: 233–41.

63. Eber SW, Armbrust R, Schroter W. Variable clinical severity of hereditary spherocytosis: relation to erythrocytic spectrin concentration, osmotic fragility, and autohemolysis. *J Pediatr* 1990; **117**: 409–16.

64. Miraglia del Giudice E, Hayette S, Bozon M *et al*. Ankyrin Napoli: a de novo deletional frameshift mutation in exon 16 of ankyrin gene (ANK1) associated with spherocytosis. *Br J Haematol* 1996; **93**: 828–34.

65. Morle L, Bozon M, Alloisio N *et al*. Ankyrin Bugey: a de novo deletional frameshift variant in exon 6 of the ankyrin gene associated with spherocytosis. *Am J Hematol* 1997; **54**: 242–8.

66. Randon J, Miraglia del Giudice E, Bozon, M *et al*. Frequent de novo mutations of the ANK1 gene mimic a recessive mode of transmission in hereditary spherocytosis: three new ANK1 variants: ankyrins Bari Napoli II and Anzio. *Br J Haematol* 1997; **96**: 500–6.

67. Eber SW, Pekrun A, Neufeldt A *et al*. Prevalence of increased osmotic fragility of erythrocytes in German blood donors: screening using a modified glycerol lysis test. *Ann Hematol* 1992; **64**: 88–92.

68. Guarnone R, Centenara E, Schischmanoff PO *et al*. Erythropoietin production and erythropoiesis in compensated and anaemic states of hereditary spherocytosis. *Br J Haematol* 1996; **92**: 150–4.

69. Delhommeau F, Cynober T, Schischmanoff PO *et al*. Natural history of hereditary spherocytosis during the first year of life. *Blood* 2000; **95**: 393–7.

70. Whitfield CF, Follweiler JB, Lopresti-Morrow L *et al*. Deficiency of alpha-spectrin synthesis in burst-forming units-erythroid in lethal hereditary spherocytosis. *Blood* 1991; **78**: 3043–51.

71. Schroter W, Kahsnitz E. Diagnosis of hereditary spherocytosis in newborn infants. *J Pediatr* 1983; **103**: 460–3.

72. Tamary H, Aviner S, Freud E *et al*. High incidence of early cholelithiasis detected by ultrasonography in children and young adults with hereditary spherocytosis. *J Pediatr Hematol Oncol* 2003; **25**: 952–4.

73. del Giudice EM, Perrotta S, Nobili B *et al*. Coinheritance of Gilbert syndrome increases the risk for developing gallstones in patients with hereditary spherocytosis. *Blood* 1999; **94**: 2259–62.

74. Economou M, Tsatra I, Athanassiou-Metaxa M. Simultaneous presence of Gilbert syndrome and hereditary spherocytosis: interaction in the pathogenesis of hyperbilirubinemia and gallstone formation. *Pediatr Hematol Oncol* 2003; **20**: 493–5.

75. Bastion Y, Coiffier B, Felman P *et al*. Massive mediastinal extramedullary hematopoiesis in hereditary spherocytosis: a case report. *Am J Hematol* 1990; **35**: 263–5.

76. Giraldi S, Abbage KT, Marinoni LP *et al*. Leg ulcer in hereditary spherocytosis. *Pediatr Dermatol* 2003; **20**: 427–8.

77. Cynober T, Mohandas N, Tchernia G. Red cell abnormalities in hereditary spherocytosis: relevance to diagnosis and understanding of the variable expression of clinical severity. *J Lab Clin Med* 1996; **128**: 259–69.

78. Michaels LA, Cohen AR, Zhao H *et al*. Screening for hereditary spherocytosis by use of automated erythrocyte indexes. *J Pediatr* 1997; **130**: 957–60.

79. King MJ, Smythe JS, Mushens R. Eosin-5-maleimide binding to band 3 and Rh-related proteins forms the basis of a screening test for hereditary spherocytosis. *Br J Haematol* 2004; **124**: 106–13.

80. Reliene R, Mariani M, Zanella A *et al*. Splenectomy prolongs in vivo survival of erythrocytes differently in spectrin/ankyrin- and band 3-deficient hereditary spherocytosis. *Blood* 2002; **100**: 2208–15.

81. Gallagher PG. Update on the clinical spectrum and genetics of red blood cell membrane disorders. *Curr Hematol Rep* 2004; **3**: 85–91.

82. Gallagher PG, Forget BG. Hematologically important mutations: band 3 and protein 4.2 variants in hereditary spherocytosis. *Blood Cells Mol Dis* 1997; **23**: 417–21.

83. Gallagher PG, Forget BG. Hematologically important mutations: spectrin and ankyrin variants in hereditary spherocytosis. *Blood Cells Mol Dis* 1998; **24**: 539–43.

84. Savvides P, Shalev O, John KM *et al*. Combined spectrin and ankyrin deficiency is common in autosomal dominant hereditary spherocytosis. *Blood* 1993; **82**: 2953–60.

85. Eber SW, Gonzalez JM, Lux ML *et al*. Ankyrin-1 mutations are a major cause of dominant and recessive hereditary spherocytosis. *Nat Genet* 1996; **13**: 214–18.

86. Gallagher PG, Sabatino DE, Basseres DS *et al*. Erythrocyte ankyrin promoter mutations associated with recessive hereditary spherocytosis cause significant abnormalities in ankyrin expression. *J Biol Chem* 2001; **276**: 41683–9.

87. Miraglia del Giudice E, Francese M, Nobili B *et al*. High frequency of de novo mutations in ankyrin gene (ANK1) in children with hereditary spherocytosis. *J Pediatr* 1998; **132**: 117–20.

88. Lux SE, Tse WT, Menninger JC *et al*. Hereditary spherocytosis associated with deletion of human erythrocyte ankyrin gene on chromosome 8. *Nature* 1990; **345**: 736–9.

89. Garbarz M, Galand C, Bibas D *et al*. A 5' splice region G→C mutation in exon 3 of the human beta-spectrin gene leads to decreased levels of beta-spectrin mRNA and is responsible for dominant hereditary spherocytosis (spectrin Guemene-Penfao). *Br J Haematol* 1998; **100**: 90–8.

90. Hassoun H, Vassiliadis JN, Murray J *et al*. Characterization of the underlying molecular defect in hereditary spherocytosis associated with spectrin deficiency. *Blood* 1997; **90**: 398–406.

91. Becker PS, Tse WT, Lux SE *et al*. Beta spectrin Kissimmee: a spectrin variant associated with autosomal dominant hereditary spherocytosis and defective binding to protein 4.1. *J Clin Invest* 1993; **92**: 612–16.

92. Agre P, Asimos A, Casella JF *et al*. Inheritance pattern and clinical response to splenectomy as a reflection of erythrocyte spectrin deficiency in hereditary spherocytosis. *N Engl J Med* 1986; **315**: 1579–83.

93. Agre P, Orringer EP, Bennett V. Deficient red-cell spectrin in severe, recessively inherited spherocytosis. *N Engl J Med* 1982; **306**: 1155–61.

94. Wichterle H, Hanspal M, Palek J *et al*. Combination of two mutant alpha spectrin alleles underlies a severe spherocytic hemolytic anemia. *J Clin Invest* 1996; **98**: 2300–7.

95. Delaunay J, Nouyrigat V, Proust A *et al*. Different impacts of alleles α^{LEPRA} and α^{LELY} as assessed versus a novel, virtually null allele of the SPTA1 gene in *trans*. *Br J Haematol* 2004; **127**: 118–22.

96. Jarolim P, Murray JL, Rubin HL *et al.* Characterization of 13 novel band 3 gene defects in hereditary spherocytosis with band 3 deficiency. *Blood* 1996; **88**: 4366–74.

97. Dhermy D, Galand C, Bournier O *et al.* Heterogenous band 3 deficiency in hereditary spherocytosis related to different band 3 gene defects. *Br J Haematol* 1997; **98**: 32–40.

98. Jarolim P, Rubin HL, Brabec V *et al.* Mutations of conserved arginines in the membrane domain of erythroid band 3 lead to a decrease in membrane-associated band 3 and to the phenotype of hereditary spherocytosis. *Blood* 1995; **85**: 634–40.

99. Alloisio N, Maillet P, Carre G *et al.* Hereditary spherocytosis with band 3 deficiency. Association with a nonsense mutation of the band 3 gene (allele Lyon), and aggravation by a low-expression allele occurring in *trans* (allele Genas). *Blood* 1996; **88**: 1062–9.

100. Yawata Y, Kanzaki A, Yawata A *et al.* Characteristic features of the genotype and phenotype of hereditary spherocytosis in the Japanese population. *Int J Hematol* 2000; **71**: 118–35.

101. Matsuda M, Hatano N, Ideguchi H *et al.* A novel mutation causing an aberrant splicing in the protein 4.2 gene associated with hereditary spherocytosis (protein 4.2 Notame). *Hum Mol Genet* 1995; **4**: 1187–91.

102. Balague C, Targarona EM, Cerdan G *et al.* Long-term outcome after laparoscopic splenectomy related to hematologic diagnosis. *Surg Endosc* 2004; **18**: 1283–7.

103. Rescorla FJ, Engum SA, West KW *et al.* Laparoscopic splenectomy has become the gold standard in children. *Am Surg* 2002; **68**: 297–301; discussion 301–2.

104. Schilling RF. Estimating the risk for sepsis after splenectomy in hereditary spherocytosis. *Ann Intern Med* 1995; **122**: 187–8.

105. Singer DB. Postsplenectomy sepsis. *Perspect Pediatr Pathol* 1973; **1**: 285–311.

106. Konradsen HB, Henrichsen J. Pneumococcal infections in splenectomized children are preventable. *Acta Paediatr Scand* 1991; **80**: 423–7.

107. Jardine DL, Laing AD. Delayed pulmonary hypertension following splenectomy for congenital spherocytosis. *Intern Med J* 2004; **34**: 214–16.

108. Wandersee NJ, Olson SC, Holzhauer SL *et al.* Increased erythrocyte adhesion in mice and humans with hereditary spherocytosis and hereditary elliptocytosis. *Blood* 2004; **103**: 710–16.

109. Bolton-Maggs PH, Stevens RF, Dodd NJ *et al.* Guidelines for the diagnosis and management of hereditary spherocytosis. *Br J Haematol* 2004; **126**: 455–74.

110. Bader-Meunier B, Gauthier F, Archambaud F *et al.* Long-term evaluation of the beneficial effect of subtotal splenectomy for management of hereditary spherocytosis. *Blood* 2001; **97**: 399–403.

111. de Buys Roessingh AS, de Lagausie P, Rohrlich P *et al.* Follow-up of partial splenectomy in children with hereditary spherocytosis. *J Pediatr Surg* 2002; **37**: 1459–63.

112. Rice HE, Oldham KT, Hillery CA *et al.* Clinical and hematologic benefits of partial splenectomy for congenital hemolytic anemias in children. *Ann Surg* 2003; **237**: 281–8.

113. Stoehr GA, Stauffer UG, Eber SW. Near-total splenectomy: a new technique for the management of hereditary spherocytosis. *Ann Surg* 2005; **241**: 40–7.

114. Gallagher PG. Hereditary elliptocytosis: spectrin and protein 4.1R. *Semin Hematol* 2004; **41**: 142–64.

115. Nagel RL. Red-cell cytoskeletal abnormalities: implications for malaria. *N Engl J Med* 1990; **323**: 1558–60.

116. Glele-Kakai C, Garbarz M, Lecomte MC *et al.* Epidemiological studies of spectrin mutations related to hereditary elliptocytosis and spectrin polymorphisms in Benin. *Br J Haematol* 1996; **95**: 57–66.

117. Palek J, Jarolim P. Clinical expression and laboratory detection of red blood cell membrane protein mutations. *Semin Hematol* 1993; **30**: 249–83.

118. Nkrumah FK. Hereditary elliptocytosis associated with severe haemolytic anaemia and malaria. *Afr J Med Sci* 1972; **3**: 131–6.

119. Pui CH, Wang W, Wilimas J. Hereditary elliptocytosis: morphologic abnormalities during acute hepatitis. *Clin Pediatr (Phila)* 1982; **21**: 188–90.

120. Coetzer T, Palek J, Lawler J *et al.* Structural and functional heterogeneity of alpha spectrin mutations involving the spectrin heterodimer self-association site: relationships to hematologic expression of homozygous hereditary elliptocytosis and hereditary pyropoikilocytosis. *Blood* 1990; **75**: 2235–44.

121. Tchernia G, Mohandas N, Shohet SB. Deficiency of skeletal membrane protein band 4.1 in homozygous hereditary elliptocytosis. Implications for erythrocyte membrane stability. *J Clin Invest* 1981; **68**: 454–60.

122. Schoomaker EB, Butler WM, Diehl LF. Increased heat sensitivity of red blood cells in hereditary elliptocytosis with acquired cobalamin (vitamin B12) deficiency. *Blood* 1982; **59**: 1213–19.

123. Jarolim P, Palek J, Coetzer TL *et al.* Severe hemolysis and red cell fragmentation caused by the combination of a spectrin mutation with a thrombotic microangiopathy. *Am J Hematol* 1989; **32**: 50–6.

124. Zarkowsky HS, Mohandas N, Speaker CB *et al.* A congenital haemolytic anaemia with thermal sensitivity of the erythrocyte membrane. *Br J Haematol* 1975; **29**: 537–43.

125. Wrong O, Bruce LJ, Unwin RJ *et al.* Band 3 mutations, distal renal tubular acidosis, and Southeast Asian ovalocytosis. *Kidney Int* 2002; **62**: 10–19.

126. Allen SJ, O'Donnell A, Alexander ND *et al.* Prevention of cerebral malaria in children in Papua New Guinea by southeast Asian ovalocytosis band 3. *Am J Trop Med Hyg* 1999; **60**: 1056–60.

127. Liu SC, Jarolim P, Rubin HL *et al.* The homozygous state for the band 3 protein mutation in Southeast Asian ovalocytosis may be lethal. *Blood* 1994; **84**: 3590–1.

128. Mentzer WC Jr, Iarocci TA, Mohandas N *et al.* Modulation of erythrocyte membrane mechanical stability by 2,3-diphosphoglycerate in the neonatal poikilocytosis/elliptocytosis syndrome. *J Clin Invest* 1987; **79**: 943–9.

129. Delaunay J, Dhermy D. Mutations involving the spectrin heterodimer contact site: clinical expression and alterations in specific function. *Semin Hematol* 1993; **30**: 21–33.

130. Gallagher PG, Forget BG. Hematologically important mutations: spectrin variants in hereditary elliptocytosis and hereditary pyropoikilocytosis. *Blood Cells Mol Dis* 1996; **22**: 254–8.

131. Tse WT, Lecomte MC *et al.* Point mutation in the beta-spectrin gene associated with alpha I/74 hereditary elliptocytosis. Implications for the mechanism of spectrin dimer self-association. *J Clin Invest* 1990; **86**: 909–16.

132. Bennett V, Baines AJ. Spectrin and ankyrin-based pathways: metazoan inventions for integrating cells into tissues. *Physiol Rev* 2001; **81**: 1353–92.

133. An X, Lecomte MC, Chasis JA *et al*. Shear-response of the spectrin dimer-tetramer equilibrium in the red blood cell membrane. *J Biol Chem* 2002; **277**: 31796–800.

134. Shahbakhti F, Gratzer WB. Analysis of the self-association of human red cell spectrin. *Biochemistry* 1986; **25**: 5969–75.

135. Zhang Z, Weed SA, Gallagher PG *et al*. Dynamic molecular modeling of pathogenic mutations in the spectrin self-association domain. *Blood* 2001; **98**: 1645–53.

136. Alloisio N, Morle L, Pothier B *et al*. Spectrin Oran (alpha II/21), a new spectrin variant concerning the alpha II domain and causing severe elliptocytosis in the homozygous state. *Blood* 1988; **71**: 1039–47.

137. Alloisio N, Wilmotte R, Morle L *et al*. Spectrin Jendouba: an alpha II/31 spectrin variant that is associated with elliptocytosis and carries a mutation distant from the dimer self-association site. *Blood* 1992; **80**: 809–15.

138. Fournier CM, Nicolas G, Gallagher PG *et al*. Spectrin St Claude, a splicing mutation of the human alpha-spectrin gene associated with severe poikilocytic anemia. *Blood* 1997; **89**: 4584–90.

139. Alloisio N, Morle L, Marechal J *et al*. Sp alpha V/41: a common spectrin polymorphism at the alpha IV-alpha V domain junction. Relevance to the expression level of hereditary elliptocytosis due to alpha-spectrin variants located in trans. *J Clin Invest* 1991; **87**: 2169–77.

140. Wilmotte R, Marechal J, Morle L *et al*. Low expression allele alpha LELY of red cell spectrin is associated with mutations in exon 40 (alpha V/41 polymorphism) and intron 45 and with partial skipping of exon 46. *J Clin Invest* 1993; **91**: 2091–6.

141. Wilmotte R, Harper SL, Ursitti JA *et al*. The exon 46-encoded sequence is essential for stability of human erythroid alpha-spectrin and heterodimer formation. *Blood* 1997; **90**: 4188–96.

142. Baklouti F, Huang SC, Tang TK *et al*. Asynchronous regulation of splicing events within protein 4.1 pre-mRNA during erythroid differentiation. *Blood* 1996; **87**: 3934–41.

143. Chasis JA, Coulombel L, McGee S *et al*. Differential use of protein 4.1 translation initiation sites during erythropoiesis: implications for a mutation-induced stage-specific deficiency of protein 4.1 during erythroid development. *Blood* 1996; **87**: 5324–31.

144. Deguillien M, Huang SC, Moriniere M *et al*. Multiple *cis* elements regulate an alternative splicing event at 4.1R pre-mRNA during erythroid differentiation. *Blood* 2001; **98**: 3809–16.

145. Gascard P, Lee G, Coulombel L *et al*. Characterization of multiple isoforms of protein 4.1R expressed during erythroid terminal differentiation. *Blood* 1998; **92**: 4404–14.

146. Hou VC, Conboy JG. Regulation of alternative pre-mRNA splicing during erythroid differentiation. *Curr Opin Hematol* 2001; **8**: 74–9.

147. Huang JP, Tang CJ, Kou GH *et al*. Genomic structure of the locus encoding protein 4.1. Structural basis for complex combinational patterns of tissue-specific alternative RNA splicing. *J Biol Chem* 1993; **268**: 3758–66.

148. Feo CJ, Fischer S, Piau JP *et al*. 1st instance of the absence of an erythrocyte membrane protein (band 4(1)) in a case of familial elliptocytic anemia. *Nouv Rev Fr Hematol* 1980; **22**: 315–25.

149. Lambert S, Zail S. Partial deficiency of protein 4.1 in hereditary elliptocytosis. *Am J Hematol* 1987; **26**: 263–72.

150. Yawata A, Kanzaki A, Gilsanz F *et al*. A markedly disrupted skeletal network with abnormally distributed intramembrane particles in complete protein 4.1-deficient red blood cells (allele 4.1 Madrid): implications regarding a critical role of protein 4.1 in maintenance of the integrity of the red blood cell membrane. *Blood* 1997; **90**: 2471–81.

151. Daniels GL, Shaw MA, Judson PA *et al*. A family demonstrating inheritance of the Leach phenotype: a Gerbich-negative phenotype associated with elliptocytosis. *Vox Sang* 1986; **50**: 117–21.

152. Reid ME, Mohandas N. Red blood cell blood group antigens: structure and function. *Semin Hematol* 2004; **41**: 93–117.

153. Winardi R, Reid M, Conboy J *et al*. Molecular analysis of glycophorin C deficiency in human erythrocytes. *Blood* 1993; **81**: 2799–803.

154. Marfatia SM, Leu RA, Branton D *et al*. Identification of the protein 4.1 binding interface on glycophorin C and p55, a homologue of the *Drosophila* discs-large tumor suppressor protein. *J Biol Chem* 1995; **270**: 715–19.

155. Chishti AH, Palek J, Fisher D *et al*. Reduced invasion and growth of *Plasmodium falciparum* into elliptocytic red blood cells with a combined deficiency of protein 4.1, glycophorin C, and p55. *Blood* 1996; **87**: 3462–9.

156. Gratzer WB, Dluzewski AR. The red blood cell and malaria parasite invasion. *Semin Hematol* 1993; **30**: 232–47.

157. Magowan C, Coppel RL, Lau AO *et al*. Role of the *Plasmodium falciparum* mature-parasite-infected erythrocyte surface antigen (MESA/PfEMP-2) in malarial infection of erythrocytes. *Blood* 1995; **86**: 3196–204.

158. Kane J, Havel R. Disorders of the biogenesis and secretion of lipoproteins containing the B apolipoproteins. In: Scriver C, Baudet A, Sly W *et al*. (eds) *The Metabolic and Molecular Bases of Inherited Disease* New York: McGraw-Hill, 1995, p. 1853.

159. Berriot-Varoqueaux N, Aggerback LP, Samson-Bouma M *et al*. The role of the microsomal triglyceride transfer protein in abetalipoproteinemia. *Annu Rev Nutr* 2000; **20**: 663–97.

160. Ceska R, Vrablik M, Horinek A. Familial defective apolipoprotein B-100: a lesson from homozygous and heterozygous patients. *Physiol Res* 2000; **49** (suppl. 1): S125–S130.

161. Narcisi TM, Shoulders CC, Chester SA *et al*. Mutations of the microsomal triglyceride-transfer-protein gene in abetalipoproteinemia. *Am J Hum Genet* 1995; **57**: 1298–310.

162. Rampoldi L, Danek A, Monaco AP. Clinical features and molecular bases of neuroacanthocytosis. *J Mol Med* 2002; **80**: 475–91.

163. Rampoldi L, Dobson-Stone C, Rubio JP *et al*. A conserved sorting-associated protein is mutant in chorea-acanthocytosis. *Nat Genet* 2001; **28**: 119–20.

164. Ueno S, Maruki Y, Nakamura M *et al*. The gene encoding a newly discovered protein, chorein, is mutated in chorea-acanthocytosis. *Nat Genet* 2001; **28**: 121–2.

165. Danek A, Jung HH, Melone MA *et al*. Neuroacanthocytosis: new developments in a neglected group of dementing disorders. *J Neurol Sci* 2005; **229–230**: 171–86.

166. Danek A, Walker RH. Neuroacanthocytosis. *Curr Opin Neurol* 2005; **18**: 386–92.

167. Margolis RL, Holmes SE, Rosenblatt A *et al.* Huntington's disease-like 2 (HDL2) in North America and Japan. *Ann Neurol* 2004; **56**: 670–4.

168. Walker RH, Rasmussen A, Rudnicki D *et al.* Huntington's disease-like 2 can present as chorea-acanthocytosis. *Neurology* 2003; **61**: 1002–4.

169. Hayflick SJ, Westaway SK, Levinson B *et al.* Genetic, clinical, and radiographic delineation of Hallervorden–Spatz syndrome. *N Engl J Med* 2003; **348**: 33–40.

170. Houlden H, Lincoln S, Farrer M *et al.* Compound heterozygous PANK2 mutations confirm HARP and Hallervorden–Spatz syndromes are allelic. *Neurology* 2003; **61**: 1423–6.

171. Pellecchia MT, Valente EM, Cif L *et al.* The diverse phenotype and genotype of pantothenate kinase-associated neurodegeneration. *Neurology* 2005; **64**: 1810–12.

172. Zhou B, Westaway SK, Levinson B *et al.* A novel pantothenate kinase gene (PANK2) is defective in Hallervorden–Spatz syndrome. *Nat Genet* 2001; **28**: 345–9.

173. Kay J, Stricker RB. Hematologic and immunologic abnormalities in anorexia nervosa. *South Med J* 1983; **76**: 1008–10.

174. Kayden HJ. The genetic basis of vitamin E deficiency in humans. *Nutrition* 2001; **17**: 797–8.

175. Frey D, Machler M, Seger R *et al.* Gene deletion in a patient with chronic granulomatous disease and McLeod syndrome: fine mapping of the Xk gene locus. *Blood* 1988; **71**: 252–5.

176. Danek A, Rubio JP, Rampoldi L *et al.* McLeod neuroacanthocytosis: genotype and phenotype. *Ann Neurol* 2001; **50**: 755–64.

177. Ho MF, Chalmers RM, Davis MB *et al.* A novel point mutation in the McLeod syndrome gene in neuroacanthocytosis. *Ann Neurol* 1996; **39**: 672–5.

178. Gallagher PG, Lux SE. Disorders of the erythrocyte membrane. In: Nathan DG, Orkins SH, Ginsburg D, Look AT (eds) *Nathan and Oski's Hematology of Infancy and Childhood*, 6th edn. Philadelphia: WB Saunders, 2003, pp. 560–684.

179. Cooper RA, Jandl JH. Bile salts and cholesterol in the pathogenesis of target cells in obstructive jaundice. *J Clin Invest* 1968; **47**: 809–22.

180. Cooper RA, Diloy Puray M, Lando P *et al.* An analysis of lipoproteins, bile acids, and red cell membranes associated with target cells and spur cells in patients with liver disease. *J Clin Invest* 1972; **51**: 3182–92.

181. Calabresi L, Pisciotta L, Costantin A *et al.* The molecular basis of lecithin:cholesterol acyltransferase deficiency syndromes. A comprehensive study of molecular and biochemical findings in 13 unrelated Italian families. *Arterioscler Thromb Vasc Biol* 2005.

182. Hovingh GK, de Groot E, van der Steeg W *et al.* Inherited disorders of HDL metabolism and atherosclerosis. *Curr Opin Lipidol* 2005; **16**: 139–45.

183. de Haan LD, Werre JM, Ruben AM *et al.* Alterations in size, shape and osmotic behaviour of red cells after splenectomy: a study of their age dependence. *Br J Haematol* 1988; **69**: 71–80.

184. Lande WM, Mentzer WC. Haemolytic anaemia associated with increased cation permeability. *Clin Haematol* 1985; **14**: 89–103.

185. Delaunay J. The hereditary stomatocytoses: genetic disorders of the red cell membrane permeability to monovalent cations. *Semin Hematol* 2004; **41**: 165–72.

186. Delaunay J, Stewart G, Iolascon A. Hereditary dehydrated and overhydrated stomatocytosis: recent advances. *Curr Opin Hematol* 1999; **6**: 110–14.

187. Vives Corrons JL, Besson I, Aymerich M *et al.* Hereditary xerocytosis: a report of six unrelated Spanish families with leaky red cell syndrome and increased heat stability of the erythrocyte membrane. *Br J Haematol* 1995; **90**: 817–22.

188. Basu AP, Carey P, Cynober T *et al.* Dehydrated hereditary stomatocytosis with transient perinatal ascites. *Arch Dis Child* 2003; **88**: F438–F439.

189. Grootenboer-Mignot S, Cretien A, Laurendeau I *et al.* Sub-lethal hydrops as a manifestation of dehydrated hereditary stomatocytosis in two consecutive pregnancies. *Prenat Diagn* 2003; **23**: 380–4.

190. Glader BE, Sullivan DW. Erythrocyte disorders leading to potassium loss and cellular dehydration. In: Lux SE, Marchesi VT, Fox CF (eds) *Normal and Abnormal Red Cell Membranes*. New York: Alan R Liss, 1979, pp. 503–13.

191. Fairbanks G, Dino JE, Snyder LM. Passive cation transport in hereditary xerocytosis. In: Kruckeberg WC *et al.* (eds) *Erythrocyte Membranes 3: Recent Clinical and Experimental Advances*. New York: Alan R Liss, 1984, pp. 205–17.

192. Clark MR, Mohandas N, Caggiano V *et al.* Effects of abnormal cation transport on deformability of desiccytes. *J Supramol Struct* 1978; **8**: 521–32.

193. Fortier N, Synder LM, Garver F *et al.* The relationship between in vivo generated hemoglobin skeletal protein complex and increased red cell membrane rigidity. *Blood* 1988; **71**: 1427–31.

194. Platt OS, Lux SE, Nathan DG. Exercise-induced hemolysis in xerocytosis. Erythrocyte dehydration and shear sensitivity. *J Clin Invest* 1981; **68**: 631–8.

195. Snyder LM, Lutz HU, Sauberman N *et al.* Fragmentation and myelin formation in hereditary xerocytosis and other hemolytic anemias. *Blood* 1978; **52**: 750–61.

196. Snyder LM, Sauberman N, Condara H *et al.* Red cell membrane response to hydrogen peroxide-sensitivity in hereditary xerocytosis and in other abnormal red cells. *Br J Haematol* 1981; **48**: 435–44.

197. Clark MR, Shohet SB, Gottfried EL. Hereditary hemolytic disease with increased red blood cell phosphatidylcholine and dehydration: one, two, or many disorders? *Am J Hematol* 1993; **42**: 25–30.

198. Glader BE, Fortier N, Albala MM *et al.* Congenital hemolytic anemia associated with dehydrated erythrocytes and increased potassium loss. *N Engl J Med* 1974; **291**: 491–6.

199. Carella M, Stewart G, Ajetunmobi JF *et al.* Genomewide search for dehydrated hereditary stomatocytosis (hereditary xerocytosis): mapping of locus to chromosome 16 (16q23–qter). *Am J Hum Genet* 1998; **63**: 810–16.

200. Stewart GW, Amess JAL, Eber SW *et al.* Thrombo-embolic disease after splenectomy for hereditary stomatocytosis. *Br J Haematol* 1996; **93**: 303–10.

201. Mentzer WC Jr, Smith WB, Goldstone J *et al.* Hereditary stomatocytosis: membrane and metabolism studies. *Blood* 1975; **46**: 659–69.

202. Eber SW, Lande WM, Iarocci TA *et al.* Hereditary stomatocytosis: consistent association with an integral membrane protein deficiency. *Br J Haematol* 1989; **72**: 452–5.

203. Kanzaki A, Yawata Y. Hereditary stomatocytosis: phenotypical

expression of sodium transport and band 7 peptides in 44 cases. *Br J Haematol* 1992; **82**: 133–41.

204. Lande WM, Thiemann PV, Mentzer WC Jr. Missing band 7 membrane protein in two patients with high Na, low K erythrocytes. *J Clin Invest* 1982; **70**: 1273–80.

205. Morle L, Pothier B, Alloisio N *et al*. Reduction of membrane band 7 and activation of volume stimulated (K$^+$, Cl$^-$)-cotransport in a case of congenital stomatocytosis. *Br J Haematol* 1989; **71**: 141–6.

206. Stewart GW, Hepworth-Jones BE, Keen JN *et al*. Isolation of cDNA coding for an ubiquitous membrane protein deficient in high Na$^+$, low K$^+$ stomatocytic erythrocytes. Blood 1992; **79**: 1593–601.

207. Fricke B, Argent AC, Chetty MC *et al*. The "stomatin" gene and protein in overhydrated hereditary stomatocytosis. *Blood* 2003; **102**: 2268–77.

208. Zhu Y, Paszty C, Turetsky T *et al*. Stomatocytosis is absent in "stomatin"-deficient murine red blood cells. *Blood* 1999; **93**: 2404–10.

209. Argent AC, Chetty MC, Fricke B *et al*. A family showing recessively inherited multisystem pathology with aberrant splicing of the erythrocyte Band 7.2b ("stomatin") gene. *J Inherit Metab Dis* 2004; **27**: 29–46.

210. Coles SE, Stewart GW. Temperature effects on cation transport in hereditary stomatocytosis and allied disorders. *Int J Exp Pathol* 1999; **80**: 251–8.

211. Christiansson A, Kuypers FA, Roelofsen B *et al*. Lipid molecular shape affects erythrocyte morphology: a study involving replacement of native phosphatidylcholine with different species followed by treatment of cells with sphingomyelinase C or phospholipase A2. *J Cell Biol* 1985; **101**: 1455–62.

212. Smith BD, Segel GB. Abnormal erythrocyte endothelial adherence in hereditary stomatocytosis. *Blood* 1997; **89**: 3451–6.

213. Gallagher PG, Chang SH, Rettig MP *et al*. Altered erythrocyte endothelial adherence and membrane phospholipid asymmetry in hereditary hydrocytosis. *Blood* 203; **101**: 4625–7.

214. Haines PG, Jarvis HG, King S *et al*. Two further British families with the "cryohydrocytosis" form of hereditary stomatocytosis. *Br J Haematol* 2001; **113**: 932–7.

215. Van Kim CL, Colin Y, Cartron JP *et al*. Rh proteins: Key structural and functional components of the red cell membrane. *Blood Rev* 2005.

216. Mouro-Chanteloup I, Delaunay J, Gane P *et al*. Evidence that the red cell skeleton protein 4.2 interacts with the Rh membrane complex member CD47. *Blood* 2003; **101**: 338–44.

217. Nicolas V, Le Van Kim C, Gane P *et al*. Rh-RhAG/ankyrin-R, a new interaction site between the membrane bilayer and the red cell skeleton, is impaired by Rh(null)-associated mutation. *J Biol Chem* 2003; **278**: 25526–33.

218. Rees DC, Iolascon A, Carella M *et al*. Stomatocytic haemolysis and macrothrombocytopenia (Mediterranean stomatocytosis/macrothrombocytopenia) is the haematological presentation of phytosterolaemia. *Br J Haematol* 2005; **130**: 297–309.

219. Stefkova J, Poledne R, Hubacek JA. ATP-binding cassette (ABC) transporters in human metabolism and diseases. *Physiol Res* 2004; **53**: 235–43.

13 Thalassemias

Nancy F. Olivieri and David J. Weatherall

Introduction

The thalassemias, a heterogeneous family of inherited disorders of hemoglobin synthesis, were first recognized independently in the USA and Italy in the years between 1925 and 1927.[1] The word "thalassemia" owes its name to an attempt, mistaken as it turned out later, to relate the diseases to Mediterranean populations; *thalassa* is from the Greek word for "sea".

It is now apparent that the thalassemias are the world's commonest monogenic diseases and are widespread among races ranging from the Mediterranean region, through the Middle East and Indian subcontinent, to Southeast Asia. Many countries in these regions have, over the last 30 years, gone through a remarkable demographic change in the pattern of their illnesses. With improvements in hygiene and public health measures, very high infant and childhood mortalities due to infection and malnutrition have fallen. In the past, babies born with serious genetic blood diseases would have been unlikely to survive the first years of life, but the scene has now changed dramatically. As these countries undergo this demographic transition, the majority of these children are now surviving long enough to come to diagnosis and to require management. And because the symptomatic treatment of thalassemia is expensive, this change in the pattern of childhood illness will place an increasing drain on the resources of countries in which the disease occurs at a high frequency.[2]

These diseases are also assuming an increasing importance in the clinical practice of pediatricians in the richer countries.

Genetics and classification

Genetic control of hemoglobin synthesis

A great deal is known about the structure, genetic regulation and synthesis of hemoglobin. Only those aspects of particular importance for an understanding of the thalassemias are summarized here. Readers are referred to more extensive reviews and monographs.[3-6]

Different hemoglobins, each adapted to the particular oxygen requirements at each stage of development, are synthesized in the embryo, fetus and adult. All hemoglobins have a similar tetrameric structure, consisting of two different pairs of globin chains, each attached to a heme moiety. Adult and fetal hemoglobins have α chains combined with β chains (HbA, $\alpha_2\beta_2$), δ chains (HbA$_2$, $\alpha_2\delta_2$) and γ chains (HbF, $\alpha_2\gamma_2$). In embryonic life, α-like chains called ζ chains combine with γ chains to produce Hb Portland ($\zeta_2\gamma_2$), or with ε chains to form Hb Gower 1 ($\zeta_2\varepsilon_2$), and α and ε chains combine to form Hb Gower 2 ($\alpha_2\varepsilon_2$). Fetal hemoglobin is itself heterogeneous; there are two kinds of γ chains, which differ in their amino acid compositions only at position 136, where they have either glycine or alanine. Those γ chains with glycine are called $^G\gamma$ chains and those with alanine $^A\gamma$ chains. The $^G\gamma$ and $^A\gamma$ chains are the products of separate ($^G\gamma$ and $^A\gamma$) loci.

The different globin chains are controlled by two main families of globin genes (Fig. 13.1). The β-like globin genes are arranged in a linked cluster on chromosome 11, which is distributed over approximately 60 kb (kilobase or 1000 nucleotide bases). They are arranged in the order 5' to 3' (left to right) ε-$^G\gamma$-$^A\gamma$-$\psi\beta$-δ-β. The symbol ψ is used to described a pseudogene, probably a burnt-out evolutionary remnant of a once-active gene. The α-like globin genes also form a cluster, in this case on chromosome 16. They are distributed in the order 5'-ζ-$\psi\zeta$-$\psi\alpha$1-α2-α1-3'.

In order to appreciate the molecular basis for the thalassemias, it is important to understand, at least in outline, something of the structure of the globin genes, how they are regulated, and how their products are synthesized and unite with heme to form hemoglobin molecules in the red cell precursors.[4,6]

Each globin gene consists of a string of nucleotide bases that are divided into coding sequences, called exons, and

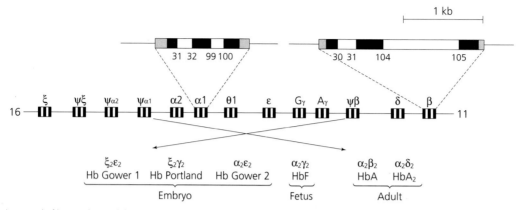

Fig. 13.1 Genetic control of human hemoglobin synthesis. The α- and β-globin gene clusters on chromosomes 16 and 11 are shown, together with the different hemoglobins produced in embryonic, fetal and adult life. In the extended representations of the α1- and β-globin genes the exons are shown in dark shading, the introns unshaded, and the 5′ and 3′ noncoding regions are shown in light shading.

noncoding regions known as intervening sequences (IVS) or introns. In the 5′ (left-hand) noncoding or flanking regions of globin genes, there are blocks of nucleotide homology, which are found in similar positions in many species. Three such regions, called promoter elements, play a major role in the transcription of the structural genes. The globin gene clusters contain other elements that play an important part in promoting erythroid-specific gene expression and in coordinating the changes in globin gene activity at different stages during development. These include enhancers, i.e., sequences that increase gene expression despite being located at a variable distance from a particular gene, and "master" regulatory sequences, called the locus control region (LCR) in the case of the β-globin gene family and HS40 in the case of the α-gene complex, which lie upstream from the globin gene clusters and are responsible for their activation in erythroid tissue. Each of these regulatory sequences has a modular structure comprising an array of short nucleotide motifs that represent binding sites for transcriptional activators or repressors, molecules involved in the activation or repression of globin gene production in different cell types and at different stages of development.

Each of these regulatory regions binds a number of erythroid-specific factors, including GATA-1 and NF-E2, thereby activating the LCR, which renders the entire β-globin gene cluster transcriptionally active. It seems likely that the LCR and HS40 regions come into apposition with the promoter regions of each of the globin genes in turn and, together with a complex collection of transcription factors and other proteins, form an initiation complex so that individual genes are transcribed.

When a globin gene is transcribed, messenger RNA (mRNA) is synthesized from one of its strands by the action of RNA polymerase. The primary transcription product is a large mRNA precursor, which contains both intron and exon sequences (Fig. 13.2). While in the nucleus this molecule undergoes a remarkable series of modifications; the introns

are removed and the exons are spliced together. This is a multistep process that requires certain structural features of the mRNA precursor, notably the nucleotides GT at the 5′ end and AG at the 3′ end of intron–exon junctions. We will discuss the importance of these sequences when we consider the mutations that cause thalassemia. The mRNAs are now modified at both their 5′ and 3′ ends and move into the cytoplasm of the red cell precursor to act as a template for globin chain production.

Amino acids are transported to the mRNA template on carrier molecules called transfer RNAs (tRNAs). There are specific tRNAs for each amino acid. The order of amino acids in a globin chain is determined by a triplet code, where three bases (codons) code for a particular amino acid. The tRNAs also contain three bases, or anticodons, that are complementary to the mRNA codons for particular amino acids. Hence the tRNAs carry amino acids to the template, find the right position by codon/anticodon base pairing, and initiate globin chain synthesis. When the first tRNA is in position, a complex is formed between several protein initiation factors and the subunits of the ribosome that is to hold the growing peptide chains together on the mRNA as it is translated. A second tRNA moves in alongside and the two amino acids are united by a peptide bond; the globin chain is now two amino acid residues long. This process is continued as the message is translated, from left to right, until a specific codon for termination is reached, whereupon the finished globin chain drops off the ribosome mRNA complex and the ribosomal subunits are recycled. The finished globin chain combines with heme and three of its fellows to form a definitive hemoglobin molecule.

The developmental switches from embryonic to fetal and fetal to adult hemoglobin production are synchronized throughout the different organs of hemopoiesis that function at various times of development.[4,6] The way in which these switches are regulated is not yet completely understood. It is believed that the LCR becomes spatially related sequentially

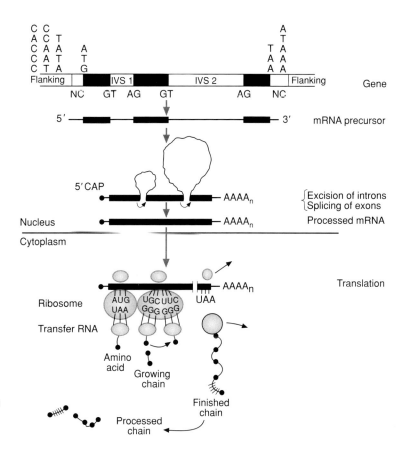

Fig. 13.2 A schematic representation of gene action and protein synthesis. Reproduced from Weatherall DJ, Clegg JB, eds. *The Thalassaemia Syndromes*, Blackwell Science Ltd, 2001.

to the ε, γ and finally δ and β chains at different times during fetal development. Why this happens is not clear, although it is possible that there are specific DNA-binding proteins involved in the activation or repression of these genes at different developmental stages.

Classification

The thalassemias can be defined as a heterogeneous group of genetic disorders of hemoglobin synthesis, all of which result from a reduced rate of production of one or more of the globin chains of hemoglobin. This basic defect results in imbalanced globin chain synthesis, which is the hallmark of all forms of thalassemia.[1]

The thalassemias can be classified at different levels. Clinically, it is useful to divide them into three groups: the severe transfusion-dependent (major) varieties; the symptomless carrier states (minor) varieties; and a group of conditions of intermediate severity that fall under the loose heading "thalassemia intermedia". This classification is retained because it has implications for both diagnosis and management.

Thalassemias can also be classified at the genetic level into the α, β, δβ or εγδβ thalassemias, according to which globin chain is produced in reduced amounts (Table 13.1). In some thalassemias, no globin chain is synthesized at all, and hence they are called α^0 or β^0 thalassemias, whereas in others

Table 13.1 Classification of the common thalassemias and related disorders.

β Thalassemia
β^+, β^0

δβ Thalassemia
$(\delta\beta)^+$ Hb Lepore thalassemia
$(\delta\beta)^0$
$(^A\gamma\delta\beta)^0$

εγδβ Thalassemia
$(\varepsilon\gamma\delta\beta)^0$

δ Thalassemia

β or δβ thalassemia associated with β-chain variants
HbS β thalassemia
HbE β thalassemia
Many others

α Thalassemia
α^+ (deletion)
α^+ (nondeletion)
α^0

Hereditary persistence of HbF
Deletion $(\delta\beta)^0$
Nondeletion $^A\gamma\beta^+$, $^G\gamma\beta^+$
Unlinked to β-globin gene cluster

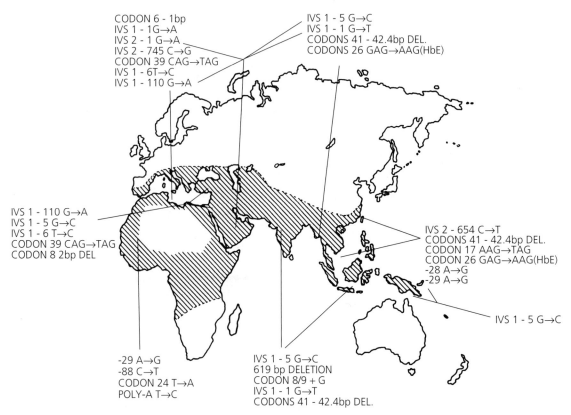

CODON 6 - 1bp
IVS 1 - 1G→A
IVS 2 - 1 G→A
IVS 2 - 745 C→G
CODON 39 CAG→TAG
IVS 1 - 6T→C
IVS 1 - 110 G→A

IVS 1 - 5 G→C
IVS 1 - 1 G→T
CODONS 41 - 42.4bp DEL.
CODON 26 GAG→AAG(HbE)

IVS 1 - 110 G→A
IVS 1 - 5 G→C
IVS 1 - 6 T→C
CODON 39 CAG→TAG
CODON 8 2bp DEL

IVS 2 - 654 C→T
CODONS 41 - 42.4bp DEL.
CODON 17 AAG→TAG
CODON 26 GAG→AAG(HbE)
-28 A→G
-29 A→G

IVS 1 - 5 G→C

-29 A→G
-88 C→T
CODON 24 T→A
POLY-A T→C

IVS 1 - 5 G→C
619 bp DELETION
CODON 8/9 + G
IVS 1 - 1 G→T
CODONS 41 - 42.4bp DEL.

Fig. 13.3 World distribution of the different mutations that cause β thalassemia. IVS, intervening sequence.

some globin chain is produced but at a reduced rate; these are designated α⁺ or β⁺ thalassemias. The δβ thalassemias, in which there is defective δ and β chain synthesis, can be subdivided in the same way, i.e., into (δβ)⁺ and (δβ)⁰ varieties.

Because the thalassemias occur in populations in which structural hemoglobin variants are also common, it is not unusual to inherit a thalassemia gene from one parent and a gene for a structural variant from the other. Furthermore, since both α and β thalassemia occur commonly in some countries, individuals may receive genes for both types. All these different interactions produce an extremely complex and clinically diverse family of genetic disorders, which range in severity from death *in utero* to extremely mild, symptomless, hypochromic anemias.

Despite their genetic complexity, most thalassemias are inherited in a mendelian recessive or codominant fashion. Heterozygotes are usually symptomless, while more severely affected patients are either homozygous for α or β thalassemia, or compound heterozygous for different molecular forms of the diseases.

Distribution

A world map of the distribution of the thalassemias is shown in Figs 13.3 and 13.4. Several detailed accounts of their frequency and population genetics have been reported.[1,7]

The α⁰ thalassemias are found predominantly in Southeast Asia and in the Mediterranean islands. The α⁺ thalassemias occur widely throughout Africa, the Mediterranean region, the Middle East, parts of the Indian subcontinent, and throughout Southeast Asia. They occur at remarkably high frequencies in some populations, achieving carrier rates of between 40 and 80%.

The β thalassemias have a distribution similar to that of the α thalassemias. With the exception of a few countries, the β thalassemias are less common in Africa, extremely frequent in some of the Mediterranean island populations, and occur at variable frequencies throughout the Middle East, the Indian subcontinent and parts of Southeast Asia. As we shall see later, the structural hemoglobin variant, HbE, is associated with the phenotype of a mild form of β thalassemia. This also reaches extremely high gene frequencies in eastern parts of India, Myanmar, and in many countries in Southeast Asia. Thus the interaction of HbE and β thalassemia, HbE thalassemia, is the most important form of the disease in these regions.

There is increasing evidence that these high gene frequencies for the different forms of thalassemia have been maintained by heterozygote advantage against severe forms

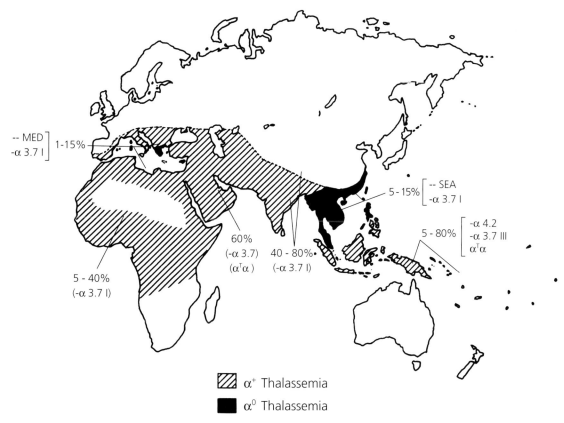

Fig. 13.4 World distribution of the different varieties of α thalassemia. The three different forms of α⁺ thalassemia due to deletions of a single α-globin gene involving the loss of 3.7 kb of the α-gene cluster are represented as types I, II and III. The common deletional forms of α⁰ thalassemia are designated MED (Mediterranean) and SEA (Southeast Asian). The percentages indicate the approximate frequency of these different genes.

of malaria, predominantly *Plasmodium falciparum*. One of the most remarkable features of the world distribution of these diseases is that in each high-frequency population there are different sets of mutations (Figs 13.3 and 13.4). This tells us that these diseases have arisen by new mutations and then been expanded very rapidly due to local selection by malaria. The fact that the mutations are so different among populations indicates that this selective force is, in evolutionary terms, quite recent, probably not more than a few thousand years.

Pathophysiology

To appreciate the pathophysiology of the thalassemias, it is necessary to understand both their molecular pathology and how globin chain imbalance causes the characteristic ineffective erythropoiesis and shortened red cell survival.

Molecular pathology

Although the basic principles are similar, the patterns of the mutations that cause α and β thalassemia are different. Because of their greater clinical importance, we consider the β thalassemias first.

Over 150 different mutations have been described in patients with β thalassemia (Fig. 13.5).[8,9] Unlike the α thalassemias, major deletions causing β thalassemia are unusual. The bulk of β-thalassemia mutations are single base changes or small deletions or insertions of one or two bases at critical points along the genes. Remarkably, they occur in both introns and exons, and outside the coding regions of the genes.

Some substitutions, called nonsense mutations, result in a single base change in an exon that generates a stop codon in the coding region of the mRNA. This, of course, causes premature termination of globin chain synthesis and leads to the production of a shortened and nonviable β-globin chain. Other exon mutations cause frameshifts, which result in one or more bases being lost or inserted so that the reading frame of the genetic code is thrown out of phase or a new stop codon is produced. Mutations within introns or exons, or at their junctions, may interfere with the mechanism of splicing the exons together after the introns have been removed during processing of the mRNA precursor. For example, single substitutions at the invariant GT or AG sequences at the intron/exon junctions prevent splicing altogether and cause β⁰ thalassemia. The sequences adjacent to the GT and AG sequences are highly conserved and are also involved in splicing; several β-thalassemia mutations involve this region

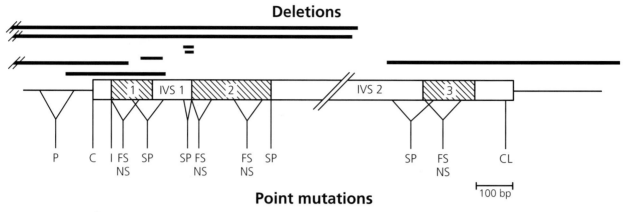

Fig. 13.5 Different classes of mutations of the β-globin gene involved in β thalassemia. FS, frameshift; NS, nonsense; SP, splicing; P, promoter; CL, polyA addition site mutations; IVS, intervening sequence.

and are associated with variable degrees of defective β-globin production. Mutations in sequences in exons that resemble consensus sequences at the intron/exon junctions may activate "cryptic" splice sites. For example, there is a sequence that resembles the IVS-1 consensus site and spans codons 24–27 of exon 1 of the β-globin gene; mutations at codons 19 (A→G), 26 (G→A), and 27 (G→T) result in both a reduced amount of mRNA due to abnormal splicing and an amino acid substitution encoded by the mRNA that is spliced normally and translated into protein. The abnormal hemoglobins produced are hemoglobins Malay, E and Knossos, each of which is associated with a mild β-thalassemia phenotype.

Single base substitutions are also found in the flanking regions of the β-globin genes. Those which involve the promoter elements downregulate β-globin gene transcription, and are usually associated with a mild form of β thalassemia. Other mutations involving the 3′ end of the β-globin mRNA interfere with its processing and produce severe β-thalassemia phenotypes.

Because there are so many different β-thalassemia mutations, it follows that many patients who are apparently homozygous for the disease are, in fact, compound heterozygotes for two different molecular lesions. Rarely, patients are encountered with forms of β thalassemia in which the HbA$_2$ level, which is usually raised in carriers, is normal. Usually this results from the coinheritance of β and δ thalassemia.

The δβ thalassemias are also divided into the (δβ)$^+$ and (δβ)^0 forms. The (δβ)$^+$ thalassemias result from misalignment of the δ and β globin genes during meiosis with the production of δβ fusion genes. These give rise to structural hemoglobin variants called the Lepore hemoglobins, after the family name of the first patient to be identified with this condition. Because the genes that direct the δβ fusion chains have δ-globin gene promoter regions that contain mutations which result in their ineffective transcription, the δβ chains are synthesized at a reduced rate and hence are associated with the phenotype of δβ thalassemia. The different forms of (δβ)^0

thalassemia all result from long deletions of the β-globin gene cluster that remove the δ and β genes, and leave either one or both the γ-globin genes intact. Longer deletions that remove the β-globin LCR and all or most of the cluster completely inactivate the gene complex and result in (εγδβ)^0 thalassemia.[9,10]

The molecular pathology and genetics of the α thalassemias are more complicated than that of β thalassemia, largely because there are two functional α-globin genes on each pair of chromosomes.[9,11,12] The normal α-globin genotype can be written αα/αα. The α^0 thalassemias result from a family of different-sized deletions that remove both α-globin genes; the homozygous and heterozygous states are designated − −/− − and − −/αα, respectively. Rarely, α^0 thalassemia may result from deletions involving a region similar to the β-globin LCR, 40 kb upstream from the α-globin gene cluster, or from short truncations of the end of the short arm of chromosome 16.

The molecular basis for the α$^+$ thalassemias is more complicated. In some cases they result from deletions that remove one of the linked pairs of α-globin genes, − α/αα, leaving the other intact, while in others both α-globin genes are intact but one of them has a mutation that either partially or completely inactivates it, α^{T}α/αα.

The deletion forms of α$^+$ thalassemia are further classified into the particular size of the underlying deletion. There are two common varieties, involving loss of either 3.7 or 4.2 kb of DNA; they are designated −α$^{3.7}$ and −α$^{4.2}$ respectively. It turns out that the former is quite heterogeneous, depending on the site of the abnormal genetic cross-over event that underlies the deletion. These deletions are thought to be due to misalignment and reciprocal cross-over between the α-globin gene segments at meiosis; this mechanism results in one chromosome with a single (− α) α gene and the opposite of the pair with a triplicated (ααα) α-gene arrangement.

Nondeletional forms of α thalassemia, in which the α-globin genes are intact, are caused by mutations that are very similar to those that cause β thalassemia. Some result from initiation or splice mutations, or the production of a highly unstable α globin that is incapable of producing a viable tetramer. Another particularly common form, found in Southeast Asia, results from a single base change in the termination codon UAA, which changes to CAA. The latter is the code for the amino acid glutamine. Hence, when the ribosomes reach this point, instead of the chain terminating, mRNA which is not normally transcribed is read through until another stop codon is reached. Thus, an elongated α-globin chain is produced that is synthesized at a reduced rate; the resulting variant is called Hb Constant Spring after the name of the town in Jamaica where it was first discovered. It occurs in about 2–5% of the population of Thailand and other regions of Southeast Asia. Because the termination codon can change to yield several different codons, this variant is only one of a family of chain-termination mutants. Another common form of nondeletional α thalassemia, which is found in the Middle East, results from a single base change in the highly conserved sequence of the 3′ coding region of the α-globin gene, AATAAA, which is changed to AATAAG. This is the signal site for polyadenylation of globin mRNA, a process that appears to stabilize its passage into the cytoplasm. This mutation results in marked reduction in α-globin chain production from the affected locus.

In addition to these common forms of α thalassemia, there is a syndrome characterized by mild α thalassemia and mental retardation (ATR) that is being recognized increasingly in many different populations. By combining clinical and molecular studies, it has been possible to subclassify this condition into two main syndromes, one encoded on chromosome 16 (ATR-16) and another on the X chromosome (ATR-X). ATR-16 is associated with relatively mild mental retardation and results from a variety of long deletions that remove the end of the short arm of chromosome 16. These may occur alone or as part of a chromosomal translocation.[10] ATR-X, which is characterized by a more severe form of mental retardation with a severe dysmorphologic picture, results from mutations of a gene on the X chromosome identified as *ATRX*.[11] The gene product is a DNA helicase that appears to be one of a family of *trans*-acting proteins involved with gene regulation through the remodeling of chromatin.[12] There is also a form of α thalassemia associated with myelodysplasia, particularly in elderly patients.[13] Recently it has been found that this condition, like ATR, is also associated with acquired somatic mutations in *ATRX*.[14]

Cellular pathology

Although the basic defect, imbalanced globin chain synthesis, is similar in all types of thalassemia, the consequences of excess α or β chain production in the β and α thalassemias are quite different.[1] Excess α chains that are produced in β thalassemia are unable to form a hemoglobin tetramer and precipitate in the red cell precursors. On the other hand, the excess of γ and β chains produced at different developmental stages in the α thalassemias are able to form homotetramers which, although unstable, are viable and form soluble hemoglobin molecules called Hb Barts (γ_4) and HbH (β_4). It is these fundamental differences in the behavior of the excess chains in the two common classes of thalassemia that are responsible for the major differences in their cellular pathology.

The β-thalassemias

The excess of α chains produced in β thalassemia is highly unstable, and rapidly precipitates and becomes associated with the membrane of red cell precursors and red cells. This phenomenon leads to extensive intramedullary destruction of red cell precursors, probably through a variety of complex mechanisms including interference with cell division and oxidative damage to the precursor membranes.[15–18] Because they contain large inclusion bodies, such red cells as do reach the peripheral blood are damaged in their passage through the spleen and their membranes also suffer severe oxidative injury due to the action of heme liberated from denatured hemoglobin and the excess of iron that accumulates in the thalassemic red cell. Thus the anemia of β thalassemia reflects a combination of ineffective erythropoiesis combined with reduced red cell survival.

Small populations of red cell precursors retain the capacity for producing γ chains of HbF in extrauterine life. In β thalassemics these cells come under intense selection; the excess of α chains is smaller because some of them combine with γ chains to produce HbF. Thus, the baseline level of fetal hemoglobin is elevated in β thalassemia. Cell selection occurs throughout the lifespan of the HbF-rich population;[1] it is also apparent that there are a number of genetic factors that modify the ability to make HbF in response to severe anemia.[19] These factors combine to produce increased levels of HbF in all forms of severe β thalassemia. Since δ-chain synthesis is unaffected in β thalassemia, heterozygotes usually have an elevated level of HbA_2, another important diagnostic feature.

The profound anemia of β thalassemia, and the production of red cell populations rich in HbF and a high oxygen affinity, combine to cause severe hypoxia and stimulate erythropoietin production. This, in turn, leads to extensive expansion of the ineffective erythroid mass with consequent bone changes, increased iron absorption, a high metabolic rate, and many of the other clinical features of severe β thalassemia. The bombardment of the spleen with abnormal red cells causes increasing splenomegaly; hence the disease may be complicated by trapping of part of the circulating red cell mass in the spleen which, together with sequestration of white cells and platelets, may produce the classical picture of severe hypersplenism.

Many of these features can be reversed by suppressing ineffective erythropoiesis by transfusion, which leads in turn to increased iron overload. The resulting pathology can

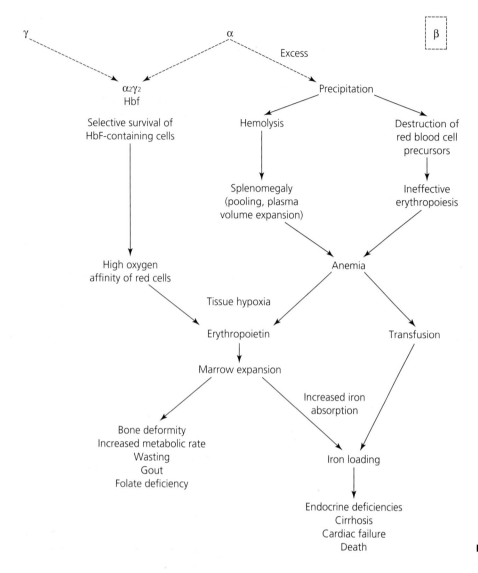

Fig. 13.6 Pathophysiology of β thalassemia.

be best appreciated against the background of normal iron metabolism.[20] In normal individuals, tight binding of plasma iron to the transport protein transferrin prevents the catalytic activity of iron in free-radical production.[21] In heavily iron-loaded patients, transferrin becomes fully saturated and a nontransferrin-bound fraction of iron becomes detectable in plasma. This may accelerate the formation of free hydroxyl radicals and results in accelerated iron loading in tissues, with consequent organ damage and dysfunction. In patients with iron overload, excess iron is deposited in both reticulo-endothelial cells (where it is relatively harmless) and paren-chymal tissue, primarily myocytes and hepatocytes (where it may cause significant damage). The toxicity of iron is mediated, in part, by its catalysis of reactions that gener-ate free hydroxyl radicals, propagators of oxygen-related damage.[21]

Clearly, therefore, it is possible to relate most of the clinical features of severe β thalassemia to the consequences of defect-ive β-globin production, the deleterious results of excess α-

globin chain synthesis on erythroid maturation and survival, and the effects of iron loading resulting from increased absorption and blood transfusion (Fig. 13.6). If these prin-ciples are appreciated, it is easy to understand why some forms of β thalassemia are associated with a much milder phenotype. Indeed, all the known factors that modify the phenotype of this disease act by reducing the amount of globin chain imbalance. They include the coinheritance of α thalassemia, the presence of a mild β-thalassemia allele, or the cosegregation of a gene that results in a higher than usual output of fetal hemoglobin.[19]

The α-thalassemias

The cellular pathology of α thalassemia, because of the prop-erties of HbH and Hb Barts, is different in many ways to that of β thalassemia.[1,11,18] As the result of the generation of these soluble tetramers there is less ineffective erythropoiesis. Particularly in the case of HbH, the tetramer tends to precipitate as cells age, with the production of inclusion bodies, and hence a major hemolytic component is a feature of the disorder. The clinical effects of the anemia are exacerbated by the fact that both HbH and Hb Barts are homotetramers and therefore cannot undergo the allosteric changes required for normal oxygen delivery. They behave, in effect, like myoglobin and are unable to give up oxygen at physiologic tensions. Hence, high levels of Hb Barts or HbH are associated with severe hypoxia.

The pathophysiology of the α thalassemias can be best understood in terms of simple gene dosage effects.[11] In the homozygous state for $α^0$ thalassemia ($--/--$) no α chains are produced. Affected infants have very high levels of Hb Barts with some embryonic hemoglobin. Although their hemoglobin concentration might be compatible with intrauterine life if the structure of their hemoglobin were normal, the fact that it is nearly all Hb Barts renders them seriously hypoxic. Most affected infants are stillborn with all the signs of gross intrauterine hypoxia. The compound heterozygous state for $α^0$ and $α^+$ thalassemia ($--/α-$) results in less chain imbalance and is compatible with survival, a condition called HbH disease. This disorder is characterized by a variable hemolytic anemia; adaptation to the level of anemia is often unsatisfactory because HbH, like Hb Barts, is unable to function as an oxygen carrier.

The heterozygous state for $α^0$ thalassemia ($--/αα$) and the homozygous state for the deletion form of $α^+$ thalassemia ($-α/-α$) are associated with a mild hypochromic anemia, very similar to β-thalassemia trait. Although a few red cells contain HbH inclusions in $α^0$-thalassemia trait, they are not observed in $α^+$-thalassemia trait, suggesting that there must be a critical level of excess β chains required to form viable $β_4$ tetramers. Interestingly, the homozygous states for the nondeletion forms of α thalassemia ($α^Tα/α^Tα$) are associated with a more severe deficiency of α chains and the clinical phenotype of HbH disease.

Clinical features

The β thalassemias

Most children with the severe forms of homozygous or compound heterozygous β thalassemia present within the first year of life, with failure to thrive, poor feeding, intermittent bouts of infection, and general malaise. These infants are pale and, in many cases, splenomegaly is already present. At this stage there are no other specific clinical signs and the diagnosis rests on the hematologic changes, outlined later. If the infant receives regular red cell transfusions, subsequent development is usually normal and further symptoms do not occur until puberty, when, if they have not received adequate chelation therapy, the signs of iron loading start to appear. If, on the other hand, the infant is not adequately transfused,

the typical clinical picture of thalassemia major develops. It follows therefore that clinical manifestations of the severe forms of β thalassemia can be described in two contexts: in the well-transfused child, and in the child with chronic anemia throughout early childhood.[1,22]

In the adequately transfused child, early growth and development are normal and splenomegaly is minimal or absent. If chelation therapy is effective, these children may enter normal puberty and continue to grow and develop normally into early adult life.[23,24]

On the other hand, if chelation therapy is inadequate, there is a gradual accumulation of iron, the effects of which start to become manifest by the end of the first decade. The normal adolescent growth spurt fails to occur and the hepatic, endocrine and cardiac complications of iron overloading give rise to a variety of symptoms, including diabetes, hyperthyroidism, hypoparathyroidism and progressive liver failure. Secondary sexual development is delayed or absent.

The commonest cause of death in iron-loaded children, which usually occurs toward the end of the second decade or early in the third decade, is iron-induced cardiac dysfunction; these patients die either in protracted cardiac failure or suddenly due to an acute arrhythmia, often precipitated by infection.

The clinical picture in inadequately transfused patients is quite different.[1] The rates of growth and development are retarded and progressive splenomegaly may cause a worsening of the anemia, and is sometimes associated with thrombocytopenia. There may be extensive bone marrow expansion leading to deformities of the skull, with marked bossing and overgrowth of the zygomata giving rise to the classical "mongoloid" appearance. These bone changes are associated with a characteristic radiologic picture that includes a lacy trabecular pattern of the long bones and phalanges, and a characteristic "hair on end" appearance of the skull. These children are prone to infection, which may cause a catastrophic drop in the hemoglobin level. Because of the massive expansion of the ineffective erythroid mass, they are hypermetabolic, run intermittent fevers, and fail to thrive. They have increased requirements for folic acid; deficiency is often associated with worsening of anemia. Because of the increased turnover of red cell precursors, hyperuricemia and secondary gout occur occasionally. There is also a bleeding tendency, which, although partly explained on the basis of thrombocytopenia, may also be exacerbated by liver damage associated with iron loading, viral hepatitis, or extramedullary hemopoiesis. If these children survive to puberty, they often develop the same complications of iron loading as well-transfused patients; in this case some of the iron accumulation results from an increased rate of gastrointestinal absorption.

The prognosis for inadequately transfused thalassemic children is poor. If they receive no transfusions, they may die within the first 2 years; if maintained at a low hemoglobin level throughout childhood, they usually die of infection or other intercurrent illness in early childhood. If they survive to reach puberty, they succumb to the effects of iron accumulation in the same way as the adequately transfused but poorly chelated child.

It should be emphasized that poor growth in children with β thalassemia is not restricted to those who are inadequately transfused or iron chelated. This problem is also observed in well-managed patients for reasons that are not entirely understood, and may include iron-induced selective central hypogonadism, impaired growth hormone responses to growth hormone-releasing hormone, delay in pubertal development, zinc deficiency, and over-intensive deferoxamine administration.

On presentation, hemoglobin values in the thalassemic child range from 2 to 8 g/dL. The red cells show marked hypochromia and variation in shape and size; there are many hypochromic macrocytes and misshapen microcytes, some of which are mere fragments of cells. There is moderate basophilic stippling and nucleated red cells are always present in the peripheral blood. After splenectomy these may appear in large numbers. The reticulocyte count is only moderately elevated. The white cell and platelet counts are normal unless hypersplenism is present. The bone marrow shows marked erythroid hyperplasia and many of the red cell precursors contain ragged inclusions, best demonstrated by staining with methyl violet, that represent α-globin precipitates.

The HbF level is always elevated and it is heterogeneously distributed among the red cells. In β^0 thalassemia there is no HbA; the hemoglobin consists of F and A_2 only. In β^+ thalassemia the level of HbF ranges from 20 to over 90%. The HbA_2 value is usually normal and of no diagnostic value. *In vitro* globin synthesis studies, involving the labeling of the globin chains with radioactive amino acids, reveals a marked degree of globin chain imbalance with an excess of α over non-α chain production.

β-Thalassemia trait

This is almost invariably asymptomatic and is characterized by mild anemia; splenomegaly is unusual. There is a slightly reduced hemoglobin level and a marked reduction in mean cell hemoglobin (MCH) and mean cell volume (MCV). The blood film shows hypochromia, microcytosis and variable basophilic stippling. In the majority of cases the HbA_2 level is elevated to about twice normal (i.e., in the 4–6% range), while there is a slight elevation of HbF in about 50% of cases. In some populations, notably those of the Mediterranean, β-thalassemia trait may be associated with a normal HbA_2 level. By far the commonest cause is the coinheritance of a gene for δ thalassemia. For genetic counseling (see later), it is vital to distinguish this condition from the different forms of α-thalassemia trait.

Intermediate forms of β thalassemia

Not all forms of homozygous or compound heterozygous β thalassemia are transfusion dependent from early life. The term "β thalassemia intermedia" is used to describe a wide spectrum of conditions, ranging from those that are almost as severe as β thalassemia, with marked anemia and growth retardation, to those which are almost as mild as β-thalassemia trait and which may only be discovered on routine hematologic examination.[19] In the more severe varieties there is obvious growth retardation, bone deformity and failure to thrive from early life and, except for a later presentation, the condition differs little from the transfusion-dependent forms of the illness. For its management this type of thalassemia intermedia should be considered to be in the same category as the severe transfusion-dependent form. On the other hand, many varieties are associated with good early growth and development, a satisfactory steady-state hemoglobin level, and mild to moderate splenomegaly. Even in these patients, several important complications may develop as these patients grow older, including increasing bone deformity, progressive osteoporosis with spontaneous fractures, leg ulcers, folate deficiency, hypersplenism, progressive anemia, and the effects of systemic iron overload due to increased intestinal absorption.

β Thalassemia associated with β-globin structural variants

Although β thalassemia has been found in association with many different β-globin chain variants, the only common disorders of this type are due to the coinheritance of HbS, HbC, or HbE.[1,3]

HbS β thalassemia

HbS β thalassemia varies considerably in its clinical manifestations, depending mainly on the nature of the associated β-thalassemia gene. HbS β^0 thalassemia, in which no HbA is produced, is often indistinguishable from sickle cell anemia. Similarly, HbS β^+ thalassemia in which the thalassemia gene results in a very low output of normal β chains, and hence a level of HbA in the 5–10% range, often runs a severe course. On the other hand, HbS β^+ thalassemia in which the β-thalassemia allele is of the mild variety, particularly those forms seen in Black populations and in which levels of HbA are in the 30–40% range, may be extremely mild and are often asymptomatic. The clinical manifestations of the sickling disorders are described in Chapter 10.

HbC β thalassemia

HbC β thalassemia occurs in West Africa and in the Mediterranean population and is characterized by a mild to moderate form of thalassemia intermedia with the typical hematologic changes of thalassemia associated with the presence of nearly 100% of target cells in the peripheral blood.

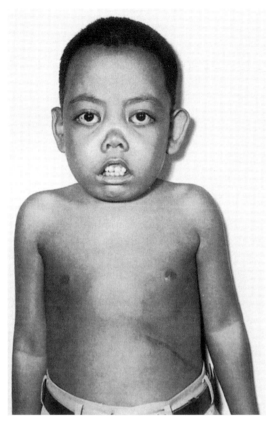

Fig. 13.7 Child with HbE β thalassemia showing the typical facial appearance of the more severe forms of the disease. This child had undergone splenectomy for worsening anemia.

HbE β thalassemia

HbE β thalassemia is a condition of major importance in eastern parts of India, Bangladesh, Myanmar, and throughout Southeast Asia. Since HbE behaves like a mild β-thalassemia allele, it is not surprising that his condition can behave like homozygous β thalassemia. However, what is difficult to explain is the remarkable clinical variability in its course. The clinical picture and complications may range from those of transfusion-dependent homozygous β thalassemia (Fig. 13.7) through the milder forms of thalassemia intermedia, as described above. The pattern of complications of the more severe forms of HbE β thalassemia are similar to those described earlier for β thalassemia major; the milder forms behave like β-thalassemia intermedia. The hemoglobin pattern depends on the nature of the associated β-thalassemia gene; in HbE β[0] thalassemia the globin is made up of F and E, whereas in HbE β[+] thalassemia there are variable amounts of HbA.

δβ Thalassemia

The common forms of (δβ)[+] thalassemia are the Hb Lepore disorders.[1,19] The homozygous state is usually characterized by a clinical disorder that is indistinguishable from β thalassemia major, although some cases run a milder course. The hemoglobin consists mainly of HbF, with up to 20% Hb Lepore. Heterozygotes for the different Hb Lepore disorders have the hematologic findings of thalassemia trait, with a hemoglobin pattern that consists of approximately 5–15% Hb Lepore and low or normal levels of HbA$_2$.

There are many different molecular varieties of (δβ)[0] thalassemia. The homozygous states are characterized by a mild to moderate form of thalassemia intermedia with typical thalassemic red cell changes and a hemoglobin pattern characterized by 100% HbF. Heterozygotes have mild thalassemic red cell changes, with levels of HbF in the 10–20% range and low-normal levels of HbA$_2$.

(εγδβ)[0] Thalassemia

This condition has not been observed in the homozygous state, presumably because it would be incompatible with fetal survival. Heterozygotes may be quite severely anemic at birth, with the clinical picture of hemolytic disease of the newborn[25] associated with hypochromic red cells and globin chain imbalance typical of β-thalassemia trait. For reasons that are not understood, anemia improves with age, hemoglobin level increasing during childhood; in adult life a blood picture typical of β-thalassemia trait but with a normal HbA$_2$ level is observed.

The α thalassemias

Homozygous α[0] thalassemia

This condition, Hb Barts hydrops syndrome, is usually characterized by death *in utero*.[1,12] These babies are either stillborn near term or, if liveborn, untreated usually only survive for a short period. The clinical picture is typical of hydrops fetalis, with marked edema and hepatosplenomegaly. The blood picture shows a hemoglobin level in the 6–8 g/dL range and the red cells are hypochromic with numerous nucleated forms. The hemoglobin consists of approximately 80% Hb Barts, with the remainder the embryonic Hb Portland. This syndrome is associated with a high frequency of toxemia of pregnancy, with postpartum bleeding, and other problems due to massive hypertrophy of the placenta. Autopsy studies show an increased frequency of fetal abnormalities, although these are not always present; in a few babies that have been rescued by exchange transfusion and maintained on regular red cell transfusions, growth and development has not always been normal.

α[0]/α[+] Thalassemia: HbH disease

This condition is characterized by a moderate degree of anemia and splenomegaly. It has a remarkably variable clinical course: while some patients become transfusion dependent, the majority are able to grow and develop normally without transfusion. The blood picture shows typical thalassemic red cell changes and the hemoglobin pattern is characterized by variable amounts of HbH, small amounts of Hb Barts, and a low-normal level of HbA$_2$. HbH may be demonstrated by incubating the red cells with a redox agent like brilliant cresyl blue, which causes it to precipitate with the formation of inclusion bodies. After splenectomy, large preformed inclusion bodies are present in many of the red cells.

α-Thalassemia trait

The clinical picture of α-thalassemia trait may result from the heterozygous state for α^0 thalassemia (– –/αα) or the homozygous state for α$^+$ thalassemia (– α/– α) as described above. These conditions are asymptomatic and the hematologic findings are characterized by a mild hypochromic anemia with a marked reduction in MCH and MCV. The hemoglobin pattern is normal and these conditions can only be diagnosed with certainty by DNA analyses. In the newborn period there are increased levels of Hb Barts, in the 5–10% range, but HbH is not demonstrable in adult life; occasional inclusions may be seen in the red cells in α^0-thalassemia carriers.

"Silent" α-thalassemia carriers

The heterozygous state for α$^+$ thalassemia (– α/αα) is associated with no hematologic abnormalities and a normal hemoglobin pattern in adult life. At birth approximately 50% of cases have slightly elevated levels of Hb Barts in the 1–3% range, but its absence does not rule out the diagnosis.

α Thalassemia mental retardation syndromes

The ATR-16 syndrome is characterized by moderate mental retardation and a very mild form of HbH disease or a blood picture resembling α-thalassemia trait. Patients with this disorder should undergo detailed cytogenetic analysis; in some cases chromosomal translocations may be found that are of importance for genetic counseling for future pregnancies. The ATR-X syndrome is characterized by severe mental retardation, seizures, an unusual facial appearance with flattening of the nose, urogenital abnormalities, and other dysmorphic features.[26] The blood picture shows a mild form of HbH disease or α-thalassemia trait, and HbH inclusions can usually be demonstrated. The mothers of these children usually have small populations of red cells that contain HbH inclusions.

Screening and prevention

There are two major approaches to the avoidance of the thalassemias. Since the carrier states for β thalassemia can be easily recognized, it is possible to screen populations and provide genetic counseling about the choice of marriage partners. If two β-thalassemia heterozygotes marry, one in four of their children will have the severe compound heterozygous or homozygous disorder. Alternatively, when heterozygous mothers are identified prenatally, the husbands may be tested; if they are also carriers, the couple may be counseled and offered the possibility of prenatal diagnosis and termination of pregnancies carrying a fetus with a severe form of β thalassemia.

Screening

If populations wish to offer marital choice, it is essential to develop premarital screening programs, best carried out in schoolchildren. It is vital to have a very well organized genetic counseling program in place and to provide both verbal advice and written information about the results of screening. The alternative approach is to screen every woman of an appropriate racial background in early pregnancy.

Probably the most cost-effective way of screening for thalassemia is through red cell indices.[27] If MCV and MCH values are found to be in the range associated with the carrier states for thalassemia, a HbA$_2$ estimation should be carried out.[5] This will be elevated in the majority of cases of β thalassemia. If the HbA$_2$ level is normal, it is essential to refer the patient to a center that can analyze the α-globin genes. It is important to distinguish between the homozygous state for α$^+$ thalassemia (– α/– α) and the heterozygous state for α^0 thalassemia (– –/αα); in the former case the patient is not at risk for having a baby homozygous for α^0 thalassemia with its attendant obstetric risks. In those rare cases in which the blood picture resembles heterozygous β thalassemia but the HbA$_2$ level is normal and the α-globin genes are intact, the differential diagnosis lies between a nondeletional form of α thalassemia and a normal-HbA$_2$ form of β thalassemia. These conditions have to be distinguished by globin chain synthesis analysis and further DNA studies.[28] It is important, of course, to carry out routine hemoglobin electrophoresis in all these cases to exclude a coexisting structural hemoglobin variant.

Prenatal diagnosis

Prenatal diagnosis of different forms of thalassemia can be carried out in several ways.[28] It can be made by studies of globin chain synthesis in fetal blood samples obtained by fetoscopy at 18–20 weeks' gestation, although this approach has now been largely replaced by fetal DNA analysis. DNA is usually obtained by chorionic villous sampling (CVS) between weeks 9 and 12 of gestation. There is a small risk of fetal loss and of the production of fetal abnormalities following this approach.[27]

The diagnostic techniques used for DNA analysis after CVS have changed rapidly over recent years.[28] The first diagnoses were carried out by Southern blotting of fetal DNA, using either restriction fragment length polymorphisms (RFLPs) combined with linkage analysis, or direct detection of mutations. More recently, following the development of the polymerase chain reaction (PCR), the identification of thalassemia mutations in fetal DNA has been greatly facilitated. For example, it can be used for the rapid detection of mutations that alter restriction enzyme cutting sites. The particular fragment of the β-globin gene is amplified, after which the DNA fragments are digested with an appropriate enzyme and separated by electrophoresis; these fragments can be detected by either ethidium bromide or silver staining of DNA bands on gels, and radioactive probes are not required.

Now that the mutations have been identified in many forms of α and β thalassemia, it is possible to detect them directly as the first-line approach to fetal DNA analysis. The development of PCR, combined with the availability of oligonucleotide probes to detect individual mutations, has opened up a variety of new approaches for improving the speed and accuracy of carrier detection and prenatal diagnosis. For example, a diagnosis can be made using hybridization of specific ^{32}P-end-labeled oligonucleotides to an amplified region of the β-globin genes dotted onto nylon membranes. Since the β-globin gene sequence of interest can be amplified more than a million-fold, thus increasing the efficiencies of probe annealing, hybridization times can be limited to 1 hour, and the entire procedure can be carried out in 2 hours.

There are many variations on the PCR approach to prenatal diagnosis. For example, in a technique called ARMS (amplification refractory mutation system), which is based on the observation that, in many cases, oligonucleotides for the 3′ mismatched residue will, under appropriate conditions, not function as primers in the PCR, it is possible to construct two specific primers.[29] The normal primer is refractory to PCR on a mutant template DNA, while the mutant sequence is refractory to PCR on normal DNA. Other modifications of PCR involve the use of nonradioactively labeled probes.

The error rate using these different approaches in most laboratories is now well below 1%.[30] Potential sources of error include maternal contamination of fetal DNA, nonpaternity and, if RFLP linkage analysis is used, genetic recombination.

More recently, other approaches have been developed for prenatal detection of the thalassemias, including the isolation of fetal cells from maternal blood and preimplantation diagnosis.[1] Although there have been a few reported successes of the prenatal diagnosis of β thalassemia and Hb Lepore thalassemia by the analysis of fetal cells isolated from the maternal circulation, this technique is still under development and is only applicable to certain forms of β thalassemia. Several laboratories have reported success with preimplantation diagnosis but this remains technically difficult; this seems to be a promising area for future development in this field.

Clinical management

Over recent years there have been major improvements in the clinical management of the severe forms of β thalassemia.[22] The development of better blood transfusion regimens, combined with effective iron-chelating therapy, has transformed the outlook for children with this disease, at least those for whom, in richer countries, this treatment is available.

Red cell transfusions

Regular red cell transfusions eliminate the complications of anemia and ineffective erythropoiesis, permit normal growth and development throughout childhood, and extend survival in thalassemia major.[20,22] The decision to initiate regular transfusions is generally based on the observation of a hemoglobin concentration less than 6 g/dL over three consecutive months, a finding usually associated with poor growth, splenic enlargement and some degree of marrow expansion. Determination of the molecular basis for severe β thalassemia is only occasionally of value in predicting a requirement for regular transfusions.[1,19] Prior to the first transfusion, iron and folate status should be assessed, a hepatitis B vaccine series should be initiated, and a complete red cell phenotype obtained so that subsequent alloimmunization may be detected.

It is important that the pretransfusion hemoglobin concentration does not generally exceed 9.5 g/dL.[31] The pretransfusion hemoglobin concentration, the volume of red cells administered, the weight of the patient, and the size of the spleen should be recorded at each visit in order to detect the development of hypersplenism.

Type of red cell concentrates

All patients should receive leukocyte-reduced red cell preparations.[32] Early clinical experience with neocytes, young red blood cells separated from older cells by density centrifugation, suggested that their use is associated with modest extensions of transfusion intervals and reduction in annual transfusional iron load.[33] However, because these potential benefits are offset by major increases in preparation expenses and donor exposure,[34] neocytes have had a minor impact on the long-term management of patients with thalassemia.

Alloimmunization

Red cell alloimmunization may be higher in patients in whom blood transfusion was begun after the age of 1 year,[32] and lower in Mediterranean patients (3–10%) compared with Asian individuals (~21%), because of differences in antigenic distribution.[35] If possible, patients with thalassemia should receive blood matched for ABO, CcDdEe, and Kell antigens.

Splenectomy

In the past, an increase in transfusion requirements due to hypersplenism was frequently observed at the age of approximately 10 years. When annual transfusion requirements exceed 200–250 mL packed cells per kilogram body weight, splenectomy significantly reduces these requirements.[36] In the modern era, with improved transfusion practices, hypersplenism is reduced and many patients do not require splenectomy.[22] Concerns that splenectomy may be associated with acceleration of iron loading in other organs remain unproven; the spleen does not appear to be a significant repository of transfused iron.[37] The biliary tract should be carefully assessed at surgery, but in the absence of disease there seems little place for prophylactic cholecystectomy. Because of the risk of postsplenectomy infection, splenectomy should usually be delayed until the age of 5 years.[22] At least 3 weeks prior to splenectomy, patients should be vaccinated with the pneumococcal and *Haemophilus influenzae* type B vaccines, and after surgery daily prophylactic penicillin should be administered at least during childhood and probably indefinitely. Erythromycin should be substituted for those who are allergic to penicillin.

Infectious complications

Hepatitis B and hepatitis C virus, HIV, human T-cell leukemia virus and cytomegalovirus may cause significant morbidity and mortality in humans.[32] Iron-induced hepatic damage may be influenced by infection with hepatitis C virus, the most frequent cause of hepatitis in thalassemic children. The clinical and pathologic responses to interferon-α in thalassemia patients with hepatitis C may be inversely related to body iron burden.[38] A 70% response rate in interferonnaive patients treated for 12 months with interferon oca and ribavirin has been reported.[39] Infection with *Yersinia enterocolitica*, which poses a risk because of its growth enhancement in iron-rich environments,[40] should be suspected in patients with iron overload who present with high fever and no obvious focus of infection. Even in the absence of a positive blood culture for *Yersinia* in this clinical setting, therapy with intravenous gentamicin and oral trimethoprim-sulfamethoxazole should be promptly instituted, and continued for at least 7 days. Transfusion-transmitted malaria remains a major hazard in many developing countries.

Iron overload and iron-chelating therapy

Iron overload is the most important consequence of lifesaving transfusions in thalassemia.[20] The only chelating agent approved for first-line therapy is deferoxamine. The standard method of deferoxamine administration today is prolonged parenteral infusion using portable ambulatory pumps (reviewed in ref. 20). Even suboptimal doses of defer-

oxamine prevent a rise in body iron during transfusion.[41] Early reports of the beneficial effects of deferoxamine therapy on survival[42,43] were confirmed by two studies from four North American centers with follow-up periods of 10–15 years.[23,24] Patients in whom most serum ferritin concentrations were maintained at less than 2500 µg/L over 15 years had an estimated cardiac disease-free survival of 91%. Similarly, patients with hepatic storage iron less than 15 mg/g liver dry weight were protected from cardiac disease, impaired glucose tolerance and diabetes mellitus. Survival in recent studies in compliant patients is reported as 95–100% at 30 years of age.[44–49]

Liver disease

The beneficial effects of deferoxamine on liver disease, the second leading cause of death in thalassemia,[42] include reduction in iron concentration and improvement in liver function even in patients with massively elevated hepatic iron concentrations.[41]

Endocrine function

Long-term deferoxamine appears to have a beneficial effect on growth, sexual maturation and other endocrine complications (reviewed in ref. 20). Normal pubertal development has been reported in approximately 50–70% of younger patients,[42] although the development of secondary amenorrhea may develop eventually in about 20% of women. Adequate deferoxamine therapy also reduces the likelihood of the development of diabetes mellitus and hypothyroidism.[24,44] A striking increase in fertility in both men and women, as well as many successful pregnancies, has been reported over the last decade.[45]

Growth

In well-transfused but inadequately chelated patients, the first evidence of iron-mediated damage to the hypothalamic–pituitary axis may be amelioration of the pubertal growth spurt, associated with delayed sexual maturation. In some patients overintensive deferoxamine administration may be a cause of poor growth.[46]

Optimal body iron in patients with thalassemia major

The magnitude of the body iron burden is the principal determinant of clinical outcome.[23,24] A balance must be struck between the risk of complications from iron overload and the toxicity of deferoxamine, which is increased in the presence of a relatively reduced body iron burden.[47] A conservative goal for iron-chelating therapy in thalassemia is maintenance

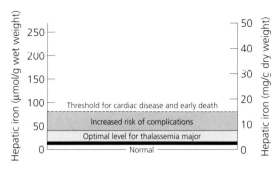

Fig. 13.8 Thresholds of hepatic iron concentration in thalassemia (see text).

of hepatic storage iron between 3.2 and 7 mg/g liver dry weight (Fig. 13.8).[20,48]

Management of iron-chelating therapy

One practical problem associated with long-term chelating therapy is the assessment of body iron. While plasma or serum ferritin concentration is the most commonly used indirect estimate of body iron stores, a concentration exceeding 4000 µg/L, the result of ferritin release from damaged cells, may not reflect body iron stores.[49] Changes above this level of serum ferritin may have limited clinical relevance. Inter-

pretation of the serum ferritin may be complicated by a variety of conditions that alter concentrations independently of changes in body iron, including ascorbate deficiency, acute and chronic infection and inflammation, hepatic disease, and ineffective erythropoiesis.[20] Because of this, in thalassemia major, variations in body iron account for only 57% of the variation in serum ferritin.[50]

In contrast, measurement of hepatic iron concentration is a quantitative, specific and sensitive method of assessing body iron burden in thalassemia (Table 13.2).[51,52] Liver biopsy represents the best means of evaluating the pattern of iron accumulation, and the inflammatory activity and histology of the liver. Liver biopsy under ultrasound guidance has a low complication rate in children,[53] and should be performed at important crossroads in the management of the child with thalassemia.

Imaging techniques including computed tomography and magnetic resonance imaging (MRI) have been used to evaluate tissue iron stores *in vitro* and *in vivo*.[51] Although MRI potentially provides the best available technique for examining the distribution of excess iron, further research is needed to develop means of making these measurements quantitative.[51] To date, MRI has been more useful as a screening technique for the detection of marked iron overload than as a means for quantitative measurement.[51] A calibration curve relating liver MRI signal to hepatic iron concentration has

Table 13.2 Assessment of body iron burden in thalassemia.

Test	Comments
Indirect (most tests widely available)	
Serum/plasma ferritin concentration	Noninvasive
	Lacks sensitivity and specificity
	Poorly correlated with hepatic iron concentration in individual patients
Serum transferrin saturation	Lacks sensitivity
Tests of 24-hour deferoxamine-induced urinary iron excretion	Less than half of outpatient aliquots collected correctly
	Ratio of stool to urine iron variable; poorly correlated with hepatic iron concentration
Imaging of tissue iron	
Computed tomography: liver	Variable correlation with hepatic iron concentration reported
Magnetic resonance	
Liver	Variable correlations with hepatic iron concentration reported
	Treatment-induced changes confirmed by liver biopsy
Heart	Only modality available to image cardiac iron stores; changes observed during chelating therapy consistent with reduction in cardiac iron
Anterior pituitary	Only modality available to image pituitary iron; signal moderately well correlated with pituitary reserve
Evaluation of organ function	Most tests lack sensitivity and specificity; may identify established organ dysfunction
Direct (most tests not widely available)	
Cardiac iron quantitation: biopsy	Imprecise due to inhomogeneous distribution of cardiac iron
Hepatic iron quantitation: biopsy	Reference method; provides direct assessment of body iron burden, severity of fibrosis and inflammation
	Safe when performed under ultrasound guidance
Superconducting susceptometry (SQUID)	Noninvasive; excellent correlation with biopsy-determined hepatic iron

Table 13.3 Monitoring of deferoxamine-related toxicity.

Toxicity	Investigations	Frequency	Alteration in therapy
High-frequency sensorineural hearing loss	Audiogram	Yearly; if patient symptomatic, immediate reassessment	Interrupt DFO immediately Directly assess body iron burden Discontinue DFO × 6 months if HIC 3.2–7 mg/g dry wt liver tissue Repeat audiogram every 3 months until normal or stable Adjust DFO to HIC (see Table 15.2)
Retinal abnormalities	Retinal examination	Yearly; if patient symptomatic, immediate reassessment	Interrupt DFO immediately Directly assess body iron burden Discontinue DFO × 6 months if HIC 3.2–7 mg/g dry wt liver tissue Review every 3 months until normal or stable Adjust DFO to HIC (see Table 15.2)
Metaphyseal and spinal abnormalities	Radiography of wrists, knees, thoraco-lumbar-sacral spine Bone age of wrist	Yearly	Reduce DFO to 25 mg/kg daily × 4/week Directly assess body iron burden Discontinue DFO × 6 months if HIC ≤ 3 mg/g dry weight liver tissue Reassess HIC after 6 months Adjust DFO to HIC (see Table 15.2)
Decline in height velocity and/or sitting height	Determination of sitting and standing heights	Twice yearly	As for metaphyseal and spinal abnormalities Regular (6-monthly) assessment by pediatric endocrinologist

DFO, deferoxamine; HIC, hepatic iron concentration.

been deduced over a clinically relevant range of hepatic iron concentrations, with a coefficient of variation of 2.1%.[54] Biomagnetic susceptometry (SQUID)[55] provides the only noninvasive measurement of tissue iron stores validated for use in clinical studies, but it is available in only a few centers worldwide.[51] Recently, attempts to assess cardiac iron using different MRI techniques have included a much-promoted "T2*" technique,[56,57] the validity and prognostic significance of which requires clarification by long-term, prospective studies.[58] The most comprehensive and valid assessment of cardiac function is still the combined information obtained from the patient's transfusion record, knowledge of adherence to a chelation regimen, and serial hepatic iron concentrations.[59]

Initiation and management of chelating therapy

Few guidelines exist with respect to the start of iron-chelating therapy. In practice, the usual approach is to begin a regimen of nightly subcutaneous deferoxamine based on the serum ferritin concentration after a period of regular transfusions, but initiation (and titration) of deferoxamine therapy is ideally based on hepatic iron concentration, determined after 1 year of regular transfusions. If a liver biopsy is not obtained, treatment with subcutaneous deferoxamine not exceeding 25–35 mg/kg body weight per 24 hours should be initiated after approximately 1 year of regular transfusions.

Balance between effectiveness and toxicity of deferoxamine (Table 13.3)

Virtually all toxicities are *dose related*, occurring only when excessive doses, or regular doses in patients with modest body iron burdens, are administered. Guidelines for safe dosage include restricting daily doses to 50 mg/kg body weight or less and twice-yearly calculation of a "toxicity" index, calculated as mean daily dose of deferoxamine (mg/kg) divided by serum ferritin concentration (μg/L), which should not exceed 0.025.[47,60,61]

Alternatives to subcutaneous infusion of deferoxamine

The most common difficulty associated with long-term therapy is erratic compliance, especially in adolescents. Regimens of intravenous ambulatory deferoxamine, in which drug is administered through implantable venous access ports,[62] circumvents tissue irritation and are associated with rapid reduction of body iron burden and good patient compliance. Such regimens have been shown to reverse cardiac dysfunction.[63]

Orally active iron-chelating agents

The expense and inconvenience of deferoxamine has led to a long-time search for an orally active iron chelator. The agent most extensively evaluated to date is deferiprone. Clinical trials that were intended to support an application for the licensing of deferiprone were terminated prematurely by their corporate sponsor in 1996 after concerns were raised by the investigators about inadequate control of body iron in many patients.[64] Because serum ferritin showed a less clear relationship to hepatic iron concentration[65] than in patients treated with deferoxamine, it may be problematic to interpret changes in serum ferritin as evidence of the effectiveness of deferiprone. In studies which determined hepatic storage iron, this exceeded 15 mg/g dry weight in 18–65% of patients treated over 2–8 years,[66] raising concerns that deferiprone may not be sufficiently effective to protect all patients from iron-induced cardiac disease.

Claims that deferiprone is a more effective cardioprotective agent than deferoxamine are not yet supported by prospective clinical data.[58,67] Continued cardiac mortality in patients receiving deferiprone has been reported,[65,68] including deaths after years of treatment, during which period an improvement in cardiac disease is regularly observed with deferoxamine.

Since 1999, deferiprone has been licensed for patients in Europe "unable to use" deferoxamine. An application submitted to North American regulators in 2002 has been unsuccessful in obtaining marketing approval to date. Reassuringly, only 16 patients truly "unable to use" deferoxamine are reported in the literature over 20 years;[69] all have been capable of being desensitized and of resuming deferoxamine safely. Non-compliance remains a serious problem however.

Deferiprone has also been administered "in combination" with deferoxamine (although this combination is not formally permitted under European licensing). Most of these are short-term studies, with periods of administration less than 2 years, report poor control of iron in most of the 39 patients. No long-term efficacy or safety data are available for combination therapy.[69a]

Toxicity of deferiprone

Reports of arthropathy in deferiprone-treated patients are somewhat confusing. Most reviews claim that this complication, "varies between ethnic groups;" subtotal destruction with an incidence of 2–10%, is reversible on stopping the drug. However, recent data suggest that both the incidence and severity of this complication varies between ethnic groups; subtotal destruction of the knee joints has now been observed in some patients. In India,[70,71] Sri Lanka,[72,73] and Lebanon,[74,75] arthropathy is reported as developing in up to 50% of patients. A lower incidence (0–18%) has been reported from other centers.[68,76–80]

Accelerated progression of hepatic fibrosis has been observed at proportions of 29%,[78] 36%,[81] 37%,[79] and 0%[82] (of all patients who underwent baseline and follow-up biopsies). In some[79,82] but not all[81] studies, liver function worsened in

deferiprone-treated patients, regardless of hepatitis C virus status, while remaining unchanged in deferoxamine-treated patients. More worrisome is the evidence of hepatocellular damage in deferiprone-treated patients emerging after many years of treatment,[68,83] consistent with the observation that the time to onset of accelerated hepatic damage might exceed 3 years.[81] The one study to report no accelerated liver damage[82] was undermined by a failure to report striking increases (32–85% over baseline) in hepatocellular iron, although this finding was reported in an earlier publication.[84] Other toxicities of deferiprone include nausea, agranulocytosis and neutropenia. In summary, it is generally accepted that deferiprone is less effective than deferoxamine in maintaining iron balance. Its potential for cardioprotection requires further prospective study.[85]

Other orally active iron chelators

The iron chelator ICL670A (Exjade; Novartis) has undergone early evaluation in a randomized, double-blind, placebo-controlled, dose-escalation study that established its short-term tolerability.[86] This was followed by Phase II and Phase III studies to examine short-term efficacy and safety,[87–89] in which hepatic iron was assessed at baseline and after 1 year of treatment. The long-term effectiveness and safety of this drug await further study.

Bone marrow transplantation

Allogeneic bone marrow transplantation offers an accepted alternative to standard clinical management. Three pretransplant characteristics are significantly associated with survival and event-free survival: (i) hepatomegaly greater than 2 cm below the costal margin; (ii) the presence of portal fibrosis on liver biopsy; and (iii) the effectiveness of therapy with deferoxamine prior to transplantation.[90] In patients in whom none of these factors were present prior to transplantation (identified as "class 1" patients), event-free survival exceeded 90%; in contrast, in those with all three ("class 3" patients), event-free survival was only 56%. In over 1000 consecutive transplants in patients aged 1–35 years, overall survival was 68%.[91] In class 1 patients, thalassemia-free survival was 90% and survival was 93%. Umbilical cord blood has been used as a source of stem cells for class 1 and 2 children.[92]

Less than 30% of patients have an available HLA-identical family donor. In a study of unrelated donors matched by high-resolution molecular HLA methods ("extended haplotypes"), 69% of patients were alive and well after 7–109 months.[93] This approach, and the use of related partially mismatched donors, is considered experimental in thalassemia.[94]

Successful transplantation liberates patients from chronic transfusions, but does not eliminate the necessity for iron-chelating therapy in all cases. Iron overload and hepatitis

C virus are independent and synergistic risk factors for progression of hepatic fibrosis and the development of cirrhosis in the "ex-thalassemic". Removal of iron by phlebotomy and deferoxamine is safe and effective in the reduction of tissue iron and the arrest of fibrosis and early cirrhosis.[95]

Many parents may be confronted with the choice between standard medical (transfusion and chelation) therapy and bone marrow transplantation. The excellent results from Italy suggest that marrow transplantation should be offered to any patient with a compatible donor. On the other hand, the choice between these therapeutic approaches may be a difficult one, since extended cardiac disease-free survival in patients regularly compliant with deferoxamine exceeds 90%, comparable to that achieved with transplantation in class 1 patients. However, while the long-term outcomes of transplantation are not fully known, and mortality is always a risk, this cost-saving procedure renders patients not merely cardiac disease-free but also thalassemia-free. Furthermore, if compliance with regular deferoxamine falters or ineffective treatments are embarked upon, survival in "medically treated" patients may be considerably less than 90%.

Experimental approaches

Augmentation of fetal hemoglobin synthesis may reduce globin chain imbalance and ameliorate the severity of the disease.[96] Several cell cycle-specific chemotherapeutic agents, and nonchemotherapeutic drugs including hematopoietic growth factors and short-chain fatty acids, stimulate HbF production *in vitro* and in animal models. Clinical trials in thalassemia have included short- and long-term administration of 5-azacytidine, hydroxycarbamide, recombinant human erythropoietin, butyric acid compounds, and combinations of these agents.[96]

5-Azacytidine successfully increased HbF levels in early studies of patients with β thalassemia but predictably causes bone marrow suppression, limiting drug administration in some patients. Consideration of its potential adverse effects shifted interest to the use of alternate therapies.[96,97]

Clinical responses associated with administration of hydroxycarbamide have been disappointing, given the recent observation that patients with certain polymorphisms and specific mutations, notably Gy-158 (c → T) and Hb Lepore, may demonstrate durable responses to hydroxycarbamide, with some patients achieving transfusion-independence.[97] Further trials may be of interest.

In patients treated with recombinant human erythropoietin therapy, total hemoglobin increased in a few, usually without observed effects on HbF synthesis.[96,97] This expensive regimen has not shown great promise in thalassemia.

Butyric acid compounds, derivatives of natural short-chain fatty acids, have offered potential therapy for the hemoglobinopathies following the observation that elevated plasma concentrations of α-amino-*n*-butyric acid in infants of diabetic mothers delayed the switch from β to γ globin around the time of birth.[98] Hematologic responses to arginine butyrate and sodium phenylbutyrate have been reported in thalassemia,[97] the most striking, for reasons that remain undefined,[99] in two siblings with homozygous Hb Lepore.

Management of other forms of thalassemia

Thalassemia intermedia

Thalassemia intermedia, a descriptive title with no clear-cut genetic meaning, is used to refer to patients with a hemoglobin level persistently below 9 g/dL who can be maintained without transfusions. The diagnosis should be made only after a considerable period of observation, and often requires revision.

At diagnosis, folate supplementation should be initiated and the hemoglobin should be determined twice monthly. A substantial decline should prompt investigations for secondary causes, including infection, folate deficiency, or hypersplenism. In patients over 4 years of age, splenectomy may be indicated prior to initiation of a program of regular transfusions. Some patients may become less tolerant of anemia with advancing age, or may develop transfusion dependency in adolescence or early adulthood. Abnormal growth, pathologic fractures, or signs of intolerance of anemia should prompt consideration of a program of regular transfusions. Spinal or nerve compression should be treated by red cell transfusion or local irradiation followed by transfusions.[100]

Iron loading is less accelerated than in thalassemia major. Daily gastrointestinal iron loading may be in the order of 3–9 mg, or about 2–5 g/year.[101] In contrast, in regularly transfused patients iron accumulation is in the range of 6–7 g/year. The coinheritance of hereditary hemochromatosis may adversely increase iron loading in thalassemia intermedia.[102] In patients with elevated serum ferritin concentrations, assessment of liver iron is indicated; if this exceeds 6 mg/g liver dry weight, deferoxamine should be initiated.

HbE β thalassemia

This is the commonest form of severe thalassemia in many Asian countries and is being seen increasingly in North America and Europe. Relatively little is known about its natural history, the reasons for its clinical diversity, or how it should be managed and it may not be possible to define its severity without a long period of observation. Until more is known about this important disease, approaches to its management should follow those recommended above for thalassemia intermedia.

The α thalassemias

All children with Hb Barts hydrops fetalis syndrome require regular blood transfusion and chelation therapy. Many patients with HbH disease can be managed conservatively with regular folate supplementation and avoidance of oxidant drugs, which tend to exacerbate their anemia. Occasionally, the hemoglobin level is such that a regular transfusion regimen, similar to that employed for severe cases of β thalassemia, may be required. Overall, the results of splenectomy are disappointing, and in a few cases it has been followed by severe thrombotic complications. Older patients may accumulate considerable amounts of iron through increased gastrointestinal absorption. Coexistence with the common form of hereditary hemochromatosis may explain more severe iron overload in occasional patients.

References

1. Weatherall DJ, Clegg JB (eds) *The Thalassaemia Syndromes*, 4th edn. Oxford: Blackwell Science, 2001.
2. Weatherall DJ, Clegg JB. Inherited haemoglobin disorders: an increasing global health problem. *Bull World Health Organ* 2001; **79**: 704–12.
3. Steinberg MH, Forget BG, Higgs DR, Nagel RL (eds) *Disorders of Hemoglobin*. New York: Cambridge University Press, 2001.
4. Weatherall DJ, Clegg JB, Higgs DR, Wood WG. The hemoglobinopathies. In: Scriver CR, Beaudet AL, Sly WS, Valle D (eds) *The Metabolic and Molecular Bases of Inherited Disease*, 8th edn. New York: McGraw Hill, 2001, pp. 4571–636.
5. Stamatoyannopoulos G, Grosveld F. Hemoglobin switching. In: Stamatoyannopoulos G, Majerus PW, Perlmutter RM, Varmus H (eds) *The Molecular Basis of Blood Disease*. Philadelphia: WB Saunders, 2001, pp. 136–82.
6. Higgs DR. Ham-Wasserman Lecture. Gene regulation in hematopoiesis: new lessons from thalassemia. *Hematology (Am Soc Hematol Educ Program)* 2004; 1–13.
7. Weatherall DJ, Clegg JB. Genetic variability in response to infection: malaria and after. *Genes Immunity* 2002; **3**: 331–7.
8. Huisman TH, Carver MFH, Baysal E. *A Syllabus of Thalassemia Mutations*. Augusta, GA: The Sickle Cell Anemia Foundation, 1997.
9. Weatherall DJ, Higgs DR, Bunch C *et al*. Hemoglobin H disease and mental retardation: a new syndrome or a remarkable coincidence? *N Engl J Med* 1981; **305**: 607–12.
10. Higgs D. Alpha thalassaemia with mental retardation or myelodysplasia. In: Weatherall DJ, Clegg JB (eds) *The Thalassaemia Syndromes*, pp. 526–49, 4th edn. Oxford: Blackwell, 2001.
11. Picketts DJ, Higgs DR, Bachoo S, Blake DJ, Quarrell OWJ, Gibbons RJ. *ATRX* encodes a novel member of the SNF2 family of proteins: mutations point to a common mechanism underlying the ATR-X syndrome. *Hum Mol Genet* 1996; **5**: 1899–907.
12. McDowell TL, Gibbons RJ, Sutherland H *et al*. Localization of a putative transcriptional regulator (ATRX) at pericentromeric heterochromatin and the short arms of acrocentric chromosomes. *Proc Natl Acad Sci USA* 1999; **96**: 13983–8.
13. Higgs DR, Wood WG, Barton C, Weatherall DJ. Clinical features and molecular analysis of acquired hemoglobin H disease. *Am J Med* 1983; **75**: 181–91.
14. Gibbons RJ, Pellagatti A, Garrick D *et al*. Identification of acquired somatic mutations in the gene encoding chromatin-remodeling factor ATRX in the alpha-thalassemia myelodysplasia syndrome (ATMDS). *Nat Genet* 2003; **34**: 446–9.
15. Shinar E, Rachmilewitz EA. Differences in the pathophysiology of hemolysis of alpha- and beta-thalassemic red blood cells. *Ann NY Acad Sci* 1990; **612**: 118–26.
16. Rund D, Rachmilewitz E. Advances in the pathophysiology and treatment of thalassemia. *Crit Rev Oncol Hematol* 1995; **20**: 237–54.
17. Schrier SL. Pathobiology of thalassemic erythrocytes. *Curr Opin Hematol* 1997; **4**: 75–8.
18. Weatherall DJ. Pathophysiology of thalassaemia. *Baillières Clin Haematol* 1998; **11**: 127–46.
19. Weatherall DJ. Phenotype–genotype relationships in monogenic disease: lessons from the thalassaemias. *Nat Rev Genet* 2001; **2**: 245–55.
20. Olivieri NF, Brittenham GM. Iron-chelating therapy and the treatment of thalassemia. *Blood* 1997; **89**: 739–61.
21. Andrews N. Disorders of iron metabolism. *N Engl J Med* 1999; **341**: 1986–95.
22. Olivieri NF. The beta-thalassemias. *N Engl J Med* 1999; **341**: 99–109.
23. Olivieri NF, Nathan DG, MacMillan JH *et al*. Survival in medically treated patients with homozygous beta-thalassemia. *N Engl J Med* 1994; **331**: 574–8.
24. Brittenham GM, Griffith PM, Nienhuis AW *et al*. Efficacy of deferoxamine in preventing complications of iron overload in patients with thalassemia major. *N Engl J Med* 1994; **331**: 567–73.
25. Kan YW, Forget BG, Nathan DG. Gamma-beta thalassemia: a cause of hemolytic disease of the newborn. *N Engl J Med* 1972; **286**: 129–34.
26. Gibbons RJ, Brueton L, Buckle VJ *et al*. Clinical and hematologic aspects of the X-linked alpha-thalassemia/mental retardation syndrome (ATR-X). *Am J Med Genet* 1995; **55**: 288–99.
27. Weatherall D, Letsky E. Genetics of haematological disorders. In: Wald N, Leck I (eds) *Antenatal and Neonatal Screening*, 2nd edn. Oxford: Oxford University Press, 2000, pp. 243–81.
28. Cao A, Rosatelli MC. Screening and prenatal diagnosis of the haemoglobinopathies. *Clin Haematol* 1993; **6**: 263–86.
29. Old JM, Varawalla NY, Weatherall DJ. Rapid detection and prenatal diagnosis of beta-thalassaemia: studies in Indian and Cypriot populations in the UK. *Lancet* 1990; **336**: 834–7.
30. Modell B, Petrou M, Layton M *et al*. Audit of prenatal diagnosis for haemoglobin disorders in the United Kingdom: the first 20 years. *Br Med J* 1997; **315**: 779–84.
31. Cazzola M, Borgna-Pignatti C, Locatelli F, Ponchio L, Beguin Y, De Stefano P. A moderate transfusion regimen may reduce iron loading in beta-thalassemia major without producing excessive expansion of erythropoiesis. *Transfusion* 1997; **37**: 135–40.
32. Prati D. Benefits and complications of regular blood

transfusion in patients with beta-thalassaemia major. *Vox Sang* 2000; **79**: 129–37.

33. Kevy SV, Jacobson MS, Fosburg M *et al.* A new approach to neocyte transfusion: preliminary report. *J Clin Apheresis* 1988; **4**: 194–7.

34. Collins AF, Dias GC, Haddad S *et al.* Comparison of a transfusion preparation of newly formed red cells and standard washed red cell transfusions in patients with homozygous β-thalassemia. *Transfusion* 1994; **34**: 517–20.

35. Singer ST, Wu V, Mignacca R, Kuypers FA, Morel P, Vichinsky EP. Alloimmunization and erythrocyte autoimmunization in transfusion-dependent thalassemia patients of predominantly Asian descent. *Blood* 2000; **96**: 3369–73.

36. Modell B, Bedoukas V. *The Clinical Approach to Thalassemia.* Orlando: Grune & Stratton, 1984.

37. Borgna-Pignatti C, de Stefano P, Bongo IG, Avato F, Cazzola M. Spleen iron content is low in thalassemia. *Am J Pediatr Hematol Oncol* 1984; **6**: 340–3.

38. Clemente MG, Congia M, Lai ME *et al.* Effect of iron overload on the response to recombinant interferon-alfa treatment in transfusion-dependent patients with thalassemia major and chronic hepatitis C. *J Pediatr* 1994; **125**: 123–8.

39. Li CK, Chan PK, Ling SC, Ha SY. Interferon and ribavirin as frontline treatment for chronic hepatitis C infection in thalassaemia major. *Br J Haematol* 2002; **117**: 755–8.

40. Adamkiewicz TV, Berkovitch M, Krishnan C, Polsinelli K, Kermack D, Olivieri NF. *Yersinia entercolitica* and beta thalassemia: a report of 15 years' experience. *Clin Infect Dis* 1998; **27**: 1367–8.

41. Barry M, Flynn DM, Letsky EA, Risdon RA. Long-term chelation therapy in thalassaemia major: effect on liver iron concentration, liver histology, and clinical progress. *Br Med J* 1974; **2**: 16–20.

42. Zurlo MG, De Stefano P, Borgna-Pignatti C *et al.* Survival and causes of death in thalassaemia major. *Lancet* 1989; **ii**: 27–30.

43. Wolfe L, Olivieri N, Sallan D *et al.* Prevention of cardiac disease by subcutaneous deferoxamine in patients with thalassemia major. *N Engl J Med* 1985; **312**: 1600–3.

44. Borgna-Pignatti C, Rugolotto S, De Stefano P *et al.* Survival and complications in patients with thalassemia major treated with transfusion and deferoxamine. *Haematologica* 2004; **89**: 1187–93.

45. Protonotariou AA, Tolis GJ. Reproductive health in female patients with beta-thalassaemia major. *Ann NY Acad Sci* 2000; **900**: 119–24.

46. Olivieri NF, Koren G, Harris J *et al.* Growth failure and bony changes induced by deferoxamine. *Am J Pediatr Hematol Oncol* 1992; **14**: 48–56.

47. Porter JB, Davis BA. Monitoring chelation therapy to achieve optimal outcome in the treatment of thalassaemia. *Baillières Best Pract Clin Haematol* 2002; **15**: 329–68.

48. Telfer PT, Prestcott E, Holden S, Walker M, Hoffbrand AV, Wonke B. Hepatic iron concentration combined with long-term monitoring of serum ferritin to predict complications of iron overload in thalassaemia major. *Br J Haematol* 2000; **110**: 971–7.

49. Worwood M, Cragg SJ, Jacobs A, McLaren C, Ricketts C, Economidou J. Binding of serum ferritin to concanavalin A: patients with homozygous beta thalassaemia and transfusional iron overload. *Br J Haematol* 1980; **46**: 409–16.

50. Brittenham GM, Cohen AR, McLaren CE *et al.* Hepatic iron stores and plasma ferritin concentration in patients with sickle cell anemia and thalassemia major. *Am J Hematol* 1993; **42**: 81–5.

51. Brittenham GM, Badman DG. Noninvasive measurement of iron: report of an NIDDK workshop. *Blood* 2003; **101**: 15–19.

52. Angelucci E, Brittenham GM, McLaren CE *et al.* Hepatic iron concentration and total body iron stores in thalassemia major. *N Engl J Med* 2000; **343**: 327–31.

53. Angelucci E, Baronciani D, Lucarelli G *et al.* Needle liver biopsy in thalassaemia: analyses of diagnostic accuracy and safety in 1184 consecutive biopsies. *Br J Haematol* 1995; **89**: 757–61.

54. St Pierre TG, Clark PR, Chua-anusorn W *et al.* Noninvasive measurement and imaging of liver iron concentrations using proton magnetic resonance. *Blood* 2005; **105**: 855–61.

55. Brittenham GM, Farrell DE, Harris JW *et al.* Magnetic-susceptibility measurement of human iron stores. *N Engl J Med* 1982; **307**: 1671–5.

56. Anderson LJ, Holden S, Davis B *et al.* Cardiovascular T2-star (T2*) magnetic resonance for the early diagnosis of myocardial iron overload. *Eur Heart J* 2001; **22**: 2171–9.

57. Jensen PD, Jensen FT, Christensen T, Eiskjaer H, Baandrup U, Nielsen JL. Evaluation of myocardial iron by magnetic resonance imaging during iron chelation therapy with deferrioxamine: indication of close relation between myocardial iron content and chelatable iron pool. *Blood* 2003; **101**: 4632–9.

58. Hershko C, Cappellini MD, Galanello R, Piga A, Tognoni G, Masera G. Purging iron from the heart. *Br J Haematol* 2004; **125**: 545–51.

59. Jessup M, Manno CS. Diagnosis and management of iron-induced heart disease in Cooley's anemia. *Ann NY Acad Sci* 1998; **850**: 242–50.

60. Porter JB, Huehns ER. The toxic effects of desferrioxamine. *Baillières Clin Haematol* 1989; **2**: 459–74.

61. Porter JB, Jaswon MS, Huehns ER, East CA, Hazell JW. Desferrioxamine ototoxicity: evaluation of risk factors in thalassaemic patients and guidelines for safe dosage. *Br J Haematol* 1989; **73**: 403–9.

62. Olivieri NF, Berriman AM, Tyler BJ, Davis SA, Francombe WH, Liu PP. Reduction in tissue iron stores with a new regimen of continuous ambulatory intravenous deferoxamine. *Am J Hematol* 1992; **41**: 61–3.

63. Davis BA, O'Sullivan C, Jarritt PH, Porter JB. Value of sequential monitoring of left ventricular ejection fraction in the management of thalassemia major. *Blood* 2004; **104**: 263–9.

64. Thompson J, Baird P, Downie J. *The Olivieri Report: The Complete Text of the Report of the Independent Inquiry Commissioned by the Canadian Association of University Teachers.* Toronto: James Lorimer and Company, 2001.

65. Hoffbrand AV, Al-Refaie F, Davis B *et al.* Long-term trial of deferiprone in 51 transfusion-dependent iron overloaded patients. *Blood* 1998; **91**: 295–300.

66. Olivieri NF, Brittenham GM, Matsui D *et al.* Iron-chelation therapy with oral deferiprone in patients with thalassemia major. *N Engl J Med* 1995; **332**: 918–22.

67. Piga A, Roggero S, Vinciguerra T, Sacchetti L, Gallo V, Longo F. Deferiprone: New Insight. *Ann New York Acad Sci* 2005; **1054**: 155–68.

68. Ceci A, Baiardi P, Felisi M *et al.* The safety and effectiveness

of deferiprone in a large-scale, 3-year study in Italian patients. *Br J Haematol* 2002; **118**: 330–6.

69. Lombardo T, Ferro G, Frontini V, Percolla S. High-dose intravenous desferrioxamine (DFO) delivery in four thalassemic patients allergic to subcutaneous DFO administration. *Am J Hematol* 1996; **51**: 90–2.

69a. Kattamis A. Combined therapy with Deferoxamine and Deferiprone. *Ann New York Acad Sci* 2005; **1054**: 175–82.

70. Agarwal MB, Gupte SS, Vasandani D *et al.* Efficacy and safety of 1,2-dimethyl-3-hydroxypyrid-4-one (L1) as an oral iron chelator in patients of beta thalassaemia major with iron overload. *J Assoc Physicians India* 1991; **39**: 669–72.

71. Agarwal MB, Gupte SS, Viswanathan C *et al.* Long-term assessment of efficacy and safety of L1, an oral iron chelator, in transfusion dependent thalassaemia: Indian trial. *Br J Haematol* 1992; **82**: 460–6.

72. Lucas GN, Perera BJ, Fonseka EA, De Silva DD, Fernandopulle M. A trial of deferiprone in transfusion-dependent iron overloaded children. *Ceylon Med J* 2000; **45**: 71–4.

73. Lucas GN, Perera BJ, Fonseka EA *et al.* Experience with the oral iron chelator deferiprone in transfusion-dependent children. *Ceylon Med J* 2002; **47**: 119–21.

74. Taher A, Chamoun FM, Koussa S *et al.* Efficacy and side effects of deferiprone (L1) in thalassemia patients not compliant with desferrioxamine. *Acta Haematol* 1999; **101**: 173–7.

75. Taher A, Sheikh-Taha M, Koussa S, Inati A, Neeman R, Mourad F. Comparison between deferoxamine and deferiprone (L1) in iron-loaded thalassemia patients. *Eur J Haematol* 2001; **67**: 30–4.

76. Mazza P, Anurri B, Lazzari G *et al.* Oral iron chelating therapy. A single center interim report on deferiprone (L1) in thalassemia. *Haematologica* 1998; **83**: 496–501.

77. Del Vecchio GC, Crollo E, Schettini F, Fischer R, De Mattia D. Factors influencing effectiveness of deferiprone in a thalassaemia major clinical setting. *Acta Haematol* 2000; **104**: 99–102.

78. Berdoukas V, Bohane T, Eagle C *et al.* The Sydney Children's Hospital experience with the oral iron chelator deferiprone (L1). *Transfus Sci* 2000; **23**: 239–40.

79. Maggio A, D'Amico G, Morabito A *et al.* Deferiprone versus deferoxamine in patients with thalassemia major: a randomized clinical trial. *Blood Cells Mol Dis* 2002; **28**: 196–208.

80. Rombos Y, Tzanetea R, Konstantopoulos K *et al.* Chelation therapy in patients with thalassemia using the orally active iron chelator deferiprone (L1). *Haematologica* 2000; **85**: 115–17.

81. Olivieri NF, Brittenham GM, McLaren CE *et al.* Long-term safety and effectiveness of iron-chelation therapy with deferiprone for thalassemia major. *N Engl J Med* 1998; **339**: 417–23.

82. Wanless IR, Sweeney G, Dhillon AP *et al.* Lack of progressive hepatic fibrosis during long-term therapy with deferiprone in subjects with transfusion-dependent beta-thalassemia. *Blood* 2002; **100**: 1566–9.

83. Cohen AR, Galanello R, Piga A, De Sanctis V, Tricta F. Safety and effectiveness of long-term therapy with the oral iron chelator deferiprone. *Blood* 2003; **102**: 1583–7.

84. Wanless IR, Sweeney G, Dhillon AP *et al.* Absence of deferiprone-induced hepatic fibrosis: a multi-center study. *Blood* 2000; **96**: 606a.

85. Neufeld EJ. Oral chelators deferasirox and deferiprone for transfusional iron overload in thalassaemia major: new data, new questions. *Blood* 2006; **107**: 3436–41.

86. Nisbet-Brown E, Olivieri NF, Giardina PJ *et al.* Effectiveness and safety of ICL670 in iron-loaded patients with thalassaemia: a randomised, double-blind, placebo-controlled, dose-escalation trial. *Lancet* 2003; **361**: 1597–602.

87. Porter J, Elliot V, Rose C *et al.* A Phase II study with ICL670 (Exjade), a once-daily oral iron chelator, in patients with various transfusion-dependent anemias and iron overload. *Blood* 2004; **104**: 872a.

88. Piga A, Galanello R, Foschini ML *et al.* Once-daily treatment with the oral iron chelator ICL670 (Exjade): results of a Phase II study in pediatric patients with β-thalassemia major. *Blood* 2004; **104**: 983a.

89. Capellini M, Bejaoui M, Perrotta S *et al.* A Phase III evaluation of once-daily, oral therapy with ICL670 (Exjade) versus deferoxamine in patients with β-thalassemia and transfusional hemosiderosis. *Blood* 2004; **104**: 984a.

90. Lucarelli G, Galimberti M, Polchi P *et al.* Bone marrow transplantation in patients with thalassemia. *N Engl J Med* 1990; **322**: 417–21.

91. Lucarelli G, Andreani M, Angelucci E. The cure of the thalassemia with bone marrow transplantation. *Bone Marrow Transplantation* 2001; **28**, Suppl 1: S11–S13.

92. Locatelli F, Rocha V, Reed W *et al.* Related umbilical cord blood transplantation in patients with thalassemia and sickle cell disease. *Blood* 2003; **101**: 2137–43.

93. La Nasa G, Giardini C, Argiolu F *et al.* Unrelated donor bone marrow transplantation for thalassemia: the effect of extended haplotypes. *Blood* 2002; **99**: 4350–6.

94. Angelucci E, Lucarelli G. Bone marrow transplantation for thalassemia. In: Nagel R (ed.) *Disorders of Hemoglobin: Genetics, Pathophysiology and Clinical Managements*. Cambridge: Cambridge University Press, 2001, pp. 1052–72.

95. Lucarelli G, Andreani M, Angelucci E. The cure of thalassemia by bone marrow transplantation. *Blood Rev* 2002; **16**: 81–5.

96. Olivieri NF, Weatherall DJ. The therapeutic reactivation of fetal haemoglobin. *Hum Mol Genet* 1998; **7**: 1655–8.

97. Lal AV, Vichinsky E. The role of fetal hemoglobin-enhancing agents in thalassemias. *Semin Hematol* 2004; **41**: 17–22.

98. Bard H, Prosmanne, J. Relative rates of fetal hemoglobin and adult hemoglobin synthesis in cord blood of infants of insulin-dependent diabetic mothers. *Pediatrics* 1985, **75**. 1143–7.

99. Olivieri NF, Rees DC, Ginder GD *et al.* Treatment of thalassaemia major with phenylbutyrate and hydroxyurea. *Lancet* 1997; **350**: 491–2.

100. Salehi SA, Koski T, Ondra SL. Spinal cord compression in beta-thalassemia: case report and review of the literature. *Spinal Cord* 2004; **42**: 117–23.

101. Pippard MJ, Weatherall DJ. Iron absorption in non-transfused iron loading anaemias: prediction of risk for iron loading, and response to iron chelation treatment, in beta thalassaemia intermedia and congenital sideroblastic anaemias. *Haematologia* 1984; **17**: 17–24.

102. Rees DC, Luo LY, Thein SL, Singh BM, Wickramasinghe S. Nontransfusional iron overload in thalassemia: association with hereditary hemochromatosis. *Blood* 1997; **90**: 3234–6.

Granulocyte Disorders

14 Disorders of granulopoiesis and granulocyte function

Arian Laurence, Pratima Chowdary and Philip Ancliff

Introduction

Granulocytes by definition include leukocytes with granules, that is, neutrophils, eosinophils and basophils. Physiologically monocytes and neutrophils act sequentially and concurrently, constituting a vital component of innate immunity. A decrease in neutrophil numbers and/or impairment of neutrophil function may result in life-threatening infections. Neutropenia is not uncommon and is usually transient with little significance. Persistent neutropenia is uncommon and can be life-threatening, but an early diagnosis and appropriate interventions can have profound impact on the life of the patient.

A disorder of phagocyte function should be considered in a child with a normal or raised neutrophil count that has a history of repeated bacterial and fungal infections. Many of the diseases discussed are either very rare or common with uncertain clinical significance. Children being investigated for these disorders should have a history of unusually severe infections involving peculiar organisms (*Serratia, Aspergillus*) in peculiar places (brain, liver) or the presence of severe childhood periodontal disease.

For the purpose of this chapter the disorders have been separated as disorders of function and disorders of numbers. Where appropriate, an attempt has been made to give a brief overview of the normal physiology of a process to explain the clinical manifestations of altered physiologic states.

Innate immunity

The immune system is an organization of various specialized cells and molecules with several key functions that aim to prevent invasion by parasitic microbes. The three lines of defense that human pathogens need to breach to cause disease are *physical barriers, innate immunity* and *adaptive immunity*. A brief overview of the physical barriers and innate immunity is presented to provide a basis for clinical consequences, secondary to disorders of granulocytes. Adaptive immunity and its disorders are presented elsewhere.

Physical barriers and antimicrobial peptides

Mechanical
Intact epithelial cells lining the respiratory, gastrointestinal and urogenital tracts and the skin prevent intrusion by their tight junctions and local physical adaptations, for instance, the mucociliary escalator in the respiratory system.

Microbiologic
Normal flora on the external surfaces prevent colonization by pathogenic and resistant strains.

Chemical defense
Proteins, peptides and other substances act by inactivating potential pathogens; examples are lysozyme in salivary secretions and azurocidin in human neutrophils, fatty acids in skin, and the acid pH of the stomach.

Antimicrobial peptides
The two major classes of antimicrobial peptides (AMPs) described in humans are defensins and cathelicidins. They protect mucosal and dry epithelial surfaces of all multicellular organisms. The protection is immediate due to rapid inactivation of potential pathogens, and the defense is as powerful as that provided by any of the body's circulating cells.[1] AMPs are produced not only by neutrophils and macrophages, but also by the epithelial cell lining of the gastrointestinal and genitourinary tracts, the tracheobronchial tree and keratinocytes. Some are produced constitutively, whereas others are induced by proinflammatory cytokines and exogenous microbial products. They act on selected molecular targets, for example phospholipid membrane peptidoglycans, resulting in disruption of cell membranes.

AMPs have a broad spectrum of activity against bacteria, fungi, viruses and frequently transformed cells. Most organisms synthesize several different types of AMP within their epithelial surfaces, creating a synergistic broad-spectrum antimicrobial cocktail. It is difficult for a microbe to change the phospholipid organization of its membrane, therefore resistance to the peptides occurs at levels that are orders of magnitude lower than those observed for conventional antibiotics.[2] Increasingly it is being recognized that AMPs are chemotactic for phagocytes, T cells and immature dendritic cells, providing evidence for their participation in alerting, mobilizing and amplifying innate and adaptive antimicrobial immunity of the host.[3]

Innate immunity

Innate immunity represents the second line of defense and is triggered rapidly without the need for prior exposure. It is immediate and stereotyped with the potential for being completely effective. Innate immunity does not have the specificity of adaptive immunity, but is capable of distinguishing self from nonself.

Immune recognition is mediated by probably hundreds of germline-encoded receptors with predetermined specificity that have evolved by natural selection. These pattern-recognition receptors identify highly conserved structures in microorganisms: pathogen-associated molecular patterns (PAMPs).[2] The best-known examples of PAMPs are bacterial lipopolysaccharide (LPS), peptidoglycan, lipoteichoic acids, mannans, bacterial DNA, double-stranded RNA and glucans. These patterns are unique to microbial pathogens, are usually essential for the survival or pathogenicity of microorganisms, and often are invariant structures shared by entire classes of pathogens; for instance, all Gram-negative bacteria have LPS. The pattern-recognition receptors are expressed on many effector cells of the immune system, most importantly on macrophages, dendritic cells and B cells.

Functionally, pattern-recognition receptors can be divided into three classes: secreted, endocytic and signaling. Secreted pattern-recognition receptors function as opsonins by binding to microbial cell walls and flagging them for recognition by the complement system and phagocytes. For example, mannan-binding lectin, on binding to microbial carbohydrates initiates the lectin pathway of complement activation. Endocytic pattern-recognition receptors occur on the surface of phagocytes; for example, macrophage mannose receptor recognizes mannose repeating sequences on microbial cell walls and mediates the uptake and delivery of the pathogen to the lysosome. Signaling receptors recognize PAMPs and activate signal-transduction pathways that induce the expression of a variety of immune-response genes. The Toll-like receptors (TLRs) are found on macrophages, dendritic cells and epithelial cells and are a well-defined family of at least ten evolutionarily conserved transmembrane receptors that appear to function exclusively as signaling receptors; for example, TLR4 recognizes bacterial lipopolysaccharide.

The effector branch has three major components. First is the release and, at times, activation of a variety of extracellular humoral mediators such as complement, cytokines, chemokines and AMPs including defensins and cathelicidin. Second is the recruitment and activation of phagocytic granulocytes, monocytes/macrophages, and in some instances natural killer cells to sites of microbial invasion. Third, there is surface expression of antigen-presenting cell-derived co-stimulatory molecules, necessary for efficient antigen presentation, leading to T-cell activation and induction of adaptive immunity. The T-helper cells in turn promote antigenic activation of B cells, and CD4 and CD8 effector T cells that produce cytokines capable of activating phagocytes to eliminate pathogens more effectively. A deficiency of innate immunity typically results in recurrent bacterial and fungal infections.

Recruitment of leukocytes to sites of inflammation

Granulocytic phagocytes represent the foot soldiers of the immune system. For a granulocyte to function, it must be able to extravasate from the bloodstream into affected tissues, adhering to inflamed endothelial cells of the venules. It must efficiently phagocytose microbes and kill them. The first half of the chapter is subdivided to consider these discrete abilities and the diseases that stem from their disruption.

Excluding tissue macrophages, most professional phagocytes of the immune system are found within the bone marrow or bloodstream. These cells must be recruited to sites of infection by a complex series of chemotactic stimuli, which not only attract the cells to infection sites but also sustain their survival and promote any necessary maturation. Cells within inflamed tissues are able to secrete a number of agents that are capable of attracting granulocytes, for example inflammatory proteins including fragments of complement (C3a, C5a), the inflammatory eicosanoid lipids (leukotrienes B_4 and C_4), and the chemokines.

Chemokines are a family of 40 small, structurally related proteins that are potent inducers of chemotaxis and maturation.[4] Chemokines are subdivided into two principal groups based on the spacing between two cysteine residues. The CC chemokines have the cysteine residues juxtaposed. An individual CC chemokine will often bind to multiple CC receptors expressed on multiple cell types. The CXC chemokines in contrast tend to bind to unique CXC receptors. A single chemokine may attract a certain cell type and induce its maturation so that the affected cell in turn recognizes a different repertoire of chemokines and moves in a different direction. In this manner a number of chemokines can regulate complex movement of cells. Table 14.1 lists a number of common chemokines and the cells they are able to recruit.

Table 14.1 An abridged list of some common chemokines.

Modern name	Original name	Receptor	Cells affected
CXC chemokines			
CXCL7	NAP-2	CXCR2	Endothelial cells, granulocytes
CXCL8	IL-8	CXCR1, CXCR2	Endothelial cells, neutrophils
CXCL10	IP-10	CXCR3	Endothelial cells, T lymphocytes
CXCL12	SDF-1	CXCR4	Endothelial cells, lymphocytes, myeloid stem cells
CC chemokines			
CCL2	MCP-1	CCR2	Endothelial cells, monocytes, T lymphocytes
CCL3	MIP-1a	CCR1, CCR5	Monocytes, T lymphocytes
CCL4	MIP-1b	CCR5	Monocytes, T lymphocytes
CCL5	RANTES	CCR1, CCR3, CCR5	Eosinophils, basophils, monocytes, T lymphocytes

NAP-2 Neutrophil Activating Protein-2
IL-8 Interleukin-8
IP-10 gamma interferon Induced Protein-10
SDF-1 Stromal cell-Derived Factor-1
MCP-1 Monocyte Chemoattractant Protein-1
MIP-1α Monocyte Inflammatory Protein-1α
MIP-1β Monocyte Inflammatory Protein-1β
RANTES Regulated upon Activation, Normal T-cell Expressed and Secreted

Table 14.2 A summary of ligands involved in leukocyte endothelial adhesion.

	Leukocyte surface	Endothelial surface	Associated disorder
Leukocyte rolling	L-selectin Carbohydrate residues	Carbohydrate residues E-selectin, P-selectin	LAD2
Leukocyte sticking, diapedesis	Integrins: LFA-1, Mac-1 (CR3)	Immunoglobulin family adhesion molecules: ICAM-1, ICAM-2	LAD1

To reach most sites of infection granulocytes must adhere to the inflamed endothelium of blood vessels and extravasate to the site of inflammation; this requires the expression of a number of adhesion molecules both on the attracted granulocyte and the target endothelial lining. Most extravasation typically occurs in the postcapillary venules. Chemokines secreted at sites of inflammation are carried across the vessel wall and coat the luminal surface of the endothelium.

Quiescent endothelial cells and neutrophils weakly express a number of selectins: E and P selectins on the endothelial cells; L selectin on the neutrophil. These proteins bind to carbohydrate residues on neighbouring cells. These weak interactions between neutrophil and endothelial cell result in a proportion of neutrophils rolling along the surface of the endothelium.

At sites of inflammation, chemokines induce the further expression of E, P and L selectins, resulting in an increased proportion of the blood neutrophils rolling along the endothelial surface.[4] Rolling leukocytes are then fixed by the binding of endothelial intercellular adhesion molecules (ICAMs) to integrin proteins on the leukocyte surface. Integrins are expressed constitutively on both the leukocyte and endothelium; after chemokine stimulation the avidity of the integrins is increased by a mechanism of "inside out" signaling involving the small G protein Rap1.[5,6] With tight adhesion to the endothelial cell wall the leukocyte extravasates toward the chemokine signal within the inflamed tissues. Phagocytes exposed to pathogens within the inflamed tissue in turn secrete more chemokines. This mechanism is common to all granulocytes and any failure of adhesion will prevent multiple cell types from reaching sites of infection. The proteins involved are summarized in Table 14.2 and Fig. 14.1.

Diseases of phagocyte adhesion and chemotaxis

Disorders of adhesion tend to result in dry and necrotic infections associated with raised white cell counts as neutrophils are unable to leave the bloodstream and form pus.

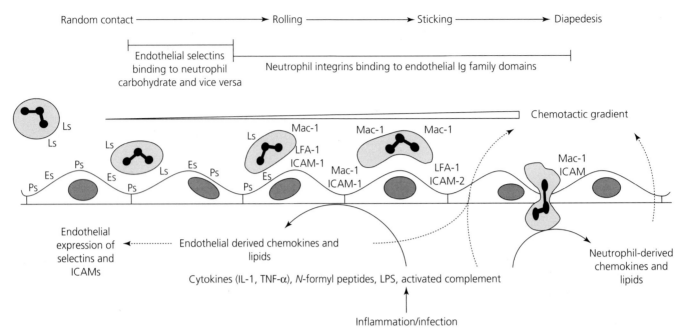

Fig. 14.1 Granulocyte chemotaxis and extravasation across the endothelium to a site of acute inflammation. Random contact and rolling is mediated by the binding of lectin receptors: Ps, P-selectin; Ls, L-selectin; Es, E-selectin to carbohydrates (not shown). Movement arrest and extravasation is mediated by the binding of immunoglobulin superfamily receptors, intercellular adhesion molecules 1 and 2 (ICAM-1 and -2), to the integrins Mac-1 (the C3bi receptor) and LFA-1 (leukocyte fixation antigen 1).

Leukocyte adhesion deficiency type 1

Leukocyte adhesion deficiency (LAD) is a rare autosomal recessive disorder of neutrophil adhesion, chemotaxis and opsonization. Approximately 100 cases have been reported. Patients express either a structurally abnormal or reduced amounts of β_2 integrin (CD18b).[7] CD18b is an essential component of the integrins LFA-1 and Mac-1 (the C3bi receptor). Absence of LFA-1 prevents neutrophils from binding tightly to inflamed vascular endothelium, a prerequisite for their migration into the interstitial tissues. Absence of C3bi receptor prevents granulocytes and monocytes from binding C3bi opsonized particles.

Affected children present with recurrent severe bacterial infections. Infections tend to involve the skin and gut. The failure to adhere to endothelium results in both a raised peripheral blood neutrophil count and infections that are dry, necrotic and lacking pus. Responsible bacteria include pneumococci and *Pseudomonas* species. Lack of monocyte function renders these children susceptible to fungal infections, typically *Aspergillus* and *Candida albicans*. Patients typically present with a delayed umbilical cord separation and associated infection of the stump. There is some variability in the severity of the disorder, with different mutations leading to a variable degree of clinical severity.[8] Children with severe disease typically die by the age of 2 years.[9,10]

The diagnosis is made by flow cytometry. Surface CD18b levels of > 11% are associated with no phenotype; 2.5–11% represents a mild phenotype; 0.3–2.5% is a moderate pheno-

type; and < 0.3% is a severe phenotype. Neutrophil function tests identifying the inability to opsonize C3bi-coated particles confirm the diagnosis. Both these investigations can be performed on cord blood allowing a prenatal diagnosis to be made.[11]

Management of mild to moderate disease requires prophylactic oral antibiotics and antifungals with parenteral antibiotic therapy for breakthrough infections. Patients with a severe phenotype should be assessed for bone marrow transplantation.

Leukocyte adhesion deficiency type 2

Four Arabic children and a Turkish child have been reported to have a variant LAD, now called LAD type 2.[12] This vanishingly rare autosomal recessive disorder is due to an inability to form sialyl Lewis X structures that form the Lewis and ABO blood group antigens and are the targets of endothelial E and P selectin binding on the neutrophil surface. LAD2 is a multisystem disorder; affected individuals have mental retardation and distinctive facies. The lack of ABO and Lewis antigens gives them a Bombay (hh) red cell phenotype. Generally the immune features of the disease are as for mild LAD1.

Leukocyte adhesion deficiency type 3

Two groups have reported children with a LAD1 picture associated with mucosal bleeding and platelet function abnormalities. These children express both β_1 and β_2 integrins but are unable to increase the avidity of their receptors in response to cell stimulation.[13] Recently, Kinashi *et al.*[14] have implicated a defect of the small G protein Rap1 as a cause of this disorder in one of the children studied. The children reported all required antibiotic prophylaxis together with management for their thrombasthenia.

Hyperimmunoglobulin E syndrome

Hyperimmunoglobulin E syndrome (HIES) is a rare heterogeneous multisystem disorder of unknown etiology. It is classically a triad of susceptibility to bacterial and fungal infections, atopy associated with a grossly raised IgE, and a connective tissue disorder.[15,16] Most cases are sporadic but a few follow an autosomal dominant (classic phenotype) or recessive (variant phenotype) inheritance pattern. Linkage analysis has identified a region involving the proximal region of 4q. area of chromosome 4.[17] T cells from HIES patients show a decreased response to candidal antigens. Although the mechanism is uncertain, some groups have implicated a reduction in interferon (IFN)-γ secretion suggesting that there is a shift from a type 1 (cellular) to a type 2 (humoral) response.[18,19] This would explain the elevated IgE and atopy that is a hallmark of the disorder; however, reduced IFN-γ secretion is not a consistent finding. Recently, Martinez *et al.* have noted that HIES T cells have a reduction in ICAM-1 expression.[20] They go on to show that this is associated with a reduction in T-cell responses and an increase in B-cell production of IgE. Any defect in ICAM-1 expression could explain the poor *in vivo* neutrophil chemotaxis.

The clinical features are characterized by recurrent skin and chest infections beginning in infancy and typically involving staphylococci, *Haemophilus influenzae* and fungi. Skin infections manifest as cold staphylococcal abscesses involving the head and neck regions. Pulmonary infections are typically cystic, leading to bronchiectasis,[21] and cysts may become colonized by fungal balls. Fungal nail infections are common. Skin and pulmonary infections may be precipitated and exacerbated by the associated atopic complications of eczema and asthma. Features of the connective tissue disorder include hyperextensible joints, scoliosis, delayed shedding of primary teeth and coarse facies. Osteopenia and long-bone fractures are common.[15]

On investigation there is a marked elevation of IgE (>2 kIU/mL) together with an eosinophilia.[22] The other immunoglobulin subtypes are often reduced. Neutrophil function tests including chemotaxis tests are usually normal suggesting an indirect effect. The differential diagnosis is that of Wiskott–Aldrich and DiGeorge syndromes together with severe simple atopy where attacks of asthma and eczema can be associated with comparable IgE levels.

Management of HIES is threefold:

- minimizing the atopic symptoms to avoid breakage of the skin;
- use of prophylactic antistaphylococcal antibiotics and antifungal agents;
- use of surgery to drain abscesses and remove lung cysts before they become colonized with fungus.[23]

A number of other therapies have been considered although none has been proven to be of benefit.[21,24] The hypo-IgG gammaglobulinemia would suggest that intravenous immunoglobulin (IVIG) may be of benefit, and this has been reported in a few cases.[25] There is a debate about the role of IgE in the disorder, and some groups have considered plasmapheresis in patients that fail to respond to antibiotics[21] (although of note, plasma from HIES patients has no inhibitory action on neutrophils from healthy donors). Finally, the reduced secretion of IFN-γ in HIES T cells has led some groups to use IFN-γ as a therapy.[26] However, this agent is unproven and has been reported to precipitate autoimmune disease in a patient with HIES.[27]

Localized juvenile periodontitis

Localized juvenile periodontitis is a rare heterogeneous group of familial disorders that present in puberty with severe alveolar bone loss around the first molars and incisors. The underlying mechanism is unclear although it should be noted that most neutrophil disorders predispose to severe periodontal disease.[28]

Localized juvenile periodontitis neutrophils have been shown to have defects in chemotaxis in response to formyl peptides, C5a and leukotrienes although none of these defects is universal.[29,30] More recently, Shibata and colleagues have identified a defect in calcium signaling.[31] The underlying defect may be exacerbated by both inhibitory and inflammatory agents secreted by bacteria known to colonize the oral cavity.[28,32] Good oral hygiene is critical to minimize tooth loss in this disorder.

Wiskott–Aldrich syndrome

Wiskott–Aldrich syndrome (WAS) is an X-linked disorder associated with mutations of the WAS protein (WASp). Children present with a spectrum of disease ranging from a mild thrombocytopenia to a severe immunodeficiency with failure to clear bacterial and viral infections leading to multiple chest infections and Epstein–Barr virus-driven lymphomas. WASp is involved in regulation of the actin cytoskeleton.[33,34] When activated, WASp is activated by the Rho family GTPases Cdc42 and Rac, in turn leading to activation of the cytoskeletal organising complex Arp 2/3. This protein complex regulates the polymerization of actin monomers to form structural filaments. WASp-deficient lymphocytes activated by the presence of antigen-presenting cells are unable to form a stable immunologic synapse

Table 14.3 A summary of the signs and symptoms of Wiskott–Aldrich syndrome.

Neonatal onset
Thrombocytopenia possibly exacerbated by increased platelet consumption

Early childhood onset
Eczema, colitis, susceptibility to pyogenic (bacterial) and opportunistic (viral, PCP) infections
Lymphopenia, abnormal B-cell function with reduced IgM and elevated IgA and IgE

Late childhood/adolescent onset
Virally precipitated B-cell lymphomas

PCP, *Pneumocystis carinii* pneumonia.

leading to inadequate stimulation and deficiencies in both cell-mediated and humoral adaptive immunity.[35] An inability to organize the cytoskeleton leads to deficiencies of phagocyte chemotaxis[36] and neutrophil phagocytosis, the latter requiring the formation of an actin cup.[37]

Patients usually present at birth with a thrombocytopenia, the platelet count typically being in the range $10–20 \times 10^9/L$ together with small platelets. The other manifestations of the disease appear with age and are summarized in Table 14.3. The disorder may be diagnosed by flow cytometry looking for the lack of WASp.

Management of WAS involves supportive care for deficiencies of both acquired and innate immunity. Splenectomy has been successful in limiting the thrombocytopenia and is still a recommended therapy in those without a suitable bone marrow donor.[38,39] Bone marrow transplantation using a sibling or matched unrelated donor remains the gold standard cure but is not available to all.[40] Gene therapy to replace the nonfunctioning gene is under investigation and has been successful in mouse models.[41,42]

Mutations of Rac2

Rac is a Rho family small G protein involved in regulation of the actin cytoskeleton. Whereas Rac1 is ubiquitously expressed, Rac2 is found only within the hematopoietic lineage. Mouse neutrophils lacking Rac2 are unable to translocate across epithelia.[43] A couple of cases of children with inactivated Rac2 have been described. Clinically they presented with a LAD1-like picture.[44] The diagnosis is made by Western blotting of neutrophil lysate for Rac2.

Acquired disorders of adherence and chemotaxis

Prematurity

Neonates are at increased risk of group B streptococcal infection with defects of chemotaxis, adherence, and phagocytosis all reported.[45] Chemotaxis and adherence defects may be due to a defect in signaling in response to chemokines. These defects are more pronounced in preterm infants. To compound this, bone marrow reserves of neutrophils are smaller resulting in a greater propensity to become neutropenic. It is unclear whether reduced antibody-mediated opsonization is an important factor.

Drugs

Corticosteroids and epinephrine (adrenaline) are associated with a decrease in neutrophil adhesion, the former by inhibiting eicosanoid metabolism.[46,47] This is usually of little significance except to note that a reduction in adhesion liberates endothelial neutrophils and artefactually raises the blood neutrophil count. In contrast agents that increase neutrophil adhesion such as amphotericin and granulocyte colony-stimulating factor (G-CSF) are associated with a neutrophil lung syndrome where neutrophil aggregates precipitate in the lung, causing respiratory insufficiency.[48,49]

A neutrophil lung syndrome may be precipitated by complement activation secondary to bacterial sepsis, thermal injury, tissue necrosis or manipulation of blood or blood products such as hemofiltration or leukopheresis. Rarely, neutrophils may be activated by the infusion of anti-neutrophil antibodies present in blood products inducing a transfusion-related lung injury (TRALI).

Hematologic disease

Children with myelodysplasia often have a predisposition to bacterial infections even in the presence of near normal neutrophil counts. Many reports have shown qualitative abnormalities in neutrophil adhesion and migration;[50] this is noted particularly in myelodysplasia with a monosomy 7.

Functional *in vitro* abnormalities of granulocytes are a common feature of chronic myeloid leukemia (CML) in chronic phase with abnormal adhesion and reduced migration common. However, this may be of limited clinical significance as patients in chronic phase are not usually susceptible to bacterial infections.

Neutrophils of donor origin in patients who have recently undergone bone marrow transplantation (BMT) may show reduced chemotaxis particularly when associated with graft-versus-host disease.[51]

Nonhematologic disease

Diabetes mellitus is commonly associated with pyogenic infections, particularly when glycemia is poorly controlled. Chemotactic and adhesion defects have both been identified in this situation.[52] Depressed neutrophil activity, mainly chemotaxis, has been reported in liver disease, burns and premature neonates.[53] Defects of chemotaxis and adhesion have been described in splenectomized patients,[54] a group known to be at risk of infections with encapsulated bacteria.

Several viral infections have been shown to inhibit monocyte chemotaxis including herpes simplex, influenza and human immunodeficiency virus (HIV).[55] Several other diseases, including α-mannosidase deficiency, myotonic dystrophy, α_1-antitrypsin deficiency, cirrhosis and sarcoidosis are also associated with diminished chemotaxis.[55]

Disorders of phagocyte opsonization and ingestion

For a target to be phagocytosed it must either contain compounds that innately bind to receptors on the phagocyte surface, such as lipopolysaccaride, or be opsonized by bound immunoglobulin or complement. Consequent disorders can be divided into those that are due to a lack of proteins that opsonize targets, such as immunoglobulin or complement proteins, or those that lack the receptors to bind opsonized targets.

Humoral disorders of opsonization

Hypogammaglobulinemias

Typically B-cell disorders may be subclass specific or affect all antibody production. Those affecting IgG are most likely to be associated with pyogenic encapsulated bacteria (*Haemophilus influenzae*, pneumococci, *Staphylococcus aureus*).

Complement disorders

Deficiencies of the classical pathway (C1, C2, C4) cause only minor infectious problems as the alternate pathway remains intact. Deficiency of C3 renders patients susceptible to encapsulated organisms (pneumococci, etc.). Deficiencies of these factors are associated with a lupus-like disorder as immune complexes are not efficiently cleared.[56] Deficiencies of C5–9 result in a lupus-like disease and susceptibility to *Neisseria* infections.[56] Patients at risk should be vaccinated for pneumococcus, *Haemophilus influenzae* and meningococcus.

Mannose-binding protein deficiency

Mannose-binding protein (MBP) binds free mannose on bacteria and triggers the complement cascade (Fig. 14.2). Five percent of the population have low MBP levels but this is of uncertain significance.[57] MBP may be important in the first year of life to bridge the gap between maternal and infant immunoglobulin. MBP deficiency may coexist with other defects of innate immunity making a mild disorder severe. A rare autosomal dominant condition that disturbs the ability

of MBP to trigger complement is associated with herpetic and *Klebsiella* infections in adults.[58]

Cellular disorders of ingestion

Targets of neutrophil phagocytosis are often opsonized with either bound antibody or fragments of complement. Neutrophils adhere to these bound proteins via specific receptors. There are a number of rare familial disorders, summarized in Table 14.4, where neutrophils lack one or more of these receptors. Excluding CR3 deficiency (LAD1), individual receptor defects confer a minor susceptibility to infection although multiple deficiencies can occur with more severe symptoms. As with MBD deficiency, these disorders may coexist with other defects of innate immunity making an otherwise mild disease severe.

Acquired disorders of opsonization and ingestion

Neutrophils of patients with myelodysplasia have been reported to have qualitative defects of phagocytosis that may contribute to the predisposition to infection seen in patients with this disorder.[50] A defect in opsonization has been noted in splenectomized patients although the mechanism is unclear.[54]

Disorders of granule contents and integrity

Once phagocytosed, microorganisms are held within the phagosome. This then fuses with various lysosomal granules containing potent digestive enzymes necessary for killing. Early myeloid cells express primary or azurophilic granules containing inflammatory proteins, digestive enzymes and bactericidal proteins. Later myelocytes develop secondary or specific granules, which contain further enzymes for cell killing including the NADPH oxidase, followed by tertiary or secretory granules that contain plasma proteins. Regulation of granule formation is performed by transcription factors. Knockout mouse studies have identified the factor C/EBPα as crucial for the formation of primary granules and C/EBPε as crucial for the formation of secondary granules. A summary of the different types of neutrophil granule contents is given in Table 14.5.

Disorders of granulation include a lack of these lysosomal granules or a failure to regulate their fusion with other granules resulting in uncontrolled mixing and inactivation of their contents.

Chédiak–Higashi syndrome (Fig. 14.3)

This is an autosomal recessive multiorgan disorder of lysosomal trafficking that presents with a tetrad of neurologic,

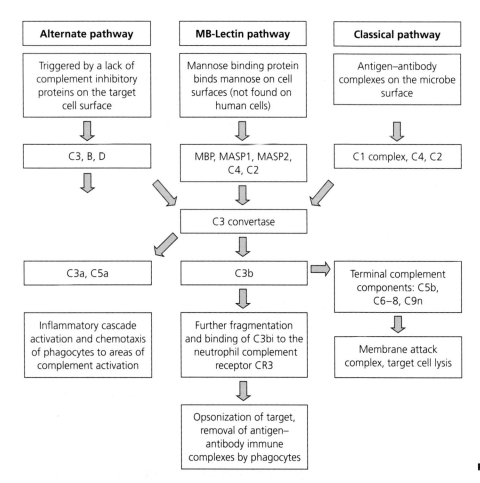

Fig. 14.2 The complement cascade.

Table 14.4 Granulocyte receptors of phagocytosis.

Receptor	Clinical association	Reference
CR3/C3bi receptor		See LAD type 1
FcγRIIIb receptor	Deficiency is common (1 in 800). GPI-linked receptor, absent in paroxysmal nocturnal hemoglobinuria. Isolated deficiency is of uncertain significance	59,60
FcγRIIa receptor	Deficiency may confer susceptibility to encapsulated bacteria, may be potentiated by FcγRIIIb deficiency	61

Table 14.5 Granule contents of mature neutrophils.

	Granule		
	Primary (azurophil)	**Secondary (specific)**	**Tertiary (secretory)**
Membrane proteins	CD63, CD68	CD11b, f-Met receptor, NADPH oxidase	CD11b, CD14, CD16, f-Met receptor, alkaline phosphatase
Granule contents	β-Glucuronidase, defensins, elastase, myeloperoxidase, lysozyme	Collagenase, gelatinase, lactoferrin, lysozyme	Albumin, B_{12}-binding protein and other plasma proteins

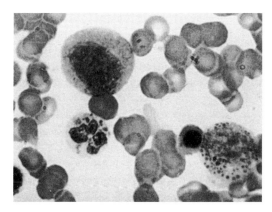

Fig. 14.3 Giant neutrophil inclusions seen in the Chédiak–Higashi syndrome. A myelocyte in the picture also shows abnormal giant granules.

Table 14.6 Clinical features of the stable phase of Chédiak–Higashi syndrome.

Organ	Signs and symptoms
Skin	Patchy oculocutaneous albinism
Central nervous system	Photophobia, nystagmus, ataxia
Peripheral nervous system	Peripheral sensorimotor neuropathy, cranial nerve lesions
Clotting	Minor bleeding problems typically presenting with easy bruising and epistaxis
Innate immunity	Multiple life-threatening bacterial (commonly *Staphylococcus aureus*) and fungal infections of the mouth, skin and lungs

coagulation, immunologic and skin pigmentation defects. The underlying defect is due to mutations in the *CHS1* or *LYST* gene.[62,63] Lack of this protein leads to fusion of heterogeneous lysosomes and the formation of giant particles with mixed contents. In neutrophils azurophilic and secondary granules fuse leading to perturbation of their contents with a reduced cathepsin G noted.[64] Similarly, cells in other affected organs show giant granules including platelets (bleeding disorder), Schwann cells (peripheral neuropathy), hepatocytes (hepatomegaly) and melanocytes (partial or patchy oculocutaneous albinism). The exact mechanism of the immune disorder is complex; neutrophils have a defect in the contents of their giant granules but also have defects of degranulation and chemotaxis. Other cells of the immune system are affected with giant granules seen in lymphocytes and monocytes. The underlying defect may also affect the plasma membrane and associated cytoskeleton as cytoskeletal and membrane fluidity defects have been reported in natural killer (NK) cells and fibroblasts.[65,66]

The clinical features and course of the disease is complex. Patients typically present early in the first decade of life with a stable phase, features of which are summarized in Table 14.6.

Children in the stable phase typically have a reduction in peripheral neutrophils due to ineffective myelopoiesis; neutrophils show the classical giant azurophilic granules. Neutrophil function tests are perturbed, with delayed degranulation and impaired chemotaxis. Platelet function tests demonstrate a storage pool defect.[67] There are diffuse abnormalities on electroencephalography, and visual evoked potentials highlight the defects of the optic chiasm. Patients commonly have a raised intracranial pressure.[55]

Patients that survive into their second decade of life develop an accelerated phase of the disease that is thought to be mediated by Epstein–Barr virus infection.[68–70] The accelerated phase is characterized by pyrexia together with pancytopenia and a diffuse polyclonal multiorgan lymphohistiocytic infiltration classically involving the liver, spleen and bone marrow.

The management of stable-phase patients includes prophylactic oral antibiotics and antifungals. Ascorbic acid has been used to try to prevent fused neutrophil granule contents from redox breakdown but its use is controversial.[71] Once a hemophagocytic syndrome has developed, chemotherapy using vincristine, corticosteroids and antithymocyte globulin has been used but with little success.[72] In the UK patients are typically started on a standard hemophagocytic lymphohistiocytosis protocol such as HLH-94, which uses a mixture of corticosteroid, etoposide and ciclosporin. The only proven curative therapy for this condition is BMT.[73]

Specific granule deficiency

This very rare neutrophil disorder is characterized by a lack of specific, or secondary, granules together with morphologic abnormalities including bilobed neutrophils. Secondary granules are lined with components of the oxidase system, vital for bacterial killing.[53] The absence of secondary granules is reflected in lactoferrin and vitamin B_{12}-binding protein levels at 3–10% of normal.[74] Similarly the neutrophil alkaline phosphatase (NAP) score is low. Primary granules are present but have abnormal morphology and an altered content with increased myeloperoxidase and decreased defensins. In many patients the gene encoding the C/EBPε transcription factor is mutated.[75] Secondary granules are also required for expression of β_2 integrins and consequently the affected neutrophils show defects in chemotaxis.

Clinically the disorder presents with recurrent and often indolent pyogenic infections of the epithelia typically presenting in infancy.[76] Therapy involves prompt use of antibiotics and antifungals together with surgical drainage of any chronic abscesses. The prognosis is relatively good, with most patients surviving to adulthood. Cytogenetic investigation and neutrophil function tests help differentiate this disorder from myelodysplasia as the latter includes defects of chemotaxis and respiratory burst together with a failure of neutrophil disaggregation following stimulation.[74]

Acquired granule disorders

Rarely an acquired loss of neutrophil granule contents can be seen in neutrophils from patients with myelodysplasia and acute myeloid leukemia.[77] This may contribute to bacterial infections seen with these disorders. In contrast, loss of some granule enzymes including alkaline phosphatase is common in myeloproliferative disorders; however, this is of uncertain significance as recurrent infections are not a significant problem in patients with chronic phase CML.

Disorders of oxidative metabolism

Granulocytes and other professional phagocytosing cells of the immune system require a potent mechanism of cell killing to combat the many microorganisms that they ingest; central to this is their ability to secrete chemically highly active reactive oxygen species (ROS). Most ROS stem from the production of free radical forms of oxygen. A free radical is a compound that contains an unpaired electron, which drives it to covalently bind to neighbouring compounds, forming adducts that often maintain the unpaired electron and trigger a cascade of chemical reactions that disrupt complex biological macromolecules. A typical cascade is summarized below, where the unpaired electron is denoted by a dot and R1, R2 represent biological macromolecules:

$$\cdot OH + R1H \rightarrow R1\cdot + H_2O$$

$$R1\cdot + O_2 \rightarrow R1OO\cdot + RH$$

$$R1OO\cdot + R2H \rightarrow R1OOH + R2.$$

Granulocyte free radical ROS include superoxide ($O_2^-\cdot$) and the hydroxyl radical ($\cdot OH$), the dot denoting the unpaired electron. The superoxide radical serves as the starting point for the production of a large assortment of other radical and nonradical ROS including oxidized halogens (OCl^-, ClO_4^-), oxides of nitrogen ($NO\cdot$), singlet oxygen ($O\cdot$) and, in turn, ozone (O_3).[78]

The NADPH oxidases provide granulocyte superoxide and are similar in structure to the mitochondrial redox transport chain, with membrane-associated proteins oxidizing NADPH at one end and the reducing potential passing via the cytochrome b_{558} complex to oxygen. The reaction can be summarized as follows:

$$2O_2 + NADPH \rightarrow 2O_2^-\cdot + NADP^+ + H^+$$

In contrast to the mitochondrial redox transport chain the reaction is not linked to the generation of ATP and so this energetically favorable reaction must be tightly regulated. Recently, this mechanism has been elucidated.[79–81] Cytochrome b_{558} exists as a heterodimer of two proteins, the glycoprotein gp91[PHOX], which contains the NADPH binding site, and a p22[PHOX], which passes the electron to oxygen to form superoxide. In order for the reaction to proceed, the oxidase must be held in place by three adaptor proteins: p40[PHOX], p47[PHOX] and p67[PHOX]. The binding of bacterial lipopolysaccharide, chemokines or opsonized particles to their specific receptors on the granulocyte surface activates downstream signaling pathways leading to the formation of phosphatidylinositol 3-phosphate (PI 3-P) and the active form of the small G protein Rac1 (Rac[GTP]). The presence of membrane PI 3-P and Rac[GTP] recruits p40[PHOX] and p47[PHOX] to the inner surface of the lysosomal membrane where the latter is serine phosphorylated. This leads to the assembly of the active NADPH oxidase.[82] The assembled oxidase induces a respiratory burst as granulocyte stores of NADPH are rapidly oxidized to NADP[+] and oxygen is converted into ROS (Fig. 14.4).

Superoxide is formed on the luminal surface of the lysosomal membrane and reacts with biologic material within the lysosomal contents. Much of this superoxide is metabolized by superoxide dismutase (SOD) into hydrogen peroxide (H_2O_2). H_2O_2 is a weak oxidant but in the presence of free metal ions or ozone can dissociate to form the potent hydroxyl radical. The presence of myeloperoxidase within lysosomes converts H_2O_2 into the potent oxidant HOCl:

$$H_2O_2 + HCl \rightarrow HOCl + H_2O$$

Eosinophils contain their own peroxidase enzyme, which can form other potent oxidizing agents including HOBr and HOSCN.[83,84]

All the ROS discussed will damage both neutrophil and bacterial proteins indiscriminately, and the NADPH oxidase can be inactivated by its own product. Granulocytes and monocytes must have a potent array of antioxidant enzymes to maintain their integrity.[85] Excess H_2O_2 that leaks back into the granulocyte cytosol is inactivated either by catalase or by the oxidation of glutathione. Glutathione is in turn restored via the oxidation of NADPH by glutathione reductase. It is of note that NADPH is important both for the formation of oxygen radicals and their removal.

Chronic granulomatous disease

Chronic granulomatous disease (CGD) (Fig. 14.5) is the product of a heterogeneous collection of inherited defects of the phagocyte respiratory burst. The overall incidence is 1 in 250 000, with autosomal recessive and X-linked inheritance being described (Table 14.7). Mutations affecting the gp91[PHOX] protein account for the majority of patients. Mutations involving the cytosolic adaptor proteins tend to carry a milder phenotype as the intact flavocytochrome leaks a small amount of superoxide in the nonstimulated state.[86]

Patients suffer recurrent and chronic infections with catalase-positive organisms. They present from the first year of life with infections of the epithelia and associated draining lymph nodes. Catalase is a ubiquitous enzyme that inactivates hydrogen peroxide, converting it to oxygen and water.

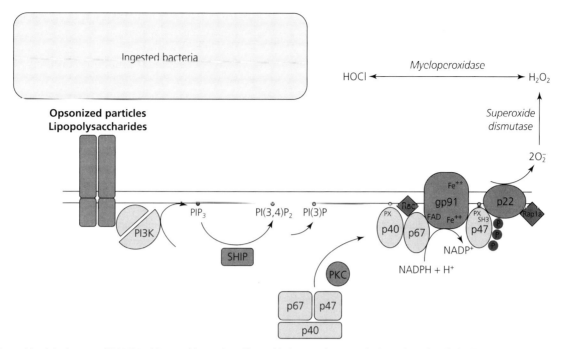

Fig. 14.4 Assembly of the lysosomal NADPH oxidase and formation of hypochlorite. On phagocytosis, lipopolysaccharide (LPS), complement and antibody receptors activate neutrophil phosphoinositol 3-kinase (PI3K), protein kinase C (PKC) and the small G proteins Rac and Rap1. The products of PI3K, phosphoinositol 3-phosphate (PIP$_3$) and phosphoinositol 3,4-bisphosphate (PI(3,4)P), recruit the adaptor proteins p40 and p47 respectively via binding to their PX domains. The adaptor proteins in turn assemble the components of the oxidase: gp91 and p22. Upon localization at the membrane, p47 is phosphorylated and activated by PKC. The activated complex secretes superoxide into the lumen of the lysosome, where it is further metabolized to hydrogen peroxide and hypochlorite.

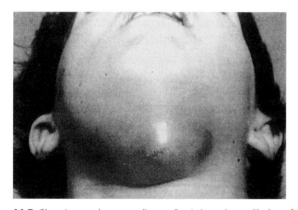

Fig. 14.5 Chronic granulomatous disease. Persisting submandibular soft tissue infection with incipient skin breakdown and chronic discharge.

Ingested catalase-negative organisms are killed by the small amount of oxygen radicals that accumulate within the phagosome. Staphylococci are responsible for half of the infections seen, *Aspergillus* is the next most common at 10–20%, and Gram-negative enteric organisms make up the remainder.[86] Neutrophils and monocytes are recruited to sites of infection but are unable to kill ingested pathogens leading to the formation of chronic granulomas. Infectious abscesses are typically found in the skin and subcutaneous tissues, the facial sinuses, liver and urethral tract. Chronic granuloma formation may lead to noninfectious complications such as hepatosplenomegaly, lymphadenopathy, hypergammaglobulinemia and a chronic diarrhea associated with an inflammatory bowel-like disease that may require immuno-

Table 14.7 Chronic granulomatous disease and mutations of NADPH oxidase.

Affected protein	Coding gene	Gene locus	Inheritance	Location and protein function	Frequency (% of cases)
gp91PHOX	CYBB	Xp21.1	X	Membrane flavocytochrome *b*	64
p22PHOX	CYBA	16p24	AR	Membrane flavocytochrome *b*	7
p47PHOX	NCF1	7q11.23	AR	Cytosolic adaptor protein	23
p67PHOX	NCF2	1q25	AR	Cytosolic adaptor protein	6

X, X-linked; AR, autosomal recessive.

suppression.[87,88] Granulomas can obstruct certain organs, such as the gastric pylorus, colon and ureters. Patients become chronically ill and their ability to withstand frequent infections gradually decreases. Death is often the result of fungal sepsis, mainly caused by *Aspergillus* species.[89]

The diagnosis is made by demonstrating an absolute lack of superoxide production in activated phagocytes; those that are able to generate 1–10% of normal superoxide are regarded as having a variant disease (vCGD). In the Nitroblue Tetrazolium test, phorbol ester-stimulated neutrophils oxidize the yellow water-soluble dye to form a blue precipitate. In the absence of an X-linked history a Western immunoblot of neutrophil protein lysate is required to identify the affected protein. Identification of the genetic defect now makes it possible to provide earlier and accurate prenatal diagnosis of CGD using fetal DNA from chorionic villi or amniocytes.

Improvements in the management of CGD are reflected in an increase in life expectancy of children with this disorder.[90] A review of the American registry estimated a 2% chance of death per year.[86] Current and future treatment strategies are listed below.

• *Prophylactic antibacterial and antifungal drugs.* The widespread use of co-trimoxazole (Septrin) has led to an improvement in life expectancy for patients with CGD.[91] Recently, co-trimoxazole has been superseded by azithromycin as this agent is better tolerated and need only be given in short courses fortnightly. The use of antibacterials has led to an increased proportion of fungal infections and hence the use of prophylactic antifungals such as itraconazole[92] or more recently voriconazole.

• *Early aggressive treatment of breakthrough infections.* The identification of breakthrough infections can be difficult as patients can remain asymptomatic. Any pyrexia or rising inflammatory markers (C-reactive protein, erythrocyte sedimentation rate) should be thoroughly investigated and intravenous antimicrobials considered. Surgical drainage or excision of granulomas may be necessary. In severe infections granulocyte transfusions offer an alternative. Granulocytes can be derived either from buffy coat collected by national blood transfusion services or ideally can be leukophoresed from donors, often friends and relatives, who have taken a single dose of granulocyte colony-stimulating factor (G-CSF) together with a corticosteroid to increase the yield.[93]

• *The use of IFN-γ.* The use of IFN-γ has been shown to reduce the frequency and severity of infection in patients with CGD.[94] The mechanism is unclear; approximately 14–28 days after a subcutaneous injection of IFN-γ there is an increase in macrophage gp91[PHOX] mRNA levels;[95] in keeping with this, IFN-γ treatment is most effective in those with the X-linked variant form of CGD. However, in a phase III trial of IFN-γ, despite showing a clinical improvement, none of the patients showed an increase in neutrophil O_2^-· production.[96] This suggests that in patients where gp91[PHOX] levels are absent or

unaffected, IFN-γ therapy may still be of value by inducing nonoxidative bacterial killing by phagocytes.

• *The use of immunosuppressives.* It seems counterintuitive to treat a disorder blighted by multiple infections with immunosuppressives, and this strategy should be used with caution. However, corticosteroids have been successfully used to disperse granulomas causing obstruction to vital organs.[97] Corticosteroids, with or without ciclosporin, have been used to treat the inflammatory bowel disease associated with CGD.

• *Bone marrow transplantation.* Bone marrow transplantation offers a potential cure for the disease but its role is controversial as patients often receive therapy with multiple unresolved infections, and the transplant-related mortality rates are high in comparison with the long-term survival benefits achieved with antimicrobial prophylaxis. With the introduction of low-intensity, nonmyeloablative regimens, transplantation may have a role in severe disease.[98]

• *Gene therapy.* CGD, along with other inherited disorders of granulocyte function, is a candidate for gene therapy as it is possible to stably infect intact genes into bone marrow stem cells using retroviral vectors. However, in contrast with the successful trials in patients with common gamma chain and adenosine deaminase deficiencies, the infected cells in CGD do not have a survival advantage over unaffected cells and are thus not able to dominate the marrow.[99]

Glucose-6-phosphate dehydrogenase deficiency

The oxidation of NADPH to NADP+ provides the electron source for the formation of superoxide (O_2^-·). Much of granulocyte NADP+ is reduced back to NADPH by the action of glucose-6-phosphate dehydrogenase (G6PD) (Fig. 14.6). G6PD deficiency is one of the world's commonest inherited diseases and results in a hemolytic anemia. Despite erythroid and neutrophil G6PD being coded by the same gene and the ubiquity of G6PD deficiency, only a very rare subgroup of patients with the hemolytic anemia have a neutrophil dysfunction.[100] G6PD levels do not decay during the short lifespan of the neutrophil and there are shunt enzymes to transfer reducing potential between NADH and NADPH. However, if erythrocyte/neutrophil G6PD levels are less than 3% there is not enough NADPH to feed the redox enzyme chain to generate superoxide.

In the few cases reported, patients are male or homozygous females with the severe Mediterranean variant of the deficiency. The critically low erythrocyte G6PD levels (typically < 1% of normal) result in a chronic hemolytic anemia that does not require precipitation by an oxidative stress as in classical G6PD deficiency. This differentiates the disorder from CGD. The neutrophil defect is similar to variant CGD, and neutrophil function tests typically show 5–30% normal oxidative activity with an initially normal respiratory burst that is cut short.

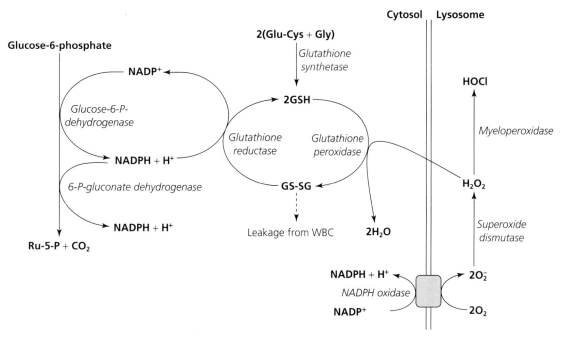

Fig. 14.6 Reduction of NADP+ by glucose-6-phosphate dehydrogenase and glutathione metabolism. NADPH is required for both the production and removal of reactive oxygen species (ROS). Most NADPH is made via the shunt pathway of glucose metabolism using the enzyme glucose-6-phosphate dehydrogenase. NADPH is used to reconstitute glutathione (GSH), which in turn is oxidized into dimers (GS–SG) by the presence of hydrogen peroxide leaking back across the lysosomal membrane into the neutrophil cytosol.

Treatment is as for CGD together with supportive therapy for the chronic hemolysis and strict avoidance of oxidative stimuli that may trigger an acute life-threatening crisis. IFN-γ is of little benefit in these patients.

Myeloperoxidase deficiency

Myeloperoxidase (MPO) deficiency is the commonest inherited disorder of neutrophil function. Inherited in an autosomal recessive fashion, partial deficiencies are seen in 1 in 2000 individuals, and complete deficiency in 1 in 4000 individuals.[101] Monocytes and macrophages are affected, but not eosinophils as their peroxidase is encoded by a different gene. MPO is required for the generation of HOCl from H_2O_2; the hypochlorite in turn reacts with amine groups to form potent microbicidal radicals. This is important for *in vitro* killing of fungi. Rarely an acquired MPO deficiency can be seen in acute myeloid leukemia (AML) M2, M3, M4. In contrast, up to 25% of sufferers of CML and myelodysplasia with excess blasts acquire an MPO deficiency.[102–104]

The disorder is surprisingly asymptomatic in both inherited and acquired forms, and prophylactic antibiotics are not indicated. This may be due to a compensatory increase in oxidative burst as HOCl destroys the neutrophil NADPH oxidase, limiting its production of superoxide.[105] Only in diabetics is MPO deficiency of concern, where it predisposes to severe *Candida* infections.

The disorder is diagnosed by demonstrating the absence of cytochemically stainable enzyme and can be identified by flow cytometry. Furthermore, some cell counters that identify neutrophils by virtue of a peroxide stain may erroneously diagnose the patients as neutropenic.[106] Neutrophil function tests are unnecessary as MPO-deficient neutrophils show normal chemotaxis, adherence, phagocytosis and degranulation. MPO-deficient neutrophils have an increased respiratory burst producing augmented amounts of H_2O_2. Affected neutrophils can kill bacteria although this may be delayed.

Disorders of oxidant scavenging

Loss of granulocyte antioxidant enzymes can potentially reduce their lifespan and potency as oxidant enzymes are destroyed by their own product. However, in contrast with their effects on red cells these disorders show little evidence of a clinically significant reduction in neutrophil lifespan or ability to clear infection. These disorders can be subdivided into two groups.

Disorders of glutathione metabolism

Glutathione (GSH) is a tripeptide containing a central cysteine. The cysteine's –SH group can be oxidizd to form glutathione dimers (GSSG). The tripeptide is synthesized from

Table 14.8 A summary of disorders of glutathione metabolism.

Enzyme	Physiologic role	Clinical significance	Other features	References
Glutathione synthetase	Synthesis of glutathione (GSH)	Abnormal neutrophil phagocytosis in severe cases. May be relieved with vitamin E	Chronic hemolysis and acidosis due to an inability to reduce oxyproline	107, 108
Glutathione reductase	Recovery of glutathione dimers (GSSG) back to GSH	Reduced respiratory burst of uncertain significance	GGPD-like intermittent hemolytic anemia precipitated by oxidative stress	109, 110
Glutathione peroxidase	Reduction of H_2O_2 to water, oxidizing GSH	CGD-like disorder, but the role of enzyme deficiency is unclear		111–114

glutamyl, cysteine and glycine by glutathione synthetase. Toxic ROS are reduced by the action of glutathione peroxidase, which in turn oxidizes GSH into GSSG. Free GSSG is able to diffuse out of the cell; to prevent its loss it is rapidly reduced back to GSH by glutathione reductase, a reaction that requires oxidation of NADPH. Thus the presence of NADPH is required both for the formation and inactivation of neutrophil ROS. Disorders of glutathione metabolism are summarized in Table 14.8.

Catalase deficiency

Catalase inactivates excess hydrogen peroxide to form oxygen and water. Roos *et al.*[115] have reported two patients with reduced levels of both erythrocyte (<2% activity) and neutrophil (10–20%) catalase activity. Neither patient had a significant problem with pyogenic infections.

Investigation of the child with a suspected disorder of phagocyte function

Phagocytes are only one component of the normal defense mechanisms against infection, and many different phagocytic defects may present in a similar clinical fashion. A good history is important to differentiate the diseases listed. It is important to note that many children develop bacterial infections and that the incidence of most of the diseases discussed is rare; it follows that most children investigated for disorders of granulocyte function are entirely normal. Prior to embarking on an extensive program of investigations the following points should be considered.
• *Nature and timing of infections.* An early presentation suggests a severe disorder with a poor prognosis. A lack of pus together with a high neutrophil count suggests a defect of adhesion. The presence of granulomas suggests CGD. The milder phagocyte disorders may reveal themselves in the second decade of life with dental disease.
• *Type of infectious organisms.* CGD is associated with infections from staphylococci and other catalase producers.

Infections with *Pneumocystis* and viruses suggest a lymphocyte immunodeficiency in addition to a phagocyte disorder as in hyperimmunoglobulin E syndrome. All of the severe diseases listed are associated with fungal infections.
• *Noninfectious symptoms.* A history of atopy is associated with hyper-IgE, whereas the granulomas of CGD cause obstruction and an inflammatory bowel disease-like picture. Disorders of glutathione metabolism and G6PD present with a hemolytic anemia. A peripheral neuropathy and minor bleeding history is associated with Chédiak–Higashi.
Figure 14.7 represents a typical algorithm for the investigation of a phagocyte disorder.

Neutrophil function tests

Examination of a peripheral blood smear should precede any attempt at investigating neutrophil function. This can identify large abnormal granules in Chédiak–Higashi disease, or bilobed nuclei with a distorted nuclear membrane in neutrophil-specific granule deficiency. The Pelger–Huët anomaly may be seen in various marrow stem cell disorders such as myelodysplasia, Döhle-body-like inclusions in the May–Hegglin anomaly, and hypersegmented neutrophils in megaloblastic anemia. Neutrophil function tests are complex, unreliable and should only be performed in a specialist center.
• A Boyden chamber consists of two chambers linked by a thin flat channel. Phagocytes are placed in one chamber and a chemoattractant is placed in the second chamber. The proportion of motile cells is then measured after a defined period of time. The test can be performed in the presence of the patient's own or control plasma.
• Rebuck skin window measures the migration of neutrophils on to a glass cover slip applied to a superficial skin abrasion. An unreliable test that has been superseded by *in vitro* tests.
• Neutrophil adhesion can be determined *in vitro* by the adherence of the cells to nylon wool; this can be done in the presence of the patient's or control plasma.
• The respiratory burst is evaluated using the nitroblue tetrazolium (NBT) reduction test. Neutrophils are activated

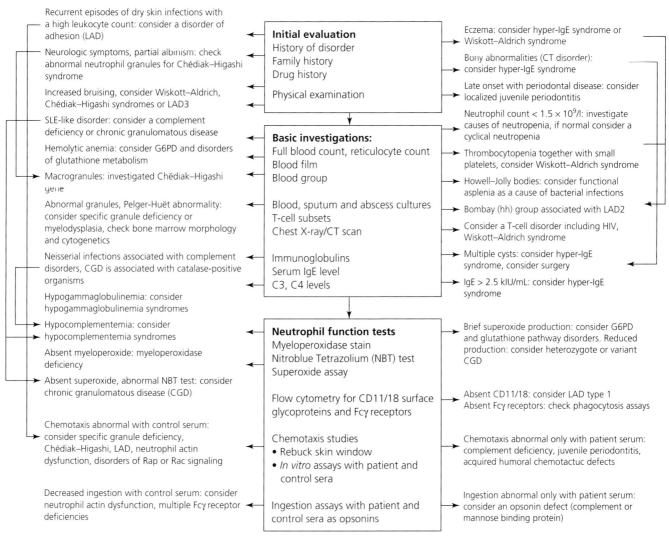

Fig. 14.7 Investigational algorithm for a neutrophil function defect.

in the presence of NBT, which produces a dark precipitate in cells producing superoxide (O_2^-). Respiratory burst activity can be measured directly as oxygen consumption, oxygen production (using cytochrome *c* reduction) or hydrogen peroxide production, and indirectly using neutrophil chemiluminescence.[116] Such tests are now available in kit form (Phagoburst) using f-Met-Leu-Phe or LPS as stimulants. ORPEGEN Pharma Heidelberg, Germany.

• Cytochemical stains and flow cytometry can be used to detect deficiencies in the enzymes myeloperoxidase and alkaline phosphatase and the lack of β_2 integrins and antibody Fc receptors.

• Bacterial and fungal phagocytosis and killing can also be measured. These tests are now available in kit form (Phagotest) using opsonized microbes. ORPEGEN Pharma Heidelberg, Germany.

• Additional tests include measurement of neutrophil degranulation and can be used to differentiate between disorders of primary and secondary granules.

Disorders of phagocyte numbers

Normal neutrophil structure and development
(Fig. 14.8)

Neutrophilic, eosinophilic and basophilic granulocytes are thought to follow similar patterns of proliferation, differentiation, maturation and storage in the bone marrow and delivery into the blood. For neutrophils the stages comprise myeloblast, promyelocyte, myelocyte, metamyelocyte, band form and mature neutrophil. The differentiation and maturation of polymorphonuclear neutrophils from a primitive stem cell involves sequential transcription of various genes and development of various organelles. Morphologically, using a light microscope, the various stages can be identified. The nuclei of immature cells with active gene transcription have open chromatin with promin-

Feature	Myeloblast	Promyelocyte	Myelocyte	Metamyelocyte	Band form	Mature neutrophil
Proliferation vs Maturation	The mitotic pool undergoes division and maturation. Currently it is believed that there are about five divisions, with possibly three at the level of the myelocyte and one each at the other levels			No evidence of cell division at these stages. There is maturation of the various components		
Size	10–18 µm	12–20 µm	12–18 µm	10–18 µm	10–16 µm	10–15 µm
Nucleus shape, position, chromatin pattern, nucleoli, nuclear membrane and color	Round to oval, eccentric/central, with fine chromatin, 2–5 nucleoli	Round to oval, eccentric/central, fine chromatin, 2–5 nucleoli	Oval or slightly indented, eccentric, partial chromatin condensation with no nucleoli	Markedly indented or U-shaped, condensed chromatin and no nucleoli	Band shaped of uniform thickness, coarse chromatin	2–5 distinct lobes joined by a filamentous strand. The chromatin is coarse
Cytoplasm colour, amount and golgi apparatus	Scanty and moderately basophilic (blue)	Moderate amounts of bluish cytoplasm, with Golgi apparatus	Moderate amounts of bluish pink cytoplasm	Plentiful amount of pink cytoplasm or finely granular cytoplasm	Plentiful amount of pink cytoplasm or finely granular cytoplasm	Plentiful amount of pink cytoplasm or finely granular cytoplasm
Granules	None	Primary (azurophilic)	Secondary or specific granules. Violet, orange–red, purple	And tertiary granules		
Morphology	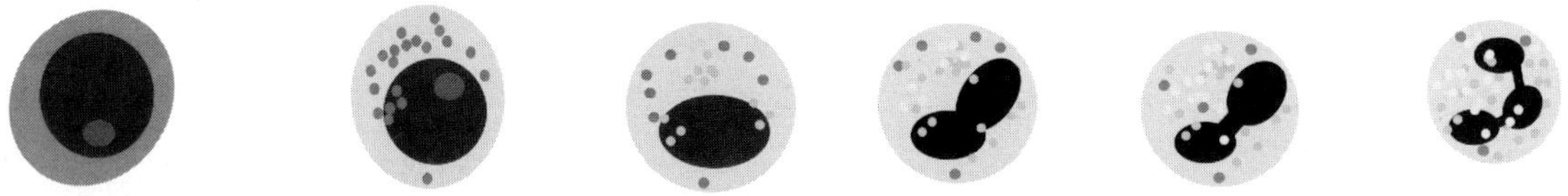					

Fig. 14.8 Neutrophil maturation.

ent nucleoli. Cytoplasmic basophilia (i.e., bluish coloration), is due to the presence of RNA and rough endoplasmic reticulum and represents active protein synthesis. Neutrophils have three types of granules with distinctive constituents, which arise chronologically. In general, cell maturation is accompanied by reduction in cell size, diminished cell volume, increased chromatin condensation of the nucleus, loss of nucleoli, appearance of cytoplasmic granules and a change in cytoplasmic basophilia. Further changes in the cell surface carbohydrates, glycoprotiens, glycolipids, and HLA antigens and granule contents occur during the entire maturation.

Neutrophil kinetics

Neutrophil kinetics describes the process of neutrophil multiplication, maturation, storage and distribution to tissues and sites of infection and tissue damage. Various methods have been employed to study these processes, for example, neutrophil depletion to assess the size and rate of mobilization of reserves; radioactive tracers to study the production, distribution and survival times; mitotic indices of marrow granulocytic cells to assess proliferative capacity; and induction of inflammatory lesions to study cell movement into the tissues. Such studies are helpful in explaining the physiological variations in neutrophil counts

and potentially explaining the mechanisms of neutropenia and risk of infections in different neutropenic states.

The three major compartments are the marrow, blood and tissue (Table 14.9). The mechanisms controlling the release of neutrophils from the bone marrow are only partially understood. A variety of compounds induce neutrophil movement into the circulation, including endotoxin, glucocorticoids, chemoattractants such as C5a, and cytokines such as tumor necrosis factor (TNF)-α. From the blood, neutrophils migrate into the lung, oral cavity, gastrointestinal tract, liver and spleen. They may be lost from mucosal surfaces, die in tissues or be phagocytosed by macrophages. The survival time in tissues is not known exactly, but is believed to be short. On average it takes 10 days for a neutrophil to mature and be released into the blood.

Neutropenia: definition

Neutropenia refers to an absolute blood neutrophil count (ANC) that is less than two standard deviations below the normal mean of the population. The neutrophil count in the peripheral blood is influenced by age, activity, and genetic and environmental factors. In infants the threshold is 1.0×10^9/L, and after the age of 1 year, the usual value is 1.5×10^9/L up to the age of 10 years, with an adult threshold of 1.8×10^9/L being applied thereafter.[119] The

Table 14.9 Neutrophil kinetics[117,118]

Compartment	Transit time (h)	Size of cell compartment ($\times 10^9$/kg)
Stem cells	Not known	Not known
Marrow: mitotic compartment		
Myeloblasts	23	0.14
Promyelocytes	26–78	0.51
Myelocytes	17–126	1.95
Marrow: maturation and storage compartment		
Metamyelocytes	8–108	2.7
Band forms	17–96	3.6
PMN	0–120	2.5
Blood		
Circulating neutrophil pool	Half-life in	0.31
Marginating neutrophil pool	blood is 6.7 h	0.39
Total blood neutrophil pool		0.70
Tissues	Not known	Neutrophil turnover rate is $0.3–1.3 \times 10^9$/kg per day

white blood cell (WBC) and neutrophil counts are lower in black people than Caucasians, and lower in Africans than in West Indians or black people in the USA. Yermite Jews also have lower counts than Caucasians.[120] A recent population-based study in Uganda showed a median absolute neutrophil count $\approx 2 \times 10^9$/L, and 90% reference ranges were quoted for different age groups: < 1 year ($0.9–4.4 \times 10^9$/L), 1–5 years ($1.0–3.9 \times 10^9$/L), 6–12 years ($0.9–3.6 \times 10^9$/L).[121] In most Afro-Caribbean adults an ANC above 1×10^9/L is considered normal, but in infants the total neutrophil count may be less than 1.0×10^9/L in as many as 20%.[122]

The severity of neutropenia can be classified as:
- mild: below the lower limit of normal but $> 1.0 \times 10^9$/L;
- moderate: $0.5–1.0 \times 10^9$/L;
- severe: $< 0.5 \times 10^9$/L;
- very severe: $< 0.2 \times 10^9$/L.

The lower limits are useful because the risk of severe infections does not increase until the neutrophil count falls below 0.5×10^9/L. The term agranulocytosis means complete absence of neutrophils and is often used to refer to severe neutropenia.

Pathophysiologic mechanisms of neutropenia

Neutropenic conditions can be distinguished according to the neutrophil pool that is predominantly affected, and are listed as follows.
- Decreased proliferation of progenitor cells, e.g., decreased number of stem cells in aplastic anemia, hostile micro-environment with decreased proliferating cells in leukemia and other infiltrative disorders, chemotherapy- or infection-induced inhibition of progenitor cells.
- Ineffective granulopoiesis/accelerated apoptosis, e.g., inherited defects of stem cells and progenitors in congenital neutropenia, acquired defect in B_{12}/folate deficiency.
- Reduced survival, e.g., increased peripheral consumption/accelerated destruction, in tissues during infections, by spleen in immune neutropenias, complement-mediated lysis in dialysis.
- Redistribution of the intravascular pool of neutrophils, e.g., endotoxin-induced margination of neutrophils.

It is of note that for a given ANC, the risk of infection is higher when the neutropenia is due to decreased production compared with increased destruction.

Severe chronic neutropenia

Severe chronic neutropenia is an inclusive term for hematologic diseases that cause severe neutropenia, that is a blood neutrophil count of $< 0.5 \times 10^9$/L for months or years. It is not a disease but a group of conditions with common clinical manifestations and both congenital and acquired causes.[123] Currently in the literature the terms "severe congenital neutropenia (SCN)" and "Kostmann syndrome" are used synonymously by some authors although others solely apply the eponymous name to those conditions believed to be of autosomal recessive inheritance as in Kostmann's original description.

The patients usually suffer infections with endogenous flora of the oropharynx, gastrointestinal tract and skin. Susceptibility to bacterial infections is variable even in patients with severe neutropenia. In SCN there is a very selective defect in the host defense mechanism with decreased neutrophils. The remaining components of innate immunity and adaptive immunity are intact and, indeed, compensatory monocytosis is not uncommon. This contrasts with chemotherapy-induced neutropenia, where innate immunity and adaptive immunity are also impaired, leading to a relatively higher incidence of infection. SCN patients present with recurrent oral ulcerations, gingivitis, recurrent upper respiratory tract infections, perirectal inflammation or minor skin infections and cellulitis. Frequent aphthous stomatitis and gingival hyperplasia lead to early loss of permanent teeth. Consequent to the sparing of the monocyte lineage, fungal infections are uncommon except as a possible complication of antibiotic therapy.[124]

Congenital neutropenias

Classification

Congenital neutropenias are a group of disorders characterized by a genetic defect that is known or postulated, con-

Table 14.10 Classification of congenital neutropenias.

Isolated congenital neutropenias
Kostmann syndrome and severe congenital neutropenia
Cyclic neutropenia

Neutropenia as part of congenital bone marrow failure syndromes, e.g.,
Fanconi anemia, dyskeratosis congenita

Congenital neutropenia as part of multisystem disorder
Shwachman–Diamond syndrome
Barth syndrome
Pearson syndrome
Glycogen storage disease type Ib (GSDIb)

Congenital neutropenia in association with defects of adaptive immunity
Severe combined immune deficiency (SCID) and reticular dysgenesis
X-linked hypogammaglobulinemia
Hyper-IgM
WHIM syndrome and myelokathexis

---

tributing to defective myelopoiesis (Table 14.10). The genetic defect might affect either the myeloid progenitors or stem cells or alter the microenvironment. Perhaps surprisingly, the neutropenia is not always present at birth. Although the age of onset is variable, symptoms can usually be traced back to the first year of life.

Common features

The congenital neutropenias have a number of common features, as summarized below.
• These are rare disorders. All modes of inheritance have been described. Patients with severe neutropenia are at risk of overwhelming infections. Clinical suspicion with early diagnosis and management can have a profound impact on the morbidity and mortality.
• Recombinant human G-CSF, cloned in 1986,[125] has revolutionized the management of these disorders. In 1987 it was shown that filgrastim selectively stimulated neutrophil production.[126] Four phase I/II trials and one phase III trial documented the safety and efficacy of G-CSF in the management of severe congenital, cyclic and idiopathic neutropenia. G-CSF elevated the neutrophil counts, and decreased or eliminated recurrent infections. More than 90% of patients respond to G-CSF.[125–128]
• The use of G-CSF and antibiotics has allowed survival into adulthood even in severely affected children.
• Genetic mutations have been identified in a proportion of the congenital neutropenias. The exact pathogenetic mechanisms, i.e., the translation of gene to disease, remain largely unclear.
• Some of the congenital neutropenias are preleukemic conditions. Currently it is not possible, at least at an early stage, to identify patients who are at high risk of transformation.

With increasing genotype and phenotype analysis, an individualized risk assessment is both possible and desirable.

Severe congenital neutropenia and Kostmann syndrome

R. Kostmann was among the first to describe severe congenital neutropenia in a Swedish family, with an apparent autosomal recessive inheritance, maturation arrest at promyelocyte/myelocyte stage, and early onset of bacterial infections with high mortality.[129] Severe congenital neutropenia is genetically heterogeneous, and inheritance patterns now recognized include sporadic, autosomal dominant, autosomal recessive and X-linked forms.[130,131] Constitutional heterozygous *ELA2* mutations are present in the majority of patients with sporadic and autosomal dominant disease, but not in the others. There is no association with other congenital abnormalities.

Clinical presentation

The disease usually presents in the first year of life with severe neutropenia, often $< 0.2 \times 10^9$/L, and recurrent infections. The infections are mostly bacterial and can present as an omphalitis immediately after birth. Fatal infections were common in the past, and in the pre-cytokine era 42% of the published cases died in the first two years of life usually from sepsis and pneumonia.[132] Bone marrow aspirate shows a maturation arrest at the promyelocyte/myelocyte stage. Promyelocytes may show dysplastic features, including atypical nuclei, vacuolization of the cytoplasm and occasional abnormal granulation. The remaining hematopoietic system is essentially normal with mild anemia of chronic disease, reactive thrombocytosis and presumably a compensatory monocytosis and eosinophilia. Immune response to vaccination is normal. IgG levels are often elevated.

Treatment of neutropenia

The neutropenia of SCN responds to G-CSF in more than 90% of the patients. Most patients respond to a dose of 3–10 µg/kg daily. Registry data suggest that 92% of patients respond to a dose of < 30 µg/kg daily with an increase in mean neutrophil count of $> 1.5 \times 10^9$/L.[132,133] Recommendations include a starting dose of 5 µg/kg daily, and incrementing by 10 µg/kg per day every 14 days, aiming for a neutrophil count of $1–5 \times 10^9$/L. Nonresponders are defined as not responding to 120 µg/kg daily, although rarely is anything achieved beyond 30 µg/kg daily. Partial responders are patients who increase their neutrophil counts to between 0.5 and 1×10^9/L. A good initial rise usually predicts good long-term improvement; loss of response with time through marrow exhaustion has not been observed with long-term therapy.

Other clinical features

Other clinical features associated with severe congenital neutropenia[134] are summarized below.

• Musculoskeletal pains and headache are commonly seen at the beginning of treatment with G-CSF, and respond well to a nocturnal dosing schedule and simple analgesics.

• Mild splenomegaly is seen in less than a fifth of patients before starting G-CSF, but the incidence increases with treatment.

• Thrombocytopenia is uncommon and should raise concerns about possible transformation to myelodysplastic syndrome (MDS)/AML, although sometimes it is associated with excessive G-CSF dosage.

• Osteopenia and osteoporosis have been documented either by dual energy X ray absorptiometry (DEXA) scan or symptomatic fractures in a small group of patients, but the true incidence and relation to G-CSF are unknown.

• Vasculitis, typically cutaneous or renal, has a 3% incidence, and is temporally related to an increase in ANC; biopsy shows leukocytoclastic vasculitis. Patients with recurrent vasculitis or organ involvement often have other autoimmune disorders, worsened by G-CSF.

• Growth and longitudinal development can be impaired, although this may merely be a manifestation of chronic illness in older cases series.

Transformation to myelodysplastic syndrome and acute myeloid leukemia

There is an excess incidence of MDS and AML in patients with severe chronic neutropenia and Shwachman–Diamond syndrome (SDS). This predisposition to hematologic malignancy is confined to SCN and SDS and has not been observed in other chronic neutropenias including cyclic and idiopathic variants. The transformation is often associated with the development of cytogenetic abnormalities (frequently partial or complete loss of chromosome 7, abnormalities of chromosome 21) and point mutations in the *ras* and G-CSF receptor genes.[135] There has been concern regarding the use of G-CSF and the excess risk of transformation in children with SCN. Epidemiologic data do not reveal an association between G-CSF dose or duration of treatment and transformation risk.[136] The current consensus is that G-CSF merely allows the most severely affected children to live long enough for the full disease phenotype to manifest rather than accelerating the progression *per se*.

The cumulative risk of development for AML/MDS by the end of year 8 of G-CSF was about 13%, based on 94 patients who had received a minimum of 8 years of G-CSF.[133] Leukemic events appear to be randomly distributed with reference to duration of observational exposure to G-CSF.

Chemotherapy alone offers no long-term survival once transformation has occurred. Although the data are largely unpublished, bone marrow transplantation (without significant AML-like chemotherapy) can achieve a surprisingly good "cure" rate, even at this stage of the disease. Transplant-related mortality was historically very high but has been reduced dramatically with antifungal prophylaxis.

Follow-up

Clinical examination and blood count are recommended every 3 months for patients on long-term therapy. Cytogenetic changes may precede overt leukemia, therefore yearly bone marrow aspirates and cytogenetic studies are recommended.

Cyclic neutropenia

Cyclic neutropenia is a rare hematologic disorder, classically described as an autosomal dominant cyclical oscillation in the neutrophil count (and to a lesser extent other cell lineages) with a regular periodicity of 21 days. A few sporadic cases have also been documented. Mutations in *ELA2* (discussed later) are seen in almost all patients with the classic 21-day periodicity. During the nadir the neutrophil count is usually $< 0.2 \times 10^9/L$ for about 3–5 days, and during the normal periods the counts are typically around the lower limit of normal.[137] The role of *ELA2* mutations is described later.

Clinical presentation

The age of onset is variable, but most patients have symptoms in infancy. During the neutropenic phase patients present with fever, malaise, aphthous stomatitis, and cervical adenopathy. Cellulitis can develop at sites of injury and in the perianal region. Fatalities secondary to spontaneous peritonitis, segmental bowel necrosis and septicemia are recorded, possibly secondary to colonic ulcers.[138,139] A wide spectrum of symptom severity, ranging from asymptomatic to life-threatening illness, can be observed even within families. Thrice weekly blood counts for 6 weeks are recommended by the Severe Chronic Neutropenia International Registry (SCNIR) to enable diagnosis, although this is difficult in children. Serial bone marrow examination shows maturation arrest at varying stages, with only early myeloid precursors being seen during the neutropenic phase.

Treatment

Cyclic neutropenia responds extremely well to G-CSF, often within 1–2 weeks of initiation of treatment. G-CSF shortens the duration of the neutropenic phase and increases the peak neutrophil count. More than 90% of patients respond and they require a smaller dose than SCN patients. The median daily dose is 2 μg/kg with a maximum of 10 μg/kg daily. There is no evidence of transformation to MDS/AML.[133,134]

ELA2 mutations in the pathophysiology of cyclic neutropenia and severe congenital neutropenia

Heterozygous mutations of the *ELA2* gene are detected in nearly all families with cyclical neutropenia and the majority of patients with sporadic and autosomal dominant severe congenital neutropenia but not in those with autosomal recessive variants.[130,131,140] Biallelic mutation of *ELA2* is unknown, and these mutations therefore do not explain the syndrome first reported by Kostmann.

ELA2 codes for neutrophil elastase (NE), the synthesis of which is confined to promyelocytes and promonocytes. NE is packaged into the azurophilic granules and appears to have an important role in both host response to infection and the inflammatory response. Pathophysiologically extracellular release of NE at sites of inflammation appears to have an important role in a variety of conditions including emphysema, cystic fibrosis and rheumatoid arthritis.

There is now plentiful genetic data supporting the role of *ELA2* mutations in the pathogenesis of cyclic neutropenia and some forms of SCN. Two major observations that strongly support an etiological role for *ELA2* mutations are firstly that they occur almost invariably in cyclic neutropenia and commonly in SCN, and none of the described mutations has been reported in a normal individual. Secondly, germline mosaic individuals who have fathered children with SCN demonstrate *ELA2* mutations in myeloid progenitors, but not neutrophils, indicating that the mutation alone is sufficient to prevent the maturation of stem cells into neutrophils.[141]

The severe neutropenia of these disorders is characteristically associated with a maturation arrest at the promyelocyte/myelocyte stage. There is no well-defined explanation for this arrest. Several hypotheses have been proposed to explain the role of abnormal NE in the development of SCN.[142,143] Protein modeling suggests that a feature common to all mutations of NE is that they can lead to destabilization of the mature protein. This destabilization may result in a gain of function or abnormal function. A recent hypothesis suggests that there is abnormal trafficking of the neutrophil elastase with increased membrane expression. Although initial studies suggested that the mutations affect different areas of the protein in cyclic and congenital neutropenia, subsequent studies demonstrated considerable overlap in the mutations with some being reported repeatedly in both cyclical and congenital neutropenia. Furthermore, the excess risk of leukemia and MDS seen in SCN is not present in cyclic neutropenia, further adding to the difficulty of understanding the mechanism of disease. One genotype–phenotype study suggested that SCN patients whose disease is the result of *ELA2* mutations represent a subset with more severe disease, with lower neutrophil counts, higher requirements for G-CSF and a higher rate of neoplastic progression.[144] However, attempts to predict the risk of malignant transformation within the group that have *ELA2* mutations appear unlikely to be successful.

Shwachman–Diamond syndrome

SDS is a rare autosomal recessive multisystem disorder, and has already been described in Chapter 3. It is the second most common cause of pancreatic insufficiency after cystic fibrosis, and probably the third most common inherited bone marrow failure syndrome after Fanconi anemia and Diamond–Blackfan anemia. It has two main characteristics: pancreatic exocrine insufficiency and neutropenia/bone marrow failure.[145] SDS typically presents in infancy as failure to thrive due to a combination of pancreatic insufficiency, feeding difficulties and recurrent infections. In milder cases, the diagnosis can be delayed until the second decade of life.

Genetics and pathophysiology

SDS appears to be caused by mutations of the previously undescribed *SBDS* gene.[146] Most patients have compound heterozygous mutations. Homozygosity for the predicted null mutations has not been reported, these presumably being embryonically lethal and implying that some functional gene product is essential. This highly conserved gene is expressed in most human cell types and encodes a 250 amino acid protein whose function is unclear, although indirect genetic evidence suggests that it may be involved in RNA processing. Presumably, there is an effect on some aspect of RNA metabolism that is essential for development of the exocrine pancreas, hematopoiesis and chondrogenesis.[147]

Hematologic abnormalities and MDS/AML

Ineffective hematopoiesis commonly presents as neutropenia. The neutropenia can be intermittent, although it is probably not truly cyclic as suggested in the past. Neutrophil dysfunction is present with impaired mobility, migration and chemotaxis. Anemia may be present at diagnosis but usually responds to the improved nutritional status associated with enzyme replacement and good gastrointestinal care. Intermittent mild thrombocytopenia is not unusual and pancytopenia develops in a significant proportion of patients. The marrow appearances include varying degrees of hypoplasia, left-shifted granulopoiesis with maturation arrest, and scattered trilineage dysplastic changes. SDS is a preleukemic stem cell disorder with a crude risk of leukemic transformation probably > 30% with prolonged (40-year) follow-up. Stable clonal cytogenetic abnormalities are not uncommon, with occasional spontaneous disappearance of large clones.[148] Cytogenetic abnormalities often involve chromosome 7; however, clones containing isochromosome 7q and del(20q) frequently wax and wane over many years in SDS and their exact prognostic value is unknown. Although the neutropenia does respond to G-CSF, most patients manage well on prophylactic antibiotics alone.

Pancreatic dysfunction

Varying severity of pancreatic dysfunction due to acinar maldevelopment is a hallmark of SDS. There is extensive fatty replacement of pancreatic acinar tissue with relatively normal ductal architecture. Secretion of lipase, amylase and trypsinogen is decreased. Malabsorption and steatorrhea are present in around 90% of the patients at diagnosis. Surprisingly, with increasing age, up to half of SDS patients show improvement in enzyme production and can just become pancreatically sufficient although remaining clearly abnormal on more formal testing.

Other abnormalities

Skeletal dysostosis produces thoracic cage and gait abnormalities. The latter can be severe and require surgical correction. Dental dysplasia (not solely related to neutropenia) and behavioral and intellectual problems are also frequent.

Pearson syndrome

This syndrome is caused by deletions in mitochondrial DNA.[149] It presents with macrocytic anemia, variable degrees of neutropenia, thrombocytopenia and exocrine pancreatic failure. The bone marrow is characteristic, with hemosiderosis, ring sideroblasts and remarkable vacuolization of erythroid and myeloid precursors, all of which point to the diagnosis and largely exclude the diagnosis of SDS, with which there can be confusion clinically.[150]

Barth syndrome

Barth syndrome is an inherited disorder, often fatal in childhood, characterized by cardiac and skeletal myopathy, short stature, neutropenia and 3-methylglutaconic aciduria.[151] The disease is caused by mutations in the X-linked G4.5 gene, which encodes for a protein involved in cardiolipin biosynthesis.[152] The mechanism of neutropenia is unknown. The neutropenia responds well to G-CSF. Early diagnosis and initiation of G-CSF is important as neutropenia and cardiomyopathy are a potentially lethal combination. There does not appear to be a risk of malignant transformation.

Glycogen storage disease type Ib

Glycogen storage disease type Ib (GSDIb) results from deficiency of the glucose 6-phosphate translocase enzyme, which transports glucose 6-phosphate into the endoplasmic reticulum for conversion to glucose. Absence of the enzyme leads to an inability to produce glucose by either gluconeogenesis or glycogenolysis, with the risk of fasting hypoglycemia and lactic acidosis. These patients suffer from severe neutropenia, neutrophil function defects and recurrent infections.[153] The mechanism of the neutropenia is again uncertain. Surprisingly, an inflammatory bowel disease is associated with the neutropenia of GSDIb. G-CSF treatment reduces the number and severity of infections and the inflammatory bowel disease improves subjectively.[154] G-CSF can lead to splenomegaly, and some patients require dose reduction. There have been two case reports of AML in patients on long-term G-CSF; affected individuals therefore need monitoring similarly to the SCN children.[155]

Neutropenia associated with primary immunodeficiency disorders

Neutropenia is a feature of congenital immunodeficiency states and a factor contributing to the increased risk of infection in many patients. The primary immunodeficiency diseases involve virtually every component of the immune system. Most of the immunodeficiency disorders are inherited as single gene defects. The disorders of primary immunodeficiency are discussed in detail in Chapter 19. A brief mention is made of disorders where neutropenia is severe or prominent.[156]

Severe combined immunodeficiency disease and reticular dysgenesis

Reticular dysgenesis is a form of severe combined immunodeficiency disease (SCID), characterized by complete failure of development of both myeloid and lymphoid stem cells. The lack of adaptive immunity with absence of phagocytes leads to severe and often fatal infections in the first year of life. Bone marrow transplantation has been reported to be curative. In the other variants neutropenia is variable, and can respond to G-CSF.

X-linked agammaglobulinemia

Severe often intermittent neutropenia is seen in about one-quarter of patients. The *XLA* gene responsible for the disorder is expressed in cells of myeloid lineage, although the mechanism of neutropenia is ill defined.

Hyper-IgM syndrome

Intermittent or chronic neutropenia is prominent and affects over half of the patients. Although an autoimmune basis has been suggested, there is no evidence of antineutrophil antibodies. A defective interaction with the microenvironment due to deficiency of CD40 ligand would appear to alter the cytokine milieu necessary for myelopoiesis. Indeed, the marrow in these patients shows a maturation arrest with vacuolated promyelocytes, indistinguishable from that seen in SCN.

Common variable immunodeficiency

Neutropenia has been noted, probably on an autoimmune basis. There is an association with hemolytic anemia and thrombocytopenia. The neutropenia has been reported to be responsive to G-CSF, and G-CSF is indicated if the patient is symptomatic in spite of IVIG and antibiotics.

Cartilage-hair-hypoplasia syndrome

This rare autosomal recessive syndrome is characterized by short limb dwarfism with hyperextensile digits, fine hair, neutropenia, lymphopenia and recurrent infections. The syndrome is due to mutation in the *RMRP* gene, which encodes the mitochondrial RNA-processing endoribonuclease.[157]

Chédiak–Higashi syndrome

The neutropenia is mild, and recurrent infections are due to the combination of neutropenia with defective microbicidal activity. It has been discussed in detail with disorders of function, above.

Myelokathexis and WHIM syndrome

Myelokathexis is a rare cause of severe leukopenia and neutropenia. It is a genetically heterogeneous disorder, and WHIM syndrome is one of the autosomally dominant inherited variants. The acronym WHIM was coined to describe an unusual form of congenital neutropenia characterized by *w*arts, *h*ypogammaglobulinemia, *i*mmunodeficiency and *m*yelokathexis (the apparent retention of mature neutrophils in the bone marrow). The pathognomonic bone marrow findings are myeloid hypercellularity with morphologic abnormalities consistent with apoptosis, which are cytoplasmic vacuolation, hypersegmented and pyknotic nuclei, and long thin strands of chromatin separating the nuclear lobes. Affected individuals typically present with recurrent infections and leucopenia. The total leukocyte counts are often $< 1 \times 10^9/L$, and absolute neutrophil counts tend to be 0.0 to $0.5 \times 10^9/L$. The clinical course is relatively benign, and indeed a significant proportion of cases are diagnosed in adulthood. There is no excess of viral infections, except for a unique susceptibility to human papillomavirus, which can occur from infancy to adolescence. Hypogammaglobulinemia can range from moderate deficiency to essentially normal levels. T- and B-cell dysfunction fluctuate in the same individual over time. No neutrophil function defects have been reported in WHIM syndrome, although some of the isolated forms appear to show functional defects.

Truncating mutations in the cytoplasmic tail of the chemokine receptor 4 (CXCR4) are the cause of WHIM syndrome.[158,159] The mutations result in prolonged activation, with enhanced chemotactic responsiveness of neutrophils to CXCL12, its natural ligand in the stroma. This results in impaired migration from bone marrow. The identification of mutations in CXCR4 in individuals with WHIM syndrome represents the first example of aberrant chemokine receptor function causing human disease, and suggests that the receptor may be important in cell-mediated immunity to human papillomavirus infection. Infection, epinephrine and steroids all cause release of neutrophils into the periphery and neutrophil survival in infections may be increased resulting from the surge of endogenous cytokines and growth factors, which would explain the relatively benign course of the disease.

Acquired neutropenias

Pathophysiologically, acquired neutropenias may be due to any of the mechanisms alluded to earlier, namely decreased proliferation of the myeloid precursors, ineffective granulopoiesis, increased peripheral destruction, or abnormal tissue distribution. Neutropenia is often the only cytopenia, but there may be a concurrent mild anemia and thrombocytopenia. In the following pages, disorders with dominant or isolated neutropenia are covered, and mention is made of disorders where neutropenia is an important component of pancytopenia (Table 14.11).

Infections

Viral infections

Viral infections are the most common cause of transient neutropenia in childhood. Viruses commonly associated with neutropenia include hepatitis A and B, herpes simplex virus, cytomegalovirus, Epstein–Barr virus (EBV), influenza A and B, measles, mumps, rubella and respiratory syncytial virus. Transient neutropenias develop in the initial 1–2 days of the illness in association with the peak viremic phase, and persist

Table 14.11 Examples of acquired neutropenias.

Neutropenia as the only or dominant cytopenia
Infections: viral, bacterial, fungal, rickettsial and protozoal
Drugs
Immune
   Neonatal alloimmune neutropenia
   Primary autoimmune neutropenia of infancy and childhood
   Secondary autoimmune neutropenia
Nutrition: anorexia nervosa, copper deficiency
Chronic idiopathic neutropenia
Neutropenia associated with complement activation

Neutropenia as part of pancytopenia
Acquired marrow failure due to decreased proliferation of progenitors in the bone marrow, e.g., aplastic anemia, marrow infiltration
Nutritional deficiency, e.g., vitamin B_{12} and folate deficiency
Splenic sequestration

for 3–7 days. The neutropenia can be severe, but rarely causes serious bacterial infection. The suggested mechanisms include: redistribution of neutrophils from the circulating to the marginating pool; aggregation and sequestration of neutrophils after activation by complement; and destruction of the neutrophils by circulating antibodies.[160] Prolonged neutropenia with or without other cytopenias is known to occur with hepatitis B, EBV, parvovirus B19, Kawasaki disease and HIV infection. Neutropenia is also seen with yellow fever, dengue fever, Colorado tick fever and sandfly fever.

Bacterial infections

Significant neutropenia and other cytopenias are seen in certain bacterial infections, where the bacteria tend to be intracellular pathogens. It is not uncommon with typhoid, paratyphoid, brucellosis and tularemia, which are all characterized by bacteria with a predilection for macrophages. Neutropenia and other cytopenias in tuberculosis are only seen in disseminated/miliary tuberculosis. Rickettsias, which are obligate intracellular Gram-negative organisms, are another important cause of neutropenia. In scrub typhus, epidemic typhus, rickettsial pox and severe cases of Rocky Mountain spotted fever, there is infection of the vascular endothelial cells of the lungs and brain, with secondary neutropenia and other cytopenias as part of a vasculitic process.

Sepsis is one of the most serious causes of neutropenia. The mechanism is due to increased destruction/utilization, impaired production and C5a-mediated sequestration in the pulmonary vasculature. This sequestration can result in the release of toxic mediators and subsequent tissue damage. Neonates are particularly susceptible to sepsis-induced neutropenia as their storage pool is small and the baseline production of granulocytes is often near maximal.

Protozoal infections

Visceral leishmaniasis is commonly associated with neutropenia and pancytopenia. Mechanisms include hypersplenism, antineutrophil antibodies and ineffective hematopoiesis.[161] Malaria and trypanosomiasis have been associated with neutropenia. The neutropenia during febrile episodes in malaria is due to margination, although severe disease presents with neutrophilia. Hypersplenism is an important cause of neutropenia in tropical hyperactive malarial splenomegaly.

Drug-induced neutropenia

Drug-induced neutropenia is rare in children, with only 10% of the cases reported in children and young adults.[162] The drugs most commonly implicated are antibiotics (beta-lactam and trimethoprim-sulfamethoxazole), antithyroid drugs, antiplatelet agents, neuroleptic and antiepileptic agents and nonsteroidal antiinflammatory agents.[163]

Mechanisms of idiosyncratic drug reactions

Immune-mediated destruction of granulocytes or their precursors

Hapten- or T-cell-mediated allergic reactions can occur when drugs act as haptens. Most drugs are small molecules with a molecular mass less than 1000 Da, and are not capable of eliciting a direct immune response. They conjugate with another macromolecule or at times directly to MHC molecules. The end result is antibody formation, complement fixation and neutrophil destruction. The antineutrophil antibodies are often identified *in vitro* only in the presence of the drug. Examples of such drugs include penicillin, propylthiouracil, aminopyrine, antithyroid drugs and gold.[164]

Drug-induced autoimmunity (e.g., with quinidine, alphamethyldopa) involves a drug inducing the formation of antineutrophil antibodies, which bind the neutrophils and cause premature destruction. Most often the antibodies disappear after the drug is withdrawn, but at times they can persist even when the drug is stopped.[165]

Dose-dependent inhibition of granulocytic precursors

Dose-dependent inhibition of granulopoiesis has been documented with beta-lactam antibiotics, carbamazepine and valproic acid. Both valproic acid and carbamazepine cause dose-dependent inhibition of the granulocyte–macrophage colony-forming unit (CFU-GM), which is pronounced at high levels and variable at low levels. Valproate, in addition to neutropenia and Pelger–Huët abnormalities, causes a spectrum of hematologic abnormalities, including aplastic anemia, other cytopenias and acquired von Willebrand disease.[166,167]

Direct toxic effect on marrow progenitors or mature cells

Clozapine accelerates apoptosis of neutrophils due to the generation of a reactive metabolite within the neutrophil. Sulfasalazine is toxic to promyelocytes at therapeutic levels in comparison with lymphocytes. With azathioprine, polymorphism of thiopurine methyltransferase increases the risk of hematologic toxicity.

Clinical presentation and management

Drug-induced neutropenia is associated with a high rate of infectious complications and is reported to have a mortality rate of approximately 10%. In drug-induced neutropenia, most studies have shown that G-CSF shortens the time to neutrophil recovery, although several authors have commented that evidence-based data are lacking to justify its use.[163,168] Given the rarity and heterogeneity of drug-induced neutropenia, it seems unlikely that an evidence-based algorithm for G-CSF use will ever be validated. However, because drug-induced neutropenia is an acute, life-threatening complication of therapy, the demonstrated safety and apparent

Table 14.12 Human neutrophil antigen (HNA) nomenclature and disease associations.

Antigens	Previous nomenclature	Glycoprotein	Allele frequency (%) in Caucasians	Disease associations
HNA-1a	NA1	FcγIIIb (CD16)	58	NAIN, AIN, TRALI
HNA-1b	NA2	FcγIIIb (CD16)	88	NAIN, AIN, TRALI
HNA-1c	SH, NA3	FcγIIIb (CD16)	5	NAIN, AIN, TRALI
HNA-2a	NB1	CD177 (NB1gp)	97	NAIN, AIN, TRALI and drug-induced neu.
HNA-3a	5b	gp70–95	97	TRALI
HNA-4a	MART	CD11b (CR3)	99	NAIN (1 case)
HNA-5a	OND	CD11a (LFA-1)	96	Not known

CR3, C3bi receptor; LFA-1, leukocyte function antigen 1; gp, glycoprotein; NAIN, neonatal alloimmune neutropenia; AIN, (primary) autoimmune neutropenia; TRALI, transfusion-related acute lung injury.
Modified with permission from Refs 169 and 170.

effectiveness of G-CSF in hastening neutrophil recovery justifies its use in this setting.

Immune neutropenia

Immune neutropenia can be subdivided into neonatal alloimmune neutropenia (NAIN), primary autoimmune neutropenia (AIN) and secondary autoimmune neutropenias. The immune neutropenias are mostly due to accelerated destruction of mature neutrophils.

Granulocyte alloantigens and the human neutrophil antigen system

Antibodies directed against granulocyte membrane antigens cause NAIN and primary AIN. The implicated antigens are highly immunogenic membrane glycoproteins. Alloantibodies to these glycoproteins are responsible for alloimmune neonatal neutropenia, nonfebrile hemolytic transfusion reactions, refractoriness to granulocyte transfusions, post-bone-marrow-transplant immune neutropenia and TRALI. Autoantibodies to the same antigens are responsible for primary and some secondary autoimmune neutropenias, and drug-induced neutropenia.

Currently there are seven well-defined clinically relevant human neutrophil antigens (HNAs), which are assigned to five glycoproteins (Table 14.12).

Granulocyte alloantigens and polymorphisms

In a recent review on platelet and granulocyte glycoprotein polymorphisms, Lucas and Metcalfe have suggested that the granulocyte membrane antigens be divided into three types:[171]

• granulocyte-specific antigens;
• the "shared" antigens, which often have a limited distribution amongst other cell types, mostly white cells; and

• the "common" antigens, which have wider distribution on other tissue and blood cells, e.g., HLA class I molecules, I and P blood groups, etc.

Granulocyte-specific antigens

HNA-1, localized to FcγRIIIb (CD16), is the most common antigen against which antibodies are detected. The Fc receptors belong to the immunoglobulin superfamily and bind to the constant domain of the antibody molecule, which is specific for each class of immunoglobulin. The most important receptors for microbial opsonization are the Fcγ receptors, which recognize IgG. The Fcγ receptors are of three types, varying in their structure, function and the types of cells they are distributed across. FcγRIII exists in two non-allelic forms, a and b. FcγRIIIb is linked to the plasma membrane via a glycosylphosphatidylinositol (GPI) anchor, has low affinity for IgG and is exclusively expressed on neutrophils. The HNA-1a, -1b and -1c antigens are all located on FcγRIIIb. HNA-1a and -1b show five nucleotide differences at the DNA level; four of these substitutions result in amino acid changes and two of them result in additional glycosylations. The immunogenicity of this receptor may be related to the high concentration of the molecules on the surface of the neutrophil, with 100 000 to 300 000 copies per neutrophil.

HNA-2a antigen is located on the NB1 glycoprotein, which is a glycosyl-phosphatidylinositol-anchored glycoprotein (gp) found on neutrophil membranes and secondary granules. NB1 gp is unusual in that it is expressed on a subpopulation of neutrophils, representing 45–65% of the total. It is encoded by the CD177 gene which has another allel- PRV-1. CD177mRNA levels are increased in polycythemia vera, hence the labelling of the second allele.[172]

Shared antigens

HNA-3a antigen is located on a 70–90-kDa neutrophil

glycoprotein, whose gene is not yet known. HNA-4a and 5a are located on neutrophil β_2-integrin. It belongs to the integrin superfamily and consists of three members sharing a common β subunit with three different α subunits. HNA-4a is the result of a polymorphism in complement receptor 3 (CR3, CD11b) and HNA-5a is the result of a polymorphism in the leukocyte function antigen 1 (LFA-1, CD11a).

Detection of antineutrophil antibodies

Screening for neutrophil antibodies is technically challenging because of the need for intact neutrophils (which have a short lifespan) as a source of antigen. A panel of donor neutrophils of known phenotype is used, so as to detect all clinically relevant antibodies. The following tests can be done on patient sera.[169]

• Granulocyte agglutination test: detects microscopic agglutination of neutrophils.

• Granulocyte immunofluorescence test (GIFT): antigen–antibody reactions are detected by fluorescence-conjugated secondary antibodies using a fluorescent microscope or flow cytometry.

• Monoclonal antibody immobilization of granulocyte antigens (MAIGA): allows detection of antibodies to specific neutrophil membrane glycoproteins, even in the presence of antibodies to HLA antigens.[173]

There are methodologic limitations to the above tests, and often the tests need to be repeated on at least two occasions to increase detection rate and decrease false positivity. The following points should also be noted.

• A minimum of two techniques should be used to detect granulocyte-specific serum antibodies, including one of the two techniques recommended, i.e., the granulocyte agglutination test and the granulocyte immunofluorescence test. The chosen techniques must enable reliable detection of clinically significant alloantibodies, including anti-HNA-1a, -1b, -1c, -2a, and -3a and be able to detect both IgG and IgM isotypes.

• At least two techniques should be available to detect cytotoxic and noncytotoxic antilymphocyte antibodies and thereby aid the distinction between granulocyte-specific antibodies, HLA class I antibodies, granulocyte/lymphocyte/monocyte-reactive antibodies and antibody mixtures.

• Further techniques, usually glycoprotein-specific assays that can be used to detect and identify granulocyte-specific antibodies in the presence of HLA class I or lymphocyte-reactive antibodies, should also be available.

Neonatal alloimmune neutropenia

NAIN is analogous to alloimmune neonatal thrombocytopenia purpura of the newborn. During gestation there is maternal sensitization to paternally derived fetal neutrophil antigens, resulting in IgG antibodies that cross the placenta and prime the fetal neutrophils for premature destruction.[174] Newborns develop transient neutropenia, the duration of which is related to the clearance of maternal IgG, on average 11 weeks (range 3–28 weeks).[175] Infectious complications include omphalitis, skin infections, pneumonia, urinary infections and septicemia. A few deaths have been reported in some case series. Treatment is supportive and G-CSF has been used with good effect.[176]

Alloantibodies to most of the neutrophil antigens have been described in association with NAIN. Anti-HNA-1a and anti-HNA-1b are the most frequent. In a study of unselected pregnant women where HNA-1a and 1b genotypes were done, genotypic fetomaternal incompatibility was seen in 20% of cases. However, only 3% of the mothers with an incompatible child developed antibodies and none of the neonates developed NAIN.[177] These observations are similar to earlier serologic data.[178,179] The exact incidence is unknown, but a rate of 1 in 6000 has been suggested based on unpublished data.

Primary autoimmune neutropenia

Primary AIN is predominantly a disorder of infancy and early childhood and is the most frequent cause of neutropenia in this age group. A study of 240 children with primary AIN has given a comprehensive picture of the clinical and laboratory features, infectious complications and natural history of the disorder.[180] The key features can be summarized as follows.

• Age: majority of children are under 3 years at diagnosis and two-thirds present between the ages of 5 and 15 months.

• Full blood count (FBC): severe neutropenia is present in two-thirds of cases, and a compensatory monocytosis in one-third.

• Bone marrow: a decreased number of mature neutrophils is the most common finding. Ten percent of the patients can show unusual features like hypocellularity, and maturation arrest at later stages of development. No cases were seen with maturation arrest at the promyelocyte stage.

• Serology: antibodies are often detected on the first occasion, but one-quarter of patients require multiple testing.

• Antibody specificity: IgG or IgM or a combination. The specificity is either HNA-1 or HNA-2 or none, with rarer cases associated with antibodies to CD11b (HNA-5a) or pan-FcγRIIIb. This is in contrast to secondary AIN, where pan-FcγRIIIb antibodies are frequently detected. Interestingly the same group in a later study showed the presence of panspecific antibodies earlier in the primary AIN, with specificity to a single antigen developing later on.[181,182]

• Clinical presentation: mild skin and upper respiratory tract infections predominate. One-tenth of patients can present with severe infections such as pneumonia, meningitis or sepsis. A significant number are asymptomatic.

- In 80% of the patients observed, the neutropenia persisted for 7–24 months. Disappearance of antibodies preceded the normalization of the counts.
- Management: symptomatic treatment with antibiotics is sufficient in most patients. Patients with recurrent infections respond well to antibiotic prophylaxis. The most severe cases require the use of regular G-CSF therapy.

Secondary immune neutropenias

The mechanism of the immune neutropenia is variable. Targeted antigens are both membrane bound and intracellular. Antibody- and T-cell-mediated destruction are important mechanisms. There is evidence of neutrophil dysfunction in a few diseases. The various diseases associated with secondary immune neutropenia will be discussed briefly below.

Evans syndrome is characterized by autoimmune hemolytic anemia with immune thrombocytopenia. Immune neutropenia is not uncommon.[183]

Neutropenia is found in about 50–60% of patients with active *systemic lupus erythematosus* (SLE), at some stage of the disease. The neutropenia is usually mild, and often acts as a marker of disease activity. Clinically, increased susceptibility to infections is a major cause of morbidity and mortality in patients with SLE. The increased risk of infections is, however, most probably related to potent immunosuppression. The pathogenesis can be multifactorial and may include both specific and nonspecific antineutrophil antibodies and direct bone marrow suppression. G-CSF can be useful for treating the neutropenia, but it has been associated with worsening of the underlying lupus.

Felty syndrome is classically described as a triad of rheumatoid arthritis, splenomegaly and neutropenia. Patients have high levels of rheumatoid factor, immune complexes, hypergammaglobulinemia and antinuclear antibodies. Recurrent pyogenic infections contribute to a significant disease mortality. There are two main mechanisms of neutropenia, antibody- and cell-mediated, the latter due to a secondary expansion of cytotoxic T cells not dissimilar to that seen in large granular lymphocytic leukemia.[143,184] The treatment is that of the underlying disease. G-CSF is effective for the treatment of neutropenia, but should be used with caution as there is increased incidence of leukocytoclastic vasculitis at 6%.

Large granular lymphocytic (LGL) leukemia is a clonal proliferation of cytotoxic T lymphocytes, characterized by neutropenia, anemia and/or thrombocytopenia. It is generally an indolent disorder of the elderly, but has been described in all age groups, including children. Clinical presentation is often with recurrent infections, B symptoms or asymptomatic cytopenia. Splenomegaly is more common than hepatomegaly. Examination of blood films shows the large granular lymphocytes, but diagnosis is usually established by peripheral blood flow cytometry demonstrating the presence of proliferation of T cells with the characteristic immunophenotype of $CD3^+CD4^-CD8^+CD16^+CD57^+$. Clonality is demonstrated by polymerase chain reaction (PCR) for T-cell receptor gene rearrangement.[143]

One-third of patients with LGL leukemia have rheumatoid arthritis and there is association with other autoimmune disorders. Indications for treatment include severe chronic neutropenia, recurrent infections or transfusion-dependent anemia. Effective medications include low-dose methotrexate, ciclosporin, prednisolone and cyclophosphamide. Interestingly, although immunosuppression ameliorates the cytopenias, cytotoxic T lymphocytes continue to be present in the peripheral blood.

Nutritional deficiencies

Neutropenia can be caused by certain nutritional deficiencies or disorders.
- Vitamin B_{12} and folate deficiency cause anemia and pancytopenia, although isolated neutropenia is uncommon.
- Copper deficiency can present with isolated neutropenia, followed by anemia and occasionally pancytopenia.[185] It was first noted in the context of total parenteral nutrition prior to the introduction of trace element supplementation. Currently it is mainly seen in the context of protein-energy malnutrition.
- Anorexia nervosa is associated with leucopenia, neutropenia and anemia in various combinations. Gelatinous transformation of the bone marrow has been reported in severe cases.[186]

Chronic idiopathic neutropenia

The term chronic idiopathic neutropenia (CIN) encompasses an ill-defined group of heterogeneous disorders characterized by persistent unexplained neutropenia. Patients rarely have serious infections. Some cases of CIN appear to be acquired, and certainly a significant proportion of CIN reported in the literature (in particular, benign neutropenia of infancy) most likely were immune in nature. CIN is also often used to describe milder probably inherited cases of neutropenia.

Neutropenia associated with complement activation

The exposure of blood to artificial membranes used in medical procedures, including dialysis, cardiopulmonary bypass, apheresis and extracorporeal membrane oxygenation may result in activation of the classical complement pathway with generation of C3a and C5a.[187] This results in increased neutrophil aggregation and adherence to endothelial surfaces, especially in the lung, with transient neutropenia and occasional cardiopulmonary symptoms.

Investigation of neutropenia

A detailed history and a few investigations tend to identify most common causes of neutropenia. The presence of other system abnormalities often necessitates investigations for rare disorders. The initial FBC will dictate further investigations by documenting either isolated neutropenia or pancytopenia. In relatively well children only a FBC, film and antineutrophil antibody screen are required at the first consultation. The following schema may be helpful.

History
- Detailed evaluation of the infection history; including the type, severity and frequency and duration of each episode.
- Age of onset of neutropenia.
- History of recent infections, medication use.
- Family history of infections.
- Any documented normal counts in the past.

Examination
- Stigmata of chronic neutropenia, in particular gingivitis.
- Congenital abnormalities.
- Hepatosplenomegaly.

Investigations
- Document severe chronic neutropenia, ANC $< 0.5 \times 10^9$/L, ideally tested at least thrice within 3 months.
- Antineutrophil antibodies to exclude primary AIN.
- If there is periodicity of infections, especially mouth, consider FBC over 6 weeks, thrice weekly, to attempt to define a 21-day oscillation (cyclic neutropenia).
- If there is a history of severe infections consider: bone marrow aspirate, serum immunoglobulins, basic lymphocyte panel; maturation arrest at the promyelocyte stage.
- History and physical examination to exclude other system involvment: no metabolic abnormalities indicates Kostmann syndrome; fatty stools, failure to thrive, abnormal pancreatic function indicate Shwachman–Diamond syndrome; hypoglycemia, hepatomegaly and glucose 6-phosphate translocase defect indicate GSDIb.

Neutrophilia

Neutrophilia is defined as an increase in the absolute neutrophil count to a level greater than two standard deviations above the mean value for normal individuals. Neutrophilia is most often secondary to an appropriate stimulus and may occur by several mechanisms.
- Demargination: a shift of neutrophils from the marginating pool to the circulating pool, which usually takes a few minutes.

- Mobilization: a shift from the marrow storage pool to the circulation, which takes a few hours.
- Increased proliferation: a maximum response can take up to a week.
- Increased survival.

The etiologic classification of neutrophilia is shown in Table 14.13.[120,188]

Eosinophils

Structure

The eosinophil is recognized by characteristic intracytoplasmic granules, the secondary or specific granules, which appear bright red by light microscopy, due to their high affinity for eosin, a negatively charged dye. The mature eosinophil is slightly larger than the neutrophil, with a diameter of 12–17 μm, and the nucleus is characteristically bilobed. The specific granules contain the basic proteins (MBP, major basic protein; ECP, eosinophil cationic protein; EDN, eosinophil-derived neurotoxin; EPO, eosinophil peroxidase), which are potent cytotoxic proteins.

Function

The eosinophil contains a potent array of proinflammatory mediators with considerable potential to initiate and sustain an inflammatory response. Eosinophils are believed to have a pathologic or physiologic role in helminth infections, allergic inflammation and tissue repair.[189]

Normal range, eosinopenia and eosinophilia

The normal eosinophil count varies with age, time of the day, exercise status, and environmental stimuli, particularly allergen exposure. The normal count is taken as $< 0.4 \times 10^9$/L, although a range of $0.015–0.65 \times 10^9$/L has been suggested, based on a study in medical students. Division of eosinophil counts is arbitrary, but a mild eosinophilia is regarded as $< 1.5 \times 10^9$/L, a moderate elevation is $1.5–5.0 \times 10^9$/L, and severe eosinophilia is $> 5.0 \times 10^9$/L. Allergic diseases generally cause a mild to moderate eosinophilia, but infection with helminths can often result in very high eosinophil count.

Eosinopenia

The causes of isolated eosinopenia are limited. In a hospital-based study, when patients with abnormal white cell counts, hematologic disorders or requiring chemotherapy were excluded, isolated eosinopenia was uncommon at 0.1% and was associated with the use of corticosteroids or severe organic disease.[190]

Table 14.13 Etiologic classification of neutrophilia.

Physiologic neutrophilia
Mediated by epinephrine and other catecholamines; due to demargination
Associated with monocytosis and lymphocytosis
Acute physical stress, including vigorous exercise, convulsions, labor, surgery, anesthesia and blood loss
Acute emotional stimuli, like panic, rage
Acute hypoxia, acute hemorrhage

Glucocorticosteroids
Mechanism is via decreased egress into the tissues
Over prolonged periods it is associated with lymphopenia and monocytopenia

Infections
Neutrophilia occurs with most acute bacterial infections, localized or systemic. It is seen less predictably with other infections, when neutrophilia is probably due to tissue damage caused either by the organism or a toxin produced by it
Neutrophilia is common in Gram-positive infections, but in Gram-negative infections there may be an initial neutropenia caused by the endotoxin, followed by extreme neutrophilia due to the various cytokines, chemokines and complement components

Tissue damage (e.g., inflammation/infarction)
Burns, electric shock, trauma, surgery
Hepatic necrosis, pancreatitis, myocardial infarction, pulmonary embolism
Connective tissue disorders including rheumatoid arthritis, gout, vasculitis, antigen–antibody complexes, complement activation, Still disease
Most acute inflammatory reactions, such as colitis, dermatitis, drug sensitivity reactions, Sweet syndrome

Drugs
Epinephrine
Glucocorticosteroids
Lithium

Tumors
Large tumor burden or secretion of colony-stimulating factors

Endocrine and metabolic emergencies
Eclampsia, diabetic ketoacidosis, Cushing syndrome, thyrotoxic crisis

Inherited neutrophilias
Familial cold urticaria, presents with fever, urticaria, and a rash characterized histologically by a neutrophil infiltrate, occurring 7 hours after exposure
Leukocyte adhesion deficiencies

Hematologic disorders
Chronic hemolysis and bleeding
Sickle cell crisis
Asplenia

Myeloproliferative disorders
Clonal hematopoietic stem cell disorders characterized by proliferation in the bone marrow of one or more of the myeloid lineages
Proliferation is associated with relatively normal maturation that is effective, resulting in increased numbers of granulocytes and/or red cells and platelets

Acute bacterial or viral infections characteristically produce eosinopenia persisting for the duration of the fever, with the exception of scarlet fever where eosinophilia is common. This can be helpful in the differential diagnosis of rashes where drug-induced rashes are often associated with eosinophilia, but not viral exanthemas.[191]

Eosinophilia

The various causes of peripheral blood eosinophilia are summarized in Table 14.14.

Basophils

Structure, development and function

The normal mature basophil is $10{-}15\ \mu m$ in diameter, has a central nucleus with two to three lobes and characteristic granules, which are large, coarse, purplish-black, usually filling the cytoplasm and often obscuring the nucleus. The primary granules are formed early in the development and contain large amounts of histamine and heparin, features that are responsible for the affinity of the granules for basic dyes.[117] Both basophils are a key component of allergic inflammation polycythaemia vera, essential thromboytosis, chronic idiopathic myelofibrosis.

Basopenia and basophilia[193]

Basophils are so infrequent in normal blood that their reduction is not likely to be noticed on inspection of blood films. In theory basopenia can be detected by automated counters since their reference ranges for basophils are $0.02{-}0.12 \times 10^9/L$. However, in practice, automated basophil counts are not very accurate and the observation of basopenia has not been found to be of great diagnostic significance.

Basophilia is commonly associated with type I hypersensitivity reactions mediated by IgE, for example drug, food and inhalant hypersensitivity, and urticaria. The inflammatory disorders ulcerative colitis and juvenile rheumatoid arthritis show an increase in basophil count in contrast to most other inflammatory disorders. Important causes of significant basophilia are clonal disorders of hematopoiesis, including CML. Basophilia is almost always present in CML and at times it can represent 20–90% of all white cells.

Monocytes

Structure, development and function

The mononuclear phagocyte system is composed of bone marrow monoblasts and promonocytes, blood monocytes

Table 14.14 Causes of peripheral blood eosinophilia.

Allergic diseases

Atopic disorders: eczema and allergic asthma show a variable eosinophilia and are the commonest causes in general pediatric practice

Drug-induced eosinophilia: drugs commonly involved are semisynthetic penicillins, nonsteroidal antiinflammatory agents and tetracyclines

Infectious disease

Helminth parasites, including nematodes, trematodes, and cestodes. Outside the Western world, invasive parasitic infections are the commonest cause of eosinophilia. The degree of eosinophilia seen is related to the magnitude and extent of tissue invasion by the parasite, but lack of eosinophilia does not exclude helminth infection. Helminths commonly involved in developed countries include ascarids, hookworms, trichinosis, visceral larva migrans and strongyloidiasis

Protozoan parasites, including *Giardia lamblia* and *Entamoeba histolytica*, do not characteristically elicit blood eosinophilia, with the exception of *Dientamoeba fragilis* and *Isospora belli*

Immunologic

Primary immunodeficiency: hyper-IgE syndrome, IgA deficiency, Wiskott–Aldrich syndrome

Rejection of transplanted kidneys, lungs or liver is associated with blood and tissue eosinophilia

Pulmonary diseases

Sarcoidosis.

Pulmonary eosinophilias[192] are group of disorders characterized by lung shadows radiologically and blood eosinophilia

Gastrointestinal diseases

Eosinophilic gastroenteritis

Rheumatologic diseases

Occasionally, eosinophilia accompanies dermatomyositis, severe rheumatoid arthritis, progressive systemic sclerosis or Sjögren syndrome

Miscellaneous diseases

Adrenal insufficiency

Atheroembolic disease

Neoplastic disorders with secondary eosinophilia

T-cell lymphomas

Hodgkin lymphoma

Acute lymphoblastic leukemia/lymphoma

Mastocytosis

Nonhematologic malignant diseases including breast, renal, lung tumors; female genital tract neoplasms; vascular tumors

Neoplastic disorders in which eosinophilia is part of a clone

Chronic myeloid leukemia

Acute myeloid leukemia

Myelodysplastic syndromes

Other myeloproliferative disorders including both basophils and eosinophils PV, ET, and CIMF

Clonal proliferations

Eosinophilic leukemia

Hypereosinophilic syndrome

and tissue macrophages. Phylogenetically it is a primitive system with a wide range of functions. Important functions include antimicrobial activity, participation in the inflammatory response, antitumor activity, processing and presenting antigens to T and B cells in adaptive immunity, regulating function of other cells, and removal of dead, senescent, foreign, or altered cells and particles.

The monocytes in peripheral blood are 10–11 μm in diameter, with a variable shape. The nucleus is large, centrally placed, oval or indented, with delicate nuclear chromatin and inconspicuous nucleoli. The cytoplasm is abundant, gray or grayish blue in color, with fine azurophilic granules and small vacuoles

Monocytopenia and monocytosis[120,194]

The mean monocyte count in adults is 0.4×10^9/L. The counts are higher in neonates, with an average count of 1.0×10^9/L. Because the monocyte is involved in many pathophysiologic processes, a modest elevation can occur in many disparate conditions.

Monocytopenia

This is commonly seen as part of marrow failure, especially in aplastic anemia. Other important causes include glucocorticosteroids, HIV and autoimmune disease.

Monocytosis

The causes of monocytosis are summarized in Table 14.15.

References

1. Zasloff M. Antimicrobial peptides of multicellular organisms. *Nature* 2002; **415**: 389–95.
2. Medzhitov R, Janeway C. Innate immunity. *N Engl J Med* 2000; **343**: 338–44.
3. Yang D, Chertov O, Oppenheim JJ. Participation of mammalian defensins and cathelicidins in anti-microbial immunity: receptors and activities of human defensins and cathelicidin (LL–37). *J Leukoc Biol* 2001; **69**: 691–7.
4. Middleton J, Patterson AM, Gardner L, Schmutz C, Ashton BA. Leukocyte extravasation: chemokine transport and presentation by the endothelium. *Blood* 2002; **100**: 3853–60.
5. Bos JL, de Bruyn K, Enserink J *et al.* The role of Rap1 in integrin-mediated cell adhesion. *Biochem Soc Trans* 2003; **31**: 83–6.
6. Caron E. Cellular functions of the Rap1 GTP-binding protein: a pattern emerges. *J Cell Sci* 2003; **116**: 435–40.
7. Crowley CA, Curnutte JT, Rosin RE *et al.* An inherited abnormality of neutrophil adhesion. Its genetic transmission and its association with a missing protein. *N Engl J Med* 1980; **302**: 1163–8.
8. Harlan JM. Leukocyte adhesion deficiency syndrome: insights

Table 14.15 Causes of monocytosis.

Reactive

Collagen vascular disease
  Systemic lupus erythematosus
  Rheumatoid arthritis
  Myositis
  Systemic vasculitis
Gastrointestinal disease
  Ulcerative colitis
  Crohn disease
  Alcoholic liver disease
  Sprue
Infections
  Acute bacterial infections on occasion
  Subacute bacterial endocarditis, syphilis
  Viruses, typically cytomegalovirus and varicella zoster virus
Nonhematologic malignancies and lymphomas
Miscellaneous
  Postsplenectomy state
  Chronic neutropenia causes compensatory monocytosis
  Hemolytic anemia and idiopathic thrombocytopenia

Clonal hematologic disorders

Acute myeloid leukemia, M4 and M5
Chronic myelomonocytic leukemia
Juvenile myelomonocytic leukemia

into the molecular basis of leukocyte emigration. *Clin Immunol Immunopathol* 1993; **67**: S16–S24.

9. Todd RF III, Freyer DR. The CD11/CD18 leukocyte glycoprotein deficiency. *Hematol Oncol Clin North Am* 1988; **2**: 13–31.

10. Arnaout MA. Structure and function of the leukocyte adhesion molecules CD11/CD18. *Blood* 1990; **75**: 1037–50.

11. Fischer A, Lisowska-Grospierre B, Anderson DC, Springer TA. Leukocyte adhesion deficiency: molecular basis and functional consequences. *Immunodefic Rev* 1988; **1**: 39–54.

12. Etzioni A, Frydman M, Pollack S *et al.* Brief report: recurrent severe infections caused by a novel leukocyte adhesion deficiency. *N Engl J Med* 1992; **327**: 1789–92.

13. Kuijpers TW, Van Lier RA, Hamann D *et al.* Leukocyte adhesion deficiency type 1 (LAD-1)/variant. A novel immunodeficiency syndrome characterized by dysfunctional beta2 integrins. *J Clin Invest* 1997; **100**: 1725–33.

14. Kinashi T, Aker M, Sokolovsky-Eisenberg M *et al.* LAD-III, a leukocyte adhesion deficiency syndrome associated with defective Rap1 activation and impaired stabilization of integrin bonds. *Blood* 2004; **103**: 1033–6.

15. Buckley RH. The hyper-IgE syndrome. *Clin Rev Allergy Immunol* 2001; **20**: 139–54.

16. Grimbacher B, Holland SM, Puck JM. Hyper-IgE syndromes. *Immunol Rev* 2005; **203**: 244–50.

17. Grimbacher B, Schaffer AA, Holland SM *et al.* Genetic linkage of hyper-IgE syndrome to chromosome 4. *Am J Hum Genet* 1999; **65**: 735–44.

18. Ohga S, Nomura A, Ihara K *et al.* Cytokine imbalance in hyper-IgE syndrome: reduced expression of transforming growth factor beta and interferon gamma genes in circulating activated T cells. *Br J Haematol* 2003; **121**: 324–31.

19. Del PG, Tiri A, Maggi E *et al.* Defective in vitro production of gamma-interferon and tumor necrosis factor-alpha by circulating T cells from patients with the hyper-immunoglobulin E syndrome. *J Clin Invest* 1989; **84**: 1830–5.

20. Martinez AM, Montoya CJ, Rugeles MT, Franco JL, Patino PJ. Abnormal expression of CD54 in mixed reactions of mononuclear cells from hyper-IgE syndrome patients. *Mem Inst Oswaldo Cruz* 2004; **99**: 159–65.

21. Leung DY, Geha RS. Clinical and immunologic aspects of the hyperimmunoglobulin E syndrome. *Hematol Oncol Clin North Am* 1988; **2**: 81–100.

22. Geha RS, Leung DY. Hyper immunoglobulin E syndrome. *Immunodefic Rev* 1989; **1**: 155–72.

23. Merten DF, Buckley RH, Pratt PC, Effmann EL, Grossman H. Hyperimmunoglobulinemia E syndrome: radiographic observations. *Radiology* 1979; **132**: 71–8.

24. Donabedian H, Alling DW, Gallin JI. Levamisole is inferior to placebo in the hyperimmunoglobulin E recurrent-infection (Job's) syndrome. *N Engl J Med* 1982; **307**: 290–2.

25. Kimata H. High-dose intravenous gamma-globulin treatment for hyperimmunoglobulinemia E syndrome. *J Allergy Clin Immunol* 1995; **95**: 771–4.

26. Jeppson JD, Jaffe HS, Hill HR. Use of recombinant human interferon gamma to enhance neutrophil chemotactic responses in Job syndrome of hyperimmunoglobulinemia E and recurrent infections. *J Pediatr* 1991; **118**: 383–7.

27. Aihara Y, Mori M, Katakura S, Yokota S. Recombinant IFN-gamma treatment of a patient with hyperimmunoglobulin E syndrome triggered autoimmune thrombocytopenia. *J Interferon Cytokine Res* 1998; **18**: 561–3.

28. Van Dyke TE, Vaikuntam J. Neutrophil function and dysfunction in periodontal disease. *Curr Opin Periodontol* 1994; **2**: 19–27.

29. Genco RJ, Van Dyke TE, Levine MJ, Nelson RD, Wilson ME. 1985 Kreshover lecture. Molecular factors influencing neutrophil defects in periodontal disease. *J Dent Res* 1986; **65**: 1379–91.

30. Offenbacher S, Scott SS, Odle BM, Wilson-Burrows C, Van Dyke TE. Depressed leukotriene B4 chemotactic response of neutrophils from localized juvenile periodontitis patients. *J Periodontol* 1987; **58**: 602–6.

31. Shibata K, Warbington ML, Gordon BJ, Kurihara H, Van Dyke TE. Defective calcium influx factor activity in neutrophils from patients with localized juvenile periodontitis. *J Periodontol* 2000; **71**: 797–802.

32. Shapira L, Champagne C, Van Dyke TE, Amar S. Strain-dependent activation of monocytes and inflammatory macrophages by lipopolysaccharide of *Porphyromonas gingivalis. Infect Immun* 1998; **66**: 2736–42.

33. Snapper SB, Rosen FS. The Wiskott–Aldrich syndrome protein (WASP): roles in signaling and cytoskeletal organization. *Annu Rev Immunol* 1999; **17**: 905–29.

34. Aspenstrom P, Lindberg U, Hall A. Two GTPases, Cdc42 and Rac, bind directly to a protein implicated in the

immunodeficiency disorder Wiskott–Aldrich syndrome. *Curr Biol* 1996; **6**: 70–5.

35. Thrasher AJ. Wasp in immune-system organization and function. *Nat Rev Immunol* 2002; **2**: 635–46.

36. Zicha D, Allen WE, Brickell PM *et al.* Chemotaxis of macrophages is abolished in the Wiskott–Aldrich syndrome. *Br J Haematol* 1998; **101**: 659–65.

37. Lorenzi R, Brickell PM, Katz DR, Kinnon C, Thrasher AJ. Wiskott–Aldrich syndrome protein is necessary for efficient IgG-mediated phagocytosis. *Blood* 2000; **95**: 2943–6.

38. Corash L, Shafer B, Blaese RM. Platelet-associated immunoglobulin, platelet size, and the effect of splenectomy in the Wiskott–Aldrich syndrome. *Blood* 1985; **65**: 1439–43.

39. Mullen CA, Anderson KD, Blaese RM. Splenectomy and/or bone marrow transplantation in the management of the Wiskott–Aldrich syndrome: long-term follow-up of 62 cases. *Blood* 1993; **82**: 2961–6.

40. Filipovich AH, Stone JV, Tomany SC *et al.* Impact of donor type on outcome of bone marrow transplantation for Wiskott–Aldrich syndrome: collaborative study of the International Bone Marrow Transplant Registry and the National Marrow Donor Program. *Blood* 2001; **97**: 1598–603.

41. Strom TS, Turner SJ, Andreansky S *et al.* Defects in T-cell-mediated immunity to influenza virus in murine Wiskott–Aldrich syndrome are corrected by oncoretroviral vector-mediated gene transfer into repopulating hematopoietic cells. *Blood* 2003; **102**: 3108–16.

42. Klein C, Nguyen D, Liu CH *et al.* Gene therapy for Wiskott–Aldrich syndrome: rescue of T-cell signaling and amelioration of colitis upon transplantation of retrovirally transduced hematopoietic stem cells in mice. *Blood* 2003; **101**: 2159–66.

43. Roberts AW, Kim C, Zhen L *et al.* Deficiency of the hematopoietic cell-specific Rho family GTPase Rac2 is characterized by abnormalities in neutrophil function and host defense. *Immunity* 1999; **10**: 183–96.

44. Ambruso DR, Knall C, Abell AN *et al.* Human neutrophil immunodeficiency syndrome is associated with an inhibitory Rac2 mutation. *Proc Natl Acad Sci USA* 2000; **97**: 4654–9.

45. Kowanko IC, Ferrante A, Maxwell GM. Effects of neutrophil migration inhibitory factors on neonatal neutrophils. *Pediatr Res* 1987; **21**: 377–80.

46. Hirata F, Schiffmann E, Venkatasubramanian K, Salomon D, Axelrod J. A phospholipase A2 inhibitory protein in rabbit neutrophils induced by glucocorticoids. *Proc Natl Acad Sci USA* 1980; **77**: 2533–6.

47. Oseas RS, Allen J, Yang HH, Baehner RL, Boxer LA. Mechanism of dexamethasone inhibition of chemotactic factor induced granulocyte aggregation. *Blood* 1982; **59**: 265–9.

48. Boxer LA, Ingraham LM, Allen J, Oseas RS, Baehner RL. Amphotericin-B promotes leukocyte aggregation of nylon-wool-fiber-treated polymorphonuclear leukocytes. *Blood* 1981; **58**: 518–23.

49. Tate RM, Repine JE. Neutrophils and the adult respiratory distress syndrome. *Am Rev Respir Dis* 1983; **128**: 552–9.

50. Martin S, Baldock SC, Ghoneim AT, Child JA. Defective neutrophil function and microbicidal mechanisms in the myelodysplastic disorders. *J Clin Pathol* 1983; **36**: 1120–8.

51. Clark RA, Johnson FL, Klebanoff SJ, Thomas ED. Defective neutrophil chemotaxis in bone marrow transplant patients. *J Clin Invest* 1976; **58**: 22–31.

52. Andersen B, Goldsmith GH, Spagnuolo PJ. Neutrophil adhesive dysfunction in diabetes mellitus; the role of cellular and plasma factors. *J Lab Clin Med* 1988; **111**: 275–85.

53. Bogomolski-Yahalom V, Matzner Y. Disorders of neutrophil function. *Blood Rev* 1995; **9**: 183–90.

54. Dahl M, Hakansson L, Kreuger A, Olsen L, Nilsson U, Venge P. Polymorphonuclear neutrophil function and infections following splenectomy in childhood. *Scand J Haematol* 1986; **37**: 137–43.

55. Brown CC, Gallin JI. Chemotactic disorders. *Hematol Oncol Clin North Am* 1988; **2**: 61–79.

56. Ruddy S. Rheumatic diseases and inherited complement deficiencies. *Bull Rheum Dis* 1996; **45**: 6–8.

57. Super M, Thiel S, Lu J, Levinsky RJ, Turner MW. Association of low levels of mannan-binding protein with a common defect of opsonisation. *Lancet* 1989; **ii**: 1236–9.

58. Summerfield JA, Ryder S, Sumiya M *et al.* Mannose binding protein gene mutations associated with unusual and severe infections in adults. *Lancet* 1995; **345**: 886–9.

59. Fromont P, Bettaieb A, Skouri H *et al.* Frequency of the polymorphonuclear neutrophil Fc gamma receptor III deficiency in the French population and its involvement in the development of neonatal alloimmune neutropenia. *Blood* 1992; **79**: 2131–4.

60. De HM, Kleijer M, van ZR, Roos D, von dem Borne AE. Neutrophil Fc gamma RIIIb deficiency, nature, and clinical consequences: a study of 21 individuals from 14 families. *Blood* 1995; **86**: 2403–13.

61. van de Winkel JG, Capel PJ. Human IgG Fc receptor heterogeneity: molecular aspects and clinical implications. *Immunol Today* 1993; **14**: 215–21.

62. Barbosa MD, Nguyen QA, Tchernev VT *et al.* Identification of the homologous beige and Chediak–Higashi syndrome genes. *Nature* 1996; **382**: 262–5.

63. Tchernev VT, Mansfield TA, Giot L *et al.* The Chediak–Higashi protein interacts with SNARE complex and signal transduction proteins. *Mol Med* 2002; **8**: 56–64.

64. Ganz T, Metcalf JA, Gallin JI, Boxer LA, Lehrer RI. Microbicidal/cytotoxic proteins of neutrophils are deficient in two disorders: Chediak–Higashi syndrome and "specific" granule deficiency. *J Clin Invest* 1988; **82**: 552–6.

65. Huynh C, Roth D, Ward DM, Kaplan J, Andrews NW. Defective lysosomal exocytosis and plasma membrane repair in Chediak–Higashi/beige cells. *Proc Natl Acad Sci USA* 2004; **101**: 16795–800.

66. Klein M, Roder J, Haliotis T *et al.* Chediak–Higashi gene in humans. II. The selectivity of the defect in natural-killer and antibody-dependent cell-mediated cytotoxicity function. *J Exp Med* 1980; **151**: 1049–58.

67. Bell TG, Meyers KM, Prieur DJ, Fauci AS, Wolff SM, Padgett GA. Decreased nucleotide and serotonin storage associated with defective function in Chediak–Higashi syndrome cattle and human platelets. *Blood* 1976; **48**: 175–84.

68. Okano M, Gross TG. A review of Epstein–Barr virus infection in patients with immunodeficiency disorders. *Am J Med Sci* 2000; **319**: 392–6.

69. Kinugawa N. Epstein–Barr virus infection in Chediak–Higashi syndrome mimicking acute lymphocytic leukemia. *Am J Pediatr Hematol Oncol* 1990; **12**: 182–6.

70. Merino F, Henle W, Ramirez-Duque P. Chronic active Epstein–Barr virus infection in patients with Chediak–Higashi syndrome. *J Clin Immunol* 1986; **6**: 299–305.

71. Weening RS, Schoorel EP, Roos D *et al.* Effect of ascorbate on abnormal neutrophil, platelet and lymphocytic function in a patient with the Chediak–Higashi syndrome. *Blood* 1981; **57**: 856–65.

72. Nair MP, Gray RH, Boxer LA, Schwartz SA. Deficiency of inducible suppressor cell activity in the Chediak–Higashi syndrome. *Am J Hematol* 1987; **26**: 55–66.

73. Fischer A, Griscelli C, Friedrich W *et al.* Bone-marrow transplantation for immunodeficiencies and osteopetrosis: European survey, 1968–1985. *Lancet* 1986; **ii**: 1080–4.

74. Lomax KJ, Malech HL, Gallin JI. The molecular biology of selected phagocyte defects. *Blood Rev* 1989; **3**: 94–104.

75. Gombart AF, Koeffler HP. Neutrophil specific granule deficiency and mutations in the gene encoding transcription factor C/EBP(epsilon). *Curr Opin Hematol* 2002; **9**: 36–42.

76. Gallin JI. Neutrophil specific granule deficiency. *Annu Rev Med* 1985; **36**: 263–74.

77. Suda T, Onai T, Maekawa T. Studies on abnormal polymorphonuclear neutrophils in acute myelogenous leukemia: clinical significance and changes after chemotherapy. *Am J Hematol* 1983; **15**: 45–56.

78. Wentworth P Jr, McDunn JE, Wentworth AD *et al.* Evidence for antibody-catalyzed ozone formation in bacterial killing and inflammation. *Science* 2002; **298**: 2195–9.

79. Sato TK, Overduin M, Emr SD. Location, location, location: membrane targeting directed by PX domains. *Science* 2001; **294**: 1881–5.

80. Zhan Y, Virbasius JV, Song X, Pomerleau DP, Zhou GW. The p40phox and p47phox PX domains of NADPH oxidase target cell membranes via direct and indirect recruitment by phosphoinositides. *J Biol Chem* 2002; **277**: 4512–18.

81. Ago T, Takeya R, Hiroaki H *et al.* The PX domain as a novel phosphoinositide-binding module. *Biochem Biophys Res Commun* 2001; **287**: 733–8.

82. Yamamori T, Inanami O, Nagahata H, Kuwabara M. Phosphoinositide 3-kinase regulates the phosphorylation of NADPH oxidase component p47(phox) by controlling cPKC/PKCdelta but not Akt. *Biochem Biophys Res Commun* 2004; **316**: 720–30.

83. Weiss SJ, Test ST, Eckmann CM, Roos D, Regiani S. Brominating oxidants generated by human eosinophils. *Science* 1986; **234**: 200–3.

84. Arlandson M, Decker T, Roongta VA *et al.* Eosinophil peroxidase oxidation of thiocyanate. Characterization of major reaction products and a potential sulfhydryl-targeted cytotoxicity system. *J Biol Chem* 2001; **276**: 215–24.

85. Dinauer MC, Nauseef WM and Newburger PE. Inherited Disorders of Phagocyte Killing. In: Scriver CR, Beaudet AL, Sly WS *et al.* (eds) *The Metabolic Basis of Inherited Disease* 2001; 4857–4863.

86. Winkelstein JA, Marino MC, Johnston RB Jr *et al.* Chronic granulomatous disease. Report on a national registry of 368 patients. *Medicine (Baltimore)* 2000; **79**: 155–69.

87. Isaacs D, Wright VM, Shaw DG, Raafat F, Walker-Smith JA. Chronic granulomatous disease mimicking Crohn's disease. *J Pediatr Gastroenterol Nutr* 1985; **4**: 498–501.

88. Southwick FS, van der Meer JW. Recurrent cystitis and bladder mass in two adults with chronic granulomatous disease. *Ann Intern Med* 1988; **109**: 118–21.

89. Gallin JI. *Disorders of Phagocytic Cells. Inflammation: Basic Principles and Clinical Correlates*, 2nd edn. New York: Raven Press, 1992.

90. Cale CM, Jones AM, Goldblatt D. Follow up of patients with chronic granulomatous disease diagnosed since 1990. *Clin Exp Immunol* 2000; **120**: 351–5.

91. Margolis DM, Melnick DA, Alling DW, Gallin JI. Trimethoprim-sulfamethoxazole prophylaxis in the management of chronic granulomatous disease. *J Infect Dis* 1990; **162**: 723–6.

92. Gallin JI, Alling DW, Malech HL *et al.* Itraconazole to prevent fungal infections in chronic granulomatous disease. *N Engl J Med* 2003; **348**: 2416–22.

93. Liles WC, Huang JE, Llewellyn C, SenGupta D, Price TH, Dale DC. A comparative trial of granulocyte-colony-stimulating factor and dexamethasone, separately and in combination, for the mobilization of neutrophils in the peripheral blood of normal volunteers. *Transfusion* 1997; **37**: 182–7.

94. Marciano BE, Wesley R, De Carlo ES *et al.* Long-term interferon-gamma therapy for patients with chronic granulomatous disease. *Clin Infect Dis* 2004; **39**: 692–9.

95. Ezekowitz RA, Dinauer MC, Jaffe HS, Orkin SH, Newburger PE. Partial correction of the phagocyte defect in patients with X-linked chronic granulomatous disease by subcutaneous interferon gamma. *N Engl J Med* 1988; **319**: 146–51.

96. Woodman RC, Erickson RW, Rae J, Jaffe HS, Curnutte JT. Prolonged recombinant interferon-gamma therapy in chronic granulomatous disease: evidence against enhanced neutrophil oxidase activity. *Blood* 1992; **79**: 1558–62.

97. Chin TW, Stiehm ER, Falloon J, Gallin JI. Corticosteroids in treatment of obstructive lesions of chronic granulomatous disease. *J Pediatr* 1987; **111**: 349–52.

98. Horwitz ME, Barrett AJ, Brown MR *et al.* Treatment of chronic granulomatous disease with nonmyeloablative conditioning and a T-cell-depleted hematopoietic allograft. *N Engl J Med* 2001; **344**: 881–8.

99. Malech HL, Choi U, Brenner S. Progress toward effective gene therapy for chronic granulomatous disease. *Jpn J Infect Dis* 2004; **57**: S27–S28.

100. Gray GR, Stamatoyannopoulos G, Naiman SC *et al.* Neutrophil dysfunction, chronic granulomatous disease, and non-spherocytic haemolytic anaemia caused by complete deficiency of glucose-6-phosphate dehydrogenase. *Lancet* 1973; **ii**: 530–4.

101. Parry MF, Root RK, Metcalf JA, Delaney KK, Kaplow LS, Richar WJ. Myeloperoxidase deficiency: prevalence and clinical significance. *Ann Intern Med* 1981; **95**: 293–301.

102. dix-Hansen K. Myeloperoxidase-deficient polymorphonuclear leucocytes (VII): incidence in untreated myeloproliferative disorders. *Scand J Haematol* 1986; **36**: 8–10.

103. dix-Hansen K, Kerndrup G, Pedersen B. Myeloperoxidase-deficient polymorphonuclear leucocytes (VI): Relation to cytogenetic abnormalities in primary myelodysplastic syndromes. *Scand J Haematol* 1986; **36**: 3–7.

104. dix-Hansen K, Kerndrup G. Myeloperoxidase-deficient polymorphonuclear leucocytes (V): relation to FAB-classification and neutrophil alkaline phosphatase activity in primary myelodysplastic syndromes. *Scand J Haematol* 1985; **35**: 197–200.

105. Nauseef WM. Myeloperoxidase deficiency. *Hematol Pathol* 1990; **4**: 165–78.

106. Kitahara M, Simonian Y, Eyre HJ. Neutrophil myeloperoxidase: a simple, reproducible technique to determine activity. *J Lab Clin Med* 1979, **93**: 232–7.

107. Spielberg SP, Boxer LA, Oliver JM, Allen JM, Schulman JD. Oxidative damage to neutrophils in glutathione synthetase deficiency. *Br J Haematol* 1979; **42**: 215–23.

108. Boxer LA, Oliver JM, Spielberg SP, Allen JM, Schulman JD. Protection of granulocytes by vitamin E in glutathione synthetase deficiency. *N Engl J Med* 1979; **301**: 901–5.

109. Loos H, Roos D, Weening R, Houwerzijl J. Familial deficiency of glutathione reductase in human blood cells. *Blood* 1976; **48**: 53–62.

110. Roos D, Weening RS, Voetman AA *et al.* Protection of phagocytic leukocytes by endogenous glutathione: studies in a family with glutathione reductase deficiency. *Blood* 1979; **53**: 851–66.

111. Baker SS, Cohen HJ. Altered oxidative metabolism in selenium-deficient rat granulocytes. *J Immunol* 1983; **130**: 2856–60.

112. Holmes B, Park BH, Malawista SE, Quie PG, Nelson DL, Good RA. Chronic granulomatous disease in females. *N Engl J Med* 1970; **283**: 217–21.

113. Matsuda I, Oka Y, Taniguchi N *et al.* Leukocyte glutathione peroxidase deficiency in a male patient with chronic granulomatous disease. *J Pediatr* 1976; **88**: 581–3.

114. Whitin JC, Cohen HJ. Disorders of respiratory burst termination. *Hematol Oncol Clin North Am* 1988; **2**: 289–99.

115. Roos D, Weening RS, Wyss SR, Aebi HE. Protection of human neutrophils by endogenous catalase: studies with cells from catalase-deficient individuals. *J Clin Invest* 1980; **65**: 1515–22.

116. Metcalfe JA, Gallin JI, Nauseef WM *et al. Laboratory Manual of Neutrophil Function.* New York: Raven Press, 1986.

117. Skubitz KM, Greer JP, Foerster J, Lukens JN (eds). Neutrophilic leucocytes. In: *Wintrobe's Clinical Hematology*, 11th edn. Lippincott Williams & Wilkins, Philadelphia 2004; 267–310.

118. Babior BM, Golde DW, Beutler E, Lichtman MA, Coller BS (eds). Production, distribution, and fate of neutrophils. In: *Williams' Hematology*, 6th edn. McGraw-Hill Medical Publishing, New York 2001; 753–760.

119. Dallman PR. Reference ranges for leukocyte counts in children. In: Nathan DG, Orkin SH, Ginsburg D and Look AT (eds) *Nathan and Oski's Hematology of Infancy and Childhood*, 6th edn. Philadelphia: WB Saunders 2003; 1848.

120. Bain BJ. *Blood Cells: A Practical Guide*, 3rd edn. Oxford: Blackwell Science, 2002.

121. Lugada ES, Mermin J, Kaharuza F *et al.* Population-based hematologic and immunologic reference values for a healthy Ugandan population. *Clin Diagn Lab Immunol* 2004; **11**: 29–34.

122. Sadowitz PD, Oski FA. Differences in polymorphonuclear cell counts between healthy white and black infants: response to meningitis. *Pediatrics* 1983; **72**: 405–7.

123. Dale DC. Introduction: severe chronic neutropenia. *Semin Hematol* 2002; **39**: 73–4.

124. Boxer L, Dale DC. Neutropenia: causes and consequences. *Semin Hematol* 2002; **39**: 75–81.

125. Nagata S, Tsuchiya M, Asano S *et al.* Molecular cloning and expression of cDNA for human granulocyte colony-stimulating factor. *Nature* 1986; **319**: 415–18.

126. Souza LM, Boone TC, Gabrilove J *et al.* Recombinant human granulocyte colony-stimulating factor: effects on normal and leukemic myeloid cells. *Science* 1986; **232**: 61–5.

127. Dale DC, Bonilla MA, Davis MW *et al.* A randomized controlled phase III trial of recombinant human granulocyte colony-stimulating factor (filgrastim) for treatment of severe chronic neutropenia. *Blood* 1993; **81**: 2496–502.

128. Bonilla MA, Gillio AP, Ruggeiro M *et al.* Effects of recombinant human granulocyte colony-stimulating factor on neutropenia in patients with congenital agranulocytosis. *N Engl J Med* 1989; **320**: 1574–80.

129. Kostmann R. Infantile genetic agranulocytosis. *Acta Paediatr* 1956; **45** (suppl. 105): 1–78.

130. Dale DC, Person RE, Bolyard AA *et al.* Mutations in the gene encoding neutrophil elastase in congenital and cyclic neutropenia. *Blood* 2000; **96**: 2317–22.

131. Ancliff PJ, Gale RE, Liesner R, Hann IM, Linch DC. Mutations in the ELA2 gene encoding neutrophil elastase are present in most patients with sporadic severe congenital neutropenia but only in some patients with the familial form of the disease. *Blood* 2001; **98**: 2645–50.

132. Zeidler C, Welte K. Kostmann syndrome and severe congenital neutropenia. *Semin Hematol* 2002; **39**: 82–8.

133. Dale DC, Cottle TE, Fier CJ *et al.* Severe chronic neutropenia: treatment and follow-up of patients in the Severe Chronic Neutropenia International Registry. *Am J Hematol* 2003; **72**: 82–93.

134. Cottle TE, Fier CJ, Donadieu J, Kinsey SE. Risk and benefit of treatment of severe chronic neutropenia with granulocyte colony-stimulating factor. *Semin Hematol* 2002; **39**: 134–40.

135. Freedman MH, Alter BP. Risk of myelodysplastic syndrome and acute myeloid leukemia in congenital neutropenias. *Semin Hematol* 2002; **39**: 128–33.

136. Freedman MH, Bonilla MA, Fier C *et al.* Myelodysplasia syndrome and acute myeloid leukemia in patients with congenital neutropenia receiving G-CSF therapy. *Blood* 2000; **96**: 429–36.

137. Dale DC, Bolyard AA, Aprikyan A. Cyclic neutropenia. *Semin Hematol* 2002; **39**: 89–94.

138. Wright DG, Dale DC, Fauci AS, Wolff SM. Human cyclic neutropenia: clinical review and long-term follow-up of patients. *Medicine (Baltimore)* 1981; **60**: 1–13.

139. Palmer SE, Stephens K, Dale DC. Genetics, phenotype, and natural history of autosomal dominant cyclic hematopoiesis. *Am J Med Genet* 1996; **66**: 413–22.

140. Horwitz M, Benson KF, Person RE, Aprikyan AG, Dale DC. Mutations in ELA2, encoding neutrophil elastase, define a 21-

day biological clock in cyclic haematopoiesis. *Nat Genet* 1999; **23**: 433–6.

141. Ancliff PJ, Gale RE, Watts MJ *et al*. Paternal mosaicism proves the pathogenic nature of mutations in neutrophil elastase in severe congenital neutropenia. *Blood* 2002; **100**: 707–9.

142. Ancliff PJ. Congenital neutropenia. *Blood Rev* 2003; **17**: 209–16.

143. Berliner N, Horwitz M, Loughran TP Jr. Congenital and acquired neutropenia. *Hematology* (*Am Soc Hematol Educ Program*) 2004; 63–79.

144. Bellanne-Chantelot C, Clauin S, Leblanc T *et al*. Mutations in the ELA2 gene correlate with more severe expression of neutropenia: a study of 81 patients from the French Neutropenia Register. *Blood* 2004; **103**: 4119–25.

145. Smith OP. Shwachman–Diamond syndrome. *Semin Hematol* 2002; **39**: 95–102.

146. Boocock GR, Morrison JA, Popovic M *et al*. Mutations in SBDS are associated with Shwachman–Diamond syndrome. *Nat Genet* 2003; **33**: 97–101.

147. Dror Y, Freedman MH. Shwachman–Diamond syndrome marrow cells show abnormally increased apoptosis mediated through the Fas pathway. *Blood* 2001; **97**: 3011–6.

148. Dror Y, Durie P, Ginzberg H *et al*. Clonal evolution in marrows of patients with Shwachman–Diamond syndrome: a prospective 5-year follow-up study. *Exp Hematol* 2002; **30**: 659–69.

149. Rotig A, Cormier V, Blanche S *et al*. Pearson's marrow-pancreas syndrome. A multisystem mitochondrial disorder in infancy. *J Clin Invest* 1990; **86**: 1601–8.

150. Pearson HA, Lobel JS, Kocoshis SA *et al*. A new syndrome of refractory sideroblastic anemia with vacuolization of marrow precursors and exocrine pancreatic dysfunction. *J Pediatr* 1979; **95**: 976–84.

151. Barth PG, Scholte HR, Berden JA *et al*. An X-linked mitochondrial disease affecting cardiac muscle, skeletal muscle and neutrophil leucocytes. *J Neurol Sci* 1983; **62**: 327–55.

152. Bione S, D'Adamo P, Maestrini E, Gedeon AK, Bolhuis PA, Toniolo D. A novel X-linked gene, G4.5 is responsible for Barth syndrome. *Nat Genet* 1996; **12**: 385–9.

153. Kannourakis G. Glycogen storage disease. *Semin Hematol* 2002; **39**: 103–6.

154. Visser G, Rake JP, Labrune P *et al*. Granulocyte colony-stimulating factor in glycogen storage disease type 1b. Results of the European Study on Glycogen Storage Disease Type 1. *Eur J Pediatr* 2002; **161** (suppl. 1): S83–S87.

155. Pinsk M, Burzynski J, Yhap M, Fraser RB, Cummings B, Ste-Marie M. Acute myelogenous leukemia and glycogen storage disease 1b. *J Pediatr Hematol Oncol* 2002; **24**: 756–8.

156. Cham B, Bonilla MA, Winkelstein J. Neutropenia associated with primary immunodeficiency syndromes. *Semin Hematol* 2002; **39**: 107–12.

157. Ridanpaa M, van Eenennaam H, Pelin K *et al*. Mutations in the RNA component of RNase MRP cause a pleiotropic human disease, cartilage-hair hypoplasia. *Cell* 2001; **104**: 195–203.

158. Diaz GA. CXCR4 mutations in WHIM syndrome: a misguided immune system? *Immunol Rev* 2005; **203**: 235–43.

159. Hernandez PA, Gorlin RJ, Lukens JN *et al*. Mutations in the chemokine receptor gene CXCR4 are associated with WHIM syndrome, a combined immunodeficiency disease. *Nat Genet* 2003; **34**: 70–4.

160. Dinauer MC. The phagocyte system and disorders of granulopoiesis and granulocyte function. In: Nathan DG, Orkin SH, Ginsburg D and Look AT (eds) *Nathan and Oski's Hematology of Infancy and Childhood*, 6th edn. Elsevier Science, 2003; 923–1010.

161. Marwaha N, Sarode R, Gupta RK, Garewal G, Dash S. Clinico-hematological characteristics in patients with kala azar. A study from north-west India. *Trop Geogr Med* 1991; **43**: 357–62.

162. Kaufman DW, Kelly JP, Jurgelon JM *et al*. Drugs in the aetiology of agranulocytosis and aplastic anaemia. *Eur J Haematol Suppl* 1996; **60**: 23–30.

163. Andres E, Kurtz JE, Maloisel F. Nonchemotherapy drug-induced agranulocytosis: experience of the Strasbourg teaching hospital (1985–2000) and review of the literature. *Clin Lab Haematol* 2002; **24**: 99–106.

164. Salama A, Schutz B, Kiefel V, Breithaupt H, Mueller-Eckhardt C. Immune-mediated agranulocytosis related to drugs and their metabolites: mode of sensitization and heterogeneity of antibodies. *Br J Haematol* 1989; **72**: 127–32.

165. Pichler WJ. Drug-induced autoimmunity. *Curr Opin Allergy Clin Immunol* 2003; **3**: 249–53.

166. Acharya S, Bussel JB. Hematologic toxicity of sodium valproate. *J Pediatr Hematol Oncol* 2000; **22**: 62–5.

167. Watts RG, Emanuel PD, Zuckerman KS, Howard TH. Valproic acid-induced cytopenias: evidence for a dose-related suppression of hematopoiesis. *J Pediatr* 1990; **117**: 495–9.

168. Sprikkelman A, de Wolf JT, Vellenga E. The application of hematopoietic growth factors in drug-induced agranulocytosis: a review of 70 cases. *Leukemia* 1994; **8**: 2031–6.

169. Stroncek D. Granulocyte antigens and antibody detection. *Vox Sang* 2004; **87** (suppl. 1): 91–4.

170. Nomenclature of granulocyte alloantigens. Short Report. ISBT Working Party on Platelet and Granulocyte Serology, Granulocyte Antigen Working Party. *Vox Sang* 1999; **77**: 251.

171. Lucas GF, Metcalfe P. Platelet and granulocyte glycoprotein polymorphisms. *Transfus Med* 2000; **10**: 157–74.

172. Stroncek DF, Caruccio L, Bettinotti M. CD177: A member of the Ly-6 gene superfamily involved with neutrophil proliferation and polycythemia vera. *J Transf Med* 2004; **2**: 8.

173. Bux J, Chapman J. Report on the second international granulocyte serology workshop. *Transfusion* 1997; **37**: 977–83.

174. Lalezari P, Nussbaum M, Gelman S, Spaet TH. Neonatal neutropenia due to maternal isoimmunization. *Blood* 1960; **15**: 236–43.

175. Bux J, Jung KD, Kauth T, Mueller-Eckhardt C. Serological and clinical aspects of granulocyte antibodies leading to alloimmune neonatal neutropenia. *Transfus Med* 1992; **2**: 143–9.

176. Gilmore MM, Stroncek DF, Korones DN. Treatment of alloimmune neonatal neutropenia with granulocyte colony-stimulating factor. *J Pediatr* 1994; **125**: 948–51.

177. Zupanska B, Uhrynowska M, Guz K *et al*. The risk of antibody formation against HNA1a and HNA1b granulocyte antigens during pregnancy and its relation to neonatal neutropenia. *Transfus Med* 2001; **11**: 377–82.

178. Bux J, Jung KD, Kauth T, Mueller-Eckhardt C. Serological and clinical aspects of granulocyte antibodies leading to alloimmune neonatal neutropenia. *Transfus Med* 1992; **2**: 143–9.

179. Verheugt FW, van Noord-Bokhorst JC, von dem Borne AE, Engelfriet CP. A family with allo-immune neonatal neutropenia: group-specific pathogenicity of maternal antibodies. *Vox Sang* 1979; **36**: 1–8.

180. Bux J, Behrens G, Jaeger G, Welte K. Diagnosis and clinical course of autoimmune neutropenia in infancy: analysis of 240 cases. *Blood* 1998; **91**: 181–6.

181. Bruin MC, von dem Borne AE, Tamminga RY, Kleijer M, Buddelmeijer L, De HM. Neutrophil antibody specificity in different types of childhood autoimmune neutropenia. *Blood* 1999; **94**: 1797–802.

182. Bruin M, Dassen A, Pajkrt D, Buddelmeyer L, Kuijpers T, De HM. Primary autoimmune neutropenia in children: a study of neutrophil antibodies and clinical course. *Vox Sang* 2005; **88**: 52–9.

183. Mathew P, Chen G, Wang W. Evans syndrome: results of a national survey. *J Pediatr Hematol Oncol* 1997; **19**: 433–7.

184. Starkebaum G. Chronic neutropenia associated with autoimmune disease. *Semin Hematol* 2002; **39**: 121–7.

185. Uauy R, Olivares M, Gonzalez M. Essentiality of copper in humans. *Am J Clin Nutr* 1998; **67** (5 suppl.): 952S–959S.

186. Devuyst O, Lambert M, Rodhain J, Lefebvre C, Coche E. Haematological changes and infectious complications in anorexia nervosa: a case-control study. *Q J Med* 1993; **86**: 791–9.

187. Watts RG. Neutropenia. In: *Wintrobe's Clinical Hematology*, 11th edn. Lippincott Williams & Wilkins, Philadelphia 2004; 1777–1800.

188. Dale DC. Neutropenia and neutrophilia. In: *Williams' Hematology*, 6th edn. McGraw-Hill Medical Publishing, New York 2001; 823–834.

189. Munitz A, Levi-Schaffer F. Eosinophils: "new" roles for "old" cells. *Allergy* 2004; **59**: 268–75.

190. Krause JR, Boggs DR. Search for eosinopenia in hospitalized patients with normal blood leukocyte concentration. *Am J Hematol* 1987; **24**: 55–63.

191. Kranke B, Richtig E, Aberer W. Exanthema with eosinopenia. *Allergy* 2002; **57**: 57–8.

192. Leitch AG. Pulmonary eosinophilias. In: *Crofton and Douglas's Respiratory Diseases*, 5th edn. Oxford: Blackwell Publishing, 2000.

193. Galli SJ, Metcalfe DD, Dvorak AM. Basophils and mast cells and their disorders. In: *Williams' Hematology*, 6th edn. McGraw-Hill Medical Publishing, 2001; 801–816.

194. Lichtman MA. Monocytosis and monocytopenia. In: *Williams' Hematology*, 6th edn. McGraw-Hill Medical Publishing, 2001; 881–886.

15 Histiocytic disorders

Amir H. Shahlaee and Robert J. Arceci

Introduction

The histiocytoses are a diverse group of hematologic disorders defined by the pathologic infiltration of normal tissues by cells of the mononuclear phagocyte system (MPS). The heterogeneity of this family of disorders, a direct result of the biologic variability of the cells of the MPS and the tissues they inhabit, makes the study of these diseases one of the most intriguing yet complex areas of modern hematology.

Advances in basic hematology and immunology over the last two decades have significantly enhanced our understanding of the histiocytic disorders. It is now accepted that the pathogenic cells central to the development of the histiocytoses arise from a common hematopoietic progenitor. More specifically, the ability to molecularly identify the hematopoietic cells has enabled us to classify the histiocytoses based on the cellular basis of the disease and to define the natural history of these disorders.[1,2] These pathologic cells phenotypically resemble immature mononuclear phagocytes at specific stages of differentiation.[77]

The Histiocyte Society, formed in 1985, has served as a forum for enhanced collaboration between international histiocytosis experts. Since its inception, the Histiocyte Society has used the cellular based classification of the histiocytoses as a guideline for therapeutic studies, which have in turn significantly advanced our ability to care for patients, improve their outcomes and advance the scientific understanding of the histiocytoses. In this chapter we use the cellular classification of histiocytic disorders, as adopted by the Histiocyte Society, to present each subgroup of this family of disorders, describe their natural history and present current therapeutic approaches and outcomes.

Histiocytes and normal immune function

The MPS is a system of cells whose primary function consists of phagocytosis of foreign material, antigen processing, and antigen presentation to lymphocytes. This system, recognized in part through the work of Metchnikoff, was originally termed the reticuloendothelial system by Ludwig Aschoff in the early part of the twentieth century.[3,4] The central cell of this system, the mononuclear phagocyte or histiocyte, represents a group of anatomically and functionally distinct cells arising from a common precursor, the hematopoietic stem cell.

Cells of the MPS have a wide range of morphologic, anatomic and functional characteristics that make classification of this system difficult. Our ability to identify and classify the cells of the MPS has advanced in parallel with developments in basic hematology and immunology. As our knowledge of the molecular biology regulating hematopoiesis has improved, we have been able to identify specific characteristics that have enabled us to classify the cells of the MPS. Mononuclear phagocytes can be divided into two major classes, macrophages and dendritic cells. This classification is based on (i) phagocytic and antigen-presenting abilities, (ii) morphologic and ultrastructural appearance, (iii) expression of common enzymes, (iv) presence of common cell surface antigens, and (v) common regulatory cytokine and transcription factor networks.

Tissue macrophages are derived from bone marrow hematopoietic precursors and can arise directly from circulating peripheral blood monocytes. These cells enter different tissues and assume tissue-appropriate morphology based on the local cytokine milieu. Once established in various tissues, macrophages typically do not have the ability to self-renew extensively except possibly under specialized microenvironments such as in the lungs and pituitary. Tissue inflammation increases the influx of monocytes, which in turn give rise to macrophages with an immunologically activated phenotype. Inflammatory stimuli can also further enhance the local replication of macrophages in cases of tissue injury.[5,6] Regardless of location, macrophage growth and differentiation is a tightly controlled process regulated by specific growth factors.

Interleukin (IL)-3, IL-4, IL-13, granulocyte–macrophage colony-stimulating factor (GM-CSF) and macrophage colony-stimulating factor (M-CSF) are all stimulatory cytokines with a major role in macrophage development and differentiation.[6] M-CSF activity is especially essential for appropriate macrophage growth and differentiation. The M-CSF receptor, a product of the *c-fms* protooncogene, is expressed by most members of the MPS. When bound by M-CSF this receptor dimerizes, leading to the activation of its kinase domain and initiation of downstream signaling pathways. The signaling cascade initiated by the binding of M-CSF to its receptor is essential for the proliferation of progenitor cells of the monocyte–macrophage lineage, differentiation and their long-term survival. Information regarding the role of M-CSF primarily arises from studies of *op/op* knockout mice, which are deficient in the M-CSF receptor.[7] Despite their severe monocyte–macrophage deficiencies, *op/op* mice maintain normal levels of dendritic cells in their spleens and skin, thus demonstrating an alternative and M-CSF-independent pathway for their development.[8,9] The GM-CSF receptor, also present on most members of the MPS, plays a critical role in normal cellular homeostasis, differentiation and function.[8] There is also a positive survival effect of stem cell factor (the ligand for the c-KIT receptor) and FLT3 ligand and its cognate receptor FLT3, as well as inhibitory roles for interferon (IFN)-α/β, transforming growth factor (TGF)-β and leukocyte inhibitory factor as critical determinants in macrophage development.[6] The phenotypic and functional heterogeneity of macrophages as a group is attributed to the tissue-specific effects of cytokine stimulation on the multipotent monocyte. Pathologic changes in this cytokine milieu play important roles in the pathogenesis of the histiocytoses.[10,14]

Macrophages are ubiquitously distributed in the body and are heavily represented in mucosal tissues and other potential portals of entry for microorganisms, where they function in both innate and adaptive immunity. They have the capacity to phagocytose foreign organisms and release inflammatory cytokines that in turn recruit other inflammation-associated cell types. Macrophages also maintain the ability to process and present antigenic portions of foreign organisms to T lymphocytes, although not as effectively as dendritic cells. Tissue macrophages have significant functional variability depending on their location within the body. Peritoneal and soft tissue macrophages, Kupffer cells, foam cells, synovial cells, osteoclasts and microglial cells are all members of this class of cells and contribute to tissue growth, repair and remodeling. A distinguishing feature of macrophages is expression of the enzymes lysozyme, α_1-antitrypsin, α_1-antichymotrypsin, aminopeptidase, peroxidase, alkaline phosphatase, α-naphthol-chloroacetate esterase and β-glucuronidase.

The second class of mononuclear phagocytes, the dendritic cells, was first described by Steinman and Cohn in 1973. These cells were named because of their unique membranous, and often branch-like, cytoplasmic aberrations (from the Greek word for tree, δενδρεον).[15] Dendritic cells are primarily located in skin, mucosa, bone marrow, spleen, thymus and lymph nodes. This group of cells also includes dendritic cells of the lymphoid follicle, the interdigitating dendritic cells of the paracortical regions of lymph nodes, and Langerhans cells of the skin and other organs. Langerhans cells, originally identified by Paul Langerhans in the late 1800s, are mononuclear cells with little cytoplasmic vacuolization and a folded or indented nucleus. Electron microscopic observation of Langerhans cells reveals the presence of Birbeck granules, a distinguishing characteristic of these cells. Birbeck granules, or X bodies, are rod-shaped, pentalaminar, cytoplasmic inclusions, typically ending in a vesicular structure that arise as a result of receptor-mediated endocytosis and are involved in antigen processing.[16]

In contrast to macrophages, dendritic cells are less phagocytic but play a central role in initiating primary T-lymphocyte antigen responses. The hallmark of dendritic cells is their conversion from immature, peripherally located sentinels capable of antigen capture and processing to mature immunostimulatory cells, a process called *maturation*. This specific characteristic of dendritic cells, in combination with their ability to migrate, provides a physical and functional link between peripheral tissues and secondary lymphoid organs where lymphocyte maturation takes place.[17] Langerhans cells and the interdigitating dendritic cells present antigens to stimulate primary T-lymphocyte responses. It is well established that the precursor to most dendritic cells is bone marrow derived but the biologic significance of this differentiation schema is still not completely defined as a significant amount of the data has been derived from *in vitro* studies.[16] Other distinguishing characteristics of mature dendritic cells include (i) high expression levels of class II major histocompatibility complex (MHC) antigens and costimulatory receptors, making them potent at antigen presentation, (ii) adenosine triphosphatase and α-mannosidase expression and (iii) distinct paranuclear and cell surface-staining pattern with peanut agglutinin that contrasts with the diffuse staining pattern demonstrated by macrophages.[16,18]

The development of methods to generate monoclonal antibodies in the 1970s and 1980s significantly enhanced our knowledge of the MPS. The F4/80 antibody, a murine pan-macrophage antibody, was one of the first well-recognized markers of the MPS. This antibody recognizes members of a gene family that includes the human epidermal growth factor (EGF) module-containing mucin-like hormone receptor 1 and CD97. The presence of this antigen on the surface of tissue macrophages and dendritic cells helped confirm the existence of a common origin for the diverse lineages that comprises the MPS. Other markers such as S-100β subunit, CD1a and Langerin, are found on Langerhans cells but are usually absent on macrophages are used clinically to distinguish

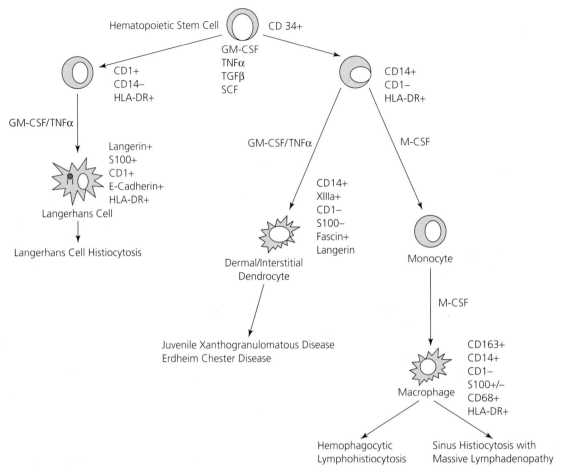

Fig. 15.1 Possible lineage relationships of hematopoietic cells and cells of the mononuclear phagocyte system along with the histiocytic disorders that arise from them. GM-CSF, granulocyte–macrophage colony-stimulating factor; M-CSF, macrophage colony-stimulating factor; SCF, stem cell factor; TGF, transforming growth factor; TNF, tumor necrosis factor. Adapted with permission from Ref. 3.

between the cells of the MPS. Conversely, monocytes and macrophages express nonspecific carcinoembryonic cross-reacting antigen, CD4 antigen, nonspecific esterase and the cell surface marker CD11c (Leu-M5). Both types of cells express class II MHC molecules and T-lymphocyte costimulatory receptors. These markers, in particular S100, CD1a and Langerin are utilized clinically to distinguish between the different histiocytic syndromes. Figure 15.1 denotes the lineage relationships thought to define the differentiation of cells of the MPS and the developmental stages from which various histiocytic disorders are believed to arise.

The development and differentiation of the cells of the MPS, much like other hematopoietic lineages, is driven by a tightly regulated pattern of gene expression governed by distinctive sets of transcription factors that control cell proliferation and differentiation. The main transcription factor families implicated in the development of this system include the *myb* family, the *Ets* family and the C/EBP family. PU.1, a member of the *Ets* family, plays a central role in monocyte–macrophage lineage as demonstrated by PU.1 knockout mice which lack functional monocytes and tissue

macrophages and display significant dendritic cell abnormalities.[19,21] This has become clearer recently as it has been shown that PU.1 regulates the expression of c-*fms*, the gene coding for the M-CSF receptor, in addition to other critical genes such as FcγRI, FcγRIIIA, scavenger receptors type 1 and 2, CD11b, CD18 and CD14.[21]

In summary, the MPS represents a continuum of functionally distinct cell types that arise from common bone marrow progenitors and differentiate along specific lineage pathways based on environmental stimuli and intrinsically regulated gene expression patterns. The result is the generation of a diverse group of cell types with distinct but often overlapping biologic functions. Understanding this biologic heterogeneity is an important key to more accurate diagnosis and treatment of the histiocytic disorders.

Modern classification of histiocytic disorders

As proposed in 1987,[1] the histiocytic disorders can be

classified into three classes based on the pathologic cells present within the lesions.

• Class I: Langerhans cell histiocytoses and other dendritic cell disorders.
• Class II: non-Langerhans cell histiocytoses primarily consisting of hemophagocytic lymphohistiocytosis.
• Class III: malignant histiocytosis.

This system was revised in 1997 by the World Health Organization's Committee on Histiocytic/Reticulum Cell Proliferations and the Reclassification Working Group of the Histiocyte Society. The central theme of this reclassification schema consisted of distinguishing the clearly malignant histiocytoses from the remaining subtypes, the so-called "disorders of varied biological behavior". Acute myelomonocytic leukemia (FAB M4), acute monocytic leukemia (FAB M5), chronic myelomonocytic leukemia and the histiocytic sarcomas are all classified in the malignant histiocytoses category. The disorders of varied biological behavior continued to be divided into dendritic cell-related disorders (class I) and macrophage-related disorders (class II). The dendritic cell-related disorders include Langerhans cell histiocytosis, the most common type in this class, in addition to other less common subtypes. Primary and secondary hemophagocytic lymphohistiocytosis, in addition to sinus histiocytosis with massive lymphadenopathy (also known as Rosai–Dorfman disease), are the two major types of macrophage-related histiocytosis discussed in this chapter. This classification schema is summarized in Table 15.1.[2] The remainder of this chapter focuses on the pathophysiology, clinical presentation, treatment and outcomes of the principal histiocytoses.

Disorders of varied biological behavior: dendritic cell-related (class I) histiocytoses

Langerhans cell histiocytosis

Biology

Langerhans cell histiocytosis (LCH) is the most common member of the dendritic cell-related histiocytic disorders. LCH includes the previously identified disorders known as eosinophilic granuloma, Abt–Letterer–Siwe disease and Hand–Schüller–Christian disease. The pathologic similarity of these disorders was first noted by Sidney Farber in 1941 and by the 1950s, as a result of the work of Lichtenstein, these disorders were collectively referred to as histiocytosis X.[16] The persistent use of this historical terminology in modern medical vernacular is indicative of its significance and utility for cataloging patient symptomatology. Regardless of the historical eponyms, the pathologic hallmark of all subtypes of LCH is the abnormal proliferation and accumulation of immature Langerhans cells along with macrophages, lymphocytes and eosinophils that together form granuloma-

Table 15.1 Classification of histiocytic disorders.

Class I: dendritic cell histiocytoses
Langerhans cell histiocytosis
Secondary dendritic cell processes
Juvenile xanthogranuloma and related disorders
    Erdheim–Chester disease
Solitary histiocytomas of various dendritic cell phenotypes

Class II: nondendritic cell histiocytoses
Primary hemophagocytic lymphohistiocytosis
    Familial hemophagocytic lymphohistiocytosis
Secondary hemophagocytic lymphohistiocytosis
    Infection associated
    Malignancy associated
Rosai–Dorfman disease (sinus histiocytosis with massive lymphadenopathy)
Solitary histiocytoma with macrophage phenotype

Class III: malignant histiocytoses
Monocyte related
Leukemias (FAB and revised FAB classification)
    Monocytic leukemia M5A and M5B
    Acute myelomonocytic leukemias M4
    Chronic myelomonocytic leukemias
Extramedullary monocytic tumor or sarcoma
Dendritic cell-related histiocytic sarcoma
Macrophage-related histiocytic sarcoma

FAB, French–American–British.

tous lesions. Although the biologic role of LCH cells in the pathogenesis of LCH remains unclear, it is now generally accepted that the close physical interaction between these cells and other cell types present in these lesions is associated with an abnormal cytokine and chemokine microenvironment that underlies the pathogenesis of LCH.

In 1973 Nezelof *et al.*[22] provided definitive evidence for the phenotypic similarity of normal Langerhans cells and LCH cells, including a description of the presence of Birbeck granules in both cell types. However, LCH cells, in contrast to normal Langerhans cells, typically lack dendritic cell extensions and have a rounded appearance with distinct cellular margins. These cells express CD1a, S100 and Langerin (CD207) but not the typical markers of more mature dendritic cells such as CD83, CD86 and DC-Lamp (Fig. 15.2). In addition, these cells express CD40 and intracellular MHC class II proteins but are inefficient antigen-presenting cells. When LCH cells are exposed *in vitro* to CD40L they acquire markers of dendritic cell maturation.[23] LCH cells also express CCR6, the receptor for the proinflammatory chemokine CCL20/MIP3α, a characteristic of immature dendritic cells. Furthermore, these cells have been shown to also secrete CCL20/MIP3α, CCL5/RANTES and CXCL11/I-TAC, all of which are believed to function in recruiting additional LCH cells, eosinophils and T cells to LCH lesions.[12] Of note, the co-expression of CCR6 and CCR7 on LCH cells has also been reported. This may be suggestive of the pathological

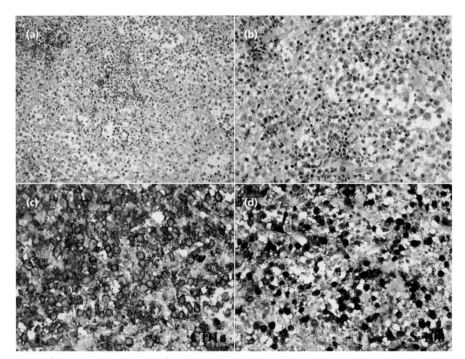

Fig. 15.2 Langerhans cell histiocytosis. Histology and immunohistochemical staining of a bone lesion (eosinophilic granuloma) characterized by (a, b) sheets of large pale Langerhans cells, many of which have prominent nuclear indentations or grooves, interspersed with large numbers of bilobed eosinophils (hematoxylin and eosin staining) (original magnification: a, ×200; b ×400). Langerhans cells strongly express CD1a (c, original magnification ×400) and S100 protein (d, original magnification ×400). Photographs courtesy of Dr John Reith, Department of Pathology, University of Florida School of Medicine, Gainesville, FL, USA.

maturational arrest of these cells.[14] Immunohistochemical and *in situ* hybridization data also demonstrate abnormal release of specific cytokines, such as GM-CSF, IL-10, TGF-α/β, IFN-γ and tumor necrosis factor (TNF)-α, by lesional cells in LCH.[13,24,25] The cytokine abnormalities noted in LCH lesions are hypothesized to magnify the local autocrine and paracrine effects of these cells, resulting in a focal "cytokine storm". These cytokines also cause local tissue damage and contribute to the systemic symptoms such as fever, skin rashes and hypotension.[16,24] Unlike hemophagocytic lymphohistiocytosis, there is no clear-cut evidence for systemic cytokine overproduction in most cases of LCH.

Despite our improved understanding of the molecular events involved in the pathophysiology of LCH, its etiology remains undetermined. Infectious, inflammatory and neoplastic mechanisms have all been postulated to play an etiologic role in LCH, but the relative contribution of each process to the development of the disease remains controversial.[10,11,16,26–28] The human androgen receptor DNA assay and analyses of T-cell receptor gene rearrangements for detecting clonality have demonstrated the clonal nature of LCH cells but not lymphocytes in lesions, a finding consistent with a neoplastic origin for LCH.[29,30] This is further supported by analyses of LCH lesions using comparative genomic hybridization and loss of heterozygosity, which reveal multiple chromosomal abnormalities.[31,32] Clinical evidence of familial cases, in addition to the increased risk of malignancy seen in patients with histiocytosis, further supports a neoplastic origin for some forms of LCH.[33,34]

However, this conclusion is tempered by several lines of evidence suggesting an inflammatory contribution to the etiology of LCH. *In vitro* studies have demonstrated an inability to grow LCH cells in culture or in immunodeficient mice, characteristics typically observed with aggressive malignancies. Studies of isolated pulmonary LCH show no consistent or uniform evidence of clonality. Immunohistochemical evidence for human herpesvirus-6 in bone lesions, in addition to differences in HLA types among patients with single-system versus multisystem LCH, might be considered suggestive of a potential inflammatory etiology for LCH, although these data remain controversial due to methodologic issues and inconsistencies.[32,35,36] Implications of the variable expression pattern of MDM2, p53 and p21 and the strong expression of TGF-β seen in LCH remain unclear.[11,37] Based on this data, most experts now agree that LCH is the result of complex interactions between environmental factors and intrinsic genetic changes leading to a clonal proliferative disorder of immature Langerhans cells with variable clinical behavior.[10,11,16,26–28,38,39] Although the pathologic findings may not be clearly different among cases of LCH, the clinical variability strongly suggests different biology and thus a possible continuum from the least to the most aggressive forms of the disease.

Incidence and epidemiology

LCH has been historically considered a disease of young children, with a peak occurrence between the ages of 1 and 3 years. A Danish study estimated the incidence of LCH in children less than 15 years old to be 0.54 per 100 000 children per year. However, this is considered to be an underestimation as a proportion of children are believed to go undiagnosed. A Swedish study has estimated an incidence of around 0.9 per 100 000.[40,41] LCH also shows a predilection for males, with a female to male ratio of 1 : 1.2–2.1.[16,41] It is also now well recognized that the incidence of LCH in adulthood is likely to be underestimated. This has been attributed to the multiple subspecialties involved in the care of patients with this disease depending on the involved organ system in addition to incorrect diagnoses.[41] This problem is now being addressed by the Histiocyte Society as more emphasis is being placed on studies of adult subjects, including the most recent adult therapeutic study, LCH A-1.

A case–control epidemiologic study has suggested associations between the diagnosis of LCH and maternal urinary tract infections as well as feeding problems, medication use and blood transfusions during the first 6 months of life.[42] A subsequent study has demonstrated a significant odds ratio for postnatal infections, diarrhea and vomiting, as well as medication use in multisystem LCH, while single-system LCH was associated with thyroid disease or a family history of thyroid disease.[43] The results of these studies are for the most part inconclusive with regard to any etiologic associations. However, it has to be pointed out that none of the studies performed has noted a geographical or seasonal clustering of cases of LCH, making a common infectious etiology unlikely.

Clinical presentation and therapy

LCH represents a wide variety of different clinical entities recognized to be pathologically the same. LCH is clinically subclassified by the degree and location of organ involvement: localized single-system disease, multifocal single-system disease and multisystem disease. The location of involvement has been shown to be of prognostic importance, with bone marrow, pulmonary, spleen and liver involvement denoted as "risk organs" while involvement of cranial bones or spine with extradural soft tissue extension is considered to be "central nervous system (CNS) risk".[44,45] This clinical classification schema currently serves as the basis for risk stratification of LCH treatment protocols.

At the time of diagnosis, a complete work-up should be performed to establish the full extent of disease and delineate risk-based therapy (Table 15.2). The work-up should include

detailed history and physical examination, complete blood count and differential, metabolic panel including liver and renal function tests, bone scan, skeletal survey and chest radiograph. Urine analysis should also be performed to assess for diabetes insipidus and possible hypothalamic–pituitary involvement. Additional studies such as water deprivation test, antidiuretic hormone levels or other endocrinologic examinations evaluating hypothalamic–pituitary function may be necessary depending on a patient's clinical presentation. Magnetic resonance imaging (MRI) of the brain with gadolinium contrast is becoming a more common part of the staging work-up of "CNS-risk" patients because of the recognition of significant CNS involvement. Bone marrow studies, computed tomography (CT) of the chest and pulmonary function tests should also be performed as clinically indicated to evaluate risk-organ involvement. The role of positron emission tomography remains undefined, but is a potentially promising imaging approach.[46]

Localized LCH involving skin, lymph node or skeleton usually carries a good prognosis. Lesions of bone, a condition often referred to as eosinophilic granuloma, usually present as a painful swelling. These lesions appear radiographically as "punched-out" sites and most commonly affect the calvarium (Fig. 15.3), although they can involve any part of the skeleton. Vertebra plana, or a collapsed vertebra, is a common presentation of this disease process (Fig. 15.4). Single bone lesions rarely need therapy beyond biopsy or curettage, except in the case of severe symptoms or danger of organ dysfunction, such as spinal cord compression or loss of vision. Treatment options for these patients with nonemergency single bone lesions that recur or remain clinically problematic after surgery include nonsteroidal antiinflammatory agents or local steroid injections and, rarely, local low-dose radiation therapy (40–80 cGy). Full surgical resection (i.e., performing a "cancer operation") of these single bone lesions, especially when other vital structures could be compromised as a result of such an operation, is not typically necessary.

Skin disease typically involves the scalp, retroauricular area, neck, upper chest, axilla and groin. This rash can vary from maculopapular to more eruptive and even nodular in appearance (Fig. 15.5). In some patients, the rash can be quite erosive and a risk factor for serious superinfection. Therapy

---

Table 15.2 Risk groups as defined by the LCH-III protocol (adapted from the Histiocyte Society LCH-III study).

Group 1: multisystem "risk" patients
Multisystem patients with involvement of one or more "risk" organs (i.e., hematopoietic system, liver, spleen or lungs)

Group 2: multisystem "low-risk" patients
Multisystem patients with multiple organs involved but without involvement of "risk" organs

Group 3: single-system "multifocal bone disease" and localized "special site" involvement
Patients with multifocal bone disease (i.e., lesions in two or more different bones)
Patients with localized special site involvement, such as "CNS-risk" lesions with intracranial soft tissue extension or vertebral lesions with intraspinal soft tissue extension

---

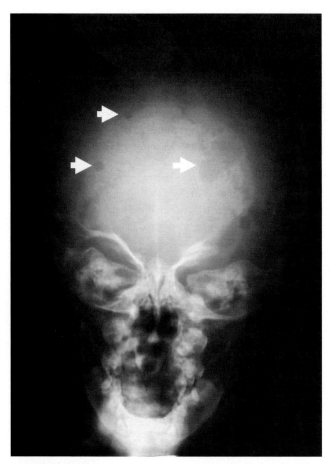

Fig. 15.3 Radiograph of skull of a patient with Langerhans cell histiocytosis showing multiple lytic lesions (white arrows).

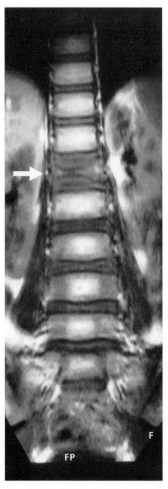

Fig. 15.4 Magnetic resonance image depicting a vertebra plana secondary to involvement of the vertebral body with Langerhans cell histiocytosis (white arrow).

for isolated skin disease typically involves topical steroids or, in some steroid-refractory cases, topical nitrogen mustard, PUVA or short-wave ultraviolet light without psoralen. Systemic steroids and vinblastine are reserved for extensive single-system disease, including skin involvement, usually with good outcomes.[38]

In contrast to localized LCH, systemic therapy is indicated in patients with multisystem LCH. The most common presentation of multifocal LCH includes diffuse skin and multifocal bone involvement. The oral cavity, lymph nodes and, to a lesser extent, the lungs, liver and brain are other common sites of involvement in this disease. Oral cavity involvement can lead to infiltrative lesions with ulceration as well as erosion of the mandible or maxilla, leading to "floating" teeth. Figure 15.6 demonstrates the characteristic CT findings of lung involvement. Diabetes insipidus, with pituitary involvement (Fig. 15.7), is the most common manifestation of CNS involvement in LCH and is reported in 5–30% of patients. The triad of lytic skull lesions, exophthalmos and diabetes insipidus, historically referred to as Hand–Schüller–Christian disease, is not commonly observed at the time of diagnosis, although the chronic waxing/waning course is frequently seen in this group of patients. Risk factors for the development of diabetes insipidus have been reported to include the presence of multisystem disease and craniofacial lesions, especially involving the orbit, ear and oral cavity.[47] In addition to acute CNS involvement, patients with LCH may develop a severe neurodegenerative process involving loss of motor functions and cognition. This syndrome characteristically involves the cerebellum, pons and midbrain, often in a symmetric pattern (Fig. 15.8).[48–50] The clinical severity of neurodegenerative-associated LCH can be independent of radiographic findings or progression.[49,51] There are currently no effective means of ameliorating the progression of this process. Liver involvement is another complication of LCH that portends a poor prognosis. Transaminitis and hyperbilirubinemia are the hallmarks of acute liver involvement in LCH. Patients with hepatic LCH or with multisystem disease appear to have a higher risk of developing sclerosing cholangitis that can, in turn, lead to hepatic fibrosis, liver failure and the need for liver transplantation.

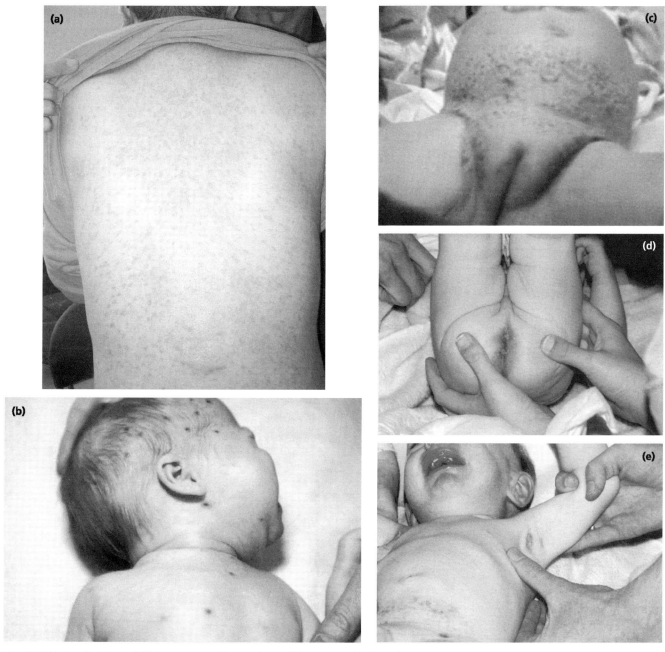

Fig. 15.5 Various depictions of skin involvement with Langerhans cell histiocytosis. (a) The back of a teenager showing slightly raised lesions. (b) Papular appearing lesion in an infant. (c) Inguinal involvement in an infant. (d) Perianal involvement in an infant. Reproduced with permission from Arceci RJ. Histiocytosis. In: Young NS, Gerson SL, High KA (eds) *Clinical Hematology*. Mosby/Elsevier, 2006. (e) Axillary, lower abdomen and oral involvement in an infant. Reproduced with permission from Ref. 39.

In addition to site of involvement, age has been thought to be an important prognostic factor in LCH, with younger patients having a significantly higher mortality rate. However, more recent clinical trial data have shown that response to initial (6–12 weeks) therapy with vinblastine and steroids is the most powerful prognostic factor, outweighing even age. Abt–Letterer–Siwe disease is a historical eponym used to describe systemic LCH characterized by extensive skin,

bone marrow, spleen, liver and lung involvement; it is usually observed in children less than 2 years old. Oral cavity and gastrointestinal involvement are other commonly seen manifestations of this severe form of LCH. Patients typically suffer from intractable fevers, failure to thrive and, in later phases of the disease, severe pancytopenia and hepatic failure leading to hemorrhage and sepsis. Abt–Letterer–Siwe disease carries a particularly poor prognosis in patients with

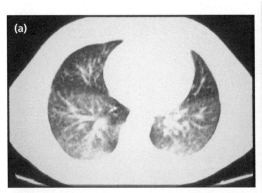

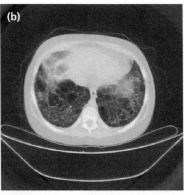

Fig. 15.6 Involvement of the lung in Langerhans cell histiocytosis. (a) Acute nodular involvement; (b) cystic changes often associated with chronic involvement. Photograph (b) courtesy of Dr William Cumming, Department of Radiology, University of Florida School of Medicine, Gainesville, FL, USA.

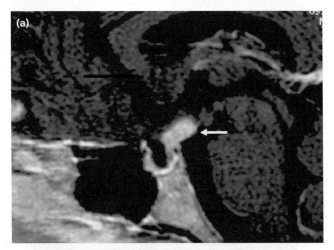

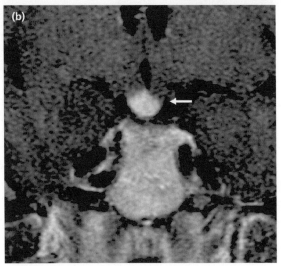

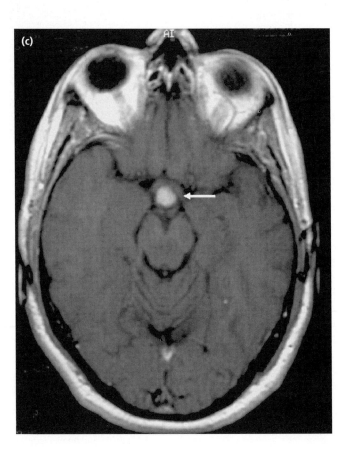

Fig. 15.7 Magnetic resonance image of pituitary involvement in Langerhans cell histiocytosis: (a) sagittal view; (b) coronal view; (c) horizontal view.

advanced hematopoietic involvement who do not show a good response to initial therapy. Patients with Abt–Letterer–Siwe disease should undergo a full evaluation for congenital and acquired immunodeficiency syndromes in addition to infectious etiologies as part of their diagnostic work-up.

It is critical that pulmonary involvement as part of multi-system disease be distinguished from isolated pulmonary LCH (PLCH). PLCH is distinguishable from other forms of LCH by its almost exclusive occurrence in young adults and close association with smoking. PLCH can cause severe inter-

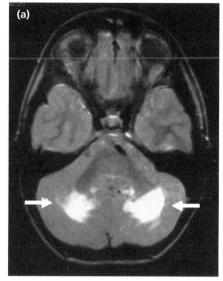

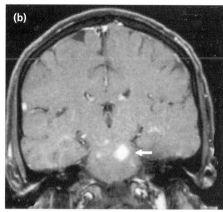

Fig. 15.8 Magnetic resonance image of neurodegenerative disease in an adult patient with Langerhans cell histiocytosis. (a) Symmetric enhancing lesions involving the cerebellar peduncles on a horizontal view; (b) enhancing lesions involving the pons on a coronal view.

stitial lung disease, cor pulmonale and eventual respiratory failure necessitating lung transplantation. The first line of therapy for PLCH remains smoking cessation, followed in some patients with steroids. The role of chemotherapy in PLCH remains uncertain as prospective data are not available. The use of 2-chlorodeoxyadenosine (2-CDA) has shown some promise in PLCH, although this therapy is reserved for patients with refractory disease and has only shown anecdotal success.[52–54] The Histiocyte Society trial for adults with LCH includes patients with PLCH.

Patients with multisystem LCH have been demonstrated to benefit from systemic chemotherapy. The current therapeutic regimens evolved from work originally performed in the 1970s and 1980s. Several studies during that time demonstrated that single-agent therapy with drugs such as methotrexate, vincristine, vinblastine, etoposide, 6-mercaptopurine and prednisone was effective treatment for LCH. These trials were subsequently followed by the larger studies (AIEOP-CNR-HX and DAL-HX 83/90), all of which used regimens with multiple agents. These studies demonstrated response rates of 60–90% using combinations of vinblastine and/or etoposide plus prednisone. These studies also demonstrated that patients with extensive disease and organ dysfunction had significantly higher mortality and recurrence rates.[38,55,56]

The AIEOP-CNR-HX and DAL-HX-83/90 studies were then followed by the first international, prospective, randomized study, LCH-I, which also represented the first international clinical trial of the Histiocyte Society. The results of this study demonstrated that patients randomized to treatment with etoposide plus steroids did not have a better outcome than those randomized to receive vinblastine plus steroids. In addition, this study revealed that response at 6 weeks was strongly predictive of overall outcome. For example, patients without a response to therapy after 6 weeks had a survival

rate of less than 40% at 5 years. Another critical outcome of this study was the confirmation of earlier work by Lahey that patients older than 2 years of age and without pulmonary, hepatosplenic or hematopoietic involvement had an excellent prognosis, with a response rate of 90% and survival of 100% at 6 years.[57,58] In comparison with the AIEOP-CNR-HX and DAL-HX 83/90 trials, LCH-I showed a higher recurrence rate and higher frequency of diabetes insipidus. This raised the question of whether more aggressive therapy in patients with high-risk disease would provide a therapeutic advantage.[59]

The second Histiocyte Society protocol, LCH-II, attempted to answer this question in a randomized fashion. The results of this study are still under analysis although preliminary evaluations led to the following conclusions:

1 response by 12 weeks of therapy is an important prognostic factor;

2 etoposide plus vinblastine and steroids does not appear to confer any benefit over therapy with vinblastine and steroids;

3 prolonged therapy may decrease the reactivation rate of LCH.

In light of the risk of therapy-associated acute myelogenous leukemia/myelodysplastic syndrome in patients treated with epipodophyllotoxins (i.e., etoposide/VP-16), this study obviated the use of etoposide in LCH. This trial also confirmed that age less than 2 years without risk-organ involvement is not an independent prognostic factor. The Histiocyte Society protocol LCH-III is attempting to determine in a randomized design whether (i) intensified induction therapy, with the addition of intermediate-dose methotrexate followed by inclusion of methotrexate in maintenance therapy, improves remission induction rates and overall outcomes and (ii) whether prolonging continuation therapy reduces the rate of disease reactivation (see Fig. 15.9 for treatment

Group 1: multisystem "risk" patients

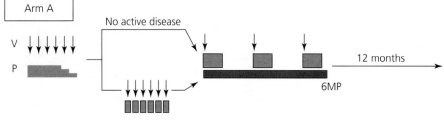

Group 1: multisystem "risk" patients

Arm A

V
P

No active disease

12 months

6MP

Intermediate response or worse

Arm B

ID-MTX/LR

No active disease

12 months

Oral MTX

Intermediate response or worse

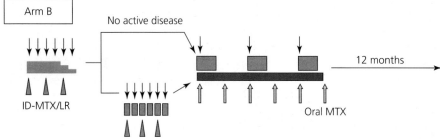

Group 2: multisystem low-risk patients

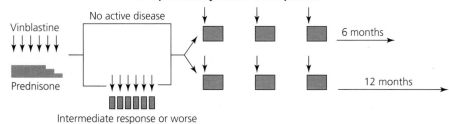

Vinblastine

Prednisone

No active disease

6 months

12 months

Intermediate response or worse

Group 3: multifocal bone disease and special sites

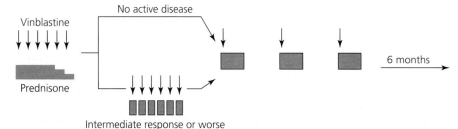

Vinblastine

Prednisone

No active disease

6 months

Intermediate response or worse

Details of chemotherapy by symbols

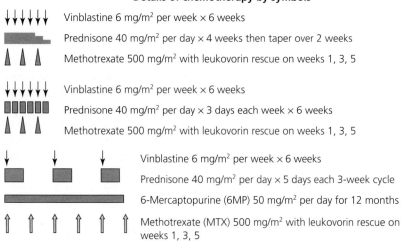

Vinblastine 6 mg/m² per week × 6 weeks

Prednisone 40 mg/m² per day × 4 weeks then taper over 2 weeks

Methotrexate 500 mg/m² with leukovorin rescue on weeks 1, 3, 5

Vinblastine 6 mg/m² per week × 6 weeks

Prednisone 40 mg/m² per day × 3 days each week × 6 weeks

Methotrexate 500 mg/m² with leukovorin rescue on weeks 1, 3, 5

Vinblastine 6 mg/m² per week × 6 weeks

Prednisone 40 mg/m² per day × 5 days each 3-week cycle

6-Mercaptopurine (6MP) 50 mg/m² per day for 12 months

Methotrexate (MTX) 500 mg/m² with leukovorin rescue on weeks 1, 3, 5

Fig. 15.9 Treatment arms for LCH-III protocol sponsored by the Histiocyte Society.

schema). Based on the results of the previous studies, etoposide is no longer recommended as initial therapy.

Despite past successes in the treatment of newly diagnosed LCH, the treatment of refractory disease remains problematic. Experience with immunosuppressive agents such as cyclosporin and antithymocyte globulin are limited and responses most commonly transient.[60] However, there is significant experience with the nucleoside analog 2-CDA, alone or in combination with cytosine arabinoside.[61–64] 2-CDA has been shown to produce a remission in more than one-third of patients with refractory disease in an international phase II study. The response rate was even better in patients with a good response to initial treatment.[38,61,63,64] 2-CDA has also shown anecdotal efficacy in the treatment of parenchymal CNS disease, although no agent has been shown to be convincingly effective in halting the progression of the neurodegenerative disease. Other approaches that have been used to treat the neurodegenerative disease associated with LCH include drugs that decrease inflammatory responses such as thalidomide and TNF inhibitors such as infliximab (Remicade) and etanercept (Enbrel).[65–67] Alemtuzumab (Campath), an anti-CD52 antibody, may also have promise in the treatment of LCH, especially in patients with advanced disease, but should be tested in prospective clinical trials because of its profound immunosuppressive effect.[68] There are case reports of hematopoietic stem cell transplantation (HSCT) in patients with refractory LCH, but the role of this therapeutic approach remains unclear in part due to difficulty in identifying matched donors and the high mortality rate in patients with significant disease-related organ dysfunction.[69] A Histiocyte Society trial is currently testing the use of a nonablative preparative regimen for HSCT.[69]

There remains a significant need for more effective agents in the treatment of patients with organ involvement and dysfunction, including those with progressive CNS, hepatic and pulmonary disease. Several new agents, including antibodies to the CD1a surface antigen as well as agents targeting cytokine receptor signaling pathways, are currently in pre-clinical/early clinical phases of development. It is anticipated that the optimization of these agents and their incorporation into routine clinical use will help increase our ability to more effectively treat patients with refractory and progressive disease.

Survivorship issues

Survivors of LCH can have significant late sequelae related to their disease after achieving remission and long-term cure. Late effects in survivors of LCH tend to be directly related to sites of original disease involvement. In one study, 42% of patients developed long-term complications, patients with multisystem disease being at highest risk. Diabetes insipidus developed in 15% of patients, CNS complications in 12% and pulmonary insufficiency in 10%.[41] Others have noted neurocognitive problems such as intellectual impairment, psychological problems and psychomotor retardation in long-term survivors of LCH.[49,50,70] The late CNS complications of LCH also include neurodegenerative changes that can be highly disabling.[48–50,71–73] The neurodegenerative disease is thought to be the result of a paraneoplastic process and pathologically is characterized by an inflammatory infiltrate dominated by CD8-positive reactive lymphocytes, microglial activation and gliosis. This contrasts with the T-cell infiltration and severe neurodegeneration surrounding CD1a infiltrates of CNS parenchyma.[48] Sclerosing cholangitis and liver failure necessitating liver transplant are also well recognized late effects of systemic LCH. The role of chemotherapy in the management of CNS and hepatic sequelae is limited as these complications appear to be related to an aberrant immune response and tissue fibrosis as opposed to active LCH.[74,75] Patients with LCH also have an increased risk of malignancy, which may be further increased when treated with etoposide or radiation as part of their therapy.[33,34,76]

It is critical for patients with LCH, especially multisystem disease, to be followed on a long-term basis at a center familiar with the care of patients with LCH. Follow-up should include imaging studies in addition to routine blood counts, liver and thyroid function testing as well as urine and electrolyte levels for assessment of diabetes insipidus. Formal neurocognitive evaluations should be done in patients with suspected or proven CNS involvement.

Non-Langerhans cell (class I) histiocytoses

Juvenile xanthogranulomatous disease and related disorders

The non-Langerhans cell (class I) histiocytic disorders represent a spectrum of disease defined by the accumulation of dendritic cells that do not meet the phenotypic criterion for diagnosis of LCH. These histiocytes, like LCH cells, phenotypically resemble a stage in the normal development of dendritic cells. It is believed that under growth factor stimulation, a common progenitor can develop along two separate differentiative pathways that can be phenotypically distinguished by the expression of CD14. The CD14-negative lineage, under the influence of TNF-α and GM-CSF, differentiates into Langerhans cells while the CD14-positive lineage can give rise to either cells of the monocyte–macrophage lineage or to interstitial/dermal dendrocytes.[77] Disorders arising from the monocyte–macrophage lineage are categorized as the class II or macrophage-related histiocytoses. However, the non-Langerhans cell (class I) histiocytoses are believed to arise from dermal dendritic cells. It is critical to emphasize that disorders arising from the dermal dendrocyte are now considered class I histiocytoses.

The non-Langerhans cell (class I) histiocytoses are histologically nonmalignant proliferative disorders that have variable

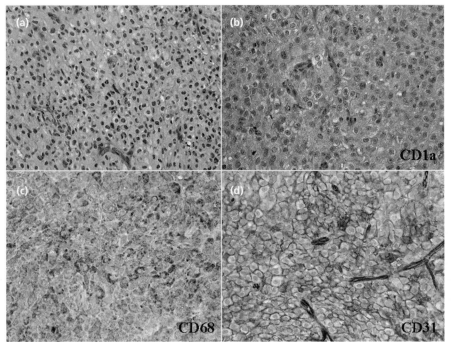

Fig. 15.10 Histopathology and immunochemical staining of juvenile xanthogranulomatous disease. (a) Juvenile xanthogranuloma characterized by oval, partially lipidized histiocytes admixed with eosinophils (hematoxylin and eosin staining) (original magnification ×200). Many juvenile xanthogranulomas also contain Touton-type multinucleated giant cells. Unlike Langerhans cell histiocytosis, juvenile xanthogranulomas do not express CD1a (b, original magnification ×400) but do express histiocyte antigens CD68 (c, original magnification ×400) and CD31 (d, original magnification ×400). Photographs courtesy of Dr John Reith, Department of Pathology, University of Florida School of Medicine, Gainesville, FL, USA.

clinical presentations. However, these disorders are all defined by the similar pathologic finding of a histiocytic proliferation that is CD1a and S100 negative but factor XIII, CD31, CD68, CD163, fascin and CD14 positive (Fig. 15.10). Clinical presentation of these disorders is variable and appears to be age dependent. It has been hypothesized that the clinical presentation of these disorders, much like LCH, depends on the variable local cytokine milieu.[78] Weitzman and Jaffe[77] have suggested that the non-Langerhans cell (class I) histiocytoses be divided into three major groups based on their clinical presentation for ease of classification: (i) disorders primarily affecting skin (cutaneous); (ii) cutaneous disorders that have a systemic component; and (iii) multisystem disorders that can also affect skin.

The juvenile xanthogranuloma (JXG) family of diseases represents the most common disorder of this subtype. Juvenile xanthogranulomatous disease is the prototypical member of this family of disorders and the most common form observed in pediatrics. The primary presentation of JXG in children is cutaneous (Fig. 15.11), although approximately 4% of children may also have systemic involvement of the CNS, liver, lungs and eyes.[79,80] JXG lesions typically self-involute, although systemic disease may sometimes necessitate chemotherapy.[77] Optimal therapy for patients with systemic JXG who need therapeutic intervention remains unclear, although LCH regimens have been most commonly used with variable responses observed.[79,81,82] Interestingly, a triple association between JXG, juvenile myelomonocytic leukemia and neurofibromatosis type I has been reported, possibly genetically linking these conditions in some patients.[83–86]

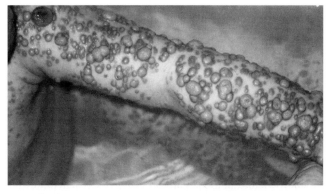

Fig. 15.11 Extensive cutaneous involvement of an infant with juvenile xanthogranulomatous disease.

Erdheim–Chester disease is also a member of the class I non-Langerhans cell histiocytoses and can often present as a systemic disease. This disease is extremely rare in the pediatric age group and patients are typically older than 50 years of age. Clinically, this disease presents with xanthoma-like skin nodules and bilateral lower extremity bone pain. Radiography shows symmetrical sclerosing bone lesions typically affecting the metaphyseal ends of long bones. Patients with disseminated disease may have severe cardiopulmonary insufficiency from parenchymal involvement of heart and lung tissues, renal insufficiency due to perinephric involvement, and CNS involvement with ataxia, diabetes insipidus and mental status changes.[87,88] This disease is frequently progressive and fatal. Limited success has been reported when treating patients with Erdheim–Chester disease with standard LCH therapy, although anecdotal cases of response to low-dose IFN-α are notable but in need of prospective confirmation.[91]

Disorders of varied biological behavior: macrophage-related (class II) histiocytoses

Hemophagocytic lymphohistiocytosis

Biology

Class II histiocytic disorders are all characterized by the abnormal accumulation of activated macrophages along with lymphocytes in tissues. The predominant member of the class II histiocytoses is hemophagocytic lymphohistiocytosis (HLH), a disorder characterized by the abnormal accumulation of T lymphocytes and macrophages in normal tissues. HLH is further subdivided as follows:

1 primary HLH (familial erythrophagocytic lymphohistiocytosis), a heritable autosomal recessive disorder;

2 secondary HLH, a sporadic disease typically associated with a preexisting inflammatory condition such as infection (infection-associated hemophagocytic syndrome), malignancy (malignancy-associated hemophagocytic syndrome) or immunosuppressive therapy (macrophage activation syndrome). Primary and secondary HLH are clinically indistinguishable. The presentation of these disorders is typically fulminant and consists of fever, cytopenias, hepatosplenomegaly, hyperbilirubinemia, hyperlipidemia, hypofibrinogenemia, coagulopathy, hemophagocytosis and CNS abnormalities such as seizures.[90,91] A family history of consanguinity and age < 2 years at time of onset are highly suggestive of primary/inherited HLH. Positive genetic testing for genes known to cause HLH establishes the diagnosis of the primary or inherited form of the disease.

The immunologic defect underlying primary HLH is low or absent natural killer (NK) cell and cytotoxic T-lymphocyte function and number.[92,95] This diminished cytotoxic function is responsible for the pathologic expansion of cellular immune responses and infiltration of tissues by inflammatory cells.

This accumulation of activated macrophages and lymphocytes in tissues is perpetuated by the release of inflammatory cytokines by both lymphocytes and antigen-presenting cells, resulting in systemic hypercytokinemia which in turn contributes to organ damage and the signs and symptoms of HLH.[96-98]

Mutations in three genes have now been identified in patients with primary HLH: *PRF1* (perforin),[99] *UNC13-D* (Munc13-4)[100] and *STX11* (syntaxin 11).[99-101] Perforin is stored in cytotoxic granules of NK cells and cytotoxic T cells and is released to the cell surface during the formation of an immunologic synapse, where it functions to create pores in the cytoplasmic membranes of target cells leading to cell death. Munc13-4 and syntaxin 11 are both involved in the stabilization and transport of cytotoxic granules in NK and T cells. Normal NK-cell and T-cell function is crucial in the clearance of infections, particularly viral infections through lysis of infected cells.[102,103] The association of *PRF1*, *UNC13-D* and *STX11* mutations with HLH and the observed NK-cell defects in patients with HLH clearly point to the central role of this pathway in the pathogenesis of HLH. Furthermore, *in vitro* NK-cell enumeration and cytotoxicity data suggest significant variability among patients with HLH that is directly related to the nature of their genetic defect.[104]

This pathophysiologic model for HLH is further supported by the reports of HLH-like syndromes in patients with other immunodeficiency diseases such as Chédiak–Higashi syndrome (*LYST*), Griscelli syndrome (*RAB27A*) and X-linked lymphoproliferative syndrome (*SH2D1A*).[105-107] Mutations in the perforin gene are thought to account for 20–58% of cases of primary HLH (Table 15.3) [101, 110–112]. Interestingly, patients with HLH with missense mutations and higher levels of perforin expression appear to have a delayed onset of symptoms relative to patients with no expression of perforin.[111]

Incidence and epidemiology

The incidence of primary HLH is estimated to be around 1 in 50 000–300 000 live births based on several retrospective epidemiologic studies.[112-114] However, these estimations may

Table 15.3 Genetic defects in primary and secondary hemophagocytic lymphohistiocytosis.

Disease	Associated gene	Gene function	Chromosomal location
FHLH-1	Unknown	Unknown	9q21.3–q22
FHLH-2	*PRF1*	Induction of apoptosis	10q21–q22
FHLH-3	*UNC13-D*	Vesicle priming	17q25
FHLH-4	*STX11*	Vesicle transport; t-SNARE	6q24
GS-2	*RAB27A*	Vesicle transport; small GTPase	15q21
CHS-1	*LYST*	Vesicle transport; not further defined	1q42.1–q42.2
XLP	*SH2D1A*	Signal transduction and activation of lymphocytes	Xq25

CHS, Chédiak–Higashi syndrome; FHLH, familial hemophagocytic lymphohistiocytosis; GS, Griscelli syndrome; XLP, X-linked lymphoproliferative syndrome.
Adapted with permission from Janka G, zur Stadt U. *Hematology (Am Soc Hematol Educ Program)* 2005; 82–8.

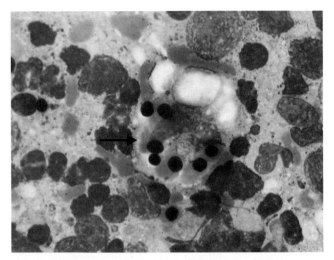

Fig. 15.12 Bone marrow biopsy from an infant presenting with pancytopenia, fever and hepatic failure shows evidence of large macrophages phagocytosing a white cell and multiple red cells (arrow). Courtesy of Dr Ying Li, Department of Pathology, University of Florida School of Medicine, Gainesville, FL, USA.

Table 15.4 Diagnostic criteria for hemophagocytic lymphohistiocytosis.*

Clinical
Fever
Hepatosplenomegaly

Laboratory
Hematologic
   Cytopenias (more than two of three lineages in peripheral blood)
   Hemophagocytosis
Biochemical
   Hypertriglyceridemia (fasting triglycerides ≥ 2 mmol/L or ≥ 3SD
     above normal)
   Hypofibrinogenemia (≤ 1.5 g/L or ≤ 3SD below normal)
   Hyperferritinemia
Immunologic
   Low or absent natural killer cell function
   Elevated soluble CD25 serum levels

Additional
Molecular demonstration of known gene mutation
Presence of familial disease

* Diagnosis requires five of the eight clinical and laboratory criteria or the identification of specific gene mutations or presence of familial disease.

under estimate the true incidence of HLH secondary to lack of familiarity of many primary physicians with this diagnosis. Interestingly, the prevalence of primary HLH is noted to be geographic in distribution, a finding attributed to the familial nature and the founder effect seen in this disease.[113,115,116]

The majority of cases of primary HLH occur within the first year of life, although cases have been reported as late as the third decade of life.[117,118] Secondary HLH, however, occurs sporadically and can be seen at any age depending on the primary initiating event. The male to female ratio of primary HLH is estimated to be 1 : 1, with some studies suggesting a slight male predominance.[113,117,118]

Clinical presentation

HLH is fatal if the diagnosis is delayed and appropriate therapy not instituted rapidly. The most common presenting symptoms include fever and hepatosplenomegaly, although rash, lymphadenopathy and CNS symptoms are common. Signs and symptoms also include cytopenias, transaminitis, coagulopathy, hypofibrinogenemia, hypertriglyceridemia, hyperferritinemia, and evidence of hemophagocytosis from bone marrow aspiration (Fig. 15.12). As significant variability in clinical presentation may impede diagnosis, specific diagnostic criteria have been established by the Histiocyte Society to aid in more expeditious diagnosis and treatment (Table 15.4).[41] In particular, some children may present with solely or primarily CNS-related symptoms; in these children a high level of suspicion on observing characteristic brain MRI changes is important in making an early diagnosis. If strong clinical suspicion is present, it is recommended that therapy be initiated even if all criteria are not fully satisfied.

In such cases, bone marrow studies should be repeated if initially negative to help establish a diagnosis by documenting hemophagocytosis. The presence of a family history positive for consanguinity or another affected sibling as well as the availability of molecular testing for gene mutations can further assist in establishing a diagnosis.

Treatment

Current therapy of HLH, as prescribed by the HLH-2004 protocol of the Histiocyte Society, consists of dexamethasone, etoposide and cyclosporin in combination with intrathecal methotrexate and prednisolone when indicated by the presence of cerebrospinal fluid pleocytosis. Antithymocyte globulin has also been used, but mostly as second-line therapy.[119] Primary HLH tends to be recurrent and does not permanently respond to chemotherapy, thus necessitating HSCT for cure.[66,120,121] However, secondary HLH, with the exception of refractory cases, can often be effectively treated with chemotherapy or immunomodulatory approaches such as intravenous immunoglobulin.[122–126] Treatment of an underlying infection or malignancy, while necessary, may be inadequate in cases of secondary HLH, necessitating HLH-type therapy. Thus, in cases of infection-associated or malignancy-associated HLH, there is often a need to sequentially treat both the HLH and the underlying disorder in order to achieve complete remission. HSCT is usually necessary in patients with recurrent secondary HLH.

The current Histiocyle Society international study, HLH-2004, is based on the HLH-94 study. The HLH-94 protocol achieved an estimated survival rate of 55% at a median of about 3 years of follow-up. This rate was slightly lower in patients with familial HLH (51%), although patients who underwent bone marrow transplantation had a 3-year survival probability of 62%. As a significant number of patients on HLH-94 died prior to receiving bone marrow transplantation, the HLH-2004 protocol has been modified so that cyclosporin is administered concurrently with dexamethasone and etoposide at the beginning of therapy with the goal of improving on the early treatment failure rate.[66]

Survivorship issues

The primary long-term sequelae of HLH are mainly related to the extent of CNS involvement. Prompt initiation of systemic therapy is critical for reducing CNS morbidity in HLH. Although the benefits of intrathecal therapy have not been clinically proven, inclusion of intrathecal therapy in patients with documented CNS disease is recommended.[91,127–129] Close follow-up of neurologic function is critical in order to assess the developmental delay that has been observed in these patients. It remains unclear if the neurologic complications are a direct result of disease involvement, therapy or infectious complications.[130] Long-term follow-up is a critical part of the care of HLH patients and should include observation for CNS effects, bone marrow transplant-related morbidities, and secondary acute myeloid leukemia related to the use of etoposide.[131]

Sinus histiocytosis with massive lymphadenopathy (Rosai–Dorfman disease)

Other members of the class II histiocytoses tend to have a more indolent course than HLH. Sinus histiocytosis with massive lymphadenopathy (SHML), also known as Rosai–Dorfman disease, is characterized by a lymphohistiocytic accumulation in the sinuses of lymph nodes without architectural effacement.[132] The proliferative macrophages seen in this disorder are typically S100 positive but CD1a negative and can be characteristically observed to wrap around intact lymphocytes or other cells, a process known as emperipolesis. SHML has a predilection for lymph nodes of the head and neck but can be seen in any organ including the CNS.[133–137] SHML more commonly occurs in patients of African ancestry; and is not typically responsive to most therapeutic approaches.[138] Recent reports have documented response to therapy with high-dose dexamethasone and also with 2-CDA.[133,139,140] Although SHML can be potentially disfiguring, it is only rarely life-threatening.

Malignant (class III) histiocytoses

This class of disorders consists of malignant histiocytosis, his-

tiocytic sarcoma and acute monocytic leukemia. For the most part, these disorders can be characterized by malignant transformation of cells of the MPS with significant cellular atypia. Those disorders characterized by malignant transformation of dendritic cells are often treated with lymphoma/leukemia protocols, including HSCT, although outcomes remain relatively poor. The wide variety of these conditions, the rarity of occurrence in pediatrics, and discussion elsewhere in this book (see Chapter 16) preclude a more detailed discussion here.

Challenges

Important landmarks have been achieved in our understanding of LCH since the first descriptions from the 1800s. We have a better understanding of the normal and abnormal responses of cells belonging to the MPS as well as of the etiology, presentation, natural history and treatment of LCH. Nevertheless, large numbers of patients remain undiagnosed or inadequately treated or simply do not respond to current therapies. The outcome for patients with LCH, particularly with refractory disease or disease involving organs such as the bone marrow, liver, lung and CNS, remains poor. The cure rate of HLH still remains close to 50%, with many survivors having significant adverse long-term sequelae. The formation of the Histiocyte Society has helped establish a framework within which collaborative studies can be undertaken. Future efforts should focus on further defining the etiology of LCH and understanding the molecular pathways with the goal of identifying molecular targets for more effective treatment and improved outcomes. Additionally, improved clinical understanding of the natural history of the histiocytoses is an important key to early diagnosis and appropriate therapy. Cooperative group clinical trials involving multidisciplinary approaches, particularly involving medical and pediatric oncologists, should help establish future improvements in outcome for patients with histiocytosis.

References

1. Writing Group of the Histiocyte Society. Histiocytosis syndromes in children. *Lancet* 1987; **i**: 208–9.
2. Favara BE, Feller AC, Pauli M *et al.* Contemporary classification of histiocytic disorders. The WHO Committee on Histiocytic/Reticulum Cell Proliferations. Reclassification Working Group of the Histiocyte Society. *Med Pediatr Oncol* 1997; **29**: 157–66.
3. Metchnikoff E. *Immunity in Infective Disease*. Cambridge: Cambridge University Press, 1905.
4. Aschoff L. Das Reticulo-Endotheliale System. *Ergebn Inn Med Kinderhulk* 1924; **26**: 1–118.
5. Hume DA, Ross IL, Himes SR, Sasmono RT, Wells CA, Ravasi

T. The mononuclear phagocyte system revisited. *J Leukoc Biol* 2002; **72**: 621–7.

6. Gordon S. Macrophages and the immune response. In: Paul WE (ed.) *Fundamental Immunology*. Philadelphia: Lippincott Williams and Wilkins, 2003, pp. 481–95.

7. Wiktor-Jedrzejczak W, Bartocci A, Ferrante AW Jr *et al*. Total absence of colony-stimulating factor 1 in the macrophage-deficient osteopetrotic (op/op) mouse. *Proc Natl Acad Sci USA* 1990; **87**: 4828–32.

8. Riches D. Monocytes, macrophages and dendritic cells of the lung. In: Murray J (ed.) *Textbook of Respiratory Medicine*. Philadelphia: WB Saunders, 2000, pp. 385–412.

9. Takahashi K, Naito M, Shultz LD, Hayashi S, Nishikawa S. Differentiation of dendritic cell populations in macrophage colony-stimulating factor-deficient mice homozygous for the osteopetrosis (op) mutation. *J Leukoc Biol* 1993; **53**: 19–28.

10. McClain KL, Natkunam Y, Swerdlow SH. Atypical cellular disorders. *Hematology (Am Soc Hematol Educ Program)* 2004; 283–96.

11. Laman JD, Leenen PJ, Annels NE, Hogendoorn PC, Egeler RM. Langerhans-cell histiocytosis: insight into DC biology. *Trends Immunol* 2003; **24**: 190–6.

12. Annels NE, Da Costa CE, Prins FA, Willemze A, Hogendoorn PC, Egeler RM. Aberrant chemokine receptor expression and chemokine production by Langerhans cells underlies the pathogenesis of Langerhans cell histiocytosis. *J Exp Med* 2003; **197**: 1385–90.

13. Egeler RM, Favara BE, van Meurs M, Laman JD, Claassen E. Differential in situ cytokine profiles of Langerhans-like cells and T cells in Langerhans cell histiocytosis: abundant expression of cytokines relevant to disease and treatment. *Blood* 1999; **94**: 4195–201.

14. Fleming MD, Pinkus JL, Fournier MV *et al*. Coincident expression of the chemokine receptors CCR6 and CCR7 by pathologic Langerhans cells in Langerhans cell histiocytosis. *Blood* 2003; **101**: 2473–5.

15. Steinman RM, Cohn ZA. Identification of a novel cell type in peripheral lymphoid organs of mice. I. Morphology, quantitation, tissue distribution. *J Exp Med* 1973; **137**: 1142–62.

16. Arceci RJ. The histiocytoses: the fall of the Tower of Babel. *Eur J Cancer* 1999; **35**: 747–67; discussion 767–9.

17. Moser M. Dendritic cells. In: William PE (ed.) *Fundamental Immunology*. Philadelphia: Lippincott Wiiliams and Wilkins, 2003, pp. 455–80.

18. Abbas A, Lichtman AH, Jordan SP. Cells and tissues of the immune system. *Cellular and Molecular Immunology*. Abbas A, Lichtman AH, Jordan SP. Fourth edition. Philadelphia: WB Saunders, 2000, pp. 17–38.

19. Guerriero A, Langmuir PB, Spain LM, Scott EW. PU.1 is required for myeloid-derived but not lymphoid-derived dendritic cells. *Blood* 2000; **95**: 879–85.

20. Anderson KL, Perkin H, Surh CD, Venturini S, Maki RA, Torbett BE. Transcription factor PU.1 is necessary for development of thymic and myeloid progenitor-derived dendritic cells. *J Immunol* 2000; **164**: 1855–61.

21. Valledor AF, Borras FE, Cullell-Young M, Celada A. Transcription factors that regulate monocyte/macrophage differentiation. *J Leukoc Biol* 1998; **63**: 405–17.

22. Nezelof C, Basset F, Rousseau MF. Histiocytosis X: histogenetic arguments for a Langerhans cell origin. *Biomedicine* 1973; **18**: 365–71.

23. Geissmann F, Lepelletier Y, Fraitag S *et al*. Differentiation of Langerhans cells in Langerhans cell histiocytosis. *Blood* 2001; **97**: 1241–8.

24. Kannourakis G, Abbas A. The role of cytokines in the pathogenesis of Langerhans cell histiocytosis. *Br J Cancer Suppl* 1994; **23**: S37–S40.

25. Emile JF, Fraitag S, Andry P, Leborgne M, Lellouch-Tubiana A, Brousse N. Expression of GM-CSF receptor by Langerhans' cell histiocytosis cells. *Virchows Arch* 1995; **427**: 125–9.

26. Nezelof C, Basset F. An hypothesis for Langerhans cell histiocytosis: the failure of the immune system to switch from an innate to an adaptive mode. *Pediatr Blood Cancer* 2004; **42**: 398–400.

27. Egeler RM, Annels NE, Hogendoorn PC. Langerhans cell histiocytosis: a pathologic combination of oncogenesis and immune dysregulation. *Pediatr Blood Cancer* 2004; **42**: 401–3.

28. Arico M, Clementi R, Caselli D, Danesino C. Histiocytic disorders. *Hematol J* 2003; **4**: 171–9.

29. Willman CL, Busque L, Griffith BB *et al*. Langerhans'-cell histiocytosis (histiocytosis X): a clonal proliferative disease. *N Engl J Med* 1994; **331**: 154–60.

30. Yu RC, Chu C, Buluwela L, Chu AC. Clonal proliferation of Langerhans cells in Langerhans cell histiocytosis. *Lancet* 1994; **343**: 767–8.

31. Murakami I, Gogusev J, Fournet JC, Glorion C, Jaubert F. Detection of molecular cytogenetic aberrations in Langerhans cell histiocytosis of bone. *Hum Pathol* 2002; **33**: 555–60.

32. Dacic S, Trusky C, Bakker A, Finkelstein SD, Yousem SA. Genotypic analysis of pulmonary Langerhans cell histiocytosis. *Hum Pathol* 2003; **34**: 1345–9.

33. Egeler RM, Neglia JP, Arico M, Favara BE, Heitger A, Nesbit ME. Acute leukemia in association with Langerhans cell histiocytosis. *Med Pediatr Oncol* 1994; **23**: 81–5.

34. Egeler RM, Neglia JP, Arico M *et al*. The relation of Langerhans cell histiocytosis to acute leukemia, lymphomas, and other solid tumors. The LCH-Malignancy Study Group of the Histiocyte Society. *Hematol Oncol Clin North Am* 1998; **12**: 369–78.

35. Glotzbecker MP, Carpentieri DF, Dormans JP. Langerhans cell histiocytosis: a primary viral infection of bone? Human herpes virus 6 latent protein detected in lymphocytes from tissue of children. *J Pediatr Orthop* 2004; **24**: 123–9.

36. Bernstrand C, Carstensen H, Jakobsen B, Svejgaard A, Henter JI, Olerup O. Immunogenetic heterogeneity in single-system and multisystem langerhans cell histiocytosis. *Pediatr Res* 2003; **54**: 30–6.

37. Schouten B, Egeler RM, Leenen PJ, Taminiau AH, van den Broek LJ, Hogendoorn PC. Expression of cell cycle-related gene products in Langerhans cell histiocytosis. *J Pediatr Hematol Oncol* 2002; **24**: 727–32.

38. Arceci RJ, Longley BJ, Emanuel PD. Atypical cellular disorders. *Hematology (Am Soc Hematol Educ Program)* 2002; 297–314.

39. Arceci RJ, Grabowski GA. Histiocytosis and disorders of the reticuloendothelial system. In: Handin RI, Lux SE, Stossel TP (eds) *Blood: Principles and Practice of Hematology*. Philadelphia: Lippincott Williams & Wilkins, 2003, pp. 921–57.

40. Carstensen H, Ornvold K. The epidemiology of LCH in children in Denmark. *Med Pediatr Oncol* 1993; **21**: 387–88.

41. Henter JI, Tondini C, Pritchard J. Histiocyte disorders. *Crit Rev Oncol Hematol* 2004; **50**: 157–74.

42. Hamre M, Hedberg J, Buckley J et al. Langerhans cell histiocytosis: an exploratory epidemiologic study of 177 cases. *Med Pediatr Oncol* 1997; **28**: 92–7.

43. Bhatia S, Nesbit ME Jr, Egeler RM, Buckley JD, Mertens A, Robison LL. Epidemiologic study of Langerhans cell histiocytosis in children. *J Pediatr* 1997; **130**: 774–84.

44. Gadner H, Grois N, Milen M, Potschger U, Thiem E. LCH-III, treatment protocol of the Third International Study for Langerhans cell histiocytosis, *Histiocyte Society*, April 2001.

45. Lahey E. Histiocytosis X: an analysis of prognostic factors. *J Pediatr* 1975; **87**: 184–9.

46. Calming U, Bemstrand C, Mosskin M, Elander SS, Ingvar M, Henter JI. Brain 18-FDG PET scan in central nervous system Langerhans cell histiocytosis. *J Pediatr* 2002; **141**: 435–40.

47. Grois N, Potschger U, Prosch H et al. Risk factors for diabetes insipidus in Langerhans cell histiocytosis. *Pediatr Blood Cancer* 2006; **46**: 228–33.

48. Grois N, Prayer D, Prosch H, Lassmann H. Neuropathology of CNS disease in Langerhans cell histiocytosis. *Brain* 2005; **128**: 829–38.

49. Grois N, Prayer D, Prosch H, Minkov M, Potschger U, Gadner H. Course and clinical impact of magnetic resonance imaging findings in diabetes insipidus associated with Langerhans cell histiocytosis. *Pediatr Blood Cancer* 2004; **43**: 59–65.

50. Grois NG, Favara BE, Mostbeck GH, Prayer D. Central nervous system disease in Langerhans cell histiocytosis. *Hematol Oncol Clin North Am* 1998; **12**: 287–305.

51. Goldberg-Stern H, Weitz R, Zaizov R, Gornish M, Gadoth N. Progressive spinocerebellar degeneration "plus" associated with Langerhans cell histiocytosis: a new paraneoplastic syndrome? *J Neurol Neurosurg Psychiatry* 1995; **58**: 180–3.

52. Vassallo R, Ryu JH. Pulmonary Langerhans' cell histiocytosis. *Clin Chest Med* 2004; **25**: 561–71, vii.

53. Vassallo R, Ryu JH, Schroeder DR, Decker PA, Limper AH. Clinical outcomes of pulmonary Langerhans'-cell histiocytosis in adults. *N Engl J Med* 2002; **346**: 484–90.

54. Shahlaee AH, Arceci RJ, Chernick V, Wilmott R. Histiocytic disorders of the lung. In: Boat T (ed.) *Kendigs Disorders of the Respiratory Tract in Children*. In press.

55. Ceci A, de Terlizzi M, Colella R et al. Langerhans cell histiocytosis in childhood: results from the Italian Cooperative AIEOP-CNR-H.X '83 study. *Med Pediatr Oncol* 1993; **21**: 259–64.

56. Gadner H, Heitger A, Grois N, Gatterer-Menz I, Ladisch S. Treatment strategy for disseminated Langerhans cell histiocytosis. DAL HX-83 Study Group. *Med Pediatr Oncol* 1994; **23**: 72–80.

57. Ladisch S, Gadner H. Treatment of Langerhans cell histiocytosis: evolution and current approaches. *Br J Cancer Suppl* 1994; **23**: S41–S46.

58. Ladisch S, Gadner H, Arico M et al. LCH-I: a randomized trial of etoposide vs. vinblastine in disseminated Langerhans cell histiocytosis. The Histiocyte Society. *Med Pediatr Oncol* 1994; **23**: 107–10.

59. Minkov M, Grois N, Heitger A, Potschger U, Westermeier T, Gadner H. Treatment of multisystem Langerhans cell histiocytosis. Results of the DAL-HX 83 and DAL-HX 90 studies. DAL-HX Study Group. *Klin Padiatr* 2000; **212**: 139–44.

60. Minkov M, Grois N, Broadbent V, Ceci A, Jakobson A, Ladisch S. Cyclosporine A therapy for multisystem langerhans cell histiocytosis. *Med Pediatr Oncol* 1999; **33**: 482–5.

61. Weitzman S, Wayne AS, Arceci R, Lipton JM, Whitlock JA. Nucleoside analogues in the therapy of Langerhans cell histiocytosis: a survey of members of the Histiocyte Society and review of the literature. *Med Pediatr Oncol* 1999; **33**: 476–81.

62. Bernard F, Thomas C, Bertrand Y et al. Multi-centre pilot study of 2-chlorodeoxyadenosine and cytosine arabinoside combined chemotherapy in refractory Langerhans cell histiocytosis with haematological dysfunction. *Eur J Cancer* 2005; **41**: 2682–9.

63. Saven A, Piro LD. 2-Chlorodeoxyadenosine: a potent antimetabolite with major activity in the treatment of indolent lymphoproliferative disorders. *Hematol Cell Ther* 1996; **38** (suppl. 2): S93–S101.

64. Stine KC, Saylors RL, Williams LL, Becton DL. 2-Chlorodeoxyadenosine (2-CDA) for the treatment of refractory or recurrent Langerhans cell histiocytosis (LCH) in pediatric patients. *Med Pediatr Oncol* 1997; **29**: 288–92.

65. Thomas L, Ducros B, Secchi T, Balme B, Moulin G. Successful treatment of adult Langerhans cell histiocytosis with thalidomide. Report of two cases and literature review. *Arch Dermatol* 1993; **129**: 1261–4.

66. Henter JI, Karlen J, Calming U, Bernstrand C, Andersson U, Fadeel B. Successful treatment of Langerhans'-cell histiocytosis with etanercept. *N Engl J Med* 2001; **345**: 1577–8.

67. McClain KL, Kozinetz CA. A phase II trial using thalidomide for Langerhans cell histiocytosis. *Pediatr Blood Cancer* 2005.

68. Jordan MB, McClain KL, Yan X, Hicks J, Jaffe R. Anti-CD52 antibody, alemtuzumab, binds to Langerhans cells in Langerhans cell histiocytosis. *Pediatr Blood Cancer* 2005; **44**: 251–4.

69. Steiner M, Matthes-Martin S, Attarbaschi A et al. Improved outcome of treatment-resistant high-risk Langerhans cell histiocytosis after allogeneic stem cell transplantation with reduced-intensity conditioning. *Bone Marrow Transplant* 2005; **36**: 215–25.

70. Haupt R, Nanduri V, Calevo MG et al. Permanent consequences in Langerhans cell histiocytosis patients: a pilot study from the Histiocyte Society Late Effects Study Group. *Pediatr Blood Cancer* 2004; **42**: 438–44.

71. Cervera A, Madero L, Garcia Penas JJ et al. CNS sequelae in Langerhans cell histiocytosis: progressive spinocerebellar degeneration as a late manifestation of the disease. *Pediatr Hematol Oncol* 1997; **14**: 577–84.

72. Whitsett SF, Kneppers K, Coppes MJ, Egeler RM. Neuropsychologic deficits in children with Langerhans cell histiocytosis. *Med Pediatr Oncol* 1999; **33**: 486–92.

73. Nanduri VR, Lillywhite L, Chapman C, Parry L, Pritchard J, Vargha-Khadem F. Cognitive outcome of long-term survivors of multisystem Langerhans cell histiocytosis: a single-institution, cross-sectional study. *J Clin Oncol* 2003; **21**: 2961–7.

74. Braier J, Ciocca M, Latella A, de Davila MG, Drajer M, Imventarza O. Cholestasis, sclerosing cholangitis, and liver transplantation in Langerhans cell histiocytosis. *Med Pediatr Oncol* 2002; **38**: 178–82.

75. Caputo R, Marzano AV, Passoni E, Fassati LR, Agnelli F. Sclerosing cholangitis and liver transplantation in Langerhans cell histiocytosis: a 14-year follow-up. *Dermatology* 2004; **209**: 335–7.

76. Egeler RM, Neglia JP, Puccetti DM, Brennan CA, Nesbit ME. Association of Langerhans cell histiocytosis with malignant neoplasms. *Cancer* 1993; **71**: 865–73.

77. Weitzman S, Jaffe R. Uncommon histiocytic disorders: the non-Langerhans cell histiocytoses. *Pediatr Blood Cancer* 2005; **45**: 256–64.

78. Zelger BW, Sidoroff A, Orchard G, Cerio R. Non-Langerhans cell histiocytoses. A new unifying concept. *Am J Dermatopathol* 1996; **18**: 490–504.

79. Dehner LP. Juvenile xanthogranulomas in the first two decades of life: a clinicopathologic study of 174 cases with cutaneous and extracutaneous manifestations. *Am J Surg Pathol* 2003; **27**: 579–93.

80. Janssen D, Harms D. Juvenile xanthogranuloma in childhood and adolescence: a clinicopathologic study of 129 patients from the Kiel pediatric tumor registry. *Am J Surg Pathol* 2005; **29**: 21–8.

81. Nakatani T, Morimoto A, Kato R *et al*. Successful treatment of congenital systemic juvenile xanthogranuloma with Langerhans cell histiocytosis-based chemotherapy. *J Pediatr Hematol Oncol* 2004; **26**: 371–4.

82. Freyer DR, Kennedy R, Bostrom BC, Kohut G, Dehner LP. Juvenile xanthogranuloma: forms of systemic disease and their clinical implications. *J Pediatr* 1996; **129**: 227–37.

83. Shin HT, Harris MB, Orlow SJ. Juvenile myelomonocytic leukemia presenting with features of hemophagocytic lymphohistiocytosis in association with neurofibromatosis and juvenile xanthogranulomas. *J Pediatr Hematol Oncol* 2004; **26**: 591–5.

84. Royer P, Blondet C, Guihard J. [Xantholeukemia in infants and Recklinghausen's neurofibromatosis.] *Sem Hop* 1958; **34**: 1504–13/P.

85. Zvulunov A, Barak Y, Metzker A. Juvenile xanthogranuloma, neurofibromatosis, and juvenile chronic myelogenous leukemia. World statistical analysis. *Arch Dermatol* 1995; **131**: 904–8.

86. Morier P, Merot Y, Paccaud D, Beck D, Frenk E. Juvenile chronic granulocytic leukemia, juvenile xanthogranulomas, and neurofibromatosis. Case report and review of the literature. *J Am Acad Dermatol* 1990; **22**: 962–5.

87. Veyssier-Belot C, Cacoub P, Caparros-Lefebvre D *et al*. Erdheim–Chester disease. Clinical and radiologic characteristics of 59 cases. *Medicine (Baltimore)* 1996; **75**: 157–69.

88. Opie KM, Kaye J, Vinciullo C. Erdheim–Chester disease. *Australas J Dermatol* 2003; **44**: 194–8.

89. Braiteh F, Boxrud C, Esmaeli B, Kurzrock R. Successful treatment of Erdheim–Chester disease, a non-Langerhans cell histiocytosis, with interferon-alpha. *Blood* 2005; Nov 1; **106**(9): 2992–4.

90. Henter JI, Elinder G, Ost A. Diagnostic guidelines for hemophagocytic lymphohistiocytosis. The FHL Study Group of the Histiocyte Society. *Semin Oncol* 1991; **18**: 29–33.

91. Henter JI, Samuelsson-Horne A, Arico M *et al*. Treatment of hemophagocytic lymphohistiocytosis with HLH-94

92. Fadeel B, Orrenius S, Henter JI. Induction of apoptosis and caspase activation in cells obtained from familial haemophagocytic lymphohistiocytosis patients. *Br J Haematol* 1999; **106**: 406–15.

93. Fadeel B, Henter JI, Orrenius S. [Apoptosis required for maintenance of homeostasis: familial hemophagocytic lymphohistiocytosis caused by too little cell death]. *Lakartidningen* 2000; **97**: 1395–1400, 1402.

94. Perez N, Virelizier JL, Arenzana-Seisdedos F, Fischer A, Griscelli C. Impaired natural killer activity in lymphohistiocytosis syndrome. *J Pediatr* 1984; **104**: 569–73.

95. Arico M, Nespoli L, Maccario R *et al*. Natural cytotoxicity impairment in familial haemophagocytic lymphohistiocytosis. *Arch Dis Child* 1988; **63**: 292–6.

96. Henter JI, Elinder G, Soder O, Hansson M, Andersson B, Andersson U. Hypercytokinemia in familial hemophagocytic lymphohistiocytosis. *Blood* 1991; **78**: 2918–22.

97. Fujiwara F, Hibi S, Imashuku S. Hypercytokinemia in hemophagocytic syndrome. *Am J Pediatr Hematol Oncol* 1993; **15**: 92–8.

98. Osugi Y, Hara J, Tagawa S *et al*. Cytokine production regulating Th1 and Th2 cytokines in hemophagocytic lymphohistiocytosis. *Blood* 1997; **89**: 4100–3.

99. Stepp SE, Dufourcq-Lagelouse R, Le Deist F *et al*. Perforin gene defects in familial hemophagocytic lymphohistiocytosis. *Science* 1999; **286**: 1957–9.

100. Feldmann J, Callebaut I, Raposo G *et al*. Munc13-4 is essential for cytolytic granules fusion and is mutated in a form of familial hemophagocytic lymphohistiocytosis (FHL3). *Cell* 2003; **115**: 461–73.

101. zur Stadt U, Schmidt S, Kasper B *et al*. Linkage of familial hemophagocytic lymphohistiocytosis (FHL) type-4 to chromosome 6q24 and identification of mutations in syntaxin 11. *Hum Mol Genet* 2005; **14**: 827–34.

102. Lowin B, Peitsch MC, Tschopp J. Perforin and granzymes: crucial effector molecules in cytolytic T lymphocyte and natural killer cell-mediated cytotoxicity. *Curr Top Microbiol Immunol* 1995; **198**: 1–24.

103. Katano H, Cohen JI. Perforin and lymphohistiocytic proliferative disorders. *Br J Haematol* 2005; **128**: 739–50.

104. Schneider EM, Lorenz I, Muller-Rosenberger M, Steinbach G, Kron M, Janka-Schaub GE. Hemophagocytic lympho-histiocytosis is associated with deficiencies of cellular cytolysis but normal expression of transcripts relevant to killer-cell-induced apoptosis. *Blood* 2002; **100**: 2891–8.

105. Introne W, Boissy RE, Gahl WA. Clinical, molecular, and cell biological aspects of Chediak–Higashi syndrome. *Mol Genet Metab* 1999; **68**: 283–303.

106. Sanal O, Ersoy F, Tezcan I *et al*. Griscelli disease: genotype–phenotype correlation in an array of clinical heterogeneity. *J Clin Immunol* 2002; **22**: 237–43.

107. Arico M, Imashuku S, Clementi R *et al*. Hemophagocytic lymphohistiocytosis due to germline mutations in SH2D1A, the X-linked lymphoproliferative disease gene. *Blood* 2001; **97**: 1131–3.

108. Trapani JA, Davis J, Sutton VR, Smyth MJ. Proapoptotic

immunochemotherapy and bone marrow transplantation. *Blood* 2002; **100**: 2367–73.

functions of cytotoxic lymphocyte granule constituents in vitro and in vivo. *Curr Opin Immunol* 2000; **12**: 323–9.

109. Goransdotter Ericson K, Fadeel B, Nilsson-Ardnor S *et al.* Spectrum of perforin gene mutations in familial hemophagocytic lymphohistiocytosis. *Am J Hum Genet* 2001; **68**: 590–7.

110. Molleran Lee S, Villanueva J, Sumegi J *et al.* Characterisation of diverse PRF1 mutations leading to decreased natural killer cell activity in North American families with haemophagocytic lymphohistiocytosis. *J Med Genet* 2004; **41**: 137–44.

111. Ishii E, Ueda I, Shirakawa R *et al.* Genetic subtypes of familial hemophagocytic lymphohistiocytosis: correlations with clinical features and cytotoxic T lymphocyte/natural killer cell functions. *Blood* 2005; **105**: 3442–8.

112. Henter JI, Elinder G, Soder O, Ost A. Incidence in Sweden and clinical features of familial hemophagocytic lymphohistiocytosis. *Acta Paediatr Scand* 1991; **80**: 428–35.

113. Ishii E, Ohga S, Tanimura M *et al.* Clinical and epidemiologic studies of familial hemophagocytic lymphohistiocytosis in Japan. Japan LCH Study Group. *Med Pediatr Oncol* 1998; **30**: 276–83.

114. Henter JI, Arico M, Elinder G, Imashuku S, Janka G. Familial hemophagocytic lymphohistiocytosis. Primary hemophagocytic lymphohistiocytosis. *Hematol Oncol Clin North Am* 1998; **12**: 417–33.

115. Ishii E, Ohga S, Imashuku S *et al.* Review of hemophagocytic lymphohistiocytosis (HLH) in children with focus on Japanese experiences. *Crit Rev Oncol Hematol* 2005; **53**: 209–23.

116. Arico M, Danesino C, Pende D, Moretta L. Pathogenesis of haemophagocytic lymphohistiocytosis. *Br J Haematol* 2001; **114**: 761–9.

117. Janka GE. Familial hemophagocytic lymphohistiocytosis. *Eur J Pediatr* 1983; **140**: 221–30.

118. Stark B, Hershko C, Rosen N, Cividalli G, Karsai H, Soffer D. Familial hemophagocytic lymphohistiocytosis (FHLH) in Israel. I. Description of 11 patients of Iranian-Iraqi origin and review of the literature. *Cancer* 1984; **54**: 2109–21.

119. Stephan JL, Donadieu J, Ledeist F, Blanche S, Griscelli C, Fischer A. Treatment of familial hemophagocytic lymphohistiocytosis with antithymocyte globulins, steroids, and cyclosporin A. *Blood* 1993; **82**: 2319–23.

120. Arico M, Janka G, Fischer A *et al.* Hemophagocytic lymphohistiocytosis. Report of 122 children from the International Registry. FHL Study Group of the Histiocyte Society. *Leukemia* 1996; **10**: 197–203.

121. Henter JI, Arico M, Egeler RM *et al.* HLH-94: a treatment protocol for hemophagocytic lymphohistiocytosis. HLH study Group of the Histiocyte Society. *Med Pediatr Oncol* 1997; **28**: 342–7.

122. Seidel MG, Kastner U, Minkov M, Gadner H. IVIG treatment of adenovirus infection-associated macrophage activation syndrome in a two-year-old boy: case report and review of the literature. *Pediatr Hematol Oncol* 2003; **20**: 445–51.

123. Fort DW, Buchanan GR. Treatment of infection-associated hemophagocytic syndrome with immune globulin. *J Pediatr* 1994; **124**: 332.

124. Freeman B, Rathore MH, Salman E, Joyce MJ, Pitel P. Intravenously administered immune globulin for the treatment of infection-associated hemophagocytic syndrome. *J Pediatr* 1993; **123**: 479–81.

125. Imashuku S, Kuriyama K, Sakai R *et al.* Treatment of Epstein–Barr virus-associated hemophagocytic lymphohistiocytosis (EBV-HLH) in young adults: a report from the HLH study center. *Med Pediatr Oncol* 2003; **41**: 103–9.

126. Larroche C, Bruneel F, Andre MH *et al.* Intravenously administered gamma-globulins in reactive hemaphagocytic syndrome. Multicenter study to assess their importance, by the immunoglobulins group of experts of CEDIT of the AP-HP. *Ann Med Interne (Paris)* 2000; **151**: 533–9.

127. Henter JI, Nennesmo I. Neuropathologic findings and neurologic symptoms in twenty-three children with hemophagocytic lymphohistiocytosis. *J Pediatr* 1997; **130**: 358–65.

128. Henter JI, Elinder G. Cerebromeningeal haemophagocytic lymphohistiocytosis. *Lancet* 1992; **339**: 104–7.

129. Haddad E, Sulis ML, Jabado N, Blanche S, Fischer A, Tardieu M. Frequency and severity of central nervous system lesions in hemophagocytic lymphohistiocytosis. *Blood* 1997; **89**: 794–800.

130. Sung L, King SM, Carcao M, Trebo M, Weitzman SS. Adverse outcomes in primary hemophagocytic lymphohistiocytosis. *J Pediatr Hematol Oncol* 2002; **24**: 550–4.

131. Henter JI, Elinder G, Lubeck PO, Ost A. Myelodysplastic syndrome following epipodophyllotoxin therapy in familial hemophagocytic lymphohistiocytosis. *Pediatr Hematol Oncol* 1993; **10**: 163–8.

132. Foucar E, Rosai J, Dorfman R. Sinus histiocytosis with massive lymphadenopathy (Rosai–Dorfman disease): review of the entity. *Semin Diagn Pathol* 1990; **7**: 19–73.

133. Rodriguez-Galindo C, Helton KJ, Sanchez ND, Rieman M, Jeng M, Wang W. Extranodal Rosai–Dorfman disease in children. *J Pediatr Hematol Oncol* 2004; **26**: 19–24.

134. Z'Graggen W, Sturzenegger M, Mariani L, Keserue B, Kappeler A, Vajtai I. Isolated Rosai–Dorfman disease of intracranial meninges. *Pathol Res Pract* 2006; **202**(3): 165–70.

135. Purav P, Ganapathy K, Mallikarjuna VS *et al.* Rosai–Dorfman disease of the central nervous system. *J Clin Neurosci* 2005; **12**: 656–9.

136. Gies U, Gruia D, Lassmann H, Bergmann M. A case of rapidly progressive Rosai–Dorfman disease restricted to the central nervous system. *Zentralbl Neurochir* 2005; **66**: 142–6.

137. Sundaram C, Uppin SG, Prasad BC *et al.* Isolated Rosai Dorfman disease of the central nervous system presenting as dural-based and intraparenchymal lesions. *Clin Neuropathol* 2005; **24**: 112–17.

138. Pulsoni A, Anghel G, Falcucci P *et al.* Treatment of sinus histiocytosis with massive lymphadenopathy (Rosai–Dorfman disease): report of a case and literature review. *Am J Hematol* 2002; **69**: 67–71.

139. Stine KC, Westfall C. Sinus histiocytosis with massive lymphadenopathy (SHML) prednisone resistant but dexamethasone sensitive. *Pediatr Blood Cancer* 2005; **44**: 92–4.

140. Tasso M, Esquembre C, Blanco E, Moscardo C, Niveiro M, Paya A. Sinus histiocytosis with massive lymphadenopathy (Rosai–Dorfman disease) treated with 2-chloro-deoxyadenosine. *Pediatr Blood Cancer* 2005; Nov 21; [Epub ahead at pnnt].

16 Acute myeloid leukemia

Leslie S. Kean, Robert J. Arceci and William G. Woods

Overview

Acute myeloid leukemia (AML) constitutes a heterogeneous group of hematologic malignancies that are derived from early hematopoietic progenitors and show myeloid, monocytic, erythroid and megakaryocytic phenotypic characteristics.[1-5] AML is the major subtype of acute leukemia in adults, but only represents 15% of newly diagnosed cases of acute leukemia in children. The complexity and challenge of AML is revealed in the fact that despite its relatively low prevalence, it nonetheless accounts for over 30% of the annual pediatric mortality attributed to leukemia.[5-8]

Before the 1970s, nearly all patients who were diagnosed with AML died of their disease. The introduction of cytara-bine (AraC) and the anthracycline class of chemotherapeutic agents to the treatment of AML in the 1960s and early 1970s marked a major milestone, and for the first time resulted in the majority of patients (60–70%) achieving a remission.[9,10] Optimization of AraC/anthracycline-based regimens resulted in greater rates of first remission (70–85%), and dose-intensification of therapy led to increased 5-year survival (Fig. 16.1). Currently, most large studies achieve 5-year event-free-survival (EFS) approaching 50%.[4,5,11-37] Although this represents a major improvement in cure, most patients with AML still die of their disease. The current focus of AML research and treatment is thus twofold. First, new therapeutic regimens are being studied that are designed both to increase the rate of first remission and to improve the "quality" of this remission, so that the risk of relapse is reduced. Second, a

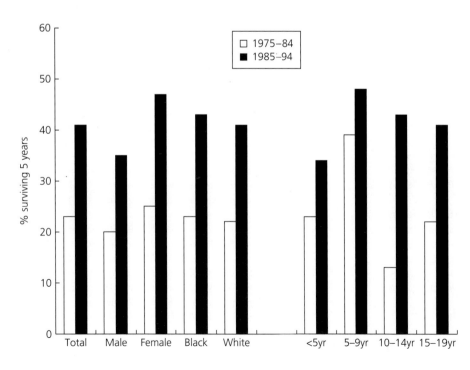

Fig. 16.1 AML 5-year relative survival rates by sex, race, age and time period, comparing SEER (Surveillance, Epidemiology and End Results) data from 1975–1984 and 1985–1994.[39]

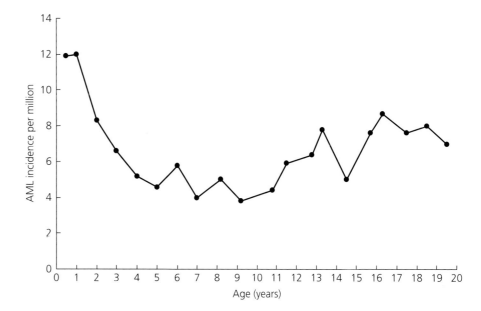

Fig. 16.2 Age-specific AML incidence rates, including all races and both sexes; data are from SEER (Surveillance, Epidemiology and End Results) 1976–1984 and 1986–1994 combined.[39]

molecular dissection of this heterogeneous class of diseases is ongoing. This will allow risk-stratification of patients based on their individual molecular defects and provide the knowledge base for future therapeutic strategies based on targeted inhibitors of the aberrant pathways that lead to the development of AML.

Epidemiology

Each year, approximately 10 000 children (ages 0–21 years) worldwide develop AML. Current epidemiologic studies predict approximately 600 new cases of AML in the USA and 100 new cases of AML in the UK per year.[38–40] This is in contrast to acute lymphocytic leukemia (ALL), which remains four times more common than AML in US children. The exception to this statistic is the neonatal period, in which AML incidence shows a relative peak. The incidence of AML is stable until the teenage years, when a small increase in incidence is noted, followed by a steadily increasing incidence during adulthood (Fig. 16.2). There is no difference in the incidence of AML in males compared with females and there has been no change in the worldwide incidence of childhood AML when statistics for the past two decades are compared.[39,40]

Racial variation can be observed in AML. In the USA, white children have historically exhibited an increased incidence compared with black children, whereas Hispanic children had the highest incidence of the three racial groups (as high as 9 cases per million in Los Angeles).[39,41] The most recent Surveillance, Epidemiology and End Results (SEER) data (years 1986–1995) demonstrated less marked differences between white and black children < 20 years, with the incidence of AML in these two populations being 6.7 and

6.4 per million, respectively.[39–41] A higher incidence of AML appears to occur in Asia (11 cases per million in China) compared with the USA, and a lower incidence in India (3.5 cases per million). The mechanisms underlying these differences have not yet been determined.

In addition to ethnicity, environmental and genetic risk factors have also been shown to influence the risk of developing AML (Tables 16.1 and 16.2).[3,38,41–52] The most common genetic risk factor is trisomy 21/Down syndrome (DS), which is associated with a 15-fold increase in the risk of leukemia (both ALL and AML) during childhood. Other genetic syndromes characterized by either chromosomal instability or cell-cycle dysregulation also increase the risk of developing AML. These include Bloom syndrome, neurofibromatosis type I and Klinefelter syndrome. Additionally, virtually all of the constitutional inborn errors of hematopoiesis are asso-

Table 16.1 Genetic risk factors in childhood AML.

Chromosomal disorders
Trisomy 21
Klinefelter syndrome
Bloom syndrome
Neurofibromatosis
Ataxia telangiectasia

Constitutional disorders of hematopoiesis
Fanconi anemia
Diamond–Blackfan syndrome
Shwachman–Diamond syndrome
Kostmann syndrome
Thrombocytopenia-absent radii syndrome
Familial thrombocytopenia

Table 16.2 Proven and potential environmental risk factors in childhood AML.

Maternal drug/cigarette/alcohol consumption
Maternal ingestion of topoisomerase II-containing foods
Ionizing radiation*
Cytotoxic chemotherapy (alkylating agents and epipodophyllotoxins)*
Petroleum products
Pesticides
Benzene*
Heavy metals

* Proven risk factors.

ciated with an increased risk of developing AML, including Fanconi anemia, Diamond–Blackfan syndrome, Kostmann disease, thrombocytopenia–absent radii syndrome, Shwachman–Diamond syndrome and familial thrombocytopenia.

Environmental risk factors for AML include both pre- and postnatal exposures (Table 16.2). Prenatally, diagnostic ionizing radiation and maternal drug and cigarette use have all been implicated.[42,44–47,49–51,53] Maternal prenatal diet may also affect the AML risk in children. Ross found that increased maternal consumption of foods containing topoisomerase 2 during pregnancy was associated with a tenfold higher risk of infant AML in a case-control study.[48] Postnatally, ionizing radiation and exposure to chemotherapeutic drugs including alkylating agents and epipodophyllotoxins both have been confirmed as increasing the risk of AML.[45,46,50,51,53–55] In addition, exposure of either the patient or the patient's parent to pesticides, petroleum products, benzene and heavy metals all have been associated with an increased risk of AML.[40,41] Although concerns persist about the possible leukemogenesis associated with exposure to electromagnetic fields, results of the case-control studies into the importance of this risk factor have been mixed. Thus, while studies from the UK,[56] Denver,[57,58] and Los Angeles[59] each supported an association between childhood leukemia and either proximity to high-voltage power lines or home wiring-configuration, other studies, based in Rhode Island,[60] Canada,[61] and Japan[62] found no such association. In addition, several small, case–control studies have shown that prenatal and postnatal electric blanket exposure was not associated with a statistically significant increase in the incidence of childhood or adult leukemia.[63,64]

Clinical manifestations at diagnosis

There is a large range of presenting signs and symptoms for pediatric AML. Life-threatening complications occur due to decreased normal hematopoiesis secondary to leukemic infiltration of the bone marrow as well as to organ dysfunction and failure as a result of leukemic infiltration.

Whereas the total white blood cell count (WBC) is often elevated in patients with AML, the number of normal, functional neutrophils is often quite low, resulting in neutropenia that places patients at increased risk for bacterial infections. Normocytic, normochromic anemia is another common hematologic abnormality that can result in headache, dizziness, fatigue, pallor and sometimes congestive heart failure. Patients with AML often present with bone pain, secondary to marrow replacement with leukemic blasts resulting in periosteal pressure. This may result in night-time waking, limp or back pain. Coagulopathy is a common presenting complication of AML, particularly in acute promyelocytic leukemia (APL) but also in acute myelomonocytic leukemia (AMML) and acute monocytic leukemia (AMoL) subtypes. The coagulopathy may result from thrombocytopenia as well as from disseminated intravascular coagulation (DIC) due either to infection or to the release of coagulant activity (e.g., thromboplastin activity) associated with the cytoplasmic granules of some AML blasts. DIC may worsen as therapy is initiated due to the increased release of these coagulant proteins associated with tumor lysis and leading to factor depletion and bleeding. Aggressive clotting factor replacement and platelet transfusions are frequently necessary to avoid catastrophic bleeding. Treatment with low-molecular weight heparin in order to inhibit microthrombi generation may be useful but remains controversial.

Organomegaly is seen in approximately half of patients with AML due to hepatic and splenic infiltration with leukemic blasts. Extramedullary leukemia (EML) is observed in 10–20% of patients, with gingival hypertrophy, lymphadenopathy, and leukemia cutis (palpable nontender nodules in the skin) being most common. Granulocytic sarcomas, or "chloromas," may involve other anatomic locations such as periorbital, paraspinal and intraorgan sites. Periorbital involvement may cause proptosis, and paraspinal chloromas invading the spinal canal may result in spinal cord compression. These manifestations are seen more commonly with the monocytic subtype of AML (M5 FAB subclass, described in detail below).

Given the large size of AML blasts and their adhesion properties, hyperleukocytosis can result in life-threatening complications. When the peripheral WBC is > 100×10^9/L, AML blasts can begin to clump, resulting in leukostasis and sludging of the blasts in small vessels. This in turn leads to cellular hypoxia, tissue infarction, and ultimately tissue hemorrhage. When this occurs in the central nervous system (CNS), the patient is at greatly increased risk for stroke and a somnolence syndrome that may progress to coma. Manifestations of hyperleukocytosis in the lungs include parenchymal infiltrates, pulmonary edema, respiratory failure and occasionally hemorrhage. Rapid lowering of the WBC is necessary, often using leukapheresis along with aggressive hydration. Definitive cytoreduction using chemotherapy should be instituted promptly, because other mechanisms for lowering

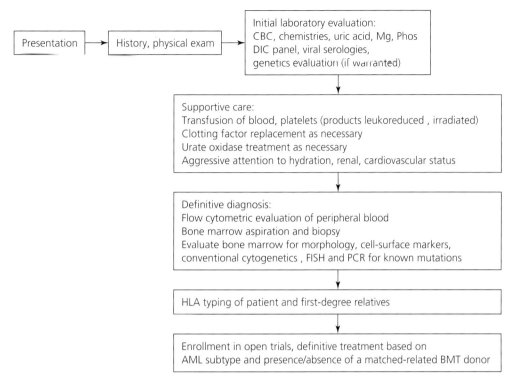

Fig. 16.3 Treatment algorithm for patients newly diagnosed with AML. BMT, bone marrow transplant; CBC, complete blood count; DIC, disseminated intravascular coagulation; FISH, fluorescence *in situ* hybridization; PCR, polymerase chain reaction.

the WBC will only provide temporary improvement. An exception to the recommendation of using leukapheresis for cytoreduction is APL. In APL, leukapheresis may activate the leukemic promyelocytes causing them to release coagulant-containing granules, thereby increasing the chance of DIC and fatal hemorrhage. Cytoreductive chemotherapy using all-*trans* retinoic acid (ATRA) and chemotherapy should instead be instituted promptly, with strong consideration for also using steroids.

After the initiation of cytoreductive therapy, tumor lysis syndrome can also lead to serious complications, especially in the setting of an initially high WBC. Treatment of hyperuricemia with the newly commercially available urate oxidase enzymes may lessen the renal complications associated with this by-product of leukemic blast lysis, but the complications of hyperphosphatemia, hypocalcemia and hyperkalemia continue to demand intensive supportive care interventions. Figure 16.3 depicts the treatment algorithm that should be followed in patients with newly diagnosed AML, from the initial patient encounter to the initiation of definitive therapy.

AML classification

AML is a heterogeneous group of diseases in which ultimate outcome varies widely. Although morphologic and cytogenetic changes (discussed below) have a major impact on outcome,

other factors may also play a role. These include initial WBC, age, race, the presence of primary versus secondary AML, and the ease with which first remission is achieved. WBC $< 100 \times 10^9$/L at diagnosis, patients greater than 1 year but less than 15 years of age, Caucasian race, the absence of secondary AML and rapid induction of complete remission (CR) are all associated with improved long-term outcome. These characteristics are often closely tied to morphologic and cytogenetic features that are increasingly appreciated as important predictors of AML prognosis.

The first comprehensive morphologic classification system for AML was the French–American–British (FAB) classification, which was established in 1976 and later revised in 1985.[65] Although this classification is based only on morphology and histochemical analysis of malignant cells (and not on either flow cytometric or molecular genetic phenotyping), it nonetheless provides a useful framework for classifying the subgroups of AML (Table 16.3). The FAB classification divides AML into eight subcategories based on morphology after staining with Wright, Wright–Giemsa, or May–Grunwald stains as well as a panel of histochemical markers. With the exception of the M6 and M7 subtypes, the original classification schema required 30% myeloblasts in the bone marrow in order to render a diagnosis of AML.

In 1997 the World Health Organization (WHO) revised the FAB classification by adding cytogenetic analysis to the classification of AML subtypes (Table 16.3).[66–70] Additionally, the WHO classification system lowered the malignant blast

Table 16.3 AML classification by both FAB and WHO criteria.

FAB

M0: minimally differentiated
M1: myeloblastic leukemia without maturation
M2: myeloblastic leukemia with maturation
M3: hypergranular promyelocytic leukemia
M4: myelomonocytic leukemia
M4Eo: variant, increase in marrow eosinophils
M5: monocytic leukemia
M6: erythroleukemia
M7: megakaryoblastic leukemia

WHO

AML with recurrent cytogenetic translocations
AML with t(8;21)(q22;q22) AML1-ETO fusion
Acute promyelocytic leukemia: AML with t(15;17)(q22q12) and
    variants PML-RARα fusion
AML with abnormal bone marrow eosinophils: inv(16)(p13q22);
    t(16;16)(p13q22): CBFβ-MYH1 fusion
AML with 11q23 MLL abnormalities

AML with multilineage dysplasia
With prior myelodysplastic syndrome
Without prior myelodysplastic syndrome

AML with myelodysplastic syndrome, therapy related
Alkylating agent-related
Epipodophyllotoxin-related
Other types

AML not otherwise categorized
AML minimally differentiated

percentage in the bone marrow needed for diagnosis of AML to 20% myeloblasts.

Although neither the FAB nor the WHO classification schemes formally utilizes flow cytometric immunophenotyping for subclassification, its clinical diagnostic use is now routine, and its use in evaluating the response to therapy is being intensely studied.[71–83] Flow cytometric detection of leukemic blasts is based on the multiparameter analysis of their aberrant pattern of expression of normal differentiation antigens. Using this approach, flow cytometry can also be used to determine quantitatively the persistence of leukemic blasts at levels as low as 1 blast per 10 000 mononuclear cells. What level of minimal-residual disease (MRD) will most accurately predict outcome is under investigation.[78,80,82,84]

Immunophenotyping studies have demonstrated significant associations between the expression of specific cell-surface markers and the WHO classification of AML subtypes. CD13, CD33, and c-Kit are the most commonly expressed myeloid markers in AML (present on the blasts of ~90% of patients). The FAB M4 subtype commonly expresses CDw14 (73% of M4 blasts expressed this antigen), CD15 (100%), CD13 (57%) and CD33 (92%). The M5 subtype shows a similar pattern of antigen expression, with the exception of CD13, which this subtype rarely expresses. In contrast, M1 and M2 blasts express lower levels of these markers, with CDw14 present in only about 14% of M1 and 19% of M2 cases. CD15 is expressed on about 38% and 44% of M1 and M2 cases, respectively. M1 and M2 blasts often express CD13, with 80% of M1 or M2 cases being positive for this marker.[71] AML blasts also frequently express lymphoid surface antigens. In a retrospective study by the Children's Cancer Group (CCG), 24% of AML cases expressed the B-lineage marker CD19 and 48% expressed one or more T-lineage cell surface antigens.[71] Expression of terminal deoxynucleotidyl transferase was much less common, being present in only 6% of AML cases. When analyzed across multiple multicenter trials over the last two decades, between 30 and 60% of AML cases express lymphoid markers.[71,76,78,82,83] There has been no definitive association with clinical outcome demonstrated due to lymphoid antigen expression in AML.

Cytogenetics and molecular markers

Cytogenetic and molecular analysis have identified molecular abnormalities that often correlate with morphologic and immunophenotypic subtypes as well as with AML prognosis.[71,85–91] Three approaches are commonly used. The first is conventional karyotyping, which demonstrates chromosome number (ploidy) as well as chromosomal structural changes such as regional amplifications and deletions, inversions or translocations. The second technique, fluorescent *in situ* hybridization (FISH), makes use of fluorescently labeled nucleic acid probes that are used to detect more subtle chromosomal abnormalities in both metaphase and interphase cell chromosomes as well as in many more leukemic cells (>500 cells routinely analyzed by FISH) than conventional cytogenetic analysis (~20 metaphase preparations routinely analyzed). FISH probes specific for distinct chromosomes, chromosomal segments or novel translocations are also a sensitive means to help establish a diagnosis or follow patients for the presence of MRD. Third, polymerase chain reaction (PCR) techniques can be used to identify specific genetic abnormalities such as inversions, deletions or translocations, based on their unique sequences. When coupled to DNA sequencing, this technique can detect single base-pair mutations in DNA, and is highly sensitive, being able to identify one mutation in as few as 100 000 bone marrow cells. Abnormal RNA transcripts, resulting from chromosomal translocations, can also be detected with high levels of sensitivity using reverse-transcription PCR (RT-PCR).

Gene expression profiling

The application of DNA microarray technology to the study of AML has already begun to reveal gene expression profiles that are both biologically important and clinically relevant.[92–105] In 2003, Yagi *et al.*[91] used microarray analysis to identify a subset of genes that were associated with AML prognosis, regardless of underlying karyotype or morphologic subtype. In 2004, Ross *et al.*[93] published the first large gene expression study of pediatric AML, which showed that expression profiles could be identified that correlate with each of the major prognostic and cytogenetic subtypes. Furthermore, this study determined that the gene clusters identified for pediatric AML subtypes also accurately predicted adult AML subtypes, underscoring the molecular similarity between AML diagnosed within a wide age range. Similar results with adult AML series are also emerging, confirming the diagnostic and prognostic power of microarray analysis. Larger studies with more AML patient samples, as well as increasingly detailed analysis of the important prognostic groups, are ongoing and should make this technology a part of standard-of-care for AML diagnosis and treatment planning in the future.

Risk-group stratification and prognostic factors

The last decade of AML research and treatment has witnessed a growing appreciation of the importance of identifying prognostic risk groups within the broader diagnosis of myeloid malignancies.[11,71,73,88,90,91,106–112] This stratification allows prediction of outcome based on the molecular phenotype at the time of diagnosis and can be used to direct different treatments. Stratification now includes several risk groups as well as treating patients with APL or infants with DS with separate therapeutic approaches.

Prognostically good cytogenetics

Several chromosomal abnormalities have emerged as predictors of good prognosis in children with AML: t(15;17)(q22;q12), inv(16)(p13q22), and t(8;21)(q22;q22).[85,86,88,89,106–108,113,114]

The t(15;17) translocation involves the fusion of the PML gene on chromosome 15 to the retinoic acid receptor alpha (RARA) on chromosome 17. It is pathognomonic of APL and absent in all other subtypes. This translocation results in recruitment of chromatin repressor complexes that involve both histone deacetylases (HDAC) and DNA methyltransferases, which in turn result in aberrant silencing of key genes in hematopoiesis.[115–120] Leukemic cells with the t(15;17) translocation are highly responsive to ATRA, which causes differentiation and apoptosis.[88,121–126] The latest results confirm that the combination of ATRA and chemotherapy results in an excellent prognosis, both in terms of success at achieving first remission (96%), survival (10-year overall survival of 89%), and EFS (76%).[126]

The inv(16) and t(8;21) translocations are characterized by disruption of *CBFβ* and *AML1* (also known as *CBFA2* or *RUNX1*) genes respectively.[108,113,114] These genes encode subunits of the core binding factor (CBF), a regulator of normal hematopoiesis. The t(8;21) translocation generates a novel fusion protein, AML1/ETO, which combines the DNA-binding properties of AML1 with the protein-binding properties of the product of the ETO gene. This fusion results in abnormal protein–protein signaling, blocking the normal function of AML1 in the transcriptional regulation of hematopoietic development. The chimeric protein continues to interact with CBFβ and bind DNA at the core enhancer sequence. However, the presence of ETO in the chimeric protein leads to the recruitment of proteins involved in transcriptional repression, similar to that observed with the PML/RARα fusion observed in APL. The inv(16) abnormality results in the creation of another fusion protein, CBFβ/MYH11, which also disrupts transcriptional regulation through CBFβ. The CBFβ/MYH11 chimeric protein continues to interact with AML1, but inhibits the binding of AML1 to DNA, functionally inactivating this crucial transcriptional regulator. These two different fusion proteins thus affect, in part, a common pathway, the core binding factor pathway, which normally functions as a transcriptional activation complex. Much work is now focused on identification of therapeutic approaches that could target these leukemia-specific fusion proteins.

The t(8;21) translocation is found predominantly in M1 and M2 AML subtypes, whereas the inv(16) mutation is seen most often in the M4 subtype associated with dysplastic eosinophilic precursors (M4Eo).[71] Patients who have inv(16)-positive AML have higher CR rates, superior EFS and better response to therapy after relapse. For this reason, most treatment approaches do not recommend allogeneic hematopoietic stem cell transplantation (HSCT) from HLA-matched family donors in first CR.[108–110] European and North American pediatric groups have extended this approach to include the t(8;21) subgroup, although there is still considerable data that indicate that allogeneic HSCT from HLA-matched family donors improves outcome for t(8;21) AML.[11,108–110]

Prognostically intermediate cytogenetics

Patients with normal cytogenetics and those with chromosomal translocations other than those described above have an intermediate prognosis. Although the patients without identifiable mutations by classic cytogenetic analysis have previously been classified as AML "not otherwise categorized" by the WHO, new data have recently emerged concerning the etiology of AML in a substantial number of these patients.[127] It was found that in approximately 30% of patients (ages 15–60 years) with primary AML and a normal karyotype, mutations occurred in the nucleophosmin (NPM) gene, which encodes a nucleocytoplasmic shuttling protein regulating the Alternative Reading Frame ARF–p53 tumor suppressor pathway.[127] Mutations often result in the aberrant cytoplasmic subcellular localization of this protein, which can be easily detected by immunohistochemical analysis. This new finding promises to have both diagnostic and prognostic significance. It may permit the identification of a new subgroup of intermediate-prognosis AML; and given that it was found to be absent in cases of secondary AML, could also be used to differentiate these two entities. The ultimate role of NPM in predicting the outcome of patients with AML and a normal karyotype will await more studies.

The *MLL* (for "mixed lineage leukemia") gene (also known as *HRX* and *ALL-1*), located on chromosome 11 (11q23), is frequently involved in translocations in AML,[55,87,90,128–130] with 65% of children diagnosed with AML before their 2nd birthday having 11q23 translocations.[87] The chimeric *MLL* gene fusions found in AML result from reciprocal translocations involving the portion of the gene encoding the amino-terminal portion of the MLL fused to the carboxy terminal region of the product of the partner gene. Nearly 50 *MLL* partner genes have been identified. These fusion proteins disrupt normal MLL function, resulting in aberrant control of hematopoiesis through its role as a transcriptional regulator. Of interest, the Hox genes, *HoxA9* and *HoxD13*, are known target genes for MLL and play roles in hematopoiesis and, when mutated, leukemogenesis.[131–135] While AML that expresses an 11q23 translocation is often of the M5 subtype, cases of M0, M1, M2 and M4 AML have also been observed. Furthermore, while the prognosis of *MLL* gene rearrangements is worse than for those with inv(16) and t(8;21) translocations, individual translocation partners can differentially influence prognosis. For example, in a study from St Jude Children's Research Hospital, the t(9;11) trans-location responded better to therapy and had a better overall outcome than other 11q23 translocations, particularly t(4;11).[130] However, the German AML Cooperative Group failed to observe a similarly good prognosis for this *MLL* fusion partner.[21,32,34,106] The basis of these differences is not known, but could reflect other underlying heterogeneity in the patients studied, including ethnic and racial differences between the European and American study populations.

Translocation between the 11q23 region and the 10p11–13 region represents an example of a translocation resulting in a particularly poor prognosis. Patients with this translocation have shorter durations of first CR and have a much higher rate of CNS relapse compared with other AML patients.[128] While the molecular mechanisms leading to this poor prognosis are still not completely understood, *MLL* fusion proteins involving two genes found on chromosome 10 (i.e., *AF10* and *ABI-1*) have both been implicated. The mechanisms by which such partner gene products influence the transforming ability of MLL remain unknown.

Prognostically poor cytogenetics

Although chromosomal translocations clearly play important

roles in leukemogenesis, abnormalities of individual chromosomes also play an important role in AML. Monosomy 7 or specific deletions of its long arm (7q–) can occur either as a single abnormality or in the context of complex karyotypic abnormalities. This abnormality, whether found in the context of myelodysplasia or AML, carries a very poor prognosis.[7,86,106,109,110] In the CCG-2891 study, only 53% of AML patients with monosomy 7 achieved remission, compared with the 78% overall remission rate. EFS for this group was 19% at 6 years compared with 39% overall. However, overall survival for patients with monosomy 7 (47% at 6 years) was no different than for the general AML population (46%). This is thought to be possibly explained by the fact that many of the relapsed monosomy 7 patients can be rescued by bone marrow transplantation, suggesting a robust graft-versus-leukemia effect.[7,11,12,136] Given the poor prognostic characteristics associated with this chromosome abnormality and the efficacy of HSCT in this population, monosomy 7 AML is an indication for stem-cell transplant in first CR, even if a matched unrelated donor is all that is available.[109,110]

Monosomy 5 and del(5q) abnormalities, while exceedingly rare in the pediatric population, also portend a poor prognosis, with decreased responsiveness to induction chemotherapy and decreased length of time in first CR if response to induction does occur. The trisomy 8 mutation is found both in isolation and also in association with complex karyotypic abnormalities. Whereas most data indicate that patients with trisomy 8 in isolation do not show a particularly aggressive disease, when combined with other cytogenetic abnormalities, trisomy 8 may contribute to poor response to therapy and poor EFS.[71,137]

FLT3

In addition to chromosomal deletions, additions and translocations, the impact of specific biologic markers of disease responsiveness or resistance to chemotherapeutic regimens is becoming increasingly important. Activating mutations of the class I receptor tyrosine kinases, including mutations in the *FLT3*, *c-KIT* and *c-fms* genes have shown promise as potent indicators of poor prognosis. *FLT3*, in particular, has been intensely studied.[111,138–145] Multiple reports have shown that the presence of internal tandem duplication of *FLT3* (FLT3/ITD) identifies pediatric and adult patients with particularly poor outcomes. These mutant *FLT3* genes result in constitutively active FLT3 tyrosine kinase activity, which contributes to leukemogenesis and chemotherapy resistance.[111,146] Indeed, remission induction in pediatric studies has been reported to be as low as 40% in patients expressing FLT3/ITD, in contrast to the overall rate of remission induction for AML, which is now reported as 70–85%.[111] While FLT3/ITD interferes with remission in some studies, there are also some AML patients who express FLT/ITD and who do well with conventional chemotherapy.[100] One hypothesis to explain this is that the effect of FLT3/ITD is modified by the presence or absence of a normal *FLT3* allele.[147] Current studies are examining the effect of the ratio of normal to mutated *FLT3* on treatment outcome to determine if an informative ratio can be used to identify those patients at highest and lowest risk for treatment failures. Future therapies are being tested in terms of targeting the FLT3 pathway for therapeutic intervention.

Principles of therapy

Historical overview

Current chemotherapeutic regimens for treating children with AML follow five treatment principles.[5]

• Aggressive induction therapy improves induction success rates as well as long-term survival.

• Consolidation or intensification therapy after remission is achieved is important for long-term disease-free survival.

• Maintenance therapy may give results comparable with the use of consolidation or intensification therapy, but it does not have a role in patients receiving aggressive postremission therapy.

• The type of treatment or prophylaxis for CNS leukemia does not appear important in influencing long-term survival.

• Targeted treatment of other extramedullary disease appears not to affect long-term survival.

The mainstay of treatment remains cytoreduction and remission induction through conventional chemotherapeutic regimens. The introduction of both AraC and anthracyclines for the treatment of AML in the early 1970s transformed a once uniformly fatal illness into one that was curable in a small percentage of patients.[9,10] Regimens employing dose intensification and improved supportive care measures have increased rates of remission induction and EFS. However, refractory AML is still the cause of death in nearly half of all children that it affects.

Chemotherapy phases consist of remission-induction therapy, CNS prophylaxis and postremission therapy. The initial trials for treatment of AML were modeled after the successful strategies for ALL: namely, intensive induction therapy to induce remission followed by a prolonged maintenance course including cranial radiation. However, unlike ALL, after an intensive consolidation/intensification phase of treatment, maintenance therapy did not lead to increased overall survival, but rather, to AML resistant to salvage therapy in the event of relapse.[16,148,149] Most current protocols have increased the intensity of induction therapy while eliminating maintenance therapy.

The Goldie–Coldman hypothesis represented a fundamental paradigm shift in the treatment of AML.[150–152] This hypothesis stated that the early use of potent combinations of non-cross-resistant drugs delivered simultaneously and in sequential rotation would provide a more potent antileukemic effect. In comparison with the first attempts at monotherapy or limited combination chemotherapy, this strategy was significantly more successful, leading to an increase in the 5-year survival estimates from less than 10% to 25–35% during the 1970s and 1980s. This approach represents the platform upon which more contemporary AML trials are built.

The first successful AML combination therapy was called "7 and 3"; it included 7 days of AraC at 100 mg/m^2/day continuous infusion and 3 days of daunorubicin at 30–60 mg/m^2/day. One or two courses of "7 and 3" induced remission (defined as < 5% AML blasts present in the bone marrow by morphologic analysis in the presence of recovery of trilineal hematopoiesis) in about 75–80% of children.[149,153] The CCG-213 trial compared "7 and 3" with a five-drug combination called "Denver," which added etoposide, thioguanine and dexamethasone to the AraC/daunorubicin backbone of the "7 and 3" regimen. There was no statistically significant difference in remission induction rate or long-term outcome with the five-drug regimen.[6,16,149,153] Dose escalation of AraC has also played an important role in improving survival of patients with AML, particularly in some good prognostic subsets.[12,108] The introduction of non-cross-resistant anthracyclines (idarubicin, mitoxantrone, amsacrine) to the AraC backbone, as well as the number of chemotherapy courses, may also have contributed to the increase in survival observed over the last decade.[9,32,154,155]

The MRC AML-10 and AML-12 trials (Fig. 16.4)

Several trials performed subsequent to the introduction of the "Denver" regimen achieved induction remission rates higher than the historical 75–80% of "7 and 3." The Pediatric Oncology Group (POG) trial 8821 used "7 and 3" plus 6-thioguanine (TAD) and reported a remission induction rate of 85%.[90] The Medical Research Council (MRC) AML-10 trial randomized patients to receive either DAT (daunorubicin/AraC/6-thioguanine) or ADE (AraC/daunorubicin/etoposide) for two courses, followed by two subsequent chemotherapeutic courses of MACE (amsacrine/AraC/etoposide) and MidAC (mitoxantrone/AraC). After these four mandatory courses of dose-intensive chemotherapy, patients were biologically randomized to allogeneic HSCT if they had an HLA matched-sibling donor, or, if not, were entered into another randomization of either no further therapy or autologous HSCT.[18,20,29,108,110] This study showed that the dose-intensive four courses of chemotherapy were highly effective in inducing first CR; no significant difference in CR was observed in children receiving either the DAT or ADE for induction therapy. Overall, AML-10 reported 92% CR after four cycles of chemotherapy; 63% of patients achieved CR after one cycle, an additional 20% achieved CR after two cycles, 7% after three cycles and 2% after four cycles. Thus, these

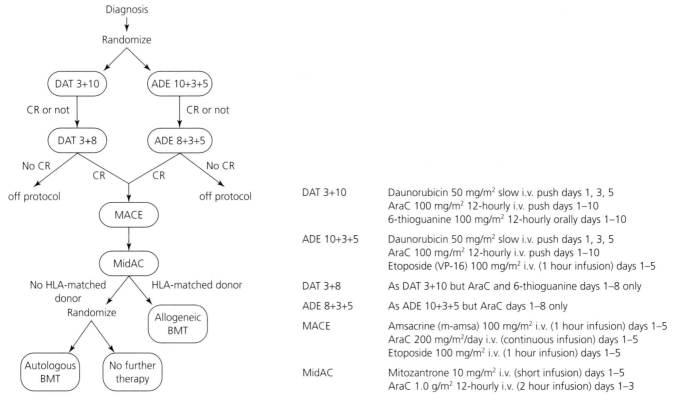

Fig. 16.4 Treatment algorithm followed by the AML-10 trial. AraC, cytarabine; BMT, bone marrow transplant; CR, complete remission.

outcomes are very similar to the results reported by both the POG-8821 and the CCG-2891 trials, which demonstrated ~80% CR after two cycles of induction chemotherapy.

Of the patients achieving CR during the MRC AML-10 trial, 6% died during induction, mostly of toxic deaths. The relapse rate was relatively low, with a 26% rate of relapse in the first year following CR, which dropped to 11% in year 2, 3% in year 3, and 2% in year 4. Overall survival in this study was also good, with a reported 59% of patients alive after 5 years. While AML-10 showed that both allogeneic and autologous HSCT reduced the risk of relapse after therapy when compared with a "no further treatment" arm, a statistically significant overall survival benefit was not detected. This was likely due to the increased number of treatment-related deaths after HSCT. However, disease-free survival (DFS) was significantly greater in the HSCT group compared with the "no further treatment" group (50% vs. 42%, $P = 0.01$).

Nearly all multicenter trials performed to date have shown a survival benefit for allogeneic HSCT compared with chemotherapy, although, like the MRC AML-10 trial, some of these studies were not sufficiently powered to reach statistical significance.[10–14,19,23,32,34–36,154,156,157] While the MRC AML-10 trial reported a survival advantage for those patients undergoing autologous HSCT, it is important to note that this survival advantage occurred when these patients were compared with those who received no more chemotherapy.

Thus, those in the autologous transplant arm received an additional cycle of intensive chemotherapy compared with those not randomized to receive the transplant. In the CCG-2891 trial, where autologous HSCT was compared with further chemotherapy, autologous transplantation did not confer a survival advantage, whereas allogeneic HSCT improved both disease-free and overall survival.[11] Similar results were found in the POG-8821 trial.[23] Although autologous HSCT may be less effective because of the reinfusion of viable leukemic cells,[158] these results also implicate a potent graft-versus-leukemia effect for AML. This concept is supported by data also reported by the CCG, which correlates graft-versus-host disease (GVHD) – as a surrogate marker for graft-versus-leukemia (GVL) – with increased survival after allotransplantation.[24]

MRC AML-10 resulted in the UK cooperative establishing three different risk groups for childhood AML.[18,29,108] The first is a good-risk group, which includes patients with favorable cytogenetic abnormalities, including t(8;21), t(15;17) and inv(16). The second is a poor-risk group, which includes those with a partial (≥ 15% leukemic blasts) or no response after course 1 of chemotherapy and those with adverse cytogenetic abnormalities, including monosomy 5, monosomy 7, del(5q), abnormalities of 3q, or complex karyotypes containing more than four chromosomal abnormalities. The remainder of patients are classified as standard-risk. MRC AML-10 noted that outcome differences for the three risk groups were significant: Good-risk patients had 78% survival from first CR, while standard-risk patients displayed 60% survival and poor-risk patients had only a 33% survival. Survival from first relapse was also significantly different between the three groups: good-risk patients had a 61% survival from relapse, while standard-risk patients only had a 17% survival and poor-risk patients displayed 0% survival from relapse. As discussed below, this risk-stratification has directed the UK collaborative group's treatment decisions in subsequent trials. While MRC AML-10 did not detect a statistically significant difference in overall survival between the three final treatment arms, there was increased DFS for autologous HSCT when compared with no further therapy. Because those receiving autologous HSCT received an additional intensive cycle of chemotherapy compared with those randomized to no further therapy, this result implied that further chemotherapy alone might also lead to increased DFS in AML. Thus, in MRC AML-12, patients were randomized to receive either four or five rounds of chemotherapy, to determine whether this extra course would produce improved survival. Early results have not confirmed an advantage in MRC12 for five courses of therapy, thus leading the MRC group to propose four dose-intensive courses of chemotherapy.[159]

The AML BFM-93 trial

The German-based BFM-87 trial also led this cooperative group to establish a risk profile for newly diagnosed AML.[160] Two prognostic groups were identified, which were based both on initial morphologic parameters as well as on the efficacy of induction therapy to produce blast cell reduction in the bone marrow on day 15. The standard risk group included FAB M1 or M2 subtypes, the presence of Auer rods, as well as FAB M3 and FAB M4Eo with ≤ 5% blasts in the bone marrow on day 15. High-risk patients included all others, plus patients initially allocated to the standard-risk group but whose day-15 bone marrow showed > 5% blasts. Patients with FAB M3 were always treated as standard risk, regardless of their blast count on day 15. The BFM-93 trial was designed to determine whether the addition of consolidation chemotherapy consisting of high-dose AraC and mitoxantrone ("HAM") could improve EFS for the high-risk patients, who had been found to do relatively poorly when treated according to BFM-87 (5-year EFS, 31%).[21,32] The trial, whose design is shown in Fig. 16.5, included two randomized study questions: (i) the relative efficacy of idarubicin versus daunorubicin in producing an induction CR; and (ii) the relative effect of "early HAM" therapy prior to consolidation or "late HAM" postconsolidation on survival and toxicity. Each of these study questions enrolled only those patients assigned to the high-risk stratification.

BFM-93 demonstrated excellent outcomes, both in CR and EFS: 82% of patients (both standard and high risk) achieved a CR, and overall 5-year EFS was 51%. While the idarubicin-

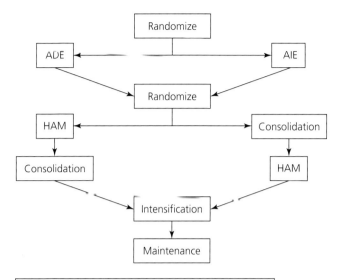

Fig. 16.5 Treatment algorithm followed by the BFM-93 trial. AraC, cytarabine.

based induction regimen showed significantly better blast reduction on day 15, the 5-year EFS and DFS for the idarubicin and daunorubicin arms were similar. Infection rates and length of pancytopenia for the idarubicin arm showed a trend toward being longer, but the differences did not reach statistical significance. The overall results of patients randomized to early versus late HAM were also similar: 5-year EFS of 52 ± 5% (early HAM) versus 45 ± 5% (late HAM) were observed. However, the timing of HAM was more important in those patients who received daunorubicin during induction rather than idarubicin: 5-year EFS of 51.9 ± 7.4% for daunorubicin plus early HAM versus 35.6 ± 7.3% for daunorubicin plus late HAM ($P = 0.05$). These results indicate that in the setting of reduced early blast reduction with daunorubicin, early escalation of dose intensity with HAM (expected to give significant blast reduction) could be an important mediator of stable remission status. Given the efficacy of HAM treatment demonstrated in BMF-93, and its acceptable toxicity profile, it was incorporated into the BFM-98 study, and its use extended to standard-risk patients as well.

The CCG-2891 trial (Fig. 16.6)

The CCG-2891 trial was the first to test in a randomized design the hypothesis that time-intensity of drug delivery might be an important approach to intensification. This

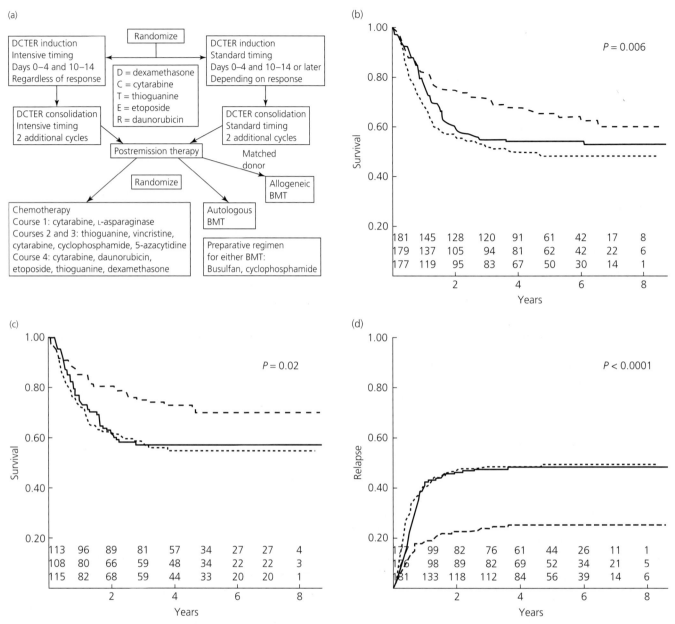

Fig. 16.6 (a) Treatment algorithm followed by CCG-2891. (b) Actuarial survival from AML remission, comparing the three postremission regimens from CCG-2891.[11] Dashed line: allogeneic human stem cell transplant (HSCT); solid line: chemotherapy; dotted line: autologous HSCT. (c) Actuarial survival from AML remission for the CCG-2891 patients who received intensive-timing induction therapy, comparing the three postremission regimens.[11] Dashed line: allogeneic HSCT; solid line: chemotherapy; dotted line: autologous HSCT. (d) Actuarial probability of relapse after AML remission, comparing the three postremission regimens from CCG-2891.[11] Dashed line: allogeneic HSCT; solid line: chemotherapy; dotted line: autologous HSCT.

hypothesis was based on previous preclinical *in vitro* studies that had documented that AML blasts show maximal recruitment and synchronization into S phase 6–8 days after cessation of AraC.[161,162] CCG-2891 therefore tested a kinetically based, timed-sequential approach to induction therapy to determine whether timing of chemotherapy delivery could produce a "better quality" first CR, which had a reduced propensity for relapse.[12,13,15,24]

CCG-2891 compared standard timing of a five-drug induction regimen called DCTER – *d*examethasone, AraC, 6-*t*hioguanine, *e*toposide, *r*ubidomycin (also known as daunorubicin) – with intensive timing of DCTER. With standard timing, the second course of DCTER was given only after hematologic recovery unless a bone marrow exam performed at day 14 showed residual leukemia (in which case, the second course was given immediately). Intensive DCTER was given on days 0–3 and repeated on days 10–13 regardless of marrow status. Remission induction rates were similar between the two arms: 78% with intensively timed therapy and 74% with conventionally timed therapy. Furthermore, induction mortality was higher with intensively timed therapy, especially prior to the institution of mandatory hospitalization during the period of pancytopenia and cytokine support with granulocyte colony-stimulating factor (G-CSF) (although these improvements in mortality were not subjected to randomized analysis). However, despite the similarities in rates of remission-induction, the 8-year EFS was significantly higher for intensive compared with standard timing (43% vs. 27% respectively, $P = 0.008$). These results suggest that not all remissions are equal, and that increased intensity of induction therapy may be one way to achieve a higher "quality" remission, that is, a remission that is more likely to continue without relapse.

Targeted therapy for APL

APL is distinguished from the other AML subtypes both by its distinct cytogenetic abnormality, t(15;17), and by the targeted therapy that is now the standard-of-care for its treatment.[163] ATRA is central to the treatment of this AML subtype, due to the ability of ATRA to induce differentiation of the APL leukemic blasts into mature granulocytes.[126,163–166] Current treatment paradigms lead to excellent results for APL in children: CR rates have most recently been reported at about 96%, with 10-year EFS of 76%.[126] The treatment of APL benefits from the ability to measure MRD with high sensitivity, by performing PCR for the disease-specific PML-RARα transcript. The ability to measure this transcript allows patients to be categorized by the presence or absence of molecular remission, and to have their treatment modified accordingly. Those in molecular remission have a high continuous CR rate, while those in molecular relapse, despite morphologic remission, almost uniformly progress.[126] For these patients, reinduction therapy followed by HSCT (either auto- or allo-transplantation) has been successful.[126,167,168] The unique biology of APL has led to important differences in the therapy for this disease compared with other AML subtypes. In addition to the efficacy of ATRA therapy, APL patients, unlike patients with other AML subtypes, have been shown to benefit from maintenance chemotherapy, as long as this maintenance therapy contains further treatment with ATRA.[126] Furthermore, in patients with APL, auto-HSCT has been shown to be beneficial, if it is performed with cells that are demonstrated by PCR to be PML-RARα-negative.[163,167–170] Thus, in one study, 7 of 7 patients receiving auto-HSCT with PML-RARα-positive marrow relapsed within 9 months, while only 1 of 8 patients transplanted with PML-RARα-negative marrow experienced a relapse.[168] In another report, 3 of 28 patients receiving PML-RARα-negative auto-HSCT subsequently relapsed while one of two patients receiving PML α-positive auto-HSCT recurred.[167] These results, although representing small numbers of patients, underscore the power of MRD detection to direct treatment for APL, and to improve outcome, even for those patients with relapsed disease. Recently, arsenic trioxide has been added to the collection of unique agents able to treat APL, and is currently in trials in both adult and pediatric patients (reviewed in refs 171–173). While the precise mechanisms by which arsenic works to induce remission in APL are not completely known, it has been shown to produce degradation of the PML-RARα fusion protein, increase cellular apoptosis and induce differentiation of the APL leukemic clone. Whether it will show increased efficacy with acceptable toxicity in pediatric patients when combined with ATRA-based therapy is currently under investigation.

Gemtuzumab ozogamicin

Current trials from both North America and Europe are testing the efficacy of gemtuzumab ozogamicin (GO), a recombinant humanized anti-CD33 monoclonal antibody linked to the genotoxic antibiotic calicheamicin, in eliminating AML blasts. CD33 is a cell-surface protein that is expressed on both normal and leukemic myeloid progenitors, but appears to be absent from the pluripotent hematopoietic stem cell. Calicheamicin belongs to a class of potent antitumor antibiotics that were originally identified by their ability to damage double-stranded DNA. This antibody–toxin conjugate is able to kill CD33+ myeloid precursors, because the CD33 molecule is internalized after binding to the monoclonal antibody, thus allowing efficient intracellular delivery of the DNA-damaging agent.[174–179] Both single-agent studies and studies in which GO was combined with conventional chemotherapeutic agents in both adults and children have documented efficacy.[178–184] This agent is now being tested in both pediatric and adult phase II/III trials.

Although GO promises to be highly efficacious in selectively targeting AML blasts, liver toxicity has occurred in adult randomized trials in combination with chemotherapy when higher doses (6 and 9 mg/m²) of this drug are used.[177,184–187] This toxicity is manifested as both hypertransaminemia and hyperbilirubinemia. There is also a risk of hepatic venoocclusive disease. In the MRC AML-15 pilot study, the addition of 6-thioguanine to a GO-containing regimen was a significant risk factor in the development of liver toxicity, when compared with other chemotherapeutic combinations.[181] This pilot study also showed that GO at 3 mg/m² was well tolerated, but that dose escalation beyond 3 mg/m² was not feasible when GO was included with the intensive combination chemotherapy regimens tested. Given these results, the new COG pilot study uses GO at 3 mg/m² in combination with an MRC-based ADE induction regimen (Fig. 16.7). A critical question will be whether GO results in improved outcome through targeting a self-renewing leukemic stem cell or whether GO will only be an effective cytoreduction agent.

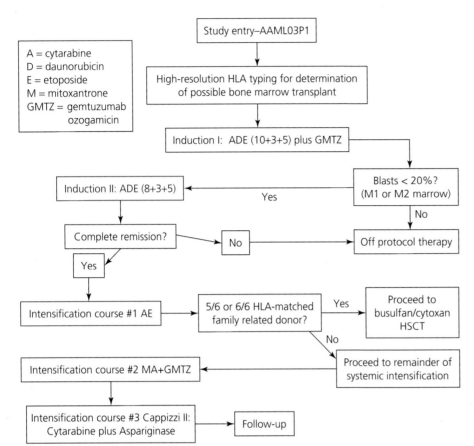

Fig. 16.7 Treatment algorithm for AAML03P1. HSCT, hematopoietic stem cell transplant. Capprizzi II includes high dose cytarabine and h-Asparaginase.

Allogeneic HSCT as consolidation therapy for AML

The most intensive postremission therapy that is available for AML is high-dose chemotherapy with or without total body irradiation (TBI) followed by stem cell transplantation. Several studies have been designed to test whether chemotherapy, autologous HSCT or matched-sibling allogeneic HSCT was more effective in increasing survival following remission with intensive induction therapy for AML.[2,3,11–13,18,20,21,23,24,31,37,153] The CCG-2891 study reported the highest compliance with receiving the assigned treatments as determined by randomization. In this study, a total of 537 children were analyzed, of whom 181 received allogeneic HSCT, 177 received autologous HSCT and 179 received chemotherapy. Allogeneic HSCT was statistically superior to either autologous HSCT or chemotherapy in terms of overall survival: 60% survival after 8 years for allogeneic HSCT versus 53% and 48% survival for chemotherapy or autologous HSCT (see Fig. 16.6b,d).[11] Results in those patients receiving intensively timed DCTER chemotherapy showed a similarly superior efficacy of allogeneic HSCT, with a 72% survival for allogeneic HSCT versus ~ 60% survival with either chemotherapy or autologous HSCT (see Fig. 16.6c).[11] These results showed a statistically significant survival difference compared with either of the other two treatments whereas survival differences for HSCT after the latter two treatments were not statistically different.

The mechanism of this improved survival after allogeneic HSCT may be related to a GVL effect. Neudorf *et al.*[24] recently showed, in an analysis of the CCG-2891 data, that grade I–II GVHD positively correlated with improved survival after allogeneic HSCT, suggesting that there was a GVL effect secondary to the GVHD. Likewise, Nordlander *et al.*[188] showed that in their single-institution experience, chronic GVHD also predicted better DFS after allogeneic HSCT for AML. Taken together, these results provide strong support for the role of an immunologic antileukemia effect and for matched sibling allogeneic HSCT in first remission for AML in children. Importantly, in the CCG studies, with the exception of t(15;17)/M3 and inv(16) AML, neither FAB subtype nor cytogenetic subtype analysis changed the positive results of allogeneic HSCT when compared with other postremission therapies.[11] The MRC cooperative group has been more cautious about using HSCT in first remission. Given the toxicity and procedure-related mortality associated with allogeneic HSCT, the MRC cooperative group currently recommends that patients in the good-risk group (which includes those with t(8;21) in addition to t(15;17) and inv(16)) do not receive HSCT until after the first relapse and induction of second remission; those in the standard- and poor-risk groups should receive HSCT in first CR if a matched sibling is available.[108,110,189] A major challenge that remains is to determine how to accrue significant numbers of patients in rare subgroups in order to rigorously test such questions.

Supportive care

Given that AML therapy is intensive and nearly myeloablative, supportive care measures have a large impact on overall survival and morbidity. Current standards of care include mandatory hospitalization for the duration of pancytopenia, with prompt initiation of an empiric antibiotic regimen for fever, which includes initial use of vancomycin for α-streptococcal coverage.[190,191] Antifungal prophylaxis is standard, as is prompt initiation of empiric antifungal treatment for prolonged fever without a source. Nutritional support is important, in addition to routine transfusional support with both platelets and packed red blood cells. The CCG-2891 study showed that cytokine support with G-CSF did not affect the incidence of grade 3 and 4 toxicities, infections, or fatal infections, and that induction remission rates, overall survival, and EFS were similar with and without G-CSF.[192] For these reasons, G-CSF is not currently a mandated component of AML supportive care. However, CCG-2891 provided data from a nonrandomized comparison that those patients who received G-CSF demonstrated a significantly shorter time to neutropenic recovery and that the use of G-CSF reduced the median length of induction by 9 days and hospital stay by 6 days.[192] Randomized trials may better determine the role of cytokine therapy in pediatric AML.

CNS prophylaxis

CNS involvement with AML occurs in approximately 20% of cases, with the highest incidence in patients with very high peripheral WBC or with M4 and M5 subtypes. All current treatment protocols for pediatric AML utilize CNS prophylaxis, either with intrathecal AraC, triple therapy including AraC, methotrexate and hydrocortisone, or, in trials performed through the BFM Cooperative group, cranial radiation. These treatments, along with high-dose systemic AraC, result in good control of CNS leukemia, with the incidence of CNS relapse reported as approximately 5%.[3,5,11,12,18,20,21,29,193] While all of the original trials included cranial radiation as part of CNS prophylaxis, current trials in the UK and the USA have eliminated this modality. The BFM Cooperative group has continued to include cranial radiation in its treatment regimens. This decision stems from a somewhat surprising result that arose from the BFM-83 trial, which showed an effect of cranial radiation on systemic rather than CNS relapse.[21,194] In this trial, a statistically significant increase was observed in the number of patients experiencing systemic relapse in the absence of cranial radiation. Of note, in the BFM trial, the difference in systemic relapse was noted only in patients who did not undergo randomization; no difference in systemic relapse was noted when cranial radiation was eliminated in the randomized cohort.

Extramedullary leukemia

Non-CNS extramedullary disease also occurs in AML. These extramedullary leukemic masses, known also as chloromas or granulocytic sarcomas, occur in a variety of anatomic locations in approximately 10% of patients with AML. The most common site is the orbit or the periorbital areas. Chloromas may also involve the spinal cord, where they can lead to symptoms related to cord compression. They are also frequently noted in the skin, and, if present in the lymphatic system, can cause multifocal lymphadenopathy. While EML is often associated with bone marrow disease, it can also present in an isolated fashion, and may precede bone marrow involvement by up to 1–2 years. EML is most commonly seen with M4 and M5 subtypes of AML, but is also seen in M1 and M2 AML.[5,30,193,195] Without systemic treatment, bone marrow involvement will eventually occur. Thus, even if diagnosed in isolation, extramedullary disease requires intensive AML therapy.[5,30,193] Several studies have shown that patients with isolated extramedullary disease do exceedingly well with AML therapy.[12,193]

Historically, when EML was present, local control in the form of radiotherapy was often added to systemic chemotherapeutic regimens. However, a recent retrospective of CCG-2891 results concluded that there was no difference in recurrence in those patients with chloromas who received radiation therapy in addition to systemic therapy and those patients who only received systemic therapy.[193] Therefore, radiation therapy is not currently recommended for patients with extramedullary AML, unless a chloroma is creating a life-threatening situation, due to obstruction or compression of vital structures.

Secondary AML

With the increasing number of survivors of other childhood cancers, there is a growing number of children and adolescents who are diagnosed with secondary AML. Known treatment-related risks of AML (primarily of the monosomy 7 subtype) include exposure to radiation or alkylating agents such as cyclophosphamide, ifosfamide, nitrogen mustard and melphalan. These secondary AML cases usually have a peak incidence 4–7 years after the initial genotoxic exposure.[54] Treatment regimens that use epipodophyllotoxins, such as VP-16, clearly lead to an increased risk of AML with 11q23 abnormalities involving the MLL gene. These MLL secondary leukemias usually develop 2–3 years following exposure.[55] Evaluation of patients treated for secondary AML on the CCG-2891 trial[54] demonstrated that these patients were older at presentation than those presenting with *de novo* AML, had lower WBC and were more likely to have preceding myelodysplastic syndrome. Patients with secondary AML had a poor induction rate (50%) and overall survival (26%). If remission was successfully achieved, patients with secondary AML demonstrated lower (but not statistically significantly different) rates of DFS (45%) compared with those in whom AML was the primary diagnosis. These results are, however, possibly misleading due to the small number of such patients.

Down syndrome and AML

Children with DS have an approximately 15-fold higher risk of developing leukemia than the general population. Furthermore, in DS children younger than 2 years old, there is a greater than 400-fold increased risk of developing megakaryoblastic leukemia compared with the general population.[3,41,196] In addition to their increased propensity to develop AML, approximately 10% of patients with DS will develop transient myeloproliferative disorder (TMD), which is clinically indistinguishable from AML.[197–199] However, TMD is distinguished from true AML by the fact that the majority of these patients undergo a spontaneous regression of their disease. Nevertheless, children with TMD may experience significant morbidity and mortality. Some patients with DS and TMD or megaloblastic leukemia may present with severe organ infiltration, particularly of the liver. Hydrops fetalis may develop in the most severe cases.

As many as 30% of DS patients with TMD will go on to develop AML.[197–204] In these cases, karyotypic evolution of the leukemic clone may be seen coincident with the development of the megakaryoblastic leukemia. The progression from TMD to AML may be explained by the multiple gene mutating hypothesis. For example, patients with DS are thought to start with "one genetic hit" given their constitutional trisomy 21. Subsequent mutations involving the GATA-1 transcription factor are found in nearly all patients with DS and TMD or megakaryoblastic leukemia. Additional chromosomal abnormalities may then develop leading to true AML.[197–204] The observation of cytogenetic evolution of the TMD clone upon progression to AML, and the fact that many more DS patients develop TMD (10%) than AML (1%), support this multiple-hit hypothesis.

Children with DS have a superior response to AML therapy when compared with other children. This was shown in the POG-8498 trial, wherein the 12 DS patients enrolled had an EFS of 100%.[196] The CCG-213 trial reported similar results, with 80% overall survival for DS children compared with 40% survival with non-DS patients.[153] In the CCG-2891 trial, DS children did better when placed on the standard arm of therapy, in contrast with the general population, which showed improved EFS when on the intensive-induction protocol. This difference was attributable to the increased tox-

icity observed in the children with DS when given intensively timed therapy.[205–210] DS children placed on the intensive-timing arm of CCG-2891 experienced 33% treatment-related mortality with only 5% persistent disease. Those patients on the standard arm showed similar results for CR induction with much less treatment-related mortality.[12] Similarly, children with DS allocated to HLA-matched-related HSCT on CCG-2891 did significantly worse than those randomized to receive chemotherapy with high-dose AraC, with an overall relapse-free survival of 67% compared with 91% in the chemotherapy arm. All of these studies have thus shown that patients with DS have an excellent DFS and overall survival with less therapy than other children with AML.

Treatment of refractory/recurrent AML

Although current treatment strategies for AML routinely yield remission rates above 80%, only about 50% of children with AML are long-term survivors.[11,19,211,212] In general, patients who relapse, or who have disease that is refractory to remission induction, are less responsive to reinduction therapies, and, if they achieve a second remission, stay in remission for shorter periods than their first remission. Only a small proportion (~20%) of these patients become long-term survivors.[213,214] Those patients who experience longer periods in CR prior to relapse (i.e., > 1 year) do better, with a 5-year survival for this population of 30–40%.[211,213] While there is no standard therapy for relapsed patients, most regimens now rely on high-dose AraC in combination with other agents, including etoposide, mitoxantrone, idarubicin, fludarabine or GO.[186,215,216] Given the poor results when chemotherapy alone is used to treat relapsed or resistant disease, allogeneic HSCT is used for these patients whenever possible. Allogeneic HSCT from HLA-matched family or unrelated donors offers the only curative therapy for such patients at this time.[217–219] Other marrow stem cell sources include cord blood or haploidentical donors, although the latter are much less studied. While allogeneic HSCT promises an increased chance at long-term survival (up to 50% in some subgroups), there is also the risk of acute and chronic treatment-related morbidity and mortality.[220–223] In most studies, the treatment-related mortality associated with alternative-donor transplants ranges from 30 to 50%.[221,224,225] Furthermore, the presence of minimal residual disease adversely affects the results of either autotransplant or allotransplant, further decreasing the efficacy for these patients with highly resistant disease.[226–232] These results underscore the need to develop novel therapies that are able to overcome chemotherapy resistance.

Late effects

With increasing numbers of pediatric patients becoming

long-term survivors of AML, there is a growing need to analyze late effects and offer appropriate treatment. Although no large study of this patient population has been published, several smaller group and single-institution retrospective analyses are available.[233–236] With respect to late effects, patients treated for AML can be most accurately divided into four groups:

- those who received chemotherapy alone;
- those receiving chemotherapy and additional cranial or cranial/spinal irradiation;
- those receiving allo-HSCT with a TBI-based preparative regimen; and
- those who received allo-HSCT with a busulfan-based preparative regimen.

All four groups have shown decreased vertical height. Those receiving cranial radiation tended to have increases in weight, while those not treated with cranial radiation had decreased weight, with this being especially prominent in post-HSCT patients. The adverse effect on growth by TBI and HSCT was thought to be multifactorial, with contributions from coexistent endocrinopathies, the effects of chronic GVHD, and the direct growth-limiting effects of radiation on the musculoskeletal system.[233] While most patients who did not receive TBI-based HSCT progressed through puberty normally and were fertile, those receiving TBI prior to HSCT exhibited high rates of infertility. Furthermore, patients receiving TBI-based HSCT also experienced an increased risk of cataracts and radiation-related dental abnormalities. Cardiac dysfunction was noted in approximately 10% of AML survivors, with the risk correlating with the cumulative dose of anthracycline received. While the number of AML survivors that have been analyzed is small, these patients have also been reported to develop second malignancies, probably due to the carcinogenic effects of both the chemotherapy and radiation-based therapy that they have received.[233] In one series,[233] approximately 18% of patients reported neurocognitive deficits, including academic difficulties, decreases in IQ, and subjective problems with immaturity, shyness and low self-esteem. Both the dose of radiation, and the age at which diagnosis and radiation therapy occurred correlated with this increased risk of neuropsychological sequelae. As these first late-effects studies have documented, given the intensive therapy that AML survivors receive in order to cure their primary disease, they are, by necessity, subject to many and varying late effects. These sequelae demand close monitoring and, as the treatment for AML becomes more effective, these effects will undoubtedly influence future therapeutic decisions.

Conclusions

The ability to achieve remission in patients with newly diagnosed AML has significantly increased over the past 40 years with a > 80% chance of achieving a first remission being a reality. However, resistant disease remains a critical barrier to long-term cure, and approximately half of all pediatric patients will still die of their primary disease. Several key concepts have emerged concerning therapy for pediatric AML:

- intensive cytoreduction is essential for disease control with currently used chemotherapeutic agents;
- timed, sequential therapy is an effective approach to treatment; and
- for most patients, postremission treatment with allogeneic HSCT offers the best chance for long-term cure when there is a matched family donor.

New targeted therapies for AML provide potentially less toxic and more effective treatment approaches. Future trials will test such targeted agents in combination with conventional chemotherapeutic regimens.

References

1. Ravindranath Y. Recent advances in pediatric acute lymphoblastic and myeloid leukemia. *Curr Opin Oncol* 2003; **15**: 23–35.
2. Lowenberg B, Downing JR, Burnett A. Acute myeloid leukemia. *N Engl J Med* 1999; **341**: 1051–62.
3. Lange BJ, Kobrinsky N, Barnard DR *et al.* Distinctive demography, biology, and outcome of acute myeloid leukemia and myelodysplastic syndrome in children with Down syndrome: Children's Cancer Group Studies 2861 and 2891. *Blood* 1998; **91**: 608–15.
4. Vormoor J, Boos J, Stahnke K, Jurgens H, Ritter J, Creutzig U. Therapy of childhood acute myelogenous leukemias. *Ann Hematol* 1996; **73**: 11–24.
5. Woods WG, Sanders JE, Neudorf S. Treatment of acute myeloid leukemia. *N Engl J Med* 1999; **340**: 1437–9.
6. Wells RJ, Arthur DC, Srivastava A *et al.* Prognostic variables in newly diagnosed children and adolescents with acute myeloid leukemia: Children's Cancer Group Study 213. *Leukemia* 2002; **16**: 601–7.
7. Barnard DR, Lange B, Alonzo TA *et al.* Acute myeloid leukemia and myelodysplastic syndrome in children treated for cancer: comparison with primary presentation. *Blood* 2002; **100**: 427–34.
8. Xie Y, Davies SM, Xiang Y, Robison LL, Ross JA. Trends in leukemia incidence and survival in the United States (1973–1998). *Cancer* 2003; **97**: 2229–35.
9. Chard RL Jr. Studies with anthracyclines in pediatric acute nonlymphocytic leukemia. *Cancer Treat Rep* 1981; **65** (suppl. 4): 77–81.
10. Capizzi RL, Poole M, Cooper MR *et al.* Treatment of poor risk acute leukemia with sequential high-dose ARA-C and asparaginase. *Blood* 1984; **63**: 694–700.
11. Woods WG, Neudorf S, Gold S *et al.* A comparison of allogeneic bone marrow transplantation, autologous bone marrow transplantation, and aggressive chemotherapy in children with acute myeloid leukemia in remission. *Blood* 2001; **97**: 56–62.

12. Woods WG, Kobrinsky N, Buckley JD *et al.* Timed-sequential induction therapy improves postremission outcome in acute myeloid leukemia: a report from the Children's Cancer Group. *Blood* 1996; **87**: 4979–89.

13. Woods WG, Kobrinsky N, Buckley J *et al.* Intensively timed induction therapy followed by autologous or allogeneic bone marrow transplantation for children with acute myeloid leukemia or myelodysplastic syndrome: a Children's Cancer Group pilot study. *J Clin Oncol* 1993; **11**: 1448–57.

14. Wells RJ, Adams MT, Alonzo TA *et al.* Mitoxantrone and cytarabine induction, high-dose cytarabine, and etoposide intensification for pediatric patients with relapsed or refractory acute myeloid leukemia: Children's Cancer Group Study 2951. *J Clin Oncol* 2003; **21**: 2940–7.

15. Wells RJ, Woods WG, Buckley JD, Arceci RJ. Therapy for acute myeloid leukemia: intensive timing of induction chemotherapy. *Curr Oncol Rep* 2000; **2**: 524–8.

16. Wells RJ, Woods WG, Buckley JD *et al.* Treatment of newly diagnosed children and adolescents with acute myeloid leukemia: a Children's Cancer Group study. *J Clin Oncol* 1994; **12**: 2367–77.

17. Weisdorf DJ, McGlave PB, Ramsay NK *et al.* Allogeneic bone marrow transplantation for acute leukaemia: comparative outcomes for adults and children. *Br J Haematol* 1988; **69**: 351–8.

18. Stevens RF, Hann IM, Wheatley K, Gray RG. Marked improvements in outcome with chemotherapy alone in paediatric acute myeloid leukemia: results of the United Kingdom Medical Research Council's 10th AML trial. MRC Childhood Leukaemia Working Party. *Br J Haematol* 1998; **101**: 130–40.

19. Suciu S, Mandelli F, de Witte T *et al.* Allogeneic compared with autologous stem cell transplantation in the treatment of patients younger than 46 years with acute myeloid leukemia (AML) in first complete remission (CR1): an intention-to-treat analysis of the EORTC/GIMEMAAML-10 trial. *Blood* 2003; **102**: 1232–40.

20. Stevens RF, Hann IM, Wheatley K, Gray R. Intensive chemotherapy with or without additional bone marrow transplantation in paediatric AML: progress report on the MRC AML 10 trial. Medical Research Council Working Party on Childhood Leukaemia. *Leukemia* 1992; **6** (suppl. 2): 55–8.

21. Ritter J, Creutzig U, Schellong G. Treatment results of three consecutive German childhood AML trials: BFM-78, -83, and -87. AML-BFM-Group. *Leukemia* 1992; **6** (suppl. 2): 59–62.

22. Ritter J, Creutzig U, Riehm HJ, Schellong G. Acute myelogenous leukemia: current status of therapy in children. *Recent Results Cancer Res* 1984; **93**: 204–15.

23. Ravindranath Y, Yeager AM, Chang MN *et al.* Autologous bone marrow transplantation versus intensive consolidation chemotherapy for acute myeloid leukemia in childhood. Pediatric Oncology Group. *N Engl J Med* 1996; **334**: 1428–34.

24. Neudorf S, Sanders J, Kobrinsky N *et al.* Allogeneic bone marrow transplantation for children with acute myelocytic leukemia in first remission demonstrates a role for graft versus leukemia in the maintenance of disease-free survival. *Blood* 2004; **103**: 3655–61.

25. Nesbit ME Jr, Buckley JD, Feig SA *et al.* Chemotherapy for induction of remission of childhood acute myeloid leukemia followed by marrow transplantation or multiagent chemotherapy: a report from the Children's Cancer Group. *J Clin Oncol* 1994; **12**: 127–35.

26. Nesbit ME Jr, Woods WG. Therapy of acute myeloid leukemia in children. *Leukemia* 1992; **6** (Suppl. 2): 31–5.

27. Klingebiel T, Creutzig U, Dopfer R *et al.* Bone marrow transplantation in comparison with conventional therapy in children with adult type chronic myelogenous leukemia. *Bone Marrow Transplant* 1990; **5**: 317–20.

28. Hurwitz CA, Mounce KG, Grier HE. Treatment of patients with acute myelogenous leukemia: review of clinical trials of the past decade. *J Pediatr Hematol Oncol* 1995; **17**: 185–97.

29. Hann IM, Stevens RF, Goldstone AH *et al.* Randomized comparison of DAT versus ADE as induction chemotherapy in children and younger adults with acute myeloid leukemia. Results of the Medical Research Council's 10th AML trial (MRC AML10). Adult and Childhood Leukaemia Working Parties of the Medical Research Council. *Blood* 1997; **89**: 2311–18.

30. Estey EH. Therapeutic options for acute myelogenous leukemia. *Cancer* 2001; **92**: 1059–73.

31. Dusenbery KE, Steinbuch M, McGlave PB *et al.* Autologous bone marrow transplantation in acute myeloid leukemia: the University of Minnesota experience. *Int J Radiat Oncol Biol Phys* 1996; **36**: 335–43.

32. Creutzig U, Ritter J, Zimmermann M *et al.* Improved treatment results in high-risk pediatric acute myeloid leukemia patients after intensification with high-dose cytarabine and mitoxantrone: results of Study Acute Myeloid Leukemia-Berlin-Frankfurt-Munster 93. *J Clin Oncol* 2001; **19**: 2705–13.

33. Creutzig U. Diagnosis and treatment of acute myelogenous leukemia in childhood. *Crit Rev Oncol Hematol* 1996; **22**: 183–96.

34. Creutzig U, Ritter J, Riehm H *et al.* Improved treatment results in childhood acute myelogenous leukemia: a report of the German cooperative study AML-BFM-78. *Blood* 1985; **65**: 298–304.

35. Creutzig U, Schellong G, Ritter J *et al.* Improved results in treatment of acute myelogenous leukemia in children: report of the German cooperative AML study BFM-78. *Haematol Blood Transfus* 1983; **28**: 46–50.

36. Buchner T, Hiddemann W, Wormann B *et al.* Double induction strategy for acute myeloid leukemia: the effect of high-dose cytarabine with mitoxantrone instead of standard-dose cytarabine with daunorubicin and 6-thioguanine: a randomized trial by the German AML Cooperative Group. *Blood* 1999; **93**: 4116–24.

37. Bostrom B, Brunning RD, McGlave P *et al.* Bone marrow transplantation for acute nonlymphocytic leukemia in first remission: analysis of prognostic factors. *Blood* 1985; **65**: 1191–6.

38. Sandler DP. Epidemiology of acute myelogenous leukemia. *Semin Oncol* 1987; **14**: 359–64.

39. Ries LAG, Smith MA, Gurney JG, Linet M, Tamra T, Young JL, Bunin GR (eds). *Cancer Incidence and Survival among Children and Adolescents: United States SEER Program 1975–1995*. National Cancer Institute, SEER Program. NIH Pub. No. 99-4649. Bethesda, MD: National Institutes of Health, 1999.

40. Greenberg RS, Shuster JL Jr. Epidemiology of cancer in children. *Epidemiol Rev* 1985; **7**: 22–48.

41. Bhatia S, Neglia JP. Epidemiology of childhood acute myelogenous leukemia. *J Pediatr Hematol Oncol* 1995; **17**: 94–100.

42. Alexander FE, Patheal SL, Biondi A *et al.* Transplacental chemical exposure and risk of infant leukemia with MLL gene fusion. *Cancer Res* 2001; **61**: 2542–6.

43. Armstrong B, Theriault G, Guenel P, Deadman J, Goldberg M, Heroux P. Association between exposure to pulsed electromagnetic fields and cancer in electric utility workers in Quebec, Canada, and France. *Am J Epidemiol* 1994; **140**: 805–20.

44. Brondum J, Shu XO, Steinbuch M, Severson RK, Potter JD, Robison LL. Parental cigarette smoking and the risk of acute leukemia in children. *Cancer* 1999; **85**: 1380–8.

45. Flodin U, Fredriksson M, Persson B, Hardell L, Axelson O. Background radiation, electrical work, and some other exposures associated with acute myeloid leukemia in a case-referent study. *Arch Environ Health* 1986; **41**: 77–84.

46. Gundestrup M, Storm HH. Radiation-induced acute myeloid leukaemia and other cancers in commercial jet cockpit crew: a population-based cohort study. *Lancet* 1999; **354**: 2029–31.

47. Robison LL, Buckley JD, Daigle AE *et al.* Maternal drug use and risk of childhood nonlymphoblastic leukemia among offspring. An epidemiologic investigation implicating marijuana (a report from the Children's Cancer Study Group). *Cancer* 1989; **63**: 1904–11.

48. Ross JA. Maternal diet and infant leukemia: a role for DNA topoisomerase II inhibitors? *Int J Cancer Suppl* 1998; **11**: 26–8.

49. Severson RK, Davis S, Heuser L, Daling JR, Thomas DB. Cigarette smoking and acute nonlymphocytic leukemia. *Am J Epidemiol* 1990; **132**: 418–22.

50. Severson RK, Buckley JD, Woods WG, Benjamin D, Robison LL. Cigarette smoking and alcohol consumption by parents of children with acute myeloid leukemia: an analysis within morphological subgroups: a report from the Children's Cancer Group. *Cancer Epidemiol Biomarkers Prev* 1993; **2**: 433–9.

51. Theriault G, Goldberg M, Miller AB, Armstrong B, Guenel P, Deadman J *et al.* Cancer risks associated with occupational exposure to magnetic fields among electric utility workers in Ontario and Quebec, Canada, and France: 1970–1989. *Am J Epidemiol* 1994; **139**: 550–72.

52. Yeazel MW, Ross JA, Buckley JD, Woods WG, Ruccione K, Robison LL. High birth weight and risk of specific childhood cancers: a report from the Children's Cancer Group. *J Pediatr* 1997; **131**: 671–7.

53. Flodin U, Fredriksson M, Persson B, Axelson O. Acute myeloid leukemia and background radiation in an expanded case-referent study. *Arch Environ Health* 1990; **45**: 364–6.

54. Rubin CM, Arthur DC, Woods WG *et al.* Therapy-related myelodysplastic syndrome and acute myeloid leukemia in children: correlation between chromosomal abnormalities and prior therapy. *Blood* 1991; **78**: 2982–8.

55. Schoch C, Schnittger S, Klaus M, Kern W, Hiddemann W, Haferlach T. AML with 11q23/MLL abnormalities as defined by the WHO classification: incidence, partner chromosomes, FAB subtype, age distribution, and prognostic impact in an unselected series of 1897 cytogenetically analyzed AML cases. *Blood* 2003; **102**: 2395–402.

56. Draper G, Vincent T, Kroll ME, Swanson J. Childhood cancer in relation to distance from high voltage power lines in England and Wales: a case-control study. *Br Med J* 2005; **330**: 1290.

57. Savitz DA, Wachtel H, Barnes FA, John EM, Tvrdik JG. Case-control study of childhood cancer and exposure to 60-Hz magnetic fields. *Am J Epidemiol* 1988; **128**: 21–38.

58. Savitz DA, Kaune WT. Childhood cancer in relation to a modified residential wire code. *Environ Health Perspect* 1993; **101**: 76–80.

59. London SJ, Thomas DC, Bowman JD, Sobel E, Cheng TC, Peters JM. Exposure to residential electric and magnetic fields and risk of childhood leukemia. *Am J Epidemiol* 1991; **134**: 923–37.

60. Fulton JP, Cobb S, Preble L, Leone L, Forman E. Electrical wiring configurations and childhood leukemia in Rhode Island. *Am J Epidemiol* 1980; **111**: 292–6.

61. McBride ML, Gallagher RP, Theriault G *et al.* Power-frequency electric and magnetic fields and risk of childhood leukemia in Canada. *Am J Epidemiol* 1999; **149**: 831–42.

62. Mizoue T, Onoe Y, Moritake H, Okamura J, Sokejima S, Nitta H. Residential proximity to high-voltage power lines and risk of childhood hematological malignancies. *J Epidemiol* 2004; **14**: 118–23.

63. Savitz DA, John EM, Kleckner RC. Magnetic field exposure from electric appliances and childhood cancer. *Am J Epidemiol* 1990; **131**: 763–73.

64. Oppenheimer M, Preston-Martin S. Adult onset acute myelogenous leukemia and electromagnetic fields in Los Angeles County: bed-heating and occupational exposures. *Bioelectromagnetics* 2002; **23**: 411–15.

65. Lilleyman JS, Hann IM, Stevens RF, Eden OB, Richards SM. French American British (FAB) morphological classification of childhood lymphoblastic leukaemia and its clinical importance. *J Clin Pathol* 1986; **39**: 998–1002.

66. Harris NL, Jaffe ES, Diebold J *et al.* The World Health Organization classification of neoplastic diseases of the hematopoietic and lymphoid tissues. Report of the Clinical Advisory Committee meeting, Airlie House, Virginia, November 1997. *Ann Oncol* 1999; **10**: 1419–32.

67. Harris NL, Jaffe ES, Diebold J *et al.* World Health Organization classification of neoplastic diseases of the hematopoietic and lymphoid tissues: report of the Clinical Advisory Committee meeting, Airlie House, Virginia, November 1997. *J Clin Oncol* 1999; **17**: 3835–49.

68. Harris NL, Jaffe ES, Diebold J *et al.* The World Health Organization classification of hematological malignancies report of the Clinical Advisory Committee Meeting, Airlie House, Virginia, November 1997. *Mod Pathol* 2000; **13**: 193–207.

69. Harris NL, Jaffe ES, Diebold J *et al.* The World Health Organization classification of neoplastic diseases of the haematopoietic and lymphoid tissues: Report of the Clinical Advisory Committee Meeting, Airlie House, Virginia, November 1997. *Histopathology* 2000; **36**: 69–86.

70. Vardiman JW, Harris NL, Brunning RD. The World Health Organization (WHO) classification of the myeloid neoplasms. *Blood* 2002; **100**: 2292–302.

71. Barnard DR, Kalousek DK, Wiersma SR *et al.* Morphologic, immunologic, and cytogenetic classification of acute myeloid leukemia and myelodysplastic syndrome in childhood: a report from the Children's Cancer Group. *Leukemia* 1996; **10**: 5–12.

72. Bradstock KF, Kirk J, Grimsley PG, Kabral A, Hughes WG. Unusual immunophenotypes in acute leukaemias: incidence and clinical correlations. *Br J Haematol* 1989; **72**: 512–18.

73. Campos L, Guyotat D, Archimbaud E *et al.* Surface marker expression in adult acute myeloid leukaemia: correlations with initial characteristics, morphology and response to therapy. *Br J Haematol* 1989; **72**: 161–6.

74. Jennings CD, Foon KA. Recent advances in flow cytometry: application to the diagnosis of hematologic malignancy. *Blood* 1997; **90**: 2863–92.

75. Jennings CD, Foon KA. Flow cytometry: recent advances in diagnosis and monitoring of leukemia. *Cancer Invest* 1997; **15**: 384–99.

76. Kuerbitz SJ, Civin CI, Krischer JP *et al.* Expression of myeloid-associated and lymphoid-associated cell-surface antigens in acute myeloid leukemia of childhood: a Pediatric Oncology Group study. *J Clin Oncol* 1992; **10**: 1419–29.

77. Launder TM, Bray RA, Stempora L, Chenggis ML, Farhi DC. Lymphoid-associated antigen expression by acute myeloid leukemia. *Am J Clin Pathol* 1996; **106**: 185–91.

78. Lo Coco F, Pasqualetti D, Lopez M *et al.* Immunophenotyping of acute myeloid leukaemia: relevance of analysing different lineage-associated markers. *Blut* 1989; **58**: 235–40.

79. Neame PB, Soamboonsrup P, Browman GP *et al.* Classifying acute leukemia by immunophenotyping: a combined FAB-immunologic classification of AML. *Blood* 1986; **68**: 1355–62.

80. Sievers EL, Lange BJ, Alonzo TA *et al.* Immunophenotypic evidence of leukemia after induction therapy predicts relapse: results from a prospective Children's Cancer Group study of 252 patients with acute myeloid leukemia. *Blood* 2003; **101**: 3398–406.

81. van der Reijden HJ, van Rhenen DJ, Lansdorp PM *et al.* A comparison of surface marker analysis and FAB classification in acute myeloid leukemia. *Blood* 1983; **61**: 443–8.

82. Griffin JD, Mayer RJ, Weinstein HJ *et al.* Surface marker analysis of acute myeloblastic leukemia: identification of differentiation-associated phenotypes. *Blood* 1983; **62**: 557–63.

83. Creutzig U, Harbott J, Sperling C *et al.* Clinical significance of surface antigen expression in children with acute myeloid leukemia: results of study AML-BFM-87. *Blood* 1995; **86**: 3097–108.

84. Langebrake C, Brinkmann I, Teigler-Schlegel A *et al.* Immunophenotypic differences between diagnosis and relapse in childhood AML: Implications for MRD monitoring. *Cytometry B Clin Cytom* 2005; **63**: 1–9.

85. Estey E, Trujillo JM, Cork A *et al.* AML-associated cytogenetic abnormalities (inv(16), del(16), t(8;21)) in patients with myelodysplastic syndromes. *Hematol Pathol* 1992; **6**: 43–8.

86. Frohling S, Skelin S, Liebisch C *et al.* Comparison of cytogenetic and molecular cytogenetic detection of chromosome abnormalities in 240 consecutive adult patients with acute myeloid leukemia. *J Clin Oncol* 2002; **20**: 2480–5.

87. Hilden JM, Smith FO, Frestedt JL *et al.* MLL gene rearrangement, cytogenetic 11q23 abnormalities, and expression of the NG2 molecule in infant acute myeloid leukemia. *Blood* 1997; **89**: 3801–5.

88. Martinez-Climent JA, Lane NJ, Rubin CM *et al.* Clinical and prognostic significance of chromosomal abnormalities in childhood acute myeloid leukemia de novo. *Leukemia* 1995; **9**: 95–101.

89. Martinez-Climent JA, Garcia-Conde J. Chromosomal rearrangements in childhood acute myeloid leukemia and myelodysplastic syndromes. *J Pediatr Hematol Oncol* 1999; **21**: 91–102.

90. Raimondi SC, Chang MN, Ravindranath Y *et al.* Chromosomal abnormalities in 478 children with acute myeloid leukemia: clinical characteristics and treatment outcome in a cooperative pediatric oncology group study POG 8821. *Blood* 1999; **94**: 3707–16.

91. Yagi T, Morimoto A, Eguchi M *et al.* Identification of a gene expression signature associated with pediatric AML prognosis. *Blood* 2003; **102**: 1849–56.

92. Coustan-Smith E, Gajjar A, Hijiya N *et al.* Clinical significance of minimal residual disease in childhood acute lymphoblastic leukemia after first relapse. *Leukemia* 2004; **18**: 499–504.

93. Ross ME, Mahfouz R, Onciu M *et al.* Gene expression profiling of pediatric acute myelogenous leukemia. *Blood* 2004; **104**: 3679–87.

94. Lindvall C, Furge K, Bjorkholm M *et al.* Combined genetic and transcriptional profiling of acute myeloid leukemia with normal and complex karyotypes. *Haematologica* 2004; **89**: 1072–81.

95. Gutierrez NC, Lopez-Perez R, Hernandez JM *et al.* Gene expression profile reveals deregulation of genes with relevant functions in the different subclasses of acute myeloid leukemia. *Leukemia* 2005; **19**: 402–9.

96. Golub TR, Slonim DK, Tamayo P *et al.* Molecular classification of cancer: class discovery and class prediction by gene expression monitoring. *Science* 1999; **286**: 531–7.

97. van Delft FW, Bellotti T, Luo Z *et al.* Prospective gene expression analysis accurately subtypes acute leukaemia in children and establishes a commonality between hyperdiploidy and t(12;21) in acute lymphoblastic leukaemia. *Br J Haematol* 2005; **130**: 26–35.

98. Haferlach T, Kohlmann A, Schnittger S *et al.* Global approach to the diagnosis of leukemia using gene expression profiling. *Blood* 2005; **106**: 1189–98.

99. Haferlach T, Schnittger S, Kern W, Hiddemann W, Schoch C. Genetic classification of acute myeloid leukemia (AML). *Ann Hematol* 2004; **83** (suppl. 1): S97–S100.

100. Lacayo NJ, Meshinchi S, Kinnunen P *et al.* Gene expression profiles at diagnosis in de novo childhood AML patients identify FLT3 mutations with good clinical outcomes. *Blood* 2004; **104**: 2646–54.

101. Valk PJ, Verhaak RG, Beijen MA *et al.* Prognostically useful gene-expression profiles in acute myeloid leukemia. *N Engl J Med* 2004; **350**: 1617–28.

102. Valk PJ, Delwel R, Lowenberg B. Gene expression profiling in acute myeloid leukemia. *Curr Opin Hematol* 2005; **12**: 76–81.

103. Ley TJ, Minx PJ, Walter MJ *et al.* A pilot study of high-throughput, sequence-based mutational profiling of primary human acute myeloid leukemia cell genomes. *Proc Natl Acad Sci USA* 2003; **100**: 14275–80.

104. Hayashi Y. Gene expression profiling in childhood acute leukemia: progress and perspectives. *Int J Hematol* 2003; **78**: 414–20.

105. Court EL, Smith MA, Avent ND *et al.* DNA microarray screening of differential gene expression in bone marrow samples from AML, non-AML patients and AML cell lines. *Leuk Res* 2004; **28**: 743–53.

106. Chang M, Raimondi SC, Ravindranath Y *et al.* Prognostic

factors in children and adolescents with acute myeloid leukemia (excluding children with Down syndrome and acute promyelocytic leukemia): univariate and recursive partitioning analysis of patients treated on Pediatric Oncology Group (POG) Study 8821. *Leukemia* 2000; **14**: 1201–7.

107. Grimwade D, Walker H, Oliver F *et al*. The importance of diagnostic cytogenetics on outcome in AML: analysis of 1,612 patients entered into the MRC AML 10 trial. The Medical Research Council Adult and Children's Leukaemia Working Parties. *Blood* 1998; **92**: 2322–33.

108. Wheatley K, Burnett AK, Goldstone AH *et al*. A simple, robust, validated and highly predictive index for the determination of risk-directed therapy in acute myeloid leukaemia derived from the MRC AML 10 trial. United Kingdom Medical Research Council's Adult and Childhood Leukaemia Working Parties. *Br J Haematol* 1999; **107**: 69–79.

109. Chen AR, Alonzo TA, Woods WG, Arceci RJ. Current controversies: which patients with acute myeloid leukaemia should receive a bone marrow transplantation? An American view. *Br J Haematol* 2002; **118**: 378–84.

110. Creutzig U, Reinhardt D. Current controversies: which patients with acute myeloid leukaemia should receive a bone marrow transplantation? A European view. *Br J Haematol* 2002; **118**: 365–77.

111. Meshinchi S, Woods WG, Stirewalt DL *et al*. Prevalence and prognostic significance of Flt3 internal tandem duplication in pediatric acute myeloid leukemia. *Blood* 2001; **97**: 89–94.

112. Webb DK, Harrison G, Stevens RF, Gibson BG, Hann IM, Wheatley K. Relationships between age at diagnosis, clinical features, and outcome of therapy in children treated in the Medical Research Council AML 10 and 12 trials for acute myeloid leukemia. *Blood* 2001; **98**: 1714–20.

113. Marcucci G, Caligiuri MA, Bloomfield CD. Molecular and clinical advances in core binding factor primary acute myeloid leukemia: a paradigm for translational research in malignant hematology. *Cancer Invest* 2000; **18**: 768–80.

114. Marcucci G, Caligiuri MA, Bloomfield CD. Core binding factor (CBF) acute myeloid leukemia: is molecular monitoring by RT-PCR useful clinically? *Eur J Haematol* 2003; **71**: 143–54.

115. Ferrara FF, Fazi F, Bianchini A *et al*. Histone deacetylase-targeted treatment restores retinoic acid signaling and differentiation in acute myeloid leukemia. *Cancer Res* 2001; **61**: 2–7.

116. Minucci S, Nervi C, Lo Coco F, Pelicci PG. Histone deacetylases: a common molecular target for differentiation treatment of acute myeloid leukemias? *Oncogene* 2001; **20**: 3110–15.

117. Insinga A, Monestiroli S, Ronzoni S *et al*. Inhibitors of histone deacetylases induce tumor-selective apoptosis through activation of the death receptor pathway. *Nat Med* 2005; **11**: 71–6.

118. Amin HM, Saeed S, Alkan S. Histone deacetylase inhibitors induce caspase-dependent apoptosis and downregulation of daxx in acute promyelocytic leukaemia with t(15;17). *Br J Haematol* 2001; **115**: 287–97.

119. Cote S, Rosenauer A, Bianchini A *et al*. Response to histone deacetylase inhibition of novel PML/RARalpha mutants detected in retinoic acid-resistant APL cells. *Blood* 2002; **100**: 2586–96.

120. Mistry AR, Pedersen EW, Solomon E, Grimwade D. The molecular pathogenesis of acute promyelocytic leukaemia: implications for the clinical management of the disease. *Blood Rev* 2003; **17**: 71–97.

121. Fenaux P, Chastang C, Chevret S *et al*. A randomized comparison of all transretinoic acid (ATRA) followed by chemotherapy and ATRA plus chemotherapy and the role of maintenance therapy in newly diagnosed acute promyelocytic leukemia. The European APL Group. *Blood* 1999; **94**: 1192–200.

122. Tallman MS, Andersen JW, Schiffer CA *et al*. All-*trans* retinoic acid in acute promyelocytic leukemia: long-term outcome and prognostic factor analysis from the North American Intergroup protocol. *Blood* 2002; **100**: 4298–302.

123. Ravindranath Y, Gregory J, Feusner J. Treatment of acute promyelocytic leukemia in children: arsenic or ATRA. *Leukemia* 2004; **18**: 1576–7.

124. Gregory J Jr, Feusner J. Acute promyelocytic leukaemia in children. *Best Pract Res Clin Haematol* 2003; **16**: 483–94.

125. Lemons RS, Keller S, Gietzen D *et al*. Acute promyelocytic leukemia. *J Pediatr Hematol Oncol* 1995; **17**: 198–210.

126. Testi AM, Biondi A, Lo Coco F *et al*. GIMEMA-AIEOPAIDA protocol for the treatment of newly diagnosed acute promyelocytic leukemia (APL) in children. *Blood* 2005; **106**: 447–53.

127. Falini B, Mecucci C, Tiacci E *et al*. Cytoplasmic nucleophosmin in acute myelogenous leukemia with a normal karyotype. *N Engl J Med* 2005; **352**: 254–66.

128. Casillas JN, Woods WG, Hunger SP, McGavran L, Alonzo TA, Feig SA. Prognostic implications of t(10;11) translocations in childhood acute myelogenous leukemia: a report from the Children's Cancer Group. *J Pediatr Hematol Oncol* 2003; **25**: 594–600.

129. Ernst P, Wang J, Korsmeyer SJ. The role of MLL in hematopoiesis and leukemia. *Curr Opin Hematol* 2002; **9**: 282–7.

130. Rubnitz JE, Raimondi SC, Tong X *et al*. Favorable impact of the t(9;11) in childhood acute myeloid leukemia. *J Clin Oncol* 2002; **20**: 2302–9.

131. Grier DG, Thompson A, Kwasniewska A, McGonigle GJ, Halliday HL, Lappin TR. The pathophysiology of HOX genes and their role in cancer. *J Pathol* 2005; **205**: 154–71.

132. Ernst P, Mabon M, Davidson AJ, Zon LI, Korsmeyer SJ. An Mll-dependent Hox program drives hematopoietic progenitor expansion. *Curr Biol* 2004; **14**: 2063–9.

133. Ernst P, Fisher JK, Avery W, Wade S, Foy D, Korsmeyer SJ. Definitive hematopoiesis requires the mixed-lineage leukemia gene. *Dev Cell* 2004; **6**: 437–43.

134. Eguchi M, Eguchi-Ishimae M, Greaves M. The role of the MLL gene in infant leukemia. *Int J Hematol* 2003; **78**: 390–401.

135. Hsu K, Look AT. Turning on a dimer: new insights into MLL chimeras. *Cancer Cell* 2003; **4**: 81–3.

136. Woods WG, Nesbit ME, Buckley J *et al*. Correlation of chromosome abnormalities with patient characteristics, histologic subtype, and induction success in children with acute nonlymphocytic leukemia. *J Clin Oncol* 1985; **3**: 3–11.

137. Wolman SR, Gundacker H, Appelbaum FR, Slovak ML. Impact of trisomy 8 (+8) on clinical presentation, treatment response, and survival in acute myeloid leukemia: a Southwest Oncology Group study. *Blood* 2002; **100**: 29–35.

138. Abu-Duhier FM, Goodeve AC, Wilson GA *et al.* FLT3 internal tandem duplication mutations in adult acute myeloid leukaemia define a high-risk group. *Br J Haematol* 2000; **111**: 190–5.

139. Abu-Duhier FM, Goodeve AC, Wilson GA, Care RS, Peake IR, Reilly JT. Identification of novel FLT-3 Asp835 mutations in adult acute myeloid leukaemia. *Br J Haematol* 2001; **113**: 983–8.

140. Abu-Duhier FM, Goodeve AC, Wilson GA, Care RS, Peake IR, Reilly JT. Genomic structure of human FLT3: implications for mutational analysis. *Br J Haematol* 2001; **113**: 1076–7.

141. Kiyoi H, Naoe T, Nakano Y *et al.* Prognostic implication of FLT3 and N-RAS gene mutations in acute myeloid leukemia. *Blood* 1999; **93**: 3074–80.

142. Kottaridis PD, Gale RE, Linch DC. Prognostic implications of the presence of FLT3 mutations in patients with acute myeloid leukemia. *Leuk Lymphoma* 2003; **44**: 905–13.

143. Kottaridis PD, Gale RE, Langabeer SE, Frew ME, Bowen DT, Linch DC. Studies of FLT3 mutations in paired presentation and relapse samples from patients with acute myeloid leukemia: implications for the role of FLT3 mutations in leukemogenesis, minimal residual disease detection, and possible therapy with FLT3 inhibitors. *Blood* 2002; **100**: 2393–8.

144. Kottaridis PD, Gale RE, Frew ME *et al.* The presence of a FLT3 internal tandem duplication in patients with acute myeloid leukemia (AML) adds important prognostic information to cytogenetic risk group and response to the first cycle of chemotherapy: analysis of 854 patients from the United Kingdom Medical Research Council AML 10 and 12 trials. *Blood* 2001; **98**: 1752–9.

145. Iwai T, Yokota S, Nakao M *et al.* Internal tandem duplication of the FLT3 gene and clinical evaluation in childhood acute myeloid leukemia. The Children's Cancer and Leukemia Study Group, Japan. *Leukemia* 1999; **13**: 38–43.

146. Zwaan CM, Meshinchi S, Radich JP *et al.* FLT3 internal tandem duplication in 234 children with acute myeloid leukemia: prognostic significance and relation to cellular drug resistance. *Blood* 2003; **102**: 2387–94.

147. Thiede C, Steudel C, Mohr B *et al.* Analysis of FLT3-activating mutations in 979 patients with acute myelogenous leukemia: association with FAB subtypes and identification of subgroups with poor prognosis. *Blood* 2002; **99**: 4326–35.

148. Perel Y, Auvrignon A, Leblanc T *et al.* Impact of addition of maintenance therapy to intensive induction and consolidation chemotherapy for childhood acute myeloblastic leukemia: results of a prospective randomized trial, LAME 89/91. Leucamie Aique Myeloide Enfant. *J Clin Oncol* 2002; **20**: 2774–82.

149. Wells RJ, Woods WG, Lampkin BC *et al.* Impact of high-dose cytarabine and asparaginase intensification on childhood acute myeloid leukemia: a report from the Children's Cancer Group. *J Clin Oncol* 1993; **11**: 538–45.

150. Goldie JH, Coldman AJ. A mathematic model for relating the drug sensitivity of tumors to their spontaneous mutation rate. *Cancer Treat Rep* 1979; **63**: 1727–33.

151. Goldie JH, Coldman AJ. Quantitative model for multiple levels of drug resistance in clinical tumors. *Cancer Treat Rep* 1983; **67**: 923–31.

152. Goldie JH, Coldman AJ, Gudauskas GA. Rationale for the use of alternating non-cross-resistant chemotherapy. *Cancer Treat Rep* 1982; **66**: 439–49.

153. Feig SA, Lampkin B, Nesbit ME *et al.* Outcome of BMT during first complete remission of AML: a comparison of two sequential studies by the Children's Cancer Group. *Bone Marrow Transplant* 1993; **12**: 65–71.

154. Creutzig U, Ritter J, Zimmermann M *et al.* Idarubicin improves blast cell clearance during induction therapy in children with AML: results of study AML-BFM 93. AML-BFM Study Group. *Leukemia* 2001; **15**: 348–54.

155. Lange BJ, Dinndorf P, Smith FO *et al.* Pilot study of idarubicin-based intensive-timing induction therapy for children with previously untreated acute myeloid leukemia: Children's Cancer Group Study 2941. *J Clin Oncol* 2004; **22**: 150–6.

156. Burnett AK, Goldstone AH, Stevens RM *et al.* Randomised comparison of addition of autologous bone-marrow transplantation to intensive chemotherapy for acute myeloid leukaemia in first remission: results of MRC AML 10 trial. UK Medical Research Council Adult and Children's Leukaemia Working Parties. *Lancet* 1998; **351**: 700–8.

157. Burnett AK, Wheatley K, Goldstone AH *et al.* The value of allogeneic bone marrow transplant in patients with acute myeloid leukaemia at differing risk of relapse: results of the UK MRC AML 10 trial. *Br J Haematol* 2002; **118**: 385–400.

158. Brenner M, Krance R, Heslop HE *et al.* Assessment of the efficacy of purging by using gene marked autologous marrow transplantation for children with AML in first complete remission. *Hum Gene Ther* 1994; **5**: 481–99.

159. Wheatley K, Clayton D. Be skeptical about unexpected large apparent treatment effects: the case of an MRC AML12 randomization. *Control Clin Trials* 2003; **24**: 66–70.

160. Creutzig U, Zimmermann M, Ritter J *et al.* Definition of a standard-risk group in children with AML. *Br J Haematol* 1999; **104**: 630–9.

161. Karp JE, Donehower RC, Burke PJ. An in vitro model to predict clinical response in adult acute myelogenous leukemia. *Semin Oncol* 1987; **14** (2 suppl. 1): 172–81.

162. Burke PJ, Karp JE, Vaughan WP. Chemotherapy of leukemia in mice, rats, and humans relating time of humoral stimulation, tumor growth, and clinical response. *J Natl Cancer Inst* 1981; **67**: 529–38.

163. Tallman MS, Nabhan C, Feusner JH, Rowe JM. Acute promyelocytic leukemia: evolving therapeutic strategies. *Blood* 2002; **99**: 759–67.

164. Bapna A, Nair R, Tapan KS *et al.* All-trans-retinoic acid (ATRA): pediatric acute promyelocytic leukemia. *Pediatr Hematol Oncol* 1998; **15**: 243–8.

165. Mann G, Reinhardt D, Ritter J *et al.* Treatment with all-trans retinoic acid in acute promyelocytic leukemia reduces early deaths in children. *Ann Hematol* 2001; **80**: 417–22.

166. Guglielmi C, Martelli MP, Diverio D *et al.* Immunophenotype of adult and childhood acute promyelocytic leukaemia: correlation with morphology, type of PML gene breakpoint and clinical outcome. A cooperative Italian study on 196 cases. *Br J Haematol* 1998; **102**: 1035–41.

167. de Botton S, Fawaz A, Chevret S *et al.* Autologous and allogeneic stem-cell transplantation as salvage treatment of acute promyelocytic leukemia initially treated with all-

trans-retinoic acid: a retrospective analysis of the European acute promyelocytic leukemia group. *J Clin Oncol* 2005; **23**: 120–6.

168. Meloni G, Diverio D, Vignetti M *et al.* Autologous bone marrow transplantation for acute promyelocytic leukemia in second remission: prognostic relevance of pretransplant minimal residual disease assessment by reverse-transcription polymerase chain reaction of the PML/RAR alpha fusion gene. *Blood* 1997; **90**: 1321–5.

169. Tallman MS, Nabhan C. Management of acute promyelocytic leukemia. *Curr Oncol Rep* 2002; **4**: 381–9.

170. Nabhan C, Mehta J, Tallman MS. The role of bone marrow transplantation in acute promyelocytic leukemia. *Bone Marrow Transplant* 2001; **28**: 219–26.

171. Chou WC, Chen HY, Yu SL, Cheng L, Yang PC, Dang CV. Arsenic suppresses gene expression in promyelocytic leukemia cells partly through Sp1 oxidation. *Blood* 2005; **106**: 304–10.

172. Douer D, Tallman MS. Arsenic trioxide: new clinical experience with an old medication in hematologic malignancies. *J Clin Oncol* 2005; **23**: 2396–410.

173. Soignet SL, Maslak P, Wang ZG *et al.* Complete remission after treatment of acute promyelocytic leukemia with arsenic trioxide. *N Engl J Med* 1998; **339**: 1341–8.

174. Zein N, Sinha AM, McGahren WJ, Ellestad GA. Calicheamicin gamma 1I: an antitumor antibiotic that cleaves double-stranded DNA site specifically. *Science* 1988; **240**: 1198–201.

175. Dinndorf PA, Andrews RG, Benjamin D, Ridgway D, Wolff L, Bernstein ID. Expression of normal myeloid-associated antigens by acute leukemia cells. *Blood* 1986; **67**: 1048–53.

176. Bernstein ID, Singer JW, Andrews RG *et al.* Treatment of acute myeloid leukemia cells in vitro with a monoclonal antibody recognizing a myeloid differentiation antigen allows normal progenitor cells to be expressed. *J Clin Invest* 1987; **79**: 1153–9.

177. Tsimberidou A, Estey E, Cortes J *et al.* Gemtuzumab, fludarabine, cytarabine, and cyclosporine in patients with newly diagnosed acute myelogenous leukemia or high-risk myelodysplastic syndromes. *Cancer* 2003; **97**: 1481–7.

178. Reinhardt D, Diekamp S, Fleischhack G *et al.* Gemtuzumab ozogamicin (Mylotarg) in children with refractory or relapsed acute myeloid leukemia. *Onkologie* 2004; **27**: 269–72.

179. Zwaan CM, Reinhardt D, Corbacioglu S *et al.* Gemtuzumab ozogamicin: first clinical experiences in children with relapsed/refractory acute myeloid leukemia treated on compassionate-use basis. *Blood* 2003; **101**: 3868–71.

180. Zwaan CM, Reinhardt D, Jurgens H *et al.* Gemtuzumab ozogamicin in pediatric CD33-positive acute lymphoblastic leukemia: first clinical experiences and relation with cellular sensitivity to single agent calicheamicin. *Leukemia* 2003; **17**: 468–70.

181. Kell WJ, Burnett AK, Chopra R *et al.* A feasibility study of simultaneous administration of gemtuzumab ozogamicin with intensive chemotherapy in induction and consolidation in younger patients with acute myeloid leukemia. *Blood* 2003; **102**: 4277–83.

182. Piccaluga PP, Martinelli G, Rondoni M *et al.* Gemtuzumab ozogamicin for relapsed and refractory acute myeloid leukemia and myeloid sarcomas. *Leuk Lymphoma* 2004; **45**: 1791–5.

183. Larson RA, Sievers EL, Stadtmauer EA *et al.* Final report of the

184. Arceci RJ, Sande J, Lange B *et al.* Safety and efficacy of gemtuzumab ozogamicin in pediatric patients with advanced CD33+ acute myeloid leukemia. *Blood* 2005; **106**: 1183–8.

185. Neumeister P, Eibl M, Zinke-Cerwenka W, Scarpatetti M, Sill H, Linkesch W. Hepatic veno-occlusive disease in two patients with relapsed acute myeloid leukemia treated with anti-CD33 calicheamicin (CMA-676) immunoconjugate. *Ann Hematol* 2001; **80**: 119–20.

186. Sievers EL, Appelbaum FR, Spielberger RT *et al.* Selective ablation of acute myeloid leukemia using antibody-targeted chemotherapy: a phase I study of an anti-CD33 calicheamicin immunoconjugate. *Blood* 1999; **93**: 3678–84.

187. Sievers EL, Larson RA, Stadtmauer EA *et al.* Efficacy and safety of gemtuzumab ozogamicin in patients with CD33-positive acute myeloid leukemia in first relapse. *J Clin Oncol* 2001; **19**: 3244–54.

188. Nordlander A, Mattsson J, Ringden O *et al.* Graft-versus-host disease is associated with a lower relapse incidence after hematopoietic stem cell transplantation in patients with acute lymphoblastic leukemia. *Biol Blood Marrow Transplant* 2004; **10**: 195–203.

189. Watson M, Buck G, Wheatley K *et al.* Adverse impact of bone marrow transplantation on quality of life in acute myeloid leukaemia patients; analysis of the UK Medical Research Council AML 10 Trial. *Eur J Cancer* 2004; **40**: 971–8.

190. Gamis AS, Howells WB, DeSwarte-Wallace J, Feusner JH, Buckley JD, Woods WG. Alpha hemolytic streptococcal infection during intensive treatment for acute myeloid leukemia: a report from the Children's cancer group study CCG-2891. *J Clin Oncol* 2000; **18**: 1845–55.

191. Creutzig U, Zimmermann M, Reinhardt D, Dworzak M, Stary J, Lehrnbecher T. Early deaths and treatment-related mortality in children undergoing therapy for acute myeloid leukemia: analysis of the multicenter clinical trials AML-BFM 93 and AML-BFM 98. *J Clin Oncol* 2004; **22**: 4384–93.

192. Alonzo TA, Kobrinsky NL, Aledo A, Lange BJ, Buxton AB, Woods WG. Impact of granulocyte colony-stimulating factor use during induction for acute myelogenous leukemia in children: a report from the Children's Cancer Group. *J Pediatr Hematol Oncol* 2002; **24**: 627–35.

193. Dusenbery KE, Howells WB, Arthur DC *et al.* Extramedullary leukemia in children with newly diagnosed acute myeloid leukemia: a report from the Children's Cancer Group. *J Pediatr Hematol Oncol* 2003; **25**: 760–8.

194. Creutzig U, Ritter J, Zimmermann M, Schellong G. Does cranial irradiation reduce the risk for bone marrow relapse in acute myelogenous leukemia? Unexpected results of the Childhood Acute Myelogenous Leukemia Study BFM-87. *J Clin Oncol* 1993; **11**: 279–86.

195. Reinhardt D, Creutzig U. Isolated myelosarcoma in children: update and review. *Leuk Lymphoma* 2002; **43**: 565–74.

196. Ravindranath Y, Abella E, Krischer JP *et al.* Acute myeloid leukemia (AML) in Down's syndrome is highly responsive to chemotherapy: experience on Pediatric Oncology Group AML Study 8498. *Blood* 1992; **80**: 2210–14.

197. Gurbuxani S, Vyas P, Crispino JD. Recent insights into the

mechanisms of myeloid leukemogenesis in Down syndrome. *Blood* 2004; **103**: 399–406.

198. Taub JW, Ravindranath Y. Down syndrome and the transient myeloproliferative disorder: why is it transient? *J Pediatr Hematol Oncol* 2002; **24**: 6–8.

199. Arceci RJ. Down syndrome, transient myeloproliferative syndrome, and leukemia: bridging development and neoplasia. *J Pediatr Hematol Oncol* 2002; **24**: 1.

200. Hitzler J, Zipursky A. GATA1 mutations as clonal markers of minimal residual disease in acute megakaryoblastic leukemia of Down syndrome: a new tool with significant potential applications. *Leuk Res* 2005; **29**(11): 1239–1240.

201. Hitzler JK, Zipursky A. Origins of leukaemia in children with Down syndrome. *Nat Rev Cancer* 2005; **5**: 11–20.

202. Lightfoot J, Hitzler JK, Zipursky A, Albert M, Macgregor PF. Distinct gene signatures of transient and acute megakaryoblastic leukemia in Down syndrome. *Leukemia* 2004; **18**: 1617–23.

203. Shen JJ, Williams BJ, Zipursky A *et al.* Cytogenetic and molecular studies of Down syndrome individuals with leukemia. *Am J Hum Genet* 1995; **56**: 915–25.

204. Zipursky A. Transient leukaemia: a benign form of leukaemia in newborn infants with trisomy 21. *Br J Haematol* 2003; **120**: 930–8.

205. Taub JW, Stout ML, Buck SA *et al.* Myeloblasts from Down syndrome children with acute myeloid leukemia have increased in vitro sensitivity to cytosine arabinoside and daunorubicin. *Leukemia* 1997; **11**: 1594–5.

206. Savasan S, Taub JW, Ravindranath Y. Down syndrome and leukemia: an overview of cytogenetic and molecular events. *Turk J Pediatr* 1997; **39**: 519–31.

207. Ravindranath Y, Taub JW. Down syndrome and acute myeloid leukemia. Lessons learned from experience with high-dose Ara-C containing regimens. *Adv Exp Med Biol* 1999; **457**: 409–14.

208. Ge Y, Jensen TL, Stout ML *et al.* The role of cytidine deaminase and GATA1 mutations in the increased cytosine arabinoside sensitivity of Down syndrome myeloblasts and leukemia cell lines. *Cancer Res* 2004; **64**: 728–35.

209. Taub JW, Ge Y. Down syndrome, drug metabolism and chromosome 21. *Pediatr Blood Cancer* 2005; **44**: 33–9.

210. Ge Y, Stout ML, Tatman DA *et al.* GATA1, cytidine deaminase, and the high cure rate of Down syndrome children with acute megakaryocytic leukemia. *J Natl Cancer Inst* 2005; **97**: 226–31.

211. Vignetti M, Orsini E, Petti MC *et al.* Probability of long-term disease-free survival for acute myeloid leukemia patients after first relapse: a single-centre experience. *Ann Oncol* 1996; **7**: 933–8.

212. Kardos G, Zwaan CM, Kaspers GJ *et al.* Treatment strategy and results in children treated on three Dutch Childhood Oncology Group acute myeloid leukemia trials. *Leukemia* 2005; **19**(12): 2063–71.

213. Estey EH. Treatment of relapsed and refractory acute myelogenous leukemia. *Leukemia* 2000; **14**: 476–9.

214. Estey E, Thall P, David C. Design and analysis of trials of salvage therapy in acute myelogenous leukemia. *Cancer Chemother Pharmacol* 1997; **40** (suppl.): S9–S12.

215. Leahey A, Kelly K, Rorke LB, Lange B. A phase I/II study of idarubicin (Ida) with continuous infusion fludarabine (F-ara-A) and cytarabine (ara-C) for refractory or recurrent pediatric acute myeloid leukemia (AML). *J Pediatr Hematol Oncol* 1997; **19**: 304–8.

216. Fleischhack G, Hasan C, Graf N, Mann G, Bode U. IDA-FLAG (idarubicin, fludarabine, cytarabine, G-CSF), an effective remission-induction therapy for poor-prognosis AML of childhood prior to allogeneic or autologous bone marrow transplantation: experiences of a phase II trial. *Br J Haematol* 1998; **102**: 647–55.

217. Webb DK, Wheatley K, Harrison G, Stevens RF, Hann IM. Outcome for children with relapsed acute myeloid leukaemia following initial therapy in the Medical Research Council (MRC) AML 10 trial. MRC Childhood Leukaemia Working Party. *Leukemia* 1999; **13**: 25–31.

218. Godder KT, Hazlett LJ, Abhyankar SH *et al.* Partially mismatched related-donor bone marrow transplantation for pediatric patients with acute leukemia: younger donors and absence of peripheral blasts improve outcome. *J Clin Oncol* 2000; **18**: 1856–66.

219. Henslee-Downey PJ. Mismatched bone marrow transplantation. *Curr Opin Oncol* 1995; **7**: 115–21.

220. Casper J, Camitta B, Truitt R *et al.* Unrelated bone marrow donor transplants for children with leukemia or myelodysplasia. *Blood* 1995; **85**: 2354–63.

221. Davies SM, Wagner JE, Shu XO *et al.* Unrelated donor bone marrow transplantation for children with acute leukemia. *J Clin Oncol* 1997; **15**: 557–65.

222. Veys PA, Meral A, Hassan A, Goulden N, Webb D, Davies G. Haploidentical related transplants and unrelated donor transplants with T cell addback. *Bone Marrow Transplant* 1998; **21** (suppl. 2): S42–S44.

223. Davies SM, Kollman C, Anasetti C *et al.* Engraftment and survival after unrelated-donor bone marrow transplantation: a report from the national marrow donor program. *Blood* 2000; **96**: 4096–102.

224. Szydlo R, Goldman JM, Klein JP *et al.* Results of allogeneic bone marrow transplants for leukemia using donors other than HLA-identical siblings. *J Clin Oncol* 1997; **15**: 1767–77.

225. Michallet M, Thomas X, Vernant JP *et al.* Long-term outcome after allogeneic hematopoietic stem cell transplantation for advanced stage acute myeloblastic leukemia: a retrospective study of 379 patients reported to the Societé Française de Greffe de Moelle (SFGM). *Bone Marrow Transplant* 2000; **26**: 1157–63.

226. Reichle A, Rothe G, Krause S *et al.* Transplant characteristics: minimal residual disease and impaired megakaryocytic colony growth as sensitive parameters for predicting relapse in acute myeloid leukemia. *Leukemia* 1999; **13**: 1227–34.

227. Venditti A, Tamburini A, Buccisano F *et al.* Clinical relevance of minimal residual disease detection in adult acute myeloid leukemia. *J Hematother Stem Cell Res* 2002; **11**: 349–57.

228. Venditti A, Maurillo L, Buccisano F *et al.* Multidimensional flow cytometry for detection of minimal residual disease in acute myeloid leukemia. *Leuk Lymphoma* 2003; **44**: 445–50.

229. Venditti A, Maurillo L, Buccisano F *et al.* Pretransplant minimal residual disease level predicts clinical outcome in patients with acute myeloid leukemia receiving high-dose chemotherapy and autologous stem cell transplantation. *Leukemia* 2003; **17**: 2178–82.

230. Venditti A, Buccisano F, Del Poeta G *et al.* Level of minimal

residual disease after consolidation therapy predicts outcome in acute myeloid leukemia. *Blood* 2000; **96**: 3948–52.

231. Yin JA, Grimwade D. Minimal residual disease evaluation in acute myeloid leukaemia. *Lancet* 2002; **360**: 160–2.

232. Raanani P, Ben-Bassat I. Detection of minimal residual disease in acute myelogenous leukemia. *Acta Haematol* 2004; **112**: 40–54.

233. Leung W, Hudson MM, Strickland DK *et al.* Late effects of treatment in survivors of childhood acute myeloid leukemia. *J Clin Oncol* 2000; **18**: 3273–9.

234. Michel G, Socie G, Gebhard F *et al.* Late effects of allogeneic bone marrow transplantation for children with acute myeloblastic leukemia in first complete remission: the impact of conditioning regimen without total-body irradiation. A report from the Societé Française de Greffe de Moelle. *J Clin Oncol* 1997; **15**: 2238–46.

235. Liesner RJ, Leiper AD, Hann IM, Chessells JM. Late effects of intensive treatment for acute myeloid leukemia and myelodysplasia in childhood. *J Clin Oncol* 1994; **12**: 916–24.

236. Leahey AM, Teunissen H, Friedman DL, Moshang T, Lange BJ, Meadows AT. Late effects of chemotherapy compared to bone marrow transplantation in the treatment of pediatric acute myeloid leukemia and myelodysplasia. *Med Pediatr Oncol* 1999; **32**: 163–9.

17 Chronic myeloid leukemia

Irene A.G. Roberts and Inderjeet S. Dokal

Epidemiology

Chronic myeloid leukemia (CML) constitutes 2–3% of all childhood leukemias and has an incidence of 0.6–1.2 per million per year in Western countries.[1–5] The incidence is higher in adolescents (age 15–19 years: 1.2 per million per year[3]) than in younger children (0–14 years: 0.6–0.8 per million per year[3,5]). This is similar to the incidence of juvenile myelomonocytic leukemia (JMML), from which CML is now usually readily distinguished because of its distinct clinical, biologic and molecular features (see Chapter 18). In all age groups CML is slightly more common in males than females, with a male to female ratio varying from just over 1.0 to 2.8.[5,6] CML is exceptionally rare in infancy, although it has been reported in a 3-month-old baby, and more than half of affected children are > 10 years old at diagnosis.[6]

Etiology

Although the molecular basis of CML has been well characterized for some time, its etiology is unknown in the vast majority of children. There is no clear evidence of a hereditary predisposition; with one exception,[7] identical twins appear to be discordant for the disease and CML is no more common in siblings of affected children. There is also no increased risk of CML in preleukemic chromosomal disorders such as Fanconi anemia and Down syndrome.

In occasional cases, an association with ionizing radiation has been described;[8] a sevenfold increase in CML, particularly in children under 5 years of age, was reported in Japan following the nuclear explosions in the 1940s. It has also been proposed that the close proximity of the *BCR* and *ABL* genes (see below) during interphase in hematopoietic cells may favor translocations between these genes.[9] The identification of a DNA repeat sequence on chromosome 9 near the *ABL* gene and on chromosome 22 near the *BCR* gene has led to

speculation that these may be involved in the genesis of the translocation.[10]

There are also reports of CML arising in children who are immunosuppressed, including one case in a child with HIV infection,[11] and following prolonged immune suppression in association with renal transplantation.[12]

Natural history

As in adults, CML in children is a triphasic disease. The majority of children present in the chronic phase,[6] the most indolent phase of the disease, which usually responds rapidly to oral chemotherapy and is readily curable by stem cell transplantation (SCT) (see below). In adults the median duration of the chronic phase in patients treated with hydroxycarbamide is around 4 years; there are no comparable data available for children. Transformation of chronic phase to accelerated phase disease is inevitable as a result of additional genetic changes to the abnormal leukemic clone responsible for chronic phase. Accelerated phase is defined on the basis of clinical, hematologic and cytogenetic features as described below. In adults the average duration of the accelerated phase is 6–18 months; comparable data are unavailable for children. CML inevitably further transforms to a rapidly progressive terminal phase known as blast crisis. This behaves as an acute leukemia: the blasts may have predominantly lymphoid morphology (lymphoid blast crisis) or myeloid morphology (myeloid blast crisis). Blast crisis is poorly responsive to chemotherapy and has a high relapse rate after transplantation. The average duration of blast crisis in adults is 3–9 months.

Molecular biology

As in CML in adults, CML in children is characterized by the presence of the Philadelphia (Ph) chromosome in all, or most,

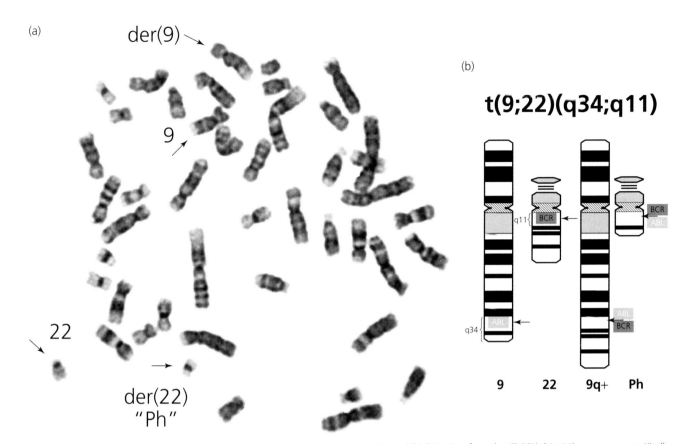

(a) der(9)

9

22

der(22)
"Ph"

(b)

t(9;22)(q34;q11)

q11
BCR

q34
ABL

BCR

ABL

ABL
BCR

9   22   9q+   Ph

Fig. 17.1 (a) Metaphase showing the normal chromosomes 9 and 22 and the 9q+ and 22q– (Ph) derivatives from the t(9;22)(q34;q11) rearrangement. Kindly provided by Andy Chase. (b) Schematic diagram of the normal chromosomes 9 and 22, and of the 9q+ and 22q– (Ph) derivatives from the t(9;22)(q34;q11). The arrows indicate the breakpoints on 9 and 22 that disrupt the *ABL* and *BCR* genes, respectively. Kindly provided by Junia Melo.

hematopoietic stem cells.[13,14] The Ph chromosome (22q–) results from the reciprocal translocation of the distal parts of the long arms of chromosomes 9 and 22 (Fig. 17.1). The translocation breakpoints disrupt genes on both chromosomes; the *ABL* (Abelson) protooncogene on chromosome 9 (9q34) and breakpoint cluster region (*BCR*) gene on chromosome 22 (22q11).[15–18] The consequence of this molecular rearrangement is the formation of an abnormal *BCR–ABL* fusion gene, which encodes a 210-kDa BCR–ABL fusion protein (Fig. 17.2). Breakpoints in *ABL* almost invariably occur upstream of exon Ib, between Ib and Ia, or between Ia and a2. The breakpoints in *BCR* usually occur within M-*bcr* (major breakpoint cluster region) (Fig. 17.2).

In around 90% of cases of CML, the Ph chromosome is readily detectable by standard cytogenetic preparations of bone marrow cells; in most of the remaining 10%, chromosomes 9 and 22 appear normal but identical patterns of *BCR–ABL* rearrangement to those found in cases of CML with the Ph chromosome can be clearly demonstrated by molecular techniques. A small proportion of children with CML (probably <5%) either have variant translocations (see below) or no evidence of *BCR–ABL* rearrangement even after extensive investigation at the molecular level.

Despite the fact that the Ph chromosome was first described in 1960 and its molecular basis determined in the 1980s, the exact role played by the novel *BCR–ABL* fusion gene in the pathogenesis of CML remains unclear. Most evidence points to *BCR–ABL* being the major factor determining the leukemic phenotype;[19–21] however, *BCR–ABL* rearrangement may not always be the initiating step in the development of CML. The identification of families in which several members have developed CML or another malignancy suggests an inherited predisposing factor;[7] the *BCR–ABL* rearrangement in these cases is likely to represent the second step in the neoplastic process. In addition, both epidemiologic data[22] and animal models of CML suggest that a minimum of two mutations are necessary for the development of chronic-phase CML.[20,21]

It is clear that the p210[BCR–ABL] fusion protein is a potent, constitutively active tyrosine kinase and, like other tyrosine kinases in hematopoietic cells, it is likely to play a direct role in stimulating cell proliferation, perhaps in an unregulated or dysregulated fashion. The functional significance of the reciprocal fusion gene, *ABL–BCR*, remains unknown.[23] The p210[BCR–ABL] fusion protein characteristic of CML is distinct from that seen in Ph-positive acute lymphoid leukemia

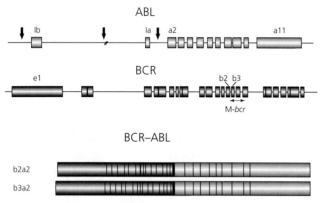

Fig. 17.2 Schematic representation of the *ABL* and the *BCR* genes disrupted in the t(9;22)(q34;q11). Exons are represented by boxes and introns by connecting horizontal lines. Breakpoints in *ABL*, illustrated as vertical arrows, almost invariably occur either upstream of exon Ib, between Ib and Ia, or between Ia and a2. The *BCR* gene contains 25 exons, including two putative alternative first (e1') and second (e2') exons. The breakpoints in *BCR* usually occur within M-*bcr* (major breakpoint cluster region), the location of which is shown by the double-headed horizontal arrows. The lower half of the figure shows the structure of the *BCR–ABL* mRNA transcripts. The breaks in M-*bcr* occur either between exons b2 (e13) and b3 (e14) or between b3 and b4 (e15), generating fusion transcripts with a b2a2 (also referred to as e13a2) or a b3a2 (also referred to as e14a2) junction, respectively. Kindly provided by Junia Melo.

(ALL), in which rearrangement of *ABL* and *BCR* results in a 185-kDa fusion protein, p185^BCR–ABL (see Chapter 20).[24]

The oncogenic potential of the p210^BCR–ABL protein resides in the fact that the normally regulated tyrosine kinase activity of the ABL protein is constitutively activated by the juxtaposition of the BCR sequences. The uncontrolled kinase activity of BCR–ABL results in altered signal transduction via interaction with a variety of effectors. The net result of this is deregulated cell proliferation, altered cell adherence and reduced apoptosis. The oncogenic potential of p210^BCR–ABL has been demonstrated in a number of *in vitro* and *in vivo* model systems. p210^BCR–ABL binds and/or phosphorylates more than 20 proteins, many of which can be directly linked to signal transduction pathways (Fig. 17.3).[25] For example, p210^BCR–ABL activates RAS, and an intact RAS protein is required for p210^BCR–ABL transformation and antiapoptotic activities.[26–28] Recent advances in our understanding of the biology of CML have been succinctly reviewed by Goldman and Melo.[29]

Biology

CML, like other hematologic malignancies, is a clonal disorder originating in a multipotent stem cell. This is clear from well-defined subpopulations of stem and progenitor cells studied by immunophenotyping and colony growth *in vitro*

and *in vivo*.[30] Thus, the Ph chromosome and/or *BCR–ABL* rearrangement can be demonstrated and expression of *BCR–ABL* is found in progenitor and mature cells of the granulocytic, erythroid and megakaryocytic lineages. In some, but not all, cases B lymphocytes and, less often, T lymphocytes have also been shown to be part of the malignant clone.[31] This suggests that leukemic transformation in these cases has occurred in a pluripotent lymphohemopoietic stem cell. In other cases, where the lymphocytes do not contain the Ph chromosome, CML may have arisen in a more mature multipotent stem cell, "sparing" the lymphoid lineage. However, the interpretation of such data is difficult and it remains uncertain whether the clonal origin of CML is truly heterogeneous or whether all cases arise in the pluripotent lymphohematopoietic stem cell, lymphocytes without the Ph chromosome representing long-lived cells arising prior to leukemic transformation. An alternative explanation, for which there is some evidence, is that in a proportion of patients with CML defective hematopoiesis precedes the acquisition of the Ph chromosome, that is, the Ph translocation may not be the initiating leukemogenic event.[32]

The clinical hallmark of CML is the hyperproliferation of the *BCR–ABL*-containing clone leading to expansion of the granulocytic compartment at all stages of maturation and variable suppression of normal hematopoiesis. Expansion of the abnormal clone presumably occurs because of failure of the normal control mechanisms that regulate hematopoiesis, perhaps as a result of activation of the β-catenin signaling pathway.[33] Interestingly, despite predominantly granulocytic hyperplasia, all lineages and classes of committed progenitor cells appear to be similarly dysregulated. Thus, in addition to granulocyte/monocyte progenitors, erythroid and megakaryocyte progenitors are also increased.

The exact mechanism(s) mediating the expansion of the *BCR–ABL*-positive clone are complex and controversial. Some studies indicate that there is increased proliferative activity of CML stem cells; others that there is increased self-renewal of more mature, committed progenitors, and this does seem more likely than myeloid expansion secondary to enhanced differentiation of progenitor cells.[30,33–35] There is also some evidence for reduced susceptibility of CML cells to apoptosis,[36] although whether this property is relevant to the myeloid expansion in CML is unclear. In addition, CML progenitors have been shown to have diminished adhesive properties, which result in reduced contact with stromal cells, possibly releasing them from physiologic inhibitory regulatory mechanisms.[37] Although the exact mechanisms remain unclear, the abnormal growth characteristics of CML cells and their progenitors are thought to be the result of the *BCR–ABL* rearrangement as suggested above. Direct evidence in support of this is provided by studies in cell lines and animal models of CML. The *BCR–ABL* gene can confer growth factor independence on previously factor-dependent cell lines.[38,39] Complementary evidence for a pathogenetic

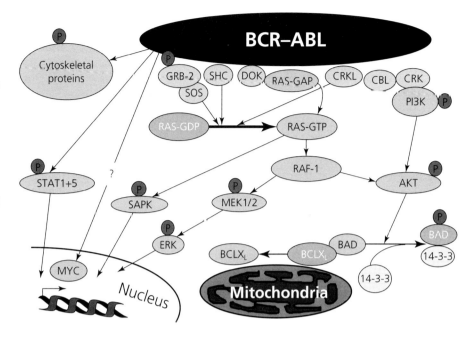

Fig. 17.3 Signal transduction pathways affected by BCR–ABL. BCR–ABL exerts its effects via its interaction with numerous proteins that are responsible for the activation or repression of gene transcription, the apoptotic pathways and cytoskeleton organization. The pathways implicated include those involving RAS, mitogen-activated protein (MAP) kinases, signal transducers and activators of transcription (STAT), phosphatidylinositol 3-kinase (PI3K), and MYC. The majority of interactions are mediated through tyrosine phosphorylation and require the binding of BCR–ABL to adaptor molecules such as growth factor receptor-bound protein 2 (GRB-2), DOK, CRK, CRK-like protein (CRKL), SRC-homology-containing protein (SHC), and casitas-B-lineage lymphoma protein (CBL). Kindly provided by Junia Melo.

role of the *BCR–ABL* rearrangement is provided by the demonstration that it is possible to induce a CML-like disorder in a mouse model by insertion of the *BCR–ABL* gene into hematopoietic cells.[20,21,35]

Clinical features

CML most commonly presents in children with nonspecific symptoms, such as fatigue, malaise and weight loss (Table 17.1).[6,40] Abdominal discomfort, due to an enlarging spleen, is also fairly common.[6,40] A recent French study of 40 children found that CML is an incidental finding in 23% of children as a result of the increased use of routine blood counts.[6] Other symptoms at presentation that occur less

Table 17.1 Clinical features at diagnosis of chronic myeloid leukemia.

Common
Fatigue
Weight loss
Abdominal discomfort/splenomegaly
Asymptomatic (incidental finding)

Uncommon
Bone pain
Bleeding
Fever
Sweating
Leukostasis (e.g., priapism)
Gout
Splenic infarction

frequently are bleeding (usually with a normal platelet count and coagulation studies) and bone pain. If there is a marked leukocytosis ($>100 \times 10^9$/L), affected children may present with symptoms of a hypermetabolic state, including fever and night sweats.[6,40]

Examination

The majority of children have mild or moderate splenomegaly; otherwise findings on examination are usually unremarkable.[6,40,41] Palpable hepatomegaly (1–2 cm) is sometimes found but gross hepatomegaly and lymphadenopathy are very uncommon unless the disease has progressed to accelerated phase or blast crisis. Signs of leukostasis (e.g., retinal hemorrhages, papilledema, priapism) are usually only seen if the leukocyte count at presentation is very high ($>300 \times 10^9$/L).[6,42] Some reports have suggested that such signs are more common in children than in adults with CML,[42] although this was not the case in the recent study of 40 children in which leukostasis was reported in only 3 (7.5%) of the children.[6] Skin nodules due to leukemic deposits (chloromas) are occasionally seen, usually in association with accelerated-phase disease or blast crisis.

Diagnosis

Peripheral blood

In chronic-phase disease the most consistent finding at presentation is the characteristic leukocytosis made up predominantly of mature granulocytic cells (neutrophils, bands and metamyelocytes) and their precursors (myelocytes and promyelocytes). In chronic-phase CML, blasts constitute < 5% of peripheral blood leukocytes. As in CML in adults, eosinophilia and basophilia are commonly present at diagnosis. The total white cell count at presentation is usually > 100 × 10^9/L; indeed, the recent French study reported a median white blood cell count at diagnosis of 242 × 10^9/L.[6] Most children have a normal or slightly increased platelet count at presentation;[6,40,41] the presence either of thrombocytopenia or of marked thrombocytosis (>1000 × 10^9/L) suggests accelerated-phase disease. By contrast, mild or moderate anemia is a presenting finding in the majority of children.[6]

Bone marrow

The marrow in CML is markedly hypercellular in all phases of the disease. In the chronic phase the increase in cellularity is mainly due to hyperplasia of granulocytic cells. A characteristic "myelocyte" peak is commonly seen at presentation, and blast cells constitute < 5% of nucleated cells in chronic-phase CML. Eosinophils, basophils and their precursors are frequently increased and are sometimes dysplastic. In addition, pseudo-Gaucher cells similar to sea-blue histiocytes are seen in a small proportion of cases. Megakaryocytes are usually present in increased numbers but they are usually morphologically normal.

The trephine biopsy is often useful in CML and should be performed at presentation if a bone marrow harvest is planned and if accelerated-phase disease is suspected. At presentation, the main features seen on biopsy in chronic phase are hypercellularity, granulocytic hyperplasia and increased megakaryocyte numbers. However, the biopsy is useful for assessing the extent of accompanying myelofibrosis and may show increases in blast cells in advanced-phase disease. Myelofibrosis is not usually prominent at presentation but it is a common feature of advanced-phase disease and may make marrow harvesting extremely difficult.

Cytogenetics

Cytogenetic studies on bone marrow at presentation show the classic Ph chromosome in around 95% of patients with chronic-phase CML. In almost all such patients, the Ph chromosome is seen in 100% of the metaphases but occasionally small numbers of cytogenetically normal cells are still detectable at presentation. Variant translocations are seen in < 5% of children in chronic phase. These are of two types: rearrangements involving two chromosomes, one of which is chromosome 22; and rearrangements involving chromosomes 22 and 9 together with at least one other chromosome. Variant translocations, and some cases that are cytogenetically normal, virtually always show *BCR* rearrangement by Southern blotting despite the absence of the Ph chromosome using classical cytogenetics.[43] Fluorescent *in situ* hybridiza-

tion (FISH) is almost as accurate at detecting the Ph chromosome *BCR–ABL* fusion gene in bone marrow from adults with CML.[44,45] More widespread introduction of FISH may make the diagnosis of CML easier, quicker and cheaper and may also render the miscellaneous rapid confirmatory tests described below redundant in CML.

There remains a very small number of children with CML who are Ph-negative and who have no evidence of *BCR–ABL* rearrangement even after extensive molecular investigation. Most, if not all, such children meet the diagnostic criteria for JMML or other types of myelodysplasia or myeloproliferative disorders (see Chapter 18). Thus, the existence of true Ph-negative CML is extremely unlikely and in adults, although of scientific interest, the distinction does not appear to be of practical clinical importance because the clinical features, laboratory findings and natural history of Ph-positive and Ph-negative, *BCR–ABL*-negative CML are so similar that their treatment is the same.[46]

A number of cytogenetic abnormalities, such as isochromosome 17q, in addition to the Ph chromosome may be seen in bone marrow cells in CML.[43] However, these changes are associated with accelerated disease or blast crisis (see below) and therefore cast doubt on the diagnosis of CML, still in chronic phase.

Miscellaneous and possible prognostic tests at diagnosis

A number of other laboratory tests are abnormal in CML and may be used to substantiate the diagnosis where cytogenetic or molecular studies are unavailable. These include reduced leukocyte alkaline phosphatase (LAP) activity (measured cytochemically as a low LAP "score") and increased vitamin B_{12}-binding protein (usually measured as a reduced serum B_{12} level). In addition, the serum uric acid is often elevated although clinical gout is unusual.

Approximately 20% of CML patients have deletions of chromosomal material of varying size on the derivative 9q+; these patients have significantly shorter survival than those who do not. Therefore assessment of derivative 9q deletion status may be a useful prognostic factor although this has not been assessed in children.[47] Assessment of telomere shortening at presentation at diagnosis also appears to be a useful prognostic factor in adults but remains to be investigated in children with CML.[48]

Accelerated-phase CML

There is no single specific feature that defines the accelerated phase. Most studies use a combination of clinical and hematologic features to classify patients as accelerated rather than chronic-phase disease. We have found the International Bone Marrow Transplant Registry definition[49] of accelerated phase

Table 17.2 International Bone Marrow Transplant Registry definition of accelerated-phase chronic myeloid leukemia.

---

*Accelerated phase is defined by the presence of **any** of:*

Clinical criteria
    Increasing splenomegaly
    Chloroma(s)
    Previous blast crisis (BM blasts > 30%)

Hematologic criteria
    WBC difficult to control or doubling in 5 days
    Hb < 10 g/dL or platelets < 100×10^9/L not responsive to treatment
    Platelets > 1000×10^9/L
    Blasts (BM or blood) > 10% but < 30%
    Blasts + promyelocytes (BM or blood) > 20%
    Basophils + eosinophils (PB) = 20%

Other criteria
    Cytogenetic abnormality in addition to single Ph chromosome
    Marrow fibrosis (stages 3–4)

BM, bone marrow; Hb, hemoglobin; PB, peripheral blood.

useful for assessing prognosis and planning management in children (Table 17.2).

One of the commonest signs is a change in the platelet count; this may manifest either as thrombocytopenia or thrombocytosis increasingly resistant to chemotherapy. Similarly, the leukocyte count may become refractory to treatment and there may be increased numbers of basophils and/or eosinophils in comparison with earlier in the disease course. Blast cells in the marrow may also increase. Many patients become anemic. In part this may be due to increasing myelofibrosis, a common feature of accelerated-phase CML, and in part due to hypersplenism in association with a larger spleen.

The progression of CML to the accelerated phase is often associated with the acquisition of new cytogenetic abnormalities. The commonest are a second Ph chromosome, isochromosome 17, trisomy 8 and trisomy 19.[43,50,51] The genes involved in the evolution of CML in adults and children have not yet been fully characterized (see below).

Blast crisis

Blast crisis is defined by the presence of > 30% blasts in peripheral blood or bone marrow. It usually evolves relatively gradually from accelerated phase, but not infrequently the switch from chronic phase is dramatic, blast cells appearing in the peripheral blood without a distinct period of "acceleration." Occasionally, children with CML present in blast crisis or relapse straight into blast crisis following allogeneic SCT. The majority of patients with blast crisis have a rapidly rising leukocyte count together with anemia and are frequently thrombocytopenic. In > 60% of cases, the blast cells have the morphologic and immunophenotypic characteristics of myeloblasts.[51,52] However, 20–30% of patients undergo lymphoid blast transformation, most commonly with a pre-B phenotype;[51–53] among adults, the median age of this subset is lower than that of patients developing myeloblastic crisis[54] but there are no large series to confirm whether or not children are more likely to undergo lymphoid rather than myeloid transformation. Classification into lymphoid versus myeloid blast crisis on morphologic grounds is often very difficult; immunophenotyping to confirm the myeloid or lymphoid characteristics of the blasts is therefore very important because this has a major impact on treatment and prognosis.

As in accelerated phase, cytogenetic changes in addition to the Ph chromosome are common.[54] As well as those affecting chromosomes 8, 17 and 19, the translocations associated with acute myeloid leukemia (AML) and ALL are sometimes seen in blastic crisis (see Chapters 16 and 20). At the molecular level, blast crisis has been variably associated with abnormalities of tumor suppressor genes, in particular *P53*, *P16* and *RB*, or protooncogenes, such as *RAS* and *MYC*, or with the generation of chimeric transcription factors, as in the *AML–EVI1* gene fusion.[55–59] It is likely, therefore, that multiple and alternative molecular defects underlie the acute transformation of the disease.

Differential diagnosis

The most important differential diagnosis in young children is JMML (see Chapter 18). JMML is seen more commonly in children < 2 years of age in contrast to CML, which occurs predominantly in children > 6 years. The profile of clinical signs is also rather different: skin rashes and lymphadenopathy are very common in JMML but rare in chronic-phase CML, while prominent splenomegaly is suggestive of CML because it is usually less marked in JMML. The laboratory features are also usually distinct: in JMML the white cell count tends to be < 100×10^9/L and there is a monocytosis, thrombocytopenia and a raised fetal hemoglobin (HbF), none of which is common in CML. The diagnosis is generally not in doubt once the bone marrow karyotype is available but the absence of the Ph chromosome in up to 10% of cases of CML may lead to diagnostic uncertainty in occasional cases.

A transient CML-like blood picture is also occasionally seen in association with severe bacterial infections, chronic Epstein–Barr virus infection and nonhematologic cancers. Similar granulocytic hyperplasia may also be found during the first year of life in 60–70% of cases of thrombocytopenia with absent radii syndrome. Finally, the blood film and marrow of children who present in lymphoid blast crisis may be difficult to distinguish from *de novo* Ph-positive ALL on morphologic grounds: molecular analysis for the p210[BCR–ABL] and p185[BCR–ABL] proteins in CML and ALL, respectively, may clarify the underlying diagnosis.

Management

Management of chronic-phase disease

General considerations

Soon after diagnosis a decision must be made about long-term treatment because there are several different options with the potential to cure or to significantly prolong survival.[60–64] The only proven cure for CML is SCT. The mortality and morbidity associated with SCT are relatively high (see below), particularly in adults. Thus, the recent development of drugs targeted to the leukemia-specific protein BCR–ABL, such as imatinib mesilate, has completely changed the management of CML in adults, as the response rate to these agents is extremely good.[60–64] However, because sustained molecular remission in response to imatinib is rare, because there is increasing evidence of primary and secondary imatinib resistance (see below), as there are very few data about imatinib in children,[65,66] and as there is no evidence yet that imatinib can cure CML, SCT remains the treatment of choice in children where an HLA-identical donor has been identified. For children without an HLA-identical sibling, the decision to transplant may be difficult if a well-matched donor is not available and in this situation imatinib is appropriate for front-line therapy. A suggested treatment algorithm is shown in Fig. 17.4.

Initial management

Discuss SCT

For children presenting in chronic phase it is rarely necessary to start treatment immediately. Except in cases where the leukocyte count is $> 100 \times 10^9/L$, treatment can be deferred for 1–2 weeks as it is important to spend time with the family explaining the natural history of the disease, particularly because it differs in so many ways from most childhood malignancies. Unlike acute leukemias, CML can only be cured by SCT. It is therefore appropriate to raise this with families and to proceed to HLA typing of family members at an early stage because the availability of an HLA-identical sibling donor has a major impact on the choice of treatment (Fig. 17.4).

Cryopreserve autologous cells

Prior to initiating treatment, hematopoietic stem cells should be collected from all children in chronic phase and cryopreserved for possible later autologous transplantation. In the majority of children, sufficient stem cells can be collected by leukapheresis (aim for $7–8 \times 10^8$ cells/kg), but where this is not possible (e.g., poor vascular access) autologous bone marrow harvesting is a satisfactory alternative (aim to cryopreserve 2×10^8 cells/kg). If stem cell harvesting is not possible prior to starting chemotherapy, it should be carried out at a later stage after control of the white count has been achieved and before SCT (this will require temporary cessation of chemotherapy; usually for 2–4 weeks or until the leukocyte count is $> 25 \times 10^9/L$).

Oral chemotherapy for initial disease control

While an HLA-identical donor is being sought and pending a decision about allogeneic SCT, oral chemotherapy should be started to bring the disease under control. For asymptomatic children the aim of chemotherapy is to "normalize" the blood count and thereby delay onset of symptoms. In symptomatic children and/or those with white cell counts $> 100 \times 10^9/L$, chemotherapy should be started promptly and most will feel considerably better after only a few days. In the rare cases presenting with symptoms of hyperviscosity, leukapheresis should be carried out as soon as possible followed by oral chemotherapy.

Several well-known oral agents are active in CML, including hydroxycarbamide, busulfan, 6-mercaptopurine and 6-thioguanine. Hydroxycarbamide has a number of advantages and is usually the best drug for initial disease control. It causes a rapid fall in both white cell and platelet counts, usually within 1–2 weeks; myelosuppressive hydroxycarbamide-associated pancytopenia is generally rapidly reversible, particularly in comparison with busulfan, and it has fewer serious side-effects. In contrast to busulfan, there is no clear evidence that hydroxycarbamide is leukemogenic or tumorigenic in humans; it does not appear to cause pulmonary fibrosis, even with long-term use and, in the doses used, it does not cause infertility. Furthermore, a history of busulfan use in adults prior to bone marrow transplantation (BMT) has been identified as one of the factors predicting a poorer outcome compared with the use of no chemotherapy or

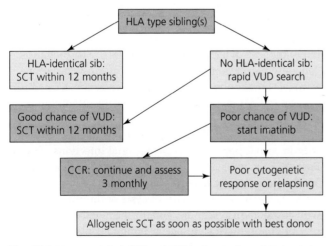

Fig. 17.4 Management of childhood CML in chronic phase. A suggested algorithm for planning the management of children with CML in first chronic phase. CCR, complete cytogenetic remission; SCT, stem cell transplantation; VUD, volunteer-unrelated donor.

hydroxycarbamide for disease control before BMT.[67] The starting dose of hydroxycarbamide is 15–20 mg/kg, increasing up to 30 mg/kg depending on response, with the aim of bringing the white cell count down below 10×10^9/L. A uricosuric agent, such as allopurinol, should be started 2–3 days before oral chemotherapy is commenced. Imatinib may be used to achieve initial disease control but is not the drug of choice for this purpose in children as it tends to achieve a response more slowly, is less well tolerated initially and may induce imatinib resistance.

Definitive management of chronic-phase CML

The options available include imatinib mesilate (STI571), allogeneic SCT, interferon (IFN)-α and experimental treatment.

Imatinib mesilate

Imatinib mesilate (previously known as STI571) is a potent tyrosine kinase inhibitor that blocks the kinase activity of BCR–ABL.[68] It also inhibits a small number of other protein kinases, including KIT (the receptor for stem cell factor) and the platelet-derived growth factor receptors (PDGFR-A and -B). The remarkable selectivity of imatinib means that it is able to inhibit the proliferation of Ph-positive hematopoietic progenitor cells while leaving normal cells relatively unscathed.[69] Imatinib probably acts mainly by binding to and stabilizing BCR–ABL in its inactive form,[70] in this way preventing phosphorylation of its downstream targets (Fig. 17.5).

Clinical trials of imatinib in adults

The first clinical trials of imatinib were completed in 2001 in IFN-refractory chronic-phase disease and in blast crisis in adults.[71,72] These trials showed a remarkable 98% complete hematologic response rate together with a 54% cytogenetic

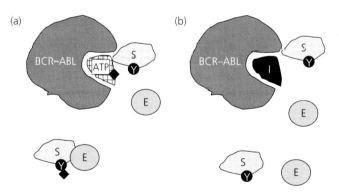

Fig. 17.5 Schematic representation of BCR–ABL inhibition by imatinib mesylate. (a) Binding of ATP by BCR–ABL facilitates phosphorylation (♦) of tyrosine residues (Y) on substrates (S), which then bind effectors (E) transmitting a downstream mitogenic signal. (b) Imatinib (I) binds to the inactive conformation of ABL in the region where ATP would normally bind thereby preventing phosphorylation of substrate tyrosines and impeding downstream signaling by BCR–ABL.

response rate for the previously treated chronic-phase patients.[71] As would be expected the results were not quite so good in accelerated-phase disease although much better than any other nontransplant approach, with a hematologic complete response rate of 78% and cytogenetic complete response rate of 17%.[73] Shortly afterwards a prospective multinational study in over 1000 adult patients of imatinib versus IFN-α plus cytarabine was published and showed a dramatic increase in the complete cytogenetic response rate in the imatinib-treated patients (74%) compared with the IFN-α/cytarabine patients (8.5%).[74] Recent data show that the frequency of major molecular responses (≥ 3 log reduction in *BCR ABL* transcript levels) was also much greater in the imatinib group compared with the IFN-α/cytarabine group.[75] The side-effects (discussed below) were modest and acceptable. More recently even higher response rates have been reported in a nonrandomized study in 114 adults with newly diagnosed chronic-phase CML, when a higher dose of imatinib was used (400 mg twice daily vs. 400 mg once daily).[76] In this study 90% of patients have achieved a complete cytogenetic response (100% Ph chromosome negative). The most important trials in adults and children are summarized in Table 17.3.

The short duration of follow-up even in the earliest studies makes it unclear if the dramatic increase in hematologic and cytogenetic response rates will translate into improved survival. Encouragingly, two recent retrospective studies suggest that imatinib does prolong survival compared with other nontransplant therapies, including IFN-α,[77,78] but it will be several years until meaningful survival data from prospective studies become available. Unfortunately, recent studies of imatinib in blast crisis confirm the poor response of myeloid blast crisis (15–23% hematologic complete response; median survival 6–8 months[78,79,80]) and even poorer response of lymphoid blast crisis.[78] Other problems with imatinib include the emergence of imatinib resistance,[81–83] side-effects,[74–76] and the very small amount of information about the effects of imatinib in children.[65,66]

Clinical trials of imatinib in children

The two published series of imatinib used to treat children with CML include 24 patients; the results are shown in Table 17.3.[65,66] These data are too preliminary to draw many conclusions. They do show that so far the response rate seems to be similar to the adult series. In addition, Champagne and colleagues carried out pharmacokinetic studies to try to estimate the optimal dose of imatinib and evaluate its safety profile in children.[66] They found that there was considerable interpatient variance in pharmacokinetic parameters.[66] However, plasma concentrations at steady state were comparable with those in adults.[66] They reported that imatinib was well tolerated over a dose range of 260–570 mg/m² (260 mg/m² is equivalent to the 400 mg daily dose in adults, and 570 mg/m² to the 800 mg daily high-dose regimen in adults.[76] The

Table 17.3 Clinical trials of imatinib in adults and children with chronic myeloid leukemia.

Trial	No. of patients			Hematologic CR	Cytogenetic CR	Molecular response	Dose per day	Discontinued*
	Total	CP1	AP					
Adult trials								
Chronic phase: newly diagnosed patients in randomized trial vs. IFN-α + cytarabine (553 randomized to imatinib)								
O'Brien (2003)[74]	553	553	0	95.3%	73.8%	39% > 3 logs reduction in BCR–ABL	400 mg	12.3%
Accelerated phase								
Talpaz (2002)[73]	181		181	69%	17%	NA	400–600 mg	43%†
Myeloid blast crisis								
Sawyers (2002)[79]			229 (BC)	15%	7%	NA	400–600 mg	NA
Chronic phase newly diagnosed: high dose								
Kantarjian (2004)[78]	114	114	0	98%	90%	28% RT-PCR negative	800 mg	10%
Pediatric trials								
Champagne (2004)[66]	20	14	6	CP 14/14 BC 2/6	CP 10/12* BC NA	NA NA	260–570 mg/m²	NA
Kolb (2003)[65]	4	4	0	4/4	4/4	RT-PCR negative 3/4	284–443 mg/m²	NA

* Reasons for discontinuation included adverse events, disease progression, death and proceeding to SCT.

† 43% of the 235 patients originally entered into the trial (only 181/235 were subsequently confirmed to be in accelerated phase but the discontinuation data are only provided for the whole group of 235 patients).

AP, acute phase; BC, blast crisis; CP, chronic phase; CR, complete remission; NA, not available; RT-PCR, reverse-transcription polymerase chain reaction.

commonest adverse effects were nausea, vomiting, fatigue, abnormal liver function tests and diarrhea. These are similar in nature to the adverse effects reported in the large adult series:[74] nausea (44%), vomiting (17%), fatigue (35%), abnormal liver function tests (43%) and diarrhea (33%); this series also reported a fairly high frequency of edema (55%), muscle cramps (38%), rash (34%) and headache (31%). Myelosuppression (anemia, thrombocytopenia and neutropenia) has been common in the adult series but little information is available in children and advice about monitoring is discussed below.

Imatinib resistance

The major limitation to the use of imatinib in children is that it is not curative, at least on the basis of current evidence. The inability of imatinib to eradicate all leukemic cells is due to imatinib resistance, which may be either primary or secondary (Table 17.4). Primary resistance to imatinib would occur in patients in whom the leukemic process is no longer entirely dependent upon BCR–ABL and could be perpetuated by BCR–ABL-independent mechanisms (see, for example, refs 84, 85). It could also occur if the quiescent pool of leukemic stem cells was insensitive to imatinib, as has recently been reported.[86]

Secondary imatinib resistance develops as a result of exposure of the leukemic cells to imatinib. Most commonly,

Table 17.4 Mechanisms of resistance of chronic myeloid leukemia to imatinib.

Primary imatinib resistance
Leukemic stem cell proliferation occurring by a BCR–ABL-independent pathway
Quiescent leukemic stem cells are insensitive to imatinib, e.g., because imatinib is not available intracellularly
BCR–ABL point mutations prior to imatinib exposure

Secondary imatinib resistance
BCR–ABL point mutations in the ABL kinase domain
BCR–ABL amplification/overexpression
Reduction of imatinib activity by production of an inhibitor (e.g., α₁-acid glycoprotein) or enzymatic modification by a P450 enzyme or overexpression of MDR1

secondary resistance is due to point mutations in the BCR–ABL kinase domain,[87–89] but resistance due to BCR–ABL amplification has also been described.[88,90] Secondary resistance may also arise due to reduction in the activity of imatinib, for instance through production of the inhibitor α₁-acid glycoprotein,[91] through reduced plasma concentrations of imatinib due to increased MDR1 overexpression,[92] or through enzymatic modification of imatinib by a P450 enzyme.[81]

Perhaps most worrying from the point of view of the use of imatinib in children is the recent evidence that mutations in the BCR–ABL kinase domain may be present in the leukemic cells before therapy with imatinib,[93,94] presumably because of the inherent genetic instability of the BCR–ABL-expressing clone and the fact that these mutations may confer a growth advantage to the mutant clone.[95] This is a very important observation as it suggests that imatinib should be used with caution in patients for whom SCT is the treatment of first choice.

Treatment of children with imatinib

At present the balance of evidence does not favor imatinib as treatment of choice for newly diagnosed children although the position may change as increasing information about imatinib becomes available. The main concerns about using imatinib as treatment of first choice are:

- there is no evidence that it can cure;
- imatinib resistance is now known to be an inherent property of the leukemic clone in some patients and in such patients imatinib would be likely to favor the outgrowth of rapidly proliferating drug-resistant clones;
- the development of chromosomal abnormalities in Ph-negative cells in 2–17% of imatinib-treated adult patients;[85,96]
- the long-term toxicity in children is completely unknown;
- some patients relapse on imatinib straight into blast crisis,[97–99] which has a much poorer outcome after SCT than chronic-phase disease;
- the outcome of SCT is better when it is carried out within a year of diagnosis.

Indications for imatinib in children with CML. The role of imatinib pre-SCT to reduce the leukemic cell burden is not clear and until evidence from clinical trials is available it seems unwise to use imatinib in this way in children. Similarly there is no proven role for imatinib as adjuvant therapy post-SCT in children especially when molecular monitoring of residual BCR–ABL cells posttransplant is so effective (see below). Where imatinib does have a role is:

- as first-line treatment for children who do not have an HLA-identical donor (see Fig. 17.4);
- for relapse after SCT where donor lymphocyte infusion (DLI) is unavailable or ineffective or families/clinicians choose this option (see below);
- for accelerated-phase CML while SCT is being arranged;
- for myeloid blast crisis following or in place of conventional chemotherapy and while SCT is being arranged.

The two studies of imatinib in children with CML suggest that imatinib should be started at a dose of 260–340 mg/m^2, rounded to the nearest 100 mg because of the formulations available. If initial disease control with hydroxycarbamide is used this should be tapered for 2–3 weeks prior to starting imatinib. Allopurinol should only be necessary if the leukocyte count is $> 20 \times 10^9$/L. We recommend monitoring the full blood count weekly for the first 6 weeks and then every 2 weeks. The leukocyte count normally starts to fall within 1–2 weeks and normalizes in 6 weeks; platelet counts normalize after 1–3 weeks. Myelosuppression occurs in around 50% of patients and is more common in accelerated phase than chronic phase. Data from adult studies suggest that the dose of imatinib should be increased if a complete cytogenetic response has not been achieved by 3–6 months.[100]

Allogeneic stem cell transplantation

Allogeneic SCT remains the only curative treatment for CML in children.[101–105] Thus, despite the efficacy and specificity of imatinib, SCT is the treatment of choice for children with CML who have an HLA-identical donor.[61,64] There are now three fairly large published series of BMT for CML in children: one from the European Group for Blood and Marrow Transplantation (EBMT) involving 314 children; a study from the Société Française de Greffe de Moëlle et de Thérapie Cellulaire (SFGM-TC) in 76 children; and an older study from Germany in 47 children.[101–103] The results of the two recent studies are summarized in Table 17.5 and the details are discussed below. There are also several studies of cord blood

Table 17.5 Outcome of allogeneic stem cell transplantation in children with chronic myeloid leukemia.

Study group	No. of patients		Overall survival (%)		LFS (%)		TRM (%)		Relapse (%)	
	CP1	AP	CP1	AP	CP1	AP	CP1	AP	CP1	AP
EBMT[103]										
Sib donor	156	26	75	46	63	35	20	16	17	49
VUD	97	35	65	39	56	34	31	46	13	20
SFGM-TC[104]										
Sib donor	42	18	73 (AP+CP)		73	32	20 (AP+CP)		15	52
VUD	5	11	27 (AP+CP)		27 (AP+CP)		69 (AP+CP)		6 (AP+CP)	

EBMT, European Group for Blood and Marrow Transplantation; SFGM-TC, Société Française de Greffe de Moëlle et de Thérapie Cellulaire; AP, accelerated phase and blast crisis; CP1, first chronic phase; LFS, leukemia-free survival; TRM, transplant-related mortality; VUD, volunteer unrelated donor.

transplantation in which a substantial proportion of children were transplanted for CML.[106–108]

Conditioning: chemotherapy vs. chemoradiotherapy
Early experience showed that the combination of high-dose cyclophosphamide and total body irradiation (TBI) is an effective conditioning regimen for cure of CML in adults and children.[67,104,105] This regimen is still used for transplants from unrelated or mismatched donors, but for transplants from an HLA-identical sibling more recent results indicate an equivalent antileukemic efficacy for cyclophosphamide in combination with busulfan,[101,109,110] thus eliminating the need for radiotherapy. Long-term toxicity may be less than with TBI regimens, although this has not yet been established. There is no benefit of additional splenic irradiation where the spleen is small or impalpable,[111] but for children in accelerated phase or blast crisis where there is significant splenomegaly (>5 cm), splenectomy prior to BMT may enable the disease to be controlled better and will facilitate engraftment, although there is no effect on overall survival.[112]

Outcome

First chronic phase. In view of the major advances in the management of relapsed chronic-phase CML (see below), the most clinically relevant measure of cure from these studies is the overall survival as most children who relapse can be cured by DLI[113–116] and possibly imatinib.[117] In the EBMT study the overall survival at 3 years was 75% for children transplanted in the first chronic phase;[101] this is similar to the SFGM study, which reported 73% event-free survival for such children.[102] The overall survival for children in first chronic phase transplanted from unrelated donors was not significantly different on multivariate analysis (65%) but the transplant-related mortality was significantly higher (31%) after unrelated donor transplantation in this study.[101] In both studies it was clear that the main cause of death, after both sibling donor and unrelated donor transplantation, was graft-versus-host disease (GVHD).

Accelerated phase and blast crisis. In advanced-phase disease the relapse rate is high, particularly when the donor is an HLA-identical sibling. In the EBMT study 49% of the advanced-phase children transplanted from a sibling donor relapsed,[101] and the hazard ratio for relapse from unrelated donors versus sibling donors was 0.38 (P < 0.01). In the SFGM study 59% of the advanced-phase children transplanted from a sibling donor relapsed and the relative risk of relapse was 5.9 for a child transplanted in advanced phase from a sibling donor (P < 0.01).[102] Because the response to DLI (or imatinib) of relapsed patients transplanted for advanced-phase disease is often temporary, it is more important to consider leukemia-free survival as a measure of cure for children transplanted in advanced-phase disease. In the EBMT study, leukemia-

free survival in children transplanted from sibling donors or unrelated donors was virtually identical: 35% and 34% respectively.[101] This is similar to the SFGM study[102] and a number of studies in adults supporting the contention that SCT for advanced-phase disease remains a worthwhile therapeutic option because leukemia-free survival of around 30% is vastly superior to the negligible chance of long-term survival without SCT.[118–120]

Predictive factors for the outcome of SCT
The principal factors determining overall survival after SCT in children with CML are:
• the phase of CML at the time of transplant, with the best results in chronic phase and the worst in accelerated phase and blast crisis, as described above;[101,102]
• the interval between diagnosis and BMT, with the best results in those transplanted within 1 year of diagnosis;[101,121–123]
• administration of methotrexate as GVHD prophylaxis: the hazard ratio in multivariate analysis in the EBMT study was 0.6 for inclusion of methotrexate (P = 0.038).[101]

Interval between diagnosis and SCT. Data from large adult series convincingly show a better outcome for patients transplanted within a year of diagnosis.[121–123] This is also likely to be true for children: the EBMT study found inferior leukemia-free survival (Relocative Risk 1.5) in children transplanted > 12 months after diagnosis, although this did not quite reach statistical significance (P = 0.064). Early transplantation also reduces the time interval in which transformation to accelerated phase or blast crisis may occur because around 10% of children progress to more advanced disease within a year of diagnosis. Thus, for children with an HLA-identical donor, SCT within 12 months of diagnosis is commonly recommended (see Fig. 17.4). However, for those without an HLA-identical donor, a better option is to treat with imatinib and monitor the response closely using sensitive molecular methods as discussed above. Where there is evidence of imatinib resistance or loss of imatinib response, SCT from a mismatched donor needs to be considered because overall long-term survival is around 40%,[124] and hence likely to be superior to chemotherapy.

Graft-versus-host disease
GVHD is the most important cause of transplant-related mortality and morbidity.[101,102,125,126] However, it appears that in CML more than any other hematologic malignancy the occurrence and clinical behavior of GVHD mediated by allogeneic donor cells is intimately linked with the "graft-versus-leukemia" (GVL) effect of the donor cells.[127–129] While it is not yet known whether these two processes are mediated by the same or distinct cell types or subtypes, it is clear that the need to maintain an effective GVL effect of allogeneic donor cells has a major impact on the choice of regimen employed to prevent GVHD after BMT for CML both in

children and in adults.[68,125,127] Broadly, the two approaches to GVHD prevention are T-cell depletion and pharmacologic immunosuppression.

T-cell depletion. A number of methods of T-cell depletion have been employed in CML. These include *ex vivo* T-cell depletion of donor marrow using antithymocyte globulin[125] or monoclonal antibodies (e.g., anti-CD6, anti-CD8, anti-CD2 or anti-CD52 (Campath-1M)), counterflow elutriation or soybean lectin agglutination, and *in vivo* T-cell depletion by intravenous infusion of antibodies such as Alemtuzumab.[130,131] There are numerous data on the impact of T-cell depletion on the outcome of BMT for CML in adults; many of these trials have included children and it is likely that the conclusions from the adult studies apply also to pediatric practice. The principal benefit of T-cell depletion is that it is highly effective in reducing the incidence and severity of GVHD both from HLA-matched siblings and alternative donors.[125,130,131] However, the benefits of T-cell depletion are achieved at the expense of a significantly increased rate of early graft rejection and relapse of CML.[131,132] The rate of relapse after sibling transplants may be as high as 60%,[131,132] and this has led several groups to abandon T-cell depletion in favor of immunosuppression, particularly in patients under 20 years of age who have a lower incidence of severe GVHD. The clear association between a low rate of GVHD and a high rate of relapse after BMT for CML (and vice versa) provides strong clinical evidence for the GVL effect of allogeneic T cells,[127–132] and has led to the development of a number of possible strategies to prevent GVHD without sacrificing important elements of GVL (see below).

Immunosuppression. There is clear evidence that combination treatment with ciclosporin and methotrexate is, apart from T-cell depletion, the most effective way of preventing GVHD.[101,133] Most regimens combine short-course methotrexate during the first 2 weeks after BMT with 6–12 months' maintenance treatment with oral ciclosporin. Acute GVHD still develops in around 30% of children treated with these regimens but in the majority of cases this is mild and responds to topical or low-dose steroids. In children who develop GVHD of severity greater than grade II the treatment of choice is high-dose steroids, usually by the intravenous route.

Graft-versus-leukemia effect

As mentioned above, GVL and GVHD are closely linked and it seems likely that similar mechanisms control both processes.[127–129] In GVHD, donor T cells recognize antigens presented by major histocompatibility complex molecules on recipient cells (in skin, gut, biliary tree, etc.) leading to the clinical features of acute and chronic GVHD. In GVL, donor T cells instead suppress or eradicate residual leukemia. Evidence for this derives not just from the clinical studies of GVHD and relapse in CML, but also directly from the demonstration of dramatic expansion of leukemia antigen-specific cytotoxic T lymphocytes coincident with the onset of durable molecular remissions of CML[128] and from animal models.[129] The target antigens for the GVL effect have not been identified but they are likely to include not only leukemia-specific antigens (e.g., BCR–ABL[134]), but also minor histocompatibility antigens expressed either ubiquitously or in a tissue-restricted fashion (e.g., those on normal lymphoid or myeloid cells).[135–137] Despite uncertainties about the exact mechanisms involved in the GVL effect, clinical protocols that utilize the GVL activity of donor T cells are already in widespread use in the treatment of children and adults with CML relapsing after SCT,[115,116,138–140] and for preemptive T-cell infusion in conjunction with transplantation of purified CD34+ cells.[141]

Management of relapse

Although the majority of patients who relapse after BMT do so into chronic-phase CML, a small proportion relapse straight into blast crisis. The options for managing relapse into chronic phase are: DLI, imatinib, IFN-α and second BMT. The most effective and least toxic options are DLI (see below) and imatinib, and there are currently no data in children to show which approach produces the best long-term outcome. The treatment of choice for an individual patient will depend upon a number of factors, including:

• the preference of the family;
• the age, size and health of a sibling donor or availability of an unrelated donor;
• whether or not the child had significant GVHD during the transplant;
• and, possibly, the stage of disease at relapse.

For example, DLI is most effective when given to patients with molecular relapse (i.e., no cytogenetic or hematologic evidence of disease) and less effective when given for frank hematologic relapse.[142] Indeed, for patients in hematologic relapse it may be preferable to aim to induce molecular remission with imatinib and then treat any further detectable disease by DLI.

Second transplant may still be contemplated for those patients resistant to both DLI (see below) and imatinib.[143–146] The available literature suggests that the second procedure should be delayed for at least 12 months after the first to reduce transplant-related mortality.[143] For children conditioned with busulfan/cyclophosphamide for the first transplant, a TBI regimen may be preferable for the second, although there is no definite evidence of greater antileukemic efficacy; for those who received TBI for the first transplant, second transplants with busulfan alone have been successful.[146] However, there is little information in the literature to guide the clinician.

For children who relapse into blast crisis, particularly myeloid blast crisis, following BMT the outlook is often, but not always, bleak. The management is that for blast crisis (see below). If chronic-phase disease is reestablished, consideration should be given to DLI or imatinib if donor cells remain detectable, or a second BMT where there is no evidence of residual donor cells.

Donor lymphocyte infusion

Since the first successful reports of DLI to treat leukemia relapsing after BMT in 1990, this approach has become part of the routine management of this difficult problem.[115,116,138–140] DLI is particularly effective in CML because of the GVL effect described above. For DLI to be successful, molecular monitoring for residual BCR–ABL-positive cells using a quantitative technique is essential as this will detect relapse before cytogenetic and hematologic relapse is apparent.[147–150] The most robust technique is quantitative reverse-transcription polymerase chain reaction (RT-PCR); many protocols are adapted to take advantage of automated analysis, such as Taqman.[151] An example of persistent and rising numbers of *BCR–ABL* mRNA transcripts detectable on serial blood samples by RT-PCR is shown in Fig. 17.6. Peripheral blood samples can be used, making serial bone marrow aspirates post-SCT unnecessary.[151] Monitoring with FISH has not been shown to be sensitive enough for this purpose. We recommend monitoring samples every 3 months for the first year and then every 6 months thereafter; any positive results should be followed up by monthly monitoring to watch for rising levels of disease.[115,152] Because a weakly positive result within the first 6 months of SCT is not predictive of relapse and neither is an occasional weakly positive result, DLI is generally only indicated when there are clearly rising levels

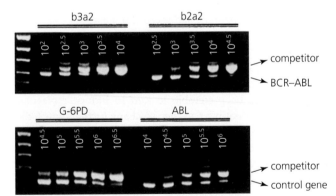

Fig. 17.6 Examples of competitive reverse-transcription polymerase chain reaction (RT-PCR) in peripheral blood leukocytes from CML patients: ethidium bromide-stained agarose gels for quantification of *BCR–ABL* (b3a2 and b2a2 junctions) and of *G6PD* and *ABL* transcripts as internal controls. Serial dilutions of a linearized competitor were added to fixed amounts of patient cDNA. The number of competitor molecules added is shown above each track. The equivalence point, at which competitor and sample bands have the same intensity, can be estimated by visual inspection or, more accurately, by densitometry. This point permits calculation of the number of target transcript molecules in the sample per unit volume of cDNA. Kindly provided by Junia Melo.

or two consecutive results of $> 0.05\%$ *BCR–ABL* compared with *ABL* transcripts.[152]

The main factors that determine the efficacy and toxicity of DLI are the cell dose and the phase of disease at the time of DLI.[153,154] There is good evidence that the success rate of DLI is higher where there is molecular or cytogenetic relapse rather than hematologic relapse, and therefore DLI should be considered as soon as any measure of recurrent disease is detected and recommended where there is evidence of disease progression.[142,153,154] There is also good evidence that escalating dose regimens that start with a low initial cell dose ($\leq 2 \times 10^7$ mononuclear cells/kg) produce the best results in terms of high efficacy with a low rate of GVHD and myelosuppression.[153,154] With escalating dose protocols each dose is normally separated by 3–4 months as this is the time required to determine the response to DLI in CML.[154] These data derive from adult studies as there are only anecdotal pediatric reports in the literature, but we have used DLI successfully for children for several years. Overall the response rate is around 90% and 70% for patients treated in molecular/cytogenetic and hematologic relapse, respectively.[115,116,138–140,142,151,153,154] For those patients who respond, the response is usually apparent by 3–6 months after DLI. Unfortunately for patients relapsing into blast crisis, the outlook is poor because most patients do not have a sustained response.[153]

Although DLI has an established role in reinducing complete remission and long-term cure, it also has significant side-effects. GVHD of greater than grade II severity occurs in around 10% of patients treated in molecular/cytogenetic relapse and in around 20% of patients treated in hematologic relapse.[155] GVHD can be fatal, although in most cases it responds to reinstitution of ciclosporin with or without steroids. Prolonged or irreversible aplasia (sometimes requiring "top up" SCT without conditioning) also occurs in around 20% of patients treated in hematologic relapse but is rarely seen in patients treated in molecular/cytogenetic relapse when an escalating dose protocol is used.[142]

Interferon-α

IFN-α was introduced as treatment for CML in adults in the early 1980s.[156] There have been seven large randomized trials in CML involving > 2000 patients, some of which have included children,[157] and several small pediatric studies.[41,158] Overall there is no significant difference between the response of children to IFN-α compared with the response of young adults. In adults the overall response rate is 70%, with around 20% of patients achieving a major or complete cytogenetic response usually within 6 months.[157] Patients who achieve a complete cytogenetic response to IFN-α ($>65\%$ Ph-chromosome-negative) live longer than those treated with hydroxycarbamide.[159] However, it is not clear whether those with a minor response or those who are nonresponders have any survival advantage with IFN-α compared with hydroxycarbamide. The role of IFN-α in the management of children with CML has reduced since imatinib became available. It should probably be considered before experimental therapy as an option for the small group of children with no suitable SCT donor who are also resistant to or intolerant of imatinib.

Mode of action

The mechanism of action of IFN-α in CML is not fully understood. It reduces cellular proliferation, at least in part due to its effects on progenitor cell–stromal cell interactions, and may have immunomodulatory effects leading to increased recognition of CML cells.[160]

Dose

The standard starting dose is 3 mega units (MU) daily by subcutaneous injection.[157] The dose should be adjusted after the first few weeks of treatment to maintain the white cell count between 2 and 4×10^9/L and platelets $> 80 \times 10^9$/L (maximum dose 5 MU daily). Response to IFN-α is assessed both by hematologic parameters and by marrow cytogenetics at 3–6-month intervals. It normally takes at least 6 months to determine whether patients are going to show a major cytogenetic response (>35% Ph-chromosome-negative) to IFN-α. IFN treatment should therefore be continued in all patients who achieve a hematologic response for at least 6 months. For children who have only a minor cytogenetic response (<35% Ph-negative), or no response by 6 months, it is unlikely that continuing IFN-α will confer a survival advantage and other treatment should be considered (allogeneic SCT, a further trial of imatinib or experimental therapy). Children who fail to achieve a hematologic response to IFN-α may be developing acceleration of disease and should be reassessed as soon as possible.

Side-effects

The commonest problems are flu-like symptoms (including fever, chills, rigors, headache, muscle aches and malaise), which usually occur during the first 2 weeks of treatment. The symptoms resolve completely on continuing therapy in most patients; however, it may be helpful to administer the IFN-α just before bedtime and to give a dose of paracetamol half an hour beforehand, particularly if fever is a prominent feature. Convulsions in association with fever have also occasionally been reported in children treated with IFN-α. Other side-effects include lethargy, depression, alopecia, rash, myelosuppression, anorexia, weight loss, abnormal liver function and autoimmune phenomena (idiopathic thrombocytopenic purpura, hypothyroidism and hemolytic anemia).

Combination treatment

Data from a French multicenter study[161] in which adult patients were randomized to IFN-α with or without cytosine arabinoside suggested that this combination can prolong survival; the 3-year survival in the IFN-cytarabine group was 86% compared with 79% for the IFN group. This difference appeared to be due to an increased proportion of patients achieving a major or complete cytogenetic response in the combination group at 12 months: 41% in the IFN-cytarabine group versus 24% in the IFN group.

Experimental treatment

There are several new drugs under clinical trial for CML (see below) which are not available yet for use in children.[62] The only situation where experimental therapy is likely to be considered in children with CML is the small group of patients who become resistant to both imatinib and IFN-α and who are unable to undergo SCT (or have relapsed after SCT and failed standard relapse therapy). In this situation two options that could be considered are autologous SCT and reduced-intensity conditioning (RIC) SCT. Whilst the exact role of autologous BMT for CML is still unclear, in adults there is considerable experience in the use of autologous stem cells.[162,163] Of the 559 transplants for CML in children reported to the EMBT since 1982, only 30 were autologous transplants, and no data on the outcome of this small group of children have been published. Nonmyeloablative RIC SCT is being investigated by a number of groups.[164,165] The results in adults are fairly promising in that transplant-related mortality seems to be low and the short-term results in chronic phase disease are encouraging.[165] However, there seems to be a high risk of GVHD even with sibling donors and the outcome for blast crisis patients is poor.[165]

Management of accelerated-phase CML and blast crisis

Accelerated-phase CML

Management of accelerated-phase CML depends on the nature of any previous treatment and the specific problems experienced by the child. Any child who develops evidence of acceleration while awaiting BMT should be transplanted at the earliest opportunity. Imatinib is the most useful drug for disease control until the transplant is carried out; for children who have relapsed on imatinib hematologic control can usually be achieved for a short time with hydroxycarbamide, 6-mercaptopurine or 6-thioguanine. The commonest manifestations of accelerated-phase disease are splenomegaly and thrombocytosis. Splenectomy is indicated for massive splenomegaly and, if SCT is planned, should preferably be carried out at least 6 weeks beforehand. Routine splenectomy and splenic irradiation prior to SCT are no longer recommended as they have not been shown to improve survival. Thrombocytosis may be difficult to control because it is sometimes resistant to imatinib and often resistant to hydroxycarbamide, or the doses required lead to unacceptable leukopenia. Fortunately, even platelet counts in excess of $1000 \times 10^9/L$ are usually well tolerated and are not usually associated with thrombosis or hemorrhage in children.[6,166] Where thrombocytosis is resistant to oral chemotherapy, IFN-α or anagrelide are often effective.[167]

Lymphoid blast crisis

The approach to treatment of lymphoid blast crisis of CML in children is similar to that of ALL. Remission induction with vincristine and steroids is successful in the majority of children.[53,168] The response to imatinib is disappointing, with a complete hematologic response in only 10–25% of patients,[72,80] and CNS relapse is common even in those with hematologic remission.[169] For those with an HLA-identical donor, allogeneic SCT is the treatment of choice following remission induction. For children in whom it is possible to proceed straight to SCT, further chemotherapy prior to SCT should not be necessary. In most cases, however, SCT is likely to be delayed for a few months and in this situation there is a choice between some form of intensification chemotherapy, as in childhood ALL protocols, or imatinib. Relapse of blast crisis within a few months is usual and SCT should not be delayed if at all possible.[72,79,80] The most appropriate CNS-directed treatment for such children is not clear. It seems wise to give regular intrathecal methotrexate, as is standard in most ALL protocols, because imatinib may not penetrate the intact blood–brain barrier.[169] Where no HLA-identical marrow donors can be identified, the options are SCT from a mismatched donor or haploidentical donor or cord blood transplantation because imatinib and maintenance chemotherapy are not curative.

Myeloid blast crisis

The remission rate for myeloid blast crisis remains poor, even with the most recent AML-type chemotherapy regimens and, in contrast to lymphoid blast crisis, vincristine and steroids are of little benefit. Several studies now show that around 50% of patients respond to imatinib but of these < 20% have a complete hematologic response and a complete cytogenetic response is uncommon.[72,79,80] Overall the median survival of adults with blast crisis on imatinib is 6–8 months.[79,80] Therefore for children with myeloid blast crisis of CML the choice lies between imatinib and AML-type chemotherapy (including daunorubicin or mitoxantrone, cytarabine and etoposide or thioguanine) as a bridge until SCT, which should be carried out as soon as possible. Where no HLA-identical marrow donors can be identified, SCT from a mismatched donor or haploidentical donor or cord blood transplantation are recommended because imatinib and maintenance chemotherapy are not curative.

Future directions

This is a very exciting time for physicians managing CML because there are several areas of clinical investigation that are likely to lead to improved management not only with respect to an increased cure rate but also to reduced toxicity. Broadly the three areas of most intense investigation are innovative forms of SCT, new drugs for imatinib-resistant CML, and immunotherapy targeted at enhancing the host immune response to BCR–ABL-expressing cells.

SCT

Because CML is a stem cell disorder, successful therapy will continue to require elimination of all of the CML clone or at least reduction in the CML clone to levels barely detectable by current techniques (around 1 in 10^5 cells). It is likely that low levels of disease can persist for long periods, and possibly indefinitely, clonal expansion being prevented by the patient's own immune response. For these reasons, SCT is likely to remain the principal therapeutic approach to CML in children. Improvement in the outcome of SCT is most likely to derive from advances in donor matching, better understanding of individual prognostic factors, GVHD prevention and treatment, increased understanding of the GVL response and the development of effective RIC regimens.

Novel drugs and new combinations

A large number of new agents are currently under investigation in adults with CML as increasing evidence points to imatinib resistance being the major limitation to cure of CML without SCT (Table 17.6). A major area of interest has been to target other signaling molecules on the downstream pathways triggered by BCR–ABL (see Fig. 17.3). This has led to the development of several new kinase inhibitors, including JAK2 inhibitors, SRC kinase inhibitors[170] and tyrphostins and farnesyl transferase inhibitors, which block the action of RAS.[171,172] In addition, safer and more effective formulations of several older drugs are being investigated as possible agents for use alone or in combination, for instance arsenicals, such as arsenic trioxide,[173–175] troxacitabine,[176] and

Table 17.6 New drugs under investigation in chronic myeloid leukemia.

Farnesyl transferase inhibitors
New kinase inhibitors, e.g., AG957, AG940, AP23464
Homoharringtonine
Nucleoside analogs, e.g., troxacitabine
Arsenicals, e.g., arsenic sulfide
Antiangiogenic agents, e.g., bevacizumab[180]
Polyethylene glycol (PEG)-IFN
Proteasome inhibitors, e.g., bortezomib[181]

polyethylene glycol (PEG)-IFN.[177] It seems most likely that a combination of agents will be necessary to cure CML as with the acute leukemias.[174,175,178,179]

Immunotherapy

There is considerable interest in the development of peptide vaccines in CML. This has the advantage that at least one leukemia-specific target antigen can be readily identified (BCR–ABL-derived peptides) and there is extremely good evidence of potent T-cell-mediated antileukemia activity both from clinical and animal models.[134,182] This approach has already reached the stage of phase II trials.[182]

Summary

- CML constitutes 2–3% of all childhood leukemias and has an incidence of 0.6–1.2 per million per year in Western countries.
- Over 90% of children with CML are Philadelphia (Ph) chromosome-positive, defined by the balanced translocation t(9q34;22q11), which causes the formation of a *BCR–ABL* fusion gene.
- Over 95% of children with CML express BCR–ABL protein, a 210-kDa constitutively active tyrosine kinase.
- CML is a triphasic disease, with an indolent chronic phase (median duration 4 years), a symptomatic accelerated phase (median duration 6–18 months) and a terminal blast crisis phase (median duration 3–9 months) that responds poorly to treatment.
- The only known cure for CML is SCT.
- SCT is the treatment of choice as it cures 65–75% of children but has a high initial transplant-related mortality.
- Relapse after SCT is fairly common but is exquisitely sensitive to donor lymphocyte infusion, which cures > 80% if given during molecular relapse.
- Children without an HLA-identical stem cell donor or who relapse after SCT usually respond to imatinib mesylate, a newly developed tyrosine kinase inhibitor with high specificity for BCR–ABL.
- Imatinib mesylate is the first of several new drugs targeted to leukemia-associated proteins in CML and currently in clinical trials but not curative when used alone due to drug resistance.
- Cure of children with CML in the future may be possible using combinations of leukemia-targeted drugs, immunotherapy and reduced-intensity conditioning SCT.

Acknowledgments

We are grateful to Andy Chase for providing Fig. 17.1a, Junia Melo for Figs 17.1b, 17.2 and 17.3, and David Swirsky for many of the morphology slides.

References

1. Horibe K, Tsukimoto I, Ohno R. Clinicopathologic characteristics of leukemia in Japanese children and young adults. *Leukemia* 2001; **15**: 1256–61.
2. Jakab Z, Balogh E, Kiss C, Olah E. Epidemiologic studies in a population-based childhood cancer registry in Northeast Hungary. *Med Pediatr Oncol* 2002; **38**: 338–44.
3. Birch JM, Alston RD, Quinn M, Kelsey AM. Incidence of malignant disease by morphological type, in young persons aged 12–24 years in England, 1979–1997. *Eur J Cancer* 2003; **39**: 2622–31.
4. Xie Y, Davies SM, Xiang Y, Robison LL, Ross JA. Trends in leukemia incidence and survival in the United States (1973–1998). *Cancer* 2003; **97**: 2229–35.
5. Clavell J, Goubin A, Auclerc MF *et al.* Incidence of childhood leukaemia and non-Hodgkin's lymphoma in France: National Registry of Childhood Leukaemia and Lymphoma 1990–1999. *Eur J Can Prev* 2004; **13**: 97–103.
6. Millot F, Traore P, Guilhot J *et al.* Clinical and biological features at diagnosis in 40 children with chronic myeloid leukemia. *Pediatrics* 2005; **116**: 140–3.
7. Tokuhata GK, Neely CL, Williams DL. Chronic myelocytic leukemia in identical twins and a sibling. *Blood* 1968; **31**: 216–25.
8. Preston DL, Kusumi S, Tomonaga M *et al.* Cancer incidence in atomic bomb survivors. Part III: leukaemia, lymphoma and multiple myeloma, 1950–1987. *Radiation Res* 1994; **137**: 68–97.
9. Neves H, Ramos C, da Silva MG, Parreira A, Parreira L. The nuclear topography of ABL, BCR, PML, and RAR alpha genes: evidence for gene proximity in specific phases of the cell cycle and stages of hematopoietic differentiation. *Blood* 1999; **93**: 1197–207.
10. Saglio G, Storlazzi CT, Giugliano E *et al.* A 76-kb duplicon maps close to the BCR gene on chromosome 22 and the ABL gene on chromosome 9: possible involvement in the genesis of the Philadelphia chromosome translocation. *Proc Natl Acad Sci USA* 2002; **99**: 9882–7.
11. Verneris MR, Tuel L, Seibel NL. Pediatric HIV infection and chronic myelogenous leukemia. *Pediatr AIDS HIV Infect* 1995; **6**: 292–4.
12. Mignozzi M, Picca S. Chronic myelogenous leukemia following kidney transplantation in a pediatric patient. *Pediatr Nephrol* 2001; **16**: 852–3.
13. Nowell PC, Hungerford DA. A minute chromosome in human granulocytic leukemia. *Science* 1960; **132**: 1497–501.
14. Rowley JD. A new consistent abnormality in chronic myelogenous leukaemia. *Nature* 1982; **243**: 290–1.
15. DeKlein A, Van Kessel AG, Grosveld G *et al.* A cellular oncogene is translocated to the Philadelphia chromosome in chronic myelocytic leukaemia. *Nature* 1982; **300**: 765–7.
16. Kurzrock R, Gutterman JU, Talpaz M. The molecular genetics of Philadelphia chromosome-positive leukemias. *N Engl J Med* 1988; **319**: 990–8.
17. Chissoe SL, Bodenteich A, Wang YF *et al.* Sequence and analysis of the human ABL gene, the BCR gene, and regions involved in the Philadelphia chromosomal translocation. *Genomics* 1995; **27**: 67–82.

18. Melo JV. The molecular biology of chronic myeloid leukemia. *Leukemia* 1996; **10**: 751–6.

19. Lugo TG, Pendergast AM, Muller AJ, Witte ON. Tyrosine kinase activity and transformation potency of bcr-abl oncogene products. *Science* 1990; **247**: 1079–82.

20. Daley GQ, Van Etten RA, Baltimore D. Induction of chronic myelogenous leukemia in mice by the P210bcr/abl gene of the Philadelphia chromosome. *Science* 1990; **247**: 824–30.

21. Kelliher MA, McLaughlin J, Witte ON, Rosenberg N. Induction of chronic myelogenous leukemia-like syndrome in mice with v-abl and BCR-ABL. *Proc Natl Acad Sci USA* 1990; **87**: 6649–53.

22. Vickers M. Estimation of the number of mutations necessary to cause chronic myeloid leukaemia from epidemiological data. *Br J Haematol* 1996; **94**: 1–4.

23. Melo JV, Gordon DE, Cross NC, Goldman JM. The ABL-BCR fusion gene is expressed in chronic myeloid leukemia. *Blood* 1993; **81**: 158–65.

24. Melo JV. The diversity of BCR-ABL fusion proteins and their relationship to leukemia phenotype. *Blood* 1996; **88**: 2375–84.

25. Sawyers C. Signal transduction pathways involved in BCR-ABL transformation. *Baillière's Clin Haematol* 1997; **10**: 223–31.

26. Sawyers CL, McLaughlin J, Witte O. Genetic requirement for Ras in the transformation of fibroblasts and hematopoietic cells by the Bcr-Abl oncogene. *J Exp Med* 1995; **181**: 307–13.

27. Cortez D, Stoica G, Pierce JH, Pendergast AM. The BCR-ABL tyrosine kinase inhibits apoptosis by activating a Ras-dependent signalling pathway. *Oncogene* 1996; **13**: 2589–94.

28. Mandanas RA, Leibowitz DS, Gharehbaghi K *et al.* Role of p21 RAS in *bcr/abl* transformation of murine myeloid cells. *Blood* 1993; **82**: 1838–47.

29. Goldman JM, Melo JV. Chronic myeloid leukemia: advances in biology and new approaches to treatment. *N Engl J Med* 2003; **349**: 1451–64.

30. Jonas D, Lubbert M, Kawasaki ES *et al.* Clonal analysis of bcr-abl rearrangement in T lymphocytes from patients with chronic myelogenous leukemia. *Blood* 1992; **79**: 1017–23.

31. Raskind W, Ferraris AM, Najfeld V, Jacobson RH, Moohr JW, Fialkow PJ. Further evidence for the existence of a clonal Ph-negative stage in some cases of Ph-positive chronic myelocytic leukemia. *Leukemia* 1993; **7**: 1163–7.

32. Eaves CJ, Eaves AC. Stem cell kinetics. *Baillière's Clin Haematol* 1997; **10**: 233–57.

33. Jamieson CH, Ailles LE, Dylla SJ *et al.* Granulocyte-macrophage progenitor as candidate leukemic stem cells in blast-crisis CML. *New Eng J Med* 2004; **351**: 657–67.

34. Gordon MY, Goldman JM. Cellular and molecular mechanisms in chronic myeloid leukaemia: biology and treatment. *Br J Haematol* 1996; **95**: 10–20.

35. Jaiswal S, Traver D, Miyamoto T, Akashi K, Lagasse E, Weissman IL. Expression of BCR/ABL and BCL-2 in myeloid progenitors leads to myeloid leukemias. *Proc Natl Acad Sci USA* 2003; **100**: 10002–7.

36. Bedi A, Zehnbauer BA, Barber J *et al.* Inhibition of apoptosis by BCR-ABL in chronic myeloid leukemia. *Blood* 1994; **83**: 2038–44.

37. Gordon MY, Dowding CR, Riley GP, Goldman JM, Greaves MF. Altered adhesive interactions with marrow stroma of haematopoietic progenitor cells in chronic myeloid leukaemia. *Nature* 1987; **328**: 342–4.

38. Harihan IK, Adams JM, Cory S. BCR-ABL oncogene renders myeloid cell line factor-independent: potential autocrine mechanism in chronic myeloid leukemia. *Oncogene Res* 1988; **3**: 387–99.

39. Sirard C, Laneuville P, Dick J. Expression of bcr-abl abrogates factor-dependent growth of human hematopoietic MO7E cells by an autocrine mechanism. *Blood* 1994; **83**: 1575–85.

40. Castro-Malaspina H, Schaison G, Briere J *et al.* Philadelphia chromosome positive chronic myelocytic leukemia in children. Survival and prognostic factors. *Cancer* 1983; **52**: 721–7.

41. Dow LW, Raimondi SC, Culbert SJ, Ochs J, Kennedy W, Pinkel DP. Response to alpha-interferon in children with Philadelphia chromosome-positive chronic myelocytic leukemia. *Cancer* 1991; **68**: 1678–84.

42. Rowe JM, Lichtman MA. Hyperleukocytosis and leukostasis: common features of childhood chronic myelogenous leukemia. *Blood* 1984; **63**: 1230–4.

43. Mitelman F. The cytogenetic scenario of chronic myeloid leukemia. *Leukemia Lymphoma* 1993; **11**: 11–15.

44. Seong DC, Kantarjian HM, Ro JY *et al.* "Hypermetaphase FISH" for quantitative monitoring of Philadelphia chromosome positive cells in chronic myelogenous leukemia patients during treatment. *Blood* 1995; **86**: 2343–9.

45. Muhlmann J, Thaler J, Hilbe W *et al.* Fluoresence in situ hybridization (FISH) on peripheral blood smears for monitoring Philadelphia chromosome-positive chronic myeloid leukemia (CML): a new strategy for remission assessment. *Genes Chrom Cancer* 1998; **21**: 90–100.

46. van de Plas DC, Grosveld G, Hagermeijer A. Review of clinical, cytogenetic and molecular aspects of Ph-negative CML. *Cancer Genet Cytogenet* 1991; **52**: 143–56.

47. Huntley BJ, Reid AG, Bench AJ *et al.* Deletions of the derivative chromosome 9 occur at the time of the Philadelphia translocation and provide a powerful and independent prognostic indicator in chronic myeloid leukemia. *Blood* 2001; **98**: 1732–8.

48. Drummond M, Lennard A, Brummendorf T, Holyoake T. Telomere shortening correlates with prognostic score at diagnosis and proceeds rapidly during progression of chronic myeloid leukemia. *Leukemia Lymphoma* 2004; **45**: 1775–81.

49. Speck B, Bortin MM, Champlin R *et al.* Allogeneic bone-marrow transplantation for chronic myelogenous leukaemia. *Lancet* 1984; **i**: 665–8.

50. Majlis A, Smith TL, Talpaz M *et al.* Significance of cytogenetic clonal evolution in chronic myelogenous leukemia. *J Clin Oncol* 1996; **14**: 196–203.

51. Kantarjian HM, Keating MJ, Talpaz M *et al.* Chronic myelogenous leukemia in blast crisis. *Am J Med* 1987; **83**: 445–54.

52. Ruff P, Saragas E, Poulos M, Weaving A. Patterns of clonal evolution in transformed chronic myelogenous leukemia. *Cancer Genet Cytogenet* 1995; **81**: 182–4.

53. Janossy G, Woodruff RK, Pippard AJ *et al.* Relation of "lymphoid" phenotype and response to chemotherapy incorporating vincristine-prednisolone in the acute phase of Ph'-positive leukemia. *Cancer* 1979; **43**: 426–34.

54. Wadhwa J, Szydlo R, Apperley JF *et al.* Factors affecting duration of survival after onset of blastic transformation of chronic myeloid leukemia. *Blood* 2002; **99**: 2304–9.

55. Sawyers C. The role of MYC in transformation by BCR-ABL. *Leukemia Lymphoma* 1993; **11**: 45–6.

56. Feinstein E, Cimino G, Gale RP *et al*. p53 in chronic myelogenous leukemia in acute phase. *Proc Natl Acad Sci USA* 1991; **88**: 6293–7.

57. Ahuja HG, Jat PS, Foti A, Bar-Eli M, Cline MJ. Abnormalities of the retinoblastoma gene in the pathogenesis of acute leukemia. *Blood* 1991; **78**: 3259–68.

58. Sill H, Goldman JM, Cross NCP. Homozygous deletions of the p16 tumor suppressor gene are associated with lymphoid transformation of chronic myeloid leukemia. *Blood* 1995; **85**: 2013–16.

59. Mitani K, Ogawa S, Tanaka T *et al*. Generation of the AML-EVI1 fusion gene in the t(3;21)(q26;q22) causes blastic crisis in chronic myelocytic leukaemia. *EMBO J* 1994; **13**: 504–10.

60. Druker BJ, O'Brien SG, Cortes J, Radich J. Chronic myelogenous leukemia. *Hematology* 2002; 111–35.

61. Thornley I, Perentesis JP, Davies SM, Smith FO, Champagne M, Lipton JM. Treating children with chronic myeloid leukemia in the imatinib era: a therapeutic dilemma. *Med Pediatr Oncol* 2003; **41**: 115–17.

62. Goldman J. Chronic myeloid leukemia – still a few questions. *Exp Hematol* 2004; **32**: 2–10.

63. Stone RM. Optimizing treatment of chronic myeloid leukemia: a rational approach. *The Oncologist* 2004; **9**: 259–70.

64. Pulsipher MA. Treatment of CML in pediatric patients: should imatinib mesylate (STI-571, Gleevec) or allogeneic hematopoietic cell transplant be front-line therapy? *Pediatr Blood Cancer* 2004; **43**: 523–33.

65. Kolb EA, Pan O, Ladanyi M, Steinherz PG. Imatinib mesylate in Philadelphia chromosome-positive leukemia of childhood. *Cancer* 2003; **98**: 2643–50.

66. Champagne MA, Capdeville R, Krailo M *et al*. Imatinib mesylate (STI571) for treatment of children with Philadelphia chromosome-positive leukemia: results from a Children's Oncology Group phase 1 study. *Blood* 2004; **104**: 2655–60.

67. Goldman JM, Szydlo R, Horowitz MM *et al*. Choice of pre-transplant treatment and timing of transplants for chronic myelogenous leukemia in chronic phase. *Blood* 1993; **82**: 2235–8.

68. Savage DG, Antman KH. Imatinib mesylate: a new oral targeted therapy. *N Engl J Med* 2002; **346**: 683–93.

69. Druker BJ, Tamura S, Buchdunger E *et al*. Effects of a selective inhibitor of the Abl tyrosine kinase on the growth of Bcr-Abl positive cells. *Nat Med* 1996; **2**: 561–6.

70. Schindler T, Bornmann W, Pellicena P, Miller WT, Clarkson B, Kuriyan J. Structural mechanism for STI-571 inhibition of abelson tyrosine kinase. *Science* 2000; **289**: 1938–42.

71. Druker BJ, Talpaz M, Resta D *et al*. Efficacy and safety of a specific inhibitor of the Bcr-Abl tyrosine kinase in chronic myeloid leukemia. *N Engl J Med* 2001; **344**: 1031–7.

72. Druker BJ, Sawyers CL, Kantarjian H *et al*. Activity of a specific inhibitor of the BCR-ABL tyrosine kinase in the blast crisis of chronic myeloid leukemia and acute lymphoblastic leukemia with the Philadelphia chromosome. *N Engl J Med* 2001; **344**: 1038–42.

73. Talpaz M, Silver RT, Druker BJ. Imatinib induces durable hematologic and cytogenetic responses in patients with accelerated phase chronic myeloid leukemia: results of a phase 2 study. *Blood* 2002; **99**: 1928–37.

74. O'Brien SG, Guilhot F, Larson RA *et al*. Imatinib compared with interferon and low-dose cytarabine for newly diagnosed chronic-phase chronic myeloid leukemia. *N Engl J Med* 2003; **348**: 994–1004.

75. Hughes TP, Kaeda J, Branford S *et al*. Frequency of major molecular responses to imatinib or interferon alfa plus cytarabine in newly diagnosed chronic myeloid leukemia. *N Engl J Med* 2003; **349**: 1423–32.

76. Kantarjian H, Talpaz M, O'Brien S *et al*. High-dose imatinib mesylate therapy in newly diagnosed Philadelphia chromosome-positive chronic phase chronic myeloid leukemia. *Blood* 2004; **103**: 2873–8.

77. Marin D, Marktel S, Szydlo R *et al*. Survival of patients with chronic phase chronic myeloid leukaemia on imatinib after failure on interferon alfa. *Lancet* 2003; **362**: 617–19.

78. Kantarjian H, Cortes J, O'Brien S *et al*. Long-term survival benefit and improved complete cytogenetic and molecular response rates with imatinib mesylate in Philadelphia chromosome-positive chronic myeloid leukemia after failure of interferon-α. *Blood* 2004; **104**: 1979–88.

79. Sawyers CL, Hochhaus A, Feldman E *et al*. Imatinib induces hematologic and cytogenetic responses in patients with chronic myelogenous leukemia in myeloid blast crisis: results of a phase II study. *Blood* 2002; **99**: 3530–9.

80. Kantarjian HM, Cortes J, O'Brien S *et al*. Imatinib mesylate (STI571) therapy for Philadelphia chromosome-positive chronic myelogenous leukemia in blast phase. *Blood* 2002; **99**: 3547–53.

81. Shah N, Tran C, Lee FY, Chen P, Norris D, Sawyers CL. Overriding imatinib resistance with a novel ABL kinase inhibitor. *Science* 2004; **305**: 399–401.

82. Deininger MW, Druker BJ. SR Circumventing imatinib resistance. *Cancer Cell* 2004; **6**: 108–10.

83. Tauchi T, Ohyashiki K. Molecular mechanisms of resistance of leukemia to imatinib mesylate. *Leuk Res* 2004; **28** (S1): S39–S45.

84. Thomas J, Wang L, Clark RE, Pirmohamed M. Active transport of imatinib into and out of cells: implications for drug resistance. *Blood* 2004; **104**: 3739–45.

85. Terre C, Eclache V, Rousselot P *et al*. Report of 34 patients with clonal chromosomal abnormalities in Philadelphia-negative cells during imatinib treatment of Philadelphia-positive chronic myeloid leukemia. *Leukemia* 2004; **18**: 1340–6.

86. Elrick LJ, Jorgensen HG, Mountford JC, Holyoake TL. Punish the parent not the progeny. *Blood* 2005; **105**: 1862–6.

87. Gorre ME, Mohammed M, Ellwood K *et al*. Clinical resistance to STI-571 cancer therapy caused by BCR-ABL gene mutation or amplification. *Science* 2001; **293**: 876–80.

88. Shah NP, Nicoll JM, Nagar B *et al*. Multiple BCR-ABL kinase domain mutations confer polyclonal resistance to the tyrosine kinase inhibitor imatinib (STI571) in chronic phase and blast crisis chronic myeloid leukemia. *Cancer Cell* 2002; **2**: 117–25.

89. Corbin AS, La Rosee P, Stoffregen EP, Druker BJ, Deininger MW. Several Bcr-Abl kinase domain mutants associated with imatinib mesylate resistance remain sensitive to imatinib. *Blood* 2003; **101**: 4611–14.

90. Hochhaus A, Kreil S, Corbin AS *et al*. Molecular and chromosomal mechanisms of resistance to imatinib (STI571) therapy. *Leukemia* 2002; **16**: 2190–6.

91. Gambacorti-Passerini C, Barni R, le Coutre P *et al.* Role of alpha1 acid glycoprotein in the in vivo resistance of human BCR-ABL (+) leukemic cells to the abl inhibitor STI. *J Natl Cancer Inst* 2000; **92**: 1641–50.

92. Mahon FX, Belloc F, Lagarde V *et al.* MDR1 gene overexpression confers resistance to imatinib mesylate in leukemia cell line models. *Blood* 2003; **101**: 2368–73.

93. Roche-Lestienne C, Soenen-Cornu V, Grardel-Duflos N *et al.* Several types of mutations of the Abl gene can be found in chronic myeloid leukemia patients resistant to STI571, and they can preexist to the onset of treatment. *Blood* 2002; **100**: 1014–18.

94. Hofmann WK, Komor M, Wassmann B *et al.* Presence of the BCR-ABL mutation E255K prior to STI571 (imatinib) treatment in patients with Ph+ acute lymphoblastic leukemia. *Blood* 2003; **102**: 659–61.

95. Yamamoto M, Kurosu T, Kakihana K, Mizuchi D, Miura O. The two major imatinib resistance mutations E255K and T315I enhance the activity of BCR/ABL fusion kinase. *Biochem Biophys Res Commun* 2004; **319**: 1272–5.

96. Cortes JE, Talpaz M, Giles F *et al.* Prognostic significance of cytogenetic clonal evolution in patients with chronic myelogenous leukemia on imatinib mesylate therapy. *Blood* 2003; **101**: 3794–800.

97. Morimoto A, Ogami A, Chiyonobu T *et al.* Early blastic transformation following complete cytogenetic response in a pediatric chronic myeloid leukemia patient treated with imatinib mesylate. *J Pediatr Hematol Oncol* 2004; **26**: 320–2.

98. Xu, Wahner AE, Nguyen PL. Progression of chronic myeloid leukemia to blast crisis during treatment with imatinib mesylate. *Arch Path Lab Med* 2004; **128**: 980–5.

99. Avery S, Nadal E, Marin D *et al.* Lymphoid transformation in a CML patient in complete cytogenetic remission following treatment with imatinib. *Leuk Res* 2004; **28** (suppl. 1): S75–7.

100. Marin D, Marktel S, Bua M *et al.* The use of imatinib (STI571) in chronic myeloid leukemia: some practical considerations. *Haematologica* 2002; **87**: 979–88.

101. Cwynarski K, Roberts IAG, Iacobelli S *et al.* Stem cell transplantation for chronic myeloid leukemia in children. *Blood* 2003; **102**: 1224–31.

102. Millot F, Esperou H, Bordigoni P *et al.* Allogeneic bone marrow transplantation for chronic myeloid leukemia in childhood: A report from the Société Française de Greffe de Moëlle et de Thérapie Cellulaire (SFGM-TC). *Bone Marrow Transplant* 2003; **32**: 993–9.

103. Creutzig U, Ritter J, Zimmermann M *et al.* Prognosis of children with chronic myeloid leukemia: A retrospective analysis of 75 patients. *Klin Pediatr* 1996; **208**: 236–41.

104. Gamis A, Haake R, McGlave P, Ramsay NKC. Unrelated-donor bone marrow transplantation for Philadelphia chromosome-positive chronic myelogenous leukemia in children. *J Clin Oncol* 1993; **11**: 834–8.

105. Dini G, Rondelli R, Miano M *et al.* Unrelated-donor bone marrow transplantation for Philadelphia chromosome-positive chronic myelogenous leukemia in children: experience in eight European countries. *Bone Marrow Transplant* 1996; **18** (suppl. 2): 80–5.

106. Gluckman E, Rocha V, Boyer-Chammard A *et al.* Outcome of cord-blood transplantation from related and unrelated donors. *N Engl J Med* 1997; **337**: 373–81.

107. Bogdanic V, Nemet D, Kastelan A *et al.* Umbilical cord blood transplantation in a patient with Philadelphia chromosome positive chronic myeloid leukemia. *Transplantation* 1993; **56**: 477–9.

108. Gluckman E, Rocha V, Arcese W *et al.* Factors associated with outcomes of unrelated cord blood transplant: guidelines for donor choice. *Exp Hematol* 2004; **32**: 397–407.

109. Clift RA, Buckner CD, Thomas ED *et al.* Marrow transplantation for chronic myeloid leukemia: a randomized study comparing cyclophosphamide and total body irradiation with busulfan and cyclophosphamide. *Blood* 1994; **84**: 2036–43.

110. Devergie A, Blaise D, Attal M *et al.* Allogeneic bone marrow transplantation for chronic myeloid leukemia in first chronic phase: a randomized trial of busulfan-cytoxan versus cytoxan-total body irradiation as a preparative regimen: a report from the French Society of Bone Marrow Graft (SFGM). *Blood* 1995; **85**: 2263–8.

111. Gratwohl A, Hermans J, Biezen AV *et al.* No advantage for patients who receive splenic irradiation before bone marrow transplantation for chronic myeloid leukemia: results of a prospective randomized study. *Bone Marrow Transplant* 1992; **10**: 147–52.

112. Kalhs P, Schwarzinger I, Anderson G *et al.* A retrospective analysis of the long-term effect of splenectomy on late infections, graft-versus-host disease, relapse and survival after allogeneic marrow transplantation for chronic myelogenous leukemia. *Blood* 1995; **86**: 2028–32.

113. Kolb HJ, Mittermuller J, Clemm C *et al.* Donor leukocyte transfusions for the treatment of recurrent chronic myelogenous leukemia in marrow transplant patients. *Blood* 1990; **76**: 2462–5.

114. Mackinnon S, Papadopoulos EB, Carabasi MH *et al.* Adoptive immunotherapy evaluating escalating doses of donor leukocytes for relapse of chronic myeloid leukemia after bone marrow transplantation: separation of graft-versus-leukemia responses from graft-versus-host disease. *Blood* 1995; **86**: 1261–8.

115. Gilleece MH, Dazzi F. Donor lymphocyte infusions for patients who relapse after allogeneic stem cell transplantation for chronic myeloid leukaemia. *Leukemia Lymphoma* 2003; **44**: 23–8.

116. Ladon D, Pieczonka A, Jolkowska J, Wachowiak J, Witt M. Molecular follow up of donor lymphocyte infusion in CML children after allogeneic bone marrow transplantation. *J Appl Genet* 2001; **42**: 547–52.

117. DeAngelo DJ, Hochberg EP, Alyea EP *et al.* Extended follow-up of patients treated with imatinib mesylate (Gleevec) for chronic myelogenous leukemia relapse after allogeneic transplantation: durable cytogenetic remission and conversion to complete donor chimerism without graft-versus host disease. *Clin Cancer Res* 2004; **10**: 5065–71.

118. Spencer A, Szydlo R, Brookes PA *et al.* Bone marrow transplantation for chronic myeloid leukemia with volunteer unrelated donors using *ex vivo* or *in vivo* T-cell depletion: major prognostic impact of HLA Class I identity between donor and recipient. *Blood* 1995; **86**: 3590–7.

119. Clift RA, Anasetti C. Allografting for chronic myeloid leukaemia. *Baillière's Clin Haematol* 1997; **10**: 319–36.

120. Clift RA, Buckner CD, Thomas ED *et al.* Bone marrow transplantation for patients in accelerated phase of chronic myeloid leukemia. *Blood* 1994; **84**: 4368–73.

121. Hansen JA, Gooley TA, Martin PJ *et al.* Bone marrow transplants from unrelated donors for patients with chronic myeloid leukemia. *N Engl J Med* 1998; **338**: 962–8.

122. Weisdorf DJ, Anasetti C, Antin JH *et al.* Allogeneic bone marrow transplantation for chronic myelogenous leukemia: comparative analysis of unrelated versus matched sibling donor transplantation. *Blood* 2002; **99**: 1971–7.

123. Passweg JR, Walker I, Sobocinski KA, Klein JP, Horowitz MM, Giralt S. Validation and extension of the EBMT Risk Score for patients with chronic myeloid leukaemia (CML) receiving allogeneic haematopoietic stem cell transplants. *Br J Haematol* 2004; **125**: 613–20.

124. Devergie A, Madrigal A, Apperley JF *et al.* European results of matched unrelated donor bone marrow transplantation for chronic myeloid leukemia. Impact of HLA Class II matching. *Bone Marrow Transplant* 1997; **20**: 11–20.

125. Zander AR, Kroger N, Schleuning M *et al.* ATG as part of the conditioning regimen reduces transplant-related mortality (TRM) and improves overall survival after unrelated stem cell transplantation in patients with chronic myelogenous leukemia (CML). *Bone Marrow Transplant* 2003; **32**: 355–61.

126. Gratwohl A, Brand R, Apperley J *et al.* Graft-versus-host disease and outcome in HLA-identical sibling transplantations for chronic myeloid leukemia. *Blood* 2002; **100**: 3877–86.

127. Barrett J. Allogeneic stem cell transplantation for chronic myeloid leukemia. *Semin Hematol* 2003; **40**: 59–71.

128. Molldrem JJ, Lee PP, Wang C *et al.* Evidence that specific T lymphocytes may participate in the elimination of chronic myelogenous leukemia. *Nat Med* 2000; **6**: 1018–23.

129. Matte CC, Cormier J, Anderson BE *et al.* Graft-versus-leukemia in a retrovirally induced murine CML model: mechanisms of T-cell killing. *Blood* 2004; **103**: 4353–61.

130. Hale G, Waldmann H. Recent results using CAMPATH-1 antibodies to control GVHD and graft rejection. *Bone Marrow Transplant* 1996; **17**: 305–8.

131. Apperley JF, Jones L, Hale G *et al.* Bone marrow transplantation for chronic myeloid leukaemia: T cell depletion with Campath-1 reduces the incidence of acute graft-versus-host disease but may increase the risk of leukaemic relapse. *Bone Marrow Transplant* 1986; **1**: 53–66.

132. Goldman JM, Gale RP, Horowitz M *et al.* Bone marrow transplantation for chronic myelogenous leukemia in chronic phase. Increased risk of relapse associated with T-cell depletion. *Ann Intern Med* 1988; **108**: 806–14.

133. Storb R, Deeg HJ, Whitehead J. Methotrexate and cyclosporine compared with cyclosporine alone for prophylaxis of acute graft versus host disease after marrow transplantation for leukemia. *N Engl J Med* 1986; **314**: 729–35.

134. Clark RE, Dodi IA, Hill SC *et al.* Direct evidence that leukemic cells present HLA-associated immunogenic peptides derived from the BCR-ABL b3a2 fusion protein. *Blood* 2001; **98**: 2887–93.

135. Mutis T, Verdijk R, Schrama E, Esendam B, Brand A, Goulmy E. Feasibility of immunotherapy of relapsed leukemia with ex vivo-generated cytotoxic T lymphocytes specific for hematopoietic system-restricted minor histocompatibility antigens. *Blood* 1999; **93**: 2336–41.

136. Molldrem JJ, Lee PP, Wang C, Champlin RE, Davis MM. A PR1-human leukocyte antigen-A2 tetramer can be used to isolate low-frequency cytotoxic T lymphocytes from healthy donors that selectively lyse chronic myelogenous leukemia. *Cancer Res* 1999; **59**: 2675–81.

137. Gao L, Bellantuono I, Elsasser A *et al.* Selective elimination of leukemic CD34(+) progenitor cells by cytotoxic T lymphocytes specific for WT. *Blood* 2000; **95**: 2198–203.

138. Kolb HJ, Mittermuller J, Clemm C *et al.* Donor leukocyte transfusions for the treatment of recurrent chronic myelogenous leukemia in marrow transplant patients. *Blood* 1990; **76**: 2462–5.

139. Mackinnon S, Papadopoulos EB, Carabasi MH *et al.* Adoptive immunotherapy evaluating escalating doses of donor leukocytes for relapse of chronic myeloid leukemia after bone marrow transplantation: separation of graft-versus-leukemia responses from graft-versus-host disease. *Blood* 1995; **86**: 1261–8.

140. Dazzi F, Szydlo RM, Cross NC *et al.* Durability of responses following donor lymphocyte infusions for patients who relapse after allogeneic stem cell transplantation for chronic myeloid leukemia. *Blood* 2000; **96**: 2712–16.

141. Elmaagacli AH, Peceny R, Steckel N *et al.* Outcome of transplantation of highly purified peripheral blood CD34+ cells with T-cell add-back compared with unmanipulated bone marrow or peripheral blood stem cells from HLA-identical sibling donors in patients with first chronic phase chronic myeloid leukemia. *Blood* 2003; **101**: 446–53.

142. Van Rhee F, Feng L, Cullis JO *et al.* Relapse of chronic myeloid leukemia after allogeneic bone marrow transplant: the case of giving donor leukocyte transfusions before the onset of hematologic relapse. *Blood* 1994; **83**: 3377–83.

143. Barrett AJ, Locatelli F, Treleaven JG *et al.* Second transplant for leukaemic relapse after bone marrow transplantation: high early mortality but favourable effect of chronic GVHD on continuing remission. *Br J Haematol* 1991; **79**: 567–74.

144. Mrsic M, Horowitz M, Atkinson K *et al.* Second HLA-identical sibling transplants for leukemic recurrence. *Bone Marrow Transplant* 1992; **9**: 269–75.

145. Arcese W, Goldman JM, D'Arcangelo E *et al.* Outcome for patients who relapse after allogeneic bone marrow transplantation for chronic myeloid leukemia. *Blood* 1993; **82**: 3211–19.

146. Cullis JO, Schwarer AP, Hughes TP *et al.* Second transplants for patients with chronic myeloid leukaemia in relapse after original transplant with T-depleted marrow: feasibility of using busulphan alone for re-conditioning. *Br J Haematol* 1992; **80**: 33–9.

147. Cross NCP, Feng L, Chase A, Bungey J, Hughes TP, Goldman JM. Competitive polymerase chain reaction to estimate the number of *BCR–ABL* transcripts in chronic myeloid leukemia patients after bone marrow transplantation. *Blood* 1993; **82**: 1929–36.

148. Radich JP, Gooley T, Bryant E *et al.* The significance of bcr-abl molecular detection in chronic myeloid leukemia patients "late," 18 months or more after transplantation. *Blood* 2001; **98**: 1701–7.

149. Olavarria E, Kanfer E, Szydlo R *et al.* Early detection of BCR–ABL transcripts by quantitative reverse transcriptase-polymerase chain

reaction predicts outcome after allogeneic stem cell transplantation for chronic myeloid leukemia. *Blood* 2001; **97**: 1560–5.

150. Emig M, Saussele S, Wittor H *et al*. Accurate and rapid analysis of residual disease in patients with CML using specific fluorescent hybridization probes for real time quantitative RT-PCR. *Leukemia* 1999; **13**: 1825–32.

151. Branford S, Hughes TP, Rudzki Z. Monitoring chronic myeloid leukaemia therapy by real-time quantitative PCR in blood is a reliable alternative to bone marrow cytogenetics. *Br J Haematol* 1999; **107**: 587–99.

152. Mughal TI, Yong A, Szydlo RM *et al*. Molecular studies in patients with chronic myeloid leukaemia in remission 5 years after allogeneic stem cell transplant define the risk of subsequent relapse. *Br J Haematol* 2001; **115**: 569–74.

153. Guglielmi C, Arcese W, Dazzi F *et al*. Donor lymphocyte infusion for relapsed chronic myelogenous leukemia: prognostic relevance of the initial cell dose. *Blood* 2002; **100**: 397–405.

154. Dazzi F, Szydlo RM, Craddock C *et al*. Comparison of single-dose and escalating-dose regimens of donor lymphocyte infusion for relapse after allografting for chronic myeloid leukemia. *Blood* 2000; **95**: 67–71.

155. Dazzi F, Szydlo RM, Apperley JF, Goldman JM. Prognostic factors for acute graft-versus-host disease after donor lymphocyte infusions. *Blood* 2002; **100**: 2673–4.

156. Kantarjian HM, Smith TI, O'Brien S, Beran M, Pierce S, Talpaz M. Prolonged survival in chronic myelogenous leukemia after cytogenetic response to interferon-α therapy. *Ann Intern Med* 1995; **122**: 254–61.

157. Richards SM. Interferon-α: results from randomized trials. *Baillière's Clin Haematol* 1997; **10**: 307–18.

158. Millot F, Brice P, Philippe N *et al*. α-Interferon in combination with cytarabine in children with Philadelphia chromosome-positive chronic myeloid leukemia. *J Pediatr Hematol Oncol* 2002; **24**: 18–22.

159. The Italian Cooperative Study Group on Chronic Myeloid Leukemia. Interferon alfa 2a as compared with conventional chemotherapy for the treatment of chronic myeloid leukemia. *N Engl J Med* 1994; **330**: 820–5.

160. Deng M, Daley GQ. Expression of interferon consensus sequence binding protein induces potent immunity against BCR/ABL-induced leukemia. *Blood* 2001; **97**: 3491–7.

161. Guilhot F, Chastang C, Michallet M *et al*. Interferon alfa-2b combined with cytarabine versus interferon alone in chronic myelogenous leukemia. *N Engl J Med* 1997; **337**: 223–9.

162. Carella AM, Cunningham I, Benvenuto F *et al*. Mobilization and transplantation of Philadelphia-negative peripheral blood progenitor cells early in chronic myelogenous leukemia. *J Clin Oncol* 1997; **15**: 1575–82.

163. Bhatia R, McGlave PB. Autologous hematopoietic cell transplantation for chronic myelogenous leukemia. *Hematol Oncol Clin North Am* 2004; **18**: 715–32.

164. Sloand E, Childs RW, Solomon S, Greene A, Young NS, Barrett AJ. The graft-versus-leukemia effect of nonmyeloablative stem cell allografts may not be sufficient to cure chronic myelogenous leukemia. *Bone Marrow Transplant* 2003; **32**: 897–901.

165. Or R, Shapira MY, Resnick I *et al*. Nonmyeloablative allogeneic stem cell transplantation for the treatment of chronic myeloid leukemia in first chronic phase. *Blood* 2003; **101**: 441–5.

166. Mitus AJ, Schafer A. Thrombocytosis and thrombocythemia. *Hematol Oncol Clin N Am* 1990; **4**: 157–78.

167. Chintagumpala MM, Kennedy LL, Steubler CP. Treatment of essential thrombocythemia with anagrelide. *J Pediatr* 1995; **127**: 495–8.

168. Rosenthal S, Canellos GP, Whang-Peng J, Gralnick HR. Blast crisis of chronic granulocytic leukemia: morphologic variants and therapeutic implications. *Am J Med* 1977; **63**: 542–7.

169. Leis JF, Stepan DE, Curtin PT *et al*. Central nervous system failure in patients with chronic myelogenous leukemia lymphoid blast crisis and Philadelphia chromosome positive acute lymphoblastic leukemia treated with imatinib (STI-571). *Leukemia Lymphoma* 2004; **45**: 695–8.

170. O'Hare T, Pollock R, Stoffregen EP *et al*. Inhibition of wild-type and mutant Bcr-Abl by AP23464, a potent ATP-based oncogenic protein kinase inhibitor: implications for CML. *Blood* 2004; **104**: 2532–9.

171. Peters DG, Hoover RR, Gerlach MJ *et al*. Activity of the farnesyl protein transferase inhibitor SCH66336 against BCR/ABL-induced murine leukemia and primary cells from patients with chronic myeloid leukemia. *Blood* 2001; **97**: 1404–12.

172. Cortes J, Albitar M, Thomas D *et al*. Efficacy of the farnesyl transferase inhibitor R115777 in chronic myeloid leukemia and other hematologic malignancies. *Blood* 2003; **101**: 1692–7.

173. La Rosee P, Johnson K, O'Dwyer ME, Druker BJ. In vitro studies of the combination of imatinib mesylate (Gleevec) and arsenic trioxide (Trisenox) in chronic myelogenous leukemia. *Exp Hematol* 2002; **30**: 729–37.

174. Yin T, Wu Y-L, Sun H-P *et al*. Combined effects of As_4S_4 and imatinib on CML cells. *Blood* 2004; **104**: 4219–25.

175. Kantarjian H, Talpaz M, Smith TL *et al*. Homoharringtonine and low-dose cytarabine in the management of late chronic-phase chronic myelogenous leukemia. *J Clin Oncol* 2000; **18**: 3513–21.

176. Giles FJ, Garcia-Manero G, Cortes JE *et al*. Phase II study of troxacitabine, a novel dioxolane nucleoside analog, in patients with refractory leukemia. *J Clin Oncol* 2002; **20**: 656–64.

177. Baccarani M, Martinelli G, Rosti G *et al*. Imatinib and pegylated human recombinant interferon-alpha2b in early chronic-phase chronic myeloid leukemia. *Blood* 2004; **104**: 4245–51.

178. Dai Y, Rahmani M, Pei XY, Dent P, Grant S. Bortezomib and flavopiridol interact synergistically to induce apoptosis in chronic myeloid leukemia cells resistant to imatinib mesylate through both Bcr/Abl-dependent and -independent mechanisms. *Blood* 2004; **104**: 509–18.

179. La Rosee P, Johnson K, Corbin AS. In vitro efficacy of combined treatment depends on the underlying mechanism of resistance in imatinib-resistant Bcr-Abl-positive cell lines. *Blood* 2004; **103**: 208–15.

180. Thomas DA, Giles FJ, Cortes J, Albitar M, Kantarjian HM. Antiangiogenic therapy in leukemia. *Acta Haematol* 2001; **106**: 190–207.

181. Cortes J, Thomas D, Koller C *et al*. Phase I study of bortezomib in refractory or relapsed acute leukemias. *Clin Cancer Res* 2004; **10**: 3371–6.

182. Cathcart K, Pinilla-Ibarz J, Korontsvit T *et al*. A multivalent bcr-abl fusion peptide vaccination trial in patients with chronic myeloid leukemia. *Blood* 2004; **103**: 1037–42.

18 Myelodysplastic syndromes

David K.H. Webb

Over 95% of children with leukemia have acute myeloid leukemia (AML) or acute lymphoblastic leukemia (ALL); the others have more chronic myeloproliferative or myelodysplastic disease. Chronic lymphocytosis in childhood is usually a response to an infection or an immunoregulatory disorder (see Chapter 19) and there have only been a handful of reports of apparent chronic lymphocytic leukemia in childhood.

The myelodysplastic syndromes (MDS) were historically characterized by a cellular marrow with peripheral pancytopenia and were first described as smouldering leukemia or preleukemia. These were predominantly disorders of late adult life and have since been well classified in the extensive adult literature.

Early reports of chronic leukemias in childhood[1,2] make no distinction between chronic myeloid leukemia (CML) and what would now be deemed MDS, and only in the last few years have any serious attempts been made to classify pediatric MDS, which differ in many important respects from the disease in adults.[3–10] The advent of more effective treatment, in particular bone marrow transplantation (BMT), has made a rational approach to diagnosis and management of increasing importance.

Historical perspective

Over 40 years ago Hardisty et al.[11] distinguished two types of chronic granulocytic leukemia in childhood. The adult type, which had a relatively long survival and was associated with the Philadelphia chromosome; and the second form, subsequently often called juvenile chronic myelomonocytic leukemia,[12] which was associated with suppurative infections, severe thrombocytopenia, a nonspecific but very characteristic skin rash and a very poor prognosis. Further interest in this rare disorder was awakened by the reports of a consistently raised fetal hemoglobin (HbF) level and fetal red cell characteristics.[13] A third chronic disorder was described

in young infants with a missing C group chromosome,[14] which was subsequently identified as chromosome 7.[15] These three conditions, dependent in part on clinical features for diagnosis, comprised the most clinically distinct myeloproliferative or myelodysplastic disorders in childhood but there was no systematic review of the associated blood and marrow morphology.

Meanwhile, the morphologic classification of MDS in adults was developed by the efforts of the French–American–British (FAB) group (see below),[17] and terms such as preleukemia tended to be abandoned in favor of the appropriate FAB type of MDS. Retrospective and more stringent analysis of cases of pediatric AML showed that a proportion of cases, perhaps 17%, had an indolent prodrome and might be called myelodysplasia.[16] More recently, an international consensus has been developed, subdividing MDS in children into a proliferative group comprising juvenile myelomonocytic leukemia (JMML), a group of adult-type MDS, and a number of very rare or secondary disorders.[18]

Incidence and epidemiology

MDS is largely a disease of the elderly and the incidence rises dramatically with increasing age.[19,20] There have been a number of recent estimates of the incidence in childhood, but these have been derived from relatively small populations and it seems probable that the incidence of the more indolent forms has been underestimated. A population-based study in Denmark estimated that the incidence of MDS approximated that of AML at 4.0 new cases per million children annually, thus representing 9% of all hematologic malignancies,[21] whereas in northern England the estimated incidence was 0.53 per million, or 1% of malignancies.[22] A report from the national UK childhood MDS registry gave an annual incidence of 1.4 per million over a 10-year period.[23] These discrepancies could be due in part to the inclusion or exclusion of more aggressive forms (e.g., refractory anemia with excess

Table 18.1 Conditions associated with the development of myelodysplasia in childhood.

Congenital disorders
Down syndrome
Trisomy 8
Neurofibromatosis type 1
Congenital bone marrow disorders
Fanconi anemia
Congenital neutropenia including Kostmann syndrome
Diamond–Blackfan anemia
Shwachman–Diamond syndrome
Familial MDS

Acquired disorders
Aplastic anemia with previous immunosuppressive therapy
Previous cytotoxic or radiation therapy

---

of blasts in transformation) as either MDS or AML rather than any true variation in incidence.

A characteristic feature of MDS in childhood is a strong association with congenital disorders and genetic syndromes (Table 18.1); in recent non-population-based reports between one-quarter and one-half of patients have shown some phenotypic abnormality. Some of these are nonspecific, such as mental retardation or small stature, but others are recognized genetic conditions. Children with Down syndrome have a 10–20-fold increased risk of development of leukemia, usually the pre-B or common type of lymphoblastic leukemia or the megakaryoblastic (M7) subtype of AML. Patients with megakaryoblastic leukemia often have a preceding phase of MDS, which may last some weeks or months. This evolving myeloid leukemia, which is fatal if untreated,[24] should not be confused with the transient abnormal myelopoiesis (TAM) seen in some newborn babies with Down syndrome and in occasional normal neonates; this condition resembles acute leukemia but usually resolves without specific treatment.[25] Constitutional trisomy 8 usually occurs in mosaic form and is associated with facial dysmorphism, skeletal abnormalities and mild-to-moderate mental retardation.[26] Trisomy 8 is a common cytogenetic finding in myeloid malignancies, and a number of patients with constitutional trisomy 8 have developed hematologic disorders including MDS.[27,28] The precise frequency of constitutional trisomy 8 and AML is unknown.

There is an increased risk of JMML in the common autosomal dominant form of neurofibromatosis,[29,30] and MDS with monosomy 7 is also associated with this disorder.[31] A number of congenital bone marrow disorders predispose to the development of AML and MDS, including congenital neutropenia, in particular Kostmann syndrome (see Chapters 3 and 14), where treatment with granulocyte colony-stimulating factor (G-CSF) may improve symptoms and obviate the need for BMT, but has been associated with risk of the development of monosomy 7 and MDS.[32] Patients with the Shwachman–Diamond syndrome of pancreatic exocrine

insufficiency and neutropenia have generalized abnormalities of hematopoiesis and are at increased risk of AML, ALL and MDS.[33,34] Patients with Fanconi anemia are at significant risk of the development of AML and MDS.[35]

There are a number of families described in the literature with no apparent congenital or genetic abnormality in whom more than one member has developed MDS or AML. MDS with monosomy 7 has been described in infant siblings,[3,36] but in other families more than one member has developed AML or MDS in later childhood or adult life, sometimes in association with a familial platelet storage pool disorder.[37] In several instances, the development of MDS has been associated with evolution of a cytogenetic abnormality in the bone marrow, most often monosomy 7 or 5.

Immunosuppressive therapy with antilymphocyte globulin and ciclosporin has improved survival in patients with acquired aplastic anemia, particularly those without a histocompatible sibling donor (see Chapter 4). However, children treated by immunosuppression are at increased risk of MDS.[38]

Secondary MDS with a predilection to development of AML was first described in patients treated for Hodgkin disease, multiple myeloma and ovarian cancer, and more recently after high-dose chemoradiotherapy and infusion of autologous bone marrow.[39,40] By contrast, secondary acute leukemia in patients who have been treated with topoisomerase II inhibitors usually occurs without any dysplastic prodrome.

Clinical features

The symptoms and signs of MDS are more insidious than those of acute leukemia, and the diagnosis may even be made incidentally. Pallor is common, bacterial infections may be a consequence of neutropenia or defective neutrophil function, and bruising may be due to thrombocytopenia or defective platelet function. Patients may also present with a prolonged history of repeated infections, which is suggestive of congenital immune deficiency. Some children with JMML develop weight loss and failure to thrive. Lymph node enlargement is unusual except in JMML. The liver and spleen may be enlarged or not palpable. A characteristic skin rash, mimicking Langerhans cell histiocytosis, may occur on the face or trunk in JMML, and occasionally in infants with other types of MDS in association with monosomy 7.

Investigations

Blood and bone marrow examination

Table 18.2 lists the recommended investigations in children with suspected MDS. The blood and bone marrow

Table 18.2 Evaluation of suspected myelodysplastic syndrome.

History
Family history of leukemia or genetic disorders
History of previous cytotoxic therapy

Examination
Associated clinical disorders
  Neurofibromatosis[a]
  Down syndrome
  Fanconi anemia
  Noonan syndrome
  Shwachman–Diamond syndrome
  Other congenital abnormalities

Laboratory tests
Full blood count and differential
Well-stained blood film
Absolute count, monocytes, basophils, eosinophils
HbF level before blood transfusion
Virology, especially parvovirus, CMV and EBV*
Bone marrow aspiration
Morphology including iron stain
Cytogenetics including FISH
In vitro cultures of CFU-GM*
Bone marrow trephine biopsy
Morphology, especially of megakaryocytes
Cellularity and fibrosis
Presence of ALIP

Observation
Consistent hematologic abnormalities over 2 months

* Investigations indicated in all cases of juvenile myelomonocytic leukemia.
ALIP, abnormally localized immature precursor cells; CFU-GM, granulocyte–macrophage colony-forming unit; CMV, cytomegalovirus; EBV, Epstein–Barr virus; FISH, fluorescence *in situ* hybridization.

appearances are extremely variable, and a list of noteworthy features is given in Table 18.3. The essential diagnostic criteria are shown in Table 18.4. It is essential to examine the blood film and bone marrow in tandem and *the blood film is often more informative in reaching a diagnosis*. A trephine biopsy of the bone marrow should be obtained in all cases and important observations include:

• overall cellularity of the bone marrow;
• relative proportions and morphology of the three cell lines, especially the megakaryocytes;
• presence of fibrosis and reticulin and of abnormally localized immature precursor cells (ALIP), which are aggregates of myeloblasts and promyelocytes in the intertrabecular region in the bone marrow biopsy.

Immunohistochemical staining of bone marrow biopsies facilitates the identification of these immature precursors[39] and deserves further systematic study in children. Other investigations, such as measurement of HbF, neutrophil function and platelet function, may serve to confirm abnormalities of development of the three cell lines. Measurement of the HbF before any transfusions of red cells may be helpful in evaluating prognosis (see below) and is essential in JMML. Immunologic abnormalities may include low immunoglobulins, autoantibodies or even abnormalities of lymphocyte subsets. It may be necessary to exclude congenital viral infections. The hematologic appearances of HIV infection in adults may mimic MDS but this presentation has not been described in children.

Lastly, the diagnosis of MDS implies the finding of consistent hematologic abnormalities over a period of time, thus excluding patients with morphologic abnormalities in association with infection, which may resolve spontaneously,

Table 18.3 Common morphologic abnormalities in myelodysplasia.

Cell lineage	Blood film	Bone marrow
Erythroid	Macrocytes Punctate basophilia Poikilocytes Normoblasts	Dyserythropoiesis Multinucleate normoblasts Cytoplasmic vacuolation Ringed sideroblasts
Megakaryocytic	Giant platelets Megakaryocyte fragments	Small megakaryocytes Abnormal nuclear morphology
Granulocytes	Hypogranular Agranular Hypersegmentation Pelger forms	Promyelocytes with sparse granules Hypogranular precursors
Monocytes	Elongated lobes Azurophilic granules	Promonocytes sometimes present
Blasts	Usually small mononuclear blasts with scanty agranular (type I) or sparsely granular (type II) blasts	

Based on Ref. 16.

Table 18.4 Diagnostic criteria for myelodysplastic syndromes in children.[23]

At least two of the following must be present:
Blood cytopenia
Bilineage dysplasia
Excess of blasts (>5%) in bone marrow
Cytogenetic clone in bone marrow

Diagnostic criteria for JMML[41]
Essential
    Monocytosis $> 1 \times 10^9$/L
    Bone marrow blasts < 20%
    Absence of t(9;22)
Plus two from:
    White blood cell count $> 10 \times 10^9$/L
    Myeloid precursors on blood film
    Cytogenetic clone in bone marrow
    Spontaneous growth of CFU-GM *in vitro*

or patients whose abnormalities progress to frank AML within weeks.

Morphologic classification: the FAB classification

The FAB classification[16] has a number of limitations, especially in childhood MDS.

• Many children with MDS have a monocytosis, which thus automatically classes them as having JMML. However, in many such cases there may be > 5% blasts in the blood without an excess of blasts in the marrow. This finding should in theory mean reclassification as RAEB (refractory anemia with excess blasts) in transformation but in most pediatric studies such cases have been included in the category of JMML.

• There are a number of patients, e.g., those with eosinophilia and dysplastic blood and bone marrows, for whom it is impossible to assign an FAB type.

• Both therapy-induced MDS and MDS occurring in association with congenital bone marrow disorders may defy classification by the scheme, the bone marrow showing hypoplasia and/or fibrosis in addition to dysplasia.

Despite these limitations, systematic morphologic classification (Table 18.5) is important to facilitate the increasing number of collaborative studies and to assess prognosis and response to treatment. There have been a number of recent reports where the FAB classification has been applied to pediatric MDS.[3,6,8,9,20] The relative frequencies of the various subtypes of MDS in children and adults, as determined by ongoing studies in the UK, are illustrated in Table 18.6, with the caveat that the results are not strictly population based.

The World Health Organization (WHO) recently published recommendations for the classification of myeloid malignancies, including MDS, and these have been modified for pediatric use (Table 18.7). It is recommended that these revised WHO criteria are used internationally in future.

Pitfalls in morphologic diagnosis of refractory cytopenias

Refractory anemia must be distinguished from congenital dyserythropoietic anemias (see Chapter 2) and megaloblastic anemia (see Chapter 6), and the presence of clonal cytogenetic abnormalities is helpful in confirming the diagnosis; without such abnormalities the diagnosis should be considered with caution.

Refractory anemia with ringed sideroblasts as a true MDS is exceptionally rare in pediatrics, with only one case identified in the UK registry; it can only be diagnosed with confidence in the presence of a cytogenetic abnormality. Congenital sideroblastic anemia, due to abnormalities of heme synthesis, is usually associated with a dimorphic blood film; abnormalities of megakaryocytes and granulocytes are not seen. Sideroblastic anemia is also a feature of

Table 18.5 FAB classification of myelodysplastic syndromes.

Type	Blood film	Bone marrow
Refractory anemia (RA)	Blasts < 1%	Blasts < 5%
RA with ringed sideroblasts (RARS)	As in RA	As in RA but > 15% of erythroblasts as ringed sideroblasts
RA with excess of blasts (RAEB)	Blasts < 5%	Blasts 5–20%
RAEB in transformation (RAEDt)	Blasts > 5% Auer rods	As RAEB but 20–30% blasts Auer rods
Juvenile myelomonocytic leukemia (JMML)	Monocytes $> 1 \times 10^9$/L Blasts < 5%*	Blasts < 20%

* JMML in children is often associated with a higher blast count in the blood, but marrow blasts should not exceed 20% and Auer rods should not be present.
Reproduced with permission from Ref. 16.

Table 18.6 Relative frequency (%) of FAB types of myelodysplastic syndrome in children based on UK experience.

RA	24
RARS	< 1
RAEB	16
RAEBt	5
JMML	50
Other/unclassified	4

For explanation of abbreviations, see Table 18.5.
Reproduced with permission from Ref. 23.

Table 18.7 Pediatric modification of WHO classification of myelodysplastic disorders.

Myelodysplastic/myeloproliferative disease
Juvenile myelomonocytic leukemia

Down syndrome disease
Transient abnormal myelopoiesis
Myeloid leukemia of Down syndrome

Myelodysplastic syndrome
Refractory cytopenia (blood blasts < 2%, marrow blasts < 5%)
Refractory anemia with excess blasts (blood blasts < 19%,
   marrow blasts 5–19%)
Refractory anemia with excess blasts in transformation
   (blood or marrow blasts 20–29%)

Reproduced with permission from Ref. 18.

mitochondrial cytopathies, a group of disorders characterized by cortical neurologic impairment, metabolic acidosis and multiorgan involvement. The most typical of these is Pearson syndrome, which is characterized by pancreatic insufficiency, neutropenia and a bone marrow showing vacuolated precursors and ringed sideroblasts.[42] Hematologic abnormalities may be the dominant and indeed the only clinical feature of mitochondrial cytopathies at presentation and thus the distinction from MDS may be difficult.[9,43] Mitochondrial cytopathies should be excluded in any patient with apparent sideroblastic anemia, and it may be necessary to look for abnormal mitochondrial DNA on several occasions and to perform a muscle biopsy to confirm the diagnosis.

MDS or AML?

The distinction between refractory anemia with an excess of blasts with or without transformation and AML is an arbitrary one because patients may present with an abnormal count but a low percentage of blasts in the marrow and develop overt AML within weeks or even days (see Chapter 16). A classical presentation of this type is the extramedullary leukemic deposit (sometimes called a chloroma) found in patients with t(8;21) and M2 AML. The diagnosis of true MDS implies a more indolent course and in a French review an essential feature for the diagnosis was the presence of consistent hematologic abnormalities without evolution to AML over a 2-month period.[9] The distinction between an MDS and typical acute leukemia presenting with a low blast count is potentially important because the latter may respond more favorably to chemotherapy. The distinction is helped by careful review of morphology, because patients with true MDS will exhibit multilineage dysplasia, and also by the cytogenetic findings: t(8;21), t(15;17), t(9;11) and inv(16) are all associated with *de novo* AML.[44]

MDS or hypoplastic anemia?

A degree of dysplasia, particularly in the red cell series, is not unusual in chronic aplastic anemia, but the hypoplastic trephine appearances, absence of ALIP and absence of cytogenetic abnormalities in aplasia should help to make the distinction apparent.

Diagnosis of juvenile myelomonocytic leukemia

There can be occasional problems in distinguishing JMML from acute monoblastic or myelomonocytic leukemia but dysplasia in the granulocyte series is marked in JMML and the bone marrow appearances do not show such a predominance of early monocytic precursors.

JMML in pediatrics is an extremely heterogeneous disease (see below) and in order to define prognosis and improve management there is a need for a systematic attempt at investigation. Additional investigations recommended in these patients, such as *in vitro* bone marrow cultures, are listed in Table 18.2 and are discussed further below. Cytomegalovirus,[45] parvovirus,[46] and Epstein–Barr virus infections,[47] particularly in infants, may mimic JMML and should be excluded by appropriate virologic investigations.

Cytogenetics

Investigation of bone marrow cytogenetics, supplemented when possible by fluorescence *in situ* hybridization (FISH), is essential in the evaluation of MDS. Cytogenetic abnormalities are found in about 50% of cases of primary MDS in both children and adults and in > 90% of patients with therapy-induced MDS.[48,49] Some of the commoner findings are listed in Table 18.8. This list is not exhaustive and is based on the adult literature. The results of cytogenetic analyses in children with JMML and MDS and included in the UK national registry are shown in Table 18.9.

The most notable distinction between the cytogenetic findings in MDS and those in AML is the predominance of whole chromosome losses or partial deletions and the relative infrequency of translocations in MDS. There are some differences in the incidence of cytogenetic abnormalities between children and adults, most notably the marked

Table 18.8 Examples of some of the more common cytogenetic findings in myelodysplastic syndrome (MDS).

Primary MDS	Secondary MDS
Chromosome loss	
Monosomy 7	Monosomy 7
Loss of Y chromosome	Loss of Y chromosome
Monosomy 17	Monosomy 17
Chromosome gain	
Trisomy 8	Trisomy 8
Partial chromosome deletion	
del 5q	del 5q
del 20q	del 7q
del 11q	del 12p
del 7q	
Translocations	
	t(1;7)(p11;p11)
	t(5;17)(p11;p11)
	t(3;3)(q21;q26)

Adapted with permission from Refs 48 and 49.

Table 18.9 Cytogenetic findings in children with juvenile myelomonocytic leukemia (JMML) and myelodysplastic syndrome (MDS) in the UK registry.

Abnormality	JMML	MDS
Normal karyotype	66%	37%
Monosomy 7	15%	32%
Other chromosome 7 abnormality	1.6%	8%
Trisomy 8	3.2%	8%
Complex	4.8%	0%
Others	9.6%	13.6%
Failed		1.3%

Reproduced with permission from Ref. 23.

predominance of monosomy 7 in pediatric MDS.[50] Monosomy 7 is also the commonest cytogenetic finding in leukemia or MDS occurring in patients with congenital bone marrow disorders. Deletions of chromosome 5q, so common in adult practice, are rare in childhood. Cytogenetic abnormalities in MDS, unlike those in AML, are not usually associated with any specific morphologic subtype. The adult exception to this is the association of loss of part of the long arm of chromosome 5 (5q– syndrome) in elderly women with macrocytic anemia, a normal or raised platelet count, and relatively prolonged survival.[51]

Cytogenetic findings have been incorporated into several scoring systems to assess prognosis and, in general, the development of more complex abnormalities is associated with a worse prognosis and/or progression to AML. Cytogenetic abnormalities are almost always found in MDS secondary to chemotherapy.

Biology and pathogenesis

Studies of variants of glucose 6-phosphate dehydrogenase and other X-linked restriction fragment length polymorphisms[52] confirm that MDS is a clonal disorder. The use of FISH in combination with cytology and immunophenotyping[53] shows that in some cases the disease arises in progenitor cells restricted to myelopoiesis and erythropoiesis while in others the lymphoid series is involved as well, thus indicating malignant transformation in a more primitive hematopoietic cell. The event(s) initiating this change remain unknown.

Many of the chromosomal abnormalities in MDS involve the loss of genetic material, particularly from the long arms of chromosomes 5 and 7 (5q and 7q).[54] The regions involved in these cytogenetic changes are rich in genes with a role in hematopoiesis and it has been postulated that both 5q and 7q may be the site of tumor-suppressor genes. Intensive investigation of the critical region 5q31–q33 is underway to try to identify a tumor suppressor gene associated with the development of the 5q– syndrome, and similar critical regions have been identified on chromosome 7. An excellent review of the significance of the cytogenetic finding of monosomy 7 in pediatric AML and MDS emphasizes its frequent occurrence in many conditions with a predisposition to leukemia, including most of the congenital bone marrow disorders.[54] The authors postulate that loss of a gene(s) located on chromosome 7 may contribute to leukemogenesis as part of a final common pathway following a number of genetic events. It remains unclear if inactivation of both alleles is essential for disease progression (i.e., a tumor suppressor gene is involved), or if there is a gene dosage effect associated with deletion of one gene only.

The literature on MDS in adults is full of reports of mutations in various protooncogenes, including p53 mutations associated with a deletion in the short arm of chromosome 17,[55] in FMS in association with deletions in the FMS locus at chromosome 5q33 and mutations in the genes of the *ras* family.[56,57] *Ras* mutations have been most extensively investigated in JMML in adults, and more recently in children. It seems probable that such genetic changes are part of a final common pathway in the development of disease rather than initiating events in MDS.

The search to identify crucial genetic changes has been accompanied by many investigations of cellular biology and cell culture in MDS. The paradox of cytopenias in the blood despite a cellular bone marrow has been debated for many years. However, investigations have shown that while cell proliferation in the bone marrow in MDS is high, with large numbers of cells entering S phase,[58] these cells rapidly undergo programmed cell death (apoptosis) and thus never enter the circulation. Both proliferation and apoptosis are influenced by the complex cytokine network in the hematopoietic microenvironment, including tumor necrosis factor (TNF)-α, transforming growth factor (TGF)-β and interleukin-1β. Increased levels of these cytokines have been demonstrated in biopsies of patients with MDS.

Factors influencing prognosis

Treatment of MDS, particularly when involving BMT, carries a significant risk of morbidity and mortality and it is thus important to determine which patients are at early risk of death from leukemia or pancytopenia and in which patients a more conservative approach might be appropriate. This search for prognostic factors has been energetically pursued in adult MDS, a disease of the elderly, where the approach to management may be justifiably conservative. Numerous attempts to assess factors influencing both survival and progression to leukemia have been made. The original Bournemouth score[59] and subsequent modifications[60,61] used the presence of cytopenias, bone marrow blasts and ALIP. Other scores have also incorporated cytogenetics.[62] Most recently, an international scoring system has been developed using cytopenias, the percentage of blasts in the bone marrow, cytogenetics, age and sex to predict evolution of AML and survival.[63] There have been few attempts to apply such systems in children and attempts have been hampered by the dominance and clinical heterogeneity of JMML and the fact that these scores do not afford sufficient discrimination between morphologic subtypes of pediatric MDS.[8]

There is little information about the risk of transformation of MDS to acute leukemia in childhood. The deterioration in JMML is associated with increasing requirement for blood products and systemic symptoms (see below), rather than development of a frank new acute leukemia. Analysis of prognostic factors in a retrospective review of 68 cases showed that age and sex were not significant prognostic factors,[8] except that in JMML as previously reported,[12] younger children had a better prognosis. Both the unmodified FAB classification and the degree of cytogenetic complexity were also of some prognostic significance. A score was developed based on objective criteria that could be measured at diagnosis; each of the following scores 1 point if present:

• platelets $< 40 \times 10^9$/L;

• cytogenetic complexity score of 2 (i.e., cases with no clonal abnormalities score 0, those with a single simple abnormality score 1 and complex abnormalities score 2);

• HbF > 10%.

The results of this scoring system in a cohort of children are shown in Fig. 18.1. In practice, most patients with a score of 0 have refractory anemia or RAEB with or without a simple cytogenetic abnormality such as monosomy 7, whereas those

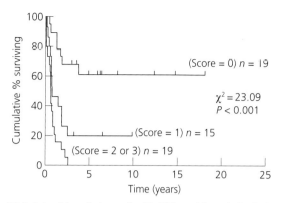

Fig. 18.1 Actuarial survival curve for 68 children with myelodysplasia based on the objective criteria scoring system described in the text. Reproduced with permission from Ref. 8.

with a score of 2 or 3 tend to have either JMML with a low platelet count and raised HbF level, or thrombocytopenia and complex cytogenetic abnormalities. Subsequent analyses have demonstrated the strongly adverse prognostic significance of monosomy 7 in refractory cytopenia and refractory anemia with excess blasts,[64,65] whilst confirming the adverse influence of older age, high HbF, and low platelet count in JMML.

Treatment

This section contains a general review of the methods of treatment available for patients with MDS; more specific recommendations about treatment are given in the individual subtype sections. There are no systematic prospective studies of treatment of pediatric MDS, and most of the information about chemotherapy is derived from studies of AML where patients with MDS have been identified retrospectively. Optimum supportive care with blood products (see Chapter 32) and appropriate management of infection (see Chapter 35) are essential for all patients.

Chemotherapy

There is limited information about the role of chemotherapy in children with MDS but it appears that response rates are inferior to those achieved in AML.[66] A comparison of 20 children treated for MDS with 31 who had AML showed that the remission rate was lower at 35% (74% in AML); resistant disease was more common, occurring in 25% (10% in AML); and 3-year survival was 15% (35% in AML); however, 8 of the patients with MDS had JMML, a subtype that in general responds poorly to chemotherapy (see below).[67] Comparison of outcome in children with classical dysplasia and those with AML with a low blast count showed that the remission rate was 30% for those with unequivocal MDS and 88% for the small number who had more typical AML; the latter group largely consisted of children with M2 or M4 AML and several had chloromas. The 4-year event-free survival was 50% for the AML patients compared with 23% in those with MDS.

In a series from the UK, children with RAEB in transformation (RAEBt) had similar survival (63%) to those with *de novo* AML when treated with the same chemotherapy. Although children with typical AML cytogenetic changes were excluded it was unclear whether all these children had stable MDS before treatment. The outcome for children with RAEB was significantly worse (28%).[65] Monosomy 7 carried a strong adverse prognosis in both groups, and after allowance for adverse cytogenetics, which were more common in MDS, survival was similar to that for children with *de novo* AML.

Low-dose cytarabine was originally used in adults with MDS in the belief that it was a differentiating agent, but it probably acts as a cytotoxic drug. Few children have been treated with low-dose cytarabine and there is no evidence that it is effective.[68] Oral cytotoxic drugs such as mercaptopurine or hydroxycarbamide have been used to reduce the leukemic burden in MDS but, as expected, they do not achieve remission.

Cytokines and differentiating agents

There is understandable interest in whether or not these agents can reduce the consequences of pancytopenia in older patients with MDS where intensive chemotherapy or BMT may not be feasible. Clinical trials are in progress to evaluate various combinations of G-CSF, granulocyte–macrophage CSF (GM-CSF), interleukin-3 (IL-3),[69] and erythropoietin sometimes in combination with low-dose cytosine arabinoside. The growth factors may improve neutropenia,[70] but there are concerns that they may accelerate progression to AML. The newly available human megakaryocyte growth and development factor, or thrombopoietin, will no doubt be evaluated in the same way.[71–73] A number of differentiating agents such as all-*trans* retinoic acid[74] have also been used in adults with little clinical benefit. There is some interest in these agents in JMML (see below). Despite this experience in adults, there is little justification for this approach in children where the aim of management is not palliation but cure.

Bone marrow transplantation

High-dose chemotherapy and/or radiotherapy with BMT is the only curative treatment for most patients with MDS. The first successful reports from BMT centers treating mainly adult patients showed a 3-year disease-free survival of about 40% for patients transplanted from an HLA-histocompatible sibling.[75,76] Children tolerate BMT better than adults, but only about 1 in 3 children in the UK have a histocompatible sibling. However, in the last few years the potential role for BMT in treatment has been expanded by the increased availability of volunteer unrelated donors and the start of programs for the use of cord blood. There is an increasing tendency to use peripheral blood stem cells (PBSC) rather than bone marrow, particularly in the context of autologous rescue from high-dose chemotherapy, and studies are in progress to evaluate allogeneic PBSC as a substitute for bone marrow.[77,78]

Choice of regimen

The choice of a preparative regimen for BMT depends on the age of the child, the diagnosis and the type of transplant. The most widely used regimen involves various combinations of total body irradiation (TBI) and cyclophosphamide, sometimes with the addition of other drugs such as cytarabine and etoposide. TBI is used in various schedules, sometimes as a single dose but more usually fractionated over 3–4 days. The most widely used chemotherapy regimen is a combination of busulfan and cyclophosphamide, which was developed originally for CML and AML.[79–81]

The choice between chemotherapy alone and regimens including TBI is in part dictated by consideration of the potential late effects of treatment, naturally an issue of extreme concern in the growing child. Although intensive chemotherapy carries the risk of significant late effects, including cardiotoxicity after anthracycline therapy, nephrotoxicity and potential sterility,[82] TBI is associated with additional complications and younger children are most vulnerable. Children who have received TBI have growth failure, which is partly due to spinal shortening and partly to hypothalamic–pituitary failure; this will be exacerbated if there is chronic graft-versus-host disease (GVHD). Delayed puberty and gonadal failure are common, and there is a variable risk of hypothyroidism, cataracts and learning problems. The combination of busulfan and cyclophosphamide has not been subjected to such rigorous long-term follow-up studies as TBI and it may induce sterility, but it is unlikely to have such a significant effect on skeletal growth and neuropsychologic development.

Randomized comparisons of chemotherapy and TBI have been performed in adults with CML[83] and AML[84] with conflicting results, but in a comparative study of adults with refractory anemia the combination of busulfan and cyclophosphamide was as satisfactory as cyclophosphamide and TBI.[84] There are no randomized pediatric trials but the combination of busulfan and cyclophosphamide has been used in children with AML,[85,86] and the two drugs in combination with melphalan are undergoing assessment in pediatric MDS.[87] Currently, therefore, it seems appropriate to use chemotherapy alone as a preparative regimen, at least in standard transplants from an HLA-identical sibling.

Type of transplant

The number of reports confined to BMT in children with MDS is small, with the exception of JMML (see below), but overall results, as for other hematologic malignancies, show that younger patients and those with less advanced disease do better.[88,89] For the many children with MDS who do not have a histocompatible sibling donor and for whom the only chance of cure may lie in BMT, it is reasonable to consider the use of alternative donors.[90] Most studies have involved the use of volunteer unrelated donors, and availability has increased significantly in recent years.[91] The chances of finding a donor depend on the patient's haplotype and ethnic group. In the last few years, cord blood has been used as a source of stem cells[92] but uncertainties remain about the risk of relapse and the stability of engraftment with this source.

Prognosis

There is a risk of relapse after BMT as after all other forms of treatment for MDS. This varies with the type and stage of MDS as well as the type of donor. The results of treatment after relapse are unsatisfactory. Donor leukocyte infusions have shown some promise in the management of relapse in CML,[93,94] presumably by induction of a graft-versus-leukemia effect. The use of such infusions is limited by the ethical issues involved in leukapheresis of young siblings but is feasible in consenting older siblings and volunteer unrelated donors. This treatment is being evaluated in other hematologic malignancies and may play a role in the management of relapsed MDS. There are anecdotal reports of successful therapy for relapsed MDS and, especially, JMML.[95]

An alternative form of high-dose therapy in MDS is the use of autologous rescue with bone marrow or blood stem cells. There have been several recent randomized trials of the use of autologous BMT (ABMT) in AML (see Chapter 17), and this form of treatment is being systematically evaluated in adults with MDS who achieve a stable remission. There are a few anecdotal reports of long-term remission after ABMT in children with MDS,[8] but the value of this form of treatment has not been established and it cannot be recommended outside a clinical trial.

It is clear that BMT is the most encouraging form of treatment for MDS, and while the choice between TBI- and chemotherapy-based regimens will depend on the age of the patient and type of transplant, it would seem possible to avoid TBI in many instances. The results from donors other than histocompatible siblings leave room for improvement but consideration of this approach is justified in children with poor prognosis of MDS or myeloproliferative syndrome.

Diagnosis and management of MDS subtypes

Refractory anemia

The diagnosis of refractory anemia is easier in the presence of a cytogenetic abnormality in the bone marrow. An expectant approach is reasonable if the patient is well, not dependent on blood products, and has no evidence of disease progression; indeed, such an approach is recommended particularly in the absence of any cytogenetic abnormality. The risk of such a policy is of course that the patient may develop acute leukemia, which is likely to be less responsive to chemotherapy than *de novo* AML. There is very little published information about the use of chemotherapy, as for AML, in refractory anemia and BMT is the treatment of choice. It is reasonable to consider early BMT in patients with a histocompatible sibling donor; in others the potential risks and benefits of an unrelated donor transplant must be carefully evaluated.

RAEB and RAEB in transformation

This category of patients includes both those with stable disease over months or years and those where the distinction from AML is a semantic one. In many national studies these patients are eligible for treatment with chemotherapy as if they had frank AML. In the absence of favorable cytogenetics such as t(8;21), such patients would in most centers be deemed eligible for BMT, at least if they have a histocompatible sibling donor. However, the use of chemotherapy where BMT is planned is contentious, and many centers recommend elective BMT without prior AML chemotherapy in stable patients. The role of unrelated donor BMT for patients with advanced MDS who have a good response to chemotherapy remains unclear.

Juvenile myelomonocytic leukemia

Clinical features and diagnosis

JMML is an extremely heterogeneous disease that is more common in boys[8,12] and in children under 2 years of age. There is an association with neurofibromatosis,[29,96] which may be found in 14% of patients, and with Noonan syndrome.[96,97]

The clinical spectrum varies from a relatively benign disease in infants with hepatosplenomegaly and monocytosis to the classical disease, usually in older children, with bleeding, thrombocytopenia, enlarged lymph nodes and splenomegaly. Progression of the disease is accompanied by wasting, fever, infections, bleeding and pulmonary infiltrations. The typical skin rash, which may precede other symptoms by months, is classically of a butterfly distribution but may be more extensive, and on biopsy shows a nonspecific infiltration with lymphocytes and histiocytes.

Hematologic findings

While the morphologic features are consistent with the FAB description of JMML and monocytosis is always present, the blood count may also show eosinophilia, basophilia and a higher number of blasts than would be acceptable for strict diagnosis of JMML on the FAB criteria. The appearance of the blood film is more diagnostic than that of the bone marrow, where abnormal monocytes and blast cells may be increased with, usually, dysplasia in all cell lines.

The original detailed hematologic description of JMML[12] has been complemented by a retrospective review of 110 cases strictly classified by the FAB criteria, except that > 5% blasts were allowed in the blood.[97] The median leukocyte count was $35 \times 10^9/L$ and exceeded $100 \times 10^9/L$ in only 7% of cases, eosinophilia was present in 8% of cases and basophilia in 28%, while over half the patients had thrombocytopenia of $< 50 \times 10^9/L$.

A characteristic feature of JMML is an increase in the HbF level,[13,98] which may increase progressively as the disease progresses, and a fetal pattern of γ-globin chain synthesis.[98] This is accompanied by a raised mean corpuscular volume, fetal pattern of 2,3-diphosphoglycerate and red cell enzyme production, red cell i/I antigen and carbonic anhydrase.[12,99] There may also be a number of immunologic abnormalities such as antinuclear antibodies and anti-IgG antibodies.[12,100]

While the diagnosis usually presents little difficulty, some patients with classical clinical features, including a grossly raised HbF, have a blood smear dominated by normoblasts, almost suggestive of erythroleukemia, while in other patients the distinction from acute myelomonocytic leukemia may be a fine one. Cytogenetic analysis in classical JMML with a grossly raised HbF is usually normal, but monosomy 7 may be found in some cases (see below).

Biology

The assumption that JMML is a clonal disorder, which is difficult to establish in the absence of cytogenetic abnormalities, has been confirmed by X-chromosome inactivation studies.[101] In addition, transplantation of cells from JMML patients can induce a JMML-like disease in irradiated severe combined immune-deficient mice.[102] The laboratory hallmark of the disease is spontaneous *in vitro* proliferation of granulocyte–macrophage colony-forming units (CFU-GM), which are formed at low cell densities and without the addition of exogenous growth factors.[103] This phenomenon has been the subject of intense study over many years and has prompted investigation of the role of a number of cytokines, including IL-1, TNF-α and GM-CSF in JMML.[104] Cells from patients with JMML cultured *in vitro* exhibit profound hypersensitivity to GM-CSF compared with those from normal controls. This appears to be a selective effect because responsiveness to other cytokines is normal, and it is postulated that the other cytokines such as TNF-α, responsible for some of the clinical features in advanced disease, are produced as a secondary response by hyperactivated monocytes.[105] Investigations are in progress to determine whether a growth factor

hypersensitivity assay, which is claimed to be both sensitive and specific for pediatric JMML, can be used in the diagnosis and monitoring of treatment.

The precise mechanism for growth factor hypersensitivity in JMML remains unknown and there is no evidence that it is associated with mutations in the GM-CSF receptor,[106] but it has been attributed to abnormalities in the GM-CSF signal transduction pathway. The proteins encoded by the *ras* family of protooncogenes play a central role in this pathway, and *ras* mutations have been demonstrated in 20–30% of patients with JMML. It is of great interest, in view of the clinical association with neurofibromatosis, that neurofibromin, the protein encoded by the NF type 1 gene (*NF1*), also plays a role in the *ras* signaling pathway, and *NF1* may function as a tumor suppressor gene in hematopoietic cells. Inactivation of neurofibromin may provide an alternative means of deregulation of the Ras signaling pathway. Investigations have shown that hematopoietic cells from knockout mice, which are homozygous for the *NF1* mutation, exhibit marked hypersensitivity to GM-CSF,[107] and that transplantation of such *NF1*-deficient hematopoietic liver cells induces a disease resembling JMML in irradiated mice.[108] The net result of this deregulated pathway is a hypersensitivity of cells to GM-CSF with proliferation of monocytes and myeloid cells, which infiltrate tissues causing bone marrow failure, and produce TNF-α and other cytokines, thus accounting for the fever, wasting and inanition characteristic of advanced JMML. Mutations in the *PTPN11* (Noonan syndrome) gene have been described in 34% of JMML patients without Noonan syndrome.[109] The gene encodes for the SHP-2 protein, involved in regulation of the mitogen-activated protein kinase (MAPK) cascade. Mutations in *ras*, *NF1*, and *PTPN11* are mutually exclusive.

Management

The essential investigations are shown in Table 18.2; particularly in the younger child with normal cytogenetics, appropriate investigations to exclude a viral infection are essential. If there is any doubt about the diagnosis of JMML, especially in young infants, a period of observation is recommended: there is no evidence that this will prejudice the efficacy of any subsequent treatment.

It is clear that older children with JMML and those with a high HbF and a low platelet count have a worse prognosis. In all reports involving significant numbers of patients, there is a small number of children who may survive for many years with minimal or no treatment; these tend to be under 2 years of age at diagnosis, with higher platelet counts and without gross elevation of HbF. Intensive chemotherapy has been notably unsuccessful in patients with aggressive JMML with high HbF and rapidly progressive disease. Despite some reports of response, true remission does not seem to be achievable and the survival in a group of 72 children with JMML who did not receive a BMT was 6%, with no difference between those patients who did and did not receive intensive treatment.[110,111]

BMT is the only curative treatment for JMML, and if the patient has no histocompatible sibling a search for an alternative donor is justified in all children, save the small minority of infants with indolent disease; the disease is difficult to eradicate by BMT,[112,113] and there is evidence that a graft-versus-leukemia effect plays an important role in cure.[114] The results of transplants from both siblings and alternative donors leave much room for improvement.[114–117] The first report of successful BMT in JMML from Seattle used a preparative regimen of TBI and cyclophosphamide. Survival in the largest case series to date of 43 children with JMML treated by BMT was 38% at 5 years for the 25 children with a sibling donor and 18% for those with an unrelated donor. The actuarial probability of relapse was 58%, and survival was superior for children whose preparative regimen did not include TBI. The combination of busulfan, cyclophosphamide and melphalan appears promising for both sibling and alternative transplants,[118,119] and is undergoing further assessment. The role of intensive chemotherapy and/or splenectomy to reduce the burden of disease before transplantation remains unclear but either form of treatment may be indicated in some patients.

The refractory nature and unique biologic features of JMML have prompted the investigation of various differentiating agents and cytokines. The most widely used has been 13-*cis*-retinoic acid, reported as producing complete or partial response in 5 of 10 children;[120] with other retinoids, it is undergoing further study. Alternative approaches being studied *in vitro* include the use of antagonists to the GM-CSF receptor[121] and the IL-1 receptor.[122]

Down syndrome and abnormal myelopoiesis

Clinical and laboratory features of transient abnormal myelopoiesis

TAM or transient myeloproliferative disease (TMD)[23,123,124] is usually discovered as an incidental finding on routine blood count in babies with Down syndrome, but has also rarely been described in normal nonmosaic infants. The precise incidence of TAM is unknown but preliminary reports from a screening program suggested that it might be found in up to 1 in 10 neonates with Down syndrome. TAM has also been diagnosed in hydropic fetuses *in utero*. Affected infants may have no associated clinical features but there is often enlargement of the liver and spleen with significant numbers of blasts in the blood, but a lesser degree of bone marrow infiltration. There is usually persistent evidence of hematopoietic maturation, with maintenance of hemoglobin, neutrophils and normal or raised platelet count in many patients. The maturing blood cells may show a degree of dysplasia. Morphologically, cytochemically and on immunophenotyping the blast cells resemble those of acute megakaryoblastic leukemia and may exhibit clonal cytogenetic abnormalities; there are no real distinctions between these blasts and those of patients with unequivocal leukemia.

Prognosis and management

The majority of patients with TAM show spontaneous improvement, which usually occurs over weeks to months but may take longer. This condition is benign in the majority of patients, but there have been a number of reports of death in the neonatal period associated with TAM; a characteristic finding at post-mortem is extensive visceral fibrosis. In general, however, supportive care is all that is needed in the majority of patients, and cytotoxic treatment should be avoided; if indicated it would be appropriate to use low-dose cytarabine in the first instance. The risk of subsequent development of myeloid leukemia after TAM has been estimated at 20–30% but these proportions need confirmation from larger prospective studies.

Postneonatal period

Virtually all cases of myeloid leukemia in Down syndrome are megakaryoblastic or erythroblastic leukemia, subtypes that are exceptionally rare in other children and usually occur in the first 4 years of life. Many cases have a long prodrome of MDS with low platelets, dysplastic cells in the blood and a low proportion of blast cells in the marrow; thus cases may be classified at various stages as having RAEB or RAEBt or AML.[125] The cytogenetic findings are also distinctive, with very few instances of the typical translocations t(8;21) or t(15;17); the commonest finding is trisomy 8.[126] The patients may remain well without treatment for weeks or months, but in contrast to TAM deterioration is inevitable and patients die if untreated.[22] There is good evidence that children with Down syndrome and AML respond very well to chemotherapy, although they exhibit more toxicity than others,[127,128] and this may be related to enhanced sensitivity to cytarabine.[129] The event-free survival for such patients is, in several series, superior to that for other children without recourse to high-dose therapy and BMT. It has been suggested that a regimen of low-dose cytarabine may afford adequate treatment,[130,131] but this approach has only been used in small numbers of patients, several of whom relapsed, and it cannot be recommended in view of the excellent results from conventional intensive therapy. There is no indication that early treatment during the prodrome of AML offers any advantage in these children, and it is usually appropriate to instigate treatment once symptoms develop.

Familial MDS and congenital bone marrow disorders

AML/MDS

There are a number of case reports from the older literature, usually reports of single families with a myeloproliferative or myelodysplastic disorder, which are imperfectly investigated compared with modern techniques, such as the large kindred described by Randall *et al.*[132] More recently a number of families have been described in which more than one member has developed AML or MDS; this may be associated with emergence of a cytogenetic abnormality in the marrow, usually involving chromosomes 7[133] or 5,[134] and in some cases with platelet storage pool deficiency.[135] From the practical point of view, it is important when examining families for suitable donors to exclude the presence of familial or genetically determined MDS.

Fanconi anemia

Patients with Fanconi anemia (see Chapter 3) have an estimated actuarial risk of developing a myeloid malignancy of 52% by the age of 40 years,[151] and may present with AML or MDS. The risk is higher in patients with clonal cytogenetic abnormalities, which most often involve chromosome 7;[136] however, clonal cytogenetic abnormalities are of little value for predicting leukemic change in the individual patient.[137,138] Treatment of Fanconi anemia by BMT[139] is likely to be more effective when undertaken early and should reduce the risk of leukemic transformation, although not of solid tumors.[141] Treatment after transformation is associated with a high risk of relapse. The results of unrelated donor transplants for patients without an HLA-compatible sibling are improving but all transplants will be more effective before development of MDS or leukemia.

Shwachman–Diamond syndrome

The Shwachman–Diamond syndrome of exocrine pancreatic insufficiency and neutropenia is a rare autosomal recessive disorder (see Chapter 3) characterized hematologically by variable neutropenia, thrombocytopenia and a raised HbF; it has been known for many years to predispose to the development of leukemia. In a review of 21 patients, MDS developed in seven and was associated in five with clonal cytogenetic abnormalities in the bone marrow; five patients progressed to AML.[34] While BMT could in theory correct the hematologic deficiency in Shwachman–Diamond syndrome, conventional BMT is too toxic and both patients in the series quoted died after transplantation, but there has been success with reduced intensity conditioning (mini BMT).

Congenital neutropenia (Kostmann syndrome)

In the last few years the use of cytokines, in particular G-CSF, has reduced the incidence of infections and improved quality of life for patients with a variety of neutropenias (see Chapter 34) and for those with severe congenital neutropenia (SCN). Treatment with G-CSF has been preferred to BMT, particularly in cases who lack a histocompatible sibling donor. Patients with SCN have previously been recognized as having a predisposition to the development of leukemia, but since the introduction of treatment with G-CSF the number of reports has increased. It is not known, however, whether this is a direct consequence of G-CSF treatment or a reflection of improved survival. Monosomy 7 and *ras* mutations have developed in the bone marrow of patients with severe congenital neutropenia undergoing malignant transformation during G-CSF therapy.[32] Mutations in the G-CSF receptor gene have been demonstrated in some patients with SCN during development of AML/MDS.[141,142] Patients treated with growth factors for SCN should be monitored with regular bone marrow examinations including cytogenetics.

MDS with eosinophilia

A raised eosinophil count is characteristic of chronic myeloproliferative disorders, JMML and the idiopathic hypereosinophilic syndrome,[144] and may, of course, be secondary to infections or infestation. There are a few reports of patients with marked eosinophilia and dysplastic blood and bone marrow whose hematologic features cannot readily be assigned to a FAB subtype; the author has arbitrarily classed such patients as having eosinophilic MDS.[4] Two such infants had hepatosplenomegaly and leukocytosis in association with t(1;5), one of whom rapidly deteriorated and the other was a long-term survivor.[145] Another 8-year-old girl described with t(5;12)(q31;p12–13) had stable eosinophilia for 7 years,[146] while the author has seen translocation t(5;12)(q31;q13) in association with marked skin infiltration in a 7-year-old boy whose clinical condition remained essentially unchanged for over 5 years.[147] Recently, successful therapy with the tyrosine kinase inhibitor imatinib has been described in a number of patients, including this child, and this approach deserves further study.[148]

Although both hydroxycarbamide and interferon therapy have been recommended in eosinophilic MDS, this has not been borne out in clinical studies, and BMT would appear to be the most appropriate form of treatment provided that there is strong evidence of a clonal disorder.

Therapy-related MDS

Clinical and laboratory features

Secondary MDS and AML were first reported in adults

treated for Hodgkin disease, but also after non-Hodgkin lymphoma, myeloma and a variety of nonhematologic solid tumors.[149] An associated genetic disease predisposing to malignancies, such as a Li–Fraumeni syndrome, cannot be confidently excluded in all cases, but preliminary investigation of the frequency of p53 mutations in 19 pediatric secondary malignancies showed a germline mutation in only 1 child, who had a family history of cancer.[150]

Two main types of secondary AML/MDS are associated with cancer treatment and each is associated with development of a characteristic pattern of cytogenetic change. Alkylating agent-induced MDS/AML tends to occur after 4–5 years, is associated with a preceding phase of MDS, and is characterized by deletions from chromosomes 5 and 7.[150] This disease is refractory to chemotherapy. The second, more recently described type of acute leukemia is related to treatment with topoisomerase II inhibitors and is associated with a shorter induction period and presentation as acute leukemia without a preceding MDS. Although secondary AML/MDS is rarer in children than adults, the correlation between type of previous therapy and clinical and chromosomal abnormalities is similar.[152]

Alkylating agent-induced AML/MDS is typified by patients treated for Hodgkin disease; the drugs implicated include cyclophosphamide, chlorambucil, procarbazine and nitrosoureas. The risk is highest with increasing numbers of treatment cycles containing alkylating agents, prolonged chemotherapy and splenectomy; it does not appear to be increased further by radiotherapy.[153] Alkylating agents are also the major risk factor in patients with other tumor types such as non-Hodgkin lymphoma: a high rate of secondary AML/MDS was observed in the first UK Children's Cancer Study Group protocol for non-Hodgkin lymphoma, in which the protocol contained nitrosoureas in addition to cyclophosphamide and epipodophyllotoxins.[154]

High-dose therapy with autologous BMT (ABMT), usually performed for patients with high-risk Hodgkin disease or non-Hodgkin lymphoma, has been recognized to be associated with an increased risk of subsequent development of MDS, but it is difficult to dissociate the risks of the ABMT from the preceding chemotherapy that such patients have almost inevitably received. Secondary MDS/AML has also recently been described in patients with aplastic anemia who have been treated with intensive immunosuppressive therapy.

Patients with secondary MDS may be asymptomatic initially when an abnormal film or blood count may prompt investigation; subsequently, as in primary MDS, symptoms of bone marrow failure develop with a mean duration of the preleukemic phase of about 11 months.

Alkylating agent-induced MDS does not always conform to the FAB subtypes. There is often a relatively low proportion of blasts at the time of diagnosis but this is accompanied by marked morphologic changes in all cell lines. There may be basophilia in both blood and bone marrow and cellularity is variable, with fibrosis in some cases producing a dilute aspirate. Clonal cytogenetic abnormalities are found in > 90% of cases and the majority involve chromosomes 5 and 7.[155,156]

Topoisomerase inhibitor-related leukemia, which may be lymphoblastic or myeloblastic, has been more systematically studied in children because of its increased incidence in children with ALL receiving intensive epipodophyllotoxin treatment.[156,157] Secondary AML was diagnosed in 21 of 734 patients treated for ALL; the overall cumulative risk was 3.8% at 6 years, but in a subgroup of children receiving drugs weekly or twice weekly the risk was > 12%. The scheduling of drug administration influenced the development of AML; the total dose, type of leukemia and radiotherapy had no influence on the risk of AML. More detailed study showed that the majority of patients had myeloid or myelomonocytic leukemia and that chromosomal translocations predominantly involved the 11q23 region, most commonly as t(9;11) or t(11;19).

Another group of therapy-related leukemias has been described in association with t(8;21), inv(16) and t(8;16) after topoisomerase inhibitor therapy, alkylating agent therapy or anthracycline therapy.[158] These do not usually have a dysplastic prodrome and the risk factors have not been so precisely defined, but there is a similar correlation between the cytogenetic findings, morphology and response to treatment, as in *de novo* AML, so that patients may respond to chemotherapy.

Management

The advent of a second cancer in a highly curable condition is, of course, a tragedy to be avoided if at all possible, and the identification of such cancers emphasizes the importance of morphology review and karyotyping in all cases of relapsed leukemia. Ideally, it is desirable to avoid this disastrous complication, and this is sometimes possible by alterations in choice of drug or scheduling, always bearing in mind that such changes must not prejudice the chance of cure.

There is relatively little reported pediatric experience in the management of secondary malignancies. It appears that the response to treatment can be predicted by the biology of the leukemia, but any remissions achieved tend to be short lived. Thus, secondary AML with chromosome 5 and 7 abnormalities is highly resistant to chemotherapy, and while remissions can be achieved with combination chemotherapy in children with 11q23 leukemia, long-term survival is extremely poor. The only exception to this poor prognosis is the small group of patients with more favorable translocations such as t(8;21), who tend to have a better response to treatment (as do those with AML).

A study of intensive chemotherapy for secondary AML showed a 2-year disease-free survival of only 8% for patients with abnormal cytogenetics, thus confirming the dismal prognosis.[66] It would appear that BMT affords the only chance of cure, and in such circumstances the use of unrelated donors is justifiable.

Conclusions

Pediatric myelodysplasias are a rare but challenging group of diseases that have only recently attracted systematic study. They frequently occur in association with other genetically determined disorders. A methodical approach to investigation and differential diagnosis is essential. The FAB classification can be applied to most cases but JMML in children is a heterogeneous disorder with unique clinical and biologic features, is resistant to chemotherapy and has a high relapse risk after BMT. A "wait and see" approach to treatment may be appropriate for children with refractory anemia or younger children with JMML, particularly in the absence of cytogenetic abnormalities. Children with MDS with an excess of blasts are eligible in many countries for inclusion in AML trials, and the role of intensive chemotherapy should thus become apparent within the next few years. BMT, the most effective treatment for MDS, should be considered in most children with a histocompatible sibling donor. The results from unrelated donor transplants still leave much room for improvement but these and other types of transplant should be considered in high-risk patients, particularly those with aggressive JMML and secondary leukemias. National and international collaboration is essential to afford a better understanding of these rare diseases.

References

1. Nix WL, Fernbach DJ. Myeloproliferative diseases in childhood. *Am J Pediatr Hematol Oncol* 1981; **3**: 397–407.
2. Smith KL, Johnson W. Classification of chronic myelocytic leukemia in children. *Cancer* 1974; **34**: 670–9.
3. Brandwein JM, Horsman DE, Eaves AC *et al*. Childhood myelodysplasia: suggested classification as myelodysplastic syndromes based on laboratory and clinical Findings. *Am J Pediatr Hematol Oncol* 1990; **12**: 63–70.
4. Chessells JM. Myelodysplasia. *Baillière's Clin Haematol* 1991; **4**: 459–82.
5. Gadner H, Haas OA. Experience in pediatric myelodysplastic syndromes. *Hematol Oncol Clin North Am* 1992; **6**: 655–72.
6. Tuncer MA, Pagliuca A, Hicsonmez G, Yetgin S, Ozsoylu S, Mufti GJ. Primary myelodysplastic syndrome in children: the clinical experience in 33 cases. *Br J Haematol* 1992; **82**: 347–53.
7. Hasle H. Myelodysplastic syndromes in childhood: classification, epidemiology and treatment. *Leukemia Lymphoma* 1994; **13**: 11–26.
8. Passmore SJ, Hann IM, Stiller CA *et al*. Pediatric myelodysplasia: a study of 68 children and a new prognostic scoring system. *Blood* 1995; **85**: 1742–50.
9. Bader-Meunier B, Mielot F, Tchernia G *et al*. Myelodysplastic syndromes in childhood: report of 49 patients from a French multicentre study. *Br J Haematol* 1996; **92**: 344–50.
10. Haas OA, Gadner H. Pathogenesis, biology, and management of myelodysplastic syndromes in children. *Semin Hematol* 1996; **33**: 225–35.
11. Hardisty RM, Speed DE, Till M. Granulocytic leukaemia in childhood. *Br J Haematol* 1964; **10**: 551–66.
12. Castro-Malaspina H, Schaison G, Passe S *et al*. Subacute and chronic myelomonocytic leukemia in children (juvenile CML). *Cancer* 1984; **54**: 675–86.
13. Weatherall DJ, Edwards JA, Donohoe WTA. Haemoglobin and red cell enzyme changes in juvenile chronic myeloid leukaemia. *Br Med J* 1968; **i**: 679–81.
14. Teasdale JM, Worth AJ, Corey MJ. A missing group C chromosome in the bone marrow cells of three children with myeloproliferative disease. *Cancer* 1970; **25**: 1468–77.
15. Sieff CA, Chessells JM, Harvey BAM, Pickthall VJ, Lawler SD. Monosomy 7 in childhood: a myeloproliferative disorder. *Br J Haematol* 1981; **49**: 235–49.
16. Bennett JM, Catovsky D, Daniel MT *et al*. Proposals for the classification of the myelodysplastic syndromes. *Br J Haematol* 1982; **51**: 189–99.
17. Blank J, Lange B. Preleukemia in children. *J Pediatr* 1981; **98**: 565–8.
18. Hasle H, Niemeyer CM, Chessells JM *et al*. A pediatric approach to the WHO classification of myelodysplasia and myeloproliferative diseases. *Leukemia* 2003; **17**: 277–82.
19. Williamson PJ, Kruger AR, Reynolds PJ, Hamblin TJ, Oscier DG. Establishing the incidence of myelodysplastic syndrome. *Br J Haematol* 1994; **87**: 743–5.
20. Aul C, Gattermann N, Schneider W. Age-related incidence and other epidemiological aspects of myelodysplastic syndromes. *Br J Haematol* 1992; **82**: 358–67.
21. Hasle H, Kerndrup G, Jacobsen BB. Childhood myelodysplastic syndrome in Denmark: incidence and predisposing conditions. *Leukemia* 1995; **9**: 1569–72.
22. Jackson GH, Carey PJ, Cant AJ, Bown NP, Reid MM. Myelodysplastic syndromes in children. *Br J Haematol* 1993; **84**: 185–6.
23. Passmore SJ, Chessells JM, Kempski H, Hann IM, Brownbill PA, Stiller CA. Pediatric MDS and JMML in the UK: a population based study of incidence and survival. *Br J Haematol* 2003; **121**: 758–67.
24. Levitt GA, Stiller CA, Chessells JM. Prognosis of Down's syndrome with acute leukaemia. *Arch Dis Child* 1990; **65**: 212–16.
25. Bain B. Down's syndrome: transient abnormal myelopoiesis and acute leukaemia. *Leukemia Lymphoma* 1991; **3**: 309–17.
26. Secker-Walker LM, Fitchett M. Constitutional and acquired trisomy. *Leukemia Res* 1995; **19**: 737–40.
27. Seghezzi L, Maserati E, Minelli A *et al*. Constitutional trisomy 8 as first mutation in multistep carcinogenesis: clinical, cytogenetic, and molecular data on three cases. *Genes Chromosomes Cancer* 1996; **17**: 94–101.
28. Hasle H, Clausen N, Pedersen B, Bendix-Hansen K. Myelodysplastic syndrome in a child with constitutional trisomy 8 mosaicism and normal phenotype. *Cancer Genet Cytogenet* 1995; **79**: 79–81.

29. Bader JL, Miller RW. Neurofibromatosis and childhood leukemia. *J Pediatr* 1978; **92**: 925–9.

30. Stiller CA, Chessells JM, Fitchett M. Neurofibromatosis and childhood leukaemia/lymphoma: a population-based UKCCSG study. *Br J Cancer* 1994; **70**: 969–72.

31. Shannon KM, Watterson J, Johnson P et al. Monosomy 7 myeloproliferative disease in children with neurofibromatosis, type 1: epidemiology and molecular analysis. *Blood* 1992; **79**: 1311–18.

32. Kalra R, Dale D, Freedman M et al. Monosomy 7 and activating *RAS* mutations accompany malignant transformation in patients with congenital neutropenia. *Blood* 1995; **86**: 4579–86.

33. Woods WG, Roloff JS, Lukens JN, Krivit W. The occurrence of leukemia in patients with the Shwachman syndrome. *J Pediatr* 1981; **99**: 425–8.

34. Smith OP, Hann IM, Chessells JM, Reeves BR, Milla P. Haematologic abnormalities in Shwachman–Diamond Syndrome. *Br J Haematol* 1996; **94**: 279–84.

35. Auerbach AD, Weiner MA, Warburton D. Acute myeloid leukemia as the first hematologic manifestation of Fanconi anemia. *Am J Hematol* 1982; **12**: 289.

36. Carroll WL, Morgan R, Glader BE. Childhood bone marrow monosomy 7 syndrome: A familial disorder? *J Pediatr* 1985; **107**: 578–80.

37. Gerrard JM, McNicol A. Platelet storage pool deficiency, leukemia, and myelodysplastic syndromes. *Leukemia Lymphoma* 1992; **8**: 277–81.

38. Socie G, Henry-Amar M, Bacigalupo A et al. Malignant tumors occurring after treatment of aplastic anemia. *N Engl J Med* 1993; **329**: 1152–7.

39. Stone RM, Neuberg D, Soiffer R et al. Myelodysplastic syndrome as a late complication following autologous bone marrow transplantation for non-Hodgkin's lymphoma. *J Clin Oncol* 1994; **12**: 2535–42.

40. Darrington DL, Vose JM, Anderson JR et al. Incidence and characterization of secondary myelodysplastic syndrome and acute myelogenous leukemia following high-dose chemoradiotherapy and autologous stem-cell transplantation for lymphoid malignancies. *J Clin Oncol* 1994; **12**: 2527–34.

41. Niemeyer CM, Fenu S, Hasle H, Mann G, Stary J, van Wering ER. Differentiating juvenile myelomonocytic leukaemia from infectious disease. *Blood* 1998; **91**: 365–7.

42. Smith OP, Hann IM, Woodward CE, Brockington M. Pearson's marrow/pancreas syndrome: haematological features associated with deletion and duplication of mitochondrial DNA. *Br J Haematol* 1995; **90**: 469–72.

43. Bader-Meunier B, Rotig A, Mielot F et al. Refractory anaemia and mitochondrial cytopathy in childhood. *Br J Haematol* 1994; **87**: 381–5.

44. Chan GC, Wang WC, Raimondi SC et al. Myelodysplastic syndrome in children: differentiation from acute myeloid leukemia with a low blast count. *Leukemia* 1997; **11**: 206–11.

45. Kirby MA, Weitzman S, Freedman M. Juvenile chronic myelogenous leukaemia; differentiation from cytomegalovirus infection. *Am J Pediatr Hematol Oncol* 1990; **12**: 292–6.

46. Hasle H, Kerndrup G, Jacobsen BB, Heergaard ED, Hornsleth A, Lillevang ST. Chronic parvovirus infection mimicking myelodysplasia syndrome in a child with subclinical immunodeficiency. *Am J Pediatr Hematol Oncol* 1994; **16**: 329–33.

47. Herrod HG, Dow LW, Sullivan JL. Persistent Epstein-Barr virus infection mimicking juvenile chronic myelogenous leukemia: Immunologic and hematologic studies. *Blood* 1983; **61**: 1098–104.

48. Third MIC Cooperative Study Group. Recommendations for a morphologic, immunologic, and cytogenetic (MIC) working classification of the primary and therapy-related myelodysplastic disorders. A report of the workshop held in Scottsdale, Arizona, USA, on February 23–25. *Cancer Genet Cytogenet* 1988; **32**: 1–10.

49. Fenaux P, Morel P, Lai JL. Cytogenetics of myelodysplastic syndromes. *Semin Hematol* 1996; **33**: 127–38.

50. Luna-Fineman S, Shannon KM, Lange BJ. Childhood monosomy 7: epidemiology, biology and mechanistic implications. *Blood* 1995; **85**: 1985–99.

51. Boultwood J, Lewis S, Wainscoat JS. The 5q– syndrome. *Blood* 1994; **84**: 3253–60.

52. Tefferi A, Thibodeau SN, Solberg LAJ. Clonal studies in the myelodysplastic syndrome using X-linked restriction fragment length polymorphisms. *Blood* 1990; **75**: 1770–3.

53. van Lom K, Hagemeijer A, Smit EME, Hahlen K, Groeneveld K, Lowenberg B. Cytogenetic clonal analysis in myelodysplastic syndrome: monosomy 7 can be demonstrated in the myeloid and in the lymphoid lineage. *Leukemia* 1995; **9**: 1818–21.

54. Johnson EJ, Scherer SW, Osborne L et al. Molecular definition of a narrow interval at 7822.1 associated with myelodysplasia. *Blood* 1996; **87**: 3579–86.

55. Pedersen-Bjergaard J, Pedersen M, Roulston D, Philip P. Different genetic pathways in leukemogenesis for patients presenting with therapy-related myelodysplasia and therapy-related acute myeloid leukemia. *Blood* 1995; **9**: 3542–52.

56. Bartram CR. Molecular genetic aspects of myelodysplastic syndromes. *Semin Hematol* 1996; **33**: 139–49.

57. Paquette RL, Landaw EM, Pierre RV et al. N-*ras* mutations are associated with poor prognosis and increased risk of leukemia in myelodysplastic syndrome. *Blood* 1993; **82**: 590–9.

58. Raza A, Gregory SA, Preisler HD. The myelodysplastic syndromes in 1996: complex stem cell disorders confounded by dual actions of cytokines. *Leukemia Res* 1996; **20**: 881–90.

59. Mufti GJ, Stevens JR, Oscier DG, Hamblin TJ, Machin D. Myelodysplastic syndromes: A scoring system with prognostic significance. *Br J Haematol* 1985; **59**: 425–33.

60. Goasguen JE, Garand R, Bizet M et al. Prognostic factors of myelodysplastic syndromes: a simplified 3-D scoring system. *Leukemia Res* 1990; **14**: 255–62.

61. Mufti GJ, Galton DAG. Myelodysplastic syndromes: natural history and features of prognostic importance. *Clinic Haematol* 1986; **15**: 953–71.

62. Morel P, Hebbar M, Lai J et al. Cytogenetic analysis has strong independent prognostic value in *de novo* myelodysplastic syndromes and can be incorporated in a new scoring system: a report on 408 cases. *Leukemia* 1993; **7**: 1315–23.

63. Greenberg P, Cox C, LeBeau MM et al. International scoring system for evaluating prognosis in myelodysplastic syndromes. *Blood* 1997; **89**: 2079–88.

64. Kardos G, Baumann I, Passmore SJ et al. Refractory anemia in childhood: a retrospective analysis of 67 patients with particular reference to monosomy. *Blood* 2003; **102**: 1997–2003.

65. Webb DK, Passmore SJ, Hann IM, Harrison G, Wheatley K,

Chessells JM. Results of treatment of children with refractory anaemia with excess blasts (RAEB) and RAEB in transformation (RAEBt) in Great Britain 1990–1999. *Br J Haematol* 2002; **117**: 33–9.

66. De Witte T, Suciu S, Peetermans M *et al*. Intensive chemotherapy for poor prognosis myelodysplasia (MDS) and secondary acute myeloid leukemia (sAML) following MDS of more than 6 months duration. A pilot study by the Leukemia Cooperative Group of the European Organisation for Research and Treatment in Cancer (EORTC-LCG). *Leukemia* 1995; **9**: 1805–11.

67. Creutzig U, Cantu-Rajnoldi A, Ritter J *et al*. Myelodysplastic syndromes in childhood. Report of 21 patients from Italy and West Germany. *Am J Pediatr Hematol Oncol* 1987; **9**: 324–30.

68. Hasle H, Kerndrup G, Yssing M *et al*. Intensive chemotherapy in childhood myelodysplastic syndrome. A comparison with results in acute myeloid leukemia. *Leukemia* 1996; **10**: 1269–73.

69. Nand S, Sosman J, Godwin JE, Fisher RI. A Phase I/II study of sequential interleukin-3 and granulocyte-macrophage colony-stimulating factor in myelodysplastic syndromes. *Blood* 1994; **83**: 357–60.

70. Negrin RS, Stein R, Doherty K *et al*. Maintenance treatment of the anemia of myelodysplastic syndromes with recombinant human granulocyte colony-stimulating factor and erythropoietin: evidence for *in vivo* synergy. *Blood* 1996; **87**: 4076–81.

71. Fanucchi M, Glaspy J, Crawford J *et al*. Effects of polyethylene glycol-conjugated recombinant human megakaryocyte growth and development factor on platelet counts after chemotherapy for lung cancer. *N Engl J Med* 1997, **336**: 404–9.

72. Molineux G, Hartley C, McElroy P, McCrea C, McNiece IK. Megakaryocyte growth and development factor accelerates platelet recovery in peripheral blood progenitor cell transplant recipients. *Blood* 1996; **88**: 366–76.

73. Basser RL, Rasko JEJ, Clarke K *et al*. Thrombopoietic effects of pegylated recombinant human megakaryocyte growth and development factor (PEG-rHuMGDF) in patients with advanced cancer. *Lancet* 1996; **348**: 1279–81.

74. Ohno R, Naoe T, Hirano M *et al*. Treatment of myelodysplastic syndromes with all-*trans* retinoic acid. Leukemia Study Group of the Ministry of Health and Welfare. *Blood* 1993; **81**: 1152–4.

75. Appelbaum FR, Barrall J, Storb R *et al*. Bone marrow transplantation for patients with myelodysplasia. Pretreatment variables and outcome. *Ann Intern Med* 1990; **112**: 590–7.

76. De Witte T, Zwaan F, Hermans J *et al*. Allogeneic bone marrow transplantation for secondary leukaemia and myelodysplastic syndrome: a survey by the Leukaemia Working Party of the European Bone Marrow Transplantation Group (EBMTG). *Br J Haematol* 1990; **74**: 151–7.

77. Bensinger WI, Clift R, Martin P *et al*. Allogeneic peripheral blood stem cell transplantation in patients with advanced hematologic malignancies: a retrospective comparison with marrow transplantation. *Blood* 1996; **88**: 2794–800.

78. Ottinger HD, Beelan DW, Scheulen B, Schaefer UW, Grosse-Wilde H. Improved immune reconstitution after allotransplantation of peripheral blood stem cells instead of bone marrow. *Blood* 1996; **88**: 2775–9.

79. Goldman JM, Glae RP, Horowitz MM *et al*. Bone marrow transplantation for chronic myelogenous leukemia in chronic phase. *Ann Intern Med* 1988; **108**: 806–14.

80. Copelan EA, Grever MR, Kapoor N, Tutschka PJ. Marrow transplantation following busulphan and cyclophosphamide for CML. *Br J Haematol* 1989; **71**: 487–91.

81. Santos GW, Tutschka PJ, Brookmeyer R *et al*. Marrow transplantation for acute nonlymphocytic leukemia after treatment with busulfan and cyclophosphamide. *N Engl J Med* 1983; **309**: 1347–53.

82. Leisner RJ, Leiper AD, Hann IM, Chessells JM. Late effects of intensive treatment for acute myeloid leukemia and myelodysplasia in childhood. *J Clin Oncol* 1994; **12**: 916–24.

83. Clift RA, Buckner CD, Thomas ED *et al*. Marrow transplantation for chronic myeloid leukemia: a randomized study comparing cyclophosphamide and total body irradiation with busulfan and cyclophosphamide. *Blood* 1994; **84**: 2036–43.

84. Blaise D, Maraninchi D, Archimbaud E *et al*. Allogeneic bone marrow transplantation for acute myeloid leukemia in first remission: A randomized trial of a busulfan-cytozan versus cytoxan-total body irradiation as preparative regimen: A report from the Groupe d'Études de la Greffe de Moëlle Osseuse. *Blood* 1992; **79**: 2578–82.

85. Anderson JE, Appelbaum FR, Schoch G *et al*. Allogeneic marrow transplantation for refractory anemia: A comparison of two preparative regimens and analysis of prognostic factors. *Blood* 1996; **87**: 51–8.

86. Michel G, Gluckman GME, Esperou-Bourdeau H *et al*. Allogeneic bone marrow transplantation for children with acute myeloblastic leukemia in first complete remission: impact of conditioning regimen without total-body irradiation: a report from the Société Française de Greffe de Moëlle. *J Clin Oncol* 1994; **12**: 1217–22.

87. Locatelli F, Pession A, Bonetti F *et al*. Busulfan, cyclophosphamide and melphalan as conditioning regimen for bone marrow transplantation in children with myelodysplastic syndromes. *Leukemia* 1994; **8**: 844–9.

88. Anderson JE, Appelbaum FR, Fisher LD *et al*. Allogeneic bone marrow transplantation for 93 patients with myelodysplastic syndrome. *Blood* 1993; **82**: 677–81.

89. Sutton L, Chastang C, Ribaud P *et al*. Factors influencing outcome in *de novo* myelodysplastic syndromes treated by allogeneic bone marrow tranplantation: A long-term study of 71 patients. *Blood* 1996; **88**: 358–65.

90. Anderson JE, Anasetti C, Appelbaum FR *et al*. Unrelated donor marrow transplantation for myelodysplasia (MDS) and MDS-related acute myeloid leukaemia. *Br J Haematol* 1996; **93**: 59–67.

91. Kernan NA, Bartsch G, Ash RC *et al*. Analysis of 462 transplantations from unrelated donors facilitated by the national marrow donor program. *N Engl J Med* 1993; **328**: 593–602.

92. Kurtzberg J, Laughlin M, Graham ML *et al*. Placental blood as a source of hematopoietic stem cells for transplantation into unrelated recipients. *N Engl J Med* 1996; **335**: 157–66.

93. Kolb H-J, Schattenberg A, Goldman JM *et al*. Graft-versus-leukemia effect of donor lymphocyte transfusions in marrow grafted patients. *Blood* 1995; **86**: 2041–50.

94. Collins RH, Shpilberg O, Droyski WR *et al*. Donor leukocyte infusions in 140 patients with relapsed malignancy after

allogeneic bone marrow transplantation. *J Clin Oncol* 1997; **15**: 433–44.

95. Worth A, Rao K, Webb DK, Chessells J, Passmore J, Veys P. Successful treatment of juvenile myelomonocytic leukaemia relapsing after stem cell transplant using donor lymphocyte infusion *Blood* 2003; **101**: 1713–14.

96. Mays JA, Neerhout RC, Bagby GC, Koler RD. Juvenile chronic granulocytic leukaemia. *Am J Dis Child* 1980; **134**: 654–8.

97. Niemeyer CM, Arico M, Basso A *et al*. Chronic myelomonocytic leukemia in childhood: a retrospective analysis of 110 cases. *Blood* 1997; **89**: 3534–43.

98. Sheridan BL, Weatherall DJ, Clegg JB *et al*. The patterns of fetal haemoglobin production in leukaemia. *Br J Haematol* 1976; **32**: 487–506.

99. Weinberg RS, Lcibowitz D, Wcinblatt ME, Kochen J, Alter BP. Juvenile chronic myelogenous leukaemia: The only example of truly fetal (not fetal-like) erythropoiesis. *Br J Haematol* 1990; **76**: 307–10.

100. Cannat A, Seligmann M. Immunological abnormalities in juvenile myelomonocytic leukaemia. *Br Med J* 1973; **i**: 71–4.

101. Busque L, Gilliland DG, Prchal JT *et al*. Clonality in juvenile chronic myelogenous leukemia. *Blood* 1995; **1**: 21–30.

102. Lapidot T, Grunberger T, Vormoor J *et al*. Identification of human juvenile chronic myelogenous leukemia stem cells capable of initiating the disease in primary and secondary SCID mice. *Blood* 1996; **88**: 2655–64.

103. Gualtieri RJ, Emanuel PD, Zuckerman KS *et al*. Granulocyte-macrophage colony-stimulating factor is an endogenous regulator of cell proliferation in juvenile chronic myelogenous leukemia. *Blood* 1989; **74**: 2360–7.

104. Freedman MH, Cohen A, Grunberger T *et al*. Central role of tumour necrosis factor, GM-CSF, and interleukin 1 in the pathogenesis of juvenile chronic myelogenous leukaemia. *Br J Haematol* 1992; **80**: 4048.

105. Emanuel PD, Shannon KM, Castleberry RP. Juvenile myelomonocytic leukemia: molecular understanding and prospects for therapy. *Mol Med Today* 1996; November: 468–75.

106. Freeburn RW, Gale RE, Wagner HM, Linch DC. Analysis of the coding sequence for the GM-CSF receptor a and b chains in patients with juvenile chronic myeloid leukemia (JCML). *Exp Hematol* 1997; **25**: 306–11.

107. Bollag G, Clapp D, Shih S *et al*. Loss of NF1 results in activation of the *Ras* signaling pathway and leads to aberrant growth in haematopoietic cells. *Nat Genet* 1996; **12**: 144–8.

108. Largaespada DA, Brannan CI, Jenkins NA, Copeland NG. Nfl deficiency causes *Ras*-mediated granulocyte/macrophage colony stimulating factor hypersensitivity and chronic myeloid leukaemia. *Nat Genet* 1996; **12**: 137–43.

109. Tartaglia M, Niemeyer CM, Fragale A *et al*. Somatic mutations in PTPN11 in juvenile myelomonocytic leukaemia, myelodysplastic syndrome and acute myeloid leukaemia. *Nat Genet* 2003; **34**: 148–50.

110. Chan HSL, Estrov Z, Weitzman SS, Freedman MH. The value of intensive combination chemotherapy for juvenile chronic myelogenous leukaemia. *J Clin Oncol* 1987; **5**: 1960–7.

111. Festa RS, Shende A, Lanzkowsky P. Juvenile chronic myelocytic leukemia: experience with intensive combination chemotherapy. *Med Pediatr Oncol* 1990; **18**: 311–16.

112. Chown SR, Potter MN, Cornish J *et al*. Matched and

113. Donadieu J, Stephan JL, Blanche S *et al*. Treatment of juvenile chronic myelomonocytic leukemia by allogeneic bone marrow transplantation. *Bone Marrow Transplant* 1994; **13**: 777–82.

114. Rassam SMB, Katz F, Chessells JM, Morgan G. Successful allogeneic bone marrow transplantation in juvenile CML: conditioning or graft-versus-leukaemia effect? *Bone Marrow Transplant* 1993; **11**: 247–50.

115. Bunin NJ, Casper JT, Lawton C *et al*. Allogeneic marrow transplantation using T cell depletion for patients with juvenile chronic myelogenous leukemia without HLA-identical siblings. *Bone Marrow Transplant* 1992; **9**: 119–22.

116. Sanders JE, Buckner CD, Thomas ED *et al*. Allogeneic marrow transplantation for children with juvenile chronic myelogenous leukemia. *Blood* 1988; **71**: 1144–6.

117. Urban C, Schwinger W, Slavc I *et al*. Busulfan/cyclophosphamide plus bone marrow transplantation is not sufficient to eradicate the malignant clone in juvenile chronic myelogenous leukemia. *Bone Marrow Transplant* 1990; **5**: 353–6.

118. Locatelli F, Niemeyer C, Angelucci E *et al*. Allogenic bone marrow transplantation for chronic myelomonocytic leukemia in childhood: a report from the European Working Group on Myelodysplastic Syndrome in childhood. *J Clin Oncol* 1997; **15**: 566–73.

119. Locatelli F, Pession A, Comoli P *et al*. Role of allogeneic bone marrow transplantation from an HLA-identical sibling or a matched unrelated donor in the treatment of children with juvenile chronic myeloid leukaemia. *Br J Haematol* 1996; **92**: 49–54.

120. Castleberry RP, Emanuel PD, Zuckerman KS *et al*. A pilot study of isotretinoin in the treatment of juvenile chronic myelogenous leukaemia. *N Engl J Med* 1994; **331**: 1680–4.

121. Iverson PO, Rodwell RL, Pitcher L, Taylor KM, Lopez AF. Inhibition of proliferation and induction of apoptosis in juvenile myelomonocytic leukemic cells by the granulocyte-macrophage colony-stimulating factor analogue E21R. *Blood* 1996; **88**: 2634–9.

122. Schiro R, Longoni D, Rossi V *et al*. Suppression of juvenile chronic myelogenous leukemia colony growth by interleukin-1 receptor antagonist. *Blood* 1994; **83**: 460–5.

123. Avet-Loiseau H, Mechinaud F, Harousseau J. Clonal hematologic disorders in Down syndrome. *J Pediatr Hematol Oncol* 1995; **17**: 19–24.

124. Zipursky A, Poon A, Doyle J. Leukemia in Down syndrome: a review. *J Pediatr Hematol Oncol* 1992; **9**: 139–49.

125. Zipursky A, Thorner P, De Harven E, Christensen H, Doyle J. Myelodysplasia and acute megakaryoblastic leukemia in Down's syndrome. *Leukemia Res* 1994; **18**: 163–71.

126. Creutzig U, Ritter J, Vormoor J *et al*. Myelodysplasia and acute myelogenous leukemia in Down's syndrome. A report of 40 children of the AML-BFM study Group. *Leukemia* 1996; **10**: 1677–86.

127. Ravindranath Y, Abella E, Krischer JP *et al*. Acute myeloid leukemia (AML) in Down's syndrome is highly responsive to chemotherapy: experience of Pediatric Oncology Group AML study *Blood* 1992; **80**: 2210–14.

128. Lie SO, Jonmundsson G, Mellander L, Siimes MA, Yssing M,

Gustafsson G. A population-based study of 272 children with acute myeloid leukaemia treated on two consecutive protocols with different intensity: best outcome in girls, infants, and children with Down's syndrome. *Br J Haematol* 1996; **94**: 82–8.

129. Taub JW, Matherty LH, Stout ML, Buck SA, Gurney JG, Ravindranath Y. Enhanced metabolism of 1-β-D-arabinofuranosylcytosine in Down syndrome cells: a contributing factor to the superior event free survival of Down syndrome children with acute myeloid leukemia. *Blood* 1996; **87**: 3395–403.

130. Zipursky A. The treatment of children with acute megakaryoblastic leukemia who have Down syndrome. *J Pediatr Hematol Oncol* 1996; **18**: 10–12.

131. Tchernia G, Lejeune F, Boccara J, Denavit M, Dommergues J, Bernaudin F. Erythroblastic and/or megakaryoblastic leukemia in Down syndrome: treatment with low-dose arabinosyl cytosine. *Pediatr Hematol Oncol* 1996; **18**: 59–62.

132. Randall DL, Reiquam CW, Githens JH, Robinson A. Familial myeloproliferative disease. *Am J Dis Child* 1965; **110**: 479–90.

133. Paul B, Reid MM, Davison EV, Abela M, Hamilton PJ. Familial myelodysplasia: progressive disease associated with emergence of monosomy. *Br J Haematol* 1987; **65**: 321–3.

134. Olopade O, Roulston D, Baker T *et al.* Familial myeloid leukemia associated with loss of the long arm of chromosome *Leukemia* 1996; **10**: 669–74.

135. Gerrard JM, Israels ED, Bishop AJ *et al.* Inherited platelet-storage pool deficiency associated with a high incidence of acute myeloid leukaemia. *Br J Haematol* 1991; **79**: 246–55.

136. Butturim A, Gale RP, Verlander PC, Adler-Brecher B, Gillio AP, Auerbach AD. Hematologic abnormalities in Fanconi anemia: an International Fanconi Anemia Registry study. *Blood* 1994; **84**: 1650–5.

137. Maaarek O, Jonveaux P, Le Coniat M, Derre J, Berger R. Fanconi anemia and bone marrow clonal chromosome abnormalities. *Leukemia* 1996; **10**: 1700–4.

138. Alter BP, Scalise A, MCombs J, Najfeld V. Clonal chromosomal abnormalities in Fanconi's anaemia: what do they really mean? *Br J Haematol* 1993; **85**: 627–30.

139. Gluckman E, Auerbach AD, Horowitz MM *et al.* Bone marrow transplantation for Fanconi anemia. *Blood* 1995; **86**: 2856–62.

140. Alter BP. Fanconi's anemia and malignancies. *Am J Hematol* 1996; **53**: 99–110.

141. Dong F, Brynes RK, Tidow N, Welte K, Lowenberg B, Touw IP. Mutations in the gene for the granulocyte colony-stimulating-factor receptor in patients with acute myeloid leukemia preceded by severe congenital neutropenia. *N Engl J Med* 1995; **333**: 487–93.

142. Dong F, Dale DC, Bonilla MA *et al.* Mutations in the granulocyte colony-stimulating factor receptor gene in patients with severe congenital neutropenia. *Leukemia* 1997; **11**: 120–5.

143. Bain BJ. Eosinophilic leukaemias and the idiopathic hypereosinophilic syndrome. *Br J Haematol* 1996; **95**: 2–9.

144. Darbyshire PJ, Shortland D, Swansbury GJ, Sadler J, Lawler SD, Chessells JM. A myeloproliferative disease in two infants associated with eosinophilia and chromosome t(1;5) translocation. *Br J Haematol* 1987; **66**: 483–6.

145. Peltier I, Le Mome PJ, Rialland X *et al.* Myelodysplastic syndrome with t(5;12)(q31;p12-p13) and eosinophilia: a pediatric case with review of literature. *J Pediatr Hematol Oncol* 1996; **18**: 285–8.

146. Jam K, Kempski HM, Reeves BR. A case of myelodysplasia with eosinophilia having a translocation t(5;12)(q31;q13) restricted to myeloid cells but not involving eosinophils. *Br J Haematol* 1994; **87**: 57–60.

147. Gotlib J, Cools J, Malone JM, Scgrier SL, Gilliland G, Coutre SE. The FIP1L1-PDGFRα fusion tyrosine kinase in hypereosinophilic syndrome and chronic eosinophilic leukaemia: implications for diagnosis, classification and management. *Blood* 2004; **103**: 2879–91.

148. Park DJ, Koeffler HP. Therapy-related myelodysplastic syndromes. *Semin Hematol* 1996; **33**: 256–73.

149. Felix CA, Hosler MR, Provisor D *et al.* The p53 gene in pediatric therapy-related leukemia and myelodysplasia. *Blood* 1996; **87**: 4376–81.

150. Le Beau MM, Àlbain KS, Larson RA *et al.* Clinical and cytogenetic correlations in 63 patients with therapy related myelodysplastic syndromes and acute non lymphocytic leukemias: further evidence for characteristic abnormalities of chromosome nos. 5 and 7. *J Clin Oncol* 1986; **4**: 325–45.

151. Rubin CM, Arthur DC, Woods WG *et al.* Therapy-related myelodysplastic syndrome and acute myeloid leukemia in children: Correlation between chromosomal abnormalities and prior therapy. *Blood* 1991; **78**: 2982–8.

152. Kaldor JM, Day NE, Clarke A *et al.* Leukemia following Hodgkin's disease. *N Engl J Med* 1990; **322**: 7–13.

153. Ingram L, Mott MG, Mann JR, Raafat F, Darbyshire PJ, Morris Jones PH. Second malignancies in children treated for non-Hodgkin's lymphoma and T-cell leukaemia with the UKCCSG regimens. *Br J Cancer* 1987; **55**: 463–6.

154. Michels SD, McKenna RW, Arthur DC, Brunning RD. Therapy-related acute myeloid leukemia and myelodysplastic syndrome: A clinical and morphologic study of 65 cases. *Blood* 1985; **65**: 1364–72.

155. Pui C, Ribeiro RC, Hancock MI *et al.* Acute myeloid leukemia in children treated with epipodophyllotoxins for acute lymphoblastic leukemia. *N Engl J Med* 1991; **325**: 1682–7.

156. Pui C, Relling MV, Rivera GK *et al.* Epipodophyllotoxin-related acute myeloid leukemia: a study of 35 cases. *Leukemia* 1995; **9**: 1990–6.

157. Quesnel B, Kantarjian H, Bjergaard JP *et al.* Therapy-related acute myeloid leukemia with t(8;21), inv(16), and t(8;16): a report on 25 cases and review of the literature. *J Clin Oncol* 1993; **11**: 2370–9.

Lymphocyte Disorders

19 Primary and acquired immunodeficiency

Andrew R. Gennery, Adam H.R. Finn and Andrew J. Cant

Overview of specific immunity

The immune system evolved to distinguish "self" from "non-self," destroying microorganisms but leaving the organism's proteins unmolested. Malfunction leads to infection and/or allergy and autoimmunity. The immune response begins when secreted protein and phagocyte defenses eliminate microorganisms. Acquired immunity acts as a slower but highly specific mechanism that retains "memory" and mounts a response of increasing magnitude and specificity at each encounter. Individuals with inherited or acquired deficiencies in their specific immunity are susceptible to unusual, abnormally frequent or severe infectious diseases. Our increased understanding of the immune responses to microbes has led to a better understanding of both primary and secondary immunodeficiency; patients with immunodeficiency have taught us much about the intricacies of immune function.

The innate immune system

Physical and chemical barriers are highly effective at excluding pathogens by antimicrobial effects or prevention of microbial attachment. On breaching these barriers, and invading tissues, pathogens are confronted by elements of the innate immune response, an early evolutionary adaptation lacking immunologic memory, so the magnitude of response is the same each time the antigen is encountered. The receptors that recognize pathogens are predetermined by germline genes and recognize a few highly conserved structures called pathogen-associated molecular patterns (PAMPs) present or abundant on or in microorganisms but not the host. After binding to these molecules, the effector cell is immediately activated, accounting for the rapid responses of the innate system. Neutrophils, monocytes and monocyte-derived cells such as macrophages, are critical phagocytic components that engulf and kill invading pathogens; monocyte-derived and professional presenting cells also process antigen and present it to lymphocytes to initiate or regulate the adaptive response. Plasma complement proteins act in a cascading sequence, binding extracellular organisms when the epithelial surfaces are breached; they enhance phagocytosis as well as causing inflammation and cell death. The first pathway to evolve was activated by foreign material in a nonspecific way (confusingly called the "alternative" activation pathway, because it was described second). In addition, mannan-binding lectin can opsonize microbes and activate the lectin pathway, and antibody–antigen (immune) complexes can activate the classical activation pathway (Fig. 19.1). Complement activation releases a series of vasoactive and proinflammatory peptides (anaphylatoxins: C3a, C4a and C5a) as well as opsonic

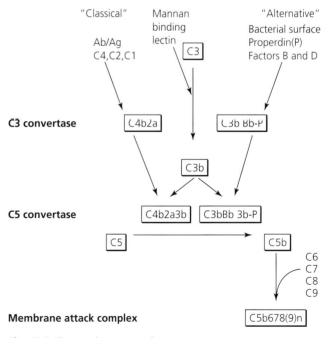

Fig. 19.1 The complement cascade.

proteins (e.g., C3b and C3bi), and culminates in the assembly of a large complex of proteins (C5b6789), which can lyse cell (or microbial cell) membranes and provoke inflammation.

Major histocompatibility complex

Major histocompatibility complex (MHC) antigens are highly polymorphic membrane glycoproteins expressed on all cell surfaces. Two classes, MHC I and MHC II, bind protein fragments in a surface groove and present them to T lymphocytes. MHC I molecules present viral or tumor proteins synthesized in the cytosol, whereas MHC II molecules present internalized and processed antigens. The MHC system is extremely polymorphic, to protect against the effects of novel pathogens, antigens of which might be ineffectively presented by monomorphic MHC and so condemn a whole species to fatal infection. Natural killer (NK) cells identify and eliminate cells, viral infected or malignant, that no longer express MHC by releasing intracellular toxic granules that promote cell death.

Recognition of antigen and heterogeneity

T and B lymphocytes of the adaptive immune response are generated in the bone marrow, thymus, lymph nodes, spleen and mucosal-associated lymphoid tissue. Each virgin lymphocyte has a unique antigen receptor, and in principle there is a lymphocyte bearing a receptor for every possible protein antigen that could be created. There are about 10^{16} different virgin B cells, each with specific antibody receptors; a similar number of virgin T cells, each with a specific receptor (TCR), are also generated from fewer than 400 TCR germline gene segments. Recombination activating genes 1 and 2 (RAG1; RAG2) cut the DNA between the gene segments which are then repaired by the normal DNA repair processes (Fig. 19.2). This remarkable diversity of T- and B-cell receptors is achieved by recombination processes that cut, splice and modify lymphocyte receptor genes. This process of extreme polymorphism, essentially random in its initial stages, generates both self-reactive lymphocytes, which are eliminated, as

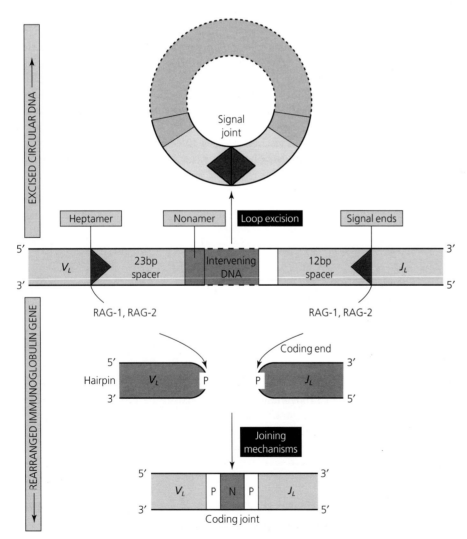

Fig. 19.2 Genetic mechanism for generating diversity in antibodies/T-cell receptors. Recombinase enzymes control recombination of a single VJ sequence at random from the many possible combinations of 70 V and 4 J sequences on the immunoglobulin light-chain gene. The heavy chain gene has 100 V, 4 D and 6 J sequences. Reproduced with permission from Ref. 106.

P, P-nucleotides

N, N-nucleotides

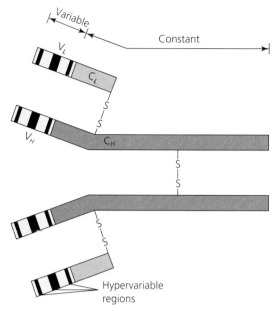

Fig. 19.3 Structure of the immunoglobin molecule. S–S, disulfide links; V, variable region; C, constant region; H, heavy chain; L, light chain. Reproduced with permission from Ref. 106.

well as lymphocytes that are effective against microorganisms and antigens. Following expression of a mature receptor, continued survival is dependent on antigen stimulation. When an antigen is encountered there is massive proliferation of T- and B-cell clones specific to that antigen.

B-lymphocyte development

B-lymphocyte receptors (BCR) are membrane-bound immunoglobulin molecules with two identical heavy (H) and two identical light (L) chains, joined by disulfide bonds (Fig. 19.3). The variable (V) domain end of the immunoglobulin molecule binds to specific antigen whereas the constant domain at the other end recruits other cells and molecules to immunoglobulin-bound antigen to effect killing and destruction. The constant (C) domain has five main forms (isotypes) that determine the immunoglobulin class (IgM, G, A, E and D). Smaller variations lead to four IgG and two IgA subclasses. Both heavy and light chains have C and V domains. There are two types of functionally identical light chains, lambda (λ) and kappa (κ).

Antibodies are immunoglobulins produced by B lymphocytes and their derivatives, plasma cells, in response to specific protein antigens. Specific serum antibodies may be present without prior exposure to the relevant antigen, so-called "natural" antibodies, resulting from cross-reactivity between antigens, particularly nonprotein (polysaccharide) antigens (e.g., ABO antibodies).

The variable region of the immunoglobulin molecule has a unique amino acid sequence, giving each antibody its unique specificity and ensuring, in principle, that there is an antibody complementary to every antigen that could be constructed. There are five main classes of immunoglobulin, each with its own structure and functions.

The immunoglobulin class or isotype is determined by the heavy chain. During B-lymphocyte development, rearrangement to bring a particular variable gene combination to lie adjacent to a different heavy chain constant region gene allows the B lymphocyte to switch to another antibody class (isotype) with the same antigen specificity. A μ chain is always produced first; class switching to other isotypes occurs later. Specific antibody diversity is created by the large number of possible combinations of variable region genes that can be selected and is increased further by a very high mutation rate in V genes and the effect of the enzyme TdT (deoxynucleotidyltransferase) during the rearrangement process.

Variable domain gene rearrangement

Variable domains of T- and B-cell antigen receptors are made by recombining segments encoded by genes from two or three "families." For immunoglobulin light chains, a variable (V) segment joins to a joining (J) segment, which joins to a C (constant) domain. A similar process occurs for the heavy chain, but using a diversity (D) segment as well as V and J segments, all joined to the heavy chain C domain. There are a number of different gene segments in each "family." Diversity is generated by varying the combination in which the V(D)J segments are arranged. Further diversity is introduced by pairing different combinations of heavy and light chain variable regions. A third way of increasing diversity is created by imprecise splicing and rejoining of different gene segments creating different nucleotides at the joining junction. These recombination events occur in the bone marrow.

T-lymphocyte development

T-lymphocyte receptor (TCR) development is similar to that of B cells, but occurs in the specialized microenvironment of the thymus. Precursor cells migrate to the thymus and undergo TCR chain rearrangements. The TCR consists of α/β or γ/δ heterodimers. Each α, β, γ and δ chain contains a variable and a constant domain. As in the BCR, variable domains are constructed from gene segments from different V, D and J "families." TCR α and γ variable domains do not contain D segments. A fundamental difference between BCR and TCR is that TCR only recognizes an antigen bound to an MHC complex. During thymic development, T cells that recognize the individual's own MHC complex are positively selected (self-MHC restricted), while those that do not undergo apoptosis (programmed cell death). Furthermore, those that recognize self antigen–MHC complexes are eliminated (negatively selected), thus preventing autoimmunity. In this way, less than 2% of T-cell precursors entering the thymus leave as mature, naive T cells.

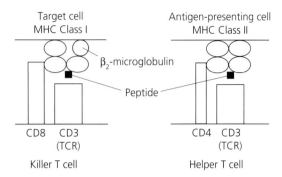

Fig. 19.4 Interactions of CD3 (T-cell receptor complex) and CD8 or CD4 with class I and class II major histocompatibility complex (MHC), respectively.

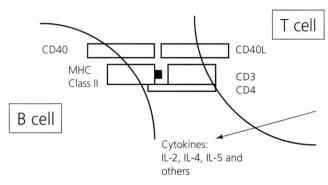

Fig. 19.5 Interactions between T and B cells: T-cell help. L, ligand; MHC, major histocompatibility complex; CD, differentiation cluster; IL, interleukin.

Antigen presentation and lymphocyte activation

Mature T and B lymphocytes circulate through blood, lymphatics and tissues "looking for" antigen specific for their receptors. Microorganisms taken up and processed by antigen-presenting cells (APCs), such as macrophages, are broken down into small peptide fragments, which are bound in the surface grooves of MHC class I or II molecules and presented at the cell surface as an antigen–MHC complex. Adaptive immune responses are generated in lymphoid tissue, where lymphocytes and APCs are mixed in high densities. Only a few hundred distinct lymphocytes will recognize each specific antigen. Although all cells can present antigens of infecting intracellular pathogens using MHC class I to CD8$^+$ cytotoxic T cells, APCs do this very effectively and also present processed antigens from extracellular organisms via MHC class II to CD4 helper T cells (Fig. 19.4). Following this, an APC surface molecule (B7) interacts with CD28 on the T cell to provide a second signal. The synchronous combination of these two signals (TCR/MHC–antigen and B7/CD28) activates the T cell causing replication of T cells bearing the same antigen-specific receptor (clonal expansion). In contrast, delivery of the first signal alone renders the T cell unable to respond to antigen (anergic). B cells express antibody (immunoglobulin) on their surface during development and recognize native (unprocessed) antigen directly. Subsequently, antibodies are secreted in large quantities by the mature B cell (plasma cell). T-cell receptors by contrast are only surface expressed and exist in a complex of coreceptors and signaling molecules. Individual lymphocytes and their progeny do not change the antigen specificity of the receptor they express. However, B cells can change the isotype of the antibody they produce (e.g., from IgM to IgG). This switching process is controlled by interactions between B and T cells via both direct receptor–ligand contact and release of soluble factors (cytokines) (Fig. 19.5). Thus, T cells are vital not only in specific cell-mediated responses but also in the regulation of most specific humoral (antibody-mediated) immune responses. More details about these processes can be found in specific texts.[1]

Primary immunodeficiency diseases

Many primary immunodeficiencies were first described as clinical syndromes, usually recognized in children who became unwell with progressive infections of particular organ systems or compartments and with certain characteristic types of pathogen. Careful investigations in such groups led, in some cases to recognition of the defect at the functional cellular level. In recent years, the molecular basis of many of the primary (genetically inherited) immunodeficiencies has been elucidated at the protein and genetic levels.[2] The identification and clarification of precise molecular mechanisms has not only enhanced understanding of the immune response but also enabled more focused treatment of primary immune deficiencies.

Specific immune defects are described below. Severe and rare conditions have tended to be elucidated first, but it is clear that many milder conditions are variants of more severe disease, and some mild defects only become manifest when other factors simultaneously impair immune function. During the late 1990s and early 21st century several new primary immunodeficiencies have been described by applying new molecular genetic techniques to groups of patients with specific unusual or recurrent infections. It has been surprising to find that defects in these pathways previously thought to have quite general regulatory or signaling roles turn out to cause propensity to infection with narrow spectra of pathogens.

T-cell and "combined" immunodeficiency

Severe combined immunodeficiency

Severe combined immunodeficiency (SCID) describes the severest form of primary immunodeficiency, where failure of both T- and B-lymphocyte function leads inevitably to death from infection within the first year of life. The different forms of SCID result from different blocks to the differentiation of

Table 19.1 Classification of severe combined immunodeficiency.

Defect	Gene defect	Inheritance	T/B/NK cells
Cytokine signaling	cδc	XL	−/+/−
	JAK 3	AR	−/+/−
	IL-7 Rα	AR	−/+/+
Defects associated with the salvage pathway of nucleotide biosynthesis	ADA deficiency	AR	T_{low}/B_{low}/NK_{low}
	PNP deficiency	AR	T_{low}/B_{low}/NK_{low}
Defects affecting signaling through the T-cell antigen receptor	CD45	AR	−/+/−
	CD3 δ	AR	−/+/−
	CD3 ε	AR	−/+/−
	ZAP 70K	AR	+/+/+ (absent CD8)
VDJ recombination defects	RAG 1 and 2	AR	−/−/+
	Artemis	AR	−/−/+
Other	Reticular dysgenesis	AR	−/−/− (+ myeloid dysfunction)
	MHC class II deficiency	AR	+/+/+ (absent CD4)

ADA, adenosine deaminase; AR, autosomal recessive; IL, interleukin; JAK, Janus-associated kinase; PNP, purine nucleoside phosphorylase; RAG, recombination activating gene; XL, X-linked.

T and, in some conditions, B and NK cells.[3] The main types of SCID can be broadly classified into five groups (Table 19.1).

Most of the SCID-associated gene mutations have now been identified, providing insight into the role of key molecules involved in lymphocyte precursor differentiation. Identifying the molecular defect in specific patients with SCID is important for prognosis, treatment, genetic counseling and increasing our knowledge about these rare diseases.

While the usual clinical features of this group of diseases are well characterized, atypical presentations and "leaky" forms with an attenuated phenotype are increasingly recognized.[4–6] Circulating T-lymphocyte numbers are usually low or absent but may be normal in certain forms (Table 19.1). Lymphocyte responses to mitogen are usually absent, but may be present in attenuated forms where immunoglobulin may also be produced. However, tests of antigen-specific T-lymphocyte proliferation and antibody production are consistently defective, and delayed hypersensitivity skin tests are negative. Patients usually have a limited diversity of T-lymphocyte receptor and immunoglobulin gene rearrangements. Thus, diagnosis may be more difficult in atypical patients.

Signaling receptor defects

Common γ-chain deficiency (X-linked SCID)
The most common form of SCID is characterized by severe lymphopenia, absence of mature T and NK lymphocytes, but normal numbers of circulating B lymphocytes. It is caused by a deficiency of the γ-chain common to the interleukin (IL)-2, IL-4, IL-7, IL-9 and IL-15 receptors.[7] Carriers show nonrandom skewed X inactivation of lymphocytes.

JAK-3 deficiency
This autosomal recessive form of SCID, phenotypically identical to the X-linked common gamma-chain deficiency, is due to mutations in the gene encoding Janus-associated kinase 3,[8] a protein that binds to the intracellular tail of the common gamma chain, and through which signals are transduced following cytokine binding.

IL-7Ra deficiency
This rarer autosomal recessive form of SCID is characterized by a T−/B+/NK+ phenotype.[9] The defect lies in the alpha chain of the interleukin 7 receptor and disrupts T cell development.

Lymphocyte metabolism defects

Adenosine deaminase deficiency
Adenosine deaminase (ADA), an enzyme of the purine salvage pathway, catalyzes the irreversible deamination of adenosine and deoxyadenosine to inosine and deoxyinosine, which are reutilized or degraded to uric acid. This pathway is particularly important for lymphocytes and erythrocytes, which have absent or low *de novo* purine synthesis. Autosomal recessive ADA deficiency results in the accumulation of toxic metabolites such as deoxyadenosine, which inhibit DNA synthesis. Gene deletion leads to very little ADA activity and a profound T and B lymphopenia and early-onset SCID. Patients present earlier than with other forms of SCID, with very low numbers of T, B and NK lymphocytes. Skeletal abnormalities (cupping deformities of the ends of the ribs, abnormalities of the transverse vertebral processes and the scapulae) are reported in up to 50% of cases.[10] Neurodevelop-

mental problems occur in some patients.[11] The diagnosis is confirmed by finding very low erythrocyte ADA activity and high levels of dATP in the urine. The clinical spectrum is broader than classical SCID; an increasing number of patients are being diagnosed in childhood with features that include sinopulmonary bacterial infections, markedly elevated IgE and/or eosinophilia, variable elevation of IgM and IgG, and autoimmune features including autoimmune hemolytic anemia and thrombocytopenia.[5]

Purine nucleoside phosphorylase deficiency
Like ADA deficiency, this extremely rare form of SCID is caused by an inherited defect in the purine pyrimidine salvage pathway. The metabolites deoxyguanosine and deoxyguanosine triphosphate are particularly toxic for thymocytes, resulting in a T-lymphocyte deficiency with relatively preserved B-lymphocyte function.[12] Recurrent infections usually begin in the first or second year, although some patients are asymptomatic until as late as 6 years of age. Additionally, patients show characteristic neurologic abnormalities, notably spastic diplegia, ataxia and dysarthria, and autoimmune problems, particularly hemolytic anemia.[13] There is a progressive fall in T-lymphocyte numbers and function, poor *in vitro* mitogen responses and negative delayed hypersensitivity skin tests. Immunoglobulin levels and antibody responses are initially normal but then fall. Serum uric acid levels are very low. The diagnosis is confirmed by demonstrating absent purine nucleoside phosphorylase activity in red cells or fibroblasts and deoxyinosine and deoxyguanosine in the urine. Without corrective treatment the prognosis is poor, with most cases dying in early childhood. Treatment by early bone marrow transplantation, if successful, corrects the immunodeficiency; its effect on the neurologic disease is uncertain.

V(D)J recombination defects
Two phenotypically identical forms of this autosomal recessive disorder have been described with absent T and B lymphocytes, but normal numbers of NK lymphocytes. The first is due to defects in the recombination activating genes (RAG) necessary for the development of T and B lymphocyte antigen receptors.[14] In the second, there is a defect in the artemis gene, necessary for rejoining DNA following V(D)J recombination, leading to *in vitro* radiosensitivity.[15] Bone marrow transplantation results are not as good as in the T⁻/B⁺ forms of SCID. "Leaky" RAG defects have been shown in some patients with Omenn syndrome.

Omenn syndrome
Omenn described 12 infants in six sibships from an inbred Irish–American kindred; all developed an infiltrating skin rash, hepatosplenomegaly and lymphadenopathy, together with diarrhea, failure to thrive and recurrent persistent infections leading to death.[16] Children usually present in early

infancy although atypical cases may be seen after the first year of life. There are normally high numbers of oligoclonal, activated, poorly functional T lymphocytes of the Th2 phenotype but absent B lymphocytes and low levels of IgA, IgG and IgM. Elevated IgE levels and eosinophilia are often present. The syndrome has been called a "leaky" form of SCID in that small numbers of very abnormal T lymphocytes "leak" past the block in T-lymphocyte development. In some cases a RAG mutation is found.[17] T cells in these patients are autologous, although the clinical picture may resemble SCID with maternofetal engraftment (see below). Molecular genetic studies to identify the origin of the dermal infiltrative T lymphocytes can differentiate the two disorders. Activated oligoclonal lymphocytes in skin provoke Langerhans cells (APC) to migrate to lymph nodes, liver and spleen where lymphoid tissue architecture is severely disrupted. Bone marrow transplantation is the only curative treatment.

SCID with maternofetal engraftment
In immunocompetent individuals, lymphocytes passing from mother to fetus are rejected by the fetal immune system. However, sensitive molecular techniques show that circulating T lymphocytes of maternal origin may be found in up to 50% of infants with SCID.[18] Maternally engrafted lymphocytes show a profoundly restricted Vβ gene usage, suggesting they have a much reduced TCR diversity and come from a small number of lymphocyte clones. They usually bear the phenotype of activated mature T lymphocytes but give markedly diminished or absent proliferative responses to phytohemagglutinin (PHA), allogeneic cells or specific antigens. Such cells may be clinically silent but in some cases can cause severe congenital graft-versus-host disease (GVHD).

Reticular dysgenesis
This rare autosomal recessive form of SCID is characterized by defective lymphoid and myeloid differentiation. Bone marrow examination confirms the absence of myeloid precursors. Platelets and red lymphocytes are formed normally but there is thrombocytopenia. This may not be a discrete entity, but the result of other forms of SCID, complicated by severe maternal engraftment and bone marrow GVHD.[18] The absence of the nonspecific cellular elements of the immune system (including neutrophils) makes the immunodeficiency even more severe than in other forms of SCID. Clinical presentation occurs earlier, as does the inevitable fatal outcome if bone marrow transplant is not performed quickly.

MHC class II deficiency
MHC class II antigens (HLA DR, DP and DQ) are expressed on APCs that present antigen to CD4⁺ T lymphocytes leading to the activation of T-helper lymphocytes specific for that antigen. Expression of MHC II in the thymus is also essential for positive selection of CD4⁺ T lymphocytes. It is therefore not surprising that lack of MHC II expression ("bare lympho-

cyte syndrome") results in a profound susceptibility to viral, bacterial, fungal and protozoal infections.[19]

MHC II deficiency, a rare autosomal recessive disease, can result from mutations in several different genes, including *MHC2TA*, *RFX5* and *RFXAP*, which code for a complex of regulatory factors controlling transcription of MHC II genes, rather than defects in the MHC II genes themselves.[20] There is little genotype/phenotype correlation.

The clinical picture resembles SCID, although sometimes infections develop slightly later. Intestinal and hepatic complications due to cryptosporidial infections are more common than in other immune defects. Neurologic manifestations caused by a range of viral infections are also well described, including coxsackievirus, adenovirus, poliovirus and meningoencephalitis.

Most patients have CD4 lymphopenia and hypogammaglobulinemia; lymphocyte proliferation responses are usually normal. The diagnosis can be confirmed flow cytometrically by showing absent or significantly reduced levels of class II molecules, for example DR, on cells that constitutively express class II (B lymphocytes and monocytes).

Affected children require treatment with replacement immunoglobulin, co-trimoxazole and antifungal prophylaxis pending bone marrow transplantation, which is the definitive treatment, although this is more difficult than for other forms of SCID.

Idiopathic CD4 lymphocytopenia

A profoundly low CD4+ lymphocyte count characterizes this poorly understood condition. Most reports have been in adults, but it occurs in children. It is regarded as a primary immunodeficiency disorder;[21] a retroviral cause has not been found despite strenuous efforts. There may be defective lymphocyte homeostasis and restricted clonality in lymphoid populations. Immunoglobulin levels and antibody responses may be normal. The CD4 cell count remains stable for a prolonged period rather than progressively declining as seen in human immunodeficiency virus (HIV) infection. Prophylaxis against *Pneumocystis carinii* infection should be given.

Other SCID syndromes

Defects in other lymphocyte surface and signaling molecules have been described in small numbers of patients. Although T and B cells are usually present, the numbers are often low and function is diminished. Such cases are being recognized in increasing numbers as molecular diagnostic testing becomes more widely available. Other atypical or unusual presentations may be due to defects in molecules already described, or to as yet unidentified molecules or mutations. More detailed texts should be consulted for specific details.

Clinical features and diagnosis of SCID

Affected babies appear well at birth, with the exception of infants with reticular dysgenesis. Most are asymptomatic

for the first few weeks of life before developing persistent respiratory tract or gut infection and failure to thrive, falling progressively away from their birth centile.[22] Chronic diarrhea caused by persistent, sometimes multiple, gastrointestinal viral infections, often with associated food intolerance, is common, as is persistent respiratory tract infection with respiratory syncytial virus or parainfluenza viruses, with failure to clear virus accompanying a persistent bronchiolitis-like illness. An insidiously progressive persistent interstitial pneumonitis should raise the suspicion of *Pneumocystis carinii* infection, often a copathogen with respiratory viruses. Other presentations include invasive bacterial infections, particularly staphylococcal or *Pseudomonas* septicemia and pneumonia, which may respond poorly to appropriate treatment. Severe invasive fungal infection is rare, but often fatal. Extensive, persistent superficial candidiasis is more common. Occasionally babies present with disseminated BCG (bacille Calmette–Guérin) or vaccine strain poliomyelitis virus. Children presenting within the first 6 months or so of life are more likely to have SCID or a severe T-lymphocyte defect.

Noninfectious manifestations mainly result from GVHD caused by foreign lymphocytes acquired either maternally *in utero* or from unirradiated transfused blood. Engraftment of transplacentally acquired maternal lymphocytes (maternofetal GVHD) sometimes, but not always, provokes GVHD, typically with a mild reticular skin rash and slightly deranged liver function tests. Fatal GVHD can follow transfusion with nonirradiated blood, white cell, lymphocyte or platelet concentrates. In these cases the skin rash is more severe, and lymphadenopathy and hepatosplenomegaly may be present. Cases may be clinically indistinguishable from Omenn syndrome, but identification of maternal cells by karyotype or DNA fingerprinting will distinguish maternofetal GVHD from Omenn syndrome. Epstein–Barr virus (EBV) infection may lead to uncontrolled B lymphoproliferative disorders.

Examination usually reveals a wasted child who has dropped through the growth centiles, with candidiasis and other infections. Skin rashes may be indicative of infection or GVHD. Lymphoid tissue is usually absent. There may be hepatomegaly.

By the time of diagnosis most infants will have several infections. Unfortunately, only interstitial pneumonitis is pathognomonic of immunodeficiency, and so infants with respiratory infection may be severely ill and needing assisted ventilation before immunodeficiency is considered: bone marrow transplantation is less successful when children are diagnosed late with significant organ damage. In a UK series, symptoms developed at a median age of 5 weeks, but diagnosis of SCID was not made until a median age of 7 months (range 4 weeks to 16 months).[23]

Lymphopenia is the most useful diagnostic clue but is often overlooked as the absolute lymphocyte count is rarely observed when a full blood count is performed. Lymphocyte counts are higher in infants than adults and the lower limit of normal can range from 2×10^9/L at birth to 4×10^9/L at 1 year (see Chapter 37 for reference values). In the UK series of 45 infants with SCID, 44 had a lymphocyte count > 2 standard deviations below the mean for age, compared with 8 in a control group all of whose counts normalized on repeat testing a few days later.[23]

Lymphocyte subset analysis demonstrates low or absent T-lymphocyte numbers; B-lymphocyte numbers may be normal. IgG levels may be normal due to transplacentally transferred maternal IgG, and many laboratories cannot distinguish between absent IgA and IgM and the low levels normally seen up to 6 months of age; hence if SCID is suspected, lymphocyte subset analysis should always be performed. Failure of lymphocyte proliferation in response to stimuli such as phytohemagglutinin helps confirm the diagnosis.

Chest radiography may demonstrate an absent thymus, and hyperinflation and/or interstitial pneumonia, if infection is present. Typical cupping and flaring of the costochondral junction is also evident in patients with ADA deficiency.

Once an immunologic diagnosis has been made the nature and extent of infection should be determined. Serology is unhelpful as infants with SCID cannot produce antibody. Viral culture and immunofluorescence studies of nasopharyngeal suction specimens, as well as electron microscopy of stool, and stool and urine viral culture, together with bacterial stool, urine and surface swab cultures are necessary. EBV, cytomegalovirus (CMV) and adenovirus must be looked for assiduously, including polymerase chain reaction (PCR) testing of blood, and in children with a respiratory disease, bronchoalveolar lavage should be performed to look for pathogens such as *Pneumocystis carinii*, bacteria and viruses. Finding a respiratory virus in a nasopharyngeal suction specimen should not preclude performing bronchoalveolar lavage as many infants have dual infections, and *Pneumocystis carinii* is usually found only in respiratory secretions and is treatable. Infants should be nursed in strict isolation to prevent nosocomial viral and fungal infections. Nutritional support is often required.

Without treatment, patients die from infection by about 12 months of age. The diagnosis of SCID is a pediatric emergency; suspected cases should be urgently referred to a designated center for assessment and treatment.

Combined immunodeficiency

Wiskott–Aldrich syndrome

This X-linked recessive condition is characterized by immunodeficiency, thrombocytopenia, eczema, an increased risk of autoimmune disorders and malignancy. It is due to defects in Wiskott–Aldrich syndrome protein (WASP), which regulates the actin skeleton of bone marrow derived cells.[24] Mutations in the WASP gene are also found in patients with X-linked thrombocytopenia (XLT),[25] and X-linked severe congenital

neutropenia.[26] Lack of a proper actin skeleton may lead to failure of polarization of T cells toward antigen-presenting cells and B cells, leading to a failure of cognate immune responses.

The classical features of bruising/bleeding, recurrent infections and eczema can each vary in severity; the eczema can be surprisingly mild. Presentation is usually in early life with bruising, petechiae and bleeding: thrombocytopenia and bleeding episodes may require platelet transfusions. Bacterial and/or viral infections of the upper and lower respiratory tract are common; opportunistic infection, such as *Pneumocystis carinii* may occur. Herpesviruses are poorly handled and may cause severe and recurrent disease. Impetigo, cellulitis and skin abscesses are common whilst molluscum contagiosum and viral warts may be very extensive. Infection exacerbates the bleeding tendency, and early death may result from bleeding. With increasing age, infective problems replace bleeding as the major cause of death. Immunization with polysaccharide vaccines are often ineffective. The median survival is 11 years. Autoimmunity, particularly hemolytic anemia and vasculitis, and lymphoreticular malignancy become more common with increasing age, and many cases are related to persistent EBV infection. Heterozygous female carriers are clinically normal and demonstrate nonrandom X-inactivation in all hematopoietic cells.

Thrombocytopenia with an abnormally small mean platelet volume (<5 fL) are pathognomonic. The severity of immunodeficiency is variable, but affects cellular and humoral responses. T lymphopenia is progressive with depressed responses to mitogens and antigens and negative delayed hypersensitivity skin tests. Serum immunoglobulins often show a very low IgM, normal IgG, and raised IgA and IgE. Antibody responses to tetanus, *Haemophilus influenzae* type B and pneumococcus are often low, as are isohemagglutinin titers. The direct Coombs test is frequently positive. *In vivo* neutrophil and monocyte chemotaxis may be impaired. Phagocytes migrate poorly to sites of inflammation and do not put out normal filopodia, dendritic cells do not present antigen effectively, lymphocytes show impaired signaling to each other, and platelets form imperfectly from megakaryocytes.[27,28] Missense mutations in exons 1–3, which lead to normal-sized or truncated protein, result in the milder phenotype of XLT, whereas most other mutations result in the classic Wiskott–Aldrich phenotype.

Acute bleeding episodes may be controlled by platelet transfusions (irradiated to prevent GVHD). Splenectomy and steroid treatment will increase the risk of infection and should be avoided if possible, although topical steroids may be required for the eczema. Intravenous immunoglobulin, with or without prophylactic antibiotics, reduces bacterial sinopulmonary infections and in high doses may help to treat autoimmune phenomena.

Even with supportive intervention, the prognosis remains poor. Immunologic and hematologic correction can be achieved by bone marrow transplantation (BMT) and despite a higher risk of EBV-driven lymphoproliferative disorders, 5-year survival is 87% after HLA-identical sibling donor BMT and 71% after unrelated donor BMT, although unlike HLA-identical sibling BMT, results for unrelated donor BMT after 5 years of age are poorer.[29]

X-linked lymphoproliferative disease (Duncan disease)

In this X-linked condition immunity is normal and the patient asymptomatic until EBV or other stimuli[30] uncover a defect in T- and B-lymphocyte interaction. There are three common clinical presentations: fulminant infectious mononucleosis (58%), dysgammaglobulinemia, often evolving to common variable immunodeficiency (31%); and EBV-driven B-lymphocyte lymphoma, usually extranodal and affecting the gastrointestinal tract or central nervous system (20%). Less common presentations are vasculitis, aplastic anemia, hemophagocytic lymphohistiocytosis or pulmonary lymphomatoid granulomatosis.[31] The prognosis is poor, with 45–96% mortality, depending on the clinical presentation; registry data indicate no survivors after 40 years of age. The gene responsible for the disease, *SH2D1A* in the Xq25 region of the X chromosome,[32] encodes a small protein, SAP – signaling lymphocyte activation molecule (SLAM)-associated protein – which is crucial for T-lymphocyte and NK cell control of EBV-infected B lymphocytes; why this causes the clinical features is unclear. Confirmation of the diagnosis involves demonstrating EBV genome in blood by PCR, together with the immune defects outlined above and an abnormal serologic response to the virus with absent antibody response to EBV nuclear antigen. The mothers of affected boys also have abnormal EBV serology, with persisting very high titers against viral capsid antigen. Protein analysis reveals absent or abnormal SAP protein in many cases, although a gene mutation is not identifiable in up to 40% of patients. Treatment with intravenous immunoglobulin on a regular basis is recommended in affected patients as passive immunization against EBV, particularly if hypogammaglobulinemia is present Hemophagocytic lymphohistiocytic episodes require treatment with immune suppression including ciclosporin, antithymocyte globulin, steroids and the HLH-94 protocol.[33] Correction of the disorder by bone marrow transplantation is the only curative treatment.

DiGeorge anomaly

This syndrome results from abnormal cephalic neural crest cell migration into the third and fourth pharyngeal arches in early embryologic development associated with a microdeletion at chromosome 22q11.2; it is also found in velocardiofacial, or Shprintzen, syndrome, which should now be considered as a part of the same spectrum.

Clinical features vary; partial forms are more common than the complete phenotype. Whilst classically recognized by the triad of congenital heart defects, immunodeficiency secondary to thymic hypoplasia and hypocalcemia secondary to parathyroid gland hypoplasia, an expanded phenotype is increasingly recognized with dysmorphic facies (low-set, abnormally formed ears, hypertelorism and anti-mongoloid slant, micrognathia, short philtrum to the upper lip and high arched palate), palatal abnormalities (cleft palate, velopharyngeal insufficiency), autoimmune phenomena, learning difficulties (particularly speech delay), renal anomalies, neuropsychiatric disorders and short stature. Conotruncal heart defects are classically associated with the syndrome, but other defects include tetralogy of Fallot, septal defects, pulmonary atresia, and aberrant subclavian vessels. Some patients have normal cardiac anatomy.

Severe T-lymphocyte immunodeficiency presenting with a SCID phenotype is rare, accounting for < 1.5% of cases. Recurrent sinopulmonary infection due to partial humoral immunodeficiency is more common;[34] significant lung damage can occur due to repeated infection. Autoimmune features are increasingly recognized, including juvenile chronic arthritis and autoimmune cytopenias. The long-term immunologic outlook is not well defined.

This diagnosis should be considered in infants with heart lesions or hypocalcemic fits. Urgent cardiac surgery is often required; blood products should be irradiated before transfusion to avoid potentially fatal GVHD in the minority of cases with total thymic aplasia. Immunologic investigations should include a lymphocyte subset analysis and a test of mitogen-induced proliferative responses (PHA). CD4$^+$ and CD8$^+$ T-cell numbers are often modestly reduced while mitogen-induced proliferation is usually normal. Antibody responses, particularly to polysaccharide antigens, are often impaired. Immunoglobulin levels may be normal but hypogammaglobulinemia may develop; occasionally such children need immunoglobulin replacement. Most individuals respond to protein antigen vaccination. It is safe to give live vaccines such as oral polio vaccine, measles, mumps, rubella vaccine, or varicella zoster vaccine as long as the CD4 count exceeds 400/mm^3, and T-lymphocyte mitogen responses are normal.[35]

When there is severe immunodeficiency children should be treated like those with SCID. Surprisingly, given that the defect is thymic, BMT may be successful; thymic transplant has also been advocated.[36]

X-linked hyper-IgM syndrome (CD40 ligand deficiency)

X-linked hyper-IgM syndrome is a T-lymphocyte immunodeficiency due to a defect in the gene encoding for the CD40 ligand glycopeptide (CD154) expressed on activated T lymphocytes. CD40L binds to CD40, expressed on B lymphocytes and monocyte/macrophage-derived cells (Fig. 19.5). Lack of binding prevents B-lymphocyte immunoglobulin isotype switching from IgM to IgA, IgG and IgE as well as activation of Kupffer cells and pulmonary macrophages. Lack of IgA and IgG results in a similar clinical picture to X-linked agammaglobulinemia (XLA), with sinopulmonary and invasive bacterial infection, but, in contrast to XLA, opportunistic infections also occur; failure of T lymphocytes to activate macrophages results in *Pneumocystis carinii* pneumonia, and repeated bowel, pancreas and biliary tree infections with *Cryptosporidium parvum* leading to sclerosing cholangitis, cirrhosis, pancreatitis and hepatic malignancy. Neutropenia with oral ulceration is seen in 50% of patients and may be cyclical. A low or absent IgA and IgG, with normal or raised IgM, should suggest the diagnosis. Autoimmune phenomena are relatively common and include hemolytic anemia, thrombocytopenia, hypothyroidism, arthritis and liver disorders.[37]

Patients should receive co-trimoxazole prophylaxis for *Pneumocystis carinii* pneumonia and immunoglobulin replacement therapy. With adequate replacement the high IgM levels may normalize. The neutropenia sometimes responds to granulocyte colony-stimulating factor (G-CSF) and intravenous immunoglobulin (IVIG). All drinking water should be boiled and filtered to lessen the risk of *Cryptosporidium parvum* infection, for which purpose antimicrobial prophylaxis is given by some practitioners although supportive evidence for this is lacking. Despite conventional treatment, many patients do not survive beyond the third decade of life, largely due to hepatic complications, but a few patients with a common variable immunodeficiency-like clinical course and no biliary or liver disease are relatively well in middle life. Bone marrow transplantation is increasingly being recommended for this condition.[38]

MHC class I deficiency

Although described before MHC class II deficiency, SCID due to abnormal expression of the A, B and C components of the MHC class I complex is much less common. MHC class I is required for development of CD8+ T lymphocytes, and affected children have low numbers of these cells. Mitogen responses are frequently normal. The genetic basis for the disease is mutations in TAP1 or 2,[39] proteins required for transport of antigen from the cytoplasm into the endoplasmic reticulum where they associate with MHC class I.

This disease has a milder clinical phenotype than MHC class II deficiency, symptoms often not beginning until late childhood. Recurrent respiratory tract infections leading to bronchiectasis and sinus problems are common. Unusual skin lesions thought to be due to vasculitis have been reported.

Diagnosis is confirmed by showing absent HLA class I expression on peripheral blood cells. Sinopulmonary infections should be promptly treated with antibiotics, physiotherapy and bronchodilators. The value of prophylactic antibiotic treatment is debated. Most cases do not require replacement immunoglobulin therapy or bone marrow transplantation.

Defects of lymphocyte apoptosis (autoimmune lymphoproliferative syndrome)

Apoptosis (programmed cell death) is important for regulating immune responses once an infection has been eliminated. Defects lead to the marked autoimmune and lymphoproliferative features that characterize autoimmune lymphoproliferative syndrome (ALPS).[40] There are a number of pathways through which apoptosis can be induced; one of the most important is via a cell surface molecule Fas (CD95). Ligation of this molecule initiates a cascade of intracellular reactions culminating in apoptosis induced by proteolytic enzymes including caspases. Mutations in several molecules in this cascade result in molecularly distinct but clinically similar forms of ALPS.

Type Ia is the most frequent form of ALPS. Fas is expressed as a trimeric surface protein. As a consequence heterozygotes with a Fas mutation in one allele develop disease because one abnormal protein chain is sufficient to impair the trimer's function, a so-called dominant-negative effect. Most of the cases described have been heterozygotes although the few homozygous cases seen have had severe disease. The clinical variability and the occurrence of asymptomatic individuals make estimates of incidence very difficult.

Many cases present in early childhood although adult presentation is also described. Symptomatic and asymptomatic cases may occur in the same families. Autoimmune disease most commonly affects the hematopoietic system. Lymphoproliferation often results in characteristically massive asymmetric lymph nodes in the anterior triangle of the neck, with splenomegaly in nearly all cases and hepatomegaly in some. Lymphoid malignancies (both Hodgkin and non-Hodgkin) are reported with increased frequency but have probably been overdiagnosed because the histologic picture of proliferation resembles malignancy: clonality studies distinguish the two.[41]

Lymphocyte counts and immunoglobulin levels are often high. Autoantibodies are usually present, a direct Coombs test is usually positive. In almost all cases 5–20% of circulating CD3+ T lymphocytes express normal α/β receptors but do not express CD4 or CD8 (so-called double-negative T lymphocytes). Many of these cells also express HLA DR (a marker of T-lymphocyte activation). CD95 is not expressed on lymphocytes even after activation with mitogens. Apoptotic assays, where cell death is measured after artificial ligation of CD95 with an antibody, confirm the ALPS defect. Mutation analysis of Fas, Fas ligand (FasL) and the appropriate caspase genes will confirm the precise molecular diagnosis.

Autoimmune phenomena usually respond to steroids and high-dose IVIG treatment. Where there is marked B-lymphocyte proliferation, administration of anti-CD20 B-cell monoclonal antibody can be very effective. Splenectomy should be avoided, as signs and symptoms often improve with time, and because of the risk of death from bacterial sepsis; however, when unavoidable, long-term antibiotic prophylaxis is mandatory. The diagnosis of lymphoma should only be made when clonality and molecular markers have confirmed this, because on conventional microscopy benign lymphoproliferation can be mistaken for malignancy and inappropriate chemotherapy given. Bone marrow transplantation has been successful in patients with severe (usually homozygous) Fas deficiency but is not usually needed for heterozygous cases.

Chronic mucocutaneous candidiasis

Chronic mucocutaneous candidiasis (CMC) describes a group of disorders characterized by chronic and recurrent candidal infection of variable severity affecting the mouth, napkin area, skin and nails. Invasive candidal infection rarely occurs. The failure of usually effective antifungal drugs to completely clear *Candida* distinguishes CMC from other conditions that predispose to candida such as secondary immunodeficiency, steroid treatment or systemic antibiotics. Most patients present in the first few months of life with persistent candidiasis of the mouth, perineum and, sometimes, esophagus. When present, esophagitis is often severe and associated with esophageal reflux and failure to thrive. In about half the patients there is an associated endocrinopathy (with, in order of frequency: hypoparathyroidism, Addison disease, pernicious anemia, hypothyroidism and diabetes mellitus), usually not apparent until the second or third decades onward. Less common autoimmune findings include hemolytic anemia, thrombocytopenia and neutropenia, chronic active hepatitis and uveitis. Cases may be familial or sporadic with recessive or dominant patterns of inheritance. Patients may also have evidence of dental enamel hypoplasia and keratopathy associated with autoimmune endocrinopathy. Some patients with CMC have defects in the *AIRE* gene associated with autoimmune polyendocrinopathy, candidiasis, ectodermal dystrophy (APECED).[42] A minority of patients suffer from invasive bacterial sepsis, opportunistic infection, autoimmune hemolytic anemia, malabsorption and chronic active hepatitis. Bronchiectasis and restrictive lung disease can occur.

Candida is often very difficult to eradicate, but can be ameliorated by long-term treatment with fluconazole or itraconazole (unless resistance develops); liver enzymes must be monitored when using these agents, particularly if there is evidence of autoimmune hepatitis. A proportion of cases improve considerably with age.

Immunodeficiency and short-limbed dwarfism

Abnormalities of T- and B-lymphocyte function are seen in a number of osteochondrodysplasias, including Shwachman–Diamond syndrome where there is neutropenia and pancreatic insufficiency, and Schimke immuno-osseous dysplasia, which features radiographic changes of spondyloepiphyseal dysplasia, nephrotic syndrome and cellular immunodeficiency. Other short-limbed dwarfisms associated with immunodeficiency are less clearly delineated.

Cartilage–hair hypoplasia is the best-described autosomal recessive variant, associated with mutations in the *RMRP* gene, encoding an RNA-editing enzyme. Severe short-limbed short stature (–11.8 SD to 2.1 SD) with radiographic appearances of metaphyseal and spondyloepiphyseal dysplasia are always present, accompanied by sparse light hair in most patients. Severe anemia and Hirschsprung disease are well-recognized associations, as are malignancies, notably lymphoma and skin carcinoma. The immunodeficiency is variable; most have T lymphopenia and impaired *in vitro* mitogen proliferative responses, but only half suffer recurrent infection.[43] Patients are excessively vulnerable to viral infections, particularly varicella zoster, EBV and other human herpesvirus infections, and the risk of infective death is 300 times greater than normal.[44] Severely affected patients should be assessed for bone marrow transplantation, which has successfully corrected the immunodeficiency.

DNA repair defects and immunodeficiency

The immune system has utilized ubiquitous cellular DNA repair mechanisms to generate the diversity of specific immune responses by V(D)J recombination. Without the ability to repair DNA damage, cells may apoptose or undergo malignant proliferation, hence individuals with defective DNA repair mechanisms have a predisposition to neurodegeneration, developmental anomalies and cancer as well as defective immunity.[45] The mechanisms are complex, with so many single-gene defects able to give rise to distinct clinical entities.

Ataxia telangiectasia

This multisystem autosomal recessive disorder is characterized by progressive cerebellar ataxia, oculocutaneous telangiectasia, variable immunodeficiency and increased risk of lymphoid malignancy. There is chromosomal instability, and cellular radiosensitivity. Diagnosis is chiefly clinical, and gait anomalies lead to referral often before telangiectasia appears. Ataxia and cerebellar signs usually appear in the second year, and although they may be delayed, are always present. Progressive neurologic degeneration usually results in severe disability by late childhood. Telangiectasia usually appears between 2 and 8 years of age, first on the bulbar conjunctivae but later elsewhere, particularly on the nose, the ears and in the antecubital and popliteal fossae. Cutaneous hypopigmentation or hyperpigmentation, atrophy and atopic dermatitis are seen. Gonadal atrophy occurs, and growth failure is also prominent in the later stages. Immunodeficiency affects 60–80% of cases but clinical manifestations are variable.

Recurrent sinopulmonary infection is common and may lead to bronchiectasis and clubbing. Lymphoreticular malignancies and carcinomas occur with increased frequency. Radiosensitivity means that treatment with radiotherapy is toxic and often lethal. Irrespective of the development of malignancy, survival beyond early adult life is unusual.[46]

Immunologic findings vary but there is progressive failure of antibody production, with poor responses to polysaccharide antigens progressing to hypogammaglobulinemia. IgM may be raised; there is lymphopenia, predominantly of CD4+ T lymphocytes, with increased numbers of T lymphocytes bearing the γ/δ receptor. Raised α-fetoprotein (abnormal in 90%) and carcinoembryonic antigen support the diagnosis. Increased chromosome breakage on exposure to ionizing radiation is found. Patients have a high incidence of translocations at the sites of the T-lymphocyte receptor and immunoglobulin heavy chain genes, which may explain the immunodeficiency. The *ATM* gene encodes for a phosphatidyl kinase that signals to proteins involved in DNA repair and cell-cycle control;[47] it is absent or inactive in ataxia telangiectasia patients.

Prophylactic antibiotics or intravenous immunoglobulin ameliorates sinopulmonary infection in some patients. As the immunodeficiency is often progressive, the need for such treatment should be reviewed regularly.

Ataxia telangiectasia-like disorder

Patients with features similar to those of ataxia telangiectasia patients but with no mutation in the *ATM* gene have been described. In some, mutations have recently been found in the Mre11 gene, part of the complex with which nibrin associates (see below) and which is one of the complexes downstream from ATM.[48]

Nijmegen breakage syndrome

Nijmegen breakage syndrome (NBS), an autosomal recessive disorder, is characterized by microcephaly, moderate mental retardation, "bird-like" facies, immunodeficiency, clinical radiation sensitivity and chromosomal instability.[49] In some cases sensitivity to cross-link damaging agents such as mitomycin C has been described, a phenomenon previously considered to be found only in Fanconi anemia.[50] Bacterial sinopulmonary infection is common.

Hypogammaglobulinemia is the most common immunologic abnormality. There is a CD4+ T lymphopenia, and diminished T-lymphocyte proliferative responses are also found. A defect in the gene encoding nibrin causes NBS.[51] Nibrin is part of a protein signal transduction cascade downstream of the ATM protein. Absence of ataxia and telangiectasia, together with normal α-fetoprotein levels distinguishes NBS from ataxia telangiectasia. Treatment with antibiotic prophylaxis or IVIG may help.

Fanconi anemia

Progressive bone marrow failure leading to pancytopenia is the main problem in this condition. There may also be skeletal malformations. Immune deficiency can occur, and selective IgA deficiency and T-lymphocyte abnormalities have been recorded. At least nine genes are implicated in the disorder, encoding for proteins that form a complex involved in sensing cross-link DNA damage, and facilitating repair.[52] In some variants, radiosensitivity is described, and it is clear that the DNA repair pathways involved in cross-linking and also double-strand break repair are connected.[50,53]

Bloom syndrome

This rare autosomal recessive disorder is associated with increased sister chromatid exchange, severe growth failure, increased malignancy and immunodeficiency. Affected individuals may develop facial telangiectasia and facial photosensitivity. Recurrent bacterial sinopulmonary infections associated with hypogammaglobulinemia, most often low IgM, may lead to bronchiectasis.[54]

Defects in DNA ligases

DNA ligases function in DNA repair. Defects in DNA ligases I[55] and IV[56] have been described in rare individuals with radiosensitive cell lines and combined immunodeficiencies and cytopenias.

Other immunodeficiencies

A number of syndromes have been described that include primary immunodeficiency as part of the phenotype. In some, the syndrome is well described, and in a few the underlying molecular defect has recently been elucidated (Table 19.2).

Anhidrotic ectodermal dysplasia, incontinentia pigmenti and defects in the NEMO signaling pathway

X-linked anhidrotic ectodermal dysplasia is associated with immunodeficiency.[57] Patients present with sparse scalp hair, conical teeth and absent sweat glands. Some suffer from recurrent sinopulmonary infection and have poor antibody responses to polysaccharide antigens, or frank hypogammaglobulinemia. Incontinentia pigmenti is a rare X-linked dominant condition characterized by developmental abnormalities in skin, hair, teeth and the central nervous system. Rare male infants with a progressive combined immunodeficiency have been described. Hypofunctional mutations in the *NEMO* gene encoding a protein required to activate the transcription factor NF-κB have been described in male patients with both X-linked anhidrotic ectodermal dysplasia and incontinentia pigmenti.[58] Defects in IRAK4, which acts

Table 19.2 Syndromes with immunodeficiency as part of the phenotype.

Disease	Gene defect	Clinical characteristics
Hoyeraal–Hreidarsson syndrome	XL DKCI (some)	Microcephaly, cerebellar hypoplasia, aplastic anemia, growth retardation, progressive immunodeficiency, hypogammaglobulinemia, lymphopenia
Netherton syndrome	AR SPINK5	Generalized infantile erythroderma, diarrhea, failure to thrive, mild lymphopenia, bamboo hairs (distinguished from Omenn syndrome and SCID with MFE)
Immune dysregulation, polyendocrinopathy, enteropathy X-linked (IPEX) syndrome	XL Foxp3 (some AR)	Infantile ichthyosiform dermatitis, protracted diarrhea, IDDM, hemolytic anemia, thyroiditis
Immunodeficiency, centromeric instability, facial dysmorphism (ICF) yndrome	AR DNMT3B	DNA methylation defect, structural abnormalities in chromosomes 1 and 9, agammaglobulinemia, normal T- and B-cell numbers. Opportunistic, viral and fungal infections

AR, autosomal recessive; IDDM, insulin-dependent diabetes mellitus; MFE, maternofetal engraftment; SCID, severe combined immunodeficiency; *XL*, X-linked.

upstream of *NEMO,* lead to recurrent invasive bacterial infection, particulary due to pneumococci.[59]

NK cell deficiency

NK cells are large granular lymphocytes that bear CD56 instead of B- or T-lymphocyte markers and kill target cells without being previously sensitized. They do not depend on MHC restriction. Isolated complete absence of NK cells is extremely rare, and is associated with severe herpesvirus infections including varicella zoster virus and CMV, together with erythrophagocytosis.[60] Defective NK function due to absence of CD16 has also been described.[61]

Disorders of B-cell function

X-linked agammaglobulinemia (Bruton tyrosine kinase deficiency)

First described by Bruton in 1952, this is caused by a defect in the Bruton tyrosine kinase (BTK) gene, which encodes a cytoplasmic enzyme that is crucial for B-lymphocyte development beyond the pre-B-lymphocyte stage. Affected boys classically show greatly reduced or absent antibody production but cell-mediated immunity is normal. These children contract abnormally severe and frequent upper and lower respiratory bacterial infections and also gastrointestinal infections, pyoderma, septic arthritis, septicemia and meningitis.[62] These are usually manifest by the second year of life as maternal antibody wanes, and are associated with growth failure. Unfortunately, diagnosis is often delayed resulting in severe chronic lung injury or other complications of invasive infection. These children are also prone to severe infection due to enteroviruses (coxsackievirus and echovirus),[63] which can cause chronic meningitis, dermatomyositis and hepatitis. Polioviruses, including the attenuated virus strains in oral

polio vaccine, can cause paralytic poliomyelitis and chronic infection (an issue for the global eradication of polio).[64]

Where there is a family history, diagnosis can be confirmed at birth by the absence or very low numbers of cells expressing the B-cell markers CD19 or CD20 in peripheral blood. Bone marrow aspirate shows pre-B-lymphocytes (containing cytoplasmic μ chains). Lymph nodes show absent follicles and germinal centers. Plasma cells are absent. Molecular genetic analysis of the BTK gene is possible in patients and carrier mothers. Nonrandom X-chromosome inactivation in B cells of carrier mothers is present. Immunoglobulin measurements only become meaningful from 6 months of age as most infants have high levels of transplacentally acquired maternal IgG and low levels of IgA, IgM and IgE before this. After this age, all types of immunoglobulin are low or absent except in mild cases where there is presumably a partial defect in BTK; however, no clear genotype–phenotype correlation has been found. Absent or abnormal BTK has been described in cases of partial antibody deficiency,[65] so the condition should be considered in such cases in boys, particularly if circulating B-lymphocyte numbers are low, and there is a family history suggesting an X-linked inheritance.

IgG replacement is the mainstay of treatment. Even on adequate therapy, infections may still occur, especially giardiasis and chronic conjunctivitis. Antecedent chronic lung damage and sinus disease may progress after initiation of treatment; respiratory tract infection should be treated with vigorous, early antibiotic therapy. If recurrent infection persists despite increased doses of immunoglobulin, prophylactic antibiotics should be given, and some practitioners use both routinely in this condition. With the widespread use of IVIG, lung disease seems less common, emphasizing the importance of early diagnosis and treatment. There is some evidence that maintaining patients at higher IgG levels reduces the risk of lung disease but not of sinus problems.[66]

Rare associations of X-linked agammaglobulinemia include

growth hormone deficiency, neutropenia, malabsorption and protein-losing enteropathy, although the basis for these problems is unclear and, specifically, it is not known if they are causally linked to BTK mutations. Progressive sensorineural hearing loss has been described with XLA, due to large deletions in the terminal part of the BTK gene that were believed to involve a contiguous gene encoding the deafness, dystonia protein, DDP.

Autosomal recessive forms of agammaglobulinemia

Hypogammaglobulinemia in girls or in children with consanguineous parents suggests the existence of an autosomal recessive genetic defect affecting B-lymphocyte differentiation. Mutations have been described so far in genes coding for μ heavy chain, Igα (part of the signal transduction complex of the B-lymphocyte antigen receptor), λ5 light chain, or BLNK (B-lymphocyte linker protein).[67] These molecules are required for early B-lymphocyte development from pro-B-lymphocyte to pre-B-lymphocyte stage. In contrast to XLA, pre-B-lymphocytes are not detectable in marrow samples from these patients. Other families have also been described in whom the molecular defect is yet to be identified. In all cases the defect is B-lymphocyte specific. The clinical picture seems to be similar to XLA.

Autosomal recessive hyper-IgM syndrome

Autosomal recessive cases of hyper-IgM syndrome are also described, with defects in isotype class switch recombination and somatic hypermutations due to defects in AID[68] or UNG genes.[69]

Common variable immunodeficiency

Common variable immunodeficiency (CVID) is a poorly defined entity or group of conditions characterized by the presence of quantitative or qualitative hypogammaglobulinemia. It has an incidence of between 1 in 10 000 and 1 in 50 000. The onset of symptoms is typically seen within the second or third decade of life but is increasingly recognized in childhood.

Familial inheritance is seen in up to 25% of cases, but phenotypic variability within and between families suggests a polygenic inheritance. Selective IgA deficiency may be one end of the spectrum of this disease.[70] Autoimmune diseases, such as rheumatoid arthritis, are also seen more commonly in these kindreds. A number of patients with CVID have mild phenotypes of other immunodeficiencies such as X-linked agammaglobulinemia, CD40 ligand deficiency or X-linked lymphoproliferative disease.[71,72]

Patients present with recurrent sinopulmonary and gastrointestinal infections. They are susceptible to *Giardia lamblia* and are at risk from enteroviral infections, causing choriomeningitis in particular; arthritis may result from chronic *Mycoplasma* infection. Other clinical manifestations include autoimmune disease, particularly autoimmune cytopenias. Nonmalignant granulomatous lymphadenopathy, hepatosplenomegaly and involvement of the gastrointestinal tract is a frequent finding in a subgroup of patients; clinical differentiation from malignancy may be difficult although histologically lesions resemble those seen in sarcoidosis. These granulomas are normally sensitive to steroid treatment. Patients with CVID have a significantly increased risk of lymphoreticular and gastrointestinal malignancies.

Hypogammaglobulinemia may vary from a failure of specific vaccine responses to panhypogammaglobulinemia. B-lymphocyte numbers are frequently normal. A significant proportion of patients have a reversed CD4/8 ratio and a generalized lymphopenia.[73] Such abnormalities at presentation should prompt a search for other defined immunodeficiencies.

The aim of treatment is prevention of further infections and end-organ damage such as bronchiectasis. Mild phenotypes may require only prophylactic antibiotics. Significant hypogammaglobulinemia requires immunoglobulin replacement therapy. Patients with significantly abnormal cell-mediated immunity should receive prophylactic co-trimoxazole. Granulomatous lesions and autoimmune phenomena may respond to steroids.

Other humoral immune defects

IgA deficiency

One in every 600–700 healthy Caucasian blood donors have absent serum and salivary IgA; the clinical significance is unclear as most are asymptomatic. However, patients with chronic lung disease and autoimmune disease found to have IgA deficiency have significant morbidity. The pathophysiology of disease in these individuals is probably multifactorial; other factors may include IgG subclass and mannan-binding lectin deficiency. Selective IgA deficiency forms part of the CVID spectrum; in infancy, low IgA may be the last manifestation of transient hypogammaglobulinemia to resolve. Acquired IgA deficiency (usually reversible) may occur as a result of drug therapies (e.g., penicillamine, phenytoin, sodium valproate, captopril). It also occurs in congenital infections and after hepatitis C infection.

If IgA deficiency is found incidentally it is unlikely to be of clinical significance. If recurrent infections are present, IgG subclass levels and specific vaccination responses should be measured. IgG subclass deficiencies are found in approximately 15% of cases.

Recurrent sinopulmonary infections are the commonest symptoms in young children. Middle ear infections can be troublesome, and recurrent lower respiratory tract infections may result in lung damage. In most children the frequency and severity of infections improves with age, regardless of the IgA level. Gastrointestinal infections, in particular with *Giardia lamblia*, are more common than in the general population. IgA deficiency is strongly associated with auto-immune disease,[74] whether or not there are recurrent infections; the mechanisms are poorly understood. There is an associated increased risk of celiac disease, a diagnosis that can only be made on intestinal biopsy as the inability to make IgA means that IgA anti-gliadin and anti-endomysial anti-bodies will be negative. An increased risk of gastrointestinal lymphoma and gastric malignancies has also been reported although the true incidence has not been well defined.

Symptomatic patients may respond to prophylactic anti-bacterial treatment, replacement Ig is almost never required. Patients with IgA deficiency may have anti-IgA antibodies, which have been reported to cause severe anaphylactoid reactions if IgA-containing preparations are given (including IVIG or blood). The risks can be minimized by choosing an immunoglobulin preparation with the lowest IgA content.

Isotype (IgA, IgM and IgG subclass) deficiency with abnormally frequent or severe infections, and/or atopy and asthma, can be diagnosed if serum levels of one or more of these isotypes repeatedly lie two standard deviations below the mean for age. There is often a poor correlation between serum levels and the severity of infections. The degree of functional antibody impairment must vary widely and other unelucidated factors are likely to be involved. Evaluation is difficult because: (i) different methods are used to measure antibody concentrations; (ii) laboratories often do not prepare age-matched normal ranges using serum from healthy children in their own assays; and (iii) isotype levels change with time in response to infections and with age so that abnormalities are often transient. IgG subclass deficiency (with normal total IgG) is common in pediatric clinics. Levels of IgG2 are low and responsiveness to unconjugated pneumococcal vaccine is often absent in children under 2 years of age. Some children develop this facet of the humoral immune system rather late and so up to the age of 5–6 years such findings may simply represent slow maturation that will resolve with time. Certain combinations of isotype deficiency are well recognized (e.g., low IgA with IgG2).

A small proportion of these children progress to develop CVID in adolescence. The management of such children is not standardized, but should be tailored to the frequency and severity of infections. Some children appear to benefit from antibiotic prophylaxis (see below). Occasional cases require IgG replacement therapy (see below), although very rarely for selective IgA deficiency alone. In our practice such children are offered immunologic review every 6–12 months in order that reassurance can be given as matters improve (as is usually the case) or appropriate treatment can be started and early Ig replacement treatment instituted in the rare cases that progress to CVID.

Specific antibody production defects

Occasionally, children with severe or recurrent infection

have normal IgA, IgM, IgG and IgG subclasses and the only humoral abnormality is an inability to make antibodies to specific antigens (in particular polysaccharides).[75] It is thus important to check child-specific antibody responses to vaccine antigens as part of the investigation for immunodeficiency. However, specific antibody deficiency can persist despite repeated immunization, whilst some individuals with persistently abnormal IgG subclasses respond well to protein and polysaccharide vaccines. IgG replacement treatment is occasionally needed but only after careful evaluation of the severity of the patients' infections, including a search for evidence of sinopulmonary damage.

Transient hypogammaglobulinemia of infancy

Serum IgG levels are higher at birth due to active transport of IgG across the placenta during the third trimester of pregnancy. Levels fall progressively, reaching a nadir at around 4–5 months and then rise toward adult levels throughout the first decade of life. In a small proportion of infants, immunoglobulin levels of one or more isotypes are low during the second half of the first year of life, later catching up and approaching normal levels.[76] This is usually uncovered during investigations for frequent infections in a baby who is often well by the time the result comes to light. It is unclear which of these infants form a distinct group as opposed to one extreme of normal. In practice, all that is usually required is reassurance and a repeat test at 18 months of age.

Disorders of phagocytic cells

Chronic granulomatous disease

Chronic granulomatous disease (CGD) is an inherited defect of the phagocyte nicotinamide adenine dinucleotide phosphate (NADPH) oxidase enzyme complex, which generates superoxide and other reactive oxygen species that are required to kill organisms ingested into phagosomes. The commonest gene defect, affecting *CYBA* (which encodes the cytoplasmic protein gp91phox), is inherited in an X-linked manner. Defects in the cytoplasmic components p67phox and p47phox are inherited in an autosomal recessive pattern, as are rare mutations in the second membrane component, p22phox.

The hallmark of the disease is acute, and potentially fatal, bacterial or fungal infection,[77] commonly acute suppurative lymphadenitis in the neck, axilla or groin. Liver abscesses, osteomyelitis, arthritis, pneumonia, skin sepsis and perianal abscesses are also seen. *Staphylococcus aureus*, *Burkholderia cepacia*, *Aspergillus* species and *Serratia marcescens* are common pathogens. Fungal infection starts with pneumonia, and progresses to pleural and spinal involvement; osteomyelitis and hepatic involvement are also seen. Once established, fungal infection is hard to treat and frequently fatal.

Noninfectious inflammatory granulomas cause bowel

disease, restrictive lung defects, genitourinary and upper gastrointestinal obstruction. Many children have a colitis, which may be clinically and histologically indistinguishable from Crohn disease. These noninfective manifestations may respond to corticosteroid treatment.[78] Female carriers of the X-linked form have an increased incidence of autoimmune diseases and mouth ulcers.

Prophylactic antibiotics and antifungals, particularly co-trimoxazole and itraconazole, reduce morbidity and mortality from bacterial infections in this disease.[79] Infections or unexplained fevers should be treated aggressively. Interferon (IFN)-γ is a useful adjunctive treatment in severe bacterial or fungal infections. White-cell infusions may be life-saving in severe infection. Registry data suggest that the outlook in early childhood has improved considerably in recent years, but considerable morbidity and mortality occurs and consideration should be given to bone marrow transplantation when a suitable donor is available.[80]

Other neutrophil disorders

These include neutropenia, Shwachman–Diamond syndrome, other enzymatic deficiencies resulting in neutrophil killing defects, Chédiak–Higashi syndrome, Griscelli syndrome, familial lymphohistiocytosis, and leukocyte adhesion deficiency, and are covered in Chapter 14.

Defects in the IL-12-dependent IFN-γ pathway

Defects in the IL-12-dependent IFN-γ pathway result in persistent, severe, invasive or intractable mycobacterial infections with bone and soft-tissue abscesses complicated by persistent discharging sinuses due to BCG (bacille Calmette–Guérin) or poorly pathogenic environmental nontuberculous mycobacteria; they are often fatal.[81] Invasive non-*Salmonella typhi* infections also occur. There is increased susceptibility to infection with human herpesviruses, respiratory syncytial virus and parainfluenza virus type 3. Infections result from a failure of upregulation of macrophage killing. The clinical picture depends on the precise molecular defect that is present. Defects have been described in a number of constituents of the IL-12-dependent IFN-γ pathway, including complete or partial IFN-γ-R1 deficiency, IL-12 p40 subunit deficiency, and complete IL-12 β1 subunit deficiency. The outcome for patients with complete IFN-γ-R1 deficiency is poor, whereas the phenotype of IL-12-deficient patients is milder with typically later onset.

Deficiency of plasma proteins

Specific complement component deficiencies (C1–C9)

Complement component deficiency is rare, although patients with defects in virtually all the proteins in the pathways have been described.[82] Deficiency is manifest as increased susceptibility to infection, collagen vascular disease or both. Many factors show "autosomal codominant" inheritance so that heterozygote individuals (with one "null" or mutated gene) have half normal levels of the component.[83] The commonest deficiency is of C2, with around 1 in 100 of the population carrying one C2 mutation and a frequency of around 1 in 10 000. It exemplifies this group of disorders; affected individuals may be asymptomatic, may suffer from a variety of autoimmune and vasculitic disorders or may develop recurrent bacteremia, particularly with encapsulated organisms such as *Streptococcus pneumoniae* and *Neisseria meningitidis*. Terminal pathway component deficiency is particularly associated with neisserial infection, and in some populations as many as 14% of children with invasive meningococcal infection may have a such a deficiency,[83] although complement deficiency accounts for less than 1% of cases of meningococcal disease in the UK.[84]

Mannose-binding lectin deficiency

Unlike eukaryotic cells, yeasts such as *Candida* species, mycobacteria and Gram-negative bacteria express high quantities of mannose-rich sugars on their surfaces. Mannose-binding lectin (MBL) is an opsonic protein synthesized in the liver, which recognizes foreign microbes by binding to such sugars, a nonspecific immune response. Low levels of MBL are found in approximately 1 in 100 individuals and most appear well. However, mutations in the MBL gene are found more frequently in individuals with severe or recurrent infections of different types suggesting that this may become important when another immune problem is present.[85] It may therefore be appropriate to measure serum levels of this protein with other investigations in these patients. Prophylactic antibiotics have been suggested for symptomatic patients.

Interaction of antibody and complement deficiencies

Defects in complement components of the early classical pathway are associated with poor antibody responses, presumably because antigen processing and presentation is impaired. Alternative pathway opsonization is less efficient in the absence of specific antibody to bacterial surfaces. There is evidence that antibody may "neutralize" surface molecules, such as sialic acid, which otherwise inhibit alternative pathway activation.

Management of complement deficiencies

Specific replacement therapies are not available. There is no evidence to support the use of fresh plasma infusions. Lifelong antibiotic prophylaxis is recommended, usually with penicillin, but compliance may be better with amoxicillin, which covers a wider range of organisms, has a longer dose interval and tastes nicer. Meningococcal, pneumococcal, and *Haemophilus influenzae* type B (Hib) vaccination to maintain protective antibody levels may help. Despite these measures we have seen breakthrough bacterial infections, which highlight the need to respond quickly to the early signs of sepsis and/or meningitis. It is our practice to see patients annually, to look for clinical signs of autoimmune disease, to look for autoantibodies and, more intermittently, to measure levels of antibody to pneumococcus, Hib and meningococcus.

Treatment of primary immunodeficiency disorders

Vaccination of the child with a potentially impaired immune response

Immunocompromised children need protection conferred by vaccination yet are less likely to be vaccinated because of false concerns about potential risks and lack of efficacy in immunodeficiency. Non-live vaccines pose no infectious risk, and live vaccines are sufficiently attenuated to be safe even in children with impaired immune responses. Thus immunodeficient children should be immunized but may require augmented dose regimens and additional vaccines not in routine universal use. BCG vaccine remains a concern in patients with significantly impaired T-cell immunity and with CGD. Measles, mumps and rubella vaccine is remarkably safe, and the balance of risk and benefit often favors use in the immunodeficient patient. Experience with varicella vaccine is growing: it may be better to expose high-risk patients to a two-dose course of attenuated vaccine virus, rather than allow their first encounter to be with the wild-type strain, although the need for passive protection with varicella zoster immunoglobulin following exposure may remain. The vaccine virus is sensitive to aciclovir, which can be used if significant vaccine-induced infection occurs. Children who have undergone bone marrow transplantation are normally re-immunised *de novo* with all antigens from around 12–18 months post BMT (Table 19.3). Conjugate rather than polysaccharide vaccines should be used in children at high risk of pneumococcal or meningococcal infection, such as those with asplenia, hyposplenism, sickle-cell disease, nephrotic syndrome or opsonic defects. Official

Table 19.3 Indications for vaccination following bone marrow transplantation (BMT).

12–18 months post BMT
T- and B-cell reconstitution
Ceased immunosuppression ≥ 6 months
Ceased pharmacologic dose of steroids ≥ 6 months

published guidelines on immunization of immunodeficient patients tend to be cautious. Expert advice should be sought in formulating immunization advice for a child with compromised immunity.[86]

Supportive care

Children with primary immunodeficiency disorders (PID) require good general pediatric care, with particular attention to growth, nutritional status, secondary dietary intolerances and psychological support. Prevention and early treatment of infections is of paramount importance. Genetic counseling is important, including carrier detection for female relatives of boys with X-linked PID.

Newborns with suspected severe PID should be isolated, and the number of persons involved with care restricted; individuals with respiratory or gastrointestinal symptoms of infection should avoid contact. Breast-feeding should be encouraged. Strict hand-washing procedures are mandatory.

Regular oral co-trimoxazole prophylaxis for *Pneumocystis carinii* is usually given for PID with reduced T-cell function (SCID, CD40L), but dapsone or atovaquone can be used, or inhaled pentamidine in older children. Co-trimoxazole prophylaxis also reduces the incidence of pyogenic infections in patients with phagocytic or humoral immunodeficiencies, in whom it is usually given once daily (30 mg/kg). Antifungal prophylaxis (usually itraconazole) may be used in patients with combined immunodeficiencies and CGD. Where the PID predisposes to infection with relatively few organisms, prophylaxis with a narrow-spectrum antibiotic should be used, for example penicillin for patients with terminal complement defects to prevent neisserial infection. Prophylactic antibiotics are commonly used for patients with minor humoral deficiencies such as symptomatic IgA deficiency. Antiviral prophylaxis with aciclovir is used in patients with cell-mediated immunodeficiency and post-BMT to prevent herpes simplex and CMV reactivation.

Passive immunization is the basis of immunoglobulin replacement therapy (see below), and specific hyperimmune globulins are available for post-exposure prophylaxis in primary or secondary immunodeficiency patients exposed to chickenpox or hepatitis B. After measles exposure, standard immunoglobulin is used. High-titer anti-respiratory syncytial virus (RSV) and monoclonal anti-RSV antibodies protect children with chronic lung disease from infection, and it therefore seems logical to use them in children with severe PIDs during the RSV season, although this has not been formally evaluated.

Recurrent infections cause severe life-limiting and life-threatening damage. Chronic lung disease leading to bronchiectasis is a serious complication, particularly in antibody deficiency states. Regular physiotherapy, sputum cultures to direct appropriate antibiotic therapy and monitoring of pulmonary function are useful. High-resolution computerized tomography may detect early damage or progression of existing lung damage. Breakthrough infections in spite of prophylactic antibiotics may be an indication for starting immunoglobulin therapy even if laboratory studies show only minor abnormalities of humoral immunity.

Treatment of infections

Infections require prompt, vigorous treatment with appropriate antibiotics. Broad-spectrum antimicrobial cover may be needed to cover unusual agents. In neutrophil disorders it is important to cover *Pseudomonas* and other Gram-negative bacilli. Systematic attempts at identification of the causative agent, including invasive diagnostic procedures such as bronchoalveolar lavage or open lung biopsy, should not prevent early treatment. Amphotericin is currently the first line of treatment for systemic fungal infection; promising new agents include voriconazole and caspofungin. Antiviral agents, such as the anticytomegalovirus agents ganciclovir and foscarnet, are particularly useful in the immunocompromised infant.

Blood product support

All blood products except IVIG and fresh frozen plasma contain viable leukocytes; when given to patients with severe T-cell deficiency or those undergoing BMT, all products should be irradiated with 20–30 Gy to prevent possible GVHD. Patients with no evidence of exposure to CMV should be given blood products from CMV antibody-negative donors. White-cell infusions, harvested from GCSF-primed donors, can be life-saving in patients with neutrophil function disorders who are not responding to antibiotics or antifungals.

Support for families and patients

Patient support organizations provide helpful information and advice; they can also arrange contact for families with the same (rare) disorders. In the UK the main one is the Primary Immunodeficiency Association (PIA) (http://www.pia.org.uk/). In the USA the main one is the Immune Deficiency Foundation (IDF) (http://www.primaryimmune.org/). Abundant information is published on the Internet but this can be confusing as much is produced without reference to expert advice.

Bone marrow transplantation

T-lymphocyte and phagocyte immunodeficiency disorders are potentially correctable by BMT;[87] patients with immediately life-threatening conditions, mainly SCID, have been treated with BMT for 30 years. An increasing understanding of the basis of PIDs, international registry data on their long-term outcome, together with greatly improved results from BMT, has led to more conditions being treated by BMT, such as Wiskott–Aldrich syndrome,[29] CD40L deficiency,[38] other

T-cell immunodeficiencies, CGD,[80] and other phagocyte deficiencies. Matched unrelated donors, particularly for non-SCID immunodeficiencies, peripheral blood and umbilical cord stem cells are being increasingly used.

Complications of bone marrow transplantation

These are covered in Chapter 3.

Matched related donor bone marrow transplantation

Usually only sibling donors can be a perfect HLA-antigen match, but when parents are consanguineous, other family members may be a full match. For SCID, prior immunosuppression ("conditioning") is not usually required. The risk of GVHD is low. Full and long-lasting immune reconstitution is usually achieved although in a few cases lack of B-lymphocyte engraftment necessitates continuing immunoglobulin therapy. Success rates are now in the order of 90% and failure is usually secondary to preexisting infection. Matched transplants for PID, where conditioning is needed to destroy a residual immune system capable of graft rejection, are also increasingly successful with survival improving from about 70% to 80%.[87]

Mismatched bone marrow transplantation

In an HLA-mismatched situation, GVHD can be prevented by removing T lymphocytes from marrow. T-lymphocyte-depleted stem cells produce precursor T lymphocytes, which are "educated" into a state of tolerance in the host thymus. Successful mismatched BMT is not as easily achieved as matched BMT. Even in SCID, the T-lymphocyte-depleted bone marrow can be rejected (or fail to take), and to prevent this, full conditioning therapy (marrow ablation) is often needed. Immune function develops more slowly, T-cell function taking 3–6 months and full immune reconstitution a year or more. B-lymphocyte function is often good following fully conditioned BMT,[88] although responses to polysaccharide antigens may remain poor.[89] The prolonged period of immunoincompetence increases the risk of opportunistic infection. Refinements of the technique over recent years have resulted in continuing improvement in results, with success rates for SCID of around 78% for T-lymphocyte-depleted grafts, and > 90% for matched sibling donors.[90] Success is dependent on the type of SCID, with better results for B⁺ SCID than the B⁻ phenotype.[91] Age at presentation also influences outcome, with very good results for those transplanted in the neonatal period, before they have contracted infections.[92]

The problems and risks of mismatched BMT together with greater availability and excellent results for unrelated donor umbilical cord stem cells mean that fewer mismatched hematopoietic stem cell (HSC) transplants are now performed.

Matched unrelated donor bone marrow transplantation

National and international registries of tissue-typed volunteers willing to donate bone marrow, as well as storage of screened umbilical cord blood donations, have greatly increased the availability of phenotypically identical HSC for transplantation. Umbilical HSC are particularly useful for infants with SCID,[93] where the inevitable delay in obtaining unrelated donor HSC may decrease the chance of successful transplantation. The relatively low stem cell numbers in umbilical donations is less of a problem for infants as their body weight is so much less than adults.

Other replacement therapies

Enzyme replacement

In ADA deficiency, purified bovine ADA conjugated with polyethylene glycol (PEG-ADA), given by regular intramuscular injection, can significantly improve immune function, but regular treatment is needed and the long-term outcome is not known. If a suitable donor is available, BMT seems the best treatment. The role of ADA replacement as an adjunct to transplantation is unclear.

Somatic gene therapy

This has been attempted in adenosine deaminase deficiency using *ADA*-transfected CD34+ autologous cells, and more recently for common γ-chain deficiency.[94] Unfortunately, insertional mutagenesis was associated with a life-threatening leukemia in 3 of the 11 patients. A number of other conditions may be amenable to gene therapy but at present BMT remains the best treatment except, perhaps, for the sickest patients for whom no matched donor is available.

Replacement of thymus function

Fetal thymus transplants, originally attempted 40 years ago but superseded by HSCT, have recently been again attempted for complete DiGeorge syndrome, with encouraging results.[95]

Replacement immunoglobulin therapy

This is the mainstay of treatment for antibody deficiency and some combined immunodeficiencies. The need for replacement immunoglobulin therapy must be evaluated on an individual patient basis. Absolute indications include quantitative defects (IgG less than the 5th centile for age or < 3 g/L in an older child) and qualitative defects (failure of response to booster vaccinations) in association with clinical features of immunodeficiency. Other indications include failure of antibiotic prophylaxis in a child with quantitatively minor

Ig abnormalities (e.g., IgA and IgG subclass deficiency) and risk of end-organ damage (e.g., bronchiectasis) in a child with any degree of antibody deficiency.

Replacement immunoglobulin must contain the full range of protective antibodies in order to provide effective prophylaxis against infections. Human plasma is used as the source, and to ensure that IVIG contains the full spectrum of protective antibody, preparations are made from pooled (5000–10 000 donors) plasma donations, albeit with an associated very small risk of transmitted infection. Pools are screened for known agents (e.g., hepatitis B and C), and cold ethanol precipitation, universally used in plasma fractionation, kills some viruses, including HIV; a further viral inactivation step such as pasteurization or nanofiltration is employed. There is a theoretical risk of transmission of variant Creutzfeldt–Jakob disease (vCJD), and to minimize this plasma is no longer sourced from the UK. Patients should be evaluated by PCR for hepatitis B and C prior to commencement of therapy, and they require regular monitoring of immunoglobulin levels and liver function tests. Any elevation in liver function tests should prompt reevaluation of their hepatitis status. Batch numbers of all products administered must be recorded to facilitate patient tracing if there is a problem with an individual batch. Switching between different preparations should be avoided unless there are good clinical reasons, to minimize the chance of subsequent problems with hypersensitivity and adverse reactions.

IVIG therapy is given in doses of 0.3–0.5 g/kg every 3 weeks, infused over 2–3 hours. Immediate reactions to IVIG include nausea, vomiting, flushing, rigors and occasionally hypertension, normally controlled by slowing the infusion rate. Severe headaches may occur hours or days later. Anaphylactoid reactions are said to be a risk in IgA-deficient patients with anti-IgA antibodies,[96] but are very rare. Subcutaneous administration of immunoglobulin is effective in adults,[97] with far fewer side-effects. Recently this has been licensed for children; the lack of need for venous access and ease of parental training for home therapy make it attractive. Only a limited volume can be given in one site, necessitating two pumps and infusions for larger children. Most families do not find the inconvenience of giving weekly doses (instead of 3-weekly for IVIG) problematic, once established at home.

Acquired (secondary) immunodeficiency diseases

Much human disease is the direct or indirect result of infection (e.g., *Helicobacter pylori* in upper gastrointestinal disease and infectious agents in atheroma). Infectious agents may cause direct or toxin-mediated tissue injury (e.g., gas gangrene, tetanus) but immune/inflammatory responses to infection cause much pathophysiology (e.g., Gram-negative bacterial septicemia, postinfectious arthritis). Many infections induce

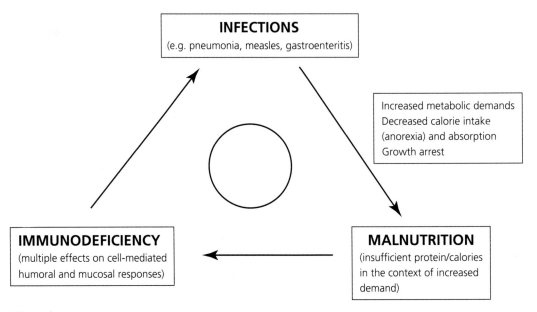

Fig. 19.6 Malnutrition cycle.

an immunodeficient state enhancing the risk of other infectious diseases. This is best exemplified by the vicious spiral of infection and childhood malnutrition (Fig. 19.6).

Even where nutrition is adequate, many childhood infections, such as measles, predispose to further infection. Secondary perioral herpes simplex infection is associated with pneumococcal pneumonia, and bacterial pneumonia may follow a viral upper respiratory prodrome. Epidemiologic studies have revealed a temporal association of outbreaks of meningococcal disease shortly after epidemics of influenza.[98]

Human immunodeficiency virus 1 and 2

The HIV epidemic has been remarkable both for the emergence of large-scale secondary immunodeficiency and the severe and unrelentingly progressive immunodeficiency it causes. HIV, an RNA lentivirus, has high replication rates even early in infection as well as high spontaneous mutation rates permitting rapid acquisition of resistance to antiviral agents.

Transmission and its prevention

In children acquisition is mainly by vertical transmission from an infected mother, either transplacentally, perinatally in the birth canal or postnatally via breast milk. Horizontal transmission from sexual activity, or infected blood products also occurs. Breast-feeding by HIV-positive mothers should be avoided in developed countries but the balance of risk and benefit may be reversed in other settings. Giving antiretroviral therapy to the mother and baby substantially reduces transmission.[99] The exact drug regimen depends on the resistance pattern of the HIV strain infection in the mother (2005 guidelines can be found at http://www.bhiva.org). Elective cesarean delivery is widely used but may not be imperative if the mother's viral load is undetectable. Low-cost measures such as vaginal viricides are useful in countries where perinatal infection is common and systemic antiviral agents are unavailable. Use of barrier contraception not only prevents the spread of HIV but also other sexually transmitted diseases, which may act as cofactors in HIV-related illness. Because these forms of intervention have the potential to prevent many cases of pediatric HIV infection there is an urgent need to institute effective programs of antenatal testing, particularly in areas of relatively high prevalence. Such programs were instituted in the UK between 2000 and 2003 and, in the context of rising rates of new HIV diagnoses particularly in heterosexuals, is resulting in prevention of significant numbers of childhood cases (http://www.hpa.org.uk/infections/topics_az/hiv_and_sti/publications/annual2004/annual2004.htm).

Manifestations

Staging of HIV disease has evolved over the years; current definitions are as shown in Table 19.4. The progression of HIV has slowed dramatically since the introduction of highly active antiretroviral therapy (HAART). The clinical features are often distinct from those seen in adults. In some children, particularly with a high viral load due to prenatal infection, there is rapid and often fatal progression during the first year of life, whereas the remainder progress heterogeneously toward severe immunosuppression usually between 5 and 10 years of age. Infections with encapsulated bacteria, in particular *Streptococcus pneumoniae*, including septicemia,

Table 19.4 Clinical staging of HIV-related disease in children.

Category	Features
N	Asymptomatic
A	Mildly symptomatic. At least two of:
	Lymphadenopathy
	Hepatomegaly
	Splenomegaly
	Parotitis
	Rash
	Ear, nose and throat infections
B	Moderately symptomatic
	Single episode of a severe bacterial infection
	Lymphocytic interstitial pneumonitis
	Anemia, neutropenia, thrombocytopenia
	Cardiomyopathy, nephropathy, hepatitis, diarrhea
	Candidiasis, severe varicella zoster or herpes simplex virus
C	Severely symptomatic
	Two serious bacterial infections
	Encephalopathy (acquired microcephaly, cognitive delay, abnormal neurology)
	Wasting syndrome (severe failure to thrive or downward-crossing two weight centiles)
	Opportunistic infections (*Pneumocystis carinii* pneumonia, cytomegalovirus, toxoplasmosis, disseminated fungal infections)
	Disseminated mycobacterial disease
	Cancer (Kaposi sarcoma, lymphomas)

Reproduced with permission from Ref. 107.

pneumonia and otitis media, are a particular problem. As immunosuppression advances, opportunistic infections including *Pneumocystis carinii* pneumonia, mycobacterial infection (both typical and atypical) and cryptosporidial diarrhea can occur, although infections such as CMV and toxoplasmosis, which are common in adults, are seen less often in children.

An insidious progressive lymphocytic intestinal pneumonitis is seen in some cases. Although really a histologic diagnosis, it is usually made in practice on clinical and radiologic evidence alone. Its etiology is obscure but may be due to chronic viral infection. It is associated with significant respiratory morbidity.[100] Neurologic disease is also well described in children with HIV, manifesting variously as developmental delay and regression, paresis and encephalopathy. Malignancies are also a feature, in particular lymphoma,[101] and growth failure can be a major problem.

The progression of the immunodeficiency can be followed by monitoring the fall in the peripheral blood count of CD4+ T lymphocytes, which are selectively infected and destroyed by HIV. The normal range for CD4 counts varies with age and so must be compared with age-appropriate normal ranges. Quantitative measurement of HIV genomic RNA by PCR in plasma is now an additional standard for monitoring disease progression and response to therapy.

Specific and adjunctive treatment

Until the mid-1990s medical management of pediatric HIV infection consisted mainly of prophylaxis and treatment of secondary infections with antimicrobial agents combined with the use of one available antiretroviral drug, azidothymidine. Co-trimoxazole is widely used for prophylaxis against *Pneumocystis carinii* pneumonia and bacterial infection, with dapsone being used as an alternative when the former is not well tolerated. The importance of appropriate neurodevelopmental, dietetic, social and psychological support for the children and their families is well established.[102] The years 1996–97 saw the arrival of HAART, when a large number of new antiretroviral agents were used in combination, with dramatic results.

Agents in general use can now be classified into three main groups:
- nucleoside analog reverse transcriptase inhibitors (RTIs), such as azidothymidine or zidovudine, didanosine, lamivudine, and stavudine, and related nucleotide reverse transcriptase inhibitors (e.g., tenofovir);
- nonnucleoside RTIs such as nevirapine and efavirenz;
- protease inhibitors such as nelfinavir and ritonavir, the latter often used in small doses in combination with other protease inhibitors such as lopinavir, promoting their effectiveness by inhibiting their metabolism.

Several other promising classes of drugs are emerging, the most advanced being fusion inhibitors such as enfuvirtide. Despite the immense success of HAART, the emergence of resistance and short- and long-term drug toxicity are major issues, as are convenience of dosing regimens and palatability. HAART is also expensive.

Children with HIV should be followed in a center providing up-to-date management and offering participation in multicenter therapeutic trials, which are essential to evaluate the best form of HAART. Children with HIV usually have parents with HIV, often affected by social deprivation and isolation. Combining medical care with psychological and social support in a family clinic is an excellent way of caring for these families[102] (http://www.medfash.org.uk/publications/documents/Recommended_standards_for_NHS_HIV_services.pdf). It should be remembered that the number of children affected indirectly by HIV, through illness or death in their parents or other family members, greatly exceeds those actually infected with the virus. The main hope for effective control and eradication of HIV infection must be through development of a vaccine.

Hyposplenism

Posttraumatic splenectomy is rare in childhood. However,

primary asplenia or hyposplenia, splenectomy for malignant, hematologic or immunologic indications, or reduced splenic function secondary to hemoglobinopathy, lymphoproliferative diseases, inflammatory bowel disease or following irradiation for BMT are seen more often. Hyposplenism is associated with an enhanced risk of fulminant bacterial infection,[103] particularly in early childhood. This is because the spleen acts as a filter for bacteria and parasitized erythrocytes. Furthermore, many disorders associated with hyposplenism or requiring splenectomy cause immunodeficiency either directly (e.g., Wiskott–Aldrich syndrome and haematologic malignancy) or through their treatment (e.g., chemotherapy or steroids).

Streptococcus pneumoniae (with a mortality of up to 60%) and *Neisseria meningitidis* cause most infections.[104] The risk of 0.42% per year is significant when viewed over a lifetime, and is four times higher in young children with congenital asplenia, where other aspects of immunity are less effective and pathogens include *Haemophilus influenzae* and Gram-negative organisms. Patients are also at enhanced risk of *Escherichia coli* infection, malaria, babesiosis and DF-2 bacillus (*Capnocytophaga canimorsus*) infection following dog bites.

The immunodeficiency is multifactorial, but largely functional. Failure to clear opsonized bacteria, lack of a B-lymphocyte reservoir, and low activity of the alternative pathway of complement, found in 10% of splenectomized and 16% of sickle-cell patients, all contribute. In older patients, IgG responses to pneumococcal vaccine are close to normal although low serum IgM levels have been reported; antipolysaccharide IgG levels decay more quickly.[105]

All children with hyposplenism should receive continuous daily oral antibiotic prophylaxis with phenoxymethylpenicillin, amoxicillin or, in allergic patients, erythromycin. Some experts use co-trimoxazole prophylaxis in children up to the age of 5 years. However, these treatments do not guarantee protection against invasive infection, so urgent medical advice should still be sought when the child is feverish or unwell so that appropriate intravenous antimicrobial therapy can be instituted if necessary.

Hyposplenic children should be immunized routinely. The polysaccharide 23-valent pneumococcal and 2- and 4-valent meningococcal vaccines are poorly immunogenic in children under 2 years of age but can be given to hyposplenic children at age 2 years. Conjugate pneumococcal vaccine is now used in preference in this group of children regardless of age by many practitioners, despite narrower serotype coverage, because of enhanced long-term protection against the commoner serotypes. Immunization should be performed prior to elective splenectomy. Serotype-specific antipneumococcal antibody levels may be measured periodically, and patients revaccinated if levels are low. Influenza vaccine can be given each autumn to reduce the risk of secondary bacterial infection.

References

1. Janeway CA, Travers P, Walport M, Shlomchick M. *Immunobiology, The Immune System in Health and Disease*, 6th edn. Edinburgh: Churchill Livingstone, 2004.
2. Chapel H, Geha R, Rosen F, for the IUIS PID classification committee. Primary immunodeficiency diseases: an update. *Clin Exp Immunol* 2003; **132**: 9–15.
3. Fischer A. Primary immunodeficiency diseases: an experimental model for molecular medicine. *Lancet* 2001; **357**: 1863–9.
4. Moshous D, Pannetier C, Chasseval R *et al.* Partial T and B lymphocyte immunodeficiency and predisposition to lymphoma in patients with hypomorphic mutations in Artemis. *J Clin Invest* 2003; **111**: 381–7.
5. Ozsahin H, Arredondo-Vega FX, Santisteban I *et al.* Adenosine deaminase deficiency in adults. *Blood* 1997; **89**: 2849–55.
6. Frucht DM, Gadina M, Jagadeesh GJ *et al.* Unexpected and variable phenotypes in a family with JAK3 deficiency. *Genes Immun* 2001; **2**: 422–32.
7. Noguchi M, Yi H, Rosenblatt HM *et al.* Interleukin-2 receptor gamma chain mutation results in X-linked severe combined immunodeficiency in humans. *Cell* 1993; **73**: 147–57.
8. Macchi P, Villa A, Giliani S *et al.* Mutations of Jak-3 gene in patients with autosomal severe combined immune deficiency (SCID). *Nature* 1995; **377**: 65–8.
9. Roifman CM, Zhang J, Chitayat D, Sharfe N. A partial deficiency of interleukin-7R alpha is sufficient to abrogate T-cell development and cause severe combined immunodeficiency. *Blood* 2000; **96**: 2803–7.
10. Cederbaum SD, Kartila I, Runoin DL *et al.* The chondro-osseous dysplasia of adenosine deaminase deficiency with severe combined immunodeficiency. *J Pediatr* 1976; **89**: 737–42.
11. Rogers MH, Lwin R, Fairbanks L, Gerritsen B, Gaspar HB. Cognitive and behavioral abnormalities in adenosine deaminase deficient severe combined immunodeficiency. *J Pediatr* 2001; **139**: 44–50.
12. Cohen A, Grunebaum E, Arpaia E *et al.* Immunodeficiency caused by purine nucleoside phosphorylase deficiency. *Immunol Allergy Clin North Am* 2000; **20**: 143–59.
13. Markert ML. Purine nucleoside phosphorylase deficiency. *Immunodefic Rev* 1991; **3**: 45–81.
14. Schwarz K, Gauss GH, Ludwig L *et al.* RAG mutations in human B cell-negative SCID. *Science* 1996; **274**: 97–9.
15. Moshous D, Callebaut I, de Chasseval R *et al.* Artemis, a novel DNA double-strand break repair/V(D)J recombination protein, is mutated in human severe combined immune deficiency. *Cell* 2001; **105**: 177–86.
16. Omenn GS. Familial reticuloendotheliosis with eosinophilia. *N Engl J Med* 1965; **273**: 427–32.
17. Villa A, Santagata S, Bozzi F *et al.* Partial V(D)J recombination activity leads to Omenn syndrome. *Cell* 1998; **93**: 885–96.
18. Muller SM, Ege M, Pottharst A, Schulz AS, Schwarz K, Friedrich W. Transplacentally acquired maternal T lymphocytes in severe combined immunodeficiency: a study of 121 patients. *Blood* 2001; **98**: 1847–51.
19. Klein C, Lisowska-Grospierre B, LeDeist F, Fischer A, Griscelli C. Major histocompatibility complex class II deficiency: clinical

manifestations, immunologic features, and outcome. *J Pediatr* 1993; **123**: 921–8.

20. Masternak K, Muhlethaler-Mottet A, Villard J, Peretti M, Reith W. Molecular genetics of the bare lymphocyte syndrome. *Rev Immunogenet* 2000; **2**: 267–82.

21. Piketty C, Weiss L, Kazatchkine M. Idiopathic CD4 lymphocytopenia. *Presse Med* 1994; **23**: 1374–5.

22. Fischer A. Severe combined immunodeficiencies (SCID). *Clin Exp Immunol* 2000; **122**: 143–9.

23. Hague RA, Rassam S, Morgan G, Cant AJ. Early diagnosis of severe combined immune deficiency syndrome. *Arch Dis Child* 1994; **70**: 260–3.

24. Aspenstrom P, Lindberg U, Hall A. Two GTPases, Cdc42 and Rac, bind directly to a protein implicated in the immunodeficiency disorder Wiskott–Aldrich syndrome. *Curr Biol* 1996; **6**: 70–5.

25. Zhu Q, Zhang M, Blaese RM *et al*. The Wiskott–Aldrich syndrome and X-linked congenital thrombocytopenia are caused by mutations of the same gene. *Blood* 1995; **86**: 3797–804.

26. Devriendt K, Kim AS, Mathijs G *et al*. Constitutively activating mutation in WASP causes X-linked severe congenital neutropenia. *Nat Genet* 2001; **3**: 313–17.

27. Westerberg L, Larsson M, Hardy SJ, Fernandez C, Thrasher AJ, Severinson E. Wiskott-Aldrich syndrome protein deficiency leads to reduced B-cell adhesion, migration, and homing, and a delayed humoral immune response. *Blood* 2005; **105**: 1144–52.

28. de Noronha S, Hardy S, Sinclair J *et al*. Impaired dendritic-cell homing in vivo in the absence of Wiskott-Aldrich syndrome protein. *Blood* 2005; **105**: 1590–7.

29. Filipovich AH, Stone JV, Tomany SC *et al*. Impact of donor type on outcome of bone marrow transplantation for Wiskott-Aldrich syndrome: collaborative study of the International Bone Marrow Transplant Registry and the National Marrow Donor Program. *Blood* 2001; **97**: 1598–603.

30. Sumegi J, Huang D, Lanyi A *et al*. Correlation of mutations of the SH2D1A gene and Epstein-Barr virus infection with clinical phenotype and outcome in X-linked lymphoproliferative disease. *Blood* 2000; **96**: 3118–25.

31. Morra M, Howie D, Grande MS *et al*. X-linked lymphoproliferative disease: A progressive immunodeficiency. *Ann Rev Immunol* 2001; **19**: 657–82.

32. Coffey AJ, Brooksbank RA, Brandau O *et al*. Host response to EBV infection in X-linked lymphoproliferative disease results from mutations in an SH2-domain encoding gene. *Nat Genet* 1998; **20**: 129–35.

33. Henter JI, Arico M, Egeler RM *et al*. HLH-94: a treatment protocol for hemophagocytic lymphohistiocytosis. HLH Study Group of the Histiocyte Society. *Med Pediatr Oncol* 1997; **5**: 342–7.

34. Gennery AR, Barge D, O'Sullivan JJ, Flood TJ, Abinun M, Cant AJ. Antibody deficiency and autoimmunity in 22q11.2 deletion syndrome. *Arch Dis Child* 2002; **86**: 422–5.

35. Moylett EH, Wasan AN, Noroski LM, Shearer WT. Live viral vaccines in patients with partial DiGeorge syndrome: clinical experience and cellular immunity. *Clin Immunol* 2004; **112**: 106–12.

36. Markert ML, Alexieff MJ, Li J, Sarzotti M *et al*. Postnatal thymus transplantation with immunosuppression as treatment for DiGeorge syndrome. *Blood* 2004; **104**: 2574–81.

37. Levy J, Espanol-Boren T, Thomas C *et al*. Clinical spectrum of X-linked hyperIgM syndrome. *J Pediatr* 1997; **131**: 47–54.

38. Gennery AR, Khawaja K, Veys P *et al*. Treatment of CD40 ligand deficiency by hematopoietic stem cell transplantation: a survey of the European experience, 1993–2002. *Blood* 2004; **103**: 1152–7.

39. de la Salle H, Hanau D, Fricker D *et al*. Homozygous human TAP peptide transporter mutation in HLA class I deficiency. *Science* 1994; **265**: 237–41.

40. Bleesing JHJ, Straus SE, Fleisher TA. Autoimmune lymphoproliferative syndrome: a human disorder of abnormal lymphocyte survival. *Pediatr Clin North Am* 2000; **47**: 1291–310.

41. Straus SE, Jaffe ES, Puck JM *et al*. The development of lymphomas in families with autoimmune lymphoproliferative syndrome with germline Fas mutation defective apoptosis. *Blood* 2001; **98**: 194–200.

42. The Finnish-German APECED Consortium. An autoimmune disease, APECED, caused by mutations in a novel gene featuring two PHD-type zinc-finger domains. Autoimmune Polyendocrinopathy-Candidiasis-Ectodermal Dystrophy Consortium. *Nat Genet* 1997; **17**: 399–403.

43. Makitie O, Kaitila I, Savilahti E. Susceptibility to infections and in vitro immune functions in cartilage-hair hypoplasia. *Eur J Pediatr* 1998; **157**: 816–20.

44. Makitie O, Kaitila I. Cartilage-hair hypoplasia: clinical manifestations in 108 Finnish patients. *Eur J Pediatr* 1993; **152**: 211–17.

45. Gennery AR, Cant AJ, Jeggo PA. Immunodeficiency associated with DNA repair defects. *Clin Exp Immunol* 2000; 121: 1–7.

46. Chun HH, Gatti RA. Ataxia-telangiectasia, an evolving phenotype. *DNA Repair (Amst.)* 2004; **3**: 1187–96.

47. Lavin MF, Shiloh Y. The genetic defect in ataxia-telangiectasia. *Ann Rev Immunol* 1997; **15**: 177–202.

48. Stewart GS, Maser RS, Stankovic T *et al*. The DNA double-strand break repair gene hMRE11 is mutated in individuals with an ataxia-telangiectasia-like disorder. *Cell* 1999; **99**: 577–87.

49. The International Nijmegen Breakage Syndrome Study Group. Nijmegen breakage syndrome. *Arch Dis Child* 2000; **82**: 400–6.

50. Gennery AR, Slatter MA, Bhattacharya A *et al*. The clinical and biological overlap between Nijmegen breakage syndrome and Fanconi anemia. *Clin Immunol* 2004; **113**: 214–19.

51. Varon R, Vissinga C, Platzer M *et al*. Nibrin, a novel DNA double-strand break repair protein, is mutated in Nijmegen breakage syndrome. *Cell* 1998; **93**: 467–76.

52. Joenje H, Patel KJ. The emerging genetic and and molecular basis of Fanconi anaemia. *Nat Rev Genet* 2001; **2**: 446–57.

53. Taniguchi T, Garcia-Higuera I, Xu B *et al*. Convergence of the Fanconi anemia and ataxia telangiectasia signaling pathways. *Cell* 2002; **109**: 459–72.

54. German J. The immunodeficiency of Bloom syndrome. In: Ochs HD, Smith CIE, Puck JM (eds) *Primary Immunodeficiency Diseases; A Molecular and Genetic Approach*. Oxford: Oxford University Press, 1997; pp. 335–8.

55. Webster AD, Barnes DE, Arlett CF, Lehmann AR, Lindahl T. Growth retardation and immunodeficiency in a patient with mutations in the DNA ligase I gene. *Lancet* 1992; **339**: 1508–9.

56. O'Driscoll M, Cerosaletti KM, Girard PM *et al.* DNA ligase IV mutations identified in patients exhibiting developmental delay and immunodeficiency. *Mol Cell* 2001; **8**: 1175–85.

57. Abinun M, Spickett G, Appleton AL, Flood T, Cant AJ. Anhidrotic ectodermal dysplasia associated with specific antibody deficiency. *Eur J Pediatr* 1996; **155**: 146–7.

58. Doffinger R, Smahi A, Bessia C *et al.* X-linked anhidrotic ectodermal dysplasia with immunodeficiency is caused by impaired NF-κB signalling. *Nat Genet* 2001; **27**: 277–85.

59. Picard C, Puel A, Bonnet M *et al.* Pyogenic bacterial infections in humans with IRAK-4 deficiency. *Science* 2003; **299**: 2076–9.

60. Orange JS. Human natural killer cell deficiencies and susceptibility to infection. *Microbes Infect* 2002; **15**: 1545–58.

61. de Vries E, Koene HR, Vossen JM *et al.* Identification of an unusual Fc gamma receptor IIIa (CD16) on natural killer cells in a patient with recurrent infections. *Blood* 1996; **88**: 3022–7.

62. Lederman HM, Winkelstein JA. X-linked agammaglobulinemia: an analysis of 96 patients. *Medicine (Baltimore)* 1985; **64**: 145–56.

63. McKinney RE Jr, Katz SL, Wilfert CM. Chronic enteroviral meningoencephalitis in agammaglobulinemic patients. *Rev Infect Dis* 1987; **9**: 334–56.

64. MacLennan C, Dunn G, Huissoon AP *et al.* Failure to clear persistent vaccine-derived neurovirulent poliovirus infection in an immunodeficient man. *Lancet* 2004; **363**: 1509–13.

65. Wood PM, Mayne A, Joyce H, Smith CI, Granoff DM, Kumararatne DS. A mutation in Bruton's tyrosine kinase as a cause of selective anti-polysaccharide antibody deficiency. *J Pediatr* 2001; **139**: 148–51.

66. Plebani A, Soresina A, Rondelli R *et al.* Clinical, immunological, and molecular analysis in a large cohort of patients with X-linked agammaglobulinemia: an Italian multicenter study. *Clin Immunol* 2002; **104**: 221–30.

67. Conley ME, Broides A, Hernandez-Trujillo V *et al.* Genetic analysis of patients with defects in early B-cell development. *Immunol Rev* 2005; **203**: 216–34.

68. Revy P, Muto T, Levy Y *et al.* Activation-induced cytidine deaminase (AID) deficiency causes the autosomal recessive form of the hyper-IgM syndrome (HIGM2). *Cell* 2000; **102**: 565–75.

69. Imai K, Slupphaug G, Lee WI *et al.* Human uracil-DNA glycosylase deficiency associated with profoundly impaired immunoglobulin class-switch recombination. *Nat Immunol* 2003; **4**: 1023–8.

70. Vorechovsky I, Cullen M, Carrington M, Hammarstrom L, Webster AD. Fine mapping of IGAD1 in IgA deficiency and common variable immunodeficiency: identification and characterization of haplotypes shared by affected members of 101 multiple-case families. *J Immunol* 2000; **164**: 4408–16.

71. Kanegane H, Tsukada S, Iwata T *et al.* Detection of Bruton's tyrosine kinase mutations in hypogammaglobulinaemic males registered as common variable immunodeficiency (CVID) in the Japanese Immunodeficiency Registry. *Clin Exp Immunol* 2000; **120**: 512–17.

72. Gilmour KC, Cranston T, Jones A *et al.* Diagnosis of X-linked lymphoproliferative disease by analysis of SLAM-associated protein expression. *Eur J Immunol* 2000; **30**: 1691–7.

73. Cunningham-Rundles C, Bodian C. Common variable immunodeficiency: clinical and immunological features of 248 patients. *Clin Immunol* 1999; **92**: 34–48.

74. Liblau RS, Bach JF. Selective IgA deficiency and autoimmunity. *Int Arch Allerg Immunol* 1992; **99**: 16–27.

75. Epstein MM, Gruskay F. Selective deficiency in pneumococcal antibody response in children with recurrent infections. *Ann Allergy Asthma Immunol* 1995; **75**: 125–31.

76. Dalal I, Reid B, Nisbet-Brown E, Roifman CM. The outcome of patients with hypogammaglobulinemia in infancy and early childhood. *J Pediatr* 1998; **133**: 144–6.

77. Fischer A, Segal AW, Seger R, Weening RS. The management of chronic granulomatous disease. *Eur J Pediatr* 1993; **152**: 896–9.

78. Cale CM, Jones AM, Goldblatt D. Follow up of patients with chronic granulomatous disease diagnosed since 1990. *Clin Exp Immunol* 2000; **120**: 351–5.

79. Finn A, Hadzic N, Morgan G, Strobel S, Levinsky RJ. Prognosis of chronic granulomatous disease. *Arch Dis Child* 1990; **65**: 942–5.

80. Seger RA, Gungor T, Belohradsky BH *et al.* Treatment of chronic granulomatous disease with myeloablative conditioning and an unmodified hematopoietic allograft: a survey of the European experience 1985–2000. *Blood* 2002; **100**: 4344–50.

81. Remus N, Reichenbach J, Picard C *et al.* Impaired interferon gamma-mediated immunity and susceptibility to mycobacterial infection in childhood. *Pediatr Res* 2001; **50**: 8–13.

82. Johnston RB Jr. The complement system in host defense and inflammation: the cutting edges of a double-edged sword. *Pediatr Infect Dis J* 1993; **12**: 933–41.

83. Tedesco F, Nürnberger W, Perissutti S. Inherited deficiencies of the terminal complement components. *Int Rev Immunol* 1993; **10**: 51–64.

84. Hoare S, El-Shazali O, Clark JE, Fay A, Cant AJ. Investigation for complement deficiency following meningococcal disease. *Arch Dis Child* 2002; **86**: 215–17.

85. Turner MW, Hamvas RMJ. Mannose-binding lectin: structure, function, genetics and disease associations. *Rev Immunogenet* 2000; **2**: 305–22.

86. Skinner R, Cant A, Davies G, Finn AHR, Foot A. *Immunisation of the Immunocompromised Child. Best Practice Statement.* London: Royal College of Paediatrics and Child Health, 2002.

87. Antoine C, Muller S, Cant A *et al.* Long-term survival and transplantation of haemopoietic stem cells for immunodeficiencies: a report of the European experience 1968–99. *Lancet* 2003; **361**: 553–60.

88. Gennery AR, Dickinson AM, Brigham K *et al.* CAMPATH-1M T-cell depleted BMT for SCID: long-term follow-up of 19 children treated 1987–98 in a single center. *Cytotherapy* 2001; **3**: 221–32.

89. Slatter MA, Bhattacharya A, Flood TJ *et al.* Polysaccharide antibody responses are impaired post bone marrow transplantation for severe combined immunodeficiency, but not other primary immunodeficiencies. *Bone Marrow Transplant* 2003; **32**: 225–9.

90. Buckley RH, Schiff SE, Schiff RI *et al.* Hematopoietic stem-cell transplantation for the treatment of severe combined immunodeficiency. *N Engl J Med* 1999; **340**: 508–16.

91. Bertrand Y, Landais P, Friedrich W *et al.* Influence of severe

combined immunodeficiency phenotype on the outcome of HLA non-identical, T-cell-depleted bone marrow transplantation. *J Pediatr* 1999; **134**; 740–8.

92. Kane L, Gennery AR, Crooks BN, Flood TJ, Abinun M, Cant AJ. Neonatal bone marrow transplantation for severe combined immunodeficiency. *Arch Dis Child* 2001; **85**; F110–F113.

93. Bhattacharya A, Slatter MA, Chapman CE *et al.* Single centre experience of umbilical cord stem cell transplantation for primary immunodeficiency. *Bone Marrow Transplant* 2005; **36**: 295–9.

94. Cavazzana-Calvo M, Lagresle C, Hacein-Bey-Abina S, Fischer A. Gene therapy for severe combined immunodeficiency. *Annu Rev Med* 2005; **56**: 585–602.

95. Markert ML, Sarzotti M, Ozaki DA *et al.* Thymus transplantation in complete DiGeorge syndrome: immunologic and safety evaluations in 12 patients. *Blood* 2003; **102**: 1121–30.

96. Misbah SA, Chapel HM. Adverse effects of intravenous immunoglobulin. *Drug Safety* 1993; **9**: 254–62.

97. Chapel HM, Spickett GP, Ericson D, Engl W, Eibl MM, Bjorkander J. The comparison of the efficacy and safety of intravenous versus subcutaneous immunoglobulin replacement therapy. *J Clin Immunol* 2000; **20**: 94–100.

98. Hubert B, Watier L, Garnerin P, Richardson S. Meningococcal disease and influenza-like syndrome: a new approach to an old question. *J Infect Dis* 1992; **166**: 542–5.

99. Connor EM, Sperling RS, Gelber R *et al.* Reduction of maternal-infant transmission of human immunodeficiency virus type 1 with zidovudine treatment. Pediatric AIDS Clinical Trials Group Protocol 076 Study Group. *N Engl J Med* 1994; **331**: 1173–80.

100. Sharland M, Gibb DM, Holland F. Respiratory morbidity from lymphocytic interstitial pneumonitis (LIP) in vertically acquired HIV infection. *Arch Dis Child* 1997; **76**: 334–6.

101. Evans JA, Gibb DM, Holland FJ, Tookey PA, Pritchard J, Ades AE. Malignancies in UK children with HIV infection acquired from mother to child transmission. *Arch Dis Child* 1997; **76**: 330–3.

102. Gibb DM, Masters J, Shingadia D *et al.* A family clinic: optimising care for HIV infected children and their families. *Arch Dis Child* 1997; **77**: 478–82.

103. Cullingford GL, Watkins DN, Watts AD, Mallon DF. Severe late postsplenectomy infection. *Br J Surg* 1991; **78**: 716–21.

104. Holdsworth RJ, Irving AD, Cuschieri A. Postsplenectomy sepsis and its mortality rate: actual versus perceived risks. *Br J Surg* 1991; **78**: 1031–8.

105. Spickett GP, Bullimore J, Wallis J, Smith S, Saunders P. Northern Region asplenia register – analysis of first two years. *J Clin Pathol* 1999; **52**: 424–9.

106. Roitt I, Delves PJ (eds). *Essential Immunology*, 10th edn. Oxford: Blackwell Science, 2001.

107. Sharland M, Gibb D, Tudor-Williams G, Walters S, Novelli V. Paediatric HIV infection. *Arch Dis Child* 1997; **76**: 293–6.

20 Clinical features and therapy of lymphoblastic leukemia

Owen P. Smith and Ian M. Hann

Acute lymphoblastic leukemia (ALL) is the commonest malignancy in children, comprising about 30–35% of all childhood cancers. Only 30 years ago this disease was fatal within 6 months in the vast majority of children.[1] In 1965, less than 1% of children with ALL were expected to be long-term survivors;[2] however, today, approximately 80% of children and adolescents with ALL are cured.[3–5] Furthermore, 20–30% of children with leukemic relapse have a long-lasting second remission with the chance of cure with second-line treatment.[6,7] This success was made possible by a series of carefully designed clinical trials both in the USA and Europe, pioneered by Pinkel and colleagues at St Jude Children's Research Hospital in Memphis, and by several groups in Europe. Despite this progress in treatment outcome, the absolute number of children with ALL who relapse and eventually die of their leukemia still exceeds the absolute number of children with newly diagnosed acute myeloid leukemia (AML). Thus, childhood ALL continues to contribute significantly to the overall mortality of childhood cancer.

Clinical characteristics

The clinical presentation of ALL is determined by the degree of marrow failure, caused by the infiltration of lymphoblasts and extramedullary organ infiltration. About two-thirds of children with ALL will have had signs and symptoms of disease for less than 4 weeks at the time of diagnosis; however, a history of some months is also compatible with the diagnosis of ALL. The first symptoms are usually nonspecific and include lethargy, unrelenting fatigue, bone pain or loss of appetite. More specific symptoms such as anemia, hemorrhage and infections are a consequence of lymphoblasts occupying the bone marrow and disturbing the residual normal hematopoiesis. Signs and symptoms of childhood ALL are listed in Table 20.1. It is to be noted that there is an association with Down syndrome, where the risk of developing ALL is at least 15-fold greater than usual.[8–11] Other associations, for example with immunodeficiency disorders, are very rare.

Once leukemia is suspected from the history and clinical symptoms, the evaluation of a blood count and especially microscopic evaluation of a blood smear allows an immediate diagnosis in many cases. However, a normal blood picture and normal blood smear do not exclude ALL. Thus, bone marrow aspiration must be performed immediately if there is any suspicion of ALL. In the past many children with a "rheumatic" presentation were erroneously treated with steroids. This practice is now thankfully far less common, as

Signs of anemia	Lethargy, weariness, fatigue, rapid exhaustion, lack of appetite Laboratory: normochromic, normocytic anemia
Signs of susceptibility to infections	Febrile illness Laboratory: reduced absolute number of neutrophils
Signs of bleeding tendency	Purpura, mucosal bleeding, haematomas and bruising Laboratory: thrombocytopenia and occasional coagulopathy
Signs of organ infiltration	Bone and joint discomfort, hepatomegaly and splenomegaly, generalized lymph node swelling, mediastinal mass and subsequent superior vena cava obstruction
Signs of systemic disease	Fever of unknown origin, weight loss, night sweats

Table 20.1 Signs and symptoms in children with acute leukemias.

Table 20.2 Differential diagnosis of acute leukemia in children and adolescents.

Aplastic anemia and other marrow failure syndromes (e.g., Fanconi disease)	Less common than leukemia, marrow aspiration, trephine biopsy and DEB test
Rheumatic disease (e.g., Still disease, rheumatic fever)	Rare, bone marrow aspiration
Osteomyelitis	Radiography, skeletal scintigraphy, bone marrow aspiration
Bone marrow dissemination of different malignancies (e.g., neuroblastoma, rhabdomyosarcoma)	Tumor markers, immunophenotyping, bone marrow aspiration, immunohistochemistry, trephine biopsy
Myeloproliferative/myelodysplastic syndrome	Bone marrow aspiration, trephine biopsy, marrow cytogenetics, hemoglobin F level
Viral and other infection (e.g., infectious mononucleosis, cytomegalovirus and *Leishmania*)	Specific serology, bone marrow aspiration
Leukemoid reaction (e.g., in whooping cough, sepsis)	Bone marrow aspiration
Transient erythroblastopenia of childhood	Normal platelet and granulocyte count, bone marrow aspiration
Idiopathic thrombocytopenic purpura	Normal neutrophil and red blood cell count, bone marrow aspiration

DEB, di epoxy butane

it masks the underlying diagnosis and may lead to temporary remissions and drug resistance.

The differential diagnosis of ALL includes infections, other pediatric malignancies that involve the bone marrow, collagen vascular diseases, and other hematologic diseases such as idiopathic thrombocytopenic purpura (ITP) and aplastic anemia (Table 20.2).

ALL may present as an incidental finding on a routine blood count of an asymptomatic child or as a life-threatening hemorrhage or infection or episode of respiratory distress, especially in children with hyperleukocytosis, e.g., in T-cell ALL (T-ALL). Lymphadenopathy is commonly present and mostly correlates with a high white blood cell count (WBC) (lymphomatous feature). In about 30–60% of children with ALL, marked hepatomegaly and/or splenomegaly is found at diagnosis. Hepatosplenomegaly also correlates with a high WBC at diagnosis.

Although ALL is primarily a disease of the bone marrow and blood, any other organ may be infiltrated by leukemic blasts. Such infiltration may be clearly apparent clinically, such as lymphadenopathy or hepatosplenomegaly. However, leukemic infiltration of other organs may be occult and detectable only by histologic or cytologic examination or diagnostic imaging.

Mediastinal manifestations

Anterior mediastinal masses, mostly within the thymus, are present in about two-thirds of children with T-ALL but are extremely rare in other immunologic subtypes (Table 20.3). Leukemic pleural effusion may be associated with mediastinal masses in some children with T-ALL.[12] Superior vena cava syndrome and severe respiratory distress may occur in these children and may lead to medical emergencies. During

Table 20.3 Basic investigations required at diagnosis of childhood acute lymphoblastic leukemia.

Blood tests
Whole blood count, including platelets, hemoglobin, red cell indices and white cell count
Differential blood count
Lactate dehydrogenase
Electrolytes
Renal function (creatinine, urea, uric acid)
Liver function tests
Coagulation screen
Viral serology (Epstein–Barr virus, varicella zoster virus, cytomegalovirus, measles)

Bone marrow diagnostics
Bone marrow aspiration (if unsuccessful, trephine biopsy)
Morphology
Immunophenotyping
Cytogenetics and DNA content, looking especially for near-haploid and hypodiploid chromosome abnormalities
Molecular genetics, including t(4;11) and t(9;22) translocations and RUNX1 amplification

CNS diagnostics
Cerebrospinal fluid: cell count, cytospin preparation, protein, glucose and culture

Cardiology
Echocardiography

Diagnostic imaging
Chest radiography
Bone radiography if indicated
Abdominal sonography for liver, spleen, kidney size (optional)

Miscellaneous
Alkaline phosphatase and myeloperoxidase are sometimes required as marrow cytochemistry

induction chemotherapy these children may develop pronounced tumor lysis syndrome.

Central nervous system manifestations

Overt central nervous system (CNS) leukemia as defined by the presence of lymphoblasts in the cerebrospinal fluid (CSF) is found in 1.5–10% of children with newly diagnosed ALL, depending on their immunologic subtype (see below). CNS leukemia is more common in children with ALL of the relatively rare mature B-cell subtype, and in T-ALL and children with high WBCs. Children with CNS leukemia at diagnosis may present with diffuse or focal neurologic signs such as increased intracranial pressure (headache, vomiting, papilledema and lethargy), mostly without nuchal rigidity. Cranial nerve involvement, mostly involving nerves III, IV, VI and VII, may be found on careful neurologic evaluation. Occasionally, VI and VII nerve palsies occur without other evidence for CNS disease. CNS leukemia presents rarely with hypothalamic involvement, resulting in excessive weight gain and behavior disturbances.[13]

Leukemic blasts may enter the CNS by hematogenous spread or more rarely by direct extension of involved skull bone marrow through bridging veins to the superficial arachnoid. With progressive CNS leukemia, the blasts eventually infiltrate the deep arachnoid and then the pia/glial membrane and eventually invade brain parenchyma. In a severe combined immunodeficiency (SCID) mouse model, histologically detectable engraftment of leukemic cells in the skull, vertebral bone marrow and meninges preceded engraftment at other sites.[14]

Most children with CNS leukemia at presentation have CNS pleocytosis as a result of the presence of leukemic blasts. These blasts can be identified with the use of cytocentrifugation and May–Grünewald–Giemsa staining. Careful morphologic evaluation is necessary to distinguish leukemic blasts from reactive blood cells, which may be seen after intrathecal chemotherapy or during CNS infection. Contamination of the CNS with blood, as indicated by the presence of red blood cells, often makes the interpretation of morphologic examination difficult or even impossible. The incidence of CNS leukemia at presentation varies considerably depending on the diagnostic criteria used.[15] In 1986, the Rome International Workshop recommended an absolute leukocyte count of $\geq 5 \times 10^6$/L with unequivocal blasts in a cytocentrifuge preparation as the definition of cerebromeningeal leukemia.[16] In most trials, patients with CNS-3 overt disease at diagnosis (see below) are treated with 24-Gy cranial radiotherapy, but this has been dropped by some groups such as St Jude's, Memphis.

While some investigators reported that a low number of blasts in the CSF at presentation did not predict later development of overt CNS leukemia or CNS relapse,[17] several other studies have shown an increased risk of CNS relapse in patients with low levels of blasts (<5 per high-power field) and those in whom the CSF lumbar puncture was traumatic at diagnosis, presumably related to seeding of leukemic.[18] CNS status Classification:
- CNS-1 (no blast cells).
- CNS-2 (leukocyte count $< 5 \times 10^6$/L with morphologically detectable blasts).
- CNS-3 (leukocyte count $\geq 5 \times 10^6$/L with morphologically detectable blasts and/or cranial nerve involvement.[19]

The adverse effect of a CNS-2 classification and a traumatic lumbar puncture appear to be abrogated by the addition of two intrathecal therapies during induction. It should be noted that additional testing for clonality/immunophenotyping does not currently improve the diagnosis.

Leukemic blasts may persist within the CNS throughout induction chemotherapy because most drugs used in the treatment of ALL inadequately penetrate the CNS, thus allowing progressive growth of lymphoblasts or the emergence of resistant clones. Cytogenetic studies and patterns of systemic relapse following the appearance of CNS disease strongly suggest that the hematologic recurrence may be due to reseeding of leukemic blasts from the CNS to the marrow.[20,21]

Spinal cord involvement due to a localized epidural leukemic infiltrate may lead to spinal cord compression with back pain, weakness of the extremities, paralysis, and bladder or bowel incontinence.[22] Gadolinium-enhanced magnetic resonance tomography (MRT) is helpful in localizing the leukemic infiltrate and in differentiating epidural hematoma and vertebral body collapse due to leukemic osteopathy. This feature is more frequently seen with the lymphomatous presentation, and also at relapse.

Genitourinary manifestations

Overt testicular disease, found by careful palpation or sonography, is rare at presentation with ALL. However, leukemic blasts have been found by testicular biopsy in as many as 25% of boys at presentation.[23] Occult testicular involvement occurred only in boys with a WBC $> 25 \times 10^9$/L. The leukemic infiltration is found mainly in the interstitium.

Clinically overt testicular relapse is usually painless and unilateral. Some boys also show involvement of intraabdominal lymph nodes. Bilateral testicular biopsy often shows an occult leukemic infiltration of the contralateral testis at the time of unilateral testicular relapse. The relatively high incidence of testicular relapse compared with, for example, ovarian relapse may be because the blood–testes barrier is analogous to the blood–brain barrier. However, the wider use of intensified multidrug regimens in recent years, including high-dose chemotherapy with methotrexate, has significantly reduced overt relapse of the testes.[3] Thus the use of bilateral testicular biopsies, which was advocated for many years in some trials,[24] is no longer recommended.[25] Current protocols have also abandoned testicular radiotherapy for patients with clinically overt testicular involvement at diagnosis, and simply recommend an upgrading of the overall chemotherapy intensity (cf. St Jude's and MRC/NCRI protocols).

Renal infiltrates may lead to oliguria or may be asymptomatic and discovered by their presentation in large kidneys shown by sonography or computed tomography (CT). The incidence of pretherapeutic renal infiltration was 18% in one BFM study but the use of rasburicase in such cases makes the need for dialysis rare nowadays.[26] Priapism is very rarely found in boys with T-ALL and the hyperleukocytosis/leukostasis syndrome.[27]

Skeletal manifestations

About 20–30% of children with ALL present with severe pain, mainly in the lower extremities, leading to a limp or refusal to walk. These children suffer nearly exclusively from B-precursor ALL and often present with a normal blood count and low number or even absence of blood lymphoblasts (aleukemic leukemia), which often results in a delayed diagnosis.[28] Up to 20% of children with ALL present with characteristic bony radiographic changes, including transverse radiolucent lines in metaphyses, subperiostal new bone formation or osteolytic lesions mimicking primary bone tumors, diffuse demineralization (osteopenia) or vertebral collapse, mimicking Langerhans cell histiocytosis.[29,30] Pathologic fractures and vertebral collapses may occur secondary to severe osteopenia (leukemic osteopathy). Osteonecrosis, especially of the hip and knee, may also produce severe bone pain and is a rare complication of antileukemic therapy, especially with steroids.[31] Children with these problems rarely need specific orthopedic maneuvers/equipment, which can in fact lead to worsening of osteopenia especially of spinal lesions.

Gastrointestinal manifestations

Specific problems of the oral cavity are common in children with acute leukemia. Infection with *Candida albicans* (oral thrush) is common at diagnosis and during polychemotherapy, and regular mouth care along with antifungal agents is an essential part of supportive care. Petechiae, hemorrhage and gum bleeding occur frequently, especially in children with severe thrombocytopenia. Mucosal ulceration is also common, especially in the presence of profound neutropenia in addition to fungal or bacterial infections, particularly with *Streptococcus viridans* (*S. mitis*, *S. sanguis*, *S. hominis*). Viral infections, mainly due to herpes simplex virus (HSV), can be a problem in neutropenic children. *Candida* or HSV esophagitis characterized by retrosternal pain rarely occurs in neutropenic children with leukemia, because of the use of effective agents such as fluconazole.

Bleeding, as reflected by gross or occult blood in the stool, is the commonest gastrointestinal manifestation of leukemia and may be due to thrombocytopenia, disseminated intravascular coagulation (DIC), infiltration with leukemic cells, or infection (e.g., with *Candida*). Massive infiltration of intraabdominal lymph nodes, especially in the right lower quadrant, is frequently found in children with mature B-cell ALL.

A characteristic syndrome of right lower quadrant pain with tenderness, abdominal tension, vomiting and sepsis is often seen during profound neutropenia due to intensive polychemotherapy (neutropenic typhlitis or necrotizing enterocolitis).[32] Sonography may show a characteristic thickening of the gut wall in the right lower quadrant.[33] Peptic ulcers of the stomach and duodenum may be occasionally seen in children with ALL, especially during steroid treatment.

Severe hemorrhage or necrotizing pancreatitis can be found in children with ALL during asparaginase treatment, and can be extremely troublesome and difficult to diagnose. Amylase is often but not always elevated, when a high lipase may assist diagnosis.[34] Management of these conditions includes bowel rest, intravenous fluids and broad-spectrum antibiotics. Surgery is rarely indicated except in rare cases of perforation or peripheral abscess formation, which is usually due to Gram-negative organisms.[35,36] The differential diagnosis must include common childhood surgical problems, including appendicitis, cholangitis and intussusception.

Impairment of liver function with or without elevated bilirubin levels may be due to liver infiltration by leukemic blasts, chemotherapy-induced hepatotoxicity, especially during treatment with asparaginase, methotrexate and purine analogs, or viral hepatitis, especially with hepatitis B or C virus.[37] Rarely, patients can present at diagnosis with severe hepatic dysfunction due to liver infiltration.

Eye manifestations

Occult ocular involvement seen on careful ophthalmologic investigation may be found in up to one-third of newly diagnosed children with ALL.[38] Virtually all ocular structures have been found to be involved.[39] Retinal hemorrhages are presumably due to thrombocytopenia and may precede intracranial hemorrhage, especially in children with the hyperleukocytosis/leukostasis syndrome.[40] Overt leukemic infiltration of the eye is uncommon at presentation and is more usually associated with leukemic relapse.[41] About half of children with leukemic eye infiltration present with overt CNS relapse.[42] Oculomotor palsies and papilledema are frequent signs of meningeal leukemia at presentation or at the time of relapse. Thus, it has been suggested that the eye could be a sanctuary site in ALL, like the CNS and testes.[43]

Under the conditions of today's intensive polychemotherapy protocols, which include high-dose chemotherapy and CNS-directed treatment, the incidence of ocular manifestations of ALL is lower than in the past, as are the incidences of CNS and testicular manifestations.[3,44]

Cardiopulmonary manifestations

Leukemic involvement of the lungs and heart is rare. However, these manifestations may cause life-threatening problems in a child with ALL. Pericardial leukemic effusions are found by echocardiographic examination in about one-third of children with T-ALL and are often associated with leukemic pleural effusion and a mediastinal mass. A life-threatening hyperleukocytosis/leukostasis syndrome may cause massive respiratory distress due to infiltration and leukostasis within the lung in patients with high WBCs. Emergency leukapheresis or exchange transfusion can rarely be required as a life-saving emergency measure in this situation but much more commonly patients will respond better to intensive chemotherapy and supportive care.[45,46]

During polychemotherapy, pulmonary complications in children with leukemia almost always have an infectious origin. Differentiation between bacterial and fungal infections, leukemic infiltrations and hemorrhage is often possible with the help of diagnostic imaging, including high-resolution CT of the lungs.[47]

Severe cardiomyopathy in children with leukemia is seen during severe septicemia or metabolic disturbance in children with high blood counts and rapid lysis of lymphoblasts (tumor lysis syndrome). Late cardiomyopathy is found after extensive treatment with anthracyclines.[48,49]

The rare ALL subtype with hypereosinophilia[50] may present with life-threatening involvement of the heart, with mural thrombi of the myocardium or Löffler endocardial fibrosis.[51]

Skin manifestations

Skin infiltration is rarely seen in children with ALL in contrast to children with monocytic leukemia. However, lymphoblasts may proliferate within the skin secondary to intradermal bleeding due to thrombocytopenia. In the rare case of congenital leukemia, skin infiltration has been reported in about 50% of neonates.[52]

Laboratory findings

Laboratory data may show a broad spectrum of abnormal findings at presentation of ALL. Normochromic (normal mean cell hemoglobin), normocytic (normal mean corpuscular volume) anemia is present in about two-thirds of children with ALL and reflects progressive bone marrow failure. The WBC is raised higher than 10×10^9/L in about half of children with newly diagnosed ALL, reflecting the proliferative capacity of their lymphoblasts. However, in about 5% of children with ALL, the WBC is less than 2×10^9/L, often without detectable lymphoblasts in the blood. Rarely, ALL presents with an aplastic blood and marrow profile and in this situation there is initial marrow recovery followed shortly therafter by frank leukemia. Hypereosinophilia in the blood is rarely found and is associated with the t(5;14) translocation.[50] This hypereosinophilia has to be differentiated from AML M4 eosinophilia, where atypical eosinophils are found in the bone marrow.

Blood blasts may not always reflect the bone marrow status of leukemia. In some patients a pathologic shift to the left of the granulocyte series, with increased numbers of promyelocytes or even myeloblasts, can be found as a result of the leukoerythroblastic response to bone marrow infiltration seen in ALL, non-Hodgkin lymphoma (NHL), granulomatous infections, osteopetrosis, and metastatic tumors (e.g., neuroblastoma, Ewing's sarcoma, rhabdomyosarcoma). Thus, the definitive diagnosis of leukemia should not be made from peripheral blood smears alone.

Thrombocytopenia ($<100 \times 10^9$/L) is present in about 80% of children with ALL at diagnosis. The platelets are morphologically normal, and thrombocytopenia is accompanied by other hematologic or physical manifestations of leukemia in the vast majority of children.[53]

Bone marrow

Inspection of bone marrow smears is essential to establish the diagnosis of leukemia. Whereas a normal bone marrow usually contains < 5% of blast cells (M1 marrow), leukemic marrow generally contains > 40% and in most cases > 80% of blasts. By arbitrary convention, > 25% blasts (M3 marrow) is required to confirm the diagnosis of acute leukemia and to distinguish leukemia from NHL with bone marrow infiltration (stage IV NHL). For cytomorphologic purposes, anterior or posterior iliac crest aspirates smeared in the same way as blood smears are required. The sternum is not used for bone marrow aspiration in children because this procedure may be hazardous, especially to young children. In very young infants, some physicians prefer the tibia, but this can also be dangerous and is rarely necessary. A "dry tap" may be caused by bone infarction, myelofibrosis or bone necrosis,[54,55] and in such cases a bone marrow trephine biopsy should be performed and the aspirate repeated.

ALL is subclassified according to morphologic, immunologic and genetic features of the leukemic blasts cells. The primary diagnosis is generally based on examination of the bone marrow aspirate; other recommended tests are detailed in Table 20.3. The cytologic appearance of the blast cells in ALL can be highly variable, even in a single specimen, and no completely satisfactory morphologic classification has been devised. The French–American–British (FAB) classification distinguishes three morphologic subtypes (L1, L2 and L3) (Table 20.4).[56] L1 lymphoblasts are predominantly small with little cytoplasm; L2 cells are larger and pleomorphic with increased cytoplasm and sometimes an irregular nuclear shape and prominent nucleoli; L3 blasts have a deep-blue

Table 20.4 FAB morphologic classification for acute lymphoblastic leukemia.

	L1	L2	L3
Size of blast	Small, uniform	Large, variable	Medium to huge, uniform
Amount of cytoplasm	Scanty	Variable	Moderate
Cytoplasmic basophilia	Moderate	Variable	Intense
Cytoplasmic vacuoles	Variable	Variable	Prominent
Nucleus	Regular, occasional clefting, homogeneous chromatin	Irregular, clefting, common heterogeneous chromatin	Regular, no clefting, finely stippled chromatin
Nuceolus	0–1, inconspicuous	1 or more, prominent	2–5, prominent
Nuclear/cytoplasmic ratio	High	Low	Low

FAB, French–American–British.

Table 20.5 Immunophenotypic classification of B-lineage acute lymphoblastic leukemia (ALL).

Marker	B-precursor ALL	Pre-B ALL	B-ALL
CD10	+	±	±
CD19	+	+	+
CD20	±	±	+
CD22	−	−	+
CD24	+	+	+
CD34	+	−	−
Cytoplasmic CD79a	+	+	+
HLA-DR	+	+	+
Cytoplasmic μ	−	+	−
sIg	−	−	+
TdT	+	±	−

sIg, surface immunoglobulin; TdT, terminal deoxynucleotidyl transferase.

cytoplasm with prominent vacuoles and homogeneous nuclear chromatin with prominent nucleoli and immunophenotypic features of immature B-cell ALL.

Granular ALL has been described as a rare variant in about 3% of cases.[28] In contrast to myeloblasts, the myeloperoxidase stain is always negative in granular ALL. Immunophenotyping reveals CD10 positivity in nearly all cases

with this morphologic subtype.[57] The usual patterns of immunophenotypes in B- and T-cell ALL are shown in Tables 20.5 and 20.6 and their relationships to cytomorphologic and cytogenetic classifications are shown in Table 20.7.

In about 10% of children with ALL, morphology alone does not produce a specific diagnosis, even with the use of cytochemical stains,[58] which can sometimes be useful (e.g., acid phosphatase staining the Golgi region in T-ALL).[59,60] The introduction of immunophenotyping and genetic classification of acute leukemias has revealed that some blasts show an ambiguous phenotype and genotype that do not allow clear differentiation between ALL and AML.[61] These leukemias have been referred to as mixed lineage,[62] biphenotypic,[63] or acute hybrid leukemias.[64] They may arise from malignant transformation of a progenitor cell capable of differentiation into more than one lineage (lineage promiscuity).[65] Alternatively, they may result from aberrant gene regulation not representative of normal hematopoiesis (lineage infidelity).[66] In B-precursor ALL, coexpression of one or more myeloid markers (e.g., CD13, CD33, CDw65) ranges from 4% to more than 20% depending on the criteria applied.[67,69] The prognostic significance of coexpression of myeloid markers is now clear: there is no impact of such changes in large modern treatment series.[68,70,71] ALL defined by morphologic and cytochemical criteria in which blast cells

Table 20.6 Immunophenotypic classification of T-cell acute lymphoblastic leukemia.

	CD1	CD2	CD3	SCD3	SCD3	CD4	CD5	CD7	CD8	TdT
Pre-T cell	−	−	+	−	−	−	−	+	−	+
Early cortical	−	+(75%)	+	−	−	−	+(90%)	+	−	+
Late cortical	+	+	+	+	+(25%)	+(90%)	+	+	+(90%)	+
Medullary	−	+	+	+	+	±	+	+	±	±

CD3, cytoplasmic CD3; SCD3, surface CD3; TdT, terminal deoxynucleotidyl transferase.

Table 20.7 Morphologic, immunologic and cytogenetic (MIC) classification of acute lymphoblastic leukemia (ALL).

MIC group	Immunologic markers								Karyotype
	FAB	CD2	CD7	CD10*	CD19	TdT	cIg	
Early B-precursor ALL	L1, L2		−	+	+	+	−	t(4;11), t(9;22)
Common ALL	L1, L2		−	+	+	+	−	6q−, near haploid, del(12) or t(9;22)
Pre-B ALL	L1		−	+	+	+	+	t(1;19), t(9;22)
B-cell ALL	L3		−	±	+	−	−	t(8;14), t(2;8), t(8;22)
Early T-precursor ALL	L1, L2	+	+		−	+		t/del(9p)
T-cell ALL	L1, L2	+	+		−	+		6q−

* CD10 is usually negative in cases of t(4;11) and positive in cases of t(9;22).

+, positive; −, negative; no symbol, not specified by MIC workshop. FAB, French–American–British classification; TdT, terminal deoxynucleotidyl transferase.

coexpress myeloid antigens most probably represents phenotypic deviations and should be classified as ALL.[72] True biphenotypic leukemias with two separate blast cell populations are very rare and have poor prognosis.

Most cases of morphologically and cytochemically undifferentiated acute leukemias can be immunophenotypically classified as either B-precursor ALL or AML M0. However, in about 2% of childhood ALL,[3] the cellular origin of blasts remains obscure.[73] These leukemias are probably derived from a very immature hematopoietic progenitor cell. In recent years, microarry gene technology has been very helpful in categorizing these cases.[74]

Cytomolecular genetics

Cytogenetic analysis of leukemic blasts provides important information in up to 90% of cases of ALL, and this information is clinically relevant for diagnosis and prognosis of childhood leukemia (Tables 20.7 and 20.8).[75] There are two major classes of cytogenetic aberrations: those that result in the visible loss or gain of chromosomal material and those that result in a balanced exchange without apparent loss or gain of DNA.[76] Loss may be characterized as partial (deletion, abbreviated as del) or complete loss of a chromosome (monosomy). Gains may refer to portions of chromosomes (e.g., duplications) or whole chromosomes (trisomy, tetrasomy). Unidentified abnormal chromosomes are labeled as markers (mar). Balanced alterations involve the reciprocal exchange of genetic material either between two or more chromosomes (translocations, t) or between various portions of one chromosome (inversions, inv).

While this type of conventional cytogenetic information (karyotypic analysis) provided information that led to the identification and localization of genes involved in leukemogenesis, there are a number of limitations. Firstly, only a few

Table 20.8 Cytogenetic abnormalities in acute lymphoblastic leukemia (ALL).

Structural chromosome changes in B-ALL
t(9;22)(q34;q11)
Cryptic t(12;21)(p13;q22)
t(1;19)(q23;p13)
t(8;14)(q24;q32) and variants
MLL rearrangements (11q23)
  t(4;11)(q21;q23)
  t(6;11)(q27;q23)
  t(9;11)(p12;q23)
  t(10;11)(p12;q23)
  t(11;19)(q23;p13.3)

Structural chromosome changes in T-ALL
t(10;14)(q24;q11)
t(7;10)(q35;q24)
t(1;14)(p15;q11)
t(7;9)(q34;q32)
t(11;14)(p15;q11)20p
t(11;14)(p13;q1)
t(7;11)(q35;p13)
t(8;14)(q24;q11)
Others

Numerical chromosomal abnormalities
Hypodiploid
Hyperdiploid (47–49 chromosomes)
Hyperdiploid (>50 chromosomes)
Near triploidy
Near tetraploidy

cells in metaphase are analyzed. Secondly, analysis is entirely dependent on the production of high-quality metaphase preparations and analysis is significantly restricted for cells that have low mitotic rates or which cannot easily be grown in culture. It is also very labor-intensive. For these reasons, and because conventional karyotypic analysis may not reveal all cytogenetic abnormalities and gene alterations, molecular cytogenetics in the form of fluorescent *in situ* hybridization (FISH) and polymerase chain reaction (PCR) have been employed to increase the sensitivity level for detection of genetic defects.[77]

Although specific cytogenetic abnormalities in ALL can be related to immunophenotype, with the exception of t(8;14)(q24;q32) and its FAB L3 variants, they do not show a close relationship to the FAB subtype. On the other hand, in AML, chromosomal abnormalities including t(8;21)(q22;q22) FAB M2, t(15;17)(q22;q21) FAB M3, inv(16)(p13;q22) FAB M4 E0, or t(9;11)(q2;q23) FAB M5 have been associated with specific morphologic features.

In terms of numeric changes, hyperdiploidy, the most frequent chromosomal abnormality in ALL, has been identified in over 40% of cases of precursor B-cell disease (Table 20.8). High hyperdiploidy (51–65 chromosomes), which occurs in approximately 27% of cases of ALL, is associated with a particularly favorable response to antimetabolite-based therapy, which translates into an event-free survival (EFS) in excess of 85%.[78] This karyotype is usually associated with other good risk features: age ≥ 1 and < 10 years, a low WBC and pre-B immunophenotype.[79] Within the high hyperdiploid group, children with chromosomal numbers between 56 and 67 do better than the subgroup with 51–55, translating into EFS values of 86% and 72% at 5 years respectively. These genes normally involve chromosomes 4, 6, 10, 14, 17, 18, 21 and X. Trisomies involving chromosomes 4, 6, 10 and 17 are associated with good prognosis, whereas trisomy 5, a rare abnormality in childhood ALL, is associated with a poor prognosis.[80]

Gene expression profiles

Recent advances in DNA microarray assay technology in association with bioinformatics has enabled gene expression profiles to be produced that categorize specific leukemias. For example, Golub *et al.*[81] analyzed 27 patients with ALL and 11 with AML and were able to define 50 of 1100 genes that allow ALL to be distinguished from AML but also B-lineage ALL from T-lineage ALL with approximately 100% accuracy. Further studies on larger numbers of ALL samples have been able to identify several prognostic cytogenetic subgroups of B-lineage ALL – hyperdiploid > 50, t(12;21), t(1;19) and *MLL* – with 95–100% accuracy. This technique may also be able to predict those patients who will do less well with combination chemotherapy regimens and therefore these patients will be candidates for more intense or experimental therapies. This molecular genetic strategy may also be powerful enough to shed further light not only on the genetic drivers of leukemogenesis but also generate a patient-specific gene fingerprint that will warrant individualized treatment approaches.

Biological subsets

Infant leukemias: 11q23

As stated above, infant leukemias tend to have a unique clinical presentation, with high circulating blast counts, massive organomegaly and CNS involvement. After neuroblastoma these are the commonest malignancies seen in infancy and they account for approximately 4% of childhood ALL and about 10% of childhood AML. Unlike older children, where ALL is the predominant leukemia, in infants ALL is only marginally more common. The majority of infant leukemias, both AML and ALL, are associated with a translocation involving 11q23 and its various partners in 50 and 80% of cases respectively. The commonest translocations involving 11q23 in ALL are t(4;11) and t(11;19) and in approximately two-thirds of cases involve the CD10-negative B-lineage precursor cell, with the rest consisting of common/pre-B types. The single most common translocation in AML involving this region occurs at t(9;11)(p22;q23) and is associated with monocytic morphology (AML M5).[82] Different types of 11q23 translocations are seen in children with ALL who have been treated with the epipodophyllotoxins etoposide and teniposide who develop secondary AML.[83]

The gene involved in these chromosomal translocations that maps to 11q23 has been cloned by a number of groups, hence the many abbreviations ascribed to it (*HRX*, *ALL-1*, *MLL*).[84] A 15-kb mRNA is transcribed from 11q23 and translates into a 430-kDa protein. This protein shares sequence homology with the *Drosophila* trithorax regulator, which plays a key role in the embryonic development of the fruit fly. The precise leukemogenic events that result from the expression of this protein have not been fully elucidated, but probably involves impairment of the transcription factor function of *MLL* as a result of which the translocation breaks the gene between the two DNA-binding regions.

B (precursor B+ and mature B) ALL: cryptic t(12;21)(p13;q22)

A translocation between the short arm of chromosome 12 and the long arm of chromosome 21 was first reported in 1994 and subsequently shown to be the commonest genetic translocation in childhood ALL, occurring in approximately 25% of patients.[75] The cryptic translocation results in the *TEL/AML1* fusion gene. The TEL protein is a member of the ETS family of transcription factors. The other target in this translocation is the *AML1* (*CBFA2*) gene, a member of the family of core-binding factor (CBF) genes. AML1 represents one of three CBFα subunits that, together with a common CBFβ subunit, comprise functional transcription factors. Both AML1 and CBFβ are involved in several translocations in AML. CBF oncoproteins, such as TEL/AML1 fusion product, modulate endogenous CBF activities, which is most likely to be relevant to leukemia transformation.[85,86]

The presence of this fusion gene defines a subgroup of children with a better-than-average prognosis and, interestingly, this may be related to sensitivity to L-asparaginase therapy. Because of the prognostic significance of this cryptic translocation, it is essential that molecular screening for the translocation be standard practice in order to improve the understanding of the management of such patients.

t(8;14)(q24;q32) and variants (L3)

The translocation t(8;14)(q24;q11) and the variant forms, t(2;8)(p13;q24) and t(8;22)(9q24;q32), are found in Burkitt lymphoma and also occur in mature B-cell or Burkitt-type ALL (FAB L3). The translocation results in the activation of the c-*myc* oncogene through juxtaposition with immunoglobulin heavy-chain loci t(8;14) or light-chain loci t(2;8) or t(8;22), the former occurring more commonly. These cases constitute about 2% of childhood ALL.

The breakpoint on chromosome 8 corresponds to the c-*myc* oncogene while those on chromosome 14, 2 and 22 correspond to heavy chain, κ and λ light chains respectively. Therefore, the translocations are always between the c-*myc* oncogene and an immunoglobulin gene. This translocation results in dysregulation of the c-*myc* gene, which is considered to be the mechanism for the mature B-cell clonal proliferation.[87] These cytogenetic abnormalities can now be detected not only by karyotyping but also by Southern blotting, PCR and FISH.[88]

Leukemia of mature B cells more frequently involves the testis, ovary, pleura, CSF, peripheral lymph nodes and pharynx, factors that in the past probably contributed to a poorer prognostic group.[89] However, more recently these patients were found to respond favorably to short-term very intensive chemotherapy compared with typical ALL therapeutic regimens, and hence urgent cytogenetic or molecular confirmation of these genetic lesions is essential to treatment planning.

t(1;19)(q23;p13)

First described in 1984, this translocation is seen in approximately 5% of childhood cases of ALL.[90] It is associated with a pre-B immunophenotype and the blasts express cytoplasmic immunoglobulin (cyμ) in a high percentage (>90%) of cases.[90] These children do well on current regimens. The identification of the translocation is sometimes difficult as it can be missed in up to 50% of cases when using conventional cytogenetic analysis. Reverse transcriptase (RT)-PCR looking for the cryptic t(1;19) is the preferred investigational tool.[91] These children more commonly present with high-risk factors such as high WBC and CNS disease.[91] Molecularly, this translocation juxtaposes the *E2A* gene with the *PBX1* gene. E2A proteins function as transcriptional activators, which are

essential for normal B-cell development.[91] The translocation creates an *E2A/PBX1* fusion gene on the der(19) chromosome. Cases of t(1;19) ALL without detection of *E2A/PBX1* fusion transcripts have been described, suggesting that this translocation is molecularly heterogeneous.

T-ALL

T-ALL accounts for approximately 12% of cases of childhood ALL and usually presents with a high WBC in males aged 6–8 years with a relatively poor prognosis. These children usually have bulky disease (hepatosplenomegaly with peripheral lymphadenopathy), some having an anterior mediastinal mass, and a WBC in excess of 100×10^9/L is not unusual.[92]

Although, T-ALL and B-ALL share some cytogenetic abnormalities, there are some characteristic changes specific to T-ALL. Numerical abnormalities such as hyperdiploidy are more frequently demonstrated in B-ALL, whereas pseudodiploidy (normal chromosomal number with structural abnormality) or near-tetraploidy (chromosomes > 65) are more frequently seen in T-ALL. These cytogenetic changes such as hyperdiploid near tetraploidy are predictive of better EFS.[92] Genetic changes in T-ALL involve the T-cell receptor (TCR) genes *TCRα* and *TCRδ*. Rearrangements involving the TCR loci occur in up to 30% of cases.[93]

Several different protooncogenes are activated by translocations in T-ALL, the commonest being stem cell leukemia (SCL) on *TAL-1* gene, which is aberrantly expressed after translocation from 1p32–33 into *TCRα/δ* or *TCRβ* locus. Most patients with SCL/TAL-1 dysregulation have one or both *TCRδ* genes deleted and express a CD3-positive, TCRα/δ-positive phenotype. The important translocations involve the *TCRα/δ* locus at 14q11 are t(1;14), t(8;14), t(10;14) and t(11;14). Those involving the *TCRβ* locus at 7q3236 include t(1;7), t(7;9), t(7;11) and t(7;19). The prognosis of patients with SCL/TAL-1 expression is indistinguishable from that of patients without it.

ALL with eosinophilia and t(5;14)(q31;q32)

Eosinophil proliferation is associated with immature B-lineage ALL with t(5;14)(q31;q32).[94] This translocation joins the interleukin (IL)-3 gene to the immunoglobulin heavy chain gene. The eosinophilia is probably reactive, i.e., through IL-3 gene activation, as the clonal cytogenetic lesion is not seen in the eosinophils themselves and serum IL-3 levels have been found to correlate with disease activity.[94]

Eosinophilia has been demonstrated in association with L1 and L2 blasts. Not all cases of ALL with eosinophilia manifest the t(5;14) chromosome rearrangement. The eosinophils may demonstrate myelodysplastic change. This type of ALL is usually more difficult to manage because of cardiac and pulmonary infiltration of eosinophils and this tends to occur more frequently in males and in older children.[94]

Aplastic/hypoplastic ALL

Transient pancytopenia and hypoplastic/aplastic bone marrow occurs in a small number of children prior to the onset of ALL, but the pathogensis is poorly understood at present. A transient recovery of normal blood counts is followed by overt leukemia in weeks to months. Dysplastic change is not seen in the blood or marrow and the blasts are usually of L1 FAB subtype and are usually CD10[+].[95] The association of a history of fever, usually with an infectious disease prodrome, and a preponderance of girls has also been noted.[95] Immunophenotype and cytogenetic analysis are not usually helpful and differentiating the marrow findings from bone marrow necrosis can be extremely difficult. It is recommended that the bone marrow should be repeated at a different site or at a later date. However, close follow-up is essential as leukemia will in time become evident.

Prognostic factors

A retrospective analysis of clinical trials established many important prognostic factors, which were subsequently applied prospectively to stratify children into different treatment groups according to their relative risk of treatment failure. Children at higher risk of relapse are treated more intensively,[3,96,97] whereas in those with a lower risk of relapse the more toxic components of treatment, such as cranial irradiation, anthracyclines, oxazaphorines and epipodophyllotoxins, are reduced or even eliminated.[96-99] Thus, treatment tailored to the individual risk of relapse is an essential prerequisite for current clinical trials. This approach greatly complicates any comparative analysis of treatment results.[100] A uniform approach to risk classification and the classification of special prognostic factors has been agreed by clinicians in the USA.[19]

Since ALL is a heterogeneous disease, there may be multiple populations of patients with different prognosis on identical treatments. Various clinical and laboratory findings at the time of diagnosis have been correlated with prognosis (Table 20.7). The relative importance of a given prognostic factor varies between different treatment protocols.[3,97,101] Intensification of treatment can eliminate the prognostic significance of some of the unfavorable features, illustrating that treatment *per se* is probably the most important risk factor in childhood ALL. Although all prognostic factors should be considered treatment-specific, certain features appear to be consistently valuable (Table 20.9).

Clinical phenotype

The initial WBC shows independent significance in most studies (Figs 20.1–20.4), with a linear relationship between the number of leukemic cells and the risk of relapse.[96,102,103] Organ infiltration is strongly correlated with WBC but has no additional prognostic significance in most trials.[104]

Age at presentation is an important prognostic factor (Figs 20.1–20.4). Whereas infants younger than 1 year of age have the worst prognosis of any age group,[3,83] children aged 2–6 years do best of all.[3,4,98] Adolescents have faired poorly in many trials and adults with ALL have a poorer outcome compared with children.[3,4,105] The prognostic importance of age may be due to the fact that, for unknown reasons, specific biologic subtypes of ALL occur more or less frequently in different age groups.

In the past, girls have had a better prognosis than boys, which is not completely explained by testicular relapse or the higher incidence of T-ALL in males. However, some recent trials do not find male sex to be an adverse prognostic factor.[5,106]

Black children, who account for about 10% of all newly diagnosed children with ALL in the USA, have been reported to have a worse prognosis than white children. This has been attributed to the higher frequency of specific biologic subtypes of ALL with a poorer prognosis in black children.[107] However, a recent trial found race to lack prognostic importance.[5]

Table 20.9 Prognostic factors in the therapy of *de novo* acute lymphoblastic leukemia.

Factor	Favorable	Unfavorable
Age	> 1 to < 6 years	< 1 year
White blood cell count (× 10⁹/L)	< 20	> 100
Response to initial 7-day prednisone monotherapy	Slow response*	Good response*
Response to initial induction therapy (bone marrow on day 14)	M1 marrow†	M2, M3 marrow†
Chromosome count	> 50	< 45
DNA index	≥ 1.16	< 1.16
Chromosomal translocations	t(12;21)	t(9;22), t(4;11)
Probability of 5-year event-free survival	> 80%	10–60%, depending on specific constellation

* Blast count of < 1 × 10⁹/L in blood after 1 week is a good response.

† M1 marrow, < 5% blasts and complete regeneration of hematopoiesis; M2 marrow, > 5% to < 25% blasts and/or incomplete regeneration of hematopoiesis; M3 marrow, > 25% blasts in the bone marrow.

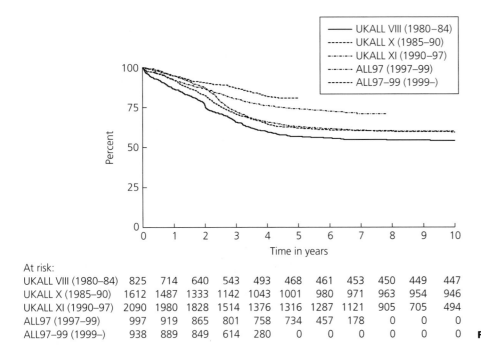

At risk:

UKALL VIII (1980–84)	825	714	640	543	493	468	461	453	450	449	447
UKALL X (1985–90)	1612	1487	1333	1142	1043	1001	980	971	963	954	946
UKALL XI (1990–97)	2090	1980	1828	1514	1376	1316	1287	1121	905	705	494
ALL97 (1997–99)	997	919	865	801	758	734	457	178	0	0	0
ALL97–99 (1999–)	938	889	849	614	280	0	0	0	0	0	0

Fig. 20.1 Event-free survival by trial.

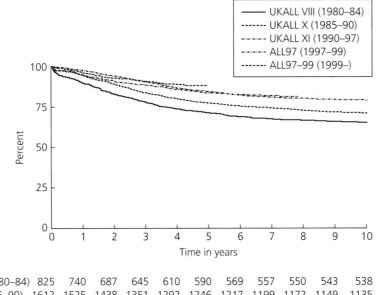

At risk:

UKALL VIII (1980–84)	825	740	687	645	610	590	569	557	550	543	538
UKALL X (1985–90)	1612	1525	1438	1351	1292	1246	1217	1199	1172	1149	1135
UKALL XI (1990–97)	2090	2039	1967	1892	1810	1765	1717	1492	1205	922	649
ALL97 (1997–99)	997	946	909	884	857	829	522	204	0	0	0
ALL97–99 (1999–)	938	901	871	643	303	0	0	0	0	0	0

Fig. 20.2 Overall survival by trial.

Cellular phenotype and genotype

The immunophenotype of lymphoblasts was thought to be the most important factor in childhood ALL. This is still true for mature B-ALL which is now treated differently from B-precursor ALL and T-ALL. However, T-ALL is no longer an unfavorable entity using contemporary risk-adapted polychemotherapy.[3,97,98]

A pre-B cell phenotype has been reported to confer a worse prognosis compared with the early pre-B phenotype.[108,109] However, results of a trial using intensive polychemotherapy revealed no difference in outcome between these two immunologic subgroups.[3] ALL derived from an even earlier B-cell precursor (CD10$^-$CD19$^+$) (pro-B ALL) has also been associated with a poor response to therapy.[110,111] However, in one study the adverse impact of this immune phenotype was

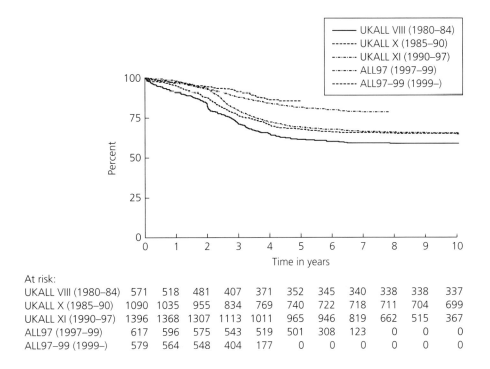

Fig. 20.3 Event-free survival by trial: standard risk (age 1–9 years and white cell count < 50).

At risk:

UKALL VIII (1980–84)	571	518	481	407	371	352	345	340	338	338	337
UKALL X (1985–90)	1090	1035	955	834	769	740	722	718	711	704	699
UKALL XI (1990–97)	1396	1368	1307	1113	1011	965	946	819	662	515	367
ALL97 (1997–99)	617	596	575	543	519	501	308	123	0	0	0
ALL97–99 (1999–)	579	564	548	404	177	0	0	0	0	0	0

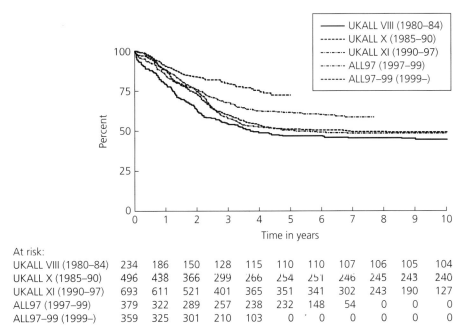

Fig. 20.4 Event-free survival by trial: high risk (age ≥ 10 years and white cell count > 50).

At risk:

UKALL VIII (1980–84)	234	186	150	128	115	110	110	107	106	105	104
UKALL X (1985–90)	496	438	366	299	266	254	251	246	245	243	240
UKALL XI (1990–97)	693	611	521	401	365	351	341	302	243	190	127
ALL97 (1997–99)	379	322	289	257	238	232	148	54	0	0	0
ALL97–99 (1999–)	359	325	301	210	103	0	0	0	0	0	0

abolished when infants were excluded from the analysis.[3] The prognostic importance of coexpression of myeloid antigens has been shown to be insignificant.[68,70,71]

Children with hyperdiploid leukemia (DNA index ≥ 1.16) were reported to have a better prognosis compared with children without this feature.[112,113] The translocation t(12;21)(p13;q22) with the *TEL-AML1* fusion transcript found in about 20% of children with ALL confers a favorable outcome with long-term survival exceeding 90%.[114,115] Children with t(9;22)[116–120] and t(4;11)[121,122] have a particularly poor

prognosis irrespective of other chromosomal translocations presenting features or treatment regimens. However, Aric *et al.*[123] identified a subset of good responding patients with low WBC and t(9;22) childhood ALL with a lower risk for relapse.

Response to treatment

Response to induction polychemotherapy[124,125] or monotherapy with steroids,[3,126,127] as measured by the absolute number of leukemic blasts in the peripheral blood on day 7 or the

Table 20.10 Methods for the detection of minimal residual leukemic cells in childhood acute lymphoblastic leukemia (ALL).

Technique	Detection limit	Applicability
Morphology and cytochemistry	10^{-1}–10^{-2}	All leukemias
Cytogenetics	10^{-1}–10^{-2}	Leukemias with microscopically detectable numeric or structural aberrations (only cells in mitosis)
Fluorescence *in situ* hybridization	10^{-1}–10^{-2}	Leukemias with known numeric or structural aberrations (interphase cells)
Flow cytometry for DNA content	10^{-1}–10^{-2}	About 30% of B-precursor ALL; < 5% of T-ALL
Flow cytometry for leukemia-associated immunophenotype	10^{-3}–10^{-4}	50–90% of ALL
PCR techniques		
DNA level		
Rearranged immunoglobulin and T-cell receptor genes	10^{-3}–10^{-6}	90% of ALL
Chromosomal aberrations with known breakpoints	10^{-4}–10^{-6}	10–20% of T-ALL, > 5% of B-ALL
RNA level		
Chromosomal aberrations resulting in leukemia-specific fusion genes and fusion mRNA	10^{-3}–10^{-5}	10–15% of B-precursor ALL

percentage of bone marrow blasts on days 7 or 14, has been defined as a new important predictor of outcome in many recent trials, again illustrating the importance of treatment response as a prognostic factor. However, the reality is that the majority of children who relapse come from the so-called good or standard risk group(s), i.e., favorable cytogenetics, low count at presentation and rapid early response to corticosteroids, and it is for this reason it is hoped that minimal residual disease monitoring will enhance response prognostic classification.[128]

Minimal residual disease and its detection

Molecular and cellular biological assays have defined the concept of minimal residual disease (MRD) where detection of "leukemia-specific" DNA or RNA or "leukemia-associated" antigens is achievable at levels of sensitivity that are much greater than those for morphologic or karyotypic analysis (Table 20.10).[129] The two most common methods used for MRD assessment are the detection of cells expressing abnormal immunophenotypes by flow cytometetry, and of leukemia-associated molecular targets, e.g., fusion transcripts such as *BCR-ABL*, *TEL/AML1* and clone-specific immunoglobulin and TCR gene rearrangements.[130] The sensitivities of these two methodologies differ: flow cytometetry can routinely detect as few as 0.01% leukemia cells in the blood or marrow, whereas PCR-based assays usually detect one leukemia cell in 10^4–10^6 normal cells and hence most investigators have used the latter technique.[131–133]

The majority of clinical MRD studies to date have been in childhood ALL both during and after treatment. Low levels or absence of MRD after completion of induction therapy appears to predict good outcome both by immunophenotyp-

ing and PCR clonality studies. However, it is important to note that quantitation of levels of MRD can differ in particular types of leukemia. A steady decrease of MRD levels during treatment is associated with a good prognosis whereas persistent high levels or increases in MRD positivity generally lead to clinical relapse. Several prospective studies have indicated that sequential sampling, preferably using a quantitative approach, allows stratification of patient risk of relapse. However, it is important to note that although this technique is a powerful and independent prognostic indicator in certain types of childhood leukemia, it has not been proven that planning treatment according to MRD results will improve outcome or decrease toxicity. Current studies such as the UK-ALL 2003 randomized protocol are addressing this very point.

Treatment of newly diagnosed ALL

Table 20.3 gives an overview of the diagnostic work-up that should be carried out in a newly diagnosed child with ALL prior to comemencing therapy. Levels of lactate dehydrogenase (LDH), liver enzymes and serum uric acid are often abnormal at presentation due to leukemic cell turnover or kidney infiltration. In children with hyperleukocytosis and a high leukemic cell burden, metabolic abnormalities such as hypercalcemia, hyperphosphatemia or hyperkalemia may not preclude the immediate start of antileukemic treatment. Renal dialysis may be required in the occasional patient with B-ALL.[134] Most children with ALL and hyperleukocytosis can be managed by careful steroid-based cytoreductive treatment and preventive measures for hyperuricemia including rasburicase.

In addition to a careful history recording previous infections, recent contact with infections and immunizations as well as baseline viral serologies are recommended, especially for measles, varicella zoster virus, cytomegalovirus and herpes simplex virus. A diagnostic lumbar puncture in most modern treatment protocols combined with intrathecal injection of methotrexate for CSF examination (cell count including the number of red cells because of possible contamination with blood) and a cytospin is required at the beginning of treatment.

Chest radiography or sonography of the mediastinum may reveal a mediastinal mass, which may lead to severe obstruction of the airways and/or the superior vena cava. Sonography of the abdomen is recommended for the determination of liver, spleen and kidney size. Before the start of treatment with potential cardiotoxic drugs, most protocols recommend echocardiography.

Antileukemic drugs

The ability of a cytotoxic drug to induce complete remission of ALL was first reported in 1948,[135] and since then a multitude of effective agents has been discovered. Despite the fact that single-agent therapy has no place in the curative treatment of ALL, knowledge of the administration and action of each of the available cytotoxic drugs is necessary so that optimal combinations and a sequential strategy can be determined. Figures 20.5 and 20.6 show the steady improvement

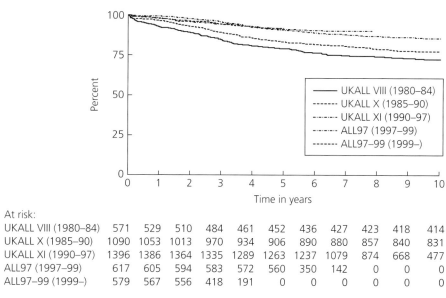

At risk:											
UKALL VIII (1980–84)	571	529	510	484	461	452	436	427	423	418	414
UKALL X (1985–90)	1090	1053	1013	970	934	906	890	880	857	840	831
UKALL XI (1990–97)	1396	1386	1364	1335	1289	1263	1237	1079	874	668	477
ALL97 (1997–99)	617	605	594	583	572	560	350	142	0	0	0
ALL97–99 (1999–)	579	567	556	418	191	0	0	0	0	0	0

Fig. 20.5 Survival by trial: standard risk (age 1–9 years and white cell count < 50).

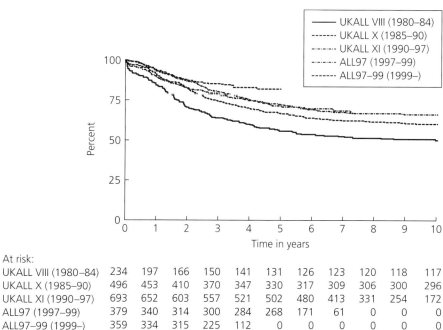

At risk:											
UKALL VIII (1980–84)	234	197	166	150	141	131	126	123	120	118	117
UKALL X (1985–90)	496	453	410	370	347	330	317	309	306	300	296
UKALL XI (1990–97)	693	652	603	557	521	502	480	413	331	254	172
ALL97 (1997–99)	379	340	314	300	284	268	171	61	0	0	0
ALL97–99 (1999–)	359	334	315	225	112	0	0	0	0	0	0

Fig. 20.6 Survival by trial: high risk (age ≥ 10 years and white cell count > 50).

in EFS and overall survival in successive MRC UK-ALL trial protocols over the past quarter of a decade.

Steroids

Of all agents currently used in ALL treatment, the adrenocorticosteroids are of utmost importance in remission induction treatment. Steroids are lympholytic via a mechanism that is as yet poorly understood but which probably involves the activation of nucleases leading to DNA fragmentation (apoptosis). The particular susceptibility of lymphoblasts to steroids permits rapid reduction of leukemic cell number with minimal myelosuppression. The steroid most often used in polychemotherapy protocols is prednisone in oral doses of 60–80 mg/m^2/day or its soluble analog prednisolone. Other steroids have essentially identical remission induction capability, although dexamethasone may provide greater control of leukemia in the CNS and other extramedullary sites.[136]

Vinca alkaloids

Vinca alkaloids, together with steroids, are the most important agents for remission induction in ALL. Vincristine in a weekly dose of 1.5 mg/m^2 (maximal dose 2.0 mg/m^2) is by far the most frequently used vinca alkaloid in ALL. Using this schedule, only mild myelosuppression is to be expected; however, neurotoxicity with paresthesia or paralytic ileus may occur, especially in older children. More frequent injections and continuous infusion increase the efficacy of vincristine but also increase the neurotoxicity considerably. Other vinca alkaloids such as vinblastine and vindesine appear to be less effective than vincristine in ALL.

L-Asparaginase

L-Asparaginase, an enzyme that cleaves asparagine into aspartic acid and ammonia, has a restricted activity against lymphoblasts. Asparaginases of two different origins are in current use, namely from *Escherichia coli* and *Erwinia carotovora* (renamed *Erwinia chrysanthemis*), and have different pharmacokinetics.[137] Side-effects result from the inhibition of protein synthesis, especially of clotting and fibrinolytic factors,[138] and anaphylactoid reactions. With polyethylene glycol (PEG)-bound asparaginase, the risk of the latter may be reduced; however, PEG binding alters the pharmacokinetics.[137] L-Asparaginase is given at various doses and schedules in modern polychemotherapy protocols.

Anthracyclines

Daunorubicin was the first anthracycline antibiotic to show significant antileukemic activity. It is a highly myelosuppressive drug and its cardiotoxicity is cumulative. Cumulative doses should not exceed 300–400 mg/m^2 in children with AL and most current schedules aim for total doses of less than 240 mg/m^2. Doxorubicin (Adriamycin) has been less extensively tested in childhood ALL but may have a similar activity and at least the same toxicity compared with daunorubicin. Of the newer anthracyclines, idarubicin has substantial antileukemic efficacy, although its relative value in comparison with daunorubicin has not been established in childhood ALL.

Folic acid antimetabolites

Folic acid antagonists initiated the revolution in treatment of childhood ALL.[135] Methotrexate, the only compound in current use, together with mercaptopurine is the basis of maintenance chemotherapy in ALL. Given intrathecally, methotrexate is the key component in CNS-directed chemotherapy. High-dose methotrexate, introduced in the 1960s, may provide effective antileukemic methotrexate concentrations in extramedullary sites, especially the CNS and testes, although its use is currently controversial.[139]

Purine antagonists

Mercaptopurine is the traditional purine antagonist in childhood ALL, whereas thioguanine is preferred in AML. Mercaptopurine remains the drug most often combined with methotrexate in virtually all continuation chemotherapy protocols in childhood ALL. Drug dosage, patient compliance and route of administration determine the antileukemic efficacy during maintenance treatment. Several pharmacologic studies show that bioavailability following oral administration of mercaptopurine is highly variable.[140,141] Large randomized trials have now shown equivalent efficacy of thioguanine and mercaptopurine but thioguanine causes more liver veno occlusive disease and thus mercaptopurine is the preferred drug.[142] Information on the new purine analogs, such as 2-deoxycoformicin, 2-chlorodeoxyadenosine and fludarabine, are scarce in childhood ALL.

Pyrimidine antagonists

Cytarabine arabinoside is the only pyrimidine antagonist used in childhood ALL. *In vitro* studies suggest that T lymphoblasts may be especially sensitive to cytarabine. High-dose cytarabine is a potent inducer of remissions in refractory and relapsed ALL, in both children and adults, and is now included in most protocols for high-risk patients.

Alkylating agents

Cyclophosphamide is the most commonly used alkylating drug for the treatment of childhood ALL. It is effective in both T-ALL and B-ALL.[44,143,144] Ifosfamide may be as effective as cyclophosphamide and is included in most modern intensive polychemotherapy protocols for B-ALL.[44,144]

Epipodophyllotoxin

The two most important epipodophyllotoxins are teniposide (VM-26) and etoposide (VP-16). These compounds interact with topoisomerase-II to prevent the reannealing of DNA after it has been disrupted by the enzyme. This in turn leads to apoptosis. VP-16 particularly is included in some poly-chemotherapy protocols for high-risk patients. However, there is some concern about the development of secondary AML but usually only when used in schedules other than short-intensive blocks.[145]

Intensive polychemotherapy approach

The major advances achieved during the past three decades in the treatment of ALL in children and adolescents have dramatically changed the prognosis for this disease, which was always fatal in the past. While treatment was purely palliative until the 1960s, the aim of current treatment protocols is cure; 70–75% of all children and adolescents with ALL can be expected to be cured of their leukemia. This altered prognosis of ALL is mainly the result of very intensive chemotherapy associated with severe suppression of both the normal hematopoietic stem cells and the immune system. Thus, the improvement of supportive measures such as packed red blood cells, effective platelet support and highly effective antimicrobial agents, including broad-spectrum antibiotics, antifungal agents and antiviral drugs, has been a prerequisite for the use of increasingly intensive polychemotherapy protocols (see below).

The aim of treatment is the elimination of the neoplastic cell clone and the restoration of normal hematopoiesis. The different phases of antileukemic treatment are delivered usually in four separate phases or blocks, called remission induction, intensification, CNS directed and continuation treatments.

Remission induction

After stabilization of the clinical status in a child with ALL (treatment of metabolic changes, infections, bleeding complications), remission induction polychemotherapy should be started without delay. The initial phase of treatment is designed to reduce the leukemic cell burden to a clinically and hematologically undetectable level. Complete remission is achieved when the marrow cellularity has returned to normal with < 5% of blasts, the blood values are within the normal range, and all clinical signs and symptoms of the disease have disappeared.

Clinical trials in the 1960s demonstrated that the combination of two antileukemic agents gives superior remission rates compared with single agents. The combination of vincristine and prednisone led to complete remission in about 90% of children with ALL.[146] The addition of a third drug, namely an anthracycline or asparaginase, increased the com-

plete remission rate to > 95%. This increased remission rate was later shown to translate into an increased long-term relapse-free survival,[96,147] thus demonstrating the importance of maximal early cell kill for the overall effectiveness of treatment. Current induction regimens therefore consist of three or more drugs. A large Children's Cancer Study Group (CCSG) report has demonstrated similar EFS in intermediate-risk ALL treated with a four- and three-drug induction if intensive reintensification was given.[105]

CNS-directed treatment is integrated in most current remission induction regimens, most often in the form of intrathecally given methotrexate or triple drug (methotrexate, cytarabine and hydrocortisone) intrathecal therapy.

Current polychemotherapy treatment protocols give a remission rate of > 95%.[3–5] Induction failures are divided equally between children with refractory leukemia and those dying from complications of leukemia or toxicity of treatment. Thus, intensive induction polychemotherapy can increase long-term survival but may result in increased short-term morbidity and mortality, especially if supportive care is suboptimal, which illustrates the delicate balance required between intensive polychemotherapy and sometimes life-threatening toxicity.

Intensification

Remission induction treatment is followed by intensification (reinduction treatment) early in remission in most current polychemotherapy regimens in order to maximize early leukemic cell kill. Intensification therapy is less standardized compared with remission induction treatment. While some regimens use single agents in high dosages, such as asparaginase, methotrexate or cytarabine, other trials rely on reinduction with the same drug combinations or related drugs to those administered during remission induction. In most trials, children with a presumed higher risk for relapse are treated with more intensive polychemotherapy compared to those with presumed standard risk. However, reintensification therapy is an important phase of therapy for all children with B-precursor ALL.[96,105]

In standard-risk patients the improvement in treatment outcome by addition of reinduction treatment early in remission was first demonstrated in the 1980s. In this randomized trial, children receiving reinduction did significantly better compared with those who did not receive re-induction therapy [probability of complete continuous remission after 5 years 84% (SD 5%) vs. 62% (SD 7%)].[3,96] The importance of reinduction treatment was also confirmed by the CCSG demonstration of 7-year EFS of 63% for standard-risk children receiving BFM-type intensification compared with 42% for children not given such treatment.[105]

The importance of intensification therapy in children with high-risk features has been confirmed in many trials.[4,5,96,148–151] In children with very high-risk features as defined by slow early response, prednisone nonresponse, or unique biologic features such as t(9;22) or t(4;11), an improved outcome could not be demonstrated with further treatment intensification.[3,152] However, a recent CCSG trial demonstrated that further prolongation and intensification of therapy (augmented protocol) improved the outcome of children with high-risk features and slow response to induction therapy as defined by an M3 marrow on day 7.[153]

CNS-directed treatment

The use of CNS-directed treatment (CNS irradiation, intrathecal chemotherapy and high-dose chemotherapy) has been considered a prerequisite for long-term leukemia-free survival. Before its introduction more than 50% of children with ALL developed overt CNS disease while in systemic remission. The concept of CNS preventive therapy is based on the premise that the CNS is a sanctuary site in which leukemic cells are protected by the blood–brain barrier from therapeutic concentrations of systemically administered antileukemic drugs.

The use of CNS irradiation as preventive therapy was first demonstrated in a series of studies at St Jude Children's Hospital in Memphis, USA.[154] Relatively low doses of craniospinal irradiation (5 or 12 Gy) demonstrated no preventive effect, whereas 24 Gy of cranial irradiation together with five doses of intrathecal methotrexate or 24 Gy of craniospinal irradiation reduced the incidence of CNS relapse from > 50% to approximately 10%.[154] Because craniospinal irradiation was associated with excessive myelosuppression due to irradiation of large parts of the bone marrow and retardation of spinal growth, cranial irradiation (24 Gy) together with intrathecal methotrexate became the standard form of CNS preventive therapy during the 1970s. The identification of brain abnormalities on CT,[155] altered intellectual and psychometric functions, and neuroendocrine dysfunction in children treated with 24 Gy of cranial irradiation and intrathecal chemotherapy prompted a reappraisal of CNS preventive treatment strategies and stimulated the search for alternative less toxic treatments.[156]

Alternatives include intrathecal chemotherapy with one or more cytotoxic drugs such as methotrexate, cytarabine with or without hydrocortisone, as well as high doses of intravenous methotrexate to overcome the blood–brain barrier. With intermediate (500 mg/m^2) or high (> 1 g/m^2) doses of methotrexate, some trials reported a higher CNS relapse rate than that observed with inclusion of cranial irradiation. The CNS relapse rate was found to depend on pretherapy risk factors, the response to treatment and the intensity of systemic chemotherapy. Thus, in the context of more intensive systemic therapy, patients at lower risk of CNS relapse may require less intensive CNS-directed therapy with lower doses of cranial irradiation or nowadays no cranial irradiation at

all. The BFM Group demonstrated that the use of 12 Gy administered in a protocol with high-dose methotrexate and intensive reinduction/consolidation therapy was as effective in the prevention of CNS disease as 18 Gy in a selected group of standard-risk patients.[3,96,104]

The optimal choice of CNS-directed therapy in childhood ALL is controversial, mostly because of the potential for adverse effects. Extensive metaanalysis of randomized trials of CNS-directed therapy have failed to demonstrate a substantial additional effect of radiotherapy, which has been dropped from therapy in all patients in the St Jude's protocols and for all but those CNS-positive at diagnosis or relapse in the UK series, with a consequent very satisfactory extremely low CNS relapse rate.[157]

CNS preventive treatment may be associated with acute neurotoxic sequelae such as headache, nausea and vomiting, and other signs of increased intracranial pressure. In addition, 5–7 weeks after cranial irradiation some children develop a characteristic subacute neurotoxic reaction, with somnolence, lethargy, anorexia, fever and irritability. This somnolence syndrome, which may be accompanied by EEG abnormalities and CSF pleocytosis, usually resolves within 1–3 weeks.[158]

Continuation treatment

Unlike most other childhood malignancies, childhood ALL requires the continuation of therapy for a long time. Early studies in which no continuation therapy was given after remission induction were associated with the rapid relapse of almost all children.[159] Furthermore, early studies demonstrated that interrupted treatment resulted in inferior results compared with continued maintenance therapy in childhood ALL.[160] In early clinical studies a variety of single agents were evaluated as maintenance agents. Drugs particularly effective as induction agents were surprisingly not useful for continuation therapy. The combination of methotrexate and mercaptopurine administered continuously is now used most widely and is a principal constituent of nearly all maintenance regimens.

Pharmacologic studies have demonstrated that the bioavailability of oral mercaptopurine and oral methotrexate is highly variable. However, a randomized trial demonstrated that for continuation therapy oral methotrexate is as effective as intramuscular methotrexate.[161] In most trials, the interindividual variation in bioavailability of mercaptopurine and methotrexate is compensated for by adjusting the dose of both drugs according to the actual WBC. The addition of vincristine and prednisone or dexamethasone to mercaptopurine and methotrexate during maintenance therapy was found to be effective in some trials[99,162] but not in others.[96] The most recent studies suggest no value to the vincristine/steroid pulses and thus further meta analysis is required.

Duration of treatment

The use of intensive induction polychemotherapy has significantly decreased the proportion of children suffering relapse after the cessation of treatment.[163] The BFM trials using very intensive induction polychemotherapy clearly demonstrated that the frequency of relapse after cessation of treatment could be reduced by further intensifying induction and reinduction polychemotherapy.[96] The relapse frequency after cessation of therapy is in the range of 15% for all children at risk in most trials.[5,164] Most of those children eventually relapsing did so within the first year off therapy.[164] In the second, third and fourth years after cessation of treatment, the risk of relapse was only about 2–3% per year. Relapses after the fourth year off therapy are extremely rare. However, very late relapses can occur. In an MRC study, 11 of 1000 long-term survivors (older than 10 years in their first remission) relapsed very late (10–24 years after diagnosis).[165] Molecular studies showed that in five patients the second presentation of ALL revealed an identical clonal immunoglobulin heavy chain or TCR gene rearrangement, thus confirming that these second presentations were true relapses rather than a second or secondary ALL. The current practice of treating children for 2–3 years with continuation chemotherapy derives from older studies in which patients were treated with less intensive polychemotherapy than in current use. For this reason, conclusions drawn from these studies on the duration of continuation may not be applicable to current treatment protocols. In an attempt to address this question, the BFM Group randomized patients to receive 18 or 24 months of treatment. A significant advantage was observed for children receiving longer treatment.[96] The MRC UKALL-VIII trial using less intensive induction polychemotherapy reported similar results between patients randomized to receive 2 or 3 years of maintenance therapy.[166]

The optimal duration of therapy may be different for boys and girls. Boys with standard-risk features of ALL demonstrated a significant relapse cascade after cessation of therapy in both BFM '86 and '90 studies (unpublished results). This confirms treatment results from CCSG 141[167] and MRC UKALL-X,[106] which both demonstrated a higher incidence of relapse after cessation of therapy in males, even after excluding boys with occult testicular disease. Thus, in the ongoing British, American and German protocols, boys with standard-risk features are treated for a total of 36 months, whereas girls receive treatment for 24 months.

Closer monitoring of early response parameters, including the assessment of MRD at regular intervals, may provide new guidelines for the optimal duration of therapy in the individual child with ALL which can be used for further stratification of therapy intensity and duration.[168,169]

However, differences in rearrangement patterns at the time of diagnosis and relapse, most probably due to clonal evaluation, have been described.[170–172] Thus, two or more junctional regions of different genes need to be monitored for detection of MRD.[170,173–175]

ALL of mature B-cell type

The lymphoblasts of about 4% of all children with ALL demonstrate features of more mature lymphocytes, a unique immunophenotype with the expression of surface immunoglobulin with light chain restriction (either κ or λ chains), and specific chromosomal translocations t(8;14), t(2;8) and t(8;22).

Clinically, mature B-ALL is characterized by a high tumor burden, especially within the abdomen, a high LDH and a high propensity to invade the CNS.[44] Differentiation between mature B-ALL (>25% B lymphoblasts in the bone marrow) and B-NHL (stage IV) (<25% lymphoblasts in the bone marrow) is arbitrary. Thus, most protocols recommend identical treatment for mature B-ALL and B-NHL stage IV.[44,144] Children with B-ALL had a poor outcome when treated with the regimen used for B-precursor ALL. Using a very intensive therapy approach, including high-dose methotrexate, cytarabine and cyclophosphamide, as well as intensive intrathecal chemotherapy, the EFS of children with mature B-ALL has increased up to greater than 80%.[44,144] The duration of treatment for B-ALL is short, usually no more than 4–6 months. Nearly all relapses, often with involvement of the CNS, occur within the first year after initial presentation.[44,144]

Infant leukemia

About 3–5% of children with ALL are infants (<12 months of age). ALL in infancy differs from that in older children with respect to clinical and biologic features and outcome of therapy (see above). At presentation, infants demonstrate a high tumor burden, including a high WBC, hepatosplenomegaly and a higher incidence of CNS leukemia compared with older children. The lymphoblasts appear to arise from a very early stage of commitment to B-cell differentiation, with an immunophenotype of CD19+CD10−, HLA-DR+ and frequent coexpression of myeloid markers such as CD13, CD33 or CD65.

Infants with ALL have an increased incidence of chromosomal abnormalities associated with a poor prognosis. Structural abnormalities of chromosome 11, especially rearrangement of band 11q23 within the *MLL* gene, are frequently observed. The t(4;11) abnormality is particularly common in infants with hyperleukocytosis. Hyperdiploidy, a common finding in ALL of older age groups, is extremely rare in infant ALL.[176,177]

Although the complete response rate of infants appears to be no different from that for older children, the eventual outcome is much poorer. The 5-year EFS in infant ALL ranges from 25 to 50% in most trials.[3] This is especially true for infants under 6 months of age.[178]

Because the pharmacokinetics of cytotoxic drugs may differ between infants and older children, the optimal dosage of polychemotherapy in infants with ALL is unclear. Most protocols recommend a reduced dosage or calculation according to body weight instead of body surface area.[3] Although polychemotherapy is generally well tolerated by infants and cranial irradiation is deferred until the second year of life, late effects of therapy are more often seen in this age group compared with older children.[179,180]

Congenital ALL, i.e., ALL diagnosed within the first 4 weeks of life, is especially rare and has to be differentiated from transient myeloproliferative disorders, which are mostly seen in children with Down syndrome.[181]

Treatment of relapsed ALL

Despite progress in treatment outcome of childhood ALL, 15–20% of children with ALL do suffer from relapse. Most relapses occur within the bone marrow, followed by the CNS, testes and other rare sites such as the eye, ovary or skin. Combined relapses may occur within bone marrow and CNS, followed by bone marrow and testes in boys. However, a leukemic relapse at any site should always be considered as a localized manifestation of a systemic disease, thus leading to careful staging procedures for other occult disease manifestations and to reinduction of systemic polychemotherapy in addition to local treatment including CNS-directed therapy.[7,182,183]

Since most, if not all, effective antileukemic drugs have already been delivered during primary polychemotherapy, treatment of relapse has to rely on combinations of the same drugs. Such an approach has been used by most groups since the early 1980s using cytotoxic drugs in intermittent blocks of polychemotherapy followed by continuation treatment for 24 months.

Careful documentation of relapse sites is of great importance in the individual child, including examination of extramedullary sites such as the CNS (lumbar puncture and diagnostic imaging of the neuroaxis), testes and eye. Bone marrow relapse is diagnosed if > 25% unequivocal lymphoblasts are found. In some patients, the immunophenotype may be different from that found at presentation (phenotypic shift).[184] Similarly, there can be differences in chromosomal aberration and in gene rearrangement patterns at the time of diagnosis and relapse due to clonal evolution.[170,171,184] In most children with CNS relapse, lymphoblast counts in the CSF are $> 5 \times 10^6/L$. In rare cases, the differentiation between reactive CSF pleocytosis and true CNS relapse may be difficult and further immunologic and cytogenetic/molecular genetic studies are warranted. In doubtful cases, another lumbar puncture is indicated after a couple of days, or several weeks if intrathecal therapy has been given. Testicular relapse is documented by biopsy or fine-needle aspiration. However, the latter technique may give false-positive results if lymphoblasts are present in the blood. A combined relapse is diagnosed if in addition to extramedullary relapse, > 5% unequivocal lymphoblasts are present in the bone marrow.[7]

Different mechanisms may be responsible for the occurrence of relapse of childhood ALL. One reason for treatment failure may be the existence of an anatomic barrier that prevents antileukemic drugs from reaching their target at therapeutically effective concentrations. This may be the reason for most CNS and testicular relapses (sanctuary sites). Another reason for relapse is drug resistance, either primary or secondary, resulting in nonresponse to treatment of early systemic relapse. Clinical resistance to antileukemic drugs is multifactorial and the cellular mechanisms are still poorly understood. Multiple drug resistance is partly due to the overexpression of p-glycoprotein, which acts as a drug-transport protein.[185] The third reason for relapse might be that cells are hidden in metabolic sanctuaries, thus being prevented from recruitment into the cell cycle (G_0 phase) and therefore not accessible to the cytotoxic drug. This may be due to either intrinsic properties of the leukemic cell or altered metabolic environmental conditions that may exist in the CNS or the testes, resulting in much lower proliferative activity. In the individual child with relapsing ALL, one or more of these possible reasons may be responsible and have different treatment implications.[7]

As in the primary treatment of childhood ALL, a number of prognostic factors have emerged from long-term observation of multicenter ALL relapse trials (Table 20.11), implying that different relapse situations should be treated differently.[7,186–188]

Very early relapse

Children relapsing at any site within the first 18 months after presentation (very early relapse) and children with any relapse of T-ALL have a dismal prognosis with chemotherapy alone.[7,189,190] Thus, if the relapsing leukemia again responds to intensive polychemotherapy, allogeneic bone marrow transplantation (BMT) in second complete remission from a related or unrelated donor is the treatment of choice in such patients.[191–194]

Early isolated bone marrow relapse

Most children with isolated bone marrow relapse within the first 6 months after cessation of therapy (early relapse) initially respond to second-line polychemotherapy. However, since prognosis is also dismal in this group,[7,195] allogeneic BMT from a related or unrelated donor is indicated in this subgroup of relapsing patients as well, preferably on a clinical trial.

CNS relapse

The CNS is the second commonest site for relapse in child-

Table 20.11 Prognostic factors in the therapy of relapsed acute lymphoblastic leukemia.

Factor	Favorable	Unfavorable
Duration of first complete remission	Late (> 6–12 months after cessation of treatment)	Early
Site of relapse	Extramedullary relapse	Bone marrow relapse
Peripheral blasts at relapse ($\times 10^9$/L)	< 10	> 10
Immunophenotype	B-precursor ALL	T-ALL, B-ALL
Cytogenetics/molecular genetics	t(12;21)	t(4;11), t(9;22)
Response to relapse treatment	Complete remission within 6 weeks	Complete remission after 6 weeks

hood ALL. The incidence of CNS relapses depends largely on the CNS-directed treatment applied in first-line treatment.[100] With adequate CNS-directed treatment, isolated and combined CNS relapses occur in < 5% of children in first remission.[3–5,101,196] As in other presumed isolated extramedullary relapses of ALL, CNS relapses should be considered a localized manifestation of systemic leukemia and thus treatment should always include intensive systemic polychemotherapy as well as local therapy. Most successful treatment regimens use intensive polychemotherapy together with extended intrathecal therapy and cranial or craniospinal irradiation at a dose dependent on the dose given during first-line treatment.[7,197,198]

A study from St Jude Children's Hospital reported a 5-year disease-free survival in second remission of > 70% in children with isolated CNS relapse. About half of all children with CNS relapse with or without concomitant bone marrow involvement have achieved long-term (>5 years) second remission and possible cure in the ongoing ALL-BFM relapse trials.[199]

Testicular relapse

Testicular relapse probably arises in a sanctuary area. In early ALL trials with less intensive polychemotherapy, up to 50% of males exhibited testicular relapse, either with or without concomitant bone marrow involvement.[200–203] The incidence of testicular relapse has been dramatically decreased after intensification of front-line regimens. In recent trials, < 5% of boys with ALL developed overt testicular relapse with or without bone marrow involvement.[3–5,196]

Treatment of testicular relapse with or without bone marrow involvement must include intensive polychemotherapy including CNS-directed therapy together with local therapy. Most trials recommend second remission radiotherapy to the scrotum and iliac region, usually with a dose of 24 Gy. Using this approach, boys with late isolated testicular relapse occurring later than 6 months after cessation of therapy may have a 70% or greater probability of cure.[7,204,205] Routine testicular biopsy at the end of first-line therapy has proved to be of no value.[206]

Late bone marrow relapse

Children with B-precursor ALL relapsing more than 6 months after cessation of therapy may experience extended second remission or even cure with a second course of intensive polychemotherapy.[7,189,207,208] A second remission can be induced by intensive polychemotherapy in > 90% of children with late bone marrow relapse,[7,207] with a second EFS of > 5 years in about 35%.[209,210] Duration of first remission[6,7,211] is the most important predictive factor for the length of second remission. In addition, a blood lymphoblast count of < 10×10^9/L[209] and a low WBC[211] at the time of relapse have been associated with a high second EFS rate. Furthermore, the presence of t(12;21) at relapse predicts a favorable outcome.[212] Most relapse trials demonstrate a superior outcome in children with combined rather than isolated bone marrow relapse.[7,208]

Relapse at other sites

Leukemia may very rarely reoccur at other sites (e.g., eye, ovary, tonsils and skin). As in other extramedullary relapses, intensive polychemotherapy including CNS-directed treatment together with appropriate local therapy is recommended in these rare situations.

Role of bone marrow transplantation

Over the past three decades, BMT has evolved as an effective treatment modality for hematologic malignancies.[213,214] In the past, much progress has been made in reducing treatment-related problems, which occur especially in older patients. However, BMT is still burdened by distinct toxic side-effects and infectious complications, resulting in a treatment-related mortality of up to 30%, depending on the source of hematopoietic stem cells.[191,213]

Graft-versus-host disease (GVHD), which is mediated by cytotoxic T lymphocytes, may cause severe morbidity and even mortality, but may also provide additional antileukemic efficacy via a graft-versus-leukemia (GVL) reaction. Attempts to separate GVHD and GVL reaction are ongoing. T-cell depletion of donor marrow results in a significant reduction in GVHD, but also in some situations an increased graft failure rate and an increased leukemic relapse rate.[191]

Matched related sibling or family donor transplantation is limited by the availability of a matched HLA-identical family member (available in ≤ 30% of children with leukemia).[191,213] This limitation may be overcome with increasing numbers of volunteer bone marrow donors on worldwide registries for matched unrelated donor transplantation. However, transplantation-related mortality after matched unrelated donor transplantation is significantly higher compared with matched sibling transplantation in the majority of published trials.[193,194] Another alternative source of hematopoietic stem cells may be cord blood; long-term results are not yet available after cord blood stem cell transplantation.[215]

Predictive factors for the outcome after allogeneic BMT may be similar, at least in part, to those seen in polychemotherapy, e.g., high-risk features at diagnosis and the duration of first remission.[192,216]

The most commonly used preparatory regimen consists of total body irradiation (TBI) and cyclophosphamide, the original Seattle regimen,[217] or TBI and etoposide.[218–220] Myeloablative chemotherapy with high-dose cytarabine followed by TBI[221] or a preparative regimen without TBI such as busulfan/cyclophosphamide[222] did not decrease relapse rates or improve overall survival.

The high cure rate of ALL in children and adolescents implies that BMT is generally reserved for children who relapse. However, under the conditions of recent risk-adapted polychemotherapy, some patients with very poor risk factors may benefit from allogeneic transplantation in first remission.

Although BMT is widely accepted as an appropriate form of therapy in second remission, the exact impact of BMT for the different subsets of children in second remission, the possible use of matched unrelated donors, and the possible impact of cord transplantation[223] are matters of intensive debate. The role of BMT has to be measured against the efficacy of polychemotherapy within controlled trials. In the absence of randomized trials, matched-pair analyses were used to try to answer some of the most important questions.[224]

In early bone marrow relapse (≤6 months after cessation of treatment), BMT increases the probability of EFS in second complete remission compared with chemotherapy.[219,225] This is especially true for T-ALL relapses and for relapses of Philadelphia-positive ALL. In these situations, the prognosis after conventional chemotherapy is dismal. Therefore, allogeneic BMT from a matched unrelated donor should be considered if no matched related donor is available.

In late bone marrow relapse (>6 months after cessation of therapy), about 35% of children with non-T-ALL may be cured by intensive polychemotherapy alone; thus allogeneic BMT is not recommended by most investigators in this

Table 20.12 Possible indications for bone marrow transplantation (BMT) in childhood acute lymphoblastic leukemia (ALL).

BMT in first complete remission
  Philadelphia chromosome-positive (*BCR/ABL*-positive) ALL
  t(4;11), near haploid, *AML1* amplification
  Poor response to treatment (e.g., no complete remission after 4 weeks of induction therapy)

BMT in second complete remission
  Early (< 6 months after cessation of therapy) bone marrow relapse
  Late bone marrow relapse with unfavorable features (*BCR/ABL*-positive ALL; *TEL/AML*-negative ALL; poor response to relapse therapy after 6 weeks)
  All relapses of T-ALL

BMT in greater than second complete remission
  All patients

situation.[225] It is expected that new technologies such as monitoring response to polychemotherapy for relapse, including monitoring of MRD, will help with the difficult decision of which child should receive allogeneic BMT in second complete remission and these tests are indeed the basis of current international relapse protocols.

The possible indications for BMT using hematopoietic stem cells are summarized in Table 20.12. Autologous stem cell transplantation has the advantage of applicability to all patients in the absence of GVHD. However, there exists a risk of reinfusing residual leukemic blasts.[226,227] In a recent matched-pair analysis, the outcome after autotransplantation was no different from intensive chemotherapy.[224] At this time there is no defined role for this procedure in therapy of ALL.

Complications of treatment

Early complications

Major complications can be expected in children who present with a high leukemic cell burden and a high proliferation capacity, such as T-ALL, B-ALL and c-ALL with hyperleukocytosis (WBC > 10 × 10⁹/L). Life-threatening metabolic complications can result from spontaneous leukemic cell turnover and chemotherapeutically induced leukemic cell death (tumor lysis syndrome), presenting with hyperuricemia, hyperkalemia and hyperphosphatemia.[228,229] Massive release of cellular nucleic acids and their conversion to uric acid may result in the precipitation of uric acid in the renal collecting system and urethers.[230,231] Careful hydration, together with the administration of allopurinol prior to chemotherapy[232–234] or application of rasburicase, help avert these metabolic complications. Potassium is released from lysed lymphoblasts and requires dialysis in some children with decreased renal function due to leukemic infiltration.[233]

In children with hyperleukocytosis (WBC > 10×10^9/L) the microcirculation may be impaired by intravascular clumping of leukemic blasts, resulting in local hypoxemia, endothelial damage, hemorrhage and infarction, especially within the CNS and lungs (hyperleukocytosis/leukostasis syndrome).[45] This syndrome is seen more often in children with AML but has been reported in children with ALL. Packed red blood cell transfusion should not be given in this situation to avoid further increasing blood viscosity and thus worsening the symptoms of hyperleukocytosis/leukostasis syndrome.[45,46]

In children with T-ALL and an enlarged mediastinal mass, life-threatening bronchial and/or cardiovascular (superior vena cava syndrome) compression may occur. Immediate application of systemic chemotherapy is necessary in this oncologic emergency.

Signs and symptoms of meningeal or intracranial involvement, such as headache, vomiting, meningism and cranial nerve palsies, are rare at presentation. Differentiation between intracranial bleeding and leukemic infiltration of the CNS is sometimes impossible even with the help of diagnostic imaging (cranial CT, MRT), especially in children with the hyperleukocytosis/leukostasis syndrome. Immediate lumbar puncture may be dangerous in this situation. Prompt administration of systemic chemotherapy should be considered.

Leukemic infiltration of the optic nerve and/or the retina is extremely rare.[235,236] Immediate systemic chemotherapy including high doses of steroids together with local radiotherapy and intrathecal therapy should be given to prevent blindness.

Supportive care

Optimal treatment of children with ALL requires appropriate supportive care, including the rational use of blood products, an aggressive approach to detection and treatment of bleeding and infectious complications, and continuous psychosocial support for the patient and family. Some of these topics are addressed elsewhere, and only the most important issues, namely the diagnosis, treatment and prophylaxis of bleeding and infectious complications, are discussed here.

Bleeding

Bleeding in children with leukemia is usually due to thrombocytopenia, the differential diagnosis including decreased production due to marrow infiltration and/or chemotherapy-induced marrow aplasia, disseminated intravascular coagulation and septicemia. In rare cases, heparin-induced thrombocytopenia has also to be considered.[237]

Thrombosis

Venous thrombosis (e.g., intracranial sinus vein thrombosis) may occur during treatment of childhood ALL, especially when asparaginase is given.[238,239] Nowak Göttl *et al.*[240] described 15 thromboembolic episodes in 243 consecutive children with

ALL. Most of these children had central venous catheters, and at least one of the following thrombophilic defects were found in all children: factor V Leiden mutation, protein C deficiency, protein S deficiency, antithrombin III deficiency and increased level of lipoprotein (a). Prophylaxis with antithrombin III and avoidance of central venous catheters during asparaginase therapy may be useful in children with defined thrombophilic disorders.[138] However, other series have failed to confirm these findings.

Infections

Infections during granulocytopenia are an important complication of intensive polychemotherapy. Most are presumably bacterial, but a significant microorganism can often not be found by standard methods. Therefore, any febrile child with leukemia and an absolute neutrophil count < 0.5×10^9/L should be considered bacteremic and treated with broad-spectrum antibiotics covering Gram-positive and Gram-negative organisms.

A variety of nonbacterial opportunistic microorganisms can invade the immunocompromised host. Fungal infections, especially *Candida* and *Aspergillus* species, are increasingly observed during prolonged periods of neutropenia and immunosuppression.[47]

The administration of the hematopoietic growth factor granulocyte colony-stimulating factor (G-CSF) to intensively treated children with high-risk ALL may reduce febrile neutropenia and culture-confirmed infections.[241] However, the evidence for regular use is weak at present.

Viral infections, especially due to varicella zoster virus (VZV), complicated by pneumonia, hepatitis and cerebral infection had a high morbidity and mortality in earlier studies.[242,243] Prophylaxis with VZV hyperimmunoglobulin[244] and treatment with aciclovir in overt VZV infection[245,246] have significantly reduced the frequency of disease. Rare cases of measles in severely compromised children with leukemia still have a high mortality and emphasize the importance of vaccination in the general population.[247–249]

In early trials, *Pneumocystis carinii*, now believed to be a fungus, was the cause of severe, often fatal interstitial pneumonia in children with leukemia receiving polychemotherapy, especially with steroids.[250] Prophylaxis with co-trimoxazole almost completely abolished the incidence of severe infection with this organism.[251]

Late complications

The improved survival of childhood ALL has focused attention on the late effects of antileukemic therapy (Table 20.13).

Gonadal

Normal sexual development can be expected in most girls regardless of the form of CNS-directed treatment.[252,253]

Table 20.13 Late sequelae of leukemia treatment.

Organ	Etiology
Gonads	
Infertility	Alkylating agents, radiotherapy
Liver	
Fibrosis/cirrhosis	Methotrexate, mercaptopurine, hepatitis B, C virus
Hepatocellular carcinoma	Hepatitis B virus
Venoocclusive disease	Busulfan, bone marrow transplantation
Lung	
Fibrosis/pneumonitis	Busulfan, radiotherapy
Kidney	
Tubulopathy (Fanconi syndrome)	Ifosfamide
Thyroid	
Tumors, hypothyroidism	Radiotherapy
Spleen	
Overwhelming sepsis	Splenectomy/radiotherapy
Bone	
Osteonecrosis	Steroids
Heart	
Cardiomyopathy	Anthracyclines, radiotherapy
Central nervous system	
Leukoencephalopathy	Radiotherapy, intrathecal chemotherapy
↓IQ, ↓cognition	Radiotherapy, intrathecal chemotherapy
↓Psychomotor skills	Radiotherapy, intrathecal chemotherapy
↓Growth	Radiotherapy, intrathecal chemotherapy
Second malignancies	Genetic predisposition; radiotherapy; alkylating agents, epipodophyllotoxins

Sexual maturation is also normal in most boys,[254,255] although gonadal dysfunction is common following testicular irradiation.[256] Testosterone replacement is recommended in this situation. Currently, there is no evidence that the progeny of survivors of childhood ALL are at increased risk of congenital abnormalities.[257]

Liver

Children receiving continuation treatment with methotrexate frequently have elevated liver function tests. After cessation of therapy these tests return to normal. Chronic liver diseases may occur in children with a history of hepatitis B or C infection.[258]

Cardiac

Anthracyclines are known to exhibit cumulative dose-related cardiotoxicity. Children receiving a cumulative anthracycline dose of 200–260 mg/m^2 are usually asymptomatic,

although in some reduced contractility has been measured after cessation of therapy.[48] Younger age, female sex and a greater cumulative dose of anthracyclines were found to be risk factors for late cardiotoxicity.[49] Additional cardiotoxicity may be caused by other cytotoxic drugs, such as high-dose cyclophosphamide and spinal or mediastinal irradiation.[259]

Central nervous system

A number of CNS sequelae have been described after different modalities of CNS-directed treatment.[180] The incidence of neuroradiologically observed structural abnormalities varies greatly between different trials and may be as high as 75%.[260–263] Four radiologically distinct forms have been identified in children with ALL: subacute leukoencephalopathy, mineralizing angiopathy, subacute necrotizing leukomyelopathy, and cortical atrophy.[264] Although a higher incidence of structural pathology was observed after more intensive CNS-directed treatment, the role of the different components of this treatment (namely high-dose systemic chemotherapy, intrathecal drug application and cranial irradiation) remains to be determined. Several trials revealed no difference in the CT abnormalities between patients receiving cranial irradiation and those who did not.[265,266]

Often a discrepancy between neurologic findings and clinical measurements of neurologic or neurocognitive function is found.[267,268] Children who receive cranial irradiation at a younger age tend to show greater neurologic decrements.[269,270] While most children in these studies had received cranial irradiation, the potential adverse sequelae with intensive intrathecal and systemic high-dose chemotherapy must also be appreciated.[271,272]

Children with CNS relapse who receive a second course of CNS-directed treatment are at particular risk of significant cerebral dysfunction, in addition to neuropsychologic deficits, seizures and leukoencephalopathy.[273,274]

Growth

Cranial irradiation with doses of 18–24 Gy may have a negative impact on final growth, depending on age at radiation, fraction schedule, type of systemic chemotherapy, and pubertal status at radiation. In general, the slowing of growth during treatment of ALL is followed by catch-up growth.[275,276] The effects of cranial irradiation on final growth are more marked in children treated at a young age[277,278] and in female patients.[279] Endocrine studies revealed growth hormone deficiencies in some of these children and treatment with growth hormone has been evaluated in some of the most severely affected children.[280]

Others

Hypothyroidism is relatively common after radiation

treatment.[281] Avascular osteonecrosis has been reported during and after treatment with high doses of corticosteroids.[282,283] The reader is directed to recent excellent reviews of the complex problem of late effects of therapy.[284,285]

Second malignancies

The risk of developing second malignancy after successful treatment of ALL is low. Two large cohort studies from the Nordic countries and the USA estimated a cumulative risk of 2.9% by 20 years[286] and 2.5% by 15 years[287] respectively. The majority of second malignancies were brain tumors, mostly gliomas, developing in the radiation field. Exposure to radiotherapy appears to be associated with a continuous risk of second neoplasm, especially within the thyroid gland.[288,289]

The use of epipodophyllotoxins has been found to be associated with a risk of secondary AML if used in schedules other than short intensive blocks,[83] a complication not observed in treatment protocols that do not contain these drugs.[290]

References

1. Zuelzer WW, Inoue S, Thompson RI *et al.* Long-term cytogenetic studies in acute leukemia of children: the nature of relapse. *Am J Hematol* 1976; **1**: 143–90.

2. Burchenal JH, Murphy ML. Long term survivors in acute leukemia. *Cancer Res* 1965; **25**: 1491–4.

3. Reiter A, Schrappe M, Ludwig W-D *et al.* Chemotherapy in 998 unselected childhood ALL patients. Results and conclusions of the multicenter trial ALL-BFM '86. *Blood* 1994; **84**: 3122–33.

4. Gaynon PS, Steinherz PG, Bleyer WA *et al.* Improved therapy for children with acute lymphoblastic leukemia and unfavorable presenting features: a follow-up report of the Children's Cancer Group Study CCG-106. *J Clin Oncol* 1993; **11**: 2234–42.

5. Rivera GK, Raimondi SC, Williams DL *et al.* Improved outcome in childhood acute lymphoblastic leukemia with reinforced early treatment and rotational combination chemotherapy. *Lancet* 1991; **337**: 61–6.

6. Buchanan GR, Rivera GK, Boyett JM *et al.* Reinduction therapy in 297 children with acute lymphoblastic leukemia in first bone marrow relapse: A Pediatric Oncology Group study. *Blood* 1988; **72**: 1286–92.

7. Henze G, Fengler R, Hartmann R *et al.* Six-year experience with a comprehensive approach to the treatment of recurrent childhood acute lymphoblastic leukemia (ALL-REZ BFM 85). A relapse study of the BFM group. *Blood* 1991; **78**: 1166–72.

8. Dordelmann M, Schrappe M, Reiter A *et al.* Down's syndrome in childhood acute lymphoblastic leukemia: clinical characteristics and treatment outcome in four consecutive BFM trials. Berlin–Frankfurt–Munster Group. *Leukemia* 1998; **12**: 645–51.

9. Pui CH, Raimondi SC, Borowitz MJ *et al.* Immunophenotypes and karyotypes of leukemic cells in children with Down syndrome and acute lymphoblastic leukemia. *J Clin Oncol* 1993; **11**: 1361–7.

10. Ragab AH, Abdel Mageed A, Shuster JJ *et al.* Clinical characteristics and treatment outcome of children with acute lymphocytic leukemia and Down's syndrome. A Pediatric Oncology Group study. *Cancer* 1991; **67**: 1057–63.

11. Robison LL, Nesbit ME Jr, Sather HN *et al.* Down syndrome and acute leukemia in children: a 10-year retrospective survey from Children's Cancer Study Group. *J Pediatr* 1984; **105**: 235–42.

12. Mainzer R, Taybi H. Thymic enlargement and pleural effusion: an unusual roentgenographic complex in childhood leukemia. *Am J Roentgenol* 1971; **112**: 35–9.

13. Greydanus DE, Burgert O, Gilchrist GS *et al.* Hypothalamic syndrome in children with acute lymphocytic leukemia. *Mayo Clin Proc* 1978; **53**: 217–22.

14. Gunther R, Chelstrom LM, Tuel Ahlgren L, Simon J, Myers DE, Uckun FM. Biotherapy for xenografted human central nervous system leukemia in mice with severe combined immunodeficiency using B43 (anti-CD19)-pokeweed antiviral protein immunotoxin. *Blood* 1995; **85**: 2537–45.

15. Lauer SJ, Kirchner PAE. Identification of leukemic cells in the cerebrospinal fluid from children with acute lymphoblastic leukemia: advances and dilemmas. *Am J Pediatr Hematol Oncol* 1989; **11**: 64–73.

16. Mastrangelo R, Poplack D, Bleyer A *et al.* Report and recommendations of the Rome workshop concerning poor-prognosis acute lymphoblastic leukemia in children: biologic bases for staging, stratification, and treatment. *Med Pediatr Oncol* 1986; **14**: 191–4.

17. Gilchrist GS, Tubergen DG, Sather HN *et al.* Low numbers of CSF blasts at diagnosis do not predict for the development of CNS leukemia in children with intermediate-risk acute lymphoblastic leukemia: a Children's Cancer Group report. *J Clin Oncol* 1994; **12**: 2594–600.

18. Mahmoud HH, Rivera GK, Hancock ML *et al.* Low leukocyte counts with blast cells in cerebrospinal fluid of children with newly diagnosed acute lymphoblastic leukemia. *N Engl J Med* 1993; **329**: 314–19.

19. Smith M, Arthur D, Camitta B *et al.* Uniform approach to risk classification and treatment assignment for children with acute lymphoblastic leukemia. *J Clin Oncol* 1996; **14**: 18–24.

20. Hustu HO, Aur RJA. Extramedullary leukemia. *Clin Haematol* 1978; **7**: 313–37.

21. Mastrangelo R, Zuelzer WW *et al.* Chromosomes in the spinal fluid: evidence for metastatic origin of meningeal leukemia. *Blood* 1970; **35**: 227–35.

22. Kataoka A, Shimizu K, Matsumoto T *et al.* Epidural spinal cord compression as an initial symptom in childhood acute lymphoblastic leukemia: rapid decompression by local irradiation and systemic chemotherapy. *Pediatr Hematol Oncol* 1995; **12**: 179–84.

23. Kim TH, Hargreaves HK, Chan WC *et al.* Sequential testicular biopsies in childhood acute lymphocytic leukemia. *Cancer* 1986; **57**: 1038–41.

24. Hudson MM, Frankel LS, Mullins J *et al.* Diagnostic value of surgical testicular biopsy after therapy for acute lymphocytic leukemia. *Pediatrics* 1985; **107**: 50–3.

25. Pui C-H, Dahl GV, Bauman MP *et al.* Elective testicular biopsy during chemotherapy for childhood leukaemia is of no clinical value. *Lancet* 1985; **ii**: 410–12.

26. Schrappe M, Beck J, Brandeis WE *et al.* Treatment of acute lymphoblastic leukemia in young age: results of multicenter study ALL-BFM 81. *Klin Padiatr* 1987; **199**: 133–8.

27. Steinhardt GF, Steinhardt E. Priapism in children with leukemia. *Urology* 1981; **18**: 604–6.

28. Ritter J, Hiddemann W. *Akute Leukämie bei Kindern*. Munich: Urban & Schwarzenberger, 1985.

29. Hughes RG, Kay HEM. Major bone lesions in acute lymphoblastic leukemia. *Med Pediatr Oncol* 1982; **10**: 67–70.

30. Kushner DC, Weinstein HJ, Kirkpatrick JA *et al.* The radiologic diagnosis of leukemia and lymphoma in children. *Semin Oncol* 1980; **15**: 316–34.

31. Murphy RG, Greenberg ML. Osteonecrosis in pediatric patients with acute lymphoblastic leukemia. *Cancer* 1990; **65**: 1717–21.

32. Katz JA, Milton L, Wagner MI *et al.* Typhlitis: an 18-year experience and postmortem review. *Cancer* 1990; **65**: 1041–7.

33. Gootenberg JE, Abbondanzo SL. Rapid diagnosis of neutropenic enterocolitis by ultrasonography. *Am J Pediatr Hematol Oncol* 1987; **9**: 222–7.

34. Weetman RM, Baehner RL. Latent onset of clinical pancreatitis in children receiving L-asparaginase therapy. *Cancer* 1974; **34**: 780–5.

35. Shamberger RC, Weinstein HJ, Levery RH *et al.* The medical and surgical management of typhlitis in children with acute nonlymphocytic (myelogenous) leukemia. *Cancer* 1986; **57**: 603–9.

36. Boddie AWJ, Bines SD. Management of acute rectal problems in leukemic patients. *J Surg Oncol* 1986; **33**: 53–6.

37. Arico M, Maggiore G, Silini E *et al.* Hepatitis C virus infection in children treated for acute lymphoblastic leukemia. *Blood* 1994; **84**: 2919–22.

38. Schachat A, Markowitz JA. Ophthalmic manifestations of leukemia. *Arch Ophthalmol* 1989; **107**: 697–700.

39. Leonardy NJ, Rupani M, Dent G, Klintworth GK. Analysis of 135 autopsy eyes for ocular involvement in leukemia. *Am J Ophthalmol* 1990; **109**: 436–44.

40. Creutzig U, Ritter J, Budde M, Sutor A, Schellong G. Early deaths due to hemorrhage and leukostasis in childhood acute myelogenous leukemia. Associations with hyperleukocytosis and acute monocytic leukemia. *Cancer* 1987; **60**: 3071–9.

41. Robb RM, Ervin LD, Sallan SE *et al.* A pathological study of eye involvement in acute leukemia childhood. *Med Pediatr Oncol* 1979; **6**: 171.

42. Lo Curto M, D'Angelo P, Lumia F *et al.* Leukemic ophthalmopathy: a report of 21 pediatric cases. *Med Pediatr Oncol* 1994; **23**: 813.

43. Ninane J, Taylor D, Day S *et al.* The eye as a sanctuary in acute lymphoblastic leukaemia. *Lancet* 1980; **i**: 452–3.

44. Reiter A, Schrappe M, Ludwig WD *et al.* Favorable outcome of B-cell acute lymphoblastic leukemia in childhood: a report of three consecutive studies of the BFM group. *Blood* 1992; **80**: 2471–8.

45. Lichtman M, Rowe J. Hyperleukocytic leukemias: rheological, clinical and therapeutic considerations. *Blood* 1982; **60**: 279–83.

46. Strauss RA, Gloster ES, Neuberg RW *et al.* Acute cytoreduction techniques in the treatment of hyperleukocytosis associated with childhood hematologic malignancies. *Med Pediatr Oncol* 1985; **13**: 346–51.

47. Ritter J, Roos N. Special aspects related to invasive fungal infections in children with cancer. *Baillière's Clin Infect Dis* 1995; **2**: 179–204.

48. Lipshultz SE, Colan SD, Sallan SE *et al.* Late cardiac effects of doxorubicin therapy for acute lymphoblastic leukemia in childhood. *N Engl J Med* 1991; **324**: 808–15.

49. Lipshultz SE, Lipsitz SR, Mone SM *et al.* Female sex and higher drug dose as risk factors for late cardiotoxic effects of doxorubicin therapy for childhood cancer. *N Engl J Med* 1995; **332**: 1738–43.

50. Meeker TC, Hardy D, Hogan T *et al.* Activation of the interleukin-3 gene by chromosome translocation in acute lymphocytic leukemia with eosinophilia. *Blood* 1990; **76**: 285–9.

51. Pereira F, Moreno H, Crist W *et al.* Loffler's endomyocardial fibrosis, eosinophilia, and acute lymphoblastic leukemia. *Pediatrics* 1977; **59**: 950–1.

52. Spier CM, Kjeldsberg CR, Marty J *et al.* Pre-B-cell acute lymphoblastic leukemia in the newborn. *Blood* 1984; **64**: 1064–6.

53. Dubansky AS, Boyett JM, Pullen J *et al.* Isolated thrombocytopenia in children with acute lymphoblastic leukemia: a rare event in a Pediatric Oncology Group study. *Pediatrics* 1989; **84**: 1068–71.

54. Eguiguren JM, Pui C-H. Bone marrow necrosis and thrombotic complications in childhood acute lymphoblastic leukemia. *Med Pediatr Oncol* 1992; **20**: 58–60.

55. Hann IM, Evans DIK, Jones PM *et al.* Bone marrow fibrosis in acute lymphoblastic leukaemia of childhood. *J Clin Pathol* 1978; **31**: 313–15.

56. Bennett JM, Catovsky D, Daniel MT *et al.* Proposals for the classification of the acute leukemias. French–American–British (FAB) co-operative group. *Br J Haematol* 1976; **33**: 451–8.

57. Cerezo L, Shuster JJ, Pullen DJ *et al.* Laboratory correlates and prognostic significance of granular acute lymphoblastic leukemia in children. A Pediatric Oncology Group study. *Am J Clin Pathol* 1991; **95**: 526–31.

58. Stass SA, Pui C-H, Dahl GV *et al.* Sudan black B positive acute lymphoblastic leukaemia. *Br J Haematol* 1984; **57**: 413–21.

59. Catovsky D, Greaves MF, Pain C *et al.* Acid-phosphatase reaction in acute lymphoblastic leukaemia. *Lancet* 1978; **i**: 749–51.

60. Ritter J, Gaedicke G, Winkler K, Beckmann H, Landbeck G. Possible T-cell origin of lymphoblasts in acid-phosphatase-positive leukaemia. *Lancet* 1975; **ii**: 75.

61. Ludwig WD, Bartram CR, Ritter R *et al.* Ambiguous phenotypes and genotypes in 16 children with acute leukemia as characterized by multiparameter analysis. *Blood* 1988; **71**: 1515–28.

62. Mirro J, Zipf TF, Pui CH *et al.* Acute mixed lineage leukemia: clinicopathologic correlations and prognostic significance. *Blood* 1985, **66**: 1115–23.

63. Perentesis J, Ramsay N, Ramsay NK *et al.* Biphenotypic leukemia: immunologic and morphologic evidence for a common lymphoid-myeloid progenitor in humans. *J Pediatr* 1983; **102**: 63–7.

64. Ben-Bassat I, Gale RP. Hybrid acute leukemia. *Leukemia Res* 1984; **8**: 929–36.

65. Greaves MF, Chan LC, Watt SM *et al.* Lineage promiscuity in hemopoietic differentiation and leukemia. *Blood* 1986; **67**: 1–11.

66. Smith LJ, Curtis JE, Senn JS *et al.* Lineage infidelity in acute leukemia. *Blood* 1983; **61**: 1138–45.

67. Fink FM, Köller U, Mayer H *et al.* Prognostic significance of myeloid-associated antigen expression on blast cells in children with acute lymphoblastic leukemia. *Med Pediatr Oncol* 1993; **21**: 340–6.

68. Ludwig WD, Harbott J, Bartram CR *et al.* Incidence and prognostic significance of immunophenotypic subgroups in childhood acute lymphoblastic leukemia: Experience of the BFM study 86. In: Ludwig WD, Thiel E (eds) *Recent Results in Cancer Research*. Berlin/Heidelberg: Springer-Verlag, 1993, pp. 269–82.

69. Pui C-H, Behm F, Crist WM *et al.* Myeloid-associated antigen expression lacks prognostic value in childhood acute lymphoblastic leukemia treated with intensive multiagent chemotherapy. *Blood* 1990, **75**: 198–202.

70. Wiersma SR, Ortega J, Sobel E *et al.* Clinical importance of myeloid-antigen expression in acute lymphoblastic leukemia of childhood. *N Engl J Med* 1991; **324**: 800–8.

71. Hann I, Vora A, Harrison G *et al.* Determinants of outcome after intensified therapy of childhood lymphoblastic leukaemia: results of MRC UKALL XI. protocol. *Br J Haematol* 2001; **113**: 103–14.

72. Catovsky D, Matutes E, Buccheri V *et al.* A classification of acute leukaemia for the 1990s. *Ann Hematol* 1991; **62**: 16–21.

73. Campana D, Hansen-Hagge TE, Matutes E *et al.* Phenotypic, genotypic, cytochemical and ultrastructural characterization of acute undifferentiated leukemia. *Leukemia* 1990; **4**: 620–4.

74. van Delft F, Saha V. Molecular techniques to improve outcome in childhood ALL. *Methods Mol Med* 2004; **91**: 111–22.

75. Romain SP, Le Coriat M, Berger R. E(12;21): a new recurrent translocation in acute lymphoblastic leukaemia. *Genes Chromosomes Cancer* 1994; **9**: 184–91.

76. Rubnitz JE, Look AT. Molecular genetics of childhood leukaemias. *J Pediatr Hematol Oncol* 1998; **20**: 1–7.

77. Ramakers-van Waerden NL, Pieters R, Loonen AH *et al.* Tel/AML1 gene fusion is related to in vitro drug sensivity for L-asparaginase in childhood acute lymphoblastic leukaemia. *Blood* 2002; **96**: 1094–9.

78. Paimonid SC, Pui C-H, Hancock ML *et al.* Heterogeneity of hyperdiploid (51–67) childhood acute lymphoblastic leukaemia. *Leukaemia* 1996; **10**: 213–24.

79. Jackson JF, Boyett J, Pallen J *et al.* Favourable prognosis associated with hyper-diploidy in children with acute lymphoblastic leukaemia correlates with extra chromosome 6. *Cancer* 1990; **66**: 1184–9.

80. Heerema NA, Sather NH, Sensel MG *et al.* Prognostic impact of trisomies 10, 17 and 5 among children with acute lymphoblastic leukaemia and high hyperdiploidy (>50 chromosomes). *J Clin Oncol* 2000; **18**: 1876–87.

81. Golub TR, Slonim DK, Tamayou P *et al.* Molecular classification of cancer: class discovery and class prediction by gene expression monitoring. *Science* 1999; **286**: 531–7.

82. Fourth International Workshop on Chromosomes in Leukaemia. A prospective study of acute non-lymphocytic leukaemia. *Cancer Genet Cytogenet* 1984; **11**: 249–360.

83. Pui C-H, Behm FG, Raimondi SC *et al.* Secondary acute myeloid leukaemia in children treated for acute lymphoid leukaemia. *N Engl J Med* 1989; **321**: 136–42.

84. Zieman-van Der Poel S, McCabe NR, Gill HJ *et al.* Identification of a gene, MLL, that spans the breakpoint in 11q23 translocations associated with human leukaemias. *Proc Natl Acad Sci USA* 1991; **88**: 10735–9.

85. Rubnitz JE. Pui C-H, Downing JR. The role of TEL fusion genes in paediatric leukaemia. *Leukaemia* 1999; **13**: 6–13.

86. Marrow M, Horton S, Kioussis D, Brady H, Williams O. TEL-AML1 promotes development of specifc haemopoietic lineages consistent with preleukaemic activity. *Blood* 2004; **103**: 890–6.

87. Siebert R, Mathiesen P, Harder S *et al.* Application of interphase fluorescence in situ hybridisation for the detection of the Burkett translocation t(8;14)(q24;q32) in B-cell lymphoma. *Blood* 1998; **91**: 984–90.

88. Mederos LE. Intermediate and high-grade diffuse non-Hodgkin's lymphoma in the working formulation. In: Jaffe ES (ed.) *Surgical Pathology of the Lymph Nodes and Related Organs*, 2nd cdn. Philadelphia: WB Saunders, 1995, pp. 283–343.

89. Hoelzer D, Ludwig W, Eckhard E *et al.* Improved outcome to adult B-cell acute lymphoblastic leukaemia. *Blood* 1996; **87**: 495–508.

90. Carroll AJ, Crist WM, Parmley RT *et al.* Pre-B cell leukaemia associated with chromosome translocations 1:19. *Blood* 1994; **63**: 721–4.

91. Hunger SP. Chromosomal translocations involving the E2A gene in acute lymphoblastic leukaemia: clinical features and molecular pathogenesis. *Blood* 1996; **87**: 1211–16.

92. Uckum FM, Sensel MG, Sun L *et al.* Biology and treatment of children T-lineage acute lymphoblastic leukaemia. *Blood* 1998; **91**: 735–46.

93. Campana D, Coustan-Smithe E. Detection of minimal residual disease in acute leukemia by flow cytometry. *Cytometry* 1999; **38**: 139–52.

94. Meekev TC, Haroy D, William C *et al.* Activation of the interleukin-3 gene by chromosomal translocation in acute lymphocytic leukaemia with eosinophilia. *Blood* 1990; **76**: 285–8.

95. Matloub YH, Brunning RD, Arthur DC *et al.* Severe aplastic anaemia preceding acute lymphoblastic leukaemia. *Cancer* 1993; **71**: 234–68.

96. Riehm H, Gadner H, Henze G *et al.* Results and significance of six randomized trials in four consecutive ALL-BFM studies. In: Büchner T, Schellong G, Hiddemann W, Ritter J (eds) *Haematology and Blood Transfusion*. Berlin/Heidelberg: Springer-Verlag, 1990, pp. 439–50.

97. Rivera CK, Pinkel D, Simone JV, Hancock ML, Crist WM. Treatment of acute lymphoblastic leukaemia: 30 years' experience at St. Jude Children's Research Hospital. *N Engl J Med* 1993; **329**: 1289–95.

98. Pullen J, Boyett J, Shuster J *et al.* Extended triple intrathecal chemotherapy trial for prevention of CNS relapse in good risk and poor-risk patients with B-progenitor acute lymphoblastic leukemia: a Pediatric Oncology Group Study. *J Clin Oncol* 1993; **11**: 839–49.

99. Veerman AJP, Hählen K, Kamps WA *et al.* High cure rate with a moderately intensive treatment regimen in non-high-risk childhood acute lymphoblastic leukaemia: results of protocol ALL VI from the Dutch Childhood Leukemia Study Group. *J Clin Oncol* 1996; **14**: 911–18.

100. Niemeyer CM, Hitchcock-Bryan S, Sallan SE *et al.* Comparative analysis of treatment programs for childhood acute lymphoblastic leukemia. *Semin Oncol* 1985; **12**: 122–30.

101. Schorin MA, Blattner S, Gelber RD *et al.* Treatment of childhood acute lymphoblastic leukaemia: results of Dana-Faber Cancer Institute Children's Acute Lymphoblastic Leukaemia Consortium Protocol 85-01. *J Clin Oncl* 1994; **12**: 740–7.

102. Lilleyman JS, Hann IM, Stevens RF *et al.* Cytomorphology of childhood lymphoblastic leukaemia: a prospective study of 2000 patients. *Br J Haematol* 1992; **81**: 52–7.

103. Steinherz PG, Siegal, Bleyer WA *et al.* Lymphomatous presentation of childhood acute lymphoblastic leukaemia: a subgroup at high risk of early treatment failure. *Cancer* 1991; **68**: 751–8.

104. Crist W, Pullen J, Dowell B *et al.* Clinical and biological features predict a poor prognosis in acute lymphoid leukaemias in infants: a Paediatric Oncology Group study. *Blood* 1986; **67**: 135–40.

105. Tubergen DG, Gilchrist GS, O'Brien RT *et al.* Improved outcome with delayed intensification for children with acute lymphoblastic leukemia and intermediate presenting features: a Children's Cancer Group phase III trial. *J Clin Oncol* 1993; **11**: 527–37.

106. Chessells JM, Richards SM, Bailey CC, Lilleyman JS, Eden OB. Gender and treatment outcome in childhood lymphoblastic leukaemia: report from the MRC UKALL trials. *Br J Haematol* 1995; **89**: 364–72.

107. Pui C-H, Boyett JM, Hancock ML, Pratt CB, Meyer WH, Crist WM. Outcome of treatment for childhood cancer in black as compared with white children. The St. Jude Children's Research Hospital experience, 1962 through 1992. *JAMA* 1995; **273**: 633–7.

108. Crist WM, Boyett J. Pre B-cell leukemia responds poorly to treatment: a Pediatric Oncology Group study. *Blood* 1984; **63**: 407–14.

109. Crist WM, Caroll AJ, Behm FG *et al.* Poor prognosis of children with pre-B acute lymphoblastic leukemia is associated with the t(1;19)(q23;q13): a Pediatric Oncology Group study. *Blood* 1990; **76**: 117–22.

110. Pui C-H, Williams DL, Melvin SL *et al.* Unfavorable presenting clinical and laboratory features are associated with CALLA-negative non-T, non-B lymphoblastic leukemia in children. *Leukemia Res* 1986; **11**: 1287–92.

111. Vannier JP, Bene MC, Faure GC *et al.* Investigation of the CD 10 (CALLA) negative acute lymphoblastic leukaemia: further description of a group with a poor prognosis. *Br J Haematol* 1989; **72**: 156–60.

112. Kaspers GJ, Smets LA, Pieters R, van Zantwijk CH, van Wering ER, Veerman AJ. Favorable prognosis of hyperdiploid common acute lymphoblastic leukemia may be explained by sensitivity to antimetabolites and other drugs: results of an in vitro study. *Blood* 1995; **85**: 751–6.

113. Raimondi SC, Pui C-H, Hancock ML, Behm FG, Filatov L, Rivera GK. Heterogeneity of hyperdiploid (51–67) childhood acute lymphoblastic leukemia. *Leukemia* 1996; **10**: 213–24.

114. McLean TW, Ringold S, Neuberg D *et al.* TEL/AML-1 dimerizes and is associated with a favorable outcome in childhood acute lymphoblastic leukemia. *Blood* 1996; **88**: 4252–8.

115. Borkhardt A, Cazzaniga G, Viehmann S *et al.* Incidence and clinical relevance of TEL/AML1 fusion genes in children with acute lymphoblastic leukemia enrolled in the German and Italian multicenter therapy trials. Associazione Italiana Ematologia Oncologia Pediatrica and the Berlin–Frankfurt–Munster Study Group. *Blood* 1997; **90**: 571–7.

116. Crist W, Carroll A, Link M *et al.* Philadelphia chromosome positive childhood acute lymphoblastic leukemia: clinical and cytogenetic characteristics and treatment outcome. A Pediatric Oncology Group study. *Blood* 1990; **76**: 489–94.

117. Beyermann B, Agthe AG, Adams H-P *et al.* Clinical features and outcome of children with first marrow relapse of acute lymphoblastic leukemia expressing BCR-ABL fusion transcripts. *Blood* 1996; **87**: 1532–8.

118. Fletscher JA, Lynch EA, Kimball VM *et al.* Translocation (9;22) is associated with extremely poor prognosis in intensively treated children with acute lymphoblastic leukemia. *Blood* 1991; **77**: 435–9.

119. Ribeiro RC, Abromowitch M, Behm F *et al.* Clinical and biologic hallmarks of the Philadelphia chromosome in childhood acute lymphoblastic leukemia. *Blood* 1987; **70**: 948–53.

120. Roberts WM, Rivera GK, Raimondi SC *et al.* Intensive chemotherapy for Philadelphia-chromosome-positive acute lymphoblastic leukaemia. *Lancet* 1994; **343**: 331–2.

121. Lampert F, Harbott J, Ludwig W-D *et al.* Acute leukemia with chromosome translocation (4;11): 7 new patients and analysis of 71 cases. *Blut* 1987; **54**: 325–35.

122. Pui C-H, Frankel LS, Carroll AJ *et al.* Clinical characteristics and treatment outcome of childhood acute lymphoblastic leukemia with the t(4;11)(q21;q23): a collaborative study of 40 cases. *Blood* 1991; **77**: 440–7.

123. Aric M, Schrappe M, Harbott J *et al.* Prednisone good response (PGR) identifies a subset of t(9;22) childhood acute lymphoblastic leukemia (ALL) at lower risk for early leukemia relapse. *Blood* 1997; **90** (suppl.): 2494–8.

124. Gaynon PS, Bleyer WA, Miller DR *et al.* Day 7 marrow response and outcome for children with acute lymphoblastic leukemia and unfavorable presenting features. *Med Pediatr Oncol* 1990; **18**: 273–9.

125. Miller DR, Coccia PF. Early response to induction therapy as a predictor of disease-free survival and late recurrence of childhood acute lymphoblastic leukemia: a report from the Children's Cancer Study Group. *J Clin Oncol* 1989; **7**: 1807–15.

126. Riehm H, Reiter A, Schrappe M *et al.* Die Corticosteroid-abhängige Dezimierung der Leukämiezellzahl im Blut als Prognosefaktor bei der akuten lymphoblastischen Leukämie im Kindesalter (Theraiestudie ALL-BFM 83). *Klin Padiatr* 1987; **199**: 151–60.

127. Schrappe M, Reiter A, Sauter S *et al.* Concept and interim result of the ALL-BFM 90 therapy study in treatment of acute lymphoblastic leukemia in children and adolescents: the significance of initial therapy response in blood and bone marrow. *Klin Padiatr* 1994; **206**: 208–21.

128. Biondi A, van Dongen JJM, Seriu T *et al.* Predictive value of minimal residual disease measurement during remission in childhood acute lymphoblastic leukemia: the results of the International-BFM Study Group (I-BFM-SG). *Blood* 1997; **10** (suppl.): 1878.

129. Pui C-H, Campana D, Evans WE. Childhood acute lymphoblastic leukaemia: current status and future prospectives. *Lancet Oncol* 2001; **2**: 597–607.

130. Pui C-H, Campana E. New definition of remission in

childhood acute lymphoblastic leukaemia. *Leukemia* 2000; **14**: 1483–5.

131. Szczepanski T, Orfao A, van der Velden V *et al*. Minimal residual disease in leukaemia patients. *Lancet Oncol* 2001; **2**: 409–17.

132. Krejki O, van der Velden V, Bader P *et al*. Level of MRD prior to stem cell transplantation. *Bone Marrow Transplant* 2003; **32**: 849–51.

133. Moppett J, Burke GA, Steward CG. The clinical relevance of detection of MRD in childhood ALL. *J Clin Pathol* 2003; **56**: 249–53.

134. Cheson B, Dutcher BS. Managing malignancy-associated hyperuricaemia with rasburicase. *J Support Oncol* 2005; **3**: 117–24.

135. Farber S, Diamond LK *et al*. Temporary remissions in acute leukemia in children produced by folic acid antagonist, 4-amionopteroyl-glutamic acid (aminopterin). *N Engl J Med* 1948; **238**: 787–96.

136. Mitchel C, Richards S, Kinsey S *et al*. Benefit of dexamethasone compared with prednisolone for childhood ALL. Results of the UK-ALL 97 randomized trial. *Br J Haematol* 2005; **129**: 734–45.

137. Boos J, Werber G, Ahlke E *et al*. Monitoring of asparaginase activity and asparagine levels in children on different asparaginase preparations. *Eur J Cancer* 1996; **32A**: 1544–50.

138. Nowak-Göttl U, Kuhn N, Wolff JE *et al*. Inhibition of hypercoagulation by antithrombin substitution in *E. coli* L-asparaginase-treated children. *Eur J Haematol* 1996; **56**: 35–8.

139. Freeman AI, Weinberg V, Jones B *et al*. Comparison of intermediate-dose methotrexate with cranial irradiation for the post-induction treatment of acute lymphocytic leukemia in children. *N Engl J Med* 1983; **308**: 477–84.

140. Lennard L, Lilleyman JS. Variable mercaptopurine metabolism and treatment outcome in childhood lymphoblastic leukemia. *J Clin Oncol* 1989; **7**: 1816–26.

141. Riccardi R, Balis FM, Poplack DG *et al*. Influence of food intake on bioavailability of oral 6-mercaptopurine in children with acute lymphoblastic leukemia. *Pediatr Hematol Oncol* 1986; **3**: 319–424.

142. Hann I, Vora A, Richards S. Results from MRC UKALL XI and ALL 97. *Leukaemia* 2000; **14**: 356–63.

143. Lauer SJ, Camitta BM, Leventhal BG *et al*. Intensive alternating drug pairs for treatment of high-risk childhood acute lymphoblastic leukemia. A Pediatric Oncology Group pilot study. *Cancer* 1993; **71**: 2854–61.

144. Patte C, Philip T, Rodary C *et al*. High survival rate in advanced-stage B-cell lymphomas and leukemias without CNS involvement with a short intensive polychemotherapy: Results from the French Pediatric Oncology Society of a randomized trial of 216 children. *J Clin Oncol* 1991; **9**: 123–32.

145. Pui C-H, Behn FG, George SL *et al*. Secondary acute myeloid leukemia in children treated for acute lymphoid leukemia. *N Engl J Med* 1989; **321**: 136–42.

146. Selawry OS, Hananian J. Vincristine Treatment of Cancer in Children. *Jama* 1963; **183**: 741–6.

147. Clavell LA, Gelber RD, Tarbell MJ *et al*. Four-agent induction and intensive asparaginase therapy for treatment of childhood acute lymphoblastic leukemia. *N Engl J Med* 1986; **315**: 657–63.

148. Henze G, Langermann HJ, Riehm H *et al*. Treatment strategy for different risk groups in childhood acute lymphoblastic leukemia: a report form the BFM Study Group. *Haematol Bluttransfus* 1981; **26**: 87–93.

149. Camitta B, Mahoney D, Leventhal B *et al*. Intensive intravenous methotrexate and mercaptopurine treatment of higher-risk non-T, non-B acute lymphocytic leukemia. *J Clin Oncol* 1994; **12**: 1383–9.

150. Raimondi SC, Behm FG, Roberson PK *et al*. Cytogenetics of childhood T-cell leukemia. *Blood* 1988; **72**: 1560.

151. Sallan SE, Gelber RD *et al*. More is better! Update of Dana-Farber Cancer Institute/Children's Hospital childhood acute lymphoblastic leukemia trials. In: Büchner T, Schellong G *et al*. (eds) *Haematology and Blood Transfusion 33. Acute Leukemias II*. Heidelberg: Springer-Verlag, 1990, p. 459.

152. Schrappe M, Reiter A, Sauter S *et al*. Risk-oriented treatment of childhood ALL. favorable outcome despite reduced intensity of treatment in trial ALL-BFM 90. *Blood* 1997; **90** (suppl.): 2488.

153. Nachman J, Sather H, Lukens J *et al*. Acute lymphocytic leukemia: clinical investigation and pathophysiology. Augmented Berlin–Frankfurt–Münster (A-BFM) chemotherapy improves event free survival (EFS) for children with acute lymphoblastic leukemia (ALL) and unfavorable presenting features who show a slow early response (SER) to induction chemotherapy. *Blood* 1997; **90** (suppl.): 2487.

154. Hill FG, Richards S, Gibson B *et al*. Successful treatment without radiotherapy: results of the CNS treatment trial MRC UKALL XI. *Br J Haematol* 2004; **124**: 33–46.

155. Peylan-Ramu N, Poplack DG, Pizzo PA *et al*. Abnormal CT scans of the brain in asymptomatic children with acute lymphocytic leukemia after prophylactic treatment of the central nervous system with radiation and intrathecal chemotherapy. *N Engl J Med* 1978; **298**: 815–18.

156. Ochs J, Rivera G, Berg R *et al*. Central nervous system morbidity following an initial isolated central nervous system relapse and its subsequent therapy in childhood acute lymphoblastic leukemia. *J Clin Oncol* 1985; **3**: 622–6.

157. Clarke M, Graynon P, Hann I *et al*. CNS-directed therapy for childhood ALL: collaborative group overview of 43 randomised trials. *J Clin Oncol* 2003; **21**: 1798–809.

158. Freeman JE, Johnston PGB *et al*. Somnolence after prophylactic cranial irradiation in children with acute lymphoblastic leukaemia. *Br Med J* 1973; **1**: 523.

159. Frei E III, Karon M, Robert H *et al*. The effectiveness of combinations of antileukemia agents in inducing and maintaining remission in children with acute leukemia. *Blood* 1965; **26**: 642–56.

160. Lonsdale D, Gehan EA, Lane DM *et al*. Interrupted vs. continued maintenance therapy in childhood acute leukemia. *Cancer* 1975; **36**: 341–52.

161. Chessells JM, Leiper AD, Richards S *et al*. Oral methotrexate is as effective as intramuscular in maintenance therapy of acute lymphoblastic leukaemia. *Arch Dis Child* 1987; **62**: 172–6.

162. Bleyer WA, Sather HN, Nickerson HJ *et al*. Monthly pulses of vincristine and prednisone prevent bone marrow and testicular relapse in low-risk childhood acute lymphoblastic leukemia: a report from the CCSG-161 Study by the Children's Cancer Study Group. *J Clin Oncol* 1991; **9**: 1012–21.

163. Childhood ALL Collaborative Group. Duration and intensity of maintenance chemotherapy in acute lymphoblastic

leukaemia: overview of 42 trials involving 12 000 randomised children. *Lancet* 1996; **347**: 1783–8.

164. George SL, Aur RJA *et al*. A reappraisal of the results of stopping therapy in childhood leukemia. *N Engl J Med* 1979; **330**: 269–73.

165. Frost L, Richards DS, Goodeve A *et al*. Late relapsing childhood lymphoblastic leukemia. *Blood* 1997; **90**: 560A.

166. Eden OB, Lilleyman JS, Richards S, Shaw MP, Peto J. Results of Medical Research Council Childhood Leukaemia Trial UKALL VIII (report to the Medical Research Council on behalf of the Working Party on Leukaemia in Childhood). *Br J Haematol* 1991; **78**: 196.

167. Miller DR, Leikin S, Palmer MF *et al*. Prognostic factors and therapy in acute lymphoblastic leukemia of childhood: CCG-141. *Cancer* 1983; **51**: 1041.

168. Steenbergen EJ, Verhagen OJ, van Leeuwen EF *et al*. Prolonged persistence of PCR-detectable minimal residual disease after diagnosis or first relapse predicts poor outcome in childhood B-precursor acute lymphoblastic leukaemia. *Leukemia* 1995; **9**: 1726–34.

169. Wasserman R, Galili N, Ito Y *et al*. Residual disease at the end of induction therapy as a predictor of relapse during therapy in childhood B-lineage acute lymphoblastic leukemia. *J Clin Oncol* 1992; **10**: 1879–88.

170. Beishuizen A, Verhoeven MA, van Wering ER, Hählen K, Hooijkaas H, van Dongen JJ. Analysis of Ig and T-cell receptor genes in 40 childhood acute lymphoblastic leukemias at diagnosis and subsequent relapse: implications for the detection of minimal residual disease by polymerase chain reaction analysis. *Blood* 1994; **83**: 2238–47.

171. Raghavachar A, Ludwig W-D, Bartram CR *et al*. Clonal variation in childhood acute lymphoblastic leukaemia at early and late relapse detected by analyses of phenotype and genotype. *Eur J Pediatr* 1988; **147**: 503–7.

172. Wright JJ, Poplack DG, Cole D *et al*. Gene rearrangements as markers of clonal variation and minimal residual disease in acute lymphoblastic leukemia. *J Clin Oncol* 1987; **5**: 735–41.

173. Baruchel A, Cayuela JM, Macintyre E, Berger R, Sigaux F. Assessment of clonal evolution at Ig/TCR loci in acute lymphoblastic leukemia by single-strand conformation polymorphism studies and highly resolutive PCR derived methods: implication for a general strategy of minimal residual disease detection. *Br J Haematol* 1995; **90**: 85–93.

174. Steenbergen EJ, Verhagen OJ, van Leeuwen EF, van den Berg H, von dem Borne AE, van der Schoot CE. Frequent ongoing T-cell receptor rearrangements in childhood B-precursor acute lymphoblastic leukemia: implications for monitoring minimal residual disease. *Blood* 1995; **86**: 692–702.

175. Steward CG, Goulden NJ, Katz F *et al*. A polymerase chain reaction study of the stability of Ig heavy-chain and T-cell receptor delta gene rearrangements between presentation and relapse of childhood B-lineage acute lymphoblastic leukemia. *Blood* 1994; **83**: 1355–62.

176. Lampert R, Harbott J, Ritterbach J. Cytogenetic findings in acute leukaemias of infants. *Br J Cancer* 1992; **66**: 20–2.

177. Pui C-H, Kane JR, Crist WM. Biology and treatment of infant leukemias. *Leukemia* 1995; **9**: 762–9.

178. Bucsky P, Reiter A, Riehm H *et al*. Die akute lymphoblastische Leukämie im Säuglingsalter: Ergebnisse aus fünf multizentrischen Therapiestudien ALL-BFM 1970–1986. *Klin Padiatr* 1988; **200**: 177–83.

179. Ochs J, Mulhern RK. Late effects of antileukemic treatment. *Pediatr Clinic North Am* 1988; **35**: 815–33.

180. Ochs JJ. Neurotoxicity due to central nervous system therapy for childhood leukemia. *Am J Pediatr Hematol Oncol* 1989; **11**: 93–105.

181. Creutzig U, Ritter J, Vormoor J *et al*. Myelodysplasia and acute myelogenous leukemia in Down's syndrome. A report of 40 children of the AML-BFM Study Group. *Leukemia* 1996; **10**: 1677–86.

182. Neale GA, Pui C-H, Mahmoud HH *et al*. Molecular evidence for minimal residual bone marrow disease in children with "isolated" extra-medullary relapse of T-cell acute lymphoblastic leukemia. *Leukemia* 1994; **8**: 768–75.

183. Rivera G, Aur RJA, Husto HO *et al*. Second central nervous system prophylaxis in children with acute lymphoblastic leukemia who relapse after elective cessation of therapy. *J Clin Oncol* 1983; **1**: 471–6.

184. Pui C-H, Raimondi SC, Mirro J *et al*. Shifts in blast cell phenotype and karyotype at relapse of childhood lymphoblastic leukemia. *Blood* 1986; **68**: 1306–10.

185. Nooter K, Sonneveld P. Multidrug resistance (MDR) genes in haematological malignancies. *Cytotechnology* 1993; **12**: 213–30.

186. Buchanan GR, Boyett JM, Pollock BH *et al*. Improved treatment results in boys with overt testicular relapse during or shortly following initial therapy for acute lymphoblastic leukemia: a Pediatric Oncology Group study. *Cancer* 1991; **68**: 48–55.

187. Bührer C, Hartmann R, Fengler R *et al*. Superior prognosis in combined compared to isolated bone marrow relapses in salvage therapy of childhood acute lymphoblastic leukemia. *Med Pediatr Oncol* 1993; **21**: 470–6.

188. Bührer C, Hartmann R, Fengler R *et al*. Importance of effective central nervous system therapy in isolated bone marrow relapse of childhood acute lymphoblastic leukemia. *Blood* 1994; **83**: 3468–72.

189. Bleyer WA, Sather H, Hammond JD *et al*. Prognosis and treatment after relapse of acute lymphoblastic leukemia and non-Hodgkin's lymphoma: 1985. A report from the Children's Cancer Study Group. *Cancer* 1986; **58**: 590–4.

190. Rivera GK, Buchanan G, Ochs J *et al*. Intensive retreatment of childhood acute lymphoblastic leukemia in first bone marrow relapse. A Pediatric Oncology Group study. *N Engl J Med* 1986; **315**: 274–8.

191. Barrett AJ, Horowitz MM, Pollock BH *et al*. Bone marrow transplants from HLA-identical siblings as compared with chemotherapy for children with acute lymphoblastic leukemia in a second remission. *N Engl J Med* 1994; **331**: 1253–8.

192. Butturini A, Rivera GK, Gaie RP *et al*. Which treatment for childhood acute lymphoblastic leukemia in second remission? *Lancet* 1987; **i**: 429–32.

193. Casper J, Camitta B, Truitt R *et al*. Unrelated bone marrow donor transplants for children with leukemia or myelodysplasia. *Blood* 1995; **85**: 2345–63.

194. Oakhill A, Pamphilon DH, Potter MN *et al*. Unrelated donor bone marrow transplantation for children with relapsed acute lymphoblastic leukaemia in second complete remission. *Br J Haematol* 1996; **94**: 574–8.

195. Pinkerton CR, Mills S, Gale *et al*. Modified Capizzi maintenance

regimen in children with relapsed acute lymphoblastic leukaemia. *Med Pediatr Oncol* 1989; **14**: 69–432.

196. Chessells JM, Bailey CC, Richards SM. Intensification of treatment and survival in all children with lymphoblastic leukemia. *Lancet* 1995; **345**: 143–8.

197. Ribeiro RC, Rivera GK, Hudson M *et al.* An intensive re-treatment protocol for children with an isolated CNS relapse of acute lymphoblastic leukemia. *J Clin Oncol* 1995; **13**: 333–8.

198. Winick NJ, Smith SD, Shuster J *et al.* Treatment of CNS relapse in children with acute lymphoblastic leukaemia: a Pediatric Oncology Group study. *J Clin Oncol* 1993; **11**: 27–278.

199. Henze G, Fengler R, Hartmann R for the BFM Relapse Study Group. Chemotherapy for relapsed childhood acute lymphoblastic leukaemia: results of the BFM Study Group. *Haematol Blood Transfusion* 1993; **36**: 374–9.

200. Bowman WP, Rhodes JA, Husto HO *et al.* Isolated testicular relapse in acute lymphocytic leukemia of childhood: categories and influence on survival. *J Clin Oncol* 1984; **2**: 924–9.

201. Eden OB, Hardisty RM *et al.* Testicular disease in acute lymphoblastic leukaemia in childhood. Report on behalf of the Medical Research Council's Working Party on Leukaemia in Childhood. *Br Med J* 1978; **1**: 334.

202. Tiedemann K, Chessells JM. Isolated testicular relapse in boys with acute lymphoblastic leukaemia: treatment and outcome. *Br Med J* 1982; **285**: 1614.

203. Wong KY, Ballard ET, Kisker CT *et al.* Clinical and occult testicular leukemia in long-term survivors of acute lymphoblastic leukemia. *J Pediatr* 1980; **96**: 569–74.

204. Chessells JM, Eden OB, Bailey C, Lilleyman JS, Richards SM. Acute lymphoblastic leukaemia in infancy: experience in MRC UKALL trials: report from the Medical Research Council Working Party on Childhood Leukaemia. *Leukemia* 1994; **8**: 1275–9.

205. Uderzo C, Zurlo G, Zanesco L *et al.* Treatment of isolated testicular relapse in childhood acute lymphoblastic leukemia: an Italian multicenter study. *J Clin Oncol* 1990; **8**: 672–7.

206. Nachman J, Palmer NF, Sather WH *et al.* Open-wedge testicular biopsy in childhood acute lymphoblastic leukaemia after two years of maintenance therapy: diagnostic accuracy and influence on outcome. A report from Children's Cancer Study Group. *Blood* 1990; **75**: 1051–5.

207. Chessells J, Leiper A, Rogers D. Outcome following late marrow relapse in childhood acute lymphoblastic leukaemia. *J Clin Oncol* 1984; **2**. 1099–1091.

208. Chessells JM, Veys P, Kempski H *et al.* Long term follow up of relapsed childhood ALL. *Br J Haematol* 2003; **123**: 396–406.

209. Bührer C, Hartmann R, Fengler R *et al.* Peripheral blast counts at diagnosis of late isolated bone marrow relapse of childhood acute lymphoblastic leukemia predict response to salvage chemotherapy and outcome. *J Clin Oncol* 1996, **14**: 2812–17.

210. Somervaille T, Hann I, Harrison G *et al.* Intraocular relapse of childhood ALL. *Br J Haematol* 2003; **121**: 280–8.

211. Sadowitz PD, Smith SD, Shuster J, Wharam MD, Buchanan GR, Rivera GK. Treatment of late bone marrow relapse in children with acute lymphoblastic leukemia: a Pediatric Oncology Group study. *Blood* 1993; **81**: 602–9.

212. Harbott J, Viehmann S, Borkhardt A, Henze G, Lampert F. Incidence of TEL/AML1 fusion gene analyzed consecutively

213. Ramsay NKC, Kersey JH. Indications for marrow transplantation in acute lymphoblastic leukemia. *Blood* 1990; **75**: 815–18.

214. Thomas ED. Marrow transplantation for malignant diseases. *J Clin Oncol* 1983; **1**: 517–31

215. Kurtzberg J, Laughlin M, Graham ML *et al.* Placental blood as a source of hematopoietic stem cells for transplantation into unrelated recipients. *N Engl J Med* 1996; **335**: 157–66.

216. Kersey JH, Weisdorf D, Kim T *et al.* Comparison of autologous and allogeneic bone marrow transplantation for treatment of high risk refractory acute lymphoblastic leukemia. *N Engl J Med* 1987; **317**: 461–7.

217. Sanders JE, Thomas ED, Buckner CD, Doney K. Marrow transplantation for children with acute lymphoblastic leukemia in second remission. *Blood* 1987; **70**: 324–6.

218. Blume KG, Forman SJ, Metter GE *et al.* Total body irradiation and high dose etoposide: a new preparatory regimen for bone marrow transplantation of patients with advanced hematologic malignancy. *Blood* 1987; **69**: 1015–20.

219. Dopfer R, Henze G, Bender-Götze C *et al.* Allogeneic bone marrow transplantation for childhood acute lymphoblastic leukemia in second remission after intensive primary and relapse therapy according to the BFM- and CoALL-protocols: results of the German Cooperative Study. *Blood* 1991; **78**: 2780–4.

220. Suttorp M, Schmitz N, Rister M *et al.* Fractionated total body irradiation plus high-dose VP-16 prior to allogeneic bone marrow transplantation in children with poor risk acute leukaemias. *Bone Marrow Transplant* 1989; **4**: 144–8.

221. Woods WG, Ramsay NKC, Haaker R *et al.* Bone marrow transplantation for acute lymphocytic leukemia utilizing total body irradiation followed by high doses of cytosine arabinoside: lack of superiority over cyclophosphamide-containing regimens. *Bone Marrow Transplant* 1990; **6**: 9–16.

222. Ringdén O, Ruutu T, Remberger M *et al.* A randomized trial comparing busulfan with total body irradiation as conditioning in allogeneic marrow transplant receipts with leukemia: a report from the Nordic Bone Marrow Transplantation Group. *Blood* 1994; **83**: 2723–30.

223. Dowey S, Armitage S, Rocha V. The London Cord Blood Bank. *Br J Haematol* 2004; **125**: 358–65.

224. Borgmann A, Schmid H, Hartmann R *et al.* Autologous bone-marrow transplants compared with chemotherapy for children with acute lymphoblastic leukaemia in a second remission: a matched-pair analysis. *Lancet* 1995; **346**: 873–6.

225. Schmid H, von Schenck U, Hartmann R, Borgmann A, Henze G. Allogeneic BMT vs. chemotherapy in late bone marrow relapsed childhood non-T/non-B ALL: results of BFM ALL relapse studies. *Bone Marrow Transplant* 1996; **18** (suppl. 2): 28–30.

226. Brenner MK, Rill DR, Moen RC *et al.* Gene-marking to trace origin of relapse after autologous bone-marrow transplantation. *Lancet* 1993; **341**: 85–6.

227. Brenner MK. Autologous bone marrow transplantation in childhood acute lymphoblastic leukaemia. *Lancet* 1995; **346**: 856–7.

228. Maidment CG, Greaves MF, Black AG *et al.* T-cell leukaemia

presenting with hyperuricaemia, acute renal failure and gout. *Clin Lab Haematol* 1983; **5**: 423–6.

229. Zusman J, Brown DM, Nesbitt ME *et al.* Hyperphosphatemia, hyperphosphaturia and hypocalcemia in acute lymphoblastic leukemia. *N Engl J Med* 1973; **289**: 1335–40.

230. Andreoli SP, Cark JH, McGuire WA *et al.* Purine excretion during tumor lysis in children with acute lymphocytic leukemia receiving allopurinol: relationship to acute renal failure. *J Pediatr* 1986; **109**: 292–8.

231. Jones DP, Stapleton FB, Pui CH *et al.* Renal dysfunction and hyperuricemia at presentation and relapse of acute lymphoblastic leukemia. *Med Pediatr Oncol* 1990; **18**: 283–6.

232. Basade M, Dhar AK, Kulkarni SS *et al.* Rapid cytoreduction in childhood leukemic hyperleukocytosis by conservative therapy. *Med Pediatr Oncol* 1995; **25**: 204–7.

233. Maurer HS, Steinherz PG, Gaynon PS *et al.* The effect of initial management of hyperleukocytosis on early complications and outcome of children with acute lymphoblastic leukemia. *J Clin Oncol* 1988; **6**: 1425–32.

234. Nelson SC, Bruggers CS, Kurtzberg J, Friedman HS. Management of leukemic hyperleukocytosis with hydration, urinary alkalinization, and allopurinol. Are cranial irradiation and invasive cytoreduction necessary? *Am J Pediatr Hematol Oncol* 1993; **15**: 351–5.

235. Lo Curto ML, Zingone A, Dini G *et al.* Leukemic infiltration of the eye: results of therapy in a retrospective multicentric study. *Med Pediatr Oncol* 1989; **17**: 134–9.

236. Murray KM, Goldman JM, Galton DA *et al.* Ocular involvement in leukaemia. Report of three cases. *Lancet* 1977; **i**: 829–31.

237. Warkentin TE, Kelton JG. Heparin-induced thrombocytopenia. *Prog Hemost Thromb* 1991; **10**: 1–34.

238. Ott N, Ramsay NKC, Pui CH *et al.* Sequelae of thrombotic or hemorrhagic complications following L-asparaginase therapy for childhood lymphoblastic leukemia. *Am J Pediatr Hematol Oncol* 1988; **10**: 191–5.

239. Priest JR, Ramsey NKC, Levitt CJ *et al.* A syndrome of thrombosis and hemorrhage complicating L-asparaginase therapy for childhood acute lymphoblastic leukemia. *J Pediatr* 1982; **100**: 984–9.

240. Nowak Göttl U, Auberger K, Göbel U *et al.* Inherited defects of the protein C anticoagulant system in childhood thrombo-embolism. *Eur J Pediatr* 1996; **155**: 921–7.

241. Welte K, Reiter A, Mempel K *et al.* A randomized phase-III study of the efficacy of granulocyte colony-stimulating factor in children with high-risk acute lymphoblastic leukemia. *Blood* 1996; **87**: 3143–50.

242. Feldman S, Hughes WT, Daniel CB *et al.* Varicella in children with cancer: seventy-seven cases. *Pediatrics* 1975; **56**: 388–97.

243. Rowland P, Wald ER, Mirro JR *et al.* Progressive varicella presenting with pain and minimal skin involvement in children with acute lymphoblastic leukemia. *J Clin Oncol* 1995; **13**: 1697–703.

244. Zaia JA, Levin MJ, Curtis AC *et al.* Evaluation of varicella-zoster immune globulin: protection of immunosuppressed children after household exposure to varicella. *J Infect Dis* 1983; **147**: 171–753.

245. Balfour HH Jr, Bean B, Kirk LE *et al.* Acyclovir halts progression of herpes zoster in immunocompromised patients. *N Engl J Med* 1983; **308**: 1448–53.

246. Prober CG, Kirk LE, Keeney RE *et al.* Acyclovir therapy of chickenpox in immunosuppressed children: a collaborative study. *J Pediatr* 1982; **101**: 622–5.

247. Gray MM, Hann IM, Glass S, Eden OB, Jones PM, Stevens RF. Mortality and morbidity caused by measles in children with malignant disease attending four major treatment centres: a retrospective study review. *Br Med J* 1987; **295**: 19–21.

248. Gururangan S, Stevens RF, Morris DJ. Ribavirin response in measles pneumonia. *J Infect* 1990; **20**: 219–21.

249. Hughes I, Jenney MEM, Newton RW, Morris DJ, Klapper PE. Measles encephalitis during immunosuppressive treatment for acute lymphoblastic leukaemia. *Arch Dis Child* 1993; **68**: 775–8.

250. Pifer LL, Hughes WT, Woods D *et al.* *Pneumocystis carinii* infection: evidence for high prevalence in normal and immunosuppressed children. *Pediatrics* 1978; **61**: 35–41.

251. Hughes WT, Rivera GK, Lott L *et al.* Successful intermittent chemoprophylaxis for *Pneumocystis carinii* pneumonitis. *N Engl J Med* 1987; **316**: 1627–32.

252. Pasqualini T, Escobar ME, Muriel FS *et al.* Evaluation of gonadal function following long-term treatment for acute lymphoblastic leukemia in girls. *Am J Pediatr Hematol Oncol* 1987; **9**: 15–22.

253. Siris ES, Leventhal BG, Vaitukaitis JL *et al.* Effects of childhood leukemia and chemotherapy on puberty and reproductive function in girls. *N Engl J Med* 1976; **294**: 1143–6.

254. Lentz RD, Bergstein J, Prem K *et al.* Postpubertal evaluation of gonadal function following cyclophosphamide therapy before and during puberty. *J Pediatr* 1977; **91**: 385–94.

255. Wallace WH, Shalet SM, Lendon M, Morris Jones PH. Male fertility in long-term survivors of childhood acute lymphoblastic leukaemia. *Int J Androl* 1991; **14**: 312–19.

256. Sklar CA, Robison LL, Kim TH *et al.* Effects of radiation on testicular function in long-term survivors of childhood acute lymphoblastic leukemia: a report from the Children's Cancer Study Group. *J Clin Oncol* 1990; **8**: 1981–7.

257. Kenney LB, Nicholson HS, Brasseux C *et al.* Birth defects in offspring of adult survivors of childhood acute lymphoblastic leukemia. *Cancer* 1996; **78**: 169–76.

258. Bessho F, Kinumaki H, Yokota S, Hayashi Y, Kobayashi M, Kamoshita S. Liver function studies in children with acute lymphocytic leukemia after cessation of therapy. *Med Pediatr Oncol* 1994; **23**: 111–15.

259. Goldberg MA, Antin JH, Guinan EC *et al.* Cyclophosphamide cardiotoxicity: An analysis of dosing as a risk factor. *Blood* 1986; **68**: 1114.

260. Habermalz E, Habermalz H, Henze G *et al.* Cranial computed tomography of 64 children in continuous complete remission of leukemia: I. Relations to therapy modalities. *Neuropediatrics* 1983; **14**: 144–8.

261. Hara T, Kishikawa T, Goya N *et al.* Central nervous system complications in childhood leukemia. *Am J Pediatr Hematol Oncol* 1984; **6**: 129–36.

262. Ochs JJ, Parvey LS, Coburn T *et al.* Serial cranial computed tomography scans in children with leukemia given two different forms of central nervous system therapy. *J Clin Oncol* 1983; **1**: 793–8.

263. Riccardi R, Brouwers P, Popblack DG *et al.* Abnormal computed tomography brain scans in children with acute

lymphoblastic leukemia: serial long-term follow-up. *J Clin Oncol* 1985; **3**: 12–128.

264. Poplack DG, Brouwers P. Adverse sequelae of central nervous system therapy. *Clin Oncol* 1985; **4**: 263.

265. Esseltine DW, Freeman CR, Dube J *et al.* Computerized tomography brain scans in long-term survivors of childhood acute lymphoblastic leukemia. *Med Pediatr Oncol* 1981; **9**: 429–38.

266. Jankovic M, Scotti G, Riccardi R *et al.* Correlation between cranial computed tomography scans at diagnosis in children with acute lymphoblastic leukaemia and central nervous system relapse. *Lancet* 1988; **ii**: 1212–14.

267. Kramer JH, Crittenden MR, Halberg FE, Wara WM, Cowan MJ. A prospective study of cognitive functioning following low-dose cranial radiation for bone marrow transplantation. *Pediatrics* 1992; **90**: 447–50.

268. Obetz WW, Smithson WA, Gilchwist GS *et al.* Neuro-psychologic follow-up study of children with acute lymphocytic leukemia. *Am J Pediatr Hematol Oncol* 1979; **3**: 207–13.

269. Christie D, Leiper AD, Chessells JM, Vargha-Khadem F. Intellectual performance after presymptomatic cranial radiotherapy for leukaemia: effects of age and sex. *Arch Dis Child* 1995; **73**: 136–40.

270. Jannoun L. Are cognitive and educational development affected by age at which therapy is given in acute lymphoblastic leukaemia? *Arch Dis Child* 1983; **58**: 953–8.

271. Chessells JM, Cox TCS, Kendall B, Cavanagh NPC, Jannoun L, Richards S. Neurotoxicity in lymphoblastic leukaemia: comparison of oral and intramuscular methotrexate and two doses of radiation. *Arch Dis Child* 1990; **65**: 416–22.

272. Meadows AT, Evans AE. Effects of chemotherapy on the central nervous system: a study of parenteral methotrexate in long-term survivors of leukemia and lymphoma in childhood. *Cancer* 1976; **37**: 1079–85.

273. Kumar P, Mulhern RK, Regine WF, Rivera GK, Kun LE. A prospective neurocognitive evaluation of children treated with additional chemotherapy and craniospinal irradiation following isolated central nervous system relapse in acute lymphoblastic leukemia. *Int J Radiat Oncol Biol Phys* 1995; **31**: 561–6.

274. Longeway K, Mulhern R, Kun L *et al.* Treatment of meningeal relapse in childhood acute lymphoblastic leukemia: II. A prospective study of intellectual loss specific to CNS relapse and therapy. *Am J Pediatr Hematol Oncol* 1990; **12**: 45–50.

275. Berglund G, Karlberg J, Mellander L *et al.* A longitudinal study of growth in children with acute lymphoblastic leukaemia. *Acta Paediatr Scand* 1985; **74**: 530–3.

276. Voorhess ML, Brecher ML *et al.* Growth in children treated for acute lymphoblastic leukaemia. *Lancet* 1988; **i**: 460.

277. Kirk JA, Raghupathy P, Vines RH *et al.* Growth failure and growth-hormone deficiency after treatment for acute lymphoblastic leukaemia. *Pediatr Hematol Oncol* 1988; **5**: 187–93.

278. Robison LL, Nesbit ME Jr. Height of children successfully treated for acute lymphoblastic leukaemia: a report from the Late Effects Committee of the Children's Cancer Study Group. *Med Pediatr Oncol* 1985; **13**: 114–21.

279. Moell C, Marky L, Hovi L *et al.* Cerebral irradiation causes blunted pubertal growth in girls treated for acute leukemia. *Med Pediatr Oncol* 1994; **22**: 375–9.

280. Rappaport R, Brauner R. Growth and endocrine disorders secondary to cranial irridation. *Pediatr Res* 1989; **25**: 561–7.

281. Pasqualim T, McCalla J, Berg S *et al.* Subtle primary hypothyroidism in patients treated for acute lymphoblastic leukemia. *Acta Endocrinol* 1991; **124**: 375–80.

282. Hanif I, Mahmoud H, Pui C-H. Avascular femoral head necrosis in pediatric cancer patients. *Med Pediatr Oncol* 1993; **21**: 655–60.

283. Pieters R, van der Schans-Dop AM, Veerman AJ *et al.* Osteonecrosis following chemotherapy for leukemia. *Eur J Haematol* 1989; **43**: 262–4.

284. Leiper AD. Non-endocrine late complications of bone marrow transplantation in children. *Br J Haematol* 2002; **118**: 3–43.

285. Dorup I, Levitt G, Sullivan I, Sorensen K. Prospective longitudinal assessment of late anthracycline cardiotoxicity after childhood cancer. *Heart* 2004; **90**: 1214–16.

286. Nygaard R, Garwicz S, Haldorsen T *et al.* Second malignant neoplasms in patients treated for childhood leukemia. A population-based cohort study from the Nordic countries. *Acta Paediatr Scand* 1991; **80**: 1220–8.

287. Neglia JP, Meadows AT, Robison LL *et al.* Second neoplasms after acute lymphoblastic leukemia in childhood. *N Engl J Med* 1991; **325**: 1330–6.

288. Tang TT, Holcenberg JS, Camitta BM *et al.* Thyroid carcinoma following treatment for acute lymphoblastic leukemia. *Cancer* 1980; **46**: 1572–6.

289. Bessho F, Ohta K, Akanuma A. Dosimetry of radiation scattered to thyroid gland from prophylactic cranial irradiation for childhood leukemia. *Pediatr Hematol Oncol* 1994; **11**: 47–53.

290. Kreissmann SG, Gelber RD, Cohen HJ, Clavell LA, Leavitt P, Sallan SE. Incidence of secondary acute myelogenous leukemia after treatment of childhood acute lymphoblastic leukemia *Cancer* 1992; **70**: 2208–13.

21 Lymphomas

O.B. Eden and Ross Pinkerton

Non-Hodgkin lymphoma

Childhood non-Hodgkin lymphoma (NHL) represents a heterogeneous group of disorders that are different from adult NHL in that they are commonly disseminated; diffuse not nodular; high grade; of mature and immature T- or B-cell lineage; and have frequent extranodal disease, marrow and central nervous system (CNS) involvement. Over the last three decades, empirical chemotherapeutic management has transformed survival, and more recently greater understanding of the biology is offering hope for improved management of resistant disease.

Epidemiology

Age-standardized incidence rates for NHL vary from 6.1 per million children (0–15 years) in the UK and Japan to 90.1 per million reported from Ibadan, Nigeria.[1] Hidden within these statistics are very different patterns of disease, particularly the incidence of B-cell lymphomas. Of all childhood cancers reported from Ibadan between 1960 and 1984, 47% were Burkitt lymphoma (BL) with an age-standardized incidence rate of 80 per million. Even higher rates have been reported from Uganda.

In endemic malarial areas of Africa, especially where BL is common, the peak age incidence is between 5 and 9 years, with a ratio of up to three boys to each girl affected. The primary tumor is most frequently in the jaw. Other areas with an NHL incidence intermediate between the African and UK experience also report high BL rates (e.g., Middle East, Latin America, Mediterranean area and North Africa), but in these regions the tumors occur more commonly in the abdomen and over a wider age range (0–9 years). The age-standardized incidence for BL in the USA it is 3.6 per million in white males, 0.4 per million in white females, 0.7 per million in black males and of a very low incidence in black girls.[1]

In western Europe, the male to female ratio for all NHL is approximately 2 : 1 and NHL constitutes 5–6% of all childhood cancers, although the relative and absolute incidence rises southwards toward the Mediterranean. In the UK the peak age incidence is between 7 and 10 years, but all ages can be affected. Over the last 30 years there appears to have been a steady increase in the overall incidence of NHL for reasons that are unclear.

Etiology and cell biology

The childhood immune system consists of many different mature functional cells as well as a wide array of precursor and stem cells. Malignancy can occur at any stage of lymphocyte ontogeny, and monoclonal antibodies have helped to define the differentiation process of both normal and malignant lymphocytes (Fig. 21.1).

Young children are constantly exposed to antigens, but unlike adults they do not have a large immune memory bank to help them recognize and repel such antigens. As a result, a large proportion of lymphoid cells during childhood are in a very active state, undergoing molecular rearrangements to produce specific immunoglobulins and other factors required for the normal immune response. For B cells to function, the genes that regulate the different components of immunoglobulin production have to be brought together or rearranged in an ordered sequence. In T cells, the genes that control T-cell antigen receptor molecules similarly need to be organized. The immunoglobulin heavy chain genes are on chromosome 14q32, the λ light chain genes on chromosome 22q11 and the κ light chain genes on chromosome 2p12.

The human T-cell receptor α-chain gene maps to chromosome 14q11–q12 and harbors the T-cell receptor δ genes between its V and J region gene sequences. The T-cell receptor β-chain locus is on chromosome 7q35. A complete product molecule requires two chains, an α from chromosome 14 and a β from chromosome 7. In normal health the rearrangement process producing the product of the receptor gene is very similar to that for immunoglobulin gene rearrangements.

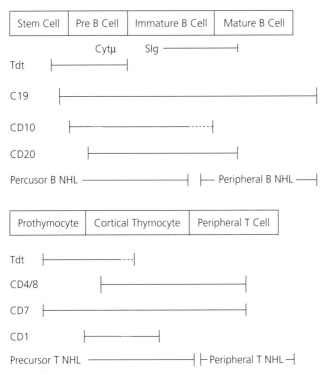

Fig. 21.1 Phenotypic features of lymphoma in relation to normal lymphocyte differentiation: T and B cells differentiate in parallel with malignant lymphoma. Cytμ, cytoplasmic immunoglobulin; NHL, non-Hodgkin lymphoma; SIg, surface immunoglobulin; Tdt, terminal deoxynucleotidyl transferase.

The enzyme terminal deoxynucleotidyl transferase is intimately involved in T-cell rearrangements but is not found in mature B-cell acute lymphoid leukemia (ALL) or lymphoma and can be used as a distinguishing marker.

Malignant change can occur when genetic defects arise secondary to deletion, mutation or translocation. This can interrupt the normal orderly rearrangement, but what actually initiates the disorganization is not clear in most instances. Accumulating evidence incriminates viruses, at least in the pathogenesis of some lymphomas. The products from the retroviruses human T-cell leukemia/lymphoma virus (HTLV)-1 and HTLV-2 rearrange genes within the host cell, thus stimulating production of interleukin (IL)-2 and its receptor, which can activate T-cell proliferation. Clonal or polyclonal proliferation provides the opportunity for a second strike, which may be necessary to produce a malignant clone. HTLV-1 is thought to play a role in the genesis of a particular form of adult T-cell leukemia/lymphoma, particularly in Japan. No viral inclusions have yet been found in childhood T-cell NHL.

More directly relevant to pediatric practice was the discovery of Epstein–Barr virus (EBV) particles in the nuclei of endemic African BL cells.[2] The finding of such viral inclusion and high antibody titers (especially to the viral capsid antigen)

to EBV in the vast majority of cases (95%) from tropical regions contrasts with those in temperate regions, where the incidence of raised titers and/or viral inclusions is only about 15–20%.[3,4] However, there is increasing evidence of aberrant expression in sporadic cases. In very high incidence regions, malaria is endemic and is thought to cause a continuous antigenic stimulus that alters responses to EBV infections, which are also endemic (nearly 100% of children have been exposed by age 3 years). EBV infection early in life is thought to enlarge the size of certain pre-B and B-cell populations and maintain them in a proliferative state, thereby rendering them more likely to genetic change. Alternatively, it has been postulated that EBV produces an immortal cell clone with genetic translocations already present, perhaps induced by another infection. The product of the *EBER* locus of the EBV genome has been implicated in oncogenesis by its antiapoptotic activity. The promoter region of this locus is a binding site for c-*myc*, which could upregulate *EBER* transcription.[5]

Repeated infections, especially of malaria (a T-cell suppressor and B-cell mutagen), malnutrition and other cofactors (e.g., use of phorbol esters as herbal medicine) result in T-cell immunosuppression (reduced CD4 : CD8 ratio and decreased number and function of EBV-specific T cells) and B-cell hyperplasia that can potentiate the effects of EBV infection. A consequent increase in number of EBV genome-positive cells during acute malaria is postulated to increase the chance of genetic changes, including the characteristic translocation involving the long arm of chromosome 8 (q23–24), usually as part of a t(8;14)(q24;q32) rearrangement, although variants including t(2;8)(p12;q24) and t(8;22)(q24;q11) are seen in about 15% of cases. The c-*myc* oncogene lies at the chromosome 8 breakpoint, while the immunoglobulin heavy chain locus and κ and λ light chain loci are at 14q32, 2p12 and 22q11, respectively. In all cases, an immunoglobulin gene enhancer is placed close to c-*myc* and induces its expression. Of great interest has been the finding that the chromosome 8 breakpoint is upstream of c-*myc* in endemic cases, whereas in the sporadic form it occurs within c-*myc* or immediately upstream. However, in all forms, the c-*myc* coding region appears to be left intact so that deregulation of the oncogene rather than mutation seems to be the consequence of the translocation. The myc-encoded protein appears to regulate the expression of target genes required for cell cycle progression through G_1 into S phase. If it is dysregulated, it leads to progression through the cell cycle and lymphoproliferation. On chromosome 14 the breakpoints involve limited D and J segments, regions prone to physiologic rearrangements during the normal sequence of VDJ recombination. Endemic cases of BL usually have low levels of surface immunoglobulin, while sporadic cases have high levels and the cells also secrete immunoglobulin. It is thought that in sporadic cases the translocations are at a later stage of B-cell differentiation. These endemic cases have a more homogeneous immunophenotype and fewer genetic abnormalities.[6] This ever-increasing knowledge of the biology of NHL has been applied to the detection of minimal residual disease using polymerase chain reaction techniques to detect specific patterns of immunoglobulin gene rearrangements.[7]

8q24 is a fragile site but what specifically initiates the translocation is not clear. A multiple-hit model is postulated for the initiation of BL. Some have speculated that genetic factors might also be involved, since familial clusters of BL have been reported,[8] and genetic factors including inherited mutations of the *c-myc* oncogene or p53, and the finding of an excess of HLA-DR7 phenotype, raise the possibility of inherent DNA repair defects or abnormal responsiveness to infection. The intriguing effect of extracts from *Euphorbia triucalli* (used as a herbal medicine) in inducing *c-myc* activation[9] further suggests that a complex interaction of environmental and genetic factors is likely.

Human immunodeficiency virus (HIV) infection as a result of profound T-helper cell depression predisposes to a variety of tumors, including intermediate- to high-grade B-cell lymphomas, Hodgkin disease, T-cell NHL and some pre-T and pre-B tumors, especially Kaposi sarcoma. Some of the resultant lymphomas appear to be polyclonal B-cell proliferations similar to those seen after intense iatrogenic immunosuppression. The characteristic feature of HIV-associated lymphomas is extranodal disease, especially of the skin, and a high incidence of EBV positivity, raising the possibility that HIV may predispose to EBV-driven proliferation.[10]

For T-cell ALL and NHL, chromosomal abnormalities are more heterogeneous. About 25% of cases of T-cell ALL involve a small deletion of the *TAL1* gene on chromosome 1 and this is sometimes associated with a t(1;14) translocation. Also, translocations can involve the locus for the α chain of the T-cell receptor gene on chromosome 14 or for the β chain on chromosome 7.[11] No clear-cut association between these changes and etiologic factors has been made but the changes can be used to detect minimal residual disease.

In anaplastic large-cell lymphoma (ALCL), a t(2;5)(p23;q35) translocation has been described.[12] This is found in occasional cases of Hodgkin disease, and current interest exists in exploring the overlap between these two conditions, and also the association of chromosome 2 anomalies in ALCL with more advanced disease and with a poorer prognosis. To date, no clear etiologic link has been made. The translocation produces a fused gene (nucleophosmin, *NPM*, from chromosome 5 and AL kinase gene, *ALK*, from chromosome 2) and a product that is primarily cytoplasmic in location. Its precise function has not been defined. Inhibitors of antiapoptotic mechanisms such as BCL-6 have been implicated in a range of lymphomas.[13] Overexpression has been described in pre-T NHL.[14]

Genetic factors may be important in NHL development, not just given the occasional familial clustering with BL but also because a number of inherited or congenital immunodeficiency syndromes are associated with NHL. These include ataxia telangiectasia (including a number of variants, especially with T-cell malignancies), Wiskott–Aldrich syndrome, Bruton agammaglobulinemia, severe combined immunodeficiency and IgA deficiency. Post-organ transplantation lymphomas representing either monoclonal or polyclonal B-cell proliferation have been referred to already. The X-linked syndrome described by Grierson and Purtillo,[15] characterized by undue sensitivity to EBV and leading to uncontrolled EBV proliferation, comprising hepatitis, encephalopathy, aplasia and malignant lymphomas, has similar features. Other chromosomal or genetic disorders associated with NHL include Klinefelter syndrome[16] and neurofibromatosis type 1.

Apart from postnatal long-term exposure to phenytoin (which can produce a benign lymphadenopathy, a self-limiting pseudolymphoma and, rarely, a true lymphoma), EBV infection for BL and the intense immunosuppression following transplantation or chemotherapy, no other environmental factors have been firmly incriminated in the causation of NHL. Although still the subject of intense investigation, prenatal or postnatal exposure to irradiation, chemicals, electromagnetic fields and electricity have not been firmly associated with NHL.

Classification

A confusing array of classifications exists for NHL. For pediatric practice there is a concerted effort to use the REAL (Revised European American Lymphoma) classification, which is an update of the Kiel scheme, incorporating immunophenotyping and dividing NHL into T- and B-cell neoplasms, and further classifying them as of high- or low-grade malignancy (Table 21.1). Virtually all childhood NHL are diffuse, with three types, namely BL (42%), T lymphoblastic (20%) and ALCL (15%), predominating.

Clinical presentation

Abdominal primary

Lymphadenopathy is a common referral to GP, general pediatrician and oncologist. The vast majority of cases are

Table 21.1 REAL classification scheme for childhood non-Hodgkin lymphoma (relative incidence in parentheses).

Burkitt (42%)
Burkitt like (4%)
Precursor B lymphoblastic (5%)
Precursor T lymphoblastic (20%)
Diffuse large B cell (3%) (primary sclerosing mediastinal 0.4%)
Peripheral T cell unspecified (1%)
Anaplastic large-cell T or "null" types (15%)

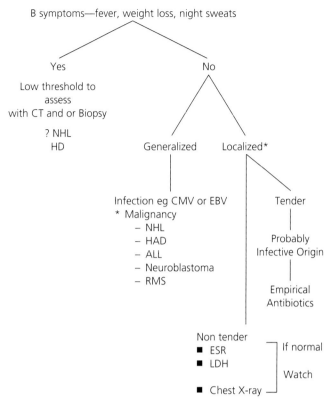

Fig. 21.2 Assessment of child with lymphadenopathy. Asterisk indicates that biopsy should only be considered if swelling is very large or rapidly increasing in size. ALL, acute lymphoid leukemia; CMV, cytomegalovirus; CT, computed tomography; EBV, Epstein–Barr virus; ESR, erythrocyte sedimentation rate; HD, Hodgkin disease; LDH, lactate dehydrogenase; NHL, non-Hodgkin lymphoma; RMS, rhabdomyosarcoma.

nonmalignant and self-remitting; with malignancies, the primary site will give a clue to likely tumor type (Fig. 21.2).

In Europe, the commonest presentation of high-grade B-cell NHL (BL or non-BL type) is an abdominal mass (30–45% of all NHL cases). There are two commonly recognized types. The first is the diffuse abdominal tumor with involvement throughout the omentum and mesentery, often including infiltration into the kidney, liver and spleen. With this type, bone marrow and CNS involvement is more common. Only a few cases present with jaw involvement, whereas in African BL this is almost universal. Abdominal involvement is also present in up to 50% of African patients presenting with jaw primaries. There is a lower incidence of bone marrow involvement in African compared with non-African BL.

The second type comprises localized tumors of the bowel wall, most commonly the terminal ileum (thought to arise in Peyer's patches), which can lead to intussusception or bleeding with or without perforation of the bowel. Patients most often present with a right iliac fossa mass and are sometimes thought to have appendicitis or an appendix mass. This type of presentation is much rarer than the rapidly growing diffuse abdominal form.

Mediastinal primary

Up to two-thirds of patients with precursor T-lymphoblastic NHL and 25–30% of all NHL present with mediastinal masses, with or without pleural effusions. Frequently, there are signs of superior vena cava obstruction, with dysphagia, dyspnea and pericardial effusion. Lymphadenopathy is usually confined to the neck and axillae. Abdominal node enlargement is uncommon. Hepatosplenomegaly is common and bone marrow and CNS infiltration may occur. Patients with mediastinal disease are at especially high risk of developing respiratory obstruction and/or distress if general anesthesia is instigated for investigations. Parenchymal lung disease is very rare except in ALCL.

Localized disease

Lymphoid swelling can occur anywhere but most commonly arises in the head and neck, including Waldeyer's ring and the facial bones (10–20%). Neck nodal tumors apparently have a lower risk of CNS spread. Some 5–10% of tumors arise in nodes or lymphoid tissue at other sites, including pharyngeal masses which are usually of B-cell origin. Rarer sites for primary tumors include bone, skin, thyroid, testis (usually lymphoblastic), orbit, eyelid, kidney (can mimic Wilms tumor) and epidural space. Bony NHL can be localized or more generalized, and is sometimes associated with hypercalcemia. Lymphoblastic lymphoma can present peripherally with skin and/or bone disease, and these tumors are usually of more mature T-cell phenotype. Subcutaneous lymphoma, often seen in very young children, is usually of precursor B-cell type. Skin involvement, either alone or combined with nodal disease, is a feature of ALCL.

CNS involvement

Primary CNS lymphomas are rare except after organ transplantation, but CNS involvement as secondary spread from disease elsewhere is quite common, particularly in lymphoblastic and advanced BL. It leads to headache, vomiting, papilledema, cranial nerve dysfunction and seizures. It is much more common at diagnosis if the bone marrow is also infiltrated, but is occasionally seen in patients with localized disease and those with large-cell histology.

Diagnostic investigations and staging

Following a full history and an extensive clinical examination, the aim of subsequent investigations is to confirm the diagnosis as accurately and as quickly as possible, and to determine the extent of disease so that appropriate therapy is started immediately. All patients should have a preliminary chest radiograph to exclude mediastinal mass and/or

Table 21.2 Characteristic features of main subgroups of non-Hodgkin lymphoma.

	B cell	Lymphoblastic	Anaplastic large cell
Primary site	Most frequently abdominal primary	Most frequently mediastinal but also nodal	Nodal ± skin
Histology	Burkitt (small noncleaved) centroblastic or B-cell immunoblastic	Lymphoblastic	Large cell
Cytomorphology	L3	L1/L2 characteristics (focal capped acid phosphatase positivity in T cell)	–
Immunomarkers	Cells display SIg$^+$ B-cell markers (CD19$^+$, CD22$^+$, CD24$^+$), Tdt negative	CD1–CD8 T-cell markers (SIg$^-$ but occasionally CyIg$^+$) (CD10$^+$ in precursor B)	CD30$^+$
Cytogenetics	t(8;14), t(2;8), t(8;22)	Heterogeneous	t(2;5)

L1, L2, L3, French–American–British (FAB) classification; SIg, surface immunoglobulin; CyIg, cytoplasmic immunoglobulin; Tdt, terminal deoxynucleotidyl transferase.

pericardial/pleural effusions, and this should certainly be done prior to any anesthetic procedure.

Biopsy

Unless the diagnosis can be made from cytologic examination of tapped pleural fluid or bone marrow, biopsy is indicated in the presence of accessible localized disease and if there is peripheral lymphadenopathy associated with a mediastinal mass. If there is truly isolated mediastinal disease, material should be obtained by percutaneous needle or mediastinoscopy. For abdominal primaries, diagnosis should be attempted by cytologic examination of ascitic fluid or by percutaneous needle biopsy. Unless there is an acute abdominal emergency (e.g., gastrointestinal obstruction or intussusception) or the primary tumor is small and resectable, laparatomy should be avoided in order to prevent the common sequelae of prolonged ileus and even ruptured abdominal wounds. In extensive disease, the most accessible tumor deposits, not necessarily the primary, should be biopsied. All tumor material should be submitted for routine histology diagnosis, full immunophenotyping profile and cytogenetics. Table 21.2 shows the characteristic diagnostic features that help to distinguish subtypes of NHL.

Bone marrow studies

The marrow should be examined from at least two, and preferably four, sites (ideally from two aspirates and two trephines). The specimens should routinely be sent for cytogenetic analysis and immunophenotyping as well as standard cytomorphology.

Lumbar puncture

Provided there is no clinical evidence of raised intracranial pressure, cerebrospinal fluid should be examined. If there are signs of raised intracranial pressure, either computed tomography (CT) or magnetic resonance imaging (MRI) should be carried out before lumbar puncture to exclude any focal deposit with consequent risk of brain shift.

Imaging

Abdominal ultrasonography is often the quickest way to define liver, spleen and kidney involvement and the extent of abdominal primaries and is adequate to stage advanced disease. It can also be carried out without sedation, whereas general anesthesia is frequently required in young children when using MRI or CT. These modalities can be reserved for confirmation of localized disease and definition if there is complete response after chemotherapy. In experienced hands ultrasound is very effective for guiding needle biopsies, especially of abdominal masses. Bone scans are only indicated if there is focal bone pain.

Blood tests

Initial investigation should include a full blood count, liver and renal function studies, serum lactate dehydrogenase (LDH) levels, and urate, calcium, phosphate and urea levels.

Staging

Table 21.3 shows the most commonly used staging system for childhood NHL. All primary mediastinal and diffuse abdominal tumors are considered to be at least stage III. Spread in NHL, unlike Hodgkin disease, is not orderly or contiguous from node to node. Therefore, there is no place for routine staging laparotomy or lymphangiography in childhood NHL.

Role of gallium and positron emission tomography

Both Ga-67 uptake and fluorodeoxyglucose (FDG) positron emission tomography (PET) are indicators of tumor viability.

Table 21.3 St Jude modified staging system for non-Hodgkin lymphoma.

Stage		Approximate percent seen in UK
I	Single tumor (extranodal) or single anatomic area (nodal). Not mediastinum or abdomen	5
II	Single tumor (extranodal) with regional node involvement. Primary gastrointestinal tumor with or without involvement of associated mesenteric nodes only On the same side of diaphragm: (i) two or more nodal areas; (ii) two single (extranodal) tumors with or without regional node involvement	20
III	On both sides of the diaphragm: (i) two single tumors (extranodal); (ii) two or more nodal areas All primary intrathoracic tumors (mediastinal, pleural, thymic), all extensive primary intraabdominal disease; all primary paraspinal or epidural tumors regardless of other sites	50
IV	Any of the above with initial CNS* or bone marrow involvement (<25%)[†]	25

* CNS disease: unequivocal blasts > 5/mm^3 in a cytocentrifuged cerebrospinal fluid specimen with or without neurologic deficits, e.g., cranial nerve pulses plus intracerebral nodal deposits.

† Distinction is arbitrarily made at 25% to distinguish between acute lymphoid leukemia and non-Hodgkin lymphoma (NHL). This may not be useful for all, e.g., in B-cell NHL there is no difference in outcome between stage III and IV disease up to a marrow infiltration of 70%.

Specificity and sensitivity of Ga-67 are only around 75%[17] but are higher with FDG-PET.[18] Only rarely does Ga-67 imaging add to initial staging in a manner that would influence therapy, i.e., upstage the patient. No large prospective study in childhood NHL has evaluated either Ga-67 imaging or FDG-PET. In adult NHL, PET appears to be a useful tool in the assessment of response, and residual positivity may predict recurrence. No such studies have been done in children. At the present time, neither Ga-67 imaging nor PET are part of standard evaluation but may be of help in determining whether residual abnormalities require biopsy. In general it would be unwise to either upstage or introduce additional therapy on the basis of such scans alone.

Prognostic factors

Therapy

With modern aggressive intensive chemotherapy regimens, the overall cure rates are 70–75% for T-cell NHL, 80–85% for B-cell NHL (ranging from 100% for stage I and II disease to 60–70% for stage IV with CNS involvement), and 60% for anaplastic large-cell tumors. Each type requires very specific treatment (see below) and the most significant prognostic factor now appears to be the choice of the right therapy, based on meticulous initial work-up and definition of tumor type. There remains doubt as to the optimal therapy for ALCL and peripheral T-cell lymphoma and even more so for the rare low-grade follicular tumors. The speed of response may be significant, especially in T-cell NHL. In a UK T-cell NHL study, Shepherd *et al.*[19] reported that for the 25% of patients in full radiologic remission at day 60, 5-year disease-free survival (DFS) was 84% compared with only 56% for patients who had some radiologic evidence of residual mediastinal thickening.

Stage

In general, the higher the stage, the worse the prognosis, although effective therapy is reducing the differential. In T-cell disease, very few relapses occur in stage I and II tumors, whereas 5-year DFS for stage III and stage IV tumors is expected to be 70% and 60% respectively.

In B-cell NHL, the figures are 95–100% for stage I and II tumors, and have greatly improved for stage III and IV tumors. The previously defined adverse prognostic features of extensive abdominal organ involvement, pleural effusions, extraabdominal disease, poor nutritional status and bulky disease no longer appear significant. The only remaining adverse clinical features in B-cell NHL are the presence of marrow infiltration of > 70% and CNS-positive disease, but even in the latter more aggressive treatment has increased survival to nearly 70% (see below). Elevated serum LDH levels in patients with stage III B-cell NHL remains an indicator of prognosis, but is of less significance with improved therapy.

Site

Patients with stage I disease with orbital or Waldeyer's ring tumors appear to fare worse than those with other localized nodal NHL, partly due to a higher CNS relapse rate. Stage II localized abdominal tumors have a better prognosis than a similarly staged nasopharyngeal tumor extending to the skull base.

Cytogenetics

Recent studies have suggested that in B-cell NHL, karyotype may be of prognostic significance.[20] In ALCL, a t(2;5) translocation was originally thought to influence outcome, but with better methods of detection this is no longer apparent.

Treatment

General principles

Frequently, patients with lymphomas present with poor nutrition, concomitant infection and metabolic problems. Of the latter, spontaneous tumor lysis, especially in stage IV T- and B-cell disease, is the commonest.[21] Hypercalaemia has been described.[22] The features of tumor lysis syndrome are hyperphosphatemia, hypocalcemia, hyperuricemia and azotemia. In order to avoid this complication, it is essential to provide high fluid intake (3 L/m^2 daily) to induce diuresis, with intravenous or oral allopurinol or urate oxidase. Policy varies regarding alkalinization of urine to keep urate and phosphate in solution (if used, it should only maintain urinary pH at about 6.5; above this level, phosphate will precipitate). With established tumor lysis syndrome, aluminum hydroxide or calcium carbonate to lower serum phosphate levels, and slow intravenous or intramuscular magnesium (intravenous calcium tends to be tissue deposited) to reverse any symptomatic tetany are usually adequate. Maintenance of adequate diuresis is essential, and if necessary furosemide may be required; although this drug raises serum urate levels, it prevents urate from being deposited within the renal tubules. However, lysis prior to therapy or signs of renal failure progression (rapidly rising urea, creatinine and, most significantly, sustained serum potassium levels > 6.5 mmol/L) warrants early instigation of dialysis to facilitate antilymphoma therapy, since the lysis will only really cease when tumor bulk has been reduced.

The use of urate oxidase revolutionized the management of tumor lysis syndrome and significantly reduced morbidity and the need for dialysis. Recombinant urate oxidase (rasburicase) has been shown to be more effective than allopurinol, although in the absence of bulk disease is probably not necessary.[23–25]

Provided patients can be acutely supported using nasogastric feeding, malnutrition at diagnosis is not now considered an adverse prognostic feature in European and North American studies, although it may still adversely affect outcome in patients with extensive disease presenting in developing countries.

Surgery should generally be reserved for taking biopsies and repeat biopsies in the presence of residual masses after intensive therapy, and sometimes for the resection of residual tumor. Extensive initial surgery is strongly contraindicated, especially in mediastinal and extensive abdominal disease. Radiotherapy probably has a place in the local control of refractory disease, in primary CNS lymphoma and for tumors in unusual primary sites (e.g., bone). It is frequently used although its value in the setting of intensive chemotherapy is unclear. CNS-positive B-cell NHL is now curable without irradiation.

Chemotherapeutic strategies

Wollner *et al.*[26] observed that lymphoblastic disease (T and precursor B) responded optimally to an intensive leukemia-type regimen (LSA2L2). In a key randomized trial, the Children's Cancer Study Group (CCSG) confirmed that LSA2L2 was better for lymphoblastic disease, whereas a shorter pulsed cyclophosphamide-based regimen (COMP; cyclophosphamide, vincristine, methotrexate, prednisolone) produced superior results in diffuse undifferentiated lymphoma (especially in extensive abdominal disease).[27,28] The latter approach has been applied successfully in large B-cell lymphomas. In ALCL, the situation is less clear and no randomized trial has shown whether T-cell leukemia regimens are inferior to more aggressive B-cell protocols.

Localized NHL (stage I and II)

For low-stage peripheral B-cell NHL, both the CCSG and Pediatric Oncology Group have reported short-course therapy (approximately 6 months) using COMP or CHOP (cyclophosphamide, doxorubicin, vincristine, prednisolone) protocols to be extremely effective.[29,30] For stage I and abdominal stage II disease, there is no need for CNS-directed therapy. All groups have attempted to reduce the risks of late cardiotoxicity by limiting or omitting anthracyclines, of infertility by omitting alkylators, or of oncogenesis by limiting exposure to anthracyclines and/or alkylators.[31–35]

The Pediatric Oncology Group[30] reported inferior results for localized precursor B or T lymphoblastic disease, and thus all other collaborative groups have excluded such disease from short-course chemotherapy protocols and instead treated them with a longer duration leukemia-type regimen, as they would for more advanced disease

Advanced-stage B-cell lymphomas

Progressively more intensive protocols introduced in the early 1980s by the Société Française d'Oncologie Pediatrique (SFOP) have achieved 60–70% cure rates for stage IV disease. Both the LMB and BFM (Berlin–Frankfurt–Münster) protocols use initial relatively low-dose cytoreductive therapy, in particular cyclophosphamide, vincristine and prednisolone (COP) before the more intensive induction regimen, which in the case of the LMB protocol consists of two courses of high-dose methotrexate, fractionated high-dose cyclophosphamide, vincristine, prednisolone and doxorubicin (COPAdM), followed by further high-dose methotrexate and continuous-infusion cytarabine. Since the first LMB study in 1981, event-free survival (EFS) has progressively increased, and therapy and duration reduced from 12 to 4–6 months

Table 21.4 Chemotherapy regimens in FAB LMB trial.

Group A (localized resected disease): COPAd × 2

*Group B (stage II unresected, stage III, stage IV < 25% marrow,
CNS negative)*
Arm B1: COP, COPAdM, COPAdM, CYM × 2, COPAdM
Arm B2: COP, COPAdM, reduced-dose COPAdM, CYM × 2
Arm B3: COP, COPAdM, COPAdM, CYM × 2
Arm B4: COP, COPAdM, reduced-dose COPAdM, CYM × 2, COPAdM
Arm C: COP, COPAdM × 2, full-dose CYVE vs. reduced-dose
CYVE + continuation

COP, low-dose cyclophosphamide, vincristine, prednisolone; COPAdM,
cyclophosphamide, vincristine, prednisolone, doxorubicin, high-dose
methotrexate; CYM, cytarabine, high-dose methotrexate; CYVE, high-
dose cytarabine, etoposide; continuation, lower-dose COPAdM, CYM.

depending on risk stratification. Identified high-risk groups include those with bone marrow involvement of > 70% (essentially B-ALL) and those with CNS involvement at diagnosis, who now receive the most intensive regimen (i.e., 8 g/m^2 of systemic methotrexate per dose) along with triple intrathecal therapy and consolidation with continuous-infusion high-dose cytarabine and etoposide (CYVE). The LMB '89 protocol yielded an EFS of 87% in patients with B-ALL without CNS involvement and 81% in those with CNS disease at presentation, which contrasts with only 19% for such patients on the LMB '81 protocol. Inevitably, there is morbidity and some mortality associated with such intensive therapy.[36] A similar progressive improvement in EFS was seen in the BFM studies, especially for patients with stage IV disease and those with B-ALL (increase in EFS from 50 to 80%), and for stage III patients with raised LDH levels who seem to benefit from an increase in consolidation methotrexate dosage from 0.5 to 5 g/m^2 per dose.[33]

The UKCCSG also adopted the short intensive course based on the French LMB '86 regimen for patients with stage IV disease and those with B-ALL.[37] At a median follow-up of 3.1 years, 68% of patients were alive in complete first remission. There was a relapse rate of 16% and a death rate due to toxicity of 11%, with five deaths from sepsis and two from sepsis with renal failure. CNS toxicity was also notable.[38] Subsequent experience with this regimen and the use of urate oxidase during induction has significanctly reduced morbidity. Various other regimens have been reported but the precise duration and dose intensity required for cure remains unclear.[39–47] The recent combined COG, UKCCSG and SFOP study (FAB LMB '96) addressed the issues of whether the total dose of cyclophosphamide given, duration of therapy or both can be reduced in standard-risk disease. For high-risk disease the high dose of cytarabine was reduced.[48] (Table 21.4)

Speed of response to initial therapy is of prognostic significance; for example, where there is no tumor reduction fol-lowing the initial COP in the LMB protocol or there is failure to remit by 3 months, intensification of therapy is indicated. However, any residual mass should be biopsied or resected since many are fully necrotic. Relapses in advanced B-cell NHL tend to occur early, within the first 1–2 years after diagnosis, and relapses beyond 3 years appear quite rare.

Although intensive second-line treatment may be effective in relapse after localized disease where minimal chemotherapy has been used, in previously heavily treated patients the outcome is bleak.[49] There may be some longterm survivors where a high-dose regimen achieves complete response and is followed by myeloablative therapy.[50] There is some evidence of graft-versus-leukemia effect in NHL, supporting the use of allogeneic transplant.[51,52] High-dose methylprednisolone may play a useful role in palliation of symptoms.[53]

The role of antibody therapy is currently under evaluation both in combination with front-line chemotherapy and as antibody-guided radiation therapy in relapsed disease. Anti-CD20 (rituximab) has been reported to produce responses in relapsed disease.[54]

Advanced-stage T-lymphoblastic NHL

Since the mid-1970s, T-cell and precursor B-cell lymphoblastic disease has been treated using sustained, progressively more intensive leukemia-type protocols; this approach was verified in the randomized CCSG trial, which demonstrated superiority of LSA2L2 over CHOP regimens.[27] The BFM group pioneered such therapy with induction, reinduction, four courses of high-dose methotrexate as CNS-directed therapy, plus cranial irradiation. The basic protocols have been proven by the test of time; systemic methotrexate dosages have been increased from 0.5 to 5 g/m^2 and the cranial irradiation dose reduced from 18 to 12 Gy. The BFM '86 study[33] reported an EFS of 79% (±5%) for 71 patients treated with a modified LSA2L2 protocol in which 10 pulses of 3 g/m^2 of methotrexate infused over 3 hours was used as CNS-directed therapy. EFS was 79% for those with stage III disease and 72% for those with stage IV disease.[34] CNS control was excellent. In the UK, a protocol identical to the Medical Research Council ALL protocol (UKALLX) has been used, consisting of a standard four-drug induction, early (week 5) and late (week 20) six-drug consolidation modules, cranial irradiation (18 Gy) plus six intrathecal methotrexate injections, plus 2 years of standard continuing therapy (including four weekly pulses of vincristine and prednisolone). The 4-year EFS for 95 patients with stage III and IV disease was 65% (±15%). Subsequently, in protocol 9004, cranial irradiation was been replaced by three pulses of high-dose methotrexate ($6–8 \text{ g/m}^2$ depending on age), with ongoing intrathecal methotrexate every 3 months during the 2 years of treatment; in 1995, a third intensification module was introduced at week 35. No increase in CNS relapses was seen in a series of over 100 patients treated using this protocol.[55,56]

Comparable results have been reported from most un-selected series, with single-center studies reporting 5-year EFS of 70–75% and collaborative unselected series 65–70%, with little difference between patients with stage III and IV disease. The BFM '90 study reported a 90% 5-year EFS and this remains the benchmark protocol.[57] The addition of high-dose cytarabine to the BFM regimen was of no value in one randomized trial.[58]

Failure to remit by day 60 with complete resolution of a mediastinal primary is an adverse prognostic sign.[19] Instigation of more intensive therapy, including high-dose chemotherapy and autologous stem cell rescue, may be justified in the presence of such residual disease. In the BFM '90 strategy, if there was < 70% tumor regression at day 33 or residual viable tumor at the end of induction, an intensified high-risk ALL regimen was used. An early UKCCSG study suggested a useful role for localized mediastinal irradiation. Although incorporated into a modified pulsed LSA2L2-like protocol with overall worse results than now seen, this randomized study showed significantly improved results in patients who received 15-Gy irradiation to the mediastinum compared with those who did not.[59] In the presence of persistent mediastinal widening, the local use of irradiation may improve results from the rather stubbornly fixed level of 65–70% now seen.

It is important to remember that in lymphoblastic disease relapses continue to occur up to 5 years from diagnosis. Greater understanding of the cell biology involved in T-cell NHL and ALL may assist in the future application of novel strategies.

Anaplastic large-cell lymphoma

Since clinicians recognized this as an entity and improved immunohistochemical and cytogenetic techniques became available, its incidence has progressively risen. What defines the prognostic features is unclear, as is how to treat its variable forms. Indeed, it is not known whether it is a single entity or a group of disorders awaiting further classification. Rashes, which are common in this condition, may resolve spontaneously, whereas other patients progress rapidly to requiring aggressive chemotherapy.[60,61] In view of these ambiguities, both sustained leukemia-type regimens, as employed for lymphoblastic disease, and B-cell lymphoma protocols have been utilized.[62–68] Using the latter approach, an overall EFS of 76% at 5 years has been achieved.[63] Less good results have been reported by the UKCCSG using the LMB regimen (65% EFS at 5 years).[66]

A collaborative retrospective European analysis has defined four prognostic groups, although one limitation is that it was based on a range of treatment protocols (Table 21.5). As the results with BFM B-NHL regimens have been the best reported, this provides the backbone of the current European trial ALCL '97. Treatment is based on the new risk grouping

Table 21.5 Risk groups in anaplastic large cell lymphoma.

Low risk
Localized disease, completely resected

Standard risk
No skin involvement
No mediastinal involvement
No liver, spleen or lung involvement

High risk
Presence of biopsy-proven skin lesions (except skin overlying an involved or isolated skin disease)
Presence of mediastinal involvement
Presence of liver, spleen or lung involvement

Patients with CNS involvement

and the study asks questions about the schedule of high-dose methotrexate and the value of continuation therapy with single-agent vinblastine. There remains controversy about the need for such aggressive therapy being given for the disease. Results with simpler COMP-based regimens appear encouraging but there are difficulties in comparing regimens due to differences in pathologic classification and the combining of disease types.

Relapsed ALCL is unusual in that prolonged remissions may be achieved with weekly vinblastine regimens, either alone or in combination.[69] High-dose therapy with autologous or allogeneic rescue has been used but its value remains unproven.

ALCL is the third largest subgroup of childhood NHL and more needs to be learned about how to stage and treat it successfully. Resources need to be pooled internationally so that the group of patients requiring more, or less, intensive approaches can be identified.

Large B-cell lymphoma

It is important that all large-cell lymphomas are not grouped together, as ALCL and large B-cell NHL are clearly distinct entities.[67,68] The tumor is generally treated with the same approach as for BL and to date results appear to be very similar. Current studies are attempting to define distinct clinical and pathologic features.[70]

Peripheral T-cell lymphoma

There are a small number of CD30-negative patients with peripheral T-cell lymphoma for whom the optimal therapy is not known.[71,72] It is probably logical to treat them in the same way as for ALCL, although T-ALL regimens have been used.

Primary mediastinal B-cell NHL

This is mostly seen in adolescents and young adults, where it mimics T-cell NHL. Bone marrow and CNS involvement are rare.[73–75] Recommended treatment is as the same as for stage III B-cell NHL. The possibility that a mediastinal lymphoma may be of B-cell rather than T-cell origin, and so may not respond to standard lymphoblastic therapy, emphasizes the need in all childhood NHLs for full pathologic confirmation plus immunophenotyping of diagnostic material.

Follicular lymphomas

These are extremely rare in childhood and are usually stage I/II.[76] Localized disease should be treated conservatively as dissemination is very rare.[77,78] With advanced disease, CHOP regimens are effective in adults, although long-term outcome is poor.

NHL following intense immunosuppression

Over the last decade an increasing incidence of lymphoproliferative disorders has been seen in organ-transplant recipients (especially in those receiving multiple immunosuppressant drugs such as ciclosporin, FK506 or mycophenolate) and in others receiving intense immunosuppression, including patients with a diverse range of diseases (e.g., chronic inflammatory bowel disease). Although many are polyclonal, EBV-driven proliferations that recede with withdrawal of the immunosuppression, others behave more aggressively or become true malignant lymphomas. Almost all appear to be B-cell disorders, although a range of pathologies is seen. These can be divided into polymorphous (usually polyclonal, EBV-driven, good prognosis) and monomorphous (variable clonality, less clear EBV association, poorer outcome). In contrast to BL, the EBV expression patterns in these proliferations consist of a mixture of cells, with latency type 1, latency type 2 or cells expressing lytic genes.[79]

In the UK a graded therapeutic response is recommended, starting wherever possible with withdrawal or drastic reduction of the immunosuppressives followed, if there is no early response, by weekly pulses of low-dose cyclophosphamide, vincristine and prednisolone (Fig. 21.3).[80] If COP therapy does not produce resolution, then standard intensive B-cell NHL therapy is initiated. Alternative strategies have been proposed, including the use of anti-B-cell monoclonal antibodies such as rituximab[81,82] and *in vitro* production of cytotoxic T lymphocytes against EBV-infected cells.[83,84]

Indications for high-dose chemotherapy with stem cell support

There are now few indications for high-dose therapy in childhood NHL. Dose intensification appears to be of value where only partial remission is achieved after induction therapy in B-cell NHL. Dose escalation with CYVE may be sufficient where complete response is not achieved with surgery.[85] Regimens such as BEAM BCNU, etoposide, cytarabine,

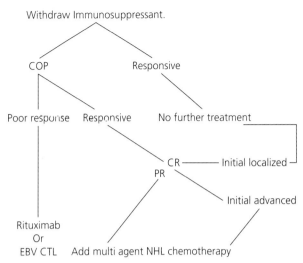

Fig. 21.3 Treatment strategy in posttransplant lymphoproliferative disorders. COP, cyclophosphamide, vincristine, prednisolone; EBV CTL, Epstein–Barr virus-specific cytotoxic T lymphocytes; CR, complete response; PR, < 50% response.

melphalan with autograft have been recommended. Relapse after localized B-cell NHL may be curable with the full LMB regimen C.

Relapse of either B- or T-cell NHL is an indication to consider allogeneic transplantation. In adults there are also suggestions of a graft-versus-lymphoma effect. The management of relapsed T-cell NHL is essentially the same as for relapsed T-ALL.

Future approaches

The evolution of humanized monoclonal antibodies and the demonstration of significant benefit using rituximab in low- and high-grade NHL in adults has encouraged their use in childhood peripheral B-cell NHL.[86,87] Current trials are evaluating both rituximab and radiolabeled anti-CD20 in relapsed and front-line regimens. Rituximab not only has a direct antitumor effect but may also chemosensitize by downregulation of BCL2. Evidence of activity in childhood NHL is limited to case reports and series of PTLPD post transplant lymphoproliferative disorders. Current trials are attempting to clarify whether rituximab should be used as part of induction or subsequent therapy. Radio-labeled anti-CD20 is also under evaluation after encouraging phase 2 studies in adults. Antisense oligonucleotide therapy has been proposed and tested in adult tumors.[88]

Hodgkin disease

It is now widely accepted that Hodgkin disease (HD) is a malignancy of uncertain cellular origin. The mononuclear HD cell and the polynucleated Reed–Sternberg cell represent the malignant cells and are derived from immature lymphoid elements. Evidence suggests that there is an EBV association in some, if not all, childhood HD.

Epidemiology

Age-standardized incidence rates for children (0–15 years) vary considerably around the world, from 0.6 per million in Japan to 10.3 per million in the Middle East, with European rates ranging from 3.3 per million (Sweden) to 6.9 per million (Italy). The UK rate is 4.1 per million.[89,90] In western industrialized countries, incidence increases with age, whereas in developing countries an earlier onset (even peaking in the first decade) is seen, as well as a much higher relative proportion of mixed cellularity cases. Incidence appears to be lower in colder latitudes where nodular sclerosis is more frequent. Genetic factors may be relevant: for example, UK children of South Asian origin have a higher incidence of early-onset mixed cellularity disease compared with those of north European Caucasian origin. In the USA there is a higher rate for black children under 10 years but for white children during adolescence. Lymphocyte predominance is more common in black than white children in North America. In northern Europe there is a bimodal pattern, with a peak at 15–30 years of age of predominantly nodular sclerotic type and a second at 45–55 years with mixed cellularity and other subtypes predominating. Boys predominate in the first decade (ratio 10 : 1) but by adolescence there is no sex difference.

Etiology

Case clusters, patterns of seasonal variation and an increased risk of developing HD in early life for children living in poor socioeconomic circumstances and among large sibships has long raised the suggestion that HD is of infectious etiology.[91–93] The bimodal peak seen in northern Europe and North America strongly resembles the epidemiology of, for example, poliovirus. The identification of EBV inclusions, especially in the early-onset mixed cellularity subtype and in cases from developing countries, has fueled speculation of a causative relationship, at least in some circumstances.[94,95] Rather like BL, other antigens and cofactors may be involved, but for at least some cases the response to such viral infection, including genetic rearrangements and initiation of inflammatory and cytokine responses, could explain the mixed pathologic pattern. There have been occasional reports of familial clusters,[96] as well as association with immunodeficiency disorders, suggesting genetic factors may be relevant for some children at least.

Cell biology and pathology

The principal malignant cell is considered to be the Reed–Sternberg (RS) cell, a large multinucleated giant cell with

Table 21.6 Rye histopathologic classification of Hodgkin disease.*

Lymphocyte predominance (7–14%)
Nodular sclerosis (17–68%)
Mixed cellularity (17–68%)
Lymphocyte depletion (0.5–20%)

* Percentages represent ranges of relative incidence reported by different pathologists in childhood series.

inclusion-like nucleoli surrounded by a clear halo. The mononuclear cells and the lacunar RS cell seen especially in the nodular sclerosing subtype are also considered to be malignant cells. However, the mere presence of these cells is not diagnostic, since on occasion they can be found in a variety of other conditions, including infectious mononucleosis and graft-versus-host disease. "Malignant" cells in the midst of a reactive collection of lymphocytes, histiocytes, plasma cells, eosinophils and fibroblasts is the characteristic pattern of HD. The cellular origin of the atypical cells in HD has been a topic of controversy for many years. Results of clonality and gene rearrangement studies on involved cells have produced conflicting results. However, it seems probable that RS cells are clonal and of B-cell origin. The absence of B-cell antigen expression may reflect defective immunoglobin transcription.[97]

Table 21.6 shows the Rye histopathologic classification scheme in universal use for HD.[98] The categories are determined by the relative proportions of RS cells, lymphocytes, sclerosis and fibrosis. There is variability in reported series of different proportions of subtypes, but mixed cellularity is seen much more commonly in younger patients and in those from developing countries.[94,99] Lymphocyte depletion is rare in the UK and northern European children, while nodular sclerosis and mixed cellularity are seen in roughly equal proportions. Nonrandom cytogenetic changes have been reported (involving chromosomes 1, 2, 7, 11, 14, 15 and 21) as well as the presence of a t(2;5) translocation in occasional cases. Whether these represent true HD or denote ALCL remains unclear.[100]

There does appear to be some correlation between patterns of presentation and histopathology. Mixed cellularity and lymphocyte-depleted forms usually present with more disseminated disease, nodular sclerosis classically with mediastinal disease in adolescents, and lymphocyte-predominant disease with focal nodal disease (characteristically in the neck or groin). Recurrence at distant sites is more common in mixed cellularity disease treated with local irradiation as sole therapy.[101] The lymphocyte-predominant nodular variety is probably best regarded as a separate entity (i.e., a variant of B-cell lymphoma) due to its unique behavior.[102]

Clinical presentation

The commonest presentation is painless cervical lymphadenopathy with or without a mediastinal mass. The cervical nodes quite characteristically fluctuate in size, often over a considerable time, giving long latent periods between first symptom/sign and diagnosis. The presence of "B symptoms" confers a less favorable prognosis, and are seen with increasing frequency in more advanced-stage disease. These symptoms comprise fever, night sweats and loss of 10% or more of body weight over the preceding 6 months, without another clear-cut explanation. Isolated disease of the spleen, liver and lung pose particular diagnostic difficulties.

Diagnostic investigations and staging

Biopsy

Adequate biopsy from the most accessible, preferably primary, tumor mass is essential. Open rather than needle biopsies are optimal, since reactive surrounding lymphadenopathy can lead to false negativity in HD and the full pattern of cellularity within the tumor needs to be reviewed in order to classify the patient properly. Careful clinical examination to detect nodal disease and organomegaly is essential as distant nodal involvement will alter the stage of disease and therefore determine therapy. Confirmation of disease extent by appropriate imaging and/or biopsy is mandatory.

Imaging

The mere size of nodes especially in the neck is no guarantee of involvement. Mediastinal disease, which is usually clinically silent, is seen in about 60% of children (proportion rises with age) and should be evaluated using posterior/anterior and lateral radiography. CT of the chest is essential to identify nodal, pleural and pulmonary disease, and will identify nodal and pulmonary deposits not seen with conventional radiography. MRI is being employed increasingly to visualize abdominal organs and nodal disease, but the gold standard imaging for HD at diagnosis remains plain chest radiography and CT of chest and abdomen. Ultrasound can be used to monitor nodal, hepatic and splenic shrinkage with therapy. Lymphangiography, a technically difficult procedure and at one time the mainstay of abdominal node detection, is now very rarely performed. Lymphangiography does enable both size and architecture of nodes to be examined but CT or MRI are as efficient as lymphangiography and much less invasive. Lymphangiography may occasionally be of value where CT/MRI are equivocal and if therapy depends on precise definition of abdominal disease. Gallium imaging, and more recently FDG-PET, have been used both to identify initial disease extent and, more importantly, to try to define disease activity at the end of treatment.[103] Abnormalities may persist on CT/MRI but subsequent clinical behavior shows that this is inactive "scarring". Residual gallium positivity, especially in the mediastinum, is highly suggestive of disease. FDG-PET is the most accurate method of defining residual disease[103] but like gallium imaging is not free of false-positive or false-negative results. If the treatment strategy involves omission of radiation therapy on the basis of complete response after chemotherapy, then PET may be useful to decide whether to biopsy residual CT/MRI abnormalities. Current paediatric studies should clarify if PET positivity alone is an indication for radiotherapy or to determine the dose administered.

Laparotomy

There is now little or no indication for primary staging laparotomy in children. Once the only truly reliable method of determining subdiaphragmatic disease and hence in formulating appropriate therapy options, especially radiation fields, it is a procedure associated with morbidity (intestinal obstruction) and even mortality (especially the lifelong risk of septic death after splenectomy). Preoperative vaccination with pneumococcal and *Haemophilus influenzae* vaccines plus lifelong prophylactic oral penicillin are essential. Death can occur up to 20 years after splenectomy from a wide range of infective agents, not just the pneumococcus. The use of combined modality therapy or chemotherapy alone for the majority of patients obviates the need for such primary staging laparatomy, especially as CT or MRI and imaging-guided biopsies can be performed if abdominal organ involvement is in doubt. With modern intensive therapy, isolated liver, spleen or other organ relapses are rare.

Bone marrow studies

Bone marrow aspirates (×2) and trephines (×2) should be performed in all patients except those with stage IA disease. Although bone marrow disease is much more common in advanced disease, an occasional patient with apparently localized disease is found to have marrow infiltration and failure to treat this appropriately leads to early recurrence. Those with B symptoms, an altered blood picture, or the rare bony disease are at higher risk of bone marrow infiltration.

Blood tests

Once the diagnosis is confirmed, useful laboratory investigations include a full blood count, erythrocyte sedimentation rate (ESR), viral titers for EBV, cytomegalovirus, measles, chickenpox and rubella status, and biochemical assessment of renal and liver function. Markers that have been reported to be useful include IL-2 receptor, soluble CD30 antigen and IL-10 levels.[104–106] However, routine use of any of these is not yet recommended. A number of risk grouping have been devised based on outcome analysis in individual studies (Table 21.7). It is important to emphasize that these relate to the specific treatment strategy applied, which may differ widely with regard to intensity of chemotherapy and irradiation.

Table 21.7 Examples of risk groupings based on multiple clinical parameters.

Stanford[105]

Poor risk = three factors, event-free survival < 70%

    Male

    Stage IIB, IIIB, IV

    Bulky mediastinum

    White cell count > 13.5

    Hemoglobin < 11.0 g/dL

SFOP[111]

Poor risk score = 3, event-free survival < 65%

    Score 1: hemoglobin < 10.5 g/dL

    Score 2: two or more of following:

        Erythrocyte sedimentation rate > 40 mm/hr

        White cell count > 12×10^9/L

        Fibrinogen > 5 g/L

        α_2-Globulin > 10 g/L

        Albumin < 35 g/L

    Score 2: nodular sclerosis

Staging

Table 21.8 shows the Ann Arbor staging scheme employed universally in HD. In most reported series low-stage disease (I and II) accounts for 50–70% of cases, while stage IV is seen in < 10% of childhood patients, and stage III in 20–40%. The variation in percentages reported in different series depends on the methods used in staging, and the rigor of clinical and imaging procedures employed.

Prognostic features

Bulky disease and poor response to initial chemotherapy remain key factors. Advanced stage in the presence of B symptoms confers adverse prognostic significance.[107] Pathologic subtype used to be more significant in predicting relapse but with modern aggressive therapy is less so, although patients with the rare lymphocyte-depleted form do fare worse than all other types. Lukes and Butler originally described two forms of lymphocyte-predominant type, a diffuse and a nodular form. The latter is a very slowly progressive disease

that may with time evolve into a more aggressive high-grade B-cell NHL.[108]

Lymphopenia is a sign of advanced disease and is consequently a less favorable feature. Neutrophilia and eosinophilia are not thought to be of prognostic significance. An elevated ESR predicts more advanced-stage disease and if found in stage I disease, unless in the presence of clearly defined and confirmed infection, should lead to a much more extensive search for occult disease. Patients with B symptoms usually have a markedly elevated ESR.

Treatment

Since Kaplan's report in 1970 of the effectiveness of 40–44 Gy in curing HD, a number of controversies have dogged the management of childhood disease.

- If irradiation is to be used, how large should the field be and what is the optimal dosage and scheduling?
- Is chemotherapy as effective as irradiation?
- Which group of patients requires combined modality therapy?
- Which combination of drugs is both efficacious and least likely to cause long-term toxicity, either alone or in combination with radiation?
- How is high-risk disease defined and treated?

In deciding treatment strategies, therapeutic groups have tried to balance the beneficial and adverse effects of each treatment modality and of individual drug toxicities.

Neck, mantle and total nodal irradiation may produce compensated or full-blown hypothyroidism, risk of thyroid malignancy, soft tissue thinning, chest and spinal deformities (short clavicles and high spinal kyphosis), and impaired spinal growth. This will depend on total dose, fraction size, field and patient's age (the younger the patient, the more likely that tissue damage will be long term). Reactive pleural and pericardial effusions, long-term fibrosis and even restrictive pericarditis have been described, as has an increased risk of coronary artery disease. Chronic radiation enteritis and retroperitoneal fibrosis are reported following abdominal radiation in HD.

Chemotherapy regimens such as MOPP (mustine, vincristine, prednisolone, procarbazine) or ABVD (Adriamycin,

Table 21.8 Ann Arbor staging system for Hodgkin disease.

Stage I	Involvement of one lymph node region (I) or a single extralymphatic organ or site (IE)
Stage II	Involvement of two or more lymph node regions on the same side of the diaphragm (II) or solitary involvement of an extralymphatic organ or site and of one or more lymph node regions on the same side of the diaphragm (IIE)
Stage III	Involvement of lymph node regions on both sides of the diaphragm (III) which may be accompanied by localized involvement of extralymphatic organ or site (IIIE) or by involvement of the spleen (IIIS) or both of these (IIISE)
Stage IV	Diffuse or disseminated involvement of one or more extralymphatic organs or tissues with or without associated lymph node enlargement

bleomycin, vinblastine, dacarbazine) are highly effective but also carry specific hazards. Azoospermia is to be expected following the dose of alkylators (mustine, procarbazine, chlorambucil or cyclophosphamide) that are generally given to cure HD. Whether there is a safe alkylator dosage is unclear. MOPP and other derivative regimens appear to have less impact on female fertility, especially in young girls, but loss of follicles may be associated with subsequent premature menopause. The ABVD regimen has much less impact on the gonads, but greater impact on pulmonary and cardiac function. The risks are compounded by the use of radiotherapy to the mediastinal region. Chemotherapy-induced second-tumor induction is a major worry in this disease where long-term survival is over 80%. This risk appears to be lower in the UKCCSG series where chlorambucil replaced mustine (ChlVPP) and most patients did not receive radiotherapy. Although ABVD was previously reported to be at low risk of inducing such tumors, anthracyclines are increasingly implicated in the causation of leukemia. Consequently, in planning any therapeutic strategy these effects and benefits must be weighed carefully. Hybrid regimens are designed to reduce the total dose of any single agent, thus reducing the incidence of infertility or cardiac problems associated with MOPP or ABVD alone.

Radiation therapy has played a major role in curative treatment of HD. With the advent of effective chemotherapy the role of radiation therapy, either combined with chemotherapy or on its own, has been reviewed and is the subject of a number of randomized trials. The dose of radiation and the field to which radiation is administered have been progressively reduced with no adverse influence on efficacies. Extended field radiation is now rarely used and total dose has been reduced to 20–30 Gy. Radiotherapy alone has been used by the UKCCSG for stage IA high cervical disease in order to avoid the effects of chemotherapy.[109]

In the HD2 II series, children with stage IA disease received involved field radiation therapy at a dose of 35 Gy as sole therapy.[101] Progression-free survival was 70%, i.e., there was a high local relapse rate. Patients with mixed cellularity disease appeared to do particularly poorly, with a progression-free survival of only 48%, although the salvage rate was very high with subsequent chemotherapy. Current practice in the UK group is that all but mixed cellularity cases still receive limited radiation therapy although an exception may be the younger child (i.e., <5 years of age) in whom the late sequelae of radiation therapy may be more marked, and in this situation the option of chemotherapy alone may be discussed with the family. In a small study using VEEP (vincristine, etoposide, epirubicin and prednisolone) as sole therapy, there was a comparatively high initial failure or relapse rate and it was concluded that this approach was not suitable particularly in patients with more advanced disease.[110]

An alternative strategy to reduce the extent of radiation is that followed by the French SFOP group, where risk stratification is based on the initial response to a nonalkylating combination of vinblastine, bleoymicin and etoposide. In those patients who have a rapid response to this low-intensity treatment, radiation therapy dose is reduced.[111] This strategy is now increasingly applied (Tables 21.9 and 21.10).[112–115]

Where alkylating agent-based chemotherapy is combined with radiation, attempts have been made to reduce the total number of cycles of MOPP or the hybrid regimen MOPP/ABVD. Follow-up of these shorter regimens is insufficient to be clear about the precise risk of infertility or cardiac dysfunction but it is likely that these are significantly lower than with previous protocols. In the UKCCSG HD1 study, patients with all stages of disease apart from stage IA received ChlVPP chemotherapy, radiation therapy being confined to those with bulky mediastinal disease (where it exceeded one-third of maximal transthoracic diameter). Using this approach the 10-year progression-free survival (and overall survival) was 85% (92%) for stage II, 73% (84%) for stage III, and 38% (71%) for stage IV. In the subsequent HD2 study, radiation therapy was omitted completely unless there was biopsy-proven residual disease following chemotherapy alone. This did not adversely affect the outcome of patients with stage II and III disease. The ChlVPP protocol appears to be associated with a lower incidence of second tumors than MOPP, with an overall risk of 3.4% at 10 years, of which 2.7% are leukemia/NHL and 0.7% solid tumor. The low risk of late second solid

Table 21.9 Examples of regimens designed to reduce late sequelae by the omission of radiotherapy.

Study	Chemotherapy	No. of patients	5-year EFS (OS)
UKCCGS HD2[101]	Chlorambucil, vincristine, procarbazine, prednisolone (ChlVPP)	217	Stage II 80% (95%) Stage III 75% (91%)
Royal Marsden[110]	Vincristine, epirubicin, etoposide, prednisolone (VEEP)	54	Stage I –III 82% (93%)
Rotterdam[118]	Mustine, vincristine, procarbazine, prednisone, epirubicin, bleomycin, vinblastine, dacarbazine (MOPP-EBVD)	46	91% (98%)
Amsterdam[119]	MOPP-ABVD	21	90% (90%)

EFS, event-free survival; OS, overall survival.

Table 21.10 Examples of reduced-dose or response-related radiotherapy strategies.

Study	Chemotherapy	Radiotherapy	No. of patients	5-year EFS (OS)
SFOP[111]	VBP → Good response ↓ Poor response ↓ ABVD → Good response ↓ Poor response	20 Gy 20 Gy 40 Gy	171 stage I, II	91% (97%)
St Jude[113]	Vinblastine, doxorubicin, methotrexate, prednisolone (VAMP/COP)	CR 15 Gy PR 25.5 Gy	100	Stage II 78% (NS) Stage III 69% (NS)
Boston[117]	Vinblastine, etoposide, prednisone, doxorubicin (VEPA)	Early CR 15 Gy Bulky or PR 25.5 Gy	34 stage II, III	Stage II 79% Stage III 70% (NS)

ABVD, doxorubicin, bleomycin, vinblastine, dacarbazine; COP, cyclophosphamide, vincristine, prednisolone; CR, complete response; EFS, event-free survival; NS, not significant; OS, overall survival; PR, partial response; VBP, vinblastine, bleomycin, prednisolone.

Table 21.11 Examples of regimens used for stage IV disease.

Study	Chemotherapy	Radiotherapy	No. of patients	5-year EFS (OS)
UKCCSG, HD 8201, 9201[122]	ChlVPP × 6–8	No irradiation except bulky mediastinum in 8201 study	67	55% (81%)
GPOH[116]	OPPA × 2 COPP × 4	+20 Gy all involved sites	84	90% (96%)
Boston[117]	VEPA × 6	+25 Gy to all involved sites	20	49% (NS)
St Jude[113]	VAMP/COP × 6	+25.5 Gy to all involved sites	44	65% (NS)
Stanford[105]	VAMP × 6	CR 15 Gy PR 25.5 Gy	64	70% (83%)

ChlVPP, chlorambucil, vincristine, procarbazine, prednisolone; COP, cyclophosphamide, vincristine, prednisolone; COPP, cyclophosphamide, vincristine, procarbazine, prednisone; CR, complete response; EFS, event-free survival; NS, not significant; OS, overall survival; OPPA, vincristine, procarbazine, prednisone, doxorubicin; PR, partial response; VAMP, vinblastine, doxorubicin, methotrexate, prednisolone; VEPA, vinblastine, etoposide, prednisone, doxorubicin.

tumors almost certainly reflects the omission of radiation therapy for the majority of patients. A randomized Pediatric Oncology Group study has demonstrated that after delivery of eight cycles of MOPP/ABVD, the addition of radiotherapy has no beneficial effect. Other studies where chemotherapy alone or reduced radiation strategies have been applied are shown in Tables 21.9 and 21.10.[116–120]

Patients with stage IV disease continue to have relatively high relapse rates, although subgroups such as those with only pulmonary involvement do better.[121,122] The best published data come from the BFM group. Using the same intensive approach with OPPA/COPP and extensive radiation therapy administered to all sites of disease,[116] the SFOP group has replicated the encouraging outcome although late sequelae are inevitable. The comparatively high salvage rate in the

UKCCSG series has led this group to persist with the current strategy of ChlVPP alone, with dose intensification, including in some cases high-dose melphalan, in the event of a poor response (Table 21.11).

Relapsed disease

The management of relapsed HD depends on the initial extent of the disease, the nature of chemotherapy, prior use of radiation therapy and time of relapse.[123,124] In the case of early-relapse high-stage disease previously treated with multimodal therapy, the outcome with second-line chemotherapy alone is poor. This is in contrast to a late relapse of localized disease treated with low-dose therapy or single-modality strategies. In the former group the use of very high-dose therapy requiring stem cell rescue has been explored but not tested in a randomized study. In single-center or national series the benefit remains unproven.[125–127]

Summary

- *Stage IA*: patients appear to be highly curable with involved field irradiation only (dosages 30–35 Gy) (although some will require salvage chemotherapy) but will develop hypothyroidism and some soft tissue thinning of the neck. Chemotherapy with or without low-dose involved field radiotherapy can be equally effective, but the number of cycles needed for cure is unclear, and exposure to alkylators and anthracyclines should be restricted.
- *Stages II and IIIA*: both short-course hybrid chemotherapy (three cycles of MOPP or ChlVPP/AVBD or VEBP) with involved field irradiation (20 Gy), and chemotherapy alone (six cycles of therapy) can be curative. However, without irradiation more chemotherapy appears to be required (i.e., six rather than three cycles) and there is probably an increased risk of sterility with therapy including alkylators, or cardiopulmonary dysfunction for that including anthracyclines and/or bleomycin. The long-term safety of the short course of chemotherapy with involved field irradiation has not been fully evaluated. The strategy of response-adapted therapy has now been adopted by groups including the COG and seems the most logical way to minimize treatment for those who do not need aggressive therapy while maintaining high cure rates in those who do. A philosophy of accepting high relapse rates on the assumption that salvage rates are high is accompanied by a high overall burden of therapy and later sequelae. This approach is unacceptable unless the initial treatment is minimal.
- *Advanced stage IIIB and IV*: hybrid chemotherapy and radiotherapy to involved sites appears to be most efficacious, but the total duration of therapy required is not clear.

Long-term sequelae of lymphoma therapy

Table 21.12 shows some of the potential sequelae of lymphoma therapy. These risks must be taken into consideration

Table 21.12 Potential long-term sequelae in children treated for lymphoma.

Secondary neoplasia
Growth impairment
Endocrine dysfunction
Infertility
Educational and psychologic dysfunction
Other organ toxicity, e.g., cardiac with anthracyclines,
    pulmonary with bleomycin
Problems with obtaining jobs and insurance, and acceptance as adopters

for both childhood NHL and HD because of the high overall cure rates now possible.

Second tumors

Hawkins *et al.*[128] reported a 1.4% rate of leukemias in patients treated for NHL within the first 6 years from diagnosis compared with 0.5% for all other tumors. This increased risk appears to be associated with a specific era of treatment, when high doses of epipodophyllotoxins were used in schedules that did not allow for adequate DNA repair and which allowed total doses in excess of 1.2 g/m^2. These second leukemias characteristically have a short latency and are associated with chromosomal translocations involving 11q23 (*MLL* gene). It is also important to note that the anthracyclines included in many lymphoma protocols are also inhibitors of topoisomerase II and are linked with therapeutically induced acute leukemia. The leukemia risk is reduced by the omission of mechlorethamine from combination regimens.[129]

Irradiation to the thyroid, especially if compensated hypothyroidism is not treated early, is associated with an increased risk of thyroid cancer.[130] The Late Effects Study Group in a follow-up study of 1380 childhood HD survivors reported an 18-fold overall increase in tumors, principally leukemias, but also a remarkable 75-fold increased risk of young women developing breast cancer at 20 years from diagnosis (17 cases compared with an expected 0.2 cases).[131] With extended follow-up of this cohort treated between 1955 and 1986, the cumulative incidence of any malignancy was 26% at 30 years. The standardized incidence ratios for breast and thyroid cancer were 56% and 36%, respectively. A significance increase in bone, colorectal, lung and gastric cancers were also documented.[132] In a recent study from Boston, the standardized incidence rates in over 6000 women diagnosed between 1970 and 1986 was 25%. Age of diagnosis was not an independent risk factor.[133]

It has been suggested that DNA repair mechanism polymorphisms (e.g., XRCCI and GSTTI) may be associated with risk of second cancers.[134]

Growth impairment

Although now rarely used, CNS-directed radiotherapy will cause the well-documented risk of induced growth hormone insufficiency.[135] Age at treatment and total plus fraction dose of radiation determine the extent of impairment. Modern protocols that omit irradiation probably avoid the risk, although high-dose intensity chemotherapy may have some direct effect on bone growth,[136] although not as great as that from irradiation of the hypothalamic–pituitary axis.

Endocrine dysfunction

Irradiation to the neck even at very low dosages (0.1 Gy) can induce thyroid dysfunction, initially with a rise in thyroid-stimulating hormone and only subsequently a fall in thyroxine.[137] Replacement therapy is almost universally required in HD patients treated with bilateral neck or mantle fields. Although many drugs used for lymphomas, especially alkylating agents, are gonadotoxic and usually disproportionately affect fertility in boys, they are not steroidogenic (secondary sexual characteristics and potency are preserved). There is much less direct effect of chemotherapy on ovarian function, although follicle numbers may be reduced (inducing premature menopause). Conversely, irradiation, especially total nodal irradiation, has a major effect on ovarian function with a requirement for lifelong hormonal replacement.[138]

Fertility

Male long-term survivors exposed to alkylating agents have a very low fertility rate, whereas females do not appear to be as severely affected, but abdominal irradiation affects fertility in both sexes,[139] depending on the dose received by the gonads. Risk of male infertility is low in the absence of alkylators.[140] As mentioned above, premature menopause is a significant risk for adolescent lymphoma survivors and is associated with exposure to alkylating agents (nine times the risk) and/or abdominal irradiation (four times the risk), even in the third decade of life.[141] The prospects for any specific pregnancy are good provided extensive irradiation involving the pelvis (specifically uterine vasculature) has not been required. In the postpubertal male, it is important that sperm cryopreservation is discussed and performed prior to chemotherapy. Recently a number of centers have considered more novel and often experimental approaches such as testicular aspiration and ovarian slice cryopreservation. It seems likely that such techniques will become more widely used as data on effectiveness emerges.[142]

Educational and psychologic functioning

The well-documented impact of cranial irradiation (in dosages of 18–24 Gy) on neuropsychologic functioning includes impairment of attention span and cognitive processing skills. Verbal IQ is frequently well preserved. Age at treatment, and possibly gender, influence the degree of impairment. The adverse impact of high-dose methotrexate remains to be clearly defined.

Apart from the physical effects of CNS-directed therapy, patients who do not adjust well to the diagnosis, its treatment and survival may have long-term schooling problems (especially attendance) and overall coping problems.

Organ dysfunction

The increasing risk of acute cardiac toxicity with increasing doses of anthracyclines is well recognized, but what is still far from clear is the true long-term risk of more moderate dose exposure. Lipshultz *et al.*[143] have shown abnormalities in patients with acute leukemia after only small doses of doxorubicin. Given that survival rates for lymphomas are high, it seems prudent to:

- limit total dose of anthracylines wherever possible;
- avoid bolus administration of anthracyclines, although it appears that for a truly protective effect infusion times in excess of 72–96 hours are required;
- consider the use of cardioprotective agents such as cardioxone, which has been shown to give a significantly reduced incidence of subclinical cardiotoxicity in patients receiving anthracyclines.[144,145]

Chest and mediastinal irradiation compounds the cardiotoxicity risk of anthracyclines. Even without chemotherapy, mediastinal irradiation has been reported to be associated with an increased early mortality risk from myocardial infarction (30 times the rate for the general population) among HD survivors[146] and with a high incidence of cardiovascular problems.[147] These risks appear to be reduced if the total irradiation dose is lowered, and combined modality therapy not involving anthracyclines is used with limited involved field irradiation.

Chest or spinal irradiation in childhood may restrict the growth of the chest wall and lungs, and subsequently progressive fibrosis may develop. For lymphomas, a much greater risk is associated with the use of bleomycin, particularly for HD. Acute toxicity is associated with high single doses, cumulative dose and exposure to high levels of oxygen.[148] The chronic toxicity of bleomycin is under further investigation as is the impact of other chemotherapies.[149]

Soft tissue hypoplasia and bony damage from high-dose local irradiation has been mentioned in the context of early HD therapy, and is another reason for the reduction, wherever possible, of total dosages used.

Future prospects

Further improvements in cure rate while minimizing lapse sequences will come from a range of strategies.

- Better use of existing drugs based on pharmacogenetics and dose individualization.[150,151]
- Better understanding of molecular phenotyping and its significance in tumor behavior.[152]
- Improved risk stratification based on response using novel imaging and minimal residual disease quantitation.[7,103,153]
- Novel molecular therapies directed toward tumor-specific targets.[88,154]

References

1. Parkin DM, Stiller CA, Bieber CA, Draper GJ, Terracini B,

Young JL (eds) *International Incidence of Childhood Cancer.* IARC Scientific Publication No. 87. Lyon: IARC, 1988.

2. Epstein MA, Achong BG, Barr YM. Virus particles in cultured lymphoblasts from Burkitt's lymphoma. *Lancet* 1964; **i**: 702–3.

3. Karajannis M, Hummel M, Oschiles I *et al.* Epstein–Barr virus infection in western European pediatric non-Hodgkin lymphomas. *Blood* 2003; **102**: 4244.

4. Thorley-Lawson D, Gross A. Persistence of the Epstein–Barr virus and the origins of associated lymphomas. *N Engl J Med* 2004; **350**: 1328–37.

5. Rossi G, Bonetti F. EBV and Burkitt's lymphoma. *N Engl J Med* 2004; **350**: 2621.

6. Barth T, Muller S, Pawlita M *et al.* Homogeneous immunophenotype and paucity of secondary genomic aberrations are distinctive features of endemic but not sporadic Burkitt's lymphoma and diffuse large B-cell lymphoma with MYC rearrangement, *J Pathol* 2004; **203**: 940–5.

7. Sabesan V, Cairo MS, Lones MA *et al.* Assessment of minimal residual disease in childhood non-Hodgkins lymphoma by polymerase chain reaction using patient specific primers. *J Pediatr Hematol Oncol* 2003; **25**: 109–13.

8. Brubaker G, Levin AG, Steel CM *et al.* Multiple cases of Burkitt's lymphoma and other neoplasms in families in the North Mara District of Tanzania. *Int J Cancer* 1980; **26**: 165–70.

9. Aya T, Kinoshita T, Imai S *et al.* Chromosome translocation and c-MYC activation by Epstein–Barr virus and *Euphorbia tirucalli* in B lymphocytes. *Lancet* 1991; **337**: 1190.

10. Hamilton-Dutoit SJ, Rea D, Raphael M *et al.* Epstein–Barr virus latent gene expression and tumor cell phenotype in acquired immunodeficiency syndrome-related NHL. Correlation of lymphoma phenotype with three distinct patterns of viral latency. *Am J Pathol* 1993; **143**: 1072–85.

11. Hecht F, Morgan R, Gemmill RM *et al.* Translocations in T-cell leukemia and lymphoma. *N Engl J Med* 1985; **313**: 758.

12. Mason DY, Bastard C, Rimokh R *et al.* CD30-positive large cell lymphomas (Ki-1 lymphomas) are associated with a chromosomal translocation involving 5q34. *Br J Haematol* 1990; **74**: 161–8.

13. Dalla-Favera R, Migliazza A, Chang CC *et al.* Molecular pathogenesis of B cell malignancy: the role to BC1-6. *Curr Top Microbial Immunol* 1999; **246**: 257–63.

14. Hyjek E, Chadburn A, Lin Y *et al.* BCL-6 protein is expressed in precursor T-cell lymphoblastic lymphoma in prenatal and postnatal thymus. *Blood* 2001; **97**: 270–6.

15. Grierson H, Purtillo DT. Epstein–Barr virus infections in males with the X-linked lymphoproliferative syndrome. *Ann Intern Med* 1987; **106**: 538–45.

16. Attard-Montalto SP, Schuller I, Lastowska MA, Gibbons B, Kingston JE, Eden OB. Non-Hodgkin's lymphoma and Klinefelter syndrome. *Pediatr Hematol Oncol* 1994; **11**: 197–200.

17. Bayar E, Matthew P, Jasty R *et al.* Anterior mediastinal mass in childhood non-Hodgkin lymphoma: dilemma of post-therapy imaging, *Med Pediatr Oncol* 2000; **34**: 157–61.

18. Montravers F, McNamara D, Landman-Parker J *et al.* FDG in childhood lymphoma: clinical utility and impact on management. *Eur J Nucl Med* 2002; **29**: 1165.

19. Shepherd SF, Aherne RP, Pinkerton CR. Childhood T-cell lymphoblastic lymphoma: does early resolution of mediastinal mass predict for final outcome? *Br J Cancer* 1995; **72**: 752–6.

20. Lones MA, Sanger WG, Le Beau MM *et al.* Chromosome abnormalities may correlate with prognosis in Burkitt/Burkitt like lymphomas of children and adolescents: report from Children's Cancer Group Study CCG-E08. *J Pediatr Hematol Oncol* 2004; **26**: 169–78.

21. Cairo M, Bishop M *et al.* Tumour lysis syndrome: new therapeutic strategies and classification. *Br J Haematol* 2004; **127**: 3–11.

22. Leblanc A, Caillaud JM, Hartmann O *et al.* Hypercalcaemia preferentially occurs in unusual forms of childhood non-Hodgkin's lymphoma, rhabdomyosarcoma and Wilms' tumour. *Cancer* 1984; **54**: 2132–6.

23. Coiffer B, Mounier N, Bologna S *et al.* Efficacy and safety of rasburicase (recombinant urate oxidase) for the prevention and treatment of hyperuricemia during induction chemotherapy, aggressive non-Hodgkin's lymphoma. *J Clin Oncol* 2003; **21**: 4402–6.

24. Goldman S, Holcenberg J, Finklestein J *et al.* A randomized comparison between rasburicase and allopurinol in children with lymphoma or leukaemia at high risk for tumour lysis. *Blood* 2001; **97**: 2998–3003.

25. Wossmann W, Schrappe M, Meyer U *et al.* Incidence of tumour lysis syndrome in children with advanced Burkitt's lymphoma/leukaemia before and after introduction of prophylactic use of urate oxidase. *Ann Hematol* 2003; **82**: 160–5.

26. Wollner N, Exelby PR, Lieberman PH. Non-Hodgkin's lymphoma in children. A progress report on the original patients treated with the LSA2L2 protocol. *Cancer* 1979; **44**: 1990–9.

27. Anderson JR, Wilson JF, Jenkin DT *et al.* Childhood non-Hodgkin's lymphoma: results of a randomised therapeutic trial comparing a 4 drug regimen (COMP) to a 10 drug regimen (LSA2L2). *N Engl J Med* 1983; **308**: 559–65.

28. Anderson JR, Jenkin RDT, Wilson JF *et al.* Long term follow up of patients treated with Comp or LSA2L2 therapy for childhood NHL: a report of CCG-551 from the Children's Cancer Study Group. *J Clin Oncol* 1993; **11**: 1024–32.

29. Meadows AT, Sposto R, Jenkin RDT *et al.* Similar efficacy of 6 and 18 months of therapy with four drugs (COMP) for localised non-Hodgkin's lymphoma of children: a report from the Children's Cancer Study Group. *J Clin Oncol* 1989; **7**: 92–9.

30. Hvizdala EV, Berard C, Callihan T *et al.* Non lymphoblastic lymphoma in children: histology and stage-related response to therapy. A Pediatric Oncology Group Study. *J Clin Oncol* 1991; **9**: 1189–95.

31. Burke A, Imerson J, Hobson R *et al.* Localised non-Hodgkins lymphoma with B-cell histology: with cyclophosphamide? A report of the United Kingdom Children's Cancer Study Group on studies NHL 8501 and NHL 9001 (1985–1996). *Br J Haematol* 2003; **121**: 586–91.

32. Jenkin RDT, Anderson JR, Chilcote RR *et al.* The treatment of localised non-Hodgkin's lymphoma in children: a report from the Children's Cancer Study Group. *J Clin Oncol* 1984; **2**: 88–97.

33. Reiter A, Schrappe M, Parwaresch R *et al.* Non-Hodgkin's lymphoma of childhood and adolescence: results of a treatment stratified for biologic subtypes and stage. A report of the Berlin–Frankfurt–Münster Group. *J Clin Oncol* 1995; **13**: 359–72.

34. Patte C, Kalifa C, Flamant F *et al.* Results of the LMT 81 protocol, a modified LSA2L2 protocol with high dose

methotrexate, on 84 children with non B-cell lymphoma. *Med Pediatr Oncol* 1992; **20**: 105–13.

35. Neth O, Seidmann K, Jansen P *et al*. Precursor B-cell lymphoblastic lymphoma in childhood and adolescence: clinical features, treatment, and results in trials NHL-BFM 86 and 90. *Med Pediatr Oncol* 2000; **35**: 20–7.

36. Patte C, Auperin A, Michon J *et al*. The Societe Francaise d'Oncologie Pediatrique LMB89 protocol: highly effective multiagent chemotherapy tailored to the tumor burden and initial response in 561 unselected children with B-cell lymphomas and L3 leukemia. *Blood* 2001; **97**: 3370–9.

37. Atra A, Gerrard M, Hobson R, Immerson J, Ashley S, Pinkerton CR on behalf of the UKCCSG and SFOP study. Improved cure rate in children with B-cell acute lymphoblastic leukaemia (B-ALL) and stage IV B cell NHL. *Br J Cancer* 1988; **77**: 2281–5.

38. Atra A, Pinkerton CR, Bouffet E *et al*. Acute neurotoxicity in children with advanced stage B-non-Hodgkins lymphoma, and B-acute lymphoblastic leukaemia treated with the United Kingdom Cancer Study group 9002/9003 protocols. *Eur J Cancer* 2004; **40**: 1346–50.

39. Rizzieri DA, Johnson JL, Niedzwiecki D *et al*. Intensive chemotherapy with and without cranial radiation for Burkitt leukaemia and lymphoma: final results of Cancer and Leukaemia Group B Study. *Cancer* 2004; **100**: 1438–48.

40. Cairo MS, Krailo M, Morse M *et al*. Long term follow up of short intensive multi agent chemotherapy without high-dose methotrexate ("Orange") in children with advanced non-lymphoblastic non-Hodgkin's lymphoma: a Children's Cancer Group report. *Leukemia* 2002; **16**: 594–600.

41. Cairo MS, Sposto R, Perkins SL *et al*. Burkitt's and Burkitt-like lymphoma in children and adolescents for review of the Children's Cancer Group experience. *Br J Haematol* 2003; **120**: 660–70.

42. Messeling PB, Broadhead R, Molyneux E *et al*. Malawi pilot study of Burkitt lymphoma treatment. *Med Pediatr Oncol* 2003; **41**: 532–40.

43. Pillon M, Di Tullio MT, Garaventa A *et al*. Long term results of the first Italian Association of Paediatric Haematology Oncology protocol for the treatment of paediatric B-cell non-Hodgkin lymphoma. *Cancer* 2004; **15**: 385–94.

44. Nicola MD, Carlo-Stella C, Mariotti J *et al*. High response rate and manageable toxicity with a intensive term chemotherapy programme for Burkitt's lymphoma. *Br J Haematol* 2004; **126**: 815–20.

45. Spreafico F, Massimino M, Luksch R *et al*. Intensive, very short-term chemotherapy for advanced Burkitt's lymphoma in children. *J Clin Oncol* 2002; **15**: 2783–8.

46. Schwenn MR, Blattner SR, Lynch E *et al*. HIC-COM: a 2 month intensive chemotherapy regimen for children with Stage III and IV Burkitt's lymphoma and B-cell acute lymphoblastic leukaemia. *J Clin Oncol* 1991; **9**: 133–8.

47. Pinkerton CR, Hann IM, Eden OB *et al*. Outcome in Stage III non-Hodgkin's lymphoma in children. How much treatment is needed? *Br J Cancer* 1991; **64**: 583–7.

48. Patte C, Gerrard M, Auperin A *et al*. Final results and prognostic factors of the randomised international trial FAB LMB 96 for the "Intermediate risk" in childhood and adolescent B-cell lymphoma [abstract]. *Pediatr Blood Cancer* 2004; **43**: 348.

49. Attarbaschi A, Dwoezak M, Steiner M *et al*. Outcome of children with primary resistant or relapsed non-Hodgkin lymphoma and mature B-cell leukaemia after intensive first-line treatment: a population-based analysis of the Austrian Cooperative Study Group. *Pediatr Blood Cancer* 2005; **44**: 70–6.

50. Ladenstein R, Pearce R, Hartman O *et al*. High-dose chemotherapy with autologous bone marrow rescue in children with poor-risk Burkitt's lymphoma: a report from the European Lymphoma Bone Marrow Transplantation Registry. *Blood* 1997; **90**: 2921–30.

51. Grigg A, Seymour J *et al*. Graft versus Burkitt's lymphoma effect after allogeneic marrow transplantation. *Leukemia Lymphoma* 2002; **43**: 889–92.

52. Peniket A, Ruiz de Elvira M, Taghipour G. An EBMT registry matched study of allogeneic stem cell transplants for lymphoma: allogeneic transplantation is associated with a lower relapse rate but higher procedure-related mortality rate than autologous transplantation. *Bone Marrow Transplant* 2003; **31**: 667–78.

53. Ryalls M, Pinkerton C, Meller S *et al*. High-dose methylprednisolone sodium succinate as a single agent in relapsed childhood acute lymphoblastic leukaemia. *Med Pediatr Oncol* 1992; **20**: 119–23.

54. Yokohama A, Tsukamoto N, Uchiumi H *et al*. Durable remission induced by rituximab-containing chemotherapy in a patient with primary refractory Burkitt's lymphoma. *Ann Hematol* 2004; **83**: 120–3.

55. Eden OB, Hann I, Imeson J *et al*. Treatment of advanced stage T-cell lymphoblastic lymphoma: results of the United Kingdom Children's Cancer Study Group protocol 8503. *Br J Haematol* 1992; **82**: 310–16.

56. Eden OB, Saha V, Hann I *et al*. Results of three consecutive UKCCSG trials for advanced stage T-cell NHL. *Med Pediatr Oncol* 1993; **21**: 550.

57. Reiter A, Schrappe M, Ludwig W *et al*. Intensive ALL-type therapy without local radiotherapy provides a 90% event-free survival for children with T-cell lymphoblastic lymphoma: a BFM group report. *Blood* 2000; **95**: 416–21.

58. Millot F, Suciu S, Philippe N *et al*. Value of high dose cytarabine during interval therapy of a Berlin-Frankfurt-Münster based protocol in increased-risk children with acute lymphoblastic leukaemia and lymphoblastic lymphoma: results of the European Organisation for Research and Treatment of Cancer 5881 randomised phase III trial. *J Clin Oncol* 2001; **19**: 1935–42.

59. Mott MG, Eden OB, Palmer MK. Adjuvant low dose radiation in childhood non-Hodgkin's lymphoma. *Br J Cancer* 1984; **50**: 463–9.

60. Paulli M, Berti E, Rosso R *et al*. CD30/Ki-1 positive lymphoproliferative disorders of the skin: clinico-pathological correlation and statistical analysis of 86 cases. *J Clin Oncol* 1995; **13**: 1343–54.

61. Sandlund JT, Pui Ch, Santana VM *et al*. Clinical features and treatment outcome for children with CD3+ large cell non-Hodgkin's lymphoma. *J Clin Oncol* 1994; **12**: 885–98.

62. Massimo M, Gasparini M, Giardini R. Ki1 (CD30) anaplastic large cell lymphoma in children. *Ann Oncol* 1995; **9**: 915–20.

63. Reiter A, Schrappe M, Tiemann M *et al*. Successful treatment strategy for Ki-1 anaplastic large cell lymphoma of childhood: a prospective analysis of 62 patients enrolled in three

consecutive Berlin-Frankfurt-Münster group studies. *J Clin Oncol* 1994; **12**: 899–908.

64. Seidemann K, Tiemann M, Schrappe M *et al*. Short-pulse non-Hodgkin lymphoma type chemotherapy is efficacious treatment for pediatric anaplastic large cell lymphoma: a report of the Berlin-Frankfurt-Münster Group Trial NHL-BFM 90. *Blood* 2001; **97**: 3699–706.

65. Raetz E, Perkins S, Davenport V *et al*. B large cell lymphoma in children and adolescents. *Cancer Treat Rev* 2003; **29**: 91–8.

66. Williams D, Hobson R, Imerson J *et al*. Anaplastic large cell lymphoma in childhood: analysis of 72 patients treated on the United Kingdom Children's Cancer Study Group chemotherapy regimens. *Br J Haematol* 2002; **117**: 812–20.

67. Mora J, Fillippa D, Thaler H *et al*. Large cell non-Hodgkin lymphoma of childhood: analysis of 78 consecutive patients enrolled in 2 consecutive protocols at the Memorial Sloan-Kettering Cancer Center. *Cancer* 2000; **88**: 186–97.

68. Cairo M, Sposto R, Hoover-Regan M *et al*. Childhood and adolescent large cell lymphoma (LCL): a review of the Children's Cancer Group experience. *Am J Haematol* **72**: 53–63.

69. Brugieres L, Quartier P, Le Deley M *et al*. Relapses of childhood anaplastic large-cell lymphoma: treatment results in a series of 41 children. A report from the French Society of Paediatric Oncology. *Ann Oncol* 2000; **11**: 53–8.

70. Wilder R, Rodrigues M, Medeiros L *et al*. International prognostic index-based outcomes for diffuse large- B cell lymphomas. *Cancer* 2002; **94**: 3083–8.

71. Berge R, De Bruin P, Oudejans J *et al*. ALK-negative anaplastic large-cell lymphoma demonstrates similar poor prognosis to peripheral T-cell lymphoma, unspecified. *Histopathology* 2003; **43**: 462–9.

72. Massimino M, Perotti D, Sperafico F *et al*. Non ALC peripheral T-cell lymphomas in children: a report on two cases and a review of literature. *Haematologica* 2000; **85**: 1109–11.

73. Lazzarino M, Orlandi E, Paulli M *et al*. Primary mediastinal B-cell lymphoma with sclerosis, an aggressive tumor with distinctive clinical and pathological features. *J Clin Oncol* 1993; **11**: 2306–13.

74. Lones MA, Perkins S, Sposto R *et al*. Large cell lymphoma arising in the mediastinum in children and adolescents is associated with an excellent outcome: a Children's Cancer Group report. *J Clin Oncol* 2000; **18**: 3845–53.

75. Seidemann K, Tiemann M, Lauterbach I *et al*. Primary mediastinal large B-cell lymphoma with sclerosis in pediatric and adolescent patients: treatment and results from three therapeutic studies. Berlin-Frankfurt-Münster Group. *J Clin Oncol* 2003; **21**: 1782–9.

76. Lorsbach R, Shay-Seymore D, Moore J *et al*. Clinicopathologic analysis of follicular lymphoma occurring in children. *Blood* 2002; **99**: 1959–64.

77. Atra A, Meller S, Stevens R *et al*. Conservative management of follicular non-Hodgkin's lymphoma in childhood. *Br J Haematol* 1998; **103**: 220–3.

78. Sapunar F, Catovsky D, Wotherspoon A *et al*. Follicular lymphoma. A series of 11 patients within minimal or no treatment and long survival. *Leukemia Lymphoma* 2000; **37**: 163–7.

79. Oudejans JJ, Jiwa M, van den Brule A *et al*. Detection of heterogeneous Epstein–Barr virus gene expression patterns within individual post transplantation lymphoproliferative disorders. *Am J Pathol* 1995; **147**: 923–33.

80. Pinkerton CR, Hann I, Weston C *et al*. immunodeficiency-related lymphoproliferative disorders: prospective data from the United Kingdom Children's Cancer Study Group Registry. *Br J Haematol* 2002; **118**: 456–61.

81. Fischer A, Blanche S, Le Bidois *et al*. Anti B-cell monoclonal antibodies in the treatment of severe B-cell lymphoproliferative syndrome following bone marrow and organ transplantation. *N Engl J Med* 1991; **324**: 1451–6.

82. Verschuuren EA, Stevens S, Van Imhoff G *et al*. Treatment of post transplant lymphoproliferative disease with rituximab: the remission, the relapse, and the complication. *Transplantation* 2002; **73**: 100–4.

83. Burns D, Crawford D. Epstein–Barr virus-specific cytotoxic T-lymphocytes for adoptive immunotherapy of post-transplant lymphoproliferative disease. *Blood Rev* 2004; **18**: 193–209.

84. Haque T, Wilkie G, Taylor C *et al*. Treatment of Epstein–Barr-virus-positive post-transplantation lymphoproliferative disease with partly HLA-matched allogeneic cytotoxic T cells. *Lancet* 2002; **360**: 436–42.

85. Philip T, Hartmann O, Michon J *et al*. Curability of relapsed childhood B-cell NHL following intensive first line therapy. *Blood* 1993; **81**; 2003–6.

86. Maloney DG. Treatment of follicular non-Hodgkin's lymphoma. *Curr Hematol Rep* 2005; **4**: 39–45.

87. Coiffier B. Treatment of diffuse large B-cell lymphoma. *Curr Hematol Rep* 2005; **4**: 7–14.

88. Webb A, Cunningham D, Cotter F *et al*. BCL-2 antisense therapy in patients with non-Hodgkin's lymphoma. *Lancet* 1997; **349**: 1137–41.

89. Gutherson N, Cole P. Epidemiology of Hodgkin's disease in the young. *Int J Cancer* 1977; **19**: 595–604.

90. Stiller CA, Parkin DM *et al*. International variations in the incidence of childhood lymphoma. *Pediatr Perinat Epidemiol* 1990; **4**: 303–24.

91. Alexander FE, Williams J, McKinney PA *et al*. A specialist leukaemia/lymphoma registry in the UK. Part 2. Clustering of Hodgkin's disease. *Br J Cancer* 1989; **60**: 948–52.

92. Guthenson N, Cole P. Childhood social environment and Hodgkin's disease. *N Engl J Med* 1981; **304**: 135–40.

93. Benharroch D, Shemer-Avni Y, Myint YY *et al*. Measles virus: evidence of an association with Hodgkin's disease. *Br J Cancer* 2004; **91**: 572–9.

94. Weinreb M, Day P, Niggli F *et al*. The role of Epistein–Barr virus sequences in Hodgkin's disease from different geographical areas. *Arch Dis Child* 1996; **74**: 27–31.

95. Gandhi MK. Epstein–Barr virus-associated Hodgkin's lymphoma. *Br J Haematol* 2004; **125**: 267–81.

96. Grufferman S, Cole P, Smith P, Lukes RJ. Hodgkin's disease in siblings. *N Engl J Med* 1979; **300**: 1006–11.

97. Marafioti T, Hummel M, Hans-Dieter F *et al*. Hodgkin and Reed-Stenberg cells represent an expansion of a single clone originating from a germinal centre B-cell with functional immunoglobulin gene rearrangements but defective immunoglobulin transcription. *Blood* 2000; **95**: 1443–50.

98. Lukes RJ, Butler JJ. The pathology and nomenclature of Hodgkin's disease. *Cancer Res* 1966; **26**: 1063–8.

99. Cavdar AO, Tacoy A, Babacan E *et al*. Hodgkin's disease in

Turkish children: a clinical and histopathological analysis. *J Natl Cancer Inst* 1977; **58**: 479–81.

100. Orscheschek K, Merz H, Hell J *et al*. Large cell anaplastic lymphoma: specific translocation t(2;5)(p23;q35) in Hodgkin's disease: indication of a common pathogenesis. *Lancet* 1995; **345**: 87–90.

101. Shankar A, Radford A, Barrett A *et al*. Does histology influence outcome in childhood Hodgkin's disease? Results from the United Kingdom Children's Cancer Study Group. *J Clin Oncol* 1997; **15**: 2622–30.

102. Pellegrino B, Terrier-Lacombe M, Oberlin O *et al*. Lymphocyte-predominant Hodgkin's lymphoma in children: therapeutic abstention after initial lymph node resection. A study of the French Society of Pediatric Oncology. *J Clin Oncol* 2003; **21**: 2948–52.

103. Burton C, Ell P, Linch D *et al*. The role of PET imaging in lymphoma. *Br J Haematol* 2004; **126**: 772–84.

104. Nadali G, Tavecchia L, Zanolin E *et al*. Serum level of the soluble form of the CD30 molecule identifies patients with Hodgkin's disease at high risk of unfavourable outcome. *Blood* 1998; **91**: 3011–16.

105. Smith R, Chen Q, Hudson M *et al*. Prognostic factors for children with Hodgkin's disease treated with combined modality therapy. *J Clin Oncol* 2003; **21**: 2026–33.

106. Sarris A, Kliche K, Pethambaram P *et al*. Interleukin-10 levels are often elevated in serum of adults with Hodgkin's disease and are associated with inferior failure-free survival. *Ann Oncol* 1999; **10**: 433–40.

107. Diechmann K, Potter R, Hofmann J *et al*. Does bulky disease at diagnosis influence outcome in childhood Hodgkin's disease and require higher radiation doses? Results from German-Austrian Pediatric multicenter trial DAL-HD90. *Int J Radiat Oncol Biol Phys* 2003; **56**: 644–52.

108. Diehl V, Sextro M, Franklin J *et al*. Clinical presentation, course and prognostic factors in lymphocyte predominant Hodgkin's disease and lymphocyte-rich classical Hodgkin's disease. Report from the European Task Force on lymphoma project on lymphocyte-predominant Hodgkin's disease. *J Clin Oncol* 1999; **17**: 776–90.

109. Barrett A, Crennan E, Barnes J *et al*. Treatment of clinical stage I Hodgkin's disease by local radiation therapy alone. A United Kingdom Children's Cancer Study Group Study. *Cancer* 1990; **66**: 670–4.

110. Shankar A, Ashley S, Atra A *et al*. A limited role for VEEP (vincristine, etoposide, epirubicin, prednisolone) chemotherapy in childhood Hodgkin's disease. *Eur J Cancer* 1998; **34**: 2058–63.

111. Landman-Parker J, Pacquement H, Leblanc T *et al*. Localized childhood Hodgkin's disease: a response-adapted chemotherapy with etoposide, bleomycin, vinblastine, and prednisone before low-dose radiation therapy. Results of the French Society of Pediatric Oncology Study MDH90. *J Clin Oncol* 2000; **18**: 1500–7.

112. Carde P, Koscielny S, Franklin J *et al*. Early response to chemotherapy: a surrogate for final outcome Hodgkin's disease patients that should influence initial treatment length and intensity? *Ann Oncol* 2002; **13**: 86–91.

113. Hudson M, Krasin M, Link MP *et al*. Risk-adapted, combined-modality therapy with VAMP/COP response-based, involved-field radiation for unfavourable pediatric Hodgkin's disease. *J Clin Oncol* 2004; **22**: 4541–50.

114. Donaldson S, Hudson N, Lamborn K *et al*. VAMP and low dose, involved field radiation for children and adolescents with favourable early stage Hodgkin's disease: results of a prospective clinical trial. *J Clin Oncol* 2002; **20**: 3081–7.

115. Dorffel W, Luders H, Ruhl U *et al*. Preliminary results of the multicentre trial GPOH-HD 95 for treatment of Hodgkin's disease in children and adolescents: analysis and outlook. *Klin Padiatr* 2003; **215**: 139–45.

116. Schellong G, Potter R, Bramswig J *et al*. High cure rates and reduced long-term toxicity in pediatric Hodgkin's disease: the German-Austrian multi centre trial DAL-DH90. The German-Austrian Pediatric Hodgkin's Disease Study Group. *J Clin Oncol* 1999; **17**: 3736–44.

117. Friedman A, Hudson M, Weinstein H *et al*. Treatment of unfavourable childhood Hodgkin's disease with VEPA and low dose, involved-field radiation. *J Clin Oncol* 2002; **20**: 3088–94.

118. Hakvoort-Cammel F, Buitendijk S, Van Den Heuvel-Eibrink M *et al*. Treatment of pediatric Hodgkin disease avoiding radiotherapy, excellent outcome with the Rotterdam-HD-84 protocol. *Pediatr Blood Cancer* 2004; **43**: 8–16.

119. Van den Berg H, Stuve W, Behrendt H *et al*. Treatment of Hodgkin's disease in children with alternating mechlorethamine, vincristine, procarbazine and prednisone (MOPP) and adriamycin, bleomycin, vinblastine and dacarbazine (ABVD) courses without radiotherapy. *Med Pediatr Oncol* 1997; **29**: 23–7.

120. Hamilton V, Norris C, Bunin N *et al*. Cyclophosphamide-based, seven drug hybrid and low dose involved field radiation for the treatment of childhood and adolescent Hodgkin disease. *J Pediatr Hematol Oncol* 2001; **23**: 84–8.

121. Atra A, Higgs E, Capra M *et al*. Isolated parenchymal lung involvement in children with Hodgkin's disease: results of the UKCCSG HD8201 and HD90 studies. *Br J Haematol* 2002; **119**: 441–4.

122. Atra A, Higgs E, Carpa M *et al*. ChlVPP chemotherapy in children with stage IV Hodgkin's disease: results of the UKCCSG HD 8201 and HD 9201 studies. *Br J Haematol* 2002; **119**: 647–51.

123. Josting A, Franklin J, May M *et al*. New prognostic score based on treatment outcome of patients with relapsed Hodgkin's lymphoma registered in the database the German Hodgkin's lymphoma study group. *J Clin Oncol* 2002, **20**: 221–30.

124. James N, Kingston J, Plowman P *et al*. Outcome of children with resistant and relapsed Hodgkin's disease. *Br J Cancer* 1992; **66**: 1155–8.

125. Baker S, Gordon B, Gross T *et al*. Autologous hematopoietic stem-cell transplantation for relapsed or refractory Hodgkin's disease in children and adolescents. *J Clin Oncol* 1999; **17**: 825–31.

126. Lieskovsky Y, Donaldson S, Torres M *et al*. High-dose therapy and autologous hematopoietic stem-cell transplantation for recurrent or refractory paediatric Hodgkins disease: results and prognostic indices. *J Clin Oncol* 2004; **15**: 4532–40.

127. Stoneham S, Ashley S, Pinkerton C *et al*. Outcome after autologous hemopoietic stem cell transplantation in relapsed

or refractory childhood Hodgkin disease *J Pediatr Hematol Oncol* 2004; **26**: 740–5.

128. Hawkins MM, Kinnier-Wilson LM, Stovall MA *et al.* Epipodophyllotoxins, alkylating agents and radiation and the risk of secondary leukaemia after childhood cancer. *Br Med J* 1992; **304**: 951–8.

129. Schellong G, Riepenhausen M, Creutzig U *et al.* Low risk of secondary leukemias after chemotherapy without mechlorethamine in childhood Hodgkin's disease. German-Austrian Paediatric Hodgkins Disease Group. *J Clin Oncol* 1997; **15**: 2247–53.

130. Ron E, Lubin JH, Shore RE *et al.* Thyroid cancer after exposure to external radiation: a pooled analysis of seven studies. *Radiat Res* 1995; **141**: 259–77.

131. Bhatia S, Robison L, Oberlin O *et al.* Breast cancer and other neoplasms after childhood Hodgkin's disease. *N Engl J Med* 1991; **325**: 1330–6.

132. Bhatia S, Yasui Y, Robison L *et al.* High risk of subsequent neoplasms continues with extended follow-up of childhood Hodgkin's disease: a report from the Late Effects Study Group. *J Clin Oncol* 2003; **21**: 4386–94.

133. Kenney L, Yasui Y, Inskip P *et al.* Breast cancer after childhood cancer: a report from the Childhood Cancer Survivor Study. *Ann Intern Med* 2004; **19**: 590–7.

134. Mertens A, Mitby P, Radloff G *et al.* XRCC1 amd glutathione-S-transferase gene polymorphisms and susceptibility to radiotherapy-related malignancies in survivors of Hodgkin disease. *Cancer* 2004; **101**: 1463–72.

135. Darzy KH, Shalet SM. Radiation induced growth hormone deficiency. *Horm Res* 2003; **59**: 1–11.

136. Robson H, Anderson E, Eden OB, Isaksson O, Shalet S. Chemotherapeutic agents used in the treatment of childhood malignancies have direct effects on growth plate chondrocyte proliferation. *J Endocrinol* 1998; **157**: 225–35.

137. Constine LS, Donaldson SS, McDougall IR. Thyroid dysfunction after radiotherapy in children with Hodgkin's disease. *Cancer* 1984; **53**: 878–83.

138. Shalet SM. Disorders of gonadal function due to radiation and cytotoxic chemotherapy in children. *Adv Intern Med Pediatr* 1989; **58**: 1–21.

139. Byrne J, Mulvihill J, Myers MH *et al.* Effects of treatment on fertility in long term survivors of childhood or adolescent cancer. *N Engl J Med* 1987; **317**: 1315–21.

140. Gerres L, Branswig J, Schlegel W *et al.* The effects of etoposide on testicular function in boys treated with Hodgkin's disease. *Cancer* 1998; **83**: 2217–22.

141. Byrne J, Fears TR, Gail MH *et al.* Early menopause in long term survivors of cancer during adolescence. *Am J Obstet Gynecol* 1992; **166**: 788–93.

142. Gosden RG, Baird DT, Wade JC, Webb R. Restoration of fertility to oophorectomised sheep by ovarian autografts stored at –196°C. *Hum Reprod* 1994; **9**: 597–603.

143. Lipshultz SE, Colan SD, Gelber RD, Perez-Atayde AR, Sallan SE, Sanders SP. Late cardiac effects of doxorubicin therapy for ALL in childhood. *N Engl J Med* 1991; **324**: 808–15.

144. Lipshultz S, Rifai N, Dalton V *et al.* The effect of dexrazoxane on myocardial injury in doxorubicin-treated children with acute lymphoblastic leukemia. *N Eng J Med* 2004; **351**: 145–53.

145. Wexler LH, Andrich MP, Venzon D *et al.* Randomised trial of the cardioprotective agent ICRF-187 in pediatric sarcoma patients treated with doxorubicin. *J Clin Oncol* 1996; **14**: 362–72.

146. Hancock SL, Donaldson S, Hoppe RT. Cardiac disease following treatment of Hodgkin's disease in childhood and adolescence. *J Clin Oncol* 1993; **11**: 1208–15.

147. Adams M, Lipsitz S, Colan S *et al.* Cardiovascular status in long term survivors of Hodgkin's disease treated with chest radiotherapy. *J Clin Oncol* 2004; **22**: 3139–48.

148. Eigen H, Wyszomierski D. Bleomycin lung injury in children. Pathophysiology and guidelines for management. *Am J Pediatr Hematol Oncol* 1985; **7**: 71–8.

149. Shaw N, Tweedale PM, Eden OB. Pulmonary function in childhood leukemia survivors. *Med Pediatr Oncol* 1989; **17**: 149–54.

150. Dieckvoss B, Stanulla M, Schrappe M *et al.* Polymorphisms within glutathione S-transferase genes in paediatric non-Hodgkin's lymphoma. *Haematologica* 2002; **87**: 709–13.

151. Yule S, Price L, McMahon A *et al.* Cyclophosphamide metabolism in children with non-Hodgkin's lymphoma. *Clin Cancer Res* 2004; **10**: 455–60.

152. Wessendorf S, Schwaenen C, Kohlhammer H *et al.* Hidden gene amplifications in aggressive B cell non-Hodgkins lymphomas detected by microarray-based comparative genome hybridisation. *Oncogene* 2003; **22**: 1425–9.

153. Busch K, Borkhart A, Reiter A. Combined polymerase chain reaction methods to detect c-myc/IgH rearrangement in childhood Burkitt's lymphoma for minimal residual disease analysis. *Haematologica* 2004; **89**: 818–25.

154. McManaway ME, Neckers LM, Loke SL *et al.* Tumour specific inhibition of lymphoma growth by an antisense oligodeoxynucleotide. *Lancet* 1990; **335**: 808–10.

Platelet Disorders

22 Inherited and congenital thrombocytopenia

Owen P. Smith

Introduction

The normal range of the platelet count in fetal life is similar to that seen in adulthood, being about $150-400 \times 10^9/L$. Neonatal thrombocytopenia, defined as a platelet count of $< 150 \times 10^9/L$ is common, with a reported frequency of approximately 0.9% in unselected newborns and 40% in infants in intensive care units.[1] The differential diagnosis of thrombocytopenia in the neonatal period is similar to thrombocytopenia in older children, with a number of exceptions including the inherited thrombocytopenias and those that arise due to pathophysiologic events unique to the antenatal and perinatal periods. It is important to remember to confirm that the low platelet count is genuine by careful inspection of the blood sample and smear before initiating further investigations. Once established, the approach to the diagnosis of the thrombocytopenia should be tailored to the individual infant and mother. For example, assessment of the child's general well-being is very important as healthy neonates usually have an immune or an inherited etiology, whereas the presence of lymphadenopathy, hepatosplenomegaly, mass lesions, hemangiomas, bruits and congenital anomalies point toward a totally different spectrum of causes. It should also be emphasized that obtaining a detailed maternal history, including bleeding problems, preeclampsia and drug ingestion in the present and any previous pregnancies, and history of viral infections (cytomegalovirus, rubella, herpes simplex and HIV) or connective tissue disease (systemic lupus erythematosus), will save time and unnecessary investigation.

In this chapter the causes of thrombocytopenia are divided into two broad categories: (i) those arising on a background of an established genetic defect (inherited thrombocytopenia) and (ii) those associated with birth (congenital thrombocytopenia).

Historic perspective

Although Donne,[2] Geber,[3] Addison,[4] and Simon[5] are said to have each independently described the platelet first in 1842, the first true description is generally credited to Max Schultze of Freiburg, who in 1865 described them as "gray, colorless spherical bodies in the blood from which, when clumped, rays of finely granular protoplasm often spread, in conjunction with fibrin coagulation."[6] In 1882, Julius Bizzozero, who coined the term *Blut Plättchen*, wrote his classic paper describing "viscous metamorphosis" of platelets in which he stated: "Platelets become granular within the lumen of an injured vessel: and this change produces a substance which activates the coagulation system to form fibrin."[7] By 1906, Wright[8] confirmed Bizzozero's theory of the origin of the platelet from bone marrow megakaryocytes by observing that the cytoplasmic pseudopodia from megakaryocytes have the same staining characteristics as platelets and concluded that the pseudopodia produced new platelets. These findings were subsequently confirmed in the late 1940s and early 1950s with the arrival of electron microscopy. Over the following three decades, steady, albeit limited, progress was made in characterizing platelet pathophysiologic states.

The 1970s witnessed the birth of the modern era of platelet and megakaryocyte research as newer methods of analysis (molecular biologic tools and *in vitro* systems) became available to study megakaryocytopoiesis and platelet structure and function. The fruits of this endeavor have been the recognition of different stages of normal megakaryocytopoiesis and a greater understanding of the molecular events responsible for dysmegakaryocytopoiesis. During this period, the cloning of cytokines that act on the megakaryocytic lineage and their clinical application was realized. The c-*mpl* proto-oncogene as the receptor of a major regulator of thrombocytopoiesis was identified and this greatly facilitated the subsequent isolation and cloning of c-*mpl* ligand or thrombopoietin (TPO) by several groups.[9] More recently, mutations in the nonmuscle myosin heavy chain II-A have been shown to be responsible for the MYH9-related disease, which is characterized by macrothrombocytopenia, granulocyte inclusions, deafness, cataracts and renal failure.[10] These three discoveries represent significant recent advances in platelet/megakaryocyte research.

Inherited thrombocytopenia

The inherited thrombocytopenias comprise a group of platelet formation abnormalities in which platelet numbers are reduced. In the vast majority of patients the platelet count is only mild to moderately reduced ($50-100 \times 10^9$/L) and therefore significant spontaneous hemorrhage tends not be problematic. There are, however, a number of notable exceptions where spontaneous bleeding is a prominent clinical feature of the syndrome:

• Wiskott–Aldrich syndrome, amegakaryocytic thrombocytopenia and thrombocytopenia with absent radii where the platelet count is usually very low;
• Bernard–Soulier and Chédiak–Higashi syndromes where there is marked platelet dysfunction.

Immune-mediated thrombocytopenia is a major differential diagnosis in children with low platelet counts and therefore making the correct diagnosis of these conditions is important, as it usually prevents the useless and potentially dangerous prescribing of immunosuppressants such as corticosteroids. Although the inherited nature of these conditions has been known for the past 30 years, the molecular basis for the thrombocytopenia has only been fully elucidated in a very small number of these conditions, in particular those arising from defects in von Willebrand factor (vWF) and its platelet receptor, glycoprotein (Gp)Ib–V–IX complex.

Hereditary thrombocytopenias are an etiologically heterogeneous group of disorders that have traditionally been classified into three groups depending on platelet volume (see Chapter 30). In this chapter they are classified into two broad categories based on the presence or absence of a concomitant platelet function abnormality (Tables 22.1 and 22.2).

Disorders with dysfunctional platelets

GpIb–V–IX complex

The GpIb–V–IX complex is one of the major adhesion receptors on the platelet surface and plays a pivotal role in primary hemostasis by mediating vWF attachment following collagen exposure on the damaged vessel wall. Its structure is well known, with each gene product possessing one or more characteristic leucine-rich domains.[11,12] Binding of vWF occurs to one or more sites within or close to a double disulfide-bonded and sulfated loop region close to the amino-terminal of the receptor during high shear conditions involving the platelet cytoskeleton. The three inherited bleeding disorders associated with gene defects within this complex are Bernard–Soulier syndrome (BSS), pseudo-von Willebrand disease (vWD) and type 2B vWD.

Bernard–Soulier syndrome (see Chapter 25)

This is the best-characterized inherited thrombocytopenia with associated abnormal platelet function.[13] Typically there is (i) moderate-to-severe thrombocytopenia (automated platelet counting usually underestimates the true platelet count as

Table 22.1 Inherited thrombocytopenia with dysfunctional platelets.

Disorder	Inheritance	Platelet feature	Platelet size	Other findings
Bernard–Soulier syndrome	AR	↓Aggregation to ristocetin	Large	Qualitative and/or quantitative defects in platelet GpIb–V–IX
Pseudo-von Willebrand disease	AD	↑ Aggregation to ristocetin	Normal	Spontaneous ↑ platelet binding of vWF due to GpIb defect
Type 2b von Willebrand disease	AD	↑ Aggregation to ristocetin	Large	Spontaneous ↑ vWF binding to platelets due to vWF defect
Montreal syndrome	AD	Spontaneous aggregation	Large	Calpain defect, pale-staining platelets, agranular megakaryocytes
Gray platelet syndrome	AR	α-Granule defect	Normal	Pale platelets due to α-granule deficiency, bone marrow fibrosis
Paris–Trousseau syndrome	AD	Giant α-granules	Normal	Chromosome 11 (del(11)(q23.3;qter))
Wiskott–Aldrich syndrome	X-linked	↓ Dense granules in some	Small	*WASP* mutations at Xp11.22–11.23, infections, eczema
X-linked thrombocytopenia	X-linked	↓ Dense granules in some	Small	*WASP* mutations at Xp11.22–11.23
XLTT	X-linked	↓ α-granules	Large	*GATA-1/FOG-1* mutations
XLTDEA	X-linked	↓ α-granules	Large	*GATA-1/FOG-1* mutations
Chédiak–Higashi syndrome	AD	↓ Aggregation to Ep and Co	Normal	Oculocutaneous albinism, recurrent infections, large white cell inclusions
Quebec syndrome	AD	↓ Aggregation to Ep	Normal	↓ Platelet P-selectin, fibrinogen, vWF, factor V, thrombospondin, osteonectin; normal platelet factor 4 and β-thromboglobulin

AR, autosomal recessive; AD, autosomal dominant; Ep, epinephrine (adrenaline); Co, collagen; vWF, von Willebrand factor protein; XLTT, X-linked thrombocytopenia/thalassemia; XLTDEA, X-linked thrombocytopenia/dyserythropoietic anemia; FOG-1, friend of GATA-1.

Table 22.2 Inherited thrombocytopenia without dysfunctional platelets.

Disorder	Inheritance	Platelet feature	Platelet size	Other findings
May–Hegglin anomaly	AD	Function studies vary	Large	Neutrophil inclusions ± hearing loss, cataracts and/or renal diseases. Gene locus: *MYH9* (22q12–13)
Epstein syndrome	AD	↓ Aggregation to Ep and Co	Large	Neutrophil inclusions ± hearing loss ± cataracts ± renal diseases. Gene locus: *MYH9* (22q12–13)
Eckstein syndrome	AD	Normal platelet function	Large	Neutrophil inclusions with features of Alport syndrome. Gene locus: *MYH9* (22q12–13)
Fechtner syndrome	AD	Function studies vary	Large	Neutrophil inclusions ± hearing loss ± cataracts ± renal diseases. Gene locus: *MYH9* (22q12–13)
Sebastian syndrome	AD	Normal platelet function	Large	Neutrophil inclusions ± hearing loss ± cataracts ± renal diseases. Gene locus: *MYH9* (22q12–13)
Thrombocytopenia with absent radii	AR	↓ Aggregation to Ep and Co	Normal	↓ Marrow megakaryocytes
Pure genetic thrombocytopenia	AD	Not known	Large	Normal morphology and platelet survival
Mediterranean thrombocytopenia	AD	Not known	Large	Dysmegakaryocytopoiesis

AR, autosomal recessive; AD, autosomal dominant; Ep, epinephrine (adrenaline); Co, collagen.

some platelets are so large), (ii) prolonged bleeding time and (iii) platelet morphology usually reveals "giant" forms as mentioned above. The platelets in this condition are incapable of interacting with vWF and hence the bleeding seen is typical of a primary hemostatic defect. While BSS platelets show normal shape change, secretion, signal transduction and aggregation in the presence of ADP, epinephrine (adrenaline), collagen and arachidonic acid, they do not aggregate with ristocetin in the presence of vWF.

BSS is inherited in an autosomal recessive manner with the underlying molecular defects due to quantitative or qualitative defects in the GpIb–V–IX complex. In homozygotes the platelets are comparable in size to those seen in MYH9-related diseases (see below). Numerous variants of BSS have been described at the molecular level, ranging from "classic" BSS, where the entire glycoprotein complex is missing from the membrane, to full platelet expression of the GpIb–V–IX complex but with a point mutation in codon 156, the crucial leucine-repeat region (Ala^{156} → Val^{156}) of the subunit GpIbα, which in turn prevents vWF binding, the so-called "Bolzano" variant.[13–15]

Pseudo-von Willebrand disease (see Chapter 27)

This is an autosomal dominant disorder characterized by mild intermittent thrombocytopenia, mild bleeding, absence of high-molecular-weight vWF multimers, and increased ristocetin-induced platelet aggregation.[13] It is caused by a mutation(s) in the major double-loop structure of GpIbα that causes a conformational change in the receptor, which in turn leads to enhanced vWF binding and hence spontaneous platelet aggregation and thrombocytopenia.[14–16] It can be differentiated from type 2B vWD, where the mutation resides in the vWF protein, by spontaneous aggregation of the patient's platelets with normal plasma (see below).

Bolin–Jamieson syndrome is a mild bleeding disorder characterized by one allele of the GpIbα gene producing a molecule about 10 kDa larger than the normal range.[17] How this defect leads to an increased bleeding susceptibility is not known.

Type 2B von Willebrand's disease

This subtype of vWD is clinically and biochemically very similar to pseudo-vWD. It is an autosomal dominant disorder, usually diagnosed by the increased platelet agglutination induced by low concentrations of ristocetin. However, it should be remembered that in some cases defects can be delineated in the absence of ristocetin. Like type 2A vWD, the mutations causing type 2B are clustered within exon 28 of the vWF gene.[18] These mutations result in gain of function, i.e., there is spontaneous binding of the mutant vWF to GpIb, with consequent loss of high-molecular-weight multimers from the plasma and a tendency to thrombocytopenia. Desmopressin (DDAVP) may result in more marked thrombocytopenia by increasing the levels of vWF multimers that have increased avidity for platelet glycoproteins and result in further exacerbations of platelet agglutination. Assessment of vWF multimer size and platelet agglutination profile distinguishes this disorder from pseudo-vWD.

Montreal platelet syndrome

This syndrome is characterized by thrombocytopenia, large platelets, spontaneous platelet aggregation, and a reduced response to thrombin-induced aggregation.[19] It can be distinguished from BSS by its autosomal dominant inheritance and normal platelet agglutinability response to ristocetin. The platelets have a quantitative and qualitative reduction of the calcium-dependent proteinase calpain that prevents them from returning to normal volume after agonist stimulation.[20,21]

Gray platelet syndrome (see Chapter 25)

This is an extremely rare syndrome that in the majority of cases is inherited in an autosomal recessive fashion. It is characterized by markedly reduced platelet α-granule content but normal dense bodies and lysosomes.[22] The name "gray platelet" comes from the bland gray agranular appearance of platelets on Wright–Giemsa-stained blood smears, which reflects the reduced number of platelet α-granules. Other features include a prolonged skin bleeding time, morphologically large platelets and highly variable platelet aggregation profiles. The platelet α-granules that are present, albeit in reduced numbers, are deficient in the storage proteins coagulation factor V, vWF, platelet factor 4, β-thromboglobulin, fibrinogen, platelet-derived growth factor (PDGF) and thrombospondin.[23] Concomitant elevation in plasma levels of platelet factor 4 and β-thromboglobulin are seen, implying that there is an abnormality in α-granule protein packaging within the megakaryocyte; this would appear to be lineage restricted to megakaryocytes as vWF biosynthesis within endothelial cells is normal.[24] Myelofibrosis is not an uncommon finding in these patients and the continuous premature release of α-granule proteins such as PDGF into the bone marrow microenvironment may be key to its development.[25] The accompanying thrombocytopenia and bleeding symptoms are usually mild. The mechanism responsible for the bleeding propensity is not fully understood but is likely to be multifactorial, involving mild impairment of platelet aggregation and adhesion together with impaired thrombin and fibrin generation as there is probably a paucity of coagulation factor V within the α-granules.[26]

Appropriate on-demand or prophylactic treatment needs to be individualized. For example, those patients with moderate thrombocytopenia and evidence of abnormal platelet aggregation are most likely to benefit from a combination of platelet transfusion and desmopressin, whereas for those with very mild thrombocytopenia and a prolonged bleeding time desmopressin alone is all that is needed.

Jacobsen or Paris–Trousseau syndrome

This is a recently described autosomal dominant syndrome that comprises mild thrombocytopenia, normal platelet lifespan, moderate hemorrhagic tendency, giant α-granules in a subpopulation of platelets, bone marrow micromegakaryocytes with enhanced megakaryocyte apoptosis, and deletion of the distal part of chromosome 11 at position 11q23, i.e., del(11)(q23.3;qter).[27] The giant α-granules fail to release their content following thrombin exposure and this may explain the moderate bleeding events seen in this disorder. The cytogenetic abnormality seen in this syndrome is probably responsible for the abnormal megakaryocytopoiesis as the two protooncogenes *ETS1* and *FL1* map to 11q23–24 and are involved in normal expression of megakaryocyte-specific genes.

Wiskott–Aldrich syndrome

Wiskott–Aldrich syndrome (WAS) is inherited as an X-linked recessive trait and is characterized by eczema, microthrombocytopenia and combined immunodeficiency.[28,29] It is often fatal by the early teens due to infection, lymphoreticular malignancy or bleeding. Hemorrhagic events are common during the first 2 years of life and the reason for this is multifactorial. For example, platelet survival is modestly reduced to half normal,[30] ineffective megakaryocytopoiesis is prominent as reflected by platelet turnover 25% that of normal with normal megakaryocyte mass,[30] and there is evidence of platelet functional abnormalities related to abnormal storage of adenine nucleotides and impaired platelet energy metabolism.[31,32]

Allogeneic bone marrow transplantation (BMT) is the treatment of choice when there is a fully matched donor available as this corrects the abnormal stem cell compartment.[33] When there is no suitable donor, splenectomy is the therapeutic first choice as this usually raises the platelet count into the normal range, improves platelet survival and normalizes platelet size.[34] It should be remembered that splenectomy in patients with WAS may produce an increased risk of overwhelming sepsis compared with other diseases where splenectomy is indicated. Splenectomy is not advocated for the other hereditary thrombocytopenic disorders as it usually gives little benefit.

Wiskott–Aldrich syndrome variants (X-linked thrombocytopenia)

This is a heterogeneous group of thrombocytopenic disorders with X-linked inheritance. Some families have microthrombocytopenia and no associated abnormalities, while others have mild eczema and impaired immune responses.[35] The thrombocytopenia is usually less severe in WAS variants and requires no treatment but in the rare case with severe thrombocytopenia splenectomy has been shown to be effective.[36]

Both WAS and WAS variants appear to be caused by different mutations of the same gene on the short arm of the X chromosome (Xp11.2), with the latter involving primarily exon 2 of the *WASP* gene.[37]

X-linked thrombocytopenia and erythropoiesis

The transcription factor GATA-1 and its cofactor FOG-1 regulate erythropoiesis and megakaryocytopoiesis.[38] Therefore it is not surprising that when mutations occur within these key regulatory proteins, platelets and red cells may be affected as seen in X-linked thrombocytopenia associated with dyserythropoietic anemia and/or thalassemia (see Table 22.1). Defects in megakaryocyte maturation with associated macrothrombocytopenia α-granule deficiency have also been observed in some of these patients.[38]

Oculocutaneous albinism (Hermanksy–Pudlak and Chédiak–Higashi syndromes)

Oculocutaneous albinism denotes a group of inherited disorders characterized by reduced or absent pigmentation of skin, hair and eyes. While the majority of these patients have an isolated platelet storage pool defect, in some an accompanying low platelet count can occur.

Hermansky–Pudlak syndrome

Hermansky–Pudlak syndrome is an autosomal recessive disorder with the classic triad of oculocutaneous albinism (tyrosinase positive), platelet dense-body or combined dense-body and α-granule storage pool deficiency, and deposits of ceroid-like material in the monocyte–macrophage system (see Chapter 24). The bleeding tendency is usually mild (related to the storage pool defect and not thrombocytopenia, as the latter is not a feature of the syndrome); however, excessive bleeding following tooth extractions and tonsillectomy is the rule. The ceroid-like deposits in the lungs, gastrointestinal tract and renal tubule cells may lead to restrictive lung disease, colitis or renal failure respectively.

Chédiak–Higashi syndrome

The features of Chédiak–Higashi syndrome include partial oculocutaneous albinism, the presence of giant granules in all granule-containing cells, neutropenia, peripheral neuropathy, and platelet storage pool deficiency that usually involves the dense bodies. Thrombocytopenia usually occurs during the accelerated phase of the disease, which involves the development of pancytopenia, hepatosplenomegaly, lymphadenopathy and extensive tissue infiltration with lymphoid cells. The accelerated phase, which is clinically similar to virus-associated hemophagocytic lymphohistiocytosis, unfortunately occurs in most patients and the majority die. The precise molecular basis of Chédiak–Higashi syndrome has not been fully elucidated and the only curable therapeutic modality is allogeneic BMT, which in one report was successful in six of seven patients grafted.[39]

Quebec syndrome

This condition is characterized by an autosomal dominant inheritance pattern, mild thrombocytopenia, an epinephrine platelet aggregation defect, and a severe posttraumatic bleeding tendency.[40] Deficiency in multimerin, a large complex multimeric protein expressed in platelet α-granules and endothelial cell Weibel–Palade bodies, is responsible for the reduced levels of α-granule proteins such as factor V, P-selectin, fibrinogen, vWF, thrombospondin and osteonectin.[40] Platelets in this disorder have unusually large amounts of urokinase-type plasminogen activator that is released on platelet activation, and whose presence in excess of the natural inhibitors of this protease accounts for the

in situ protein degradation in the α-granules.[41] The platelet aggregation defect is most striking with epinephrine, the mechanism of which remains to be elucidated.

RUNX1–thrombocytopenia–leukemia syndrome

RUNX1 (also known as AML1 and CBFA2), a hematopoietic transcription factor, is mutated in affected members of families with autosomal dominant thrombocytopenia in association with platelet dense-body storage pool deficiency.[42] These individuals are predisposed to the development of acute myeloid leukemia and, to a lesser extent, solid organ tumors. Although the thrombocytopenia is usually mild $(80–100 \times 10^9/L)$, bleeding is the norm as the platelets are functionally impaired. The mechanism of the thrombocytopenia is most likely related to low TPO receptor levels on megakaryocytes.[42]

Disorders without dysfunctional platelets

MYH9-related disease

These are rare autosomal dominant macrothrombocytopenic disorders with characteristic Döhle body-like cytoplasmic inclusions in the granulocytic series.[43] They are distinguished from each other by different clinical and laboratory features, such as sensorineural hearing loss, cataract, nephritis and white cell inclusions. Mutations in the *MYH9* gene encoding the nonmuscle myosin heavy chain IIA have been identified in all these syndromes.[43] These conditions are now felt to be most likely a single disorder with a continuous clinical spectrum, varying from mild macrothrombocytopenia with granulocyte inclusions to a severe form complicated by hearing loss, cataract and renal failure. *MYH9* expression patterns most likely differ in each MYH9-related disease, accounting for the diverse phenotype observed (see Table 22.2). Outlined below are the classical descriptions of what we now call the MYH9-related disease.

May–Hegglin anomaly

This is an autosomal dominant disorder characterized by giant platelets, variable thrombocytopenia and Döhle-like inclusions within granulocytic cells, including monocytes.[44,45] These structures are blue on Wright–Giemsa staining (denoting RNA), spindle-shaped, occur singly in each cell, and have a distinctive ultrastructure of 7–10 nm filaments of remnant rough endoplasmic reticulum oriented in parallel in the long axis.[46] A small percentage of patients have persistent leukopenia, which has been associated with occasional infections, and in one case neutrophil chemotaxis and chemokinetic responses were impaired.[46] Platelet function has been reported to be normal in some and impaired in others.[23,47–50] Troublesome primary hemostatic bleeding,[47] which is seen in approximately 40% of these patients, is felt to be most likely secondary to the degree of thrombocytopenia at the time of hemorrhage.

Alport syndome

This is associated with sensorineural deafness (usually high tone), hematuria, cataracts and progressive renal failure.[51] The disorder is a heterogeneous group, with the majority having autosomal dominant inheritance. Many variants of Alport syndrome have been described, the commonest being associated with hyperprolinemia. The genetic basis of this syndrome is believed to involve deletions or rearrangements in the α5(IV) collagen gene (*COL4A5* locus) located on Xq22.3.[52] Three variants have been described with associated thrombocytopenia. It is not known whether the gene defect seen in "classic" Alport syndrome is linked to the thrombocytopenia seen in the variants described below.

Epstein and Eckstein syndromes

Epstein syndrome was first described in 1972 in a family with features of Alport syndrome, macrothrombocytopenia, and defective platelet aggregation and secretion in response to ADP and collagen.[53] Three years later, Eckstein syndrome was reported and described to have all the features that characterized Epstein syndrome but in contrast had normal platelet function.[54]

Fechtner syndrome

This is characterized by the same morphologic features as those seen in Sebastian platelet syndrome (see below) but in addition is associated with deafness, cataracts and renal failure.[55] The white cell inclusion bodies (Fechtner inclusions) are characteristic of the syndrome and resemble toxic Döhle bodies (seen with infection and malignancies) and May–Hegglin granulocyte inclusions. They can be differentiated by light and electron microscopy as Fechtner inclusion bodies are smaller and lighter-staining than those seen in May–Hegglin granulocytes and are composed of dispersed filament, ribosome and endoplasmic reticulum. Fechtner inclusion bodies lack the parallel bundles of fine filaments seen in May–Hegglin inclusions.[56]

While these syndromes are associated with a mild-to-moderate bleeding tendency, significant hemorrhagic morbidity is usually encountered following trauma, dental extraction and other forms of surgery and platelet concentrates are the main therapeutic intervention. It should be remembered that the progressive renal failure seen in these patients usually adds to the hemorrhagic tendency and is also the main etiologic factor contributing to overall morbidity and indeed mortality.

Sebastian platelet syndrome

Sebastian platelet syndrome resembles May–Hegglin anomaly but the Döhle body-like inclusions seen in granulocytes are different in that they are smaller and ultrastructural analysis shows them to consist of ribosomes and dispersed filaments without an enclosing membrane. They are detected by light microscopy only if the blood smear is stained within 4 hours after venepuncture,[57] which implies that this syndrome is probably an underreported cause of hereditary thrombocytopenia.[58] This syndrome is felt to be a variant of Fechtner syndrome without the associated Alport syndrome features.[57] It is inherited in an autosomal dominant manner and while the bleeding tendency is considered to be mild to moderate, hemorrhagic deaths have been reported.[59]

Inherited bone marrow failure syndromes

Thrombocytopenia with absent radii (see Chapter 3)

This is a rare autosomal recessive disorder that is usually diagnosed at birth as the vast majority of these patients are thrombocytopenic and have the pathognomonic physical signs of bilateral absent radii or indeed other orthopediac anomalies involving the ulna, humerus and tibia.[60] Other skeletal abnormalities involving the ulnae, fingers and lower limbs are also seen but are much rarer.[61] Thrombocytopenia with absent radii (TAR) differs from Fanconi anemia in several ways: the absent radii are accompanied by the presence of thumbs, the thrombocytopenia is the only cytopenia, there is absence of spontaneous or clastogenic stress-induced chromosomal breakage, and evolution of aplastic anemia and leukemia has not been reported.[61] It is not uncommon for these children to be anemic and have transient white cell counts at presentation (the former is felt to be secondary to bleeding as it is always accompanied by a reticulocytosis and the latter usually subsides by 6 months of age). The striking morphologic feature within the bone marrow is the absence or greatly reduced numbers of megakaryocytes with normal granulopoietic and erythroid compartments.[62,63] Although the precise pathophysiologic defect responsible for TAR is not known, signaling through the TPO receptor c-mpl is abnormal.[60] The restoration of platelet count seen following sibling allogeneic BMT supports the idea that the thrombopoietic defect lies within the hematopoietic stem cell compartment rather than being a deficiency of TPO or another platelet humoral factor.[64]

The majority of children with TAR have recurrent significant bleeding episodes in the first 6 months of life. Intracerebral and gastrointestinal hemorrhage are the usual cause of mortality with previously 1 in 4 of these children dying by 4 years of age.[61] However, the majority of these deaths occurred in the first year of life. The severity of the bleeding problem is related to the degree of thrombocytopenia, which in the majority of children is usually $< 20 \times 10^9/L$, and in some there is evidence of qualitative platelet defects (storage pool and abnormal aggregation profiles).[61,65] The mainstay of treatment is the judicious use of single donor platelet concentrates, aiming to keep the platelet count above $20 \times 10^9/L$, especially in the first year of life as this is the time of maximum morbidity and mortality. This more aggressive platelet transfusion approach should dramatically reduce the unacceptable hemorrhagic mortality and morbidity rate. If the patient survives the first year of life, survival appears to be normal.[61] All elective reconstructive orthopedic surgery should be postponed during the first few years of life.

Prenatal diagnosis of TAR is possible, with absent radii easily visualized with radiography and/or ultrasound and thrombocytopenia diagnosed following fetal blood sampling obtained by fetoscopy or cordocentesis.[66,67] This relatively recent advance in obstetric care allows for the possibility of prophylactic antenatal management.

Amegakaryocytic thrombocytopenia (see Chapter 3)

This is an extremely rare disorder of infancy and early childhood. In the majority of cases it results from a mutation in the TPO receptor c-*mpl* and as a consequence megakaryocytes do not proliferate following TPO ligation.[60] The thrombocytopenia is nonimmune and usually severe and early bone marrow examination shows a normal karyotype, absence or greatly reduced numbers of megakaryocytes, with normal granulopoietic and erythroid elements.[68] Some patients have macrocytic red cells with increased expression of i antigen and elevated hemoglobin F levels,[69] implying that the pathophysiologic trigger occurs at the stem cell level. The inheritance pattern in the majority of cases is X-linked, the remainder being autosomal recessive. Patients with amegakaryocytic thrombocytopenia can be broadly divided into two groups, those with physical anomalies and those without. The pattern of somatic anomalies is not unlike that seen with Fanconi anemia; however, in those children tested, there was no evidence of DNA repair abnormality. The presence of anomalies influences outcome; projected median survivals are 6 years for those with no anomalies and 2 years when anomalies are present.[69] Those with isolated thrombocytopenia usually die from hemorrhagic complications whereas those with aplasia, which usually occurs after a relatively long period of thrombocytopenia, succumb to infection and bleeding.[61] Amegakaryocytic thrombocytopenia is considered to be a leukemia predisposition syndrome.[61,70]

Platelet transfusions are the main therapeutic intervention following diagnosis. Treatment with corticosteroids alone or in combination with androgens, the cytokines, granulocyte-macrophage colony stimulating factor and IL-11 have been disappointing, and splenectomy has no role. Encouraging platelet responses following the administration of IL-3 have been reported[68] and clinical trial results with TPO are eagerly awaited. Allogeneic BMT offers the only probable chance of cure, although gene therapy in which insertion of an artificial TPO receptor intended to convey a growth advantage in stem cells has now begun.

Fanconi anemia (see Chapter 3)

This is a premalignant disorder, inherited as an autosomal recessive trait, with genetic heterogeneity and a gene frequency of about 1 in 600.[71] Thrombocytopenia is usually the first cytopenia to appear, followed by granulocytopenia and ultimately severe aplasia, which occurs in the majority of patients.[72] The average age of onset of the hematologic abnormalities varies, with boys developing pancytopenia earlier than girls at 6.6 years and 8.8 years, respectively, with ranges from 18 months to 22 years.[73] The diagnosis of Fanconi anemia should always be considered in a child with an isolated cytopenia even when somatic anomalies are absent as a significant number of these cases are physically normal.

Trisomy syndromes

Moderately severe thrombocytopenia is seen in some cases of trisomy 18,[74] trisomy 13,[75] and to a lesser extent trisomy 21.[75] Both trisomy 13 and 18 are usually diagnosed at birth as the associated abnormalities are usually quite striking. The majority of these cases die in the neonatal period from non-hemorrhagic sequelae.[76]

Pure genetic thrombocytopenia

This is an autosomal dominant macrothrombocytopenic disorder characterized by a chronic low platelet count, normal platelet half-life, normal platelet function (aggregation and adhesion), normal skin bleeding time, absent platelet-associated immunoglobulins, and a morphologically normal bone marrow megakaryocyte compartment.[77] Although the molecular lesion causing the thrombocytopenia has not been elucidated, platelet isotope studies using homologous and autologous platelets are highly suggestive that there is a pure production defect within the bone marrow.[77,78] The majority of cases are detected following routine blood tests carried out for nonhematologic indications. The diagnosis is usually considered when there is a negative surrogate marker profile for inherited thrombocytopenia and is confirmed with isotope studies using the tracer ^{111}In-oxine and autologous platelets, which show a normal platelet lifespan.[78] The dose of radioactive ^{111}In necessary to perform the study is approximately 50 kBq (1.5 µCi)/kg, which is negligible and perfectly acceptable in children, although not all pediatricians are comfortable with this view. Failure to differentiate this pure genetic thrombocytopenia from the commoner immune thrombocytopenias may expose the child to potentially toxic and unnecessary expensive therapeutics such as corticosteroids, chemotherapy and immunoglobulin. As the majority of these patients have platelet counts in the region of $50-100 \times 10^9/L$ with normal skin bleeding times, the hemorrhagic potential for spontaneous bleeding is low and only rises at menses or following trauma or surgery.[78]

Mediterranean macrothrombocytopenia

This type of macrothrombocytopenia was initially reported from Australia in blood donors with Greek and Italian ancestry and has subsequently been shown to be present in the North African immigrant population in France.[79,80] The thrombocytopenia is mild with platelet counts ranging between 100 and $150 \times 10^9/L$ and platelet morphology showing only a mild increase in platelet size. Inheritance is autosomal dominant and the low platelet count is very rarely if ever associated with troublesome bleeding.[81] The defect is felt to be in the demarcatory membrane system by which megakaryocytes divide up their cytoplasm into platelets, although the precise mechanism by which this is achieved remains to be elucidated.

Congenital thrombocytopenia

Congenital thrombocytopenia is defined as a low platelet count at birth that does not result from the association of a specific gene defect; it accounts for the majority of cases of neonatal thrombocytopenia. However, thrombocytopenia is a common finding in sick neonates, and since the introduction of automated cell counters it is now considered a relatively common (~ 1%) finding in apparently normal infants. In the vast majority of cases the thrombocytopenia results from increased platelet destruction, which can arise by several mechanisms, the majority of which are not known. It is helpful to consider etiologic factors contributing to neonatal thrombocytopenia in terms of whether the insult is maternal (Table 22.3), infant (Table 22.4) or placentally based.

Maternal factors

Immune thrombocytopenia

Immune-mediated thrombocytopenia is usually seen in term babies who are clinically well and may be responsible for one-third of cases of thrombocytopenia seen in the general neonatal population.[1] There are two broad categories of conditions: those mediated by an alloimmune mechanism and those with associated autoimmune phenomena.

Table 22.3 Congenital thrombocytopenias: maternal factors.

Immune thrombocytopenia
Neonatal alloimmune thrombocytopenia
Maternal autoimmune thrombocytopenia

Intrauterine infections (TORCH syndromes)
Toxoplasmosis
Rubella
Cytomegalovirus
Herpes simplex
Other (including HIV and parvovirus B19)

Preeclampsia/hypertension

Drugs

Table 22.4 Congenital thrombocytopenias: infant and placental factors.

Infant factors
Disseminated intravascular coagulation
Primary microangiopathic hemolytic anemias
   Hemolytic–uremic syndrome
   Thrombotic thrombocytopenic purpura
Giant hemangioma syndrome (Kasabach–Merritt syndrome)
Hypercoagulable states
   Birth asphyxia
   Cyanotic congenital heart disease
   Respiratory distress syndrome
   Necrotizing enterocolitis
   Bacterial infection
   Rhesus hemolytic disease
   Anticoagulant deficiency (homozygous antithrombin,
      protein C and S deficiency)
   Heparin-induced thrombocytopenia
Rare bone marrow diseases
   Transient abnormal myelopoiesis
   Hemophagocytic lymphohistiocytosis
   Osteopetrosis
   Congenital leukemia
   Metastatic neuroblastoma

Placental factors
Infarction
Angiomas (chorioangiomas)
Lupus anticoagulant/anticardiolipin antibodies

Neonatal alloimmune thrombocytopenia (see Chapter 30)
This arises following maternal sensitization to paternal antigens present on fetal platelets.[82] It occurs in approximately 1 in 1500–2000 births, with the mother having a normal platelet count and a negative history of bleeding.[83,84] The maternal alloantibody produced does not react with the mother's platelets but crosses the placenta and destroys fetal platelets. The paternal-derived fetal platelet antigen target against which the maternal alloantibody is directed is usually HPA-1a (also called P1[A1] or Zw[a]), which is present on the platelets of 98% of the population and is responsible for neonatal immune thrombocytopenia (NAIT) in approximately 80% of cases.[83] The second commonest platelet antigen involved in NAIT is HPA-5b (also called Br[a], Zav[a] or Hc[a]).[85] While NAIT is in other ways analogous to hemolytic disease of the newborn due to Rhesus or ABO incompatibility (see Chapter 8), in NAIT the first child is usually affected with thrombocytopenia.[82] Given that 2% of the population is HPA-1a negative, it is somewhat surprising that the frequency of NAIT is lower than would be predicted from the prevalence of the alloantigen.[84,86] The most likely reason for this discrepancy is that certain HLA types are more likely to be associated with alloantibody formation, e.g., women who have the HLA-DR3 alloantigen account for the majority of affected cases of HPA-1a-induced NAIT.[84,87–89] A similar finding is seen with the Br[a] alloantigen and HLA-DRw6.[90]

NAIT typically presents as an isolated severe thrombocytopenia in an otherwise healthy child at birth. Severe thrombocytopenia may be present early in gestation and at least 20% of cases suffer intracranial hemorrhage (ICH),[91] some sustaining it *in utero*, which usually results in long-term severe neurologic sequelae such as porencephalic cysts and optic hypoplasia [92,93] Widespread petechial hemorrhage is present in more than 90% of cases, while cephalohematomas, hematuria and gastrointestinal bleeding occur in a significantly smaller number of children. Typically, the platelet count spontaneously returns into the normal range within 3 weeks after birth.

Neonates with alloimmune thrombocytopenia usually have platelet counts $< 20 \times 10^9$/L. Making the distinction from autoimmune causes is usually facilitated by the maternal platelet count, in that the mother has no thrombocytopenia nor is there any history of immune thrombocytopenic purpura (ITP). The diagnosis of NAIT is usually confirmed by platelet antigen typing of the parents, showing the antigen to be absent on the mother's platelets and present on the father's platelets, or by demonstrating antibody activity to the antigen in the mother's serum using indirect immunofluorescence assay[93,94] or enzyme-linked immunoassay.[96] It should be remembered that failure to detect a platelet-specific alloantibody in the maternal serum does not exclude the diagnosis,[96,97] and testing for NAIT does not require testing of the baby.

The mainstay of treatment for affected infant is washed, irradiated, maternal platelet concentrates.[98–100] The reason for washing the platelets is to remove antibody-laden plasma,[96,97] while irradiation destroys maternal lymphocytes that are capable of stimulating transfusion-associated graft-versus-host disease.[101] Both unrelated matched and maternal platelets can be administered; however, the latter are preferred because of their certain compatibility, availability and, perhaps most importantly, safety. With *de novo* cases of NAIT, platelets can be rapidly procured from the mother and following washing and gamma-irradiation given to the infant in a matter of a few hours. Random donor platelets should be given to infants who are actively bleeding while awaiting maternal platelets. In less severe cases, high-dose (1 g/kg) immunoglobulin therapy on two consecutive days will usually increase the platelet count within 2 days of administration.[101–104] In those cases of known NAIT where elective cesarean section is the preferred route of delivery, platelets are usually collected from the mother a few days before surgery; if this is deemed logistically problematic, then platelets can be collected early in the pregnancy or indeed when the mother is not pregnant and frozen for use at a later stage.[105] Alternatively, nonmaternal HPA-1a-negative platelets can be ordered in advance from a blood bank.

All children born to a father homozygous for the implicated antigen will harbor the antigen, whereas half of the offspring will have it if there is paternal heterozygosity. This has important implications for future pregnancies as imaging with ultrasound early in the pregnancy will indicate if intervention is required. Sampling fetal blood at 20 weeks' gestation allows accurate assessment of the platelet count and fetal alloantigen genotyping can also be carried out on the sample.[106,107] Knowing the fetal platelet count and whether intracranial bleeding is present usually dictates the most appropriate therapeutic intervention. For example, a fetus with severe thrombocytopenia and high risk of ICH will probably benefit from antigen-negative platelets transfused weekly.[96] At the other end of the clinical spectrum, a fetus who is at risk of NAIT, who has mild thrombocytopenia and a normal cranial ultrasound may equally benefit from maternal high-dose immunoglobulin therapy alone.[108,109] It should be noted, however, that there is no published randomized trial comparing the more aggressive approach of intrauterine platelet transfusion with the least aggressive therapeutic modality of maternal immunoglobulin infusion. Elective cesarean section is recommended for all affected mature fetuses as this optimizes postnatal management.[110]

Maternal autoimmune thrombocytopenia (see Chapter 30)
Autoimmune thrombocytopenia (AIT) is due to the passive transfer of autoantibodies from mothers with isolated ITP or it may be seen in association with conditions that have immune dysregulatory features, such as maternal systemic lupus erythematosus, hypothyroidism and lymphoproliferative states.[111,112] Unlike NAIT, the specificity of the platelet antibody seen in AIT is to antigen(s) common to maternal and fetal platelets.[113] Approximately 1 in 10 000 pregnancies are complicated by maternal ITP.[114] The risk of significant infant morbidity and mortality is minimal as the infant platelet count is rarely $< 50 \times 10^9$/L and ICH rarely if ever occurs; when it does, it is not related to birth trauma.[114,115] It is also clear that there is no correlation between the platelet count and level of autoantibody seen in the mother to the severity of thrombocytopenia observed in the infant; in fact, it has been well documented that women with normal platelet counts following splenectomy for ITP still deliver babies who are thrombocytopenic.[116] AIT needs to be distinguished from incidental or "gestational" thrombocytopenia, where the thrombocytopenia is usually mild (70–100 $\times 10^9$/L) with no history of bleeding or thrombocytopenia outside pregnancy and the platelet count swiftly returns to normal following delivery.[117,118] Infants born to mothers with "gestational" thrombocytopenia never or extremely rarely have a low platelet count.

The bleeding manifestations, including the risk of ICH, in children of mothers with AIT is significantly less than in children with NAIT.[114,115,119] These infants are usually very well and born at term. The neonatal platelet count often falls after birth to a nadir on days 1–3 and it is during this time that bleeding occurs.[120] Spontaneous recovery of the infant platelet count is usually observed within 3 weeks after birth.

However, if the platelet count is $< 20 \times 10^9/L$ or if there is significant bleeding, then intravenous immunoglobulin (1 g/kg) should be given on two consecutive days; if this fails to raise the platelet count, then a short course of prednisolone (2–4 mg/kg daily by mouth) for 7–14 days should be added.[121] The mother's immune thrombocytopenia should be treated in accordance with the severity of the platelet count and not for a theoretical risk estimate of bleeding in the baby. As there are no reliable maternal predictors of severe thrombocytopenia in the infant, prenatal treatment of the mother with immunoglobulin and/or steroids does not make therapeutic sense.[122] Birth is usually by spontaneous vaginal delivery and cesarean section should only be contemplated in those pregnancies where problems are anticipated or if there is a history of a previous complicated delivery.

Intrauterine infections (TORCH syndromes)
(see Chapters 30 and 35)

Intrauterine viral infections rarely produce thrombocytopenia ($< 20 \times 10^9/L$) and therefore therapeutic intervention in the form of platelet concentrate and/or antiviral therapy is only indicated when there is active bleeding or surgical intervention is being considered. The mechanism(s) responsible for thrombocytopenia secondary to intrauterine infection is not fully understood but is probably multifactorial, including megakaryocyte injury with decreased platelet production, splenic removal, liver dysfunction and platelet–endothelial cell injury. In the vast majority of cases, the platelet count returns into the normal range within 2–4 weeks after birth but may persist to 4 months of age.[123] The well-established intrauterine infections that cause congenital thrombocytopenia are outlined below.

Toxoplasmosis
Contracted during pregnancy, toxoplasmosis can result in serious damage to the fetus, including hydrocephaly, intracranial calcification, chorioretinitis and neurologic manifestations. Fortunately, as maternal screening for toxoplasmosis in pregnancy and good antenatal treatment is now available, the severe form is less frequently seen. Subclinical forms are now more frequently encountered, with chorioretinitis occurring in approximately one-third of cases. Thrombocytopenia is seen in one-quarter of cases of congenital toxoplasmosis and in approximately 20% of these cases the platelet count is $< 50 \times 10^9/L$.[123] Blood eosinophilia is also a common hematologic manifestation of this disease.

Congenital rubella
This is always due to a primary infection occurring in the first 3 months of pregnancy. The risk of serious malformation is highest if the infection is contracted in the first trimester. Mild-to-moderate thrombocytopenia is seen in approximately 20% of affected cases.[124] Hemolytic anemia and dermal

extramedullary hematopoiesis, which resembles the skin manifestation seen in congenital leukemia (so-called "blueberry muffin"), and other hematologic abnormalities are seen.

Cytomegalovirus
Like the other herpes viruses, especially herpes simplex (types I and II), cytomegalovirus (CMV) can cause thrombocytopenia in the fetus and newborn. Approximately 1 in 5000 births have evidence of CMV inclusion disease, characterized by hypotrophy, jaundice, hepatosplenomegaly, thrombocytopenia, anemia, microcephaly, intracerebral calcification and/or chorioretinitis. While most newborns congenitally infected with CMV are asymptomatic, symptoms and sequelae are much more likely to occur in infants congenitally infected as a result of the mother's primary infection during pregnancy than in those infected from reactivation of latent virus.[125] In two studies, thrombocytopenia was observed in 36% and 77% of infants infected with CMV, respectively;[125] in the former study, the platelet count was $< 50 \times 10^9/L$ in more than one-third of infants.[125]

Herpes simplex
Herpes simplex infection only causes problems to the fetus when the mother has a primary infection prior to 20 weeks' gestation. The risk of congenital malformation is very low; however, the frequency of fetal loss may be as high as 25% if the mother is infected during this time period. Thrombocytopenia is a well-established hematologic abnormality associated with congenital herpes simplex infection.[126]

Other causes
Other causes of intrauterine viral-induced neonatal thrombocytopenia include human immunodeficiency virus (HIV)[127,128] and parvovirus B19.[129] Estimates of the rates of HIV transmission from mother to newborn range from 20 to 60% depending on the study.[130] The risk is reduced significantly when the mother is asymptomatic but increases with the length of time that she is seropositive.[130] Thrombocytopenia is rarely if ever the first clinical manifestation of congenital HIV and, like parvovirus B19 infection, thrombocytopenia seems to be less frequently seen than with the other well-established causes of intrauterine viral-induced thrombocytopenia.[127–129]

Maternal preeclampsia

The association of neonatal thrombocytopenia and maternal preeclampsia and maternal hypertension is a controversial one. As there are more premature infants born to mothers with hypertensive disorders of pregnancy, it is most likely that the increased rate of thrombocytopenia seen in these infants is more a reflection of how sick and premature the child is at birth, rather than a direct result of the maternal hypertension. Very few of these infants have severe thrombocytopenia and ICH is exceedingly rare.[114]

Maternal use of drugs

Drug-induced thrombocytopenia in the mother may also affect the neonate and when it occurs is usually mediated by immune destruction of platelets.[114] It should be stressed that maternal use of drugs is an extremely rare cause of low platelets in the newborn and the drugs that have been implicated include anticonvulsants (valproic acid, phenytoin, carbamazepine), quinidine and possibly thiazides and hydralazine.[114]

Infant factors

Disseminated intravascular coagulation
(see Chapters 29 and 30)

Disseminated intravascular coagulation (DIC) is an acquired hemostatic syndrome usually seen in association with well-defined clinical disorders. It is characterized by consumption of procoagulant and natural anticoagulant proteins, which contributes to a state of mixed hemorrhage and thrombosis. The classic laboratory markers are thrombocytopenia, prolonged thrombin, prothrombin (PT) and activated partial thromboplastin (APTT) times, elevated D-dimers, and reductions in plasma levels of fibrinogen, factors II, V and VIII, protein C and antithrombin. The causes of DIC in infants and children are legion (see Chapters 29 and 30).

As a general axiom in medicine, when a pathologic syndrome is secondary to another primary disease state, the appropriate therapy should be directed when at all possible toward the underlying disease in order to correct the associated problem. For example, the appropriate treatment of the thrombotic DIC seen shortly after birth in children with homozygous protein C deficiency is replacement with protein C concentrate. As the plasma protein C level comes into the normal range following protein C concentrate infusion, the laboratory markers of DIC are corrected and resolution of skin purpura then becomes apparent.[131] The same clinical and laboratory response is seen following administration of protein C in children with severe acquired protein C deficiency secondary to meningococcemia.[132] Supportive treatment in the form of clotting factor replacement (fresh frozen plasma [FFP] 15 mL/kg to maintain PT below 17 s), cryoprecipitate (1 bag/5 kg to maintain fibrinogen above 1 g/L) and platelets (5 bags/m^2 to keep the count above 50×10^9/L) is usually administered as initial therapy, especially when there is evidence of active surface bleeding.[133] Use of heparin and natural anticoagulant concentrates (antithrombin and protein C) should also be considered.

Primary microangiopathic hemolytic anemias
(see Chapter 29)

Microangiopathic hemolytic anemia (MAHA) is a term that describes intravascular destruction of red cells in the presence of an abnormal microcirculation. In a significant number of clinical syndromes associated with MAHA there is also thrombocytopenia. The thrombocytopenia results from platelet activation and thus platelet thrombi formation, while the red cell fragmentation is a consequence of the shearing force produced by the abnormal flow within the abnormal microvasculature in concert with the microthrombi. The hallmark of MAHA is red cell fragmentation, polychromasia and thrombocytopenia on the blood smear, with absent haptoglobulins, hemoglobinuria and elevated serum lactate dehydrogenase and bilirubin levels. The PT and APTT are usually within the normal range as are the plasma levels of clotting factors V and VIII.

Hemolytic–uremic syndrome (see Chapter 29)
Hemolytic–uremic syndrome (HUS), with its classic triad of MAHA, low platelets and renal failure, is usually seen in infants and children following seasonal epidemics of gastroenteritis caused by *Escherichia coli* (0157:H7 strain) producing verotoxin. It is one of the commonest causes of renal failure in childhood and while the precise pathogenic mechanism responsible for it is not fully understood, renovascular endothelial damage is probably a key event in promoting platelet activation and fibrin deposition that ultimately leads to microthrombi formation.[134] The other important contributing factor may be elevated levels of abnormal vWF multimer released from the damaged endothelium, which enhance platelet aggregation and adhesion.[135,136] Treatment is essentially supportive with early renal dialysis allowing for better control of fluid and electrolyte balance. Unlike the situation in thrombotic thrombocytopenia purpura (see below), the role of plasma infusions and plasma exchange remains to be proven and therefore they are not used in the treatment of classic HUS.[137]

Thrombotic thrombocytopenic purpura
While Moschcowitz initially described thrombotic thrombocytopenic purpura (TTP) in a 16-year-old girl,[138] it is more commonly seen in young adults, with < 20% of all patients reported to be under 21 years of age.[137] It is characterized by MAHA, low platelets, fluctuating neurologic symptoms, fever and renal failure. However, severe thrombocytopenia, intravascular hemolysis with many red cell fragments on the blood smear, and neurologic symptoms and signs constitute the characteristic TTP clinical triad. Unlike HUS, the pathophysiologic mechanisms involved in TTP (acquired or inherited forms) are now beginning to be understood and are most likely caused by severe deficiency of the vWF cleavage protease ADAMTS-13.[139] Deficiency of this protease results in the presence of unusually large vWF multimers in the circulation, causing platelet activation with resultant platelet thrombi formation.[139,140] TTP should not be considered as a single disorder but as a heterogeneous group or a

spectrum of disease with at least four clinically distinguishable subtypes:[140]

- single-episode TTP (occurs *de novo* and seldom if ever recurs);
- intermittent TTP (characterized by occasional relapses at infrequent intervals);
- secondary TTP (usually seen in association with recognized clinical entities such as BMT, chemotherapy, pregnancy and infection, e.g., HIV);
- chronic relapsing TTP (frequent episodes occurring at regular intervals).

The commonest form seen in infancy and childhood is the chronic relapsing variety, which may be different from its adult counterpart as there is usually no end-organ damage and only very small quantities of FFP (without plasma exchange) are needed to reverse the anemia and thrombocytopenia.[141] However, the vWF multimer profile, characterized by the presence of unusually large vWF multimers, seen in both chronic relapsing types is similar, making it most likely that they are indeed the same disease state.[142,143]

The mainstay of treatment is plasma exchange with FFP or plasma devoid of the large vWF multimers (cryosupernatant or solvent detergent treated). Plasma infusions have also been shown to be efficacious, but plasma exchange is now considered the therapeutic modality of choice as controlled clinical trials have shown it to have superior efficacy.[144] Plasma exchange is continued until the platelet count and lactate dehydrogenase level return into the normal range. For those patients who do not respond to first-line treatment, a variety of other therapeutic approaches can be considered. These include corticosteroids, immunosuppression (vincristine, azathioprine, immunoglobulins), antiplatelet-aggregating agents (aspirin, dipyridamole) and splenectomy. It should be stated that all of these approaches have been reported to be successful anecdotally and not in a controlled clinical setting.

Giant hemangioma syndrome (Kasabach–Merritt syndrome)

Kasabach–Merritt syndrome (KMS) is the association of giant cavernous hemangiomas and DIC.[145] The consumptive coagulopathy seen in approximately 25% of cases of KMS is usually low grade and compensated. However, acceleration into the fulminant form, characterized by hypofibrinogenemia, raised D-dimers, red cell microangiopathy and severe thrombocytopenia, is not uncommon. This transformation can arise without an identifiable precipitating cause but it is usually accompanied by an expansion of the vascular tumor. The tumors are usually present at birth, grow in size over the first few months of life and then gradually recede. Therefore, the thrombocytopenia and indeed hemostatic failure that can be seen with these tumors may not be manifest until well into infancy. Most of the hemangiomas are cutaneous; however

"hidden" visceral tumors, especially splenic, should always be included in the differential diagnosis of a child with unexplained thrombocytopenia with or without evidence of compensated intravascular coagulopathy as these forms of KMS have a high mortality rate if appropriate therapeutic measures are not undertaken.[146,147] Computed tomography or magnetic resonance imaging is useful, but platelets labeled with ^{111}In-oxine is probably a more sensitive modality in delineating the size and number of hemangiomas present.

Fortunately, spontaneous regression of these tumors occurs in the majority of patients.[146] A number of therapeutic approaches can be instituted in those who fail to undergo spontaneous regression and depend on the severity of the hemostatic failure and anatomic location and size of the hemangiomas. Treatment modalities that have been used with varying success include corticosteroids,[147,148] surgical resection,[147,148] α-interferon,[149] embolization,[150,151] and radiotherapy.[152] Replacement therapy with platelets, fibrinogen concentrate, FFP, cryoprecipitate and antifibrinolytic drugs and antiplatelet agents have a role in the fulminant phase of severe forms. In situations where there is no obvious systemic hemorrhage but at the same time there is ongoing significant consumptive coagulopathy, it may be worth considering withholding platelet concentrate infusions. Blocking platelet function may also be a possibility, as there is now some evidence to suggest that degranulation with release of angiopoietins from endogenous and exogenous platelets as they become activated within the vascular tumor adds "fuel to the fire" and promotes further vascular tumor growth.

Hypercoagulable states (see Chapter 31)

Consumptive thrombocytopenia, mainly secondary to DIC following thrombin generation, can be the first manifestation of an acquired or inherited hypercoagulable state. The clinical hallmark in a significant number of these disorders is an inappropriate thrombotic event(s). It should be remembered, however, that venous and arterial thrombotic events in young children and neonates are rare, but when they do occur can be associated with morbidity and significant mortality such as limb loss and organ impairment. Most events occur in the neonatal period and while the majority are usually associated with indwelling vascular catheters,[153] other etiologic factors, both inherited and acquired, characteristic of the neonatal period may predispose to hypercoagulability and these are discussed below.

Birth asphyxia

Birth asphyxia as reflected by low Apgar scores is strongly associated with neonatal thrombocytopenia.[154,155] The mechanism responsible for the low platelet count has not been fully elucidated but consumption secondary to thrombin generation/DIC is probably the key event as hypoxia is known to upregulate tissue factor expression, reduce thrombomodulin activity and enhance plasminogen activator inhibitor-1 production by endothelial cells.[156]

Cyanotic congenital heart disease

The same mechanism probably plays a role in the thrombocytopenia seen in association with polycythemia in some cases of cyanotic congenital heart disease; however, other factors such as increased platelet destruction on abnormal anatomic vascular beds[157] and an artifactual low platelet count secondary to a high hematocrit may also be operating.

Respiratory distress syndrome

A significant number of infants with respiratory distress syndrome also develop thrombocytopenia,[158] which is usually accompanied by evidence of DIC. Postmortem findings in some infants who die from respiratory distress syndrome show pulmonary microvascular thrombosis[114] and again, like most of the other perinatal conditions seen in association with thrombocytopenia, the precise mechanism(s) responsible for the low platelet count in respiratory distress syndrome is not known. The degree of thrombocytopenia may be exacerbated with treatment as it is known that mechanical ventilation can induce mild thrombocytopenia in newborn infants.[159]

Necrotizing enterocolitis

The majority of infants with necrotizing enterocolitis have evidence of thrombocytopenia. In one study, 90% of infants studied had a platelet count $< 150 \times 10^9/L$ and over half a platelet count $< 50 \times 10^9/L$. Over 50% of the severe thrombocytopenic group had bleeding complications, with one-third having serious sequelae that were felt to be a contributing factor to infant mortality. A significant number of the severe cases had evidence of DIC.[160] Increased platelet destruction is thought to be the principal mechanism contributing to necrotizing enterocolitis-associated thrombocytopenia.

Bacterial infections

Thrombocytopenia is frequently seen in septic infants and probably results from consumptive coagulopathy, especially in those with bacterial infections.[75,161,162] Immune-mediated platelet destruction as well as impaired platelet production secondary to bone marrow infection have also been shown to contribute to the thrombocytopenia.[163] A low platelet count is usually seen after the onset of infectious symptoms and resolution of the platelet count occurs promptly when infection control is achieved.[164-167]

Rhesus hemolytic disease

Severe Rhesus hemolytic disease of the newborn may be associated with thrombocytopenia, especially in the setting of liver dysfunction and DIC.[168-170] The mechanism of the thrombocytopenia has not been fully elucidated but is probably multifactorial, involving hyperbilirubinemia, phototherapy, consumptive coagulopathy and the immune process. The thrombocytopenia usually improves during the first week of life and following exchange transfusion.[171] It should be remembered that exchange transfusion itself may cause thrombocytopenia, a process felt to be due to a dilutional effect, which can be prevented in some infants by using whole blood.[170,171]

Protein C and S deficiency

Hereditary protein C (PC) and protein S (PS) deficiency (homozygosity or compound heterozygosity) are associated with a high venous thromboembolic risk at birth or in the first few months of life.[131,172] The first clinical manifestation is usually necrotic purpura mainly affecting the extremities, and in some cases massive large-vessel thrombosis (renal and iliac veins, vena cava) can also be a presenting feature. Laboratory markers of DIC are usually present within the first week of life. Low levels of PC and PS are also usually seen in DIC associated with other etiologies, especially infection, and therefore it is important to make the correct diagnosis of hereditary PC or PS deficiency because optimum therapy involves factor replacement (protein C concentrate in PC deficiency or FFP in PS deficiency) and heparin in the acute phase and oral anticoagulation in the long term. Within hours of factor replacement, restoration of plasma coagulation proteins and platelets levels is apparent.[172,173] Homozygotes for antithrombin deficiency producing functional defects are also associated with a high risk of venous thromboembolic disease; however, only one case of thrombosis presenting in childhood has been reported.[174] Like PC deficiency, emergency or elective therapy involves antithrombin concentrate and heparin infusions.[175] Heterozygotes for PC, PS and antithrombin deficiency generally do not experience thrombosis until adolescence or early adulthood.

Heparin-induced thrombocytopenia

Heparin-induced thrombocytopenia constitutes the severest adverse effect of heparin therapy. It is of highly variable incidence, depending on the type of heparin used and whether the patient was infected/inflamed at the time of administration, but generally varies between > 1% and < 15% of patients receiving unfractionated heparin.[176] There are two types of heparin-induced thrombocytopenia:
- type I occurs within 1–2 days, is nonimmune and is usually totally benign;
- type II usually occurs after a latent period of 7–14 days, is immune mediated and is associated with paradoxical thrombosis/thromboembolism.[177]

Fortunately, the latter is an extremely rare event in neonates; nevertheless, when an infant is receiving heparin, no matter how small the dose, whether to keep a catheter patent or in total parenteral nutrition, a watchful eye should always be kept on the daily platelet count.

Rare bone marrow diseases

Transient abnormal myelopoiesis (see Chapters 16 and 18)
Transient abnormal myelopoiesis associated with Down syndrome (trisomy 21) or trisomy 21 mosaicism is a clonal disorder usually affecting children under 3 months of age. It is classically manifest as a myeloproliferative syndrome, with hepatosplenomegaly, elevated white cell count, normal hemoglobin and commonly thrombocytopenia. Blood smear examination usually reveals increased numbers of eosinophils and basophils but also blast cells that in the majority resemble megakaryoblasts.[178] Essentially, transient abnormal myelopoiesis looks like congenital leukemia; however, spontaneous remission is usually seen. Approximately 1 in 4 of these children develop megakaryoblastic leukemia by their third birthday.[179]

Hemophagocytic lymphohistiocytosis (see Chapter 15)
Hemophagocytic lymphohistiocytosis is a rare, probably autosomal recessive disorder of the monocyte–macrophage lineage. It usually occurs within the first 6 months of life and is characterized by fever, maculopapular rash, jaundice, hepatosplenomegaly, lymphadenopathy, pancytopenia, hypofibrinogenemia, hypertriglyceridemia and abnormal liver chemistry. Bone marrow examination shows numerous macrophages actively engulfing bone marrow elements including platelets. This disorder is usually rapidly fatal and allogeneic BMT offers the only real chance of cure.[180] Infection-associated hemophagocytic syndrome, especially in the immunocompromised host, can also present with thrombocytopenia as can the systemic variety of Langerhans cell histiocytosis; however, older children are those usually affected.[180]

Osteopetrosis
Variable cytopenias and a leukoerythroblastic blood smear are not uncommon features of autosomal recessive osteopetrosis (severe form). This usually presents during the first few months of life as failure to thrive, hypocalcemia, thrombocytopenia and anemia with or without infection. Generalized hyperostosis leads to bone marrow cavity obliteration and thus induces extramedullary hematopoiesis, which results in hepatosplenomegaly. Allogeneic BMT is the optimal therapeutic option for the severe disease as a significant number of these children die early in childhood.

Congenital leukemia
Congenital leukemia is a rare disease, usually of the myelomonoblastic, monoblastic or megakaryoblastic phenotype.[181] Nodular skin infiltration, the so-called "blueberry muffin" appearance, and hepatosplenomegaly are not uncommon associations. Thrombocytopenia alone or in association with other cytopenias is usually present at diagnosis.

Metastatic neuroblastoma
Metastatic neuroblastoma may also cause cytopenias secondary to marrow infiltration. Neuroblastoma cells are usually easily identifiable on marrow smears as they usually appear in tight groups and/or rosettes. While thrombocytopenia occurs in metastatic neuroblastoma, thrombocytosis is more common as a presenting hematologic abnormality.[182]

Placental factors

Placental infarction, which is not uncommon in women with circulating lupus anticoagulants and anticardiolipin antibodies, together with circulating lupus (chorioangiomas) can lead to thrombocytopenia which is usually present early in neonatal life. The mechanism(s) responsible for the thrombocytopenia has not been fully elucidated but is probably the end result of localized DIC within the abnormal vascular bed.

Conclusions

The inherited and congenital thrombocytopenias represent a very diverse group of disorders ranging from those with little or no hemorrhagic problems to those where significant mortality occurs within the neonatal period if appropriate therapy is not initiated. The inherited thrombocytopenias are very rare disorders compared with the congenital or acquired thrombocytopenias and making the correct diagnosis at the outset is very important as it usually avoids the prescribing of unnecessary and potentially toxic therapies. The differential diagnosis of neonatal thrombocytopenia differs enormously depending on the general well-being of the infant and therefore a detailed maternal history and neonatal examination are essential in making a speedy diagnosis. Platelet concentrate transfusions are the mainstay of therapy in the inherited group, whereas treating the underlying cause in the congenital group usually raises the platelet count into the normal range.

The past 25 years have witnessed remarkable progress in the understanding, at the molecular level, of the mechanism(s) by which platelet production and survival is controlled. More recently, the molecular basis of MYH9-related disease has been elucidated. Despite these impressive breakthroughs, much remains to be learned about the molecular defects responsible for the majority of inherited thrombocytopenias. No doubt, the next 25 years will see not only the isolation of the rogue genes responsible for these conditions but also gene therapies for these disorders will become a reality.

References

1. Dreyfus M, Kaplan C, Verdy E *et al*. Frequency of immune thrombocytopenia in newborns. A prospective study. *Blood* 1997; **89**: 4402–6.

2. Donne AD. L'origine des globules der san, de leur mode de formation et de leur fin. *CR Acad Sci* 1842; **14**: 366–71.

3. Geber F. *Elements of General and Minute Anatomy of Man and Mammals.* London: G Gulliver, 1942.

4. Addison W. On the colorless corpuscles and on the molecules and cytoblasts in the blood. *London Med Gas (NS)* 1842; **30**: 144–8.

5. Simon F. Physiologische und pathologische antropochemic mit Berucksiehtigung der eigentlichen Zoochemie. *Handbuch derangewandten medizinischen chemie nach dem neusten Standpunkte der wissengraft and nach zahlreichen eigenen untersuehungen. Theil II.* Berlin: Forstner, 1842.

6. Wintrobe MM. Early beginnings. In: *Hematology: the Blossoming of a New Science. A Story of Inspiration and Effort.* Philadelphia: Lea & Febiger, 1985, pp. 28–9.

7. Bizzozero J. Uber einen neuen Formbestandtheil des Blutes und die rolle bei der Thrombose und der Blutgrinning. *Virchows Arch A* 1882; **90**: 264.

8. Wright JH. The origin and nature of blood plates. *Boston Med Surg J* 1906; **154**: 643–5.

9. Eaton D. The purification and cloning of human thrombopoietin. In: Kuter DJ, Hunt P, Sheridan W, Zucker-Franklin D (eds) *Thrombopoiesis and Thrombopoietins: Molecular, Cellular, Preclinical and Clinical Biology.* Totowa, NJ: Humana Press, 1997, pp. 135–42.

10. D'Apolito M, Guarnieri V, Boncristiano M, Zelante L, Savoia A. Cloning of the murine non-muscle myosin heavy chain IIA gene ortholog of human MYH9 responsible for May–Hegglin, Sebastian, Fechtner, and Epstein syndromes. *Gene* 2002; **286**: 215–22.

11. Clemetson KH, Clemetson JM. Platelet GpIb–V–IX complex: structure, function, physiology and pathology. *Semin Thromb Hemost* 1995; **21**: 130–6.

12. Tuddenham EGD, Cooper DN. The von Willebrand factor and von Willebrand disease. In: Tuddenham EGD, Cooper DN (eds) *The Molecular Genetics of Haemostasis and its Inherited Disorders.* Oxford: Oxford University Press, 1994, pp. 374–401.

13. Clemetson KH, Clemetson JM. Molecular abnormalities in Glanzman's thrombasthenia, Bernard–Soulier syndrome and platelet type von Willebrand's disease. *Curr Opin Hematol* 1994; **1**: 388–93.

14. Lopez JA. The platelet glycoprotein Ib-IX. *Blood Coag Fibrinol* 1994; **5**: 97–118.

15. Roth GJ. Developing relationships: arterial platelet adhesion, glycoprotein Ib, and leucine-rich glycoproteins. *Blood* 1991; **77**: 5–19.

16. Miller JL, Cunningham D, Lyle VA, Finch CN. Mutation in the gene encoding the α chain of platelet glycoprotein Ib in platelet-type von-Willebrand disease. *Proc Natl Acad Sci USA* 1991; **88**: 4761–5.

17. Bolin RB, Okumura T, Jamieson GA. New polymorphism of platelet membrane glycoproteins. *Nature* 1977; **269**: 69–70.

18. Bowen DF, Hampton KK. von Willebrand disease and its diagnosis. In: Poller L, Ludlam CA (eds) *Recent Advances in Blood Coagulation.* Edinburgh: Churchill Livingstone, 1997, pp. 201–19.

19. Milton JG, Frojmovic MM, Tracy SS, White JG. Spontaneous platelet aggregation in an hereditary giant platelet syndrome (MPS). *Am J Pathol* 1984; **4** (2): 336–45.

20. Okita JR, Frojmovic MM, Kristopeit S, Wong T, Kunicki TJ. Montreal platelet syndrome: a defect in calcium-activated neutral proteins (calpain). *Blood* 1989; **74**: 715–21.

21. Milton JG, Frojmovic MM. Shape-changing agents produce abnormally large platelets in a hereditary "giant platelet syndrome (MPS)". *J Lab Clin Med* 1979; **93**: 154–9.

22. Bennett JS, Shattil SJ. Congenital qualitative platelet disorders. In: Williams WJ (ed.) *Hematology.* New York: McGraw Hill, 1990, pp. 1407–19.

23. Jantunen E. Inherited giant platelet disorders. *Eur J Haematol* 1994; **53**: 191–6.

24. Gebrane-Younes J, Martin Cramer E, Orcel L, Caen JP. Gray platelet syndrome. Dissociation between abnormal sorting in megakaryocyte alpha-granules and normal sorting in Weibel–Palade bodies of endothelial cells. *J Clin Invest* 1993; **92**: 3023–8.

25. Jantunen E, Hanninen A, Naukkarinen A, Vornanen M, Lahtinen R. Gray platelet syndrome with splenomegaly and signs of extramedullary hematopoiesis. *Am J Hematol* 1994; **46**: 218–24.

26. George JN, Nurden AT, Phillips DR. Molecular defects in interactions of platelets with the vessel wall. *N Engl J Med* 1984; **311**: 1084–9.

27. Breton-Gorius J, Favier R, Guichard J *et al.* A new congenital dysmegakaryopoietic thrombocytopenia (Paris–Trousseau) associated with giant α-granules and chromosome 11 deletion at 11q23. *Blood* 1995; **85**: 1805–14.

28. Aldrich RA, Steinberg AG, Campbell DC. Pedigree demonstrating a sex-linked recessive condition characterised by draining ears, eczematoid dermatitis and bloody diarrhea. *Pediatrics* 1954; **13** (2): 133–9.

29. Cooper MD, Chase HP, Lowman JT *et al.* Wiskott–Aldrich syndrome: an immunologic deficiency disease involving the afferent limb of the immunity. *Am J Med* 1968; **44**: 499–513.

30. Ochs HD, Slichter SJ, Harker LA *et al.* The Wiskott–Aldrich syndrome: studies of lymphocytes, granulocytes and platelets. *Blood* 1980; **55**: 243–52.

31. Grottum KA, Hovig T, Holmsen H *et al.* Wiskott–Aldrich syndrome: qualitative platelet defects and short survival. *Br J Haematol* 1969; **17**: 373–7.

32. Verhoeven AJM, Oostrum IEA, van Haarlem H. Impaired energy metabolism in platelets from patients with Wiskott–Aldrich syndrome. *Thromb Haemost* 1989; **61**: 10–15.

33. Mullen CA, Anderson KD, Blaese M. Splenectomy and/or bone marrow transplantation in the management of Wiskott–Aldrich syndrome: long term follow-up of 62 cases. *Blood* 1993; **82**: 2961–5.

34. Lum LG, Tubergen DG, Corash L, Blaese M. Splenectomy in the management of the thrombocytopenia of the Wiskott–Aldrich syndrome. *N Engl J Med* 1980; **302**: 892–5.

35. Stomorken H, Hellum B, Egeland T *et al.* X-linked thrombocytopenia and thrombocytopathia: attenuated Wiskott–Aldrich syndrome. Functional and morphological studies of platelets and lymphocytes. *Thromb Haemost* 1991; **65**: 300–5.

36. Ata M, Fisher OD, Holman CA. Inherited thrombocytopenia. *Lancet* 1965; **i**: 119–21.

37. Zhu Q, Zhang M, Bles RM *et al.* The Wiskott–Aldrich syndrome

and X-linked congenital thrombocytopenia are caused by mutations of the same gene. *Blood* 1995; **86**: 3797–802.

38. Balduini CL, Pecci A, Loffredo G *et al*. Effects of the R216Q mutation of GATA-1 on erythropoiesis and megakaryocytopoiesis. *Thromb Haemost* 2004; **91**: 129–40.

39. Haddad WM, Haddad E, Le Deist F, Blanche S *et al*. Treatment of Chediak–Highasi syndrome by allogeneic bone marrow transplantation: report of 10 cases. *Blood* 1995; **85**: 3328–42.

40. Hayward CP, Cramer EM, Kane WH *et al*. Studies of a second family with the Quebec platelet disorder: evidence that the degradation of the alpha-granule membrane and its soluble contents are not secondary to a defect in targeting proteins to alpha-granules. *Blood* 1997; **89**: 1243–53.

41. Kahr WH, Zheng S, Sheth PM *et al*. Platelets from patients with the Quebec platelet disorder contain and secrete abnormal amounts of urokinase-type plasminogen activator. *Blood* 2001; **98**: 257–65.

42. Heller PG, Glembotsky AC, Gandhi MJ *et al*. Low Mpl receptor expression in a pedigree with familial platelet disorder with predisposition to acute myelogenous leukemia and a novel AML1 mutation. *Blood* 2005; **105**: 4664–70.

43. Canobbio I, Noris P, Pecci A, Balduini A, Torti M. Altered cytoskeletal organisation in platelets from patients with MYH9 related disease. *J Thromb Haemost* 2005; **3**: 1026–35.

44. Hegglin R. Gleichzeitige knostitutionelle Veranderungen an Neutrophylen und Thrombozyten. *Helv Med Acta* 1945; **12**: 439–44.

45. Godwin HA, Ginsburg AD. May–Hegglin anomaly: a defect in megakaryocyte fragmentation? *Br J Haematol* 1974; **26**: 117–24.

46. Cabrera JR, Fonton G, Lorente F *et al*. Defective neutrophil mobility in the May–Hegglin anomaly. *Br J Haematol* 1981; **47**: 337–41.

47. Buchanan JG, Buchanan JG, Pearce L, Wetherley-Mein G *et al*. The May–Hegglin anomaly. A family report and chromosome study. *Br J Haematol* 1964; **10**: 508–14.

48. Hamilton RW, Shaikh BS, Ottie JN *et al*. Platelet function, ultrastructure and survival in the May–Hegglin anomaly. *Am J Clin Pathol* 1980; **74**: 663–71.

49. Davis JW, Wilson SJ. Platelet survival in the May–Hegglin anomaly. *Br J Haematol* 1966; **12**: 61–4.

50. Greinacher A, Bux J, Kiefel V *et al*. May–Hegglin anomaly: a rare cause of thrombocytopenia. *Eur J Pediatr* 1994; **53**: 191–6.

51. Alport CA. Hereditary familial congenital haemorrhagic nephritis. *Br Med J* 1927; **1**: 504–5.

52. Ars E, Tazon-Vega B, Ruiz P *et al*. Male-to-male transmission of X-linked Alport syndrome in a boy with a 47, XXY karyotype. *Eur J Hum Genet* 2005; **13** (9): 1040–6.

53. Epstein CJ, Sahud MA, Piel CF *et al*. Hereditary macrothrombocytopenia, nephritis and deafness. *Am J Med* 1972; **52**: 299–310.

54. Eckstein JD, Filip DJ, Watts JC. Hereditary thrombocytopenia, deafness and renal disease. *Ann Intern Med* 1975; **82**: 639–45.

55. Peterson LC, Rao KV, Crosson JT, White JG. Fechtner syndrome: a variant of Alport's syndrome with leucocyte inclusion and macrothrombocytopenia. *Blood* 1985; **65**: 397–406.

56. Gershoni-Baruch R, Viener A, Lichtig C. Fechtner syndrome: clinical and genetic aspects. *Am J Med Genet* 1988; **31**: 357–67.

57. Greinacher A, Niewenhuis HK, White JG. Sebastian platelet syndrome: a new variant of hereditary macrothrombocytopenia with leukocyte inclusions. *Blut* 1990; **61**: 282–8.

58. Pujol-Moix N, Muniz-Diaz E, Moreno-Torres MLB, Hernandez A, Madox P, Domingo A. Sebastian platelet syndrome. *Ann Hematol* 1991; **62**: 235–7.

59. Greinacher A, Muller-Eckhart C. Hereditary types of thrombocytopenia with giant platelets and inclusion bodies in the leukocytes. *Blut* 1990; **60**: 53–9.

60. Van den Qudenrijn S, Bruin, M, de Hass M, von dem Borne AE. From gene to disease: from thrombopoietin receptor gene defects to congenital amegakaryocytic thrombocytopenia. *Ned Tijdschr Geneeeskd* 2002; **146**: 469–71.

61. Alter BP. Inherited bone marrow failure syndrome. In: Handin RI, Stossel TP, Lux SE (eds) *Blood: Principles and Practice of Hematology*. Philadephia: JB Lippincott, 1995, pp. 227–91.

62. Bessman JD, Harrison RL, Howard LC, Peterson D. The megakaryocyte abnormality in thrombocytopenia-absent radius syndrome. *Blood* 1983; **62**: 143–8.

63. Homans AC, Cohen JL, Mazur EM. Defective megakaryocytopoiesis in the syndrome of thrombocytopenia with absent radii. *Br J Haematol* 1988; **70**: 205–10.

64. Brochstem JA, Shank B, Kernan NA, Terwillinger JW, O'Reilly RJ. Marrow transplantation for thrombocytopenia-absent radii syndrome. *J Pediatr* 1992; **121**: 587–9.

65. Day HJ, Holmsen H. Platelet adenine nucleotide "storage pool deficiency" in thrombocytopenia absent radii syndrome. *JAMA* 1972; **221**: 1053–6.

66. Filkins K, Russo J, Bilinki I, Diamond N, Searle B. Prenatal diagnosis of thrombocytopenia absent radius syndrome using ultrasound and fetoscopy. *Prenat Diagn* 1984; **4**: 139–44.

67. Daffos F, Forestier F, Kaplan C, Cox W. Prenatal diagnosis and management of bleeding disorders with fetal blood sampling. *Am J Obstet Gynecol* 1988; **158**: 939–42.

68. Guinan EC, Lee Y, Lopez KD *et al*. Effects of interleukin-3 and granulocyte-macrophage colony-stimulating factor on thrombopoiesis in congenital amegakaryocytic thrombocytopenia. *Blood* 1993; **81**: 1691–8.

69. Van Oostrom CG, Wilms RHH. Congenital thrombocytopenia associated with raised concentrations of haemoglobin F. *Helv Paediatr Acta* 1978; **33**: 59–64.

70. O'Gorman Hughes DW. Aplastic anemia in childhood. III. Constitutional aplastic anaemia and related cytopenias. *Med J Aust* 1974; **1**: 519–26.

71. Schroeder-Kurt TM, Auerbach AD, Obe G. *Fanconi Anemia. Clinical, Cytogenetic and Experimental Aspects*. Berlin: Springer-Verlag, 1989, p. 264.

72. Minagi HJ, Steinbach H. Roentgen appearance of anomalies associated with hypoplastic anemia of childhood: Fanconi's anemia and congenital hypoplastic anemia (erythrogenesis imperfecta). *Am J Roentgenol* 1966; **97**: 100–5.

73. McIntosh S, Breg WR, Lubiniecki AS. Fanconi's anemia: the preanemic phase. *Am J Pediatr Hematol Oncol* 1979; **1**: 107–10.

74. Rabinowitz JG, Mosely JE, Mitty HA, Hirshorn K. Trisomy-18, esophageal atresia, anomalies of the radius and congenital hypoplastic thrombocytopenia. *Radiology* 1967; **89**: 488–91.

75. De Alarcon PA. Thrombopoiesis in the fetus and newborn. In: Stockman JA, Pochedly C (eds) *Developmental and Neonatal Hematology*. New York: Raven Press, 1988, pp. 103–30.

76. Oski FA, De Angelis CD, Feigin RD, Warshaw JB (eds)

Principles and Practice of Pediatrics, 6th edn. Philadelphia: JB Lippincott, 1990.

77. Najean Y, Lecompte T. Genetic thrombocytopenia with autosomal dominant transmission. *Br J Haematol* 1990; **74**: 203–8.

78. Najean Y, Lecompte T. Hereditary thrombocytopenia in childhood. *Semin Thromb Hemost* 1995; **21**: 294–304.

79. Von Behrens WC. Mediterranean thrombocytopenia. *Blood* 1975; **46**: 199–208.

80. Najean Y. The congenital thrombocytopenias due to a production defect. In: Sutor AH, Thomas KB (eds) *Thrombocytopenia in Childhood*. Basel: Roche Schattauer, 1994, pp. 199–208.

81. Guerois G, Gruel Y, Petit A *et al.* Familial macrothrombocytopenia. *Curr Stud Hematol Blood Transfus* 1988; **55**: 153–61.

82. Pearson HA, Shulman NR, Marder VJ, Cone TE. Isoimmune neonatal thrombocytopenic purpura: clinical and therapeutic considerations. *Blood* 1964; **23**: 154–77.

83. Blanchette VS, Peters MA, Pegg-Feige K. Alloimmune thrombocytopenia. Review from a neonatal intensive care unit. *Curr Stud Hematol Blood Transfus* 1986; **52**: 87–96.

84. Mueller-Eckhardt C, Kiefel V, Grubert A *et al.* 348 cases of suspected neonatal alloimmune thrombocytopenia. *Lancet* 1989; **i**: 363–6.

85. Kaplan C, Morel-Kopp MC, Kroll H *et al.* HPA-5b (Br^a) neonatal alloimmune thrombocytopenia. Clinical and immunological analysis of 39 cases. *Br J Haematol* 1991; **78**: 425–9.

86. Blanchette VS, Chen L, Salomon de Friedberg Z, Hogan VA, Trudel E, Decary F. Alloimmunization to the Pl^{A1} platelet antigen: results of a prospective study. *Br J Haematol* 1990; **74**: 209–15.

87. Reznikoff-Etievant MF, Kaplan C, Durieux I, Huchet J, Salmon C, Neter A. Alloimmune thrombocytopenia, definition of a group at risk: a prospective study. *Curr Stud Hematol Blood Transfus* 1988; **55**: 119–25.

88. De Wall LP, Van Dalen CM, Englefriet CP, von dem Borne AEG. Alloimmunisation against the platelet-specific Zw^a antigen, resulting in neonatal thrombocytopenia or post-transfusion purpura, is associated with the supertypic DR-w52 antigen including DR3 and DRw6. *Hum Immunol* 1986; **17**: 45–53.

89. Reznikof Etievant MR, Dangu C. ALA-B8 antigens and anti-Pl^{A1} and alloimmunisation. *Tissue Antigens* 1981; **18**: 66–72.

90. Mueller-Eckhardt C, Kiefel V. HLA-DRw6, a new immune response marker for immunisation against the platelet alloantigen Br^a. *Vox Sang* 1986; **50**: 94–9.

91. Bussel J, Berkowitz R, McFarland J. *In-utero* platelet transfusion for alloimmune thrombocytopenia. *Lancet* 1988; **ii**: 506.

92. Herman JH, Jumbelic MI, Ancona RJ, Kickler TS. *In utero* cerebral hemorrhage in alloimmune thrombocytopenia. *Am J Pediatr Hematol Oncol* 1986; **8**: 312–17.

93. Davidson JE, McWilliam RC, Evans TJ, Stephenson JB. Porencephaly and optic hypoplasia in neonatal isoimmune thrombocytopenia. *Arch Dis Child* 1989; **64**: 858–60.

94. Mueller-Eckhardt C, Kayser W, Forster C, Muller-Eckhardt G, Ringenberg C. Improved assay for detection of platelet-specific Pl^{A1} antibodies in neonatal immune thrombocytopenia. *Vox Sang* 1982; **43**: 76–81.

95. Kiefel V, Santoso S, Katzmann B, Mueller-Eckhardt C. A new platelet-specific alloantigen Br^a. Report of 4 cases with neonatal alloimmune thrombocytopenia. *Vox Sang* 1988; **54**: 101–6.

96. Kaplan C, Daffos F, Forestier F. Management of alloimmune thrombocytopenia: antenatal diagnosis and *in-utero* transfusion of maternal platelets. *Blood* 1988; **72**: 340–3.

97. McFarland JG, Frenzke M, Aster RH. Testing of maternal sera in pregnancies at risk for neonatal alloimmune thrombocytopenia. *Transfusion* 1989; **29**: 128–33.

98. Adner MM, Fisch GR, Starobin SG, Aster RH. Use of "compatible" platelet transfusions in the treatment of congenital isoimmune thrombocytopenic purpura. *N Engl J Med* 1969; **280**: 244–7.

99. Katz J, Hodder FS, Aster RS, Bennetts GA, Cairo MS. Neonatal isoimmune thrombocytopenia. The natural course and management and the detection of maternal antibody. *Clin Pediatr* 1984; **23**: 159–62.

100. Sanders MR, Graeber JE. Post-transfusion graft-versus-host-disease in infancy. *J Pediatr* 1990; **117**: 159–63.

101. Sidiropoulos D, Straume B. The treatment of neonatal thrombocytopenia with intravenous immunoglobulin (IgG i.v.). *Blut* 1984; **48**: 383–6.

102. Derycke M, Dreyfus M, Ropert JC, Tchernia G. Intravenous immunoglobulin for neonatal isoimmune thrombocytopenia. *Arch Dis Child* 1985; **60**: 667–9.

103. Suarez CR, Anderson C. High-dose intravenous gamma-globulin (IVIG) in neonatal immune thrombocytopenia. *Am J Hematol* 1987; **26**: 247–53.

104. Massey GV, McWilliams NB, Mueller DG, Napolitano A, Mauer HM. Intravenous immunoglobulin in the treatment of neonatal isoimmune thrombocytopenia. *J Pediatr* 1987; **111**: 133–5.

105. McGill M, Mayhaus C, Hoff R, Carey P. Frozen maternal platelets for neonatal thrombocytopenia. *Transfusion* 1982; **27**: 341–7.

106. McFarland JG, Aster RH, Bussel JB, Gianopoulos JG, Derbes RS, Newman PJ. Prenatal diagnosis of neonatal alloimmune thrombocytopenia using allele specific oligonucleotide probes. *Blood* 1991; **78**: 2276–82.

107. Kuijpers RW, Faber NM, Kanhai HH, von dem Borne AE. Typing of fetal platelet alloantigens when platelets are not available. *Lancet* 1990; **336**: 1391.

108. Bussel JB, Berkowitz RL, McFarland JG, Lynch L, Chitkara U. Antenatal treatment of neonatal alloimmune thrombocytopenia. *N Engl J Med* 1988; **319**: 1374–8.

109. Lynch L, Bussel JB, McFarland JG, Chitkara U, Berkowitz RL. Antenatal treatment of alloimmune thrombocytopenia. *Obstet Gynecol* 1992; **80**: 67–71.

110. Anon. Management of alloimmune neonatal thrombocytopenia. *Lancet* 1989; **i**: 137–9.

111. Kapatkin S, Stick N, Kapatkin MB, Siskind GW. Cumulative experience in the detection of antiplatelet antibody in 234 patients with idiopathic thrombocytopenic purpura, systemic lupus erythematosus and other clinical disorders. *Am J Med* 1972; **52**: 776–85.

112. de Swiet M. Maternal alloimmune disease and the fetus. *Arch Dis Child* 1985; **60**: 749–97.

113. Dixon RH, Rosse WF. Platelet antibody in autoimmune thrombocytopenia. *Br J Haematol* 1975; **31**: 129–37.

114. George D, Bussel JB. Neonatal thrombocytopenia. *Semin Thromb Hemost* 1995; **21**: 276–93.

115. Burrows RF, Kelton JG. Low fetal risks in pregnancies associated with idiopathic thrombocytopenic purpura. *Am J Obstet Gynecol* 1990; **163**: 1147–50.

116. Barbui T, Cortelazzo S, Viero P, Buelli M, Casarotto C. Idiopathic thrombocytopenic purpura and pregnancy. Maternal platelet count and antiplatelet antibodies do not predict the risk of neonatal thrombocytopenia. *La Ric Clin Lab* 1985; **15**: 139–45.

117. Burrows RF, Kelton JG. Incidentally detected thrombocytopenia in healthy mothers and their infants. *N Engl J Med* 1988; **319**: 142–5.

118. Aster RH. "Gestational" thrombocytopenia. A plea for conservative management. *N Engl J Med* 1990; **323**: 264–6.

119. Sauels P, Bussel JB, Braitman LE *et al.* Estimation of the risk of thrombocytopenia in the offspring of pregnant women with presumed immune thrombocytopenia purpura. *N Engl J Med* 1990; **323**: 229–35.

120. Kapatkin M, Porges RF, Karpatkin S. Platelet counts in infants of women with autoimmune thrombocytopenia: effects of steroid administration to the mother. *N Engl J Med* 1981; **52**: 776–85.

121. Bussel JB, Kaplan C, McFarland J. Recommendations for the evaluation and treatment of neonatal autoimmune and alloimmune thrombocytopenia. *Thromb Haemost* 1991; **65**: 631–5.

122. Blanchette VS, Sacher RA, Ballem PJ, Bussel JB, Imbash P. Commentary on the management of autoimmune thrombocytopenia during pregnancy and the neonatal period. *Blut* 1989; **59**: 121–6.

123. Hohlfield P, Forestier F, Kaplan C *et al.* Fetal thrombocytopenia: a retrospective survey of 5,914 fetal blood samplings. *Blood* 1994; **84**: 1851–6.

124. Cooper LZ, Green RH, Krugman S. Neonatal thrombo-cytopenic purpura and other manifestations of rubella contracted *in utero*. *Am Dis Child* 1965; **110**: 416–19.

125. Boppana SB, Pass RF, Britt WJ, Stagno S, Alford CA. Symptomatic congenital cytomegalovirus infection: neonatal morbidity and mortality. *Pediatr Infect Dis J* 1992; **11**: 93–9.

126. Malbrunot C, Boue A. Herpes. In: Boue A (ed.) *Fetal Medicine, Prenatal Diagnosis and Management*. Oxford: Oxford University Press, 1995, pp. 233–40.

127. Rigaud M, Leibovitz E, Quee CS *et al.* Thrombocytopenia in children infected with human immunodeficiency virus: long-term follow-up and therapeutic considerations. *J Acquir Immune Defic Syndr* 1992; **5**: 450–5.

128. Mandlebrot L, Schlienger I, Bongain A *et al.* Thrombocytopenia in pregnant women infected with human immunodeficiency virus. Maternal and neonatal outcome. *Am J Obstet Gynecol* 1994; **171**: 252–7.

129. Srivastava A, Bruno E, Briddell R *et al.* Parvovirus B19-induced perturbation of human megakaryocytopoiesis *in vitro*. *Blood* 1990; **76**: 1997–2004.

130. Malbrunot C, Boue A. AIDS. In: Boue A (ed.) *Fetal Medicine, Prenatal Diagnosis and Management*. Oxford: Oxford University Press, 1995, pp. 242–6.

131. Dreyfus M, Magny JF, Bridey F. Treatment of homozygous protein C deficiency and neonatal purpura fulminans with a purified protein C concentrate. *N Engl J Med* 1991; **325**: 1565–8.

132. Smith OP, White B, Vaughan D *et al.* Use of protein C concentrate, heparin and haemodiafiltration in meningococcus-induced purpura fulminans. *Lancet* 1997; **350**: 1590–3.

133. Hilgartner NW, Corrigan JJ Jr. Coagulation disorders. In: Miller DR, Baehnwer RL (eds) *Blood Diseases of Infancy and Childhood*. St Louis: CV Mosby, 1995, pp. 924–86.

134. Kaplan BS, Cleary TG, Obrig TG. Recent advances in understanding the pathogenesis of hemolytic uremic syndrome. *Pediatr Nephrol* 1990; **4**: 276–83.

135. Beningi A, Boccardo P, Nons M *et al.* Urinary excretion of platelet-activating factor in haemolytic-uraemic syndrome. *Lancet* 1992; **339**: 835–6.

136. Moake JL, McPherson PD. Abnormalities of von Willebrand factor multimers in TTP and HUS. *Am J Med* 1989; **87** (suppl. 3N): 9N–15N.

137. McSherry KJ, Sills RH. Acquired microangiopathic haemolytic anaemias. *Int J Paediatr Haematol Oncol* 1994; **1**: 25–112.

138. Moschcowitz E. Hyaline thrombosis of the terminal arterioles and capillaries: a hitherto undescribed disease. *Proc N Y Pathol Soc* 1924; **24**: 21–4.

139. Schneppenheim R, Budde U, Hassenpflug W, Obser T. Severe ADAMTS-13 deficiency in childhood. *Semin Hematol* 2004; **41**: 83–9.

140. Moake JL. Thrombotic thrombocytopenic purpura. Pathophysiologic and therapeutic studies. In: Brubaker DB, Simpson MB Jr (eds) *Dynamics of Hemostasis and Thrombosis*. Bethesda, MD: American Association of Blood Banks, 1995, pp. 123–32.

141. Upshaw JD Jr. Congenital deficiency of a factor in normal plasma that reverses microangiopathic hemolysis and thrombocytopenia. *N Engl J Med* 1978; **298**: 1350–2.

142. Miura M, Koizumi S, Nakamura K *et al.* Efficacy of several plasma components in a young boy with chronic thrombocytopenia and hemolytic anemia who responds repeatedly to normal plasma infusions. *Am J Hematol* 1984; **17**: 307–19.

143. Chintagumpala M, Hurwitz R, Moake J *et al.* Chronic relapsing thrombotic thrombocytopenic purpura in infants with large von Willebrand factor multimers during remission. *J Pediatr* 1992; **120**: 49–53.

144. Rock GA, Shumak KH, Buskard NA *et al.* Comparison of plasma exchange with plasma infusion in the treatment of thrombotic thrombocytopenic purpura. *N Engl J Med* 1991; **325**: 393–7.

145. Kasabach HH, Merritt KK. Capillary hemangioma with extensive purpura: report of a case. *Am J Dis Child* 1940; **59**: 1063–70.

146. Berman B, Lim HW-P. Concurrent cutaneous and hepatic haemagiomata in infancy. Report of a case and review of the literature. *J Dermatol Surg Oncol* 1978; **4**: 869–73.

147. Enjolras O, Riche MC, Merland JJ, Escande JP. Management of alarming hemangiomas in infancy. A review of 25 cases. *Pediatrics* 1990; **85**: 491–498.

148. Kushner BJ. The treatment of periorbital infantile hemangiomas with intralesional steroids. *Plast Reconstr Surg* 1985; **76**: 517–26.

149. Ezekowitz RÀB, Mulliken JB, Folkman J. Interferon alpha-2a therapy for life-threatening hemagiomas in infancy. *N Engl J Med* 1992; **326**: 1456–63.

150. Argenta LC, Bishop E, Cho KL, Andrews AF, Coran AG. Complete resolution of life-threatening haemangioma by embolisation and corticosteroids. *Plast Reconstr Surg* 1982; **70**: 739–44.

151. Stanley P, Gomperts E, Woolley MM. Kasabach–Merritt syndrome treated by therapeutic embolisation with polyvinyl alcohol. *Am J Pediatr Hematol Oncol* 1986; **8**: 308–11.

152. Schild SE, Buskrit SJ, Frick LM, Cupps RE. Radiotherapy for large symptomatic hemangiomas. *Int J Radiat Oncol Biol Phys* 1991; **21**: 729–35.

153. David M, Andrew M. Venous thromboembolism complications in children: a critical review of the literature. *J Pediatr* 1993; **123**: 337–42.

154. Chessells JM, Wigglesworth JS. Coagulation studies in severe birth asphyxia. *Arch Dis Child* 1971; **46**: 253–6.

155. Chadd MA, Elwood PC, Grey OP, Muxworthy SM. Coagulation studies in hypoxic fullterm newborn infants. *Br Med J* 1971; **4**: 516–18.

156. van Hinsbergh VWM. The vessel wall and hemostatis. In: van Hinsbergh VWM (ed.) *Vascular Control of Hemostasis*. Australia: Harwood Academic Publishers, 1996, pp. 1–9.

157. Henriksson P, Varendh G, Lundstrom NR. Haemostatic defects in cyanotic congenital heart disease. *Br Heart J* 1979; **41**: 23–7.

158. Segal ML, Goetzman BW, Schick JB. Thrombocytopenia and pulmonary hypertension in perinatal aspiration syndromes. *J Pediatr* 1980; **96**: 727–30.

159. Ballin A, Koren G, Kohelet D *et al.* Reduction of platelet counts induced by mechanical ventilation in newborn infants. *J Pediatr* 1987; **111**: 445–9.

160. Hutter JJ, Hathaway WE, Wayne ER. Hematologic abnormalities in severe neonatal necrotising enterocolitis. *J Pediatr* 1976; **88**: 1026–31.

161. Castle V, Andrew M, Kelton J, Giron D, Johnston M, Carter C. Frequency and mechanism of neonatal thrombocytopenia. *J Pediatr* 1986; **108**: 749–55.

162. Naiman JL. Disorders of platelets. In: Oski FA, Naiman J (eds) *Hematologic Problems of the Newborn*. Philadelphia: WB Saunders, 1982, pp. 175–222.

163. Desforges JF, O'Connell LG. Hematologic observations of the course of erythroblastosis fetalis. *Blood* 1955; **10**: 802–10.

164. Tate DY, Carlton GT, Johnson D *et al.* Immune thrombo-cytopenia in severe neonatal infections. *J Pediatr* 1981; **98**: 449–53.

165. Mehta P, Vasa R, Neumann L, Karpartkin M. Thrombo-cytopenia in the high risk infant. *J Pediatr* 1980; **97**: 791–4.

166. Zipursky A, Jaber HM. The haematology of bacterial infection in newborn infants. *Clin Haematol* 1978; **7**: 175–93.

167. Mondanlou HD, Ortiz OB. Thrombocytopenia in neonatal infection. *Clin Pediatr* 1981; **20**: 402–7.

168. Chessells JM, Wigglesworth JS. Haemostatic failure in babies with rhesus isoimmuisation. *Arch Dis Child* 1971; **46**: 38–45.

169. Andrew M. The hemostatic system in the infant. In: Nathan DG, Oski FA (eds) *Hematology of Infancy and Childhood*, 4th edn. Philadelphia: WB Saunders, 1993, pp. 115–53.

170. Andrew M, Castle V, Saigal S, Carter C, Kelton JG. Clinical impact of neonatal thrombocytopenia. *J Pediatr* 1987; **110**: 457–64.

171. Andrew M, Vegh P, Caco C *et al.* A randomised, controlled trial of platelet transfusions in thrombocytopenic premature infants. *J Pediatr* 1993; **123**: 285–91.

172. Mahasandana C, Suvatte V, Marlar RA. Neonatal purpura fulminans associated with homozygous protein S deficiency. *Lancet* 1990; **335** (8680): 61–2.

173. White B, Livingstone W, Murphy C, Hodgson A, Rafferty M, Smith OP. An open-label study of the role of adjuvant hemostatic support with protein C replacement therapy in purpura fulminans-associated meningococcemia. *Blood* 2000; **96**: 3719–24.

174. Boyer C, Wolf M, Vendrenne J. Homozygous variant of antithrombin III: AT III Fontaineblue. *Thromb Haemost* 1986; **56**: 18–21.

175. Schwartz RS, Bauer KA, Rosenberg RD, Kavanaugh EJ, Davies DC, Bogdanoff DA. Clinical experience with antithrombin III concentrate in treatment of congenital and acquired deficiency of antithrombin. *Am J Med* 1989; **87**: 53S.

176. Bick RL. Heparin-induced thrombocytopenia and paradoxical thromboembolism: diagnostic and therapeutic dilemmas. *Clin Appl Thromb Hemost* 1997; **3**: 63–5.

177. Spadone D, Clark F, James E, Laster J, Hoch J, Silver D. Heparin-induced thrombocytopenia in the newborn. *J Vasc Surg* 1992; **15**: 306–11.

178. Iselius L, Jacobs P, Morton, N. Leukaemia and transient leukaemia in Down syndrome. *Hum Genet* 1990; **85**: 477–81.

179. Zipursky A, Poon A, Doyle J. Hematologic and oncologic disorders in Down's syndrome. In: Lott I, McCoy E (eds) *Down Syndrome: Today's Health Care Issues*. New York: John Wiley & Sons, 1991, pp. 42–56.

180. Pritchard J, Malone M. Histiocyte disorders. In: Peckham M, Pinedo HM, Veronesi U (eds) *Oxford Textbook of Oncology*. Oxford: Oxford University Press, 1995, pp. 1878–94.

181. Koller U, Haas HA, Ludwig W-D. Phenotypic and genotypic heterogeneity in infant acute leukaemia. II. Acute nonlymphoblastic leukaemia. *Leukemia* 1989; **3**: 708–12.

182. Roald B, Ninane J. Neuroblastoma. In: Peckham M, Pinedo HM, Veronesi U (eds) *Oxford Textbook of Oncology*. Oxford: Oxford University Press, 1995, pp. 1992–2000.

23 Idiopathic thrombocytopenic purpura

Paul Imbach

Idiopathic thrombocytopenic purpura (ITP) is a bleeding disorder that occurs as either an acute self-limiting condition or a recurrent or chronic autoimmune disorder. Synonyms for this condition are immune or autoimmune thrombocytopenic purpura (AITP; often used for chronic ITP in adults), Morbus Werlhof and purpura hemorrhagica. Pathophysiologically, it is characterized by early platelet destruction due to antibody binding and subsequent removal of platelets by the mononuclear phagocytic system. ITP also presents in association with other disorders such as infections or connective tissue diseases, or as thrombocytopenia after bone marrow transplantation. Moreover, ITP may also occur with alloimmune platelet destruction as observed in neonatal purpura and posttransfusion purpura. Finally, drug-induced ITP is seen more frequently in adults than in children.

History

In 1735, Werlhof described a bleeding disorder which he called morbus maculosus hemorrhagicus.[1] In 1883, Krauss observed decreased platelets and in 1890 Hayem performed the first platelet count and found a low number of platelets in the disease. The first splenectomy in ITP was successfully performed in Prague in 1916.[2] Subsequently, splenectomy became the main treatment for chronic ITP despite a lack of knowledge concerning the pathophysiologic role of the spleen in this disorder.

Since 1950 there has been increasing clinical evidence for an immunopathogenetic mechanism of ITP. In 1951, Harrington et al.[3,4] observed that newborns of mothers with chronic ITP often had a transient decrease in their platelet count, suggesting the transfer of a humoral antiplatelet factor from the mother to her baby. Harrington developed classical transient ITP after self-administration of plasma from a patient with ITP, as did other volunteers (Fig. 23.1A). Later, Shulman et al.[5] showed that the thrombocytopenic factor was associated with the 7S IgG fraction of ITP plasma and,

importantly, that this factor binds to autologous as well as homologous platelets. Since 1975, laboratory techniques have demonstrated elevated platelet-associated IgG in the majority of patients with thrombocytopenia.[6] In 1980, Imbach et al.[7] observed that the intravenous administration of intact 7S IgG, fractionated and pooled from single blood donors, raises the platelet count in patients with acute and chronic ITP (Fig. 23.1B). Two years later Salama et al.[8] described the use of anti-D-immunoglobulin in ITP.

In 1982, Van Leeuwen et al.[10] provided the first evidence for autoantibodies in chronic ITP. They reported that 32 of 42 eluates from ITP platelets would bind to normal but not to thrombasthenic platelets. Since these latter platelets are deficient in glycoproteins (Gp) IIb and IIIa, they postulated that ITP patients have autoantibodies to one of these glycoproteins. In 1987, two assays were developed that can detect both platelet-associated and free plasmic autoantibodies: the immunobead assay[11] and the monoclonal antibody-specific immobilization of platelet antigens (MAIPA) assay.[12]

In 1991, Semple and Freedman[13] documented that chronic ITP was associated with a CD4+ T-helper cell defect in which peripheral blood T cells secrete interleukin (IL)-2 on stimulation with autologous platelets. In 2000/2001, the role of phagocytosis and the Fcγ receptor in ITP was elucidated by the group of Ravetch.[14,15]

Incidence

ITP is diagnosed more frequently than any other form of destructive thrombocytopenia. In its acute form, it affects mostly children, while the chronic form is frequently seen in young adults. By arbitrary definition chronic ITP starts after the disease has been present for > 6 months. ITP is more common in white than black children and its severity and duration may display geographic variations.

Of children with ITP, 80–90% have an acute transient bleeding episode that resolves within a few days or weeks

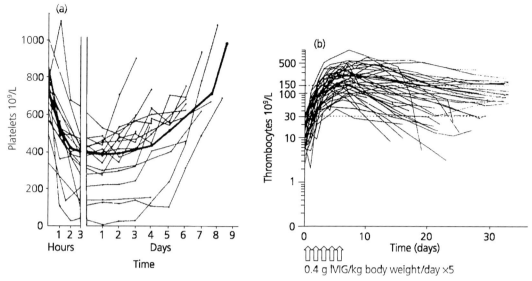

Fig. 23.1 (a) Platelet counts of volunteers after infusion of plasma from patients with immune thrombocytopenic purpura (ITP). (b) Platelet counts of 42 children with ITP during and after intravenous immunoglobulin (IVIG) treatment. Reproduced with permission from Ref. 9.

and, by definition, ends within 6 months. A prospective registry has documented a higher rate of acute ITP in boys than girls (54.8% vs. 45.2%) on all continents worldwide.[16] The male/female ratio was highest in infants and decreased with age.[17] Peak occurrence is between 2 and 5 years of age. There is frequently a history of viral or bacterial infection or vaccination 1–6 weeks prior to the onset of acute ITP. The onset of bleeding is often abrupt and is associated with a platelet count $< 20 \times 10^9$/L.

Chronic ITP in children manifests with similar clinical features to those seen in adults, i.e., the onset is usually insidious and there is a predominance among females.[16,18,19] Chronic ITP occurs significantly less frequently in infants (23.1%) than in children over 10 years of age (47.3%).[17]

The recurrent form of ITP is defined as episodes of thrombocytopenia at intervals of > 3 months and occurs in 1–4% of children with ITP.[20,21]

Familial ITP is a rare disorder[22–27] and the precise nature of inheritance remains unclear.

Pathogenesis

The clinical signs and symptoms of ITP are caused by an increased rate of premature platelet destruction, which occurs preferentially in the spleen, liver, bone marrow and lung. The severity of thrombocytopenia thus reflects the balance between platelet production by megakaryocytes and the accelerated clearance of sensitized platelets. Thrombocytopenic bleeding occurs when the platelet counts fall below $10–50 \times 10^9$/L.

The pathogenesis of acute ITP is regarded as a consequence of inappropriate immune recovery after an infection.

Circulating antigens or antibodies may alter the platelet membrane. Alternatively, immune complexes derived from primary or underlying disease processes may nonspecifically adsorb to platelet surfaces, resulting in opsonization and destruction of young platelets (Fig. 23.2).[27–31] Chronic ITP is attributed to autoantibodies directed against platelet constituents such as glycoproteins. Corroborating these findings, labeling studies[32,33] of autologous or homologous platelets using ^{51}Cr or ^{111}In-oxine have shown that platelet survival is decreased in patients with ITP.[34–39]

Platelet antigen and autoantibody

The main epitope for ITP-associated antibody binding lies on either the platelet GpIIb–IIIa or the GpIb–IX complex.[11,12,41,42] There is also evidence that some antibodies implicated in ITP bind to glycolipids.[43] The sensivity of platelet-associated antibody assays is 49–66% and the specificity 78–95%.[44–46] In a controlled laboratory study,[47] platelet and plasma samples from 67 children and 23 adults with chronic ITP were evaluated for glycoprotein autoantibodies. As shown in Table 23.1, platelet-associated autoantibodies were detected in 26 of 36 (72.2%) children with thrombocytopenia of the chronic form and in 15 of 31 (48.4%) with a history of ITP but normal platelet counts at the time of sampling. Of 23 adults with chronic ITP, 12 of 18 (66.7%) with thrombocytopenia displayed platelet-associated antibodies. A significant correlation was noted between the platelet-associated autoantibody level and the patient's age at the time of diagnosis. Children with high platelet-associated autoantibody levels were older, with a mean age of 12.4 years (range 8–17 years) compared with an average age of 7.1 years (range 1–16) for children with moderate or negative autoantibody levels.

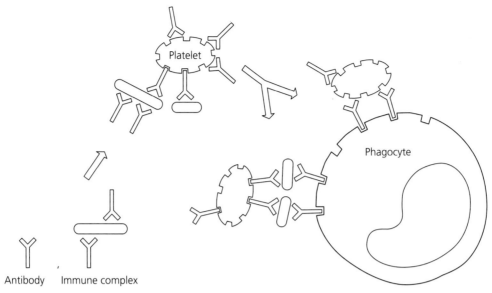

Fig. 23.2 Pathogenic aspects of platelet opsonization and phagocytosis. Reproduced with permission from Ref. 40.

Table 23.1 Antiglycoprotein antiplatelet autoantibody in chronic immune thrombocytopenic purpura (ITP).

	Ongoing ITP*	Prior ITP†
Children (n = 67)		
Autoantibody level‡ elevated	26/36	15/31
Autoantibody level‡ negative	10/36	16/31
Adults (n = 23)		
Autoantibody level‡ elevated	12/18	4/5
Autoantibody level‡ negative	6/18	1/5

* Ongoing ITP: platelet count at time of sampling < 150 × 10⁹/L.
† Prior ITP: history of platelet count < 50 × 10⁹/L for at least 6 months but with normal counts, without therapy, at the end of sampling.
‡ Autoantibody level: ratio of patient autoantibody value to that of the mean control value plus 3 standard deviations.
Reproduced with permission from Ref. 47.

These data suggest that there may be different forms of childhood ITP. Younger children with moderate autoantibody levels appear to have an increased likelihood of spontaneous remission or compensated disease with a platelet count > 20–150 × 10⁹/L. The course of adolescents with high autoantibody levels seems similar to that of adults, in whom spontaneous remission or compensation of ITP is unusual. In the above study,[47] children with a history of chronic ITP but normal platelet counts at the time of blood sampling had elevated autoantibody levels. This suggests a compensated form of ITP. However, recurrence of disease is likely to occur if this balance is altered by factors that decrease platelet production (i.e., viral infection) or that increase autoantibody production and/or platelet consumption.

Furthermore, the offspring of a mother with the compensated stage of ITP and platelet autoantibodies may be at risk of neonatal thrombocytopenia.

Platelet destruction

The mechanisms of platelet destruction are outlined in Fig. 23.2. The rapid destruction of platelets is due to either autoantibodies that bind via the antigenic site or immune complexes that bind via Fc receptors on platelets. These opsonized cells are rapidly removed by cells of the mononuclear phagocytic system. The quantity of antibodies correlates with the degree of thrombocytopenia.[48] Phagocytosis of platelets has been demonstrated by *in vivo* studies using reticuloendothelial blockade with monoclonal anti-Fc receptor antibodies.[49] The role of complement is documented by increased platelet-associated C4 and C3. *In vitro* studies show binding of C4 and C3 followed by platelet lysis after incubation of platelets with patients' plasma and fresh serum.[50]

For effective platelet destruction, there must be sufficient antigens and autoantibodies on platelets. The specific anatomic configuration of the spleen is optimal for engulfment and subsequent phagocytosis.[51] In some patients with ITP, the reticuloendothelial system of the liver may also be efficient in removing platelets. In the bone marrow, thrombopoiesis and intramedullary platelet destruction could be concomitantly inhibited as there is antibody production[52] and antibody binding to platelets and megakaryocytes.[53] In addition, platelet kinetic studies showing decreased platelet delivery into the bloodstream suggest that intramedullary events may also be critical for clinical disease in many patients with ITP.[39,54,55]

In addition, at the level of apoptosis, Fas (CD95) antibodies

Table 23.2 Defects related to cellular immunity in chronic immune thrombocytopenic purpura.

Antigen-specific autoantibodies[60,61]	↑
Lymphocyte defects	
Phenotype	
CD19+ or CD20+CD5+ B cells[13,62]	↑
CD3+DR+ T cells[13,63,64]	↑
CD3+CD57+ T cells[65]	↑
CD3−CD57+ NK cells[65]	↑
Function	
PHA stimulation of PBMC[13,63,64,66,67]	Normal or ↑
Platelet induced IL-2 secretion[13,68]	↑
T-cell-mediated autoantibody production[69]	↑
T-suppressor cells[70]	↓
NK-mediated cytolysis[71,72]	↓

PHA, phytohemagglutinin; PBMC, peripheral blood mononuclear cell; NK, natural killer.

Reproduced with permission from Ref. 59.

result in prolonged persistence of lymphocytes and autoantibody production in patients with ITP as well as in those with autoimmune lymphoproliferative syndrome.[56–58]

Immune regulation

Normally, the immune response to an antigenic challenge is well regulated. Initiated by antigen-presenting cells, the pathways of humoral and cell-mediated immunity are activated via cell–cell interactions and lymphokine production resulting, among other events, in the generation of cytotoxic T-effector cells and the secretion of specific antibodies. Regulatory mechanisms, possibly involving suppressor T cells and antiidiotypic antibodies, downmodulate the degree and duration of the immune response to a specific stimulus.

In ITP, the maintenance of self-tolerance and the effective immune response may be altered in the presence of an inflammatory process directed at another target cell than platelets. As shown in Table 23.2 and Fig. 23.3, multiple defects related to cellular immunity have been described in patients with ITP.[13,59–74] Enhanced serum levels of HLA-DR molecules have been detected.[75–77] In acute ITP, the transient increase in surface expression of HLA-DR molecules may be induced by proinflammatory cytokines such as interferon (IFN)-γ. As a consequence of immune activation, increased serum levels of IL-2 have been observed in various autoimmune disorders, including ITP.[71,78–83] In parallel, high levels of IL-10 have also been detected. IL-10 is a potent stimulator of human B cells[84] and downmodulates the production of inflammatory cytokines by T cells (Th1) and monocytes/macrophages.[85] Increased serum concentrations of IL-2, IFN and/or IL-10 reflecting *in vivo* T-cell activation have been observed in patients with chronic ITP, but not in those with

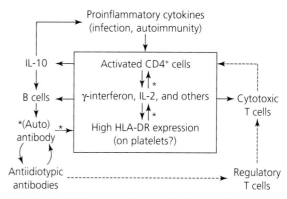

Fig. 23.3 Model of the immunopathogenesis of acute and chronic immune thrombocytopenic purpura (ITP). Dotted line represents hypothetical feedback. * Only in chronic ITP. Reproduced with permission from Ref. 88.

the acute form.[71,86] Moreover, an increased serum concentration of IL-2 in chronic ITP correlates significantly with *in vitro* IL-2 secretion by platelet-stimulated T-helper cells.[71]

The difference in serum detection of IFN-γ, IL-2 and IL-10 expression suggests that different mechanisms operate in the pathogenesis of chronic versus acute ITP. It has been proposed that acute ITP may be due to a cross-reactive immune response directed against an infectious agent.[87] In contrast, chronic ITP may be perpetuated by a constant HLA-DR-stimulated immune response with enhanced cytokine production, increased activation of T cells, increased production of specific autoantibodies (Fig. 23.3) and disturbed apoptosis by prolonged persistence of lymphocytes.[56,57] Therefore, both forms of ITP appear to result from an altered feedback mechanism critical for the termination of an immune response.

Clinical features and diagnosis

In the majority of children with acute ITP, thrombocytopenia occurs within 1–3 weeks after an infectious disease. Commonly, the infection is a bacterial or nonspecific viral (upper respiratory or gastrointestinal) infection. ITP may also occur after rubella, rubeola, chickenpox or live virus vaccination. The hemorrhagic manifestations depend on the degree of thrombocytopenia (Table 23.3) and are individually different. Common first signs of bleeding are easy bruising and skin petechiae. These signs occur with platelet counts below 20×10^9/L. Severe mucosal bleeding, hematuria and genital bleeding usually occur with platelet counts below 10×10^9/L. Adolescent girls may have prolonged menorrhagia. Intracranial hemorrhage (ICH) occurs in 0.5–1% of hospitalized children with ITP and is fatal in one-third.[89] The risk is greater during the initial days of thrombocytopenia but can occur at any time in ongoing ITP[90] and is also observed under various therapies. Salicylate-containing medications or antihistamines may increase the risk of bleeding.[89]

Table 23.3 Staging due to platelet count and clinical manifestation and intervention guidelines in children with immune thrombocytopenic purpura.

Stage	Symptoms	Platelet count (× 10⁹/L)	Management
1	Normal daily life	> 20–150	Consent for observation
2	Troublesome bleeding	> 10–20	Punctual intervention to reach stage 1
3	Bleeding, ↓ hemoglobin	< 20	Intervention

The characteristic features of history, physical examination and laboratory analysis are summarized in Table 23.4. Apart from bleeding and thrombocytopenia, there should be no other abnormal physical findings. Bone marrow examination is not necessary in patients displaying the typical signs and symptoms of ITP. In one study, 127 children with ITP diagnosed clinically were subjected to bone marrow examination but only five (4%) had abnormal cytologic findings not compatible with the diagnosis of ITP, and on closer examination all five had additional atypical features on presentation.[91] Importantly, bone marrow examination is indicated for establishing the diagnosis in patients who fail to respond to treatment after 3–6 months.

Differential diagnosis

Initially, ITP has to be differentiated from other forms of thrombocytopenic bleeding disorders (Table 23.5). The bleeding manifestations in ITP are similar in presentation to the findings in patients with thrombocytopenia associated, for example, with bone marrow hypoproliferation. A decreased mean platelet volume suggests marrow hypoproduction of platelets or indicates findings characteristic of Wiskott–Aldrich syndrome. If there is anemia and leukocyte abnormalities, a bone marrow examination is required to rule out marrow diseases such as acute leukemia, aplastic anemia, myelodysplasia, lymphoma or metastatic disease. Autoimmune hemolysis, if suspected, can be confirmed by a Coombs test. If risk factors are present for human immunodeficiency virus (HIV) infection, serologic testing must be performed. Thrombotic thrombocytopenic purpura and hemolytic–uremic syndrome can be distinguished by the presence of hemolysis, a negative Coombs test, and microangiopathic red cell changes. Disseminated intravascular coagulation is associated with characteristic coagulation abnormalities. Splenomegaly may indicate hypersplenism.

Clinical course

Independent of treatment, complete remission of ITP occurs in 80–90% of children within 6 months and in over 90% within 3–37 years (Fig. 23.4).[18,19,93–95] The 3–5% of children

Table 23.4 Elements of the history, physical examination and peripheral blood analysis in a child with suspected immune thrombocytopenic purpura.

History
Bleeding symptoms
  Type of bleeding
  Severity of bleeding
  Duration of bleeding
  History of prior bleedings
Systemic symptoms
  Especially of recent (within 6 weeks) infectious illness
  Exposure or vaccination or recurrent infections suggesting immunodeficiency
  Symptoms of an autoimmune disorder
Medications
  Heparin, sulfonamides and quinidine/quinine, which may cause thrombocytopenia
  Aspirin, which may exacerbate bleeding
Risk of HIV infection, including maternal HIV status
Family history of thrombocytopenia or hematologic disorder
In an infant < 6 months old, include perinatal and maternal history
Comorbid conditions, which may increase the risk of bleeding
Lifestyle, including vigorous and potentially traumatic activities

Physical examination
Bleeding signs
  Type of bleeding (including retinal hemorrhages)
  Severity of bleeding
Liver, spleen and lymph nodes
Evidence of infection
Presence of dysmorphic features suggestive of congenital disorder, including skeletal anomalies, auditory acuity
Exclude specific congenital syndromes
  Fanconi syndrome
  Thrombocytopenia with absent radii
  Wiskott–Aldrich syndrome
  Alport syndrome (and its variants)
  Bernard–Soulier syndrome
  May–Hegglin anomaly
  Gray platelet syndrome

Peripheral blood analysis
Thrombocytopenia: platelets are normal in size or may appear larger than normal, but consistently giant platelets (approaching the size of red blood cells) should be absent
Normal red blood cell morphology
Normal white blood morphology, normal reticulocyte count

Reproduced with permission from Ref. 92.

who do not display remission have chronic ITP (Table 23.6). Children who have chronic ITP are mostly over 7 years of age and are rarely those with postinfectious ITP. Recurrent ITP, defined as periodic episodes of thrombocytopenia at intervals of > 3 months, occurs in 4% of children with acute ITP.[20,21] In children with persistent ITP of 3–6 months' duration, additional laboratory testing is indicated (Table 23.7).

ICH occurs in 0.5–1% of hospitalized children with ITP and is fatal in one-third despite treatment with corticosteroids[89]

Table 23.5 Differential diagnosis in childhood thrombocytopenia.

	Onset	MPV	PAlgG	Coagulation	Marrow	Other
Destructive thrombocytopenia						
ITP	Sudden	Increased	Increased	ND	ND	–
Wiskott–Aldrich	Insidious	Decreased*	Increased	ND	ND	–
HIV-ITP	Variable	Increased	Increased	ND	ND	HIV positive*
DIC, TTP, HUS	Sudden	Increased	Increased	Diagnostic*	ND	–
Hypersplenism	Insidious	Increased	ND	ND	ND	Splenomegaly*
ALPS	Insidious	Increased	Increased	ND	ND	Fas (CD95) low
Decreased production						
Amegakaryocytic	Insidious	Decreased	ND	ND	Diagnostic*	± Radius*
Aplastic anemia	Insidious	Decreased	ND	ND	Diagnostic*	–
Myelodysplasia	Insidious	Decreased	ND	ND	Diagnostic*	–
Acute leukemia	Insidious	Decreased	ND	ND	Diagnostic*	–
Lymphoma	Insidious	Decreased	ND	ND	Diagnostic*	–
Metastatic disease	Insidious	Decreased	Variable	ND	Diagnostic	–

* Characteristic.

ALPS, autoimmune lymphoproliferative syndrome; DIC, disseminated intravascular coagulation; HIV, human immunodeficiency virus; HUS, hemolytic–uremic syndrome; ITP, immune thrombocytopenic purpura; MPV, mean platelet volume; ND, nondiagnostic; PAlgG, plasma-associated IgG; TTP, thrombotic thrombocytopenic purpura.

Table 23.6 Summary of the clinical course of immune thrombocytopenic purpura from a series of 12 reports.*

No. of children	Remission at 6 months without treatment[†]	Remission at 6 months[‡]	ICH (fatal)	Other deaths	Persisten ITP after 6–12 months'	Spontaneous remission	Deaths
1693	389/467 (83%)	1207/1597 (76%)	16 (13) 0.9% (0.7%)	4 (0.2%)	179 (10.6%)	66/179 (37%)	3 (2%)

* Data from Refs 93, 95, 96–105.

† Number of patients managed without specific initial therapy. The response rate for untreated patients is greater than the overall response at 6 months because of selection of patients with good prognostic features for no treatment.

‡ A different denominator from the original number of patients indicates that some patients were not followed long enough to be included in the estimate. ICH, intracranial hemorrhage.

Reproduced with permission from Ref. 92.

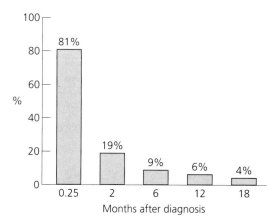

Fig. 23.4 Clinical course of immune thrombocytopenic purpura (ITP) in children. Percentage of children with ITP and platelet counts < 20 × 10⁹/L at 2, 6, 12 and 18 months after diagnosis. Swiss Canadian retrospective analysis (*n* = 554). Reproduced with permission from Ref. 106.

Table 23.7 Routine testing in addition to initial laboratory analysis in children with persistent immune thrombocytopenic purpura of 3–6 months' duration.

Bone marrow analysis, endocrine function, urine analysis, abdominal ultrasound

Antinuclear antibody, direct antiglobin, lupus anticoagulant, platelet antigen-specific antibodies, serum immunoglobulins with IgG subclasses, platelet function test, coagulation studies

Viral serology (HIV, CMV, EBV, VZV, rubeola, parvovirus B19 and others)

CMV, cytomegalovirus; EBV, Epstein–Barr virus; HIV, human immunodeficiency virus; VZV, varicella zoster virus.

or intravenous immunoglobulin (IVIG).[107] Postsplenectomy sepsis constitutes the other major cause of death in children with ITP (Table 23.6). Only limited observational data are available regarding the complications of ICH. In a review of

531

14 children with ICH, Woerner *et al.*[89] reported that four children died and two others may have had neurologic long-term effects. Of 30 children with ICH described in a retrospective study by the American Society of Hematology,[92] this complication occurred in 12 patients (40%) within 12 days after diagnosis, including in two with a history of head trauma. ICH in the other 18 patients occurred after 1 month to 5 years of diagnosis, and was typically associated with the administration of glucocorticoids and/or splenectomy subsequent to a lack of remission. At least 24 of these 30 patients were reported prior to 1981 when the benefits of IVIG therapy in ITP were initially described.[7] This finding argues against immunosuppression and/or splenectomy in the long-term treatment of ITP.

Unlike ITP in adults, persistent thrombocytopenia is uncommon in children. In the 12 series summarized in Table 23.6, ITP resolved in 1207 (76%) of the 1597 children. Clinical features of the presenting illness and parameters associated with an increased risk of chronic persistent thrombocytopenia included a history of purpura for more than 2–4 weeks before diagnosis,[93,94,96–98,107] female sex,[93,95,99,100] age over 10 years,[95,99,100] and a platelet count at presentation in excess of 20×10^9/L.[95] The fate of children with chronic ITP is uncertain, although about one-third appear to have spontaneous remission several months to many years after diagnosis (Fig. 23.4).[93,108–111]

Management

General aspects

Parents and the child/adolescent with ITP are often worried about bleeding. They are concerned by low platelet counts and perturbed by lifestyle restrictions.[112] On the other hand, the physician knows the low risk of severe bleeding but cannot indicate prognostic risk factors and the real origin of the disorder. The Intercontinental Childhood ITP Study (ICIS) Registry II entitled "Frequency, location and timing of hemorrhage in children with newly diagnosed ITP"[113] collected 1015 children prospectively. From this cohort, 629 children initially had platelet counts $\leq 20 \times 10^9$/L: 20/629 (3.2%) had severe bleeding, 150 (23.6%) moderate and 459 (73%) mild or no bleeding, which is in accordance with the British assessment[114] and the single-center analysis in the USA.[115] Some experienced hematologists[116,117] and the British guidelines[114] would only give medical treatment to a patient with severe or troublesome bleeding.

With this in mind, treatment is indicated in children either at risk, or with overt signs, of bleeding. Table 23.3 summarizes the recommendations for the treatment of ITP in children according to a staging system. Hospitalization is required for severe bleeding regardless of the platelet count. Treatment is indicated for a child with troublesome bleeding

and a platelet count below 20×10^9/L (stage 2). The goal is to reach stage 1, where no active intervention/treatment but observation is recommended. In stage 1, the physician should obtain consent from the individual patient/parents for observation in the presence of normal daily life. Therapeutic measures in the acute management of ITP should be maintained until bleeding has ceased and the platelet count has reached hemostatic levels (i.e., $> 20 \times 10^9$/L). However, continued treatment beyond this defined point is not indicated. Moreover, it also seems unnecessary to treat patients without signs of bleeding and with platelet counts in excess of $10–20 \times 10^9$/L.

Recent insight into the immunopathogenesis of ITP (see above) has formed the clinical base for novel therapeutic strategies. The therapy of ITP focuses on measures modulating the immune response and includes IVIG,[7,118] anti-Rh(D) immunoglobulin,[119] monoclonal anti-CD20 antibody (rituximab),[120] and eventually IFN-α.[121] Immunosuppressive treatment with corticosteroids[122–124] is used as an alternative therapeutic strategy and cytostatic agents,[125–132] splenectomy,[93–100,107–109,133–136] and other treatment possibilities are only indicated in special situations. The mechanisms of action of the therapies employed in ITP have been recently reviewed by Cines and Blanchette.[137]

The following recommendations focus on children with bleeding symptoms (stage 2 or 3; see Table 23.3) and are generally in accordance with the practical guidelines of the American Society of Hematology for diagnosis and treatment of ITP.[92]

There is a considerable amount of convincing evidence-based data available on incidence, demographics, natural history and management of ITP. Retrospective case series,[92] surveys,[138,139] guidelines,[140,141] assessments,[114] reports from expert meetings,[142] and consensus conferences[143,144] are the sources of information for patient management. As a result of the heterogeneity of ITP and various controversies, current practice does not always follow the recommendations. Prospective evidence-based studies are needed. Since 1997 the ICIS group has been establishing an international network of physicians and scientists collaborating in prospective databases and studies (see www.unibas.ch/itpbasel) that will define less heterogeneous patient subgroups for controlled treatment efficacy trials. Indeed, the first results are promising.[16,17,145,146] The ongoing Pediatric and Adult Registry of Chronic ITP database for children and adults with ITP has the objective of defining subgroups within ITP on the basis of natural history, genetics, quality of life and other criteria. One of the side studies will focus on genetic differences. In these studies, polymorphisms and variations of genes[147,148] in patients with ITP, which might be involved in loss of tolerance and unbalanced immune responses, have shown variants in IL-1 haplotypes and association with autoimmune disease.

Table 23.8 Immediate response rate (platelet count $> 20 \times 10^9$/L) to different treatment regimens.[150,151]

Randomized group	Rapid responders (≥ 72 hours) (%)
No treatment	9/16 (56)
Intravenous anti-Rh(D) 25 µg/kg for 2 days	31/38 (82)
Corticosteroids 4 mg/kg daily for 7 days	45/57 (79)
Intravenous immunoglobulin 1 g/kg daily for 2 days	50/53 (94)
Intravenous immunoglobulin 0.8 g/kg once	34/35 (97)

Acute bleeding

Acute bleeding in children with ITP (stage 2 or 3; see Table 23.3) may warrant a rapid increase in platelets. As a follow-up of earlier studies,[149] two Canadian multicenter studies prospectively analyzed children diagnosed with acute ITP and platelet counts below 20×10^9/L.[150,151] The first study compared treatment using IVIG or corticosteroids with no intervention.[150] The second trial randomized treatment with IVIG, oral corticosteroids or intravenous anti-Rh(D).[151] The results are summarized in Table 23.8, which details specifically the effect of each therapeutic regimen within 72 hours after initiation. Both studies demonstrated that IVIG produced the fastest recovery to safe, hemostatic platelet counts. Treatment with corticosteroids 4 mg/kg body weight given daily for 7 days was recommended as the second choice. However, long-term corticosteroid treatment in children should be avoided due to unacceptable side-effects. In addition, the second study found that a single dose of IVIG 0.8 g/kg was sufficient and comparable to the more traditional larger dose of 2 g/kg given over 48 hours. Treatment with the lower IVIG dose decreases the duration and cost of hospitalization. Based on these findings, the American Society of Hematology panel recommends the use of IVIG in preference to corticosteroids for the treatment of children with ITP.[92]

Table 23.9 summarizes studies of the effectiveness of corticosteroids, IVIG and anti-Rh(D), and Table 23.10 shows standard treatment regimens and dosages.

Emergency treatment

Severe life-threatening bleeding justifies intervention, including IVIG (0.8–1 g/kg per dose), high-dose intravenous methylprednisolone 30 mg/kg or dexamethasone 1–2 mg/kg, and platelet transfusions. The latter should be given as a third line of treatment because transfused platelets may survive longer *in vivo* after IVIG and/or corticosteroid administration. Emergency splenectomy in urgent life-threatening bleeding is not recommended.[92]

Mild bleeding and long-term bleeding problems

Children with a history of mild bleeding or recurrent bleeding should receive treatment aimed at maintaining their platelet count at a level that renders them free of symptoms (stage 1; see Tables 23.3 and 23.10). This level is individual and patients at increased risk of hemorrhage (i.e., those playing contact sports, undergoing surgery, etc.) may benefit from additional therapy. Recommended treatment modalities are IVIG (0.4–0.8 g/kg at 2–8 week intervals) or corticosteroids (2–4 mg/kg for 4 days). Children and adolescents who fail to respond to IVIG or corticosteroids, i.e., do not maintain safe platelet counts, may benefit from one of the following treatment regimens (see below): anti-Rh(D), IFN-α or, in special circumstances, plasma exchange, protein A immunoadsorption of antibodies or administration of cytostatic agents. The role of ascorbic acid in the treatment of ITP remains uncertain.

Prolonged response to long-term cyclic treatment versus natural course of ITP

The long-term effects of treatment in ITP must be interpreted with caution, since the natural history of ITP in children and in some young adults is one of gradual spontaneous resolution.[106,110,111,158] Several studies have reported that patients with chronic ITP display long-lasting recovery (sustained platelet counts $> 20 \times 10^9$/L) when treated with repeated courses of IVIG (Table 23.10)[160–162] with a high-dose cyclic dexamethasone regimen or with methylprednisolone.[124,157,159,163] Andersen[124] treated 10 adults with persistent symptomatic ITP with six cycles of oral dexamethasone (40 mg/day for 4 days every 4 weeks). All patients demonstrated a therapeutic response with platelet counts $> 100 \times 10^9$/L for at least 6 months after completion of treatment. Adult patients tolerated this treatment well. In contrast, children with chronic ITP given a comparable dexamethasone regimen demonstrated not only a less impressive response to treatment but also suffered significant side-effects (fatigue, weight gain, difficulty in sleeping, significant behavioral changes, hyperadrenocorticism, transient increase of blood glucose levels).[164] Based on these observations, there is a need for adequately controlled studies to determine whether long-term or cyclic treatments can alter the natural course of chronic ITP in children.

Refractory ITP

A minority of children have the refractory chronic form of ITP with bleeding problems (stage 2 or 3; see Table 23.3). The aim of management is to reach stage 1 ITP with minimal intervention and to prevent bleeding. If bleeding is not under control, other medical treatment options (see below and Table 23.12) or splenectomy has to be considered.

Table 23.9 Effectiveness of corticosteroids, intravenous immunoglobulin (IVIG) and anti-Rh(D).

	Study population				Outcome			
Reference	Number	Age	Follow-up	Randomized treatment arms	Outcome measure	Outcome result	Adverse effects
152	27	6 years (mean)	NR	Prednisone (2 mg/kg daily for 21 days)	Median time to platelet count of 150 x 10^9/L	21 days	NR
				No treatment		60 days ($P \le 0.3$)	NR
153	93	6 months to 16 years	> 6 months	Prednisone (60 mg/m^2 daily for 21 days, then tapered)	Proportion with platelet count > 30 and > 100 x 10^9/L, and negative Rumpel–Leede test	Prednisone > placebo ($P < 0.01$)	NR
				Placebo			
154	27	< 11 years	28 days	Prednisone (2 mg/kg daily for 14 days, then tapered to day 21)	Platelet count, bleeding time, clinical bleeding score at day 0–28	Prednisone > placebo ($P < 0.05$) only at day 7	Increased appetite, weight gain
				Placebo			
149	94	< 16 years	1 year	Prednisone (60 mg/m^2 daily for 21 days, follow-up protocol for poor response/remissions)	Proportion with platelet count > 100 x 10^9/L	77%	77% with weight gain or acne
				IVIG (0.4 g/kg daily for 5 days, follow-up protocol for poor response/remissions)		83% (no difference)	22% with headache, fever, vomiting, vertigo
155	61	2–12 years	> 6 months	Prednisone (0.5 mg/kg daily for 1 month or until platelet normalization)	Proportion with platelet count > 150 x 10^9/L	62%	NR
				Prednisone (1.5 mg/kg daily for 1 month or until platelet normalization)		81% ($P < 0.05$)	NR
156	160	< 15 years	> 12 months	Prednisone (0.25 mg/kg daily for 3 weeks)	Proportion with platelet count > 100 x 10^9/L for > 3 months	71%	NR
				Prednisone (1 mg/kg daily for 3 weeks)		77% (no difference)	NR

Ref.	Age range	Follow-up	Treatment regimen	Outcome measure	Results	Adverse effects
157	2 months to 15 years	> 6 months	Methylprednisolone (10 mg/kg i.v. daily for 5 days) Prednisone (2 mg/kg daily for 4 weeks) IVIG (0.4 g/kg daily for 5 days)	Mean platelet count on days 1–14	Methylprednisolone = IVIG > prednisone ($P < 0.001$)	NR NR NR
158	2 months to 11 years	> 6 months	Methylprednisolone (30 mg/kg p.o. daily for 3 days, then 20 mg/kg daily for 4 days) IVIG (0.4 g/kg daily for 5 days)	Proportion with platelet count > 150 x 10^9/L at 3 days and 6 months	60%, 90% (no difference) 60%, 75%	NR NR
150	7 months to 14 years	180 days	Prednisone (4 mg/kg daily for 7 days, then tapered to day 21) IVIG (1 g/kg daily for 2 days) No therapy	Median time to platelet count > 20, > 50 x 10^9/L	2 days, 4 days 1 day, 2 days ($P < 0.01$ vs. prednisone) 4 days, 16 days ($P < 0.1$ vs. either treatment)	Weight gain, behavioral change, 75% with nausea, vomiting, headache, fever
151	6 months to 18 years	6–32 months	Prednisone (4 mg/kg daily for 7 days, then tapered to day 21) IVIG (1 g/kg daily for 2 days) IVIG (0.8 g/kg once only) Anti-Rh(D) (25 µg/kg daily for 2 days)	Median time to platelet count > 20, > 50 x 10^9/L	2 days, 3 days 2 days, 2 days 1 day, 2 days ($P < 0.05$ vs prednisone) 2 days, 2.5 days ($P < 0.05$ vs. both IVIG regimens)	None 16–18% with fever, nausea, vomiting, headache 24% with hemoglobin < 10 g/dL
159	2 months to 17 years	6 months	Methylprednisolone (30 mg/kg p.o. daily for 7 days) Methylprednisolone (50 mg/kg p.o. daily for 7 days) IVIG (0.5 g/kg daily for 5 days)	Mean platelet count on days 0–30	Mean > 100 x 10^9/L by day 4. No difference among groups	Increased appetite and Cushingoid appearance Increased appetite and Cushingoid appearance 1 patient with aseptic meningitis, 2 with headache, vomiting

NR, not reported.
Reproduced with permission from Ref. 92.

Table 23.10 Standard treatment modalities for children with immune thrombocytopenic purpura.

Intravenous immunoglobulin (IVIG)
Initial treatment: 0.8 g/kg once. Repeat the same dose if platelet count is < 30×10^9/L on day 3 (72 hours after first infusion)
In emergency bleeding: 1–2 times 0.8 g/kg, eventually together with corticosteroids and platelet transfusion Treatment in chronic ITP: 0.4 g/kg once every 2–8 weeks

Corticosteroids
Prednisone 4 mg/kg daily orally or intravenously for 7 days, then tapering over a 7-day period
In emergency bleeding: methylprednisolone 8–12 mg/kg i.v. or dexamethasone 0.5–1.0 mg/kg i.v. or orally, together with IVIG or platelet transfusion

Anti-Rh(D) antibody
50 μg/kg i.v.

Specific treatment modalities

Standard treatment (see Table 23.10)

Immunoglobulin

IVIG treatment of children with ITP (platelet count < 20×10^9/L) resulted in a quicker and more extensive increase in platelet counts compared with patients receiving corticosteroid therapy.[7,149–151,161,162] Importantly, a single daily dose of IVIG 0.8 g/kg appears to have the identical initial effect as five IVIG doses of 0.4 g/kg or two IVIG doses of 1.0 g/kg given each day.[151] Adverse effects noted with IVIG include flu-like symptoms such as headache, backache, nausea and fever.[150,151,165,166] Aseptic transient meningitis is a rare complication.[160] It is important to use quality-controlled, commercially available (not experimental) intact 7S IgG preparations from which there is no risk of hepatitis infection.[167–170]

Mechanism of action
Following the observation that IVIG is clinically effective, it was hypothesized that the inhibition of platelet destruction by phagocytosis may have resulted from blockade of Fc receptors (FcRs).[171,172] FcRs are expressed on a range of cells and are functionally important for scavenging immunoglobulin-sensitized cells such as platelets. The plausibility of this explanation is underscored by the finding that anti-Rh(D)-coated erythrocytes also show prolonged survival with IVIG treatment.[172] A decrease in leukocyte counts or the size of the various lymphocyte subpopulations is inversely proportional to the platelet counts during IVIG treatment.[173,174] These observations suggest that not only FcRs on mononuclear phagocytes but also those on other cells are affected by IVIG infusion. In a murine model of passive ITP, Samuelsson et al.[175] demonstrated that IVIG requires the presence of the inhibitory low-affinity IgG receptor Fcγ RIIB and that monocytes from IVIG-treated mice begin to express Fcγ RIIB at increased levels within 4 hours of IVIG exposure. Since the humoral immune response *in vivo* works in concert with the cellular immune response and vice versa, IVIG could modulate the synthesis and release of cytokines from FcR-bearing lymphocytes and monocytes.[59,176,177] *In vitro*, IgG administration induces downregulation of IL-6, IL-2, IL-10, IFN-γ and tumor necrosis factor (TNF)-β in lipopolysaccharide-stimulated monocytes, and reduces IL-2 receptor expression in activated lymphocytes.[178,179] In ITP, overproduction of IL-4 has been reported in one study,[180] while high levels of IL-2, IL-10, IFN-γ and TNF-α have been described in other studies.[76,181] Availability of FcRs may be altered by IgG dimers or larger complexes in the IVIG preparations, or by erythrocyte alloantibodies.[182] Inhibition of complement activation by IVIG is another possible mechanism of action.[183] In addition, at the level of apoptosis,[56,57] antiidiotypic Fas (CD95) antibodies in IVIG stop the prolonged persistence of lymphocytes and autoantibody production in patients with ITP as well as in those with autoimmune lymphoproliferative syndrome.[184]

Long-term effects following IVIG administration (Table 23.11) may be induced by antiidiotypic antibodies. As mentioned above, antibodies against GpIIb–IIIa and GpIb–IX can be identified in 70–80% of children and adults with chronic ITP.[11,47] It has been demonstrated that IVIG contains antiidiotypic antibodies against anti-GpIIb–IIIa autoantibodies and these inhibit the binding of autoantibodies to platelet GpIIb–IIIa.[185] Thus, restoration of the balance within the antiidiotype network or, alternatively, suppression of secretion of antiidiotypic antibodies may lead to long-term improvement of ITP.[186–188] In this context, it is of note that the size of the donor pool from which IVIG is prepared may be relevant, as the chance that a given antibody idiotype is recognized and bound by a complementary antiidiotypic antibody is obviously dependent on the donor-pool size.[189]

Table 23.11 Studies showing long-term improvement for therapy with intravenous immunoglobulin.

Study	Total in study	Long-term improvement
Children		
Imholz et al.[161]	42	22 (52%)
Bussel et al.[190]	12	5 (42%)
Adults		
Bussel et al.[191]	40	16 (40%)
Godeau et al.[192]	18	7 (39%)

Corticosteroids

The mechanism of action of corticosteroids in ITP remains uncertain. Corticosteroids may inhibit the phagocytosis of antibody-bearing platelets[193] and may suppress antibody production by B lymphocytes.[194,195] Other indirect mechanisms may account for the beneficial therapeutic effect of corticosteroids: maintenance of capillary integrity[196–203] or inhibition of vascular prostacyclin synthesis leading to normalization of the possible prolonged bleeding time in ITP.[204,205]

In randomized clinical trials,[150,151] the median time to achieve a platelet count $> 50 \times 10^9/L$ was 4 days if patients received prednisone 4 mg/kg daily for 7 days. In contrast, children receiving no treatment displayed comparable platelet counts only 16 days after onset of disease. The higher dosage of steroids (4 mg/kg daily) is preferable to the classical dose of 2 mg/kg daily of oral prednisone for 21 days[122,154–156] because the side-effects are fewer and less extensive. Methylprednisolone in very high doses for several days (10–30 mg/kg oral or intravenous methylprednisolone daily) has been administered in uncontrolled studies and resulted in a dramatic increase in platelet counts with long-term improvement in some but not all patients.[123,159,163,206–209] Adverse effects include signs and symptoms of hypercortisolism, such as facial swelling, weight gain, hyperglycemia, hypertension and behavioral abnormalities. Long-term application of high corticosteroid dosages has the risk of growth retardation and cataracts,[210] and should thus be avoided. Sustained corticosteroid doses of 0.5–0.7 mg/kg daily may suppress platelet formation as well.[211,212]

Anti-Rh(D) immunoglobulin

The rationale for using anti-Rh(D) as a therapeutic measure in ITP is based on the hypothesis that an increase in platelet count following IVIG therapy may be due to competitive inhibition of the monocyte/phagocyte system as effected by the preferential sequestration of autologous erythrocytes sensitized by alloantibodies present in the IgG preparations. Indeed, a clinical trial by Salama *et al.*[213] demonstrated a clinical effect. Administration of anti-Rh(D) globulin to Rh-positive patients with ITP resulted in a significant increase in platelet counts ($> 20 \times 10^9/L$) in 6 of 10 patients. Other uncontrolled studies have demonstrated that anti-Rh(D) treatment may increase the platelet count in approximately 80% of Rh-positive children.[214–217] However, a controlled clinical study showed that anti-Rh(D) therapy was less effective in comparison with IVIG or corticosteroids, demonstrating a prolonged delay in achieving platelet counts of $20 \times 10^9/L$ as well as $50 \times 10^9/L$.[151] The therapeutic effect of antiRh(D) usually lasts for 1–5 weeks and appears to depend on the presence of an intact spleen.

The recommended dose is 50 µg/kg intravenously. Adverse effects include alloimmune hemolysis. With this

Table 23.12 Treatment options in refractory immune thrombocytopenic purpura (see text for dosage and other details).

Current treatment options
Vinca alkaloids
Azathioprine
Cyclophosphamide
Cyclic high-dose corticosteroids
Danazol
Plasmapheresis or protein A immunoadsorption
Ascorbic acid (vitamin C)
Splenectomy

Recent treatment options
Treatment influencing antigenemia
Treatment influencing the T-cell immune response: ciclosporin, CTLA-4-Ig
Treatment influencing the B-cell immune response: anti-CD20 monoclonal antibody (rituximab), anti-CD52 monoclonal antibody (alemtuzumab), interferon-α
Other options: thrombopoietin, autologous hematologic stem cell transplantation

treatment, children develop a positive direct Coombs test, which is accompanied by a transient decrease in hemoglobin concentration for 1–2 weeks.[151,216] The higher single dose of 75 µg/kg seems to increase platelet count as rapidly as IVIG. However, a higher rate of the adverse effect of hemolysis has to be taken into consideration.

Treatment of refractory ITP

If standard treatment is ineffective, the following options for refractory ITP should be considered (Table 23.12) (for overview of mechanisms of action see Cines and Blanchette[137]).

Conventional treatment options

Vinca alkaloids

The use of vinca alkaloids in ITP is based on the observation that the administration of vincristine and vinblastine can cause lymphocytopenia and suppression of antibody production. The increase in platelets after treatment with vincristine or vinblastine lasts 1–3 weeks in two-thirds of patients.[125,126,218–226]

The recommended dose of vincristine is 1–1.5 mg/m^2 intravenously (maximal single dose 2 mg) every 1–2 weeks. Combination with oral corticosteroid 1–2 mg/kg daily for 3 days may enhance the effect. For vinblastine the recommended dosage is 6 mg/m^2 intravenously every 1–2 weeks. Adverse effects include neuropathy, constipation, leukopenia and fever. The infusion of vinblastine-loaded platelets has not shown convincing results.[220]

Azathioprine

Azathioprine, an immunosuppressive drug, was the first

compound reported to be effective in chronic ITP refractory to glucocorticoid treatment and splenectomy; 50–70% of patients may achieve an improvement. Continuous treatment for 4 months appears to be necessary before a patient is considered unresponsive. The recommended dose is 50–300 mg/m^2 by mouth daily. Adverse effects are mainly leukopenia and the risk of developing malformations during pregnancy.

Cyclophosphamide
Of patients treated with cyclophosphamide, 60–80% will respond with an increase in platelet count.[127–132] Although of similar therapeutic potency as azathioprine, cyclophosphamide has more severe side-effects. The recommended dose is 3–8 mg/kg by mouth daily. Adverse effects are leukopenia, alopecia, infertility, teratogenicity and urinary bladder hemorrhage.

Cyclic high-dose methylprednisolone
Cyclic high-dose methylprednisolone (20–30 mg/kg i.v.) or dexamethasone (1 mg/kg orally) can be given on three to four consecutive days every 4 weeks for 4 months.[124,157,159,163] However, both the adverse effects and response rates of these high-dose corticosteroid regimens are disappointing in children.[164]

Danazol
The use of danazol, an androgenic steroid with minimal virilizing effects, was suggested for the treatment of ITP because one of the documented side-effects is thrombocytosis. There is a broad range of response to danazol in patients with ITP (10–80%).[232–249] The recommended dose is 100–150 mg/m^2 orally three times daily. Adverse effects include weight gain, headache, hair loss, liver dysfunction, myalgia, amenorrhea, some virilization and even thrombocytopenia.

Plasma exchange and protein A immunoadsorption
Plasma exchange[250–252] and protein A immunoadsorption[253–256] are *ex vivo* physical measures to remove antiplatelet antibodies. In 20–30% of patients with chronic ITP, plasma exchange may transiently result in a response. In one report using protein A immunoadsorption to remove antiplatelet antibodies, 16 of 72 patients demonstrated a sustained platelet increase.[253] This extracorporeal treatment is required daily for 3–5 days.

Ascorbic acid (vitamin C)
Although a response rate of 15% has been reported, the role of ascorbic acid in the treatment of ITP remains to be determined.[257–264] The recommended dose is 1–1.5 g/m^2 by mouth daily.

Splenectomy
Splenectomy as a therapeutic intervention in children with ITP should be restricted to those with uncontrollable bleeding. Recent studies document the decline in rates of splenectomy.[109,190,208] Splenectomy is indicated in children in whom thrombocytopenia has persisted for over 1 year in association with substantial bleeding episodes. In 16 reports (277 children in total), 72% of patients with ITP achieved a remission following surgical splenectomy.[93–100,107–109,133–136]

Elective splenectomy in children with chronic ITP is only recommended if platelet counts remain below 10×10^9/L in the absence of treatment (IVIG, corticosteroids, anti-RhD) for more than 14 days or in instances of severe and repetitive hemorrhage. It is paramount that children are immunized against *Haemophilus influenzae*, pneumococci and meningococci prior to splenectomy.[265]

Adverse effects
The important late effect of splenectomy is the increased risk of fatal bacterial infections, particularly in children below 5 years of age; a fatality rate of 1 in 300–1000 patient-years has been calculated.[265–267] The difficulty is therefore to decide whether the adverse effects of splenectomy outweigh its potential benefits since spontaneous recovery from ITP has been observed many years after diagnosis.[108,268]

Recent treatment options
New therapeutic developments have the main goal of influencing the altered immune response associated with ITP.

Treatment influencing antigenemia
Platelet counts were improved after antibacterial eradication of *Helicobacter pylori* and a positive urea breath test for *H. pylori* associated with gastritis or peptic ulcer disease in patients with chronic ITP.[269,270] Downmodulation of antigenemia may also be the reason for the improvement seen during antiviral treatment in patients with HIV-related thrombocytopenia.[271]

Treatment influencing the T-cell immune response

Ciclosporin
In child or adult patients with normal renal function, ciclosporin causes a dose-dependent increase in platelet count.[272–274] The dose of ciclosporin should be adjusted according to the serum level and with the aim of achieving a safe thrombocyte count. In this way, low-dose ciclosporin treatment with less adverse effects may be possible.[272–274] In one study, the long-term response rate in refractory idiopathic ITP was 11 of 20 patients (five complete responses, six partial responses) after discontinuation of treatment.[274] No large study exists.

CTLA-4-Ig
CTLA-4-Ig, a fusion protein between CTLA-4 and the immunoglobulin Fc portion, aims to block T-cell costimulation.[275] This treatment was successfully used in patients with

psoriasis. Such a drug may also be effective in other auto-immune disorders driven by dysregulated T cells, including ITP, but no data are yet available.

Treatment influencing the B-cell immune response

Anti-CD20 monoclonal antibody (rituximab)
(for overview see ref. 120)
The human/mouse anti-B-cell monoclonal antibody rituximab is a κ immunoglobulin with murine light- and heavy-chain variable sequences and human constant sequences.[276] The chimeric molecule binds to the CD20 antigen on B cells and mediates its lysis by immune effector cells. Among other autoantibody-producing disorders, refractory ITP and Evans syndrome benefit from rituximab.[277] With three to four courses of rituximab (375 mg/m^2 i.v. per week for 4 weeks), approximately two-thirds of patients had an increase in platelet count and some had long-lasting responses (>6 months). Adverse events during treatment were transient and mild, and comprised fever, chill, headache, dizziness, asthenia, nausea, vomiting and hypotension. No infections were noted.

Anti-CD52 monoclonal antibody (alemtuzumab)
CD52 antigen is present on lymphocytes and monocytes.[278,279] Monoclonal antibody directed against CD52 (alemtuzumab) is effective in clearing B lymphocytes. Of 21 children and adults with hemolytic anemia, pure red cell aplasia, ITP or Evans syndrome, 15 showed a response to treatment with alemtuzumab; some patients had a sustained response.[280] Adverse effects during treatment included fever and chill. Serious adverse effects can potentially occur with alem-tuzumab, such as profound lymphocytopenia (with potential for opportunistic infection), intravenous hemolysis, systemic venous thrombosis, or thrombotic thrombocytopenic purpura.

Interferon-α
Uncontrolled studies with IFN-α showed a response rate of 25% in children and adults with chronic ITP.[121,281] However, it may not be feasible to conduct the essential controlled trials needed to establish the efficacy of IFN in ITP because the drug is associated with significant adverse effects, a difficult mode of application (300 000 units i.m. three times weekly for 4 weeks) and is expensive.

Other options
Thrombopoietin may be effective in those patients with ITP and megakaryocyte involvement (depletion by specific antibodies). Initial data have shown favorable responses.[282]

Autologous hematologic stem cell transplantation has been performed in 12 adult patients with severe refractory ITP.[283] Four patients achieved complete remission and two patients partial remission. This approach must be considered experimental.

References

1. Jones HW, Tocantins LM. The history of purpura hemorrhagica. *Ann Med Hist* 1933; **5**: 349.
2. Kasnelson P. Verschwinden der hämorrhagischen Diathese bei einem Falle von essentieller Thrombopenie (Frank) nach Milzexstirpation. *Wien Klin Wochenschr* 1916; **29**: 1451.
3. Harrington WJ, Minnich V. Demonstration of a thrombocytopenic factor in the blood of patients with thrombocytopenic purpura. *J Lab Clin Med* 1951; **38**: 1–10.
4. Harrington WJ, Sprague CC, Minnich V, Moore CV, Aulvin RC, Dubach R. Immunologic mechanisms in idiopathic and neonatal thrombocytopenic purpura. *Ann Intern Med* 1953; **38**: 433–69.
5. Shulman NR, Marder VJ, Weinrach RS. Similarities between known antiplatelet antibodies and the factor responsible for thrombocytopenia in idiopathic purpura: physiologic, serologic and isotopic studies. *Ann NY Acad Sci* 1965; **124**: 499–542.
6. Dixon RH, Rosse WF. Platelet antibody in immune thrombocytopenia. *Br J Haematol* 1975; **31**: 129–34.
7. Imbach P, d'Appuzzo V, Hirt A *et al.* High-dose intravenous gammaglobulin for idiopathic thrombocytopenic purpura in childhood. *Lancet* 1981; **i**: 1228–31.
8. Salama A, Mueller-Eckhardt C, Kiefel V. Effect of intravenous immunoglobulin in immune thrombocytopenia. *Lancet* 1983; **ii**: 193–5.
9. Imbach P. Harmful and beneficial antibodies in immune thrombocytopenic purpura. *Clin Exp Immunol* 1994; **97** (suppl. 1): 25–30.
10. van Leeuwen EF, van der Ven JTH, Engelfriet CP, von dem Borne AEG. Specificity of autoantibodies in autoimmune thrombocytopenia. *Blood* 1982; **59**: 23–6.
11. McMillan R, Tani P, Millard F, Berchtold L, Renshaw L, Woods VL. Platelet-associated and plasma anti-glycoprotein autoantibodies in chronic ITP. *Blood* 1987; **70**: 1040–5.
12. Kiefel V, Santoso S, Weisheit M, Mueller-Eckhardt C. Monolocal antibody-specific immobilization of platelet antigens (MAIPA): a new tool for the identification of platelet-reactive antibodies. *Blood* 1987; **70**: 1722–6.
13. Semple JW, Freedman J. Increased anti-platelet T helper lymphocyte reactivity in patients with autoimmune thrombocytopenic purpura. *Blood* 1991; **78**: 2619–25.
14. Ravetch JV, Lanier LL. Immune inhibitory receptors. *Science* 2000; **290**: 84–9.
15. Samuelson A, Towers TL, Ravetch JV. Anti-inflammatory activity of IVIG mediated through the inhibitory Fc receptor. *Science* 2001; **291**: 484–6.
16. Kühne T, Imbach P, Bolton-Maggs PHB *et al.* for the Intercontinental Childhood ITP Study Group. Newly diagnosed idiopathic thrombocytopenic purpura in childhood: an observational study. *Lancet* 2001; **358**: 2122–5.
17. Kühne T, Imbach P. A propsective comparative study of 2540 infants and children with newly diagnosed idiopathic thrombocytopenic purpura (ITP) from the Intercontinental Childhood ITP Study Group (ICIS). *J Pediatr* 2003; **143**: 605–8.
18. Hirsch EO, Dameshek W. Idiopathic thrombocytopenia. *Arch Intern Med* 1951; **88**: 701.

19. Simons SM, Main CA, Yaish HM *et al*. Idiopathic thrombocytopenic purpura in children. *J Pediatr* 1975; **87**: 16.

20. Dameshek W, Ebbe S. Recurrent acute idiopathic thrombocytopenic purpura. *N Engl J Med* 1963; **269**: 647.

21. Figueroa M, Gehlsen J, Hammond D *et al*. Combination chemotherapy in refractory immune thrombocytopenic purpura. *N Engl J Med* 1993; **328**: 1226–9.

22. Ata M, Fisher OD, Holman CA. Inherited thrombocytopenia. *Lancet* 1965; **i**: 119.

23. Chiaro JJ, Ayut D, Bloom GE. X-linked thrombocytopenic purpura. I. Clinical and genetic studies of a kindred. *Am J Dis Child* 1972; **123**: 565.

24. Roberts MH, Smith MH. Thrombocytopenic purpura: a report of four cases in one family. *Am J Dis Child* 1950; **79**: 820.

25. Schaar FE. Familial idiopathic thrombocytopenic purpura. *J Pediatr* 1963; **62**: 546.

26. Bithell TC, Didisheim GE, Wintrobe MM. Thrombocytopenia inherited as an autosomal dominant trait. *Blood* 1965; **25**: 231.

27. Stuart MJ, Tomar RH, Miller ML *et al*. Chronic idiopathic thrombocytopenic purpura: a familial immunodeficiency syndrome? *JAMA* 1978; **239**: 939.

28. Lightsey AL, Koenig HM, McMilan R, Stone JR. Platelet-associated immunoglobulin G in childhood idiopathic thrombocytopenic purpura. *J Pediatr* 1979; **94**: 201–4.

29. Lightsey AL, McMilan R. The role of spleen in "autoimmune" blood disorders. *Am J Pediatr Hematol Oncol* 1979; **1**: 331.

30. McIntosh S, Johnson C, Hartigan P *et al*. Immunoregulatory abnormalities in children with thrombocytopenic purpura. *J Pediatr* 1981; **99**: 525.

31. Myllylä G, Vaheri A, Vesikari T *et al*. Interaction between human blood platelets, viruses and antibodies. IV. Post-rubella thrombocytopenic purpura and platelet aggregation by rubella antigen-antibody interaction. *Clin Exp Immunol* 1969; **4**: 323.

32. Panel on Diagnostic Application of Radioisotopes in Hematology. International Committee for Standardization in Hematology. Recommended methods for radioisotope platelet survival studies. *Blood* 1977; **50**: 1137–44.

33. Panel on Diagnostic Applications of Radionuclides in Hematology. Recommended method for indium-111 platelet survival studies. *J Nucl Med* 1988; **29**: 564–6.

34. Branehog I, Kutti J, Weinfeld A. Platelet survival and production in idiopathic thrombocytopenic purpura (ITP). *Br J Haematol* 1974; **27**: 127–43.

35. Harker LA, Finch CA. Thrombokinetics in man. *J Clin Invest* 1969; **48**: 963–74.

36. Aster RH, Keene WR. Sites of platelet destruction in idiopathic thrombocytopenic purpura. *Br J Haematol* 1969; **16**: 61–73.

37. Heyns AP, Lotter MG, Badenhorst PN *et al*. Kinetics and sites of destruction of 111-indium-oxine-labeled platelets in idiopathic thrombocytopenic purpura: a quantitative study. *Am J Hematol* 1982; **12**: 167–77.

38. Schmidt KG, Rasmussen JW. Kinetics and distribution *in vivo* of 111-In-labeled autologous platelets in idiopathic thrombocytopenic purpura. *Scand J Haematol* 1985; **34**: 47–56.

39. Ballem PJ, Segal GM, Stratton JR, Gernsheimer T, Adamson JW, Slichter S. Mechanisms of thrombocytopenia in chronic autoimmune thrombocytopenic purpura. Evidence for both impaired platelet production and increased platelet clearance. *J Clin Invest* 1987; **80**: 33–40.

40. Imbach P, Morell A. Idiopathic thrombocytopenic purpura (ITP): immunomodulation by intravenous immunoglobulin. *Int Rev Immunol* 1989; **5**: 181–8.

41. Kiefel V, Santoso S, Kaufmann E *et al*. Autoantibodies against platelet glycoprotein Ib/IX: a frequent finding in autoimmune thrombocytopenic purpura. *Br J Haematol* 1991; **79**: 256–62.

42. McMillan R. Antigen-specific assays in immune thrombocytopenic. *Transfus Med Rev* 1990; **4**: 136–43.

43. Koerner TAW, Weinfeld HM, Bullard LSB, Williams LCJ. Antibodies against platelet glycosphingolipids: detection in serum by quantitative HPTLC-autoradiography and association with autoimmune and alloimmune processes. *Blood* 1989; **74**: 274–84.

44. Brighton TA, Evans S, Castaldi PA *et al*. Prospective evaluation of the clinical usefulness of an antigen-specific assay (MAIPA) in idiopathic thrombocytopenic purpura and other immune thrombocytopenias. *Blood* 1996; **88**: 194–201.

45. Warner MN, Moore JC, Warkentin TE *et al*. A prospective study of protein-specific assay used to investigate idiopathic thrombocytopenic purpura. *Br J Haematol* 1999; **104**: 442–7.

46. McMillan R, Wang L, Tani P. Prospective evaluation of the immunobead assay for the diagnosis of adult chronic immune thrombocytopenic purpura (ITP). *J Thromb Haemost* 2003; **1**: 485–91.

47. Imbach P, Tani P, Berchtold W *et al*. Different forms of chronic ITP in children defined by antiplatelet autoantibodies. *J Pediatr* 1991; **118**: 535–9.

48. Kurata Y, Curd JG, Tamerius JD, McMillan R. Platelet-associated complement in chronic ITP. *Br J Haematol* 1985; **60**: 723–33.

49. Clarkson SB, Bussel HB, Kimberly RP, Valinsky JE, Nachman RL, Unkeless JC. Treatment of refractory immune thrombocytopenic purpura with anti-Fcg-receptor antibody. *N Engl J Med* 1986; **314**: 1236–9.

50. Tsubakio T, Tani P, Curd JG, McMillan R. Complement activation *in vitro* by antiplatelet antibodies in chronic immune thrombocytopenic purpura. *Br J Haematol* 1985; **63**: 293–300.

51. McMillan R, Longmire RL, Yelenosky R, Donnell RL, Armstrong S. Quantitation of platelet-binding IgG produced *in vitro* by spleens from patients with idiopathic thrombocytopenic purpura. *N Engl J Med* 1974; **291**: 812–17.

52. McMillan R, Yelenosky RJ, Longmire RL. Antiplatelet antibody production by the spleen and bone marrow in immune thrombocytopenic purpura. In: Battisto JR, Streinlein JW (eds) *Immunoaspects of the Spleen*. Amsterdam: North Holland Biomedical Press, 1976, pp. 227–37.

53. McMillan R, Luiken GA, Levy R, Yelenosky R, Longmire RL. Antibody against megakaryocytes in idiopathic thrombocytopenic purpura. *JAMA* 1978; **239**: 2460–2.

54. Heyns AP, Badenhorst PN, Lotter MG, Pieters H, Wessels P, Kotze HF. Platelet turnover and kinetics in immune thrombocytopenic purpura: results with autologus 111-In-labeled and homologous 51-Cr-labeled platelets differ. *Blood* 1986; **67**: 86–92.

55. Stoll D, Cines DB, Aster RH, Murphy S. Platelet kinetics in patients with idiopathic thrombocytopenic purpura and moderate thrombocytopenia. *Blood* 1985; **65**: 584–8.

56. Nagata S. Apoptosis by death factor. *Cell* 1997; **88**: 355–65.

57. Hengartner MO. The biochemistry of apoptosis. *Nature* 2000; **407**: 770–6.

58. Prasad NK, Papoff G, Zeuner A *et al.* IVIG-mediated amelioration of murine ITP via FcgammRIIB is independent of SHIP1, SHP-1, and Btk acitivity. *Blood* 2003; **102**: 558–60.

59. Semple JW, Freedman J. Abnormal cellular immune mechanisms associated with autoimmune thrombocytopenia. *Transfus Med Rev* 1995; **9** (4): 327–38.

60. Fujisawa K, O'Toole TE, Tani P *et al.* Autoantibodies to the presumptive cytoplasmic domain of platelet glycoprotein IIIa in patients with chronic immune thrombocytopenic purpura. *Blood* 1991; **77**: 2207–13.

61. Kekomaki R, Dawson B, McFarland J *et al.* Localization of human platelet autoantigen to the cysteine-rich region of glycoprotein IIIa. *J Clin Invest* 1991; **88**: 847–54.

62. Mizutani H, Furubayashi T, Kashiwagi H *et al.* B cells expressing CD5 antigen are markedly increased in peripheral blood and spleen lymphocytes from patients with immune thrombocytopenic purpura. *Br J Haematol* 1991; **78**: 474–9.

63. Ware R, Howard TA. Elevated numbers of gamma-delta (γδ+) lymphocytes in children with immune thrombocytopenic purpura. *J Clin Immunol* 1994; **11**: 237–47.

64. Garcia-Suarez J, Prieto A, Manzano L *et al.* T lymphocytes from autoimmune thrombocytopenic purpura show a defective activation and proliferation after cytoplasmic membrane and intracytoplasmic mitogenic signals. *Am J Hematol* 1993; **44**: 1–8.

65. Garcia-Suarez J, Prieto A, Ryes E. Severe chronic autoimmune thrombocytopenic purpura is associated with an expansion of CD56⁺CD3⁻ natural killer cell subset. *Blood* 1993; **82**: 1538–45.

66. Quagliata F, Karpatkin S. Impaired lymphocyte transformation and capping in autoimmune thrombocytopenic purpura. *Blood* 1979; **53**: 341–9.

67. Garcia-Suarez J, Prieto A, Reyes E *et al.* The clinical outcome of autoimmune thrombocytopenic purpura patients is related to their T cell immunodeficiency. *Br J Haematol* 1993; **84**: 464–70.

68. Ware RE, Howard TA. Phenotypic and clonal analysis of T lymphocytes in childhood immune thrombocytopenic purpura. *Blood* 1993; **82**: 2137–42.

69. Semple JW, Allen D, Gross P *et al.* CD19+ Blymphocytes from patient with chronic autoimmune thrombocytopenic purpura (ATP) require CD4+ T cell contact for antiplatelet autoantibody production. *Platelets* 1994; **5** (5) 290.

70. Hymes KB, Karpatkin S. *In vitro* suppressor T lymphocyte dysfunction in autoimmune thrombocytopenic purpura associated with complement fixing antibody. *Br J Haematol* 1990; **74**: 330–5.

71. Semple JW, Bruce S, Freedman J. Suppressed natural killer cell activity in patients with chronic autoimmune thrombocytopenic purpura. *Am J Hematol* 1991; **37**: 258–62.

72. Gardiner RA, Smith JG. A study of natural killer cells and interferon-gamma in patients with immune thrombocytopenic purpura. *Blood* 1990; **76**: 206A.

73. Mizutani H, Tsubakio T, Tomiyama Y *et al.* Increased circulating Ia-positive T cells in patients with idiopathic thrombocytopenic purpura. *Clin Exp Immunol* 1987; **67**: 191–7.

74. Semple JW, Freedam J. Increased anti platelet T helper lymphocyte reactivity in patients with autoimmune thrombocytopenic purpura. *Blood* 1991; **78**: 474.

75. Boshkov LK, Kelton JG, Halloran PF. HLA-DR expression by platelets in acute idiopathic thromocytopenic purpura. *Br J Haematol* 1992; **81**: 552–7.

76. Semple JW, Milev Y, Cosgrave D *et al.* Differences in serum cytokine levels in acute and chronic autoimmune thrombocytopenic purpura: relationship to platelet phenotype and antiplatelet T cell reactivity. *Blood* 1996; **87**: 4245–54.

77. Santoso S, Kalb R, Kiefel V, Mueller-Eckhardt C. The presence of messenger RNA for HLA class I in human platelets and its capability for protein biosynthesis. *Br J Haematol* 1993; **84**: 451.

78. Nepom G. Erlich H. MHC class-II molecules and autoimmunity. *Annu Rev Immunol* 1991; **9**: 493.

79. Bottazzo GF, Dean BM, McNally JM, McKay EH, Swift PGF, Gamble DR. In situ characterization of autoimmune phenomena and expression of HLA molecules in the pancreas in diabetes mellitus. *N Engl J Med* 1985; **313**: 353.

80. Traugott U, Scheinberg LC, Raine CS. On the presence of Ia-positive endothelial cells and astrocytes in multiple sclerosis lesions and its relevance to antigen presentation. *J Neuroimmunol* 1985; **8**: 1.

81. Trotter JL. Serial studies of serum interleukin-2 in chronic progressive multiple sclerosis patients: occurrence of bursts and effects of cyclosporine. *J Neuroimmunol* 1990; **28**: 1.

82. Tebib JG, Boughaba H, Letroublon MC. Serum IL-2 level in rheumatoid arthritis: correlation with joint destruction and disease progression. *Eur Cytokine Network* 1991; **2**: 239.

83. Huang Y-P, Perrin LH, Miescher PA, Zubler RH. Correlation of T and B cell activities *in vitro* and serum IL-2 levels in systemic lupus erythematosus. *J Immunol* 1991; **141**: 827.

84. DeFrance T, Vandeviliet B, Briere F, Durand I, Rousset F, Banchereau J. Interleukin 10 and transforming growth factor β cooperate to induce anti-CD40-activated naive human B cells to secrete immunoglobulin A. *J Exp Med* 1992; **175**: 671.

85. Howard M, Muchamuel T, Audrade S, Mennon S. Anti-inflammatory effect of IL-10. *J Exp Med* 1993; **177**: 1205.

86. Garcia-Suarez J, Prieto A, Reyes E, Manzano L, Arribalzago K, Alverez Mon M. Abnormal γ-IFN and α-TNF secretion in purified CD2⁺ cells from autoimmune thrombocytopenic purpura (ATP) patients: their implication in the clinical course of the disease. *Am J Hematol* 1995; **49**: 271.

87. Kaplan C, Morinet F, Carton J. Virus-induced autoimmune thrombocytopenia and neutropenia. *Semin Hematol* 1992; **1**: 34.

88. Imbach P, Kühne T, Holländer G. Immunologic aspects in the pathogenesis and treatment of immune thrombocytopenic purpura in children. *Curr Opin Pediatr* 1997; **9**: 35–40.

89. Woerner SJ, Abildgaard CF, French BN. Intracranial hemorrhage in children with idiopathic thrombocytopenic purpura. *Pediatrics* 1981; **67**: 453.

90. Lilleyman JS. Intracranial hemorrhage in idiopathic thrombocytopenic purpura. *Arch Dis Child* 1994; **71**: 251–3.

91. Halperin DS, Doyle JJ. Is bone marrow examination justified in idiopathic thrombocytopenic purpura? *Am J Dis Child* 1988; **142**: 509.

92. George JN, Woolf SH, Raskob GE *et al.* Idiopathic thrombocytopenic purpura: a practice guideline developed by explicit methods for the American Society of Hematology. *Blood* 1996; **88**: 3–40.

93. Ramos MEG, Newman AJ, Gross S. Chronic thrombocytopenia in childhood. *J Pediatr* 1978; **92**: 584.

94. Venetz U, Willi P, Hirt A, Imbach P, Wagner HP. Chronische idiopathische thrombozytopenische Purpura im Kindesalter. *Helv Paediatr Acta* 1982; **37**: 27.

95. Lusher JM, Zuelzer WW. Idiopathic thrombocytopenic purpura in childhood. *J Pediatr* 1966; **68**: 971.

96. Benham ES, Taft LI. Idiopathic thrombocytopenic purpura in children: results of steroid therapy and splenectomy. *Aust Paediatr J* 1972; **8**: 311.

97. Hoyle C, Darbyshire P, Eden OB. Idiopathic thrombocytopenia in childhood. *Scott Med J* 1986; **31**: 174.

98. Robb LG, Tiedeman K. Idiopathic thrombocytopenic purpura: predictors of chronic disease. *Arch Dis Child* 1990; **65**: 502.

99. Simons SM, Main CA, Yaish HM, Rutzky J. Idiopathic thrombocytopenic purpura in children. *Pediatrics* 1975; **87**: 16.

100. Zaki M, Hassanein AA, Khalil AF. Childhood idiopathic thrombocytopenic purpura: report of 60 cases from Kuwait. *J Trop Pediatr* 1990; **36**: 10.

101. Komrower GM, Watson GH. Prognosis in idiopathic thrombocytopenic purpura of childhood. *Arch Dis Child* 1954; **29**: 502.

102. Choi SI, McClure PD. Idiopathic thrombocytopenic purpura in childhood. *Can Med Assoc J* 1967; **97**: 562.

103. Walker RW, Walker W. Idiopathic thrombocytopenia, initial illness and long term follow up. *Arch Dis Child* 1984; **59**: 316.

104. Lammi AT, Lovric VA. Idiopathic thrombocytopenic purpura: an epidemiologic study. *Pediatrics* 1973; **83**: 31.

105. den Ottolander GJ, Gratama JW, deKoning J, Brand A. Longterm follow-up study of 168 patients with immune thrombocytopenia. *Scand Haematol* 1984; **32**: 101.

106. Imbach P, Akatsuka J, Blanchette V *et al.* Immun-thrombocytopenic purpura as a model for pathogenesis and treatment of autoimmunity. *Eur J Pediatr* 1995; **154**: 60–4.

107. Imbach P, Berchtold W, Hirt A *et al.* Intravenous immunoglobulin versus oral corticosteroids in acute immune thrombocytopenic purpura in childhood. *Lancet* 1985; **ii**: 464–8.

108. Tamary H, Kaplinsky C, Levy I *et al.* Chronic childhood idiopathic thrombocytopenia purpura: long-term follow-up. *Acta Paediatr* 1994; **83**: 931.

109. Reid MM. Chronic idiopathic thrombocytopenic purpura: incidence, treatment and outcome. *Arch Dis Child* 1995; **72**: 125.

110. Aronis S, Platokouki H, Mitsika A, Haidas S, Constantopoulos A. Seventeen years of experience with chronic idiopathic thrombocytopenic purpura in childhood. Is therapy always better? *Pediatr Hematol Oncol* 1994; **11**: 487–98.

111. Aronis S, Platokouki H, Mitsika A, Haidas S, Constantopoulos A. Treatment of chronic idiopathic thrombocytopenic purpura. *Pediatr Hematol Oncol* 1995; **12**: 409–10.

112. Lilleyman JS. Medical nemesis and childhood ITP. *Br J Haematol* 2003; **123**: 586–9.

113. Buchanan GR, Kuehne T, Bolton-Maggs PHB *et al.* Intercontinental Childhood ITP Study Group (ICIS). Severe hemorrhage in children with newly-diagnosed idiopathic thrombocytopenic purpura (ITP). Presented at the Pediatric Academic Societies' Annual Meeting, Washington, DC, May 14–17, 2005.

114. Bolton-Maggs PHB, Moon I. Assessment of UK practice for management of acute childhood idiopathic thrombocytopenic purpura against published guidelines. *Lancet* 1997; **350**: 620–3.

115. Buchanan GR, Adix L. Outcome measures and treatment end points other than platelet count in childhood idiopathic thrombocytopenic purpura. *Semin Thromb Hemost* 2001; **27**: 277–85.

116. Lilleyman JS. Management of childhood idiopathic thrombocytopenic purpura. *Br J Haematol* 1999; **105**: 871–5.

117. Bolton-Maggs PHB. Idiopathic thrombocytopenic purpura. *Arch Dis Child* 2000; **83**: 220–2.

118. Imbach P, Blanchette V, Nugent D, Kühne T. *Immune Thrombocytopenic Purpura: Immediate and Long-term Effects of Intravenous Immunoglobulin. Advances in IVIG Research and Therapy.* London: Parthenon Publishing Group, 1996.

119. Andrew M, Blanchette VS, Adams M *et al.* A multicenter study of the treatment of childhood chronic idiopathic thrombocytopenic purpura with anti-D. *J Pediatr* 1991; **120**: 522–7.

120. Imbach P. Refractory idiopathic immune thrombocytopenic purpura in children: current and future treatment options. *Pediatr Drugs* 2003; **5**: 795–801.

121. Proctor SJ, Jackson G, Carey P *et al.* Improvement of platelet counts in steroid-unresponsive idiopathic immune thrombocytopenic purpura after short-course therapy with recombinant alpha 2b interferon. *Blood* 1989; **74**: 1894–7.

122. Sartorius JA. Steroid treatment of idiopathic thrombocytopenic purpura in children. Preliminary results of a randomized cooperative study. *Am J Pediatr Hematol Oncol* 1984; **6**: 165.

123. Ozsoylu S, Irken G, Karabent A. High-dose intravenous methylprednisolone for acute childhood idiopathic thrombocytopenic purpura. *Eur J Haematol* 1989; **42**: 431.

124. Andersen JC. Response of resistant idiopathic thrombocytopenic purpura to pulsed high-dose dexamethasone therapy. *N Engl J Med* 1994; **330**: 1560–4.

125. Facon T, Caulier MT, Wattel E, Jouet JP, Bauters F, Fenaux P. A randomized trial comparing vinblastine in slow infusion and by bolus i.v. injection in idiopathic thrombocytopenic purpura: a report on 42 patients. *Br J Haematol* 1994; **86**: 678.

126. Alm YS, Harrington WJ, Seelman RC, Eytel CS. Vincristine therapy of idiopathic and secondary thrombocytopenias. *N Engl J Med* 1974; **291**: 376.

127. Pizzuto J, Ambriz R. Therapeutic experience on 934 adults with idiopathic thrombocytopenic purpura: multicentric trial of the cooperative Latin American group on hemostasis and thrombosis. *Blood* 1984; **64**: 1179.

128. Laros RK, Penner JA. Refractory thrombocytopenic purpura treated successfully with cyclophosphamide. *JAMA* 1971; **215**: 445.

129. Verlin M, Laros RK, Penner JA. Treatment of refractory thrombocytopenic purpura with cyclophosphamide. *Am J Hematol* 1976; **1**: 97.

130. Weinerman B, Maxwell I, Hryniuk W. Intermittent cyclophosphamide treatment of autoimmune thrombocytopenia. *Can Med Assoc J* 1974; **111**: 1100.

131. Srichaikul T, Boonpucknavig S, Archararit N, Chaisiri-pumkeeree W. Chronic immunologic thrombocytopenic purpura. Results of cyclophosphamide therapy before splenectomy. *Arch Intern Med* 1980; **140**: 636.

132. Reiner A, Gernsheimer T, Slichter SJ. Pulse cyclophosphamide therapy for refractory autoimmune thrombocytopenic purpura. *Blood* 1995; **85**: 351.

133. Brooks PL, O'Shea MJ, Pryor JP. Splenectomy in the treatment of idiopathic thrombocytopenic purpura. *Br J Surg* 1969; **56**: 861.

134. Grosfeld JL, Naffis D, Boles ET Jr, Newton WA Jr. The role of splenectomy in neonatal idiopathic thrombocytopenic purpura. *J Pediatr Surg* 1970; **5**: 166.

135. Zarella JT, Martin LW, Lampkin BC. Emergency splenectomy for idiopathic thrombocytopenic purpura in children. *J Pediatr Surg* 1978; **13**: 243.

136. Davis PW, Williams DA, Shamberger RC. Immune thrombocytopenia: surgical therapy and predictors of response. *J Pediatr Surg* 1991; **26**: 407.

137. Cines DB, Blanchette VS. Immune thrombocytopenic purpura. *N Engl J Med* 2002; **346**: 995–1008.

138. Vesely S, Buchanan GR, Cohen A *et al*. Self-reported diagnostic and management strategies in childhood idiopathic thrombocytopenic purpura: results of a survey of practicing pediatric hematology/oncology specialists. *J Pediatr Hematol Oncol* 2000; **22**: 55–61.

139. Vesely S, Buchanan GR, Adix L *et al*. Self reported initial management of childhood idiopathic thrombocytopenic purpura: results of a survey of members of the American Society of Pediatric Hematology/Oncology, 2001. *J Pediatr Hematol Oncol* 2003; **25**: 130–3.

140. Eden OB, Lilleyman JS. Guidelines for management of idiopathic thrombocytopenic purpura. The British Paediatric Haematology Group. *Arch Dis Child* 1992; **67**: 1056–8.

141. British Committee for Standards in Haemotology, General Haematology Task Force. Guidelines for the investigation and management of idiopathic thrombocytopenic purpura in adults, children and in pregnancy. *Br J Haematol* 2003; **120**: 574–96.

142. Imbach P, Kühne T, Blanchette VS (eds). State-of-the art expert report of the Intercontinental Childhood ITP Study Group ICIS. *J Pediatr Hematol Oncol* 2003; **25** (suppl. 1): S1–S84.

143. Elinder G, Blanchette VS (eds). Immune thrombocytopenic purpura from bench to bedside. Proceedings of a Swedish–Canadian Symposium. *Acta Paediatr* 1998; **87** (suppl. 424).

144. Anon. Intravenous immunoglobulin: prevention and treatment of disease. NIH Consensus Development Conference statement, May 21–23, 1990. Bethesda, MD: Office of Medical Applications of Research, National Institutes of Health, 1990.

145. Buchanan GR, Kühne T, Bolton-Maggs P *et al*. Frequency, location and timing of severe hemorrhage in children with newly-diagnosed idiopathic thrombocytopenic purpura: a study of the Intercontinental Childhood ITP Study Group. *Blood* 2003; **102**: 298a.

146. Kühne T, Blanchette V, Smith O *et al*. on behalf of the Intercontinental Childhood ITP Study Group. Splenectomy in childhood idiopathic thrombocytopenic purpura: results of the Splenectomy Registry. *Blood* 2003; **102**; 78b.

147. Foster CB, Zhu S, Erichsen HC *et al*. Polymorphisms in inflammatory cytokines and Fcgamma receptors in childhood chronic immune thrombocytopenic purpura: a pilot study. *Br J Haematol* 2001; **113**: 596–9.

148. Chanock S, Wacholder S. One gene and one outcome? No way. *Trends Mol Med* 2002; **8**: 266–9.

149. Imbach P, Wagner HP, Berchtold W *et al*. Intravenous immunoglobulin versus oral corticosteroids in acute immune thrombocytopenic purpura in childhood. *Lancet* 1985; **ii**: 464.

150. Blanchette VS, Luke B, Andrew M *et al*. A prospective, randomized trial of high-dose intravenous immune globulin G therapy, oral prednisone therapy, and no therapy in childhood acute immune thrombocytopenic purpura. *J Pediatr* 1993; **123**: 989.

151. Blanchette V, Imbach P, Andrew M *et al*. Randomized trial of intravenous immunoglobulin G, intravenous anti-D, and oral prednisone in childhood acute immune thrombocytopenic purpura. *Lancet* 1994; **344**: 703.

152. McWilliams NB, Maurer HM. Acute idiopathic thrombocytopenic purpura in children. *Am J Hematol* 1979; **7**: 87.

153. Sartorius JA. Steroid treatment of idiopathic thrombocytopenic purpura in children. Preliminary results of a randomized cooperative study. *Am J Pediatr Hematol Oncol* 1984; **6**: 165.

154. Buchanan GR, Holtkamp CA. Prednisone therapy for children with newly diagnosed idiopathic thrombocytopenic purpura. A randomized clinical trial. *Am J Pediatr Hematol Oncol* 1984; **6**: 355.

155. Mazzucconi MG, Francesconi M, Fidani P *et al*. Treatment of idiopathic thrombocytopenic purpura: results of a multicentric protocol. *Haematologia* 1985; **70**: 329.

156. Bellucci S, Charpak Y, Chastang C, Tobelem G. Low doses v conventional doses of corticoids in immune thrombocytopenic purpura (ITP). Results of a randomized clinical trial in 160 children, 223 adults. *Blood* 1988; **71**: 1165.

157. Khalifa AS, Tolba KA, El-Alfy MS, Gadallah M, Ibrahim FH. Idiopathic thrombocytopenic purpura in Egyptian children. *Acta Haematol* 1993; **90**: 125.

158. Ozsoylu S. Treatment of chronic ITP. *Pediatr Hematol Oncol* 1995; **12**: 407–10.

159. Albayrak D, Islek I, Kalayci AG, Gürses N. Acute immune thrombocytopenic purpura: a comparative study of very high oral doses of methylprednisolone and intravenously administered immune globulin. *J Pediatr* 1994; **125**: 1004.

160. Kattamis AC, Shankar S, Cohen AR. Neurologic complications of treatment of childhood acute immune thrombocytopenic purpura with intravenously administered immunoglobulin G. *J Pediatr* 1997; **130**: 281–3.

161. Imholz B, Imbach P, Baumgartner C *et al*. Intravenous immunoglobulin (i.v. IgG) for previously treated acute or for chronic idiopathic thrombocytopenic purpura (ITP) in childhood: a prospective multicenter study. *Blut* 1988; **56**: 63.

162. Warrier IA, Lusher JM. Intravenous gammaglobulin (gamimune) for treatment of chronic idiopathic thrombocytopenic purpura (ITP): a two-year follow-up. *Am J Hematol* 1990; **33**: 184.

163. Ozsoylu S, Sayli TR, Ozturk G. Oral megadose methylprednisolone versus intravenous immunoglobulin for acute childhood idiopathic thrombocytopenic purpura. *Pediatr Hematol Oncol* 1993; **10**: 317.

164. Nugent D, English M, Hawkins D, Pendergrass T, Tarantino M. High dose dexamethasone therapy for pediatric patients with refractory immune-mediated thrombocytopenic purpura (ITP). *Blood* 1994; **94**: 731A.

165. Duhem C, Dicato MA, Ries F. Side-effects of intravenous immune globulins. *Clin Exp Immunol* 1994; **97** (suppl. 1): 79.

166. Thomas MJ, Misbah SA, Chapel HM, Jones M, Elrington G, Newsom-Davis J. Hemolysis after high-dose intravenous Ig. *Blood* 1993; **82**: 3789.

167. Centers for Disease Control and Prevention. Outbreak of hepatitis C associated with intravenous immunoglobulin administration, United States, October 1993 June 1994. *MMWR* 1994; **43**: 505.

168. Bjoro K, Froland SS, Yun Z, Samdal H, Haaland T. Hepatitis C infection in patients with primary hypogammaglobulinemia after treatment with contaminated immune globulin. *N Engl J Med* 1994; **331**: 1607.

169. Yu MW, Mason BL, Guo ZP *et al*. Hepatitis C transmission associated with intravenous immunoglobulins. *Lancet* 1995; **345**: 1173.

170. Schiano TD, Bellary SV, Black M. Possible transmission of hepatitis C virus infection with intravenous immunoglobulin. *Ann Intern Med* 1995; **122**: 802.

171. Salama A, Mueller-Eckhardt C, Kiefel V. Effect of intravenous immunoglobulin in immune thrombocytopenia. *Lancet* 1983; **ii**: 193–5.

172. Fehr J, Hofmann V, Kappeler U. Transient reversal of thrombocytopenia in idiopathic thrombocytopenic purpura by high-dose intravenous gamma globulin. *N Engl J Med* 1982; **306**: 1254–8.

173. Dammacco F, Jodice G, Campobasso N. Treatment of adult patients with ITP with intravenous immunoglobulin: effect on T cell subsets and PWM induced antibody synthesis *in vitro*. *Br J Haematol* 1986; **62**: 125–35.

174. Macey MG, Newland AG. CD4 and CD8 subpopulation changes during high dose intravenous immunoglobulin treatment. *Br J Haematol* 1990; **76**: 513–20.

175. Samuelsson A, Towers TL, Ravetch JV. Anti-inflammatory activity of IVIG mediated through the inhibitory Fc receptor. *Science* 2001; **291**: 484–6.

176. Leung DYM, Cotran RS, Kurf-Jones E, Burns JC, Newburger JW, Pober JS. Endothelial cell activation and high interleukin-secretion in the pathogenesis of acute Kawasaki disease. *Lancet* 1989; **ii**: 1298–302.

177. Ross C, Hansen MB, Schyberg T, Berk K. Autoantibodies to crude human leukocyte interferon (IFN), native human IFN, recombinant human IFN alpha 2b and human IFN gamma in healthy blood donors. *Clin Exp Immunol* 1990; **32**: 695–701.

178. Andersson JP, Andersson UG. Human intravenous immunoglobulin modulates monokine production *in vitro*. *Immunology* 1990; **71**: 372–6.

179. Andersson UG, Björk L, Skansen-Saphir U, Andersson JP. Down-regulation of cytokine production and interleukin-2 receptor expression by pooled human IgG. *Immunology* 1993; **79**: 211–16.

180. Nugent D, Wang Z, Sandborg C, Berman M. Reduced levels of IL-4 in immune mediated thrombocytopenia (ITP): role of cytokine imbalances in autoimmune disease. *Immunohematology* 1988; **2**: 65A.

181. Garcia-Suarez J, Prieto A, Reyes E *et al*. Abnormal γIFN and αTNF secretion in purified CD2+ cells from autoimmune thrombocytopenic purpura (ATP) patients. Their implication in the clinical course of the disease. *Am J Hematol* 1995; **49**: 271–6.

182. Templeton JG, Cocker JE, Crawford RJ *et al*. Fcγ-receptor blocking antibodies in hyperimmune and normal pooled gammaglobulin. *Lancet* 1985; **i**: 1337.

183. Basta M, Langlois PF, Marques M *et al*. High dose intravenous immunoglobulin modifies complement-mediated *in vivo* clearance. *Blood* 1989; **74**: 326–33.

184. Prasad NK, Papoff G, Zeuner A *et al*. Therapeutic preparations of normal polyspecific IgG (IVIg) induce apoptosis in human lymphocytes and monocytes: a novel mechanism of action of IVIg involving the Fas apoptotic pathway. *J Immunol* 1998; **161**; 3781–90.

185. Berchtold P, Dale GL, Tani P, McMillan R. Inhibition of autoantibody binding to platelet glycoprotein IIb/IIa by anti-idiotypic antibodies in intravenous gammaglobulin. *Blood* 1989; **74**: 2414–17.

186. Rossi F, Kazatchkine MD. Anti-idiotypes against autoantibodies in pooled normal human polyspecific Ig. *J Immunol* 1989; **143**: 4104–9.

187. Dietrich G, Kazatchkine MD. Normal immunoglobulin G (IgG) for therapeutic use (intravenous Ig) contain anti-idiotypic specificities against an immunodominant, disease-associated, cross-reactive idiotype of human anti-thyroglobulin autoantibodies. *J Clin Invest* 1990; **85**: 620–5.

188. Dietrich S, Kaverl SV, Kazatchkine MD. Modulation of autoimmunity by intravenous globulin through interaction with the functions of the immune/idiotypic network. *Clin Immunol Immunopathol* 1992; **62**: 873–81.

189. Roux KH, Tankersley DL. A view of the human idiotypic repertoire. Electron microscopic and immunologic analyses of spontaneous idiotype–anti-idiotype dimers in pooled human IgG. *J Immunol* 1990; **84**: 2136–43.

190. Bussel JB, Schulman I, Hilgartner MW, Barandun S. Intravenous use of gammaglobulin in the treatment of chronic immune thrombocytopenic purpura as a means to defer splenectomy. *J Pediatr* 1983; **103**: 651.

191. Bussel JB, Pham LC, Aledort L, Nachman R. Maintenance treatment of adults with chronic refractory immune thrombocytopenic purpura using repeated intravenous infusions of gammaglobulin. *Blood* 1988; **72**: 121–7.

192. Godeau B, Bierling P, Oksenhendler E, Castaigne S, Dexoninck E, Wechsler B. High-dose dexamethasone therapy for resistant autoimmune thrombocytopenic purpura. *Am J Hematol* 1996; **51**: 334.

193. McMillan R, Longmire RL, Tavassoli M *et al*. *In vitro* platelet phagocytosis by splenic leucocytes in idiopathic thrombocytopenic purpura. *N Engl J Med* 1974; **290**: 249.

194. Dixon R, Rosse W. Platelet antibody in autoimmune thrombocytopenia. *Br J Haematol* 1975; **31**: 129.

195. McMillan R, Longmire R, Yelenosky R. The effect of corticosteroids on human IgG synthesis. *J Immunol* 1976; **116**: 1592.

196. Robson HN, Duthie JJR. Capillary resistance and adrenocortical activity. *Br Med J* 1950; **2**: 971.

197. Labran C. Etude de l'action vaso-constrictrice de la prednisone. *Rev Fr Etude Clin Biol* 1963; **8**: 765.

198. Hutter JJ, Hathaway WE. Prednisone-induced hemostasis in a platelet function abnormality. *Am J Dis Child* 1975; **129**: 641.

199. Alexander M, van den Bogaert N, Fondu P. Le pronostic et le traitement du purpura thrombopénique idiopathique de l'enfant. *Arch Fr Pediatr* 1976; **33**: 329.

200. Johnson SA. Endothelial supporting function of platelets. In: Johnson SA (ed.) *The Circulating Platelet*. New York: Academic Press, 1971, p. 283.

201. Kitchens CS, Weiss L. Ultrastructural changes of endothelium associated with thrombocytopenia. *Blood* 1975; **46**: 567.

202. Kitchens CS, Weiss L. Amelioration of endothelial abnormalities by prednisone in experimental thrombocytopenia in the rabbit. *J Clin Invest* 1977; **60**: 1129.

203. Kitchens CS, Pendergast JF. Human thrombocytopenia is associated with structural abnormalities of the endothelium that are ameliorated by glucocorticoid administration. *Blood* 1986; **67**: 203.

204. Senyi A, Blajchman MA, Hirsch J *et al*. The experimental corrective effect of hydrocortisone on the bleeding time in thrombocytopenic rabbits. Presented at the American Society of Hematology, 18th Annual Meeting, 1975, p. 80A.

205. Blajchman MA, Senyi AF, Hirsch J *et al*. Shortening of the bleeding time in rabbits by hydrocortisone caused by inhibition of prostacyclin generation by the vessel wall. *J Clin Invest* 1979; **63**: 1026.

206. Gaulier MT, Rose C, Roussel MT, Huart C, Bauters F, Fenaux P. Pulsed high-dose dexamethasone in refractory chronic idiopathic thrombocytopenic purpura: a report on 10 cases. *Br J Haematol* 1995; **91**: 477–9.

207. del Principe D, Menichelli A, Mori PG *et al*. Phase II trial of methylprednisolone pulse therapy in childhood chronic thrombocytopenia. *Acta Haematol* 1987; **77**: 226.

208. van Hoff J, Ritchey AK. Pulse methylprednisolone therapy for acute childhood idiopathic thrombocytopenic purpura. *J Pediatr* 1988; **113**: 563.

209. Adams DM, Kinney TR, Obranksirupp E, Ware RE. High-dose oral dexamethasone therapy for chronic childhood idiopathic thrombocytopenic purpura. *J Pediatr* 1996; **128** (2): 281–3.

210. Saag KG, Koehnke R, Caldwell JR *et al*. Low dose long-term corticosteroid therapy in rheumatoid arthritis: an analysis of serious adverse effects. *Am J Med* 1994; **96**: 115.

211. Cohen P, Gardner FH. The thrombocytopenic effect of sustained high-dosage prednisone therapy in thrombocytopenic purpura. *N Engl J Med* 1961; **265**: 611.

212. Giles AH, Shellshear ID. Unwanted corticosteroid effects in childhood bone marrow failure, renal failure and brain damage: case report. *NZ Med J* 1975; **81** (539): 424–7.

213. Salama A, Kiefel V, Mueller-Eckhardt C. Effect of IgG and Rho(D) in adult patients with chronic autoimmune thrombocytopenia. *Am J Hematol* 1986; **22**: 241–50.

214. Becker T, Kuenzlen E, Salama A *et al*. Treatment of childhood idiopathic thrombocytopenic purpura with Rhesus antibodies (antiD). *Eur J Pediatr* 1986; **145**: 166.

215. Bussel JB, Graziano JN, Kimberly RP, Pahwa S, Aledort LM. Intravenous anti-D treatment of immune thrombocytopenic purpura: analysis of efficacy, toxicity, and mechanism of effect. *Blood* 1991; **77**: 1884.

216. Andrew M, Blanchette VS, Adams M *et al*. A multicenter study of the treatment of childhood chronic idiopathic thrombocytopenic purpura with anti-D. *J Pediatr* 1992; **120**: 522.

217. Borgna-Pignatti C, Battisti L, Zecca M, Locatelli F. Treatment of chronic childhood immune thrombocytopenic purpura with intramuscular anti-D immunoglobulins. *Br J Haematol* 1994; **88**: 618.

218. Ahn YS, Byrnes JJ, Harrington WJ *et al*. The treatment of idiopathic thrombocytopenia with vinblastine-loaded platelets. *N Engl J Med* 1978; **298**: 1101.

219. Cervantes F, Rozman C, Feliu E, Montserrat E, Diumenjo C, Granena A. Low-dose vincristine in the treatment of corticosteroid-refractory idiopathic thrombocytopenic purpura (ITP) in nonsplenectomized patients. *Postgrad Med J* 1980; **56**: 711.

220. Kelton JG, McDonald JWD, Barr RM *et al*. The reversible binding of vinblastine to platelets: implications for therapy. *Blood* 1981; **57**: 431.

221. Ahn YS, Harrington WJ, Mylvaganam R, Allen LM, Pall LM. Slow infusion of vinca alkaloids in the treatment of idiopathic thrombocytopenic purpura. *Ann Intern Med* 1984; **100**: 192.

222. Manoharan A. Slow infusion of vincristine in the treatment of idiopathic thrombocytopenic purpura. *Am J Hematol* 1986; **21**: 135.

223. Simon M, Jouet J, Fenaux P, Pollet J, Walter M, Bauters F. The treatment of adult idiopathic thrombocytopenic purpura. Infusion of vinblastine in ITP. *Eur J Haematol* 1987; **39**: 193.

224. Linares M, Cervero A, Sanchez M *et al*. Slow infusion of vincristine in the treatment of refractory thrombocytopenic purpura. *Acta Haematol* 1988; **80**: 173.

225. Fenaux P, Quiquandon I, Caulier MT, Simon M, Walter MP, Bauters F. Slow infusions of vinblastine in the treatment of adult idiopathic thrombocytopenic purpura: a report on 43 cases. *Blut* 1990; **60**: 238.

226. Manoharan A. Targeted-immunosuppression with vincristine infusion in the treatment of immune thrombocytopenia. *Aus NZ J Med* 1991; **21**: 405.

227. Bouroncle BA, Doan CA. Refractory idiopathic thrombocytopenic purpura treated with azathioprine. *N Engl J Med* 1966; **275**: 630.

228. Bouroncle BA, Doan CA. Treatment of refractory idiopathic thrombocytopenic purpura. *JAMA* 1969; **207**: 2049.

229. Sussman LN. Azathioprine in refractory idiopathic thrombocytopenic purpura. *JAMA* 1967; **202**: 259.

230. Quiquandon I, Fenaux P, Caulier MT, Pagniez D, Huart JJ, Bauters F. Re-evaluation of the role of azathioprine in the treatment of adult chronic idiopathic thrombocytopenic purpura: a report on 53 cases. *Br J Haematol* 1990; **74**: 223.

231. Hilgartner MW, Lanzkowsky P, Smith CH. The use of azathioprine in refractory idiopathic thrombocytopenic purpura in children. *Acta Paediatr Scand* 1970; **59**: 409.

232. Ahn YS, Harrington WJ, Simon SR, Mylvaganam R, Pall LM, So AG. Danazol for the treatment of idiopathic thrombocytopenic purpura. *N Engl J Med* 1983; **308**: 1396.

233. Buelli M, Cortelazzo S, Viero P *et al*. Danazol for the treatment of idiopathic thrombocytopenic purpura. *Acta Haematol* 1985; **74**: 97.

234. McVerry BA, Auger M, Bellingham AJ. The use of danazol in the management of chronic immune thrombocytopenic purpura. *Br J Haematol* 1985; **61**: 145.

235. Almargo D. Danazol in idiopathic thrombocytopenic purpura. *Acta Haematol* 1985; **74**: 120.

236. Ambriz R, Pizzuto J, Morales M, Chavez G, Guillen C, Aviles A. Therapeutic effect of danazol on metrorrhagia in patients with idiopathic thrombocytopenic purpura (ITP). *Nouv Rev Fr Hematol* 1986; **28**: 275.

237. Mazzucconi MG, Francesconi M, Falcione E *et al.* Danazol therapy in refractory chronic immune thrombocytopenic purpura. *Acta Haematol* 1987; **77**: 45.

238. Manoharan A. Danazol therapy in patients with immune cytopenias. *Aus NZ J Med* 1987; **17**: 613.

239. Schreiber AD, Chien P, Tomaski A, Cines DB. Effect of danazol in immune thrombocytopenic purpura. *N Engl J Med* 1987; **316**: 503.

240. Kotlarek-Haus S, Podolak-Dawidziak M. Danazol in chronic idiopathic thrombocytopenic purpura resistant to corticosteroids. *Folia Haematol* 1987; **114**: 768.

241. Ahn YS, Mylvaganam R, Garcia RO, Kim CI, Palow D, Harrington WJ. Low-dose danazol therapy in idiopathic thrombocytopenic purpura. *Ann Intern Med* 1987; **107**: 177.

242. Nalli G, Sajeva MR, Maffe GC, Ascari E. Danazol therapy for idiopathic thrombocytopenic purpura (ITP). *Haematologia* 1988; **73**: 55.

243. Alm YS, Rocha R, Mylvaganam R, Garcia R, Duncan R, Harrington WJ. Long-term danazol therapy in autoimmune thrombocytopenia: unmaintained remission and age-dependent response in women. *Ann Intern Med* 1989; **111**: 723.

244. Edelmann DZ, Knobel B, Virag L, Meytes D. Danazol in nonsplenectomized patients with refractory idiopathic thrombocytopenic purpura. *Postgrad Med J* 1990; **66**: 827.

245. Flores A, Carles J, Junca J, Abella E. Danazol therapy in chronic immune thrombocytopenic purpura. *Eur J Haematol* 1990; **45**: 109.

246. Arrowsmith JB, Dreis M. Thrombocytopenia after treatment with danazol. *N Engl J Med* 1986; **314**: 585.

247. Rabinowe SN, Miller KB. Danazol-induced thrombocytopenia. *Br J Haematol* 1987; **65**: 383.

248. Laveder F, Marcolongo R, Zamboni S. Thrombocytopenic purpura following treatment with danazol. *Br J Haematol* 1995; **90**: 970.

249. Weinblatt ME, Kochen J, Ortega J. Danazol for children with immune thrombocytopenic purpura. *Am J Dis Child* 1988; **142**: 1317.

250. Marder VJ, Nusbacher J, Anderson FW. One-year follow-up of plasma exchange therapy in 14 patients with idiopathic thrombocytopenic purpura. *Transfusion* 1981; **21**: 291.

251. Blanchette VS, Hogan VA, McCombie NE *et al.* Intensive plasma exchange therapy in ten patients with idiopathic thrombocytopenic purpura. *Transfusion* 1984; **24**: 388.

252. Bussel JB, Saal S, Gordon B. Combined plasma exchange and intravenous gammaglobulin in the treatment of patients with refractory immune thrombocytopenic purpura. *Transfusion* 1988; **28**: 38.

253. Snyder HW, Cochran SK, Balint JP *et al.* Experience with protein A-immunoadsorption in treatment-resistant adult immune thrombocytopenic purpura. *Blood* 1992; **79**: 2237.

254. Balint JP Jr, Snyder HW Jr, Cochran SK, Jones FR. Long-term response of immune thrombocytopenia to extracorporeal immunoadsorption. *Lancet* 1991; **337**: 1106.

255. Guthrie TH, Oral A. Immunethrombocytopenic purpura: a pilot study of staphylococcal protein A immunomodulation in refractory patients. *Semin Hematol* 1989; **26**: 3.

256. Balint J, Quagliata F, Cochran SK, Jones FR. Association of antiplatelet IgG antibody levels with response to extracorporeal protein A/silica immunoadsorption in ITP patients. *Am J Hematol* 1995; **50**: 74–5.

257. Brox AG, Howson Jan K, Fauser AA. Treatment of idiopathic thrombocytopenic purpura with ascorbate. *Br J Haematol* 1988; **70**: 341.

258. Toyama K, Ohyashiki K, Nehashi Y, Ohyashiki JH. Ascorbate for the treatment of idiopathic thrombocytopenic purpura. *Br J Haematol* 1990; **75**: 623.

259. Win N, Matthey F, Davies SC. Ascorbate for the treatment of idiopathic thrombocytopenic purpura. *Br J Haematol* 1990; **75**: 626.

260. Verhoef GEG, Boonen S, Boogaerts MA. Ascorbate for the treatment of refractory idiopathic thrombocytopenic purpura. *Br J Haematol* 1990; **74**: 234.

261. Godeau B, Bierling P. Treatment of chronic autoimmune thrombocytopenic purpura with ascorbate. *Br J Haematol* 1990; **75**: 289.

262. Novitzky N, Wood L, Jacobs P. Treatment of refractory immune thrombocytopenic purpura with ascorbate. *South Afr Med J* 1992; **81**: 44.

263. Van der Beek-Boter JW, Van Oers MHJ, Von dem Borne AEKG, Klaassen RJL. Ascorbate for the treatment of ITP. *Eur J Haematol* 1992; **48**: 61.

264. Jubelirer SJ. Pilot study of ascorbic acid for the treatment of refractory immune thrombocytopenic purpura. *Am J Hematol* 1993; **43**: 44.

265. Lortan JE. Clinical annotation. Management of asplenic patients. *Br J Haematol* 1993; **84**: 566.

266. Styrt B. Infection associated with asplenia: risks, mechanisms, and prevention. *Am J Med* 1990; **88**: 5N–33N.

267. Schilling RF. Estimating the risk for sepsis after splenectomy in hereditary spherocytosis. *Ann Intern Med* 1995; **122**: 187.

268. Dickermann JD. Splenectomy and sepsis: a warning. *Pediatrics* 1979; **63**: 938–41.

269. Gasbarini A, Franceschi F, Tartaglione R *et al.* Regression of autoimmune thrombocytopenia after eradication of *Helicobacter pylori*. *Lancet* 1998; **352**: 878.

270. Emilia G, Longo G, Luppi M *et al. Helicobacter pylori* eradication can induce platelet recovery in idiopathic thrombocytopenic purpura. *Blood* 2001; **97**: 812–14.

271. Ellaurie M, Burns E, Bernstein L *et al.* Thrombocytopenia and human immunodeficiency virus in children. *Pediatrics* 1988; **82**: 905–8.

272. Imbach P, Luginbühl L, Späth P *et al.* Cyclosporin A (CyA) and intravenous immunoglobulin (i.v. IgG) in chronic immune thrombocytopenic purpura (ITP) in childhood: a clinical and immunological study (progress report). In: Schindler R (ed.) *Cyclosporin in Autoimmune Disease.* 1985, pp. 268–9.

273. Kappers-Klunne MC, van't Veer MB. Cyclosporin A for the treatment by cyclosporin in refractory autoimmune haematological disorders. *Br J Haematol* 2001; **114**: 121–5.

274. Emilia G, Morselli M, Luppi M *et al.* Long-term salvage therapy with cyclosporin A in refractory idiopathic thrombocytopenic purpura. *Blood* 2002; **99**: 1482–5.

275. Abrams JR, Lebwohl MG, Guzzo CA *et al.* CTLA4Ig-mediated blockade of T-cell costimulation in patients with psoriasis vulgaris. *J Clin Invest* 1999; **103**: 1243–52.

276. Reff ME, Carner K, Chambers KS *et al.* Depletion of B cells in vivo by a chimeric mouse human monoclonal antibody to CD20. *Blood* 1994; **83**: 435–45.

277. Stasi R, Pagana A, Stipa E *et al.* Rituximab chimeric anti-CD20 monoclonal antibody treatment for adults with chronic idiopathic thrombocytopenic purpura. *Blood* 2001; **98**: 952–7.

278. Gilleece MH, Dexter TM. Effect of Campath-1H antibody on human hematopoietic progenitors in vitro. *Blood* 1993; **82**: 807–12.

279. Hale G. Synthetic peptide mimotope of the CAMPATH-1 (CD52) antigen, a small glycosylphosphatidylinositol-anchored glycoprotein. *Immunotechnology* 1995; **1**: 175–87.

280. Willis F, Marsh JC, Bevan DH *et al.* The effect of treatment with Campath-1H in patients with autoimmune cytopenias. *Br J Haematol* 2001; **114**: 891–8.

281. Hrstkova H, Bajer M, Michalek J. Recombinant human interferon alpha-2a therapy in children with chronic immune thrombocytopenic purpura. *J Pediatr Hematol Oncol* 2002; **24**: 299–303.

282. Rice L, Nichol JL, McMillan R. Cyclic immune thrombocytopenia responsive to thrombopoietic growth factor therapy. *Am J Hematol* 2001; **68**: 210–14.

283. Huhn RD, Read EJ, Rick M *et al.* Intensive immunosuppression with high-dose cyclophosphamide and autologous CD34⁺ selected hematopoietic cell support for chronic refractory autoimmune thrombocytopenia [abstract]. *Blood* 1999; **94**: 178.

24 Thrombocytosis

Christof Dame

Introduction

Thrombocytosis occurs in up to 15% of hospitalized infants and children. In almost all cases, platelet counts are elevated secondary to infection, anemia, surgery, chronic inflammatory disorders, malignancies, or pharmaceutical agents (reactive thrombocytosis).[1–4] In contrast, essential thrombocytosis is very rare in children and is subdivided into nonfamilial and familial forms. Since essential thrombocytosis is a myeloproliferative disorder, such as chronic myelogenous leukemia, polycythemia vera and idiopathic myelofibrosis (agnogenic myeloid metaplasia), in any child with newly recognized thrombocytosis the question should be addressed whether thrombocytosis is reactive or a sign of a primary hematopoietic disorder. It is also necessary to analyze the immediate risk of the child developing thrombosis or hemorrhage, and to decide how this risk should be managed. To answer these questions, fundamental knowledge of the pathogenesis, clinical manifestation, diagnosis, prognosis, and treatment of essential and reactive thrombocytosis is required.

Definition and classification of thrombocytosis

Thrombocytosis in children is defined by an elevated platelet count, as in adults. A normal platelet count of $150-450 \times 10^9/L$ is generally accepted for healthy preterm and term neonates, infants, children, and adolescents. However, the definition of thrombocytosis varies, from a platelet count $> 400 \times 10^9/L$ to one $> 1000 \times 10^9/L$.[5] In order to consider the characteristics and clinical implications of thrombocytosis and to compare published data, the following arbitrary classification of thrombocytosis has been chosen in most recent publications.
- Mild thrombocytosis: platelet count > 450 and $< 700 \times 10^9/L$.
- Moderate thrombocytosis: platelet count > 700 and $< 900 \times 10^9/L$.
- Severe thrombocytosis: platelet count $> 900 \times 10^9/L$.
- Extreme thrombocytosis: platelet count $> 1000 \times 10^9/L$.[5,6]

Thrombocytosis is classified into an essential (primary) and a reactive (secondary) form. Essential thrombocytosis is a myeloproliferative disorder, caused by monoclonal or polyclonal abnormalities of hematopoietic cells or by abnormalities in the biology of thrombopoietin (Tpo), the primary regulator of megakaryopoiesis. Reactive thrombocytosis is caused by stimulated megakaryopoiesis in the absence of a chronic myeloproliferative/dysplastic disorder of hematopoiesis. Reactive thrombocytosis is associated with various hematologic or nonhematologic diseases, and platelet counts normalize after resolution of the underlying medical condition.

Symptoms of thrombocytosis in childhood

Regardless of its pathogenic origin, thrombocytosis can cause thrombosis (particularly in the vena cava, subclavian vein, renal vein, or intracerebral vessels), hemorrhage (particularly epistaxis) and vasomotor complications (especially headache, visual symptoms, light-headedness, seizures). These complications are much less likely to occur in reactive than in essential thrombocytosis. However, many children remain asymptomatic, even in extreme thrombocytosis with platelet counts in excess of $1000 \times 10^9/L$.[1,7,8]

Diagnostic features of thrombocytosis

Counting of platelets

A gold standard for the method of blood sampling (venous or capillary blood sample) or platelet counting (automated cell counter, counting under the microscope) is still not defined. If an abnormal platelet count has been found by automated cell counting, analysis of a blood smear is necessary to exclude morphologic abnormalities of platelets or other blood cells, such as abnormal platelet granules, cytoplasmic fragments, red cell fragments, or extremely microcytic red blood cells.[6]

Other diagnostic features of thrombocytosis

In most children with thrombocytosis, clinically apparent symptoms of an active underlying systemic disease or medical condition causing stimulated megakaryopoiesis may be evident. However, in single cases, it can be very difficult to differentiate between essential and reactive forms of thrombocytosis. The initial laboratory analysis of complete blood count, including examination of the peripheral blood smear, and of serum ferritin concentration is helpful to differentiate the origin of thrombocytosis. These tests allow exclusion of iron deficiency, hyposplenism or asplenia (Howell–Jolly bodies), and inflammatory or infectious conditions (neutrophilic leukocytosis, increased numbers of neutrophilic band forms and/or metamyelocytes, neutrophilic vacuolization, toxic granules) as indices for reactive thrombocytosis. If these tests are unrevealing, additional measurements of C-reactive protein, interleukin (IL)-6, plasma fibrinogen, and analysis of erythrocyte sedimentation rate may help further decision-making, although their specificity for differentiating various forms of thrombocytosis is low.[9] The measurement of the plasma concentration of Tpo is generally not helpful for distinguishing reactive from essential forms of thrombocytosis, although differences in the regulation and clearance of Tpo do exist.[10–14]

Before ascribing thrombocytosis to an essential disorder of megakaryopoiesis, which is largely a diagnosis of exclusion, repeated complete blood counts and extended diagnostics are necessary, including the analysis of platelet counts from family members.[15,16] As in adults, the gold standard diagnostic criteria for essential thrombocytosis remain those proposed by the Polycythemia Vera Group, summarized in Table 24.1.[6,17,90] Besides the morphologic (reticulin staining) and genetic/cytogenetic analysis of a bone marrow specimen (exclusion of Philadelphia chromosome, Bcr/Abl fusion protein, chromosomal translocation), many other diagnostic features have been studied. These include measurement of reticulated platelets, culture of megakaryocyte colonies (megakaryocytic colony-forming units), clonal analysis using X-chromosome inactivation patterns, analysis of Tpo receptor expression on platelets and/or megakaryocyte progenitor cells, and measurement of various megakaryopoietic growth factors or cytokines, particularly Tpo and transforming growth factor (TGF)-β. The analysis of such diagnostic features has significantly contributed to a better understanding of the pathogenesis of essential thrombocytosis, but a hallmark feature for essential thrombocytosis has still not been identified.[18] Of note, preliminary data suggest that in adults the combined presence of decreased Tpo expression on megakaryocytes, marked bone marrow megakaryocyte proliferation, and increased bone marrow angiogenesis is highly

Table 24.1 Diagnostic criteria for essential thrombocytosis: 'A' criteria are diagnostic; 'B' criteria are confirmative.

A1	Platelet count > 600 × 10^9/L and no known cause of reactive thrombocytosis
A2	Increase in and clustering of mature giant megakaryocytes with hyperploid nuclei
A3	No preceding or allied other subtype of myeloproliferative disorder or myelodysplastic syndrome
B1	Normal or elevated leukocyte alkaline phosphatase score, normal erythrocyte sedimentation rate, no fever
B2	Normal or slightly increased cellularity and no or minimal reticulin fibrosis
B3	Splenomegaly on palpation or spleen length > 11 cm* on diagnostic imaging procedure
B4	Spontaneous erythroid colony and/or spontaneous megakaryocyte colony formation in bone marrow progenitor assays

* A spleen length above two standard deviations of normal may fulfil this criterion in children.
Reproduced with permission from Ref. 6.

sensitive and specific in distinguishing essential from reactive thrombocytosis.[19] Currently, there is no evidence to suggest that these features have the same or even a higher diagnostic value in children than in adults, because some of them can be normal in children with essential thrombocytosis.[6,8]

Physiology of stimulated platelet production

Tpo is the key regulator of megakaryopoiesis and plays a pivotal role in normal platelet production.[20] Developmental changes or abnormalities in the biology of Tpo and its receptor (Tpo-R) have significant implications for the pathogenesis of thrombocytosis in children. The human *Tpo* gene is located on chromosome 3q26–27.[21] The full-length Tpo protein is composed of 332 amino acids and characterized by two distinct domains plus an additional 21-amino acid secretory leader sequence. The N-terminal receptor-binding domain shares 20% sequence identity plus 25% sequence homology with erythropoietin (Epo) ("Epo-like" domain).[22,23] This domain is essential for the signaling and the proliferative activity of the molecule.[24] The C-terminal domain specifically characterizes the Tpo molecule (Tpo glycan domain). The human full-length Tpo protein is highly glycosylated and has an apparent molecular mass of approximately 70 kDa (68–85 kDa as analyzed in SDS page electrophoresis).[25] The *Tpo* gene is primarily expressed in the liver and to a lower extent in the kidneys, bone marrow, and other organs.[24,26–29] Tpo acts by binding to its specific receptor and through the JAK-STAT (members of the Janus tyrosine kinase family and members of the Stat family of transcription factors) signal transduction pathway.[30]

The human *Tpo-R* gene is located on chromosome 1p34.[31] Since Tpo-R was characterized some years before Tpo was identified as its ligand, the *Tpo-R* gene is still named with the acronym c-*Mpl* (for *c*ellular homolog of a retrovirus complex inducing *m*yeloproliferative *l*eukemia).[32] Tpo-R belongs to the cytokine receptor family and is composed of a 466-amino acid extracellular ligand-binding domain, which includes two cytokine receptor motifs, a 22-residue transmembrane domain, and a 122-amino acid cytoplasmic domain.[31] The distal cytokine receptor motif of the extracellular domain is responsible for ligand binding. In the absence of Tpo, it inhibits the constitutive signaling activity of the membrane proximal cytokine receptor motif.[33] The juxta-membrane WSXWS motif (tryptophan-serine-X-tryptophan-serine, where X represents any amino acid), which is a common motif in each member of the cytokine receptor family, is thought to be responsible for maintaining the proper structural conformation of the extracellular domain as well as for internalization and signal transduction. The intracellular domain, which contains the highly conserved box 1 and box 2 motifs, is crucial for full biological activity of Tpo-R.[34] Although precise data are not available, it is assumed that megakaryocyte progenitor cells display a significantly higher number of Tpo-Rs on their surface than platelets, which display approximately 220 receptors per cell.[35] Among hematopoietic cells, the Tpo-R is expressed on CD34+ cells, pluripotent early hematopoietic progenitor cells, megakaryocytes, and platelets.[36] Tpo acts on the commitment of early hematopoietic stem and progenitor cells into lineage-specific differentiation, and it stimulates the proliferation of committed megakaryocyte progenitor cells and the differentiation of megakaryoblasts to megakaryocytes.[37,38] However, Tpo seems not to be required for megakaryocyte proplatelet formation, the final step in thrombopoiesis.[39]

Hepatic Tpo production is primarily constitutive.[35,40] Circulating Tpo is regulated by binding to Tpo-R-bearing cells. Functional Tpo-Rs remove Tpo by absorption and internalization of the cell surface complex. Thereby, under normal conditions circulating Tpo concentrations are inversely proportional to the mass of megakaryocytes and platelets. The concept of end-cell-mediated regulation of Tpo is illustrated in Fig. 24.1. Accordingly, circulating Tpo concentrations are elevated if thrombocytopenia results from reduced megakaryopoiesis.[41] In contrast, Tpo concentrations are normal or slightly elevated if thrombocytopenia results from platelet destruction.[42,43] However, there is evidence that hepatic Tpo production can be upregulated in response to hepatic growth factor and IL-6.[44–47] These regulatory mechanisms are specific, since other factors such as IL-1β, IL-11, tumor necrosis factor (TNF)-α, interferon (IFN)-α, IFN-β or IFN-γ do not modulate Tpo production in human hepatoma cells.[44,48]

Besides Tpo, other cytokines or hematopoietic growth factors such as granulocyte–macrophage colony-stimulating factor (GM-CSF), IL-3, IL-6, IL-11, and leukemia inhibitory factor contribute directly to megakaryopoiesis, each of them with a specific activity at certain steps in this process.[49] Most recently, the role of IL-1 in megakaryopoiesis has been further elucidated. IL-1β stimulates directly the formation of megakaryocytic colony-forming units (CFU-Meg).[50] Moreover, in megakaryocytic progenitor cells IL-1β stimulates the expression of both Tpo and transcription factors, such as the zinc finger protein GATA-1 and the basic leucine zipper NF-E2, which are involved in the proliferation and differentiation of megakaryocyte progenitor cells.[51]

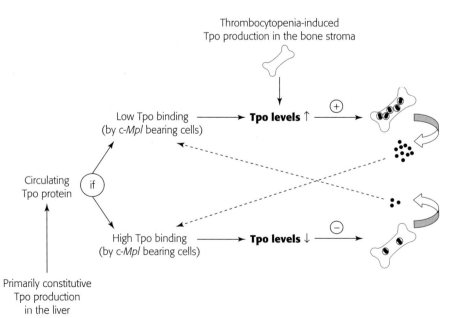

Fig. 24.1 Model of the regulation of circulating thrombopoietin (Tpo) concentrations. The model is based on the concept of end-cell-mediated regulation by the mass of c-*Mpl* (Tpo receptor)-bearing cells and a mainly constitutive Tpo production in the liver and kidneys. In the bone marrow, stromal cells contribute to Tpo production if thrombocytopenia occurs. This model implicates an autoregulatory loop mechanism as illustrated by the dashed lines. Modified with permission from Ref. 125.

Essential thrombocytosis

Pathogenesis

Essential thrombocytosis is classified as a chronic myeloproliferative disorder of hematopoiesis, resulting in uncontrolled platelet production as the major hematologic abnormality.[52] Essential thrombocytosis can be a monoclonal or polyclonal disorder. In adults, the risk of thromboembolic complications seems to be higher in cases of monoclonality.[53] Since essential thrombocytosis is extremely rare in childhood, data on pathogenesis have been obtained nearly exclusively in adults.

During recent years, research on the pathogenesis of essential thrombocytosis has focused on the role of Tpo in this disorder. In adolescents and adults with essential thrombocytosis, normal or even slightly elevated circulating Tpo concentrations have been measured, although decreased Tpo concentrations would be expected as a consequence of the elevated mass of Tpo-R-bearing megakaryocytes and platelets.[11,12,14,54–56] The findings of "inadequately high" circulating Tpo concentrations raises the question of abnormal Tpo production or a defect in Tpo clearance from the plasma. In contrast to familial forms of thrombocytosis, structural defects in the *Tpo* or c-*Mpl* gene locus have not yet been found in children or adults with nonfamilial essential thrombocytosis.[8,57–59] However, the expression of c-Mpl on megakaryopoietic progenitors and platelets can be decreased in essential thrombocytosis.[55,60–62] Thereby, defective clearance of circulating Tpo and subsequent Tpo excess result in the stimulation of megakaryopoiesis.[55,62] However, neither "inadequately high" (or even elevated) Tpo concentrations nor reduced Tpo clearance are specific for essential thrombocytosis, and both have also been described in polycythemia vera.[60,63] In polycythemia vera, reduced Tpo clearance may be caused by the posttranslational hypoglycosylation of c-Mpl protein with derailment of membrane localization.[64]

Spontaneous formation of CFU-Meg colonies is another well-known phenomenon in serum-free hematopoietic progenitor cell assays from both adults and children with nonfamilial essential thrombocytosis.[65–67] Megakaryopoiesis can be additionally stimulated, and increased sensitivity of these CFU-Meg colonies to Tpo has been observed.[68,69] One pathogenic factor leading to the increased sensitivity of CFU-Meg to cytokines may be a decreased response to TGF-β, which normally suppresses megakaryocyte growth.[70] Reduced Smad4 (Sma- and Mad-related protein-4) expression in CFU-Meg may cause the lack of megakaryopoietic suppression by TGF-β.[71] While the proliferation of megakaryopoietic progenitor cells cannot be inhibited by antibodies directed against IL-3, IL-6, GM-CSF or Tpo, blocking of c-Mpl reduces the proliferation rate of megakaryopoietic progenitor cells *in vivo*.[72,73] This phenomenon has been described as "a paradox, Tpo-independent, but c-Mpl-dependent modulation" of megakaryopoietic progenitors in essential thrombocytosis.[52] As in adults, children with nonfamilial essential thrombocytosis show spontaneous formation of CFU-Meg, which can be (at least in some children) combined with spontaneous formation of erythroid progenitors (erythroid burst-forming units), indicating that two different cell lines or a bi-potent erythromegakaryocytic progenitor are affected in this disorder.[66,67]

The role of the bone marrow microenvironment in the pathogenesis of essential thrombocytosis is not completely elucidated. In bone marrow stromal cells, expression of *Tpo* is regulated by proteins released from platelet α-granules. Specifically, platelet-derived growth factor and fibroblast growth factor-2 stimulate *Tpo* mRNA expression, whereas platelet factor-4, thrombospondin and TGF-β suppress *Tpo* mRNA expression.[74–76] However, in adults, *Tpo* mRNA expression in bone marrow and mononuclear cells isolated from peripheral blood does not significantly differ from that of patients with myelofibrosis or controls.[75] Neither (serum) Tpo concentrations nor platelet counts correlate with measured transcripts.[77]

It is unclear whether stimulated angiogenesis in the bone marrow stroma has a primary pathogenic implication or whether it is a secondary phenomenon of essential thrombocytosis.[19] Recently published data indicate that the expression of hematopoietically relevant genes, such as the polycythemia rubra vera-1 (*PRV-1*) gene or the gene of the transcription factor *NF-E2*, can be changed in essential thrombocytosis.[61,78–80] Adult PRV-1-positive patients with essential thrombocytosis seem to have a significantly increased risk for vascular complications compared with PRV-1-negative patients.[81]

Most recently, data obtained in mice with mutations of the c-*Myb* gene indicate a fundamental role of this transcription factor in the development of thrombocytosis.[82] C-Myb is a helix–loop–helix basic-leucine zipper protein that controls the proliferation of immature progenitors and interacts with ubiquitous transcriptional coactivators, such as CBP and p100. *C-Myb* mutant mice, bearing single amino acid substitutions in the c-Myb DNA-binding domain or within the leucine zipper domain, referred to as *Plt3* and *Plt4* alleles of c-*Myb*,[83] exhibit excessive megakaryopoiesis in both the presence and absence of Tpo (c-*mpl* −/− or *Tpo* −/− background).[82] The half-life of platelets in these mice is normal, and *in vivo* labeling studies have confirmed the enhanced rate of platelet production. Although the development of CFU-Meg is independent of Tpo, GM-CSF stimulates megakaryocyte progenitors carrying the *Plt3* or *Plt4* mutant c-*Myb* genes. These cells are also hyperresponsive to other cytokines, such as stem cell factor, IL-3 and Epo.[82] Future studies might show whether mutations of c-*Myb* are relevant for thrombocytosis in humans.

Clinical and laboratory features of essential thrombocytosis in childhood

In children, the annual incidence of newly diagnosed essential thrombocytosis is about 1 per 10 million, 60 times lower than the rate in adults.[84,85] Based on the criteria of the Polycythemia Vera Study Group, about 75 children with essential thrombocytosis have been reported between 1966 and 2005.[8,66,85–89] Clinical and laboratory features of essential thrombocytosis in childhood are summarized in Table 24.2 and compared with those characteristic of reactive thrombocytosis. Familial forms occur in 40–55% of children with essential thrombocytosis. Approximately two-thirds of children with essential thrombocytosis have platelet counts in excess of $1000 \times 10^9/L$. In childhood, the median age at diagnosis of essential thrombocytosis is 11 years. Similar to adults, about 30% of patients experience thromboembolic or hemorrhagic complications at the time of diagnosis or later; 20% of initially asymptomatic children suffer these complications later.[85,86] Splenomegaly has been found in 50% and hepatomegaly in 25% of children with essential thrombocytosis. As far as longitudinal analysis is available, 10% of patients died due to the underlying hematopoietic disorder and another 5% developed other myeloproliferative disorders.[86]

The risk of hemorrhage may increase with extreme thrombocytosis ($>1500 \times 10^9/L$).[90] Hemostasis is altered in about 20% of patients with essential thrombocytosis, as indicated by a prolonged bleeding time, prothrombin time, and partial thromboplastin time. Platelet function is also often diminished due to increased proteolysis of large von Willebrand factor multimers.[86] In adults, clot lysis is reduced and a higher amount of plasminogen activator inhibitor 1 is released from platelets.[91] Adult patients with essential thrombocytosis also show an increased prevalence of anti-phospholipid antibodies, which may be associated with thrombosis.[92]

Morphologic abnormalities of platelets include giant platelets, platelet conglomerates, bizarre forms, megakaryocytic fragments, and hypogranularity. Ultrastructural abnormalities include reduced numbers of pseudopodia and α-granules. Bone marrow examination reveals hypercellularity, mostly with an elevated number of megakaryocytes. These cells also display hyperploidy, dysplasia, or giant forms. Histologic criteria, such as stimulated angiogenesis, reduced c-Mpl expression on megakaryocytes, and increased proliferation

Table 24.2 Characteristics of essential (primary) and reactive (secondary) thrombocytosis in childhood.

Criteria	Essential thrombocytosis	Reactive thrombocytosis
Age-dependent occurrence	Mostly 11 years*	Mostly < 2 years*
Incidence per year	1 per million children	> 600 per million children
Duration of thrombocytosis	Months, years, or permanently	Days, weeks or months; temporary
Splenomegaly	Often	Rare
Fever	No	Often
Bleeding disorders and thrombosis	Often in monoclonal essential thrombocytosis, rare in familial thrombocythemia	Extremely rare
Frequent laboratory findings	Prolonged bleeding time, increased PT and PTT in 20%; increased praevalence of anti-phospholipid antibodies	Increased vWF, fibrinogen, proinflammatory cytokines, and C-reactive protein if reactive thrombocytosis is caused by infection
Platelet count	Mostly > $1000 \times 10^9/L$	Mostly < $800 \times 10^9/L$
Platelet morphology	Large or small, dysmorphic	Large, but normal morphology
Platelet function	Abnormal	Normal
Bone marrow	Increased megakaryocyte number with abnormal morphology	Increased megakaryocyte number, normal morphology
Pathogenic mechanisms	Clonal defect in hematopoietic or megakaryopoietic progenitors, decreased c-Mpl expression and/or hyperreactivity to Tpo. In some familial forms, mutations in the Tpo or c-Mpl gene locus	Increased Tpo production or release of megakaryopoietic growth factors, particularly IL-6

* Relevant only for primary thrombocytosis in childhood.[86]

IL, interleukin; PT, prothrombin time; PTT, partial thromboplastin time; Tpo, thrombopoietin; vWF, von Willebrand factor.

Reproduced with permission from Ref. 6.

of megakaryocytes, are helpful in distinguishing essential from reactive thrombocytosis.

Familial forms of essential thrombocytosis

Familial, mostly recessive, but also autosomal dominant or (rarely) X-linked forms of essential thrombocytosis should be classified as a separate entity.[93,94] In familial thrombocytosis, mutations in the *Tpo* gene locus have been identified. These mutations occur typically in the 5' untranslated region. They result in functional loss of untranslated open reading frames, causing increased translational efficiency for the mutant *Tpo* mRNA and overproduction of Tpo. Of note, hematocrit values and leukocyte counts are normal in these individuals.[95–98] Familial thrombocytosis can also be caused by mutations in the c-*Mpl* gene. Recently, a mutation in the transmembrane domain of c-Mpl resulting in the activation of intracellular signaling has been identified as causing familial thrombocytosis in a Japanese family.[99] Another mutation in the Tpo-binding domain of c-Mpl causes decreased c-Mpl function and reduced Tpo absorption by platelets, resulting in overstimulation of megakaryopoiesis.[100] Currently known germline mutations in the *Tpo* and c-*Mpl* gene loci are summarized in Table 24.3. However, in other individuals with familial thrombocytosis, *Tpo* or c-*Mpl* mutations have been excluded, suggesting that one or more additional genes are involved in the origin of familial thrombocytosis.[101,102]

In children with familial thrombocytosis, platelet counts are lower than in nonfamilial essential thrombocytosis. Splenomegaly is less frequent, and almost no thrombotic or hemorrhagic complications occur.[86] Therefore, strategies to reduce platelet numbers in familial thrombocytosis are much more conservative. The clinical and pathogenic differences may restore the terms "familial thrombocythemia" or "familial thrombocytosis" to describe this subgroup of essential thrombocytosis.

Treatment options in nonfamilial essential thrombocytosis

Cytoreductive treatment for mild (nonfamilial) essential thrombocytosis, defined as the absence of bleeding or thrombosis in the patient's history and a platelet count $< 1500 \times 10^9/L$, is not recommended, since the incidence of thrombosis or hemorrhage is not significantly different from that of an age- and sex-matched control population.[103] Low-dose acetylsalicylic acid has been used to reduce platelet aggregation in adolescents and some children with recurrent thromboses and seems to be safe, if the platelet count is $< 1500 \times 10^9/L$.[7,87,104,105] To prevent major arterial or venous thrombotic complications, children with dehydration should be efficiently rehydrated to reduce blood viscosity.

Children and adolescents with a platelet count in excess of $1500 \times 10^9/L$ may have an indeterminate risk of thrombotic or bleeding complications, but considered. In this group, cytoreductive treatment is also not generally recommended. If the platelet count is $> 1500 \times 10^9/L$, the use of low-dose acetylsalicylic acid is controversial, since in adults no significant benefit of this treatment in preventing thrombosis has been shown and reduced platelet aggregation is loosely associated with an increased risk of gastrointestinal bleeding.[52] In patients at high risk for thrombotic or hemorrhagic complications, defined as extreme thrombocytosis plus previous hemorrhage, previous thrombosis or medical conditions with increased risk for these complications, cytoreductive therapy may be indicated.

Table 24.3 Summary of currently identified mutations in the *Tpo* and c-*Mpl* gene locus causing familial forms of essential thrombocytosis.

Variant	Functional implication	Tpo concentration	Platelet count ($\times 10^9/L$)	Reference
***Tpo* gene locus** (NCBI accession no. D32046)				
ΔG 3252 (exon 3, 5'UTR)	Increased translation efficacy of Tpo	6.04–26.03 fmol/mL	847–1600	95, 96
G→T 3271 (exon 3, 5'UTR)	Increased translation efficacy of Tpo	5.6–8 fmol/mL	1095–1380	150
G→C 3315 (intron 3, 5'UTR)	Increased translation efficacy of Tpo	74–1180 pg/mL	530–1280	97
A→G 3320 (intron 3, 5'UTR)	Increased translation efficacy of Tpo	430–980 pg/mL	700–1000	98
***C-Mpl* gene locus** (NCBI accession no. M90102)				
G→T 117	Decreased c-Mpl function	Not done	"Significantly higher"	100
Lys → Asn 39				
(ligand-binding domain)				
G→A 1514	Activation of intracellular signaling	Not done	>600–1300	99
Ser→Asn 505				
(transmembrane domain)				

Note that the Tpo protein translation start site is the eighth initiation codon (exon/intron 3). Mutations in this region disturb normal arrangements and result in the functional loss of open reading frames, causing increased translation efficacy of Tpo gene expression.
UTR, untranslated region.

Hydroxycarbamide, an antimetabolite that impairs DNA repair by inhibiting ribonucleotide reductase in all cell lines, may be one effective agent. Hydroxycarbamide has been demonstrated in a clinical trial to produce a significant reduction (from 24 to 4%) in the incidence of thrombotic complications in patients of all ages with essential thrombocytosis.[106] The initial dose of hydroxycarbamide is 15 mg/kg daily, subdivided in two doses. Doses should then be decreased or increased in order to achieve a balance between a platelet count of $150–400 \times 10^9$/L and undesired effects such as neutropenia and anemia. Hydroxycarbamide should not be used in women of childbearing age, during pregnancy and during breast-feeding. However, the risk of leukemic transformation after long-term treatment with hydroxycarbamide in children and young adults is still a major concern, and its use is controversial.[7,16,107] Two recent studies reported no increased incidence of leukemic or neoplastic transformation after long-term treatment (5–14 years) with hydroxycarbamide in 25 young adults (18–49 years) with essential thrombocytosis and in nine children (5.7–13.7 years) with severe sickle cell disease treated for a median of 14 months (range 12–46 months).[108,109]

Anagrelide, an oral imidazo-quinazoline derivative that reduces platelet counts by interfering with megakaryocyte maturation, may be an alternative agent for treating essential thrombocytosis in children and young adults.[86,110–113] In young adults, anagrelide has been administered at 2–4 mg/day in four doses, with increases of 0.5 mg/day every 5–7 days up to a maximal dose of 10 mg/day. The median maintenance dose is 2.5 mg/day.[111] One 16-month-old infant was treated with an initial dose of 0.02 mg/kg daily, which was progressively increased up to 1.5 mg/day.[114] A long-term analysis of the use of anagrelide in young adults with essential thrombocytosis showed good tolerability but complications were still high, with thrombosis in 20%, major bleeding in 20%, and anemia in 24% of patients. Complete normalization of platelet counts may be required in order to minimize the residual risk for thrombosis or hemorrhage.[111] Anagrelide has no known leukemogenic potential. Therefore, anagrelide is increasingly considered as first-line therapy for nonfamilial essential thrombocytosis in children.[7]

As previously reviewed, other platelet-lowering agents such as busulfan, IFN-α, radio-phosphorus, or dipyridamole have been used only in single children or young adults, and cannot be recommended in general.[1] Platelet apheresis has been used to reduce platelet counts in adults with severe acute thrombotic or hemorrhagic complications or platelet counts $> 1500 \times 10^9$/L, but this treatment option has not yet been proven in randomized controlled trials and there is no experience in treating children or adolescents.[2,90]

In children and adolescents, the decision for treating essential thrombocytosis should be made primarily by weighing up the potential risks of all treatment options (particularly the leukemogenic or myelosuppressive side-effects of cytoreductive therapy) and the expected benefit in terms of preventing thrombotic or hemorrhagic complications.[16] Laboratory examinations prior to this decision should include the determination of proteins C and S, antithrombin, anti-cardiolipin antibodies, homocysteine, and mutations of factors II and V.[52] If a platelet-lowering treatment is indicated, it is highly recommended that these patients are enrolled in controlled studies because careful long-term follow-up will help to clarify the natural course of essential thrombocytosis in children and to develop best management strategies.

Reactive thrombocytosis

Pathophysiology

Reactive thrombocytosis results from increased megakaryopoiesis associated with various hematologic (nonproliferative) or nonhematologic diseases. Megakaryopoietic activity can be stimulated up to 10-fold of normal.[115] The proinflammatory cytokine IL-6 plays a major role in the pathogenesis of reactive thrombocytosis by direct stimulation of megakaryocyte progenitor cells and by upregulation of Tpo production. *In vitro* experiments have showed that IL-6 increases *Tpo* gene expression in human hepatocytes and murine liver endothelial cells, and *in vivo* studies have confirmed that reactive thrombocytosis induced by bacterial lipopolysaccharides results from increased hepatic Tpo production.[44–46,116] The effects of IL-6 on both megakaryocyte progenitor cells and Tpo-producing cells may explain why in reactive thrombocytosis circulating Tpo concentrations do not correlate inversely with the mass of Tpo-R-bearing cells.[12,117,118]

The analysis of circulating Tpo concentrations has helped to elucidate in detail the role of Tpo in reactive thrombocytosis associated with infectious diseases. In the first week, when platelet counts are still normal, *Tpo* is upregulated like acute-phase proteins; circulating Tpo concentrations peak on day 4 ± 2, before they gradually decrease. When increasing platelet counts peak in the second or third week, Tpo concentrations normalize.[10] In postoperative thrombocytosis, Tpo plasma concentrations also rise before platelet counts increase. Previously increased IL-6 concentrations again suggest its direct stimulation of Tpo production in hepatocytes.[119] In malignancies, stimulation of megakaryopoiesis may result from Tpo production in tumor cells, particularly in hepatoblastoma, but also to a lesser extent in neuroblastoma, lymphoma, and others.[120,121]

Clinical and laboratory features of reactive thrombocytosis

Reactive thrombocytosis has an estimated incidence of 3–15% among hospitalized children. Typical clinical and laboratory findings in reactive thrombocytosis are summarized in

Table 24.4 Clinical features of reactive thrombocytosis in children: only studies containing more than 130 children are considered.

	Sutor & Hank (1992),[151] Germany	Vora & Lilleyman (1993),[123] UK	Yohannan et al. (1994),[124] Saudi-Arabia	Heng & Tan (1998),[2] Singapore	Chen et al. (1999),[3] Taiwan	Matsubara et al. (2004),[4] Japan
Number of children (platelet count)	227 ($>500 \times 10^9$/L)	458 ($>500 \times 10^9$/L)	663 ($>500 \times 10^9$/L)	135 ($>600 \times 10^9$/L)	220 ($>500 \times 10^9$/L)	456 ($>500 \times 10^9$/L)
Age	72% < 2 years	Median 13 months	Mostly < 5 years*	Mostly < 1 year	Mostly < 2 years	Mostly < 2 years
Boys to girls ratio	1	1.1	1.6	1.7	1.7	1.3
Infections	39%	38%	37%	78%	50%	68%
Surgery/trauma/burns	15%	20%	15%		13%	3.3%
Anemia	12%	6%	14.8% plus 19.3%*		3.7%	6.4%
Gastroesophageal reflux	6.5%					
Autoimmune diseases	4%	9%	2%		3.6%	2%
Kawasaki syndrome				–†	6.4%	9%
Low birthweight (<2500 g)	2.1%			3.2%	3.2%	9.2%

Further conditions (<3% of children with thrombocytosis) included neoplasia, drug-associated thrombocytosis, stress, allergies, metabolic disease and others.

* Without infants; country with high prevalence of hereditary hemolytic anaemia.

† The majority of children with autoimmune disease suffered from Kawasaki syndrome.

Reproduced with permission from Ref. 6.

Table 24.2.[122] Variations in the reported incidence may result from differences in the definition of thrombocytosis, the study setting (hospitalized patients, outpatients, or both), the epidemic occurrence of certain infections, or other factors (Table 24.4).[4,5] In 72–86% of children with reactive thrombocytosis, platelet counts range between 500 and 700×10^9/L (mild thrombocytosis). Moderate thrombocytosis (platelet count $700–900 \times 10^9$/L) has been found in approximately 6–8% of children with reactive thrombocytosis, and only 0.5–3% have a platelet count $> 1000 \times 10^9$/L.[2,4,5,123,124]

The incidence of reactive thrombocytosis in childhood shows an age-dependent pattern. The highest incidence has been found in children up to 24 months old (Table 24.4). Platelet counts $> 500 \times 10^9$/L have been found in 13% of neonates at birth; during the first month, thrombocytosis occurred in 36% of neonates, most of them low birthweight infants (<2500 g) and/or neonates who suffered from infection. At this age, 10% of the studied neonates had platelet counts of $600–700 \times 10^9$/L, while 4% had platelet counts $> 700 \times 10^9$/L. In the second month, 8% of infants had platelet counts $> 700 \times 10^9$/L. The incidence of reactive thrombocytosis returned to 13% in the group of infants aged 6–11 months. Afterwards, the incidence gradually decreased to only 0.6% in children 11–15 years old.[4]

The higher susceptibility for thrombocytosis during the neonatal period may result from various physiologic phenomena. During the ontogeny of medullary hematopoiesis, *Tpo* is expressed at high levels in the bone marrow.[26] Circulating Tpo concentrations are significantly higher in fetuses and neonates than in children and adults.[43,125] During

postnatal development, circulating Tpo concentrations underlie age-dependent changes. They increase after birth, with a peak on the second day, before they return to levels found in cord blood by the end of the first month. Later, Tpo concentrations gradually decrease until the end of the first year of life, where they are still somewhat higher than in adults.[126] Moreover, neonatal megakaryocytic progenitor cells have a higher sensitivity to Tpo compared with cells obtained in adults.[127,128] In small-for-gestational age infants (birthweight below the 10th percentile), additional factors may be relevant for overwhelming platelet production and thrombocytosis, particularly after fetal distress or eclampsia with or without initial neonatal thrombocytopenia.

Clinical conditions frequently associated with reactive thrombocytosis are listed in Table 24.5. Bacterial or viral infections (acute or chronic) are the most common cause for reactive thrombocytosis (37–78%) at any age during childhood. Within this group, infections of the respiratory tract account for 60–80% of thrombocytosis, followed by infections of the gastrointestinal and urinary tracts.[129,130] No relationship has been found between thrombocytosis and the prognosis or antibiotic treatment of the infection. Reactive thrombocytosis occurs in about 50% of children with bacterial meningitis after the first week of treatment, but has no influence on the neurologic outcome of surviving patients. Patients who died developed thrombocytopenia instead of thrombocytosis.[131]

In 1–21% of children, megakaryopoiesis is stimulated secondary to tissue damage (trauma, burns, major surgery).[4,5] Platelet counts usually peak between the first and second

Table 24.5 Clinical conditions frequently associated with reactive thrombocytosis in childhood.

Infections (bacterial, viral; acute, chronic)
Respiratory tract
Gastrointestinal tract
Urinary tract
Meningitis

Tissue damage
Trauma, burns
Major surgery, particularly splenectomy

Splenectomy, hyposplenism, asplenia

Anemia
Iron deficiency
Hemolytic anemia

Acute blood loss
Others, such as thalassemia after splenectomy

Prior hypoxemia and respiratory distress syndrome

Autoimmune diseases or chronic inflammation
Kawasaki disease
Inflammatory bowel diseases
Rheumatoid diseases
Henoch–Schönlein purpura

Renal diseases
Renal failure
Nephrotic syndrome

Malignancies
Hepatoblastoma
Lymphoma (Hodgkin and non-Hodgkin)
Leukemia
Neuroblastoma
Others, such as sarcoma

Prematurity, small-for-gestational age infants, prior fetal and neonatal stress

Drug-induced thrombocytosis
Epinephrine
Corticosteroids
Ciclosporin
Vinca alkaloids
Miconazole
Penicillamine
Meropenem
Imipenem
Aztreonam
Methadone and hydantoin exposure during gestation
Zidovudine treatment in the neonatal period

Others

Response to exercise
Gastroesophageal reflux
Caffey disease

postoperative week. After splenectomy, reactive thrombocytosis results from reduced platelet storage and decreased removal by the reticuloendothelial system.[5]

Increased IL-6 serum concentrations in splenectomized adults with thalassemia again suggest a role for IL-6 in the pathogenesis of thrombocytosis; in addition, an increased platelet aggregability has been reported.[132,133] In children, thromboembolic complications after splenectomy are very rare, but have been reported in association with immune hemolytic anemia and portal hypertension.[5]

Anemia accounts for 6–12% of reactive thrombocytosis in children. Hemolytic anemia and anemia due to iron deficiency are most frequently associated with reactive thrombocytosis. Their incidence varies with the ethnic origin of the study population and the age of the children studied (Table 24.4). Iron deficiency occurs in 4–6% of children with thrombocytosis, most frequently in infants. Within a study group of children with iron deficiency, reactive thrombocytosis was found in up to one-third of them.[134] The relationship between iron deficiency and thrombocytosis is likely to be complex, and there is increasing evidence that it is not caused by cross-reactivity between Epo and Tpo.[135] Thrombocytosis has also been observed in infants with bleeding due to vitamin K deficiency or other bleeding disorders, and in the recovery from severe hemodilution in open-heart surgery.[5]

Autoimmune diseases (juvenile rheumatoid arthritis, inflammatory bowel disease, polyarteritis nodosa, Kawasaki disease) account for 4–11% of reactive thrombocytosis in childhood (Table 24.4). Among them, Kawasaki syndrome is the major cause of reactive thrombocytosis in children under 7 years old, while other diseases occur mainly in children aged 11 years or older. As in adults, a direct correlation between IL-6 concentrations and both the activity of the underlying inflammatory disease and platelet counts has been described.[136] In active inflammatory bowel disease, Tpo concentrations are also elevated but do not correlate with thromboembolic complications. The lack of a direct correlation between Tpo and platelet counts, and the fact that the increase in Tpo concentrations precedes thrombocytosis, is highly suggestive that megakaryopoiesis is stimulated by both Tpo and other megakaryopoietic growth factors.[137] Children with Henoch–Schönlein purpura show typically mild thrombocytosis. The coincidence of reactive thrombocytosis and abdominal pain due to hemorrhage and thrombosis should be noticed.[5,138]

About 1–3% of children exhibit thrombocytosis at the diagnosis of a malignancy.[1,139] Elevated Tpo concentrations have been reported in malignant Tpo-producing liver tumors, particularly hepatoblastoma and hepatocellular carcinoma.[120] Less frequently, thrombocytosis can also be associated with acute lymphocytic leukemia (3.2% of children diagnosed).[140]

Reactive thrombocytosis can also be related to treatment with several pharmaceutical agents. Epinephrine (adrenaline), corticosteroids, ciclosporin, vinca alkaloids, miconazole, penicillamine, imipenem, and meropenem are claimed or known to cause or promote thrombocytosis in children.[5,141–143] Epinephrine and stress increase the platelet count by shifting stored platelets from the spleen to the circulation.[144] Of children treated with corticosteroids and/or vinca alkaloids for a malignancy (solid tumor, acute lymphocytic leukemia), 90% develop thrombocytosis during therapy.[5]

Transient thrombocytosis has been described in neonates after intrauterine exposure to methadone, hydantoin, or psychopharmaceutical drugs.[5] It has been speculated that reactive thrombocytosis is caused by rebound megakaryopoiesis after suppression of fetal Tpo production. Such a rebound phenomenon is also obvious in neonates receiving antiretroviral treatment with zidovudine due to maternal HIV infection. After initial thrombocytopenia or normal platelet counts, platelets can rise to $> 1000 \times 10^9/L$.[145]

In children, reactive thrombocytosis can be also associated with various other diseases, such as allergies, metabolic diseases, myopathies, or neurofibromatosis.[5]

Complications of reactive thrombocytosis in childhood

In childhood, reactive thrombocytosis does not usually result in thromboembolic or hemorrhagic complications (<1–2%). However, such complications occur after splenectomy or if the underlying disease is associated with additional thrombotic risk factors.[146] Thromboembolism, for example, occurs more frequently in (auto)splenectomized children with thalassemia or congenital spherocytosis who have persistent hemolysis, increased platelet reactivity, low protein C, and antithrombin concentrations,[147] or who suffer the sequelae of thalassemia such as cardiomyopathy, diabetes, hepatopathy, and portal hypertension.[148] Furthermore, neonates and infants have a higher thromboembolic risk if central venous catheters are placed or other thrombophilic conditions are present, such as maternal diabetes, maternal antiphospholipid syndrome, septicemia, intrauterine growth retardation, or cardiac malformation.[149]

Indications for treatment of reactive thrombocytosis

Reactive thrombocytosis in children does not justify general prophylaxis with anticoagulants or platelet aggregation inhibitors, even if the platelet count is greater than $1000 \times 10^9/L$. There is no evidence for the efficacy of prophylaxis against thromboembolic complications in asymptomatic children with reactive thrombocytosis. Individually tailored thrombosis prophylaxis and additional laboratory screening for thrombophilia should be considered if additional thrombotic risk factors exist or if thromboembolic events are reported in family history. The underlying disease (e.g., iron deficiency) should be treated rather than the platelet count.

Only if thrombosis occurs repeatedly is reduction of platelet aggregation and platelet count indicated.[146]

Acknowledgment

This chapter is dedicated to Professor Anton Heinz Sutor (1938–2004), formerly of the Department of Paediatrics, University of Freiburg, Germany. With great enthusiasm and the highest clinical and scientific skill, he contributed significantly for over 30 years to the understanding of thrombocytosis in childhood

References

1. Sutor AH. Thrombocytosis in childhood. *Semin Thromb Hemost* 1995; **21**: 330–9.
2. Heng JT, Tan AM. Thrombocytosis in childhood. *Singapore Med J* 1998; **39**: 485–7.
3. Chen HL, Chiou SS, Sheen JM, Jang RC, Lu CC, Chang TT. Thrombocytosis in children at one medical center of southern Taiwan. *Acta Paediatr Taiwan* 1999; **40**: 309–13.
4. Matsubara K, Fukaya T, Nigami H et al. Age-dependent changes in the incidence and etiology of childhood thrombocytosis. *Acta Haematol* 2004; **111**: 132–7.
5. Sutor AH. Thrombocytosis. In: Lilleyman JS, Hann IM, Blanchette VS (eds) *Pediatric Hematology*, 2nd edn. London: Churchill Livingstone, 1999, pp. 455–64.
6. Dame C, Sutor AH. Primary and secondary thrombocytosis in childhood. *Br J Haematol* 2005; **129**: 165–77.
7. Randi ML, Putti MC. Essential thrombocythaemia in children: is a treatment needed? *Expert Opin Pharmacother* 2004; **5**: 1009–14.
8. Randi ML, Putti MC, Pacquola E, Luzzatto G, Zanesco L, Fabris F. Normal thrombopoietin and its receptor (c-mpl) genes in children with essential thrombocythemia. *Pediatr Blood Cancer* 2005; **44**: 47–50.
9. Tefferi A, Ho TC, Ahmann GJ, Katzmann JA, Greipp PR. Plasma interleukin-6 and C-reactive protein levels in reactive versus clonal thrombocytosis. *Am J Med* 1994; **97**: 374–8.
10. Ishiguro A, Suzuki Y, Mito M et al. Elevation of serum thrombopoietin precedes thrombocytosis in acute infections. *Br J Haematol* 2002; **116**: 612–18.
11. Uppenkamp M, Makarova E, Petrasch S, Brittinger G. Thrombopoietin serum concentration in patients with reactive and myeloproliferative thrombocytosis. *Ann Hematol* 1998; **77**: 217–23.
12. Wang JC, Chen C, Novetsky AD, Lichter SM, Ahmed F, Friedberg NM. Blood thrombopoietin levels in clonal thrombocytosis and reactive thrombocytosis. *Am J Med* 1998; **104**: 451–5.
13. Hou M, Andersson PO, Stockelberg D, Mellqvist UH, Ridell B, Wadenvik H. Plasma thrombopoietin levels in thrombocytopenic states: implication for a regulatory role of bone marrow megakaryocytes. *Br J Haematol* 1998; **101**: 420–4.
14. Cerutti A, Custodi P, Duranti M, Noris P, Balduini CL.

Thrombopoietin levels in patients with primary and reactive thrombocytosis. *Br J Haematol* 1997; **99**: 281–4.

15. Ruggeri M, Tosetto A, Frezzato M, Rodeghiero F. The rate of progression to polycythemia vera or essential thrombocythemia in patients with erythrocytosis or thrombocytosis. *Ann Intern Med* 2003; **139**: 470–5.

16. Schafer AI. Thrombocytosis. *N Engl J Med* 2004; **350**: 1211–19.

17. Michiels JJ, Kutti J, Stark P *et al*. Diagnosis, pathogenesis and treatment of the myeloproliferative disorders essential thrombocythemia, polycythemia vera and essential megakaryocytic granulocytic metaplasia and myelofibrosis. *Neth J Med* 1999; **54**: 46–62.

18. Harrison CN. Current trends in essential thrombocythaemia. *Br J Haematol* 2002; **117**: 796–808.

19. Mesa RA, Hanson CA, Li CY *et al*. Diagnostic and prognostic value of bone marrow angiogenesis and megakaryocyte c-Mpl expression in essential thrombocythemia. *Blood* 2002; **99**: 4131–7.

20. Kaushansky K. Thrombopoietin: the primary regulator of platelet production. *Blood* 1995; **86**: 419–31.

21. Sohma Y, Akahori H, Seki N *et al*. Molecular cloning and chromosomal localization of the human thrombopoietin gene. *FEBS Lett* 1994; **353**: 57–61.

22. Lok S, Kaushansky K, Holly RD *et al*. Cloning and expression of murine thrombopoietin cDNA and stimulation of platelet production in vivo. *Nature* 1994; **369**: 565–8.

23. Geddis AE, Linden HM, Kaushansky K. Thrombopoietin: a pan-hematopoietic cytokine. *Cytokine Growth Factor Rev* 2002; **13**: 61–73.

24. Bartley TD, Bogenberger J, Hunt P *et al*. Identification and cloning of a megakaryocyte growth and development factor that is a ligand for the cytokine receptor Mpl. *Cell* 1994; **77**: 1117–24.

25. Gurney AL, Kuang WJ, Xie MH, Malloy BE, Eaton DL, de Sauvage FJ. Genomic structure, chromosomal localization, and conserved alternative splice forms of thrombopoietin. *Blood* 1995; **85**: 981–8.

26. Wolber EM, Dame C, Fahnenstich H *et al*. Expression of the thrombopoietin gene in human fetal and neonatal tissues. *Blood* 1999; **94**: 97–105.

27. Sungaran R, Markovic B, Chong BH. Localization and regulation of thrombopoietin mRNA expression in human kidney, liver, bone marrow, and spleen using in situ hybridization. *Blood* 1997; **89**: 101–7.

28. Dame C, Wolber EM, Freitag P, Hofmann D, Bartmann P, Fandrey J. Thrombopoietin gene expression in the developing human central nervous system. *Dev Brain Res* 2003; **143**: 217–23.

29. Ehrenreich H, Hasselblatt M, Knerlich F *et al*. A hematopoietic growth factor, thrombopoietin, has a proapoptotic role in the brain. *Proc Natl Acad Sci USA* 2005; **102**: 862–7.

30. Gurney AL, Wong SC, Henzel WJ, de Sauvage FJ. Distinct regions of c-Mpl cytoplasmic domain are coupled to the JAK-STAT signal transduction pathway and Shc phosphorylation. *Proc Natl Acad Sci USA* 1995; **92**: 5292–6.

31. Mignotte V, Vigon I, Boucher de Crevecoeur E, Romeo PH, Lemarchandel V, Chretien S. Structure and transcription of the human c-mpl gene (MPL). *Genomics* 1994; **20**: 5–12.

32. Vigon I, Mornon JP, Cocault L *et al*. Molecular cloning and characterization of MPL, the human homolog of the v-mpl oncogene: identification of a member of the hematopoietic growth factor receptor superfamily. *Proc Natl Acad Sci USA* 1992; **89**: 5640–4.

33. Sabath DF, Kaushansky K, Broudy VC. Deletion of the extracellular membrane-distal cytokine receptor homology module of Mpl results in constitutive cell growth and loss of thrombopoietin binding. *Blood* 1999; **94**: 365–7.

34. Drachman JG, Miyakawa Y, Luthi JN *et al*. Studies with chimeric Mpl/JAK2 receptors indicate that both JAK2 and the membrane-proximal domain of Mpl are required for cellular proliferation. *J Biol Chem* 2002; **277**: 23544–53.

35. Fielder PJ, Gurney AL, Stefanich E *et al*. Regulation of thrombopoietin levels by c-mpl-mediated binding to platelets. *Blood* 1996; **87**: 2154–61.

36. Debili N, Wendling F, Cosman D *et al*. The Mpl receptor is expressed in the megakaryocytic lineage from late progenitors to platelets. *Blood* 1995; **85**: 391–401.

37. de Sauvage FJ, Hass PE, Spencer SD *et al*. Stimulation of megakaryocytopoiesis and thrombopoiesis by the c-Mpl ligand. *Nature* 1994; **369**: 533–8.

38. Kaushansky K, Lok S, Holly RD *et al*. Promotion of megakaryocyte progenitor expansion and differentiation by the c-Mpl ligand thrombopoietin. *Nature* 1994; **369**: 568–71.

39. Choi ES, Hokom M, Bartley T *et al*. Recombinant human megakaryocyte growth and development factor (rHuMGDF), a ligand for c-Mpl, produces functional human platelets in vitro. *Stem Cells* 1995; **13**: 317–22.

40. Cohen-Solal K, Villeval JL, Titeux M, Lok S, Vainchenker W, Wendling F. Constitutive expression of Mpl ligand transcripts during thrombocytopenia or thrombocytosis. *Blood* 1996; **88**: 2578–84.

41. Kuter DJ, Rosenberg RD. The reciprocal relationship of thrombopoietin (c-Mpl ligand) to changes in the platelet mass during busulfan-induced thrombocytopenia in the rabbit. *Blood* 1995; **85**: 2720–30.

42. Ichikawa N, Ishida F, Shimodaira S, Tahara T, Kato T, Kitano K. Regulation of serum thrombopoietin levels by platelets and megakaryocytes in patients with aplastic anaemia and idiopathic thrombocytopenic purpura. *Thromb Haemost* 1996; **76**: 156–60.

43. Cremer M, Dame C, Schaeffer HJ, Giers G, Bartmann P, Bald R. Longitudinal thrombopoietin plasma concentrations in fetuses with alloimmune thrombocytopenia treated with intrauterine PLT transfusions. *Transfusion* 2003; **43**: 1216–22.

44. Wolber EM, Jelkmann W. Interleukin-6 increases thrombopoietin production in human hepatoma cells HepG2 and Hep3B. *J Interferon Cytokine Res* 2000; **20**: 499–506.

45. Wolber EM, Fandrey J, Frackowski U, Jelkmann W. Hepatic thrombopoietin mRNA is increased in acute inflammation. *Thromb Haemost* 2001; **86**: 1421–4.

46. Kaser A, Brandacher G, Steurer W *et al*. Interleukin-6 stimulates thrombopoiesis through thrombopoietin: role in inflammatory thrombocytosis. *Blood* 2001; **98**: 2720–5.

47. Yamashita K, Matsuoka H, Ochiai T *et al*. Hepatocyte growth factor/scatter factor enhances the thrombopoietin mRNA expression in rat hepatocytes and cirrhotic rat livers. *J Gastroenterol Hepatol* 2000; **15**: 83–90.

48. Wolber EM, Haase B, Jelkmann W. Thrombopoietin production in human hepatic cell cultures (HepG2) is resistant to IFN-

alpha, IFN-beta, and IFN-gamma treatment. *J Interferon Cytokine Res* 2002; **22**: 1185–9.

49. Begley CG, Basser RL. Biologic and structural differences of thrombopoietic growth factors. *Semin Hematol* 2000; **37**: 19–27.

50. Yang M, Li K, Chui CM *et al*. Expression of interleukin (IL) 1 type I and type II receptors in megakaryocytic cells and enhancing effects of IL-1beta on megakaryocytopoiesis and NF-E2 expression. *Br J Haematol* 2000; **111**: 371–80.

51. Chuen CK, Li K, Yang M *et al*. Interleukin-1beta up-regulates the expression of thrombopoietin and transcription factors c-Jun, c-Fos, GATA-1, and NF-E2 in megakaryocytic cells. *J Lab Clin Med* 2004; **143**: 75–88.

52. Tefferi A. Recent progress in the pathogenesis and management of essential thrombocythemia. *Leuk Res* 2001; **25**: 369–77.

53. Harrison CN, Gale RE, Machin SJ, Linch DC. A large proportion of patients with a diagnosis of essential thrombocythemia do not have a clonal disorder and may be at lower risk of thrombotic complications. *Blood* 1999; **93**: 417–24.

54. Allen AJ, Gale RE, Harrison CN, Machin SJ, Linch DC. Lack of pathogenic mutations in the 5′-untranslated region of the thrombopoietin gene in patients with non-familial essential thrombocythaemia. *Eur J Haematol* 2001; **67**: 232–7.

55. Horikawa Y, Matsumura I, Hashimoto K *et al*. Markedly reduced expression of platelet c-mpl receptor in essential thrombocythemia. *Blood* 1997; **90**: 4031–8.

56. Pitcher L, Taylor K, Nichol J *et al*. Thrombopoietin measurement in thrombocytosis: dysregulation and lack of feedback inhibition in essential thrombocythaemia. *Br J Haematol* 1997; **99**: 929–32.

57. Harrison CN, Gale RE, Wiestner AC, Skoda RC, Linch DC. The activating splice mutation in intron 3 of the thrombopoietin gene is not found in patients with non-familial essential thrombocythaemia. *Br J Haematol* 1998; **102**: 1341–3.

58. Kiladjian JJ, Elkassar N, Hetet G, Briere J, Grandchamp B, Gardin C. Study of the thrombopoitin receptor in essential thrombocythemia. *Leukemia* 1997; **11**: 1821–6.

59. Wiestner A, Padosch SA, Ghilardi N *et al*. Hereditary thrombocythaemia is a genetically heterogeneous disorder: exclusion of TPO and MPL in two families with hereditary thrombocythaemia. *Br J Haematol* 2000; **110**: 104–9.

60. Harrison CN, Gale RE, Pezella F, Mire Sluis A, MacHin SJ, Linch DC. Platelet c-mpl expression is dysregulated in patients with essential thrombocythaemia but this is not of diagnostic value. *Br J Haematol* 1999; **107**: 139–47.

61. Kralovics R, Buser AS, Teo SS *et al*. Comparison of molecular markers in a cohort of patients with chronic myeloproliferative disorders. *Blood* 2003; **102**: 1869–71.

62. Li J, Xia Y, Kuter DJ. The platelet thrombopoietin receptor number and function are markedly decreased in patients with essential thrombocythaemia. *Br J Haematol* 2000; **111**: 943–53.

63. Le Blanc K, Andersson P, Samuelsson J. Marked heterogeneity in protein levels and functional integrity of the thrombopoietin receptor c-mpl in polycythaemia vera. *Br J Haematol* 2000; **108**: 80–5.

64. Moliterno AR, Spivak JL. Posttranslational processing of the thrombopoietin receptor is impaired in polycythemia vera. *Blood* 1999; **94**: 2555–61.

65. Li Y, Hetet G, Maurer AM, Chait Y, Dhermy D, Briere J. Spontaneous megakaryocyte colony formation in myeloproliferative disorders is not neutralizable by antibodies against IL3, IL6 and GM-CSF. *Br J Haematol* 1994; **87**: 471–6.

66. Randi ML, Putti MC, Fabris F, Sainati L, Zanesco L, Girolami A. Features of essential thrombocythaemia in childhood: a study of five children. *Br J Haematol* 2000; **108**: 86–9.

67. Florensa L, Zamora L, Besses C *et al*. Cultures of myeloid progenitor cells in pediatric essential thrombocythemia. *Leukemia* 2002; **16**: 1876–7.

68. Mi JQ, Blanc-Jouvan F, Wang J *et al*. Endogenous megakaryocytic colony formation and thrombopoietin sensitivity of megakaryocytic progenitor cells are useful to distinguish between essential thrombocythemia and reactive thrombocytosis. *J Hematother Stem Cell Res* 2001; **10**: 405–9.

69. Axelrad AA, Eskinazi D, Correa PN, Amato D. Hypersensitivity of circulating progenitor cells to megakaryocyte growth and development factor (PEG-rHu MGDF) in essential thrombocythemia. *Blood* 2000; **96**: 3310–21.

70. Zauli G, Visani G, Catani L, Vianelli N, Gugliotta L, Capitani S. Reduced responsiveness of bone marrow megakaryocyte progenitors to platelet-derived transforming growth factor beta 1, produced in normal amount, in patients with essential thrombocythaemia. *Br J Haematol* 1993; **83**: 14–20.

71. Kuroda H, Matsunaga T, Terui T *et al*. Decrease of Smad4 gene expression in patients with essential thrombocythaemia may cause an escape from suppression of megakaryopoiesis by transforming growth factor-beta1. *Br J Haematol* 2004; **124**: 211–20.

72. Kimura T, Kaburaki H, Tsujino T, Ikeda Y, Kato H, Watanabe Y. A non-peptide compound which can mimic the effect of thrombopoietin via c-Mpl. *FEBS Lett* 1998; **428**: 250–4.

73. Taksin AL, Couedic JPL, Dusanter-Fourt I *et al*. Autonomous megakaryocyte growth in essential thrombocythemia and idiopathic myelofibrosis is not related to a c-mpl mutation or to an autocrine stimulation by Mpl-L. *Blood* 1999; **93**: 125–39.

74. Sungaran R, Chisholm OT, Markovic B, Khachigian LM, Tanaka Y, Chong BH. The role of platelet alpha-granular proteins in the regulation of thrombopoietin messenger RNA expression in human bone marrow stromal cells. *Blood* 2000; **95**: 3094–101.

75. Hirayama Y, Sakamaki S, Matsunaga T *et al*. Concentrations of thrombopoietin in bone marrow in normal subjects and in patients with idiopathic thrombocytopenic purpura, aplastic anemia, and essential thrombocythemia correlate with its mRNA expression of bone marrow stromal cells. *Blood* 1998; **92**: 46–52.

76. Sakamaki S, Hirayama Y, Matsunaga T *et al*. Transforming growth factor-beta1 (TGF-beta1) induces thrombopoietin from bone marrow stromal cells, which stimulates the expression of TGF-beta receptor on megakaryocytes and, in turn, renders them susceptible to suppression by TGF-beta itself with high specificity. *Blood* 1999; **94**: 1961–70.

77. Wang JC, Hashmi G. Elevated thrombopoietin levels in patients with myelofibrosis may not be due to enhanced production of thrombopoietin by bone marrow. *Leuk Res* 2003; **27**: 13–17.

78. Teofili L, Martini M, Luongo M *et al*. Overexpression of the polycythemia rubra vera-1 gene in essential thrombocythemia. *J Clin Oncol* 2002; **20**: 4249–54.

79. Catani L, Vianelli N, Amabile M *et al*. Nuclear factor-erythroid

2 (NF-E2) expression in normal and malignant megakaryocytopoiesis. *Leukemia* 2002; **16**: 1773–81.

80. Liu E, Jelinek J, Pastore YD, Guan Y, Prchal JF, Prchal JT. Discrimination of polycythemias and thrombocytoses by novel, simple, accurate clonality assays and comparison with PRV-1 expression and BFU-E response to erythropoietin. *Blood* 2003; **101**: 3294–301.

81. Johansson P, Ricksten A, Wennstrom L, Palmqvist L, Kutti J, Andreasson B. Increased risk for vascular complications in PRV-1 positive patients with essential thrombocythaemia. *Br J Haematol* 2003; **123**: 513–16.

82. Metcalf D, Carpinelli MR, Hyland C *et al.* Anomalous megakaryocytopoiesis in mice with mutations in the c-Myb gene. *Blood* 2005; **105**: 3480–7.

83. Carpinelli MR, Hilton DJ, Metcalf D *et al.* Suppressor screen in Mpl–/– mice: c-Myb mutation causes supraphysiological production of platelets in the absence of thrombopoietin signaling. *Proc Natl Acad Sci USA* 2004; **101**: 6553–8.

84. Hasle H. Incidence of essential thrombocythaemia in children. *Br J Haematol* 2000; **110**: 751.

85. Jensen MK, de Nully Brown P, Nielsen OJ, Hasselbalch HC. Incidence, clinical features and outcome of essential thrombocythaemia in a well defined geographical area. *Eur J Haematol* 2000; **65**: 132–9.

86. Dror Y, Blanchette VS. Essential thrombocythaemia in children. *Br J Haematol* 1999; **107**: 691–8.

87. Kudo K, Horibe K, Iwase K, Kondo M, Kojima S. [Clinical features of essential thrombocythemia in three children.] *Rinsho Ketsueki* 2000; **41**: 1164–70.

88. Michiels JJ, Van Genderen PJ. Essential thrombocythemia in childhood. *Semin Thromb Hemost* 1997; **23**: 295–301.

89. Yang RC, Qian LS. Essential thrombocythaemia in children: a report of nine cases. *Br J Haematol* 2000; **110**: 1009–10.

90. Greist A. The role of blood component removal in essential and reactive thrombocytosis. *Ther Apheresis* 2002; **6**: 36–44.

91. Posan E, Ujj G, Kiss A, Telek B, Rak K, Udvardy M. Reduced in vitro clot lysis and release of more active platelet PAI-1 in polycythemia vera and essential thrombocythemia. *Thromb Res* 1998; **90**: 51–6.

92. Harrison CN, Donohoe S, Carr P, Dave M, Mackie I, Machin SJ. Patients with essential thrombocythaemia have an increased prevalence of antiphospholipid antibodies which may be associated with thrombosis. *Thromb Haemost* 2002; **87**: 802–7.

93. Kikuchi M, Tayama T, Hayakawa H, Takahashi I, Hoshino H, Ohsaka A. Familial thrombocytosis. *Br J Haematol* 1995; **89**: 900–2.

94. Stuhrmann M, Bashawri L, Ahmed MA *et al.* Familial thrombocytosis as a recessive, possibly X-linked trait in an Arab family. *Br J Haematol* 2001; **112**: 616–20.

95. Ghilardi N, Skoda RC. A single-base deletion in the thrombopoietin (TPO) gene causes familial essential thrombocythemia through a mechanism of more efficient translation of TPO mRNA. *Blood* 1999; **94**: 1480–2.

96. Kondo T, Okabe M, Sanada M *et al.* Familial essential thrombocythemia associated with one-base deletion in the 5′-untranslated region of the thrombopoietin gene. *Blood* 1998; **92**: 1091–6.

97. Wiestner A, Schlemper RJ, van der Maas AP, Skoda RC. An activating splice donor mutation in the thrombopoietin gene causes hereditary thrombocythaemia. *Nat Genet* 1998; **18**: 49–52.

98. Jorgensen MJ, Raskind WH, Wolff JF, Bachrach HR, Kaushansky K. Familial thrombocytosis associated with overproduction of thrombopoietin due to a novel splice donor site mutation [abstract]. *Blood* 1998; **92**: 205a.

99. Ding J, Komatsu H, Wakita A *et al.* Familial essential thrombocythemia associated with a dominant-positive activating mutation of the c-MPL gene, which encodes for the receptor for thrombopoietin. *Blood* 2004; **103**: 4198–200.

100. Moliterno AR, Williams DM, Gutierrez-Alamillo LI, Salvatori R, Ingersoll RG, Spivak JL. Mpl Baltimore: a thrombopoietin receptor polymorphism associated with thrombocytosis. *Proc Natl Acad Sci USA* 2004; **101**: 11444–7.

101. Fujiwara T, Harigae H, Kameoka J *et al.* A case of familial thrombocytosis: possible role of altered thrombopoietin production. *Am J Hematol* 2004; **76**: 395–7.

102. Kralovics R, Skoda RC. Molecular pathogenesis of Philadelphia chromosome negative myeloproliferative disorders. *Blood Rev* 2005; **19**: 1–13.

103. Ruggeri M, Finazzi G, Tosetto A, Riva S, Rodeghiero F, Barbui T. No treatment for low-risk thrombocythaemia: results from a prospective study. *Br J Haematol* 1998; **103**: 772–7.

104. van Genderen PJ, Prins FJ, Michiels JJ, Schror K. Thromboxane-dependent platelet activation in vivo precedes arterial thrombosis in thrombocythaemia: a rationale for the use of low-dose aspirin as an antithrombotic agent. *Br J Haematol* 1999; **104**: 438–41.

105. Michiels JJ. Aspirin and platelet-lowering agents for the prevention of vascular complications in essential thrombocythemia. *Clin Appl Thromb Hemost* 1999; **5**: 247–51.

106. Cortelazzo S, Finazzi G, Ruggeri M *et al.* Hydroxyurea for patients with essential thrombocythemia and a high risk of thrombosis. *N Engl J Med* 1995; **332**: 1132–6.

107. Cheung MC, Hicks LK, Pendergrast J. Thrombocytosis. *N Engl J Med* 2004; **350**: 2524–5; author reply 2524–5.

108. Finazzi G, Ruggeri M, Rodeghiero F, Barbui T. Efficacy and safety of long-term use of hydroxyurea in young patients with essential thrombocythemia and a high risk of thrombosis. *Blood* 2003; **101**: 3749.

109. Benkerrou M, Delarche C, Brahimi L *et al.* Hydroxyurea corrects the dysregulated L-selectin expression and increased H_2O_2 production of polymorphonuclear neutrophils from patients with sickle cell anemia. *Blood* 2002; **99**: 2297–303.

110. Silverstein MN, Petitt RM, Solberg LA Jr, Fleming JS, Knight RC, Schacter LP. Anagrelide: a new drug for treating thrombocytosis. *N Engl J Med* 1988; **318**: 1292–4.

111. Storen EC, Tefferi A. Long-term use of anagrelide in young patients with essential thrombocythemia. *Blood* 2001; **97**: 863–6.

112. Lackner H, Urban C, Beham-Schmid C, Benesch M, Kerbl R, Schwinger W. Treatment of children with anagrelide for thrombocythemia. *J Pediatr Hematol Oncol* 1998; **20**: 469–73.

113. Chintagumpala MM, Kennedy LL, Steuber CP. Treatment of essential thrombocythemia with anagrelide. *J Pediatr* 1995; **127**: 495–8.

114. Hankins J, Naidu P, Rieman M, Wang W, Kaushansky K, Rodriguez-Galindo C. Thrombocytosis in an infant with high thrombopoietin concentrations. *J Pediatr Hematol Oncol* 2004; **26**: 142–5.

115. Klinger MH, Jelkmann W. Role of blood platelets in infection and inflammation. *J Interferon Cytokine Res* 2002; **22**: 913–22.

116. Cardier JE. Effects of megakaryocyte growth and development factor (thrombopoietin) on liver endothelial cells in vitro. *Microvasc Res* 1999; **58**: 108–13.

117. Hsu HC, Tsai WH, Jiang ML *et al*. Circulating levels of thrombopoietic and inflammatory cytokines in patients with clonal and reactive thrombocytosis. *J Lab Clin Med* 1999; **134**: 392–7.

118. Cerutti A, Custodi P, Duranti M, Cazzola M, Balduini CL. Circulating thrombopoietin in reactive conditions behaves like an acute phase reactant. *Clin Lab Haematol* 1999; **21**: 271–5.

119. Folman CC, Ooms M, Kuenen BB *et al*. The role of thrombopoietin in post-operative thrombocytosis. *Br J Haematol* 2001; **114**: 126–33.

120. Komura E, Matsumura T, Kato T, Tahara T, Tsunoda Y, Sawada T. Thrombopoietin in patients with hepatoblastoma. *Stem Cells* 1998; **16**: 329–33.

121. Sasaki Y, Takahashi T, Miyazaki H *et al*. Production of thrombopoietin by human carcinomas and its novel isoforms. *Blood* 1999; **94**: 1952–60.

122. Kutti J, Wadenvik H. Diagnostic and differential criteria of essential thrombocythemia and reactive thrombocytosis. *Leukemia Lymphoma* 1996; **22** (suppl. 1): 41–5.

123. Vora AJ, Lilleyman JS. Secondary thrombocytosis. *Arch Dis Child* 1993; **68**: 88–90.

124. Yohannan MD, Higgy KE, al-Mashhadani SA, Santhosh-Kumar CR. Thrombocytosis. Etiologic analysis of 663 patients. *Clin Pediatr (Phila)* 1994; **33**: 340–3.

125. Dame C. Developmental biology of thrombopoietin in the human fetus and neonate. *Acta Paediatr Suppl* 2002; **91**: 54–65.

126. Ishiguro A, Nakahata T, Matsubara K *et al*. Age-related changes in thrombopoietin in children: reference interval for serum thrombopoietin levels. *Br J Haematol* 1999; **106**: 884–8.

127. Murray NA, Watts TL, Roberts IA. Endogenous thrombopoietin levels and effect of recombinant human thrombopoietin on megakaryocyte precursors in term and preterm babies. *Pediatr Res* 1998; **43**: 148–51.

128. Sola MC, Du Y, Hutson AD, Christensen RD. Dose–response relationship of megakaryocyte progenitors from the bone marrow of thrombocytopenic and non-thrombocytopenic neonates to recombinant thrombopoietin. *Br J Haematol* 2000; **110**: 449–53.

129. Wolach B, Morag H, Drucker M, Sadan N. Thrombocytosis after pneumonia with empyema and other bacterial infections in children. *Pediatr Infect Dis J* 1990; **9**: 718–21.

130. Garoufi A, Voutsioti K, Tsapra H, Karpathios T, Zeis PM. Reactive thrombocytosis in children with upper urinary tract infections. *Acta Paediatr* 2001; **90**: 448–9.

131. Kilpi T, Anttila M, Kallio MJ, Peltola H. Thrombocytosis and thrombocytopenia in childhood bacterial meningitis. *Pediatr Infect Dis J* 1992; **11**: 456–60.

132. Chuncharunee S, Archararit N, Hathirat P, Udomsubpayakul U, Atichartakarn V. Levels of serum interleukin-6 and tumor necrosis factor in postsplenectomized thalassemic patients. *J Med Assoc Thai* 1997; **80** (suppl. 1): S86–S91.

133. Nagasue N, Inokuchi K, Kobayashi M, Kanashima R. Platelet aggregability after splenectomy in patients with normosplenism and hypersplenism. *Am J Surg* 1978; **136**: 260–4.

134. Dickerhoff R, von Ruecker A. Thrombozytose im Kindesalter. Differentialdiagnose und klinische Bedeutung. *Paediatrische Praxis* 1991; **41**: 25–8.

135. Geddis AE, Kaushansky K. Cross-reactivity between erythropoietin and thrombopoietin at the level of Mpl does not account for the thrombocytosis seen in iron deficiency. *J Pediatr Hematol Oncol* 2003; **25**: 919–20; author reply 920.

136. de Benedetti F, Massa M, Robbioni P, Ravelli A, Burgio GR, Martini A. Correlation of serum interleukin-6 levels with joint involvement and thrombocytosis in systemic juvenile rheumatoid arthritis. *Arthritis Rheum* 1991; **34**: 1158–63.

137. Papa A, Danese S, Piccirillo N *et al*. Thrombopoietin serum levels in patients with inflammatory bowel disease with and without previous thromboembolic events. *Hepatogastroenterology* 2003; **50**: 132–5.

138. Al Mazyad AS. Polyarteritis nodosa in Arab children in Saudi Arabia. *Clin Rheumatol* 1999; **18**: 196–200.

139. Chan KW, Kaikov Y, Wadsworth LD. Thrombocytosis in childhood: a survey of 94 patients. *Pediatrics* 1989; **84**: 1064–7.

140. Blatt J, Penchansky L, Horn M. Thrombocytosis as a presenting feature of acute lymphoblastic leukemia in childhood. *Am J Hematol* 1989; **31**: 46–9.

141. Oral R, Akisu M, Kultursay N, Vardar F, Tansug N. Neonatal *Klebsiella* pneumonia sepsis and imipenem/cilastatin. *Indian J Pediatr* 1998; **65**: 121–9.

142. Koksal N, Hacimustafaoglu M, Bagci S, Celebi S. Meropenem in neonatal severe infections due to multiresistant gram-negative bacteria. *Indian J Pediatr* 2001; **68**: 15–19.

143. Hsu HL, Lu CY, Tseng HY *et al*. Empirical monotherapy with meropenem in serious bacterial infections in children. *J Microbiol Immunol Infect* 2001; **34**: 275–80.

144. Chamberlain KG, Tong M, Penington DG. Properties of the exchangeable splenic platelets released into the circulation during exercise-induced thrombocytosis. *Am J Hematol* 1990; **34**: 161–8.

145. Bruel H, Chabrolle JP, el Khoury E *et al*. [Thrombocytosis and cholestasis in a newborn treated with zidovudine.] *Arch Pediatr* 2001; **8**: 893–4.

146. Sutor AH. Screening children with thrombosis for thrombophilic proteins. Cui bono? *J Thromb Haemost* 2003; **1**. 886–8.

147. Shebl SS, el-Sharkawy HM, el-Fadaly NH. Haemostatic disorders in nonsplenectomized and splenectomized thalassaemic children. *East Mediterr Health J* 1999; **5**: 1171–7.

148. Borgna PC, Carnelli V, Caruso V *et al*. Thromboembolic events in beta thalassemia major: an Italian multicenter study. *Acta Haematol* 1998; **99**: 76–9.

149. Edstrom CS, Christensen RD. Evaluation and treatment of thrombosis in the neonatal intensive care unit. *Clin Perinatol* 2000; **27**: 623–41.

150. Ghilardi N, Wiestner A, Kikuchi M, Ohsaka A, Skoda RC. Hereditary thrombocythaemia in a Japanese family is caused by a novel point mutation in the thrombopoietin gene. *Br J Haematol* 1999; **107**: 310–16.

151. Sutor AH, Hank D. Thrombosen bei Thrombozytosen im Kindesalter. In: Sutor AH (ed.) *Thrombosen im Kindesalter. Risikofaktoren, Diagnose, Prophylaxe, Therapie*. Basel: Roche, 1992, pp. 113–36.

25 Platelet function disorders

Alan D. Michelson

Normal platelet function

Platelets are small cells of great importance in many pathophysiologic processes including thrombosis, hemorrhage, inflammation, antimicrobial host defense, and tumor growth and metastasis.[1] The mammalian platelet is derived from the cytoplasm of megakaryocytes. Polyploid megakaryocytes and their progeny, nonnucleated platelets, are found only in mammals.[2] In all other animal species, cells involved in hemostasis and blood coagulation are nucleated. The evolutionary event or events that resulted in the appearance of mammalian megakaryocytes and platelets, as well as the biologic advantage of this system, remains unknown.[2]

Megakaryocytes are descended from pluripotent stem cells and undergo multiple DNA replications without cell divisions by the unique process of endomitosis.[3] On completion of endomitosis, polyploid megakaryocytes begin a rapid cytoplasmic expansion phase characterized by the development of an elaborate demarcation membrane system and the accumulation of cytoplasmic proteins and granules essential for platelet function. During the final stages of development, the megakaryocyte cytoplasm undergoes massive reorganization into beaded cytoplasmic extensions called proplatelets.[3]

Platelets circulate in a concentration of $150–400 \times 10^9/L$ and have a lifespan of 7–10 days. Human platelets are 2–4 μm in diameter and contain granules (α, dense, lysosomes), mitochondria, and endoplasmic reticulum. The contents of α-granules include P-selectin, von Willebrand factor (VWF), β-thromboglobulin (β-TG), platelet factor (PF)4, factor V, platelet-derived growth factor (PDGF), transforming growth factor β, plasminogen activator inhibitor 1, thrombospondin, fibrinogen, fibronectin, multimerin, albumin, and IgG.[4] The contents of dense granules include ATP, ADP, Ca^{2+}, serotonin, CD63, and LAMP 2.[4]

Formation of the hemostatic plug at sites of vascular injury begins with the arrest of circulating platelets on exposed collagen and continues with the recruitment of additional platelets into a growing platelet mass that will eventually be stabilized with cross-linked fibrin.[5] Formation of a platelet plug can be thought of as occurring in three phases: initiation, extension, and perpetuation (Fig. 25.1).[5] Initiation occurs when circulating platelets arrest and are activated by exposed collagen and VWF, allowing the accumulation of a platelet monolayer that supports thrombin generation and the formation of platelet aggregates. Key to this phase of platelet activation is the presence of receptors on the platelet surface that can bind to collagen (integrin $\alpha_2\beta_1$ and glycoprotein (Gp)VI) and VWF (GpIb–IX–V and integrin $\alpha_{IIb}\beta_3$) and initiate intracellular signaling.[5] Extension occurs when additional platelets accumulate on the initial monolayer, a process for which $\alpha_{IIb}\beta_3$ activation is certainly essential but not necessarily sufficient. Key to this phase is the presence on the platelet surface of receptors that can respond rapidly to locally generated thrombin, secreted ADP, and released thromboxane $(Tx)A_2$ to activate phospholipase C, increase cytosolic Ca^{2+} concentration, and suppress synthesis of cyclic AMP (cAMP).[5] Most of the receptors involved in these events are members of the superfamily of G protein-coupled receptors (Fig. 25.2). Perpetuation refers to the late events of platelet plug formation, when the intense but short-lived signals arising from G protein-coupled receptors have faded and the receptors responsible have been desensitized.[5] These late events stabilize the platelet plug and prevent premature disaggregation (Fig. 25.1). Perpetuation is less well understood than initiation and extension, but recent studies point to a central role for outside-in signaling through cell surface integrins and to the signals generated by receptor tyrosine kinases, including members of the Eph and Axl families.[5] Platelets localize, amplify, and sustain the coagulant response at the injury site[6] and release procoagulant platelet-derived microparticles.[7]

Platelet function in the newborn

Healthy newborns maintain normal circulating platelet counts,

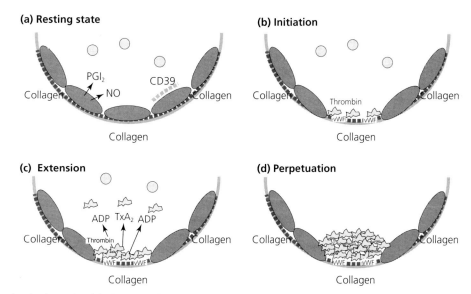

Fig. 25.1 Steps in platelet plug formation. (a) Prior to vascular injury, platelets are maintained in the resting state by a combination of inhibitory factors that place a "threshold" that must be surmounted in order for platelets to be activated. These factors include prostaglandin (PG)I$_2$ and nitric oxide (NO) released from endothelial cells, and CD39, an ADPase on the surface of endothelial cells that hydrolyzes any small amounts of ADP that might otherwise cause inappropriate platelet activation. (b) The development of the platelet plug is initiated by the exposure of collagen and the local generation of thrombin. This causes platelets to adhere via collagen and von Willebrand factor (VWF) and spread on the connective matrix, forming a monolayer. (c) Afterwards, the platelet plug is extended as additional platelets are activated via the release or secretion of thromboxane (Tx)A$_2$, ADP, and other platelet agonists, most of which are ligands for G protein-coupled receptors on the platelet surface. (d) Finally, close contacts between platelets in the growing hemostatic plug, along with a fibrin meshwork, help to perpetuate and stabilize the platelet aggregate. Reproduced with permission from Ref. 5.

Fig. 25.2 Overview of platelet activation via G protein-coupled receptors (GPCR) and G proteins. A number of agonists activate platelets via GPCRs on the platelet surface. Although the details differ from one receptor to the next, critical responses include G$_q$-mediated activation of phospholipase C (PLC)β isoforms to allow an increase in cytosolic Ca^{2+}, activation of phospholipase A$_2$ (PLA$_2$) and protein kinase C (PKC), and G$_{12}$-mediated guanine nucleotide exchange on Rho family members to support rearrangement of the platelet cytoskeleton (shape change). Activated PGI$_2$ receptors (IP) stimulate adenylyl cyclase, raising platelet cAMP levels, and causing a generalized inhibition of platelet responses to agonists. G$_i$ family members support the suppression of adenylyl cyclase by platelet agonists and may couple their receptors to other effector pathways as well, including those which activate phosphatidylinositol 3-kinase (PI3K)γ and the Ras family member Rap1B. Reproduced with permission from Ref. 5.

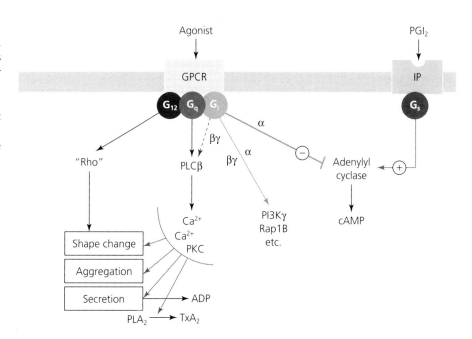

and have a platelet ultrastructure that does not differ from that of adults.[8] However, *in vitro* assessments of intrinsic platelet function have demonstrated transient hyporesponsiveness that is most marked in platelets from preterm infants (Fig. 25.3).[9,10] Decreased responses were originally considered to be the result of platelet activation and degranulation during labor and delivery, but more recent studies of platelet activation markers have not supported this hypothesis.[9,10] Decreased activation responses are due to relative deficiencies of phospholipid metabolism, calcium mobilization, granule secretion, and aggregation.[8] These result in turn from differences in intrinsic signal transduction in the neonatal

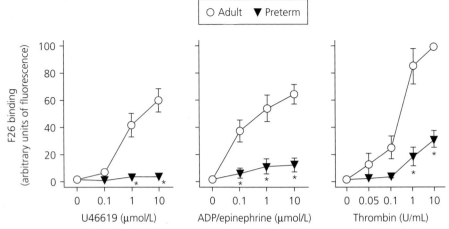

Fig. 25.3 The platelets of very low birthweight preterm neonates are less reactive than adult platelets, as determined by the activation-dependent binding of fibrinogen to the GpIIb–IIIa complex. Whole-blood flow cytometry was used to analyze the platelet surface binding of monoclonal antibody F26 (directed against a conformational change in fibrinogen bound to the GpIIb–IIIa complex) after stimulation with either U46619 (thromboxane A$_2$ agonist), the combination of ADP and epinephrine, or thrombin. The fluorescence intensity of adult platelets incubated with maximal thrombin (10 U/mL) was assigned a value of 100 units. Data are mean ± SEM, $n = 5$. Asterisks indicate $P < 0.05$ (by paired Student's t test) for platelets of preterm neonates compared with adult platelets. Reproduced with permission from Ref. 10.

platelet compared with those in the adult. In contrast, there is enhanced platelet adhesion due to the presence in neonatal plasma of larger, more functionally potent VWF multimers. These ultra-large multimers result from decreased concentrations of VWF-cleaving protease in neonatal plasma, and are associated with shorter bleeding times and platelet function analyzer (PFA)-100 closure times in neonates.[8] In the immediate newborn period this enhanced platelet adhesion may compensate for the decreased intrinsic platelet activation in healthy neonates, but may leave sick neonates at increased risk of bleeding.

Clinical approach to platelet function disorders

The characteristic clinical features that differentiate primary hemostatic disorders (platelet function disorders, thrombocytopenia, von Willebrand disease) from coagulation disorders (e.g., hemophilia) are listed in Table 25.1. Three of these clinical features are particularly helpful.

1 Petechiae are a very strong pointer toward a primary hemostatic disorder and away from a coagulation disorder.

2 Hemarthroses are a very strong pointer toward a coagulation disorder and away from a primary hemostatic disorder.

3 In the setting of an injury, immediate excessive bleeding suggests a primary hemostatic disorder (because the initial platelet plug does not form correctly), whereas delayed bleeding suggests a coagulation disorder (because the lack of a well-formed fibrin clot results in gradual breakdown of the initial platelet plug).[11]

Clinical history

Bleeding

Spontaneous bleeding, or excessive bleeding during or after an injury, is suggestive of an underlying hemostatic disorder. The clinician must obtain a history of the patient's responses to hemostatic challenges: surgery (including circumcision), dental procedures (especially tooth extractions), trauma, injections, menses, labor and delivery, and tooth brushing. Immediate bleeding suggests a primary hemostatic disorder, whereas delayed bleeding suggests a coagulation disorder (Table 25.1).

Table 25.1 Characteristic clinical features that differentiate primary hemostatic disorders from coagulation disorders.

	Primary hemostatic disorder	Coagulation disorder
Prototypic disorders	Thrombocytopenia, platelet function disorder, von Willebrand disease*	Hemophilia
Bleeding	Immediate	Delayed
Petechiae	Yes	No
Hemarthroses	No	Yes
Intramuscular hematomas	Uncommon	Common
Epistaxes	Common	Uncommon
Menorrhagia	Common	Uncommon

* In the uncommon type 3 von Willebrand disease, the factor VIII level is low enough for the clinical features to be those of a combined primary hemostatic and coagulation disorder.

Reproduced with permission from Ref. 11.

Easy bruising is common in hemostatic disorders, but does not help distinguish disorders of platelet number and function from other disorders of hemostasis. However, epistaxes, gingival bleeding, and menorrhagia are all more common in primary hemostatic disorders than in coagulation disorders. The age of onset of the excessive bleeding may help to distinguish inherited bleeding disorders from acquired bleeding disorders.

Gender and family history

Some disorders of platelet number and function are X-linked recessive (e.g., Wiskott–Aldrich syndrome) and therefore present almost exclusively in males. Other disorders of platelet number and function are autosomal recessive (e.g., Bernard–Soulier syndrome and Glanzmann thrombasthenia) or autosomal dominant (e.g., May–Hegglin anomaly). Hemophilia A (factor VIII deficiency) and hemophilia B (factor IX deficiency) are common X-linked recessive coagulation disorders that occur almost exclusively in males.

Medications

The history of the patient's intake of medications is important. A platelet function defect can be caused by many drugs, including aspirin, nonsteroidal antiinflammatory drugs (NSAIDs), ADP receptor antagonists (clopidogrel, ticlopidine), GpIIbIIIa antagonists (abciximab, tirofiban, eptifibatide), dipyridamole, cilostazol, antimicrobial agents (β-lactam antibiotics, nitrofurantoin, hydroxychloroquine, miconazole), cardiovascular drugs (propranolol, nitroprusside, nitroglycerin, furosemide, calcium channel blockers), ethanol, and food items and supplements (ω-3 fatty acids, vitamin E, onions, garlic, ginger, cumin, turmeric, clove, black tree fungus, *Ginkgo*).[12]

Medical history

A history of renal disease, liver disease, myeloproliferative disorder, acute leukemia, myelodysplastic syndrome, or dysproteinemia suggests a platelet function defect.

Physical examination

Hemorrhage

Petechiae very strongly suggest a primary hemostatic disorder rather than a coagulation disorder (see Table 25.1). Petechiae can also be a sign of vasculitis or, in a sick patient, bacteremia (including meningococcemia) and disseminated intravascular coagulation. In contrast, hemarthroses very strongly suggest a coagulation disorder rather than a primary hemostatic disorder (see Table 25.1). Intramuscular hematomas are more typical of a coagulation disorder than a primary hemostatic disorder.

Other physical signs

Oculocutaneous albinism is observed in Hermansky–Pudlak syndrome and Chédiak–Higashi syndrome. Deafness and cataracts suggest Fechtner syndrome. Deafness and hypertension occur in Epstein syndrome. Cardiac defects, delayed development, otorhinolaryngologic manifestations, psychiatric disturbances, and mental retardation suggest the velocardiofacial syndrome associated with Bernard–Soulier syndrome.

Clinical tests

Blood smear

Giant platelets are observed in Bernard–Soulier syndrome, May–Hegglin anomaly, Fechtner syndrome, Sebastian syndrome, Epstein syndrome, and Montreal platelet syndrome. Agranular gray platelets are observed in the gray platelet syndrome. Döhle bodies are observed in the neutrophil cytoplasm in May–Hegglin anomaly. Neutrophil inclusions are also observed in Sebastian syndrome. Giant cytoplasmic granules are observed in neutrophils, monocytes, and lymphocytes in Chédiak–Higashi syndrome, but these granules may be more easily recognized in leukocyte precursors in the bone marrow rather than in leukocytes in the peripheral blood.[11]

Platelet aggregation

In Glanzmann thrombasthenia, the platelets do not aggregate in response to ADP, epinephrine (adrenaline), arachidonic acid, or collagen, but do agglutinate in response to ristocetin. In Bernard–Soulier syndrome, the platelets do not agglutinate in response to ristocetin but do aggregate in response to all other agonists. Patients with storage pool disease or defects in platelet secretion show decreased platelet aggregation or absence of the second wave of aggregation in response to ADP, epinephrine, arachidonic acid, or collagen. Some patients with storage pool disease cannot be reliably diagnosed by standard platelet aggregometry;[13] the diagnosis is made by measuring the granule adenine nucleotides by biochemical assays or by labeling the platelets with the fluorescent dye mepacrine and then measuring platelet fluorescence by microscopy or flow cytometry.[14,15]

Bleeding time

Although both thrombocytopenia and platelet function defects of sufficient degree usually result in a prolonged bleeding time, this test has a limited role in clinical medicine.[16]

Other tests

Other tests that may be clinically useful in patients with platelet function disorders include the PFA-100,[17] the VerifyNow rapid platelet function analyzer,[18] the cone and plate(let) analyzer,[19] and flow cytometry.[20] The PFA-100 may be useful as a screening test for primary hemostasis[17] instead of the bleeding time. Other tests used in the specific diagnosis of platelet function disorders are discussed below in the context of each disorder.

Differential diagnosis

The presence of a platelet function disorder can usually be determined from the clinical history, physical examination (Table 25.1), complete blood count (including examination of the blood smear), platelet aggregation and, if necessary, tests for von Willebrand disease (ristocetin cofactor, VWF antigen, factor VIII coagulant).[11]

The list of specific causes of platelet function defects is long (Tables 25.2 and 25.3). However, acquired defects are the commonest and the underlying medical condition is usually evident. With the exception of storage pool disease, inherited platelet function defects, at least the well-characterized ones, are all rare. These rare disorders usually require specialized

Table 25.2 Causes of inherited platelet function defects.

Adhesion
Bernard–Soulier syndrome
von Willebrand disease

Agonist receptors
Integrin $\alpha_2\beta_1$ (collagen receptor) deficiency
GpVI (collagen receptor) deficiency
P2Y$_{12}$ (ADP receptor) deficiency
Thromboxane A$_2$ receptor deficiency

Signaling pathways
G$_{\alpha q}$ deficiency
Phospholipase C β_2 deficiency
Cyclooxygenase deficiency
Thromboxane synthetase deficiency
Lipooxygenase deficiency
Defects in calcium mobilization

Secretion
Storage pool disease
Hermansky–Pudlak syndrome
Chédiak–Higashi syndrome
Gray platelet syndrome
Quebec syndrome
Wiskott–Aldrich syndrome

Aggregation
Glanzmann thrombasthenia
Congenital afibrinogenemia

Platelet–coagulant protein interaction
Scott syndrome

Table 25.3 Causes of acquired platelet function defects.

Drugs and other causes
Uremia
Liver disease
Extracorporeal perfusion
Acquired storage pool deficiency
Antiplatelet antibodies
Acute leukemias and myelodysplastic syndromes
Myeloproliferative disorders

research laboratories to make a specific diagnosis, with the exception of Bernard–Soulier syndrome and Glanzmann thrombasthenia, which are easily diagnosed by platelet aggregometry and flow cytometry.

Inherited disorders of platelet function

Based on the normal function of platelets, inherited disorders of platelet function can be considered to be defects in adhesion, agonist receptors, signaling pathways, secretion, aggregation, or platelet–coagulant protein interaction (Table 25.2). Table 25.4 presents the essential characteristics of the principal inherited disorders of platelets.

Adhesion defects

Bernard–Soulier syndrome

In 1948, Bernard and Soulier described a severe hereditary bleeding disorder characterized by a prolonged bleeding time, moderate thrombocytopenia with giant and morphologically abnormal platelets, normal clot retraction but defective prothrombin consumption.[21] Subsequent investigation of similar cases showed that the platelets aggregated normally with ADP, epinephrine, collagen, and all other platelet agonists, but were not agglutinated by VWF or ristocetin.[22] In contrast to von Willebrand disease, in which the defective response to ristocetin is due to deficiency of plasma VWF, in Bernard–Soulier syndrome it is the platelet membrane that is defective, lacking receptors for VWF. Specifically, there is a defect in the GpIb–IX–V complex, of which the individual subunits (GPIbα, GpIbβ, GpIX, and GpV) are members of the "leucine-rich" family of glycoproteins.[23] This complex carries a binding site for VWF on the outermost extracellular portion of the GpIbα subunit. VWF binding to GpIbα is induced *in vitro* by ristocetin, and occurs *in vivo* as a result of the conformational change in VWF that results from the prior binding of VWF to the vascular subendothelium.[23] This platelet–VWF–subendothelium interaction is an essential step in the initial adhesion of platelets to damaged blood vessels, particularly at the shear rates that occur in small

Table 25.4 Essential characteristics of the principal inherited disorders of platelets.

	Bleeding syndrome	Platelet count × 10^9/L	Platelet ultrastructure	Associations	Functional abnormality	Inheritance	Structural defects and gene affected
Bernard–Soulier syndrome	Moderate to severe	20–100	Giant platelets	DiGeorge/velocardiofacial syndrome*	Abnormal adhesivity, no agglutination with ristocetin or botrocetin, retarded response to thrombin	AR (1 report of AD)	GpIb-IX GpIbα (chr. 17) GpIbβ (chr. 22) GpIX (chr. 3)
May–Hegglin anomaly	Mild	30–100	Large size	Neutrophil inclusions	No consistent defects	AD	Nonmuscle myosin heavy chain MYH9
Fechtner syndrome (FS), Sebastian syndrome (SS)	Mild	30–100	Large size, large vacuoles	Hereditary nephritis and hearing loss (FS) Leukocyte inclusions (FS, SS)	No consistent defects	AD	Nonmuscle myosin heavy chain MYH9
Epstein syndrome	Mild	5–100	Large size, large vacuoles	Hereditary nephritis and hearing loss	Impaired response to collagen (not consistent)	AD	Unknown
Montreal platelet syndrome	Moderate to severe	5–40	Large size	None	Spontaneous agglutination, decreased aggregation with thrombin	AD	Unknown, reduced calpain activity
Platelet-type von Willebrand disease	Moderate	Normal or decreased	Platelet size heterogeneity	Absence of high molecular weight VWF multimers in plasma	Increased sensitivity to agglutination by ristocetin	AD	GPIbα
$\alpha_2\beta_1$ collagen receptor	Mild	Normal	Normal	Modification in receptor density with hormonal status	Decreased response to collagen	?	Probably α_2 (chr. 5)
GpVI collagen receptor	Mild	Normal	Normal	Function dependent on FcR γ chain	Decreased response to collagen	?	Probably GpVI (chr. 19)
P2Y$_{12}$ ADP receptor	Mild	Normal	Normal	None known, but receptor found in brain	Small and unstable aggregates with ADP	Probably AR	P2Y$_{12}$ receptor defect (chr. 3)
Thromboxane (TX)A$_2$ receptor	Mild	Normal	Normal	None known	Absence of response to TXA$_2$ and analogs, diminished response to collagen	AD	TXA$_2$ receptor

(continued p. 568)

Table 25.4 (continued)

	Bleeding syndrome	Platelet count × 10⁹/L	Platelet ultrastructure	Associations	Functional abnormality	Inheritance	Structural defects and gene affected
Signaling[†]	Mild	Normal	Normal	None known	Diminished aggregation and secretion to multiple agonists	Not reported	Phospholipase C β2 $G_{\alpha q}$ protein
Cyclooxygenase[‡]	Moderate	Decreased on occasion	Normal	None known	No aggregation with arachidonic acid, diminished response to collagen and ADP	Probably AR	Cyclooxygenase
Gray platelet syndrome	Mild	30–100	Empty α-granules	Myelofibrosis	Sometimes normal, can be decreased with thrombin, epinephrine and collagen	AR or AD	Unknown but prevents storage of α-granule proteins
Quebec syndrome	Moderate to severe	~100	Subnormal content of α-granules	None known	Absent aggregation with epinephrine	AD	Multimerin. Increased urokinase-type plasminogen activator in α-granules with degraded proteins
Wiskott–Aldrich syndrome	Mild to severe	10–100	Small size, fewer granules	Usually eczema, infections Immunodeficiency	Decreased aggregation and secretion with multiple agonists	X-linked	WASP protein (a signaling molecule)
Hermansky–Pudlak (HP), Chédiak–Higashi (CH) syndromes§	Mild to moderate	Normal	Reduced number of abnormal dense granules Giant granules (CH)	Oculocutaneous albinism Ceroid-lipofuscinosis (HP) Infections (CH)	Decreased aggregation and secretion with multiple agonists	AR	Proteins involved in vesicle formation and trafficking
Glanzmann thrombasthenia	Moderate to severe	Normal	Normal	Possible increased bone thickening and low fertility (β₃)	Absent aggregation with all agonists, clot retraction often defective	AR	α_{IIb} and β_3 (chr. 17q21–23)
Scott syndrome	Moderate to severe	Normal	Normal	Defects extend to other blood cells	Low expression of procoagulant activity and microparticle release	AR	Unknown

* Condition associated with loss of GpIbβ gene in chromosome 22q11 deletion.

† Two examples only are given.

‡ Other enzyme deficiencies have been reported (e.g., thromboxane synthetase, lipooxygenase).

§ Other types of storage pool disease are described in the text.

AD, autosomal dominant; AR, autosomal recessive; chr., chromosome; VWF, von Willebrand factor.

Reproduced with permission from Ref. 58.

arteries and capillaries, and it is the failure of this initial step in platelet plug formation which accounts for the bleeding tendency of Bernard–Soulier syndrome.

The thrombocytopenia of Bernard–Soulier syndrome is chiefly due to a shortened platelet lifespan, which may be an end result of the deficiency of the sialic acid-rich glycoprotein. Unstimulated platelets also have a high basal prothrombinase activity.[24] The partial defect of thrombin binding and aggregation reported by Jamieson and Okumura[25] suggested that the GpIb–IX–V complex carries a thrombin receptor, and this has subsequently been confirmed and shown to be distinct from the VWF receptor.[23] The abnormally deformable membrane of platelets in this syndrome[26] is evidently also related to the GpIb–IX–V deficiency, since this complex plays an important part in linking the plasma membrane to the cytoskeleton of the platelet.[23]

Clinical features

Bernard–Soulier syndrome is an extremely rare autosomal recessive disorder. It is clinically indistinguishable from Glanzmann thrombasthenia and, like it, usually presents early in life with multiple petechiae and ecchymoses, and bleeding from mucous membranes and superficial grazes and cuts. Epistaxes and menorrhagia are among the commonest symptoms and can present difficult problems in management. Several children have died from uncontrollable bleeding, and the original patient of Bernard and Soulier, who presented with epistaxis and anal hemorrhage at the age of 15 days, had numerous bleeding episodes during his first 7 years, after which hemorrhage occurred less frequently and usually only after injury; he died at the age of 28 from a cerebral hemorrhage following a bar-room brawl.[27] As in Glanzmann thrombasthenia, clinical severity may vary widely between affected family members.

Laboratory diagnosis

The platelet count is usually only moderately reduced (commonly $50–100 \times 10^9$/L), but the bleeding time and PFA-100 closure time are very prolonged. The giant platelets may not be recognized as such by electronic cell counters, leading to spuriously low counts, but their presence in the blood film will suggest the diagnosis. It is difficult to prepare platelet-rich plasma for aggregation and other tests because the large dense platelets tend to sediment with the red and white cells. The failure to agglutinate in response to ristocetin (even in the presence of normal plasma or VWF), together with the normal or even increased aggregation response to ADP, epinephrine and collagen, and the demonstration of normal VWF in the patient's plasma, further establishes the diagnosis, which can be confirmed by demonstrating the deficiency of GpIb–IX–V complex in the platelet membrane. This can be achieved by biochemical methods such as polyacrylamide gel electrophoresis or by the use of specific monoclonal antibodies in flow cytometric or immunochemical tests.

Molecular genetics

Mutations in GpIbα, GpIbβ, and GpIX but not GpV have been described in Bernard–Soulier syndrome.[22] Most of the described mutations have been homozygous, resulting from consanguinity in the parents of the affected individual. An exception is the seemingly frequent association of the velocardiofacial syndrome with hemizygous mutation of GpIbβ as a cause of Bernard–Soulier syndrome. Velocardiofacial syndrome is a congenital disorder characterized by variable manifestations of cardiac defects, delayed development, otorhinolaryngologic manifestations, psychiatric disturbances, and mental retardation. The disorder results from deletion of the region of chromosome 22 (22q11.2) that includes the gene encoding GpIbβ.[23] Thus, it is important to be alert to the concomitant presence of cardiac disorders and potentially subtle IQ and facial abnormalities when evaluating patients with Bernard–Soulier syndrome.

Detection of heterozygotes and prenatal diagnosis

Most heterozygotes for Bernard–Soulier syndrome in whom platelet size has been examined possess larger than normal platelets, despite generally normal hemostatic parameters. In a recent evaluation of causes of autosomal dominant macrothrombocytopenia in Italy, Savoia *et al.*[28] found that a predominance of affected individuals were heterozygotes for Bernard–Soulier syndrome. Quantitation of the GpIb–IX–V complex in small volumes of whole blood by means of monoclonal antibodies and flow cytometry[20] provides the most suitable method for detecting heterozygotes and for prenatal diagnosis. Prenatal blood sampling may carry a high risk to the affected fetus, as in the case of Glanzmann thrombasthenia. In those few cases in which the genetic defect has been identified, early prenatal diagnosis by chorionic villous sampling may be feasible.

von Willebrand disease

Von Willebrand disease is not primarily an inherited disorder of platelet function but an inherited disorder of VWF. However, because of the key role of VWF in platelet adhesion via its binding to the GpIb–IX–V complex (see above), von Willebrand disease results in a platelet adhesion defect. Thus it can present clinically with mucocutaneous bleeding, petechiae, and a prolonged bleeding time (see Table 25.1). Von Willebrand disease is discussed in detail in Chapter 27. Of particular relevance here is the rare platelet-type or "pseudo" von Willebrand disease which, like Bernard–Soulier syndrome, results not from an abnormality in VWF but from an abnormality in the platelet GpIb–IX–V complex. However, unlike Bernard–Soulier syndrome, in this autosomal dominant disease there is an unusual gain of function phenotype with facilitated binding of plasma VWF to platelets and increased platelet agglutination in the presence of low amounts of ristocetin. The mutations giving rise to this disorder are $Gly^{233} \rightarrow Val$ and $Met^{239} \rightarrow Val$.[22] These amino acid substitutions occur within the disulfide-bonded double-loop region of GpIbα. It has been speculated that these mutations induce conformational changes that mimic those induced by high shear. Because the mutated GpIbα binds VWF multimers spontaneously, the VWF multimers are cleared from the plasma. The result is a clinical condition that resembles type 2B von Willebrand disease. In this latter disease, mutations within the VWF monomer result in an abnormal protein that binds spontaneously to platelets. Platelet-type von Willebrand disease varies from clinically mild to severe. Most have patients have moderately prolonged bleeding times and a degree of thrombocytopenia, probably due to platelet aggregation *in vivo*, and some have an increased platelet volume (see Table 25.4). Platelet agglutination by low-dose ristocetin is increased, and indeed the patient's platelets are usually agglutinated by the addition of normal plasma or VWF in the absence of ristocetin. The distinction from type 2B von Willebrand disease depends on the demonstration of binding of normal VWF to isolated platelets: lower concentrations of ristocetin are required for binding to platelets from patients with platelet-type von Willebrand disease than to either normal platelets or those from patients with type 2B von Willebrand disease.

Agonist receptor defects

Integrin α₂β₁ deficiency

Nieuwenhuis *et al.*[29] reported the case of a young woman who had suffered from easy bruising and menorrhagia since her teens, with a constantly prolonged bleeding time, whose platelets failed to respond by aggregation, secretion or thromboxane synthesis to collagen (although they responded normally to other agonists) or to adhere to purified type I or type III collagen or subendothelial microfibrils. These investigators found that her platelet membranes were deficient in GpIa, which together with GpIIa forms the integrin α₂β₁ (VLA-2), an important collagen receptor (Table 25.4).[30] Although no corresponding abnormality could be found in the platelets of this patient's parents, sister or son, the defect seems likely to have been genetically determined. A similar patient has subsequently been described with a lifelong bleeding tendency and a decreased reaction with collagen, in whom GpIa deficiency was associated with a lack of platelet thrombospondin.[31] The symptoms and platelet defect disappeared at the time of the menopause, perhaps suggesting that they were related to hormonal influences.

P2Y₁₂ deficiency

Platelets possess two receptors for ADP: P2Y₁, which mediates ADP-induced Ca^{2+} mobilization and shape change; and P2Y₁₂, which results in stabilization of platelet aggregation.[30]

Both P2Y₁ and P2Y₁₂ belong to the seven-transmembrane-domain family of G protein-linked receptors. Deficiency of the P2Y₁₂ receptor has been reported (Table 25.4).[32] Such patients are of particular interest because their platelets show identical functional changes to those of normal platelets treated with clopidogrel or ticlopidine, suggesting that P2Y₁₂ is the molecular target for these antiplatelet drugs. So far, no human pathology of the P2Y₁ receptor has been reported.

Thromboxane A₂ receptor deficiency

Defective platelet aggregation to TXA₂ resulting from an $Arg^{60} \rightarrow Leu$ mutation in the TXA₂ receptor has been reported (Table 25.4).[33]

Defective response to epinephrine

The aggregatory response of normal platelets to epinephrine is variable and decreased responsiveness may be inherited without conferring any hemostatic failure.[34,35] It can therefore be argued that tests of epinephrine-induced aggregation are best avoided in the investigation of bleeding disorders, or at least discounted in the absence of other demonstrable abnormalities. However, Stormorken *et al.*[36] reported a 16-year-old boy who had had frequent bleeding episodes since early childhood and whose platelets completely failed to aggregate in response to epinephrine. Like the hemostatically normal subjects studied by Scrutton *et al.*,[34] his platelets had normal α₂-adrenergic receptors. The exact nature of the defect was not established.

Signaling pathway defects

Platelet pathologies may also be present in the intracellular signal transduction pathways into which surface receptors are locked.[22] This heterogenous group of disorders (see Tables 25.2 and 25.4) present as mild bleeding disorders and defects of platelet aggregation that affect individual stimuli more than others. For example, patients have been reported with impaired Ca^{2+} mobilization, defective inositol 1,4,5-trisphosphate production, and reduced phosphorylation of the protein plekstrin by protein kinase C. One patient was selectively deficient in the phospholipase C β₂ isoform, thereby highlighting its role in platelet activation. Another patient had a specific decrease in platelet membrane $G_{\alpha q}$ and platelets that responded less well to several agonists including decreased activation of $\alpha_{IIb}\beta_3$.[37] Rare patients with congenital deficiencies of cyclooxygenase, prostaglandin H synthetase 1, thromboxane synthetase, lipoxygenase, glycogen 6 synthetase, or ATP metabolism have been reported and lead to platelet function abnormalities that often resemble those seen in storage pool disease or after aspirin ingestion (see Tables 25.2 and 25.4).[22] These reports of abnormalities in signaling pathways represent the first of what may eventually prove to be a long list of rare congenital disorders of platelets. The key to identifying these disorders will be improved diagnostic methods, perhaps including the simultaneous assessment of a wide range of genes by microarraybased technology.[22]

Secretion defects

Storage pool disease

This term was first applied to deficiency of the platelet dense bodies, the site of the storage pool of adenine nucleotides and of 5-HT (serotonin). Following the suggestion of Weiss et al.,[38] its use has been extended to include deficiency of the α-granules. Pure dense body deficiency is therefore now designated δ-storage pool deficiency (δ-SPD), pure deficiency of α-granules (gray platelet syndrome) α-SPD, and combined deficiency of both types of organelle αδ-SPD.

Dense body deficiency

Laboratory diagnosis

The definitive diagnosis of δ-SPD depends on demonstration of the dense body deficiency, biochemically, morphologically or by flow cytometry. The bleeding time, or PFA-100 closure time, is usually moderately prolonged, and the platelet aggregation pattern commonly reflects the defect of secretion, although it will not clearly distinguish dense body deficiency from other secretory disorders. The typical features are normal primary aggregation in response to ADP and epinephrine, but without a second wave, a marked defect of aggregation and ATP secretion in response to collagen, and a normal response to arachidonic acid, which serves to exclude a defect of thromboxane generation.[39] However, this typical pattern may not be seen in milder cases: Nieuwenhuis et al.[13] studied over 100 patients with long bleeding times and a deficiency of total platelet ADP and 5-HT, of which about half were congenital in origin, and found that about one-quarter had a normal aggregation pattern with ADP, epinephrine and collagen, while only one-third showed a pattern completely typical of a secretory defect. The hallmarks of δ-SPD are therefore actual deficiency of the dense bodies and their contents. Dense bodies can be enumerated in platelets by either electron microscopy or fluorescence microscopy after incubation with the fluorescent dye mepacrine, which is taken up and localized in the dense bodies.[40] δ-SPD can be accurately diagnosed by a simple, rapid, one-step flow cytometric assay for mepacrine uptake.[14,15] Biochemical evidence of dense body deficiency depends on measurement of the platelet content of adenine nucleotides and 5-HT and their uptake and secretion. The storage pool of nucleotides in the dense bodies (which is largely deficient in δ-SPD) has an ATP/ADP ratio of about 2 : 3, while that of the metabolic pool in the cytosol is about 8 : 1. In δ-SPD,

therefore, the ATP/ADP ratio of whole platelets (normally 1.5–2.5 : 1) is much increased, approximating to that of the metabolic pool alone of normal platelets.[41] The defective secretion of adenine nucleotides can also be demonstrated by lumiaggregometry after thrombin activation.

Clinical associations

Dense body deficiency has been observed in a number of families as an isolated platelet defect, and also occurs as an integral part of two well-defined syndromes in association with albinism and lysosomal abnormalities: Hermansky–Pudlak and Chédiak–Higashi syndromes. The nonalbino group (idiopathic δ-SPD) shows considerable heterogeneity with respect to both heredity and the degree of dense body deficiency, and patients are usually more mildly affected than albino patients. While in several families the isolated defect appears to be transmitted as an autosomal dominant trait, others exhibit recessive inheritance. In contrast to the albino patients, whose platelets are profoundly deficient in both dense body membranes and contents, the idiopathic nonalbino group shows various degrees of dissociation between these two features.

Hermansky–Pudlak syndrome is an autosomal recessive disorder characterized by the triad of tyrosinase-positive oculocutaneous albinism, a lifelong moderate bleeding tendency, and the presence of ceroid-like pigment in cells of the reticuloendothelial system (see Table 25.4). The pigment was first observed in bone marrow macrophages but may also be deposited in the lungs and intestine, where it leads to pulmonary fibrosis and inflammatory bowel disease, as well as in the buccal mucosa and urinary bladder. The bleeding tendency is primarily attributable to the deficiency of platelet dense bodies. The dense body deficiency is more severe than that in nonalbino patients and affects both membranes and contents,[42,43] suggesting that the defect is a structural one, involving dense body formation in the megakaryocyte. Heterozygotes are clinically unaffected, and their platelets contain normal amounts of adenine nucleotides and aggregate normally. Hermansky–Pudlak syndrome is common in Puerto Rico. The defect is in the *HPS1* or *HPS2* genes.[22]

Chédiak–Higashi syndrome, an autosomal recessive disorder of lysosome formation in neutrophils and other cells (Table 25.4). Thrombocytopenia is common and is the chief cause of the bleeding tendency, but dense body deficiency is also characteristic.[22] As in Hermansky–Pudlak syndrome, granulophysin (CD63) is deficient, indicating a defect of dense body membrane formation. Like the neutrophils, the platelets contain large abnormal granules. The defect is in the *CHS* gene on chromosome 13.[22]

Wiskott–Aldrich syndrome is an X-linked recessive disorder characterized by thrombocytopenia, small platelets, eczema, and recurrent infections secondary to immune deficiency (see Table 25.4).[22] In addition, the platelets also have a dense body deficiency.[22] The genetic defect in Wiskott–Aldrich syndrome results from a defect in the 502-amino acid protein termed WASP (Wiskott–Aldrich syndrome protein). Wiskott–Aldrich syndrome is more fully described in Chapter 19.

α-Granule deficiency (gray platelet syndrome)

Unlike dense body deficiency, a pure deficiency of α-granules occurs in only a single hereditary disorder, named by Raccuglia[44] as gray platelet syndrome (Table 25.4), based on the appearance of the agranular platelets on a stained blood smear. This extremely rare hereditary platelet disorder, which shows either autosomal recessive or autosomal dominant inheritance, is sometimes surprisingly mild clinically, considering the profound nature of the structural and biochemical platelet defect. Epistaxes, menorrhagia and prolonged bleeding after serious injury are the commonest symptoms.

Laboratory findings

The bleeding time is usually moderately prolonged. Unlike most other defects of platelet function, the first diagnostic clue comes from examination of the blood film, which reveals the characteristic gray agranular platelets. The platelet count is usually slightly below normal and mean platelet volume is increased. The profound α-granule deficiency can be confirmed by electron microscopy, which also shows normal numbers of dense bodies and mitochondria and numerous large vesicles. The latter probably represent both abortive α-granules and elements of the open canalicular system. Small abnormal granules may also be seen, recognizable as α-granule precursors by their content of fibrinogen and VWF, and also by the specific proteins, including P-selectin, in their membranes.[45]

Gray platelets have been shown to be profoundly deficient in many of the proteins normally contained in α-granules, including 2-TG, PF4, thrombospondin, PDGF, VWF and factor V,[46,48] all of which are synthesized within the megakaryocyte. The defect is one of packaging of these endogenous proteins within the organelles rather than of protein synthesis, as shown by normal or even slightly elevated plasma levels of 2-TG and PF4. It has been suggested that this failure of packaging may lead to the premature release of PDGF and PF4 from the megakaryocyte, so accounting for the myelofibrosis observed in some of these patients,[49] and perhaps for the pulmonary fibrosis which has also been described.[50] However, this failure of packaging does not extend to the plasma proteins, including fibrinogen, fibronectin, immunoglobulins and albumin, which are taken up essentially normally into α-granule precursors.

Gray platelets typically show a partial defect of aggregation and dense body secretion, particularly in response to thrombin and collagen. This appears to be due to a defect of phosphoinositide hydrolysis and cytosolic calcium transport,[51,52] associated with an increased rate of transport of calcium into membrane vesicles;[53] this in turn may be related to an abnormality of the monomeric GTP-binding protein Rap-1, which is normally expressed in intracellular membranes from gray platelets but abnormally phosphorylated by cAMP.[54]

Gray platelet syndrome has not yet been diagnosed prenatally, but Wautier and Gruel[55] were able to exclude the condition in the 19-week fetus of a woman with gray platelet syndrome by demonstrating normal platelet β-TG content and ultrastructure.

Combined storage pool deficiency

A proportion of patients with the nonalbino variety of hereditary dense body deficiency also have various degrees of α-granule deficiency, i.e., αδ-SPD.[56] The clinical severity does not appear to be significantly greater in patients with the combined deficiency than in those with pure δ-SPD. An apparent association with acute myeloid leukemia has been reported in two families with SPD: two affected members of the family with mild αδ-SPD had leukemia,[56] while a large family with apparent δ-SPD (in whom α-granules were not studied) included seven patients with myeloid leukemias, of whom at least four had a preexisting platelet disorder.[57] It may be that both these families were expressing defects in a protooncogene that regulates the maturation of both granulocytes and megakaryocytes.

Quebec syndrome

Quebec syndrome (see Table 25.4) is an autosomal dominant bleeding disorder that was first described in two French-Canadian families.[58] Originally thought to involve factor V, Quebec syndrome platelets in fact have a severe deficiency of multimerin, a high-molecular-mass multimeric protein that is stored as a complex with factor V in α-granules. In this syndrome, platelets typically show protease-related degradation of many α-granule proteins (including P-selectin) even though α-granule ultrastructure is preserved.[59] Platelets in this disorder have unusually large amounts of urokinase-type plasminogen activator that is released on platelet activation, and whose presence in excess of the natural inhibitors of this protease accounts for the in situ protein degradation in the α-granules.[60] For unknown reasons, the platelet aggregation deficiency is most striking with epinephrine. Thrombocytopenia is sometimes observed.

Aggregation defects

Glanzmann thrombasthenia

In 1918, Glanzmann provided the first description of a hereditary disorder of platelet function, characterized by a prolonged bleeding time and impaired clot retraction in the presence of a normal platelet count.[58] The defect is now known to be characterized by a global defect in platelet aggregation as a result of a deficiency of integrin $\alpha_{IIb}\beta_3$ (GpIIb–IIIa, CD41/CD61).

Clinical features

Glanzmann thrombasthenia is an autosomal recessive disorder, rare in a global context but relatively more common in those communities where consanguineous marriages are frequent. It cannot be distinguished on clinical grounds alone from other congenital platelet disorders or severe von Willebrand disease. It commonly presents in infancy or early childhood with multiple bruises following minimal or unrecognized trauma, or with crops of petechiae or ecchymoses. George *et al.*[61] reported the incidence and severity of bleeding symptoms in a series of 177 patients. Epistaxes are very common, and may be difficult to control with local measures, and may even be life-threatening. Gingival hemorrhage is a frequent result of the shedding of deciduous teeth, or even of tooth brushing, and is likely to lead to iron deficiency. Large muscle hematomas and hemarthroses seldom occur, but menorrhagia is virtually inevitable and may present a serious hazard in pubertal girls. Serious accidental and surgical trauma can be life-threatening. Although the failure of platelet aggregation *in vitro* is always virtually complete, clinical severity correlates poorly with the nature and degree of the molecular abnormality, with even siblings sometimes being very differently affected.[61]

Laboratory diagnosis

The essential diagnostic features are normal platelet count and morphology associated with a complete failure of platelet aggregation in response to all agonists (e.g., ADP, epinephrine, collagen, arachidonic acid, thrombin); this is because Glanzmann thrombasthenia is the result of a defect in integrin $\alpha_{IIb}\beta_3$ which, as the fibrinogen receptor, is the final common pathway for platelet aggregation.[58] However, platelet agglutination with ristocetin is normal because this process is not dependent on integrin $\alpha_{IIb}\beta_3$ interactions with fibrinogen but on GpIb–IX–V interactions with VWF. After the platelet aggregation defect has been demonstrated, the diagnosis of Glanzmann thrombasthenia can be confirmed, and in the case of unusual variants extended, by measuring the amounts of integrins α_{IIb} and β_3 in the platelet surface membrane. The methods available for this include one- and two-dimensional polyacrylamide gel electrophoresis, crossed immunoelectrophoresis using specific antibodies, and binding assays or flow cytometry with monoclonal antibodies to the constituent glycoproteins. The last of these has the advantage of being simply performed on very small volumes of whole blood,[62] making it particularly appropriate for prenatal diagnosis (see below) or the investigation of small children. Clot retraction, platelet fibrinogen and PF3 availability are all defective in Glanzmann thrombasthenia, but contribute no more to the diagnosis when the defective

platelet aggregation and deficiency of integrin $\alpha_{IIb}\beta_3$ has been demonstrated.

Molecular genetics

A normal tertiary structure of integrin $\alpha_{IIb}\beta_3$ is required for its receptor activity, as demonstrated by patients with variant forms of Glanzmann thrombasthenia who have qualitative defects of $\alpha_{IIb}\beta_3$ that result in an inability to bind fibrinogen. Nevertheless, the majority of patients have severely decreased platelet surface expression of $\alpha_{IIb}\beta_3$.[58] Large gene deletions are rare, while splice defects and nonsense mutations in the α_{IIb} and β_3 genes are common. The gene encoding α_{IIb} spans 17 kb and comprises 30 exons. The gene encoding β_3 spans 46 kb and is composed of 15 exons. The genes colocalize to 17q21–23.

Detection of heterozygotes

Heterozygotes for Glanzmann thrombasthenia usually have no significant bleeding symptoms and no demonstrable defect of platelet aggregation. However, their platelet surface expresses about half the normal number of copies of integrin $\alpha_{IIb}\beta_3$, thus providing a means of carrier detection by flow cytometry, gel electrophoresis, or fibrinogen binding. None of these methods is completely reliable, but in kindreds in which the precise genetic defect has been identified, unequivocal carrier detection can be provided using DNA probes specific for the abnormal DNA sequence or by the detection of deletions by polymerase chain reaction analysis.[63]

Prenatal diagnosis

Since platelet integrin $\alpha_{IIb}\beta_3$ has reached adult levels by 18 weeks of gestation, its expression and functional integrity can be determined on fetal blood samples.[64,65] These methods are applicable to families with the classical form of the disease, characterized by integrin $\alpha_{IIb}\beta_3$ deficiency, and can even detect the heterozygous state *in utero*,[55] but are less appropriate for the prenatal diagnosis of disease variants. In such cases, prenatal blood testing depends on the demonstration of a defect in aggregation[66] or fibrinogen binding.[67] When the molecular genetic abnormality is known, diagnosis can be performed at 8–10 weeks' gestation by chorionic villous sampling and the use of appropriate DNA probes. Fetal sampling for the prenatal diagnosis of Glanzmann thrombasthenia carries a high risk to the affected fetus of death from continuing hemorrhage.[66,68]

Abnormalities of platelet coagulant activity

Scott syndrome

Scott syndrome is a rare inherited disorder of Ca^{2+}-induced phospholipid scrambling, leading to abnormal assembly of the prothrombinase complex on blood cells including platelets (see Table 25.4).[58] When activated, Scott syndrome platelets are unable to translocate phosphatidylserine from the inner to the outer phospholipid leaflet of the membrane bilayer, with the result that they cannot assemble the prothrombinase (factors Va/Xa) and tenase (factors VIIIa/IXa) enzyme complexes. The resultant lack of thrombin generation is sufficient to induce a bleeding diathesis. Stimuli that induce this phosphatidylserine translocation under physiologic conditions include a thrombin and collagen mixture and complement C5b–9. Microvesiculation and the diffusion of the procoagulant activity into the circulation may accompany surface phosphatidylserine expression, which can be readily measured by flow cytometry using fluorescein isothiocyanate (FITC)-conjugated annexin V. Microvesicle formation is also deficient in Scott syndrome. The defect in Scott syndrome may be related to capacitative Ca^{2+} entry into cells, and the subsequent regulated activation of the scramblase enzyme thought to be responsible for phosphatidylserine mobilization.[69–71]

MYH9-related disease

May–Hegglin anomaly, Sebastian syndrome, Fechtner syndrome, and Epstein syndrome are autosomal dominant macrothrombocytopenias distinguished by different combinations of clinical and laboratory signs, such as sensorineural hearing loss, cataract, nephritis, and polymorphonuclear Döhle-like bodies (see Table 25.4). Mutations in the *MYH9* gene encoding nonmuscle myosin heavy chain IIA have recently been identified in all these syndromes.[72] May–Hegglin anomaly, Sebastian syndrome, Fechtner syndrome, and Epstein syndrome are therefore not distinct entities but rather a single disorder with a continuous clinical spectrum, varying from mild macrothrombocytopenia with leukocyte inclusions to a severe form complicated by hearing loss, cataracts, and renal failure. For this new nosologic entity, the term "MHY9-related disease" has been proposed,[72] which identifies patients at risk of developing renal, hearing, and/or visual defects.

Miscellaneous disorders

Various platelet abnormalities have been reported in hereditary disorders of connective tissue, including Ehlers–Danlos and Marfan syndromes and osteogenesis imperfecta, but the bleeding tendency in these disorders is more likely to result from the connective tissue abnormality. In Ehlers–Danlos syndrome, for example, skin collagen has been shown to be defective in aggregating normal platelets.[73] The bleeding tendency is most severe in type IV Ehlers–Danlos syndrome, in which type III collagen, the most potent type of collagen in activating the platelets, is deficient.[74] Defective platelet aggregation has been described in Bartter syndrome but is due to a plasma factor, the probable consequence of the underlying metabolic disturbance.[75] Biochemical and/or

functional abnormalities of the platelets have been described in Down syndrome, adenosine deaminase deficiency and idiopathic scoliosis, but none of these conditions is associated with abnormal bleeding.

Acquired disorders of platelet function

Abnormalities of platelet function occur in a wide range of acquired conditions, often in association with other hemostatic defects including both thrombocytopenia and disorders of blood coagulation. It may therefore be difficult to assess the relative importance of several observed abnormalities in the pathogenesis of the bleeding tendency. In most acquired disorders of platelet function, the nature of the platelet abnormality is much less clear-cut than in the genetic disorders of platelet function. A predominantly clinical rather than pathogenetic classification is therefore appropriate (see Table 25.3).

Drugs and other agents

Aside from the deliberate use of platelet inhibitory drugs as antithrombotic agents, interference with platelet function may occur as a side-effect of drugs used for other purposes. The defects induced are usually of minor degree and observed only on laboratory testing. The following account is largely confined to those drugs and agents that have been recognized as potential causes of clinical bleeding (Table 25.5).

Cyclooxygenase inhibitors

Aspirin irreversibly acetylates serine 529 of cyclooxygenase (COX)-1, resulting in inhibition of TXA_2 generation by platelets and prostacyclin by endothelial cells.[76] Because platelets lack the synthetic machinery to generate significant amounts of new COX, aspirin-induced COX-1 inhibition lasts for the lifetime of the platelet. In contrast, endothelial cells retain their capacity to generate new COX and recover normal function shortly after exposure to aspirin. Aspirin results in absence of the second wave of aggregation with ADP and failure of aggregation and secretion in response to collagen and arachidonic acid. It is therefore important to ensure abstention from aspirin for at least 10 days before platelet function testing for diagnostic purposes. Aspirin ingestion is a common cause of platelet dysfunction, and may occasionally precipitate gastrointestinal or other hemorrhage, particularly in susceptible individuals. Aspirin is therefore contraindicated in patients with known bleeding disorders. Since aspirin crosses the placenta and can contribute to neonatal bleeding,[8] it should if possible be withheld during the week before delivery. Compared with aspirin, other NSAIDs, including indometacin,

Table 25.5 Drugs that affect platelet function.

Cyclooxygenase inhibitors
Aspirin
Nonsteroidal antiinflammatory agents (indometacin, phenylbutazone, ibuprofen, sulfinpyrazone, sulindac, meclofenamic acid, naproxen, diflunisal, piroxicam, tolmetin, zomepirac)

ADP receptor antagonists
Ticlopidine
Clopidogrel

GpIIb–IIIa antagonists
Abciximab
Tirofiban
Eptifibatide

Drugs that increase platelet cyclic AMP or cyclic GMP
Prostaglandin I_2 and analogs
Phosphodiesterase inhibitors (dipyridamole, cilostazol, caffeine, theophylline, aminophylline)
Nitric oxide and nitric oxide donors

Antimicrobials
Penicillins
Cephalosporins
Nitrofurantoin
Hydroxychloroquine
Miconazole

Cardiovascular drugs
β-Adrenergic blockers (propranolol)
Vasodilators (nitroprusside, nitroglycerin)
Diuretics (furosemide)
Quinidine

Anticoagulants
Heparin

Thrombolytic agents
Streptokinase, tissue plasminogen activator, urokinase

Psychotropics and anesthetics
Tricyclic antidepressants (imipramine, amitriptyline, nortriptyline)
Phenothiazines (chlorpromazine, promethazine, trifluoperazine)
Local anesthetics
General anesthesia (halothane)

Chemotherapeutic agents
Mithramycin
BCNU
Daunorubicin

Miscellaneous agents
Dextrans and hydroxyethyl starch
Aminocaproic acid
Antihistamines
Ethanol
Radiographic contrast agents
Food items and food supplements (ω-3 fatty acids, vitamin E, onions, garlic, ginger, cumin, turmeric, clove, black tree fungus, *Ginkgo*)

Reproduced with permission from Ref. 12.

phenylbutazone and sulfinpyrazone, have a similar but reversible, and therefore less prolonged, effect on platelet function.

ADP receptor antagonists

The thienopyridines clopidogrel (Plavix) and ticlopidine (Ticlid) inhibit platelet function by antagonism of the $P2Y_{12}$ ADP receptor.[77] In patients treated with a thienopyridine, platelet aggregation responses to several agonists, including ADP, collagen, epinephrine, and thrombin, are inhibited to various extents depending on agonist concentrations. Significant inhibition of platelet aggregation is observed after 2–3 days of therapy with a maximal effect at 4–7 days.[77] The platelet inhibitory effect persists to some extent for 7–10 days after therapy is discontinued. Because of this prolonged effect, these drugs need to be discontinued for 7–10 days prior to elective surgery. Ticlopidine and, to a lesser extent, clopidogrel are rarely associated with thrombotic thrombocytopenic purpura.[77]

GpIIb–IIIa antagonists

GpIIb–IIIa antagonists abciximab (ReoPro), eptifibatide (Integrilin) and tirofiban (Aggrastat) inhibit fibrinogen binding to GpIIb–IIIa (integrin $\alpha_{IIb}\beta_3$, CD41/CD61), the final common pathway of platelet aggregation.[78] Platelet aggregation induced by all agonists (with the exception of ristocetin, which is not a true agonist) is therefore inhibited. Abciximab may have additional mechanisms of action through binding to integrins $\alpha_v\beta_3$ (vitronectin receptor) and $\alpha_M\beta_2$ (Mac-1, CD11b/CD18).[78] Bleeding secondary to these intravenous drugs is responsive to platelet transfusion, but this is usually unnecessary with eptifibatide and tirofiban because of their shorter half-life.[79] In addition to their platelet inhibitory effect, thrombocytopenia is a potential side-effect of GpIIb–IIIa antagonists.[79]

Antimicrobials

Many of the β-lactam antibiotics, particularly the penicillins, can cause a bleeding tendency by interfering with platelet function. This side-effect, which may persist for up to 12 days after withdrawal of the drug,[80] is seen only with high-dosage regimes. Patients in renal failure are at particular risk, since high drug concentrations resulting from impaired clearance may coexist with other hemostatic defects. Thrombocytopenia-induced bleeding in patients on chemotherapy for malignant disease may be exacerbated by antibiotic-induced platelet dysfunction. Both penicillins and cephalosporins have been shown to inhibit platelet adhesion, aggregation and secretion *in vitro*: the underlying mechanisms appear to involve the inhibition of agonist binding to membrane receptors and impairment of thromboxane synthesis and calcium mobilization.[81,82] The platelet inhibitory effect of β-lactam antibiotics is influenced by plasma albumin concentration: platelet binding of the antibiotic and the impact on platelet responses are inversely related to albumin concentration.[83] In addition to the β-lactam antibiotics, other antimicrobials shown to inhibit platelet function include nitrofurantoin,[84] hydroxychloroquine,[85] and miconazole.[86]

Cardiovascular drugs

The following cardiovascular drugs have been reported to inhibit platelet function: β-blockers (propranolol, pindolol, atenolol, metoprolol), furosemide, nitroprusside, nitroglycerin, isosorbide dinitrate, and quinidine.[12]

Heparin

The main platelet-related complication of heparin therapy is heparin-induced thrombocytopenia (see Chapter 31).[87] In addition, unfractionated heparins have been found to bind to the platelet membrane and to inhibit platelet function in certain experimental systems, possibly by inducing a refractory state following partial activation. These effects might contribute to the bleeding tendency of heparin overdosage. Heparin fractions of low molecular weight and high antithrombin affinity are the least likely to bind to platelets[88] and interfere with platelet function,[89] and this may partly account for the lower incidence of bleeding complications seen with low molecular weight than with unfractionated heparin.[90]

Thrombolytic agents

The major complication following the administration of thrombolytic agents (streptokinase, urokinase, recombinant tissue plasminogen activator (rt-PA)) is hemorrhage, which arises from multiple mechanisms including the effect of plasmin on the plasma coagulation system and platelets, and the dissolution of blood clots providing local hemostasis.[12] The bleeding time in patients receiving rt-PA may be prolonged.[91] *In vitro*, plasmin induces several effects in platelets: initial platelet activation followed by inhibition, cleavage of membrane glycoproteins, inhibition of TXA_2 production, and disaggregation of platelet clumps.[92] Urinary metabolites of TXA_2 are increased during thrombolytic therapy with rt-PA or streptokinase, indicating *in vivo* activation of platelets.[93,94] Other factors contributing to platelet inhibition in patients receiving thrombolytic therapy include radiographic contrast media and elevated levels of fibrin(ogen) degradation products.[12]

Miscellaneous agents

Other drugs that have been reported to inhibit platelet function include tricyclic antidepressants (imipramine, amitriptyline,

nortriptyline), phenothiazines (chlorpromazine, promethazine, trifluoperazine), chemotherapeutic agents (mithramycin, BCNU, daunomycin), local anesthetics, halothane, sodium valproate, dextrans, hydroxyethyl starch, aminocaproic acid, antihistamines, ethanol, and radiographic contrast agents.[12] The following food items and supplements have been reported to inhibit platelet function: ω-3 fatty acids, vitamin E, onions, garlic, ginger, cumin, turmeric, clove, black tree fungus and *Ginkgo*.[12]

Uremia

Although coagulation defects and thrombocytopenia may both occur in patients in renal failure, defective platelet function is the main cause of bleeding. This commonly presents as purpura, epistaxis or bleeding from the gums, although serious internal hemorrhage may also occur, and renal biopsy or surgical procedures present a special hazard. The bleeding time is typically prolonged, and abnormalities have been reported in a variety of aspects of platelet function, including aggregation,[95] adhesion to subendothelium[96] (perhaps related to reduction in platelet membrane GpIb[97]), elevation of cytoplasmic free calcium,[98] and thromboxane formation.[99] The aggregation defect correlates poorly with the severity of the renal failure, but can be at least partially corrected by hemodialysis or peritoneal dialysis.[100,101] No general agreement has been reached on the identity of the dialysable component responsible for the effect on the platelets; urea,[102] guanidinosuccinic acid,[103] and phenolic acids[104] have all been incriminated. Various defects of arachidonate metabolism have been described in uremic patients, leading to both impaired generation of TXA_2[99] and increased prostacyclin production.[105]

Liver disease

The hemostatic failure of liver disease results chiefly from defective synthesis of clotting factors, but low-grade intravascular coagulation and increased fibrinolysis may also occur. Defective platelet aggregation may be another contributory factor: acquired storage pool deficiency is a likely mechanism, and defects of thromboxane synthesis[106] and membrane glycoproteins[107] have also been reported. Although patients with liver disease usually have normal or raised levels of VWF, desmopressin has been found to shorten the prolonged bleeding time[108] as well as improving the results of coagulation tests.

Extracorporeal perfusion

Bleeding during and after cardiopulmonary bypass has many contributory causes, including defective surgical hemostasis, but transient thrombocytopenia and platelet dysfunction are important in the etiology.[109] The platelet dysfunction results in marked prolongation of the bleeding time during the procedure, with gradual normalization during the subsequent 2–4 hours. The platelet dysfunction is attributable to a combination of platelet activation and membrane damage from contact with the bypass apparatus, decreased available thrombin, contact activation, complement activation, plasmin, fibrin(ogen) degradation products, hypothermia, and heparin.[109] Excessive perioperative bleeding can be reduced by aprotinin, (to a lesser extent) desmopressin, and (possibly) platelet transfusions.[109]

Acquired storage pool deficiency

An acquired storage pool deficiency has been reported in a number of different clinical settings including autoimmune disease, disseminated intravascular coagulation, hemolytic–uremic syndrome/thrombotic thrombocytopenic purpura, severe burns and valvular heart disease.[12]

Antiplatelet antibodies

Many patients with immune thrombocytopenic purpura have autoantibodies directed against determinants on GpIIb–IIIa or GpIb. Such antibodies have also been detected in patients with acquired bleeding disorders and long bleeding times but normal platelet counts, resulting in platelet function defects resembling those of Glanzmann thrombasthenia[110] and Bernard–Soulier syndrome.[111] Similarly, acquired antibodies directed against GpIa can result in a platelet function defect.[112] In patients with immune thrombocytopenic purpura, the antibody-induced functional defect can persist after recovery of the platelet count.

Acute leukemias and myelodysplastic syndromes

Platelet dysfunction can occur in acute leukemias (especially myeloid) and myelodysplastic syndromes.[12] Defects of aggregation and secretion have been described and attributed variously to storage pool deficiency and defects of secretory mechanisms,[113] impaired thromboxane production,[114] and deficiency of thrombin-binding sites on the platelet membrane.[115]

Myeloproliferative disorders

Hemorrhagic symptoms and arterial thromboses are common in adults with myeloproliferative disorders, and both may occur in the same patient.[12] The most common bleeding symptoms are large superficial ecchymoses, epistaxes and hemorrhage from the gastrointestinal tract. Thrombosis usually involves either the cerebral arteries or the peripheral arteries of the limbs. The platelet defects that have been described are not specifically associated with any one of the adult myeloproliferative disorders; similar defects have been observed in essential thrombocythemia, polycythemia vera, chronic granulocytic leukemia, and myelofibrosis.[12] All these conditions are rare in childhood, particularly the first two, but when they do occur they may also be associated with functional platelet disorders. Structural platelet abnormalities are commonly seen in the myeloproliferative disorders, and among the disturbances of platelet function that have been described are:

- defects of aggregation, particularly in response to epinephrine;[116]
- storage pool deficiency;[117]
- defects of arachidonate metabolism;[118]
- defects of platelet coagulant activities;[119]
- resistance to the action of the antiaggregatory prostaglandin D_2;[120]
- various abnormalities of platelet membrane glycoproteins.[121]

Michelson[122] studied four children with juvenile (Ph-negative) chronic myeloid leukemia (CML) and with Ph-positive adult CML, all of whom (in contrast to age-matched controls and adults with Ph-positive CML) showed two subpopulations of platelets, positive and negative respectively, for both GpIb and GpIIb–IIIa. Berndt *et al.*[123] described the case of a 9-year-old girl with a myelodysplastic syndrome characterized by monosomy 7, thrombocytopenia and giant platelets, who had had a bleeding tendency from the age of 5. She was also found to have two populations of platelets, the majority being large and deficient in GpIb–IX complex and the minority normal. Some of the platelet abnormalities that have been observed in myeloproliferative disorders would be expected to lead to abnormal bleeding and others to predispose to thrombotic episodes, but in practice the laboratory findings have been found to correlate poorly with the clinical course of the disease.

Treatment of platelet function disorders

General principles

Platelet function disorders are often mild bleeding disorders. The general principles of treatment of platelet function defects are as follows.

- Avoidance of major body contact activities.
- Avoidance of drugs that interfere with platelet function (e.g., aspirin and other NSAIDs) and other components of the hemostatic system.
- Avoidance of intramuscular injections.
- Good dental care (to minimize gum bleeding and avoid tooth extraction).
- Local hemostatic measures.
- Oral iron (to prevent or treat iron deficiency secondary to blood loss).
- Oral contraceptive pills may be necessary for the control of menorrhagia.

- Immunizations can be given subcutaneously with direct pressure using ice. If necessary, Stimate can be given (see below).
- Consideration should be given to the wearing of a medical bracelet or necklace with the words "platelet function defect" inscribed and/or the patient should carry an information card to that effect.

Antifibrinolytic agents

- Oral aminocaproic acid, an inhibitor of plasminogen activator, is often useful for oral bleeding.
- In Quebec syndrome, the bleeding responds to antifibrinolytic agents rather than to platelet transfusions, because platelets in this disorder have unusually large amounts of urokinase-type plasminogen activator that is released on platelet activation, and whose presence in excess of the natural inhibitors of this protease accounts for the *in situ* protein degradation in α-granules.[60]

Desmopressin (DDAVP)

- Desmopressin, either intravenously or by nasal spray (Stimate), is often helpful for patients with a platelet function defect.[124]
- There should be a major response by 30 min with a maximum response at 90 min.
- Plasma levels last at least 8–10 hours.
- Desmopressin can be repeated every 12 hours, but tolerance may occur after 72 hours.
- The beneficial effect of desmopressin in platelet function disorders may be related to increased release of factor VIII and VWF from endothelial Weibel–Palade bodies and/or a poorly characterized direct effect on platelets.[124]

Activated factor VII

- NovoSeven (intravenous activated factor VII) is effective in many platelet function disorders.[125,126]
- The beneficial effect of activated factor VII may be via a tissue factor-dependent mechanism and/or a tissue factor-independent, platelet-dependent mechanism.[125]

Platelet transfusion

- If necessary, platelet transfusions (preferably HLA-matched) can be given for major bleeding episodes. The platelet transfusion will temporarily correct the platelet function defect.
- Platelets should be available for transfusion during any surgery.
- There is evidence that leukocyte depletion of platelet and red cell concentrates by filtration reduces the likelihood of alloimmunization as well as of febrile transfusion reactions.[127]

- A major problem with platelet transfusion in Bernard–Soulier syndrome and Glanzmann thrombasthenia is alloimmunization, with patients forming antibodies against the glycoproteins missing from their own platelets. Some of these antibodies may recognize epitopes on active sites of the glycoproteins involved in adhesion and aggregation, thus rendering transfused platelets refractory as well as leading to their accelerated destruction. Therefore, platelet transfusions in Bernard–Soulier syndrome and Glanzmann thrombasthenia should be reserved for life-threatening emergencies.
- Platelet concentrates are the treatment of choice in platelet-type von Willebrand disease, because the defect is in the platelets. Both desmopressin and cryoprecipitate should be avoided in platelet-type von Willebrand disease because the resultant increase in circulating large VWF multimers may result in worsening thrombocytopenia.

Treatment of the platelet function defect of uremia

- The most effective therapeutic measure is correction of the hematocrit, either by red cell transfusions[128] or by administration of human recombinant erythropoietin.[129] The beneficial effect on hemostasis of correcting the anemia in uremic patients remains to be fully explained; the mechanical effect of red cells in influencing flow conditions so as to promote interaction of platelets with the vessel wall[130] is probably part of the explanation, but erythropoietin treatment also appears to diminish the inhibitory effect of uremic plasma on platelet adhesion and aggregation.[131,132]
- Conjugated estrogens have also been shown to correct the bleeding time of uremic patients.[133,134] The effect lasts for several days and appears to depend on reduction of endothelial synthesis of nitric oxide.[135]
- The platelet aggregation defect correlates poorly with the severity of the renal failure, but can be at least partially corrected by hemodialysis or peritoneal dialysis.[100,101]

Bone marrow transplantation

- Bone marrow transplantation is used in children with severe diseases such as Chédiak–Higashi syndrome,[136] Wiskott–Aldrich syndrome[137] and, occasionally, Glanzmann thrombasthenia.[138]
- The risks of bone marrow transplantation confine its use to cases in which severe bleeding cannot be adequately controlled by more conservative measures.

Gene therapy

Diseases such as Bernard–Soulier syndrome and Glanzmann thrombasthenia are good candidates for gene therapy and progress is being made in this regard.[139]

Acknowledgment

The author acknowledges the contribution of the late Professor Roger M. Hardisty.

References

1. Michelson AD (ed.) *Platelets*. New York: Academic Press/Elsevier Science, 2002.
2. Levin J. The evolution of mammalian platelets. In: Michelson AD (ed.) *Platelets*. New York: Academic Press/Elsevier Science, 2002, pp. 3–19.
3. Italiano JE, Hartwig JH. Megakaryocyte development and platelet formation. In: Michelson AD (ed.) *Platelets*. New York: Academic Press/Elsevier Science, 2002, pp. 21–35.
4. Reed GL. Platelet secretion. In: Michelson AD (ed.) *Platelets*. New York: Academic Press/Elsevier Science, 2002, pp. 181–95.
5. Woulfe D, Yang J, Prevost N, O'Brien PJ, Brass LF. Signal transduction during the initiation, extension, and perpetuation of platelet plug formation. In: Michelson AD (ed.) *Platelets*. New York: Academic Press/Elsevier Science, 2002, pp. 197–213.
6. Bouchard BA, Butenas S, Mann KG, Tracy PB. Interactions between platelets and the coagulation system. In: Michelson AD (ed.) *Platelets*. New York: Academic Press/Elsevier Science, 2002, pp. 229–53.
7. Nieuwland R, Sturk A. Platelet-derived microparticles. In: Michelson AD (ed.) *Platelets*. New York: Academic Press/Elsevier Science, 2002, pp. 255–65.
8. Israels SJ, Rand ML, Michelson AD. Neonatal platelet function. Semin Thromb Hemost 2003; **29**: 363–72.
9. Rajasekhar D, Kestin AS, Bednarek FJ, Ellis PA, Barnard MR, Michelson AD. Neonatal platelets are less reactive than adult platelets to physiological agonists in whole blood. *Thromb Haemost* 1994; **72**: 957–63.
10. Rajasekhar D, Barnard MR, Bednarek FJ, Michelson AD. Platelet hyporeactivity in very low birth weight neonates. *Thromb Haemost* 1997; **77**: 1002–7.
11. Michelson AD. The clinical approach to disorders of platelet number and function. In: Michelson AD (ed.) *Platelets*. New York: Academic Press/Elsevier Science, 2002, pp. 541–5.
12. Rao AK. Acquired disorders of platelet function. In: Michelson AD (ed.) *Platelets*. New York: Academic Press/Elsevier Science, 2002, pp. 701–26.
13. Nieuwenhuis HK, Akkerman JW, Sixma JJ. Patients with a prolonged bleeding time and normal aggregation tests may have storage pool deficiency: studies on one hundred six patients. *Blood* 1987; **70**: 620–3.
14. Gordon N, Thom J, Cole C, Baker R. Rapid detection of hereditary and acquired platelet storage pool deficiency by flow cytometry. *Br J Haematol* 1995; **89**: 117–23.
15. Wall JE, Buijs-Wilts M, Arnold JT *et al.* A flow cytometric assay using mepacrine for study of uptake and release of platelet dense granule contents. *Br J Haematol* 1995; **89**: 380–5.
16. Lind SE. The bleeding time. In: Michelson AD (ed.) *Platelets*. New York: Academic Press/Elsevier Science, 2002, pp. 283–9.
17. Francis JL. Platelet function analyzer (PFA)-100. In: Michelson AD (ed.) *Platelets*. New York: Academic Press/Elsevier Science, 2002, pp. 325–35.
18. Steinhubl SR, Kereiakes DJ. Ultegra rapid platelet function analyzer. In: Michelson AD (ed.) *Platelets*. New York: Academic Press/Elsevier Science, 2002, pp. 317–23.
19. Varon D, Savion N. Cone and plate(let) analyzer. In: Michelson AD (ed.) *Platelets*. New York: Academic Press/Elsevier Science, 2002, pp. 337–45.
20. Michelson AD, Barnard MR, Krueger LA, Frelinger AL III, Furman MI. Flow cytometry. In: Michelson AD (ed.) *Platelets*. New York: Academic Press/Elsevier Science, 2002, pp. 297–315.
21. Bernard J, Soulier JP. Sur une nouvelle varieté de dystrophhie thrombocytaire hémorrhagipare congenitale. *Semaine Hôpitaux Paris* 1948; **24**: 3217–23.
22. Nurden AT, Nurden P. Inherited disorders of platelet function. In: Michelson AD (ed.) *Platelets*. New York: Academic Press/Elsevier Science, 2002, pp. 681–700.
23. Lopez JA, Berndt MC. The GPIb–IX–V complex. In: Michelson AD (ed.) *Platelets*. New York: Academic Press/Elsevier Science, 2002, pp. 85–104.
24. Bevers EM, Comfurius P, Nieuwenhuis HK *et al.* Platelet prothrombin converting activity in hereditary disorders of platelet function. *Br J Haematol* 1986; **63**: 335–45.
25. Jamieson GA, Okumura T. Reduced thrombin binding and aggregation in Bernard–Soulier platelets. *J Clin Invest* 1978; **61**: 861–4.
26. White JG, Burris SM, Hasegawa D, Johnson M. Micropipette aspiration of human blood platelets: a defect in Bernard–Soulier's syndrome. *Blood* 1984; **63**: 1249–52.
27. Bernard J. History of congenital hemorrhagic thrombocytopathic dystrophy. *Blood Cells* 1983; **9**: 179–93.
28. Savoia A, Balduini CL, Savino M *et al.* Autosomal dominant macrothrombocytopenia in Italy is most frequently a type of heterozygous Bernard–Soulier syndrome. *Blood* 2001; **97**: 1330–5.
29. Nieuwenhuis HK, Akkerman JW, Houdijk WP, Sixma JJ. Human blood platelets showing no response to collagen fail to express surface glycoprotein Ia. *Nature* 1985; **318**: 470–2.
30. Clemetson KJ. Platelet receptors. In: Michelson AD (ed.) *Platelets*. New York: Academic Press/Elsevier Science, 2002, pp. 65–84.
31. Kehrel B, Balleisen L, Kokott R *et al.* Deficiency of intact thrombospondin and membrane glycoprotein Ia in platelets with defective collagen-induced aggregation and spontaneous loss of disorder. *Blood* 1988; **71**: 1074–8.
32. Hollopeter G, Jantzen HM, Vincent D *et al.* Identification of the platelet ADP receptor targeted by antithrombotic drugs. *Nature* 2001; **409**: 202–7.
33. Hirata T, Ushikubi F, Kakizuka A, Okuma M, Narumiya S. Two thromboxane A2 receptor isoforms in human platelets. Opposite coupling to adenylyl cyclase with different sensitivity to Arg60 to Leu mutation. *J Clin Invest* 1996; **97**: 949–56.
34. Scrutton MC, Clare KA, Hutton RA, Bruckdorfer KR. Depressed responsiveness to adrenaline in platelets from apparently normal human donors: a familial trait. *Br J Haematol* 1981; **49**: 303–14.
35. Gaxiola B, Friedl W, Propping P. Epinephrine-induced platelet aggregation. A twin study. *Clin Genet* 1984; **26**: 543–8.

36. Stormorken H, Gogstad G, Solum NO. A new bleeding disorder: lack of platelet aggregatory response to adrenaline and lack of secondary aggregation to ADP and platelet activating factor (PAF). *Thromb Res* 1983; **29**: 391–402.

37. Gabbeta J, Yang X, Kowalska MA, Sun L, Dhanasekaran N, Rao AK. Platelet signal transduction defect with Galpha subunit dysfunction and diminished Galphaq in a patient with abnormal platelet responses. *Proc Natl Acad Sci USA* 1997; **94**: 8750–5.

38. Weiss HJ, Witte LD, Kaplan KL *et al.* Heterogeneity in storage pool deficiency: studies on granule-bound substances in 18 patients including variants deficient in alpha-granules, platelet factor 4, beta-thromboglobulin, and platelet-derived growth factor. *Blood* 1979; **54**: 1296–319.

39. Ingerman CM, Smith JB, Shapiro S, Sedar A, Silver MJ. Hereditary abnormality of platelet aggregation attributable to nucleotide storage pool deficiency. *Blood* 1978; **52**: 332–44.

40. Rendu F, Nurden AT, Lebret M, Caen JP. Relationship between mepacrine-labelled dense body number, platelet capacity to accumulate 14C-5-HT and platelet density in the Bernard–Soulier and Hermansky–Pudlak syndromes. *Thromb Haemost* 1979; **42**: 694–704.

41. Hardisty RM, Mills DC. The platelet defect associated with albinism. *Ann NY Acad Sci* 1972; **201**: 429–36.

42. Weiss HJ, Lages B, Vicic W, Tsung LY, White JG. Heterogeneous abnormalities of platelet dense granule ultrastructure in 20 patients with congenital storage pool deficiency. *Br J Haematol* 1993; **83**: 282–95.

43. Shalev A, Michaud G, Israels SJ *et al.* Quantification of a novel dense granule protein (granulophysin) in platelets of patients with dense granule storage pool deficiency. *Blood* 1992; **80**: 1231–7.

44. Raccuglia G. Gray platelet syndrome. A variety of qualitative platelet disorder. *Am J Med* 1971; **51**: 818–28.

45. Cramer EM, Vainchenker W, Vinci G, Guichard J, Breton-Gorius J. Gray platelet syndrome: immunoelectron microscopic localization of fibrinogen and von Willebrand factor in platelets and megakaryocytes. *Blood* 1985; **66**: 1309–16.

46. Gerrard JM, Phillips DR, Rao GH *et al.* Biochemical studies of two patients with the gray platelet syndrome. Selective deficiency of platelet alpha granules. *J Clin Invest* 1980; **66**: 102–9.

47. Levy-Toledano S, Caen JP, Breton-Gorius J *et al.* Gray platelet syndrome: alpha-granule deficiency. Its influence on platelet function. *J Lab Clin Med* 1981; **98**: 831–48.

48. Nurden AT, Kunicki TJ, Dupuis D, Soria C, Caen JP. Specific protein and glycoprotein deficiencies in platelets isolated from two patients with the gray platelet syndrome. *Blood* 1982; **59**: 709–18.

49. Breton-Gorius J, Vainchenker W, Nurden A, Levy-Toledano S, Caen J. Defective alpha-granule production in megakaryocytes from gray platelet syndrome: ultrastructural studies of bone marrow cells and megakaryocytes growing in culture from blood precursors. *Am J Pathol* 1981; **102**: 10–19.

50. Facon T, Goudemand J, Caron C *et al.* Simultaneous occurrence of grey platelet syndrome and idiopathic pulmonary fibrosis: a role for abnormal megakaryocytes in the pathogenesis of pulmonary fibrosis? *Br J Haematol* 1990; **74**: 542–3.

51. Rendu F, Marche P, Hovig T *et al.* Abnormal phosphoinositide metabolism and protein phosphorylation in platelets from a patient with the grey platelet syndrome. *Br J Haematol* 1987; **67**: 199–206.

52. Srivastava PC, Powling MJ, Nokes TJ, Patrick AD, Dawes J, Hardisty RM. Grey platelet syndrome: studies on platelet alpha-granules, lysosomes and defective response to thrombin. *Br J Haematol* 1987; **65**: 441–6.

53. Enouf J, Lebret M, Bredoux R, Levy-Toledano S, Caen JP. Abnormal calcium transport into microsomes of grey platelet syndrome. *Br J Haematol* 1987; **65**: 437–40.

54. Enouf J, Corvazier E, Papp B *et al.* Abnormal cAMP-induced phosphorylation of rap 1 protein in grey platelet syndrome platelets. *Br J Haematol* 1994; **86**: 338–46.

55. Wautier JL, Gruel Y. Prenatal diagnosis of platelet disorders. *Baillières Clin Haematol* 1989; **2**: 569–83.

56. Lages B, Shattil SJ, Bainton DF, Weiss HJ. Decreased content and surface expression of alpha-granule membrane protein GMP-140 in one of two types of platelet alpha delta storage pool deficiency. *J Clin Invest* 1991; **87**: 919–29.

57. Gerrard JM, Israels ED, Bishop AJ *et al.* Inherited platelet-storage pool deficiency associated with a high incidence of acute myeloid leukaemia. *Br J Haematol* 1991; **79**: 246–55.

58. Nurden AT, Nurden P. Inherited disorders of platelet function. In: Michelson AD (ed.) *Platelets*. New York: Academic Press/Elsevier Science, 2002, pp. 681–700.

59. Hayward CP, Cramer EM, Kane WH *et al.* Studies of a second family with the Quebec platelet disorder: evidence that the degradation of the alpha-granule membrane and its soluble contents are not secondary to a defect in targeting proteins to alpha-granules. *Blood* 1997; **89**: 1243–53.

60. Kahr WH, Zheng S, Sheth PM *et al.* Platelets from patients with the Quebec platelet disorder contain and secrete abnormal amounts of urokinase-type plasminogen activator. *Blood* 2001; **98**: 257–65.

61. George JN, Caen JP, Nurden AT. Glanzmann's thrombasthenia: the spectrum of clinical disease. *Blood* 1990; **75**: 1383–95.

62. Michelson AD. Flow cytometry: a clinical test of platelet function. *Blood* 1996; **87**: 4925–36.

63. Newman PJ, Seligsohn U, Lyman S, Coller BS. The molecular genetic basis of Glanzmann thrombasthenia in the Iraqi-Jewish and Arab populations in Israel. *Proc Natl Acad Sci USA* 1991; **88**: 3160–4.

64. Seligsohn U, Mibashan RS, Rodeck CH, Nicolaides KH, Millar DS, Coller BS. Prenatal diagnosis of Glanzmann's thrombasthenia. *Lancet* 1985; **ii**: 1419.

65. Kaplan C, Patereau C, Reznikoff-Etievant MN, Muller JY, Dumez Y, Kesseler A. Antenatal PLA1 typing and detection of GP IIb-IIIa complex. *Br J Haematol* 1985; **60**: 586–8.

66. Champeix P, Forestier F, Daffos F, Kaplan C. Prenatal diagnosis of a molecular variant of Glanzmann's thrombasthenia. *Curr Stud Hematol Blood Transfus* 1988; **55**: 183.

67. Warkentin TE, Powling MJ, Hardisty RM. Measurement of fibrinogen binding to platelets in whole blood by flow cytometry: a micromethod for the detection of platelet activation. *Br J Haematol* 1990; **76**: 387–94.

68. Seligsohn U, Mibashan RS, Rodeck CH, Nicolaides KH, Millar DS, Coller BS. Prevention program of type I Glanzmann thrombasthenia in Israel: prenatal diagnosis. *Curr Stud Hematol Blood Transfus* 1988; **55**: 174–9.

69. Dachary-Prigent J, Pasquet JM, Fressinaud E, Toti F, Freyssinet JM, Nurden AT. Aminophospholipid exposure, microvesiculation and abnormal protein tyrosine phosphorylation in the platelets of a patient with Scott syndrome: a study using physiologic agonists and local anaesthetics. *Br J Haematol* 1997; **99**: 959–67.

70. Zhou Q, Sims PJ, Wiedmer T. Expression of proteins controlling transbilayer movement of plasma membrane phospholipids in the B lymphocytes from a patient with Scott syndrome. *Blood* 1998; **92**: 1707–12.

71. Martinez MC, Martin S, Toti F *et al.* Significance of capacitative Ca^{2+} entry in the regulation of phosphatidylserine expression at the surface of stimulated cells. *Biochemistry* 1999; **38**: 10092–8.

72. Seri M, Pecci A, Di Bari F *et al.* MYH9-related disease: May–Hegglin anomaly, Sebastian syndrome, Fechtner syndrome, and Epstein syndrome are not distinct entities but represent a variable expression of a single illness. *Medicine* 2003; **82**: 203–15.

73. Karaca M, Cronberg L, Nilsson IM. Abnormal platelet–collagen reaction in Ehlers–Danlos syndrome. *Scand J Haematol* 1972; **9**: 465–9.

74. Pope FM, Martin GR, Lichtenstein JR *et al.* Patients with Ehlers–Danlos syndrome type IV lack type III collagen. *Proc Natl Acad Sci USA* 1975; **72**: 1314–16.

75. Solomon LR, Bobinski H, Astley P, Goldby FS, Mallick NP. Bartter's syndrome: observations on the pathophysiology. *Q J Med* 1982; **51**: 251–70.

76. Patrono C, Coller B, FitzGerald GA, Hirsh J, Roth G. Platelet-active drugs: the relationships among dose, effectiveness, and side effects. *Chest* 2004; **126**: 234S–264S.

77. Curtin R, Cox D, Fitzgerald D. Clopidogrel and ticlopidine. In: Michelson AD (ed.) *Platelets.* New York: Academic Press/Elsevier Science, 2002, pp. 787–801.

78. Agah R, Plow EF, Topol EJ. GPIIb–IIIa antagonists. In: Michelson AD (ed.) *Platelets.* New York: Academic Press/Elsevier Science, 2002, pp. 769–85.

79. Michelson AD. GPIIb–IIIa antagonists. In: *Hematology 2000.* San Francisco: American Society of Hematology Education Program, 2000, pp. 228–33.

80. Brown CH III, Natelson EA, Bradshaw W, Williams TW Jr, Alfrey CP Jr. The hemostatic defect produced by carbenicillin. *N Engl J Med* 1974; **291**: 265–70.

81. Shattil SJ, Bennett JS, McDonough M, Turnbull J. Carbenicillin and penicillin G inhibit platelet function in vitro by impairing the interaction of agonists with the platelet surface. *J Clin Invest* 1980; **65**: 329–37.

82. Burroughs SF, Johnson GJ. Beta-lactam antibiotic-induced platelet dysfunction: evidence for irreversible inhibition of platelet activation in vitro and in vivo after prolonged exposure to penicillin. *Blood* 1990; **75**: 1473–80.

83. Sloand EM, Klein HG, Pastakia KB, Pierce P, Prodouz KN. Effect of albumin on the inhibition of platelet aggregation by beta-lactam antibiotics. *Blood* 1992; **79**: 2022–7.

84. Rossi EC, Levin NW. Inhibition of primary ADP-induced platelet aggregation in normal subjects after administration of nitrofurantoin (furadantin). *J Clin Invest* 1973; **52**: 2457–67.

85. Cummins D, Faint R, Yardumian DA, Dawling S, Mackie I, Machin SJ. The in-vitro and ex-vivo effects of chloroquine sulphate on platelet function: implications for malaria prophylaxis in patients with impaired haemostasis. *J Trop Med Hyg* 1990; **93**: 112–15.

86. Ishikawa S, Manabe S, Wada O. Miconazole inhibition of platelet aggregation by inhibiting cyclooxygenase. *Biochem Pharmacol* 1986; **35**: 1787–92.

87. Chong BH. Heparin-induced thrombocytopenia. In: Michelson AD (ed.) *Platelets.* New York: Academic Press, 2002, pp. 571–91.

88. Horne MK III, Chao ES. The effect of molecular weight on heparin binding to platelets. *Br J Haematol* 1990; **74**: 306–12.

89. Salzman EW, Rosenberg RD, Smith MH, Lindon JN, Favreau L. Effect of heparin and heparin fractions on platelet aggregation. *J Clin Invest* 1980; **65**: 64–70.

90. Levine MN, Hirsh J, Gent M *et al.* Prevention of deep vein thrombosis after elective hip surgery. A randomized trial comparing low molecular weight heparin with standard unfractionated heparin. *Ann Intern Med* 1991; **114**: 545–51.

91. Gimple LW, Gold HK, Leinbach RC *et al.* Correlation between template bleeding times and spontaneous bleeding during treatment of acute myocardial infarction with recombinant tissue-type plasminogen activator. *Circulation* 1989; **80**: 581–8.

92. Coller BS. Platelets and thrombolytic therapy. *N Engl J Med* 1990; **322**: 33–42.

93. Fitzgerald DJ, Catella F, Roy L, FitzGerald GA. Marked platelet activation in vivo after intravenous streptokinase in patients with acute myocardial infarction. *Circulation* 1988; **77**: 142–50.

94. Kerins DM, Roy L, FitzGerald GA, Fitzgerald DJ. Platelet and vascular function during coronary thrombolysis with tissue-type plasminogen activator. *Circulation* 1989; **80**: 1718–25.

95. Di Minno G, Martinez J, McKean ML, De La RJ, Burke JF, Murphy S. Platelet dysfunction in uremia. Multifaceted defect partially corrected by dialysis. *Am J Med* 1985; **79**: 552–9.

96. Castillo R, Lozano T, Escolar G, Revert L, Lopez J, Ordinas A. Defective platelet adhesion on vessel subendothelium in uremic patients. *Blood* 1986; **68**: 337–42.

97. Sloand EM, Sloand JA, Prodouz K *et al.* Reduction of platelet glycoprotein Ib in uraemia. *Br J Haematol* 1991; **77**: 375–81.

98. Ware JA, Clark BA, Smith M, Salzman EW. Abnormalities of cytoplasmic Ca^{2+} in platelets from patients with uremia. *Blood* 1989; **73**: 172–6.

99. Remuzzi G, Benigni A, Dodesini P *et al.* Reduced platelet thromboxane formation in uremia. Evidence for a functional cyclooxygenase defect. *J Clin Invest* 1983; **71**: 762–8.

100. Stewart JH, Castaldi PA. Uraemic bleeding: a reversible platelet defect corrected by dialysis. *Q J Med* 1967; **36**: 409–23.

101. Remuzzi G, Livio M, Marchiaro G, Mecca G, de Gaetano G. Bleeding in renal failure: altered platelet function in chronic uraemia only partially corrected by haemodialysis. *Nephron* 1978; **22**: 347–53.

102. Eknoyan G, Wacksman SJ, Glueck HI, Will JJ. Platelet function in renal failure. *N Engl J Med* 1969; **280**: 677–81.

103. Horowitz HI, Stein IM, Cohen BD, White JG. Further studies on the platelet-inhibitory effect of guanidinosuccinic acid and its role in uremic bleeding. *Am J Med* 1970; **49**: 336–45.

104. Rabiner SF, Molinas F. The role of phenol and phenolic acids on the thrombocytopathy and defective platelet aggregation of patients with renal failure. *Am J Med* 1970; **49**: 346–51.

105. Kyrle PA, Stockenhuber F, Brenner B *et al.* Evidence for an increased generation of prostacyclin in the microvasculature

and an impairment of the platelet alpha-granule release in chronic renal failure. *Thromb Haemost* 1988; **60**: 205–8.

106. Laffi G, La Villa G, Pinzani M *et al.* Altered renal and platelet arachidonic acid metabolism in cirrhosis. *Gastroenterology* 1986; **90**: 274–82.

107. Ordinas A, Maragall S, Castillo R, Nurden AT. A glycoprotein I defect in the platelets of three patients with severe cirrhosis of the liver. *Thromb Res* 1978; **13**: 297–302.

108. Mannucci PM, Vicente V, Vianello L *et al.* Controlled trial of desmopressin in liver cirrhosis and other conditions associated with a prolonged bleeding time. *Blood* 1986; **67**: 1148–53.

109. Smith BR, Rinder HM, Rinder CS. Cardiopulmonary bypass. In: Michelson AD (ed.) *Platelets.* New York: Academic Press/Elsevier Science, 2002, pp. 727–41.

110. Niessner H, Clemetson KJ, Panzer S, Mueller-Eckhardt C, Santoso S, Bettelheim P. Acquired thrombasthenia due to GPIIb/IIIa-specific platelet autoantibodies. *Blood* 1986; **68**: 571–6.

111. Stricker RB, Wong D, Saks SR, Corash L, Shuman MA. Acquired Bernard–Soulier syndrome. Evidence for the role of a 210,000-molecular weight protein in the interaction of platelets with von Willebrand factor. *J Clin Invest* 1985; **76**: 1274–8.

112. Deckmyn H, Chew SL, Vermylen J. Lack of platelet response to collagen associated with an autoantibody against glycoprotein Ia: a novel cause of acquired qualitative platelet dysfunction. *Thromb Haemost* 1990; **64**: 74–9.

113. Cowan DH, Graham RC Jr, Baunach D. The platelet defect in leukemia. Platelet ultrastructure, adenine nucleotide metabolism, and the release reaction. *J Clin Invest* 1975; **56**: 188–200.

114. Woodcock BE, Cooper PC, Brown PR, Pickering C, Winfield DA, Preston FE. The platelet defect in acute myeloid leukaemia. *J Clin Pathol* 1984; **37**: 1339–42.

115. Ganguly P, Sutherland SB, Bradford HR. Defective binding of thrombin to platelets in myeloid leukaemia. *Br J Haematol* 1978; **39**: 599–605.

116. Schafer AI. Bleeding and thrombosis in the myeloproliferative disorders. *Blood* 1984; **64**: 1–12.

117. Malpass TW, Savage B, Hanson SR, Slichter SJ, Harker LA. Correlation between prolonged bleeding time and depletion of platelet dense granule ADP in patients with myelodysplastic and myeloproliferative disorders. *J Lab Clin Med* 1984; **103**: 894–904.

118. Schafer AI. Deficiency of platelet lipoxygenase activity in myeloproliferative disorders. *N Engl J Med* 1982; **306**: 381–6.

119. Walsh PN, Murphy S, Barry WE. The role of platelets in the pathogenesis of thrombosis and hemorrhage in patients with thrombocytosis. *Thromb Haemost* 1977; **38**: 1085–96.

120. Cooper B, Schafer AI, Puchalsky D, Handin RI. Platelet resistance to prostaglandin D2 in patients with myeloproliferative disorders. *Blood* 1978; **52**: 618–26.

121. Clezardin P, McGregor JL, Dechavanne M, Clemetson KJ. Platelet membrane glycoprotein abnormalities in patients with myeloproliferative disorders and secondary thrombocytosis. *Br J Haematol* 1985; **60**: 331–44.

122. Michelson AD. Flow cytometric analysis of platelet surface glycoproteins: phenotypically distinct subpopulations of platelets in children with chronic myeloid leukemia. *J Lab Clin Med* 1987; **110**: 346–54.

123. Berndt MC, Kabral A, Grimsley P, Watson N, Robertson TI, Bradstock KF. An acquired Bernard–Soulier-like platelet defect associated with juvenile myelodysplastic syndrome. *Br J Haematol* 1988; **68**: 97–101.

124. Cattaneo M, Mannucci PM. Desmopressin. In: Michelson AD (ed.) *Platelets.* New York: Academic Press/Elsevier Science, 2002, pp. 855–66.

125. Poon M-C. Factor VIIa. In: Michelson AD (ed.) *Platelets.* New York: Academic Press/Elsevier Science, 2002: pp. 867–73.

126. Almeida AM, Khair K, Hann I, Liesner R. The use of recombinant factor VIIa in children with inherited platelet function disorders. *Br J Haematol* 2003; **121**: 477–81.

127. Perrotta PL, Snyder EL. Platelet storage and transfusion. In: Michelson AD (ed.) *Platelets.* New York: Academic Press/Elsevier Science, 2002, pp. 877–905.

128. Fernandez F, Goudable C, Sie P *et al.* Low haematocrit and prolonged bleeding time in uraemic patients: effect of red cell transfusions. *Br J Haematol* 1985; **59**: 139–48.

129. Moia M, Mannucci PM, Vizzotto L, Casati S, Cattaneo M, Ponticelli C. Improvement in the haemostatic defect of uraemia after treatment with recombinant human erythropoietin. *Lancet* 1987; **ii**: 1227–9.

130. Turitto VT, Baumgartner HR. Platelet interaction with subendothelium in a perfusion system: physical role of red blood cells. *Microvasc Res* 1975; **9**: 335–44.

131. Zwaginga JJ, IJsseldijk MJ, de Groot PG *et al.* Treatment of uremic anemia with recombinant erythropoietin also reduces the defects in platelet adhesion and aggregation caused by uremic plasma. *Thromb Haemost* 1991; **66**: 638–47.

132. Zwaginga JJ, IJsseldijk MJ, de Groot PG, Vos J, Bos Kuil RL, Sixma JJ. Defects in platelet adhesion and aggregate formation in uremic bleeding disorder can be attributed to factors in plasma. *Arterioscler Thromb* 1991; **11**: 733–44.

133. Liu YK, Kosfeld RE, Marcum SG. Treatment of uraemic bleeding with conjugated oestrogen. *Lancet* 1984; **ii**: 887–90.

134. Livio M, Mannucci PM, Vigano G *et al.* Conjugated estrogens for the management of bleeding associated with renal failure. *N Engl J Med* 1986; **315**: 731–5.

135. Remuzzi G, Perico N, Zoja C, Corna D, Macconi D, Vigano G. Role of endothelium-derived nitric oxide in the bleeding tendency of uremia. *J Clin Invest* 1990; **86**: 1768–71.

136. Haddad E, Le Deist F, Blanche S *et al.* Treatment of Chediak–Higashi syndrome by allogenic bone marrow transplantation: report of 10 cases. *Blood* 1995; **85**: 3328–33.

137. Filipovich AH, Stone JV, Tomany SC *et al.* Impact of donor type on outcome of bone marrow transplantation for Wiskott–Aldrich syndrome: collaborative study of the International Bone Marrow Transplant Registry and the National Marrow Donor Program. *Blood* 2001; **97**: 1598–603.

138. Bellucci S, Damaj G, Boval B *et al.* Bone marrow transplantation in severe Glanzmann's thrombasthenia with antiplatelet alloimmunization. *Bone Marrow Transplant* 2000; **25**: 327–30.

139. Wilcox DA, White GC. Gene therapy for platelet disorders: studies with Glanzmann's thrombasthenia. *J Thromb Haemost* 2003; **1**: 2300–11.

SECTION

7 Coagulation Disorders

26 Hemophilia A and B

Judith Smith and Owen P. Smith

Introduction

Hemophilia is unique among diseases for two main reasons. Firstly, it is generally well known to members of the public because of its connection with the royal families of Europe, in particular those descendants of Queen Victoria who were associated with the Russian and Spanish royal families. The presence of this genetic defect within these families subsequently had catastrophic social, personal and political effects. Secondly, the history of hemophilia shows that there was parallel progress in understanding the causes of the disease, diagnosis of the disease as well as improved therapy, and indeed cure of the disease, a situation unrivalled in any other human illness.

Historical perspective

The word "hemophilia" is derived from two Greek words, *haima* meaning blood and *philein* meaning to love.[1] Despite the inappropriateness of this description of excess bleeding, the word "hemophilia" continues to be used in patients with an inherited predisposition to blood loss. It is interesting that this inherited blood disease is not mentioned in early Egyptian, Roman and Greek medical literature.[2]

The first documented account of an inherited bleeding disorder was in the 2nd century AD. The Babylonian Talmud describes the decision of Rabbi Juddah that the son of a woman whose three previous sons had bled to death following circumcision be excused from the rite.[3] Although further descriptions by Arabic physicians appear in the 12th century, it was not until the 18th century that the first reports on a possible genetic basis and effective treatment with blood transfusion appeared.[4] By the 1950s fresh frozen plasma was the main step in treatment, and then in the mid 1960s Poole and Shannon made the first major advance in hemophilia treatment care with the discovery that factor (F)VIII was concentrated in cryoprecipitate.[5] This discovery made it possible for blood banks to prepare a potent "wet" concentrate and, together with the advances made by the plasma industries in preparing coagulation factor concentrate, hemophilia care was thus dramatically altered from solely hospital-based management to one where treatment could be administered at home immediately following trauma or at the first sign of bleeding. The next major innovation was prophylaxis, which resulted in markedly reduced hospitalizations and the incidence of crippling deformities in children and adolescents with hemophilia A and B. Advances in recombinant DNA technology led to the cloning of the FVIII and FIX genes in the early 1980s. Today we have several recombinant FVIII and one FIX gene products and all have been shown to be safe, effective and extremely well tolerated in children. The next milestone in the history of hemophilia treatment clearly will be cure of the disease with gene therapeutics.

Hemophilia A and B (factor VIII and factor IX deficiency)

The term "hemophilia", originally applied to a lifelong hemorrhagic disorder, was by the early 1950s classified into two distinct disease types based on specific plasma protein deficiencies. FVIII deficiency (hemophilia A) and FIX deficiency (hemophilia B) are inherited as sex-linked recessive disorders, with a prevalence in all racial groups of approximately 1 in 10 000 and 1 in 50 000 respectively.[6]

After von Willebrand's disease, hemophilia A and B are considered the commonest but also the most severe forms of congenital bleeding disorder, with FVIII deficiency being five times more prevalent than FIX deficiency. The reason for the relatively high incidence of FVIII deficiency is partly due to the high mutation rate and the X-linked pattern of inheritance. In approximately one-third to half of newly diagnosed infants with hemophilia A there is no family history of the disorder and the hemophilia has resulted from spontaneous (*de novo*) mutations. Following activation by FXa and thrombin, FVIIIa acts as a cofactor for FIXa in the formation of FXa. It is not surprising therefore that the clinical syndromes associated with hemophilia A and B are phenotypically identical.

Laboratory criteria have varied in different classifications and in an effort to standardize this the Scientific and Standardization Committee of the International Society of Thrombosis and Haemostasis recently recommended revised criteria for the classification of hemophilia based on biological FVIII:C and FIX:C levels as follows.[7]
- Severe hemophilia: FVIII/FIX concentration < 0.01 IU/mL (<1% of normal).
- Moderate hemophilia: FVIII/FIX concentration 0.01–0.05 IU/mL (2–5% of normal).
- Mild hemophilia: FVIII/FIX concentration 0.05–0.4 IU/mL (5–40% of normal).

Clinical presentation

The clinical manifestations of both hemophilia A and B are similar, depending on the concentration of the deficient clotting factor (Table 26.1). Patients with severe hemophilia (FVIII:C or FIX:C levels < 0.01 IU/mL) usually present in the first 2 years of life with spontaneous bleeding involving joints and muscles. Spontaneous bleeding involving the central nervous system, head and neck, and the gastrointestinal tract are well-recognized but less frequent complications. Children with severe hemophilia may also present with excessive bleeding after minor trauma, postoperatively (Fig. 26.1), or after intramuscular childhood vaccinations. Moderate hemophilia (FVIII:C or FIX:C levels 0.01–0.05 IU/mL) usually results in bleeding at time of hemostatic challenge (trauma, surgery or dental extractions) but occasionally spontaneous

bleeding occurs. The bleeding that occurs in mild hemophilia (FVIII:C or FIX:C > 0.05 IU/mL) is usually restricted to hemostatic challenge and these patients are often not diagnosed until teenage years or adulthood.

Making the diagnosis

FVIII and FIX deficiency are associated with prolongation of the activated partial thromboplastin time, which corrects on mixing studies. The prothrombin time and thrombin clotting time are normal. The diagnosis is made on specific clotting assays that assess the activity of FVIII (FVIII:C) or FIX (FIX:C). These assays should be repeated on separate occasions to confirm the diagnosis. A variant of FVIII deficiency is associated with normal FVIII:C as measured by the standard (one-stage) clotting assay but reduced FVIII by alternative assays (chromogenic or two-stage clotting assay).[8,9] The measurement of FVIII by chromogenic assay is becoming part of first-line investigation in most hemophilia comprehensive care centers. In centers where this practice is not established, the chromogenic assay should be considered in children in the following situations: (i) a family history of FVIII deficiency where the affected individuals have a normal one-stage FVIII:C assay, or (ii) children with a normal one-stage FVIII:C assay where there is a high clinical suspicion of hemophilia.

Differential diagnosis

The differential diagnosis of FVIII deficiency includes von Willebrand's disease (vWD). One of the functions of von Willebrand factor (vWF) is to bind and protect circulating FVIII from proteolytic degradation. vWD is caused by a defect in vWF and consequently these patients may have a

Table 26.1 Bleeding manifestations with different severities of hemophilia A and B.

Type of bleeding	IU/mL		
	Severe (<0.1)	Moderate (0.1–0.4)	Mild (0.5–4.0)
Age of onset	<1 year	<2 years	>2 years
Hemarthroses			
Spontaneous	++++	++	–
Following minor trauma	++++	+++	–
Muscle hematoma	++++	++	–
Central nervous system	++*	+	–
Hematuria	++++	++	–
Surgery	++++	+++	++
Dental extraction	++++	+++	++
Trauma to soft tissue			
Mild	++++	++	–
Significant	++++	+++	+

++++, usual; +++, common; ++, not unusual; +, can occur; –, rare.

(a)

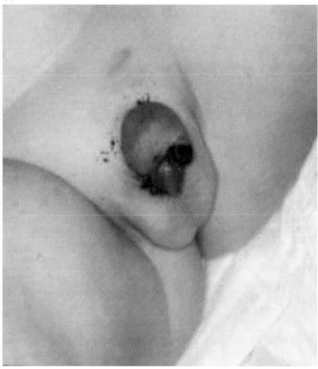

(b)

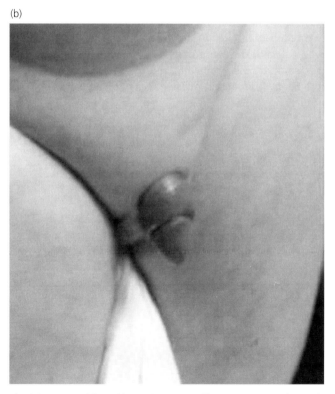

Fig. 26.1 Hemophilia A. (a) Postcircumcisional hematoma in an infant with no family history of hemophilia. Mutational analysis showed the presence of IVS 22. (b) Full hematoma resolution 1 week later following replacement with recombinant FVIII.

reduced FVIII:C level. vWD is assessed by the measurement of vWF antigen and function. The gold standard vWF functional assay is the ristocetin cofactor assay. This measures the ability of the patient's vWF to agglutinate normal platelets in the presence of ristocetin.

Occasionally children may have vWD despite normal vWF assays. This occurs in a subtype of vWD called type 2 Normandy, which is caused by an isolated defect in the ability of vWF to bind circulating FVIII. These patients have normal vWF as measured by standard vWF antigen and functional (ristocetin cofactor) assays. The diagnosis of type 2 Normandy vWD is made on the basis of an assay that assesses the ability of the patient's vWF to bind to FVIII, with or without the identification of a mutation within the relevant region of the vWF gene.

Genetics, carrier testing and genetic counseling

Hemophilia is inherited in an X-linked recessive manner. If a male with hemophilia has children, all the daughters will be carriers and no son will be affected. If a female hemophilia carrier has children, there will be a 50% chance that each male child will have hemophilia and a 50% chance of a female child being a carrier. It should be noted that female carriers of severe hemophilia mutations frequently have reduced FVIII:C or FIX:C levels (0.2–0.5 IU/mL, normal > 0.5 IU/mL). Rarely, females who are carriers of hemophilia mutations may have levels as low as affected males within the family due to nonrandom inactivation of the X chromosome, inheritance of a mutated FVIII gene from both maternal and paternal chromosomes, or Turner syndrome.

FVIII and FIX gene defects may be divided into several categories: (i) gross gene rearrangements, (ii) insertions/deletions, and (iii) single-base substitutions resulting in missense mutations, nonsense mutations or mRNA splicing defects. There are in excess of 2500 reported mutations in FVIII and FIX genes. The single most important defect is an inversion involving the noncoding sequence (intron) 22 of the FVIII gene that results in approximately 50% of all cases of severe FVIII deficiency. This intron contains a CpG island associated with two additional transcripts, F8A and F8B. F8A is transcribed in the opposite direction to the FVIII gene and there are two additional copies of the F8A transcript approximately 400 kb telomeric of the FVIII gene. Homologous recombination occurs between the F8A transcript within intron 22 and one of the two extragenic homologs of this sequence. The recombination occurs during the meiotic division of spermatogenesis. This results in the translocation of the gene sequences involved in exons 1–22 away from exons 23–26. The most common type of the inversion involves the distal homolog.

An additional inversion is responsible for 5% of cases of severe FVIII deficiency. This occurs as a result of homologous recombination between a sequence within intron 1 and a similar sequence telomeric of the FVIII gene. There is evidence to suggest that large deletions, nonsense mutations and gross gene rearrangements such as the inversion 22 mutation are associated with a higher risk of inhibitor formation.[10]

Strategies for the identification of carrier status include family pedigree, measurement of FVIII:C and FIX:C levels, linkage analysis and direct mutation analysis. A detailed family pedigree may identify obligate carriers. Daughters of men with hemophilia are obligate carriers, as are women with two children with hemophilia, or one child with hemophilia and another maternal relative with hemophilia. FVIII:C or FIX:C levels should be measured in the potential carrier to identify those at risk of bleeding. However, the measurement of factor levels alone is an unreliable guide to carrier status. Direct mutation analysis has now replaced linkage analysis as the investigation of choice when the mutation can be identified in affected males within the family. The identification process is simplified by the common occurrence of an inversion within intron 22 in severe FVIII deficiency. When direct mutation analysis is unavailable, linkage analysis may be informative in the determination of carrier status. Antenatal diagnosis using chorionic villous sampling at 10–14 weeks or amniocentesis at 15–20 weeks can be used to determine both the sex and presence of the family-specific hemophilia mutation if known.[11]

With recent advances in molecular laboratory techniques, it is now possible to give each individual patient and family member very reliable genetic information. To enable these genetic data to be used for the benefit of the patient with hemophilia or to influence reproductive choices, genetic counseling should be initiated as early as possible. Comprehensive genetic counseling addresses a wide range of issues, but different levels of genetic counseling can be provided according to circumstances. According to Miller,[12] the basic requirements for providing genetic counseling in hemophilia include knowledge of inheritance patterns, what tests are available, and personnel able to interpret results. The main aims of genetic counseling are to help people make informed choices about their own and their family's well-being, ensure informed consent for testing is obtained, and that the discussion includes information about:
- hemophilia, its prognosis and therapeutic options;
- inheritance pattern of hemophilia;
- tests for diagnosing hemophilia and carrier status;
- implications for future and existing children.

The importance of informed consent is particularly relevant when discussing the issue of genetic testing in children. It is recognized that genetic tests can only be performed on people who give informed consent after appropriate counseling. It is recommended that all children with hemophilia have their phenotype established as this provides valuable information regarding the risk of developing inhibitors and may allow information to be given to different family members.[13]

The area of particular difficulty revolves around testing female children who are potential carriers of hemophilia. This subject raises ethical conflict about who should give consent, when it should be raised, and how to consider the child's best interests. The 1989 Children's Act in the UK states that the child's views should be taken into consideration along with his/her intellectual capacity to give informed consent. In some circumstances it may be appropriate to carry out genetic testing for hemophilia in a child younger than 16 years providing the implications of the test are understood. If young children are genetically tested for hemophilia before they are competent to give informed consent, they are denied the right to refuse the test and the knowledge gained from that test. Despite these possible pitfalls, every opportunity should be taken to discuss carrier status with potential carriers and their families. What is more straightforward and agreed is that all potential carriers of hemophilia have their coagulation factor levels tested in infancy. This information will determine if the child is at increased risk of bleeding and treatment plans can be put in place.

Treatment

Development of factor concentrates

Although the first description of effective treatment of hemophilia with blood transfusion is as far back as 1840,[14] it was not until the 1950s that the widespread use of plasma pioneered by Mcfarlane and his colleagues at Oxford came into being. Prior to this, plasma from pigs and cows was used with good effect, although allergic reactions were frequent and often severe and thus limited its widespread use. The main problem with human plasma is that it contains only small amounts of antihemophilic globulin (FVIII) and therefore large quantities of plasma needed to be infused in order to achieve a desired effect. The early work of Cohn in developing fractionation of plasma with variation in temperature and concentrations of saline and alcohol led to the development of fairly crude concentrates of human FVIII and these were used by a number of hemophilia physicians in Europe and North America.

In 1964, Judith Poole serendipitously discovered "cryoprecipitate", which she found to be rich in antihemophilic factor.[5] This simple process involved the rapid freezing of fresh plasma, which was then allowed to thaw at 4°C; this results in the formation of a sludge called cryoprecipitate. The reason why hemophilia physicians were excited about cryoprecipitate was that a small volume contained high concentrations of antihemophilic globulin and thus made it possible for blood banks to prepare it and patients to store it in their homes. Hemophilia care was dramatically altered from hospital-based management to one where treatment could be administered at home immediately following trauma or at the first sight of bleeding. This major therapeutic innovation markedly reduced hospitalization and the incidence of crippling deformities. Following this discovery the plasma fractionation industry went a step further, developing lyophilized clotting factor concentrates. These concentrates were now in powder form and could be stored in the home; when needed for active treatment, the addition of water was all that was required prior to administration. Again, a very small volume of concentrate was needed to arrest bleeding and this was very important when dealing with small children. The initial big drawback of this high-technology blood product was cost. The thousands of donors that needed to be recruited to supply the plasma essential for producing these lyophilized concentrates had to be paid.

By the early 1970s, the widespread availability of lyophilized FVIII concentrates offered considerable advantages in terms of storage and ease of administration and this had a dramatic effect on the natural history of the disease. The median life expectancy for people with severe hemophilia was 11 years in the 1920s; by the 1970s the median life expectancy approached that of normal males. The following decade saw the arrival in the developed world of ultra-pure forms of FVIII and FIX. These newer concentrates were produced from even larger numbers of donors. Soon complications became apparent, particularly viral transmission. The first case of acquired immunodeficiency syndrome (HIV) in hemophilia patients was reported in 1982. Prior to the mid 1980s most patients who received factor concentrates developed hepatitis C. The scientific response, driven by the biotechnology industry, to this disastrous happening was swift. The aim was to develop recombinant FVIII as it was felt that a synthetic product would solve not only the problem of contaminating viruses but also the problems of quality and supply, especially to developing countries. Remarkably, within 18 months of beginning this work two large scientific teams using two different cloning strategies not only cloned the FVIII gene but also demonstrated expression of the gene and the recombinant protein had the same biologic function as FVIII derived from human plasma.

Treatment with factor concentrates

Acute bleeds

Hemorrhagic complications in moderate and severe hemophilia may become obvious after birth, especially if the child is circumcised. Severity and type of bleeding is related to the absolute concentration of circulating plasma VIII:C (Table 26.1). A minimum effective level of FVIII and FIX for hemostasis is about 30–50%. Those with severe deficiency (<1%) usually experience repeated and often spontaneous hemorrhages, most commonly hemarthroses; if not treated adequately, this will develop into chronic synovitis, resulting in target joint formation with eventual crippling arthropathy. While muscular skeletal bleeding is by far the commonest clinical event, other spontaneous hemorrhagic manifestations occur frequently and may be life-threatening (Table 26.1).

Successful treatment in acute or potentially acute (pre surgery) bleeding is usually achieved with adequate and prompt factor replacement therapy. The level of factor concentrate required to achieve adequate hemostasis will depend on the type of bleeding. It should be remembered that the initial plasma half-life of infused FVIII:C is 3–6 hours during equilibration with the extravascular space; thereafter the plasma half-life will be approximately 12 hours. As stated above, the amount of factor concentrate given will depend on the type of bleed and also on the weight of the child: FVIII 1 IU/kg raises plasma FVIII:C by 2% so that

Units of FVIII concentrate required = weight (kg) × desired level (%) × 0.5.

For the majority of soft tissue bleeds and hemarthroses, FVIII levels of around 50% may be adequate. If the bleed is more severe and a longer period of treatment is anticipated, then the desired level should be around 70%. Increasing the level above 50% is sufficient to treat major soft tissue or visceral bleeds and cover minor surgical procedures. With major surgery, a preoperative level of 100% is considered mandatory by most hemophilia physicians and thereafter daily prophylactic levels of 50–100% for approximately 7–12 days are sufficient to facilitate wound healing. With severe or pharyngeal and central nervous system bleeding, 100% correction is also required, and treatment is usually continued for a more protracted period of time. Indeed, in patients with an intracerebral bleed it may be necessary to continue treatment until imaging reveals that the brain lesion has fully resolved (Table 26.2).

As with FVIII treatment, the dosage and frequency of FIX administration is governed by the type of bleeding and its plasma half-life (18–24 hours). Unlike FVIII, recovery of infused FIX is lower than expected, presumably because FIX is absorbed at sites in the vascular endothelium recently shown to be collagen IV. Thus these patients require approximately twice the amount per dose once daily to treat bleeding, i.e., weight (kg) × desired level (%) × 1. The exception is on the first day of surgery, when a twice-daily dose is usually administered to achieve the desired level.

It is important to note that the recovery of recombinant FIX (BeneFIX, Genetics Institute-Baxter Hyland) is less than that of plasma-derived FIX. Thus, to raise a given individual's plasma concentration by 1% the recombinant product should be given in doses of 1.2 IU/kg and not 1 IU/kg as for the plasma-derived products.

Prophylaxis

Recurrent hemarthroses are the major cause of morbidity in children with severe FVIII and FIX deficiency. For children with severe hemophilia and no evidence of inhibitors, the unwanted musculoskeletal complications of severe

Type of bleed	Desired plasma level after treatment	Duration of treatment
Major bleed CNS or bleed involving peripheral nerve Ileopsoas/retroperitoneal	100% rise + commence CI	See note
Tongue/neck/retropharyngeal Gastrointestinal Preoperative treatment	100% rise + commence CI	
Joint (hemarthrosis) Muscle	50–70%	See note
Mucosal	50–70% and tranexamic acid	
Minor bleed	50%	
Dental extraction	50% and tranexamic acid	
Dental filling	30%	
Laceration requiring sutures	40% until sutures removed	
Hematuria	High fluid intake ± 50%	

Table 26.2 Treatment of specific bleeds: desired factor levels in plasma after treatment.

Note: duration of treatment depends on the severity of the injury, type of surgery and the clinical findings on daily examination.

CI, continuous infusion.

Reproduced with permission from Ref. 15.

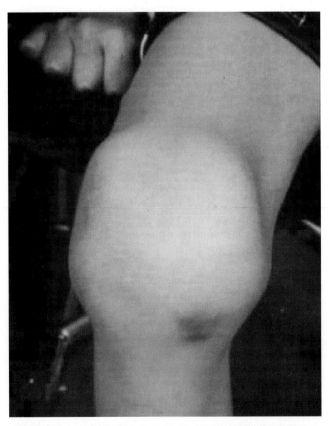

Fig. 26.2 Hemophilia B. Chronic severe hemophilic arthropathy of the right knee joint. The quadriceps muscle is severely wasted. This adolescent was only treated intermittently with plasma throughout the first 5 years of life.

hemophilia can be effectively prevented by the early initiation of a program of long-term prophylaxis. Prophylactic factor concentrates given on a regular basis significantly reduce the incidence of hemarthrosis,[16,17] and when commenced early in life long-term joint damage (Fig. 26.2) can be avoided[18] or in some cases reversed.[17] Although there is still some debate with regard to prophylaxis versus on-demand treatment, more long-term studies are now available to support the benefits of an early initiated prophylaxis program.[19,20] The World Health Organization[21] and the World Federation of Hemophilia therefore now recommend that primary prophylaxis be commenced between 1 and 2 years of age in those with severe hemophilia and should continue until around 20 years of age.

The primary prophylaxis regimen (Malmö protocol) was pioneered and tested in Sweden in the 1960s and involves the infusion of FVIII 20–40 IU/kg on alternate days (minimum three times per week) for FVIII deficiency, and FIX 20–40 IU/kg twice weekly for FIX deficiency. The treatment is usually commenced at around 1 year of age and continued until at least 20 years but usually lifelong. The results of this protocol have been reported[14,21] and demonstrate that all children treated with this regimen maintained perfect musculoskeletal status. Outcome measures included orthopedic and radiologic joint scores. Although very effective, this protocol is demanding on peripheral veins, is very time-consuming for families, may result in compliance issues, and is very expensive. Many modifications have been made to this protocol, such as starting primary prophylaxis with once-weekly infusions and dose escalation based on frequency of bleeds and tolerance of the child.[20]

The efficacy of such an approach is largely influenced by the level of compliance. Compliance with any long-term medical regimen is challenging and in pediatrics especially, noncompliance can be a major barrier to successful treatment outcomes. Hacker *et al.*[22] demonstrated a 58.8% compliance rate in a group of 38 children with hemophilia who had commenced prophylaxis. The major barrier to compliance in this cohort, as self-reported by the families, was the time-consuming nature of prophylaxis (52%); the uncooperative nature of the child was cited as the most significant challenge in 16% and venous access was reported as the most significant barrier in 13% of participants.

It is important when discussing the issue of prophylaxis with parents that they are aware of the potential problems associated with this therapy and that this is balanced with the evidence supporting prophylaxis. Due to the advances in pediatric hemophilia care, both life-threatening bleeding and chronic bleeding are preventable. Consequently, the traditional approach of measuring morbidity and mortality are no longer practical in the design of clinical trials for children with hemophilia. One option is to use more subjective constructs with direct relevance to patients, such as health-related quality-of-life measurements. Much work has been done to develop quality-of-life assessment tools in children with hemophilia[23–26] and this would certainly seem to be the most appropriate way of measuring the impact of medical advances and treatment outcomes in children with hemophilia.

Desmopressin

Desmopressin (1-deamino-8-D-arginine vasopressin, DDAVP) is a synthetic analog of L-arginine vasopressin that produces a two- to eight-fold increase in circulating plasma FVIII:C levels.[27] The mechanism responsible for this effect is unclear but most likely includes the release of vWF from endothelial stores (Weibel–Palade bodies), with subsequent stabilization of plasma FVIII:C. The therapeutic efficacy of desmopressin in reducing blood product requirements in patients with mild hemophilia was first reported over 20 years ago.[28] Concerns about viral transmission associated with blood products have resulted in desmopressin becoming the therapeutic treatment of choice for patients with mild FVIII deficiency. However, the increase in endogenous plasma FVIII:C to therapeutic levels does not occur in all patients and cannot be predicted. Nolan *et al.*[29] report a response rate of 77% in children, while Revel-Vilk *et al.*[30] report a response rate of 57%. It is therefore now considered mandatory that all patients with mild or moderate FVIII deficiency be assessed for desmopressin responsiveness at the time of diagnosis to decide whether it will provide a therapeutic response in the event of bleeding or surgery.[31–35] Revel-Vilk *et al.* also point out that the association between desmopressin response and age is unclear; they report a lower response rate in younger

children (<6 years), and in the younger nonresponders a subsequent response to rechallenge with desmopressin after a mean of 6.3 years.[30] They conclude that in their study group repeating the desmopressin challenge increased the response rate from 57 to 71%.

We believe that it is clearly preferable to assess desmopressin response at diagnosis so as to facilitate the development of a treatment strategy for each patient. Failure to adhere to these guidelines will likely increase the risk of morbidity or mortality associated with surgical intervention or bleeding episodes in patients who have a suboptimal response to desmopressin.

Desmopressin can be administered intravenously (0.3 µg/kg), subcutaneously (0.3 mcg/kg) or intranasally (150–300 µg), with peak values occurring at 60, 90 and 120 min respectively after treatment. Contraindications are a history of seizures, congestive heart failure, polydipsia and type 2B vWD. The commonest side-effects of desmopressin are facial flushing, mild headache and minor changes in blood pressure. More serious side-effects include fluid retention, hyponatremia and seizures.[36] It has been suggested that desmopressin is dangerous in children under 18 months old[37] as there is increased risk of cerebral irritation. However, Revel-Vilk *et al.*[30] would advocate the use of desmopressin in this age group where there is a reasonable chance of benefit and that fluid intake be minimized.

The use of desmopressin in FIX deficiency has been reported.[38,39] Both these groups show that desmopressin appears to be useful in preventing and treating bleeding episodes in FIX deficiency despite the fact that plasma FIX levels are not increased by desmopressin. Ehl's hypothesis that desmopressin could cause changes that bypass the need for normal FIX levels, namely supraphysiologic levels of FVIII and stimulation of vWF, remains open to debate.[38]

Central venous access devices

As outlined above, the World Health Organization/World Federation of Hemophilia now recommend that prophylaxis with FVIII and FIX concentrate be commenced in children with severe hemophilia between 1 and 2 years of age. The intravenous administration of factor concentrate twice or three times per week is fraught with difficulty in the majority of young children when using only peripheral veins. Similarly, immune tolerance therapy using large doses of factor concentrate, up to twice daily for 12–24 months for children with inhibitors to FVIII/FIX (see below), is almost impossible without the use of central venous access devices. These can be fully implantable (Port-a-Cath, Deltac, USA) or partly externalized (single or double lumen Quintan Catheters). The use of a port is preferable to an external device because it causes fewer limitations to the child's lifestyle and it has been suggested that there is a lower infective risk.[40,41] However, despite the obvious attractions of these devices, their routine use for prophylaxis and immune tolerance therapy has not gained universal acceptance because of the potential risks of hemorrhage,[41] thrombosis,[42] and infection,[43–46] all of which may lead to a high rate of morbidity and permanent removal of the device. Infection is cited as the reason for removal of a port in up to 69.9% of all port removals.[48] The rate of infection is higher in children with inhibitors according to Ljung,[49] and a reasonable conclusion that he and others make based on different experience is that patients with inhibitors can expect one Port-a-Cath infection per 6–12 months of use. He goes on to conclude that in the best of hands, the patient with a Port-a-Cath, without inhibitors and on regular prophylaxis, will have a maximum of one catheter-related infection in approximately 10 years.

Although there is no consensus on their use, it is our practice that long-term indwelling devices are necessary to facilitate the modern intensive treatment of congenital coagulation disorders. There are complications, as outlined above, particularly infections, but with improved management of the perioperative period and regular frequent reeducation, particularly in those children with inhibitors, many of these complications may be avoided.

The decision to use an indwelling port to facilitate venous access merits careful and individual discussion. As well as explaining the benefits and complications to the parents and child, an indication should be given as to the amount of instruction necessary to ensure competency in caring for the port. Parents and, if relevant, the child need to be taught appropriate sterile techniques to ensure safe access of the device. General consensus with regard to catheter-site sterile technique or catheter flushing have not been reached and most institutions follow local policy. However, there are a number of general issues regarding care of the access device that have been recognized.

- Strict handwashing procedure and aseptic technique should be followed.[50]
- If a local anesthetic cream is used, this should be removed with soap and water prior to aseptic technique being performed.[51]
- Cleansing of the skin prior to puncture should be with 2% chlorhexidine as this has been shown to be a more effective cleansing agent than povidone-iodine or 70% alcohol.[50,52,53]
- Ports must be flushed after each use or at least monthly[54] with either saline[55,56] or heparin in the lowest concentration possible. Baranowski[57] recommends 5 mL of heparin 10 units/mL solution to be safe and effective.
- Once the port is accessed, the needle should not be rocked or tilted. Needles should be removed as soon as possible after every infusion. If the needle is left in place, it should be changed every 7 days.[57]
- To reduce potential for blood backflow when de-accessing the port, positive pressure should be maintained on the syringe while clamping the infusion set.[58]
- Syringes smaller than 10 mL should not be used as they generate pressures greater than 172 kPa (~25 pounds per square inch) and this can cause venous damage and catheter rupture.[58,59]

More recently Santagastino *et al.*[60] have reported on the use of arteriovenous fistulae (AVF) as a reliable means of vascular assess in children with hemophilia. They report on the creation of 31 proximal AVF in 27 children with severe hemophilia. Complication rates were minimal, with bleeding in 16%, thrombotic complications in 3% and infections in none. This group report that 96% of their study cohort achieved functional AVF that are still regularly used for home treatment over a median period of 29 months. The results of this study would support and encourage the creation of AVF as the first option for achieving permanent venous access in children with severe hemophilia, although longer follow-up is warranted to determine the potential development of late complications.

Complications of treatment

The risk of blood-borne infections associated with plasma-derived products was demonstrated to catastrophic effect with the infection of the hemophilia population with HIV and hepatitis C in the 1980s. This risk relates to the fact that these products are produced from plasma pools containing up to 20 000 donors.[61,62] Plasma-derived factor concentrates are currently tested for a variety of known infectious agents, such as HIV, hepatitis C, hepatitis B, hepatitis A and parvovirus, and usually undergo dual and complementary viral inactivation steps. However, there is a residual risk of infection from nonenveloped viruses (which are not effectively inactivated by current viral inactivation steps), variant Creutzfeldt–Jakob disease (CJD) and unknown infectious agents. Due to the residual risk of blood-borne infections associated with factor concentrates and blood transfusions, it is recommended that all nonimmune patients with inherited bleeding disorders are vaccinated against hepatitis A and B.

Variant CJD is caused by an abnormal prion protein and is likely to have resulted from the consumption of beef infected with a related prion disease called bovine spongiform encephalopathy (BSE). At present, 170 people have died from variant CJD, the vast majority of cases occurring in UK residents. The risk of variant CJD is currently the subject of concern for hemophilia populations in the UK, France and other European countries. This is due to the development of vCJD in British and French donors whose plasma was used in the production of factor concentrates. There have been two probable cases of variant CJD transmission by blood transfusion, although there have been no reports of either variant CJD in patients with hemophilia or transmission of variant CJD by factor concentrate.[63]

One of the most serious complications of hemophilia is the development of an inhibitor, which is usually an IgG antibody with the capacity to neutralize the function of FVIII or FIX. The prevalence of inhibitors is approximately 30% in severe hemophilia and 1–7% in severe FIX deficiency. Inhibitor development is a well-recognized but uncommon complication of mild and moderate FVIII deficiency, and represents only 10% of inhibitors seen with FVIII deficiency.

Inhibitors and their treatment

The development of inhibitors to therapeutic factor concentrates in children with hemophilia A and B is a troublesome complication, with an incidence approaching 33% of those with hemophilia A and 3% of those with hemophilia B.[64] The median age for the development of inhibitors in severe FVIII deficiency is approximately 2 years after a median of 9–12 days of exposure. The first 50 exposure days represent the most significant inhibitor risk and thereafter there is a continuous but low risk of subsequent inhibitor formation. Risk factors for inhibitor development include race (black population have a higher risk than white), genotype (large gene deletions, major gene rearrangements or nonsense mutations), and family history.[9] Recent studies have suggested that both early exposure to FVIII and the use of recombinant rather than plasma-derived FVIII is associated with a higher risk of inhibitor formation.[65,66] However, further studies are required to validate these data.

The development of inhibitors may be detected by routine laboratory screening for inhibitor or by the identification of a poor clinical or routine laboratory response to factor replacement therapy. The Bethesda assay is the standard for the measurement of inhibitor titer. FVIII inhibitors are measured using a Nijmegen modification of the Bethesda assay. Patients should be screened for inhibitors every 6 months, or in the setting of a poor clinical or laboratory response to therapy. Inhibitors are classified as low or high responding. A low-responding inhibitor is defined as a peak historical inhibitor titer of < 5 Bethesda units (BU)/mL with a low or very attenuated response to FVIII/FIX administration. These patients frequently continue to respond to factor therapy, albeit at higher or more frequent dosing schedules. Conversely, high-responding inhibitors are defined as a peak historical inhibitor titer of > 5 BU/mL or a brisk anamnestic response to FVIII challenge. These patients will usually not respond to FVIII replacement therapy at times of bleeding and alternative treatments are required, such as FVIIa or activated prothrombin complex concentrates. Patients can convert from low- to high-titer inhibitor over time.

The management of acute bleeding episodes in children with inhibitors depends on the severity of bleed and whether they are low- or high-responding inhibitors. In low-responding inhibitors the use of FVIII and FIX at higher doses and more frequent intervals may be effective. Otherwise, recombinant FVIIa (90 μg/kg every 2 hours) or activated prothrombin complex concentrates (FEIBA 50–100 IU/kg every 6–12 hours) is usually effective in achieving hemostasis. It should be stated that recombinant FVIIa, at least in the developed world, has revolutionized the treatment of patients with severe FVIII deficiency and high-responding inhibitors.[67] Hemostasis is achieved by promoting tissue factor–FVIIa assembly at the site of vessel injury. Recombinant FVIIa may also cause activation of FIX and FX on the surface of activated platelets.[68] Effective hemostasis occurs without significant activation of the systemic coagulation cascade unlike other FVIII and FIX bypassing agents. Recombinant FVIIa has been used successfully in adults for the treatment of serious bleeding disorders and in the prevention of surgical bleeding. Few adverse events have been reported with therapy.[69]

As is the case in FVIII deficiency, most inhibitors in severe FIX deficiency occur after relatively few exposure days. A unique feature of FIX inhibitors is the association with allergic reactions (including anaphylaxis) in response to FIX infusion. The risk of allergic reaction is higher in patients with large gene deletions or rearrangements, and those who have or may have these mutations usually receive the first 20 treatments in hospital.[70] The principles of management of bleeding episodes in these patients include the use of FIX concentrate (for low-titer inhibitors in the absence of allergic reactions), FVIIa and activated prothrombin complex concentrates (in the absence of allergic reactions and anamnestic responses).[71] The response to immune tolerance therapy in children with FIX inhibitors is inferior to that for FVIII inhibitors.

Early recognition of the presence of an inhibitor allows a planned treatment program, avoiding further use of FVIII or FIX concentrate until the inhibitor has reached its nadir and then initiating immune tolerance therapy. Immune tolerance protocols have been developed that are successful in approximately 80% of children.[72–75] Higher success rates are seen when the inhibitor titer is allowed to decline to a low level, preferably < 10 BU, before commencing immune tolerance therapy. In addition, central venous access is necessary to facilitate the administration by parents of frequent high-dose factor concentrate.[46,76,77] Recombinant FVIIa has been used successfully in adults and children with severe FVIII deficiency and inhibitors who are undergoing surgery.[78,79] It is crucial that perioperative hemostasis is achieved with an agent that is safe and effective.

The optimal dose and interval for immune tolerance has not been determined and different regimens have been used, varying from 50 IU/kg three times per week to 300 IU/kg daily. Adjunctive therapies may be used and include any or all of the following: intravenous immunoglobulins, cyclophosphamide and protein A immunoadsorption. The most important predictor of success is the inhibitor titer prior to commencing immune tolerance, with a titer of < 10 BU/mL associated with a higher and quicker response rate.[80] Time to tolerance ranges from a few months to 2 years. If no response has been achieved at 2 years, then treatment is usually discontinued. Immune tolerance is continued until there is no evidence by inhibitor titer, recovery, and half-life.[81] Successful immune tolerance with a return to standard FVIII or FIX prophylaxis has been shown to be cost-effective when analyzed as part of total lifetime treatment costs.[82] The use of recombinant FVIIa in patients with high-responding inhibitors has been shown to significantly increase the cost of treatment.[83] However, this must be counterbalanced by the efficacy of recombinant FVIIa in preventing serious morbidity and mortality from bleeding episodes.[82,83] A significant minority of patients will fail immune tolerance therapy and recombinant FVIIa will continue to be the treatment of choice in these patients for the management of surgery and acute bleeding.

The use of rituximab (a monoclonal antibody against CD20)[84] or intermediate-purity FVIII (i.e., containing vWF) may prove effective in patients unresponsive to standard immune tolerance regimens. At present their use is deemed experimental.

Inhibitory activity in patients with hemophilia usually occurs on a background of severe disease. However, when it occurs in the setting of mild or moderate disease there are a number of unique features. The development of inhibitors usually occurs outside the pediatric age group, with a median age of 30 years. The presence of the inhibitor usually results in a change in the bleeding phenotype. Patients experience severe spontaneous bleeding whereas previously they only bled after trauma or surgery. This is caused by the cross-reactivity of the inhibitor against endogenous mutated FVIII, which frequently results in a reduction of baseline FVIII to < 1%, although occasionally FVIII levels may remain unchanged despite laboratory evidence of inhibitor and the onset of more severe bleeding symptoms.[85] Another distinctive feature of the bleeding phenotype of these patients is that they frequently have a bleeding profile similar to acquired hemophilia, with a higher incidence of soft tissue, gastrointestinal or urogenital bleeding. The response to immune tolerance is inferior to that of patients with severe hemophilia; at present the role of immune tolerance is a controversial issue in these patients, especially in the older age group. The management of acute bleeding episodes is similar to that in patients with severe hemophilia who develop inhibitors. However, desmopressin may be effective especially in patients whose baseline factor level does not reduce and in whom the inhibitor does not appear to cross-react with endogenous FVIII.

Comprehensive care approach

In order to improve the quality of life of patients with bleeding disorders, with their great variety of other clinical problems, hemostatic treatment alone is far from sufficient and a more comprehensive approach involving a multidisciplinary team is now considered best practice. The team is composed of diverse specialists and health-care professionals delivering comprehensive care on a 24-hour basis. In practice this involves a core team of hemophilia center medical staff, hemophilia nurses, hemophilia physiotherapist, hemophilia social worker and hemophilia center laboratory.[86] To deliver comprehensive care effectively, the involvement of other specialist services is also necessary, i.e., dental surgery, general surgery, counseling services and clinical psychology, and genetics service. It is advisable that all children with severe and moderate hemophilia have assess to comprehensive care services and that these children must have a comprehensive care review at least every 6 months.

Social care

Hemophilia identification cards

In conjunction with a diagnosis, a patient with hemophilia should be issued with a registration card that states the type and severity of disorder that the child has and contact details of their hemophilia treatment center.

Vaccinations

Children with hemophilia can be vaccinated like other children but the vaccinations must be given subcutaneously not intramuscularly.[87] If there is concern regarding the efficacy and uptake of specific vaccinations given via the subcutaneous route, then the vaccine should be administered after the child has received prophylaxis or treatment. It is recommended that all children with hemophilia be vaccinated against hepatitis A and B.[88]

School

It is important that parents inform school staff that a child has hemophilia. The staff from the hemophilia center can help to support the parents with this if necessary. If the child is on an adequate prophylaxis program, there should be no need for further resources within the school.

Leisure activities

A child with hemophilia who is on an adequate prophylaxis program can enjoy most sporting activities. Despite this some parents are apprehensive about allowing their children to play sports. Legitimate concerns do arise, especially in competitive or team events, but it is important to remember that participation in sports is an important part of an individual's life. Being active contributes to physical fitness and can influence the psychologic and emotional development of a growing child.

The National Hemophilia Foundation[89] has classified different sporting activities into three categories in order to help evaluate their risk–benefit in children with hemophilia.

- Category 1: most individuals with hemophilia can safely participate in these sports (e.g., cycling, fishing, hiking, swimming, tai chi).
- Category 2: the physical, social and psychologic benefits often outweigh the risks in these sports. The majority of sports fall into this category (e.g., basketball, karate, mountain biking, roller-blading, rowing, skiing, soccer, tennis, weight-lifting).
- Category 3: the risks outweigh the benefits in these sports. The nature of these activities make them dangerous even for those without hemophilia (e.g., boxing, hockey, lacrosse, motorcycling, rock climbing, rugby, wrestling).

Transition from pediatric to adult services

The adolescent years are full of tremendous social, psychological and emotional changes. Transition from a pediatric to an adult care setting should be the purposeful and planned movement of adolescents and young adults with hemophilia from child to adult-centered health-care systems. The timing of this transfer depends on physical and psychological maturity because adolescence, despite the familiarity of the term, proves difficult to define. Adolescence is a critical juncture for the development of positive health behaviors and it is important that certain barriers to adolescent independence are recognized and addressed. These barriers may be personal (i.e., maturity level, self-image, self-confidence, gaps in education), family-related (i.e., cultural, sibling issues, parental issues), or institutional (i.e., learned dependence, lack of formalized transition programs or family-centered care).

Conclusions

Significant advances in hemophilia A and B over the past quarter of a century have made hemophilia the paradigm of a human disease, where the application of not only molecular genetics but also innovations in medical, surgical and psychosocial practices have had significant impact in terms of diagnosis, treatment and, hopefully in the next decade, cure. By then gene therapeutics will have become a reality.

References

1. Hopff F. *Ueber die Haemophilie oder die Evbliche Frulage zu Tödtlichen Blutungan (inaug – abhand lung)*. Würzburg: Carl Wilhelm Becker, 1828.
2. Owen CA. A history of blood coagulation. In: Nichols WL, Walter Bowie EJ (eds). Rochester, MN: Mayo Foundation for Medical Education and Research, 2001, pp. 117–32.
3. Rosner FL. Haemophilia in the Talmud and Rabbinic writings. *Ann Intern Med* 1969; **70**: 833–7.
4. Otto JC. An account of an haemorrhagic disposition existing in certain families. *Med Repository* 1803; **6**: 1–4.
5. Poole JG, Gershgold EJ, Pappenhagen AR. High-potency anti-haemophilic factor concentrate prepared from cryoglobulin. *Nature* 1964; **203**: 312–13.
6. Rosendaal FR, Briet E. The increasing prevalence of haemophilia. *Thromb Haemost* 1990; **63**: 145.
7. White GC, Rosendaal F, Aledort LM, Lusher JM, Rothchild C, Ingeslev J. Definitions in haemophilia. Recommendations of the Scientific Subcommittee of FVIII and FIX of the SSC of ISTH. *Thromb Haemost* 2001; **85**: 560.
8. Parquet-Gernez A, Mazurie C, Goudemand M. Functional and immunological assays of FVIII in 133 haemophiliacs: characterization of a subgroup of patients with mild haemophilia A and discrepancy in 1- and 2-stage assays. *Thromb Haemost* 1998; **59**: 202–6.
9. Rudzki Z, Duncan EM, Casey GJ *et al.* Mutations in a subgroup of patients with mild haemophilia A and discrepancy between the one-stage and two-stage factor VIII:C methods. *Br J Haematol* 1996; **94**: 400–6.
10. Resource site: HAMSTeRS version 4. *Nucl Acids Res* 1998; **26**: 216–19.
11. Giannelli F, Green PM. The molecular basis of haemophilia A and B. *Baillière's Clin Haematol* 1996; **9**: 211–28.
12. Miller R. *Genetic counselling for haemophilia*. Treatment for haemophilia No. 25. Montreal: World Federation of Haemophilia, 2002.
13. Ludlam CA, Pasi KJ, Bolton-Maggs P *et al.* A framework for genetic service provision for haemophilia and other inherited bleeding disorders. *Haemophilia* 2005; **11**: 145–63.
14. Lane S. Haemorrhagic diathesis: successful transfusion of blood. *Lancet* 1840; **i**: 185–8.
15. Batorova A, Martinowitz U. Intermittent injections vs. continuous infusion of factor VIII in haemophilia patient undergoing major surgery. *Br J Haematol* 2000; **110**: 715–20.
16. Nilsson IM, Berntorp E, Lofqvist T, Pettersson H. Twenty-five years experience of prophylactic treatment in severe haemophilia A and B. *J Intern Med* 1992; **232**: 25–32.
17. Liesner RJ, Khair K, Hann IM. The impact of prophylactic treatment on children with severe haemophilia. *Br J Haematol* 1996; **92**: 973–8.
18. Petrini P, Lindvall N, Egberg N, Blomback M. Prophylaxis with factor concentrates in preventing hemophilic arthropathy. *Am J Pediatr Hematol Oncol* 1991; **13**: 280–7.
19. Blanchette VS. Prophylaxis in haemophilia: a comprehensive perspective. *Haematologica* 2004; **89** (suppl. 1): 29–35.
20. Berntorp E, Astermark J, Bjorkman S *et al.* Consensus perspectives on prophylactic therapy for haemophilia: summary statement. *Haemophilia* 2003; **9** (suppl. 1): 1–4.
21. Löfqvist T, Nilsson IM, Berntorp E, Petterson H. Haemophilia prophylaxis in young patients: a long term follow-up. *J Intern Med* 1997; **241**: 395–400.
22. Hacker MR, Geraghty S, Manco-Johnson M. Barriers to compliance with prophylaxis therapy in haemophilia. *Haemophilia* 2001; **7**: 392–6.
23. Manco-Johnson M, Morrissey-Harding G, Edelman-Lewis B, Oster G, Larson P. Development and validation of a measure of disease-specific quality of life in young children with haemophilia. *Haemophilia* 2004; **10**: 34–41.
24. Von Mackensen S, Bullinger M for Haemo-Qol group. Development and testing of an instrument to assess the quality

of life of children with haemophilia in Europe (Haemo-Qol). *Haemophilia* 2004; **10** (suppl. 1): 17–25.

25. Young NL, Bradley CS, Blanchette V *et al*. Development of health-related quality of life measure for boys with haemophilia: the Canadian Haemophilia Outcomes-Kids Life Assessment Tool (CHO-KLAT). *Haemophilia* 2004; **10** (suppl. 1): 34–43.

26. Gringeri A, Von Mackensen S, Auerswad G *et al.* for the Haemo-Qol study. Health status and health-related quality of life of children with haemophilia from six west European countries. *Haemophilia* 2004; **10** (suppl. 1): 26–33.

27. Mannucci PM, Aberg M, Nilsson IM, Robertson B. Mechanism of plasminogen activator and factor VIII increase after vasoactive drugs. *Br J Haematol* 1975; **30**: 81–93.

28. Mannucci PM, Ruggeri ZM, Pareti FI, Capitano A. 1-Deamino-8-D-arginine vasopressin: a new pharmacological approach to the management of haemophilia and von Willebrand disease. *Lancet* 1977; **i**: 869–72.

29. Nolan B, White B, Smith J *et al*. Desmopressin: therapeutic limitations in children and adults with inherited coagulation disorders. *Br J Haematol* 2000; **109**: 865–9.

30. Revel-Vilk S, Blanchette VS, Sparling C, Stain AM. DDAVP challenge tests in boys with mild/moderate haemophilia. *Br J Haematol* 2002; **117**: 947–51.

31. Mannucci PM. Desmopressin: a nontransfusional form of treatment for congenital and acquired bleeding disorders. *Blood* 1988; **72**: 1449–55.

32. Cattaneo M. Review of clinical experience of desmopressin in patients with congenital and acquired bleeding disorders. *Eur J Anaesthesiol* 1997; **14** (suppl. 14): 10–14.

33. United Kingdom Haemophilia Centre Directors' Organisation. Guidelines for the diagnosis and management of von Willebrand disease. *Haemophilia* 1997; **3** (suppl. 2): 1–8.

34. United Kingdom Haemophilia Centre Directors' Organisation Executive Committee. Guidelines on therapeutic products to treat haemophilia and other hereditary coagulation disorders. *Haemophilia* 1997; **3**: 63–77.

35. Poon M-C, Lillicrap DP, Israels SJ and the Association of Haemophilia Clinic Directors of Canada. Haemophilia and von Willebrand disease consensus statements on current management. 1. Diagnosis, comprehensive care concept, and assessment. *Can Med Assoc J* 1995; **153**: 19–25.

36. Francis JD, Leary T, Nibilett DJ. Convulsions and respiratory arrest in association with desmopressin administration for the treatment of a bleeding tonsil in a child with borderline haemophilia. *Acta Anaesthesiol Scand* 1999; **43**: 870–3.

37. Sutor AH. Desmopressin (DDAVP) in bleeding disorders of childhood. *Semin Thromb Haemost* 1998; **24**: 555–66.

38. Ehl S, Severin T, Sutor AH. DDAVP treatment in children with haemophilia B. *Br J Haematol* 2000; **111**: 1260–2.

39. Kavakli K, Aydinok Y, Karapinar D, Balkan C. DDAVP treatment in children with haemophilia B. *Br J Haematol* 2001; **114**: 731.

40. Blanchette VS, Al-Musa A, Stain AM, Ingram J, Fille RM. Central venous access devices in children with hemophilia: an update. *Blood Coag Fibrinol* 1997; **8** (suppl. 1): S11–S14.

41. Warrier I, Baird-Cox K, Lusher JM. Use of central venous catheters in children with haemophilia: one haemophilia treatment centre experience. *Haemophilia* 1997; **3**: 194–8.

42. Liesner RJ, Vora AJ, Hann IM, Lilleyman JS. Use of central venous catheters in children with severe congenital coagulopathy. *Br J Haematol* 1995; **91**: 203–7.

43. Vidler V, Richards M, Vora A. Central venous catheter associated thrombosis in severe haemophilia. *Br J Haematol* 1999; **104**: 461–4.

44. Blanchette VS, Al-Musa A, Stain AM, Filler RM, Ingram J. Central venous access catheters in children with haemophilia. *Blood Coag Fibrinol* 1996; **7** (suppl. 1): S39–S44.

45. Ragni MV, Hord JD, Blatt J. Central venous catheter infection in haemophiliacs undergoing prophylaxis or immune tolerance with clotting factor concentrate. *Haemophilia* 1997; **3**: 90–5.

46. Collins PW, Khair KS, Liesner R, Hann IM. Complications experienced with central venous catheters in children with congenital bleeding disorders. *Br J Haematol* 1997; **99**: 206–8.

47. Domm JA, Hudson MG, Janco RL. Complications of central venous access devices in paediatric haemophilia patients. *Haemophilia* 2003; **9**: 50–6.

48. Valentino LA, Ewenstein B, Navickis RJ, Wilkes MM. Central venous access devices in haemophilia. *Haemophilia* 2004; **10**: 134–46.

49. Ljung R. Central venous lines in haemophilia. *Haemophilia* 2003; **9** (suppl. 1): 88–93.

50. O'Grady NP, Alexander M, Dellinger EP *et al*. Guidelines for the prevention of intravascular catheter related infections. *MMWR Recomm Rep* 2002; **51**: 1–29.

51. Perkins JL, Johnson VA, Osip JM *et al*. The use of implantable venous access devices in children with haemophilia. *J Pediatr Hematol Oncol* 1997; **19**: 339–44.

52. Maki DG, Ringer M, Alvarado CJ. Prospective randomised trial of povidone-iodine, alcohol and chlorhexidine for prevention of infection associated with central venous and artial catheters. *Lancet* 1991; **338**: 339–43.

53. Chaiyakunapruk N, Veenstra DL, Lipsky BA, Saint S. Chlorhexidine compared with povidone-iodine solution for vascular catheter-site care: a meta-analysis. *Ann Intern Med* 2002; **136**: 792–801.

54. Pieters PC, Pyle M, Tisnado J. Catheter care. In: *Venous Catheters: A Practical Manual*. New York: Thieme, 2003, pp. 234–48.

55. Smith S, Dawson S, Hennessey R, Andrew M. Maintenance of the patency of indwelling central venous catheters: is heparin necessary? *Am J Pediatr Hematol Oncol* 1991; **13**: 141–3.

56. LeDuc K. Efficacy of normal saline solution versus heparin solution for maintaining patency of peripheral intravenous catheters in children. *J Emerg Nurs* 1997; **23**: 306–9.

57. Baranowski L. Central venous access devices: current technologies, uses and management strategies. *J Intravenous Nurs* 1993; **16**: 167–94.

58. Ewenstein BM, Valentino LA, Journeycake JM *et al*. Consensus recommendations for use of central venous access devices in haemophilia. *Haemophilia* 2004; **10**: 629–48.

59. Conn C. The importance of syringe size when using implanted vascular access devices. *J Vasc Access Network* 1993; **3**: 11–18.

60. Santagastino E, Gringeri A, Berardinelli L, Beretta C, Muca-Perja M, Mannucci PM. Long term safety and feasibility of arteriovenous fistulae as vascular access in children with haemophilia: a prospective study. *Br J Haematol* 2003; **123**: 502–6.

61. Darby SC, Rizza CR, Doll R *et al*. Incidence of AIDS and excess of mortality associated with HIV in haemophiliacs in the United Kingdom: report on behalf of the Directors of Haemophilia

Centres in the United Kingdom (UKHCDO). *Br Med J* 1998; **298**: 1064–8.

62. Lee C, Dusheiko G. The natural history and antiviral treatment of hepatitis C in haemophilia. *Haemophilia* 2002; **8**: 322–9.

63. Bird SM. Attributable testing for abnormal prion protein, database linkage, and blood-borne vCJD risks. *Lancet* 2004; **364**: 1362–4.

64. Hay CR, Baglin TP, Collins PW, Hill FG, Keeling DM. The diagnosis and management of factor VIII and IX inhibitors: a guideline from the UK Haemophilia Centre Doctors' Organisation (UKHCDO). *Br J Haematol* 2000; **111**: 78–90.

65. Lorenzo JL, Lopez A, Altisent C *et al.* Incidence of factor VIII inhibitors in severe haemophilia: the importance of patient age. *Br J Haematol* 2001; **113**: 600–3.

66. Van der Bom JG, Mauser-Bunschoten EP, Fisher K *et al.* Age at first treatment and immune tolerance to factor VIII in severe haemophilia. *Thromb Haemost* 2003; **89**: 475–9.

67. Hedner U. Treatment of patients with factor VIII and factor IX inhibitors with special focus on the use of recombinant factor VIIa. *Thromb Haemost* 1999; **82**: 531–9.

68. Hoffman M, Monroe DM III, Roberts HR. Activated factor VII activates factors IX and X on the surface of activated platelets: thoughts on the mechanism of action of high dose activated factor VII. *Blood Coag Fibrinol* 1998; **9** (suppl. 1): S61–S65.

69. Roberts HR. Clinical experience with activated factor VII: focus on safety aspects. *Blood Coag Fibrinol* 1998; **9** (suppl. 1): S115–S118.

70. High KA. Factor IX: molecular structure, epitopes, and mutations associated with inhibitor formation. In: Aledot LM, Hoyer LW, Lusher JM *et al.* (eds) *Inhibitors to Coagulation Factors.* New York: Plenum Press, 1995, pp. 79–86.

71. Warrier I, Lenk H, Saidi P *et al.* Nephrotic syndrome in haemophilia B patients with inhibitors. *Haemophilia* 1998; **4**: 248–51.

72. Kreuz W, Ehrenforth S, Funk M *et al.* Immune tolerance therapy in paediatric haemophiliacs with factor VIII inhibitors: 14 years follow-up. *Haemophilia* 1995; **1**: 24–32.

73. Mauser-Bunschoten EP, Niewenhuis HK, Roosendaal G, van den Berg HM. Low-dose immune tolerance induction in haemophilia A patients with inhibitors. *Blood* 1995; **86**: 983–8.

74. Di Michele DM. Immune tolerance: a synopsis of the international experience. *Haemophilia* 1998; **4**: 568–73.

75. Brackmann HH, Effenberger E, Hess L, Schwaab R, Oldenburg J. NovoSeven in immune tolerance therapy. *Blood Coag Fibrinol* 2000; **11** (suppl. 1): S39–S44.

76. Ljung R, van den Berg M, Petrini P *et al.* Port-A-Cath usage in children with haemophilia: experience of 53 cases. *Acta Paediatr Scand* 1998; **87**: 1051–4.

77. Smith OP, Hann IM. RVIIa therapy to secure haemostasis during central line insertion in children with high-responding FVIII inhibitors. *Br J Haematol* 1996; **92**: 973–8.

78. Lusher J, Ingerslev J, Roberts H, Hedner U. Clinical experience with recombinant factor VIIa. *Blood Coag Fibrinol* 1998; **9**: 119–28.

79. Smith OP, Hann IM. rVIIa therapy to secure haemostasis during central line insertion in children with high responding factor VIII inhibitors. *Br J Haematol* 1996; **92**: 1002–4.

80. Diagnosis and management of factor VIII and factor IX inhibitors: a guideline from the United Kingdom Haemophilia Centre Doctors' Organisation (UKHCDO). *Br J Haematol* 2000; **111**: 78–90.

81. Kreuz W, Mentzer D, Auerswald G *et al.* Successful immunetolerance therapy of FVIII inhibitor in children after changing from high to intermediate purity FVIII concentrate. *Haemophilia* 1996; **2** (suppl. 1): 19.

82. Colowick AB, Bohn RL, Avorn J, Ewenstein BM. Immune tolerance induction in hemophilia patients with inhibitors: costly can be cheaper. *Blood* 2000; **96**: 1698–702.

83. Bollard CM, Teague LR, Berry EW, Ockelford PA. The use of central vemous catheters (portacaths) in children with haemophilia. *Haemophilia* 2000; **6**: 66–70.

84. Mathias M, Khair K, Hann I *et al.* Rituximab in the treatment of alloimmune factor VIII and factor IX antibodies in two children with severe haemophilia. *Br J Haematol* 2004; **125**: 366.

85. Goudemand J. Haemophilia. Treatment of patients with inhibitors: cost issues. *Haemophilia* 1999; **5**: 397–401.

86. The Haemophilia Alliance. A national specification for haemophilia and related conditions. Available at www.haemophiliaalliance.org.uk

87. Ljung R. Care of the child with haemophilia. In: *Textbook of Haemophilia.* Malden, MA: Blackwell Publishing, 2005, pp. 120–4.

88. Makris M, Conlon CP, Watson HG. Immunization of patients with bleeding disorders. *Haemophilia* 2003; **9**: 541–6.

89. National Haemophilia Foundation. Haemophilia: sports and exercise. Available at www.hemophilia.org

27 von Willebrand disease

David Lillicrap

Introduction

The disorder now recognized to be the most common inherited bleeding condition in humans, von Willebrand disease (VWD), was originally described by Erik von Willebrand in 1926.[1] He described a severe mucocutaneous bleeding problem in a large family residing in the Aland Islands in the Gulf of Bothnia. The propositus was a 5-year-old girl who later bled to death during her fourth menstrual period. An investigation of this disorder revealed a normal coagulation time, a normal platelet count and a prolonged bleeding time. During the next four decades, it was believed that this condition was most likely due to either a vascular defect or to some form of platelet dysfunction. It was not until the 1960s that an abnormality in von Willebrand factor (VWF) was implicated in the pathogenesis of the disorder, and even then the failure to differentiate VWF from factor VIII (FVIII) further complicated studies until their eventual definitive separation through genetic cloning in the mid-1980s.[2,3]

Estimates of the prevalence of VWD have varied from about 1% of the general population[4] to 125 clinically relevant cases per million population. Nevertheless, even in the surveys in which the higher prevalence figures have been obtained, the affected individuals have been documented to have some, albeit mild, clinical evidence of a hemostatic defect.[4] VWD has been reported in subjects from all ethnic backgrounds, although several localized concentrations of severe disease have been documented in, for example, Israel, Sweden and Iran.

In surveys performed on VWD populations, about 80% of cases have the mild type 1 form of the disorder. The remainder have various type 2 forms of the condition (Table 27.1). The severe type 3 form of the disease is rare, with a prevalence of about 1 per million.

As more is learned about the underlying genetic pathogenesis of VWD, the inheritance pattern of the condition continues to be revised. Most cases of types 1, 2A, 2B and 2M

Table 27.1 Classification of von Willebrand disease (VWD) subtypes based on the 1994 recommendations of the VWD Subcommittee of the Scientific and Standardization Committee of the International Society on Thrombosis and Haemostasis.

Type of VWD	Definition and prevalence
Type 1 (~80%)	Partial quantitative deficiency of normal von Willebrand factor (VWF)
Type 2 (~20%)	Qualitative defects of VWF
Type 2A	Qualitative variants with decreased platelet-dependent function associated with the absence of high-molecular-weight multimers
Type 2B	Qualitative variants with increased binding affinity for platelet glycoprotein Ib
Type 2M	Qualititative variants with decreased platelet-dependent function associated with normal VWF multimer pattern
Type 2N	Qualitative variants with reduced binding of FVIII
Type 3 VWD (prevalence ~1 per million)	Complete absence of VWF

Reproduced with permission from Ref. 5.

disease represent autosomal dominant conditions with type 1 disease exhibiting incomplete phenotypic penetrance and variable expressivity. In contrast, types 2N and 3 VWD are recessive conditions with patients having been documented to be either homozygous or compound heterozygous for mutations within the VWF gene.

Biosynthesis and function

The gene that encodes VWF is located on the short arm of chromosome 12.[3] The VWF gene is a large and complex locus encompassing 175 kb of DNA and comprising 52 exons.[6] A further level of genetic complexity is introduced by the presence of a partial pseudogene sequence on chromosome 22,

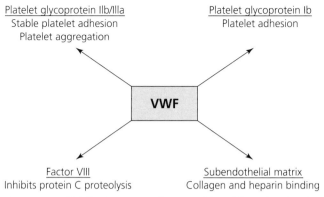

Platelet glycoprotein IIb/IIIa
Stable platelet adhesion
Platelet aggregation

Platelet glycoprotein Ib
Platelet adhesion

VWF

Factor VIII
Inhibits protein C proteolysis

Subendothelial matrix
Collagen and heparin binding

Fig. 27.1 Multiple binding partners for von Willebrand factor (VWF) and the functional role of these interactions.

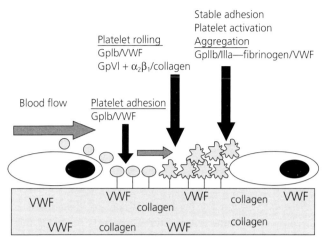

Fig. 27.2 Role of von Willebrand factor (VWF) in mediating the initial events in the hemostatic process. Platelets, rolling along the endothelial cell surface, are tethered to the site of endothelial cell injury through the binding of subendothelial VWF to the glycoprotein (Gp)Ib receptor. The platelets are subsequently activated and the GpIIb–IIIa complex is exposed on the platelet surface. Interaction of fibrinogen and VWF with GpIIb–IIIa consolidates the platelet adhesive event and initiates platelet aggregation.

corresponding to the region between exons 23 and 34 on chromosome 12. Expression of the gene is limited to two cell types, vascular endothelial cells[7] and megakaryocytes.[8] The primary translation product of the gene is a pre-pro-VWF protein that has a short amino-terminal signal peptide, an approximately 100-kDa propeptide involved in multimer assembly, and a mature subunit composed of 2050 amino acid residues. The pro-VWF molecule consists of four repeated domains (A–D) that constitute more than 90% of the sequence.[9]

Following translation, the pre-pro-VWF molecule undergoes a series of complex posttranslational modifications. These include signal peptide cleavage, dimerization, glycosylation, sulfation and eventual multimerization and propeptide cleavage in the Golgi. The fully processed protein is then sorted into one of two pathways involving either constitutive secretion from the cell of synthesis or storage in specialized organelles, the Weibel–Palade bodies of endothelial cells or α-granules of platelets. Following appropriate stimuli, such as thrombin deposition or platelet activation, VWF is released from these storage sites into the plasma, where it circulates with a molecular mass ranging from 500 to 20 000 kDa depending on the extent of subunit multimerization.[10] Following secretion, VWF is tethered to cell surface P-selectin where, under the influence of shear flow, the high-molecular-weight VWF multimers undergo partial proteolysis by the ADAMTS13 protease between amino acid residues tyrosine 1605 and methionine 1606 in the A2 domain of the protein.[11]

VWF is a multifunctional adhesive protein that binds to several different ligands in plasma and the subendothelial matrix (Fig. 27.1). It has two major physiologic roles.
1 As a carrier protein for the procoagulant cofactor FVIII. This has the consequence that low levels of VWF result in correspondingly low levels of FVIII due to its accelerated proteolytic degradation by activated protein C.[12]
2 It has an essential role in the initial cellular stages of the hemostatic process, platelet adhesion, platelet aggregation and eventual platelet plug formation (Fig. 27.2). VWF secreted from the basolateral surface of endothelial cells is adherent to the subendothelial matrix and interacts with the platelet receptor glycoprotein (Gp)Ib to initiate platelet adhesion and platelet activation.[13] The GpIIb–IIIa complex is then exposed and VWF plays an additional role in binding to this receptor and facilitating the process of platelet aggregation.[14]

Laboratory evaluation

The laboratory findings of this common bleeding condition are highly variable, ranging from the complete absence of VWF in type 3 VWD to minimal alterations in VWF and FVIII levels in patients with type 1 VWD. Indeed, due to the incomplete penetrance and variable expressivity of this trait, many individuals may have inherited mutant VWF alleles but fail to manifest any clinical or laboratory abnormalities.

Screening tests for von Willebrand disease

A number of rapid and inexpensive hematologic screening studies should be performed in the initial evaluation for possible VWD. The complete blood count may show evidence of iron-deficiency anemia due to chronic blood loss, and type 2B VWD is often associated with a mild thrombocytopenia. If the plasma VWF level is significantly reduced (below about 0.35 units/mL), the correspondingly low level of FVIII may result in a prolonged activated partial thromboplastin time (APTT).

Finally, the bleeding time may be prolonged.[15] However, it is important to note that many patients with proven VWD have a normal APTT and bleeding time and that the results of these screening studies must be interpreted in the context of the patient's clinical history. Although some hematologists no longer use the bleeding time in their diagnostic work-up of potential VWD, its use is still justified to evaluate the presence of one of the differential diagnoses for VWD, platelet dysfunction. Recently, a new analyzer that evaluates platelet function under conditions of high shear stress, the PFA-100, has also been incorporated into the screening investigations for VWD diagnosis.[16]

Tests for the VWF–FVIII complex

VWF and FVIII circulate in plasma as a noncovalent bimolecular complex, and the critical laboratory tests for VWD must include an evaluation of both these proteins. Plasma FVIII coagulant levels are measured using a standard APTT-based assay, utilizing FVIII-deficient plasma. Plasma VWF should be assessed in two ways: a quantitative immunologic assay and a functional test that evaluates its platelet-dependent interaction.

The two common VWF immunoassays (measuring VWF:Ag) used in clinical laboratories involve either a Laurell rocket immunoelectrophoretic assay or an enzyme-linked immunosorbent assay (ELISA). The former protocol is limited by a sensitivity of about 0.1 units/mL and a tendency to over-estimate the levels of VWF in type 2 variants due to the excess of low-molecular-weight forms of the protein. In comparison, most ELISA assays detect to a level of 0.01 units/mL and are unaffected by type 2 variant plasmas.

The functional activity of plasma VWF can be evaluated by testing its interactive role with platelets or collagen. The antibiotic ristocetin induces the binding of VWF to the GpIb receptor on platelets and is used in the laboratory to quantify the functional activity of plasma VWF in the ristocetin cofactor assay (VWF:RCo).[17] Ristocetin was withdrawn from clinical use because of its *in vivo* association with thrombocytopenia, presumably due to the clearance of ristocetin-induced platelet aggregates.[18] The other test that utilizes ristocetin is the ristocetin-induced platelet agglutination (RIPA) assay that evaluates the sensitivity of a patient's platelets to low-dose ristocetin. This test is especially useful in identifying individuals with type 2B VWD in whom the platelet membranes are 'overloaded' with the high-affinity mutant VWF resulting in increased sensitivity to ristocetin concentrations below 0.6 mg/mL.[19] In some laboratories, the binding of VWF to collagen is quantified in an ELISA as the functional test of choice.[20] This test has been shown to be highly dependent on, among other things, the type of collagen used in the assay.

The normal plasma level of VWF is about 10 μg/mL (equivalent to 1 unit/mL), with a wide normal population range of 50–200% of the mean value (0.5–2.0 units/mL). Several important genetic and environmental influences must be kept in mind when interpreting the results of VWF plasma

Table 27.2 Influence of ABO blood group on factor VIII (FVIII) and von Willebrand factor (VWF) levels: 95% lower confidence limits in 58 children with group O and nongroup O blood types.

	Group O	Nongroup O
FVIII:C (units/mL)	0.57	0.80
VWF:Ag (units/mL)	0.37	0.50
VWF:RCo (units/mL)	0.42	0.51

Data derived from Ref. 22.

estimations. The best-characterized genetic influence relates to an ABO blood group effect;[21] FVIII and VWF levels of blood group O individuals are approximately 25% lower than those with blood groups A, B and AB (Table 27.2). The major environmental influence on VWF and FVIII levels is their involvement in the acute-phase response. The plasma levels of both proteins will increase by three- to five-fold during acute physiologic stress and at times such as the later stages of pregnancy. The plasma levels of these proteins can vary so widely over time from a variety of influences (e.g., hormone levels in women) that at least two (and optimally three) sets of laboratory results should be obtained from patients prior to confirming or refuting the diagnosis of VWD (Fig. 27.3).

The final laboratory evaluation required to characterize VWD involves the assessment of the circulating molecular weight profile of VWF.[23] As mentioned above, VWF circulates in the plasma in the form of a heterogeneous mixture of multimers ranging in size from 500 to 20 000 kDa. The high-molecular-weight multimeric forms of the protein are the most effective in mediating the platelet interactive functions of VWF and it is these forms that are absent in some type 2 forms of VWD. The molecular weight profile of plasma VWF is most often evaluated using an SDS-PAGE electrophoretic assay (Fig. 27.4). The most recent advances in this assay have combined nonradioactive chemoluminescent detection of VWF multimers with densitometric analysis of multimer bands in efforts both to simplify and enhance the objectivity of the assay.

Von Willebrand disease classification

The VWD Subcommittee of the Scientific and Standardization Committee of the International Society of Thrombosis and Haemostasis proposed the currently accepted classification of VWD in 1994 (see Table 27.1).[5] This involves three major categories.

• Type 1 disease comprises about 80% of cases and presents with a partial, mild-to-moderate quantitative reduction of VWF levels. The VWF in type 1 disease is qualitatively normal.

• Type 3 disease, the other quantitative defect, occurs with a frequency of about 1 per million and represents a virtual absence of VWF.

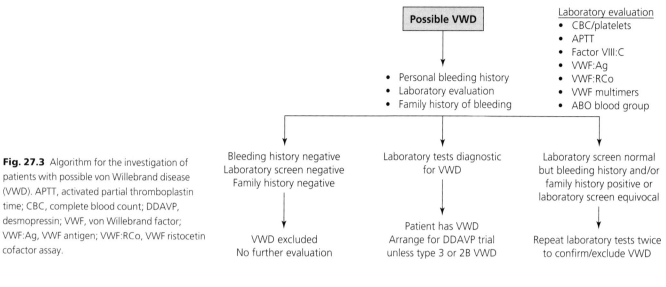

Fig. 27.3 Algorithm for the investigation of patients with possible von Willebrand disease (VWD). APTT, activated partial thromboplastin time; CBC, complete blood count; DDAVP, desmopressin; VWF, von Willebrand factor; VWF:Ag, VWF antigen; VWF:RCo, VWF ristocetin cofactor assay.

Possible VWD

Laboratory evaluation
• CBC/platelets
• APTT
• Factor VIII:C
• VWF:Ag
• VWF:RCo
• VWF multimers
• ABO blood group

• Personal bleeding history
• Laboratory evaluation
• Family history of bleeding

Bleeding history negative
Laboratory screen negative
Family history negative

Laboratory tests diagnostic for VWD

Laboratory screen normal but bleeding history and/or family history positive or laboratory screen equivocal

VWD excluded
No further evaluation

Patient has VWD
Arrange for DDAVP trial unless type 3 or 2B VWD

Repeat laboratory tests twice to confirm/exclude VWD

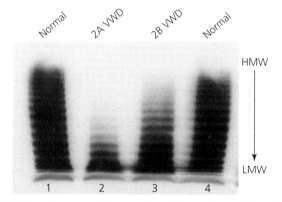

Fig. 27.4 Multimer analysis in two patients with type 2 von Willebrand disease (VWD). Lanes 1 and 4 represent normal plasma multimer patterns. Lane 2 shows the plasma von Willebrand factor (VWF) multimers for a patient with type 2A VWD and lane 3 the plasma VWF multimers for a patient with type 2B VWD. HMW, high molecular weight; LMW, low molecular weight.

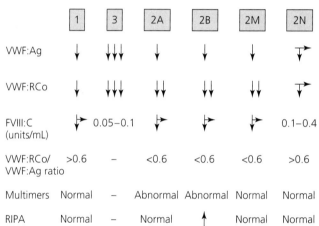

	1	3	2A	2B	2M	2N
VWF:Ag	↓	↓↓↓	↓	↓	↓	↓→
VWF:RCo	↓	↓↓↓	↓↓	↓↓	↓↓	↓→
FVIII:C (units/mL)	↓→	0.05–0.1	↓→	↓→	↓→	0.1–0.4
VWF:RCo/ VWF:Ag ratio	>0.6	–	<0.6	<0.6	<0.6	>0.6
Multimers	Normal	–	Abnormal	Abnormal	Normal	Normal
RIPA	Normal	–	Normal	↑	Normal	Normal

Fig. 27.5 Classification and results of laboratory studies in the common forms of von Willebrand disease. RIPA, ristocetin-induced platelet agglutination; VWF, von Willebrand factor; VWF:Ag, VWF antigen; VWF:RCo, VWF ristocetin cofactor assay.

• The various type 2 forms of the disease involve the synthesis of qualitatively mutant forms of the protein that manifest abnormalities in multimerization, platelet and FVIII binding (Fig. 27.5). Type 2 forms of VWD account for about 20% of diagnosed cases.

Type 1 von Willebrand disease

While this is clearly the most common form of the disease, it is also the most problematic to diagnose with certainty. Plasma levels of VWF (both VWF:Ag and VWF:RCo) and FVIII can range from about 0.05 to 0.45 units/mL in this condition and the caveat raised above concerning acute-phase influences is especially pertinent to the diagnosis of this subtype of VWD. The situation concerning the role of blood group O in type 1 VWD remains controversial, but it may be

that this is one of several genetic modifiers that contribute to this phenotype. It is important to note that only some patients with this disorder will have abnormal hemostatic screening studies (i.e., prolonged APTT and bleeding times). Recent attempts to clarify the diagnosis of this condition have focused on three factors:

• a personal history of excessive mucocutaneous bleeding;
• evidence of a family history of the condition;
• laboratory demonstration of VWF deficiency.

Without documentation of all three of these features, the diagnosis of type 1 VWD is rendered less definitive, although with the incomplete penetrance of the phenotype it should be recognized that lack of a family history is not unusual.

The genetic basis for type 1 VWD is currently under intense investigation and recent information suggests that the phenotype is most often due to a large variety of missense

Table 27.3 Clinical definitions of a significant bleeding trait.

Recurrent nosebleeds requiring medical treatment (packing, cautery, desmopressin, etc.) or leading to anemia

Oral cavity bleeding lasting for at least 1 hour, restarting over the next 7 days or requiring medical treatment

Bleeding from skin lacerations lasting for at least 1 hour, restarting over the next 7 days or requiring medical treatment

Prolonged bleeding associated with, or following, dental extraction or other oral surgery

Menorrhagia requiring medical attention or leading to anemia

Spontaneous gastrointestinal bleeding requiring medical treatment or leading to anemia, unexplained by local causes

Prolonged bleeding from other skin or mucous membrane surfaces requiring medical treatment

mutations within the VWF gene. The most common of these changes appears to be a tyrosine to cysteine mutation at codon 1584 that is present in 10–20% of type 1 patients.[24] A variety of transcriptional and splicing mutants have also been documented in type 1 patients. In contrast to these findings, some type 1 VWD patients have no obvious mutations in their VWF genes and may have mutations at other genetic loci implicated in VWF biosynthesis.

Patients with type 1 VWD exhibit an increase in mucocutaneous bleeding. The most common features are nosebleeds, easy bruising, bleeding from trivial cuts and excessive menstrual bleeding. Prolonged and delayed-onset bleeding following tooth extractions and oral surgery is also a common feature. Bleeding into soft tissues and joints does not occur unless provoked by trauma. Unfortunately, as with many aspects of this disease, definitive documentation of these clinical characteristics is not always straightforward, and an attempt should be made to enhance the objectivity of these historic details with the use of a validated bleeding questionnaire (Table 27.3).

Type 3 von Willebrand disease

Unlike most other forms of the disease (aside from type 2N), the inheritance pattern of type 3 disease best fits that of a recessive condition, with both carriers being asymptomatic. However, there is a growing realization that in some type 3 families, one parent has documented evidence of type 1 VWD, illustrating the heterogeneous nature of the inheritance of this disease subtype.

Type 3 patients manifest a clinically severe phenotype. Not only do they exhibit the same mucocutaneous bleeding features seen in type 1 disease (in a more pronounced fashion) but, due to their very low levels of plasma FVIII (<0.10 units/mL), they also experience the joint and soft tissue bleeds seen in patients with hemophilia A. In the laboratory, this condition is characterized by prolongation of the APTT and bleeding time, undetectable levels of VWF:Ag and VWF:RCo, and FVIII levels < 0.10 units/mL.

Molecular genetic studies of type 3 patients indicate that this phenotype is the result of a variety of null mutations including gross deletions, frameshift and nonsense mutations in their VWF genes. In some instances, these mutations are associated with the development of alloantibodies to VWF that seriously complicate treatment.[25,26]

Type 2 von Willebrand disease

The current classification divides these qualitative variants into those that affect the platelet-dependent function of VWF and those that reduce binding to FVIII. The clinical features are similar to those seen in type 1 disease.

Type 2A

Type 2A disease is characterized by the presence of VWF that lacks the large- and intermediate-sized multimers of the protein. This defect appears to result from either an inherent inability to form the higher molecular-weight multimers (Group I mutations) or the synthesis of multimers that are more susceptible to ADAMTS13-mediated proteolysis (Group II mutations).[27] This subtype accounts for approximately 15% of VWD cases in most populations and segregates within families as an autosomal dominant trait.

Type 2A disease can initially be suspected from a disproportionately low VWF:RCo level relative to the VWF:Ag (ratio <0.6). The FVIII level may be low or normal. Ristocetin-induced platelet agglutination is reduced and the multimer profile will show a loss of high, and sometimes intermediate, molecular-weight forms in both the plasma and platelet lysates.

The molecular genetic basis of type 2A VWD has been well characterized, with the majority of mutations being missense changes in the region of the VWF gene encoding the A2 protein domain (Fig. 27.6).[28] The remainder of the type 2A mutations disrupt the generation of dimers or multimers.

Type 2B

Type 2B VWD represents an interesting gain-of-function mutant form of the disease. In this condition, the mutant form of VWF binds with greater affinity to the GpIb receptor on platelets, resulting in the selective depletion from the plasma of the highest multimeric forms of VWF.[18,29] The increased binding of the mutant VWF to platelets also results in the formation of circulating platelet aggregates and subsequent thrombocytopenia. Thus, type 2B VWD should be

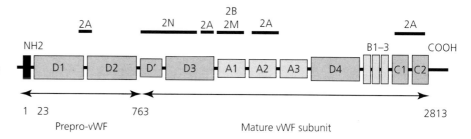

Fig. 27.6 Repeating multidomain structure of the von Willebrand factor (VWF) protein. The regions of the protein comprising the pre-pro-polypeptide and mature VWF subunits are indicated at the bottom of the diagram (numbers refer to amino acid residues). Regions of the protein where the causative mutations for types 2A, 2B, 2M and 2N von Willebrand disease are found are shown above the protein diagram.

considered in the differential diagnosis of inherited forms of thrombocytopenia.

As with type 2A disease, in patients with type 2B VWD the VWF:RCo will likely be disproportionately low relative to the VWF:Ag, but with this subtype there is increased sensitivity to low-dose ristocetin-induced platelet agglutination (ristocetin concentrations <0.7 mg/mL). On multimeric analysis, the highest molecular-weight forms are absent from the plasma, while in platelets the multimer pattern is normal (reflecting increased binding of the mutant VWF to the platelet surface).

Also like type 2A disease, this variant exhibits an autosomal dominant mode of inheritance. The mutations in type 2B disease have been well characterized and represent a variety of different missense mutations in the region of the VWF gene encoding the GpIb binding region of the protein, the A1 domain.[30]

A disorder known as platelet-type VWD (PT-VWD) exhibits identical clinical and laboratory features to those of type 2B VWD.[31] This condition is caused by mutations in the GpIbα gene that affect the region of the receptor that binds to VWF.[32] Type 2B VWD and PT-VWD can be differentiated either by specialized tests that distinguish enhanced ristocetin-induced binding of VWF to washed patient platelets or by genetic analysis of the A1 domain-encoding region of the VWF gene (exon 28) and the GpIbα gene. Because of the identical nature of the screening laboratory studies in these conditions, their relative frequencies are unknown, although it is assumed that PT-VWD is significantly less prevalent in most populations.

Type 2M

This type 2 variant form of VWD is characterized by the same disproportionate reduction in VWF:RCo levels relative to VWF:Ag seen in type 2A and 2B disease, but in type 2M VWD the plasma and platelet multimers are normal and ristocetin-induced platelet agglutination is reduced. In those cases in which the disease-causing mutation has been identified, this has been a missense alteration in the same region of the VWF gene in which the type 2B mutations are localized, the A1 domain.[33] Thus, type 2M VWD represents the result of loss-of-function mutations that adversely influence the binding of VWF to the platelet GpIb receptor.

Type 2N

This VWD subtype represents an important patient population that can be confused with other conditions in which the only laboratory abnormality is a low plasma FVIII level. Unlike the other type 2 forms of VWD, type 2N VWD exhibits a recessive mode of inheritance.

Type 2N disease has been described as an autosomal form of hemophilia A.[34] The bleeding tendency is relatively mild and on laboratory investigation often the only abnormality is a low FVIII level of 0.10–0.40 units/mL. The definitive diagnosis of type 2N disease requires one of two strategies:[35] the demonstration of reduced FVIII binding in a microtiter plate-based assay or demonstration of the disease-causing mutations in the regions of the gene encoding the N-terminal D'/D3 FVIII-binding domain of the protein (exons 18–25).

Clinical management

As this is the most common inherited bleeding condition, with a prevalence of up to 1% of the population, physicians of all types are faced with the management of patients with VWD. It should be evident from the discussion of the laboratory features of the disease and its classification that one of the most problematic areas of management is definitive diagnosis of the disorder. While type 3 and type 2 forms of the disorder should be readily identifiable (with access to an experienced coagulation laboratory), the diagnosis of type 1 disease still poses significant problems.[36] Assigning an incorrect diagnostic label of VWD to a patient can be difficult to revise and may result in confusion and inappropriate management decisions. In addition, the wider implications of this diagnostic label, including its potential social stigma and health insurance implications, should be considered before pronouncing any individual to be affected with VWD. The converse of this problem concerns the young child or male individual (no menstrual experience) who has yet to undergo a sufficient hemostatic challenge to manifest a bleeding tendency that would suggest the diagnosis of VWD.

VWD is an inherited disorder and, as such, genetic counseling is appropriate in affected families. However, the incomplete penetrance and variable expressivity of the disorder significantly complicate the prediction of phenotypic consequences. Furthermore, the relatively mild nature of the bleeding problems, except in type 3 disease, obviates the need to consider prenatal testing. Although there is no suggestion that infants who have potentially inherited VWD need to be delivered routinely by cesarean section, they should not be subjected to prolonged or complicated (vacuum extraction or mid-cavity forceps) vaginal deliveries.

Prophylactic and therapeutic treatment of bleeding

Adjunctive therapies

In addition to treatments that specifically address the VWF deficit, there are several adjunctive therapies that are effective at reducing blood loss in these patients. The antifibrinolytic agents, tranexamic acid and aminocaproic acid, have been used as highly efficacious agents either alone or as complements to desmopressin (DDAVP) and blood component therapy in both prophylactic and therapeutic situations. They should be administered 2 hours prior to an anticipated hemostatic challenge and continued for 7–10 days after the challenge. The therapeutic oral doses are 25 mg/kg every 6–8 hours for tranexamic acid and 100–200 mg/kg every 6 hours for aminocaproic acid. Both agents are also available as intravenous preparations and tranexamic acid has also been demonstrated to be effective as a mouthwash.[37] Both drugs are usually well tolerated, aside from occasional mild gastrointestinal upset. Estrogen therapy has also been shown to be an effective measure in reducing menstrual bleeding and the frequency and magnitude of nosebleeds.

Desmopressin

Desmopressin (1-deamino-8-D-arginine vasopressin, DDAVP) is a synthetic analog of the antidiuretic hormone vasopressin.[38] Its infusion increases plasma VWF and FVIII levels by two- to eight-fold within 1 hour of administration.[39] This effect is presumed to be due to the release of VWF from endothelial cell stores (Weibel–Palade bodies) with secondary stabilization of additional FVIII.

Desmopressin can be administered by the intravenous, subcutaneous or intranasal route.[40] Peak responses will be achieved within 30 and 90 min with the intravenous and intranasal routes, respectively. The usual parenteral dose is 0.3 μg/kg (to a maximum of 20 μg), infused intravenously in 10–50 mL of normal saline over about 20 min. The dose of the highly concentrated intranasal preparation is 150 μg for children under 50 kg and 300 μg for larger children. It should be noted that another intranasal preparation of desmopressin is available for the treatment of diabetes insipidus. However, this is a low-concentration compound and does not result in significant increments to the plasma VWF and FVIII levels.

Desmopressin is a safe and generally very effective hemostatic agent. Its only common side-effects are facial flushing, mild headache and minimal changes to blood pressure and heart rate. All these effects can be minimized by increasing the duration of the infusion and administering the drug with the patient lying down. The most serious side-effects that can develop are severe hyponatremia and seizures.[41,42] Children under 2 years of age are especially prone to this complication and their fluid intake should be reduced to maintenance levels for the 24 hours following desmopressin administration. In addition, with repeated doses of the drug, serial monitoring of the serum sodium should be undertaken.

The other limitation to this agent is the development of tachyphylaxis with repeated administration. When given at repeated intervals of 24 hours or shorter, the magnitude of VWF and FVIII increments achieved often falls to approximately 70% of that documented with the initial dose.[43] This is presumably related to a partial "exhaustion" of the endothelial cell stores. The reduced VWF increments obtained with repeated desmopressin infusion are only a relative limitation to its use for several consecutive days and it will often still be effective in this clinical setting.

The plasma VWF and FVIII response should be evaluated in every patient with a therapeutic trial of the agent, preferably prior to the first treatment. This is necessary as not all patients, particularly those with severe type 1 or type 2 VWD, respond adequately to this therapy.[44] This therapeutic trial should also include testing for VWF and FVIII levels at 4 hours post administration as some VWF mutants may show a significantly reduced plasma half-life.

Desmopressin can be used as a prophylactic or therapeutic agent in a wide variety of clinical circumstances, including the treatment of epistaxis and menstrual bleeding, and prior to dental procedures and minor surgery. Major surgical procedures and life-threatening bleeds should be treated with blood component therapy (see below).

Most patients with mild/moderate type 1 VWD should respond satisfactorily to desmopressin infusion, and for this common form of the disease the concomitant use of desmopressin and antifibrinolytic therapy should be sufficient for most clinical situations. In contrast, desmopressin has only been reported very rarely to be effective in type 3 patients and should not be considered the treatment of choice for this population. The therapeutic effect of desmopressin in the type 2 variant forms of VWD is variable. Some type 2A patients are very adequately treated and this patient group will be evident from a therapeutic trial infusion. In type 2B patients the situation is more controversial. While infusion of desmopressin consistently results in transient thrombocytopenia in these patients, several investigators have documented an excellent hemostatic effect from this treatment.[45,46] In addition, the theoretical concern of desmopressin-induced thrombosis due to potential platelet aggregate formation has not been documented. Finally, desmopressin has been used in type 2N VWD patients where it has been found to increase both VWF and FVIII levels between two- and nine-fold.[47] However, due to the fact that the VWF being released is a FVIII-binding mutant, the duration of the FVIII increment is only about 3 hours. This suggests that for type 2N patients, desmopressin should only be used in clinical situations where a brief transient rise in FVIII is required.

Blood component therapy

Treatment of VWD with blood component transfusion is required for major dental and surgical procedures, following trauma and to treat life-threatening bleeding. Cryoprecipitate, the standard component used for VWD therapy during the 1970s and 1980s, is no longer the material of choice. No effective viral attenuation process has yet been devised for cryoprecipitate and thus the risk of viral transmission has relegated this blood component to a rare alternative therapy in this condition.

The blood components currently used are plasma-derived, intermediate-purity FVIII concentrates (i.e., Humate-P and Alphanate) that have undergone a variety of viral inactivation steps to prevent viral infection.[48–50] The latest high-purity and ultra-high-purity FVIII concentrates, such as the monoclonally purified concentrates and recombinant FVIII, have a very low VWF content and are not useful in this context. Interestingly, although these intermediate-purity FVIII concentrates are frequently used with good effect in VWD, their regulatory approval for this purpose is highly variable.

Most dosing recommendations for the treatment of VWD with blood component infusions are based on FVIII unit increments (intermediate-purity FVIII concentrates are now often labeled with both FVIII:C and VWF:RCo potencies). This practice relates to the demonstration that FVIII replacement appears to be critical for hemostasis in most surgical bleeding situations. The dose of the intermediate-purity concentrate required to elevate plasma FVIII to the required level is calculated in the same way as recommended for hemophilia A (i.e., desired FVIII increment × weight in kg × 0.4) (see Chapter 26). A FVIII level of 1 unit/mL should be the target for major surgery and life-threatening bleeds and 0.5 unit/mL for minor surgical and dental procedures. Plasma FVIII levels can be monitored to assess treatment response and, with a VWF half-life of ~18 hours, repeat infusions should be given every 12–24 hours. Repeat infusions of these concentrates in VWD patients can result in supraphysiologic FVIII levels and there has been a suggestion that these high FVIII levels may contribute to a risk for venous thrombosis in this setting.[51] Dosing recommendations for the prevention or treatment of mucocutaneous bleeding are less well resolved, but might be better based on VWF:RCo unit dosing. Unfortunately, there are no studies that demonstrate the benefit of follow-up after therapy using any particular laboratory test.

In the rare event that infusion with an intermediate-purity concentrate is ineffective at stopping bleeding, transfusion with either platelet concentrates[52] or cryoprecipitate has been used as an effective second-line treatment.

Finally, there have been successful preclinical trials of recombinant VWF and interleukin-11 preparations, but at this stage it is too early to assess the relative advantages and likely clinical application of these compounds.

References

1. von Willebrand EA. Hereditar pseudohemofili. *Finska Lakarsallskapets Handl* 1926; **67**: 7–112.
2. Sadler JE, Shelton-Inloes BB, Sorace JM, Harlan JM, Titani K, Davie EW. Cloning and characterization of two cDNAs coding for human von Willebrand factor. *Proc Natl Acad Sci USA* 1985; **82**: 6394–8.
3. Ginsburg D, Handin RI, Bonthron DT *et al.* Human von Willebrand factor (VWF): isolation of complementary DNA (cDNA) clones and chromosomal localization. *Science* 1985; **228**: 1401–3.
4. Rodeghiero F, Castaman G, Dini E. Epidemiological investigation of the prevalence of von Willebrand's disease. *Blood* 1987; **69**: 454–9.
5. Sadler JE. A revised classification of von Willebrand disease. *Thromb Haemost* 1994; **71**: 520–5.
6. Mancuso DJ, Tuley EA, Westfield LA *et al.* Structure of the gene for human von Willebrand factor. *J Biol Chem* 1989; **264**: 19514–27.
7. Wagner DD, Marder VJ. Biosynthesis of von Willebrand protein by human endothelial cells: processing steps and their intracellular localization. *J Cell Biol* 1984; **99**: 2123–30.
8. Sporn LA, Chavin SI, Marder VJ, Wagner DD. Biosynthesis of von Willebrand protein by human megakaryocytes. *J Clin Invest* 1985; **76**: 1102–6.
9. Shelton-Inloes B, Titani K, Sadler J. cDNA sequences for human von Willebrand factor reveal five types of repeated domains and five possible protein sequence polymorphisms. *Biochemistry* 1986; **25**: 3164–71.
10. Ruggeri Z, Zimmerman T. The complex multimeric composition of factor VIII/von Willebrand factor. *Blood* 1981; **57**: 1140–3.
11. Dong JF, Moake JL, Nolasco L *et al.* ADAMTS-13 rapidly cleaves newly secreted ultralarge von Willebrand factor multimers on the endothelial surface under flowing conditions. *Blood* 2002; **100**: 4033–9.
12. Koedam JA, Meijers JCM, Sixma JJ, Bouma BN. Inactivation of human factor VIII by activated protein C. Cofactor activity of protein S and protective effect of von Willebrand factor. *J Clin Invest* 1988; **82**: 1236–43.
13. Savage B, Saldivar E, Ruggeri ZM. Initiation of platelet adhesion by arrest onto fibrinogen or translocation on von Willebrand factor. *Cell* 1996; **84**: 289–97.
14. Ruggeri ZM. Mechanisms of shear-induced platelet adhesion and aggregation. *Thromb Haemost* 1993; **70**: 119–23.
15. Mannucci PM, Pareti FI, Holmberg L, Nilsson IM, Ruggeri ZM.

Studies on the prolonged bleeding time in von Willebrand's disease. *J Lab Clin Med* 1976; **88**: 662–73.

16. Fressinaud E, Veyradier A, Truchaud F *et al*. Screening for von Willebrand disease with a new analyzer using high shear stress: a study of 60 cases. *Blood* 1998; **91**: 1325–31.

17. Howard MA, Firkin BG. Ristocetin: a new tool in the investigation of platelet aggregation. *Thromb Haemost* 1971; **26**: 362–9.

18. Gangarosa EJ, Johnson TR, Ramos HS. Ristocetin-induced thrombocytopenia: site and mechanism of action. *Arch Intern Med* 1960; **105**: 83–9.

19. Cooney KA, Lyons SE, Ginsburg D. Functional analysis of a type 2B von Willebrand disease missense mutation: increased binding of large von Willebrand factor multimers to platelets. *Proc Natl Acad Sci USA* 1992; **89**: 2869–72.

20. Casonato A, Pontara E, Bertomoro A, Sartorello F, Cattini MG, Girolami A. Von Willebrand factor collagen binding activity in the diagnosis of von Willebrand disease: an alternative to ristocetin co-factor activity? *Br J Haematol* 2001; **112**: 578–83.

21. Gill JC, Endres-Brooks J, Bauer PJ, Marks WJJ, Montgomery RR. The effect of ABO blood group on the diagnosis of von Willebrand disease. *Blood* 1987; **69**: 1691–5.

22. Dean JA, Blanchette VS, Carcao MD *et al*. von Willebrand disease in a pediatric-based population: comparison of type 1 diagnostic criteria and use of the PFA-100 and a von Willebrand factor/collagen-binding assay. *Thromb Haemost* 2000; **84**: 401–9.

23. Hoyer LW, Rizza CR, Tuddenham EGD, Carta CA, Armitage H, Rotblat F. Von Willebrand factor multimer patterns in von Willebrand's disease. *Br J Haematol* 1983; **55**: 493–507.

24. O'Brien LA, James PD, Othman M *et al*. Founder von Willebrand factor haplotype associated with type 1 von Willebrand disease. *Blood* 2003; **102**: 549–57.

25. Shelton-Inloes B, Chehab F, Mannucci P, Federici A, Sadler E. Gene deletions correlate with the development of alloantibodies in von Willebrand's disease. *J Clin Invest* 1987; **79**: 1459–65.

26. Ngo K, Glotz Trifard V, Koziol J *et al*. Homozygous and heterozygous deletions of the von Willebrand factor gene in patients and carriers of severe von Willebrand disease. *Proc Natl Acad Sci USA* 1988; **85**: 2753–7.

27. Lyons SE, Bruck ME, Bowie EJW, Ginsburg D. Impaired intracellular transport produced by a subset of type 2A von Willebrand disease mutations. *J Biol Chem* 1992; **267**: 4424–30.

28. Inbal A, Seligsohn U, Kornbrot N *et al*. Characterization of three point mutations causing von Willebrand disease type 2A in five unrelated families. *Thromb Haemost* 1992; **67**: 618–22.

29. Ruggeri ZM, Pared FI, Mannucci PM, Ciavarella N, Zimmerman TS. Heightened interaction between platelets and factor VIII/von Willebrand factor in a new subtype of von Willebrand's disease. *N Engl J Med* 1980; **302**: 1047–51.

30. Cooney KA, Nichols WC, Bruck ME *et al*. The molecular defect in type 2B von Willebrand disease. Identification of four potential missense mutations within the putative GpIb binding domain. *J Clin Invest* 1991; **87**: 1227–33.

31. Miller JL, Castella A. Platelet-type von Willebrand's disease: characterization of a new bleeding disorder. *Blood* 1982; **60**: 790–4.

32. Bryckaert MC, Pietu G, Ruan C *et al*. Abnormality of glycoprotein Ib in two cases of "pseudo"-von Willebrand's disease. *J Lab Clin Med* 1985; **106**: 393–400.

33. Mancuso DJ, Kroner PA, Christopherson PA, Vokac EA, Gill JC, Montgomery RR. Type 2M: Milwaukee-1 von Willebrand disease: an in-frame deletion in the Cys509–Cys695 loop of the von Willebrand factor A1 domain causes deficient binding of von Willebrand factor to platelets. *Blood* 1996; **88**: 2559–68.

34. Mazurier C. von Willebrand disease masquerading as haemophilia A. *Thromb Haemost* 1992; **67**: 391–6.

35. Nesbitt IM, Goodeve AC, Guilliatt AM, Makris M, Preston FE, Peake IR. Characterisation of type 2N von Willebrand disease using phenotypic and molecular techniques. *Thromb Haemost* 1996; **75**: 959–64.

36. Batlle J, Torea J, Rendal E, Fernandez MF. The problem of diagnosing von Willebrand's disease. *J Intern Med* 1997; **740** (suppl.): 121–8.

37. Sindet-Pedersen S, Ramstrom G, Bernvil S, Blomback M. Hemostatic effect of tranexamic acid mouthwash in anticoagulant-treated patients undergoing oral surgery. *N Engl J Med* 1989; **320**: 840–3.

38. Mannucci PM. Desmopressin: a nontransfusional hemostatic agent. *Annu Rev Med* 1990; **41**: 55–64.

39. Rodeghiero F, Castaman G, Di Bona E, Ruggeri M. Consistency of responses to repeated DDAVP infusions in patients with von Willebrand's disease and hemophilia A. *Blood* 1989; **74**: 1997–2000.

40. Rose EH, Aledort LM. Nasal spray desmopressin (DDAVP) for mild hemophilia A and von Willebrand disease. *Ann Intern Med* 1991; **114**: 563–8.

41. Humphries JE, Siragy H. Significant hyponatremia following DDAVP administration in a healthy adult. *Am J Hematol* 1993; **44**: 12–15.

42. Weinstein RE, Bona RD, Altman AJ *et al*. Severe hyponatremia after repeated intravenous administration of desmopressin. *Am J Hematol* 1989; **32**: 258–61.

43. Mannucci PM, Bettega D, Cattaneo M. Patterns of development of tachyphylaxis in patients with haemophilia and von Willebrand disease after repeated doses of desmopressin (DDAVP). *Br J Haematol* 1992; **82**: 87–93.

44. Federici AB, Mazurier C, Berntorp E *et al*. Biologic response to desmopressin in patients with severe type 1 and type 2 von Willebrand disease: results of a multicenter European study. *Blood* 2004; **103**: 2032–8.

45. Fowler WE, Berkowitz LR, Roberts HR. DDAVP for type 2B von Willebrand disease. *Blood* 1989; **74**: 1859–60.

46. Casonato A, Sartori MT, De Marco L, Girolami A. 1-Desamino-8-D-arginine vasopressin (DDAVP) infusion in type 2B von Willebrand's disease: shortening of bleeding time and induction of a variable pseudothrombocytopenia. *Thromb Haemost* 1990; **64**: 117–20.

47. Mazurier C, Gaucher C, Jorieux S, Goudemand M. Biological effect of desmopressin in eight patients with type 2N (Normandy) von Willebrand disease. *Br J Haematol* 1994; **88**: 849–54.

48. Rodeghiero F, Castaman G, Meyer D, Mannucci PM. Replacement therapy with virus-inactivated plasma concentrates in von Willebrand disease. *Vox Sang* 1992; **62**: 193–9.

49. Mannucci PM, Chediak J, Hanna W *et al*. Treatment of von Willebrand disease with a high-purity factor VIII/von Willebrand factor concentrate: a prospective, multicenter study. *Blood* 2002; **99**: 450–6.

50. Lillicrap D, Poon MC, Walker I, Xie F, Schwartz BA for the Association of Hemophilia Clinic Directors of Canada. Efficacy and safety of the factor VIII/von Willebrand factor concentrate, haemate-P/humate-P: ristocetin cofactor unit dosing in patients with von Willebrand disease. *Thromb Haemost* 2002; **87**: 224–30.

51. Mannucci PM. Venous thromboembolism in von Willebrand disease. *Thromb Haemost* 2002; **88**: 378–9.

52. Castillo R, Monteagudo J, Escolar G, Ordinas A, Magallion M, Villar JM. Hemostatic effect of normal platelet transfusion in severe von Willebrand disease patients. *Blood* 1991; **77**: 1901–5.

28 Rare congenital hemorrhagic disorders

Nigel S. Key and Margaret A. Heisel-Kurth

Introduction

The focus of this chapter is the inherited coagulation disorders associated with factor deficiency states that may produce bleeding from inadequate thrombin generation and/or inadequate inhibition of fibrinolysis. The more prevalent disorders hemophilia A and B and von Willebrand disease are discussed separately in Chapters 26 and 27, respectively. Inherited defects of platelet number or function, which may similarly present with hemorrhagic manifestations, are also addressed separately in Chapter 25.

In considering these rare factor deficiency states, a number of common themes emerge.

1 Bleeding is generally less severe than the hemophilias at an equivalent factor activity level.

2 The pattern of bleeding may have a somewhat different anatomic distribution than the hemophilias (Fig. 28.1).[1] Some types of bleeding may be characteristic of a particular deficiency state, for example postsurgical bleeding on mucosal surfaces in factor (F)XI deficiency or intracranial bleeding and impaired wound healing in FXIII deficiency.

3 The prevalence of these disorders individually is substantially lower than that of the hemophilias, and generally in the order of 1 in 500 000 to 1 in 2 million of the population (Table 28.1). Since even large hemophilia centers are unlikely to follow more than a handful of patients, only cooperative national registries and surveys can adequately address the clinical manifestations and outcomes in these patients.

4 Unlike the X-linked recessive mode of inheritance of the hemophilias, the majority of these disorders are inherited in an autosomal recessive fashion. In certain cultures where

Table 28.1 Characteristics of coagulation factors and their deficiency states.

	Chromosomal location	Molecular mass (kDa)	No. of chains (active)	Half-life	Plasma concentration (µg/mL)	No. of Gla domains	No. of described mutations	Prevalence	Hemostatic levels (% reference range)
FVII	13	50	2	4–6 h	0.5	10	>130	1 in 500 000	15–20
FX	13	59	2	40–60 h	10	11	~70	1 in 1 million	15–20
FII	11	72	2	3–4 days	100	10	~40	1 in 2 million	20–30
FV	1	330	2	36 h	10	–	~30	1 in 1 million	15–25
FV/FVIII									
ERGIC-53	18	330 (FV)	2 (FV)	36 h (FV)	10 (FV)		>15 (ERGIC)	1 in 2 million	15–20
MCFD2	2	330 (FVIII)	2 (FVIII)	10–14 h (FVIII)	0.1 (FVIII)		>5 (MCFD2)		
FXI	4	160	2	52 h	5	–	>50	1 in 1 million	15–20
FXIII (2 genes)	6 (A chain) 1 (B chain)	320	4	11–14 days	60	–	>50	1 in 2 million	2–5
Fibrinogen (3 genes)	4 (α, β, and γ chains)	340	6	2–4 days	3000	–	>300 (dysfibrinogenemia) >30 (hypofibrinogenemia)	1 in 1 million	50 mg/dL

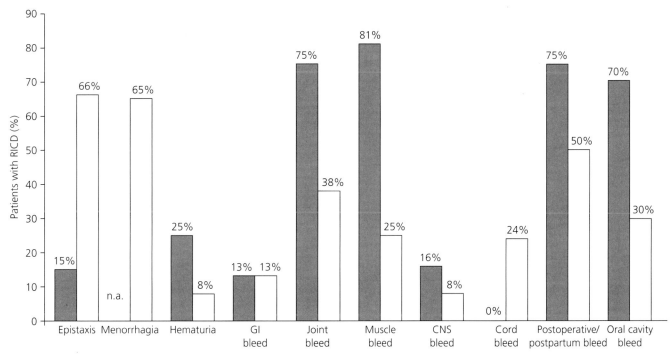

Fig. 28.1 Bleeding symptoms in patients with recessively inherited coagulation disorders (RICD) versus patients with hemophilia. Percentage of Iranian patients (*n* = 750) presumably homozygous for RICD who experienced a given bleeding symptom at least once (open bars) compared with Iranian hemophilia A patients with comparable factor VIII deficiency (<10% in plasma) (shaded bars). CNS, central nervous system; GI, gastrointestinal; n.a., not applicable. Reproduced with permission from Ref. 1.

consanguineous marriage is practiced, the prevalence may be higher. Additionally, in certain populations a founder effect for a particular genotype encoding deficiency and/or dysfunction of an individual clotting factor may account for a higher regional prevalence of that disorder, as may be the case for example with FXI deficiency.

5 The range of factor concentrates available to treat patients with rare bleeding disorders is limited, and when available is usually limited to plasma-derived products. Therefore, all patients should receive prophylactic hepatitis A and B vaccination, and all treatment decisions should be weighed against the risk of contracting blood-borne infection from fresh frozen plasma (FFP) or cryoprecipitate that have not undergone bactericidal or virucidal treatment.

6 In some disorders, a paradoxical thrombotic propensity has been identified with distinct genotypes, and occasionally a thrombotic and hemorrhagic phenotype (e.g., in certain forms of dysfibrinogenemia) may coexist.

Unlike the hemophilias, where the classification system of mild, moderate and severe cases is defined by and correlates with baseline FVIII:C or FIX:C levels, no similar categorization exists for the other rare bleeding disorders. Indeed, in some rare inherited deficiency states, such as FVII or FXI deficiency, there is rather poor correlation between plasma clotting factor activity and clinical manifestations. Thus, there is a tendency to resort to the mendelian terminology of

heterozygote for those presumed to carry one affected allele, and homozygote/compound heterozygote for those presumed to carry two affected alleles. Somewhat arbitrarily, circulating plasma activity levels of less than 20% (0.20 units/mL) for FII:C, FVII:C, FV:C, FX:C, or FXI:C are often assumed to represent homozygosity or compound heterozygosity.[2] Conversely, it may be very difficult to distinguish a heterozygote carrier from an unaffected individual on the basis of clotting factor level alone. These difficulties are compounded by the imprecision of the assay at low levels of clotting factor activity and by potential variability between assays depending on the particular reagents, as illustrated by the one-stage assay for FVII:C, where vastly different results may be seen depending on whether a human or nonhuman thromboplastin is used. Although simultaneous measurement of immunologic levels of the deficient factor in plasma may help to minimize these discrepancies, an accurate diagnosis of "heterozygote" or "homozygote" (e.g., for genetic counseling purposes) will ultimately depend on genotype analysis. Globally speaking, heterozygous carriers of these rare coagulation factor deficiency states tend to be asymptomatic and may be undetectable by routine coagulation screening assays since, as a rule, the prothrombin time (PT) and activated partial thromboplastin time (APTT) assays are prolonged only with deficiency of the constituent clotting factor activity of 30% or less of the normal reference range. Here again, however, there are some notable exceptions, such as dysfibrinogenemia, which may be clinically manifest in heterozygotes and thus by definition is considered to follow an autosomal dominant pattern of inheritance. Heterozygotes for dysfibrinogenemia may also be apparent on screening assays such as the thrombin clotting time (TCT).

Deficiency states for essentially all individual clotting factors have been created in laboratory mice using gene knockout technology. In many cases, the human phenotype is recapitulated, although there are several notable discrepancies. For example, while FV gene knockout mice (FV$^{-/-}$) do not survive to birth, the analagous defect in humans is apparently compatible with life.

Influence of developmental hemostasis on the presentation of congenital hemorrhagic disorders

A child with an inherited hemorrhagic disorder may come to medical attention in several ways. First, a positive family history may prompt the clinician to order the appropriate screening assay(s). However, since the majority of these disorders adhere to an autosomal recessive pattern of inheritance, they are much more likely than the hemophilias to present unexpectedly. A hemorrhagic event is thus a frequent mode of presentation, as is the incidental discovery of abnormal coagulation screening tests prior to a planned procedure. In the latter instance, it is important to be aware of the physiologic differences in coagulation factor levels between newborns and older infants. A number of coagulation factors are physiologically decreased at birth, and may not reach adult levels for several months or years.[3] Since coagulation proteins do not cross the placenta, fetal and newborn levels of these proteins are dependent on the fetus for synthesis. The first coagulation protein levels may be detected at 10 weeks' gestation and gradually increase with gestational age. At birth, newborns have normal adult plasma levels of fibrinogen, FV, FVIII, FXIII, and von Willebrand antigen. Essentially all the other coagulation factors, inhibitors and fibrinolytic factors are decreased at birth and variably increase in the first days and months of life to normal adult levels.[3] Administration of vitamin K in the neonatal period is critical to ensure prompt normalization of the vitamin K-dependent factors. Premature infants can be expected to have lower plasma levels of all coagulation factors compared with term newborns. The physiologic decreased synthesis associated with prematurity is frequently complicated by accelerated consumption of coagulation factors related to the postnatal complications that are so prevalent in these babies.

For all these reasons, it may be extremely difficult to determine whether there is a true inherited deficiency state in very young children with abnormal screening coagulation assays and low factor levels. This dilemma may only be resolved by repeated testing over a period of weeks or months. For a more detailed treatise on assessment of bleeding in the neonate, the reader is referred to Chapter 30.

Congenital deficiency states producing isolated prolongation of the prothrombin time

The PT measures what was formerly known as the "extrinsic" pathway of coagulation, in addition to the final common pathway. "Thromboplastin", consisting of re-lipidated full-length tissue factor (TF) apoprotein and anionic phospholipid vesicles, is added to citrated platelet-poor plasma; on recalcification, coagulation is initiated and the clotting time recorded optically or mechanically. TF binds to plasma FVIIa; this "extrinsic tenase" complex then activates both FIX and FX to initiate coagulation both *in vitro* and *in vivo*. Sequestration of TF by confinement to the surface of cells in the extravascular space is one mechanism by which the initiation of coagulation is regulated *in vivo*. Recently, however, evidence exists that very small quantities of intravascular TF may be present even in healthy subjects, where it may play a role in propagating the growth of a hemostatic plug.[4] So far, no TF deficiency states have been identified in humans.

Causes of a prolonged PT associated with a normal APTT and TCT include vitamin K deficiency, ingestion of oral anticoagulants/rodenticides that act as vitamin K antagonists, and liver disease. Once these acquired disorders have been ruled out and it has been demonstrated that a 1 : 1 mix of patient plasma and normal plasma leads to correction of the PT, FVII deficiency is a likely possibility. Acquired isolated FVII deficiency is very rare but has been reported.

Factor VII deficiency

Structure and function

The gene for FVII is located on chromosome 13. FVII zymogen is synthesized in the liver as a single polypeptide chain, and is converted to the active two-chain protease (FVIIa) as the result of cleavage of a single bond, Arg^{152}–Ile^{153}. In contrast to TF$^{-/-}$ animals, which do not survive to term due to abnormal embryonic vascular development and hemorrhage, FVII$^{-/-}$ mice develop normally *in utero*. However, intraabdominal bleeding within the first 24 hours of life leads to the demise of about half these animals, and the survivors usually succumb to intracranial bleeding shortly thereafter, with none surviving longer than 45 days.

Approximately 1% of the total FVII in plasma circulates in the active serine protease form (FVIIa, 10–100 pmol/L). Controversy still exists as to which enzyme is responsible for basal activation of FVII *in vivo*, although there is evidence implicating FIXa. In the absence of its cofactor TF, FVIIa is a very weak enzyme. Moreover, unlike other similar vitamin K-dependent serine proteases (e.g., FXa, thrombin), FVIIa is not rapidly inactivated in plasma by antithrombin, and has a circulating half-life that varies from 1.5 hours in children to 2.5 hours in adults. The relatively long half-life was a critical factor in the clinical development of recombinant (r)FVIIa for therapeutic management of bleeding in the hemophilias, and more recently in other noncoagulopathic conditions associated with excessive bleeding.

Inheritance and prevalence

FVII deficiency is inherited as an autosomal recessive disorder. Homozygotes or compound heterozygotes for approximately 130 described mutations in the FVII gene, the majority of which are missense, may manifest a bleeding tendency. Several polymorphisms in the human FVII gene may also contribute to lowering of plasma FVII:C levels. For example, homozygotes for the Arg353Gln polymorphisms are typically found to have about half-normal FVII:C levels.

Among the rare inherited hemorrhagic disorders, FVII deficiency is considered to be one of the more common, with an estimated prevalence of 1 in 300 000 to 1 in 500 000. FVII deficiency accounted for almost half of the 294 cases reported to the North American Rare Bleeding Disorders Registry.[2]

Clinical and laboratory features

There is a relatively poor correlation between FVII:C and the clinical bleeding manifestations. In general, however, individuals with FVII:C < 1% will usually manifest abnormal bleeding, although not necessarily in early life. Individuals with FVII:C > 15–20% (0.15–0.20 units/mL) are frequently asymptomatic even after surgery or trauma, indicating that the levels of FVII required to maintain hemostasis are less than for FVIII or FIX. For this reason, FVII deficiency is not uncommonly diagnosed incidentally as the result of a prolonged PT rather than because of bleeding manifestations.

For many years, it was thought that certain genotypes encoding FVII deficiency might paradoxically predispose to thrombosis, possibly through defective inhibition of the complex of TF with mutant FVIIa by the TF pathway inhibitor (TFPI). However, subsequent data from the International Registry of FVII Deficiency comprising more than 500 patients suggest that while thrombosis may occur, it is not associated with any particular genotype and is rather uncommon. The conclusion seems to be that although FVII deficiency does not necessarily predispose to thrombosis, neither does it protect affected individuals from thrombosis during times of high risk.[5]

Laboratory diagnosis of FVII deficiency is established by finding a low plasma FVII:C in a one-stage assay using FVII-deficient substrate plasma (preferably using a human thromboplastin) and/or by quantification of FVII antigen by an immunologic method such as enzyme-linked immunosorbent assay (ELISA). Both type I (CRM⁻) and type 2 (CRM⁺) variants may be encountered. In the North American registry, the median FVII:C in 49 presumed homozygotes was 0.08 units/mL. Bleeding events, 84% of which were spontaneous, were predominantly mucocutaneous (60%), followed by musculoskeletal (21%), gastrointestinal (16%) or genitourinary (3%).[2] Epistaxis and menorrhagia were particularly common.[2,5] Interestingly, these registries failed to confirm the observation reported in earlier series that neonatal intracranial hemorrhage is a common manifestation of FVII deficiency.

Treatment

Possible treatment options for bleeding in FVII-deficient patients include FFP, prothrombin complex concentrates (PCCs), plasma-derived FVII concentrates, and rFVIIa. Fibrin glues and antifibrinolytic agents may also be used for topical bleeding control and for bleeding affecting mucosal surfaces, respectively. Several plasma-derived FVII concentrates that are subjected to viral inactivation are available in Europe but not the USA.[6,7] The recommended dose is 20–40 units/kg. Virally inactivated FFP at a dose of 10 mL/kg every 6 hours is a reasonable alternative but, here again, these products are no longer available in the USA. Perhaps the most logical and attractive option is rFVIIa. The usual recommended dose is 15–25 µg/kg every 4–6 hours. Trough FVII:C levels should be maintained above 15–20% to ensure adequate hemostasis. PCCs are generally not recommended for the treatment of FVII-deficient patients, primarily because of concerns for thrombosis.[8] The development of an inhibitor to FVII as a result of treatment is a very rare occurrence, but has been described in a few patients with FVII deficiency treated with rFVIIa.

Congenital deficiency states producing isolated prolongation of the activated partial thromboplastin time

The APTT is performed by incubating the test plasma with an inert negatively charged substance (e.g., kaolin, celite, or ellagic acid) that acts as an activator for the contact system, ultimately generating FXIa. Negatively charged phospholipids, devoid of TF (i.e., "partial thromboplastin"), are then added, the sample is recalcified, and the clotting time recorded. The contact system comprises three zymogen serine proteases (FXII, prekallikrein, and FXI) and one cofactor molecule, high-molecular-weight kininogen. In plasma, FXI circulates in a complex with high-molecular-weight kininogen. The APTT is sensitive to deficiencies of all four components of the contact pathway, and to deficiencies of the components of the "intrinsic tenase" complex (i.e., FVIII and FIX). It is also sensitive to more significant deficiencies of clotting factors in the final common pathway.

The APTT may be prolonged by lupus inhibitors, auto-antibodies to a specific procoagulant (e.g., FVIII), circulating anticoagulants (e.g., heparin, low-molecular-weight heparins, direct thrombin inhibitors), and acquired causes of multiple coagulation factor deficiencies such as disseminated intra-vascular coagulation (DIC), liver disease, and oral anticoagu-lants/vitamin K deficiency. Commercial APTT reagents vary in their sensitivity to heparin, lupus inhibitors, and indi-vidual factor deficiency states. The initial evaluation of a pro-longed APTT should include a 1 : 1 mixing study. Correction during this step rules out a lupus inhibitor or circulating anticoagulant and points toward a single or multiple clotting factor deficiency state. It is imperative to correlate the results of laboratory studies with the patient's clinical manifest-ations (or lack thereof) in reaching a final diagnosis as to the cause of a prolonged APTT.

Factor XII, prekallikrein and high-molecular-weight kininogen deficiency

Deficiency of any one of these factors may be associated with an incidentally discovered prolonged APTT, but in all cases there is no associated bleeding disorder. This observation implies that these molecules must have an alternative func-tion. Indeed, the kininogens (high-and low-molecular-weight) are needed for the generation of the vasoactive peptide bradykinin. The contact activation system may also play profibrinolytic and antithrombotic roles in vascular biol-ogy. However, since they are not associated with a bleeding diathesis, further discussion of these functions is beyond the scope of this chapter.

Factor XI deficiency

Previously, the term "hemophilia C" was used to describe FXI deficiency, although this is now obsolete. It has been suggested that because some heterozygotes may experience bleeding despite seemingly adequate factor levels, the term "partial deficiency" for FXI should be used to describe these subjects.

Structure and function

FXI is a 160-kDa homodimer consisting of two 80-kDa poly-peptides connected by a single disulfide bond. Activation occurs following a single proteolytic cleavage at Arg^{369}–Ile^{370} in each chain, but FXIa remains a dimeric molecule, with each monomer comprising a heavy and a light chain. Although this activation step can be executed by FXIIa *in vitro*, it is believed that activation by thrombin on the surface of platelets is the more important physiologic mechanism *in*

vivo. FXIa activates FIX, ultimately leading to more thrombin generation. Thus, the role of FXI is to sustain thrombin forma-tion after the initiation phase of coagulation (i.e., TF–FVIIa complex formation) has been extinguished by TFPI. The high concentration of thrombin generated in this FXI-dependent manner is also necessary to activate the inhibitor known as thrombin-activated fibrinolysis inhibitor (TAFI). Activated TAFI inhibits the breakdown of fibrin clots by plasmin; thus, the second function of FXIa is antifibrinolytic.

Inheritance and prevalence

FXI deficiency is usually considered to be inherited as an autosomal recessive disorder. The gene for FXI is located on chromosome 4. Although the liver is probably the primary site of synthesis, other cells including megakaryocytes may contribute. About 50, predominantly missense, mutations in the FXI gene have been identified. The vast majority of affected individuals have a type I deficiency phenotype with concordant reduction of FXI:C and FXI:Ag; dysfunctional molecules causing a type II pattern are rather uncommon. Individuals who are homozygous or compound heterozy-gous usually have FXI:C levels that range from < 1 to 20%, whereas heterozygotes express FXI:C activities in the 20–70% range.

$FXI^{-/-}$ mice are born in the expected numbers, mature normally, and enjoy a normal lifespan. Despite the expected APTT prolongation, they do not experience spontaneous bleeding, and it is difficult to demonstrate that bleeding is excessive even after standard hemostatic challenges, such as tail transection.

FXI deficiency occurs at a frequency of about 1 per million of the general population. However, in several ethnically distinct populations, it may be found with much greater fre-quency due to a founder gene effect. Most informative among these is the Ashkenazi (European origin) Jewish population, in which the prevalence of heterozygosity for FXI deficiency is 8–9%, with a homozygote frequency of 0.2%. Although there are four well-defined "Jewish" mutations, the Jewish type II and Jewish type III mutations are the most common. Type II is a nonsense mutation (Glu117Stop) leading to a stop codon in exon 5, whereas type III is a missense mutation (Phe283Leu) in exon 9. Compound heterozygosity for type II and type III mutations is the most common genotype in severely affected individuals, and homozygosity for either type II or type III accounts for the majority of the remaining cases in this ethnic group. Type II homozygotes typically express FXI:C levels of ≤ 1%, type III homozygotes a level of ≈ 10%, and compound II/III heterozygotes a level of 3–5%. Interestingly, while the type III mutation is largely confined to Ashkenazi Jews, the type II mutation is found in both Ashkenazi and Iraqi Jews. It has been suggested that the latter mutation arose in a single ancestral population, probably in the era between the 6th century BC and the 1st century AD, whereas the type III mutation probably arose no earlier than the 15th century AD.[9] Other founder mutations have been described in French Basques and in England.

Clinical and laboratory features

It has been repeatedly recognized that there is a lack of correlation between FXI:C levels and the severity of bleeding manifestations, with many mildly deficient patients exhibiting as many symptoms as severely deficient patients. This may be explained by (i) the coexistence of phenotypic modifiers of the bleeding tendency such as von Willebrand disease; (ii) the presence of small quantities of FXI synthesized in platelets; or (iii) the fact that FXI:C assays based on the APTT may be insensitive to the other functions of FXI, such as in fibrinolysis. That being said, FXI deficiency leads to injury-related bleeding in most patients with severe deficiency and in about half of patients with a partial deficiency. Surgery or injury at sites with high fibrinolytic activity, including the oropharynx, nasal cavity and urinary tract, are particularly likely to be complicated by bleeding. It has been estimated that about 70% of FXI-deficient patients (~90% with severe deficiency and ~60% with partial deficiency) will experience excessive bleeding after tonsillectomy in the absence of prophylactic therapy.[10] This observation is probably explained by a partial or complete absence of the antifibrinolytic contribution of FXI described above. Unlike the hemophilias, spontaneous bleeding such as hemarthrosis and intramuscular hemorrhage are uncommon, although affected women (of any severity) may experience menorrhagia. However, the risk of maternal bleeding during vaginal delivery may not be invariable, and it may be reasonable to withhold prophylactic plasma replacement therapy unless bleeding occurs. Acquired autoantibodies causing FXI deficiency are very rare but have been described and should also be considered in the differential diagnosis.

Patients with previously recognized FXI deficiency may present with bleeding after surgery or injury, associated with a prolonged APTT that corrects on mixing with normal plasma. In this situation, one-stage assays for FVIII:C and FIX:C will usually be indicated in addition to FXI:C, but the likelihood of FXI deficiency is increased in a patient of Ashkenazi Jewish ancestry, and when bleeding is from the oropharynx, nose, or urogenital tract following surgery. Increasingly, however, the diagnosis of FXI deficiency is made on an asymptomatic individual with a prolonged APTT. In areas with a high Ashkenazi Jewish population, routine preoperative screening using the APTT has been advocated.

Until recently, little was known about the epidemiology of inhibitor formation in FXI deficiency. However, among Ashkenazi Jews, one-third of patients homozygous for the type II (Glu117stop) mutation developed FXI inhibitors following treatment with plasma, whereas no inhibitors were identified in patients with other genotypes.[11]

Treatment

One implication of the lack of correlation of FXI:C levels with bleeding tendency is that prophylactic hemostatic therapy is indicated for invasive procedures in the majority of patients, especially if these procedures involve an anatomic site with a high intrinsic fibrinolytic potential. Against this has to be balanced the risk of inhibitor formation in patients known to be homozygous for the Glu117Stop mutation, where plasma products should be used judiciously to minimize the risk of inhibitor formation.[11]

Currently available options for raising plasma FXI levels include FFP (preferably a virally inactivated product) and FXI concentrates, two of which are manufactured in Europe but not available in the USA.[6,7] A reasonable target FXI:C for surgery is > 30% for minor procedures and > 45% for more invasive procedures. This may entail the administration of quite large volumes of FFP. These guidelines may have to be adjusted according to a given individual's history of bleeding propensity with surgery. Of note, FXI concentrates, while offering the advantage of a lesser risk of viral transmission, have been associated with arterial and venous thrombosis and DIC, particularly when given at doses greater than the recommended maximum of 30 units/kg, and to elderly patients.

Antifibrinolytic agents such as ε-aminocaproic acid and tranexamic acid are excellent choices for dental work and other mucosal surface procedures, either administered alone or in combination with FFP. As always, however, antifibrinolytic agents should be avoided when bleeding originates from the upper urinary tract. Similarly, there may be a role for topical fibrin administered at the time of surgery. Finally, there have been anecdotal reports of the successful use of rFVIIa to control bleeding in FXI-deficient patients who have developed inhibitors to FXI.

Congenital deficiency states affecting the final common pathway of coagulation

The final common pathway of coagulation begins with the enzymatic conversion of FX to FXa, either via the intrinsic tenase complex, consisting of FIXa and its cofactor FVIIIa, or via the extrinsic tenase complex, comprising FVIIa and TF. During physiologic hemostasis, the initial activation of FX is mediated by the TF–FVIIa complex. After this burst of FXa formation has been extinguished by TFPI, further propagation of coagulation via additional FX activation is dependent on the intrinsic tenase (FIXa–FVIIIa) complex. Thereafter, activated FX, in association with its cofactor FVa, forms the "prothrombinase complex" which proteolytically cleaves and activates prothrombin to thrombin. All these enzymatic reactions depend on the presence of a suitable anionic phospholipid surface, generally provided by the activated platelet membrane, and on calcium. Thrombin has many important functions in hemostasis, including platelet activation, feedback activation of FV, FVIII and FXI, and activation of fibrinogen and FXIII.

The TCT is the simplest of the coagulation screening assays. Excess human or bovine thrombin is added to citrated platelet-poor plasma in order to convert fibrinogen to fibrin, and the clotting time is recorded. Notably this reaction is neither phospholipid nor calcium dependent. Possible causes of a prolonged TCT include congenital or acquired quantitative or qualitative fibrinogen disorders (afibrinogenemia, hypofibrinogenemia, or dysfibrinogenemia), direct and indirect thrombin inhibitors (including heparin), acquired inhibitory antibodies to thrombin, and inhibition of fibrin polymerization by monoclonal immunoglobulin or light chains or fibrin degradation products. Notably, vitamin K antagonists and lupus inhibitors do not influence the TCT.

Screening laboratory evaluation in deficiencies affecting the final common pathway will therefore be reflected by a prolonged PT and APTT but normal TCT (FX, FV, prothrombin deficiency), or by a prolonged PT, APTT and TCT (quantitative or qualitative fibrinogen defects). The Russell viper venom time (RVVT) is a useful adjunctive assay in this situation. Russell viper venom is a metalloproteinase found in the venom of *Vipera russelli* that enzymatically activates FX in a phospholipid and Ca^{2+}-dependent fashion. Therefore, the RVVT is prolonged in deficiencies affecting all the final common pathway factors (fibrinogen, prothrombin, FV, FX) but is normal in deficiencies of contact factors (FXII, FXI, prekallikrein, high-molecular-weight kininogen) or factors in the intrinsic (FVIII/FIX) or extrinsic (FVII) tenase complexes.

Factor X deficiency

Structure and function

FX is synthesized in the liver as a 59-kDa two-chain zymogen. Posttranslational modifications include vitamin K-dependent γ-carboxylation of 11 Glu residues in the membrane-binding (Gla) region of the light chain. Like other vitamin K-dependent factors, this step is essential for full procoagulant function and may be inhibited by oral anticoagulants, in dietary vitamin K deficiency, or in hemorrhagic disease of the newborn. The gene for FX is located on the long arm of chromosome 13, close to that for FVII.

Both the extrinsic and intrinsic tenase complexes activate FX by cleavage of the Arg^{194}–Ile^{195} bond, concurrently releasing an activation peptide of 52 amino acids from the heavy chain. The primary substrate for FXa is prothrombin, but activation of FV, FVIII, and FVII may also be partially dependent on FXa generation *in vivo*.

Approximately 30% of $FX^{-/-}$ embryos die *in utero* in midgestation. Although the remaining animals are born alive, they die in the perinatal period from intraabdominal bleeding or in the neonatal period from intracranial hemorrhage. Thus, complete FX deficiency does not appear to be compatible with survival into adulthood.

Inheritance and prevalence

FX deficiency is inherited in an autosomal recessive fashion, and affects about 1 per million of the population. Heterozygotes are generally asymptomatic. About one-third of affected individuals exhibit a type 1 deficiency, while the rest have a type 2 pattern, with FX:Ag levels that are preserved or at least significantly above the level of FX:C. This finding is explained by the fact that missense mutations, frequently affecting the catalytic domain, tend to predominate. Although a small number of mutations leading to stop codons have been identified, nonsense mutations are not reported, suggesting that like the murine model a total absence of FX may be incompatible with life. Perhaps for the same reason, the development of an alloantibody inhibitor to FX as a result of exposure to FX concentrates or plasma has not been reported.

Clinical and laboratory features

Patients with severe FX deficiency tend be among the most, if not the most, severely affected of the rare coagulation deficiency states. In the Iranian series of 32 patients, 18 had "severe" disease (FX:C <1%), nine had "moderate" disease (FX:C 1–5%), and five had "mild" disease (FX:C 6–10%).[12] Mucosal bleeding, especially epistaxis, was prevalent (72% of the entire cohort). Menorrhagia occurred in about 50% of affected women, and gastrointestinal bleeding was reported by about two-thirds of patients with severe disease. Umbilical cord bleeding, typically occurring at 7–10 days after birth, was reported in about 30%, predominantly in patients with severe disease. Central nervous system (CNS) bleeding was reported in about 10%. Unlike many of the other rare factor deficiency states, hemarthroses and muscle hematomas were relatively common (~75%) in those with moderate or severe disease, and in this respect the disorder is more similar to the hemophilias. In the North American Registry, the type of bleeding manifestations were similar, although patients were defined as "homozygotes" when FX:C was < 20% (in fact, more than half of these had a FX:C of <1%, and the median for the whole group was 13%).[2] This registry did emphasize that 80% of bleeding episodes were spontaneous rather than traumatic in origin. Women with severe FX deficiency may experience recurrent miscarriage, and uterine bleeding and premature labor during pregnancy, but successful outcomes are also reported.

The major differential diagnosis of isolated FX deficiency is an acquired deficiency occurring as a complication of AL (light chain) amyloidosis. This interesting association appears to be explained by adsorption of FX to amyloid fibrils, and is described in 10–15% of patients with this disorder. Bleeding may be severe but generally responds to splenectomy. While very rare, acquired inhibitors to FX have been described, often as a complication of a respiratory infection. Here again, bleeding complications may be severe.

Laboratory evaluation in patients with FX deficiency reveals prolongation of PT, APTT, and RVVT, all of which correct on mixing. The TCT is normal. In addition to functional clotting assays, it is recommended that an immunologic assay for FX be performed to distinguish type 1 and type 2 deficiency states.

Treatment

Treatment options for patients with FX deficiency include FFP or PCC; there is no purified FX concentrate. FFP can be administered at a dose of 10–15 mL/kg, followed by 5–10 mL/kg every 24 hours, monitoring trough FX:C levels. Nonactivated PCCs (for specific products see ref. 7) may be preferable to activated PCCs that contain both FX and FXa, but are more expensive. The target FX:C for hemostasis is generally 15–20% and because of the exceptionally long half-life of FX (40–60 hours), alternate-day treatment may be adequate. The FX content of PCCs is variable but generally in the range 50–150 units per 100 units of FIX;[6] 1 unit/kg of FX is expected to elevate FX:C by about 1.5%. Perhaps somewhat surprising from a mechanistic standpoint, rFVIIa has been shown to be effective in anecdotal cases of bleeding in acquired FX deficiency. Particularly for mucosal bleeds, antifibrinolytic agents, alone or in combination with FFP, may be useful, although their use with PCCs is discouraged due to increased thrombotic risk. Fibrin glues are a reasonable option for topical bleeding in a temporarily dry field.

Factor V deficiency

Structure and function

FV is a pro-cofactor that circulates in plasma at a concentration of 20 nmol/L (10 µg/mL). FV is a large molecule (330 kDa) that shares significant structural homology with FVIII and ceruloplasmin. The FV gene is located on chromosome 1, and FV is principally synthesized by hepatocytes. About 20% of the total FV in blood is stored in α-granules of platelets. Platelet-associated FV is both synthesized in megakaryocytes and taken up from plasma by megakaryocytes. On activation by thrombin, FVa (consisting of heavy and light chains) functions as the cofactor for FXa in the membrane-bound prothrombinase complex. FVa is inactivated by activated protein C in the presence of its cofactor, protein S. This inactivation process is slowed by the substitution of Glu for Arg^{506} in the FVa molecule, known as the FV Leiden mutation, which leads to a prevalent thrombophilic phenotype in Caucasian populations.

Deletion of the FV gene in knockout mice is incompatible with life. About half of $FV^{-/-}$ embryos die *in utero* as a result of an abnormality in the yolk sac vasculature, while the remainder die from massive neonatal hemorrhage. In humans, however, FV:C levels <1% appear to be compatible with survival into adulthood. It has been argued that there may be residual trace amounts of functional FV in severely affected individuals, although major homozygous deletions affecting large portions of the FV molecule have been described. Overall, it remains unresolved whether complete FV deficiency is compatible with survival in humans.

Inheritance and prevalence

Factor V deficiency is a rare autosomal recessive disorder that affects about 1 per million of the population. The number of described discrete mutations underlying FV deficiency is still relatively small (in the order of 30), and no founder mutations have been described. About three-quarters of affected patients have a type 1 deficiency.

Clinical and laboratory features

Severe FV deficiency (formerly referred to as "parahemophilia") is a moderately severe bleeding disorder that, like most of the recessively inherited deficiencies, is not associated with as much musculoskeletal morbidity as severe hemophilia A or B. Bleeding events are frequently spontaneous. Homozygotes generally manifest very low FV:C levels, usually < 5% and frequently < 1%. Heterozygotes will generally have FV:C levels in the range 20–55%.[2]

In the Iranian series of 35 patients with FV:C levels between 1 and 10%, mucocutaneous bleeding events were the most frequent complication, with epistaxis, menorrhagia and oropharyngeal bleeding in 50–60%.[13] Postoperative and postpartum bleeding were reported by about 40%, while hemarthrosis and muscle hematomas were reported by 25–30% of subjects. CNS bleeding was recorded in only two patients (6%) and gastrointestinal, genitourinary, and umbilical cord bleeding were quite uncommon, occurring in < 10%.[13] A very similar distribution of bleeding was reported in 37 patients with FV deficiency in the North American Registry.[2] A recent series describing the outcome of pregnancy in five homozygous and 17 heterozygous females with FV deficiency reported that significant postpartum bleeding requiring FFP was relatively common in the severely affected, but not in the heterozygous carriers. Fetal outcomes were generally excellent.[14] Oral contraceptives were beneficial in modulating the severity of menorrhagia in affected homozygous women.

Inhibitors to FV may occur in FV-deficient patients who have been exposed to FFP. In the North American Registry, an inhibitor was reported in 1 of 37 (3%) subjects.[2] Distinct from the entity of acquired alloantibodies to FV in patients with severe inherited deficiency is acquired FV deficiency due to an acquired autoantibody to FV in previously normal individuals. The incidence of these antibodies may be underappreciated. Classically, development of these inhibitors has been linked to exposure to topical bovine thrombin contaminated by immunogenic bovine FV, usually following cardiac surgery, and particularly when there have been multiple or recurrent exposures. The resulting cross-reactive anti-human FV inhibitory antibodies may be associated with anti-bovine prothrombin, thrombin, and/or FV inhibitors. However, they may also develop after surgery in the absence of topical thrombin exposure, with underlying malignancy, or with no identifiable precipitating factors. Although very rare in children, acquired FV autoantibodies have been described and should be considered in the differential diagnosis of inherited deficiency.

Laboratory evaluation of FV deficiency reveals prolongation of both APTT and PT but normal TCT. The RVVT is also prolonged. In the absence of a FV inhibitor, mixing studies with normal plasma demonstrate full correction. One-stage clotting assays and immunoassays demonstrate reduction in FV:C and FV:Ag, respectively. It is important to be aware of the entity of combined FV and FVIII deficiency (see below). In these patients, both FV:C and FVIII:C are typically in the 5–20% range. Therefore, it is worthwhile to consider measuring the FVIII:C level to rule out this disorder.

Treatment

No FV concentrate is available. Therefore, FFP 15–20 mL/kg is usually recommended for treatment of bleeding or surgical prophylaxis, followed by 5 mL/kg every 12–24 hours.[6] The target FV:C for hemostasis is 15–25%. Antifibrinolytic agents may be used alone or with FFP if needed for mucocutaneous bleeding episodes, such as nosebleeds. Platelet transfusions may be used as a source of FV, and may be particularly useful in patients with FV inhibitors, in whom soluble FV may be rapidly inactivated.

Prothrombin (factor II) deficiency

Structure and function

Prothrombin is a 72-kDa protein containing 10 γ-carboxyglutamic acid residues that is synthesized in the liver and in very small amounts in the brain. Activation of prothrombin by FXa results in the cleavage of two peptide bonds (after residues 271 and 320), with release of thrombin from the amino-terminal membrane-binding portion of the molecule that remains attached to the cell. Thrombin may then activate fibrinogen, FV, FVIII, FXI, FXIII, TAFI and platelets. Recently, it was demonstrated that thrombin also has a myriad of functions in inflammation, vascular reactivity, cell mitogenesis, and tissue repair mediated through a family of transmembrane protease-activated receptors expressed on platelets, leukocytes, endothelial cells, and smooth muscle cells.[15] Finally, thrombin, once bound to the endothelial cofactor thrombomodulin, loses its procoagulant activity and instead becomes an anticoagulant via activation of zymogen protein C.

The gene encoding prothrombin is on chromosome 11. The majority of FII$^{-/-}$ mice die *in utero*, and the few surviving to term die very shortly after birth from hemorrhage into the abdominal cavity and elsewhere.

Inheritance and prevalence

Prothrombin deficiency is very rare, occurring at an estimated frequency of 1 per 2 million of the population. Two major phenotypes can be defined by measurement of FII:C and FII:Ag levels. Firstly, the type 1 deficiency, with concomitantly reduced activity and antigen levels, is usually referred to as hypoprothrombinemia, whereas type 2 deficiency, characterized by reduced activity with normal to borderline low antigen, is known as dysprothrombinemia.[16] However, like FX deficiency, no individuals with a complete FII deficiency have been described, consistent with the murine model suggesting that total prothrombin deficiency is incompatible with life.

Like most of the rare coagulation factor deficiencies, patients with more severe deficiencies of prothrombin are either homozygous for a particular mutation or compound heterozygous for two distinct mutations. Patients who are compound heterozygotes for hypoprothrombinemia and dysprothrombinemia are also described. Mutation homozygosity tends to be more common in the offspring of consanguineous marriages and/or when there is a founder effect in a remote or isolated population.

Clinical and laboratory features

In the North American Registry, 10 subjects who were presumed to be "homozygous" for prothrombin deficiency were described.[2] Median FII:C was 3%, with a range from < 1 to 18%. Whether these patients had a type 1 or type 2 phenotype was not described. Parenthetically, other authorities consider that FII:C and FII:Ag levels should be < 10% in patients who are homozygotes/compound heterozygotes for hypoprothrombinemia, and that FII:C levels should be in the range 1–20% for homozygotes/compound heterozygotes for dysprothrombinemia.[16] The North American Registry reported that 60% of bleeding events were unprovoked, with mucocutaneous sites (40%) and hemarthroses/muscle hematomas (26%) being approximately equally represented.[2] Intracranial bleeds were recorded in 20% of those with FII:C levels < 1%, although numbers were small. The propensity of prothrombin-deficient patients to develop musculoskeletal hemorrhage was also reported in the Italian/Iranian series[17] and in an earlier summary of reported cases.[16] Both series also noted that severe umbilical cord bleeding may occur, often as a presenting feature.

Bleeding manifestations may occur in less severely affected individuals. Mucocutaneous hemorrhage was experienced by 83% of presumed heterozygotes (median FII:C of 25%, range 21–35%).[2]

Laboratory evaluation reveals prolongation of the PT, APTT and RVVT with a normal TCT. The abnormal screening tests may in fact be relatively modestly prolonged compared with FV or FX deficiency of the same degree. The *Echis carinatus* assay utilizes the venom from the saw-scaled viper to activate prothrombin in a FV- and phospholipid-independent manner. It is abnormal in hypoprothrombinemia and in the majority of dysprothrombinemias. A one-stage clotting assay and immunologic prothrombin assay should be performed to establish the diagnosis, and to distinguish hypoprothrombinemia and dysprothrombinemia.

The principal condition to be considered in the differential diagnosis of congenital prothrombin deficiency is the (acquired) lupus anticoagulant–hypoprothrombinemia syndrome. In this disorder, patients (particularly children) may present with acute bleeding manifestations, frequently mucocutaneous, following a viral infection. The PT, APTT, and RVVT are prolonged and the APTT does not correct on mixing, with further evaluation revealing the presence of a lupus anticoagulant. However, since lupus anticoagulants are generally not associated with hemorrhagic manifestations *per se*, the clinician should measure factor activity levels, which will demonstrate an isolated prothrombin deficiency that is occasionally very profound. Both FII:C and FII:Ag are equally reduced. These prothrombin autoantibodies both possess lupus anticoagulant activity and lead to accelerated clearance of prothrombin *in vivo*. However, since they are nonneutralizing *in vitro*, a quantitative Bethesda inhibitor assay is usually uninformative. Most patients spontaneously improve over several weeks, but occasionally intervention with immunosuppressives (e.g., steroids and/or immunoglobulin) or hemostatic agents (e.g., PCC with or without plasma exchange) may be required.

Treatment

There is no purified prothrombin concentrate, but FFP or PCC are suitable alternatives. The hemostatic level of FII:C is probably somewhat higher than FVII or FX, and a target of 30% is appropriate for most situations. Like FX, prothrombin has a long half-life in plasma so that after an initial loading dose, daily or even alternate-day dosing is sufficient. As a guideline, it can be assumed that the prothrombin content in PCC is about 1 unit per unit of FIX, and that 1 unit/kg of prothrombin will raise the FII:C level by 1%.[8]

Fibrinogen abnormalities

Structure and function

Fibrinogen (sometimes referred to in older literature as "factor 1") circulates in plasma as a 340-kDa homodimer. It is also found in platelet α-granules. Each fibrinogen monomer consists of three structurally distinct polypeptides, known as the Aα, Bβ, and γ chains. Although a separate gene codes for each polypeptide, all three genes are located in close proximity on chromosome 4. All three peptides are synthesized in the liver and, to a lesser extent, megakaryocytes.

Thrombin cleaves and releases fibrinopeptides A and B from the Aα and Bβ chains respectively. The fibrin monomers so formed can then begin to polymerize to form an insoluble fibrin gel. Finally, fibrin polymers are stabilized by FXIIIa-mediated cross-linking of fibers. The TCT detects fibrin polymerization well before the onset of action of FXIIIa; therefore the TCT is normal in patients with FXIII deficiency. Fibrinogen has another important function in hemostasis, namely to act as the cross-linking ligand for glycoprotein IIb–IIIa on activated platelets during aggregation.

Mice lacking the Aα chain of fibrinogen (Fib$^{-/-}$) are unable to assemble functional fibrinogen molecules and are phenotypically afibrinogenemic with markedly abnormal clotting studies, yet they survive to adulthood. This observation is likely explained by a degree of inherent redundancy in this arm of the hemostatic system, whereby other ligands, such as von Willebrand factor, are able to substitute for fibrinogen in platelet adhesion and aggregation. It is furthermore presumed that thrombin-dependent activation of platelets to form platelet-rich hemostatic plugs can compensate for the lack of fibrin formation *in vivo*. It has been shown that the sequence of cellular infiltration into wounds is abnormal in Fib$^{-/-}$ mice, and the tensile strength of wounds is diminished, even though wound healing does ultimately occur.

Inheritance and prevalence

Afibrinogenemia is inherited in an autosomal recessive manner with an estimated prevalence of about 1 per million. In humans, the vast majority of afibrinogenemic patients have been found to have truncating mutations in the gene for the fibrinogen α-chain. Hypofibrinogenemia and dysfibrinogenemia represent heterozygous carrier states and therefore may be inherited from generation to generation in the absence of consanguinity. Only a few patients with dysfibrinogenemia are homozygotes. Genetic mutations leading to dysfibrinogenemia result in alterations of fibrinopeptide release, fibrin polymerization, fibrin cross-linking, or resistance to plasmin digestion during fibrinolysis.[18] The latter mutations tend to be associated with a thrombotic phenotype, as expected. As an example of the complexity of the dysfibrinogenemias, some mutations can result in the formation of abnormal fibrin (leading to bleeding) while at the same time rendering the fibrin resistant to fibrinolysis (leading to thrombosis). In all, more than 300 mutations accounting for dysfibrinogenemia have been described.

Clinical and laboratory features

Although perhaps representing a continuum with hypofibrinogenemia from a clinical standpoint, afibrinogenemia is usually defined as a condition in which plasma fibrinogen levels are undetectable both by a functional assay (most commonly the Clauss method) and an immunoreactive assay. The sensitivity of these assays is generally in the order of 5–10 mg/dL. However, in the North American Registry, afibrinogenemia was defined as fibrinogen activity < 50 mg/dL.[2] Hypofibrinogenemia refers to a disorder in which there is a quantitative reduction in the amount of circulating fibrinogen, below the usual reference range of 150–350 mg/dL. As alluded to above, however, there may be overlapping definitions of patients with fibrinogen levels in the range 5–50 mg/dL, depending on the study. In hypofibrinogenemia, there is a parallel reduction in functional and immunoreactive fibrinogen levels, whereas dysfibrinogenemia refers to the presence of abnormal fibrinogen molecules in the circulation. In this disorder, the functional (Clauss) fibrinogen level is generally significantly lower than the fibrinogen antigen level. If the antigen level is itself below the normal range, the terminology "hypodysfibrinogenemia" has been used by some authors. Also, in contrast to the other rare inherited coagulation disorders, dysfibrinogenemia is considered to be inherited in an autosomal dominant fashion.

In afibrinogenemia, all routine screening assays (PT, APTT, RVVT and TCT) are abnormally prolonged. In hypofibrinogenemia, the PT is usually more likely to be prolonged than the APTT, but the TCT and reptilase time are generally the most sensitive screening assays. Reptilase (batroxobin) is a snake venom from the South American pit viper *Bothrops atrox*. It converts fibrinogen to fibrin but, unlike thrombin, it only cleaves and releases fibrinopeptide A, and is insensitive to the presence of heparin, heparin-like compounds or direct thrombin inhibitors in the test sample. This property can be exploited to distinguish contaminating anticoagulants from a true fibrinogen abnormality, since only in the latter instance will the reptilase time be prolonged.

Platelet aggregation studies using standard reagents may be abnormal in patients with severe reductions in plasma fibrinogen. This is explained by insufficient cross-linking of aggregating platelets *in vitro*. It is likely, however, that other ligands such as von Willebrand factor are capable of substituting for fibrinogen in this role *in vivo*.

Patients with afibrinogenemia, who are genetically homozygous or compound heterozygous for mutations in one or more fibrinogen chains, tend to have more severe manifestations than hypofibrinogenemic individuals, many of whom are asymptomatic unless subjected to trauma or surgery.[2] Overall, like Fib$^{-/-}$ mice, afibrinogenemic humans experience a bleeding disorder that is significantly milder than severe hemophilia. In the Iranian series of 55 patients with afibrinogenemia,[19] bleeding from the umbilical cord was found to be the most common site of hemorrhage (85%), followed by muscle hematomas, epistaxis, menorrhagia, and oral cavity bleeding (all ~70%). Hemarthrosis occurred in 54%, while CNS bleeds occurred in 10%. Gastrointestinal and genitourinary bleeding was notably absent. Hemorrhagic corpus luteal cysts and recurrent abortion are relatively frequent in afibrinogenemic women, and placental abruption may be a problem even if implantation has been successful. Thrombotic episodes, a recurring observation in several studies of afibrinogenemia, were recorded in only 4% of patients in the Iranian series.[19] Thromboses may occur independently of fibrinogen replacement therapy. It has been postulated that the lack of a "fibrin sink" for thrombin clearance leads to high circulating thrombin and a tendency to induce thrombosis via platelet activation.

The clinical manifestations of dysfibrinogenemia are protean and frequently difficult to predict. About half of affected individuals remain asymptomatic while one-quarter develop thrombotic manifestations, and the remainder have a tendency to bleed abnormally.[18] Both arterial and venous thrombotic events have been reported in dysfibrinogenemia. In yet other patients, bleeding and thrombosis can both occur at different times. To some extent, genotyping of the mutation in a specialized facility can assist in predicting the clinical phenotype, if the patient presents incidentally.[18] If, on the other hand, the patient has come to attention because of a clinical history of bleeding or thrombosis, it is likely that their future risk with surgery will be somewhat easier to predict, and will dictate the need for appropriate hemostatic or antithrombotic prophylaxis.

The differential diagnosis of inherited fibrinogen abnormalities include acquired forms of hypofibrinogenemia and dysfibrinogenemia, as well as other causes of a prolonged TCT that have already been discussed. The most frequent causes of acquired hypofibrinogenemia or dysfibrinogenemia include DIC and advanced liver disease or hepatocellular carcinoma, where hypersialylated forms of fibrinogen may produce a dysfunctional molecule. Rarely, a primary hyperfibrino(geno)lytic state may produce significant hypofibrinogenemia in the absence of other markers of DIC, such as thrombocytopenia or reduction of circulating antithrombin levels. Certain drugs, such as asparaginase, may also lead to hypofibrinogenemia.

Treatment

The mainstays of treatment or prophylaxis for bleeding in the fibrinogen defects are cryoprecipitate and antifibrinolytic agents. In some countries, virally inactivated plasma-derived fibrinogen concentrates are available.[6,7] The target plasma level for fibrinogen should be > 100 mg/dL until hemostasis is achieved, then 50 mg/dL until wound healing is complete. In an average-sized adult, one bag of cryoprecipitate, which contains about 250 mg of fibrinogen, is expected to raise the fibrinogen level by 6–8 mg/dL, with a half-life of 2–4 days in the absence of accelerated consumption. In the case of a dysfibrinogenemia associated with excessive bleeding, one strategy is to raise the fibrinogen level by at least 100 mg/dL over baseline.[8] Longer-term prophylaxis may be reasonable in certain situations, for example in a patient who has suffered an intracranial hemorrhage, targeting a fibrinogen level > 50 mg/dL. Similarly, in a pregnant woman with afibrinogenemia who has suffered multiple miscarriages, maintenance of a trough fibrinogen level > 50 mg/dL throughout pregnancy, increasing to > 100 mg/dL at the time of delivery, may improve the outcome.

Antifibrinolytic agents are a logical adjunct for bleeding associated with hypofibrinogenemic states, but are probably best avoided in dysfibrinogenemias associated with thrombosis. Fibrin glues may be useful for control of topical hemorrhage if a temporarily dry wound can be secured to allow their application.

Multiple congenital deficiency states

Apart from the chance occurrence of two inherited factor deficiency states that may occur sporadically, there are some disorders resulting from a single gene defect that may manifest as deficiency of more than one clotting factor. These include combined FV and FVIII deficiency, and deficiency of all the vitamin K-dependent factors.

Combined FV and FVIII deficiency

Structure and function

Combined FV and FVIII deficiency is a fascinating disorder for which the molecular basis has only been recently elucidated. Most affected subjects have a mutation in the gene for endoplasmic reticulum golgi intermediate compartment (ERGIC)-53, a protein that facilitates cellular export of certain glycosylated proteins (including FV and FVIII) from the endoplasmic reticulum during their synthesis. The gene for ERGIC-53 (also known as LMAN-1) is located on chromosome 18. A second defect accounts for about one-third of cases; here the defective protein is called MCFD2, the gene for which is on chromosome 2.

Inheritance and prevalence

This disorder is inherited in an autosomal recessive fashion, and is primarily found in Jews of Sephardic and Middle Eastern origin in Israel and in other countries in which consanguinity is common. Approximately 150 cases are described in the literature.

Clinical and laboratory features

In 27 Iranian patients with combined FV and FVIII deficiency, epistaxis, menorrhagia and postsurgical bleeding were the most common manifestations, but occasional hemarthroses and muscle hematomas were described.[20] Typically, both PT and APTT are prolonged, and correct on mixing. Plasma levels of FV:C and FVIII:C are usually in the range 5–30%, with antigen levels equivalently reduced. Heterozygotes generally have normal, or very slightly reduced, plasma levels of FV:C and FVIII:C, and are asymptomatic.

Treatment

Although FVIII concentrates are widely available, there is no FV concentrate. Therefore, some combination of FFP and FVIII concentrate is probably the most logical approach to bleeding in these patients.

Combined deficiency of all vitamin K-dependent factors

Structure and function

Combined inherited deficiency of vitamin K-dependent FII, FVII, FIX, FX, protein C and protein S is a very rare bleeding disorder. Mutations in the γ-glutamyl carboxylase (γ-GC) enzyme lead to impaired posttranslational γ-carboxylation of glutamic acid residues in the Ca^{2+}-dependent membrane-binding (Gla) domain of these proteins. The gene encoding γ-GC is located on chromosome 2. Alternatively, combined deficiency of these zymogens may result from inherited deficiency of vitamin K epoxide reductase (VKOR), a microsomal enzyme responsible for recycling the oxidized form of the cofactor for γ-GC (vitamin K epoxide).

Not surprisingly, $γ-GC^{-/-}$ mice do not survive, and manifest skeletal abnormalities, reflecting the fact that some bone proteins such as osteocalcin and matrix Gla-protein also depend on vitamin K-dependent posttranslational modification.

Inheritance and prevalence

This combined deficiency state is inherited in an autosomal recessive fashion. It is very rare, with less than 20 affected families described.

Clinical and laboratory features

The severity of the factor deficiencies in a given kindred is quite variable. Some homozygotes exhibit coagulation factor activities of < 5%, whereas others range from 20 to 60%. Heterozygotes are generally asymptomatic. Umbilical cord hemorrhage and CNS bleeding may occur as the presenting features in severely deficient subjects. Mucocutaneous hemorrhage and hemarthroses are described. In some pedigrees with severe factor deficiencies there are associated skeletal deformities, including nasal hypoplasia and defective bone ossification. Laboratory studies reveal marked prolongation of PT, APTT, and RVVT with correction on mixing. One-stage clotting assays for all the vitamin K-dependent factors are low, with modest if any reduction of antigen levels. Since VKOR is one of the pharmacologic targets of coumarins, it is important to rule out intentional or unintentional poisoning by these agents, or severe vitamin K deficiency. Evaluation of the subject's parents may be useful in demonstrating partial (heterozygous) deficiency.

Treatment

In some families, high-dose oral vitamin K may partially or even completely correct coagulation factor levels in individuals with mild or moderate deficiencies. If this is the case, long-term use may be needed. In the absence of correction, FFP or PCC may be administered either on demand for bleeding, or prophylactically several times weekly.

Congenital deficiency states not associated with any abnormality in screening coagulation assays

Factor XIII deficiency

Structure and function

FXIII is a zymogen that is activated by thrombin in the presence of Ca^{2+}. FXIIIa is a transglutaminase that cross-links α- and γ-fibrin chains through γ-glutamyl-ϵ-lysine bonds. Cross-linked fibrin forms a more stable clot that is more resistant to fibrinolysis. By covalently attaching α_2-plasmin inhibitor (also called α_2-antiplasmin) to the fibrin clot, FXIIIa further enhances resistance to fibrinolysis.

FXIII is composed of two enzymatically active A subunits (encoded on chromosome 6) and two carrier B subunits (encoded on chromosome 1). The molecular mass of the heterotetrameric A_2B_2 entity is 320 kDa. FXIII-A is synthesized in megakaryocytes, monocytes, and macrophages, whereas FXIII-B is synthesized in hepatocytes. Activation of A chains by thrombin follows proteolytic cleavage of the Arg^{37}–Gly^{38} bond.

FXIII-A$^{-/-}$ mice are normal at birth and mature to adulthood, although there is gradual attrition due to death from hemoperitoneum, hemothorax, and massive subcutaneous hemorrhage. Pregnant females die in gestation due to massive uterine bleeding in mid-pregnancy.

Inheritance and prevalence

FXIII deficiency is inherited as an autosomal recessive disorder with a prevalence of less than 1 per 2 million of the population. Most patients are homozygous for FXIII-A deficiency, and always with a type 1 deficiency state, with concomitantly low FXIII:C and FXIII-A:Ag levels. Bleeding is unusual in individuals with FXIII:C > 5%.

Clinical and laboratory features

The diagnosis of FXIII deficiency is suggested by characteristic clinical features, especially umbilical cord bleeding, a family history of consanguinity, and normal screening coagulation studies, including PT, APTT, and TCT.

Umbilical cord bleeding occurring a few days after birth is a common mode of presentation (~ 80%), as is bleeding at circumcision. Ecchymoses occur in about 50% and CNS bleeding in 20–30%, frequently at a very early age. About 25% of patients with FXIII deficiency manifest defective wound healing. Affected women, like those with afibrinogenemia, experience menorrhagia, hemoperitoneum during ovulation, and recurrent pregnancy loss. Like individuals severely deficient in prothrombin and FX, FXIII-deficient patients may experience hemarthroses and muscle hematomas (~25%).

Screening for FXIII deficiency is usually performed using a qualitative assay of fibrin clot solubility in 5 mol/L urea or 1% monochloroacetic acid. This poorly standardized test is probably sensitive to FXIII levels < 3%. Diagnosis is confirmed usually by immunologic measurement of FXIII-A and FXIII-B subunit antigens; generally the former are very low, while the latter are only modestly reduced.

Treatment

Two plasma-derived FXIII concentrates are marketed, although one of these, manufactured by Bio Products Laboratory (UK), is available only in the UK. Fibrogammin P is available more widely, including in the USA on an Investigational New Drug (IND) license from the Food and Drug Administration.[6] The recommended dose is 10–20 units/kg for prophylaxis and 50–75 units/kg for treatment of bleeding. Other potential sources of FXIII include FFP, cryoprecipitate and platelets.

Long-term prophylaxis is recommended for all patients with severe FXIII deficiency because of the high incidence of intracranial hemorrhage. Because FXIII has an extremely long half-life, administration of concentrate or plasma/cryoprecipitate is required infrequently, generally every 4–6 weeks. This should be adjusted to maintain trough FXIII levels at 3% or more. Prophylaxis can also facilitate a successful pregnancy outcome in FXIII-deficient women. Inhibitor alloantibodies to FXIII may occur rarely as a result of exposure to concentrates, necessitating immune suppression, plasmapheresis, and/or high-dose FXIII concentrate.

α_2-plasmin inhibitor deficiency

Structure and function

α_2-plasmin inhibitor (α_2-PI) is a serine protease inhibitor (SERPIN) of about 70 kDa that is synthesized in the liver and probably the kidneys. Its function appears to be threefold: inhibition of plasmin enzymatic activity, competitive inhibition of plasmin(ogen) binding to fibrin, and FXIIIa-dependent covalent cross-linking to fibrin α-chains. The net effect is therefore antifibrinolytic. The gene for α_2-PI is located on chromosome 17.

α_2-PI$^{-/-}$ mice are normally fertile and viable. They demonstrate a normal hemostatic response to tail transection, but by other *in vivo* thrombosis models can be shown to have modestly accelerated fibrinolysis of intravascular fibrin thrombi.

Inheritance and prevalence

α_2-PI deficiency is transmitted in an autosomal recessive fashion. It appears to be extremely rare, with fewer than 20 reported cases. Both type 1 and type 2 deficiency states are described.

Clinical and laboratory features

In contrast to α_2-PI$^{-/-}$ mice, homozygous patients with this disorder have a severe bleeding disorder characterized by delayed-onset hemorrhage after vascular injury. Presentation is in childhood, sometimes with umbilical cord bleeding. Postsurgical and posttraumatic bleeding are common, as is deep tissue bleeding including muscle hematomas, hemarthrosis and, somewhat uniquely, intramedullary hematoma formation in the diaphyses of long bones. Heterozygous carriers probably have little, or at most a mild, bleeding tendency.[21]

Treatment

Antifibrinolytic agents are the mainstay of therapy for bleeding in α_2-PI deficient individuals. Failing this, FFP may be used as a source of the SERPIN. Solvent-detergent treated plasma should not be used, as the process inhibits the functional activity of α_2-PI. The half-life of α_2-PI is about 2.5 days, but for infused concentrates is much shorter.

Plasminogen activator inhibitor-1 deficiency

Structure and Function

Plasminogen activator inhibitor (PAI)-1 is a 45-kDa SERPIN that rapidly inactivates tissue-type plasminogen activator (tPA) and urokinase-type plasminogen activator (u-PA). PAI-1 is found in a variety of cells, including platelets, vascular endothelial cells, and other vascular and nonvascular cells.

PAI-1$^{-/-}$ mice manifest mild hyperfibrinolysis and enhanced resistance to venous thrombosis, but no abnormal bleeding or rebleeding after injury. Interestingly, α_2-AP$^{-/-}$PAI-1$^{-/-}$ mice do demonstrate prolonged immediate-onset bleeding after tail transection, as well as a more profound hyperfibrinolytic state than is seen with either variant alone.

Inheritance and prevalence

The prevalence of PAI-1 deficiency is unknown, and indeed there are less than 20 homozygous deficient individuals described in the literature. It is therefore presumed to be extremely rare.

Clinical and laboratory features

Unlike the murine model, homozygous PAI-1-deficient individuals do manifest delayed rebleeding, often severe, after surgery or trauma. Intracranial bleeding, hemarthrosis, and extensive ecchymoses may occur, but spontaneous hemorrhage (with the possible exception of menorrhagia in affected females) is unusual. Heterozygotes appear to be asymptomatic. It is recommended that PAI-1 antigen and activity be measured in both plasma and serum to include the PAI-1 contributed by platelets.

Treatment

The antifibrinolytic agents tranexamic acid and ε-aminocaproic acid are the mainstays of treatment. Theoretically, transfusion of FFP or platelets would be a reasonable alternative for refractory bleeding events.

Connective tissue disorders: Ehlers–Danlos syndrome

Inherited disorders of connective tissue are a consequence of defects in the quantity and/or structure of extracellular matrix proteins, including collagen, elastin, fibrillin, and non collagenous extracellular matrix proteins such as basement membrane proteins and proteoglycans. Although bleeding complications have been associated with several connective tissue disorders, the most common condition associated with bleeding manifestations is Ehlers–Danlos syndrome (EDS).[22]

EDS is a heterogeneous disorder caused by an inherited abnormality of collagen. It is characterized by varying degrees of skin elasticity, joint hypermobility and tissue fragility. At least 10 different variants of EDS have been described, and these were reclassified in 1997 into six major types based on symptoms, physical characteristics and certain molecular and/or histologic findings (Table 28.2).[23]

The diagnosis of EDS is based primarily on clinical symptoms, physical examination (skin and musculoskeletal system), and family history. A scoring system focusing on joint

Table 28.2 Classification of Ehlers–Danlos syndrome (EDS).

New	Former	OMIM	Inheritance
Classical type	Gravis (EDS type I)	130000	AD
	Mitis (EDS type II)	130010	AD
Hypermobility type	Hypermobile (EDS type III)	130020	AD
Vascular type	Arterial-ecchymotic (EDS type IV)	130050 (225350) (225360)	AD
Kyphoscoliosis type	Ocular-scoliotic (EDS type VI)	225400 (229200)	AR
Arthrochalasia type	Arthrochalasia multiplex congenita (EDS types VIIA, VIIB)	130060	AD
Dermatosparaxis type	Human dermatosparaxis (EDS type VIIC)	225410	AR
Other forms	X-linked EDS (EDS type V)	305200	XL
	Periodontitis type (EDS type VIII)	130080	AD
	Fibronectin-deficient EDS (EDS type X)	225310	?
	Familial hypermobility syndrome (EDS type XI)	147900	AD
	Progeroid EDS	130070	?
	Unspecified forms	–	–

AD, autosomal dominant; AR, autosomal recessive; XL, X-linked.
Reproduced with permission from Ref. 23.

hypermobility, abnormal scar formation, and hemorrhagic symptoms has been successfully used to screen patients for EDS.[24] A skin biopsy is recommended to evaluate for molecular genetic and/or histologic abnormalities, and to rule out the vascular form of EDS. In many patients, particularly those with the hypermobility (the most common) variant, the biopsy is uninformative.

The presentation of EDS depends on the variant but typically includes musculoskeletal, skin, and cardiovascular manifestations, although other organ systems may also be affected (intestine, lung, uterus, eye, etc.). The most common symptoms (according to organ system) are as follows.
• Musculoskeletal: hypermobile joints, recurrent dislocation, ligament and tendon injury, early-onset degenerative joint disease, flat feet, club feet, scoliosis, temporomandibular joint disease, and early dental loss.
• Skin: velvety or doughy texture, fragility with tearing, poor wound healing, wide dystrophic scars, papyraceous-appearing scars, subcutaneous nodules on pressure points and wound dehiscence following surgery.
• Vascular: mitral valve prolapse, aortic root dilation, aneurysm of the aorta, rupture or dissection of mid-sized arteries, and early-onset varicose veins.
• Other: recurrent hernias, bladder diverticuli, intestinal rupture, recurrent pneumothorax, scoliosis, detached retina, scleral fragility, rectal prolapse, and uterine prolapse or rupture.

Described bleeding manifestations include easy bruising, soft-tissue hematomas, recurrent nosebleeds, intraoperative or postoperative dental or surgical bleeding, gastrointestinal and pulmonary hemorrhage, mennorhagia, and bleeding with childbirth. Not uncommonly, children with EDS are suspected to be victims of child abuse because of prominent bruising.

The etiology of bleeding in these patients is probably multifactorial, and includes increased vascular fragility and poor wound healing. Abnormal subendothelial collagen that is less adhesive for platelets and/or associated platelet function abnormalities and other inherited factor (VIII, IX, XI and XIIII) deficiency states may also contribute to the bleeding propensity.

Evaluation of a patient who has clinical evidence of a connective tissue disorder and bleeding symptoms should include PT, APTT, TCT, and von Willebrand studies. The bleeding time, although technically problematic, may be the only abnormal coagulation study in these patients. Further evaluation, including specific factor assays and more specific platelet function studies such as platelet aggregation, may be indicated based on bleeding symptoms and the results of preliminary screening studies.

Treatment should include the avoidance of aspirin, nonsteroidal antiinflammatory drugs, and other medications that might increase the risk of bleeding. Attention should be paid to surgical technique, including choice of suture material, and postoperative care can be important in preventing surgical bleeding and wound dehiscence. If there is an associated inherited coagulation abnormality, this should be treated aggressively with appropriate replacement therapy.

Despite these general recommendations some patients with EDS have significant bleeding particularly related to surgery and trauma. Many have been treated with intravenous or intranasal desmopressin and/or oral or intravenous antifibrinolytic agents. With surgery or trauma where serious bleeding occurs that is not responsive to desmopressin, or where desmopressin is contraindicated, intermediate-purity FVIII concentrates such as Humate-P have been used successfully to control bleeding. Anecdotally, rFVIIa has also been used successfully in rare instances.

Fortunately, the majority of patients with EDS have minor bleeding issues. Consideration of EDS as a possible cause of postoperative or posttraumatic bleeding is often overlooked because the clinical manifestations of EDS are frequently not recognized. In addition there is a paucity of clinical studies examining treatment options for these patients. Therefore, most therapeutic regimens are based on limited and anecdotal experience.

References

1. Mannucci PM, Duga S, Peyvandi F. Recessively inherited coagulation disorders. *Blood* 2004; **104**: 1243–52.

2. Acharya SS, Coughlin A, DiMichele DM and the North American Rare Bleeding Disorders Registry. Rare bleeding disorder registry: deficiencies of factors II, V, VII, X, XIII, fibrinogen and dysfibrinogenemias. *J Thromb Haemost* 2004; **2**: 248–56.

3. Andrew M, Paes B, Johnston M. Development of the hemostatic system in the neonate and young infant. *Am J Pediatr Hematol Oncol* 1990; **12**: 95–104.

4. Giesen PL, Nemerson Y. Tissue factor on the loose. *Semin Thromb Hemost* 2000; **10**: 139–43.

5. Mariani G, Dolce A, Marchetti G, Bernardi F. Clinical picture and management of congenital factor VII deficiency. *Haemophilia* 2004; **10** (suppl. 4): 180–3.

6. Di Paola J, Nugent D, Young G. Current therapy for rare factor deficiencies. *Haemophilia* 2001; **7** (suppl. 1): 16–22.

7. Kasper CK, Costa e Silva M. Registry of clotting factor concentrates. World Federation of Hemophilia monograph. Available at http://www.wfh.org/Content_Documents/FF_Mongraphs/FF-6_English_Registry_5ed.pdf. Accessed March 30, 2005.

8. Bolton-Maggs PH, Perry DJ, Chalmers LA *et al.* The rare coagulation disorders: review with guidelines for management from the United Kingdom Haemophilia Centre Doctors' Organization. *Haemophilia* 2004; **10**: 593–628.

9. Goldstein DB, Reich DE, Bradman N, Usher S, Seligsohn U, Peretz H. Age estimates of two common mutations causing factor XI deficiency: recent genetic drift is not necessary for elevated disease incidence among Ashkenazi Jews. *Am J Hum Genet* 1999; **64**: 1071–5.

10. Bolton-Maggs PH, Young Wan-Yin B, McCraw AH, Slack J, Kernoff PB. Inheritance and bleeding in factor XI deficiency. *Br J Haematol* 1998; **69**: 521–8.

11. Salomon O, Zivelin A, Livnat T *et al.* Prevalence, causes, and characterization of factor XI inhibitors in patients with inherited factor FXI deficiency. *Blood* 2003; **101**: 4783–8.

12. Peyvandi F, Mannucci PM, Lak M *et al.* Congenital factor X deficiency: spectrum of bleeding symptoms in 32 Iranian patients. *Br J Haematol* 1998; **102**: 626–8.

13. Lak M, Sharifian R, Peyvandi F, Mannucci PM. Symptoms of inherited factor V deficiency in 35 Iranian patients. *Br J Haematol* 1998; **103**: 1067–9.

14. Girolami A, Scandellari R, Lombardi AM, Girolami B, Bortoletto E, Zanon E. Pregnancy and oral contraceptives in factor V deficiency: a study of 22 patients (five homozygotes and 17 heterozygotes) and review of the literature. *Haemophilia* 2005; **11**: 26–30.

15. Coughlin SR. Protease-activated receptors in vascular biology. *Thromb Haemost* 2001; **86**: 298–307.

16. Girolami A, Scarano L, Saggiorato G, Girolami B, Bertomoro A, Marchiori A. Congenital deficiencies and abnormalities of prothrombin. *Blood Coag Fibrinol* 1998; **9**: 557–69.

17. Akhavan S, Mannucci PM, Lak M *et al.* Identification and three-dimensional structural analysis of nine novel mutations in patients with prothrombin deficiency. *Thromb Haemost* 2000; **84**: 989–97.

18. Roberts HR, Stinchcombe TE, Gabriel DA. The dysfibrinogenaemias. *Br J Haematol* 2001; **114**: 249–57.

19. Lak M, Keihani M, Elahi F, Peyvandi F, Mannucci PM. Bleeding and thrombosis in 55 patients with inherited afibrinogenaemia. *Br J Haematol* 1999; **107**: 204–6.

20. Peyvandi F, Tuddenham EGD, Akhtari AM, Lak M, Mannucci PM. Bleeding symptoms in 27 Iranian patients with the combined deficiency of factor V and factor VIII. *Br J Haematol* 1998; **100**: 773–6.

21. Favier R, Aoki N, De Moerloose P. Congenital α_2-plasmin inhibitor deficiencies: a review. *Br J Haematol* 2001; **114**: 4–10.

22. De Paepe A, Malfait F. Bleeding and bruising in patients with Ehlers–Danlos syndrome and other collagen vascular disorders. *Br J Haematol* 2004; **127**: 491–500.

23. Beighton P, De Paepe A, Steinmann B, Tsipouras P, Wenstrup RJ. Ehlers–Danlos syndromes: revised nosology, Villefranche, 1997. Ehlers–Danlos National Foundation (USA) and Ehlers–Danlos Support Group (UK). *Am J Med Genet* 1998; **77**: 31–7.

24. Holzberg M, Hewan-Lowe KO, Olansky AJ. The Ehlers-Danlos syndrome: Recognition, characterization, and importance of a milder variant of the classic form, *J Am Ac Derm* 1998; **19**: 656–66.

29 Acquired disorders of hemostasis

Elizabeth A. Chalmers, Michael D. Williams and Angela Thomas

Developmental hemostasis during childhood

Many features of the hemostatic system appear to be age dependent. This is most apparent during the neonatal period, where differences can be observed in the levels of many hemostatic proteins compared with adult values.[1,2] Considerable "maturation" of the hemostatic system occurs during the first 6 months of life even in preterm infants.[1–3] Despite this a number of differences persist throughout childhood and adolescence.[4] The availability of normal reference ranges for children of different ages is therefore crucial for accurate diagnosis in this age group and is also important in the management of clinical problems, particularly where therapeutic agents interact with the hemostatic system.[5,6]

The development of microtechniques during the early 1980s provided the first opportunity for the detailed study of the hemostatic system in neonates and young children. Using this technology, Andrew *et al.*[4] performed a comprehensive analysis of coagulation and fibrinolytic parameters across three different age ranges in healthy children undergoing minor elective day surgery. Comparison of the results obtained demonstrated the presence of important differences in the mean levels of many procoagulant proteins, coagulation inhibitors and fibrinolytic proteins.

Based on these data mean plasma concentrations of vitamin K-dependent factors (II, VII, IX and X) and the contact factors XI, XII and V are all 15–20% lower in children than in adults (Table 29.1). In contrast, concentrations of fibrinogen, factor (F)VIII and von Willebrand factor (vWF) are similar to adult values throughout childhood. The inhibitor antithrombin is increased by approximately 10% while α_2-macroglobulin is almost doubled and heparin cofactor II reduced by 10–20% (Table 29.2). Free protein S levels are similar to adult values, while mean protein C levels remain significantly reduced even in the 11–16 year age range (Table 29.2).[4] Plasma concentrations of some fibrinolytic proteins are also affected by age and while plasminogen and α_2-antiplasmin levels are similar in adults and children, plasminogen activator inhibitor (PAI)-1 is increased and tissue plasminogen activator (tPA) decreased so that overall fibrinolytic capacity appears reduced during childhood (Table 29.3).

Despite reduced levels of several procoagulant proteins, routine coagulation screening tests such as prothrombin time (PT) and activated partial thromboplastin time (APTT) show relatively minor differences compared with adult values, which reflects the relative insensitivity of these tests to minor changes in procoagulant concentrations (Table 29.1).[4]

While the data published by Andrew *et al.* still provide extremely comprehensive information on the nature of the hemostatic system during childhood, they were generated in the 1980s and do not therefore reflect current technology. All reference ranges, regardless of patient characteristics, are both instrument and reagent dependent and it is generally recommended that all laboratories establish their own in-house reference ranges. Caution is therefore required when interpreting individual results in children against previously published ranges. This was highlighted recently by Monagle *et al.*[7] who demonstrated the presence of significant differences in data derived in a group of children using currently available technology compared with data published previously by Andrew *et al.*

Normal ranges for the skin bleeding time have also been established using a number of different methods.[8] The shortest bleeding times appear to occur in neonates and very young infants. In older children the data are conflicting, with bleeding times that are both longer and shorter than adult values having been reported (Table 29.1).[5,8,9]

From a clinical point of view it has been of interest to try to assess the effects of these differences in the hemostatic system on overall thrombin regulation. Data from *in vitro* studies based on traditional models of thrombin generation have shown that thrombin generation is reduced by around 20%

Table 29.1 Reference values for coagulation tests in healthy children aged 1–16 years compared with adults.

	1–5 years	6–10 years	11–16 years	Adult
PT (s)	11 (10.6–11.4)	11.1 (10.1–12.1)	11.2 (10.2–12.0)	12 (11.0–14.0)
INR	1.0 (0.96–1.04)	1.01 (0.91–1.11)	1.02 (0.93–1.10)	1.10 (1.0–1.3)
APTT (s)	30 (24–36)	31 (26–36)	32 (26–37)	33 (27–40)
Fibrinogen (g/L)	2.76 (1.70–4.05)	2.79 (1.57–4.0)	3.0 (1.54–4.48)	2.78 (1.56–4.0)
Bleeding time (min)	6 (2.5–10)*	7 (2.5–13)*	5 (3–8)*	4 (1–7)
FII (units/mL)	0.94 (0.71–1.16)*	0.88 (0.67–1.07)*	0.83 (0.61–1.04)*	1.08 (0.70–1.46)
FV (units/mL)	1.03 (0.79–1.27)	0.90 (0.63–1.16)*	0.77 (0.55–0.99)*	1.06 (0.62–1.50)
FVII (units/mL)	0.82 (0.55–1.16)*	0.85 (0.52–1.20)*	0.83 (0.58–1.15)*	1.05 (0.67–1.43)
FVIII (units/mL)	0.90 (0.59–1.42)	0.95 (0.58–1.32)	0.92 (0.53–1.31)	0.99 (0.50–1.49)
vWF (units/mL)	0.82 (0.60–1.20)	0.95 (0.44–1.44)	1.00 (0.46–1.53)	0.92 (0.50–1.58)
FIX (units/mL)	0.73 (0.47–1.04)*	0.75 (0.63–0.89)*	0.82 (0.59–1.22)*	1.09 (0.55–1.63)
FX (units/mL)	0.88 (0.58–1.16)*	0.75 (0.55–1.01)*	0.79 (0.50–1.17)*	1.06 (0.70–1.52)
FXI (units/mL)	0.97 (0.56–1.50)	0.86 (0.52–1.20)	0.74 (0.50–0.97)*	0.97 (0.67–1.27)
FXII (units/mL)	0.93 (0.64–1.29)	0.92 (0.60–1.40)	0.81 (0.34–1.37)*	1.08 (0.52–1.64)
PK (units/mL)	0.95 (0.65–1.30)	0.99 (0.66–1.31)	0.99 (0.53–1.45)	1.12 (0.62–1.62)
HMWK (units/mL)	0.98 (0.64–1.32)	0.93 (0.60–1.30)	0.91 (0.63–1.19)	0.92 (0.50–1.36)
FXIIIa (units/mL)	1.08 (0.72–1.43)*	1.09 (0.65–1.51)*	0.99 (0.57–1.40)	1.05 (0.55–1.55)
FXIIIs (units/mL)	1.13 (0.69–1.56)*	1.16 (0.77–1.54)*	1.02 (0.60–1.43)	0.97 (0.57–1.37)

All factors except fibrinogen are expressed as units/mL, where pooled plasma contains 1.0 unit/mL. All data are expressed as the mean, followed by the upper and lower boundary encompassing 95% of the population. Between 20 and 50 samples were assayed for each value for each age group. Some measurements were skewed due to a disproportionate number of high values. The lower limit, which excludes the lower 2.5% of the population, is given.
* Values significantly different from adult values.
APTT, activated partial thromboplastin time; FVIII, FVIII procoagulant; HMWK, high-molecular-weight kininogen; INR, international normalized ratio; PK, prekallikrein; PT, prothrombin time; vWF, von Willebrand factor.
Reproduced with permission from Ref. 4.

Table 29.2 Reference values for the inhibitors of coagulation in healthy children aged 1–16 years compared with adults.

	1–5 years	6–10 years	11–16 years	Adult
ATIII (units/mL)	1.11 (0.82–1.39)	1.11 (0.90–1.31)	1.05 (0.77–1.32)	1.0 (0.74–1.26)
α_2-M (units/mL)	1.69 (1.14–2.23)*	1.69 (1.28–2.09)*	1.56 (0.98–2.12)*	0.86 (0.52–1.20)
C1E-Inh (units/mL)	1.35 (0.85–1.83)*	1.14 (0.88–1.54)	1.03 (0.68–1.50)	1.0 (0.71–1.31)
α_1-AT (units/mL)	0.93 (0.39–1.47)	1.00 (0.69–1.30)	1.01 (0.65–1.37)	0.93 (0.55–1.30)
HCII (units/mL)	0.88 (0.48–1.28)*	0.86 (0.40–1.32)*	0.91 (0.53–1.29)*	1.08 (0.66–1.26)
Protein C (units/mL)	0.66 (0.40–0.92)*	0.69 (0.45–0.93)*	0.83 (0.55–1.11)*	0.96 (0.64–1.28)
Protein S				
Total (units/mL)	0.86 (0.54–1.18)	0.78 (0.41–1.14)	0.72 (0.52–0.92)	0.81 (0.60–1.13)
Free (units/mL)	0.45 (0.21–0.69)	0.42 (0.22–0.62)	0.38 (0.26–0.55)	0.45 (0.27–0.61)

All values are expressed in units/mL, where for all factors pooled plasma contains 1.0 unit/mL, with the exception of free protein S, where the mean is 0.4 units/mL. All values are given as a mean, followed by the lower and upper boundary encompassing 95% of the population. Between 20 and 30 samples were assayed for each value for each age group. Some measurements were skewed due to a disproportionate number of high values. The lower limits, which exclude the lower 2.5% of the population, are given.
* Values significantly different from adult values.
α_2-M, α_2-macroglobulin; ATIII, antithrombin III; α_1-AT, α_1-antitrypsin; C1E-Inh, C1 esterase inhibitor; HCII, heparin cofactor II.
Reproduced with permission from Ref. 4.

during childhood compared with adult values.[10] Despite this, for any given hemostatic challenge there does not appear to be an increased risk of hemorrhagic problems during childhood. Conversely, the total capacity to inhibit thrombin, as assessed *in vitro* using ^{125}I-labeled thrombin, is increased due to increased binding to α_2-macroglobulin[11,12] and may contribute to the relatively low incidence of thrombosis during childhood.[13–16]

Table 29.3 Reference values for the fibrinolytic system in healthy children aged 1–16 years compared with adults.

	1–5 years	6–10 years	11–16 years	Adult
Plasminogen (units/mL)	0.98 (0.78–1.18)	0.92 (0.75–1.08)	0.86 (0.68–1.03)*	0.99 (0.77–1.22)
tPA (ng/mL)	2.15 (1.0–4.5)*	2.42 (1.0–5.0)*	2.16 (1.0–4.0)*	4.90 (1.40–8.40)
α_2-AP (units/mL)	1.05 (0.93–1.17)	0.99 (0.89–1.10)	0.98 (0.78–1.18)	1.02 (0.68–1.36)
PAI (units/mL)	5.42 (1.0–10.0)	6.79 (2.0–12.0)*	6.07 (2.0–10.0)*	3.60 (0–11.0)

For α_2-AP, values are expressed as units/mL, where pooled plasma contains 1.0 unit/mL. Values for tPA are given as ng/mL. Values for PAI are given as units/mL, where 1 unit of PAI activity is defined as the amount of PAI that inhibits 1 unit of human single-chain tPA. All values are given as the mean, followed by the lower and upper boundary encompassing 95% of the population (boundary).

* Values significantly different from adult values.

α_2-AP, α_2-antiplasmin; PAI, plasminogen activator inhibitor; tPA, tissue plasminogen activator.

Reproduced with permission from Ref. 4.

Evaluation of a bleeding child

When a child presents with bleeding or bruising, the main differential diagnoses are physiologic or accidental bleeding, nonaccidental injury or a bleeding diathesis. Clinical presentation and medical history, including response to any previous hemostatic challenges, are key to differentiating between these conditions. A history of any medications or other remedies taken should be included. In an ill child, bleeding is often acquired and due to more than one defect of the hemostatic mechanism. The underlying disorder such as renal failure, liver disease or sepsis may well be apparent. In a well child, bleeding, whether congenital or acquired, is more often due to a single defect such as thrombocytopenia or a coagulation factor deficiency. A family history of unusual bleeding in parents, siblings and other relatives or a family history of a specific diagnosis may be helpful in determining whether the child is likely to have an inherited disorder. X-linked disorders are usually but not exclusively seen in boys and age at presentation will influence the differential diagnosis and, in the case of congenital disorders, tends to be inversely associated with the severity of the disease.

The site and pattern of bleeding may indicate the most likely underlying hemostatic defect. Defects of platelets, both quantitative and qualitative, result predominantly in mucocutaneous bleeding. This can be manifest as petechial hemorrhages, ecchymoses, recurrent or prolonged epistaxis and menorrhagia in girls. Thrombocytopenia is commonly acquired and mucocutaneous bleeding in a well child, possibly following a viral infection, may indicate idiopathic thrombocytopenic purpura. In a sick child, the thrombocytopenia may be part of disseminated intravascular coagulation (DIC), with bleeding and oozing from multiple sites, or secondary to bone marrow failure or infiltration by malignant disease. Acquired coagulation protein defects are less common in well children but do occur in vitamin K deficiency, and occasionally hypoprothrombinemia resulting in bleeding can be seen with a lupus anticoagulant. Bleeding from wounds or puncture sites and significant mucocutaneous bleeding are seen in sick children secondary to complex coagulopathies that occur with liver disease and DIC. Examination will indicate the general health and systemic well-being of the child and will confirm the pattern of bleeding. Stigmata of underlying disease or physical signs associated with specific congenital disorders may be evident.

Screening tests in a bleeding child should include a full blood count and blood film, PT, APTT and fibrinogen. In a sick child, liver and renal function may be evaluated and other markers of DIC such as D-dimers measured. In a well child with mucocutaneous bleeding, vWF antigen and activity may be informative, particularly if the screen is normal. Further investigations will depend on initial results in association with clinical and family history.

Disseminated intravascular coagulation

DIC is a common acquired coagulopathy which in children is usually an acute event and related to a systemic disorder. Definitions have sought to encompass the various aspects of this syndrome, including it being an acquired condition characterized by intravascular activation of coagulation including both procoagulant and fibrinolytic activation and causing thrombohemorrhagic effects that may result in end-organ damage.[16,17] DIC remains a significant cause of morbidity and mortality in children and adults but progress in understanding the pathogenesis of this syndrome has provided novel approaches to diagnosis and treatment.[18]

Etiology

There are a number of disease processes that may result in DIC in children (Table 29.4). Infection remains the commonest cause of DIC. Bacterial infections predominate, with no difference being noted in the frequency of Gram-negative and Gram-positive organisms:[19] meningococcal meningitis remains one of the most frequent causes of severe DIC in

Table 29.4 Causes of disseminated intravascular coagulation in children.

Infection
Malignancy, e.g., acute leukemia
Trauma, e.g., head injury, burns
Organ destruction, e.g., acute pancreatitis
Severe immune reaction, e.g., ABO-incompatible blood transfusion
Hepatic failure
Vascular abnormality, e.g., Kasabach–Merritt syndrome

children. Viruses (most commonly cytomegalovirus, varicella and hepatitis), protozoa and systemic fungi are also recognized triggers for this disorder. DIC in association with childhood malignancy is relatively uncommon except in acute promyelocytic leukemia and tumor lysis syndromes.[20] Chronic localized DIC is infrequent in children and almost exclusively occurs in association with giant hemangiomas. Kasabach–Merritt syndrome has its peak incidence in early infancy but may present later in childhood; although the diagnosis is usually obvious, occult hemangiomas can occur and should be excluded in the presence of a significant unexplained coagulopathy.[21]

Pathophysiology

These diverse disease conditions lead to the triggering of DIC through a number of mechanisms that occur simultaneously.[17,18,22] Thrombin generation occurs via the tissue factor –FVIIa system[23,24] and results in the deposition of fibrin: it seems likely that endogenous tissue factor pathway inhibitor cannot regulate this process once triggered.[25] The natural anticoagulant pathways such as the antithrombin and protein C systems are impaired, with reduced plasma levels of antithrombin and decreased activation of protein C being consistent features of DIC.[26–28] Thrombin generation thereby increases, leading to excessive fibrin formation and consumption of coagulation factors and platelets. Circulating plasmin results in the generation of fibrin(ogen) degradation products that interfere with fibrin polymerization and platelet function, leading to additional hemorrhagic problems; however, fibrinolysis is largely suppressed due to a sustained increase in PAI-1.[29] Fibrin deposition leads to microvascular and, less frequently, large-vessel thrombosis with impaired perfusion and subsequent organ damage.

The interaction between the coagulation and inflammatory pathways has become increasingly recognized as an integral component in the pathogenesis of DIC. Cytokines and proinflammatory mediators can induce coagulation through tissue factor expression; activated coagulation proteases such as thrombin, fibrin and FXa bind with protease-activated receptors on cell surfaces to stimulate inflammation through the release of proinflammatory cytokines.[30,31] In addition, impairment of the anticoagulant pathways diminishes the regulatory effect that proteins such as activated protein C have on cytokine release, thereby adding to the inflammatory response.[32] These processes have wide-ranging systemic consequences, including vasodilatation, capillary leak and shock.

Clinical features

The most obvious clinical manifestation of overt DIC remains hemorrhage. Spontaneous bruising, petechiae from localized pressure, oozing from venipuncture sites, and continued bleeding from sites of trauma or from surgical wounds are relatively common; internal hemorrhage can involve the gastrointestinal tract, central nervous system or other organs and be life-threatening in itself. Microvascular thrombosis is a common and underdiagnosed manifestation of DIC which although more difficult to recognize clinically may lead to irreversible end-organ damage.

Acute infectious purpura fulminans is an uncommon but severe form of DIC seen in children in which purpura is followed by the development of skin bullae and necrosis. These features are identical to those seen in homozygous protein C or protein S deficiency and are the result of acquired deficiencies of these natural anticoagulants. The condition is most often seen in children with meningococcal septicemia but is also associated with chickenpox and streptococcal infection.[33]

The spectrum of DIC is wide: whereas overt DIC occurring in a patient with one of the associated conditions detailed in Table 29.4 can usually be recognized clinically, nonovert DIC is detected only by changes in laboratory parameters as it reflects hemostatic dysfunction rather than frank decompensation and is not accompanied by the clinical signs of hemorrhage or thrombosis.

Laboratory diagnosis

There is no one laboratory test that is diagnostic of DIC and the laboratory diagnosis is therefore based on the demonstration of activation of both the procoagulant and fibrinolytic systems accompanied by anticoagulant consumption. Serial testing is often necessary to establish the diagnosis of DIC; diagnosis can be made difficult by the reactive nature of such proteins as fibrinogen and FVIII, which are often elevated in ill patients; similarly, markers of fibrin(ogen) degradation are often elevated in trauma and after surgery.

In fulminant DIC the diagnosis is usually obvious, with prolongation of all coagulation screening tests together with thrombocytopenia, increased fibrin degradation and reduced plasma levels of anticoagulants, particularly antithrombin and protein C. In less severe forms of DIC, screening tests such as APTT and PT can be less reliable: thrombocytopenia is an important marker, particularly when there is a downward trend in the platelet count, as is evidence of increased fibrin degradation, with D-dimer tests being more specific for fibrin than tests for fibrinogen degradation products.

The limitations of routine laboratory tests in the diagnosis of DIC can be overcome by the use of more sensitive tests of thrombin and plasmin generation,[17] including prothrombin activation fragment 1 and 2, fibrinopeptide A and thrombin–antithrombin (TAT) complexes which reflect thrombin activation, and plasmin–antiplasmin complexes which reflect fibrinolytic activity. However, the majority of these assays remain limited to research laboratories and are not available in most routine coagulation laboratories.

A new development in the diagnosis of DIC has been waveform analysis of the APTT performed using a specific coagulation analyzer, in which a specific waveform profile has been shown to correlate with overt and nonovert DIC.[34]

Pragmatically, the laboratory diagnosis of DIC is therefore usually made using a combination of tests that are readily available in most hospitals and which can be performed quickly and serially as necessary. These include PT, APTT, fibrinogen, D-dimers and platelet count. A scoring system that incorporates these tests has been proposed for use in the diagnosis of overt and nonovert DIC.[16]

Management

The single most important aspect of the treatment of DIC remains treatment of the associated disease condition. Even with prompt and aggressive treatment, DIC may continue to evolve, with the affected child requiring intensive supportive therapy in order to reduce morbidity and mortality. Optimum supportive measures remain controversial, with recent treatment modalities incorporating the advances that have been made in understanding the pathophysiology of this condition.

Blood component replacement therapy continues to be the mainstay of most treatment strategies and should be used only in patients with either clinical bleeding or prior to invasive procedures, and not merely to correct clotting test abnormalities. The choice of product, timing of administration, and efficacy of treatment remain unclear. Fresh frozen plasma (FFP) is a source of procoagulant proteins and anticoagulants and is usually given in a dose of 10–15 mL/kg. Cryoprecipitate (10 mL/kg) provides higher concentrations of fibrinogen and FVIII and is useful when hypofibrinogenemia exists. In the absence of randomized clinical trials, it is generally accepted that platelet counts should be maintained $> 50 \times 10^9$/L and plasma fibrinogen > 1 g/L. If fluid volume is problematic, consideration should be given to the use of coagulation factor concentrates or exchange transfusion. There is no clinical or laboratory evidence to support the historical assertion that the use of blood component therapy worsens DIC by "adding fuel to the fire".

Alternative or additional treatment strategies have centered on the use of anticoagulant therapy and more recently on the replacement of the natural anticoagulants protein C

and antithrombin. Heparin has not been shown in controlled clinical trials to have had a significant effect on the outcome in DIC,[35] although its use in specific circumstances has been advocated.[17] The safety of heparin treatment in patients who are at risk of bleeding remains an obvious concern. Given the pathophysiology of DIC, an alternative target for anticoagulation has involved tissue factor activity; however, no survival benefit has been demonstrated in the single randomized clinical trial examining the use of recombinant tissue factor pathway inhibitor.[36]

A number of small studies of the use of antithrombin concentrate in adults and children with DIC have previously shown improvement in laboratory and clinical parameters[37–39] but use in patients with DIC associated with sepsis has been shown to have no significant effect on reduction in mortality.[40] Neither antithrombin concentrate nor heparin are therefore currently indicated in the routine management of children with DIC.

Protein C concentrate has been used with varying success in the treatment of purpura fulminans associated with meningococcal septicemia, a condition in which acquired protein C deficiency occurs.[41,42] However, activation of protein C *in vivo* is dependent on functional endothelial cell surface receptors, which can be greatly reduced in sepsis.[43] It is therefore uncertain as to the role of the other treatment modalities that have been used in conjunction with protein C concentrate, including hemofiltration and heparin, and further randomized trials would be helpful in determining its effect.

Replacement therapy with recombinant activated protein C concentrate has been shown to have a positive effect in reducing mortality in adults with severe sepsis, reducing 28-day mortality from 31% to 25%,[44] improving clotting test abnormalities and being associated with less organ failure in treated patients.[45] Interaction with the inflammatory pathways (see section on pathophysiology) may well be a contributory factor in these trial results. However, both the recent antithrombin III and activated protein C trials have been criticized,[46] and there remains no clear indication for the use of these products in DIC. No such studies have been performed in children and efficacy and safety of these treatments in this age group are unknown.

Vitamin K deficiency

Vitamin K is a fat-soluble vitamin, first identified over 50 years ago by the Danish biochemist Hendrik Dam, who observed bleeding in chicks fed a cholesterol-free diet.[47] Vitamin K is critical for the posttranslational modification of a number of diverse proteins. In its reduced form, vitamin K is a cofactor for the activation of the microsomal enzyme γ-glutamyl carboxylase, promoting the conversion of protein-bound glutamate residues (Glu) to γ-carboxyglutamate residues (Gla). The presence of Gla residues confers unique physiologic properties for calcium-mediated binding to negatively charged phospholipid surfaces, a requirement for effective hemostasis.[48] In the absence of vitamin K these precursor proteins are functionally inactive and circulate in their decarboxylated form (PIVKA, i.e., protein induced by vitamin K absence or antagonism).

Vitamin K-dependent proteins are present in a wide variety of tissues, including plasma (procoagulant factors II, VII, IX and X; anticoagulants protein C and protein S; protein Z), bone (osteocalcin or bone Gla-protein), kidney, lung, testes, spleen and placenta.[49,50]

Vitamin K exists in two naturally occurring forms. Phylloquinone (vitamin K_1) is the main dietary source of vitamin K and is present predominantly in leafy green vegetables and a small number of vegetable oils.[51] The menaquinones (vitamin K_2) exist in a number of molecular forms that are restricted in the diet and largely synthesized by intestinal bacteria.

Etiology

Vitamin K deficiency beyond infancy is relatively uncommon and is almost always a secondary event resulting from inadequate intake or absorption, poor utilization of vitamin K, or vitamin K antagonism. Because of the wide dietary distribution of phylloquinones, after infancy inadequate vitamin K intake is generally the result of unsupplemented total parenteral nutrition often combined with the prolonged administration of broad-spectrum antibiotics.[52] Conditions associated with malabsorption are the commonest cause of vitamin K deficiency in the pediatric age group. Vitamin K deficiency secondary to malabsorption due to absence of bile salts, either from intrahepatic or extrahepatic biliary obstruction, responds to vitamin K replacement. In contrast, in primary hepatocellular disease, liver parenchymal cells may not be capable of utilizing vitamin K even when present in adequate amounts. However, inadequate bile salt secretion may be a contributing factor and partial correction may follow vitamin K administration.

The commonest cause of vitamin K antagonism is warfarin therapy, which inhibits vitamin K epoxide reductase, resulting in the accumulation of the epoxide metabolite. There is a hepatic NAD(P)H-dependent pathway for vitamin K reduction that is fairly insensitive to warfarin.[53] Thus, vitamin K can bypass the enzyme, epoxide reductase, in situations requiring reversal of the warfarin effect. Second- and third-generation cephalosporins can also produce hypoprothrombinemia by inhibiting vitamin K epoxide reductase,[54] but these antibiotics are relatively weak vitamin K antagonists and probably only pose a risk in the presence of coexisting predisposing factors such as malnourishment with compromised vitamin K status.[55,56]

Clinical features

Although laboratory evidence of vitamin K deficiency is quite common in the predisposing conditions described above, clinical bleeding is relatively infrequent and when it occurs is usually mild to moderate and typified by bruising, oozing from venipuncture sites and, rarely, internal bleeding. The underlying cause can usually be identified from the history and physical examination. In patients with liver disease, impaired synthesis of coagulation factors may coexist with vitamin K deficiency, increasing the severity of the coagulopathy. At-risk children who require an invasive procedure such as liver or jejunal biopsies should have a coagulation screen prior to the procedure and should receive appropriate vitamin K replacement in the event of a correctable abnormality.

Laboratory diagnosis

FVII has a short half-life and is the first of the vitamin K-dependent procoagulants to become deficient, resulting in an isolated prolongation of the PT.[57] Levels of FII, FIX and FX then decline, prolonging the APTT. Both the PT and APTT are corrected by a 1 : 1 mix with normal plasma. These screening test abnormalities are not specific for vitamin K deficiency and confirmatory tests may be both necessary and helpful in some patients. Specific factor assays may help distinguish isolated vitamin K deficiency from congenital factor deficiency, liver disease or DIC. Measurement of decarboxy-prothrombin (PIVKA II), which is increased in vitamin K deficiency, is a more specific test.[58–60] It is extremely sensitive and able to detect the early subclinical deficiency state. PIVKA II has a long half-life and can be used to diagnose vitamin K deficiency even after vitamin K therapy has normalized the PT.

The diagnosis of isolated vitamin K deficiency can also be confirmed if administration of a therapeutic dose of vitamin K is followed by a fall in the PT, which can occur in as short a period as 30 min if the vitamin is given intravenously.[61,62] The rapid correction of vitamin K deficiency following parenteral administration of vitamin K has led to the hypothesis that undercarboxylated prothrombin may be stored in vitamin K deficiency states, which can then be rapidly carboxylated and secreted following replacement therapy.[63]

Treatment

Appropriate treatment of vitamin K deficiency is dictated by the urgency of the clinical situation. Where there is no or only minor bleeding and in the presence of normal absorption, oral vitamin K is effective but correction of the PT is slower than following parenteral administration. Parenteral vitamin K results in the most rapid correction of vitamin K deficiency and may be administered by either the intravenous or subcutaneous route. Severe anaphylaxis can occur following intravenous vitamin K and it is important that the preparation is diluted appropriately and infused slowly. The intramuscular route may result in painful hematoma formation and should be avoided.

Patients who are bleeding secondary to vitamin K deficiency and who require rapid correction of their coagulopathy should receive parenteral vitamin K and should also be given factor replacement therapy. Options for replacement therapy include FFP, prothrombin complex concentrate (PCC) or a four-factor concentrate.[64] FFP in a dose of 10–15 mL/kg will raise the levels of vitamin K-dependent factors by 0.1–0.2 units/mL. Virally inactivated FFP should be used wherever possible. PCCs have the advantage of rapid administration in low volume but do not contain FVII and additional supplementation with either FFP or recombinant FVIIa may also be required. Four-factor concentrates containing all the vitamin K-dependent factors may ultimately offer the best therapeutic option; however, at present these products are not licensed for use in children and there is only limited clinical data available on their use in this area.

Prophylaxis

Vitamin K 1 µg/kg is considered an adequate daily requirement.[65] Consideration should be given to the use of vitamin K supplementation in children at high risk of developing deficiency.

There is a surprising paucity in the literature of evidence-based guidelines in this area. The best researched of the disorders predisposing to vitamin K deficiency is cystic fibrosis, but even here there is no clear consensus on the need for routine vitamin K supplementation.[66] Studies suggest that vitamin K deficiency is probably unusual in patients with cystic fibrosis not receiving vitamin K supplements, but a negative effect may be masked by the current common use of vitamin K supplements in this patient group.[66] A literature review identified the children at greatest risk as those with:

- severe noncholestatic or cholestatic liver disease;
- major small bowel resection for intestinal complications;
- pulmonary disease necessitating long-term use of antibiotics;
- pancreatic insufficiency.

This review suggested that these categories of patients receive vitamin K prophylaxis until evidence from future studies identifies risk factors.[66] The Consensus Conference of the Cystic Fibrosis Foundation on Nutritional Assessment and Management in Cystic Fibrosis (1990) made dosage recommendations but there are few data on the effectiveness of specific regimens.[67] Wilson et al.[68] demonstrated that an oral fat-soluble vitamin combination containing modest amounts of vitamin K failed to reduce PIVKA levels in all children with cystic fibrosis and pancreatic insufficiency,

and van Hoorn et al.[69] have suggested that doses in excess of 1 mg/day may be required to prevent potential vitamin K deficiency-related complications.

Hemostatic complications of liver disease

Hepatic failure

Given the importance of the liver in the synthesis and clearance of components of the coagulant and fibrinolytic systems, it is not surprising that liver disease is often accompanied by abnormal hemostasis that contributes to both hemorrhage and thrombosis in affected individuals. Although the disease processes vary in neonates, children and adults, the pathophysiology of abnormal hemostasis is similar in these age groups.

Pathophysiology

Liver disease affects the procoagulant and anticoagulant pathways and the fibrinolytic sysytem, and contributes to thrombocytopenia and impaired platelet function.[70,71] As the liver is the main or sole site of synthesis of procoagulant proteins, liver failure will cause a progressive reduction in synthesis of these proteins, with the exception of FVIII, which is also produced by endothelial cells.[72] The liver is also the site for the postribosomal carboxylation of the vitamin K-dependent proteins, this process being impaired in liver failure and resulting in dysfunctional FII, FVII, FIX, FX and proteins C, S and Z.

Plasma fibrinogen levels fall in acute hepatic failure, with increased consumption and clearance also thought to contribute to impaired synthesis. Dysfibrinogenemia is a common feature of acute and chronic liver failure, resulting from an increased number of sialic acid residues in the fibrinogen molecule and leading to impaired fibrin polymerization.[73,74] All proteins of the fibrinolytic system except tPA and PAI-1 are synthesized in the liver and their plasma levels fall in liver failure. However, plasma tPA levels are increased in liver failure, with PAI-1 levels increased in acute but not chronic liver failure.[75,76] Acute liver failure is therefore associated with a hypofibrinolytic state and chronic liver failure with a hyperfibrinolytic state.

Failure of the hepatic reticuloendothelial system to clear activated coagulation factors together with localized activation due to hepatocellular damage may result in DIC and a further impairment of hemostasis, though the presence of DIC in liver disease remains controversial.[77] Impaired protein synthesis also results in reduced plasma levels of the natural anticoagulants, which may contribute to thrombotic events in children with liver failure.

Thrombocytopenia of varying degree is common in liver disease and is multifactorial, its causes including splenic sequestration, consumption and reduced platelet production. Platelet function is abnormal and results from a number of mechanisms, including impaired platelet signal transduction,[78] increased production of platelet inhibitors,[79] and defective platelet–vessel wall interaction.[80]

Clinical features

The overall result of the hemostatic changes is a tendency toward a hemorrhagic state in children with liver failure. Spontaneous hemorrhage is relatively uncommon but bruising and hemorrhage following invasive procedures is common. Epistaxis can occur, as can hemorrhage from the gastrointestinal tract. Coagulation abnormalities exacerbate bleeding from varices or ulcers, which may be life-threatening. Diagnostic procedures such as liver biopsy can result in significant hemorrhage in patients with a coagulopathy,[81] laboratory coagulation results alone being a poor predictor of bleeding in individual patients.

The extent to which the hemostatic systems are disturbed is related to the severity of hepatocellular damage that has resulted in liver failure. The PT is a sensitive marker of liver dysfunction and is the first screening test to become abnormal, reflecting a fall in plasma FVII levels, and is followed by decreases in the other vitamin K-dependent factors. More extensive damage leads to a reduction in nonvitamin K-dependent factors and a prolongation of the APTT. At this time, fibrinogen levels are usually normal or increased due to the acute-phase response. Increasing liver failure will result in a further fall in all procoagulants and natural anticoagulants, an increasing PT and APTT, falling fibrinogen levels and evidence of dysfibrinogenemia. Markers of thrombin and plasmin generation appear, such as TAT complexes and D-dimers. Thrombocytopenia is a common feature of liver failure, platelet counts usually ranging between 50 and 150×10^9/L.

Management

Apart from local measures, treatment is largely supportive in order to allow the liver to recover from the underlying insult or to enable the patient to undergo liver transplantation. Vitamin K supplementation should be administered. Blood product support should not be given unless the child is bleeding or requires an invasive procedure: in these circumstances FFP and cryoprecipitate can be used and platelet counts maintained above 50×10^9/L. Platelet increment and platelet survival are often reduced because of splenic sequestration, leading to increased requirements for platelet transfusion.

PCCs should be avoided where possible due to the increased risk of activation and thrombosis. Desmopressin has been used in patients with liver failure and coagulopathies, although its efficacy remains to be confirmed.[82]

Recombinant activated FVII (rFVIIa, NovoSeven) has recently been successfully used to correct the PT and maintain hemostasis in patients undergoing liver biopsy and there are increasing numbers of anecdotal reports of its use as adjuvant therapy to correct bleeding in patients with liver failure.[83,84]

Liver transplantation

Orthotopic liver transplantation is often the only effective treatment for children with acute or chronic end-stage liver failure. The procedure itself may add to existing hemostatic defects and can result in severe hemorrhage or, less commonly, arterial or venous thrombosis.[85–87]

Whereas bleeding during the first (preanhepatic) stage of the transplant is likely to be of surgical origin, hemorrhage in the second (anhepatic) stage of the transplant is associated with increased fibrinolysis secondary to the impaired clearance of tPA. A second burst of fibrinolysis then follows in the final (postanhepatic) stage following graft reperfusion, caused by increased tPA release from the graft endothelial cells. PAI-1 levels fall in the anhepatic stage and begin to normalize during the postanhepatic stage. Other processes that contribute to the hemostatic impairment include DIC, thrombocytopenia and the release of heparin-like factors from the graft.[85,88]

Preoperative coagulation tests are poor predictors of bleeding during liver transplantation and intraoperative monitoring of hemostasis has therefore been widely used to rationalize the use of appropriate blood components and drug therapy during surgery. As well as blood counts and coagulation screening tests, thromboelastography has been used as an overall measure of both coagulation and fibrinolysis, though doubts remain as to its value in the absence of severe bleeding. Indeed, there are no well-defined evidence-based guidelines for the use of blood component therapy during liver transplantation, and conflicting evidence exists as to the value of intraoperative coagulation testing.[89,90]

Antifibrinolytic therapy with tranexamic acid and aprotonin has been successful in reducing blood product support during surgery,[91–94] although the use of such drugs continues to vary between different liver transplant centers.

The introduction of rFVIIa has been reported to have reduced hemorrhage and blood product requirements in liver transplantation though further studies involving randomized trials are required to support these findings.[87,95,96] A large randomized and controlled study has shown that the use of rFVIIa during major liver resections has not influenced red cell transfusion requirement.[97]

Following liver transplantation there is an increased risk of hepatic artery thrombosis, which occurs in 2–20% of transplant patients with children having a higher incidence of this complication than adults.[98] Thrombosis usually occurs 4–10 days after transplant, the mechanism involving a relative delay in the recovery of the natural anticoagulants compared with procoagulant proteins, resulting in a transient prothrombotic state.[99,100] Fulminant graft necrosis often occurs, and this is also seen in the less frequent complication of portal vein thrombosis.

Hemostatic complications of renal disease

Renal disease can have a significant effect on hemostasis and result in hemorrhage or thrombosis, depending on the disease mechanism involved. In addition, treatments such as dialysis and renal transplantation can also be associated with particular hemostatic impairment.[101]

Nephrotic syndrome

Proteinuria, hypoalbuminemia and edema remain the characteristic features of this syndrome. The association between thromboembolic disease and nephrotic syndrome is well recognized both in children and in adults, occurring in up to 35% of patients.[102,103] Heavy proteinuria, membranous glomerulopathy and uncontrolled or refractory disease are risk factors for thrombosis; deep vein thrombosis, renal vein thrombosis and pulmonary embolus are the most frequent sites for thrombosis. Arterial thrombosis can also occur, though less frequently than venous disease.

A number of hemostatic defects occur in nephrotic syndrome and the etiology of thrombosis is demonstrably multifactorial.[104] Platelet aggregation and adhesion are increased, hyperfibrinogenemia is a constant finding and plasma antithrombin levels are reduced, with high levels of protein C often reported.[101,105] Effects on fibrinolysis remain unclear, both hypofibrinolysis and hyperfibrinolysis having been observed.[106,107] In addition, the contributory role of such factors as low-density lipoproteins requires further study.[108]

Coagulation tests are not predictive of the risk of thromboembolism in nephritic syndrome.[109] Heparin and warfarin are effective treatments for established thrombosis, with thrombolytic therapy being used infrequently.[103] Prophylactic anticoagulation has been proposed for high-risk nephrotic syndrome,[110] this being continued until the resolution of proteinuria.

Chronic renal failure

Bleeding is a well-known complication of chronic renal failure (CRF) that caused significant morbidity and mortality prior to the introduction of renal dialysis.[111] However, CRF should also be regarded as a prothrombotic state, and numerous studies have been undertaken to determine the pathogenesis of bleeding and thrombosis in this condition.

Bleeding is often mild and mucosal in origin, although surgery and invasive procedures can result in excessive hemorrhage. The bleeding diathesis is mainly due to defective platelet function and impaired platelet–vessel wall interaction, partly caused by uremic toxins.[112] Various and sometimes conflicting defects of platelet aggregation, adhesion and secretion have been described,[113–115] as has impaired interaction of vWF and platelet glycoprotein IIb–IIIa. Plasma vWF levels are increased in uremia, and this increase may compensate for any intrinsic platelet defect(s). Production of prostacyclin and nitric oxide by the vascular endothelium are increased in CRF, further contributing to impaired platelet aggregation and adhesion.[116,117] Activation of coagulation and fibrinolysis may also result in platelet dysfunction.[115,118]

In the absence of heparin the characteristic coagulation abnormalities in uremic children are a prolonged bleeding time with a normal or mildly reduced platelet count and normal coagulation screening tests. The hematocrit affects the bleeding time and an increase in hematocrit by red cell transfusion or erythropoietin therapy may result in a partial improvement in this parameter.[119,120] Desmopressin infusion and cryoprecipitate can result in temporary improvement in the bleeding time in some but not all patients with CRF.[121,122] The efficacy of platelet transfusions in uremic bleeding remains unproven.

Although children with CRF are at risk of bleeding, uremia can also be considered a prothrombotic state and thrombosis is a significant cause of morbidity and mortality in such patients. Again, the etiology of thrombosis is multifactorial, with hyperfibrinogenemia, high levels of vWF, increased thrombin generation and reduced plasma levels of natural anticoagulants identified as risk factors.[101] Increased platelet activation is seen with hemodialysis and can be considered a further contributory thrombophilic factor.[123–125] It is possible that the platelet dysfunction in uremia compensates for this prothrombotic state, and that the correction of platelet function may then increase the potential risk of thrombosis. Warfarin remains effective treatment for established thrombosis in CRF.

Hemolytic–uremic syndrome

Hemolytic–uremic syndrome (HUS) comprises microangiopathic hemolytic anemia, thrombocytopenia and acute renal dysfunction. The severity of the syndrome is variable but it remains the commonest cause of acute renal failure in children. The commonest, epidemic form of HUS (D+) follows infection with verotoxin-producing organisms, over 90% of cases being due to *Escherichia coli* and typically presenting with a prodromal illness of acute diarrhea or bloody diarrhea.[126] Sporadic (D–) HUS is not associated with preceding diarrhea and occurs much less commonly in children, with an incidence of about 1 per million children in the UK. Various causes of this atypical form have been described including drug exposure, other infective organisms and complement factor H deficiency.[127]

The pathogenesis of HUS is complex and follows injury to the renal endothelial cell and to circulating platelets.

Intravascular activation of coagulation occurs leading to fibrin deposition in the glomerular capillaries.[128,129] Fibrinolysis is also activated, though an overall decrease in plasma fibrinolytic potential secondary to high PAI-1 levels has been reported.[128,130] Platelet adhesion and aggregation are increased, and an imbalance in thromboxane and prostaglandin has been described.[131] Plasma levels of vWF antigen are increased and multimeric analysis may be normal or abnormal.[132,133] In contrast to thrombotic thrombocytopenic purpura, ADAMTS-13 (von Willebrand cleaving protease) deficiency has not been demonstrated in D+ HUS,[134,135] confirming different pathogenetic mechanisms in these two conditions.

Routine hematology investigations show a microangiopathic anemia, with thrombocytopenia a consistent finding. Severe thrombocytopenia is unusual and in D+ HUS both anemia and thrombocytopenia are of short duration; prolonged thrombocytopenia (>10 days) is an adverse prognostic factor, as is a raised neutrophil count on presentation. Coagulation tests are usually normal, with D-dimer levels either normal or only mildly increased.

Treatment for D+ HUS remains largely supportive with no evidence to show that FFP or plasma exchange improves outcome. Blood transfusion should be given on clinical indication and platelet transfusion avoided whenever possible. The management of D– HUS is more controversial, with plasma infusion and plasma exchange being used in selected patients.[127]

Cardiovascular-related hemostatic problems

Congenital heart disease

Conflicting data exist regarding the presence, mechanism and severity of hemostatic defects in children with congenital heart disease (CHD). The majority have been described in children with cyanotic CHD in association with secondary polycythemia.[136–146] In a study of 41 children, Henriksson *et al.*[138] concluded that hemostatic defects were common in the presence of cyanotic CHD and frequently involved deficiencies of FV and the vitamin K-dependent factors II, VII, IX and X. The mechanism was postulated to be reduced hepatic synthesis due to hypoxia, as a consequence of high blood viscosity, and there was no evidence of activation of the coagulation system. Other studies suggest that the coagulation system is activated and that low-grade DIC contributes to the observed abnormalities.[139,146]

In contrast, other investigators have demonstrated normal coagulation parameters in cyanotic CHD and it has been suggested that some of the previously documented abnormalities may have been artifactual due to failure to correct *in vitro* for the presence of polycythemia.[143,146] In support of this, a recent prospective study of 22 children with both cyanotic

and acyanotic CHD failed to demonstrate any difference in baseline preoperative concentrations of procoagulant proteins and inhibitors when compared with age-related normal ranges.[147] However, there was an increase in baseline TAT complex levels, which has been confirmed in other studies analyzing TAT together with other sensitive markers of coagulation activation.[148,149] This suggests that thrombin generation is increased in at least a proportion of patients but not to such an extent as to result in significant consumption of coagulation proteins.

Mild-to-moderate thrombocytopenia and abnormalities of platelet function have also been recorded in cyanotic CHD but again the mechanisms are poorly understood.[139,142,145,150,151] Coagulation and platelet abnormalities appear less common in acyanotic CHD; however, Gill *et al.*[152] demonstrated loss of high-molecular-weight multimers of vWF in children with a number of noncyanotic defects (atrial septal defect, ventricular septal defect and aortic stenosis), which normalized after successful cardiac surgery. Again, the mechanism is unclear but may involve platelet or endothelial cell activation.

In long-term follow-up of children who have undergone Fontan-type operations, variable coagulation defects have been reported including reduced levels of procoagulant and anticoagulant proteins.[153] These abnormalities are thought to occur as a consequence of abnormal hemodynamics resulting in subclinical hepatic dysfunction.

Noonan syndrome is a rare inherited disorder characterized by dysmorphic facies, CHD, short stature and a bleeding tendency. Various coagulation defects have been described in this condition, the most common being FXI deficiency although von Willebrand disease and abnormalities of platelet function are also reported. As yet the mechanism underlying this association in Noonan syndrome is not defined but may relate to the underlying disorder rather than the congenital heart defect.[154,155]

Although children with CHD rarely have hemorrhagic problems in day-to-day life, they may be at increased risk of bleeding during surgery, which highlights the need to correct potential underlying hemostatic defects preoperatively.

Cardiopulmonary bypass surgery

Hemorrhage remains an important problem both during and after cardiopulmonary bypass (CPB) surgery in children and the etiology is likely to be multifactorial in virtually all cases. Contributing factors include hemodilution of procoagulant proteins, thrombocytopenia and platelet dysfunction, activation of the coagulation and fibrinolytic systems with DIC, and iatrogenic anticoagulant effects (Table 29.5).[156] Whereas platelet dysfunction is thought to be the most important factor in adults, hemodilution of procoagulant proteins and problems relating to anticoagulant monitoring are probably more important in children.[157,158]

In one study, 22 children with CHD undergoing CPB had

Table 29.5 Causes of bleeding associated with cardiopulmonary bypass.

Preoperative coagulation defects
Hemodilution
Consumption (disseminated intravascular coagulation)
Thrombocytopenia
Platelet dysfunction
Heparin effects

samples collected for analysis of hemostatic proteins at various time points before, during and after bypass.[147] Significant hemodilution was demonstrated following initiation of CPB, with a reduction in the concentration of all hemostatic proteins by an average of 56% (range 50–70%). In some cases this resulted in reduction in procoagulant proteins to a level below that generally considered necessary for normal hemostasis. Although there was little further fall in levels during surgery, following completion of bypass the concentrations of certain procoagulants (FII, FV, FVII, FIX, FXI and FXII) remained significantly reduced 24 hours after the procedure. Platelet counts were also significantly reduced after bypass (mean $117 \times 10^9/L$; range $65–172 \times 10^9/L$).

Evidence of increased thrombin generation and increased fibrinolysis are also apparent during CPB and DIC may therefore contribute to hemorrhagic problems.[147,148,159] As well as thrombocytopenia, qualitative platelet defects develop during CPB, resulting in prolongation of the bleeding time independent of the actual platelet count. Platelet dysfunction is thought to be due to platelet contact with the synthetic surfaces of the bypass circuit and the effects of hypothermia. These functional abnormalities develop soon after commencement of bypass and are progressive, such that after 2 hours on bypass the bleeding time may exceed 30 min.[160] However, this effect is transient and normalization is reported after 2–4 hours in adult studies.[160] The nature of the platelet function defect remains controversial and results in keeping with platelet activation, as well as abnormalities of platelet membrane glycoproteins, have been described.[160–163] It has also been suggested that the problem may relate to an *in vivo* shortage of platelet agonists rather than to an actual intrinsic platelet defect.[164]

Anticoagulation with heparin is an important part of the CBP procedure. Current protocols utilize unfractionated heparin monitored with the activated clotting time (ACT), aiming to maintain the ACT above a predefined level (usually >400–450 s). At the end of the bypass procedure, heparin is reversed using protamine sulfate. It is clear, however, that the ACT correlates poorly with actual heparin levels as assessed by anti-FXa assays and this may result in suboptimal anticoagulant control in a significant number of cases.[147,165] The response to heparin may also be affected by the reduction in antithrombin levels that occur during the bypass procedure.[166]

Another potential complication of heparin therapy in this setting is heparin-induced thrombocytopenia (HIT). Although HIT appears less common in children than in adults, the incidence of this complication may be underestimated.[167–169] Although HIT typically develops five or more days after the initiation of heparin therapy, the onset can be more rapid where there has been prior heparin exposure.[170] This typically occurs in children who have undergone cardiac catheterization prior to surgery or in those undergoing a second surgical procedure involving CPB. Paradoxically, patients with HIT are at increased risk of thromboembolic complications, which can be arterial or venous and are often life-threatening. Patients with HIT who develop thrombotic complications and those with a prior history of HIT who require further anticoagulation have been treated with a variety of agents, including danaparoid, hirudin and argatroban.[167,171,172]

Bleeding in the context of CPB is often a multifactorial process and strategies aimed at the prevention and management of excessive bleeding need to take account of all the potential mechanisms involved. Correction of hemostatic defects with FFP, cryoprecipitate and platelets remains an important aspect of management, although there is no evidence base on which to recommend an optimal approach to replacement therapy. Adequate reversal of heparin with protamine sulfate following completion of CPB is also important. In addition, a number of other pharmacologic agents have been, or are currently in the process of being, investigated in an attempt to reduce perioperative and postoperative blood loss in this patient group. Recent interest has centered on the use of two agents, aprotinin and rFVIIa.

Aprotinin is a serine protease inhibitor that nonspecifically inhibits coagulation, fibrinolysis and complement activation.[173,174] A number of studies have now been completed in children and although early results were conflicting, more recent studies have generally shown a beneficial effect using various different end points.[174–176] In a large study published by Chauhan *et al.*,[175] 300 children with CHD were prospectively randomized to receive aprotinin plus ε-aminocaproic acid, ε-aminocaproic acid alone, or no treatment. Their results showed that all parameters, including blood loss at 24 hours and both red cell and platelet requirements, were improved in the aprotinin plus ε-aminocaproic acid group.[175] Questions remain regarding the optimal dose regimen and whether there is a benefit to adding an antifibrinolytic agent and these issues are the subject of ongoing studies.

rFVIIa (NovoSeven) is a hemostatic agent that was first developed for the treatment of hemophilia patients with inhibitors.[177] Following intravenous injection, rFVIIa enhances hemostasis by increasing thrombin generation on activated platelets. Preliminary data in small numbers of children with excessive bleeding following cardiac surgery have demonstrated potential benefits.[178,179] Further randomized studies are now required to define the place of this agent in the prevention and management of bleeding in this setting and to establish optimal dosing strategies.

Extracorporeal membrane oxygenation

Hemorrhage, particularly intracranial hemorrhage (ICH), is also a significant complication of extracorporeal membrane oxygenation (ECMO) and is an important predictor of outcome in this procedure.[180] ECMO facilitates the transfer of oxygen into blood across a semipermeable membrane and is used in a variety of conditions complicated by severe cardiorespiratory failure.[181] As with CPB, the etiology of bleeding is probably multifactorial, with thrombocytopenia, platelet dysfunction, coagulation abnormalities and problems relating to anticoagulant control all contributing. ICH is more frequent in the neonatal age group, which may reflect additional problems relating to immaturity of the hemostatic system as well as problems related to cerebral blood flow.[182]

McManus *et al.*[183] examined coagulation factors prior to and following the initiation of ECMO in 19 children and demonstrated the presence of preexisting coagulation defects (defined as reduced levels of two or more coagulation factors) in 68% of cases prior to ECMO. In addition, despite the use of coagulation factors in the circuit prime, which would be expected to compensate at least to some extent for the effect of hemodilution, 53% of patients had similar coagulation abnormalities after the start of ECMO. Four patients (three neonates and one older child) developed ICH and in this subgroup deficiencies in more than five coagulation factors were noted. McManus *et al.* concluded that a high proportion of cases have significant preexisting coagulation defects that are inadequately corrected by the circuit prime fluid at the onset of ECMO. Evidence of coagulation activation has also been demonstrated in term infants undergoing ECMO, particularly during the first 24 hours of the procedure; as with CPB, the ACT shows a poor correlation with actual heparin levels, which may increase the risk of both hemorrhagic and thrombotic problems.[184–186]

Hemostatic complications of metabolic disease

Gaucher disease

Gaucher disease is an inherited autosomal recessive condition caused by a deficiency of the enzyme glucocerebrosidase, which results in accumulation of glucocerebroside in cells of the monocytes/macrophage system. Bleeding manifestations are common in such patients and are partly caused by thrombocytopenia due to splenomegaly but platelet function abnormalities have also been described.[187] In addition, low levels of several coagulation factors, including FII, FV, FVII, FX, FIX, FXI and FXII, have been reported with

prolonged PT and APTT values in 38% and 42% of patients, respectively.[188,189] However, FXI deficiency in some cases may be an independent abnormality as both inherited FXI deficiency and Gaucher disease are common in Ashkenazi Jews.[190]

Bleeding is generally mild despite the apparent severity of the coagulation abnormalities and in most cases correlates best with the degree of thrombocytopenia. The pathophysiology of the coagulopathy remains poorly understood but does not appear to reflect impaired synthesis due to hepatic dysfunction. The effect of enzyme replacement therapy with aglucerase also appears variable, with partial correction of the coagulation disturbance recorded by Hollak *et al.*[188] while Billet *et al.*[191] did not find any effect.

Acquired inhibitors of coagulation

Acquired inhibitors of coagulation can be divided into those which inhibit specific coagulation factors (e.g., FVIII and FIX) and those which are nonspecific and interfere with other aspects of the coagulation cascade (e.g., lupus anticoagulants). Inhibitors characteristically prolong one or more of the coagulation screening tests, which will shorten as the plasma is serially diluted, rather than lengthen as happens in deficiency states.

Inhibitors of specific coagulation proteins

Factor VIII and factor IX inhibitors

Specific inhibitors are a well-recognized complication of replacement therapy in the management of congenital factor deficiencies and are most frequently seen in hemophilia A. FVIII and FIX inhibitors in children without hemophilia are uncommon but have been reported in a few cases sometimes in association with malignancy or possibly recent use of high-dose penicillin.[192–195] The pattern of bleeding is variable, with some cases being diagnosed incidentally or in association with only mild-to-moderate bleeding symptoms, while others present with severe life-threatening hemorrhage.

Management of bleeding in children with acquired antibodies to FVIII or FIX is similar to that used for children with hemophilia who develop inhibitors and may involve the administration of high-dose FVIII or FIX; alternative therapies include porcine FVIII, PCCs or rFVIIa.[196,197] Treatment aimed at the eradication of these antibodies may not always be required as some seem to disappear spontaneously. In cases where there are significant hemorrhagic problems, early introduction of immunosuppressive therapy with intravenous immunoglobulin may be beneficial. Steroids and cytotoxic agents (e.g., cyclophosphamide) have also been used successfully in some children with persisting antibodies, but may be associated with significant side-effects.[192,195]

von Willebrand factor inhibitors

Acquired inhibitors to vWF are again extremely rare in children but have been reported in association with other autoantibodies and in children with Wilm tumor.[198,199] Recognition of von Willebrand disease in Wilm tumor is important as some treatment protocols utilize early surgery. These antibodies usually disappear spontaneously following successful treatment of the tumor; however, in the event of treatment being required, desmopressin or replacement therapy with factor concentrate containing high-molecular-weight vWF multimers may be indicated.[200]

Factor V inhibitors

Acquired FV inhibitors in children have been most commonly reported following surgery in which fibrin sealant containing bovine thrombin has been used to improve hemostasis.[201,202] Only occasionally have they been reported in other situations, typically following major surgery. The development of a FV inhibitor is characterized by prolongation of both the PT and APTT on routine postoperative coagulation monitoring which may be associated with excess bleeding. While many of these antibodies appear to be transient, reexposure to the same fibrin sealant product can result in the reappearance of the antibody and lead to severe hemorrhagic problems.[202]

When treatment is required due to acute bleeding, FFP is the only available source of FV but may result in problems with fluid overload. Alternative strategies include the use of plasmapheresis, high-dose intravenous immunoglobulin and rFVIIa.[202,203]

Other inhibitors

Antibodies with specificity against FX, FXI and other contact factors have also been reported and can result in hemorrhagic problems but appear to be extremely rare in the pediatric age group.[204–206]

Antiphospholipid antibodies

Antiphospholipid antibodies comprise a family of antibodies reactive with epitopes on proteins that are complexed to negatively charged phospholipid. They can be detected *in vitro* in solid-phase immunoassays, where they are generally called anticardiolipin antibodies, or in phospholipid-dependent coagulation tests, where the term "lupus anticoagulant" is usually applied. Lupus anticoagulants prolong phospholipid-dependent clotting assays, usually the APTT, which does not correct on mixing. To confirm that there is a lupus anticoagulant present, guidelines recommend a test such as the dilute Russell's viper venom time with a platelet neutralization procedure.[207]

Although antiphospholipid antibodies can be associated with increased thrombotic risk, they are detected incidentally in a significant proportion of healthy subjects and particularly in children. The thrombotic risk associated with such incidental antiphospholipid antibodies is relatively low,[208] the antibody often being secondary to a viral infection that resolves spontaneously.[209,210] Systemic lupus erythematosus (SLE) is rare in children but where it is associated with antiphospholipid antibodies, the risk of thrombosis is significantly increased. A positive test for lupus anticoagulant is more predictive of thrombosis than a positive test for anticardiolipin antibodies, increasing the risk of thrombosis 16- to 25-fold.[211]

A number of studies have examined the prevalence of antiphospholipid antibodies in children presenting with thrombosis who do not have SLE. Manco Johnson and Nuss[212] found antiphospholipid antibodies in 19 of 78 (24%) children who presented with thrombosis at a single institution over a 7-year period. Only five fulfilled the necessary criteria for a diagnosis of SLE, while the other 14 were classified as having the antiphospholipid syndrome. The association of childhood thrombosis with antiphospholipid antibodies in the absence of SLE has been recognized in a number of other small case series and, in particular, it has been suggested that there may be a significant association with childhood stroke.[213–217] Children with the antiphospholipid syndrome may also exhibit some of the other clinical features defined in adults with this condition, including chorea, livedo reticularis and thrombocytopenia.[218]

With regard to management, standard anticoagulant protocols should be employed in the initial treatment of acute thombotic events in children with antiphospholipid antibodies. The subsequent duration and intensity of warfarin therapy and the role, if any, of steroids and immunosuppressive agents in such patients remain uncertain.

Another syndrome that is now fairly well recognized is the association of a lupus anticoagulant with acquired protein S deficiency, resulting in DIC and purpura fulminans following varicella infection.[219] Autoantibodies to protein S result in a transient free protein S deficiency, probably as a result of increased clearance of protein S from the circulation. Fragment 1 + 2 levels are increased in keeping with DIC. Although most cases involve microvascular thrombosis and purpura fulminans, large-vessel thrombosis including deep vein thrombosis and stroke has also been reported. This is a rare condition and the optimal management strategy is not yet defined. Anticoagulant therapy with heparin has been used successfully in some cases but the use of protein S replacement therapy with FFP requires further evaluation to establish a beneficial effect.

Although the vast majority of children with clinically symptomatic antiphospholipid antibodies have thrombotic events, hemorrhagic problems are occasionally seen in association with the presence of a concomitant autoimmune thrombocytopenia or coagulation factor deficiency. In the latter situation, the so-called hemorrhagic lupus anticoagulant syndrome has most commonly been observed in association with acquired hypoprothrombinemia.[220,221] Typical features of this syndrome include the sudden onset of bleeding symptoms of variable severity in a child with no past history of bleeding problems, who may have had a recent viral infection. Laboratory studies show a prolonged APTT with evidence of a lupus anticoagulant and reduced prothrombin levels. The syndrome usually resolves spontaneously within 3 months and does not generally require treatment, although steroids have been given in some cases. In the presence of significant bleeding, the use of PCCs should be considered.

References

1. Andrew M, Paes B, Milner R *et al.* Development of the coagulation system in the full term infant. *Blood* 1987; **70**: 165–72.
2. Andrew M, Paes B, Milner R *et al.* Development of the human coagulation system in the healthy premature infant. *Blood* 1988; **72**: 1651–7.
3. Salvonaara M, Riikonen P, Vahtera E, Mahlamaki E, Heinonen K. Development of selected coagulation and anticoagulants in preterm infants by the age of six months. *Thromb Haemost* 2004; **92**: 688–96.
4. Andrew M, Vegh P, Johnston M, Bowker J, Ofosu F, Mitchell L. Maturation of the hematopoietic system during childhood. *Blood* 1988; **80**: 1998–2005.
5. Andrew M. Developmental hemostasis: relevance to hemostatic problems during childhood. *Semin Thromb Hemost* 1995; **21**: 341–56.
6. Kuhle S, Male C, Mitchell L. Developmental hemostasis: pro- and anticoagulant systems during childhood. *Semin Thromb Hemost* 2003; **29**: 329–37.
7. Monagle P, Ignjatovic V, Barnes C *et al.* Reference ranges for hemostatic parameters in children. *Thromb Haemost* 2003; **1** (suppl. 1): P0076.
8. Sutor AH. The bleeding time in paediatrics. *Semin Thromb Haemost* 1998; **24**: 531–43.
9. Sanders J, Holtkamp C, Buchanan G. The bleeding time may be longer in children than in adults. *Am J Hematol Oncol* 1990; **12**: 314–18.
10. Andrew M, Mitchell L, Vegh P, Ofosu F. Thrombin regulation in children differs from adults in the absence and presence of heparin. *Thomb Haemost* 1994; **72**: 836–42.
11. Schmidt B, Mitchell L, Ofosu FA, Andrew M. Alpha-2-macroglobulin is an important progressive inhibitor of thrombin in neonatal and infant plasma. *Thromb Haemost* 1989; **62**: 1074–7.
12. Mitchell L, Piovella F, Ofosu F, Andrew M. Alpha-2-macroglobulin may provide protection from thomboembolic events in antithrombin III deficient children. *Blood* 1991; **78**: 2299–304.
13. David M, Andrew M. Venous thromboembolism complications in children: a critical review of the literature. *J Pediatr* 1993; **123**: 337–46.
14. Andrew M. Developmental hemostasis: relevance to thromboembolic complications in pediatric patients. *Thromb Haemost* 1995; **74**: 415–25.
15. Chalmers EA. Epidemiology of childhood thrombosis. *Thromb Res* 2006 (in press).
16. Taylor FB Jr, Toh CH, Hoots K, Wada H, Levi M. Towards a definition, clinical and laboratory criteria and a scoring system for disseminated intravascular coagulation. *Thromb Haemost* 2001; **86**: 1327–30.
17. Bick RL. Disseminated intravascular coagulation. A review of etiology, pathophysiology, diagnosis, and management: guidelines for care. *Clin Appl Thromb Hemost* 2002; **8**: 1–31.
18. Levi M. Current understanding of disseminated intravascular coagulation. *Br J Haematol* 2004; **124**: 567–76.
19. Bone RC. Gram-positive organisms and sepsis. *Arch Intern Med* 1994; **154**: 26–34.
20. Tallman MS, Kwaan HD. Reassesssing the hemostatic disorder associated with acute promyelocytic leukaemia. *Blood* 1992; **79**: 543–53.
21. Hall GW. Kasabach–Merritt syndrome: pathogenesis and management. *Br J Haematol* 2001; **112**: 851–62.
22. Toh CH, Dennis M. Disseminated intravascular coagulation: old disease, new hope. *Br Med J* 2003; **327**: 974–7.
23. Biemond BJ, Levi M, ten Cate H *et al.* Complete inhibition of endotoxin-induced coagulation activation in chimpanzees with a monoclonal Fab fragment against factor VII/VIIa. *Thromb Haemost* 1995; **73**: 223–30.
24. Shimura M, Wada H, Wakita Y *et al.* Plasma tissue factor and tissue factor pathway inhibitor levels in patients with disseminated intravascular coagulation. *Am J Hematol* 1997; **55**: 169–74.
25. Gando S, Kameue T, Morimoto Y, Matsuda M, Hayakawa M, Kemmotsu O. Tissue factor production not balanced by tissue factor pathway inhibitor in sepsis promotes poor prognosis. *Crit Care Med* 2002; **30**: 1729–34.
26. Esmon CT. The regulation of natural anticoagulant pathways. *Science* 1987; **235**: 1348–52.
27. Mesters RM, Mannucci PM, Coppola R, Keller T, Ostermann H, Kienast J. Factor VIIa and antithrombin III activity during severe sepsis and septic shock in neutropenic patients. *Blood* 1996; **88**: 881–6.
28. Esmon CT. Role of coagulation inhibitors in inflammation. *Thromb Haemost* 2001; **86**: 51–6.
29. Biemond BJ, Levi M, ten Cate H *et al.* Plasminogen activator and plasminogen activator inhibitor I release during experimental endotoxaemia in chimpanzees: effect of interventions in the cytokine and coagulation cascades. *Clin Sci* 1995; **88**: 587–94.
30. Coughlin SR. Thrombin signalling and protease-activated receptors. *Nature* 2000; **407**: 258–64.
31. Van der Poll T, de Jonge E, Levi M. Regulatory role of cytokines in disseminated intravascular coagulation. *Semin Thromb Hemost* 2001; **27**: 639–51.
32. Okajima K. Regulation of inflammatory responses by natural anticoagulants. *Immunol Rev* 2001; **184**: 258–74.
33. Francis RB. Acquired purpura fulminans. *Semin Thromb Hemost* 1990; **16**: 310–25.
34. Toh CH, Giles AR. Waveform analysis of clotting test optical profiles in the diagnosis and management of disseminated intravascular coagulation (DIC). *Clin Lab Haematol* 2002; **24**: 321–7.

35. Feinstein DI. Diagnosis and management of disseminated intravascular coagulation: the role of heparin therapy. *Blood* 1982; **60**: 284–7.

36. Abraham E, Reinhart K, Opal S *et al*. Efficacy and safety of tifacogin (recombinant tissue factor pathway inhibitor) in severe sepsis: a randomised controlled trial. *JAMA* 2003; **290**: 238–47.

37. Hanada T, Abe T, Takita H. Antithrombin III concentrates for treatment of disseminated intravascular coagulation in children. *Am J Pediatr Hematol Oncol* 1985; **7**: 3–8.

38. Fuse S, Tomita H, Yoshida M, Hori T, Igarashi C, Fujita S. High dose of intravenous antithrombin III without heparin in the treatment of disseminated intravascular coagulation and organ failure in four children. *Am J Hematol* 1996; **53**: 18–21.

39. Eisele B, Lamy M, Thijs LG *et al*. Antithrombin III in patients with severe sepsis. A randomised, placebo-controlled, double-blind, multicenter trial plus a meta-analysis on all randomised, placebo-controlled, double-blind trials with antithrombin III in severe sepsis. *Intensive Care Med* 1998; **24**: 663–72.

40. Warren BL, Eid A, Singer P *et al*. Caring for the critically ill patient. High dose antithrombin III in severe sepsis: a randomised controlled trial. *JAMA* 2001; **286**: 1869–78.

41. Rivard GE, David M, Farrell C. Treatment of purpura fulminans in meningococcemia with protein C concentrate. *J Pediatr* 1995; **126**: 646–52.

42. Smith OP, White B, Vaughan D *et al*. Use of protein C concentrate, heparin and haemofiltration in meningococcus induced purpura fulminans. *Lancet* 1997; **359**: 1590–3.

43. Faust SN, Levin M, Harrison OB *et al*. Dysfunction of endothelial protein C activation in severe meningococcal sepsis. *N Engl J Med* 2001; **345**: 408–16.

44. Bernard GR, Vincent JL, Laterre PF *et al*. Efficacy and safety of recombinant human activated protein C for severe sepsis. *N Engl J Med* 2001; **344**: 699–709.

45. Vincent JL, Angus DC, Artigas A *et al*. Effects of drotrecogin alfa (activated) on organ dysfunction in the PROWESS trial. *Crit Care Med* 2003; **31**: 834–40.

46. Wiedermann CJ, Kaneider NC. Comparison of mechanisms after post-hoc analyses of the drotrecogin alfa (activated) and antithrombin III trials in severe sepsis. *Ann Med* 2004; **36**: 194–203.

47. Dam H. Cholesterinstoffwechsel in Hühnereiern and Hühnchen. *Biochem Z* 1929; **215**: 475–92.

48. Jackson CM, Nemerson Y. Blood coagulation. *Annu Rev Biochem* 1980; **49**: 765–811.

49. Vermeer C. Comparison between hepatic and nonhepatic vitamin K-dependent carboxylase. *Haemostasis* 1986; **16**: 239–45.

50. Shearer M. Vitamin K and vitamin K dependent proteins. *Br J Haematol* 1990; **75**: 156–62.

51. Booth SL, Suttie JW. Dietry intake and adequacy of vitamin K. *J Nutr* 1998; **128**: 785–8.

52. Suttie JW. Vitamin K and human nutrition. *J Am Diet Assoc* 1992; **92**: 585–90.

53. Wallin R, Martin LF. Vitamin K-dependent carboxylation and vitamin K metabolism in liver: effects of warfarin. *J Clin Invest* 1985; **76**: 1879–84.

54. Lipsky JJ. Review: antibiotic-associated hypopro-thrombinaemia. *J Antimicrob Chemother* 1988; **21**: 281–300.

55. Cohen H, Scott SD, Mackie IJ *et al*. The development of hypoprothrombinaemia following antibiotic therapy in malnourished patients with low serum vitamin K levels. *Br J Haematol* 1988; **68**: 63–6.

56. Shearer MJ, Bechtold H, Andrassy K *et al*. Mechanism of cephalosporin induced hypoprothrombinemia: relation to cephalosporin side chain, vitamin K metabolism and vitamin K status. *J Clin Pharmacol* 1988; **28**: 88–95.

57. Suzuki G, Iwata G, Sutor AH. Vitamin K deficiency during the perinatal and infantile period. *Seminars in Thrombosis & Hemostasis* 2001; **27**: 93–8.

58. Blanchard RA, Furie BC, Kruger SF, Waneck G, Jorgensen MJ, Fune B. Immunoassays of human prothrombin species which correlate with functional coagulant activities. *J Lab Clin Med* 1983; **101**: 242–55.

59. Motohara K, Kuroki Y, Kan H, Endo F, Matsuda I. Detection of vitamin K deficiency by use of an enzyme-linked immunosorbent assay for circulating abnormal prothrombin. *Pediatr Res* 1985; **19**: 354–7.

60. Widdershoven J, van Munster P, De Abreu R *et al*. Four methods compared for measuring des-carboxy-prothrombin (PIVKA II). *Clin Chem* 1987; **33**: 2074–8.

61. Sutor AH, Kunzer W. Time interval between vitamin K administration and effective haemostasis. In: Suzuki S, Hathaway WE, Bonnar J, Sutor AH (eds) *Perinatal Thrombosis and Haemostasis*. Berlin: Springer-Verlag, 1991, pp. 257–62.

62. Sutor AH. Vitamin K deficiency bleeding in infants and children. *Semin Thromb Hemost* 1995; **21**: 317–29.

63. Sakkinen PA, Dickerman JD, Colletti RB, Sadowski JA, Golden EA, Bovill EG. Severe acquired vitamin K deficiency: a hypothesis for rapid response to therapy. *Blood Coag Fibrinol* 2000; **11**: 309–11.

64. Duguid J, O'Shaughnessy DF, Atterbury C *et al*. Guidelines for the use of fresh frozen plasma, cryoprecipitate and cryosupernatant. *Br J Haematol* 2004; **126**: 11–28.

65. Department of Health. *Report on Health and Social Subjects No. 41: Dietary Reference Values for Food Energy and Nutrients for the United Kingdom*. London: HMSO, 1991.

66. Durie PR. Vitamin K and the management of patients with cystic fibrosis. *Can Med Assoc J* 1994; **151**: 933–6.

67. Ramsey BW, Farrell PM, Pencharz P and the Consensus Committee. Nutritional support and the management in cystic fibrosis. *Am J Clin Nutr* 1992; **55**: 108–16.

68. Wilson DC, Rashid M, Durie PR *et al*. Treatment of vitamin K deficiency in cystic fibrosis: effectivness of a daily fat-soluble vitamin combination. *J Pediatr* 2001; **138**: 851–5.

69. Van Hoorn JHL, Hendricks JJE, Vermeer C, Forget PP. Vitamin K supplements in cystic fibrosis. *Arch Dis Child* 2003; **88**: 974–5.

70. Amitrano L, Guardascione MA, Brancaccio V, Balzano A. Coagulation disorders in liver disease. *Semin Liver Dis* 2002; **22**: 83–96.

71. Lisman T, Leebeek FWG, de Groot PG. Haemostatic abnormalities in patients with liver disease. *J Hepatol* 2002; **37**: 280–7.

72. Hollestelle MJ, Thinnes T, Crain K *et al*. Tissue distribution of factor VIII gene expression in vivo: a closer look. *Thromb Haemost* 2001; **86**: 855–61.

73. Green G, Thomson JM, Dymock JW, Poller L. Abnormal fibrinogen polymerisation in liver disease. *Br J Haematol* 1976; **34**: 425–39.

74. Soria J, Soria C, Ryckewaert JJ, Samama M, Thomson JM, Poller L. Study of acquired dysfibrinogenaemia in liver disease. *Thromb Res* 1980; **19**: 29–41.

75. Leiper K, Croll A, Booth NA, Moore NR, Sinclair T, Bennett B. Tissue plasminogen activator, plasminogen activator inhibitors and activator–inhibitor complex in liver disease. *J Clin Pathol* 1994; **47**: 214–17.

76. Pernambuco JR, Langley PG, Hughes RD, Izumi S, Williams R. Activation of the fibrinolytic system in patients with fulminant liver failure. *Hepatology* 1993; **18**: 1350–6.

77. Ben Ari Z, Osman E, Hutton RA, Burroughs AK. Disseminated intravascular coagulation in liver cirrhosis: fact or fiction? *Am J Gastroenterol* 1999; **94**: 2977–82.

78. Laffi G, Marra F, Failli P, Ruggiero M, Cecchi E, Carloni V. Defective signal transduction in platelets from cirrhotics is associated with increased cyclic nucleotides. *Gastroenterology* 1993; **105**: 148–56.

79. Albornoz L, Bandi JC, Otaso JC, Laudanno O, Mastai R. Prolonged bleeding time in experimental cirrhosis: role of nitric oxide. *J Hepatol* 1999; **30**: 456–60.

80. Pasche B, Ouimet H, Francis S, Loscalzo J. Structural changes in platelet glycoprotein IIb/IIIa by plasmin: determinants and functional consequences. *Blood* 1994; **83**: 404–14.

81. Piccinino F, Sagnelli E, Pasquale G, Giusti G. Complications following percutaneous liver biopsy. A multicentre retrospective study on 68276 biopsies. *J Hepatol* 1986; **2**: 165–73.

82. Burroughs AK, Matthews K, Qadiri M et al. Desmopressin and bleeding time in patients with cirrhosis. *Br Med J* 1985; **291**: 1377–81.

83. Chuansumrit A, Treepongkaruna S, Phuapradit P. Combined fresh frozen plasma with recombinant factor VIIa in restoring hemostasis for invasive procedures in children with liver diseases. *Thromb Haemost* 2001; **85**: 748–9.

84. Papatheodoridis GV, Chung S, Keshav S, Pasi J, Burroughs AK. Correction of both prothrombin time and primary haemostasis by recombinant factor VII during therapeutic alcohol injection of hepatocellular cancer in liver cirrhosis. *J Hepatol* 1999; **31**: 747–50.

85. Porte RJ. Coagulation and fibrinolysis in orthotopic liver transplantation: current views and insights. *Semin Thromb Hemost* 1993; **19**: 191–6.

86. Ozier Y, Steib A, Ickx B et al. Haemostatic disorders during liver transplantation. *Eur J Anaesthesiol* 2001; **18**: 208–18.

87. Silva MA, Muralidharan V, Mirza DF. The management of coagulopathy and blood loss in liver surgery. *Semin Hematol* 2004; **41** (suppl. 1): 132–9.

88. Dzik WH, Arkus CF, Jenkins RL, Stump DC. Fibrinolysis during liver transplantation in humans: role of t-PA. *Blood* 1988; **71**: 1090–5.

89. Kang Y Transfusion based on clinical coagulation monitoring does reduce hemorrhage during liver transplantation. *Liver Transplant Surg* 1997; **3**: 655–9.

90. Reyle-Hahn M, Roissant R. Coagulation techniques are not important in directing blood product transfusion during liver transplantation. *Liver Transplant Surg* 1997; **3**: 663–5.

91. Neuhaus P, Bechstein WO, Lefèbre B, Blumhardt G, Slama K. Effect of aprotonin on intraoperative bleeding and fibrinolysis in liver transplantation. *Lancet* 1989; **ii**: 924–5.

92. Boylan JF, Klinck JR, Sandler AN et al. Tranexamic acid reduces blood loss, transfusion requirements, and coagulation factor use in primary orthotopic liver transplantation. *Anesthesiology* 1996; **85**: 1043–8.

93. Findlay JY, Rettke SR, Ereth MH, Plevak DJ, Krom RA, Kufner RP. Aprotonin reduces red cell transfusion in orthotopic liver transplantation: a prospective, randomised, double-blind study. *Liver Transplant* 2001; **7**: 802–7.

94. Dalmau A, Sabaté A, Maylin K et al. The prophylactic use of tranexamic acid and aprotonin in orthotopic liver transplantation: a comparative study. *Liver Transplant* 2004; **10**: 279–84.

95. Markiewicz M, Kalicinski P, Kaminski A et al. Acute coagulopathy after reperfusion of the liver graft in children: correction with recombinant activated factor VII. *Transplant Proc* 2003; **35**: 2318–19.

96. Meijer K, Hendiks-Herman GD, De-Wolf JThM et al. Recombinant factor VIIa in orthotopic liver transplantation: influence on parameters of coagulation and fibrinolysis. *Blood Coag Fibrinol* 2003; **14**: 169–74.

97. Lodge JPA, Jones S, Oussoult Zoglou E et al. Recombinant coagulation factor VIIa in major liver resection: a randomised, placebo-controlled, double-blind trial. *Anesthesiology* 2005; **102**: 269–75.

98. Cienfuegos JA, Dominiquez RM, Tanelchoff PJ et al. Surgical complications in the post operative period of liver transplantation in children. *Transplant Proc* 1984; **16**: 1230–5.

99. Harper PL, Edgar PF, Luddington RJ et al. Protein C deficiency and portal vein thrombosis in liver transplantion on children. *Lancet* 1988; **ii**: 924–7.

100. Stahl RL, Duncan A, Hooks MA, Henderson MJ, Millikan WJ, Warren MD. A hypercoagulable state follows orthotopic liver transplantation. *Hepatology* 1990; **12**: 553–8.

101. Rabelink TJ, Zwaginga JJ, Koomans HA, Sixma JJ. Thrombosis and hemostasis in renal disease. *Kidney Int* 1994; **46**: 287–96.

102. Llach F. Hypercoagulability, renal vein thrombosis and other thrombotic complications of nephrotic syndrome. *Kidney Int* 1985; **28**: 429–39.

103. Andrew M, Brooker LA. Hemostatic complications in renal disorders of the young. *Pediatr Nephrol* 1996; **10**: 88–99.

104. Schlegel N. Thromboembolic risks and complications in nephrotic children. *Semin Thromb Hemost* 1997; **23**: 271–80.

105. Citak A, Emre S, Sâirin A, Bilge I, Nayir A. Hemostatic problems and thromboembolic complications in nephrotic children. *Pediatr Nephrol* 2000; **14**: 138–42.

106. Al-Mugeiren MM, Gader AM, al-Rasheed SA, Bahakim HM, al-Momen AK, al-Salloum A. Coagulopathy of childhood nephrotic syndrome: a reappraisal of the role of natural anticoagulants and fibrinolysis. *Haemostasis* 1996; **26**: 304–10.

107. Colle JP, Mishal Z, Lesty C et al. Abnormal fibrin clot architecture in nephritic patients is related to hypofibrinolysis: influence of plasma biochemical modifications. A possible mechanism for high thrombotic tendency? *Thromb Haemost* 1999; **82**: 1482–9.

108. Soulat T, Loyau S, Baudouin V et al. Evidence that modifications of Lp(a) in vivo inhibit plasmin formation on fibrin: a study with individual plasmas presenting natural variations of Lp(a). *Thromb Haemost* 1999; **82**: 121–7.

109. Robert A, Olmer M, Sampol J, Gugliotta J, Casanova P. Clinical

correlation between hypercoagulability and thrombo-embolic phenomena. *Kidney Int* 1987; **31**: 830–5.

110. Bellow R, Atkins RC. Membranous nephropathy and thromboembolism. Is prophylactic anticoagulation warranted? *Nephron* 1993; **63**: 249–54.

111. Remuzzi G. Bleeding in renal failure. *Lancet* 1988; **i**: 1205–8.

112. Boccardo P, Remuzzi G, Galbusera M. Platelet function in renal failure. *Semin Thromb Hemost* 2004; **30**: 579–89.

113. Di Minno G, Martínez J, McKean M, De La Rosa J, Burke JF, Murphy S. Platelet dysfunction in uraemia. Multifaceted defect partially corrected by dialysis. *Am J Med* 1985; **79**: 552–9.

114. Soslau G, Brodsky I, Putatunda B, Parker J, Schwartz AB. Selective reduction of serotonin storage and ATP release in chronic renal failure patient platelets. *Am J Hematol* 1990; **35**: 171–8.

115. Mezzano D, Tagle R, Panes O *et al*. Hemostatic disorder of uremia: the platelet defect, main determinant of the prolonged bleeding time, is correlated with indices of activation of coagulation and fibrinolysis. *Thromb Haemost* 1996; **76**: 312–21.

116. Remuzzi G, Cavenaghi A, Mecca G, Donati M, de Gaetano G. Prostacyclin-like activity and bleeding in renal failure. *Lancet* 1977; **ii**: 1195–7.

117. Remuzzi G, Perico N, Zoja C, Corna D, Macconi D, Vigano G. Role of endothelium-derived nitric oxide in the bleeding tendency of uremia. *J Clin Invest* 1990; **86**: 1768–71.

118. Mezzano D, Panes O, Muñoz B *et al*. Tranexamic acid inhibits fibrinolysis, shortens the bleeding time and improves platelet function in patients with chronic renal failure. *Thromb Haemost* 1999; **82**: 1250–4.

119. Livio M, Marchesi D, Remuzzi G, Gotti E, Mecca G, de Gaetano G. Uraemic bleeding: role of anaemia and beneficial effect of red cell transfusions. *Lancet* 1982; **ii**: 1013–15.

120. Moia M, Vizzotto L, Cattaneo M, Mannucci PM, Casati S, Ponticcelli C. Improvement in the hemostatic defect in uremia after treatment with recombinant human erythropoietin. *Lancet* 1987; **ii**: 1227–9.

121. Mannucci PM, Remuzzi G, Pusineri F *et al*. Desamino-8-arginine vasopressin shortens the bleeding time in uremia. *N Engl J Med* 1983; **308**: 8–12.

122. Zeigler ZR, Megaludis A, Fraley DS. Desmopressin effects on platelet rheology and von Willebrand factor activities in uremia. *Am J Hematol* 1992; **39**: 90–5.

123. Sirolli V, Strizzi L, Di Stante S, Robuffo I, Procopio A, Bonomini M. Platelet activation and platelet–erythrocyte aggregates in end-stage renal disease patients on hemodialysis. *Thromb Haemost* 2001; **86**: 834–9.

124. Bonomini M, Dottori S, Amoroso L, Arduini A, Sirolli V. Increased platelet phosphatidylserine exposure and caspase activation in chronic uremia. *J Thromb Haemost* 2004; **2**: 1275–81.

125. Zwaginga JJ. Hemodialysis, erythropoietin and megakaryopoiesis: factors in uremic thrombocytopathy and thrombophilia. *J Thromb Haemost* 2004; **2**: 1272–4.

126. Milford DV, Taylor CM, Guttridge B, Hall SM, Rowe B, Kleanthous H. Haemolytic uraemic syndrome in the British Isles 1985–88: association with verotoxin producing *Escherichia coli*. Part I. Clinical and epidemiological aspects. *Arch Dis Child* 1990; **65**: 716–21.

127. Allford SL, Hunt BJ, Rose P, Machin SJ. Guidelines on the diagnosis and management of the thrombotic

microangiopathic haemolytic anaemias. *Br J Haematol* 2003; **120**: 556–73.

128. Nevard CHF, Jurd KM, Lane DA, Philippou H, Haycock GB, Hunt BJ. Activation of coagulation and fibrinolysis in childhood diarrhoea-associated haemolytic uraemic syndrome. *Thromb Haemost* 1997; **78**: 1450–5.

129. Van Geet C, Proesmans W, Arnout J, Vermylen J, Declerck PJ. Activation of both coagulation and fibrinolysis in childhood haemolytic uremic syndrome. *Kidney Int* 1998; **54**: 1324–30.

130. Bergstein JM, Riley M, Bang NU. Role of plasminogen-activator inhibitor type 1 in the pathogenesis and outcome of the haemolytic uraemic syndrome. *N Engl J Med* 1992; **327**: 755–9.

131. Siegler RL. Prostacyclin in the haemolytic uremic syndrome. *J Nephrol* 1993; **6**: 64–9.

132. Rose PE, Enayat SM, Sunderland R, Short PE, Williams CE, Hill FGH. Abnormalities of factor VIII related protein multimers in the haemolytic uraemic syndrome. *Arch Dis Child* 1984; **59**: 1135–40.

133. Sutor AH, Thomas KB, Prüfer FH, Grohmann A, Brandis M, Zimmerhackl LB. Function of von Willebrand factor in chidren with diarrhea-associated haemolytic-uremic syndrome (D+ HUS). *Semin Thromb Hemost* 2001; **27**: 287–92.

134. Hunt BJ, Lämmle B, Nevard CHF, Haycock GB, Furlan M. Von Willebrand factor-cleaving protease in childhood diarrhoea-associated haemolytic uraemic syndrome. *Thromb Haemost* 2001; **85**: 975–8.

135. Veyradier A, Obert B, Houillier A, Meyer D, Girma JP. Specific von Willebrand factor-cleaving protease in thrombotic microangiopathies: a study of 111 cases. *Blood* 2001; **98**: 1765–72.

136. Jootar S, Archararit N, Suvachittanont O. Hemostatic defect in cyanotic and acyanotic congenital heart disease. *J Med Associ Thai* 1988; **71**: 382–7.

137. Suarez CR, Menendez CE, Griffin AJ, Ow EP, Walenga M, Fareed J. Cyanotic congenital heart disease in children: hemostatic disorders and relevance of molecular markers of hemostasis. *Semin Thromb Hemost* 1984; **10**: 285–9.

138. Henriksson P, Varendh G, Lundstrom NR. Haemostatic defects in cyanotic congenital heart disease. *Br Heart J* 1979; **41**: 23–7.

139. Goldschmidt B. Blood coagulation and platelet abnormalities in cyanotic congenital heart disease. *Lancet* 1973; **i**: 607.

140. Ihenacho HNC, Breeze GR, Fletcher DJ, Stuart J. Consumption coagulopathy in congenital heart disease. *Lancet* 1973; **i**: 231–4.

141. Wedemeyer AL, Edson JR, Krivit W. Coagulation in cyanotic congenital heart disease. *Am J Dis Child* 1972; **124**: 656–60.

142. Iolster NJ. Blood coagulation in children with cyanotic congenital heart disease. *Acta Paediatr Scand* 1970; **59**: 551–7.

143. Naiman JL. Clotting and bleeding in cyanotic congenital heart disease. *Pediatrics* 1970; **76**: 333–5.

144. Ekert H, Gilchrist GS, Stanton R, Hammond D. Hemostasis in cyanotic congenital heart disease. *J Pediatr* 1970; **76**: 221–30.

145. Komp DM, Sparrow AW. Polycythemia in cyanotic heart disease: a study of altered coagulation. *J Pediatr* 1970; **76**: 231–6.

146. Johnson CA, Abildgaard CF, Schulman I. Absence of coagulation abnormalities in children with cyanotic heart disease. *Lancet* 1968; **ii**: 660–2.

147. Chan AKC, Leaker M, Burrows FA *et al*. Coagulation and fibrinolytic profile of paediatric patients undergoing cardiopulmonary bypass. *Thomb Haemost* 1997; **77**: 270–7.

148. Boisclair MD, Lane DA, Philippou H *et al.* Mechanisms of thrombin generation during surgery and cardiopulmonary bypass. *Blood* 1993; **82**: 3350–7.

149. Turner-Gomes S, Lui LB, Saysana N, Dewar L, Williams WG, Ofosu F. Increased thrombin generation in cyanotic congenital heart disease. *Thromb Haemost* 1997; **78**: P2481.

150. Rinder CS, Gaal D, Student LA, Smith BR. Platelet–leukocyte activation and modulation of adhesion receptors in pediatric patients with congenital heart disease undergoing cardiopulmonary bypass. *J Thorac Cardiovasc Surg* 1994; **107**: 280–8.

151. Maurer HM, McCue CM, Robertson LW, Haggins JC. Correction of platelet dysfunction and bleeding in cyanotic congenital heart disease by simple red cell volume reduction. *Am J Cardiol* 1975; **35**: 831–5.

152. Gill JC, Wilson AD, Endres-Brooks J, Montgomery RR. Loss of the largest von Willebrand factor multimers from the plasma of patients with congenital cardiac defects. *Blood* 1986; **67**: 758–61.

153. Tomita H, Yamada O, Ohuchi H *et al.* Coagulation profile, hepatic dysfunction and haemodynamics following Fontan type operations. *Cardiology in the Young* 2001; **11**: 62–6.

154. Sharland M, Patton MA, Talbot S, Chitolie A, Bevan DH. Coagulation factor deficiencies and abnormal bleeding in Noonan's syndrome. *Lancet* 1992; **339**: 19–21.

155. Singer ST, Hurst D, Addiego JE. Bleeding disorders in Noonan syndrome: three cases and review of the literature. *J Pediatr Hematol Oncol* 1997; **19**: 130–4.

156. Tempe DK, Virmani S. Coagulation abnormalities in patients with congenital heart disease. *J Cardiothorac Vasc Anaesth* 2002; **16**: 752–65.

157. Woodman RC, Harker LA. Bleeding associated with cardiopulmonary bypass. *Blood* 1990; **76**: 1680–97.

158. Harker LA. Bleeding after cardiopulmonary bypass. *N Engl J Med* 1986; **314**: 1446–8.

159. Saatvedt K, Lindberg H, Michelen S, Pedersen T, Geiran OR. Activation of the fibrinolytic, coagulation and plasma kallikrein-kinin systems during and after open heart surgery in children. *Scand J Clin Lab Invest* 1995; **55**: 359–67.

160. Harker LA, Malpass TW, Branson HE, Hessel EA, Slitcher SA. Mechanism of abnormal bleeding in patients undergoing cardiopulmonary bypass. Acquired transient platelet dysfunction associated with selective α-granule release. *Blood* 1980; **56**: 824–34.

161. Rinder CS, Mathew JP, Rinder HM, Bonan J, Ault KA, Smith BR. Modulation of platelet surface adhesion receptors during cardiopulmonary bypass. *Anesthesiology* 1991; **75**: 563–70.

162. George JN, Pickett EB, Saucerman S *et al.* Platelet surface glycoproteins. Studies on resting and activated platelets and platelet membrane microparticle in normal subjects, and observations in patients during adult respiratory distress syndrome and cardiac surgery. *J Clin Invest* 1986; **78**: 340–7.

163. Malpass TW, Hanson SR, Savage B, Hessel EA II, Harker LA. Prevention of acquired transient defect in platelet plug formation by infused prostacyclin. *Blood* 1981; **57**: 736–40.

164. Kestin AS, Valeri R, Khuri SF *et al.* The platelet function defect in cardiopulmonary bypass. *Blood* 1993; **82**: 107–17.

165. Andrew M, MacIntyre B, MacMillan J *et al.* Heparin thearpy during cardiopulmonary bypass in children requires ongoing quality control. *Thromb Haemost* 1993; **70**: 937–41.

166. Hashimoto K, Yamagishi M, Sasaki T, Nakano M, Kurosawa H. Heparin and antithrombin levels during cardiopulmonary bypass: correlation with subclinical plasma coagulation. *Ann Thorac Surg* 1994; **58**: 799–805.

167. Severin T, Sutor AH. Heparin induced thrombocytopenia in paediatrics. *Semin Thromb Hemost* 2001; **27**: 293–9.

168. Alsoufi B, Boshkov LK, Kirby A *et al.* Heparin induced thrombocytopenia in pediatric cardiac surgery: an emerging cause of morbidity and mortality. *Seminars in Thoracic & Cardiovascular Surgery. Pediatric Cardiac Surgery Annual* 2004; **7**: 155–71.

169. Klenner AF, Lubenow N, Raschke R, Greinacher A. Heparin induced thrombocytopenia in children: 12 new cases and review of the literature. *Thromb Haemost* 2004; **91**: 719–24.

170. Warkentin TE, Kelton JG. A 14 year study of heparin induced thrombocytopenia. *Am J Med* 1996; **101**: 502–7.

171. Cetta F, Graham LC, Wrona LL, Arruda MJ, Walenga JM. Argatroban use during pediatric interventional cardiac catheterization. *Cathet Cardiovasc Intervent* 2004; **61**: 147–9.

172. Warkentin TE, Greinacher A. Heparin induced thrombocytopenia: recognition, treatment and prevention. The Seventh ACCP Conference on Antithrombotic Therapy. *Chest* 2004; **126**: 311S–337S.

173. Penkoske PA, Entwistle LM, Marchak BE, Seal RF, Gibb W. Aprotinin in children undergoing repair of congenital heart defects. *Ann Thorac Surg* 1995; **60** (suppl.): S529–32.

174. McDonough J, Gruenwald C. The use of aprotinin in pediatric patients: a review. *J Extracorporeal Technol* 2003; **35**: 346–9.

175. Chauhan S, Kumar BA, Rao BH. Efficacy of aprotinin, epsilon aminocaproic acid or combination in cyanotic congenital heart disease. *Ann Thorac Surg* 2000; **70**: 1308–12.

176. Bulutcu FS, Ozbek U, Polat B, Yacin Y, Karaci AR, Bayindir O. Which may be effective to reduce blood loss after cardiac operations in cyanotic children: tranexamic acid, aprotinin or combination? *Paediatr Anaesth* 2005; **15**: 41–6.

177. Scharrer I. Recombinant factor VIIa for patients with inhibitors to factor VIII or IX or factor VII deficiency. *Haemophilia* 1999; **5**: 253–9.

178. Tobias JD, Simsie JM, Weinstein S, Schechter W, Kartha V, Michler R. Recombinant factor VIIa to control excessive bleeding following surgery for congenital heart disease in pediatric patients. *J Intensive Care Med* 2004; **19**: 270–3.

179. Razon Y, Erez E, Vidne B *et al.* Recombinant factor VIIa (NovoSeven) as a hemostatic agent after surgery for congenital heart disease. *Paediatr Anaesth* 2005; **15**: 235–40.

180. Cook LN. Update on extracorporeal membrane oxygenation. *Paediatr Respir Rev* 2004; **5** (suppl. A): S329–S337.

181. Walker G, Liddell M, Davis C. Extracorporeal life support: state of the art. *Paediatr Respir Rev* 2003; **4**: 147–52.

182. Graziam LJ, Gringlas M, Baumgart S. Cerebrovascular complications and neurodevelopmental sequelae of neonatal ECMO. *Clin Perinatol* 1997; **24**: 655–75.

183. McManus ML, Kevy SV, Bower LK, Hickey PR. Coagulation factor deficiencies during initiation of extracorporeal membrane oxygenation. *Pediatrics* 1995; **126**: 900–4.

184. Urlesberer B, Zobel G, Zenz W *et al.* Activation of the clotting system during extracorporeal membrane oxygenation in term infants. *J Pediatr* 1996; **129**: 264–8.

185. Green TP, Isham-Schopf B, Steinhorn RH, Smith C, Irmiter RJ. Whole blood activated clotting time in infants during extracorporeal membrane oxygenation. *Crit Care Med* 1990; **18**: 494–8.

186. Chalmers EA, Kasem K, Allen G, Rafferty I, Davis C. Heparin monitoring during paediatric ECMO. *Thromb Haemost* 2001; **86** (suppl.): P279.

187. Gillis S, Hyman E, Abrohamov A, Elstein D, Zimran A. Platelet function abnormalities in Gaucher disease patients. *Am J Hematol* 1999; **61**: 103–6.

188. Hollak CEM, Levi M, Berends F, Aerts JMFG, van Oers MHJ. Coagulation abnormalities in type I Gaucher disease are due to low grade activation and can be partially restored by enzyme supplementation therapy. *Br J Haematol* 1997; **96**: 470–6.

189. Katz K, Tamary H, Lahav J, Soudry M, Cohen IJ. Increased operative bleeding during orthopaedic surgery in patients with type I Gaucher disease and bone involvement. *Bulletin of the Hospital for Joint Diseases* 1999; **58**: 188–90.

190. Seligsohn U, Zitman D, Many A, Klibansky C. Co-existence of factor XI (plasma thromboplastin antecedent) deficiency and Gaucher's disease. *Isr J Med Sci* 1976; **12**: 1448–52.

191. Billet HH, Rizvi S, Sawitsky A. Coagulation abnormalities in patients with Gaucher's disease: effect of therapy. *Am J Hematol* 1996; **51**: 234–6.

192. Shapiro SS, Jultin M. Acquired inhibitors to blood coagulation factors. *Semin Thromb Hemost* 1975; **1**: 336–85.

193. Miller K, Neely JE, Krivit W, Edson JR. Spontaneously acquired factor IX inhibitor in a nonhemophiliac child. *J Pediatr* 1978; **93**: 232–4.

194. Green D, Lechner K. A survey of 215 non-hemophilic patients with inhibitors to factor VIII. *Thromb Haemost* 1981; **45**: 200–3.

195. Nakashima K, Miyahara T, Fujii S, Kaku K, Matsumoto N, Kaneko T. Spontaneously acquired factor VIII inhibitor in a 7-year-old girl. *Acta Haematol* 1982; **68**: 58–62.

196. Hedner U, Glazer S, Falch J. Recombinant activated factor VII in the treatment of bleeding episodes in patients with inherited and acquired bleeding disorders. *Transfus Med Rev* 1993; **7**: 78–83.

197. Hay CRM, Lozier JN, Santagostino E *et al*. Porcine factor VIII therapy in patients with congenital hemophilia and inhibitors: efficacy, patient selection and side effects. *Semin Hematol* 1994; **31**: 20–5.

198. Jonge Poerink-Stockschlader AB, Dekker I, Risseeuw-Appel IM, Hahlen K. Acquired Von Willebrand disease in children with a Wilms' tumor. *Med Pediatr Oncol* 1996; **26**: 238–43.

199. Michiels JJ, Budde U, van der Planken M, van Vliet HH, Schroyens W, Berneman Z. Acquired von Willebrand syndromes: clinical features, aetiology, pathophysiology, classification and management. *Best Pract Res Clin Haematol* 2001; **14**: 401–36.

200. Coppes MJ, Zandvoort SWH, Sparling CR, Poon AO, Weitzman S, Blanchette VS. Acquired von Willebrand disease in Wilms' tumor patients. *J Clin Oncol* 1992; **10**: 422–7.

201. Carroll JF, Moskowitz KA, Edwards NM, Hickey TJ, Rose EA, Budzynski AZ. Immunologic assessment of patients treated with bovine fibrin as a hemostatic agent. *Thromb Haemost* 1996; **76**: 925–31.

202. Muntean W, Zenz W, Edlinger G, Beitzke A. Severe bleeding due to factor V inhibitor after repeated operations using fibrin sealant containing bovine thrombin. *Thromb Haemost* 1997; **77**: 1223.

203. Muntean W, Zenz W, Finding W, Zobel G, Beitzke A. Inhibitor to factor V after exposure to fibrin sealant during cardiac surgery in a two-year-old child. *Acta Paediatr* 1994; **83**: 84–7.

204. Reece E, Clyne L. Spontaneous factor XI inhibitors: seven additional cases and a review of the literature. *Arch Intern Med* 1984; **144**: 525–9.

205. Johnson CA, Schroer RJ, Moore A. Acquired inhibitor to contact activation in an 18-month-old female. *Am J Pediatr Hematol Oncol* 1985; **7**: 191–3.

206. Matsunaga AT, Shafer FE. An acquired inhibitor to factor X in a pediatric patient with extensive burns. *J Pediatr Hematol Oncol* 1996; **18**: 223–6.

207. Greaves M, Cohen H, Machin SJ, Mackie I. Guidelines on the investigation and management of the antiphospholipid syndrome. *Br J Haematol* 2000; **109**: 704–15.

208. Finazzi G, Brancaccio V, Moia M *et al*. Natural history and risk factors for thrombosis in 360 patients with antiphospholipid antibodies: a four-year prospective study from the Italian Registry. *Am J Med* 1996; **100**: 530–6.

209. Burke CD, Miller L, Handler S, Cohen A. Preoperative history and coagulation screening in children undergoing tonsillectomy. *Pediatrics* 1992; **89**: 691–5.

210. Uthman IW, Gharavi AE. Viral infections and antiphospholipid antibodies. *Semin Arthritis Rheum* 2002; **31**: 256–63.

211. Berube C, Mitchell L, Silverman E *et al*. The relationship of antiphospholipid antibodies to thromboembolic events in pediatric patients with systemic lupus erythematosus: a cross-sectional study. *Pediatr Res* 1998; **44**: 351–6.

212. Manco Johnson MJ, Nuss R. Lupus anticoagulant in children with thrombosis. *Am J Hematol* 1995; **48**: 240–3.

213. Angelim L, Ravelli A, Caporali R, Martini A. Antiphospholipid antibodies in children with idiopathic cerebral ischaemia. *Lancet* 1994; **344**: 1232.

214. Olson JC, Konkol RJ, Gill JC, Dobyns WB, Coull BM. Childhood stroke and lupus anticoagulant. *Pediatr Neurol* 1994; **10**: 54–7.

215. Ravelli A, Martini A, Burgio RG, Falcini F, Taccetti G. Antiphospholipid antibody syndrome as a cause of venous thrombosis in childhood. *J Pediatr* 1994; **124**: 831–2.

216. Nuss R, Hays T, Manco Johnson M. Childhood thrombosis. *Pediatrics* 1995; **96**: 291–4.

217. Takanashi J, Sugita K, Miyazato S, Sakao E, Miyamoto H, Niimi H. Antiphospholipid antibody syndrome in childhood strokes. *Pediatr J Neurol* 1995; **13**: 323–6.

218. von Scheven E, Athreya BH, Rose CD, Goldsmith DP, Morton L. Clinical characteristics of the antiphospholipid antibody syndrome in children. *J Pediatr* 1996; **129**: 339–45.

219. Manco Johnson MJ, Nuss R, Key N *et al*. Lupus anticoagulant and protein S deficiency in children with postvaricella purpura fulminans or thrombosis. *J Pediatr* 1996; **128**: 319–23.

220. Becton DL, Stine KC. Transient lupus anticoagulants associated with hemorrhage rather than thrombosis: the hemorrhagic lupus anticoagulant syndrome. *J Pediatr* 1997; **130**: 998–1000.

221. Gran E, Real E, Pastor E, Ivorra J, Quecedo E. Prothrombin deficiency and hemorrhage associated with a lupus anticoagulant. *Am J Hematol* 1997; **54**: 85.

30 Bleeding in the neonate

Elizabeth A. Chalmers

Neonatal hemostasis: developmental aspects

Normal hemostasis reflects a highly complex process that is dependent on a series of interactions between hemostatic proteins, endothelial cells and platelets. The hemostatic system is profoundly influenced by age, and this is particularly apparent in the newborn period, when significant differences are observed compared with older children and adults. While many of these differences are quantitative, qualitative changes are also present, particularly with regard to platelet function. Despite what is often regarded as the functional immaturity of the hemostatic system at birth, the healthy term infant experiences few hemostatic problems. This contrasts with the situation in the sick preterm infant, where additional acquired abnormalities may rapidly alter the hemostatic balance, contributing to both hemorrhagic and thrombotic problems.

Normal coagulation data for fetuses and newborns

The unique nature of the neonatal hemostatic system necessitates the use of specific normal ranges for this age group. In addition, the hemostatic system during fetal and neonatal life is constantly changing as it evolves toward what we regard as a fully mature system, and sequential reference ranges are therefore required to take account of both the gestational and postnatal age of the infant. Such reference ranges not only provide information regarding the physiology of the neonate but are absolutely crucial for diagnostic and monitoring purposes.

The International Society for Thrombosis and Haemostasis (ISTH) Scientific and Standardisation Subcommittee on Neonatal Haemostasis has previously published recommendations regarding the establishment of normal ranges for neonates, which deal with various issues including the selection of subjects for investigation, sample type, collection and storage, laboratory methodology and data analysis.[1] Nevertheless, research in this area remains difficult and data are not infrequently published based on cord blood sampling, which may not always reflect the situation in the neonate.

Based on the work of several authors, reference ranges have been published previously for most of the components of the coagulation system in both term and preterm infants at sequential stages of postnatal development.[2–5] These include ranges for screening tests, procoagulant proteins, inhibitors of coagulation and proteins involved in fibrinolysis (Tables 30.1 and 30.2; see also Tables 37.6, 37.7, 37.32 and 37.33).

Much of these data were derived by Andrew et al., who used a standard protocol whereby venous blood samples were obtained from healthy term and preterm infants (30–36 weeks gestation), all of whom had received 1 mg of intramuscular vitamin K at least 12 hours before the first blood sample. Standardized procedures were then followed for the collection, storage and analysis of these samples, which were obtained sequentially, at predetermined time points over a 6-month period.[2–4] Although this still represents the most comprehensive set of pubished data for this age group, much of this work was performed in the late 1980s and early 1990s and does not therefore reflect current technology. As all reference ranges are both instrument and reagent dependent, ideally laboratories processing neonatal samples should derive at least limited in-house reference ranges, which may then be used in conjunction with published values to interpret results.

It has not been possible to establish ranges from an adequate number of healthy premature infants born at < 30 weeks gestation, and information relating to this period currently relies on the availability of samples obtained by fetoscopy. Reverdiau-Moalic et al.[6] published data on 285 healthy fetuses analyzed between 19 and 38 weeks gestation and compared their results with a cohort of normal full-term neonates and an adult control group (Table 30.3). Fetal samples were obtained by direct puncture of the umbilical vein under ultrasound guidance. It is of interest that in the 30–38-week

Table 30.1 Reference values for the components of the fibrinolytic system in healthy full-term infants during the first 6 months of life compared with adult values. All values are given as a mean followed by the lower and upper boundary encompassing 95% of the population (in brackets).

Fibrinolytic component	Day 1 mean (boundary)	Day 5 mean) (boundary	Day 30 mean (boundary)	Day 90 mean (boundary)	Day 180 mean (boundary)	Adult mean (boundary)
Plasminogen (unit/mL)*	1.95 (1.25–2.65)	2.17 (1.41–2.93)	1.98 (1.26–2.70)	2.48 (1.74–3.22)	3.01 (2.21–3.81)	3.36 (2.48–4.24)
tPA[†] (ng/mL)	9.6 (5.0–18.9)	5.6 (4.0–10.0)[¶]	4.1 (1.0–6.0)[¶]	2.1 (1.0–5.0)[¶]	2.8 (1.0–6.0)[¶]	4.9 (1.4–8.4)
α_2-AP (unit/mL)[‡]	0.85 (0.55–1.15)	1.00 (0.70–1.30)[¶]	1.00 (0.76–1.24)[¶]	1.08 (0.76–1.40)[¶]	1.11 (0.83–1.39)[¶]	1.02 (0.68–1.36)
PAI (unit/mL)[§]	6.4 (2.0–15.1)	2.3 (0.0–8.1)[¶]	3.4 (0.0–8.8)[¶]	7.2 (1.0–15.3)	8.1 (6.0–13.0)	3.6 (0.0–11.0)

* Plasminogen units are those recommended by the Committee on Thrombolytic Agents.

† tPA, tissue plasminogen activator.

‡ α_2-AP, α_2-antiplasmin. Values are expressed as unit/mL, where pooled plasma contains 1.0 unit/mL.

§ PAI, plasminogen activator inhibitor. Values are given as unit/mL, where 1 unit of PAI activity is defined as the amount of PAI that inhibits 1 international unit of human single-chain tPA.

¶ Indicates values that are indistinguishable from those of the adult.

Reproduced with permission from Ref. 6.

Table 30.2 Reference values for the components of the fibrinolytic system in healthy premature infants during the first 6 months of life compared with adult values.

Fibrinolytic component	Day 1 mean (boundary)	Day 5 mean (boundary)	Day 30 mean (boundary)	Day 90 mean (boundary)	Day 180 mean (boundary)	Adult mean (boundary)
Plasminogen (unit/mL)	1.70 (1.12–2.48)[†]	1.91 (1.21–2.61)[†]	1.81 (1.09–2.53)	2.38 (1.58–3.18)	2.75 (1.91–3.59)[†]	3.36 (2.48–4.24)
tPA (ng/mL)	8.48 (3.00–16.70)	3.97 (2.00–6.93)*	4.13 (2.00–7.79)*	3.31 (2.00–5.07)*	3.48 (2.00–5.85)*	4.96 (1.46–8.46)
α_2-AP (unit/mL)	0.78 (0.40–1.16)	0.81 (0.49–1.13)[†]	0.89 (0.55–1.23)[†]	1.06 (0.64–1.48)*	1.15 (0.77–1.53)	1.02 (0.68–1.36)
PAI (unit/mL)	5.4 (0.0–12.2)*[†]	2.5 (0.0–7.1)*	4.3 (0.0–10.9)*	4.8 (1.0–11.8)	4.9 (1.0–10.2)*[†]	3.6 (0.0–11.0)

For explanation of abbreviations see footnotes for Table 30.1.

* Denotes values that are indistinguishable from those of the adult.

† Denotes values that are different from those of the full-term infant.

Reproduced with permission from Ref. 6.

gestation cohort, lower values were observed for the majority of the procoagulant proteins compared with the levels recorded in the study by Andrew *et al.*[3] of preterm infants of equivalent gestation. One possible explanation for this apparent discrepancy is that the birth process itself may affect the coagulation system.

Coagulation proteins

Procoagulants

Coagulation proteins do not cross the placental barrier but are synthesized in the fetus from around the 10th week of gestation onwards.[7] Both the absolute and relative concentrations of coagulation proteins in the neonate differ from adult values and are dependent to a varying extent on both the gestational and postnatal age of the infant (see Tables 37.6 and 37.32).

The vitamin K-dependent factors (II, VII, IX and X) are the most extensively studied of all the procoagulant proteins.

Mean levels in the term infant are around 50% of normal adult values and are variably reduced further in the premature infant. The postnatal maturation pattern is nonuniform, with factor VII (FVII) levels reaching the adult range by 5 days, while the other factors increase gradually over the first 6 months of life. Although within the normal adult range, mean levels remain reduced throughout infancy.

The four contact factors, XI, XII, prekallikrein (PK) and high-molecular-weight kininogen (HMWK), are reduced to around 30–50% of normal at term. HMWK increases rapidly, whereas the other factors show a more gradual increase. Analogous to the vitamin K-dependent factors, all four are within the adult range at 6 months, but average levels remain lower than comparative adult values.

Factor VIII (FVIII) levels on day 1 are indistinguishable from normal adult values and remain so throughout the neonatal period. von Willebrand factor (vWF) levels are increased at birth and although they decline slightly, remain high compared with adult values until around 3 months of age. The persistent elevation of vWF beyond the immediate

Table 30.3 Reference values for coagulation screening tests and coagulation factors in fetuses (19–38 weeks gestation), neonates and adults.

	Fetuses (weeks gestation)			Newborns (*n* = 60)	Adults (*n* = 40)
	19–23 (*n* = 20)	24–29 (*n* = 22)	30–38 (*n* = 22)		
PT (s)	32.5 (19–45)	32.2 (19–44)**	22.6 (16–30)**	16.7 (12.0–23.5)*	13.5 (11.4–14.0)
PT (INR)	6.4 (1.7–11.1)	6.2 (21–10.6)**	3.0 (1.5–5.0)*	1.7 (0.9 2.7)*	1.1 (0.8–1.2)
APTT (s)	168.8 (83–250)	154.0 (87–210)**	104.8 (76–128)**	44.3 (35–52)**	33.0 (25–39)
TCT (s)	34.2 (24–44)*	26.2 (24–28)	21.4 (17.0–23.3)	20.4 (15.2–25.0)**	14.0 (12–16)
Factor					
I (g/L, Von Clauss)	0.85 (0.57–1.50)	1.12 (0.65–1.65)	1.35 (1.25–1.65)	1.68 (0 95–2.45)**	3.0 (1.78–4.50)
I Ag (g/L)	1.08 (0.75–1.50)	1.93 (1.56–2.40)	1.94 (1.30–240)	2.65 (1.68–3.60)**	3.5 (2.50–5.20)
IIC (%)	16.9 (10–24)	19.9 (11–30)*	27.9 (15–50)**	43.5 (27–64)**	98.7 (70–125)
VIIC (%)	27.4 (17–37)	33.8 (18–48)*	45.9 (31–62)	52.5 (28–78)**	101.3 (68–130)
IXC (%)	10.1 (6 14)	9.9 (5–15)	12.3 (5–24)**	31.8 (15–50)**	104.8 (70–142)
XC (%)	20.5 (14–29)	24.9 (16–35)	28.0 (16–36)**	39.6 (21–65)**	99.2 (75–125)
VC (%)	32.1 (21–44)	36.8 (25–50)	48.9 (23–70)**	89.9 (50–140)	99.8 (65–140)
VIIIC (%)	34.5 (18–50)	35.5 (20–52)	50.1 (27–78)**	94.3 (38–150)	101.8 (55–170)
XIG (%)	13.2 (8–19)	12.1 (6–22)	14.8 (6–26)**	37.2 (13–62)**	100.2 (70–135)
XIIC (%)	14.9 (6–25)	22.7 (6–40)	25.8 (11–50)**	69.8 (25–105)**	101.4 (65–144)
PK (%)	12.8 (8–19)	15.4 (8–26)	18.1 (8–28)**	35.4 (21–53)**	99.8 (65–135)
HMWK (%)	15.4 (10–22)	19.3 (10–26)	23.6 (12–34)**	38.9 (28–53)**	98.8 (68–135)

Values are the mean, followed in parentheses by the lower and upper boundaries including 95% of the population.

Ag, antigenic value; APTT, activated partial thromboplastin time; C, coagulant activity; HMWK, high-molecular-weight kininogen; INR, international normalized ratio; PK, prekallikrein; PT, prothrombin time; TCT, thrombin clotting time.

* *P* < 0.05.

** *P* < 0.01.

Reproduced with permission from Ref. 8.

postnatal period suggests that its level is more than just a reactive response to the birth process. In addition, vWF, which is made up of a series of multimeric forms of differing molecular weights, is characterized in the neonatal period by an excess of unusually large multimers, which are not seen in older children or adults with pathologic states.[8,9] These multimers appear to be functionally more active, as indicated by increased platelet aggregation in response to ristocetin.[10] vWF collagen binding activity has also been shown to be increased in early neonatal life.[11]

Mean levels of factor V (FV) are within the normal adult range at birth and show a further minor increase by day 5. Fibrinogen levels are normal in both term and preterm neonates. A transient increase in fibrinogen is observed at day 5 but thereafter levels are stable throughout the neonatal period. Fetal fibrinogen is not identical to adult fibrinogen, having an increased content of sialic acid, similar to the situation seen in patients with chronic liver disease. The functional significance of fetal fibrinogen is unknown; however, the thrombin clotting time (TCT) is normal provided calcium is included in the buffering system.[12] FXIII is 70% of normal at birth and increases to adult levels by day 5.

Many of the coagulation factors are gestationally dependent and are further reduced in the preterm infant.[3,4] There is, however, evidence of an accelerated maturation pattern in

these infants, and levels of coagulation proteins are usually similar by 6 months of age.

Of the commonly used screening tests the prothrombin time (PT) is only minimally prolonged in the normal term infant and shortens within the first month of life (see Tables 37.6 and 37.32). This contrasts with the activated partial thromboplastin time (APTT), which can be markedly prolonged, particularly in the preterm infant. This is largely due to the reduced levels of contact factors, which have a disproportionate effect on APTT compared with FVIII and FIX. The normal range for the APTT is also significantly influenced by the choice of activating reagent.[2,3] The TCT, as mentioned above, is normal if calcium is added to the buffering system; otherwise it is prolonged, reflecting the effect of fetal fibrinogen.

Inhibitors

The direct inhibitors of thrombin are antithrombin III (ATIII), heparin cofactor II (HCII) and α_2-macroglobulin (α_2-M). ATIII and HCII are around 50% of normal at birth and gradually increase thereafter to reach adult levels by around 3 and 6 months, respectively (see Tables 37.7 and 37.33). In contrast, α_2-M is increased at birth and continues to rise postnatally: levels at 6 months are approximately twice normal adult values.

The indirect inhibitors, protein C and protein S, which are vitamin K dependent, are both reduced to < 50% of normal at birth, which parallels the reduction in the vitamin K-dependent procoagulants (see Tables 37.7 and 37.33). Although the concentration of each protein increases postnatally, the mean protein C concentration remains significantly reduced during infancy, and adult concentrations are not reached until the early teenage years. Protein C, like fibrinogen, circulates in a fetal form that is characterized by a relative increase in the proportion of the single-chain form compared with the double-chain form.[13,14] This does not, however, appear to affect the function of the molecule. Protein S in adult plasma is normally present in both free and bound forms, with only the free form being active. The inactive bound form is complexed to the C4b-binding protein. C4b-binding protein is virtually absent in neonatal plasma and protein S therefore circulates entirely in its active free form.[15,16]

Tissue factor pathway inhibitor (TFPI) or extrinsic pathway inhibitor (EPI) has not been as comprehensively investigated as the other naturally occurring coagulation inhibitors. Nevertheless, available data indicate that levels in cord plasma are reduced at birth to around 65% of adult values.[17–19]

Effects on thrombin regulation

The results of a number of *in vitro* studies looking at thrombin regulation in neonatal and cord plasma have indicated that the capacity of neonatal plasma to generate thrombin is reduced to around 50% of adult values, which is analogous to the situation seen in an adult on therapeutic anticoagulant therapy.[20] In addition, Patel *et al.*[21] have demonstrated that even when fibrin is formed, the activity of clot-bound thrombin from cord plasma is reduced compared with that from adult plasma. Both of these effects appear to be related to reduced levels of prothrombin. To what extent these *in vitro* thrombin generation assays mirror the situation *in vivo* remains open to debate. Thrombin generation assays based on coagulation activation via the extrinsic pathway using small amounts of lipidated tissue factor have been developed and are postulated to be more physiologic than conventional assays.[22] Using this type of assay, Cvirn *et al.* have assessed thrombin generation using low levels of TFPI and antithrombin, and have demonstrated both an increased rate of thrombin generation and an increase in the total amount of thrombin generated, which suggests that thrombin generation in newborn plasma may be less impaired than previously throught.[23] This is also supported by data showing an absence of any defects on thromboelastography in healthy neonates.[24] While these results require further evaluation they do offer an explanation for the apparent adequacy of hemostasis despite low levels of procoagulant proteins.

Thrombin inhibition mediated by the direct thrombin inhibitors (ATIII, HCII and α_2-M) is slower in neonatal plasma, but the overall capacity is similar to that seen in adults.[25] This occurs despite the reduced levels of ATIII, which appear to be offset by the increased concentration of α_2-M and increased thrombin binding to HCII.[26–29]

These *in vitro* studies, although providing information on the overall capacity of neonatal plasma either to generate or inhibit thrombin, do not assess the extent to which thrombin generation is actually occurring *in vivo*. This can be quantified *in vivo* by measuring activation peptides, such as prothrombin fragment 1+2 (F1+2), fibrinopeptide A and thrombin–antithrombin (TAT) complexes, which are released at different stages of the coagulation process. Using these activation peptides as markers, it has been possible to demonstrate that the coagulation system is activated in the period immediately following delivery.[25,30]

Fibrinolysis

The fibrinolytic system in the neonate, as with the coagulation system, can be regarded as physiologically immature, with the levels of all major fibrinolytic proteins showing age-dependent variation. The generation of plasmin from plasminogen is the most important step in the fibrinolytic system and is analogous to the generation of thrombin from prothrombin in the coagulation system.

Plasminogen is converted to plasmin by several activators, including tissue plasminogen activator (tPA) and urokinase plasminogen activator (uPA). The inhibitors of the fibrinolytic system include the plasminogen activator inhibitors, of which PAI-1 is the best characterized, and α_2-antiplasmin (α_2-AP), which acts directly on plasmin. α_2-M can also inhibit plasmin but is less important than α_2-AP.

Normal ranges for the major proteins involved in fibrinolysis have been published for both term and preterm infants (Tables 30.1 and 30.2).[2–4,31] At birth plasminogen levels are around 50% of adult values in the term infant and slightly lower than this in preterm infants. Plasminogen remains reduced throughout the neonatal period, increasing toward normal adult levels by 6 months. Mean α_2-AP levels are around 80% of normal at birth but neonatal and adult ranges do overlap. The levels of both tPA and PAI-1 appear to be transiently increased on day 1 of life in both term and preterm infants. These levels are higher than those documented in cord plasma and it is presumed that both tPA and PAI-1 are released from endothelial cells at the time of delivery.[32]

As well as being reduced at birth, plasminogen is present in a "fetal" form. Fetal plasminogen has an increased concentration of sialic acid, similar to that found in fetal fibrinogen, and has also been shown to contain increased amounts of mannose. The physiologic significance of these differences from adult plasminogen are unclear. Summaria[33] failed to document any significant difference in the rate of plasmin generation in fetal and adult plasminogen. However, Edelberg *et al.*[34] documented both reduced functional activity and decreased binding to cellular receptors.

Various studies have demonstrated that the fibrinolytic system, like the coagulation system, is transiently activated at birth.[35–38] Although activated, the overall rate of plasmin generation in neonatal plasma is reduced compared with adult values.[32] This is thought to relate mainly to the reduced concentration of plasminogen; however, a contribution from a dysfunctional plasminogen molecule, as discussed above, cannot be completely ruled out.

The reduced ability to generate plasmin, theoretically at least, suggests that the neonate may have an impaired ability to lyse thrombi. What part this plays in the overall pathogenesis of thrombotic problems in the neonate is unknown. There are, however, important implications for the use of thrombolytic agents in the neonatal period, and it is clear from *in vitro* studies using fibrin clots derived from cord plasma that there is an impaired response to thrombolysis, which again appears to relate to the reduced concentration of plasminogen.[39–41]

Platelets

Fetal platelet production is first observed toward the end of the first trimester, and platelet levels are usually within the normal adult range by the middle of the second trimester.[42–45] Thrombocytopenia in both the term and preterm infant is therefore defined as a platelet count of $<150 \times 10^9/L$. The mean platelet volume (MPV) is also within the normal adult range at birth, although in one study the MPV was reported to be lower in preterm infants compared with term infants.[46–48]

Thrombopoietin (Tpo) is known to be the most important regulator of platelet production in humans. Tpo and its receptor c-mpl can be detected in the human fetus in the early stages of fetal development.[49] Tpo mRNA transcripts have been detected as early as 6 weeks gestation, with the highest concentrations detected in fetal liver tissue.[50] Tpo levels in healthy nonthrombocytopenic term infants are reported to be higher than in nonthrombocytopenic adults.[49,51]

Studies on platelet production have been hampered by difficulties in obtaining bone marrow samples to assess megakaryocyte numbers and function. Murray *et al.* have developed a novel assay system to study megakaryocyte precursor development in neonatal peripheral blood, and have shown that circulating megakaryocyte (MK) precursors measured in this assay reflect the bone marrow MK population. Using this assay it has been possible to define reference ranges for circulating MK precursors in healthy term neonates and also to show that preterm babies have increased numbers of circulating MK precursors.[52]

Platelet function

Until relatively recently the investigation of neonatal platelet function was limited by sampling issues, and much of the available data were inconsistent and derived from the analysis of cord blood. The recent development of new investigational tools has facilitated the analysis of blood samples from both term and preterm neonates, and new data are beginning to define both the characteristics and mechanisms involved in neonatal platelet function.[53–55]

Platelet aggregometry is a well-established and widely used technique for the assessment of platelet function in all age groups. Unfortunately, aggregometry requires relatively large sample volumes, and there have been limited studies, particularly in preterm and very-low-birthweight (VLBW) infants, and results have not always been consistent. Nevertheless, data derived largely from studies using cord blood or samples from term neonates demonstrate that neonatal platelets are hyporesponsive to a number of specific agonists including adenosine diphosphate (ADP), epinephrine (adrenaline), collagen and thrombin.[53–55] By contrast, the response to ristocetin is enhanced compared with adult platelets.

A number of mechanisms have been proposed to account for these responses. The reduced response to epinephrine is likely to be the result of reduced numbers of α_2-adrenoceptors on neonatal platelets, while the response to collagen is thought to reflect impaired calcium mobilization. The enhanced ristocetin-induced aggregation reflects the high levels and increased activity of vWF in neonates.

Although the bleeding time remains the gold standard for assessment of the platelet–vessel wall interaction, it is a technique with significant limitations. Special templates are available for use in neonates, and using this device the bleeding time in the neonate is reported to be shorter than in adults.[56] It has been postulated that the shortened bleeding time reflects increased levels of vWF antigen and activity together with the increased red cell size and increased hematocrit. Bleeding times in VLBW infants have been reported to be longer than those of healthy term babies, and correlate with the presence of a low hemacocrit.[57]

The use of the bleeding time in neonates will, however, be subject to the same limitations as in older age groups, namely lack of standardization, etc., and has not been shown to date to correlate with a bleeding risk.[57,58]

The Platelet Function Analyzer-100 (PFA-100) is an *in vitro* method for the assessment of primary hemostasis. This assay utilizes citrated whole blood and measures the time taken for a platelet plug to occlude a standard aperture under conditions of high shear stress. Closure times can be assessed using membranes coated with collagen/epinephrine or collagen/ADP. Cord blood samples from term neonates have shorter closure times than samples from older children and adults, and therefore appear to correlate with reported bleeding times.[59,60] These shorter closure times have been shown to correlate with increased vWF activity.[61]

The analysis of platelet function using whole-blood flow cytometry has a number of advantages over other techniques, in particular that the analysis can be carried out on very small sample volumes and is therefore very applicable to the study of neonates. In a study performed on peripheral blood samples from 30 healthy neonates using whole-blood flow cytometry to look at platelet activation markers, Rajasekhar *et al.*[62] demonstrated reduced reactivity to the agonists thrombin and ADP/epinephrine in both term and preterm neonates compared with adult platelets.[63] The issue of when neonatal hyporeactivity resolves is not well defined, with some authors describing normal function by day 10 while others have indicated that hyporesponsivness may continue beyond the neonatal period.[64,65]

Neonatal bleeding problems

Clinical considerations

Bleeding problems are commonly observed in neonatal practice, particularly in the neonatal intensive care unit (NICU) setting. Although the pathophysiology of these problems is often complex, hemostatic failure, due to either platelet abnormalities or a coagulopathy, may be causal or contributory in at least a proportion of cases. Thrombocytopenia is probably the most commonly observed cause of bleeding in this age group but coagulation defects are also common, and the two problems frequently coexist. Although the vast majority of hemostatic problems are likely to reflect acquired disorders, a number of relatively uncommon inherited conditions can also present at this time. Appropriate diagnosis and management of these conditions is highly dependent on prompt recognition of clinically abnormal bleeding and the initiation of appropriate investigations.

A number of clinical considerations are important in the investigation of a neonate who is bleeding and has a suspected underlying hemostatic problem. Foremost of these is probably the clinical setting in which the bleeding occurs.

Bleeding in an otherwise well term neonate is suggestive of an immune-mediated thrombocytopenia or an inherited coagulation disorder, whereas in a sick preterm neonate a nonimmune thrombocytopenia or a consumptive coagulopathy with disseminated intravascular coagulation (DIC) is more likely. Obstetric complications, and perinatal problems associated with delivery can also affect the hemostatic system resulting in coagulation activation and DIC. The presence of a family history of a bleeding disorder or of a previously affected infant can be an important diagnostic pointer. Finally, both maternal and neonatal drugs, particularly with regard to vitamin K metabolism, may be highly relevant at this time.

Laboratory investigations

Initial screening investigations usually comprise a full blood count and a baseline coagulation screen (PT, APTT, TCT and fibrinogen). Based on the pattern of abnormalities observed the results of these initial screening tests can then be used to guide the direction of additional investigations (Table 30.4). Where further investigation is required this may include specific factor assays, which as discussed previously must be interpreted using appropriate age-adjusted reference ranges. In certain circumstances more specialized techniques may be required to investigate for less common defects including abnormalities of platelet function.

Sampling problems are common in the newborn period and it is particularly important that samples for coagulation testing avoid contamination or activation prior to analysis. As discussed previously, the levels of many hemostatic proteins are low during the neonatal period, which affects routine screening tests, and it is therefore very important that these results are interpreted in conjunction with age-adjusted normal ranges. In addition, the high neonatal hematocrit

Table 30.4 Laboratory investigation of neonatal coagulation disorders.

	PT	APTT	Fibrinogen	Platelets	Diagnostic tests/ other useful tests
Inherited disorders					
Hemophilia A	N	↑	N	N	FVIII assay
Hemophilia B	N	↑	N	N	FIX assay
vWD (type III)	N	↑	N	N/↓	FVIII/vWF assays
FVII	↑	N	N	N	FVII assay
FX	↑	↑	N	N	FX assay
Fibrinogen	N/↑	N/↑	↓	N	Fibrinogen assay
FXIII	N	N	N	N	FXIII screen/assay
Acquired disorders					
DIC	↑	↑	↓	↓	D-dimers
Vitamin K deficiency	↑	N/↑	N	N	FII, VII, IX, X
Liver disease	↑	↑	N/↓	N/↓	Factor assays

APTT, activated partial thromboplastin time; DIC, disseminated intravascular coagulation; vWD, von Willebrand disease.

N, normal; ↑, increased; ↑, decreased.

results in a minor degree of spurious prolongation of coagulation times, which may be relevant in polycythemic infants.

Inherited disorders of coagulation

Hemophilia A and B

Hemophilias A and B are inherited bleeding disorders that result from deficiencies of the procoagulant proteins FVIII and FIX, respectively. They are inherited as X-linked recessive disorders and together with von Willebrand disease (vWD) account for > 95% of all inherited bleeding disorders.[66] Current estimates of incidence of these disorders indicate that 1 in 10 000 males are affected by severe hemophilia A, and 1 in 50 000 males by severe hemophilia B.[67] Both FVIII and FIX play a crucial role in the activation of the coagulation cascade and result in clinically indistinguishable bleeding disorders of variable severity.

Hemophilia can be classified as severe, moderate or mild, based either on clinical bleeding criteria or on laboratory measurement of FVIII and FIX levels. Laboratory criteria have varied in different classifications, and in an effort to standardize this the Scientific Subcommittee of the ISTH have recommended revised criteria for the classification of hemophilia based on biologic FVIII:C and FIX:C levels, as follows.[68]
- Severe hemophilia: FVIII/FIX level < 0.01 IU/mL (< 1% of normal).
- Moderate hemophilia: FVIII/FIX level 0.01–0.05 IU/mL (2–5% of normal).
- Mild hemophilia: FVIII/FIX level 0.05–0.40 IU/mL (5–40% of normal).

For the majority of patients, this classification should provide a good indication of the likely frequency and severity of bleeding episodes. However, issues persist regarding the ability of laboratories to satisfactorily classify patients, which reflects ongoing problems with the precision and accuracy of routine FVIII and FIX assays.[69]

Clinical features

Hemophilias A and B are the commonest inherited bleeding disorders to present during the neonatal period.[70] A number of cohort studies have focused on the initial presentation of children with hemophilia and include data on the incidence of bleeding during the first month of life.[71–74] Older studies suggest that bleeding in the neonatal period is a relatively infrequent event. In a large historical study published in 1966, Baehner and Strauss reviewed clinical data on 192 infants with hemophila registered at a single center.[71] In this study less than 10% of severely affected neonates and less than 2.5% of those with mild or moderate disease had a clinical event resulting in a diagnosis being made within the first month of life. Subsequent cohort studies from Sweden, North America

Table 30.5 Percentage of newborn infants diagnosed or presenting with bleeding during the first month of life.

Reference	Years	Number	Diagnosis	Bleeding
Baehner and Strauss[71]	1952–1966	192	< 10%	5%
Ljung et al.[72]	1960–1987	140	52%	20%
Conway and Hilgarter[73]	1974–1989	56	68%	33%
Chambost et al.[74]	1980–1994	599	58%	15%*

* *De novo* cases only.

and France have recorded different results, with over 50% of neonates being diagnosed during the neonatal period and a much higher percentage than previously recorded having clinically significant bleeding (Table 30.5).[72–74]

In a cohort of Swedish hemophiliacs diagnosed between 1960 and 1987, 28/140 (20%) were recorded as having abnormal bleeding in the immediate neonatal period (i.e., within 7 days of birth).[72,75] In a similar study from North America, 68.4% of severe hemophiliacs were diagnosed within the first month of life, and in almost half of these cases the diagnosis was made after the initiation of appropriate investigations for abnormal bleeding.[73] Similarly, in a more recent French cohort study, 58% of cases were diagnosed neonatally and 15% of *de novo* cases had abnormal bleeding.[74]

The higher incidence of reported bleeding compared with historic studies presumably reflects, at least in part, a greater awareness of the condition and improved recognition of abnormal bleeding symptoms but also suggests that previous figures underestimate the risk of bleeding at this time. One possible explanation for the particularly high incidence of bleeding in the North American cohort is the relatively frequent documentation of bleeding following circumcision, which was commonly carried out during the first few weeks of life during the period of this study.

The pattern of bleeding in neonates with hemophilia is different to that typically observed in older children, in whom muscle and joint bleeds predominate. Many neonatal bleeds are iatrogenic in origin, and continued oozing or excessive hematoma formation following venipuncture, heel stab sampling or the administration of intramuscular vitamin K are characteristic.[71–74]

In a large retrospective review of the published literature Kulkarni and Lusher examined bleeding episodes reported in 349 newborns from a total of 66 publications.[76] Puncture bleeds accounted for 16% of the total, whereas joint bleeds were rarely observed (1%). Postsurgical bleeding, particularly following circumcision, was also common, occurring in 30% of reported cases. Umbilical bleeding, typical of fibrinogen and FXIII deficiency, is relatively uncommon in neonates with hemophilia. Other less common sites of bleeding include gastrointestinal hemorrhage and intraabdominal bleeding.[77,78]

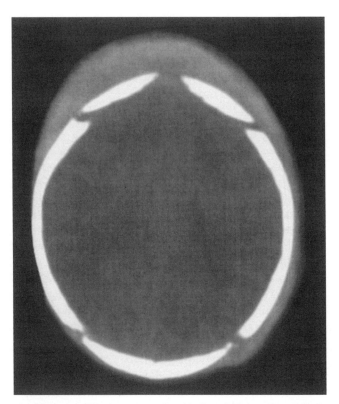

Fig. 30.1 Cephalhematoma in a 2-day-old infant with severe hemophilia A.

Cranial bleeding, which includes both intracranial hemorrhage (ICH) and extracranial hemorrhage (ECH), is potentially the most serious bleeding manifestation observed in the neonatal period and accounted for 41% of all reported bleeding episodes in the literature review of Kulkarni and Lusher. Despite the apparently frequent reporting of this complication the actual incidence of cranial bleeding is not well defined. In a second literature review covering 1964–1996, Kulkarni and Lusher identified 102 neonates with cranial bleeds and hemophilia in a total of 33 publications.[79] From a subgroup of five larger studies these authors calculated a cumulative incidence of cranial hemorrhage of 3.58%. There was, however, considerable variation in the incidence of bleeding between these studies, which included both retrospective and clinical trial data, and were therefore potentially subject to bias. Definition of the true incidence of cranial bleeding will thus require further large prospective cohort studies.

In the survey by Kulkarni and Lusher, ICH was more common than ECH and subdural hemorrhage was the most frequently observed site.[79] The mean age at diagnosis was 4.5 days, and although the majority of reported cases were severe hemophiliacs, bleeding also occurred in moderate and mildly affected cases. While the presentation of cranial bleeding in this age group may be acute and dramatic, clinical features may equally be subtle and nonspecific. ICH may present with seizures and focal neurologic signs or simply with lethargy, poor feeding or vomiting. ECH due to subgaleal

bleeding or cephalhematoma formation (Fig. 30.1) can also be potentially life-threatening, usually due to massive blood loss although cerebral compression has also been reported.[80–82]

The outcome of cranial bleeding is not always adequately recorded but it is clear that a significant proportion of cases go on to develop long-term sequelae with neurodevelopmental problems. In their literature review of cranial bleeding, Kulkarni and Lusher found that overall mortality was 7% with long-term morbidity of 38%, but outcome data were only recorded in 28 cases.[79] In a survey of 30 cases of ICH in children with hemophilia, which included 11 neonates, psychomotor retardation and cerebral palsy were reported in 59% and neonates appeared to show a poorer outcome than older children.[83] It has also been reported that some of these cases may be at risk of recurrent ICH.[80]

Perinatal management

Current opinion on the management of a known or suspected carrier of hemophilia suggests that if the fetus is male, the initial approach to delivery should be governed by obstetric factors and that there is no contraindication to vaginal delivery.[46,55,56,72,84] This is generally followed by advice regarding the avoidance of instrumental delivery (i.e., forceps, vacuum extraction and the use of scalp electrodes), and early recourse to cesarean delivery is recommended where there is a failure of labor to progress. A survey of obstetric practice in North America has indicated that these recommendations do largely reflect current practice, which is also likely to be the case in the UK.[85] It is also usually advised that a cord blood sample is obtained for diagnostic purposes and that intramuscular (i.m.) vitamin K prophylaxis is withheld until hemophilia is excluded.[76,86] If a neonate is shown to have hemophilia vitamin K should be given via an oral regimen.

Diagnosis

On baseline coagulation screening both hemophilia A and B typically result in an isolated prolongation of the APTT, which in an otherwise healthy male infant is highly suggestive of the diagnosis (Table 30.4). Confirmation of the diagnosis requires measurement of FVIII and FIX levels respectively. As FVIII levels are within the normal adult range or mildly increased at birth it is usually possible to confirm a diagnosis of hemophilia A regardless of the severity of the condition or the gestational age of the infant. The only exception to this is mild hemophilia A, where an initial result at the lower end of normal may warrant repeat screening when the infant is older.

The same is not true of hemophilia B, where levels of FIX, as with all vitamin K-dependent factors, are reduced at birth and are further reduced in preterm infants. It is therefore possible to make a diagnosis of severe and moderate hemophilia B at birth but confirmation of mildly affected cases is problematic due to overlap with the normal range, necessitating repeat testing at around 6 months of age or molecular analysis if the genetic defect in the family is known.

It is estimated that in up to one-third of newly diagnosed hemophiliacs a positive family history of hemophilia will be lacking.[71,73] Many of these cases arise as a consequence of a new mutation affecting either the male propositus or more often a female carrier in whom there may be no personal history of bleeding problems. Even where there is a positive family history of hemophilia, published data suggest that women are not always aware of their carrier status, which may have an impact on both their management and the timing of investigations of a potentially affected child.[73,87]

In the absence of a positive family history the diagnosis of hemophilia may go unsuspected in the neonatal period. It is therefore important that neonates presenting with signs of abnormal bleeding are appropriately investigated for the presence of inherited bleeding disorders including hemophilia, and that these investigations include not only baseline coagulation screening tests (PT, APTT), but also appropriate factor assays.

Published case reports both in the past and more recently suggest that there is often a failure to recognize abnormal bleeding and that appropriate investigations are often delayed or misinterpreted, which inevitably results in a failure to manage such cases appropriately.[80,88] In a series of eight cases of intracranial hemorrhage published by Yoff and Buchanan in 1988, the diagnosis of hemophilia was delayed in six cases, sometimes for a period of several months.[80] Similarly, Myles *et al.* in 2001 reported two infants presenting with intracranial hemorrhage in whom neurosurgery was undertaken before a definitive diagnosis was reached.[88] Occasionally, the diagnosis can be further confused by the coexistence of an acquired coagulopathy, for example DIC or vitamin K deficiency.[89]

Neonatal management

In the developed world recombinant FVIII and FIX products are now the treatment of choice for infants with hemophilia. Where recombinant products are not available a high-purity, plasma-derived product may be used instead. Recombinant FVIII concentrates can be subdivided into first-, second- and third-generation products, which differ in terms of the presence or absence of human and animal proteins in the manufacturing process and in the final product.[90] There remains only a single commercially available recombinant FIX concentrate, which contains no human or animal proteins in the final product. There are only limited data available on the pharmacokinetics of replacement therapy in neonates, which suggests that the half-life of FVIII may be less than in older children.[91] Careful monitoring is therefore recommended where replacement therapy is required.

The use of cranial ultrasound scanning to detect early intracranial hemorrhage and the administration of short-term primary prophylaxis to minimize bleeding related to birth trauma are two aspects of neonatal hemophilia management that remain controversial.[92] Recent surveys in both the UK and North America have reported significant variations in practice in this area, which reflects the uncertainties and the lack of evidence-based guidelines.[93,94]

von Willebrand disease

vWD is the commonest inherited bleeding disorder, with an estimated prevalence of 0.8–1.3%.[95,96] vWD is caused by either a quantitative or qualitative deficiency of von Willebrand factor (vWF). In most families vWD is inherited as an autosomal dominant disorder and the bleeding tendency is usually mild. vWF is physiologically increased in the neonatal period and high-molecular-weight multimeric forms are also disproportionately increased at this time.[8]

Clinical features

Due to the protective effect of physiologically raised levels of vWF, bleeding in the neonatal period secondary to vWD is a relatively uncommon event. Nevertheless bleeding may occur, particularly in severe type III disease and in some cases of type II vWD. Bleeding in type II vWD may occur in association with thrombocytopenia in the type IIb subgroup.[97,98] Both superficial bleeding problems and ICH have been reported in affected neonates.[99]

Diagnosis

Type III vWD is confirmed by recording low or virtually absent levels of both FVIII and vWF antigen and activity. Some cases of type II vWD may also be diagnosed in the neonate where there is reduced vWF activity. Type IIb vWD can also be recognized at this time due to the presence of thrombocytopenia, and should be included in the differential diagnosis of congenital thrombocytopenia.[97,98] Most other forms of vWD are masked by physiologically elevated levels of vWF and cannot be diagnosed neonatally other than by molecular analysis. In most cases where there is a family history of mild type IV vWD, screening can be delayed until around 6 months of age.[86]

Management

Current guidelines on the treatment of bleeding in vWD recommend the use of a viricidally treated FVIII concentrate that contains both FVIII and vWF.[90,99,100] Recombinant vWF has been developed but clinical trials have not been completed.[101] The use of desmopressin (DDAVP) should be avoided in the neonatal period due to the risk of hyponatremia.[86] Platelets may also be required in the management of bleeding in type IIb disease.

Rare inherited bleeding disorders

The rare inherited bleeding disorders comprise a group of recessively inherited conditions that include deficiencies of FI (fibrinogen), FII (prothrombin), FV, FVII, FX, FXI, FXIII and the combined deficiencies of FV/FVIII and of FII/FVII/FIX and FX. All of these disorders are extremely rare and the reported prevalence of homozygous defects ranges from around 1 in 500 000 for FVII deficiency to 1 in 2 million for FII (prothrombin) deficiency.[102] The pattern of inheritance is autosomal recessive, and clinical manifestations are most severe in homozygous or compound heterozygous states. Due to the mode of inheritance these disorders are more frequently observed in countries where consanguineous marriage is common.

The rarity of these conditions has meant that information on the most common bleeding manifestations and on optimal management strategies has lagged behind that for the more common inherited bleeding disorders. In recent years data, mainly from Iran and Italy, have expanded our knowledge of these conditions, and more recently preliminary data have also been published from a North American Registry.[102–104] In addition, significant advances have been made in our understanding of the genetic abnormalities that underlie these disorders.[105]

Disorders of fibrinogen

Congenital abnormalities of fibrinogen reflect both quantitative and qualitative defects. These include afibrinogenemia, hypofibrinogenemia and the dysfibrinogenemias.[106] Both afibrinogenemia and hypofibrinogenemia are inherited as autosomal recessive disorders, and the estimated prevalence of afibrinogenemia is 1 in 1 million.[102] Afibrinogenemia and the more severe forms of hypofibrinogenemia may present neonatally. Bleeding from the umbilical cord is the most frequently reported problem, but mucosal bleeding may also occur.[104,107,108] ICH is described in afibrinogenemia, but the age of onset in these reports is unclear.[107,108]

The dysfibrinogenemias are a heterogeneous group of disorders, which unlike most of the other rare disorders are inherited in an autosomal dominant manner. Clinically they may be asymptomatic or associated with either hemorrhagic or thrombotic problems, and are unlikely to present in the neonatal period although they may be diagnosed at this time due to the presence of a family history or following investigation of an abnormal coagulation result.

Diagnosis

Fibrinogen levels are within the normal adult range at birth.[2,3] In afibrinogenemia the PT, APTT and TCT are markedly prolonged and fibrinogen levels are undetectable using both functional (Claus) and antigenic assays.[109] In hypofibrinogenemia the PT, APTT and TCT are prolonged in proportion to the fibrinogen level, which is usually in the range 0.20–0.80 g/L. The TCT is the most sensitive screening test for dysfibrinogenemias and characteristically the fibrinogen level is higher using an antigenic assay.[109]

Management

Fibrinogen concentrate is now generally recommended as the treatment of choice for the management of bleeding in afibrinogenemia and hypofibrinogenemia, and a number of viricidally inactivated concentrates are available.[90,110] A fibrinogen level of 0.5 g/L is thought to represent the minimum level for hemostasis but it is usually suggested that fibrinogen levels are increased to 1 g/L in order to secure hemostasis in the bleeding patient.[110] Fibrinogen has a half-life of 3–5 days, which facilitates relatively infrequent dosing. In the absence of fibrinogen concentrate, cryoprecipitate and fresh frozen plasma (FFP) provide alternative sources of fibrinogen. Fibrin glue and antifibrinolytic medication may also be helpful.

Primary prophylaxis in afibrinogenemia is not generally advised due to the paucity of data. In the event of severe bleeding (e.g., ICH), secondary prophylaxis with the aim of maintaining a fibrinogen level of above 0.5 g/L is thought to be appropriate.[110]

Deficiencies of FII, FV, FVII, FX, FXI and combined FV/FVIII deficiency

Bleeding manifestations have been recorded in the neonatal period in each of these disorders, both in individual case reports and in the larger case series reported from Iran and other groups.[102–104] The pattern of bleeding observed includes umbilical hemorrhage, bleeding post-circumcision, soft-tissue hematomas, gastrointestinal bleeding and ICH.[102] Umbilical bleeding, which is an uncommon manifestation in hemophilia, was documented in 0–28% of cases in the Iranian series and was most commonly seen in cases of FX deficiency (28%) and combined FV/FVIII deficiency (22%).

Severe bleeding manifestations, particularly ICH, appear most common in association with FVII and FX deficiency. In one series, 12/75 (9%) infants with FVII deficiency had ICH; however, this very high incidence has not been confirmed in other series.[102,103,111,112] In the Iranian series, FX deficiency was associated with the most severe bleeding symptoms and the highest frequency of ICH.[102] In FV deficiency, bleeding manifestations do not always correlate well with the plasma FV level and may depend more on platelet FV levels. Similarly a poor correlation between clinical bleeding and plasma factor levels has also been recorded in FVII and FXI deficiency.

Diagnosis

Compared with adult values, plasma levels of factors II, VII, X and XI are all reduced at term and are further reduced in the preterm infant. Thus while it will be possible to diagnose the most severe deficiency states in the newborn period, infants with higher levels may require follow-up testing in order to clarify the diagnosis. Similarly it is not usually possible to diagnose heterozygous deficiencies in the newborn period. This contrasts with FV, which is within the normal adult range at birth, so it should be possible to diagnose both heterozygous and homozygous deficiencies at birth.

Management

Treatment of bleeding episodes should be with a specific factor concentrate if available (e.g., FVII and FXI), or with prothrombin complex concentrate (PCC) (e.g., FII and FX) or fresh frozen plasma (FFP).[110] FXI concentrate and PCC should be used with care in the neonatal period because of the risk of coagulation activation with these products. Recombinant FVIIa has been used as an alternative to plasma-derived FVII for the treatment of inherited FVII deficiency.[113] In the absence of factor concentrates or where their use is considered inappropriate, consideration should also be given to the use of viricidally treated FFP if available.

Factor XIII deficiency

FXIII, or fibrin-stabilizing factor, is the final enzyme to be activated in the coagulation cascade and is responsible for cross-linking fibrin.[114] Congenital deficiency of FXIII is a rare autosomal recessive disease. The homozygous form was initially described in 1960 and the estimated prevalance of this disorder is 1 in 1 000 000.[102] The condition results in a moderate-to-severe bleeding disorder associated in some cases with defective wound healing.

Clinical features

Infants with severe homozygous FXIII deficiency in which the FXIII level is < 1 IU/dL, are at greatest risk of bleeding problems and classically present in the neonatal period with delayed bleeding from the umbilical cord, which is reported in up to 80% of cases.[115,116] The time to presentation ranges from 1 to 19 days. Although characteristic, this pattern of bleeding is not pathognomonic, as around 50% of neonates with afibrinogenemia and other rare disorders also present in this way. Bleeding following circumcision and ICH has also

been recorded. The risk of ICH is lifelong and occurs in up to a third of untreated patients.

Diagnosis

FXIII deficiency does not prolong any of the routine screening tests and must be investigated specifically. The urea solubility test is a useful screening test for severe homozygous deficiency states but will not detect mild deficiencies or heterozygotes. The diagnosis is confirmed by measuring FXIII activity levels.

Management

Neonates diagnosed with FXIII deficiency with levels of < 3 IU/dL should be commenced on a prophylactic replacement regimen, preferably using a viricidally treated FXIII concentrate. Initially a dose of 10 IU/kg every 4 weeks should be adequate, and subsequent monitoring should be performed in order to maintain a pretreatment trough level of > 3 IU/dL.[110,117] If FXIII concentrate is not available, cryoprecipitate or FFP can also be used.

Combined deficiency of vitamin K-dependent coagulation factors

Hereditary combined deficiency of the vitamin K-dependent coagulation factors is an extremely rare autosomal recessive bleeding disorder, which has been described in < 20 kindreds worldwide. The condition is due to mutations affecting either the γ-glutamyl carboxylase enzyme or the vitamin K epoxide reductase enzyme complex (VKOR).[118,119] These defects result in the secretion of inadequately carboxylated FII, FVII, FIX and FX, which as a consequence have poor hemostatic function. Failure of γ-carboxylation also affects a number of other proteins including protein C, protein S, protein Z, osteocalcin, the matrix Gla protein, and the growth arrest specific protein.

Clinically the condition is associated with a variable bleeding phenotype. In severely affected individuals the onset of bleeding may be in the neonatal period, and bleeding from the umbilical stump and ICH have both been reported.[118,119] Skeletal abnormalities, similar to those reported in association with warfarin-induced embryopathy, are also reported.[120]

In affected individuals both the PT and APTT are typically prolonged in association with a variable reduction in the activity levels of the vitamin K-dependent coagulation factors. The condition must be distinguished from acquired vitamin K deficiency, and measurement of fasting serum vitamin K may be helpful. Molecular studies may also be useful.

Some individuals will show partial or complete improvement in factor levels following the administration of vitamin K. Vitamin K is therefore indicated in all cases at diagnosis, and ongoing vitamin K prophylaxis may be required to prevent bleeding.[121] In those who are unresponsive to vitamin K or in the presence of bleeding, factor replacement may be required. Both FFP and factor concentrates have been used in the management of such cases. As before, the use of viricidally inactivated products is usually advised.

Acquired disorders of coagulation

Disseminated intravascular coagulation

The term "disseminated intravascular coagulation" is used to describe an acquired disorder that involves abnormal thrombin generation and always occurs as a secondary event to another disease entity. DIC is common during the neonatal period, particularly in preterm and VLBW infants.[122] DIC in the neonatal period may occur as a consequence of both fetal and neonatal disorders and is also seen in association with certain obstetric complications (Table 30.6). As in older children and adults, DIC is often associated with increased mortality.

Pathophysiology

Although DIC is often seen as a hemostatic disorder, activation of coagulation with increased and abnormal thrombin generation is only part of a complex process that involves inflammatory pathways as well as endothelial cell activation and dysfunction.[123] Failure to regulate this process results in massive uncontrolled thrombin generation, with widespread fibrin deposition and consumption of coagulation proteins and platelets. This is discussed in more detail in Chapter 29.

Table 30.6 Conditions associated with neonatal disseminated intravascular coagulation.

Fetal/neonatal disorders
Hypoxia–acidosis: birth asphyxia, respiratory distress syndrome
Infection
Meconium aspiration
Aspiration of amniotic fluid
Necrotizing enterocolitis
Brain injury
Hypothermia
Hemolysis
Giant hemangioma (Kasabach–Merritt syndrome)
Homozygous protein C/S deficiency
Malignancy

Maternal/obstetric disorders
Severe preeclampsia
Placental abruption
Intrauterine death

Clinical features

The clinical spectrum of neonatal DIC varies greatly from low-grade subclinical DIC to fulminant DIC with bleeding and thrombosis. Superficial bruising, purpura and iatrogenic bleeding from venipuncture and central line insertion sites are relatively common. More serious hemorrhagic problems can also occur, and both pulmonary and intraventricular hemorrhage in preterm infants may be exacerbated by the presence of thrombocytopenia and an uncompensated coagulopathy. Where there is extensive large vessel and microvascular thrombosis this may contribute to end-organ damage and multiorgan failure.

Diagnosis

The diagnosis of fulminant neonatal DIC is usually fairly straightforward and is characterized by prolongation of routine coagulation screening tests (PT, APTT and TCT), combined with thrombocytopenia and evidence of increased fibrin(ogen) degradation products (FDPs) (Table 30.4). Examination of a peripheral blood film may also reveal the presence of red cell fragmentation.

A normal coagulation screen does not, however, exclude the presence of a consumptive coagulopathy. This reflects the wide clinical spectrum of DIC, and early nonovert DIC may be more difficult to diagnose, particularly in the neonatal period.[124] With the development of new therapeutic modalities early diagnosis of DIC may become increasingly important, and in adult practice this has led to the development of diagnostic algorithms for the detection of early nonovert DIC.[125]

The platelet count is almost universally reduced in DIC and has been found to be a useful predictor of a coagulopathy in high-risk neonates.[126] Thrombocytopenia is, however, extremely common in neonatal practice and is often due to failure of production rather than consumption. The PT and APTT are less predictive and can be normal in early DIC.[124] Prolongation of the TCT, which reflects both reduced fibrinogen and the effect of increased FDPs, is again often absent in the early stages.

Evidence of increased fibrin degradation is an important component of the diagnosis of DIC. The D-dimer assay, which measures fragments generated following digestion of fibrin, is now used routinely in many laboratories as a measure of FDPs.[127] D-dimer levels should, however, be interpreted with caution in the neonatal period because raised levels have been found in both term and preterm infants and may initially reflect a degree of coagulation activation at birth.[128]

Although not routinely performed for diagnostic purposes, reduced levels of procoagulant proteins and inhibitors, especially ATIII and protein C, can be observed in high-risk infants, a proportion of which will go on to develop overt DIC.[129,130] El Beshlawy *et al.* demonstrated reduced levels of AT, protein C and protein S in 100% of neonates with hypoxic-ischemic damage, 50% of whom went on to develop overt DIC.[129]

Management

DIC is a secondary phenomenon and it therefore follows that an important aspect of management is reversal of the underlying disease process. In the critically ill preterm infant this may be difficult to achieve; however, failure to remove the underlying procoagulant stimulus will result in ongoing uncontrolled thrombin generation. Beyond this, evidence-based guidelines for other specific treatment modalities are currently lacking and reflect the difficulty of conducting randomized controlled trials in this area.

Currently there is considerable interest in the use of activated protein C for the management of DIC associated with severe sepsis. Recombinant activated protein C (drotrecogin alfa [activated]) has already been shown to be beneficial in the management of severe sepsis in adults.[131] Activated protein C limits thrombin generation via degradation of the coagulation cofactors FVa and FVIIIa and also has profibrinolytic and antiinflammatory effects. Data on the use of this agent in pediatric practice are currently limited to case reports and a single phase 3 study, which included only five children under one year of age.[132,133] The latter study did, however, provide preliminary data on safety and pharmacokinetics and was able to demonstrate a reduction in the level of D-dimers and an increase in both AT and protein C following treatment.[133] Further placebo-controlled trials addressing the efficacy of this novel agent in children are currently ongoing.

Supportive therapy with FFP, cryoprecipitate and platelets to maintain adequate hemostasis remains an important aspect of the management of this condition. Although the use of blood products and the thresholds set for transfusion are largely empirical, it would appear reasonable to institute replacement therapy, particularly where there is an increased risk of bleeding. Guidelines for the transfusion of platelets suggest that the platelet count should be maintained above $50 \times 10^9/L$ by the transfusion of platelet concentrates (10–15 mL/kg).[134] FFP (10–15 mL/kg) can be used to replace hemostatic proteins, including the coagulation inhibitors ATIII, protein C and protein S.[86] Cryoprecipitate (5–10 mL/kg) is a better source of fibrinogen, which should be maintained above 1 g/L. PCCs, although used in the past, are not currently indicated due to the risks of further coagulation activation and thrombosis. Red cell concentrates are also frequently required, and exchange transfusion may be indicated to avoid problems from volume overload.

Studies looking at the efficacy of blood product replacement therapy in neonatal DIC have yielded conflicting results.[135–138] In one small controlled study 33 neonates with DIC were randomized to receive either exchange transfusion, FFP and platelets, or no therapy directed specifically at the coagulopathy, but the results failed to demonstrate any difference in either the resolution of DIC or in survival.[138] Other studies have shown improvement in coagulation profiles and variable improvement in clinical outcome.[135–137] In a recent study Hyytianen[139] demonstrated reduced thrombin generation in a group of neonates following the administration of FFP but the effect on clinical outcome was not reported.

Experimental data from animal studies support the use of both heparin and ATIII concentrates in the treatment of DIC.[140,141] There are, however, only limited data on the use of heparin in neonates with DIC.[142] Gobel *et al.* reported a reduction in the duration of ventilation in a group of neonates with DIC and respiratory distress sundrome treated with heparin compared with placebo but the results were not statistically significant and there was no difference in mortality.[142] ATIII levels are reduced in the neonatal period and are further reduced in the presence of DIC. Because the effectiveness of heparin depends on adequate levels of ATIII it has been postulated that the administration of heparin plus ATIII might be more efficacious than heparin alone. Again, there are few published data on the use of ATIII with heparin in the pediatric age group, with only one small nonrandomized study dealing exclusively with neonates, which failed to document any major benefit. Therefore, neither heparin nor ATIII, alone or in combination, are currently recommended for the routine treatment of neonatal DIC.[143]

Vitamin K deficiency bleeding

The clinical features of hemorrhagic disease of the newborn (HDN) were first described by Towsend in 1894,[144] but it was only some years later that the link with vitamin K deficiency was established. The term HDN has now been replaced by vitamin K deficiency bleeding (VKDB), which highlights the fact that bleeding in the newborn may be due to causes other than vitamin K deficiency and that VKDB may occur beyond the neonatal period.[145] For further information on vitamin K see Chapter 29.

Pathophysiology of VKDB

Levels of the vitamin K-dependent coagulation proteins are physiologically reduced at birth and are functionally inactive in the presence of vitamin K deficiency.[2] In the absence of vitamin K prophylaxis, prothrombin activity has been shown to decrease on days 2–4 of life.[146] The tendency of the neonate to become vitamin K deficient is in part due to the limited stores available at birth. The neonate has a very small hepatic reserve of vitamin K, stored almost exclusively as vitamin K_1.

655

Circulating vitamin K levels are low or undetectable at birth, with maternal:cord vitamin K ratios of between 20 : 1 and 40 : 1.[147] These findings reflect the limited passage of vitamin K across the placental barrier. The reasons for the apparent protection of the neonate from high levels of vitamin K are not well understood because there is no immediately clear biologic advantage.[148]

The situation is further aggravated by the variable but limited content of vitamin K in breast milk, the small volume intake during the first few days of life, and perhaps also by the presence initially of a sterile gut. Vitamin K requirements in the neonate are estimated to be around 1 µg/kg/day; however, breast milk often contains levels as low as 1–2 µg/L, with even lower levels in colostrum.[149,150] This is not the situation in formula-fed infants, who achieve significantly higher concentrations of vitamin K by 3–4 days of age and are therefore relatively protected and rarely develop VKDB in the absence of other factors.[151]

Clinical features

VKDB is generally divided into three forms: early, classical and late. This classification reflects differences not only in the clinical presentation but also in the associated risk factors and prophylactic strategies.[152,153]

Early VKDB

This is the least common form of the disorder, with the onset of bleeding occurring within the first 24 hours of life. The bleeding pattern is variable but can be serious and ICH does occur. This form of VKDB is typically, but not exclusively, associated with the ingestion during pregnancy of drugs that can cross the placenta and interfere with vitamin K metabolism. Warfarin, anticonvulsants and the antituberculous drugs rifampicin and isoniazid have all been implicated.[154]

Warfarin is the classic drug that can enter the fetal circulation and cause hemorrhagic problems via reduced carboxylation of vitamin K-dependent proteins. In addition to hemorrhagic problems, warfarin is teratogenic following exposure in early pregnancy.[155] With the increasing use of low-molecular-weight heparin, warfarin is less frequently prescribed during pregnancy but is still used in some countries for the management of women with artificial heart valves. Where warfarin is prescribed during pregnancy it is generally advised that it is avoided between weeks 6 and 12 of gestation due to the risk of teratogenicity and close to term due to the risk of neonatal bleeding.[156]

The risk of VKDB following ingestion of anticonvulsant drugs, particularly phenytoin, phenobarbitone and carbamazepine, is poorly defined. Using PIVKA (protein induced by vitamin K absence or antagonism)-II to assess vitamin K deficiency, Cornelissen *et al.* demonstrated detectable PIVKA II (i.e., vitamin K deficiency) in cord blood from 54% of neonates on anticonvulsant therapy compared with 20% in the control group.[157] The mechanism whereby anticonvulsant drugs cause this problem is not well understood, but is thought to involve the induction of hepatic microsomal oxidase enzymes, which result in increased degradation of vitamin K.

Classical VKDB

Estimates of the frequency of classical VKDB in the absence of vitamin K prophylaxis vary considerably (0.25–1.7%) and depend particularly on the method of feeding employed in the study population.[158–162] The condition typically presents between days 2 and 5 with bruising, purpura and gastrointestinal hemorrhage in infants who appear otherwise well. They are almost exclusively breast-fed but may have had problems feeding. Bleeding from the umbilicus and mucous membranes is also common, but ICH appears to be relatively infrequent.

Late VKDB

Although classical VKDB had been recognized for many years, the first reports of late VKDB were not published until 1967.[163,164] The onset of bleeding occurs after the first week of life, with a peak incidence between 2 and 8 weeks. It has been proposed that the upper age limit should be extended from 3 to 6 months following the recognition of cases occurring after 15 weeks of age.[165] Unlike classical VKDB, in late VKDB ICH is seen in around 50% of cases and is associated with significant morbidity and mortality.

Breast-feeding and failure to receive vitamin K at birth are frequently documented risk factors. Late VKDB is also seen in association with underlying conditions that result in malabsorption, and it can be the presenting feature of cystic fibrosis, celiac disease, α_1-antitrypsin deficiency and biliary atresia. In other cases it is thought that transient, mild abnormalities of liver function may contribute to cholestasis and temporarily reduced vitamin K absorption.[166,167]

Again, it is difficult to estimate the frequency of late VKDB in unprotected populations but figures ranging from 4.4 per 100 000 births in the UK to 72 per 100 000 in Japan have been published.[168] Recently a study from Vietnam reported an unexpectedly high incidence of late VKDB of 116 per 100 000 births, which highlights the fact that VKDB remains a very significant problem in the developing world.[169]

Laboratory diagnosis

Vitamin K deficiency results in prolongation initially of the PT and subsequently the APTT as well (Table 30.4). The diagnosis is confirmed by finding reduced levels of the vitamin K-dependent factors FII, FVII, FXI and FX.

Vitamin K prophylaxis

Prophylactic strategies differ depending on the type of

VKDB. In an attempt to reduce *early VKDB*, guidelines have been published previously for the management of pregnant women with epilepsy. In addition to advice regarding the choice of anticonvulsant medication, these suggest the need for both the immediate administration of parenteral vitamin K (1 mg) to the neonate and the use of oral vitamin K (20 mg/day) during the last 4 weeks of pregnancy.[170] The latter recommendation is based on the finding of absent PIVKA II in the cord blood of women who received antenatal oral prophylaxis.[170,171] This advice has, however, more recently been challenged by new data from both the UK and North America where there did not appear to be an increased incidence of bleeding in infants where maternal antenatal vitamin K administration had been omitted.[172,173]

Classical VKDB can be effectively prevented by the postnatal administration of a single dose of vitamin K. Various studies have shown that a single oral dose is as effective as parenteral administration.

The prevention of *late VKDB* is less straightforward and has been a major source of controversy over the last 20 years or so. It was apparent by the early 1980s that, while a single oral dose of vitamin K provided adequate protection against classical VKDB, it did not prevent late VKDB.[174] In a study by McNinch and Tripp in 1991, 27 cases of VKDB were identified, of whom 20 had received no vitamin K prophylaxis and 7 oral prophylaxis.[175] The latter presented significantly later (median 38 days) than those who had not had any prophylaxis (median 13.5 days). The solution appeared to be the use of a single dose of i.m. vitamin K at birth for all newborn infants.

In 1992 the safety of this form of prophylaxis was called into question by the case–control study of Golding *et al.*, who reported an increased incidence of childhood leukemia and cancer following intramuscular vitamin K at birth.[176] Although subsequently a number of well-designed studies have failed to support Golding's original findings, concerns over the potential risks of intramuscular vitamin K have been associated with significant variations in practice in different parts of the world.[177–181]

Following Golding's original study, the American Academy of Pediatrics recommended the continued use of intramuscular vitamin K, whereas the British Paediatric Association recommended that oral vitamin K supplements should be given to newborn infants, with repeated doses for breast-fed infants.[182,183] There followed a general trend in the UK and other parts of Europe toward oral vitamin K prophylaxis, but compliance with the triple dose regimen was initially variable, and in 1994 Croucher and Azzopardi reported that > 10% of breast-fed infants did not receive a second dose of vitamin K and < 40% received a third dose.[162]

Although oral vitamin K prophylaxis continues to be widely practiced, especially in Europe, the optimal formulation and dosing regimen remains to be defined.[184] It does, however, appear that regimens consisting of multiple doses

are more effective, particularly for breast-fed infants.[185,186] With regard to vitamin K formulations, in 1998 guidelines in the UK recommended the use of the Konakion mixed micellular preparation for oral prophylaxis. However, subsequent data published in 2003 failed to show that this formulation was superior to older vitamin K preparations for the prevention of late VKDB.[187,188]

Treatment

Once VKDB has been confirmed, intravenous vitamin K should be administered to correct the deficiency. In suspected cases a therapeutic trial of vitamin K may be given while factor assays are pending. Vitamin K should be administered by slow intravenous or subcutaneous injection but not by the intramuscular route in the presence of a coagulopathy. Following parenteral administration of 1 mg of vitamin K_1, the vitamin K-dependent proteins start to increase after 20–30 minutes and should normalize over a few hours.[189]

In the presence of significant bleeding, factor replacement therapy may also be required with either viricidally inactivated FFP, PCC (FII, FIX, FX) or a four-factor concentrate containing all the vitamin K-dependent factors.[86]

Liver disease

Although some degree of hepatic impairment is not uncommon in the neonatal period, fulminant hepatic failure is a relatively rare event. Recognized causes of neonatal hepatic failure include viral infections, metabolic disorders, mitochondrial cytopathies, storage disorders and shock.[190] The usual division into acute and chronic liver failure is somewhat arbitrary in the neonate; however, it is recognized that the onset of hepatic dysfunction may occur *in utero* or develop in the perinatal period. Lesser degrees of hepatic impairment may occur in conjunction with sepsis, hypoxia and the use of total parenteral nutrition.

Pathophysiology

The pathophysiology of the coagulopathy in neonatal liver disease is multifactorial but is not significantly different from that seen in older children and adults. Reduced synthesis of procoagulant proteins plays an important role and is further aggravated in the neonatal period by the immaturity of the liver and the physiologically reduced levels of many coagulation proteins. Reduced clearance of activated coagulation factors by the hepatic reticuloendothelial system, activation of fibrinolysis, impaired utilization of vitamin K and thrombocytopenia also contribute.[191–194]

Clinical and laboratory features

The pattern of bleeding is variable and reflects the severity of the coagulopathy. Laboratory features include prolongation of both the PT and APTT, and in fulminant hepatic failure the TCT also becomes prolonged in association with reduced levels of fibrinogen (see Table 37.32). The main differential diagnosis is vitamin K deficiency and DIC, and specific factor assays and analysis of fibrinogen/fibrin degradation products may be helpful.

Management

Management of the coagulopathy in liver disease is purely supportive. As mentioned above, neonatal liver failure is a relatively infrequent event and there are few published data on the efficacy of blood product support. In the presence of clinical bleeding, replacement therapy with FFP, cryoprecipitate and platelet concentrates may restore normal hemostasis, at least temporarily. Occasionally, exchange transfusion may be required if there are problems with fluid overload. As in DIC, PCCs should be avoided due to the risks of thrombosis. If there is evidence of cholestasis, the administration of vitamin K supplements may also be helpful.

Cardiopulmonary bypass

Neonates with congenital heart disease (CHD) who require early corrective surgery involving cardiopulmonary bypass (CPB) are at increased risk of both hemorrhagic and thrombotic complications.[195–198] Excessive bleeding may occur both perioperatively and postoperatively and is correlated with the duration of the bypass procedure. The actual incidence of major nonsurgical bleeding is difficult to define and is dependent on the criteria used but is likely to be higher in neonates than in older children.

The pathophysiology of nonsurgical post-CPB hemorrhage is complex and several contributing mechanisms are recognized (see also Chapter 29).[195,196] Although the mechanisms involved are similar in neonates and older children, the relative importance of each is influenced by age, particularly during the neonatal period, when the hemostatic system is physiologically immature.

The presence of a preoperative coagulation defect would be expected to increase the risk of bleeding associated with surgery. There are conflicting reports in the literature regarding the presence of underlying coagulation defects in CHD in older children.[197,198] In cyanotic CHD, some of the previously noted abnormalities may have been artefactual, secondary to polycythemia; however, it is likely that a low-grade consumptive coagulopathy exists in some cases. Abnormalities in acyanotic CHD have also been documented and include the loss of high-molecular-weight vWF multimers, which return to normal after surgery.[199] Chan et al. documented normal procoagulant and inhibitor levels in a group of 22 children (1–15 years) prior to CPB.[200] This contrasts with data from a neonatal study in 1992, in which 53% of infants,

aged between 1 and 30 days, had reduced procoagulant levels preoperatively compared with age-matched controls.[201] It was postulated that these abnormalities were due to impaired hepatic maturation secondary to poor organ perfusion or severe cyanosis. It was not, however, possible in this study to predict which neonates were more likely to have a preoperative coagulopathy.

Following the onset of CPB there is a very predictable decrease in the levels of virtually all hemostatic proteins, which occurs secondary to hemodilution. Mean plasma concentrations of procoagulant proteins and inhibitors are reduced by around 50% of pre-CPB values.[200,201] There is a similar reduction in the fibrinolytic proteins plasminogen and α_2-AP. These changes have a significant effect on the regulation of thrombin, and in vitro studies have demonstrated that the capacity to generate thrombin is reduced by 50%. This contrasts with the in vitro plasma thrombin inhibitory capacity, which, despite the reduced inhibitor levels, is relatively spared.[202] It has been suggested that this may be one reason why the risk of hemorrhagic complications post-CPB is relatively greater than the risk of thrombosis.

Compared with data from adult studies, the effect of hemodilution in neonates is profound. This reflects the greater degree of dilution in the neonate's circulating blood volume, which is estimated to be 5–10 times greater than that seen in an adult. The resulting global reduction in procoagulant proteins combined with the physiologic immaturity of the coagulation system may result in concentrations lower than those generally considered necessary for adequate hemostasis. The situation is further aggravated in the presence of reduced preoperative levels.

In addition to the effects of hemodilution, there is also evidence that both the coagulation and fibrinolytic systems are activated during CPB, which may result in a low-grade consumptive coagulopathy. Using prothrombin F1+2 and TAT as markers of thrombin generation, studies in both neonates and older children have shown that levels increase during CPB despite the use of heparin.[200,203] Inadequate anticoagulation and tissue damage during surgery are thought to contribute. In support of the latter it has recently been suggested that it is predominantly the extrinsic pathway rather than the contact system that triggers coagulation activation during CPB.[204] tPA and D-dimers are also increased during bypass indicating activation of the fibrinolytic system. In most studies levels fall again postoperatively in keeping with "fibrinolytic shutdown."[200,205]

Optimal anticoagulation during CPB is crucial to the successful outcome of the procedure. Current protocols use standard heparin, monitored intraoperatively using the activated clotting time (ACT) and reversed by protamine sulfate at the end of the procedure. Inadequate heparinization may cause excess fibrin deposition and consumption of coagulation factors whereas overanticoagulation increases the risk of bleeding. Despite the importance of anticoagulation, there are few or no data relating to the use of heparin in neonates undergoing CPB and current regimens are based on data from adult studies.

Current evidence suggests that neonates clear standard heparin faster than adults.[206] In addition, physiologically reduced concentrations of ATIII, which decrease further during bypass due to hemodilution, are likely to impair heparin activity. The use of increased doses of heparin with or without the addition of ATIII supplements might therefore be expected to improve anticoagulation and reduce thrombin generation.[207] It is also clear that use of the ACT to monitor heparin therapy during CPB is unsatisfactory because it is significantly influenced by other factors, particularly hemodilution, and correlates poorly with plasma heparin levels as measured by either antithrombin or anti-FXa assays.[208,209]

Thrombocytopenia develops at the onset of bypass, again largely due to the effect of hemodilution. Platelet function defects also occur and lead to prolongation of the bleeding time independent of the platelet count. Although contributing to bleeding problems, platelet dysfunction, particularly in neonates, is probably less important than the changes in the coagulation system. This contrasts with the situation in adults, where acquired platelet dysfunction is usually the main cause of hemorrhage. The pathophysiology of platelet dysfunction in CBP remains controversial. Partial platelet degranulation and defects of platelet membrane glycoproteins have all been described, and it has been suggested that the problem is "extrinsic" and due to inadequate availability of platelet agonists.[196,210]

Thrombocytopenia following CPB surgery may also be due to the development of heparin-induced thrombocytopenia, which is probably underdiagnosed in pediatric practice.[211,212] It is not, however, clear to what extent this immune-mediated complication affects infants during the first month of life.

Management of bleeding after CPB is complex and requires careful assessment of the likely causes. Replacement therapy with FFP, cryoprecipitate and platelets may be required to correct hemostatic defects. Adequate reversal of heparin with protamine sulfate is also important. Various measures can also be undertaken in an attempt to prevent excessive blood loss. These include the use of fibrin sealants, which can improve local hemostasis during surgery, and the serine protease inhibitor aprotinin.[213–216] A literature review on the use of aprotinin following cardiac surgery concluded that a number of beneficial effects had been observed in neonates following high-dose aprotinin, including attenuation of the inflammatory response, a reduction in postoperative blood loss and a reduction in overall hospital stay.[216]

Recombinant factor VIIa (rFVIIa) (NovoSeven) is a hemostatic agent that was first developed for the treatment of hemophilia patients with inhibitors.[217] Following intravenous injection rFVIIa enhances hemostasis by increasing thrombin generation on activated platelets. There has been considerable interest in the use of rFVIIa in patients with a variety of acute hemorrhagic problems and there have been a small number of reports of its use in neonatal practice.[218] Preliminary data on the management of bleeding in children undergoing cardiac surgery have demonstrated potential benefits, and further randomized studies are ongoing at the present time.[219]

Neonatal thrombocytopenia

Incidence

Data from fetal blood sampling indicate that the fetal platelet count is within the normal adult range from as early as 15–18 weeks gestation and neonatal thrombocytopenia is therefore defined as a platelet count of $< 150 \times 10^9/L$.[42,44] The incidence of neonatal thrombocytopenia is highly dependent on the population studied. In large population-based studies of unselected term neonates the reported incidence of thrombocytopenia is 1–5%.[44,220–223]

Severe thrombocytopenia (platelets $<50 \times 10^9/L$) is less common. In a large prospective study, where platelet counts were determined from $> 15\,000$ cord blood samples, only 19 cases (0.12%) were $< 50 \times 10^9/L$.[220] Six infants in this study had a platelet count of $< 20 \times 10^9/L$, all of whom had an underlying diagnosis of neonatal alloimmune thrombocytopenia (NAIT).

The situation in sick neonates is somewhat different and in this context thrombocytopenia is relatively common. In a 1-year prospective study of 807 infants admitted to a regional neonatal intensive care unit (NICU), Castle *et al.* documented thrombocytopenia in 22% of cases.[224] A similar incidence was recently recorded in a similar study from Pakistan, where 24% of all NICU admissions were thrombocytopenic.[225]

Etiology and mechanisms of thrombocytopenia

As with thrombocytopenia in other age groups, neonatal thrombocytopenia may relate to inadequate platelet production or a shortened platelet lifespan, often due to increased peripheral destruction or sequestration. Although it has been recognized for many years that a large number of maternal, perinatal and neonatal problems may be associated with the presence of neonatal thrombocytopenia, until recently relatively little was understood about the actual mechanisms involved.[224] This particularly applies to nonimmune thrombocytopenias, where the presence of a low platelet count is often attributed to the presence of a low-grade consumptive coagulopathy with DIC.

Studies focusing on the natural history of neonatal thrombocytopenia have highlighted specific patterns of thrombocytopenia and, in conjunction with data on megakaryocyte numbers and thrombopoietin (Tpo) levels, have helped to define the pathophysiology of this problem.[226,227] Revised classifications of neonatal thrombocytopenia have therefore been proposed, which define thrombocytopenia in terms of the time of onset, which is likely to relate to specific underlying mechanisms and disorders (Table 30.7).

In the majority of thrombocytopenic neonates the platelet count is low at birth or falls within the first 72 hours of life. Although a small proportion will be due to immunologic causes or other specific problems, the majority are the result of impaired platelet production, which is reflected in reduced numbers of megakaryocytes and increased levels of Tpo. The natural history of this type of thrombocytopenia is for the

Table 30.7 Classification of fetal and neonatal thrombocytopenias.

Fetal	**Alloimmune**
	Congenital infection (e.g., CMV, *Toxoplasma*, rubella, HIV)
	Aneuploidy (e.g., trisomies 18, 13, 21 or triploidy)
	Autoimmune (e.g., ITP, SLE)
	Severe Rhesus disease
	Congenital/inherited (e.g., Wiskott–Aldrich syndrome)
Early-onset neonatal (<72 hours)	**Placental insufficiency** (e.g., PET, IUGR, diabetes)
	Perinatal asphyxia
	Perinatal infection (e.g., *Escherichia coli*, GBS, *Haemophilus influenzae*)
	Disseminated intravascular coagulation
	Alloimmune
	Autoimmune (e.g., ITP, SLE)
	Congenital infection (e.g., CMV, *Toxoplasma*, rubella, HIV)
	Thrombosis (e.g., aortic, renal vein)
	Bone marrow replacement (e.g., congenital leukemia)
	Kasabach–Merritt syndrome
	Metabolic disease (e.g., propionic and methylmalonic acidemia)
	Congenital/inherited (e.g., TAR, CAMT)
Late-onset neonatal (>72 hours)	**Late-onset sepsis**
	Necrotizing enterocolitis
	Congenital infection (e.g., CMV, *Toxoplasma*, rubella, HIV)
	Autoimmune
	Kasabach–Merritt syndrome
	Metabolic disease (e.g., propionic and methylmalonic acidemia)
	Congenital/inherited (e.g., TAR, CAMT)

CAMT, congenital amegakaryocytic thrombocytopenia; CMV, cytomegalovirus; GBS, group B *Streptococcus*; HIV, human immunodeficiency virus; ITP, idiopathic thrombocytopenic purpura; IUGR, intrauterine growth restriction; PET, preeclampsia; SLE, systemic lupus erythematosus; TAR, thrombocytopenia with absent radii. Most frequently occurring conditions are emboldened.
Reproduced with permission from Ref. 227.

platelet count to fall to a nadir at around day 5 and then increase spontaneously thereafter.[226,227] Thrombocytopenia that develops after the first 72 hours of life is frequently associated with sepsis and necrotizing enterocolitis. This type of thrombocytopenia is often severe and persistent and is due to a combination of impaired production and increased consumption.[226,227]

Clinical features

The most serious potential risk associated with neonatal thrombocytopenia is ICH/IVH, and a number of studies have shown an association between thrombocytopenia, IVH and other adverse outcomes.[228,229] Such infants are often extremely sick, and whether such adverse outcomes are directly related to the presence of thrombocytopenia or can be improved by platelet transfusion remains controversial.

Platelet transfusion therapy

Outside of specific immune-mediated forms of neonatal thrombocytopenia (see below), platelet transfusion remains the most important therapeutic option for the management of neonatal thrombocytopenia. Despite this there is evidence of considerable variation in clinical practice and an absence of controlled trial data on which to base guidelines.[230,231] At present there are no data to suggest that platelet transfusion reduces the risk of neonatal bleeding, especially IVH.[232] Currently therefore a threshold for transfusion of $20–30 \times 10^9$/L is suggested for nonbleeding term and preterm neonates, with higher thresholds for VLBW infants and those who are bleeding[226] (Table 30.8).

Other potential therapeutic options: hematopoietic growth factors

There is considerable interest in the possibility of using hematopoietic growth factors as a method of either preventing or treating neonatal thrombocytopenia. Tpo and interleukin-11 (IL-11) are the two factors that have been investigated as potential therapeutic candidates.[233] Tpo is the major regulator of platelet production but, to date, information about the clinical use of recombinant Tpo remains limited. Although recombinant Tpo is a potent stimulator of megakaryocyte precursors there is a delay of 5–7 days before the platelet count increases, which may limit its clinical usefulness.[234] In addition, Tpo has been associated with the development of anti-Tpo antibodies, and recent attention has therefore been focused on the development of Tpo-mimetic peptides, which are small molecules with thrombopoietic activity but that do not share sequence homology with endogenous Tpo.[235]

IL-11 is able to exert an effect on platelet production and may also have a beneficial effect in sepsis, but again there

Table 30.8 Guidelines for platelet transfusion thresholds for neonates.

Platelet count (× 10⁹/L)	Nonbleeding neonate	Bleeding neonate	NAITP (proven or suspected)
<30	Consider transfusion in all patients	Transfuse	Transfuse (with HPA-compatible platelets)

30–49	Do not transfuse if clinically stable
	
	Consider transfusion if:
	
	  < 1000 g and < 1 week of age
	  Clinically unstable (e.g., fluctuating BP
	    or perfusion)
	  Previous major bleeding (e.g., petechiae,
	    puncture-site oozing, or bloodstained
	    ET secretions)
	  Concurrent coagulopathy
	  Requires surgery or exchange transfusion
		Transfuse	Transfuse (with HPA-compatible platelets if any bleeding)

50–99	Do not transfuse	Transfuse	Transfuse (with HPA-compatible platelets if major bleeding present)
> 99	Do not transfuse	Do not transfuse	Do not transfuse

BP, blood pressure; ET, endotracheal; HPA, human platelet antigen; NAITP, neonatal alloimmune thrombocytopenia.
Reproduced with permission from Ref. 227.

are currently no clinical data available to support its use in clinical practice.[233]

Specific types of thrombocytopenia

Neonatal alloimmune thrombocytopenia

NAIT occurs as a result of transplacental passage of maternally derived IgG antibodies directed against paternal antigens on fetal platelets. These antibodies result in immune-mediated platelet destruction leading to fetal thrombocytopenia, which may develop *in utero* as early as 20 weeks gestation. The pathophysiology of the condition is therefore analogous to hemolytic disease of the newborn.

In addition to ABO and human leukocyte antigen (HLA) class I antigens, platelets express specific human platelet antigens (HPA, groups 1–5), which represent antigens associated with platelet membrane glycoproteins. In Caucasian populations, HPA-1a (PLA-1) is the commonest human platelet antigen (expressed by almost 98% of the population) and is responsible for the majority of cases of NAIT.[236] HPA-5b (Br) and HPA-3a (Bak) are less frequently involved, while in other ethnic groups antigens such as HPA-4 (Yuk/Pen) are more frequently implicated.[237]

In a recent study from North America HPA alloantibody specificity was reported from 1162 cases of NAIT investigated at a reference center over a 12-year period.[238] In this study HPA-1a accounted for 79% of cases, while HPA-5b, HPA-3a and HPA-1b were reported in 9%, 2% and 4% of cases, respectively. Interestingly a number of cases with multiple HPA-specific alloantibodies were also identified.[238]

NAIT has very rarely been reported in association with other platelet alloantibodies including anti-Nak(a) and anti-Duv(a+) and also in association with HLA alloantibodies.[239–243]

Recent estimates from screening studies in predominantly white populations suggest that the prevalence of clinically significant NAIT is around 1 in 2000 live births.[236,244] Thus, although around 2.5% of Caucasian women are HPA-1a negative and are therefore potentially at risk, platelet antigen incompatibility does not invariably result in alloimmunization, and alloimmunization, in turn, does not always result in clinically apparent disease.[245] The immune response in this condition is in part related to the maternal HLA phenotype, with HLA-Dw52a associated with an increased risk of sensitization.[246]

In contrast to the situation in Rhesus hemolytic disease, first pregnancies are affected in around 50% of cases.[236,247] The risk of recurrence in future pregnancies is almost 100% where the father is homozygous for the HPA 1a antigen and 50% in the heterozygous state.[247] Maternal antibodies can cross the placenta from 14 weeks gestation, and fetal thrombocytopenia has been documented as early as 20 weeks gestation.

In the neonatal period the typical feature of NAIT is moderate-to-severe thrombocytopenia in an otherwise well infant in the absence of any history of maternal thrombocytopenia. The severity of the thrombocytopenia is variable and although the reasons for this are incompletely understood the platelet antigen specificity and antiplatelet antibody titer are probably important factors.[248,249]

The most serious complication is ICH, which occurs in up to 20% of all cases, with around 10% occurring *in utero*.[250,251] ICH can be clinically silent and it is important that any infant suspected of having NAIT should have a cranial ultrasound scan performed. In addition to ICH, superficial hemorrhage, anemia and gastrointestinal bleeding are also relatively frequent. The risk of bleeding in NAIT is further aggravated by impaired platelet function, which occurs as a consequence of antibody blocking the glycoprotein IIb–IIIa complex.[252]

The degree of thrombocytopenia is typically most marked on the first day of life and is followed by a gradual return to normal over a period of around 2–4 weeks. Mortality associated with NAIT is estimated at 10–15%, with the majority of deaths occurring as a consequence of ICH. In addition, neurodevelopmental sequelae in survivors of ICH are frequent and often severe, and include cerebral palsy, seizures, hydrocephalus and mental retardation.[253,254]

Laboratory confirmation of NAIT is based on the demonstration of maternal antibody with specificity for paternal antigens. In populations of European origin, rapid typing of maternal platelets for the HPA-1a antigen and screening of maternal serum for evidence of anti-HPA-1a alloantibodies should be undertaken first and will provide confirmation in the majority of cases of NAIT. If these results are negative, platelet phenotyping of both parents and screening of maternal serum for alloantibodies against other platelet-specific antigens as well as HLA and ABO antigens should also be performed. Paternal zygosity studies are important for the prediction of recurrent NAIT in future pregnancies. Although the estimated prevalence of this condition is in the order of 1 in 2000 live births, recent data from both the UK and Ireland based on confirmed clinical cases of NAIT suggest that the condition remains underdiagnosed.[255,256]

NAIT is a self-limiting condition; however, until the platelet count recovers, the affected neonate is at significant risk of life-threatening hemorrhage. Once the diagnosis has been confirmed, the most important aspect of management is the rapid administration of compatible, antigen-negative platelets, which, in the majority of cases, result in an increase in the platelet count.[257] Transfusion of compatible platelets may have to be repeated until the infant's own platelet count recovers.

Platelets may be obtained from either accredited HPA-typed donors or alternatively the infant's mother is a potential source of compatible platelets because, by definition, she will be negative for the causative antigen.[257,258] In suspected NAIT where the diagnosis has yet to be confirmed donor platelets that are HPA-1a and HPA-5b negative should be used until the results of serologic investigations are complete. In the event that maternal platelets are required these may be prepared from either a whole blood donation or by platelet pheresis. Regardless of the method of collection, maternal platelets should be plasma depleted (by washing or centrifugation) prior to administration to remove platelet alloantibodies and should also be irradiated to reduce the risk of engraftment of maternal lymphocytes and subsequent graft-versus-host disease.[259,260] It is also recommended that, unless there is extreme clinical urgency, these platelets undergo standard virologic screening prior to use.

Where NAIT is anticipated, which usually occurs following a previously affected pregnancy, antigen-negative platelets should be prepared in advance of delivery either from the mother or from a specifically identified antigen-negative donor. As discussed above, the commonest causative antigen in NAIT is HPA-1a, and many larger donor centers now have a registry of known HPA-1a negative donors who can undergo platelet pheresis if required. Very occasionally it may be necessary to use frozen platelets.[261,262] The only indication for the use of random donor platelets in this condition is life-threatening hemorrhage while awaiting antigen-negative platelets.

While high-dose intravenous immunoglobulin (IVIG) therapy has been shown to be of benefit in increasing the platelet count in NAIT, its effect is usually delayed and is less predictable than that of antigen-negative platelets and should only be used in addition to compatible platelet transfusion.[263,264] IVIG also has the disadvantage of exposing the infant to a pooled blood product, and this should be taken into consideration when planning therapy. While IVIG may have a part to play in management, there is no evidence to support the use of corticosteroids.

NAIT, although rare, is potentially life-threatening, and prevention is therefore an important aspect of the overall management of the condition. Screening for HPA-1a phenotypes during pregnancy, which can facilitate the identification of unsuspected cases in a first pregnancy, remains controversial and is not routine practice. Currently, preventive strategies are therefore aimed at reducing the risk of recurrence in future pregnancies following identification of an affected fetus/neonate.[265–268] There is, however, no consensus on the optimal management strategy. One option is regular maternal IVIG (1 g/kg per week), with or without additional corticosteroids, commenced following documentation of fetal thrombocytopenia with subsequent monitoring of the fetal platelet count by percutaneous umbilical blood sampling a few weeks later. Results achieved with this form of therapy are conflicting and it is likely that a significant percentage of cases will not respond adequately.[269–272] The major alternative strategy is cordocentesis with regular platelet transfusion, which effectively increases the fetal platelet count but carries a significant risk of procedural complications.[273] To minimize the risks from regular cordocentesis it has been suggested that regular platelet transfusions should be reserved for cases in which medical management with IVIG has demonstrably failed. Avoidance of trauma at the time of delivery is an important aspect of management, and early elective delivery by cesarean section is generally advocated.

Neonatal autoimmune thrombocytopenia

In the presence of maternal autoimmune thrombocytopenia Idiopathic thrombocytopenic purpura (ITP or other autoimmune conditions), placental transfer of idiopathic thrombocytopenic purpura IgG antibodies may result in neonatal thrombocytopenia. The antibodies in this context are directed against antigens common to both maternal and neonatal platelets.

The prevalence of maternal ITP is estimated at between 1 and 5 per 10 000 pregnancies; however, clinically significant neonatal thrombocytopenia is relatively uncommon. Data from three published series that looked at chronic maternal thrombocytopenia recorded significant neonatal thrombocytopenia (platelets $< 50 \times 10^9$/L) in 25 of 182 cases (14%) and only 2 (1%) documented cases of ICH.[274] Two other recent studies have confirmed that the risk of life-threatening hemorrhage remains low and is typically less than 1%.[275,276]

Unlike NAIT the platelet nadir usually occurs a few days post-delivery and bleeding problems *in utero* or at delivery are rare. It should be noted that the count can be normal at birth and fall subsequently, necessitating serial platelet counts. The condition is self-limiting and the count has usually normalized by 2–3 months of age. Where the platelet count is $< 50 \times 10^9$/L, treatment options include IVIG and corticosteroids. IVIG 1 g/kg per day for 2 days is effective in the majority of cases and produces a relatively rapid response.[277,278] The response to platelet transfusion is generally poor and this should only be used in infants with life-threatening hemorrhagic problems.[259]

Management of the fetus in the presence of maternal ITP remains controversial and there is no evidence that any maternal therapy increases the fetal platelet count. There is no correlation between maternal and neonatal platelet counts, and the severity of thrombocytopenia in a previous infant is the best predictor of the likelihood of thrombocytopenia in a subsequent pregnancy.[279]

Current management strategies for maternal ITP are mostly conservative, and attempts to assess the platelet count by fetal scalp sampling or fetal blood sampling have been abandoned in most centers due to the procedural risks associated with these techniques.[280,281] Routine cesarean section for maternal ITP has not been shown to improve fetal outcome and, as the risk of neonatal hemorrhage is low, the route of delivery can be determined primarily by obstetric factors.[275,279,282]

Maternal systemic lupus erythematosus (SLE) may be associated with transplacental passage of other antibodies, including anti-SSA/Ro-SSB/La antibodies, and infants are therefore at risk of other complications in addition to thrombocytopenia.[283] Neonatal lupus erythematosus comprises a number of clinical manifestations including skin rashes, complete heart block, thrombocytopenia, hepatomegaly and abnormal liver function.[283,284] Bleeding due to severe thrombocytopenia has been treated successfully with IVIG.[284]

Inherited thrombocytopenia

The inherited thrombocytopenias represent a heterogeneous group of disorders, most of which are very rare.[285] Neverthe-

Table 30.9 Inherited thrombocytopenia classified by platelet size.

Small platelets
Wiskott–Aldrich syndrome
X-linked thrombocytopenia

Normal platelets
Congenital amegakaryocytic thrombocytopenia
Amegakaryocytic thrombocytopenia with absent radii
Familial platelet disorder/acute myeloid leukaemia
Thrombocytopenia with radioulnar synostosis

Large platelets
MYH-9 related disease
Bernard–Soulier syndrome
Mediterranean thrombocytopenia
Gata-1 mutation
Velocardiofacial syndrome
Gray platelet syndrome
Paris–Trousseau thrombocytopenia
Jacobsen syndrome

less, these disorders can present with bleeding early in life but are often overlooked, at least during initial investigations. In addition to thrombocytopenia these conditions can also be associated with defects in platelet function or with other somatic abnormalities.[286] The genetic defects responsible for many of these conditions have recently been defined, and this has also resulted in the description of new disorders.[287,288] Various systems have been proposed for the classification of inherited thrombocytopenias, the most useful of which are based on inheritance pattern, platelet size or the presence of other associated features[285] (Table 30.9). The Italian Gruppo di Studio delle Piastrine has proposed a series of diagnostic algorithms for the investigation of inherited thrombocytopenia based on readily accessible clinical and laboratory parameters.[289] The application of this type of approach may aid in the diagnosis of these conditions although it is likely that a proportion of cases may still not fulfil the criteria for any known condition.

Other nonimmune thrombocytopenias

Fetal congenital infection is frequently associated with thrombocytopenia. In addition to increased destruction, reduced platelet production and splenic pooling all contribute to the thrombocytopenia in this situation. In a study looking at the platelet counts of fetuses with known congenital infections, thrombocytopenia was documented in congenital rubella in 20%, toxoplasmosis in 26% and cytomegalovirus (CMV) in 36% of cases.[44] Thrombocytopenia in this study was most marked in cases of CMV infection. In general, however, congenital infections are an uncommon cause of severe ($< 20 \times 10^9$/L) thrombocytopenia. HIV infection can also lead to thrombocytopenia but this is an uncommon presentation in the neonatal period.[290]

Chromosomal abnormalities are another well-recognized but relatively uncommon cause of neonatal thrombocytopenia.[245] The platelet count is usually only mildly reduced and clinical bleeding is uncommon. The diagnosis is almost always obvious due to the presence of characteristic associated abnormalities. In one study of fetal thrombocytopenia, 43 of 247 cases were due to chromosomal abnormalities.[44] These cases included trisomy 13, 18 and 21, Turner syndrome and triploidy, of which trisomy 18 was the commonest cause with 26 of 30 (87%) cases affected. In only one infant (triploidy) was a platelet count of $< 50 \times 10^9/L$ recorded. The mechanism of thrombocytopenia is incompletely understood but is thought to involve defects in megakaryocyte maturation.

Fanconi anemia is also recessively inherited and typically presents with marrow hypoplasia in association with a variable pattern of coexisting congenital abnormalities. There is increased sensitivity to DNA damage by alkylating agents and ionizing radiation and the diagnosis can be confirmed by performing chromosome breakage studies. Although thrombocytopenia is often an early hematologic finding, it only rarely manifests during the neonatal period.[291]

Rarer causes of thrombocytopenia include giant hemangiomas (Kasabach–Merritt syndrome) and extensive thrombosis, both of which result in platelet consumption. Very rarely, congenital leukemia, neuroblastoma and histiocytosis may present with thrombocytopenia in the neonatal period as a consequence of marrow infiltration.

References

1. Hathaway W, Corrigan J. Report of the Scientific and Standardisation Subcommittee on Neonatal Haemostasis: normal coagulation data for fetuses and newborn infants. *Thromb Haemost* 1991; **65**: 323–5.
2. Andrew M, Paes B, Milner R *et al.* Development of the coagulation system in the full term infant. *Blood* 1987; **70**: 165–72.
3. Andrew M, Paes B, Milner R *et al.* Development of the coagulation system in the healthy premature infant. *Blood* 1988; **72**: 1651–7.
4. Andrew M, Paes B, Johnston M. Development of the hemostatic system in the neonate and young infant. *Am J Pediatr Hematol Oncol* 1990; **112**: 95–104.
5. Corrigan JJ Jr. Normal haemostasis in fetus and newborn. Coagulation. In: Polin RA, Fox WW (eds) *Neonatal and Fetal Medicine. Physiology and Pathophysiology*. Philadelphia: WB Saunders, 1992, pp. 1368–71.
6. Reverdiau-Moalic P, Delahousse B, Body G, Bardos P, Leroy J, Gruel Y. Evolution of blood coagulation activators and inhibitors in the healthy human fetus. *Blood* 1996; **88**: 900–6.
7. Cade JF, Hirsh J, Martin M. Placental barrier to coagulation factors: its relevance to the coagulation defect at birth and to haemorrhage in the newborn. *Br Med J* 1969; **2**: 281–3.
8. Katz JA, Moake JL, McPherson PD *et al.* Relationship between human development and disappearance of unusually large von Willebrand factor multimers from plasma. *Blood* 1989; **73**: 1851–8.
9. Weinstein MJ, Blanchard R, Moake JL, Vosburgh E, Moise K. Fetal and neonatal von Willebrand (VWF) is unusually large and similar to the VWF in patients with thrombotic thrombocytopenic purpura. *Br J Haematol* 1989; **72**: 68–72.
10. Ts'ao CH, Green D, Schultz K. Function and ultrastructure of platelets of neonates: enhanced ristocetin aggregation of neonatal platelets. *Br J Haematol* 1976; **32**: 225–33.
11. Thomas KB, Sutor AH, Altinkaya N, Grohmann A, Zehenter A, Leititis JU. von Willebrand factor-collagen binding activity is increased in newborns and infants. *Acta Paediatr* 1995; **84**: 697–9.
12. Hamulyak K, Nieuwenhuizen W, Devillee PP, Hemker HC. Reevaluation of some properties of fetal fibrinogen purified from cord blood of normal newborns. *Thromb Res* 1983; **32**: 301–20.
13. Greffe BS, Marlar RA, Manco Johnson M. Neonatal protein C: molecular composition and distribution in normal term infants. *Thromb Res* 1989; **56**: 91–8.
14. Greffe BS, Manco Johnson MJ, Marlar RA. Molecular forms of human protein C: comparison and distribution in human adult plasma. *Thromb Haemost* 1989; **62**: 902–5.
15. Schwarz HP, Muntean W, Watzke H, Richter B, Griffin JH. Low total protein S antigen but high protein S activity due to decreased C4b-binding protein in neonates. *Blood* 1988; **71**: 562–5.
16. Moalic P, Gruel Y, Body G, Foloppe P, Dalahousse B, Leroy J. Levels and plasma distribution of free and C4b-bound protein S in human fetuses and full term newborns. *Thromb Res* 1988; **49**: 471–80.
17. Warr TA, Warn-Crammer BJ, Rao LVM, Rapaport SL. Human plasma extrinsic pathway inhibitor activity: standardisation of assay and evaluation of physiological variables. *Blood* 1989; **74**: 201–6.
18. Weissbach G, Harenberg J, Wendisch J, Pargac N, Thomas K. Tissue factor pathway inhibitor in infants and children. *Thromb Res* 1994; **73**: 441–6.
19. Tay SP, Cheong SK, Boo NY. Circulating TF, TFPI and D-dimer in umbilical cord blood of normal term neonates and adult plasma. *Blood Coagul Fibrinolysis* 2003; **14**: 125–9.
20. Andrew M, Schmidt B, Mitchell L, Paes B, Ofosu F. Thrombin generation in newborn plasma is critically dependent on the concentration of prothrombin. *Thromb Haemost* 1990; **63**: 27–30.
21. Patel, P, Weitz J, Brooker LA, Paes B, Mitchell L, Andrew M. Decreased thrombin activity of fibrin clots prepared in cord plasma compared with adult plasma. *Pediatr Res* 1996; **39**: 826–30.
22. Butenus S, Van't Veer C, Mann KG. "Normal" thrombin generation. *Blood* 1999; **94**: 2169–78.
23. Cvirn G, Gallistl S, Leschnik B, Muntean W. Low tissue factor pathway inhibitor (TFPI) together with low antithrombin allows sufficient thrombin generation in neonates. *J Thromb Haemost* 2003; **1**: 263–8.
24. Kettner SC, Pollack A, Zimpfer M *et al.* Heparinase-modified thromboelastography in term and preterm neonates. *Anesth Analg* 2004; **98**: 1650–2.
25. Andrew M. Developmental hemostasis: relevance to

hemostatic problems during childhood. *Semin Thromb Hemostas* 1995; **21**: 341–56.

26. Schmidt B, Mitchell L, Ofosu FA, Andrew M. Alpha-2-macroglobulin is an important progressive inhibitor of thrombin in neonatal and infant plasma. *Thromb Haemost* 1989; **62**: 1074–7

27. Andrew M, Mitchell L, Berry L *et al.* An anticoagulant dermatan sulfate proteoglycan circulates in the pregnant woman and her fetus. *J Clin Invest* 1992; **89**: 321–6.

28. Liu L, Dewar L, Song Y *et al.* Inhibition of thrombin by antithrombin III and heparin cofactor II *in vivo*. *Thromb Haemost* 1995; **73**: 405–12.

29. Ling X, Delorme M, Berry L *et al.* Alpha 2-macroglobulin remains as important as antithrombin III for thrombin regulation in cord plasma in the presence of endothelial cell surfaces. *Pediatr Res* 1995; **37**: 373–8.

30. Dati F, Pelzer H, Wagner C. Relevance of markers of hemostasis activation in obstetrics/gynecology and pediatrics. *Semin Thromb Hemost* 1998; **24**: 443–8.

31. Corrigan J. Neonatal thrombosis and the thrombolytic system. Pathophysiology and therapy. *Am J Pediatr Hematol Oncol* 1988; **10**: 83–91.

32. Corrigan JJ, Sluth JJ, Jetter M *et al.* Newborns' fibrinolytic mechanism: components and plasmin generation. *Am J Hematol* 1989; **32**: 273–8.

33. Summaria L. Comparison of human normal, full-term, fetal and adult plasminogen by physical and chemical analyses. *Haemostasis* 1989; **19**: 266–73.

34. Edelberg JM, Enghild JJ, Pizzo SV, Gonzalez-Gronow M. Neonatal plasminogen displays altered cell surface binding and activation kinetics: correlation with increased glycosylation of the protein. *Clin Invest* 1990; **86**: 107–12.

35. Suaraz CR, Walenga J, Mangogna LC, Fareed J. Neonatal and maternal fibrinolysis: activation at time of birth. *Am J Hematol* 1985; **19**: 365–72.

36. Kolindewala JK, Das BK, Dube E *et al.* Blood fibrinolytic activity in neonates: effect of period of gestation, birth weight, anoxia and sepsis. *Indian Pediatr* 1987; **24**: 1029–33.

37. Runnebaum IB, Maurer SM, Daly L *et al.* Inhibitors and activators of fibrinolysis during and after childbirth in maternal and cord blood. *J Pediatr Med* 1989; **17**: 113–19.

38. Pinacho A, Paramo JA, Ezcurdia M, Rocha E. Evaluation of the fibrinolytic system in full term neonates. *Int J Clin Lab Res* 1995; **25**: 149–52.

39. Andrew M, Brooker L, Leaker M, Paes B, Weitz J. Fibrin clot lysis by thrombolytic agents is impaired in newborns due to a low plasminogen concentration. *Thromb Haemost* 1992; **68**: 325–30.

40. Reis M, Zenker M, Klinge J, Keuper H, Harms D. Age related differences in a clot lysis assay after adding different plasminogen activators in a plasma milieu *in vitro*. *Am J Pediatr Hematol Oncol* 1995; **17**: 260–4.

41. Ries M, Klinge J, Rauch R, Keuper H, Harms D. The role of alpha 2-antiplasmin in the inhibition of clot lysis in newborns and adults. *Biol Neonate* 1996; **69**: 298–306.

42. Forestier F, Daffos F, Galacteros F Bardakjian J, Rainaut M, Beuzard Y. Haematological values of 163 normal fetuses between 18 and 30 weeks gestation. *Pediatr Res* 1986; **20**: 342–6.

43. Forestier F, Daffos F, Catherine N, Renard M, Andreux JP. Developmental hematopoiesis in the normal human fetal blood. *Blood* 1991; **77**: 2360–3.

44. Hohlfeld P, Forestier F, Kaplan C, Tissot JD, Daffos F. Fetal thrombocytopenia: a retrospective survey of 5,194 fetal blood samplings. *Blood* 1994; **84**: 1851–6.

45. Pahal GS, Jauniaux E, Kinnon C, Thrasher AJ, Rodeck CH. Normal development of human fetal haemopoiesis between eight and seventeen weeks gestation. *Am J Obstet Gynecol* 2000; **183**: 1029–34.

46. Kipper SL, Sieger L. Whole blood platelet volumes in newborn infants. *J Pediatr* 1982; **101**: 763–6.

47. Arad ID, Alpan G, Sznajderman SD, Eldor A. The mean platelet volume (MPV) in the neonatal period. *Am J Perinatol* 1986; **3**: 1–3.

48. Patrick CH, Lazarchick J, Stubbs T, Pittard WB. Mean platelet volume and platelet distribution width in the neonate. *Am J Pediatr Hematol Oncol* 1987; **9**: 130–2.

49. Sola MC, Juul SE, Meng YG *et al.* Thrombopoietin (Tpo) in the fetus and neonate: Tpo concentrations in preterm and term neonates, and organ distribution of Tpo and its receptor (c-mpl) during human fetal development. *Early Hum Dev* 1999; **53**: 239–50.

50. Murray NA, Watts TL, Roberts IA. Thrombopoietin in the fetus and neonate. *Early Hum Dev* 2000; **59**: 1–12.

51. Murray NA, Watts TL, Roberts IA. Endogenous thrombopoietin levels and effect of recombinant thrombopoietin on megakaryocyte precursors in term and preterm babies. *Pediatr Res* 1998; **43**: 148–51.

52. Murray NA, Roberts IA. Circulating megakaryocytes and their progenitors (BFU-MK and CFU-MK) in term and preterm neonates. *Br J Haematol* 1995; **89**: 41–6.

53. Michelson AD. Platelet function in the newborn. *Semin Thromb Hemost* 1998; **24**: 507–12.

54. Israels SJ. Platelet function in term and preterm neonates. *Semin Thromb Hemost* 2003; **29**: 363–72.

55. Saxonhouse MA. Platelet function in term and preterm neonates: correlation with bleeding risk. *Clin Perinatol* 2004; **31**: 15–28.

56. Andrew M, Paes B, Brwker J, Vegh P. Evaluation of an automated bleeding time device in the newborn. *Am J Hematol* 1990; **35**: 275–7.

57. Sola MC. The relationship between hematocrit and bleeding time in very low birth weight infants during the first week of life. *J Perinatol* 2001; **21**: 368–71.

58. Del Vechio A, Sola MC. Performing and interpreting the bleeding time in the neonatal intensive care unit. *Clin Perinatol* 2000; **27**: 643–54.

59. Israels SJ. Evaluation of primary haemostasis in neonates with a new in vitro platelet function analyser. *J Paediatr* 2001; **138**: 116–19.

60. Boudewijns M, Raes M, Peeters V *et al.* Evaluation of platelet function on cord blood in 80 healthy term neonates using the Platelet Function Analyser (PFA-100); shorter in vitro bleeding times in neonates than adults. *Eur J Paediatr* 2003; **162**: 212–13.

61. Roschitz B, Sudi K, Kostenberger M, Muntean W. Shorter PFA-100 closure times in neonates than in adults: role of red cells, white cells, platelets and von Willebrand factor. *Acta Paediatr* 2002; **90**: 664–70.

62. Rajasekhar D, Kestin A, Bednarek F, Ellis P, Barnard M, Michelson A. Neonatal platelets are less reactive than adult

665

platelets to physiological agonists in whole blood. *Thromb Haemost* 1994; **72**: 957–63.

63. Rajasekhar D, Barnard MR, Bednarek FJ, Michelson AD. Platelet hyporeactivity in very low birth weight neonates. *Thromb Haemost* 1997; **77**: 1002–7.

64. Gatti L, Guarneri D, Caccamo ML, Gianotti GA, Marini A. Platelet activation in the newborn detected by flow cytometry. *Biol Neonate* 1996; **70**: 322–7.

65. Hezard N. Unexpected persistence of platelet hyporeactivity beyond the neonatal period: a flow cytometric study in neonates, infants and older children. *Thromb Haemost* 2003; **90**: 116–23.

66. Mannucci PM, Tuddenham EG. The hemophilias: from royal genes to gene therapy. *N Engl J Med* 2001; **344**: 1773–9.

67. Rosendaal FR, Briet E. The increasing prevalence of haemophilia. *Thromb Haemost* 1990; **63**: 145.

68. White GC, Rosendaal F, Aledort LM, Lusher JM, Rothchild C, Ingeslev J. Definitions in haemophilia. Recommendations of the Scientific Subcommittee of FVIII and FIX of the SSC of ISTH. *Thromb Haemost* 2001; **85**: 560.

69. Preston FE, Kitchen S, Jennings I, Woods TAL, Makris M. SSC/ISTH classification of haemophilia: can haemophilia centre laboratories achieve the new criteria. *J Thromb Haemost* 2004; **2**: 271–4.

70. Smith PS. Congenital coagulation protein deficiencies in the perinatal period. *Semin Perinatol* 1990; **14**: 384–92.

71. Baehner RL, Strauss HS. Hemophilia in the first year of life. *N Engl J Med* 1966; **275**: 524–8.

72. Ljung R, Lindgren AC, Petrini P, Tengborn L. Normal vaginal delivery is to be recommended for haemophilia carrier gravidae. *Acta Paediatr* 1994; **83**: 609–11.

73. Conway JH, Hilgarter MW. Initial presentations of pediatric hemophiliacs. *Arch Pediatr Adolesc Med* 1994; **148**: 589–94.

74. Chambost H, Gaboulaud V, Coatmelec B, Rafowicz A, Schneider P, Calvez T. What factors influence the age at diagnosis of hemophilia? Results of a French cohort study. *J Pediatr* 2002; **141**: 548–52.

75. Ljung R, Petrini P, Nilsson IM. Diagnostic symptoms of severe and moderate haemophilia A and B. *Acta Paediatr Scand* 1990; **79**: 196–200.

76. Kulkarni R, Lusher J. Perinatal management of neonates with haemophilia. *Br J Haematol* 2001; **112**: 264–74.

77. Jannoccone G, Pasquino AM. Calcifying splenic hematoma in a hemophilia newborn. *Pediatr Radiol* 1981; **10**: 183–5.

78. Reish O, Nachum E, Naor N, Ghoshen J, Merlob P. Hemophilia B in a neonate: unusual early spontaneous gastrointestinal bleeding. *Am J Perinatol* 1994; **11**: 192–3.

79. Kulkarni R, Lusher JM. Intracranial and extracranial hemorrhages in newborns with hemophilia. *J Pediatr Hematol Oncol* 1999; **21**: 289–95.

80. Yoffe G, Buchanan GR. Intracranial haemorrhage in newborn and young infants with hemophilia. *J Pediatr* 1988; **113**: 333–6.

81. Plauche WC. Subgaleal hematoma. A complication of instrumental delivery. *JAMA* 1980; **244**: 1597–8.

82. Amar AP, Aryan HE, Meltzer HS, Levy ML. Neonatal subgaleal hematoma causing brain compression: report of two cases and review of the literature. *Neurosurgery* 2003; **52**: 1470–4; discussion 1474.

83. Klinge J, Auberger K, Auerswald G, Brackmann HH, Mauz-Korholz C, Kreuz W. Prevalence and outcome of intracranial haemorrhage in haemophiliacs: a survey of the paediatric group of the German Society for Thrombosis and Haemostasis (GTH). *Eur J Pediatr* 1999; **158**: S162–5.

84. Walker ID, Walker JJ, Colvin BT, Letsky EA, Rivers R, Stevens R, on behalf of the Haemostasis and Thrombosis Task Force. Investigation and management of haemorrhagic disorders in pregnancy. *J Clin Pathol* 1994; **47**: 100–8.

85. Kulkarni R, Lusher JM, Henry RC, Kallens DJ. Current practices regarding new-born intracranial haemorrhage and obstetrical care and mode of delivery of pregnant haemophilia carriers: a survey of obstetricians, neonatologists and haematologists in the United States, on behalf of the National Hemophilia Foundation's Medical and Scientific Advisory Council. *Haemophilia* 1999; **5**: 410–15.

86. Williams MD, Chalmers EA, Gibson BES. Guideline: the investigation and management of neonatal haemostasis and thrombosis. *Br J Haematol* 2002; **119**: 295–309.

87. MacLean PE. Impact of unaware carriership on the clinical presentation of haemophilia. *Haemophilia* 2004; **10**: 560–4.

88. Myles LM, Massicotte P, Drake J. Intracranial hemorrhage in neonates with unrecognised hemophilia A: a persisting problem. *Pediatr Neurosurg* 2001; **34**: 94–7.

89. Schmidt B, Zipursky A. Disseminated intravascular coagulation masking neonatal hemophilia. *J Pediatr* 1986; **109**: 886–8.

90. UKHCDO. Guideline for the selection and use of therapeutic products to treat haemophilia and other hereditary bleeding disorders. *Haemophilia* 2003; **9**: 1–23.

91. Gale RF, Hird MF, Colvin BT. Management of a premature infant with moderate haemophilia A using recombinant factor VIII. *Haemophilia* 1998; **4**: 850–3.

92. Buchanan GR. Factor concentrate prophylaxis for neonates with hemophilia. *J Paediatr Hematol Oncol* 1999; **21**: 254–5.

93. Tarantino MD, Larson A, DiMichelle D. Management strategy for newborns born to haemophilia carriers: a survey of haemophilia treatment centre physicians. *Haemophilia* 2002; **8**: 536.

94. Chalmers EA, Williams MD, Richards M *et al.* Management of neonates with inherited bleeding disorders: a survey of current UK practice. *Haemophilia* 2005; **11**: 186–7.

95. Rodeghiero F, Castaman G, Dini E. Epidemiological investigations of the prevalence of von Willebrand's disease. *Blood* 1987; **69**: 454–7.

96. Werner EJ, Emmett H, Tucker E, Giroux D, Schults J, Abshire T. Prevalence of von Willebrand's disease in children: a multiethnic study. *J Pediatr* 1993; **123**: 893–8.

97. Gazengel C, Fischer A, Schlegel N *et al.* Treatment of type 3 von Willebrand's disease with solvent/detergent treated factor VIII concentrates. *Nouv Rev Fr Hematol* 1988; **30**: 225–7.

98. Donner M, Kristoffersson AC, Lenk H *et al.* Type IIB von Willebrand's disease: gene mutations and clinical presentation in nine families from Denmark, Germany and Sweden. *Br J Haematol* 1992; **82**: 58–65.

99. Zeitler P, von Stockhausen HB. Type IIB von Willebrand Jurgens syndrome as the cause of neonatal thrombocytopenia. *Klin Padiatrie* 1998; **210**: 85–8.

100. Pasi KJ, Collins PW, Keeling DM *et al.* Management of von Willebrand disease: a guideline from the UK Haemophilia

Centre Doctors' Organization. *Haemophilia* 2004; **10**: 218–31.

101. Fischer BE, Schlokat U, Mitterer A *et al.* Structural analysis of recombinant von Willebrand factor produced at industrial scale fermentation of transformed CHO cells co-expressing recombinant firm. *FEBS Lett* 1995; **375**: 259–62.

102. Peyvandi F, Mannucci PM. Rare coagulation disorders. *Thromb Haemost* 1999; **82**: 1207–14.

103. Peyvandi F, Duga S, Akhavan S, Mannucci PM. Rare coagulation deficiencies. *Haemophilia* 2002; **8**: 308–21.

104. Acharya SS, Coughlin A, DiMichelle DM and the North American Rare Bleeding Disorder Study Group. Rare bleeding disorder registry: deficiencies of factors II, V, VII, X, XIII, fibrinogen and dysfibrinogenemias. *J Thromb Haemost* 2004; **2**: 248–56.

105. Mannucci PM, Duga S, Peyvandi F. Recessively inherited coagulation disorders. *Blood* 2004; **104**: 1243–52.

106. Mammen EF. Fibrinogen abnormalities. *Semin Thromb Hemost* 1983; **9**: 1–9.

107. Fried K, Kaufman S. Congenital afibrinogenemia in 10 offspring of uncle–niece marriages. *Clin Genet* 1980; **17**: 223–7.

108. Lak M, Keihani M, Elahi F, Peyvandi F, Mannucci PM. Bleeding and thrombosis in 55 patients with inherited afibrinogenaemia. *Br J Haematol* 1999; **107**: 204–6.

109. Mackie IJ, Kitchen S, Machin SJ, Lowe GD. Guidelines on fibrinogen assays. *Br J Haematol* 2003; **121**: 396–404.

110. Bolton-Maggs PHB, Perry DJ, Chalmers EA *et al.* The rare coagulation disorders: review with guidelines for management. *Haemophilia* 2004; **10**: 1–36.

111. Ragni MV, Lewis JH, Spero JA, Hasiba U. Factor VII deficiency. *Am J Hematol* 1981; **10**: 79–88.

112. Mariani G, Mazzucconi MG. Factor VII congenital deficiency. Clinical picture and classification of the variants. *Haemostasis* 1983; **13**: 169–77.

113. Wong WY, Huang WC, Miller R, McGinty K, Whisnant JK. Clinical efficacy and recovery levels of recombinant FVIIa in the treatment of intracranial haemorrhage in severe neonatal FVII deficiency. *Haemophilia* 2000; **6**: 50–4.

114. Lorand L, Losowsky MS, Miloszewski KJM. Human factor XIII: Fibrin stabilizing factor. *Prog Haemost Thromb* 1980; **5**: 245–90.

115. Abbondanzo SL, Gootenberg JE, Lofts RS, McPherson RA. Intracranial hemorrhage in congenital deficiency of factor FXIII. *Am J Pediatr Hematol Oncol* 1988; **10**: 65–8.

116. Merchant RH, Agarwal BR, Currimbhoy Z, Pherwani A, Avasthi B. Congenital factor XIII deficiency. *Ind Pediatr* 1992; **29**: 831–6.

117. Brackmann HH, Egbring R, Ferster A *et al.* Pharmacokinetics and tolerability of Factor XIII concentrates prepared from human placenta or plasma: a cross over randomised study. *Thromb Haemost* 1995; **74**: 622–5.

118. Brenner B, Sanchez-Vega B, Wu SM, Lanir N, Stafford DW, Solera J. A missense mutation in the gamma-glutamyl carboxylase gene causes combined deficiency of all vitamin K dependent blood coagulation factors. *Blood* 1998; **92**: 4554–9.

119. Oldenburg J, von Brederlow B, Fregin A. Congenital deficiency of vitamin K dependent coagulation factors in two families presents as a genetic defect of the vitamin K epoxide reductase complex. *Thromb Haemost* 2000; **84**: 937–41.

120. Brenner B, Tavori S, Zivelin A *et al.* Hereditary deficiency of

121. Ghosh K, Shetty S, Mohanty D. Inherited deficiency of multiple vitamin K dependent coagulation factors and coagulation inhibitors presenting as haemorrhagic diathesis, mental retardation and growth retardation *Am J Hematol* 1996; **52**: 67.

122. Suzuki S. Hypercoagulability and DIC in high risk infants. *Semin Thromb Hemost* 1998; **24**: 463–6.

123. Bick RL. Disseminated intravascular coagulation: a review of aetiology, pathophysiology, diagnosis and management: guidelines for care. *Clin Appl Thromb Haemost* 2002; **8**: 1–31.

124. Schmidt B, Vegh P, Johnston M, Andrew M, Weitz J. Do coagulation screening tests detect increased generation of thrombin and plasmin in sick newborn infants? *Thromb Haemost* 1993; **69**: 418–21.

125. Taylor FB, Toh CH, Hoots W, Wada H, Levi M. Towards definition, clinical and laboratory criteria and a scoring system for disseminated intravascular coagulation. *Thromb Haemost* 2001; **86**: 1327–30.

126. Schmidt BK, Vegh P, Andrew M, Johnston M. Coagulation screening tests in high risk neonates: a prospective cohort study. *Arch Dis Child* 1992; **67**: 1196–7.

127. Francis CW, Marder VJ. A molecular model of plasmin degradation of cross linked fibrin. *Semin Thromb Hemost* 1982; **8**: 25–35.

128. Hudson IRB, Gibson BES, Brownlie J, Holland BM, Turner TL, Webber RW. Increased concentrations of D-Dimers in newborn infants. *Arch Dis Child* 1990; **65**: 383–9.

129. El Beshlawy A, Hussein HA, Abou-Elew HH, Abdel Kader MS. Study of protein C, S and antithrombin in hypoxic newborns. *Pediatr Crit Care Med* 2004; **5**: 163–6.

130. Aronis S. Indications of coagulation and/or fibrinolytic system activation in healthy and sick very low birth weight infants. *Biol Neonate* 1998; **74**: 337–44.

131. Bernard GR, Vincent JL, Laterre PF. Efficacy and safety of recombinant human protein C for severe sepsis. *N Engl J Med* 2001; **344**: 699–709.

132. Rawiocz M, Sitkowska B, Rudzinska I, Kornacka MK, Bochenski P. Recombinant human activated protein C for severe sepsis in a neonate. *Med Sci Monitor* 2002; **8**: CS90–94.

133. Barton P. Safety, pharmacokinetics and pharmacodynamics of drotrecogin alpha (activated) in children with severe sepsis. *Pediatrics* 2004; **113**: 7–17.

134. BCSH. Guidelines for the use of platelet transfusions. *Br J Haematol* 2003; **122**: 10–23.

135. Hambleton G, Appleyard W. Controlled trial of fresh frozen plasma in asphyxiated low birth-weight infants. *Arch Dis Child* 1973; **48**: 31–5.

136. Turner T, Prowse CV, Prescott RJ, Cash JD. A clinical trial on the early detection and correction of haemostatic defects in selected high-risk neonates. *Br J Haematol* 1981; **47**: 65–75.

137. Turner T. Randomized sequential control trial to evaluate effect of purified factor II, VII, IX and X concentrate, cryoprecipitate and platelet concentrate in the management of preterm low birth weight and mature asphyxiated infants with coagulation defects. *Arch Dis Child* 1981; **51**: 810–15.

138. Gross SJ, Filston HC, Anderson JC. Controlled study of treatment for disseminated intravascular coagulation in the neonate. *J Pediatr* 1982; **100**: 445–8.

139. Hyytiainen S. Fresh frozen plasma reduces thrombin formation in newborn infants. *J Thromb Haemost* 2003; **1**: 1189–94.

140. Hauptmann JG, Hassouna HI, Bell TG, Penner JA, Emerson TE. Efficacy of antithrombin III in endotoxin-induced disseminated intravascular coagulation. *Circ Shock* 1988; **25**: 111–22.

141. Du Toit HJ, Coetzee AR, Chalton DO. Heparin treatment in thrombin induced disseminated intravascular coagulation in the baboon. *Crit Care Med* 1991; **19**: 1195–200.

142. Gobel U, von Voss H, Jurgens H *et al.* Efficiency of heparin in the treatment of newborn infants with respiratory distress syndrome and disseminated intravascular coagulation. *Eur J Pediatr* 1980; **133**: 47–9.

143. von Kries R, Stannigel H, Gobel U. Anticoagulant therapy by continuous heparin antithrombin III infusion in newborns with disseminated intravascular coagulation. *Eur J Pediatr* 1985; **144**: 191–4.

144. Towsend CW. The hemorrhagic disease of the newborn. *Arch Pediatr* 1894; **11**: 559–65.

145. Sutor AH, von Kries R, Cornelissen EAM, McNinch AW, Andrew M. Vitamin K deficiency bleeding in infancy. *Thromb Haemost* 1999; **81**: 456–61.

146. Aballi AJ, Lamerens S. Coagulation changes in the neonatal period and in early infancy. *Pediatr Clin North Am* 1962; **9**: 785–817.

147. Shearer MJ, Crampton OE, McCarthy PT, Mattock MB. Vitamin K1 in plasma: relationship to vitamin K status, age, pregnancy, diet and disease. *Haemostasis* 1986; **16** (suppl. 5): 83.

148. Israels LG, Israels ED. Observations on vitamin K deficiency in the fetus and newborn: has nature made a mistake? *Semin Thromb Hemost* 1995; **21**: 357–63.

149. Food and Nutrition Board, Commission on Life Sciences, National Research Council. *Recommended Dietary Allowances*, 10th edn. Washington: National Academy Press, 1988, p. 111.

150. Greer FR, Marshall S, Cherry J *et al.* Vitamin K status of lactating mothers, human milk and breast feeding infants. *Pediatrics* 1991; **88**: 751–6.

151. Widdershoven J, Lambert W, Motohara K *et al.* Plasma concentrations of vitamin K1 and PIVKA-II in bottle fed and breast fed infants with and without vitamin K prophylaxis. *Eur J Pediatr* 1988; **148**: 139–42.

152. Sutor AH. Vitamin K deficiency bleeding in infants and children. *Semin Thromb Hemost* 1995; **21**: 317–29.

153. Greer FR. Vitamin K deficiency and hemorrhage in infancy. *Clin Perinatol* 1995; **22**: 759–77.

154. Astedt B. Antenatal drugs affecting vitamin K status of the fetus and newborn. *Semin Thromb Hemost* 1995; **21**: 364–70.

155. Ginsberg JS, Hirsh J, Turner DCH, Levine MN, Burrows R. Risks to the fetus of anticoagulant therapy during pregnancy. *Thromb Haemost* 1989; **61**: 197–203.

156. Bates SM, Greer IA, Hirsh J, Ginsberg JS. Use of antithrombotic agents during pregnancy: the Seventh ACCP Conference on Antithrombotic and Thrombolytic Therapy. *Chest* 2004; **126**: 627S–644S.

157. Cornelissen M, Steegers-Theunissen R, Kollee L *et al.* Increased incidence of neonatal vitamin K deficiency resulting from maternal anticonvulsant therapy. *Am J Obstet Gynecol* 1993; **168**: 923–7.

158. American Academy of Pediatrics: Committee on Nutrition. Vitamin K compounds and water soluble analogs: use in

159. Sutherland JM, Glueck HI, Gleser G. Hemorrhagic disease of the newborn. *Am J Dis Child* 1967; **113**: 524–33.

160. Keenan WJ, Jewett T, Glueck H. Role of feeding and vitamin K in hypoprothrombinemia of the newborn. *Am J Dis Child* 1971; **121**: 271–7.

161. von Kries R, Shearer MJ, Goebel U. Vitamin K in infancy. *Eur J Pediatr* 1988; **147**: 106–12.

162. Croucher C, Azzopardi D. Compliance with recommendations for giving vitamin K to newborn infants. *Br Med J* 1994; **308**: 894–5.

163. Chan MCK, Boon WH. Late haemorrhagic disease of Singapore infants. *J Singapore Paediatr Soc* 1967; **9**: 72–81.

164. Lovric VA, Jones RF. The haemorrhagic syndrome of early childhood. *Aust Ann Med* 1967; **16**: 173–5.

165. Sutor AH, Dagres N, Neiderhoff H. Late form of vitamin K deficiency bleeding in Germany. *Klin Paediatr* 1995; **207**: 89–97.

166. von Kries R, Reifenhauser A, Gobel U, McCarthy P, Shearer MJ, Barkhan P. Late onset haemorrhagic disease of the newborn with temporary malabsorption of vitamin K1. *Lancet* 1985; i: 1035.

167. Matsuda L, Nishiyama S, Motohara K, Endo F, Ogata T, Futagoishi Y. Late neonatal vitamin K deficiency associated with subclinical liver dysfunction in human milk fed infants. *J Pediatr* 1989; **114**: 602–5.

168. von Kries R, Hanawa Y. Neonatal vitamin K prophylaxis: Report of the Scientific and Standardization Subcommittee on Perinatal Haemostasis. *Thromb Haemost* 1993, **69**: 293–5.

169. Danielsson N, Hoa DP, Thang NV, Vos T, Loughnan PM. Intracranial haemorrhage due to late onset vitamin K deficiency bleeding in Hanoi province, Vietnam. *Arch Dis Child* 2004; **89**: F546–F550.

170. Delgado-Escueta AV, Janz D. Consensus guidelines: preconception counselling, management, and care of the pregnant woman with epilepsy. *Neurology* 1992; **42** (suppl. 5): 149–60.

171. Cornelissen M, Steegers-Theunissen R, Kollee L *et al.* Supplementation of vitamin K in pregnant women receiving anticonvulsant therapy prevents neonatal vitamin K deficiency. *Am J Obstet Gynecol* 1993; **168**: 884–8.

172. Hey E. Effect of maternal anticonvulsant treatment on neonatal blood coagulation. *Arch Dis Child* 1999; **81**: F208–F210.

173. Choulika S, Grabowski E, Holmes LB. Is antenatal vitamin K prophylaxis needed for pregnant women taking anticonvulsants? *Am J Obstet Gynecol* 2004; **190**: 882–3.

174. Ekelund H. Late haemorrhagic disease in Sweden 1987–89. *Acta Paediatr Scand* 1991; **80**: 966–8.

175. McNinch AW, Tripp JH. Haemorrhagic disease of the newborn in the British Isles: two year prospective study. *Br Med J* 1991; **303**: 1105–9.

176. Golding J, Greenwood R, Birmingham K, Mott M. Childhood cancer, intramuscular vitamin K and pethidine given during labour. *Br Med J* 1992; **305**: 341–6.

177. Ekelund H, Finnstrom O, Gunnarskog J, Kallen B, Larsson Y. Administration of vitamin K to newborn infants and childhood cancer. *Br Med J* 1993; **301**: 89–91.

178. Klebanoff MA, Read JS, Mills JH, Shiono PH. The risk of

therapy and prophylaxis in pediatrics. *Pediatrics* 1961; **28**: 501–7.

childhood cancer after neonatal exposure to vitamin K. *N Engl J Med* 1993; **329**: 905–8.

179. Olsen JH, Hertz H, Blinkenberg K, Verder H. Vitamin K regimens and incidence of childhood cancer in Denmark. *Br Med J* 1994; **308**: 895–6.

180. Ansell P, Bull D, Roman E. Childhood leukaemia and intramuscular vitamin K: findings from a case-control study. *Br Med J* 1996; **313**: 204–5.

181. von Kries R, Gobel U, Hachmeister A, Kaletsch U, Michaelis J. Vitamin K and childhood cancer: a population based case-control study in Lower Saxony, Germany. *Br Med J* 1996; **313**: 199–203.

182. Vitamin K prophylaxis in infancy. Report of an expert committee. London: British Paediatric Association, 1992.

183. Merenstein K, Hathaway WE, Miller RW, Paulson JA, Rowley DL. Controversies concerning vitamin K and the newborn. *Pediatrics* 1993; **91**: 1001–2.

184. Sutor AH. New aspects of vitamin K prophylaxis. *Semin Thromb Hemost* 2003; **29**: 373–6.

185. Cornelissen M, von Kries R, Loughnan P, Schubiger G. Prevention of vitamin K deficiency bleeding: efficacy of different multiple oral dose schedules of vitamin K. *Eur J Paediatr* 1997; **156**: 126–30.

186. Hansen KN, Minousis M, Ebbesen F. Weekly oral vitamin K prophylaxis in Denmark. *Acta Paediatr* 2003; **92**: 802–5.

187. Hall R, Bull MP. *Vitamin K for All Babies*. London: Department of Health, 1998 (CMO (98)11/CNO (98) 7).

188. Von Kries R, Hachmeister A, Gobel U. Oral mixed micellar vitamin for the prevention of late vitamin K deficiency bleeding. *Arch Dis Child* 2003; **88**: F109–F112.

189. Sutor AH, Kunzer W. Time interval between vitamin K administration and effective hemostasis. In: Suzuki S, Hathaway WE, Bonnar J, Sutor AH (eds) *Perinatal Thrombosis and Haemostasis*. Berlin: Springer, 1991, pp. 257–62.

190. Shneider BL. Neonatal liver failure. *Curr Opin Pediatr* 1996; **8**: 495–501.

191. Blanchard RA, Furie BC, Jorgensen M *et al.* Acquired vitamin K dependent carboxylation deficiency in liver disease. *N Engl J Med* 1981; **305**: 242–8.

192. Joist JH. Hemostatic abnormalities in liver disease. In: Coleman RW, Hirsh J (eds) *Hemostasis and Thrombosis*. Philadelphia: JB Lippincott, 1982, pp. 861–72.

193. Kelly D, Summerfield J. Hemostasis in liver disease. *Semin Liver Dis* 1987; **7**: 182–91.

194. Mammen EF. Coagulation defects in liver disease. *Med Clin North Am* 1994; **78**: 545–54.

195. Bick RL. Hemostasis defects associated with cardiac surgery, prosthetic devices, and other extracorporeal circuits. *Semin Thromb Hemost* 1985; **11**: 249–80.

196. Woodman RC, Harker LA. Bleeding complications associated with cardiopulmonary bypass. *Blood* 1990; **76**: 1680–97.

197. Johnson CA, Abildgaard CF, Schulman I. Absence of coagulation abnormalities in children with cyanotic congenital heart disease. *Lancet* 1968; **ii**: 660–2.

198. Inenacho HNC, Breeze GR, Fletcher DJ, Stuart J. Consumption coagulopathy in congenital heart disease. *Lancet* 1973; **i**: 231–4.

199. Gill JC, Wilson AD, Endres-Brooks J, Montgomery RR. Loss of the largest von Willebrand factor multimers from the plasma of patients with congenital cardiac defects. *Blood* 1986; **67**: 758–61.

200. Chan AKC, Leaker M, Burrows FA *et al.* Coagulation and fibrinolytic profile of paediatric patients undergoing cardiopulmonary bypass. *Thromb Haemost* 1997; **77**: 270–7.

201. Kern FH, Morana NJ, Sears JJ, Hickey PR. Coagulation defects in neonates during cardiopulmonary bypass. *Ann Thorac Surg* 1992; **54**: 541–6.

202. Turner-Gomes SO, Mitchell L, Williams WG, Andrew M. Thrombin regulation in congenital heart disease after cardiopulmonary bypass operations. *J Thorac Cardiovasc Surg* 1994; **107**: 562–8.

203. Saatvedt K, Lindberg H, Michelsen S, Pedersen T, Geiran OR. Activation of the fibrinolytic, coagulation and plasma kallikrein-kinin systems during and after open heart surgery in children. *Scand J Clin Lab Invest* 1995; **55**: 359–67.

204. Boisclair MD, Lane DA, Philippou H *et al.* Mechanisms of thrombin generation during surgery and cardiopulmonary bypass. *Blood* 1993; **82**: 3350–7.

205. Petaja J, Peltola K, Sairanen H *et al.* Fibrinolysis, antithrombin III, and protein C in neonates during cardiac operations. *J Thorac Cardiovasc Surg* 1996; **112**: 665–71.

206. Gruenwald CE, Andrew M, Burrows FA, Williams WG. Cardiopulmonary bypass in the neonate. *Adv Card Surg* 1993; **4**: 137–56.

207. Turner-Gomes S, Nitschmann E, Andrew M, Williams WG. Additional heparin affects thrombin generation during cardiopulmonary bypass. *Thromb Haemost* 1993; **69**: 1167.

208. Andrew M, MacIntyre B, MacMillan J *et al.* Heparin therapy during cardiopulmonary bypass in children requires ongoing quality control. *Thromb Haemost* 1993; **70**: 937–41.

209. Gu YJ, Huyzen RJ, van-Oeveren W. Intrinsic pathway-dependent activated clotting time is not reliable for monitoring anticoagulation during cardiopulmonary bypass in neonates. *J Thorac Cardiovasc Surg* 1996; **111**: 677–8.

210. Kestin AS, Valeri R, Khuri SF *et al.* The platelet function defect of cardiopulmonary bypass. *Blood* 1993; **82**: 107–17.

211. Frost J, Mureebe L, Russo P, Russo J, Tobias JD. Heparin-induced thrombocytopenia in the pediatric intensive care unit population. *Pediatr Crit Care Med* 2005; **6**: 216–19.

212. Alsoufi B. Heparin induced thrombocytopenia in cardiac surgery: an emerging cause of morbidity and mortality. *Semin Thorac Cardiovasc Surg* 2004; **71**: 155–71.

213. Kjaergard HK, Fairbrother JE. Controlled clinical studies of fibrin sealant in cardiothoracic surgery: a review. *Eur J Cardiothorac Surg* 1996; **10**: 727–33.

214. Codispoti M, Mankad PS. Significant merits of a fibrin sealant in the presence of coagulopathy following paediatric cardiac surgery: randomised controlled trial. *Eur J Cardiothorac Surg* 2002; **22**: 200–5.

215. Penkoske PA, Entwistle LM, Marchak BE, Seal RF, Gibb W. Aprotinin in children undergoing repair of congenital heart defects. *Ann Thorac Surg* 1995; **60** (suppl.): S529–S532.

216. McDonough J, Gruenwald C. The use of aprotinin in pediatric patients: a review. *J Extracorporeal Technol* 2003; **35**: 346–9.

217. Scharrer I. Recombinant factor VIIa for patients with inhibitors to factor VIII or IX or factor VII deficiency. *Haemophilia* 1999; **5**: 253–9.

218. Veldman A, Fischer D, Voigt B *et al.* Life-threatening hemorrhage in neonates: management with recombinant activated factor VII. *Intensive Care Med* 2002; **28**: 1635–7.

219. Razon Y, Erez E, Vidne B *et al*. Recombinant factor VIIa (NovoSeven) as a hemostatic agent after surgery for congenital heart disease. *Paediatr Anaesth* 2005; **15**: 235–40.

220. Burrows RF, Kelton JG. Fetal thrombocytopenia and its relation to maternal thrombocytopenia. *N Engl J Med* 1993; **329**: 1463–6.

221. Dreyfus M, Kaplan C, Verdy E *et al*. Frequency of immune thrombocytopenia in newborns: a prospective study. Immune Thrombocytopenia Working Group. *Blood* 1997; **89**: 4402–6.

222. Sainio S, Jarvenpaa AL, Renlund M *et al*. Thrombocytopenia in term infants: a population based study. *Obstet Gynecol* 2000; **95**: 441–6.

223. Uhrynowska M, Niznikowska-Marks M, Zupanska B. Neonatal and maternal thrombocytopenia: incidence and immune background. *Eur J Haematol* 2000; **64**: 42–6.

224. Castle V, Andrew M, Kelton J, Johnston M, Carter C. Frequency and mechanism of neonatal thrombocytopenia. *J Pediatr* 1986; **108**: 749–55.

225. Aman I. The study of thrombocytopenia in sick neonates. *J Coll Physicians Surg Pak* 2004; **14**: 282–5.

226. Sola MC, Rimsza LM. Mechanisms underlying thrombocytopenia in the neonatal intensive care unit. *Acta Paediatr Suppl* 2002; **438**: 66–73.

227. Roberts IA, Murray NA. Thrombocytopenia in the newborn. *Curr Opin Pediatr* 2003; **15**: 17–23.

228. Andrew M, Castle V, Saigal S, Carter C, Kelton KG. Clinical impact of neonatal thrombocytopenia. *J Pediatr* 1987; **110**: 457–64.

229. Kahn DJ, Richardson DK, Billet HH. Association of thrombocytopenia and delivery method with IVH among very low birth weight infants. *Am J Obstet Gynecol* 2002; **186**: 109–16.

230. Kahn DJ. Inter-NICU variation in rates and management of thrombocytopenia among very low birthweight infants. *J Perinatol* 2003; **23**: 312–16.

231. Murray NA. Platelet transfusion in the management of severe thrombocytopenia in the neonatal intensive care unit. *Transfus Med* 2002; **12**: 35–41.

232. Andrew M, Vegh P, Caco C *et al*. A randomized controlled trial of platelet transfusions in thrombocytopenic premature infants. *J Pediatr* 1993; **123**: 285–91.

233. Sola MC. Evaluation and treatment of severe and prolonged thrombocytopenia in neonates. *Clin Perinatol* 2004; **31**: 1–14.

234. Sola MC, Christensen RD, Hutson AD *et al*. Pharmacokinetics, pharmacodynamics and safety of administering recombinant pegylated recombinant megakaryocyte growth and development factor to newborn rhesus monkeys. *Pediatr Res* 2000; **47**: 208–14.

235. Li J, Yang C, Xia Y *et al*. Thrombocytopenia caused by the development of antibodies to thrombopoietin. *Blood* 2001; **98**: 3241–8.

236. Mueller-Eckhart C, Kiefel V, Gribert A *et al*. 348 cases of suspected neonatal alloimmune thrombocytopenia. *Lancet* 1989; **i**: 363–6.

237. Matsui K, Ohsaki E, Goto A, Koresawa M, Kigasawa H, Shibata Y. Perinatal intracranial hemorrhage due to severe neonatal alloimmune thrombocytopenic purpura (NAITP) associated with anti-Yukb (HPA-4a) antibodies. *Brain Dev* 1995; **17**: 352–5.

238. Davoren A. Human platelet antigen-specific alloantibodies implicated in 1162 cases of neonatal alloimmune thrombocytopenia. *Transfusion* 2004; **44**: 1220–5.

239. Skacel PO, Stacey TE, Tidmarsh CEF *et al*. Maternal alloimmunization to HLA, platelet and granulocyte specific antigens during pregnancy: its influence on cord blood granulocyte and platelet counts. *Br J Haematol* 1989; **71**: 119–23.

240. Kankirawatana S, Kupatawintu P, Juji T *et al*. Neonatal alloimmune thrombocytopenia due to anti-Nak(a). *Transfusion* 2001; **41**: 375–7.

241. Julla V, Meunier M, Brement M *et al*. A new platelet polymorphism Duv(a) localised within the RGD binding domain of glycoprotein IIIa is associated with neonatal alloimmune thrombocytopenia. *Blood* 2002; **99**: 4449–56.

242. Moncharmont P, Dubois V, Obegi C *et al*. HLA antibodies and neonatal alloimmune thrombocytopenia. *Acta Haematol* 2004; **111**: 215–20.

243. Saito S, Ota M, Komatsu Y *et al*. Serologic analysis of three cases of neonatal alloimmune thrombocytopenia associated with HLA antibodies. *Transfusion* 2003; **43**: 908–17.

244. Blanchette V, Chen L, de Fridberg ZS, Hogan VA, Trudel E, Decary F. Alloimmunisation to the PLA-1 platelet antigen: results of a prospective study. *Br J Haematol* 1990; **74**: 209–15.

245. Udom-Rice I, Bussel JB. Fetal and neonatal thrombocytopenia. *Blood Rev* 1995; **9**: 57–64.

246. Valentin N, Vergracht A, Bignon JD *et al*. HLA-DRW52a is involved in alloimmunisation against PLA-1 antigen. *Hum Immunol* 1990; **27**: 73–9.

247. Shulman NR, Jordan JV. Platelet immunology. In: Coleman RW, Hirsh J, Marder VJ, Salzman EW (eds) *Hemostasis and Thrombosis*. Philadelphia: JB Lippincott, 1987, p. 477.

248. Glade-Bender J, McFarlane JG, Kaplan C *et al*. Anti-HPA-3a induces severe neonatal alloimmune thrombocytopenia. *J Pediatr* 2001; **138**: 862–7.

249. Kaplan C. Alloimmune thrombocytopenia of the fetus and the newborn. *Blood Rev* 2002; **16**: 69–72.

250. Reznikoff-Etievant MF, Kaplan C, Muller JY, Daffos F, Forestier F. Alloimmune thrombocytopenias, definition of a group at risk: a prospective study. *Curr Stud Hematol Blood Transfus* 1988; **55**: 119–24.

. Lipitz S, Ryan G, Murphy MF *et al*. Neonatal alloimmune thrombocytopenia due to anti-PLAT (Anti-HPA-1a): Importance of paternal and fetal platelet typing for assessment of fetal risk. *Prenat Diagn* 1992; **12**: 955–8.

52. Kunicki TJ, Beardsley DS. The alloimmune thrombocytopenias: neonatal alloimmune thrombocytopenic purpura and post-transfusion purpura. *Prog Hemost Thromb* 1989; **9**: 203–32.

253. Bonacossa IA, Jocelyn LJ. Alloimmune thrombocytopenia of the newborn: neurodevelopmental sequelae. *Am J Perinatol* 1996; **13**: 211–15.

254. Murphy MF, Hambley H, Nicolaides K, Waters AH. Severe fetomaternal alloimmune thrombocytopenia presenting with fetal hydrocephalus. *Prenat Diagn* 1996; **16**: 1152–5.

255. Davoren A, McParland P, Barnes CA, Murphy WG. Neonatal alloimmune thrombocytopenia in the Irish population: a discrepancy between observed and expected cases. *J Clin Pathol* 2002; **55**: 289–92.

256. Murphy MF, Verjee S, Greaves M. Inadequacies in the post natal management of fetomaternal alloimmune thrombocytopenia (FAIT). *Br J Haematol* 1999; **105**: 123–6.

257. McIntosh S, O'Brien RT, Schwartz AD, Pearson HA. Neonatal isoimmune purpura: response to platelet infusions. *J Pediatr* 1973; **82**: 1020–7.

258. Ranasinghe E, Walton JD, Hurd CM *et al.* Provision of platelet support for fetuses and neonates affected by severe fetomaternal alloimmune thrombocytopenia. *Br J Haematol* 2001; **113**: 40–2.

259. Blanchette VS, Kuhne T, Hume H, Hellmann J. Platelet transfusion therapy in newborn infants. *Transfus Med Rev* 1995; **3**: 215–30.

260. BCSH Blood Transfusion Task Force. Guidelines on gamma irradiation of blood components for the prevention of transfusion associated graft versus host disease. *Transfus Med* 1996; **6**: 261–71.

261. McGill M, Mayhaus C, Hoff R *et al.* Frozen maternal platelets for neonatal thrombocytopenia. *Transfusion* 1987; **27**: 347–9.

262. Lee K, Beaujean F, Bierling P. Treatment of severe fetomaternal alloimmune thrombocytopenia with compatible frozen thawed platelet concentrates. *Br J Haematol* 2002; **117**: 482–3.

263. Sidiropoulos D, Straume B. The treatment of neonatal isoimmune thrombocytopenia with intravenous immunoglobulin (IgG IV). *Blut* 1984; **48**: 383–6.

246. Kaplan C, Morel-Kopp MC, Clemenceau S *et al.* Fetal and neonatal alloimmune thrombocytopenia: current trends in diagnosis and therapy. *Transfus Med* 1992; **2**: 265–71.

265. Forestier F, Hohlfeld P. Management of fetal and neonatal thrombocytopenia. *Biol Neonate* 1998; **74**: 395–401.

266. Ahya R, Turner ML, Urbaniak SJ, SNAIT Study Team. Fetomaternal alloimmune thrombocytopenia. Review. *Transfus Apher Sci* 2001; **25**: 139–45.

267. Kaplan C. Platelet alloimmunity: the fetal/neonatal alloimmune thrombocytopenia. *Vox Sang* 2002; **83** (suppl. 1): 289–91.

268. Jolly MC, Letsky EA, Fisk NM. The management of fetal alloimmune thrombocytopenia. *Prenat Diagn* 2002; **22**: 96–8.

269. Lynch L, Bussel JB, McFarland JG, Chitkara U, Berkowwitz RL. Antenatal treatment of alloimmune thrombocytopenia. *Obstet Gynecol* 1992; **80**: 67–71.

270. Kroll H, Giers G, Bald R *et al.* Intravenous IgG during pregnancy for fetal alloimmune thrombocytopenic purpura. *Thromb Haemost* 1993; **69**: 997, poster 1625.

271. Kanhai HH, Porcelijn L, van Zoeren D *et al.* Antenatal care in pregnancies at risk of alloimmune thrombocytopenia: report of 19 cases in 16 families. *Eur J Obstet Gynecol Reprod Biol* 1996; **68**: 67–73.

272. Kornfeld I, Wilson RD, Ballem P, Wittmann BK, Farquharson DF. Antenatal invasive and noninvasive management of alloimmune thrombocytopenia. *Fetal Diagn Ther* 1996; **11**: 210–17.

273. Murphy MF, Metcalfe P, Waters AH, Ord J, Hambley H, Nicolaides K. Antenatal management of severe fetomaternal thrombocytopenia: HLA incompatibility may affect responses to fetal platelet transfusions. *Blood* 1993; **81**: 2174–9.

274. Bussel JB, Druzin ML, Clues DB, Samuels P. Thrombocytopenia in pregnancy. *Lancet* 1991; **337**: 251.

275. Bussel JB. Immune thrombocytopenia in pregnancy: autoimmune and alloimmune. *J Reprod Immunol* 1997; **37**: 35–61.

276. Gill, KK, Kelton JG. Management of idiopathic thrombocytopenic purpura in pregnancy. *Seminars in Hematology* 2000; **37**: 275–89.

277. Ballin A, Andrew M, Ling E, Perlman M, Blanchette V. High dose intravenous gammaglobulin therapy for neonatal idiopathic autoimmune thrombocytopenia. *J Pediatr* 1988; **112**: 789–92.

278. Blanchette V, Andrew M, Perlman M, Ling E, Ballin A. Neonatal autoimmune thrombocytopenia: role of high-dose intravenous immunoglobulin G therapy. *Blut* 1989; **59**: 139–44.

279. Kelton JG. Idiopathic thrombocytopenic purpura complicating pregnancy. *Blood Rev* 2002; **16**: 43–6.

280. Christiaens G, Helmerhorst F. Validity of intrapartum diagnosis of fetal thrombocytopenia. *Am J Obstet Gynecol* 1987; **157**: 864–5.

281. Pielet B, Socol M, MacGregor S, Ney J, Dooley S. Cordocentesis: an appraisal of risks. *Am J Obstet Gynecol* 1988; **159**: 1497–500.

282. Cook RL, Miller RC, Katz VL, Cefalo RC. Immune thrombocytopenic purpura in pregnancy: a reappraisal of management. *Obstet Gynecol* 1991; **78**: 567–83.

283. Buyon JP, Rupel A, Clancy RM. Neonatal lupus syndromes. *Lupus* 2004; **13**: 705–12.

284. Chunharas A, Nuntnarumit P, Hongeng S, Chaunsumrit A. Neonatal lupus erythematosus: clinical manifestations and management. *J Med Assoc Thai* 2002; **85** (suppl. 4): S1302–S1308.

285. Drachman JG. Inherited thrombocytopenia: when a low platelet count does not mean ITP. *Blood* 2004; **103**: 390–8.

286. Cattaneo M. Inherited platelet based bleeding disorders. *J Thromb Haemost* 2003; **1**: 1628–36.

287. Balduini CL, Iolascon A, Savoia A. Inherited thrombo-cytopenias: for genes to therapy. *Haematologica* 2002; **87**: 860–80.

288. Geddis AE, Kaushansky K. Inherited thrombocytopenias: toward a molecular understanding of platelet production. *Current Opinion in Pediatrics* 2004; **16**: 15–22.

289. Balduini CL, Cattaneo M, Fabris F *et al.* on behalf of the Italian Gruppo di Studio delle Piastrine. Inherited thrombocytopenias: a proposed diagnostic algorithm from the Italian Gruppo di Studio delle Piastrine. *Haematologica* 2003; **88**: 582–92.

290. Mandelbrot L, Schlienger I, Bongain A *et al.* Thrombocytopenia in pregnant women infected with human immunodeficiency virus: maternal and neonatal outcome. *Am J Obstet Gynecol* 1994; **171**: 252–7.

291. Landmann E, Bluetters-Sawatzki R, Schindler D, Gortner L. Fanconi anemia in a neonate with pancytopenia. *J Pediatr* 2004; **145**: 125–7.

31 Thromboembolic complications in children

Mary Bauman and M. Patricia Massicotte

Introduction

Normal infants and children have a number of physiologic hemostatic differences compared with adults, including unique protective mechanisms resulting in an overall decreased incidence of thrombosis. However, children who are now being cured of their primary illnesses (congenital heart disease, prematurity, cancer) are increasingly developing thromboembolic complications as sequelae to new surgical techniques and medical therapies that are facilitating these cures. Unfortunately, systemic venous and arterial thromboembolic complications have associated mortality and morbidity.

Systemic venous thromboembolic events (SVTE) in children most often occur due to interaction of multiple risk factors, with the presence of a central venous line (CVL) appearing to be one of the strongest risk factors. Systemic arterial thromboembolic events (SATE) in children most often occur as a result of the placement of an arterial line. Both SVTE and SATE require rapid diagnosis and institution of therapy to prevent thrombus extension or embolism, which could result in mortality or morbidity. There are few well-designed clinical studies providing sensitive and specific diagnostic regimens and safe efficacious therapeutic regimens that should be instituted (in the absence of contraindications) once thrombosis is confirmed.

This chapter discusses the hemostatic differences between children and adults (developmental hemostasis), and the epidemiology, clinical presentation, and evidence-based approaches to diagnosis and therapy (treatment and prevention) of SVTE and SATE in children. Diagnostic recommendations are based on the sensitivity and specificity of the chosen diagnostic method. Therapeutic recommendations for thrombosis are based on the strength of the published evidence supporting the recommendation. Therapeutic recommendations for thrombosis are graded according to the strength of the evidence supporting the recommendation. The grading system used is that described by the American College of Chest Physicians for antithrombotic guidelines.[1] Grade 1 recommendations have demonstrated a clear benefit for the intervention in the patient population; grade 2 recommendations are far less certain. The recommendations (grade 1, 2) are additionally supported by the level of evidence, where A represents multiple randomized trials with clear treatment effect or a metaanalysis, B represents single randomized trials, and C represents observational studies.

Developmental hemostasis

The hemostatic system in neonates and children has a number of differences compared with that of adults. Normal levels for age of the components of hemostasis have been determined and published.[2–4] The levels of the hemostatic factors approach adult levels by the time of puberty. The main differences are:
- decreased levels of contact factors (FXII and FXI);
- decreased levels of vitamin K-dependent factors (FII, FVII, FIX and FX);
- decreased thrombin generation;
- downregulated fibrinolytic system (decreased plasminogen);
- altered levels of inhibitor proteins of coagulation;
- decreased protein C, protein S and antithrombin;
- increased α_2-macroglobulin;
- decreased levels of inhibitors of fibrinolysis (plasminogen activator inhibitor, PAI).

Children are relatively protected from the development of thrombosis as a result of several unique mechanisms including:
- reduced capacity to generate thrombin;[5,6]
- increased capacity of α_2-macroglobulin to inhibit thrombin;[7]
- enhanced antithrombotic potential by the vessel wall.[8,9]

Systemic venous thromboembolism
(Table 31.1)

Epidemiology

The epidemiology of SVTE has been studied in three international registries (UK, Netherlands and Canada).[10–12] The

largest pediatric age groups for developing thrombosis are children of < 3 months and teenagers.

Etiology

The most common causative factors of SVTE are the presence of a CVL and the presence of serious diseases such as cancer, trauma/surgery, congenital heart disease and systemic lupus

Table 31.1 Venous thromboembolism: incidence, diagnosis and therapeutic considerations.

Thromboembolic event (TE)	Incidence	Diagnosis	Pretherapy considerations	Therapy
Systemic venous TE (SVTE): symptomatic and asymptomatic	General population: 0.07 per 10 000 in adults[2,4–7]	*Clinical symptoms*: Pain, redness, swelling of limb *Diagnostic*: US (albeit poor sensitivity). If US negative and clinical suspicion high proceed to venography or MRV. Neck vessels are sensitive to US	INR, PTT, hemoglobin, platelets, urea, creatinine *Rule out*: Current or potential for bleeding, hemorrhagic stroke, and recent surgery resulting in increased bleeding risk Head US in infants < 3 months to rule out intracranial hemorrhage	*Treatment recommendations*: LMWH/UFH therapy of 3 months' duration *Neonates*: follow with radiographic testing to ensure no extension of thrombus; if extension, treatment recommended Warfarin is not recommended in children < 12 months of age, except for mechanical heart valves Thrombolytic therapy (tPA, rUK) is recommended for therapy only where there is potential for loss of life, organ or limb
Pulmonary embolism (PE)	1.7–32%	*Clinical symptoms*: Chest pain, shortness of breath, hypoxia, atrial fibrillation, cardiovascular collapse *Diagnostic*: V/Q scan, MRI/MRV, spiral CT, angiogram	As above. NB: if cardiovascular collapse, proceed to **urgent** therapy	As above for SVTE Consider thrombolytic therapy or thrombectomy if cardiorespiratory compromise
Central venous line-related venous TE	Infants < 1 year of age: 0–30% ~35% in children; ALL, TPN, NS	As above for SVTE	As above for SVTE	As above for SVTE
Right atrial TE	No data	*Clinical symptoms*: Asymptomatic but may result in PE/cardiac failure *Diagnostic*: Cardiac echocardiogram, CC clinical diagnosis: currently no validated outcome measure	As above for SVTE	As above for SVTE Consider thrombectomy or thrombolytic therapy if cardiorespiratory compromise
Postthrombotic syndrome	12–62%	*Clinical diagnosis*: Currently no validated outcome measure		No effective treatment (custom-measured compression stockings may provide symptomatic relief)

ALL, acute lymphoblastic leukemia; CC, cardiac catheterization; CT, computed tomography; INR, international normalized ratio; LMWH, low-molecular-weight heparin; MRI, magnetic resonance imaging; MRV, magnetic resonance venography; NS, nephrotic syndrome; PTT, partial thromboplastin time; rUK, recombinant urokinase; tPA, tissue plasminogen activator; TPN, total parenteral nutrition; UFH, unfractionated heparin; US, ultrasound; V/Q, ventilation/perfusion scan.

erythematosus (SLE).[4,13–15] The role of congenital prothrombotic states in SVTE remains controversial. Idiopathic SVTE is rare in infants, children and teenagers.

Incidence

The incidence of SVTE in children is decreased compared with that in adults (2.5–5%).[12–21] The true incidence of pulmonary embolism (PE) among infants and children is unknown, and current studies probably underestimate the reported incidence.[14,22–25] There are two cross-sectional studies using ventilation/perfusion (V/Q) scans to detect PE, reporting incidences of 12% and 28% in children requiring home total parenteral nutrition (TPN) and children with nephrotic syndrome, respectively.[23,24] Right atrial thrombosis has been described usually in the presence of a CVL. The incidence is unknown.[26,27] Clinically overt symptoms include cardiac failure, PE, loss of CVL patency, and persistent sepsis. Over 50% of thromboses occur in the upper venous system secondary to the use of CVLs.[28,29]

Clinical symptoms

Acute symptoms

The acute symptoms of SVTE are:
- mortality, usually due to PE, estimated at 2%;[12]
- morbidity;
- loss of CVL patency;
- swelling, pain and discoloration of the related limb;
- swelling of the face and head with superior vena cava syndrome;
- respiratory compromise with PE and right atrial thrombosis.

Long-term outcomes

Various features can develop in the longer term as a result of SVTE, including the following.
1 Prominent collateral circulation in the skin:
(a) face, back, chest and neck as sequelae of upper VTE;
(b) abdomen, pelvis, groin and legs as sequelae of lower VTE.
2 Repeated loss of CVL patency:
(a) repeated requirement for CVL replacement;
(b) eventual loss of venous access.
3 CVL-related sepsis, chylothorax, chylopericardium, recurrent VTE (estimated to occur in 6% of children with SVTE[30]) necessitating long-term anticoagulation and associated bleeding risk.

Postthrombotic syndrome

Postthrombotic syndrome (PTS) is a serious long-term outcome of SVTE consisting of pain, swelling, limb discoloration and ulceration resulting from damage to venous valves in deep vessels. PTS that is clinically significant occurs in approximately 10–20% of children.[31] There is no properly validated outcome measure for PTS in children.

SVTE related to a CVL

CVLs are used in short-term intensive care, in hemodialysis or for long-term supportive care for children requiring TPN or therapy for cancer.

Etiology

Several mechanisms may play a role in the development of CVL-related VTE, including damage to the vessel wall by the CVL or by substances infused through the CVL (TPN, chemotherapy),[32,33] disrupted blood flow, and thrombogenic catheter materials.[34]

Types of CVL-related SVTE (Fig. 31.1)

Three types of CVL-related VTE are described in the literature.
1 A clot at the tip of a CVL, which impairs infusion or withdrawal of blood.
2 Fibrin sleeves that are not adherent to vessel walls but may occlude CVLs.[35]
3 CVL-related venous thromboembolic events that adhere to vessel walls, with partial or complete obstruction of vessels in which the CVL is located.[35]

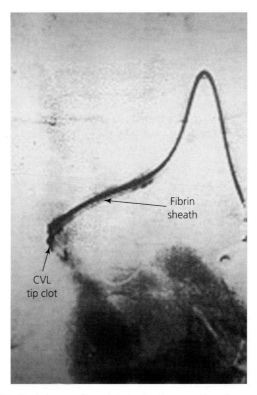

Fig. 31.1 Central venous line-related systemic venous thromboembolism.

Incidence

A CVL-related SVTE may be symptomatic or asymptomatic.

Symptomatic CVL-related SVTE

The incidence of symptomatic CVL-related SVTE has been recorded as 11% in a heterogeneous group (cardiac, cancer, other) of children.[36] Asymptomatic CVL-related SVTE occurred in 37% of children with acute lymphoblastic leukemia (upper limb CVL),[37] and an incidence of 45% was reported in children in intensive care with a lower limb CVL.[27] The incidence in other pediatric patient populations is not accurately known.

Asymptomatic CVL-related SVTE

Asymptomatic SVTE are clinically important in children and require therapy. Many are diagnosed on routine radiographic studies, with most children remaining asymptomatic.

Increasing evidence demonstrates that CVL-related venous thromboembolic events are associated with CVL-related sepsis. In a metaanalysis, prophylactic unfractionated heparin (UFH) reduced CVL-related SVTE (RR 0.43, 95% confidence interval (CI) 0.23–0.78), decreased bacterial colonization (RR 0.18, 95% CI 0.06–0.60) and likely CVL-related bacteremia (RR 0.26, 95% CI 0.07–1.03).[14] In addition, CVL-related VTE is the most common source for PE in children,[15] which may be fatal.[14] In children, PE is frequently not diagnosed during life due to the subtlety of symptoms in the presence of primary illnesses that can cause sudden cardiorespiratory compromise.

Finally, long-term sequelae of CVL-related VTE occur in 10–20% of children,[12,14] destroying the underlying venous system and potentially limiting life-saving therapy because of the absence of venous access. Case reports have documented sudden death resulting from rupture of an intrathoracic vessel, considered to be due to a previous CVL placement.[38]

Diagnosis of SVTE (including right atrial thrombosis and pulmonary embolus)
(Fig. 31.2 and Table 31.1)

There is no evidence to support screening for SVTE in any high-risk groups.[39] Diagnosis entails the following steps.
1 Clinical assessment of symptoms:
(a) pain, swelling or discoloration of an arm or leg;
(b) altered patency of CVL.
2 Chest radiography if CVL in place to determine if the CVL is in a good position and not fractured.
3 Ultrasound scan of the neck and intrathoracic vessels should be obtained. If the ultrasound is negative, and the clinical suspicion is high for VTE, the child should have a venogram.
4 Venogram: magnetic resonance imaging (MRI)/magnetic resonance venography (MRV) of the intrathoracic vessels to rule out VTE.

Sensitivity of imaging studies for diagnosis of SVTE

There are currently no studies evaluating the sensitivity of MRI/MRV for venous thrombosis. With asymptomatic SVTE, ultrasound was demonstrated to have a sensitivity of only 20% for intrathoracic thrombosis, yet it diagnosed jugular thrombi that were missed on venography.[37] No studies have yet determined the sensitivity and specificity of any form of testing used to diagnose pulmonary embolus.

Right atrial thrombosis is diagnosed on transthoracic echocardiography, although this is not as sensitive as transesophageal echocardiography in teens or children with large chest dimensions (obesity, pectus).

Treatment recommendations for SVTE
(Fig. 31.2 and Table 31.1)

Anticoagulation should be instituted in the absence of contraindications (active bleeding, very high risk of bleeding) if a symptomatic proximal SVTE, pulmonary embolism or right atrial thrombosis is clinically suspected and until diagnosis can be confirmed. In addition anticoagulation therapy should be considered if an asymptomatic proximal SVTE is diagnosed during radiographic imaging performed for other reasons (i.e., diagnosis of malignancy, echocardiography to determine cardiac anatomy, cardiac catheterization).

Thrombolysis should be strongly considered in the case of PE or massive SVTE where risk of loss of life, organ or limb is diagnosed.

First-event SVTE

"Heparin therapy" should be used as initial treatment. Intravenous unfractionated heparin should be infused and the dose titrated to achieve therapeutic levels (see monitoring). (Grade 1C recommendation; see above). Initial treatment with heparin should continue for 5–10 days (Grade 1C) prior to proceeding with warfarin or longer-term LMWH. Duration of anticoagulant therapy is extrapolated from adults, and 3 months of therapy is recommended (Grade 2C).

SVTE secondary to risk factor(s)

If risk factors persist, such as the presence of a CVL, L-asparaginase therapy, lupus anticoagulant or nephritic syndrome, continue anticoagulant therapy in prophylactic or therapeutic doses until the risk factor is resolved (Grade 2C). *Caution*: Do not use thrombolytic therapy routinely for SVTE due to the risk of major bleeds associated with its use (Grade 2C).

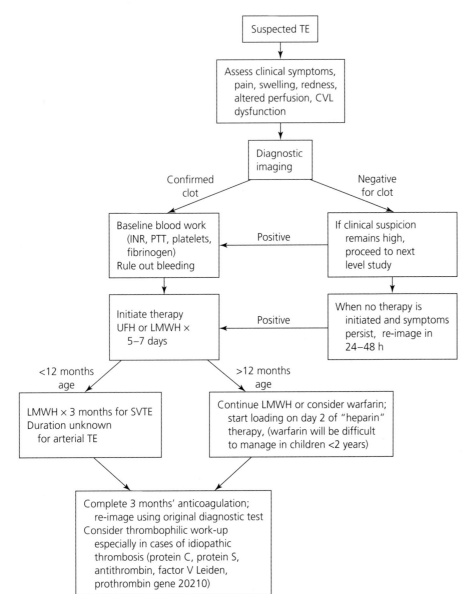

Fig. 31.2 Diagnostic and therapeutic protocol for systemic venous thromboembolism (SVTE). CVL, central venous line; INR, international normalized ratio; LMWH, low-molecular-weight heparin; PTT, partial thromboplastin time; TE, thromboembolism; UFH, unfractionated heparin.

Recurrent SVTE secondary to risk factor(s) while on anticoagulant therapy

Continue anticoagulation for an additional 3 months from the diagnosis of recurrent thrombosis or until removal of the precipitating risk factor.

CVL-related SVTE

If the CVL is not required or is nonfunctioning, remove the catheter following a minimum of 3–5 days of anticoagulant therapy (Grade 2C) to reduce the risk of embolism. Treat with heparin therapy as per first-event SVTE (see above). Treat with anticoagulant therapy for 3 months. If the CVL is functioning and is still required, it may be left in place (Grade 2C).

Idiopathic SVTE

Treat with heparin therapy as per first-event SVTE (see above). Treat with anticoagulant therapy for a minimum of 6 months (Grade 2C).

Recurrent SVTE

Treat with heparin therapy as per first-event SVTE (see above). Treat with anticoagulant therapy for an indefinite duration (Grade 2C).

Treatment of SVTE in neonates

Administer heparin therapy or follow with radiographic monitoring to ensure no extension of thrombus. If the thrombus extends, treat with heparin therapy using UFH or LMWH for 10 days to 3 months (Grade 2C).

CVL prophylaxis

Primary prophylaxis is not recommended (Grade 1B) in any clinical situation at present.

Systemic arterial thromboembolic events
(Table 31.2)

Epidemiology

The epidemiology of SATE has not been well studied.

Etiology

The most common etiology is the presence of an arterial line.[39] Arterial lines placed in the femoral artery or peripheral arteries often result in SATE.
- Arterial lines placed in the umbilical artery may result in aortic thrombosis.
- Femoral arterial catheters are placed in infants and children for therapeutic or diagnostic cardiac catheterization and often result in femoral arterial thrombosis.
- Peripheral arterial catheterization is carried out in critically ill infants and children for blood pressure monitoring and can result in vessel thrombosis.
- Occlusion of the radial artery rarely results in loss of the hand if the ulnar artery is patent.

Clinical symptoms

Differential diagnoses within 24 hours of arterial catheter placement are vascular spasm or SATE. Symptoms of vascular spasm or SATE include decreased or absent pulses, pale or mottled limb and decreased capillary refill. Vascular spasm usually resolves within a few hours with no therapy. SATE only resolves with anticoagulation therapy, and should be confirmed by ultrasound.

Outcomes

SATE is associated with mortality or morbidity in children. Short-term morbidity may include tissue ischemia followed by tissue necrosis and nonviability of the affected organ or limb. If vascular occlusion persists, loss of limb function, and occasionally surgical limb amputation, organ and tissue damage, are reported. Additionally, symptoms of SATE may occur at remote sites due to embolic events.

Long-term morbidities include leg length discrepancy, muscle wasting, claudication and loss of arterial access. Loss of access will present significant morbidity for children who require multiple interventional cardiac catheterizations.[40,41]

Classification

SATE unrelated to catheter use

Arterial thrombotic events are reported in the presence of congenital familial hyperlipidemia. Acquired conditions that are risk factors for development of SATE include Takayasu

Table 31.2 Arterial thromboembolism: incidence, diagnosis and therapeutic considerations.

Arterial thromboembolic event (TE)	Incidence	Diagnosis	Pretherapy considerations	Therapy
Femoral artery TE secondary to CC	Femoral artery 40% with no prophylaxis post-CC, 5% with prophylaxis	*Clinical*: Pain, swelling, pale, cool pulseless leg. Handheld Doppler may be used to assess pulses. Black leg may indicate irreversible tissue ischemia *Diagnostic*: US (albeit poor sensitivity). If US negative and clinical suspicion high proceed to MRA or angiogram	As for SVTE in Table 31.1	As for SVTE in Table 31.1 Duration of therapy unknown
Peripheral artery TE	Unknown	As above with arterial TE secondary to CC	As for SVTE in Table 31.1	As for SVTE in Table 31.1 Duration of therapy unknown
Umbilical artery (UA) TE secondary to UA catheter	1% symptomatic 3–59% on autopsy 10–90% incidental finding on ultrasound	*Clinical*: Pale, cool, pulseless lower limb(s) Renal dysfunction	As for SVTE in Table 31.1	As for SVTE in Table 31.1 Duration of therapy unknown

CC, cardiac catheterization; MRA, magnetic resonance angiography; US, ultrasound.

arteritis, Kawasaki disease, congenital heart disease and arterial thrombosis in transplanted organs.[42]

SATE secondary to arterial catheters

Umbilical artery catheters

Umbilical artery catheters (UACs) are used in critically ill neonates for supportive care and hemodynamic monitoring. Vascular complications include local thrombosis of the aorta. The use of UACs with end holes results in less aortic thrombosis compared with catheters with side holes.[43] Thromboembolism to organs or limbs may result causing compromise or nonviability of the limb, and necrotizing enterocolitis.

There is no evidence that catheter tip location influences the incidence of thromboembolic events.[44–49] Peripheral arterial lines may result in local thrombosis (see Peripheral artery catheterization, below).

Prophylaxis
• Low-dose heparin infusion (1–5 units/h) through the UAC should be used to improve patency[50–53] and UAC-related SATE (Grade 2A recommendation; see above).
• Intermittent flushes with heparin are ineffective in preventing UAC occlusion.[54]

Cardiac catheterization

Cardiac catheterization (CC) is used in children with congenital and acquired heart disease for diagnostic or therapeutic purposes. Most often, the superficial femoral artery is cannulated. In rare situations, the brachial artery is accessed.[55] The incidence of local thrombosis secondary to CC, without periprocedural heparin prophylaxis (after removal of the arterial sheath), is 40%, and with heparin prophylaxis is 5%.[56] There are a number of risk factors affecting the incidence of SATE, including:
• age (infants have a higher risk);
• duration of procedure;
• catheter to vessel proportion;
• larger sheath size than recommended for a given weight and body surface area;
• use of balloon dilatation;
• repeated catheter manipulations;
• increased hematocrit.[56–61]

Recommendations for prophylaxis
If CC is performed using arterial access, the following guidelines are recommended.
• Intravenous UFH therapy (Grade 1A) as a bolus of 100–150 units/kg during CC (Grade 2B).[56]
• Acetylsalicylic acid (ASA) alone for thromboprophylaxis for CC should not be used (Grade 1B).[62]

Peripheral artery catheterization

Peripheral artery catheterization (PAC) is used in children in an intensive care setting for monitoring as well as blood sampling.[30] Complications include thrombotic occlusion of the vessel and loss of patency of the arterial catheter,[63] with clinical symptoms as follows:
• decreased temperature;
• pale color;
• increased capillary refill time;
• blood pressure differential > 10 mmHg between limbs.

Prophylaxis
• Infuse continuous heparin 1 unit/mL through the peripheral arterial catheter to improve catheter patency (Grade 1A).[61,64–67]
• There are no studies establishing the safety and efficacy of any agent (including low-dose heparin infusion) for the prevention of SATE due to PAC.

Diagnosis (Fig. 31.2)

The gold standard test to diagnose SATE is angiography, but this is difficult to perform in children with existing critical illness.[68,69] The newer contrast agents are less hypertonic than those used previously allowing safer use in younger children. Other objective tests have not been tested in children for sensitivity and specificity: Doppler ultrasound and handheld Doppler at the bedside may be useful to determine absent pulses. Blood pressure differential between two limbs of at least 10 mmHg[68] may also indicate SATE.

Treatment recommendations (Fig. 31.2 and Table 31.2)

Acute SATE secondary to catheter placement (UAC, CC or PAC)

Remove the arterial catheter from any anatomic location immediately if arterial occlusion is suspected (pale or cyanosed skin, decreased or absent pulses, increased capillary time). Treatment options include anticoagulation, thrombolysis or thrombectomy.
• Therapeutic doses of intravenous heparin are effective in 70% of cases of SATE,[70] and should be administered in the absence of contraindications (Grade 1C) (see Unfractionated heparin therapy, below).
• If life, organ or limb is threatened due to arterial thrombosis, in the absence of contraindications, thrombolysis therapy should be considered (Grade 1C) (see Thrombolytic therapy, below).
• In selected cases of femoral artery thrombosis, surgical intervention should be carried out (e.g., in cases where there is a contraindication to thrombolytic therapy or where organ or limb loss is imminent) (Grade 2C).
• Thrombolytic therapies that have been used successfully after CC include streptokinase,[70–74] urokinase,[70] and tissue

Table 31.3 Thrombolytic dosing.

Agent	Load	Maintenance	Monitoring
Urokinase	4400 units/kg	4400 units/kg/h for 6–12 h	Fibrinogen, TCT, PT, APTT
Tissue plasminogen activator	None	0.1–0.6 mg/kg/h for 6 h	Same

APTT, activated partial thromboplastin time; PT, prothrombin time; TCT, thrombin clotting time.

plasminogen activator (tPA).[75–77] The incidence of major bleeding has been reported to be as high as 30% (Table 31.3).[78]

• The risk of bleeding may be reduced by pretreating children about to receive tPA with 10 mL/kg fresh frozen plasma (FFP), and limiting the tPA infusion (0.5 mg/kg/h) to 6 hours maximum.

• If thrombectomy is used in small children, there is high risk of arterial reperfusion injury.

• If arterial occlusion persists despite UFH therapy, thrombolytic therapy should be started if no contraindications are present (active bleeding, disseminated intravascular coagulation, central nervous system bleed). UFH therapy should be initiated postembolectomy to prevent vascular reocclusion (Grade 1C).

Surgical management for long-term outcomes of SATE

Reconstructive surgery should be considered if there is clinically significant claudication accompanied by muscle wasting and/or shortening of the limb. Options for reconstructive surgery include thrombectomy with autogenous saphenous vein patch angioplasty, direct angioplasty, segmental resection with end-to-end anastomosis, and interposition bypass grafting.[79]

Before reconstructive surgery, the vascular anatomy of the affected leg should be established using Doppler ultrasound and possibly angiography via the contralateral femoral artery.

Medical treatment: anticoagulant agents

Practical tips for managing anticoagulation in children

Before initiating anticoagulation therapy, obtain the patient's weight (kg) and take a sample of blood for hemoglobin, platelets, international normalized ratio (INR), APTT, urea and creatinine. Note that "heparin" is a descriptive term referring to all heparins, including UFH and LMWH.

Certain precautions must be taken when dealing with an anticoagulated child.

• Avoid intramuscular injections and arterial punctures if possible. If necessary, use extended periods (minimum 5 min, firm pressure) of external pressure to decrease bleeding.

• If analgesia is required, avoid antiplatelet agents (e.g., ibuprofen). Acetaminophen (paracetamol) is acceptable.

• If long-term warfarin is to be used (>12 months) (e.g., in case of mechanical heart valves), bone densitometry studies at baseline and then every 12 months should be considered to assess for possible osteoporosis.[80] There are no data in humans on the effect of LMWH therapy on bone mineral density.[81–83]

• Age-appropriate education should be given to the child regarding anticoagulation risk, benefit and monitoring, and this will decrease complications associated with therapy.[84–88]

Anticoagulant agents

Unfractionated heparin

The advantage of using UFH in children is its short half-life (4 hours), which permits rapid cessation of anticoagulation by simply discontinuing the infusion, and gives the ability to rapidly reverse anticoagulant effects by using protamine sulfate when immediate reversal is necessary.

Caution: UFH is supplied in multidose vials in increasing concentrations with similar packaging. Extreme caution should be used when dispensing heparin doses to ensure the correct concentration is being used to avoid administering an overdose.

Mode of action and guidelines for administration

The anticoagulant activities of heparin are mediated by catalysis of antithrombin. In children, antithrombin (AT) levels may be low, reflecting physiologic, congenital and/or acquired etiologies. To achieve a heparin effect, the addition of AT may be necessary, as either FFP (1 unit/mL) or AT concentrate. Heparin dosing and monitoring guidelines are adapted from adults. Dosing of heparin in children will probably differ from adults, but further studies are needed to delineate this.[6,89]

It is important to note the following.

• Monitor hemoglobin and platelets daily due to the risk of developing heparin-induced thrombocytopenia.

• A dedicated intravenous line is necessary for UFH infusions; this intravenous line must not be stopped for other medications, in order to maintain constant heparin levels.

Table 31.4 Heparin dosing nomogram.[39,153]

APTT (s)	Anti-factor Xa (units/mL)	Heparin hold (min)	Heparin rate change	After 4h repeat APTT
<50	<0.1	0	Increase 20%	4 h
50–59	0.1–0.34	0	Increase 10%	4 h
60–85	0.35–0.70	0	0	24 h
86–95	0.71–0.89	0	Decrease 10%	4 h
96–120	0.90–1.20	30 min	Decrease 10%	4 h
>120	>1.20	60 min	Decrease 15%	4 h

APTT, activated partial thromboplastin time.

Intravenous dosing (Table 31.4)

1 In cases of acute PE or acute SVTE, a bolus of UFH should be administered by using 75 units/kg over 10 min followed by an age-appropriate infusion.

2 Maintenance heparin doses are age dependent:
(a) infants (28 weeks' gestational age to 12 months of age), 28 units/kg/h;
(b) children > 12 months of age, 20 units/kg/h.[90]

Subcutaneous dosing

• Therapeutic UFH may be administered subcutaneously.[91]

• The daily dose (units/kg/h) is divided into two doses and is given subcutaneously every 12 hours.

• Dosing is calculated using the formula below:

Dose = patient weight × age-dependent dose of heparin (i.e., 20 units/k/hr for children > 12 months of age or 28 units/kg/hr for children < 12 months of age) × the number of hours to be covered (maximum = 12 hours)

UFH as a "bridge" anticoagulant

Reversal of anticoagulant therapy for invasive procedures[92,93] can be carried out using UFH as a "bridge" anticoagulant in children who are receiving LMWH or warfarin and who are at high risk for thromboembolic disease.

Monitoring

If possible, an anti-FXa and an APTT should be drawn within 24 hours of initiating therapy to ensure that the APTT is accurately reflecting the UFH concentration. Therapeutic levels need to be achieved and maintained for effective anticoagulant therapy. It has been shown that APTT (s) and anti-FXa levels (units/mL) correspond in 70% of children but rarely in children < 12 months of age.[94] Among infants and children, if the APTT and anti-FXa levels do not correspond, then UFH therapy should be monitored using anti-FXa levels.

• APTT or anti-FXa level (venous sample not from arterial or central venous line) should be drawn 4–6 hours after initiation of therapy. Once in the therapeutic range, monitor APTT or anti-FXa at least every 24 hours as the bioavailability of UFH is poor.

• Adjust the UFH infusion to maintain anti-FXa at 0.35–

Table 31.5 Reversal of heparin therapy.

Time since end of infusion, or last heparin dose	Protamine per 100 units unfractionated heparin dosed (maximum 50 mg/dose)
<30 min	1 mg
30–60 min	0.5–0.75 mg
61–120 min	0.375–0.5 mg
>120 min	0.25–0.375 mg

Reproduced with permission from Ref. 1.

0.7 units/mL or an APTT that corresponds to the therapeutic anti-FXa range in the treating institution.[90,91]

• Subcutaneous UFH is monitored using either the APTT or anti-FXa level measured at 6 hours after the subcutaneous dose and adjusted according to the nomogram shown in Table 31.4.

Table 31.4 is an example of a heparin-dosing nomogram where the therapeutic APTT is 60–85 s.

Reversal and antidote for UFH (Table 31.5)

If anticoagulation with UFH needs to be discontinued for clinical reasons, termination of the UFH infusion will usually suffice because of the rapid clearance of UFH. If an immediate effect is required, consider administering protamine sulfate. Intravenous protamine sulfate neutralizes heparin activity by virtue of its positive charge within 5 minutes of administration. The dose of protamine sulfate required to neutralize UFH is based on the dose of UFH received in the previous 2 hours as shown in Table 31.5.

Caution: the maximum dose of protamine sulfate, regardless of the amount of UFH received, is 50 mg.

• Administration should not exceed a rate of 5 mg/min of a 10 mg/mL concentrated solution.

• Hypersensitivity reactions may occur in children with known hypersensitivity reactions to fish, and those who have received protamine-containing insulin or previous protamine therapy.

• Perform an APTT 15 min after administration to determine the effect of administration.[1]

Table 31.6 Enoxaparin dosing nomogram: initial dose.[105,106]

	Age ≤2 months	Age ≥2 months to 18 years
Initial prophylactic dose	0.75 mg/kg/dose s.c. every 12 h or 1.5 mg/kg/dose s.c. once daily	0.5 mg/kg/dose s.c. every 12 h or 1 mg/kg/dose s.c. once daily
Initial treatment dose	1.5 mg/kg/dose s.c. every 12 h	1 mg/kg/dose s.c. every 12 h
Maximum suggested dose	3 mg/kg/dose s.c. every 12 h	2 mg/kg/dose s.c. every 12 h

The therapeutic level of anti-factor Xa for Enoxaparin treatments is 0.5–1 units/mL.[91,153]

Heparin-induced thrombocytopenia

There are case reports of heparin-induced thrombocytopenia (HIT) in children from ages 3 months to 15 years.[95–101] Many infants and children in neonatal or pediatric intensive care units who are exposed to heparin have multiple reasons for thrombocytopenia and/or thrombosis, thus a high index of suspicion is required to diagnose HIT. During heparin therapy, the platelet count should be measured daily. If platelet counts decrease by more than 50% from baseline and clinical suspicion for HIT is high, then *all* sources of heparin should be discontinued and a HIT screen should be sent.

Danaparoid, hirudin and argatroban may be used as alternatives to heparin in children with HIT, although there is a paucity of dosing data.[81,97,99,102,103]

Low-molecular-weight heparin

The use of LMWH should be considered in most children requiring anticoagulation. The potential advantages of LMWH for children include:
• minimal monitoring required due to good bioavailability (important in pediatric patients with poor or nonexistent venous access);
• lack of interference by other drugs or diet, unlike warfarin;
• reduced risk of HIT;
• probable reduced risk of osteoporosis with long-term use compared with heparin.

Dosing guidelines

The following are guidelines for initiating and monitoring enoxaparin therapy; modifications for individual clinical circumstances may be necessary. The dosage guidelines given in Table 31.6 apply to enoxaparin only and cannot be directly extrapolated to other LMWH products. The following precautions must be taken.
• LMWH is cleared renally. The blood creatinine level should be measured prior to initiating LMWH therapy. If renal compromise/failure is present, LMWH may be used cautiously.[104–108]
• Side-effects associated with subcutaneous administration of LMWH are bleeding and bruising and hematoma formation at the administration site. Firm pressure for 3–5 min at the administration site will minimize these side-effects. Do not massage the site after administration.

Monitoring

Therapeutic range doses of LMWH are extrapolated from adults and are based on anti-FXa levels. The guidelines for therapeutic LMWH suggest maintaining an anti-FXa level of 0.5–1.0 units/mL in a sample taken 4–6 hours following a subcutaneous injection. Anti-FXa levels reflect the pharmacodynamic activity of the LMWH but do not accurately reflect its antithrombotic activity.[106] Table 31.7 provides guidelines for dose adjustment of enoxaparin.

Table 31.7 Enoxaparin dosing nomogram: dose adjustment.[105,153]

Anti-FXa level	Hold next dose?	Change dose?	Next anti-FXa level?
<0.35 units/mL	No	Increase by 25% (round up to whole number*)	4 hours after next morning dose
0.35–0.49 units/mL	No	Increase by 10% (round up to whole number*)	4 hours after next morning dose
0.5–1 units/mL	No	0	Once a week at 4 hours after morning dose
<1.2 units/mL	No	Decrease by 20% (round down to whole number*)	4 hours after next morning dose
			Hold dose. Do a trough level. If trough < 0.5 units at 10 h post-dose, administer scheduled dose at 20% of previous dose

Note: the above nomogram assumes that there is no bleeding or renal compromise.

* When adjusting doses of enoxaparin, dose adjustments can be ordered in 1.0-mg increments (if monitoring results are available on a daily basis) to achieve targeted anti-FXa level.

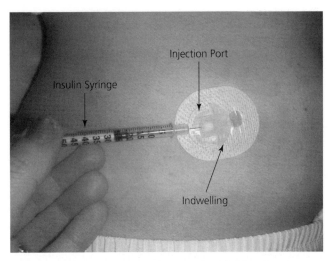

Fig. 31.3 Insuflon catheter *in situ* demonstrating administration of low-molecular-weight heparin with an insulin syringe.

Monitor anti-FXa levels monthly and adjust dose accordingly. This is necessary in the pediatric population as children gain weight and outgrow current doses; also it avoids drug accumulation over time in renal compromise.[109]

Practical tips for administration of LMWH therapy in infants and children

• Administration of enoxaparin using an insulin syringe with a short ultrafine ($^5/_{16}$ inch, 8 mm) needle is easy for parents/guardians as well as health professionals; 1 mg of drug corresponds to 1 unit on the syringe. This may assist in reducing measuring error and side-effects such as bleeding, bruising and hematoma formation at the administration site. Similarly, an insulin syringe may be used for all LMWH with accurate calculations for dose measurement. The calculation for conversion is 0.01 ml = 1 unit on an insulin syringe.

• An Insuflon catheter (Fig. 31.3) may be used for subcutaneous therapy. This device is an indwelling subcutaneous vinyl catheter that is inserted into the subcutaneous tissue and which may remain in place for 3–7 days.

• Firm pressure should be applied to the heparin administration site for a minimum of 5 min following each dose.

• The Insuflon port site must be monitored closely for any bleeding, bruising, leakage or subcutaneous hematoma formation. If any of these are present, the Insuflon must be changed before administering the next dose. The use of an insulin syringe allows easier administration of drug through the port.

• The goal is to assist the parent or guardian to become independent in the safe administration of their child's heparin therapy and facilitate early discharge from hospital.

Reversal and antidote of LMWH

Unless immediate reversal is necessary, withholding two doses will suffice to reverse the anticoagulant affect. If immediate reversal of effect is required, protamine sulfate reverses 80% of the anti-FXa activity of LMWHs.[110]

Warfarin

The INR ranges for children are extrapolated from the recommendations for adult patients, which is not appropriate due to the differences in the coagulation cascade between children and adults. However, there are no clinical trials that have assessed the optimal INR ranges for children based upon clinical outcomes. The recommended target INR for treatment of VTE is 2.5 (range 2.0–3.0), and 3.0 (range 2.5–3.5) for most children with mechanical heart valves.[111]

Monitoring

Frequent monitoring of oral anticoagulant therapy in children is required due to a number of factors affecting warfarin metabolism, including diet, medications and primary medical problems. Warfarin administration in children requires close supervision, with frequent dose adjustments by experts in anticoagulation.[112,113] Breast-fed infants are very sensitive to oral anticoagulants due to the low concentrations of vitamin K in breast milk.[114–117] It is recommended that these children receive daily vitamin K supplements in the form of 50 mL of commercial formula. In addition, variations in daily intake for infants and young children increase the challenge of managing warfarin in this population. As an alternative, LMWH therapy may be considered. Some children are resistant to oral anticoagulants due to impaired absorption. Similarly, infants and children who are receiving infant or pediatric nutritional formulas will be resistant to oral anticoagulants as these preparations are routinely enhanced with Vitamin K. These challenges that are associated with managing warfarin therapy have resulted in the recommendation that warfarin should not be used in children under 12 months of age, except in infants with mechanical heart values.

Initial warfarin loading dose (Table 31.8)

The child should be tolerating a full diet prior to initiating warfarin therapy. Most children will overshoot the target INR if full feeds are not tolerated. In children who are not tolerating full feeds, LMWH may be used until dietary toler-

Table 31.8 Warfarin dosing nomogram: loading phase.[103]

INR	Action
Following the initial loading dose, if the resultant INR is:	
1.1–1.4	Repeat initial dose
1.5–2.9	50% of initial dose
>3.0	Hold until INR < 2.5 then restart at 50% less than the previous dose

Note: these dose reductions are critical to avoid "overshooting" the target range. INR, international normalized ratio.

Table 31.9 Warfarin dosing nomogram: maintenance phase for target international normalized ratio (INR) of 2.5[154]

INR	Action
1.1–1.4	Check for compliance; if compliant increase dose by 20%
1.5–1.9	Dose increase by 10%
2.0–3.0	No change
3.1–3.5	Dose decrease by 10%
>3.5–4.0	Administer one dose at 50% less than maintenance dose. Then restart at 20% less than the maintenance dose
4.1–5.0	Hold × 1 dose then restart at 20% less than maintenance dose
>5.0	Consider reversal with vitamin K

Note: in the case of mechanical heart valves where the target INR is 3.0, the above nomogram may be used by adjusting the INR range up by 0.5. For example, the INR range of 1.1–1.4 would correspond to 1.6–1.9 with a dose adjustment increase of 20%.

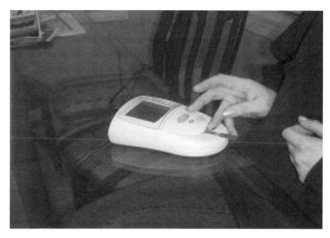

Fig. 31.4 Coaguchek (Roche Diagnostics) monitor for measuring INR using capillary whole blood samples.

ance is achieved. This practice will result in accomplishing the warfarin maintenance phase safely and efficiently.

• In most children, the loading dose is 0.2 mg/kg p.o. as a single daily dose, with a maximum of 5 mg.[103]

• In children with liver dysfunction or post-Fontan procedure, the loading dose should be reduced to 0.1 mg/kg p.o. as a single daily dose.

Practical tips for managing warfarin therapy in children

• If the INR is > 3.0 after the first or second loading dose, withhold warfarin, repeat the INR, then restart at 50% of the previous dose, providing the child is tolerating feeds.

• If the INR is not greater than 1.5 after two loading doses, increase the dose by 50% and follow the nomogram given in Table 31.8.

Long-term warfarin: maintenance dosing guidelines

The dosing guidelines for long-term maintenance of warfarin are given in Table 31.9. These apply primarily to medically stable patients already established on long-term maintenance therapy. Medically unstable patients or those completing the loading protocol may respond differently. Close monitoring with individualized dose adjustment of such patients is essential until they are clearly established on maintenance therapy.

Point-of-care testing using INR monitors

Whole-blood monitors provide an effective means of monitoring INRs in children on long-term oral anticoagulant therapy when there is a needle phobia or poor venous access. The INR is measured using a capillary blood sample. Point-of-care INR monitors have been evaluated in children and were shown to be acceptable and reliable for use in the outpatient laboratory and at-home settings.[82,83,106]

The amounts of capillary blood required for INR testing in

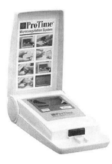

Fig. 31.5 PROTIME Monitor (ITC) used to check INR using capillary whole blood samples.

the Coaguchek monitor (Fig. 31.4) and the PROTIME monitor (Fig. 31.5) are 10 μL and 27 μL, respectively.

Warfarin reversal for outpatients with INR > 6.0

It is helpful to discharge the child with a prescription for vitamin K to treat elevated INRs at home. A vitamin K elixir is available in some centers, although an ampoule of vitamin K 10 mg for intravenous use may be given orally. Oral administration of vitamin K is found to be most effective[118] The nomogram given in Table 31.10 is based on adult recommendations. Repeat the INR within 24 hours.[119]

Reversal and antidote of warfarin

• For nonurgent reversal of warfarin withhold three doses (for children with mechanical valves consider subcutaneous unfractionated heparin 60 hours after the first dose is withheld).

• When urgent reversal is needed (e.g., in case of major bleeding or interventional procedure), administer FVIIa 50 units/kg i.v. (there are no safety or efficacy data) or FFP 20 mL/kg i.v.

• In case of nonurgent reversal, give vitamin K_1 0.5–2 mg orally, depending upon the patient's size. The administra-

Table 31.10 Vitamin K dosing nomogram.

Child's weight	INR	Vitamin K dose
≤20 kg	6–10	0.5 mg orally
≤20 kg	>10	1.0 mg orally
>20 kg	6–10	1.0 mg orally
>20 kg	>10	2.0 mg orally

Note: dosing recommendations assume no active bleeding. If there is active bleeding, increase dose by 100% and consider fresh frozen plasma. Doses greater than those noted in the table should be used with caution in children with mechanical heart valves.

tion of vitamin K intravenously or intramuscularly has been shown to be less efficacious than oral administration unless gut absorption is severely compromised.

Thrombolytic therapy

Systemic thrombolytic therapy is indicated for clinical situations where there is potential loss of life, organ or limb, such as arterial occlusions, massive PE, or PE not responding to heparin therapy.[120] It may also be indicated for acute extensive SVTE.[120] The contraindications to thrombolytic therapy must be considered; however, in some patients the need for thrombolytic therapy may necessitate treatment in spite of contraindications. If possible, before the use of thrombolytic therapy, discuss with the family the high incidence of major bleeding (30%).

Contraindications

Thrombolytic therapy has various contraindications.
• Active bleeding.
• Significant potential for local bleeding (e.g., tumor surrounding vessel with clot), general surgery within the previous 10 days, neurosurgery within the previous 3 weeks.
• Hypertension.
• Arteriovenous (AV) malformations.
• Recent severe trauma.
Caution: streptokinase is not recommended in children due to potential anaphylactic reactions. Urokinase has recently been released in recombinant form.

Prior to commencing thrombolytic therapy

A range of measures must be taken before embarking on thrombolytic therapy.
• Complete blood count, platelet count, APTT, fibrinogen, cross-match and type for 1 unit of packed red blood cells (PRBC).
• Children have less plasminogen compared with adults. Before thrombolytic therapy, ensure plasminogen levels are adequate to achieve the desired lytic effect by administering FFP at 10–20 mL/kg.

• Admit to the pediatric intensive care unit or a designated floor identified for thrombolytic therapy.
• Consider sedation depending on the child and clinical circumstances.
• Place a sign at the head of the bed indicating that the patient is receiving thrombolytic therapy.
• Notify the blood bank to ensure cryoprecipitate is available.
• Ensure good venous access for drug administration and for monitoring purposes.

Thrombolytic dosing and therapy guidelines

During thrombolytic infusion, UFH 10–20 units/kg/h should be administered concurrently with either the tpa or urokinase (lytic drug of choice) infusion. If the patient is not already on heparin, start heparin infusion but do not give a bolus dose (Table 31.3). If catheter-directed local thrombolytic therapy is used, it is suggested that the dose is decreased by 50%. In children, there is no evidence for increased efficacy or safety with local dosing.

The following therapeutic guidelines should be observed.
• No intramuscular injections during therapy.
• Minimal manipulation of the patient, e.g., no bathing or physiotherapy.
• Avoid concurrent use of warfarin or antiplatelet agents (e.g., aspirin, dipyridamole, clopidogrel).
• No urinary catheterization, rectal temperature measurements, or arterial punctures.
• Take blood samples from a superficial vein or indwelling catheter. If blood sampling is difficult, insert an indwelling catheter for blood samples prior to thrombolytic therapy.
• Reevaluate radiographically following 6 hours of infusion (for arterial thrombi use the return of pulses and blood pressure to preinvestigation values).
• Monitor the response to thrombolytic therapy by the PT/INR, APTT and fibrinogen level if bleeding and every 6–8 hours after the start of infusion.
• Expect the fibrinogen concentration to decrease by at least 20–50%; maintain the fibrinogen concentration at approximately 1 g/L by infusions of cryoprecipitate (1 unit/5 kg bodyweight).
• If there is no change in the fibrinogen concentration, check D-dimers to ensure that a thrombolytic state has been established.
• Maintain the platelet count $> 50–100 \times 10^9$/L.

Prothrombotic disorders

Congenital prothrombotic disorders

The need to screen for prothrombotic disorders in children with major illnesses, who are undergoing an invasive procedure or who have confirmed thrombosis, especially in the presence of clinical risk factors, remains uncertain. In general, homozygous deficiency of antithrombin, protein C and protein S will present in the neonatal period. Large family studies in patients with protein C, protein S, antithrombin, FV Leiden and prothrombin gene 20210 defects found negligible rates of SVTE in children <15 years of age.[121] However, cross-sectional disease-oriented studies estimate the prevalence of congenital prothrombotic disorders in children with secondary SVTE to be 13–78%, depending on the population of children studied.[122] FV Leiden homozygosity may be associated with SVTE in children.[123–129] Venous and arterial thrombotic events are reported more in the presence of congenital familial hyperhomocysteinemia.

• Most children with prothrombin gene mutation 20210 do not develop thrombosis until adult life.[121]

• Excessive plasma levels of homocysteine due to homozygous deficiencies of enzymes such as cystathionine β-synthase or methylenetetrahydrofolate reductase may be associated with severe SVTE in children.[130,131]

• Increased plasma levels of lipoprotein(a) in children have been reported in cohorts of children with SVTE.[132]

Acquired prothrombotic disorders

Prothrombotic states can arise as the result of other conditions or therapies.

• The incidence of SVTE in children with nephrotic syndrome is at least 10% when using objective radiographic methods.[133]

• There is an association between antiphospholipid antibodies and SVTE in children.

• The use of L-asparaginase and steroids in acute lymphoblastic leukemia therapy has been associated with VTE. possibly due to decreased antithrombin levels.

Heart disease in children and thrombosis

A number of different cardiac surgical procedures are used to palliate congenital heart disease. The shunts that are placed during these procedures vary in diameter, flow characteristics and composition, and are associated with the development of thrombosis. These include the following.

• Norwood procedure (Blalock–Taussig shunt, right ventricle–pulmonary artery conduit): Blalock–Taussig shunts are often as small as 2.5–3.0 mm, which results in abnormal blood flow.

• Glenn procedure (bicaval pulmonary): gortex is often used as the synthetic material for the extracardiac shunts.

• Sanno procedure (extracardiac right ventricle–pulmonary artery conduit).

• Fontan procedure (extracardiac shunt either fenestrated (right-to-left dynamic cardiac connection)) or nonfenestrated (no right-to-left dynamic cardiac connection). Blood flow is often very slow in the shunts placed during the Fontan procedure. A review of the literature revealed up to 20% incidence of

thromboembolic complications (shunt thrombosis, stroke and pulmonary embolism) in children following the Fontan procedure.

Primary prophylaxis in children with cardiac shunts

Norwood procedure

For children undergoing this procedure the recommended prophylactic regimen is intraoperative heparin followed by either aspirin (5 mg/kg/day) or no further anticoagulant therapy (Grade 2C). The duration of therapy, and the need for ongoing aspirin therapy are unknown.[39]

Glenn procedure

Current clinical practices vary, and include both no anticoagulation and heparin followed by aspirin. There is no evidence to support a preference for either of these approaches at this time.

Fontan procedure

The results of a multicenter randomized controlled trial comparing ASA (5 mg/kg daily) and heparin followed by warfarin (target INR 2.5) in children post-Fontan procedure are being analyzed.[39,134,135] The recommendation is aspirin (5 mg/kg daily) or therapeutic heparin followed by vitamin K antagonists to achieve a target INR of 2.5 (range 2–3) (Grade 2C).

Mechanical prosthetic heart valves in children

Cardiac valvular disease occurs as an isolated congenital event, as part of complex coronary heart disease, or as a result of treatments for an underlying cardiac disorder. Thrombosis of the valve or embolization to the central nervous system are both serious complications of mechanical prosthetic heart valves.[136–143] Currently, mechanical prosthetic heart valves are usually used in the mitral and aortic position while biologic prosthetic heart valves are used for tricuspid or pulmonary valve replacements in children.

Randomized controlled trials in adults with mechanical prosthetic heart valves have clearly delineated the need for oral anticoagulants with an INR of 2.5–3.5.[144–146] Antiplatelet agents have a role if there is more than one valve or a thromboembolism has occurred with a therapeutic INR.[147] There are no randomized controlled trials in children, only case series. In the absence of oral anticoagulants, and in the presence of no therapy or antiplatelet therapy alone, the incidence of thromboembolism is unacceptably increased in some studies.[148,149] Only oral anticoagulants consistently maintained the incidence of thromboembolism at <5% per patient year, which is similar to that for adults.[148,150–152]

With the use of oral vitamin K antagonists, major bleeding was <3.5% per patient year. Aspirin in combination with oral anticoagulants may be helpful in high-risk patients such as those with prior thromboembolism, atrial fibrillation, a large left atrium and/or multiple mechanical prosthetic heart valves.

Treatment recommendation

The following regimen is recommended for children with mechanical prosthetic heart valves.
• Oral anticoagulation to maintain a target INR of 2.5 (Grade 1C+).
• In children where additional antithrombotic therapy is required due to failure of vitamin K antagonists or there is a contraindication to full-dose vitamin K antagonists, use aspirin (6–20 mg/kg daily) (Grade 2 C).

Conclusions

Venous and arterial thrombosis is being increasingly diagnosed in children. The serious sequelae, including mortality and morbidity, result in the recommendation of therapy in children with thrombosis. However, the anticoagulant and thrombolytic agents used in children have had few properly designed studies to determine their age-related pharmacokinetics and provide estimates of safety and efficacy. The recommendations for the use of these agents – dosing, monitoring, duration and intensity – are based on results from adult studies. This extrapolation is inappropriate and may be exposing children to improper intensity and duration of antithrombotic agents. The difficulty in performing pediatric clinical trials should not preclude properly designed clinical studies in cohorts of children at risk for thrombosis or with thrombosis, to determine the safety and efficacy of prophylaxis and therapy.

References

1. Monagle P, Chan A, Massicotte P, Chalmers E, Michelson A. Antithrombotic therapy in children. *Chest* 2004; **126**: 645S–687S.
2. Andrew M, Paes B, Johnston M. Development of the hemostatic system in the neonate and young infant. *Am J Pediatr Hematol Oncol* 1990; **12**: 95–104.
3. Andrew M, Paes B, Milner R *et al.* Development of the human coagulation system in the healthy premature infant. *Blood* 1988; **72**: 1651–7.
4. Andrew M, Paes B, Milner R *et al.* Development of the human coagulation system in the full-term infant. *Blood* 1987; **70**: 165–72.
5. Andrew M, Schmidt B, Mitchell L, Paes B, Ofosu F. Thrombin generation in newborn plasma is critically dependent on the concentration of prothrombin. *Thromb Haemost* 1990; **63**: 27–30.
6. Andrew M, Mitchell L, Vegh P, Ofosu F. Thrombin regulation in children differs from adults in the absence and presence of heparin. *Thromb Haemost* 1994; **72**: 836–42.
7. Ling X, Delorme M, Berry L *et al.* alpha 2-Macroglobulin remains as important as antithrombin III for thrombin regulation in cord plasma in the presence of endothelial cell surfaces. *Pediatr Res* 1995; **37**: 373–8.
8. Xu L, Delorme M, Berry L, Brooker L, Mitchell L, Andrew M. Thrombin generation in newborn and adult plasma in the presence of an endothelial surface. 1991; **65**: 1230.
9. Nitschmann E, Berry L, Bridge S *et al.* Morphological and biochemical features affecting the antithrombotic properties of the aorta in adult rabbits and rabbit pups. *Thromb Haemost* 1998; **79**: 1034–40.
10. van Ommen CH, Heijboer H, Buller HR, Hirasing RA, Heijmans HS, Peters M. Venous thromboembolism in childhood: a prospective two-year registry in The Netherlands. *J Pediatr* 2001; **139**: 676–81.
11. Gibson BES, Chalmers EA, Bolton-Maggs P, Henderson DJ, Boshkov RL. Thromboembolism in childhood: a prospective 2 years study in the United Kingdom (February 2001–February 2003). *J Thromb Haemost*, Vol. 1, Suppl. 1: 2003.
12. Monagle P, Adams M, Mahoney M *et al.* Outcome of pediatric thromboembolic disease: a report from the Canadian Childhood Thrombophilia Registry. *Pediatr Res* 2000; **47**: 763–6.
13. Andrew ME, Monagle P, deVeber G, Chan AK. Thromboembolic disease and antithrombotic therapy in newborns. *Hematology (Am Soc Hematol Educ Program)* 2001; 358–74.
14. Massicotte MP, Dix D, Monagle P, Adams M, Andrew M. Central venous catheter related thrombosis in children: analysis of the Canadian Registry of Venous Thromboembolic Complications. *J Pediatr* 1998; **133**: 770–6.
15. Andrew M, Massicotte MP, deVeber G *et al.* 1-800-NO-CLOTS: A quaternary care solution to a new tertiary care disease: childhood thrombophilia. *J Thromb Haemost* 1997; **77** (suppl. 1): 727.
16. Castaman G, Rodeghiero F, Dini E. Thrombotic complications during L-asparaginase treatment for acute lymphocytic leukemia. *Haematologica* 1990; **75**: 567–9.
17. Wise RC, Todd JK. Spontaneous, lower-extremity venous thrombosis in children. *Am J Dis Child* 1973; **126**: 766–9.
18. Bernstein D, Coupey S, Schonberg SK. Pulmonary embolism in adolescents. *Am J Dis Child* 1986; **140**: 667–71.
19. Coon WW, Willis PWI, Keller JB. Venous thromboembolism and other venous disease in the Tecumseh community health study. *Circulation* 1973; **48**: 839–46.
20. Gjores J. The incidence of venous thrombosis and its sequelae in certain districts in Sweden. *Acta Chir Scand* 1956; **206** (suppl.): 1–10.
21. Carter C, Gent M. The epidemiology of venous thrombosis. In: Colman R, Hirsh J, Marder V, Salzman E (eds) *Hemostasis and Thrombosis. Basic Principles and Clinical Practice*. Philadelphia: JB Lippincott, 1982, pp. 805–19.
22. Ament J, Newth CJ. Deep venous lines and thromboembolism. *Pediatr Pulmonol* 1995; **20**: 347–8.
23. Hoyer PF, Gonda S, Barthels M, Krohn HP, Brodehl J. Thromboembolic complications in children with nephrotic syndrome. Risk and incidence. *Acta Paediatr Scand* 1986; **75**: 804–10.

24. Dollery CM, Sullivan ID, Bauraind O, Bull C, Milla PJ. Thrombosis and embolism in long-term central venous access for parenteral nutrition. *Lancet* 1994; **344**: 1043–5.

25. Uderzo C, Faccini P, Rovelli A *et al*. Pulmonary thromboembolism in childhood leukemia: 8-years' experience in a pediatric hematology center. *J Clin Oncol* 1995; **13**: 2805–12.

26. Marsh D, Wilkerson SA, Cook LN, Pietsch JB. Right atrial thrombus formation screening using two-dimensional echocardiograms in neonates with central venous catheters. *Pediatrics* 1988; **81**: 284–6.

27. Krafte-Jacobs B, Sivit CJ, Mejia R, Pollack MM. Catheter-related thrombosis in critically ill children: comparison of catheters with and without heparin bonding. *J Pediatr* 1995; **126**: 50–4.

28. Andrew M, David M, Adams M *et al*. Venous thromboembolic complications (VTE) in children: first analyses of the Canadian Registry of VTE. *Blood* 1994; **83**: 1251–7.

29. Schmidt B, Andrew M. Neonatal thrombosis: report of a prospective Canadian and international registry. *Pediatrics* 1995; **96**: 939–43.

30. Randolph AG, Cook DJ, Gonzales CA, Andrew M. Benefit of heparin in peripheral venous and arterial catheters: systemic review and meta-analysis of randomized controlled trials. *Br Med J* 1998; **316**: 969–75.

31. Choi M, Andrew M. Post-thrombotic syndrome in children with previous deep vein thrombosis. *Blood* 2000.

32. Chidi CC, King DR, Bales ET Jr. An ultrastructural study of the intimal injury by an indwelling umbilical catheter. *J Pediatr Surg* 1983; **18**: 109.

33. Wakefield A, Cohen Z, Rosenthal A *et al*. Thrombogenicity of total parenteral nutrition solutions: II. Effect on induction of endothelial cell procoagulant activity. *Gastroenterology* 1989; **97**: 1220–8.

34. Pottecher T, Forrler M, Picardat P, Krause D, Bellocq JP, Otteni JC. Thrombogenicity of central venous catheters: prospective study of polyethylene, silicone and polyurethane catheters with phlebography or post-mortem examination. *Eur J Anaesthesiol* 1984; **1**: 361–5.

35. Williams EC. Catheter-related thrombosis. *Clin Cardiol* 1990; **13**: VI34–6.

36. Massicotte MP, Julian JA, Gent M *et al*. An open-label randomized controlled trial of low molecular weight heparin for the prevention of central venous line related thrombotic complications in children: the PROTEKT trial. *Thromb Res* 2003; **109**: 101–8.

37. Male C, Chait P, Ginsberg J *et al*. Comparison of venography and ultrasound for the diagnosis of deep vein thrombosis in the upper body in children: a substudy of the PARKAA trial. *Thromb Haemost* 2002; **87**: 593–8.

38. Nowak-Gottl U, Von Kries R, Gobel U. Neonatal symptomatic thromboembolism in Germany: two year survey. *Arch Dis Child* 1997; **76**: F163–F167.

39. Monagle P, Chan A, Massicotte P, Chalmers E, Michelson A. Antithrombotic therapy in children. *Chest* 2004; **126**: 645S–87S.

40. Wigger HJ, Bransilver BR, Blanc WA. Thromboses due to catheterization in infants and children. *J Pediatr* 1970; **76**: 1–11.

41. Kern IB. Management of children with chronic femoral artery obstruction. *J Pediatr Surg* 1977; **12**: 83–90.

42. Durongpisitkul K, Gururaj VJ, Park JM, Martin CF. The prevention of coronary artery aneurysm in Kawasaki disease: a meta-analysis on the efficacy of aspirin and immunoglobulin treatment. *Pediatrics* 1995; **96**: 1057–61.

43. Price V, Massicotte MP. Arterial thromboembolism in the pediatric population. *Semin Thromb Hemost* 2003; **29**: 557–65.

44. Fletcher MA, Brown DR, Landers S, Seguin J. Umbilical arterial catheter use: report of an audit conducted by the Study Group for Complications of Perinatal Care. *Am J Perinatol* 1994; **11**: 94–9.

45. Gilhooly J, Lindberg J, Reynolds J. Survey of umbilical artery catheter practices. *Clin Res* 1986; **34**: 142–3.

46. Kempley ST, Bennett S, Loftus BG, Cooper D, Gamsu HR. Randomized trial of umbilical arterial catheter position: clinical outcome. *Acta Paediatr* 1993; **82**: 173–6.

47. Krueger TC, Neblett WW, O'Neill JA, MacDonell RC, Dean RH, Thieme GA. Management of aortic thrombosis secondary to umbilical artery catheters in neonates. *J Pediatr Surg* 1985; **20**: 328–32.

48. Stringel G, Mercer S, Richler M, McMurray B. Catheterization of the umbilical artery in neonates: surgical implications. *Can J Surg* 1985; **28**: 143–6.

49. Malloy MH, Cutter GR. The association of heparin exposure with intraventricular hemorrhage among very low birth weight infants. *J Perinatol* 1995; **15**:185–91.

50. Boros SJ, Thompson TR, Reynolds JW, Jarvis CW, Williams HJ. Reduced thrombus formation with silicone elastomere (silastic) umbilical artery catheters. *Pediatrics* 1975; **56**: 981–6.

51. Bosque E, Weaver L. Continuous versus intermittent heparin infusion of umbilical artery catheters in the newborn infant. *J Pediatr* 1986; **108**: 141–3.

52. Horgan MJ, Bartoletti A, Polansky S, Peters JC, Manning TJ, Lamont BM. Effect of heparin infusates in umbilical arterial catheters on frequency of thrombotic complications. *J Pediatr* 1987; **111**: 774–8.

53. Ankola PA, Atakent YS. Effect of adding heparin in very low concentration to the infusate to prolong the patency of umbilical artery catheters. *Am J Perinatol* 1993; **10**: 229–32.

54. Barrington KJ. Umbilical artery catheters in the newborn: effects of heparin. *Cochrane Database Syst Rev* 2000; (2):CD000507.

55. Stanger P, Heymann MA, Tarnoff H, Hoffman JI, Rudolph AM. Complications of cardiac catheterization of neonates, infants, and children. A three-year study. *Circulation* 1974; **50**: 595–608.

56. Freed MD, Keane JF, Rosenthal A. The use of heparinization to prevent arterial thrombosis after percutaneous cardiac catheterization in children. *Circulation* 1974; **50**: 565–9.

57. Vitiello R, McCrindle BW, Nykanen D, Freedom RM, Benson LN. Complications associated with pediatric cardiac catheterization. *J Am Coll Cardiol* 1998; **32**: 1433–40.

58. Saxena A, Gupta R, Kumar RK, Kothari SS, Wasir HS. Predictors of arterial thrombosis after diagnostic cardiac catheterization in infants and children randomized to two heparin dosages. *Cathet Cardiovasc Diagn* 1997; **41**: 400–3.

59. Bulbul ZR, Galal MO, Mahmoud E *et al*. Arterial complications following cardiac catheterization in children less than 10kg. *Asian Cardiovasc Thorac Ann* 2002; **10**: 129–32.

60. Rao PS, Thapar MK, Rogers JH Jr *et al*. Effect of intraarterial injection of heparin on the complications of percutaneous arterial catheterization in infants and children. *Cathet Cardiovasc Diagn* 1981; **7**: 235–46.

61. Butt W, Shann F, McDonnell G, Hudson I. Effect of heparin concentration and infusion rate on the patency of arterial catheters. *Crit Care Med* 1987; **15**: 230–2.

62. Freed MD, Rosenthal A, Fyler D. Attempts to reduce arterial thrombosis after cardiac catheterization in children: use of percutaneous technique and aspirin. *Am Heart J* 1974; **87**: 283–6.

63. Scheer B, Perel A, Pfeiffer UJ. Clinical review: complications and risk factors of peripheral arterial catheters used for haemodynamic monitoring in anaesthesia and intensive care medicine. *Crit Care* 2002; **6**: 199–204.

64. Sellden H, Nilsson K, Larsson LE, Ekstrom-Jodal B. Radial arterial catheters in children and neonates: a prospective study. *Crit Care Med* 1987; **15**: 1106–9.

65. Rais-Bahrami K, Karna P, Dolanski EA. Effect of fluids on life span of peripheral arterial lines. *Am J Perinatol* 1990; **7**: 122–4.

66. Heulitt MJ, Farrington EA, O'Shea TM, Stoltzman SM, Srubar NB, Levin DL. Double-blind, randomized, controlled trial of papaverine-containing infusions to prevent failure of arterial catheters in pediatric patients. *Crit Care Med* 1993; **21**: 825–9.

67. Tarry WC, Moser AJ, Makhoul RG. Peripheral arterial thrombosis in the nephrotic syndrome. *Surgery* 1993; **114**: 618–23.

68. Andrew M, David M, deVeber G, Brooker LA. Arterial thromboembolic complications in paediatric patients. *Thromb Haemost* 1997; **78**: 715–25.

69. Schmidt B, Andrew M. Neonatal thrombotic disease: prevention, diagnosis, and treatment. *J Pediatr* 1988; **113**: 407–10.

70. Ino T, Benson LN, Freedom RM, Barker GA, Aipursky A, Rowe RD. Thrombolytic therapy for femoral artery thrombosis after pediatric cardiac catheterization. *Am Heart J* 1988; **115**: 633–9.

71. Wessel DL, Keane JF, Fellows KE, Robichaud H, Lock JE. Fibrinolytic therapy for femoral arterial thrombosis after cardiac catheterization in infants and children. *Am J Cardiol* 1986; **58**: 347–51.

72. Kirk CR, Qureshi SA. Streptokinase in the management of arterial thrombosis in infancy. *Int J Cardiol* 1989; **25**: 15–20.

73. Brus F, Witsenburg M, Hofhuis WJ, Hazelzet JA, Hess J. Streptokinase treatment for femoral artery thrombosis after arterial cardiac catheterisation in infants and children. *Br Heart J* 1990; **63**: 291–4.

74. Kothari SS, Kumar RK, Varma S, Saxena A. Thrombolytic therapy in infants for femoral artery thrombosis following cardiac catheterisation. *Indian Heart J* 1996; **48**: 246–8.

75. Levy M, Benson LN, Burrows PE *et al*. Tissue plasminogen activator for the treatment of thromboembolism in infants and children. *J Pediatr* 1991; **118**: 467–72.

76. Zenz W, Muntean W, Beitzke A, Zobel G, Riccabona M, Gamillscheg A. Tissue plasminogen activator (alteplase) treatment for femoral artery thrombosis after cardiac catheterisation in infants and children. *Br Heart J* 1993; **70**: 382–5.

77. Ries M, Singer H, Hofbeck M. Thrombolysis of a modified Blalock–Taussig shunt with recombinant tissue plasminogen activator in a newborn infant with pulmonary atresia and ventricular septal defect. *Br Heart J* 1994; **72**: 201–2.

78. Gupta AA, Leaker M, Andrew M *et al*. Safety and outcomes of thrombolysis with tissue plasminogen activator for treatment of intravascular thrombosis in children. *J Pediatr* 2001; **139**: 682–8.

79. Chaikof EL, Dodson TF, Salam AA, Lumsden AB, Smith RBI. Acute arterial thrombosis in the very young. *J Vasc Surg* 1992; **16**: 428–35.

80. Massicotte P, Julian J, Webber C, Charpentier K. Osteoporosis: a potential complication of long term warfarin therapy. *J Thromb Haemost* 1999: (suppl.) 1333a.

81. Avioli LV. Heparin-induced osteopenia: an appraisal. *Adv Exp Med Biol* 1975; **52**: 375–87.

82. Sackler JP, Liu L. Heparin-induced osteoporosis. *Br J Radiol* 1973; **46**: 548–50.

83. Murphy MS, John PR, Mayer AD, Buckels JA, Kelly DA. Heparin therapy and bone fractures. *Lancet* 1992; **340**: 1098.

84. Bibace R, Walsh M. Development of children's concepts of illness. *Pediatrics* 1980; **66**: 912–17.

85. Bush P, Ozias J, Walson P, Ward R. Ten guiding principles for teaching children and adolescents about medicines. *Clin Ther* 1999; **21**: 1280–4.

86. Ferris T, Dougherty D, Blumenthal D, Perrin J. A report card on quality improvement for children's health care. *Pediatrics* 2001; **107**: 143–55.

87. Hart C, Chesson R. Children as consumers. *Br Med J* 1998; **316**: 1600–4.

88. Towle A, Godolphin W. Framework for teaching and learning informed shared decision making. *Br Med J* 1999; **319**: 766–9.

89. Schmidt B, Ofosu FA, Mitchell L, Brooker LA, Andrew M. Anticoagulant effects of heparin in neonatal plasma. *Pediatr Res* 1989; **25**: 405–8.

90. Andrew M, Marzinotto V, Massicotte P *et al*. Heparin therapy in pediatric patients: a prospective cohort study. *Pediatr Res* 1994; **35**: 78–83.

91. Cheng A, Williams B, Sivarajan B. *The HSC Handbook of Pediatrics*, 10th edn. Toronto: Elsevier Saunders, 2003.

92. Bauman M, Mitchell L, Chan AK, deVeber G, Massicotte MP. Very low dose warfarin for primary and secondary prophylaxis in children: a prospective cohort study of 20 children. *J Thromb Haemost* 2003; **1** (suppl. 1): P0063.

93. Bauman M, Chan AK, Mitchell L, deVeber G, Massicotte MP. Reversal of warfarin or low molecular weight heparin (LMWH) using subcutaneous unfractionated heparin (UFH) in pediatric outpatients with an ongoing high risk for thrombosis and requiring invasive procedures: a prospective cohort study of 146 children. *J Thromb Haemost* 2003; **1** (suppl. 1): P0048.

94. Kuhle S, Eulmeskian P, Massicotte PM *et al*. Poor correlation between APTT, anti-Xa levels and heparin dose in children receiving therapeutic doses of unfractionated heparin. *J Thromb Haemost* 2003; **1** (suppl. 1): P0060.

95. Potter C, Gill JC, Scott JP, McFarland JG. Heparin-induced thrombocytopenia in a child. *J Pediatr* 1992; **121**: 135–8.

96. Klement D, Rammos S, Kries R, Kirschke W, Kniemeyer HW, Greinacher A. Heparin as a cause of thrombus progression. Heparin-associated thrombocytopenia is an important differential diagnosis in paediatric patients even with normal platelet counts. *Eur J Pediatr* 1996; **155**: 11–14.

97. Murdoch IA, Beattie RM, Silver DM. Heparin-induced thrombocytopenia in children. *Acta Paediatr* 1993; **82**: 495–7.

98. Magnani HN. Heparin-induced thrombocytopenia (HIT):

an overview of 230 patients treated with orgaran (Org 10172). *Thromb Haemost* 1993; **70**: 554–61.

99. Severin T, Sutor AH. Heparin-induced thrombocytopenia in pediatrics. *Semin Thromb Hemost* 2001; **27**: 293–9.

100. Smugge M. Heparin induced thrombocytopenia in children. *Pediatrics* 2002; **10** (Issue 1): e10.

101. Newall F, Barnes C, Ignjatovic V, Monagle P. Heparin-induced thrombocytopenia in children. *J Ped Child Health* 2003; **39**: 289–92.

102. Kuhle S, Koloshuk B, Marzinotto V *et al*. A cross-sectional study evaluating post thrombotic syndrome in children. *Throm Res* 2003; **11**: 227–33.

103. Crowther M, Ginsberg J, Kearon C, Harrison L, Massicotte MP, Hirsh J. A randomized trial comparing 5 mg and 10 mg warfarin loading doses. *Arch Intern Med* 1998; **159**: 46–8.

104. Greaves M. Limitations of the laboratory monitoring of heparin therapy. Scientific and Standardization Committee Communications: on behalf of the Control of Anticoagulation Subcommittee of the Scientific and Standardization Committee of the International Society of Thrombosis and Haemostasis. *Thromb Haemost* 2002; **87**: 163–4.

105. Massicotte P, Adams M, Marzinotto V, Brooker LA, Andrew M. Low-molecular-weight heparin in pediatric patients with thrombotic disease: a dose finding study. *J Pediatr* 1996; **128**: 313–18.

106. Massicotte MP, Adams M, Leaker M, Andrew M. A nomogram to establish therapeutic levels of the low molecular weight heparin (LMWH), clivarine in children requiring treatment for venous thromboembolism (VTE). *J Thromb Haemost* 1997; **1** (suppl. 1): 282.

107. Kuhle S, Massicotte MP, Andrew M *et al*. A dose-finding study of Tinzaparin in pediatric patients. *Blood* 2002; **100** (Issue 11): 279a.

108. Hirsh J, Levine MN. Low molecular weight heparin. *Blood* 1992; **79**: 1–17.

109. Dix D, Andrew M, Marzinotto V *et al*. The use of low molecular weight heparin in pediatric patients: a prospective cohort study. *J Pediatr* 2000; **136**: 439–45.

110. Massonet-Castel S, Pelissier E, Bara L *et al*. Partial reversal of low molecular weight heparin (PK 10169) anti Xa activity by protamine sulfate: in vitro and in vivo study during cardiac surgery with extracorporeal circulation. *Haemostasis* 1986; **16**: 139.

111. Spevak PJ, Freed MD, Castaneda AR, Norwood WI, Pollack P. Valve replacement in children less than 5 years of age. *J Am Coll Cardiol* 1986; **8**: 901–8.

112. Andrew M, Marzinotto V, Brooker LA *et al*. Oral anticoagulation therapy in pediatric patients: a prospective study. *Thromb Haemost* 1994; **71**: 265–9.

113. Streif W, Andrew M, Marzinotto V *et al*. Analysis of warfarin therapy in pediatric patients: a prospective cohort study of 319 patients. *Blood* 1999; **94**: 3007–14.

114. Shearer MJ, Rahim S, Barkhan P, Stimmler L. Plasma vitamin K1 in mothers and their newborn babies. *Lancet* 1982; **ii**: 460–3.

115. Greer FR, Mummah-Schendel LL, Marshall S, Suttie JW. Vitamin K1 (phylloquinone) and vitamin K2 (menaquinone) status in newborns during the first week of life. *Pediatrics* 1988; **81**: 137–40.

116. Haroon Y, Shearer MJ, Rahim S, Gunn WG, McEnery G, Barkhan P. The content of phylloquinone (vitamin K1) in human milk, cows' milk and infant formula foods determined by high-performance liquid chromatography. *J Nutr* 1982; **112**: 1105–17.

117. Von Kries R, Shearer M, McCarthy PT, Haug M, Harzer G, Gobel U. Vitamin K1 content of maternal milk: influence of the stage of lactation, lipid composition, and vitamin K1 supplements given to the mother. *Pediatr Res* 1987; **22**: 513–17.

118. Crowther M, Douketis J, Schnurr T *et al*. Oral vitamin K lowers the International Normalized Ratio more rapidly than subcutaneous vitamin K in the treatment of warfarin-associated coagulopathy: a randomized, controlled trial. *Ann Intern Med* 2002; **137**: 251–4.

119. Wilson SE, Watson HG, Crowther MA. Low-dose oral vitamin K therapy for the management of asymptomatic patients with elevated international normalized ratios: a brief review. *Can Med Assoc J* 2004; **170**: 821–4.

120. Andrew M, Monagle P, Brooker L. Thrombolytic therapy. In: *Thromboembolic Complications During Infancy and Childhood*. Hamilton, BC: Decker, 2000, pp. 357–84.

121. Andrew M, Monagle P, Brooker L. Developmental hemostasis: relevance to thromboembolic complications in pediatric patients. In: *Thromboembolic Complications During Infancy and Childhood*. Hamilton, BC: Decker, 2000, pp. 5–46.

122. Nowak-Gottl U, Koch HG, Aschka I *et al*. Resistance to activated protein C (APCR) in children with venous or arterial thromboembolism. *Br J Haematol* 1996; **92**: 992–8.

123. Idriss FS, Nikaidoh H, King LR, Swenson O. Arteriovenous shunts for hemodialysis in infants and children. *J Pediatr Surg* 1971; **6**: 639–44.

124. Chan AKC, Coppes M, Adams M, Andrew M. Right atrial thrombosis in pediatric patients: analysis of the Canadian registry of venous thromboembolic complications. *Pediatric Res* 1997; **39**: 154A.

125. Ross P Jr, Ehrenkranz R, Kleinman CS, Seashore JH. Thrombus associated with central venous catheters in infants and children. *J Pediatr Surg* 1989; **24**: 253–6.

126. Berman W Jr, Fripp RR, Yabek SM, Wernly J, Corlew S. Great vein and right atrial thrombosis in critically ill infants and children with central venous lines. *Chest* 1991; **99**: 963–7.

127. Wacker P, Oberhansli I, Didier D, Bugmann P, Bongard O, Wyss M. Right atrial thrombosis associated with central venous catheters in children with cancer. *Med Pediatr Oncol* 1994; **22**: 53–7.

128. Korones DN, Buzzard CJ, Asselin BL, Harris JP. Right atrial thrombi in children with cancer and indwelling catheters. *J Pediatr* 1996; **128**: 841–6.

129. Andrew M, Brooker LA. Hemostatic complications in renal disorders of the young. *Pediatr Nephrol* 1996; **10**: 88–99.

130. Paramo JA, Rifon J, Lloren R, Casares J, Paloma MJ, Rocha E. Intra- and postoperative fibrinolysis in patients undergoing cardiopulmonary bypass surgery. *Haemostasis* 1991; **21**: 58–64.

131. Rehan V, Seshia MM. Complications of umbilical vein catheter. *Eur J Pediatr* 1994; **153**: 141.

132. Kooiman AM, Kootstra G, Zwierstra RP. Portal hypertension in children due to thrombosis of the portal vein. *Neth J Surg* 1982; **34**: 97–103.

133. Brady L, Magilavy D, Black DD. Portal vein thrombosis associated with antiphospholipid antibodies in a child. *J Pediatr Gastroenterol Nutr* 1996; **23**: 470–3.

134. Monagle P, Karl TR. Thromboembolic problems after the Fontan operation. *Semin Thorac Cardiovasc Surg Pediatr Card Surg Annu* 2002; **5**: 36–47.

135. Monagle P, Cochrane A, McCrindle B, Benson L, Williams W, Andrew M. Thromboembolic complications after fontan procedures: the role of prophylactic anticoagulation. *J Thorac Cardiovasc Surg* 1998; **115**: 493–8.

136. Brown JW, Dunn JM, Spooner E, Kirsh MM. Late spontaneous disruption of a porcine xenograft mitral valve. Clinical, hemodynamic, echocardiographic, and pathological findings. *J Thorac Cardiovasc Surg* 1978; **75**: 606–11.

137. Geha AS, Laks H, Stansel HC Jr *et al.* Late failure of porcine valve heterografts in children. *J Thorac Cardiovasc Surg* 1979; **78**: 351–64.

138. Silver MM, Pollock J, Silver MD, Williams WG, Trusler GA. Calcification in porcine xenograft valves in children. *Am J Cardiol* 1980; **45**: 685–9.

139. Dunn JM. Porcine valve durability in children. *Ann Thorac Surg* 1981; **32**: 357–68.

140. Williams WG, Pollack JC, Geiss DM, Trusler GA, Fowler RS. Experience with aortic and mitral valve replacement in children. *J Thorac Cardiovasc Surg* 1981; **81**: 326–33.

141. Miller D, Stinson E, Oyer P *et al.* The durability of porcine xenograft valves and conduits in children. *Circulation* 1982; **66** (Issue 2, Pt 2): I172–I185.

142. Odell J. Calcification of porcine bioprostheses in children. In: Cohn L, Gallucci V (eds) *Cardiac Bioprostheses: Proceedings of the Second International Symposium.* New York: Yorke Medical Books, 1982, p. 231.

143. Williams DB, Danielson GK, McGoon DC, Puga FJ, Mair DD, Edwards WD. Porcine heterograft valve replacement in children. *J Thorac Cardiovasc Surg* 1982; **84**: 446–50.

144. Turpie AG, Gent M, Laupacis A *et al.* A comparison of aspirin with placebo in patients treated with warfarin after heart-valve replacement. *N Engl J Med* 1993; **329**: 524–9.

145. Rajah S, Sreeharan N, Joseph A *et al.* Prospective trial of dipyridamole and warfarin in heart valve patients. *Acta Thera (Brussels)* 1980; **6**: 54A.

146. Sullivan JM, Harken DE, Gorlin R. Effect of dipyridamole on the incidence of arterial emboli after cardiac valve replacement. *Circulation* 1969; **39** (5 suppl. 1): I149–I153.

147. Stein PD, Alpert JS, Copeland J, Dalen JE, Goldman S, Turpie AG. Antithrombotic therapy in patients with mechanical and biological prosthetic heart valves. *Chest* 1995; **108** (4 suppl.): 371S–379S.

148. Solymar L, Rao PS, Mardini MK, Fawzy ME, Guinn G. Prosthetic valves in children and adolescents. *Am Heart J* 1991; **121**: 557–68.

149. Sade R, Ballenger JF, Hohn A *et al.* Cardiac valve replacement in children: comparison of tissue with mechanical prostheses. *J Thorac Cardiovasc Surg* 1979; **78**: 123–7.

150. Harada Y, Imai Y, Kurosawa H, Ishihara K, Kawada M, Fukuchi S. Ten-year follow-up after valve replacement with the St. Jude Medical prosthesis in children. *J Thorac Cardiovasc Surg* 1990; **100**: 175–80.

151. Milano A, Vouhe PR, Baillot-Vernant F *et al.* Late results after left-sided cardiac valve replacement in children. *J Thorac Cardiovasc Surg* 1986; **92**: 218–25.

152. Woods A, Vargas J, Berri G, Kreutzer G, Meschengieser S, Lazzari MA. Antithrombotic therapy in children and adolescents. *Thromb Res* 1986; **42**: 289–301.

153. Bauman M, Massicotte P. Pediatrics. In: O'Shaughnessy D, Makris M, Lillicrap D (eds) *Practical Hemostasis and Thrombosis*, 2nd edn. Oxford: Blackwell Publishing, 2005.

154. Preter M, Tzourio C, Amen A, Bousser MG. Long term prognosis in cerebral venous thrombosis: followup of 77 patients. *Stroke* 1996; **27**: 243–6.

SECTION

8

Supportive Therapy

32

Blood components and fractionated plasma products: preparation, indications and administration

Nancy Robitaille and Heather A. Hume

Blood component transfusion is an integral part of the treatment plan of many of the children and adolescents cared for by the pediatrician or the pediatric hematologist/oncologist. Physicians responsible for the transfusion of blood components should have a basic understanding of the components they prescribe, including the method of preparation, contents, the correct storage conditions, indications and contraindications for use, and procedures for administration. Physicians prescribing blood components should also be knowledgeable about the potential adverse effects of these products including requirements for further modifications of certain components, such as gamma-irradiation or the provision of components at low risk for cytomegalovirus (CMV) transmission, to meet special patient needs. These aspects of blood transfusion therapy are addressed in Chapter 33.

Blood component preparation

Blood components are prepared from blood collected by whole blood (WB) or apheresis donations. WB donations are separated into red blood cell (RBC), plasma (including cryoprecipitate) and platelet components. Automated apheresis procedures may be used to collect platelets, granulocytes or plasma, and more recently RBCs. Plasma protein products, such as albumin, immunoglobulins for intramuscular or intravenous injection and concentrated coagulation factors are prepared by more extensive processing of large pools of donor plasma obtained from WB or plasmapheresis donations. In many countries, the use of human-derived coagulation factor concentrates has been partially or totally replaced by recombinant products.

Preparation of components from whole blood donations

WB is collected into sterile blood bags that contain a premeasured amount of anticoagulant/preservative (AP) solution.

Standard blood bags contain enough AP solution to collect and store 450–500 mL (±10%) of WB. If smaller amounts of WB are to be collected, for example in pediatric autologous blood donations, the amount of AP solution must be adjusted appropriately. Because RBCs, platelets and plasma have different specific gravities they can be separated from each other by differential centrifugation. Generally WB is collected into a primary bag with one, two or three satellite bags depending on the components to be prepared. The satellite bags are attached to the primary bag with integral tubing so that components can be prepared in a closed system that maintains sterility. Two different production methods are regularly used to prepare platelets from whole blood donations: the buffy coat (BC) and the platelet-rich plasma (PRP) methods. The BC method has been used predominantly in Europe while the PRP method is used in North America. Platelets prepared by the BC method are pooled by the blood supplier, using platelets from four to six WB donations to make one pooled BC unit. Platelets prepared by the PRP are usually supplied to hospitals as single units.

Anticoagulant/preservative solutions

Two types of anticoagulant/preservative solutions, namely additive or nonadditive, may be used for blood component collection and storage. Using nonadditive solutions, the entire amount of the AP solution is present in the primary collection bag, whereas the use of additive solutions consists of collecting WB into the primary bag containing an anticoagulant solution and adding the constituents necessary for RBC preservation to the RBCs following separation of the RBCs from the plasma and platelets.

An AP solution for WB or RBC units must fulfill three requirements:
- prevent coagulation of the stored blood unit;
- maintain RBC viability and function;
- be nontoxic when reinfused into the recipient.

WB can only be stored in nonadditive AP solutions; RBCs

Table 32.1 Contents of selected anticoagulant/preservative solutions. Adapted from information supplied by the manufacturers.

Content (g/volume)	CPDA-1 (63 mL)	Adsol™ system		Nutricel™ system		SAG-M	
		Primary bag CPD (63 mL)	Additive AS-1 (100 mL)	Primary bag CP2D (63 mL)	Additive AS-3 (100 mL)	Primary bag CPD (63 mL)	Additive
Trisodium citrate	1.66	1.66	–	1.66	0.588	1.66	–
Dextrose	2.01	1.61	2.20	3.22	1.10	1.61	0.820
Citric acid	0.206	0.206	–	0.206	0.042	0.206	–
Monobasic sodium phosphate	0.140	0.140	–	0.140	0.276	0.140	–
Adenine	0.017	–	0.027	–	0.030	–	0.017
Mannitol	–	–	0.75	–	–	–	–
Sodium chloride	–	–	0.90	–	0.410	0.525	0.877
Shelf-life of RBC units (days)[a]	35	–	35–42	–	35–42	–	35–42
Shelf-life of WB units	35	28		28		28	

[a] Shelf-life varies from country to country according to licencing authorities.

AS, additive solution; CPDA-1, citrate-phosphate-dextrose-adenine anticoagulant.

SAG-M, sodium chloride, adenine, glucose, mannitol.

may be stored in nonadditive or additive AP solutions. All AP solutions contain dextrose, which is a source of metabolic energy; phosphate, which acts as a buffer; and citrate, which, based on its ability to chelate calcium, serves as an anticoagulant. Most contain adenine to maintain the RBC adenine nucleotide pool. Mannitol, which is part of some additive solutions, prevents the hemolysis of RBCs, which can occur in a plasma-poor medium. Licensing of AP solutions, including the accepted duration of RBC storage (the "shelf-life"), depends on the ability of the AP solution to assure 75% recovery of transfused RBCs 24 hours after infusion; hemolysis should be less than 1%.[1,2] RBCs in AP solutions generally have a shelf-life of 42 days, while RBCs stored in citrate-phosphate-dextrose-adenine anticoagulant (CPDA)-1 have a shelf-life of 35 days. In addition to a longer shelf-life for RBCs, the advantages of additive solutions are a lower hematocrit in the RBC unit (which facilitates infusion) and the possibility of extracting larger amounts of plasma (which then can be used for the production of pooled fractionated plasma products) from the original WB unit. Their one disadvantage is a concern (albeit theoretical) about their safety for large volume transfusions in the neonate (see below). The contents of some of the most commonly used AP solutions for RBC storage are shown in Table 32.1.

Increasingly, additive solutions for platelets, rather than plasma, are being used for the storage of platelets, especially where the BC method of platelet preparation is used. As for RBCs, additive solutions for platelets allow the removal of larger amounts of plasma and may increase the shelf-life by improving storage conditions while maintaining viability and hemostatic functions.[3] The decreased amounts of plasma in RBCs and platelets preserved in additive solutions could lead to fewer allergic reactions and increased ease of introduction of pathogen inactivation systems (see below).

The separation of WB into the most commonly used blood components using additive solutions and either the BC or PRP method is shown in Fig. 32.1.[4]

Preparation of components by apheresis techniques

Automated apheresis instruments use computer-controlled technology to draw and anticoagulate blood, separate the blood components either by centrifugation or filtration, collect the desired component, and recombine the remaining components for return to the donor. Automated apheresis procedures are routinely used to separate and collect platelets, granulocytes and plasma. Each apheresis collection can procure larger quantities of one of these components than can be extracted from a single whole blood donation. Because RBC loss for the donor is minimal, repeat donations can be performed at more frequent intervals than is permissible for WB donations. Recently, it has also become possible to collect RBC units using apheresis procedures. Similar to the advantages of apheresis collections for other components, an advantage of this technique is the possibility (depending on donor size and donation intervals) of collecting the equivalent of two WB-derived RBC units in one collection procedure.

Prestorage leukocyte reduction of cellular blood components

Several countries now use only WB, RBC and platelet products that have had the majority of leukocytes removed at the time of preparation, so-called prestorage leukocyte reduction. Other countries use these products only selectively for certain patient populations. Leukocytes are removed from WB or WB-derived components by specially designed

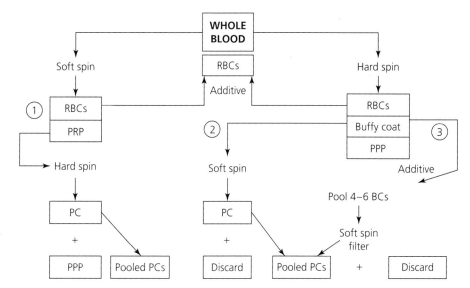

Fig. 32.1 Three ways of preparing platelets from whole blood (see text), BC, buffy coat; PRP, platelet-rich plasma; RBCs, red blood cells; PC, platelet concentrate; PPP, platelet-poor plasma. Reproduced with permission from Reference 4.

leukocyte reduction filters. Leukocytes are removed from apheresis products either by filtration or as an integral part of the apheresis production procedure. The current AABB and US Food and Drug Administration define a leukocyte-reduced component as one with a residual leukocyte count of less than 5×10^6 per unit of RBCs or apheresis (or apheresis equivalent) platelet concentrate.[5] European standards are more stringent and require a leukocyte count less than 1×10^6 per unit.[6]

Leukocyte reduction was introduced in the UK in 1999 primarily as a potential way to avoid prion transmission. However, a recent study suggests that leukocyte reduction may reduce but will not eliminate (in an animal model) transmissible spongiform encephalopathies infectivity.[7] Established advantages of leukocyte reduction (and the reasons for the introduction of universal leukocyte reduction in other countries) include the reduction in febrile non-hemolytic reactions,[8] the prevention of CMV transmission[9] and the prevention of human leukocyte antigen (HLA) alloimmunization.[10,11] A possible reduction in the risk of postoperative infection[12] and post-operative mortality[13,14] is still debated – further research is needed to establish clearly whether or not these are definite advantages of leukocyte reduction.

Pathogen reduction

The risk of the transmission of infectious diseases, in particular human immunodeficiency virus (HIV) and hepatitis C virus, has decreased dramatically over the past 20 years by careful attention to donor selection and improvement in infectious disease testing of donated blood (see Chapter 33). However, this has occurred gradually, and in parallel there has been research to develop the capability to inactivate pathogens in blood components. Efficacious techniques to

inactivate pathogens in pooled fractionated plasma products have been available for many years but until recently there were no techniques that could be applied to cellular components and still preserve the function of these components.

Technologies for pathogen inactivation or reduction of RBCs and platelets are in various stages of clinical trials and/or have received licensure in some countries.[15,16] Two methods of pathogen reduction for plasma are in routine clinical use in Europe: treatment of individual units with methylene blue and solvent/detergent treatment of plasma pools.[17]

Whole blood

Description and storage

A unit of WB has a volume of approximately 510 mL (450 mL WB plus 63 mL CPDA-1) and a hematocrit of 0.30–0.40. It must be stored at 1–6°C and, if collected into CPDA-1, has a shelf-life of 35 days. Within 24 hours of collection the platelets as well as the granulocytes in the unit are dysfunctional and after a few days of storage the labile coagulation factors FV and FVIII have fallen to suboptimal levels.

Indications for transfusion

Theoretically, the transfusion of WB could be used in situations such as rapid, massive blood loss, which require the simultaneous restoration of oxygen-carrying capacity and blood volume. However, in most cases, the resuscitation of such patients can be achieved by the use of RBC concentrates and crystalloids or colloid solutions (either albumin or non-blood-derived colloid solutions such as pentastarch or hexastarch). Should plasma coagulation factor replacement become necessary, the levels of coagulation factors V and VIII in stored WB are rarely sufficient to correct the corresponding deficiencies. Given these considerations, most centers preparing blood components provide little or no WB (except possibly autologous blood) but rather separate WB donations into the more commonly required blood components. Should both coagulation factors and RBCs be required, components are given separately or, in specific situations (e.g., exchange transfusion in the neonate), can be given in the form of reconstituted WB (i.e., the combination, in one blood bag, of an RBC unit and a plasma unit).[18] Debate has existed over the advantages of the use of fresh WB for surgery with cardiopulmonary bypass in neonates. This issue is discussed in the section Red blood cells.

Dosage and administration

WB should not be used unless the donor and recipient are ABO-identical (for use in neonates, see below). The volume of transfusion depends on the clinical situation. In an adult, 1 unit of WB will increase the recipient's hemoglobin (Hb) concentration by approximately 10 g/dL. In pediatric patients, a WB transfusion of 8 mL/kg will result in a similar increase. WB must be administered through a blood filter, either a standard 170 to 260 μm macroaggregate filter or a microaggregate filter. After an initial slow drip (to allow observation for immediate, severe transfusion reactions), the rate of infusion should be as fast as clinically indicated or tolerated, and in all cases must be completed within 4 hours of removal from a temperature-controlled refrigerator (to avoid bacterial contamination).

Red blood cells

Description and storage

RBC concentrates are usually prepared from WB donations (Fig. 32.1) although some blood suppliers now also prepare RBC components using apheresis techniques. RBC concentrates can be further modified for use in specific clinical settings. Characteristics of the various RBC preparations, including their contents and storage conditions, are summarized in Table 32.2.

Indications for transfusion

There are only two valid reasons for transfusing RBCs to children: the most common is to correct an inadequate (or avoid an imminent inadequacy of) oxygen-carrying capacity that is caused by an inadequate RBC mass; the second and rarer indication is to suppress endogenous hemoglobin (Hb)/RBC production in selected thalassemia or sickle-cell disease patients.

Indices of oxygen delivery and tissue oxygenation may accurately indicate the need to transfuse RBCs; however, invasive monitoring is required to generate these indices. Decisions about RBC transfusions are usually made on the basis of easily available but less precise clinical data. Although Hb concentration is certainly one important factor to consider in the decision to administer an RBC transfusion, most experts agree that it is not the only factor; in certain situations such as acute hemorrhage without volume replacement, it may even be misleading. As discussed in detail in several reviews, healthy adults and children have an impressive capacity to increase oxygen delivery to tissues.[20–23] A recent study (albeit in a small number of patients/volunteers) demonstrated that healthy adults subjected to acute normovolemic hemodilution were able to tolerate an Hb concentration of 5 g/dL with no adverse effects.[24] It seems reasonable to assume that this would also be the case for otherwise healthy adolescents and older children.

Studies on indications for RBC transfusions in infants and children

Although there are published clinical guidelines for allogeneic red blood cell transfusions in the pediatric/neonatal population,[25–28] they are poorly substantiated by randomized, controlled trials. A systematic review of the literature addressing allogeneic RBC and plasma transfusions in children (excluding studies addressing neonates or very young infants, or patients with thalassemia or sickle-cell disease) was published in 1997.[22] The literature search identified only three randomized, controlled trials of allogeneic RBC blood transfusion therapy in children.[29–31] Two addressed transfusion issues in the treatment of leukemic children in the 1970s[29,30] and one reported on RBC use in African children with severe anemia and malaria.[31] We performed a similar search using the same keywords that were used in 1997 for the period 1996–2004. No additional randomized, controlled trials on allogeneic RBC transfusion in children were identified. Thus, despite the large numbers of RBC transfusions administered to children, there is a remarkable paucity of scientific data on which to base RBC transfusion decisions. Recommendations and guidelines for RBC transfusions in children are, therefore, for the most part based on expert opinion and experience and not on scientific studies.

RBC transfusions for acute blood loss

In the presence of acute hemorrhage it is important to remember that the first priorities are to correct the hypovolemia (with crystalloids and/or colloids) and to attempt to stop the bleeding. In patients with hematologic problems, the latter will often include the need to correct thrombocytopenia and/or deficiencies of coagulation factors, treatment to decrease bleeding from damaged mucosal barriers (e.g., with

Table 32.2 Characteristics of various preparations of red blood cells.

Component	Preparation	Minimum Hb content*	Approximate volume	Hematocrit	Approximate leukocyte count	Storage	Indication(s)
RBCs in CPDA-1	WB with 200–250 mL of plasma removed	45 g	250 mL	0.70–0.75 L/L	10^9–10^{10}	35 days at 1–6°C	Standard RBC component (see text)
RBCs in AS	WB with most of the plasma removed and AS 100 mL added	45 g	350 mL	0.50–0.60 L/L	10^9–10^{10}	35–42 days at 1–6°C†	Standard RBC component (see text)
RBCs, buffy coat poor in AS	WB with most of the plasma and some leukocytes removed and AS 100 mL added	43 g	300 mL	0.50–0.70 L/L	$<10^9$	35–42 days at 1–6°C†	Standard RBC component or history of repeated febrile and/or allergic reactions
RBCs, leukocyte-reduced by filtration	RBCs in CPDA-1 or AS (with or without BC removed) and leukoreduced by filtration	40 g	Approx. same as non-LR component	CPDA-1: 0.70–0.75 L/L AS: 0.50–0.60 L/L	<1–5×10^6	Prestorage LR: as for non-LR components. Post-storage LR: for immediate infusion	Standard RBC component in some countries History of repeated febrile nonhemolytic reactions Prevention of HLA alloimmunization and/or CMV transmission
RBCs, washed	RBCs in AS or CPDA-1 washed then resuspended with USP	40 g	Variable depending on quantity of USP used for resuspension	Variable depending on quantity of USP used for resuspension	10^8–10^9 if prepared from non-LR component or as per LR component	24 h at 1–6°C‡	History of repeated febrile and/or allergic reactions unresponsive to BC-poor or LR RBCs Prevention of severe allergic reactions or anaphylaxis due to anti-IgA
RBCs, frozen-deglycerolized	RBCs frozen with glycerol (a cryoprotectant); thawed and deglycerolized by washing before transfusion. Resuspended in USP	36 g	Variable depending on quantity of USP used for resuspension	Variable depending on quantity of USP used for resuspension	10^8–10^9 if prepared from non-LR component or as per LR component	May be stored frozen for up to 10 years After thawing: storage at 1–6°C for 24 h‡	Prolonged storage of autologous units or allogeneic units with rare RBC phenotypes

* Council of Europe Standards.[19]

† Shelf-life varies from country to country depending on licencing authorities.

‡ There are now systems that allow washing or thawing of RBC units in a closed system so that storage may be extended to 7–14 days.

AS, additive solution; BC, buffy coat; CPDA-1, citrate–phosphate–dextrose–adenine anticoagulant; CMV, cytomegalovirus; HLA, human leukocyte antigen; LR, leukoreduced; RBC, red blood cell; USP, 0.9% sodium chloride injection; WB, whole blood.

Table 32.3 Classification of hemorrhagic shock in pediatric patients based on systemic signs.

System	Class I: very mild hemorrhage (<15% TBV loss)	Class II: mild hemorrhage (15–25% TBV loss)	Class III: moderate hemorrhage (26–39% TBV loss)	Class IV: severe hemorrhage (≥40% TBV loss)
Cardiovascular	Heart rate normal or mildly increased	Tachycardia	Significant tachycardia	Severe tachycardia
	Normal pulses	Peripheral pulses may be diminished	Thready peripheral pulses	Thready peripheral pulses
	Normal blood pressure	Normal blood pressure	Hypotension	Significant hypotension
	Normal pH	Normal pH	Metabolic acidosis	Significant acidosis
Respiratory	Rate normal	Tachypnea	Moderate tachypnea	Severe tachypnea
Central nervous system	Slightly anxious	Irritable, confused, combative	Irritable or lethargic, diminished pain response	Coma
Skin	Warm, pink	Cool extremities, mottling	Cool extremities, mottling or pallor	Cold extremities, pallor or cyanosis
	Capillary refill brisk	Delayed capillary refill	Prolonged capillary refill	Prolonged capillary refill
Renal	Normal urine output	Oliguria, increased specific gravity (urine)	Oliguria, increased BUN	Anuria

BUN, blood urea nitrogen; TBV, total blood volume.
Reproduced with permission from Ref. 33.

antifibrinolytics) and/or reversal of the effects of anticoagulant therapy. In patients with normal or near-normal Hb levels prior to the onset of hemorrhage, RBC transfusions are usually only necessary if the patient remains unstable following volume resuscitation. However, careful ongoing evaluation of children with acute blood loss is essential as the signs of shock may initially be subtle in the child. If acute hemorrhage totals more than 15% of blood volume, signs of circulatory failure (tachycardia, decrease of intensity of peripheral pulses, delayed capillary refill and cool extremities) will be observed. However, hypotension will not be present until 25–30% or more of the child's blood volume is lost.[32] It is also important to realize that in the setting of rapid ongoing hemorrhage with hypovolemia, the Hb concentration may not be an accurate indication of the actual RBC mass, so that the clinical evaluation of the blood loss is critical. The classification of hemorrhagic shock in children based on systemic signs is shown in Table 32.3.[33] Guidelines for the resuscitation of pediatric patients with acute blood loss have been published and should be followed.[34]

RBC transfusions for acute hemolysis

Unlike acute hemorrhage, where the patient suffers from both hypovolemia and a decreased RBC mass, patients with acute hemolysis are usually normovolemic. The Hb concentration therefore more accurately reflects RBC mass. The decision to administer an RBC transfusion depends upon a combination of factors, including ongoing clinical evaluation,

presence or absence of underlying cardiovascular disease, actual Hb concentration, rate of decrease in Hb concentration and possibility of alternate treatments (e.g., corticosteroids for IgG autoimmune hemolytic anemia). The management of a patient with acute severe hemolytic anemia due to the presence of a warm autoantibody presents a particularly difficult challenge to the hematologist. There are two potential problems: the first concerns the provision of appropriate blood should transfusion be necessary, and the second is the possibility of hemolysis of the transfused blood because most autoantibodies also react with transfused allogeneic RBCs. If the autoantibody is present in the patient's plasma (as well as on the surface of the patient's red cells), it is usually impossible to provide cross-match-compatible blood and, in patients who have been previously transfused or pregnant, the autoantibody may mask the presence of clinically significant alloantibodies. With respect to the second problem, transfused RBCs will have a shortened survival in patients with autoimmune hemolytic anemia but immediate transfusion reactions are rare.[35] If possible then, in this setting the choice of blood to administer and the decision to administer an RBC transfusion should be made in consultation with a transfusion medicine physician, because special serologic techniques might be indicated in order to identify clinically significant alloantibodies, and decisions about transfusing cross-match-incompatible blood will often have to be made. However, life-saving RBC transfusions should not be withheld from patients with autoantibodies even if such blood is cross-match-incompatible.[35]

RBC transfusion for chronic anemia

The majority of patients for whom a pediatric hematologist/ oncologist will consider administering an RBC transfusion have a slowly developing subacute or chronic anemia. In this setting, decisions regarding RBC transfusion rarely need to be taken rapidly. It is therefore possible to consider several factors in the decision to administer an RBC transfusion or series of transfusions and to involve the patient and/or the patient's parents in the decision. Factors to be considered should include:

• presence or absence of symptoms and/or abnormal physical signs and the likelihood that these are due to anemia;
• presence or absence of underlying diseases, particularly cardiac diseases, which may decrease the patient's capacity for cardiovascular compensation;
• likely evolution of the underlying disease causing the anemia;
• likely evolution of the anemia and its consequences with or without transfusion in both the short and long term;
• possibility of using alternate, safer therapies for the treatment of the anemia.

In general, when deciding to administer an RBC transfusion the above factors are often more important than the Hb concentration *per se*. For example, patients with Diamond–Blackfan anemia unresponsive to corticosteroids are usually placed on a chronic transfusion program with minimum pretransfusion Hb levels of 6–7 g/dL in order to maintain growth and an acceptable long-term quality of life. In contrast, young, otherwise healthy children with severe iron deficiency anemia may temporarily tolerate Hb levels as low as 4 g/dL provided they are being monitored and iron therapy has been initiated. Patients with anemia due to chronic kidney disease are usually treated with iron supplementation and recombinant erythropoietin.

RBC transfusions for patients receiving chemotherapy for leukemia or solid tumors are often given according to a predetermined protocol based on Hb level alone. However, there is no scientific basis to this practice, and in the absence of appropriate studies, clinical judgment as to the benefit:risk ratio should be used for these patients too.

The transfusion support of children with sickle-cell disease or clinically significant thalassemia syndromes requires several special considerations as discussed below.

RBC transfusions for sickle-cell disease

The administration of RBC transfusions in the management and/or prevention of the complications of sickle-cell disease (SCD) is so frequent that almost all adult HbSS patients and many HbSC or HbS/β-thalassemia patients have been transfused at least once and often multiple times. RBC transfusions are administered to SCD patients for two reasons: to increase oxygen-carrying capacity in the anemic patient

and/or to replace the abnormal HbS by normal HbA. Depending on the complication and goal of transfusion, RBC transfusions may be administered as simple transfusions or exchange transfusions, with either being used acutely or in a chronic transfusion program.[36,37]

Simple RBC transfusions (10–20 mL/kg) are used acutely to treat major splenic sequestration and aplastic crises. In acute splenic sequestration, the spleen rapidly increases in size, leading to sequestration of blood within it. In young children, the splenic sequestration may be sufficiently severe to lead to life-threatening hypovolemic shock. Parvovirus B19 infection in patients with SCD results in temporary aplasia, which may be severe, with hemoglobin levels of 4 g/dL or less. RBC transfusions are also used episodically to manage acute chest syndrome, acute stroke or severe anemia with infection, in particular malaria. Management of leg ulcers and acute or recurrent priapism with RBC transfusion is more controversial.

Transfusions are not indicated for uncomplicated painful crises. However, occasionally an exaggerated hemolysis, associated with an episode of pain, may herald the onset of multiorgan failure syndrome, which appears to respond to RBC transfusion.

The necessity of RBC transfusion prior to surgery in the SCD patient (either simple transfusion to attain a certain total Hb level or exchange transfusion to reduce the HbS level) has been debated in the literature. A large multicenter study comparing an aggressive transfusion regimen (decreasing HbS level less than 0.30%) to a conservative regimen (increasing the Hb level to 10 g/dL without consideration of the HbS concentration) in HbSS or S/β-thalassemia patients showed no difference in perioperative complications between the two groups.[38] However, transfusion-related complications were twice as common (14%) in the exchange transfusion arm, compared with the simple transfusion arm (7%). These data confirm the safety of using simple transfusions to raise the Hb level to 10 g/dL for common surgical interventions such as tonsillectomy, cholecystectomy, splenectomy and orthopedic procedures in these patients. The role of blood transfusion in SCD patients undergoing very minor procedures (such as myringotomy) or for patients with HbSC disease has not been well studied.

In children with cerebral vascular accidents (CVAs) associated with SCD, the administration of regular RBC transfusions to maintain an HbS level below 0.30% in the first 2 years after the CVA and below 0.50% thereafter has been shown to prevent recurrent CVAs.[39–41] Moreover, it has been shown that a transfusion program in children with SCD who have abnormal results on transcranial Doppler ultrasonography can reduce the risk of a first CVA by 90%.[42] A study to determine if these transfusions could be stopped after 30 months (STOP 2,[42a]) showed that discontinuation of transfusion in children whose Doppler readings had become normal resulted in a high rate of reversion to abnormal readings and stroke. Another potential indication for a chronic transfusion program is the presence of silent cerebral infarct (SCI) on magnetic resonance imaging (MRI). The Silent Cerebral Infarct Transfusion Trial (SIT) is a multicenter, randomized, controlled study that is investigating whether prophylactic transfusion therapy in children with SCI will result in reduction in the proportion of patients with clinically evident stroke or new or progressive SCI.[43] Chronic transfusion programs may also be indicated in selected patients with severe or recurrent acute chest syndrome or recurrent, debilitating painful episodes.

A major problem in the transfusion support of SCD patients is RBC alloimmunization due partly to the racial (and hence RBC phenotype) differences between the donor (often mainly Caucasian) and recipient populations.[44] Alloimmunization rates as high as 47% have been reported in adult patients with SCD.[45] A number of experts therefore recommend providing blood that is phenotypically matched (in addition to ABO and D antigens) for at least C, c, E, e and Kell antigens,[36,46,47] and this is now standard practice in many comprehensive sickle-cell programs.

RBC units for transfusion to SCD patients should be screened for the presence of HbS and transfused only if negative. This will avoid confusion when the goal of transfusion is to decrease the HbS level to a predetermined level and will prevent the use of blood from a donor with undiagnosed HbSC disease.

In vitro, the viscosity of HbS has been shown to increase to potentially clinically significant levels if the hematocrit exceeds 0.35 L/L.[48] Therefore, when transfusing SCD patients, especially in the presence of high HbS levels, the hematocrit should not be allowed to increase above 0.35 L/L. Neurologic events, including headache, seizures and CVA, have been described after exchange transfusion in SCD.[49] It has been postulated that some of these events may have been caused by hyperviscosity, although other factors may also have been important in at least some of the patients.

A rare but potentially fatal complication occurring in patients with SCD is a hyperhemolytic transfusion reaction. Patients typically present about a week following an RBC transfusion and, in addition to evidence of hemolysis, may have symptoms of an acute painful crisis.[50–53] Both donor and recipient red blood cells are destroyed, and reticulocytopenia may be a feature of the syndrome. Further transfusions can exacerbate the hemolysis and should be avoided if at all possible; alternative treatment with steroids and intravenous immunoglobulin (IVIG) may be life-saving.[53–55]

SCD patients in chronic transfusion programs will develop secondary iron overload. The net amount of iron infused can be decreased by using partial exchange transfusion.[56] Another option is the use of automated erythrocytopheresis to delay or even prevent the development of hemochromatosis.[57–59] Chelation therapy is an effective treatment of iron overload but compliance can be problematic

RBC transfusions for β-thalassemia

Before the introduction of RBC transfusion therapy for β-thalassemia major in the 1950s, β-thalassemia major was a uniformly fatal disease. Initially, children were transfused only to hemoglobin levels of 5–6 g/dL, a level sufficient to ensure survival but insufficient to suppress the exuberant erythroid bone marrow hyperplasia characteristic of this disorder. Consequently, patients survived into their second decade but developed severe skeletal deformities, osteoporosis and splenomegaly. So-called hypertransfusion regimens, in which endogenous erythroid production is suppressed by maintaining a minimum pretransfusion hemoglobin level of 9–10 g/dL, were therefore gradually introduced in the 1960s and 1970s, and remain the commonest approach today.[60,61] During the 1980s, investigators evaluated the possibility of further improving the quality of life of thalassemic patients by introducing a "supertransfusion" regimen in which the minimum pretransfusion hemoglobin level was kept entirely within the normal range.[62] However, this regimen led, not surprisingly, to a significant increase in transfusion requirements and has since been abandoned by most physicians caring for thalassemia patients.

Another approach investigated during the 1980s was the possibility of decreasing transfusion exposure and increasing transfusion intervals through the use of young RBCs. These "neocytes," with an average age of 12–21 days, can be collected by erythrocytapheresis or by fractionation of standard whole blood units using a cell processor. The studies performed in the 1980s reported only modest decreases of 12–16% in transfusion requirements; the use of neocyte transfusions was therefore abandoned.[63,64] In the mid-1990s, the use of a newly developed neocyte-separation set (Neocel System, Cutter Biological, Berkeley, CA) was reported.[65,66] Using this system, there is a 15–20% reduction in transfused iron load. Nevertheless, the costs of this system are higher and donor exposure per transfusion episode is approximately doubled.

Chronic transfusions in β-thalassemia patients will lead to iron overload and its associated complications, mainly liver disease, endocrine complications and cardiomyopathy.[60,61,67] Chelation therapy with subcutaneous deferoxamine has been the standard treatment for years but its cost and mode of administration can interfere with compliance. Recently two oral iron chelators, deferiprone and deferasirox, have been licensed for use in some countries. The availability of these oral agents may change the approach to the management of iron over-load in the future.[67]

One of the most difficult decisions facing physicians treating patients with thalassemia is the necessity of instituting a chronic RBC transfusion program for patients with thalassemia intermedia and hemoglobin levels of 6–7 g/dL. In addition to the considerations discussed above for patients with chronic anemia, the physician must take into account the fact that nontransfused thalassemia intermedia patients may develop bone deformities due to bone marrow erythroid hyperplasia, and even without RBC transfusions, these patients may develop clinically significant hemochromatosis secondary to the increased intestinal iron absorption induced by their inefficient erythropoiesis.[60] If a transfusion program is embarked upon, the goals of transfusion therapy are the same as those outlined above for thalassemia major patients. The transfusion intervals can usually be longer, although it may be more difficult to completely suppress endogenous erythropoiesis in thalassemia intermedia patients than in thalassemia major patients.

Blood group choice, dosage and administration

Acceptable choices of ABO blood groups for RBC, plasma and platelet transfusions in children are shown in Table 32.4. For RBC transfusions, these choices are based on the principle that the recipient plasma must not contain antibodies (anti-A/B) corresponding to donor A and/or B antigens. For plasma transfusions, donor plasma must not contain A/B antibodies corresponding to recipient A/B antigens, and as far as possible this rule should also be followed for platelet transfusions (see Platelets below). Patients who are RhD-antigen positive may receive RhD-positive or -negative RBCs; patients who are RhD negative should receive only RhD-negative RBCs (except possibly in life-threatening hemorrhagic emergencies if RhD-negative blood is not available). The choice of ABO blood group for RBC as well as platelet and plasma transfusion is more complicated for allogeneic hematopoietic progenitor cell transplantation patients receiving transplants from ABO-mismatched donors. Recommended choices of ABO group for blood components for these patients are shown in Table 32.5.[68]

All pediatric patients who are likely to receive multiple RBC transfusions should have an extended RBC phenotype prior to the first RBC transfusion. In addition to ABO and RhD phenotyping, an extended RBC phenotype usually includes the determination of the other common Rhesus antigens (C, c, E and e) as well as the common antigens of the Kell, Kidd, Duffy and MNS blood group systems. Patients for whom this should be done include those with congenital or acquired aplastic anemia, autoimmune hemolytic anemia, SCD, thalassemia major or intermedia, or other transfusion-dependent congenital anemias and patients undergoing hematopoietic progenitor cell transplantation. Knowing a patient's extended RBC phenotype will assist in the identification of irregular RBC antibodies should they develop. In addition, RBC units matched for antigens other than ABO and RhD may be desirable for patients with thalassemia syndromes or SCD to prevent the development of alloantibodies (see above).[36,46,47,69]

The quantity of blood administered in simple RBC transfusions depends on the hematocrit of the RBC unit, the pre-

Table 32.4 Choice of ABO blood groups for red blood cell (RBC), plasma and platelet transfusions in children.

Recipient blood group		Acceptable ABO group of blood component to be transfused		
		RBCs*	Plasma	Platelets[†]
O	First choice	O	O	O
	Second choice	None	A, B, AB	A, B, AB
A	First choice	A	A	A
	Second choice	O	AB	AB
B	First choice	B	B	B
	Second choice	O	AB	AB
AB	First choice	AB	AB	AB
	Second choice	A, B, O	None	See footnote

* The choices of ABO blood groups for RBC transfusion may not be appropriate for newborns and infants < 4 months of age in whom the potential presence of maternal anti-A/B must also be considered.
† In emergency situations platelets in plasma with A/B antibodies against recipient A/B antigens may be transfused. However, where possible such units should not be used unless the anti-A/B is of low titer and/or the plasma has been removed. This is especially important for infants and young children (see text).

transfusion Hb level and the patient's weight. If the patient's Hb level is 5 g/dL or greater, and blood stored in an additive solution (hematocrit 0.50–0.60 L/L) is used, 15 mL/kg is usually administered. This can be expected to raise the hemoglobin level by approximately 2 g/dL. To obtain the same result using blood stored in CPDA-1 (hematocrit 0.70–0.75 L/L), a transfusion of 10 mL/kg is needed. For patients who weigh < 20 kg, the volume of an entire RBC unit is too large to be administered during one transfusion. In order to minimize donor exposure, attempts should be made to use the entire unit, either by giving two or three small transfusions over a 24-hour period if the unit is opened in a non-sterile manner, or by entering the unit using a sterile docking device and transfusing appropriately sized aliquots before the unit's original expiry date.

If the anemia has developed slowly and the hemoglobin level is < 5 g/dL, it may be necessary to administer RBC transfusions more slowly and/or in smaller quantities to avoid precipitating cardiac failure from circulatory overload. A transfusion regimen for the treatment of children with severe anemia of gradual onset without clinical signs of cardiac decompensation has been published.[70] The authors successfully treated 22 such children using RBCs with a hematocrit of 0.70–0.80 L/L at a continuous infusion rate of 2 mL/kg/h until the desired Hb level was achieved. If a severely anemic child has signs of cardiac decompensation, a partial exchange transfusion should be performed.

Table 32.5 Transfusion support for patients undergoing ABO-mismatched allogeneic hematopoietic progenitor cell (HPC) transplantation.

Recipient	Donor	Mismatch type	Phase I* All components	RBCs	Phase II† First-choice platelets	Next-choice platelets§	FFP	Phase III‡ All components
A	O	Minor	Recipient	O	A	AB, B, O	A, AB	Donor
B	O	Minor	Recipient	O	B	AB, A, O	B, AB	Donor
AB	O	Minor	Recipient	O	AB	A, B, O	AB	Donor
AB	A	Minor	Recipient	A	AB	A, B, O	AB	Donor
AB	B	Minor	Recipient	B	AB	B, A, O	AB	Donor
O	A	Major	Recipient	O	A	AB, B, O	A, AB	Donor
O	B	Major	Recipient	O	B	AB, A, O	B, AB	Donor
O	AB	Major	Recipient	O	AB	A, B, O	AB	Donor
A	AB	Major	Recipient	A	AB	A, B, O	AB	Donor
B	AB	Major	Recipient	B	AB	B, A, O	AB	Donor
A	B	Minor & major	Recipient	O	AB	A, B, O	AB	Donor
B	A	Minor & major	Recipient	O	AB	B, A, O	AB	Donor

* Phase I: from the time when the patient/recipient is prepared for HPC transplantation.

† Phase II: from the initiation of myeloablative therapy until:

For RBC, DAT direct antiglobulin test is negative and antidonor isohemagglutinins are no longer detectable.

For FFP, recipient's erythrocytes are no longer detectable (i.e., the forward typing is consistent with donor's ABO group).

‡ Phase III: after the forward and the reverse type of the patient are consistent with donor's ABO group.

§ Platelet concentrates should be selected in the order presented.

Reproduced with permission from Ref. 68.

Guidelines for performing partial manual exchange transfusions have been published.[56,71] Alternatively, where available, automated red blood cell exchanges can be performed even in critically ill pediatric patients.[57,72,73]

RBC units must be administered through a blood filter, either a standard 170 to 260-μm macroaggregate filter or a microaggregate filter or, if the unit was not leukocyte-reduced prestorage, a leukocyte-reduction filter may be used. RBC transfusions must be completed within 4 hours from the time the unit is removed from a temperature-controlled refrigerator.

Special considerations for newborns

Indications for RBC transfusions

Very-low-birthweight (VLBW) infants frequently require small-volume (10–20 mL/kg) RBC transfusions. In the early 1990s, it was estimated that approximately 80% of infants weighing < 1.5 kg born in the USA received RBC transfusions in the first weeks of life.[74] Currently, transfusion practices and/or requirements for VLBW infants appear to be changing. In a recent observational clinical study from a single institution, the authors report that over a 9-year period (1989 to 1997), with the use of more restrictive transfusion guidelines, the number and volume of transfusions per infant weighing < 1000 g decreased by 71% and donor exposure by 80%; 25% of infants weighing < 1000 g born in 1995–1997 were never transfused compared with 3% born 1989–1991.[75]

There are three major factors contributing to small-volume RBC transfusion requirements in VLBW infants.

1 *The rapid decline in Hb levels that occurs in the first weeks of life.* In the healthy term infant, the mean cord blood Hb level is 16.8 g/dL, rising to 18.4 g/dL in venous blood by 24 hours of life and then gradually decreasing to a mean nadir of 11.5 g/dL (with a lower limit of normal of 9.0 g/dL) at 2 months of life.[76] Because this decline in Hb level occurs in all neonates, and in term infants, at least, is not associated with any adverse events, it is called the physiologic anemia of infancy. In preterm infants Hb levels at birth are slightly lower than those of term infants (14.5 g/dL and 15.0 g/dL at 28 and 34 weeks gestation, respectively), and the decline in Hb level occurs earlier and is more pronounced. For example, the hemoglobin concentration may drop to 8.0 g/dL in neonates with birthweights of 1.0–1.5 kg, and to 7.0 g/dL in neonates with birthweights below 1.0 kg.[76] Erythropoietin levels in preterm infants at the time of the nadir of hemoglobin levels are lower than those usually found in children or adults with similar hemoglobin levels and therefore probably explain, at least partly, the drop in hemoglobin levels.[77]

2 *The associated respiratory illnesses often present in these infants.* Early in life VLBW infants are at risk for respiratory distress syndrome, which in some may lead to bronchopulmonary dysplasia with continuing requirements for respiratory support. Even relatively stable infants may develop cardiorespiratory irregularities such as apnea and/or bradycardia. The necessity of maintaining hemoglobin values at a predetermined level in infants with these problems is somewhat controversial and has been the subject of several studies and review articles.[78,79]

3 *Phlebotomy losses.* Because of the need for laboratory monitoring of ill neonates and the relatively large volumes of blood required in relation to these tiny infants' total blood volumes, phlebotomy losses contribute significantly to the need for RBC transfusions in VLBW infants. Care must be taken to avoid blood overdraw. A recent study estimated that the mean volume of blood overdraw for all blood tests was 19% in a neonatal intensive care unit, and this could account for 5–15% of the RBC transfusion received by VLBW infants.[80]

Adhering to strict transfusion guidelines can reduce the need for transfusions.[75,81] Several guidelines for small-volume RBC transfusions for newborns have been published in recent years.[25–27,82–84] Two sets of guidelines are shown in Tables 32.6 and 32.7. However, controlled trials evaluating

Table 32.6 British guidelines for RBC transfusion thresholds for infants under 4 months of age.

Anemia in the first 24 hours	Hb 12.0 g/dL (Hct 0.36)
Cumulative blood loss in 1 week, neonate requiring intensive care	10% blood volume
Neonate receiving intensive care	Hb 12.0 g/dL
Acute blood loss	10% blood volume
Chronic oxygen dependency	Hb 11.0 g/dL
Late anemia, stable patient	Hb 7.0 g/dL

Reproduced with permission from Ref. 25.

Table 32.7 Suggested guidelines (USA publication) for RBC transfusion thresholds for infants under 4 months of age.

Hematocrit	Threshold criteria for RBC transfusion
<0.35 L/L	Patient is on mechanical ventilation requiring fraction of inspired oxygen ($F_{\mathrm{i}O_2}$) > 40% or mean arterial pressure > 9 cmH$_2$O Patient has hypotension

<0.28 L/L	Patient is on mechanical ventilation but $F_{\mathrm{i}O_2}$ is < 40% and mean arterial pressure is < 9 cmH$_2$O
	Patient has been weaned from mechanical ventilation, but still has a significant oxygen requirement (>40%)
	Patient has signs of anemia such as:
	  Unexplained apnea, 12 spells per day or two spells per day that require bag-mask resuscitation
	  Unexplained heart rate greater than 165/min for more than 48 hours
	  Unexplained poor weight gain, <10 g/kg daily over 1 week with adequate caloric intake
	  Unexplained lethargy

<0.20 L/L	No signs of anemia are required

Modified with permission from Ref. 84.

transfusion thresholds are rare. A multicenter randomized, controlled trial "Prematures in Need of Transfusion" (PINT) investigating whether a higher Hb transfusion threshold is superior to a lower one with respect to morbidity and mortality in extremely low-birthweight (<1000 g) infants has recently been completed. In a preliminary presentation, the investigators reported that the higher Hb transfusion threshold was not superior, suggesting that conservative transfusion regimens may be safely used in preterm infants.[85]

There are three clinical settings in which newborns may require large-volume RBC transfusion: exchange transfusion, surgery with cardiopulmonary bypass or during treatment with extracorporeal membrane oxygenation (ECMO). The mechanics, blood product choice and complications associated with each of these procedures have been thoroughly reviewed.[25,86]

Practical considerations

RBC units for transfusion to neonates are often chosen exclusively from group O donors, although ABO isogroup (or compatible) units can be used providing the technologists preparing the blood are experienced in the choice of units for those patients in whom the potential presence of maternal A and/or B antibodies needs to be considered. RBC units stored in any of the currently available storage media, including additive solutions, are suitable for small-volume (<20 mL/kg) RBC transfusions.[87] Several studies have demonstrated the safety of assigning a fresh (<5 days old) RBC unit to a neonatal patient at the time of his/her first small-volume RBC transfusion and, using a sterile connection device, of continuing to use this same unit up to its normal expiry date for subsequent small-volume RBC transfusions.[88] Precise descriptions for preparing small-volume RBC aliquots for neonates have been published.[89,90]

In settings of large-volume RBC transfusion, replacement of plasma coagulation factors is often also required so that WB or reconstituted WB, that is, an RBC unit mixed with a unit of fresh frozen plasma (FFP) or frozen plasma (FP), is usually used. For WB, or the RBC unit for reconstituted WB, the choice of ABO group is the same as that described above for small-volume RBC transfusions. The ABO group of the FFP or FP must also be compatible with the baby's RBCs (see Table 32.4). This may mean that the ABO groups of the RBC unit and the FFP or FP unit are different; for example, for a group A baby with maternal anti-A in his plasma, a unit of reconstituted WB would be prepared using a group O RBC unit and a group A FFP or FP unit. To limit donor exposure, some physicians use group O whole blood in this setting, although units from group O donors with high anti-A titers should not be used.

WB units or RBC units for large-volume transfusions should be relatively fresh, i.e., not > 5–7 days old. The main reason for this precaution is the high potassium concentration in stored WB or RBC units. While this does not pose a problem in the setting of small-volume transfusions (<20 mL/kg) administered slowly (over 3 or 4 hours), the potassium content of stored blood, when administered rapidly and in large volumes, may be lethal for a neonatal patient.[91]

The debate over the use of WB versus reconstituted blood in surgery with cardiopulmonary bypass (CPB) in neonates and infants is still not resolved. In one prospective, controlled study the use of very fresh WB (<48 h storage) postoperatively resulted in less bleeding in patients younger than 2 years old undergoing complex procedures and, additionally, in neonates a decrease in the rate of reexploration for bleeding.[92] However, in a more recent randomized, controlled trial the use of fresh whole blood (<48 h) for cardiopulmonary bypass priming in neonates had no advantage over reconstituted whole blood, and fresh whole blood was associated with an increased length of stay in the intensive care unit and an increased perioperative fluid overload at 48 hours.[93]

A screening test for the presence of a sickling Hb should be performed and found to be negative on RBC or WB units for large-volume transfusions in neonates.[94]

Finally, there are at least theoretical concerns that the constituents of additive solutions may be harmful to newborns if infused in large quantities, as could occur with exchange transfusion, CPB surgery or ECMO. In these situations it is recommended that the additive solutions be removed either by washing the RBCs or by centrifuging the unit and removing the supernatant.[87] The packed RBCs are then reconstituted in saline, albumin, FFP or FP as required. Alternately RBCs collected in nonadditive solutions may be used.

Strategies to decrease RBC allogeneic donor exposures

The first and possibly the most important strategy in limiting donor exposure is to administer an RBC blood transfusion only in the presence of an appropriate indication. The risks versus the anticipated benefits should be individually considered for every transfusion a physician orders. A second and equally simple strategy is to ensure the optimum utilization of each blood unit. When transfusing RBC units to very small patients, attempts should be made to use the whole unit (see above). In some situations, described below, allogeneic donor exposure may be avoided or limited using additional, special strategies.

Autologous transfusions

Autologous blood transfusion, that is, the collection and reinfusion of the patient's own blood, can be used for selected pediatric surgical patients. Three types of autologous blood transfusion can be used in surgical patients:

• preoperative blood collection and storage with reinfusion intraoperatively or postoperatively;

• immediate preoperative phlebotomy (following anesthetic induction) accompanied by normovolemic hemodilution with colloids or crystalloids;

• intraoperative salvage and reinfusion of shed blood.

Guidelines for the use of autologous blood transfusion in the surgical setting have been published.[95–99]

The majority of the published experience with autologous blood transfusion for pediatric patients addresses the use of preoperative autologous blood deposit (PAD). For both adults and children, PAD is considered most appropriate for patients predicted to have significant postoperative longevity who are scheduled to undergo a procedure in which there is a significant likelihood of transfusion and for whom the PAD procedure is likely to be well tolerated.[95–102] PAD is usually reserved for older pediatric patients, for example adolescents undergoing orthopedic procedures, in particular spinal fusion.[103–105] In this setting, preoperative collection of autologous blood is clearly feasible and decreases the need for allogeneic blood transfusion.

There are published reports describing the use of predeposit autologous blood collections in smaller and younger pediatric patients (with several patients 3 years old or younger and/or weighing as little as 10–12 kg).[106–108] Autologous blood collection is feasible in these patients but consideration must be given to several aspects unique to the pediatric setting. These include both psychologic factors such as the creation of an appropriate environment and the need for parental encouragement and commitment to the program, as well as technical considerations such as the use of local anesthesia at the venipuncture site, the use of needles smaller than the standard size (this can be accomplished using a sterile connection device), and the need to adjust the amount of anticoagulant in the collection bag according to the amount of blood collected. In the published reports, deposit of autologous blood appears to decrease the requirements for allogeneic blood transfusion in these smaller patients. However, the decision to embark on such a program should be individualized and should include a realistic prediction of whether or not sufficient blood can be collected to avoid the need for allogeneic blood transfusion.

Pediatric patients participating in autologous predeposit programs should receive iron supplementation, beginning if possible at least 3 weeks before the first donation and continuing into the postoperative period. Although the risks of autologous blood transfusion are less than those associated with allogeneic transfusion, autologous blood is not entirely risk free. Many experts therefore recommend using the same criteria for the transfusion of autologous blood as for allogeneic blood.[28]

The use of acute normovolemic hemodilution and intraoperative RBC salvage in adult patients has been extensively reported.[98,99] There are some studies examining the use of these two modalities in children.[109–112] While these approaches to decrease the requirement for allogeneic blood transfusion in pediatric patients will probably prove to be useful in selected patients, their exact roles remain to be defined.

The use of placental blood as a type of autologous blood transfusion for neonates has been investigated. A simple way to administer placental blood at birth is to slightly delay cord clamping. Most (but not all) studies show a clinical, or a theoretical, benefit for delayed cord clamping in preterm infants.[113–118] A second method, namely the collection, storage and reinfusion of placental blood, is obviously considerably more complicated and currently must be considered experimental.[119–123]

Erythropoietin

The efficacy of recombinant human erythropoietin (rHuEpo) for the correction of the anemia of chronic renal failure is now well established in both pediatric and adult patients.[124] In pediatrics, outside of the setting of uremia, the role for rHuEpo has been most extensively studied in preterm infants with anemia of prematurity. Despite a relatively large number of studies (reviewed in Refs 79 and 125), this indication remains controversial. It is generally agreed that rHuEpo is not indicated for infants with birthweights > 1300 g because they rarely require RBC transfusions. It also appears unlikely that rHuEpo can avoid the requirement for RBC transfusion in VLBW infants, for example those with birthweights < 800 g. In infants with birthweights between 800 and 1300 g, rHuEpo administration (in association with relatively large amounts of iron supplementation) does enhance erythropoiesis, and in several studies has decreased the number and/or quantity of RBC transfusions. However, these studies have not convincingly shown that donor exposures would in fact be decreased. If stringent transfusion guidelines are followed, methods to decrease iatrogenic blood loss are implemented and dedicated RBC units reused up to their expiry date, there is unlikely to be a role for routine use of erythropoietin in preterm neonates.

In October 2002, the American Society of Hematology and the American Society of Clinical Oncology jointly published guidelines for the use of erythropoietin in adult patients with anemia associated with cancer, chemotherapy, radiotherapy or bone marrow failure. These guidelines recommend that erythropoietin be a treatment option for patients with an Hb level of 10 g/dL or less.[126] Similar guidelines have recently been published in Europe.[127,128] However, the systematic reviews on which these recommendations were made were based on studies in adults. This, plus the differences in normal Hb concentrations between children and adults, means that these guidelines cannot be extrapolated to children. Definitive guidelines for the use of rHuEpo in pediatric oncology and hematopoietic progenitor transplant patients are therefore yet to be defined. Likewise there are no definitive guidelines for rHuEpo in the treatment of children undergoing surgical procedures.

Directed donations and limited-exposure blood donor programs

A directed blood donation is one in which an individual, at the request of a patient, or in the case of a child, a parent, donates blood that is reserved specifically for the subsequent transfusion of the requesting patient. When parents wish to be directed donors for their children, or request other family members or friends to do so, it is presumably because they believe that blood from such donors is less likely to be a source of transfusion-transmitted diseases than blood from an anonymous volunteer blood donor pool. Whether or not this is in fact true has been a source of controversy in the literature.[129,130] The few studies that have been performed suggest that directed donations are neither more nor less safe than donations from volunteer anonymous donors.[131–133]

Apart from the question of safety with respect to the transmission of viral infections, there are additional safety issues to consider when parents give blood for their children. In the case of neonates, blood from biologic mothers poses a potential danger because their plasma may contain HLA antibodies that could react with HLA antigens on the infant's leukocytes and/or platelets leading to neutropenia, thrombocytopenia and/or transfusion-related acute lung injury. *In utero* the placenta provides a natural barrier to these antibodies, one that obviously would be bypassed with a blood transfusion. For this reason, it has been suggested that biologic mothers should not provide blood components containing plasma for their neonates and that maternal red cells and platelets be given as washed products.[134]

Biologic fathers may also pose certain difficulties. A father may possess a red cell antigen, not inherited by his infant, to which the mother may have developed an IgG antibody. These antibodies cross the placenta but obviously would cause no harm *in utero*. Most such antibodies are easily detected by routine pretransfusion testing. However, should such an antibody be directed against an uncommon or private antigen, it may not be detected by routine pretransfusion testing if this does not include a full antiglobin cross-match.

Another potential risk of parental blood transfusion is chimerism and graft-versus-host disease. For patients of all ages (including adults), all cellular blood components obtained from biologic relatives must be irradiated before transfusion (see Chapter 33).

Finally, as for all allogeneic blood transfusions, there remain the risks related to alloimmunization, allergic reactions and bacterial contamination (see Chapter 33). In addition, as for autologous donations, it is possible that the added complexity of providing directed donations could lead to an increased frequency of errors.[135]

One situation in which directed blood donors may provide an increased level of safety is a limited-donor blood program. For example, a single donor can often provide all the RBC and/or plasma needs of a small pediatric patient ineligible for autologous donation who must undergo elective surgery for which multiple blood units are normally required.[136] Likewise, the RBC transfusion requirements of small pediatric patients with chronic anemia, for example Diamond–Blackfan anemia or β-thalassemia major, may be supplied from a small pool of two to four donors.[137] While the feasibility and success of such limited-donor programs in decreasing the number of donor exposures in small pediatric patients has been demonstrated, there are no data to support or refute the superiority with respect to safety of these programs.

Plasma

Description and storage

Plasma for transfusion is prepared from a WB donation by separation following centrifugation (see Fig. 32.1). Larger volumes of plasma may be collected using automated apheresis techniques. A typical unit of plasma has a volume around 250 mL if obtained from a WB donation or approximately 500 mL when obtained by plasmapheresis. Methylene blue-treated frozen plasma (MBFP) and solvent/detergent-treated frozen plasma (SDFP) units have a similar volume to that of a regular unit of WB-derived plasma.

Immediately following collection from a normal donor, plasma contains approximately 1 unit/mL of each of the coagulation factors as well as normal concentrations of other plasma proteins. Coagulation factors V and VIII, known as the labile coagulation factors, are not stable in plasma stored for prolonged periods at 1–6°C so plasma is usually stored in the frozen state at –18°C or lower. Plasma frozen within 8 hours of collection, known as fresh frozen plasma (FFP), contains about 87% of the FVIII present at the time of collection and according to standards in most countries must contain at least 0.70 IU/mL of FVIII. Several countries also use plasma frozen within 24 hours of collection, known as frozen plasma (FP). FVIII levels in FP are approximately 70–75% of the levels present at the time of collection. The levels of FV as well as the levels of other coagulation factors are not significantly decreased from baseline in plasma frozen within 24 hours of collection.[138,139] MBFP contains less FVIII than FFP (minimum levels of 0.5 IU/mL) and approximately the same levels of other coagulation factors. FVIII levels in SDFP are somewhat higher than those in MBFP and approximately the same as in those FP.[17,140] The levels of the anticoagulant protein S are lower in SDFP than in other frozen plasma products.[17] Depending on the exact temperature at which plasma is stored, the relevant national requirements/regulations, and the precise product, frozen plasma can be stored for periods from 3 to 24 months.

Indications and contraindications for transfusion

A systematic review of allogeneic transfusions in children or infants > 4 months of age published in 1997 identified only three controlled trials addressing FFP use in this group.[22] Two examined the use of FFP for pediatric hemolytic uremic syndrome.[141,142] Both trials failed to identify any benefit of FFP infusions with respect to mortality or long-term renal outcome measures. The other examined the use of FFP as one of the components of reconstituted WB to replace blood losses following open heart surgery.[92] More recently, a systematic review of randomized, controlled trials of FFP use in adults and children identified a total of 57 trials.[143] As noted by the authors, most enrolled small numbers of patients (and few of even these small numbers of patients were children) and few provided adequate information on the ability of the trial to detect meaningful differences in the outcomes between the two patient groups. Thus, as for RBC transfusion, guidelines for administering FFP transfusions to children (as indeed is also the case for adults) are not evidence-based but are based on expert opinion.[25–28,144–147] Most guidelines (with the exception of the recently published UK guidelines[147]) refer only to FFP. This term will be used in the remainder of this section although unless noted otherwise the other frozen plasma products (FP, MBFP and SDFP) can usually be used interchangeably with FFP.

There is broad, general consensus that the appropriate use of FFP is limited almost exclusively to the treatment or prevention of clinically significant bleeding due to a deficiency of one or more plasma coagulation factors. Such situations potentially include the presence of:
- a diminution of coagulation factors due to treatment with vitamin K antagonists;
- severe liver disease;
- disseminated intravascular coagulation (DIC);
- massive transfusion;
- isolated congenital coagulation factor deficiencies for which a safer and/or more appropriate product does not exist.

The use of FFP in each of these settings is discussed below.

FFP is also used in plasma exchange (PE) in the treatment of thrombotic thrombocytopenic purpura (TTP)/hemolytic–uremic syndrome (HUS), when PE is indicated. The use of FP, MBFP and SDFP rather than FFP for TTP/HUS has not been fully evaluated.

There is a consensus among the experts who develop the guidelines that FFP is *not* indicated in the following situations:
- intravascular volume expansion or repletion (where crystalloids, synthetic colloids or purified human albumin solutions are preferred);
- correction or prevention of protein malnutrition (where synthetic amino acid solutions are preferred);
- correction of hypogammaglobulinemia (where purified human immunoglobulin concentrates are preferred);
- treatment of hemophilia A or B and von Willebrand

disease (where desmopressin or virus-inactivated plasma-derived or recombinant factor concentrates are preferred);

- treatment of any other isolated congenital procoagulant or anticoagulant factor deficiency for which a virus-inactivated plasma-derived or recombinant factor concentrate exists;
- treatment of HUS unless plasma exchange is indicated;
- as replacement fluid in therapeutic apheresis procedures for disorders other than TTP/HUS unless proven to be beneficial.

Reversal of warfarin effect

Patients who are anticoagulated with warfarin are deficient in the functional vitamin K-dependent coagulation factors II, VII, IX, X and proteins C and S. Reversal of the warfarin effect prior to elective surgery can usually be accomplished by stopping warfarin 4 days before the procedure. Selected patients at high risk of thrombosis may require heparin coverage. For children with an international normalized ratio (INR) > 8.0 and no significant bleeding vitamin K at a dose of 30 μg/kg (given orally or intravenously) may be used. In the presence of significant bleeding, immediate reversal with FFP, prothrombin complex concentrates or recombinant FVIIa may be required.[25,147–148]

Severe liver disease

Severe liver disease is associated with multiple abnormalities of hemostasis and coagulation including thrombocytopenia from hypersplenism, decreased circulating levels of coagulation factors, and abnormal fibrinogen due to impaired hepatic synthesis.[149]

Patients with severe liver disease usually have significantly abnormal coagulation studies that raise questions about the need for plasma transfusion. Most guidelines recommend that patients who are neither bleeding nor about to undergo an invasive procedure should not receive plasma merely to correct abnormal coagulation tests. One exception to this may be patients with life-threatening acute fulminant hepatitis and extremely elevated INRs who are awaiting emergency liver transplantation. These patients are sometimes given prophylactic plasma transfusions. However, no studies have specifically addressed this issue, and it is difficult to determine whether or not such transfusions actually improve the outcome of this devastating disease.

The INR at which liver biopsy can be safely performed has not been established and may be different in those with liver failure compared with those without liver disease. For patients with acquired multiple coagulation deficiencies, Canadian guidelines published in 1997 do not recommend prophylactic FFP administration prior to invasive procedures, including liver biopsy, unless the INR is > 2.0.[28] By contrast, more recently published British reviews suggest that in practice clinicians wish to have an INR < 1.4 before liver biopsy.[147] If FFP is used to prepare a patient with liver failure for liver biopsy coagulation studies need to be repeated before biopsy as the coagulopathy in liver disease does not always respond to FFP.

Disseminated intravascular coagulation

Acute DIC is characterized by the abnormal consumption of coagulation factors and platelets and may lead to thrombocytopenia, hypofibrinogenemia and increased prothrombin time (PT), INR and/or activated partial thromboplastin time (APTT) with uncontrollable bleeding from wound and puncture sites. Retrospective and uncontrolled evidence suggests that the transfusion of plasma, along with other blood components, may be useful in limiting hemorrhage. The efficacy of treatment with FFP (or cryoprecipitate or platelets) has not been studied in randomized, controlled trials but would seem reasonable, and is generally recommended in guideline documents, for patients with DIC who are bleeding or at risk for bleeding and who have laboratory evidence of a significant depletion of coagulation factors. This assumes, of course, that aggressive measures are simultaneously undertaken to overcome the triggering disease. Plasma transfusion is generally not recommended in acute DIC in the absence of bleeding (or risk of significant bleeding) nor for the treatment of chronic DIC.[28,147,150,151]

Massive transfusion

Massive transfusion is usually defined as the replacement of a patient's total blood volume with stored blood within a period of 24 hours. However, even within this definition, the degree and rapidity of blood loss can be quite variable as are the underlying etiologies and associated complications. When plasma-poor red cells are used, clinically significant fibrinogen deficiency, that is, a fibrinogen level of 1.0 g/L or lower, occurs after a blood loss of about 150% of the patient's total blood volume. Decreases of prothrombin, FV, platelets (platelet count < 50 × 10^9/L) and FVIII to critical levels will occur after blood loss in excess of two blood volumes.[152] Previous recommendations advocated routine transfusion of plasma to reduce the risk of abnormal bleeding due to coagulation factor depletion during massive transfusion. However, there is no evidence to support the routine or prophylactic administration of plasma in this scenario.[153] Thus, assessment of the need for replacement of coagulation factors by FFP transfusion should be guided by both the ongoing clinical evaluation of the patient and laboratory measurements of hemostasis. A thorough review of the pathophysiology of coagulopathy in massively transfused patients has been recently published.[154]

Congenital coagulation factor deficiencies

Plasma has long been used to treat congenital deficiencies of

Table 32.8 Reference values for coagulation tests in healthy full-term infants during the first 6 months of life.

Test	Day 1		Day 30		Adult	
	M	B	M	B	M	B
PT (s)	13.0	10.1–15.9*	11.8	10.0–14.3*	12.4	10.8–13.9
INR	1.0	0.53–16.2	0.79	0.53–1.26	0.89	0.64–1.17
APTT (s)	42.9	31.3–54.5	40.4	32.0–55.2	33.5	26.6–40.3
Coagulation factors						
Fibrinogen (g/L)	2.83	1.67–3.99*	2.70	1.62–3.78*	2.78	1.56–4.00
V (units/mL)	0.72	0.34–1.08	0.98	0.62–1.34	1.06	0.62–1.50
VII (units/mL)	0.66	0.28–10.4	0.90	0.42–1.38	1.05	0.67–1.43
VIII (units/mL)	1.00	0.50–1.78*	0.91	0.50–1.57*	0.99	0.50–1.49
vWF (units/mL)	1.53	0.50–2.87	1.28	0.50–2.46	0.92	0.50–1.58
IX (units/mL)	0.53	0.15–0.91	0.51	0.21–0.81	1.09	0.55–1.63
X (units/mL)	0.40	0.12–0.68	0.59	0.31–0.87	1.06	0.70–1.52
XI (units/mL)	0.38	0.10–0.66	0.53	0.27–0.79	0.97	0.67–1.27

All coagulation factors except fibrinogen are expressed as units/mL, where pooled plasma contains 1.0 unit/mL. All values are expressed as mean (M), followed by the lower and upper boundary encompassing 95% of the population (B).
* Values indistinguishable from those of the adult.
APTT, activated partial thromboplastin time; INR, international normalized ratio; PT, prothrombin time; VIII, FVIII procoagulant; vWF, von Willebrand factor.
Adapted with permission from Ref. 153.

hemostatic or anticoagulant proteins. However, more appropriate alternatives such as recombinant factor concentrates now exist for most of these disorders. Physicians with special expertise in pediatric hemostasis or thrombosis should supervise the care of children with these disorders and the choice of products for their treatment. These disorders are discussed in detail in Chapters 26–28.

Special considerations for newborns

The approach to determining the indications for FFP transfusion in the newborn is the same as that for the older patient; that is, FFP is indicated for the treatment of clinically significant bleeding, or its prevention in the case of an invasive procedure, due to a decrease in one or more coagulation factors, where a safer, appropriate, alternative therapy does not exist.[25,26,147] In particular, specific factor concentrates should be used in neonates with congenital coagulation factor deficiencies, if available. As for older patients, FFP is not indicated for the treatment of volume expansion or resuscitation alone. However, the application of these underlying principles to decisions concerning FFP administration may be more difficult in newborns than older patients for a number of reasons. First, it may be difficult to obtain blood specimens of the quality and quantity necessary to obtain reliable laboratory measurements of coagulation parameters in tiny, critically ill preterm infants. Secondly, newborns and infants under 6 months of age have relatively lower levels of the vitamin K-dependent coagulation factors (factors II, VII, IX and X), as well as the four contact factors and the

vitamin K-dependent coagulation inhibitors.[155,156] PT and APTT are correspondingly prolonged. Normal values for coagulant and anticoagulant proteins as well as coagulation tests in healthy, full-term and preterm infants are shown in Tables 32.8 and 32.9, respectively. These values usually reach adult levels by 6 months of age. On the one hand, these differences in the newborn versus the older infant and child may render the correlation of laboratory values to the clinical situation difficult; on the other hand, it is likely that the coagulant and anticoagulant factors that are already relatively low in newborns are more rapidly depleted in situations such as acute hemorrhage or DIC. It may thus be reasonable to administer FFP transfusion relatively sooner in these situations to newborns and infants under 6 months of age than in older infants and children.

In most countries, newborns receive vitamin K prophylactically at birth. Newborns who do not receive vitamin K prophylaxis and who are breast-fed may develop the classic form of hemorrhagic disease of the newborn (HDN). A late form of HDN may occur in newborns with a variety of diseases that can compromise the supply of vitamin K. First-line treatment is the subcutaneous or intravenous administration of vitamin K (see also Chapter 30). Clinically significant bleeding may require FFP treatment, and life-threatening bleeding may require treatment with coagulation factor concentrates. The latter should only be used in consultation with an expert in pediatric hemostatic disorders.

In addition to the contraindications for FFP transfusion listed above, in the newborn FFP should not be used as a fluid for hematocrit adjustment in erythrocyte transfusions nor as

Table 32.9 Reference values for coagulation tests in healthy preterm infants during the first 6 months of life.

Test	Day 1		Day 30		Adult	
	M	B	M	B	M	B
PT (s)	13.0	10.6–16.2*	11.8	10.0–13.6*	12.4	10.8–13.9
INR	1.0	0.61–1.7	0.79	0.53–1.11	0.89	0.64–1.17
APTT (s)	53.6	27.5–79.4	44.7	26.9–62.5	33.5	26.6–40.3
Coagulation factors						
Fibrinogen (g/L)	2.43	1.50–3.73*	2.54	1.50–4.14*	2.78	1.56–4.00
V (units/mL)	0.88	0.41–1.48	1.02	0.48–1.56	1.06	0.62–1.50
VII (units/mL)	0.67	0.21–1.13	0.83	0.21–1.45	1.05	0.67–1.43
VIII (units/mL)	1.11	0.50–2.13*	1.11	0.50–1.99*	0.99	0.50–1.49
vWF (units/mL)	1.36	0.78–2.10	1.36	0.66–2.16	0.92	0.50–1.58
IX (units/mL)	0.35	0.19–0.65	0.44	0.13–0.80	1.09	0.55–1.63
X (units/mL)	0.41	0.11–0.71	0.56	0.20–0.92	1.06	0.70–1.52
XI (units/mL)	0.30	0.08–0.52	0.43	0.15–0.71	0.97	0.67–1.27

All factors except fibrinogen are expressed as units/mL, where pooled plasma contains 1.0 unit/mL. All values are expressed as mean (M), followed by the lower and upper boundary encompassing 95% of the population (B).
* Values indistinguishable from those of the adult.
APTT, activated partial thromboplastin time; INR, international normalized ratio; PT, prothrombin time; VIII, FVIII procoagulant; vWF, von Willebrand factor.
Adapted with permission from Ref. 154.

a replacement fluid in partial exchange transfusion for the treatment of neonatal hyperviscosity syndrome (because these two situations essentially represent the use of FFP as volume replacement). Also, the use of prophylactic FFP to prevent periventricular–intraventricular hemorrhage in preterm neonates is not recommended as this has been shown to confer no benefit.[25,157]

FFP is used in newborns to prepare reconstituted whole blood when this product is indicated.

Dosage and administration

Compatibility tests before plasma transfusion are not necessary. Plasma should be ABO compatible with the recipient's RBCs (see Table 32.4). The Rh group need not be considered.[25] However, when large volumes of FFP are given to RhD-negative females of childbearing potential (such as in intensive plasma exchange) some authors recommend the prevention of RhD immunization by the use of RhD immune globulin.[25,158] Although RBCs are hemolyzed during freezing, sensitization can rarely occur because FFP contains a small amount of red cell stroma.

FFP may be thawed in a waterbath at 30–37°C (the unit must be placed in a watertight protective plastic overwrap to prevent bacterial contamination) or in a microwave specifically designed for this purpose.

The dose of FFP depends on the clinical situation and the underlying disease process. When FFP is given for coagulation factor replacement, the dose is 10–20 mL/kg. This dose will usually raise the level of coagulation factors by

approximately 20% immediately after infusion,[159,160] although in situations where coagulation factors are being actively consumed larger doses may be necessary. FFP is transfused through a standard 170–260 μm blood filter and is usually administered over 2–4 hours or as rapidly as the patient's clinical situation dictates. Posttransfusion monitoring of the patient's coagulation status (PT, APTT and/or specific coagulation factor assays) is important for optimal treatment. Information on *in vivo* properties of coagulation factors, which may guide plasma transfusion therapy, is summarized in Table 32.10.[159,160]

Platelets

Description and storage

A platelet concentrate (PC) may be prepared from a WB donation using the platelet-rich plasma (PRP) or buffy coat (BC) method of preparation (see Fig. 32.1), or by an apheresis procedure using a variety of different systems. PCs prepared from WB using the PRP method contain a minimum of 5.5 × 10^10 platelets/unit suspended in approximately 50 mL of plasma. PRP-PCs are usually supplied to hospitals as single units. The hospital blood bank then supplies these units to the wards singly, or more often after pooling an appropriate number of units. BC platelets are pooled together by the blood supplier before issuing to hospitals; pools usually consist of platelets derived from four or five WB donations. The platelet content and unit volume are approximately the same

Factor	Plasma concentration required for hemostasis*	Half-life of transfused factor[††]	Recovery in blood (as % of amount transfused)
I (fibrinogen)	1.0 g/L	3–6 days	50
II	0.4 IU/mL	2–5 days	40–80
V	0.10–0.25 IU/mL	12 h	80
VII	0.05–0.20 IU/mL	2–7 h	70–80
VIII	0.10–0.40 IU/mL	8–12 h	60–80
IX	0.10–0.40 IU/mL	18–24 h	40–50
X	0.10–0.15 IU/mL	2 days	50
XI	0.15–0.30 IU/mL	3 days	90–100
XIII	0.01–0.05 IU/mL	6–10 days	5–100
VWF	0.25–0.50 IU/mL	3–5 h	–

Table 32.10 *In vivo* properties of blood clotting factors.

For treatment of recessively inherited (rare) coagulation disorders the reader is also referred to Ref. 160.

* Upper limit usually refers to surgical hemostasis.

†† Refers to the half-life following FFP transfusion.

Adapted with permission from Ref. 159.

as would be present in a corresponding number of PRP-PCs. The number of platelets in an apheresis unit depends on the production method and may vary with national/regional requirements. The volume of plasma is determined according to the amount necessary to maintain platelet viability given the platelet content; it is a maximum of 1.5×10^9 platelets/mL plasma. Typically an apheresis unit intended for transfusion to an adult patient will contain $300–400 \times 10^9$ platelets in 250–300 mL of plasma. Alternately, as noted above, platelets (either apheresis platelets or BC platelets) may be stored in platelet storage media. PCs are stored at 22–24°C with continuous gentle agitation. In most jurisdictions PCs may only be stored for a maximum of 5 days. However, if bacterial detection has been performed (see Chapter 33) and platelet viability has been proven, some countries now permit a 7-day storage period.[161]

Indications for transfusion

Platelet transfusions are mainly indicated to treat or prevent hemorrhages in thrombocytopenic patients or patients with dysfunctional platelets.

Decreased platelet production

Decreased platelet production occurs in children with congenital or acquired aplastic anemia, bone marrow infiltration with leukemic or other malignant cells and/or following myeloablative chemotherapy. The majority of studies addressing the indications for platelet transfusions for patients with decreased platelet production have been performed in patients with acute leukemia. It is, however, reasonable to use results of these studies to guide platelet transfusion therapy for the majority of patients with hypoproliferative thrombocytopenia.

Prior to the availability of platelets for transfusion, hemorrhage in patients with leukemia and severe thrombocytopenia was frequently fatal. In a report from the National Cancer Institute in the USA, hemorrhage was considered to have been the major cause of death in 52% of 414 acute leukemic patients studied from 1954 to 1963.[162] With the introduction of plastic blood collection systems in the late 1960s, platelets became available for the treatment of patients with thrombocytopenic bleeding. By the 1980s, deaths due to hemorrhage gradually decreased to the point that only 3% of adults with acute nonlymphoblastic leukemia (ANLL) had lethal hemorrhagic complications.[163]

In the 1970s and 1980s several studies (reviewed in Ref. 164) addressed the issue of prophylactic versus therapeutic platelet transfusions for thrombocytopenic patients with acute leukemia. These studies demonstrated that platelets given prophylactically do decrease the incidence of significant bleeding episodes in patients with leukemia, but they did not demonstrate a longer survival in patients transfused prophylactically versus those transfused only in the presence of active bleeding. Despite this, several experts began to recommend the use of prophylactic platelet transfusions,[165–168] and this is now the main indication for platelet transfusion in hematology-oncology patients.[169,170]

In the reviews cited above, published in the late 1970s and early 1980s, and advocating the use of prophylactic platelet transfusions for patients with leukemia, it was often suggested that the platelet count be maintained above 20×10^9/L. This figure appears to have been derived from a much-quoted study by Gaydos *et al.* published in 1962.[171] In this study gross hemorrhage was visible on < 1% of days at all platelet levels > 20×10^9/L and on 4% of days where platelet counts were $10–20 \times 10^9$/L. When this study was performed the platelet inhibitory effects of aspirin were not yet appreciated and many of these patients were probably receiving aspirin, which could also have contributed to the observed bleeding. The authors concluded that no clear "threshold" platelet count could be identified; nevertheless the study appears to have been the basis for the practice that developed in the 1980s of using a platelet count trigger of $20 \times 10^9/L$ for prophylactic transfusion.

In the late 1980s and the early 1990s, due to the increased awareness of transfusion-transmitted diseases and the cost and difficulty of maintaining adequate supplies of platelet concentrates, the necessity of maintaining a minimum platelet count of $20 \times 10^9/L$ in all patients with decreased platelet production began to be questioned. At a Consensus Development Conference addressing platelet transfusion therapy sponsored by the National Institutes of Health in the USA in 1986, the panel concluded that patients with severe thrombocytopenia may benefit from prophylactic transfusions but that the commonly used threshold value of $20 \times 10^9/L$ may sometimes be safely lowered.[172] During the 1990s a number of studies were performed investigating the safety of lowering the trigger for prophylactic platelet transfusions for patients with thrombocytopenia due to decreased platelet production but without other risk factors for bleeding.[164,173–180] All investigators concluded that this practice is safe, and a lower threshold for prophylactic platelet transfusions is now advocated in several published reviews and guidelines for platelet transfusion.[181,182] However, there is not complete consensus with respect to which factors may actually constitute increased risk for bleeding, and there remain concerns about the lack of accuracy when counting very low numbers of platelets. Most current guidelines are similar to those published in 2003 by the British Committee for Standards in Haematology which state the following.
• A threshold of $10 \times 10^9/L$ is as safe as higher levels for patients without additional risk factors. Risk factors include sepsis, concurrent use of antibiotics or other abnormalities of hemostasis.
• For patients without any risk factors, a threshold of $5 \times 10^9/L$ may be appropriate if there are concerns that alloimmunization could lead to platelet refractoriness. However, accurate counting of low platelet numbers may create difficulties when trying to reduce the threshold below $10 \times 10^9/L$.
• A specific threshold for transfusion may not be appropriate for patients with chronic stable thrombocytopenia who are best managed on an individual basis depending on the degree of hemorrhage.[182]

Prophylactic platelet transfusions are also indicated for thrombocytopenic patients undergoing invasive procedures. At least one study suggests that major surgical procedures can be safely performed in leukemic patients at platelet counts of $50 \times 10^9/L$.[183] However, there are limited published data concerning appropriate platelet counts for patients with hematologic or other malignancies undergoing common invasive procedures such as the insertion of permanent indwelling central venous catheters or lumbar punctures.

Most authors recommend a platelet count $\geq 40 \times 10^9/L$ for these procedures. It is possible that lower levels may be adequate when these procedures are performed by experienced personnel.[184–188] Bone marrow aspiration and biopsy can be safely performed (with respect to local bleeding) at any platelet level by providing adequate surface pressure at the procedure site.

Increased platelet destruction

Patients with thrombocytopenia due to autoimmune thrombocytopenic purpura (AITP) should only be treated with platelet transfusions in the presence of central nervous system or other life-threatening bleeding.[189,190] Before surgical procedures, such as splenectomy or cesarean section, the platelet count can usually be raised preoperatively, using corticosteroids or intravenous immunoglobulins, to levels sufficient to assure adequate hemostasis. A variety of conditions other than AITP (e.g., septicemia, trauma, obstetrical complications) may result in platelet consumption that is sufficiently severe to require platelet transfusion. Platelet increment and survival are usually decreased in these patients and a larger number of units administered at more frequent intervals may be necessary.

Massive transfusion

The average adult patient will have a platelet count $< 50 \times 10^9/L$ after losing two blood volumes.[153,155] Depending on the underlying etiology of the bleeding, the thrombocytopenia may be dilutional from platelet loss through hemorrhage and/or due to platelet consumption. Platelet transfusion therapy should be based on a consideration of several factors including platelet count, an assessment of the role of the thrombocytopenia in the observed bleeding and the estimated hemostatic platelet count necessary for the patient's given clinical situation.[146,152] Most guidelines do recommend administering platelet transfusions to maintain a platelet count of at least 50×10^9 in an actively bleeding patient.[25,26,146,182]

Platelet dysfunction

Platelet dysfunction, possibly requiring platelet transfusion, is most commonly encountered in three situations: in patients taking platelet inhibitory drugs; following surgery with cardiopulmonary bypass pump (CBP); and during ECMO.

Platelet inhibitory drugs, such as aspirin, nonsteroidal antiinflammatory agents and newer platelet aggregation inhibitors such as clopidogrel bisulfate and ticlopidine hydrochloride, and glycoprotein (Gp)IIb/IIIa receptor antagonists, should be avoided in thrombocytopenic patients and, if possible, in all patients before invasive procedures. Treatment with desmopressin acetate or antifibrinolytics may be helpful in selected patients on aspirin or other nonsteroidal antiinflammatory medications who are bleeding or who require invasive procedures.[191,192] The published literature examining the role of platelet transfusions in patients taking platelet aggregation inhibitors has recently been summarized; the authors concluded that studies do suggest a role for therapeutic platelet transfusions in bleeding patients with recent exposure (within 7 days) to these medications but do not support the use of prophylactic platelet transfusions.[193] GpIIb/IIIa receptor antagonists have relatively short half-lives (a few hours to 48 hours) so that platelet transfusion support, if required, would only be over that time frame.

Patients who have undergone surgery with CBP may have a dilutional and/or consumptive thrombocytopenia, although the platelet count usually remains above 100×10^9/L. Platelet dysfunction lasting 4–6 hours post-CBP has been well documented.[194,195] Nevertheless, studies have not shown any benefit for the use of prophylactic platelet transfusions for patients undergoing CBP.[196] Platelet transfusions should be reserved for those patients who, following CBP, have excessive bleeding thought to be due to platelet function abnormalities and/or thrombocytopenia. Platelet dysfunction and thrombocytopenia also occur during ECMO.[197] It is usually recommended to maintain the platelet count above 100×10^9/L in patients during ECMO.[25,26]

Patients with congenital thrombopathies (e.g., Glanzmann thrombasthenia) may occasionally require platelet transfusions. These patients should be managed by a subspecialist with expertise in this area.

Special considerations for newborns

Newborns should receive platelet transfusions in the same clinical settings as described above for older children. However, because newborns frequently manifest thrombocytopenia and because preterm infants are at risk for periventricular/intraventricular hemorrhage, it is possible that the platelet level at which prophylactic platelet transfusions should be administered to newborns is higher than that recommended for other patients. Only one prospective randomized study, published in 1993, has addressed this issue. In that study prophylactic platelet transfusions sufficient to maintain platelet counts $> 150 \times 10^9$/L failed to influence the incidence or extension of intraventricular hemorrhage.[198] No other prospective controlled trials have addressed this issue. The authors of a retrospective study published in 2002 concluded that a neonatal prophylactic transfusion trigger threshold of $< 30 \times 10^9$/L is likely to represent "safe" practice for the majority of neonatal intensive care unit patients (i.e., stable preterm neonates).[199]

With only such limited evidence-based information available, definitive guidelines for platelet transfusions in newborns cannot be formulated, and published guidelines actually vary considerably in their recommendations.[25,26,84,200] One recommended set of guidelines is summarized in Table 32.11.

Table 32.11 Suggested guidelines for platelet transfusions in neonates.

Platelet count $< 30 \times 10^9$/L in a neonate with neonatal alloimmune thrombocytopenia

Platelet count $< 30 \times 10^9$/L with failure of platelet production

Platelet count $< 50 \times 10^9$/L in a stable preterm infant:*
   with active bleeding
   prior to invasive procedure with failure of platelet production

Platelet count $< 100 \times 10^9$/L in a sick preterm infant:†
   with active bleeding
   prior to invasive procedure with disseminated intravascular coagulation

---

* British guidelines suggest a platelet count of $< 20 \times 10^9$/L for term infants.[179]

† British guidelines do not state specific recommendations in these situations.[179]

Adapted with permission from Ref. 26.

Prospective, randomized, controlled trials are needed to firmly establish optimal platelet transfusion thresholds in neonates.

Neonates with thrombocytopenia due to maternal platelet alloantibodies should receive platelet transfusions from donors lacking the antigen corresponding to the maternal antibody in order to maintain platelet counts $\geq 30 \times 10^9$/L.[26] In emergency situations if antigen negative platelets are unavailable (or, pending the availability of antigen negative platelets) transfusion of a platelet concentrate from an random donor may lead to an adequate platelet increment.[200a]

Product choice, dosage and administration

Platelets possess intrinsic ABH antigens and extrinsically absorbed A and B antigens.[198] Nevertheless, ABO-incompatible platelets (i.e., platelets with A and/or B antigens given to a donor with a corresponding antibody) are usually clinically effective. However, there are several reports of acute intravascular hemolysis following the transfusion of platelet concentrates containing ABO antibodies incompatible with the recipient's RBCs.[201,202] Therefore, ABO-matched platelets should be used in pediatric patients, especially for neonates and small children where the volume of plasma may be relatively large with respect to the patient's total blood volume. If ABO-matched platelets are not available, units with plasma compatible with the recipient's RBCs should be chosen. If this is also not possible, units with low titers of anti-A or -B should be selected or alternatively the plasma can be removed from platelet concentrate (i.e., use a volume-reduced platelet concentrate).[25]

Platelets do not carry Rh antigens.[201] However, the quantity of RBCs in platelet concentrates is sufficient to induce RhD sensitization even in immunosuppressed cancer patients. Hence, as far as possible, platelets from an RhD-negative donor should be used for RhD-negative patients. If platelets from an RhD-positive donor, or platelets from a donor of unknown RhD phenotype, are given to an RhD-negative recipient, administration of anti-D immunoprophylaxis should be considered, especially for female patients.[25,181] The amount of anti-D immunoglobulin necessary to prevent sensitization depends on the number of contaminating RBCs in the platelet concentrates. A dose of 25 μg (125 IU) of anti-D immunoglobulin will protect against 1 mL of RBCs.[203] An adult dose of platelets usually contains less than 2 mL of RBCs. If available, it is preferable to use a preparation of anti-D that can be administered intravenously.

Studies have not been performed to determine the most appropriate platelet doses for pediatric platelet transfusions, and recommended doses do vary. North American guidelines generally recommend a dose of 5–10 mL/kg of either WB-derived or apheresis PCs, with the larger dose (i.e., 10 mL/kg) being used in neonates and the smaller dose (5 mL/kg) being used in infants and children.[26] Practically speaking, when using WB-derived PCs (that have not been previously pooled) this corresponds to approximately one WB-derived PC per 10 kg body weight. UK guidelines recommend slightly higher doses, namely 10–20 mL/kg for children weighing less than 20 kg.[182]

In adults the question of the optimal platelet dose (i.e., the number of platelets administered per platelet transfusion), particularly in the setting of prophylactic transfusions for patients with hypoproliferative thrombocytopenia, is currently a subject of debate and ongoing clinical trials.[204–206] Potential advantages of lower doses (i.e., $< 300 \times 10^9$ platelets per transfusion) include the use of fewer platelet thereby potentially reducing donor exposure and costs, while potential advantages of higher doses include longer intervals between platelet transfusions.[207,208] To date studies with small numbers of patients that lower doses do not lead to an increased risk of serious or life-threatening bleeding but further studies are required before definitive statements can be made. Currently, a standard platelet dose for an adult is $300–600 \times 10^9$ platelets/dose; alternatively, a dose can be more specifically calculated.[182] Patients with platelet consumption (e.g., with septicemia or DIC) or splenomegaly may require larger doses of platelets.

Platelet concentrates may be volume reduced before infusion. However, this extra manipulation leads to platelet loss and, if not carefully performed, may adversely affect platelet function and/or be a cause of bacterial contamination. Volume reduction should therefore be limited to patients who require severe volume restriction or situations where ABO-incompatible platelets are the only available product. Many patients requiring platelet transfusions should receive irradiated products only. Indications for irradiation of PCs (and other blood components) are discussed in Chapter 33. PCs must be filtered using a standard 170–260 μm filter. PCs must be filtered, using either a standard 170–260 μm filter, or if the unit has not been leukoreduced prestorage, a bedside leukoreduction filter (depending upon the requirement for leukoreduction). Platelet counts should always be performed following platelet transfusion to assure that the platelet count has increased as expected. This is particularly important for platelet transfusions given before surgery or invasive procedures.

Platelet refractoriness

The response to a platelet transfusion, known as the corrected platelet count increment (CCI), is determined using the following formula, which takes into account the recipient's body surface area and number of platelets transfused:

$$CCI = \frac{[(\text{Posttransfusion} - \text{pretransfusion}) \text{ platelet count } (\times 10^9/\text{L})] \times \text{body surface area } (\text{m}^2)}{\text{Number of platelets transfused } (\times 10^{11})}$$

In general, a platelet transfusion is considered successful if the CCI is $> 7.5 \times 10^9/\text{L}$ within 10–60 min of a transfusion and $> 4.5 \times 10^9/\text{L}$ if measured 18–24 h after transfusion.

Refractoriness to platelet transfusions is defined as a consistently inadequate response to platelet transfusion, for instance, a CCI of $< 5 \times 10^9/\text{L}$ following two separate transfusions of an adequate number of platelets. Refractoriness may be due to immune causes (i.e., the presence in the recipient of HLA- or platelet-specific alloantibodies) or nonimmune causes, such as infection, DIC, splenomegaly, medications (in particular amphotericin B, vancomycin, antithymocyte globulin) and hematopoietic progenitor cell transplantation.[209–211]

If platelet refractoriness is suspected, the first steps in the management of the patient are to assure that ABO-identical platelets are used and to carefully assess the patient for nonimmune causes. The use of fresh as opposed to stored platelets may result in increased CCIs, particularly in clinically unstable patients.[209] If no increment in platelet count is observed following the transfusion of ABO-identical platelets, the recipient should be phenotyped for HLA class I antigens and screened for the presence of HLA class I antibodies. If an HLA alloimmunization is confirmed, the usual approach is then to transfuse single-donor, apheresis, HLA-matched platelets using the best HLA match available.[212] Other approaches include the selection of platelets on the basis of HLA antibody (e.g., a patient with an HLA-B27 antibody would receive platelets from an HLA-B27-negative donor) or the use of platelet cross-matching.[182,213–215] The rare patient with platelet-specific alloantibodies should be treated with platelets lacking the corresponding antigen. The use of antifibrinolytic agents such as ε-aminocaproic acid may also be helpful in these patients (as well as in nonrefractory patients).[216] Some alloimmunized patients may lose their antibodies over time and again become responsive to random donor platelet transfusions.[217,218]

The management of alloimmunized patients who do not

respond to the above measures is problematic. It is unlikely to be of benefit to administer prophylactic platelet transfusions to such patients. In the presence of clinically significant bleeding, approaches such as the use of larger and/or more frequent random-donor platelet transfusions may be attempted. The administration of intravenous immunoglobin may result in improved posttransfusion platelet increments but does not usually increase platelet survival.[219]

Granulocytes

Description and storage

To assure clinical efficacy, granulocyte concentrates for transfusion to adults should contain a minimum of 10^{10} and preferably closer to 10^{11} polymorphonuclear cells (PMNs)/unit. To obtain this number of PMNs, concentrates are prepared by automated leukapheresis using an erythrocyte sedimenting agent such as hydroxyethyl starch to enhance the efficacy of separation of granulocytes from erythrocytes. Donors are usually stimulated with oral corticosteroids before collection, but even with this only about 10% of collections contain an adequate PMN dose. Stimulation of donors with granulocyte colony-stimulating factor (G-CSF) in addition to corticosteroids results in collections with PMN counts closer to 10^{11}/dose.[220] However, the use of corticosteroids and G-CSF in donors, particularly unrelated donors, does require special ethical considerations. The platelet and RBC content varies with the collection method. The plasma volume is 200–400 mL. Granulocyte function deteriorates rapidly during storage. Thus, granulocytes should be transfused as soon as possible following collection, preferably within 12 hours, and should not be given if stored for > 24 hours. For the time between collection and infusion, granulocyte concentrates should be stored at 20–24°C and kept unagitated.[221]

Indications for transfusion

There is no evidence to support the role of prophylactic granulocyte transfusions, and even the use of granulocyte transfusions in established bacterial or fungal infections remains controversial.[222] However, the use of G-CSF-stimulated granulocyte transfusions may be reasonable in the following situations.

• A resistant severe clinical infection in a neutropenic (neutrophil count < 0.2–0.5 × 10^9/L) patient who has shown no response to aggressive antibiotic treatment with no recovery in neutrophil count expected for more than 7 days.
• Severe infections, e.g., systemic fungal infections/necrotizing fasciitis or severe neutropenic typhlitis progressing on appropriate antifungal or broad-spectrum antibiotics, in neutropenic patients where no recovery in neutrophil count is expected for more than 7 days.[220]

Nevertheless, at least one study using G-CSF-stimulated donors found no difference in survival between such patients treated with granulocyte transfusions and those not receiving granulocyte transfusions.[223] Thus, given the lack of adequate trials upon which to base decisions for this costly and logistically difficult treatment, which also includes medicating donors, further appropriate trials should be performed to determine the indications for granulocyte transfusions.[223,224]

Special considerations for newborns

Newborns normally have a transient neutrophilia in the first week of life, with mean normal absolute neutrophil counts ranging from 11.0×10^9/L at birth to 5.5×10^9/L at 1 week of life.[225] Septic newborns frequently develop neutropenia, defined in the first days of life of a newborn as an absolute neutrophil count < 3.0×10^9/L. A Cochrane Database Systematic Review to determine the efficacy and safety of granulocyte transfusions as adjuncts to antibiotics for the treatment of sepsis in neonates with neutropenia was published in 2003.[226] Four eligible studies were identified, three comparing granulocyte transfusions versus no transfusion and one comparing granulocyte transfusions versus intravenous gammaglobulin. The reviewers concluded that there is inconclusive evidence from randomized, controlled trials to support or reject the use of granulocyte transfusions in this setting to reduce mortality and morbidity. Septic, neutropenic newborns may respond to treatment with G-CSF.[227] Thus, the role for granulocyte transfusion in newborns also remains unclear.

Dosage and administration

Once the decision to administer granulocyte transfusions has been made, they are administered daily until there is evidence of recovery of peripheral neutrophil counts or clinical evidence of recovery from the infection. In order to provide granulocyte transfusions daily for several days and to assure both adequate viral testing of donors and/or units and administration of units within 24 hours of collection, special arrangements need to be made with the blood supplier. For neonates and small children, a daily infusion of 1–2 × 10^9 PMN/kg should be given, and for larger children an absolute dose of at least 2–3 × 10^{10} PMNs.[25,26] As there is significant RBC contamination, units must be ABO compatible and if possible RhD negative for RhD-negative recipients, and must undergo the usual compatibility testing. Because there is also a large amount of plasma the donor should ideally be ABO isogroup with the recipient. Patients should be tested for the presence of HLA (and if possible neutrophil) antibodies before the first granulocyte transfusion and periodically during a prolonged course of transfusions. Alloimmunization frequently occurs in patients receiving granulocyte transfusions and may render the transfusions ineffective and/or be associated with adverse reactions including respiratory distress.[228] For patients with HLA- and/or granulocyte-specific alloantibodies, only granulocytes from HLA- and/or neutrophil antigen-compatible donors should be used. In patients receiving amphotericin B the granulocyte transfusion should be separated in time as far as possible from the amphotericin B infusion to decrease the possibility of adverse pulmonary reactions.[229] Granulocytes must be transfused through a standard 170 μm blood filter. A leukoreduction filter must not be used and microaggregate filters are also not recommended. The transfusion is usually administered over 2–3 hours.

Cryoprecipitate

Description and storage

Cryoprecipitate is the precipitate formed when FFP is thawed at a temperature between 1 and 6°C. The precipitate is then refrozen within 1 hour in 5–40 mL of the donor plasma and stored at –18°C or less for a period of up to 1 year. Each unit of cryoprecipitate contains at least 80 units of FVIII and 150 mg of fibrinogen, and usually contains 40–60 mg of fibronectin, 40–70% of the von Willebrand factor and 30% of the FXIII present in the original unit of plasma.

Indications for transfusion

The majority of situations in which cryoprecipitate has been used in the past, in particular as treatment for hemophilia A and von Willebrand disease, can now usually be managed with alternative, safer products (see Chapters 26 and 27). Cryoprecipitate has also been used to treat bleeding due to congenital deficiencies of fibrinogen or FXIII. Virus-inactivated plasma-derived concentrates are now commercially available for these disorders, although they are not licensed in all countries. If unavailable, cryoprecipitate may be used. Cryoprecipitate was also used as a source of fibrinogen for fibrin glue, but again there are now virally inactivated fibrin glue products. Finally, cryoprecipitate was previously used to treat bleeding in patients with uremia. These patients are now treated with dialysis, desmopressin and erythropoietin. Currently, the main indication for cryoprecipitate therapy is to control bleeding due to acquired fibrinogen deficiency, for example in severe liver disease, DIC or certain obstetrical disorders.[25,26,147]

Dosage and administration

Compatibility testing of cryoprecipitate units is unnecessary. However, cryoprecipitate does contain anti-A and -B so the use of ABO-compatible units is preferable, especially when the infused volume is large relative to the recipient's red cell mass. The RhD group need not be considered. The number of units of cryoprecipitate required is usually based on the amount necessary to obtain a hemostatic level of fibrinogen, that is, a fibrinogen level > 0.8–1.0 g/L. If the units are carefully pooled this can usually be accomplished by the transfusion of 1 unit/5–10 kg recipient weight.

Cryoprecipitate is prepared for transfusion by thawing at 30–37°C and mixing the thawed precipitate with 10–15 mL of sodium chloride 0.9%, if necessary, according to the amount of plasma in the cryoprecipitate unit. The required number of units is then pooled. Thawed cryoprecipitate should be kept at room temperature and transfused immediately after thawing. If not transfused immediately, recommended storage temperatures (i.e., room temperature versus 4°C) and storage times (4 24 hours) vary among countries. Cryoprecipitate is transfused through a standard 170–260 μm blood filter and is administered as rapidly as the patient's clinical situation permits.

Albumin

Preparation and storage

Albumin is derived from large pools of donor plasma obtained from either WB or plasmapheresis donations. It is prepared by the cold alcohol fractionation process (Cohn fractionation) followed by heat treatment at 60°C for 10 hours. Its composition is 96% albumin and 4% other plasma proteins. In North America, albumin is available as a 25% solution in distilled water or as a 5% solution in saline. Outside North America other similar concentrations are used in some jurisdictions (e.g., 20% and 4.5%). The 25% and 5% preparations have a physiologic pH and a sodium content of about 145 mmol/L (145 mEq/L). The 5% solution is osmotically and oncotically equivalent to plasma, while the 25% solution is osmotically and oncotically 5-fold greater than plasma. These products can be stored for up to 5 years at 2–10°C.

Indications for transfusion

Indications for albumin use generally fall into two categories: the treatment of patients with hypoalbuminemia or patients requiring intravascular volume expansion. Albumin should not be used to treat either mild hypoalbuminemia or a nutritional deficiency. However, albumin may be beneficial in the treatment of nephrotic syndrome resistant to diuretics[230] or after large-volume paracentesis.[231,232] Patients requiring intravascular volume expansion can be treated with crystalloids (e.g., saline or Ringer's lactate), synthetic colloid (e.g., pentastarch, hexastarch or dextran) or albumin (a human plasma-derived colloid).

A meta-analysis published by the Cochrane Injuries Group Albumin Reviewers in 1998 concluded that there was no evidence that albumin reduced mortality in critically ill patients with hypovolemia, burns or hypoalbuminemia, and there was a strong suggestion that it could increase mortality.[233] On the other hand, authors of two other meta-analyses came to different conclusions: one group examined the effects of resuscitation with albumin-containing fluid on the risk of death in a general population of patients and did not find a significant increase in the risk of death, while the other concluded that albumin may reduce morbidity in critically ill patients.[234,235] In 2004, a randomized, controlled trial comparing albumin and saline for fluid resuscitation in critically ill adult patients (the SAFE study) was published.[236] This study showed that in a heterogeneous population of adult patients in intensive care units the use of either 4% albumin or normal saline for fluid resuscitation results in similar outcomes at 28 days. The investigators did note that there were subgroups where there were suggestions of differences and further studies are needed (e.g., patients with trauma and brain injury where saline may be preferable, and patients with septic shock and hypovolemia where albumin may be preferable). Following the publication of this study, the Cochrane Review was updated and this time the reviewers concluded that there is no evidence that albumin reduces mortality in critically ill patients with burns and hypoalbuminemia, although they noted, as did the SAFE investigators, that there remain subsets of patients for whom albumin use should be further evaluated.[237] Finally, there continues to be debate about the safety/efficacy of albumin versus synthetic colloids (and of different synthetic colloids).[238] Most studies evaluating the use of volume expanders do not include pediatric patients, so that the optimal treatment of crystalloids versus synthetic colloids versus albumin in neonates and children remains even less clear in pediatric patients than in adults. However, at least two (albeit small) studies suggest that crystalloids or synthetic volume expanders are safe and efficacious in neonates or young infants, and presumably the results of adult studies can be extrapolated to older children.[239–241]

Dosage and administration

Albumin does not need to be administered through a filter. Dosage and rate of infusion depend upon the patient's clinical condition. In shock the usual dosage of 5% albumin is 500 mL in adults and 10–20 mL/kg in children. The 25% solution should not be used in dehydrated patients unless it is supplemented by the infusion of crystalloid solutions.

Immunoglobulins

Plasma-derived immunoglobulins are available as nonspecific or specific antibody preparations for either intramuscular or intravenous use. All are prepared by fractionation from large pools of human plasma and all undergo efficacious viral removal/inactivation procedures. Intramuscular immunoglobulin, commonly known as human immune serum globulin (ISG), is prepared by cold alcohol fractionation (Cohn fractionation). ISG is approximately 95% IgG with the remaining 5% consisting of other plasma proteins. ISG is for intramuscular use only; it must not be administered intravenously as it contains aggregated IgG complexes that can activate complement causing adverse reactions if administered intravenously. The commonest use of ISG is for hepatitis A or measles prophylaxis. Several specific intramuscular human immune globulin preparations are available. They are identical to ISG except that they have high titers to an infectious agent or the RhD antigen. The most commonly used preparations are hepatitis B immune globulin and varicella zoster immune globulin for the prevention of hepatitis B and varicella zoster infections, respectively, and RhD immune globulin for the prevention of RhD alloimmunization.

IVIG preparations are virtually free of immunoglobulin complexes and therefore safe for intravenous infusion. The protein content of IVIG preparations is > 95% IgG. Several nonspecific IVIG preparations are commercially available. They differ in the manufacturing processes used for immunoglobulin purification and for viral inactivation/removal and in their formulations, but for practical purposes are generally therapeutically equivalent. Some contain less IgA than others and are therefore preferentially chosen if treating a patient with anti-IgA. Licensed indications for IVIG administration vary among products and countries. Licensed indications include the use of IVIG as replacement therapy in primary immunodeficiency states and some secondary immunodeficiency states, including HIV infection in children and acquired hypogammaglobulinemia, and as an immunomodulating agent to treat patients with autoimmune thrombocytopenic purpura or Kawasaki disease.[242,243]

IVIG is also commonly used for the treatment of several disorders that are not labelled indications. There is good or reasonably good evidence for the efficacy of IVIG in some of these indications, such as Guillain–Barré syndrome, chronic inflammatory demyelinating polyneuropathy, refractory myasthenia gravis, hemolytic disease of the newborn and neonatal alloimmune thrombocytopenia (selected women during pregnancy and severely thrombocytopenic newborns for whom appropriate platelet concentrates are not immediately available).[242–248] The use of IVIG in other disorders for which it has been advocated is often based on the rationale that the disorder has a known or suspected autoimmune pathophysiology and the presence in the literature of anecdotal reports of efficacy. In these cases decisions as to the appropriate use of this expensive treatment are often problematic. A recent Cochrane Database Systematic Review evaluated the evidence for the use of IVIG for suspected or proven infection in neonates; the reviewers concluded that, at the present time, there is insufficient evidence to support the routine use of IVIG in this situation.[249]

There are intravenous immunoglobulin preparations with high-titer antibodies against infectious disease agents, such as cytomegalovirus or hepatitis B, which may be indicated for the prevention of the corresponding infections in selected patients (e.g., transplant recipients).[250,251] Intravenous anti-D preparations are also available, and in addition to their use to prevent RhD alloimmunization may also be used in the treatment of selected patients with autoimmune thrombocytopenic purpura.[252,253]

References

1. Hess JR, Greenwakt TG. Storage of red blood cells: new approaches. *Transfus Med Rev* 2002; **16**: 283–95.

2. Högman CF, Meryman HT. Storage parameters affecting red blood cell survival and function after transfusion. *Transfus Med Rev* 1999; **13**: 275–96.

3. Gullikson H. Additive solutions for the storage of platelets. *Transfus Med* 2000; **10**: 257–64.

4. Biomedical Excellence for Safer Transfusion (BEST) Collaborative. Platelets from pooled buffy coats: an update. *Transfusion* 2005; **45**: 634–9.

5. AABB. Process control. In: *Standards for Blood Banks and Transfusion Services*, 23rd edn. Bethesda, MD: American Association of Blood Banks Press, 2004, pp. 10–65.

6. Council of Europe. Red cells, leucocyte-depleted. In: *Guide to the Preparation, Use and Quality Assurance of Blood Components*, 11th edn. Germany: Council of Europe Publishing Strasbourg, 2005, pp. 109–12.

7. Gregori L, McCombie N, Palmer D *et al.* Effectiveness of leucoreduction for removal of infectivity transmissible spongiform encephalopathies from blood. *Lancet* 2004; **264**: 529–31.

8. Vamvakas EC, Blajchman MA. Universal WBC reduction: the case for and against. *Transfusion* 2001; **41**: 691–712.

9. Preiksaitis JK. The cytomegalovirus-"safe" blood product: is leukoreduction equivalent to antibody screening? *Transfus Med Rev* 2000; **14**: 112–36.

10. The Trial to Reduce Alloimmunization to Platelets Study Group. Leukocyte reduction and ultraviolet B irradiation of platelets to prevent alloimmunization and refractoriness to platelets transfusions. *N Engl J Med* 1997; **337**: 1861–9.

11. Seftel MD, Growe GH, Petraszko T *et al.* Universal prestorage leukoreduction in Canada decreases platelet alloimmunization and refractoriness. *Blood* 2004; **103**: 333–9.

12. Fergusson D, Khanna MP, Tinmouth A *et al.* Transfusion of leukoreduced red blood cells may decrease postoperative infections: two meta-analyses of randomized controlled trials. *Can J Anaesth* 2004; **51**: 417–25.

13. Vamvakas EC. WBC-containing allogeneic blood transfusion and mortality: a meta-analysis of randomized controlled trials. *Transfusion* 2003; **43**: 963–73.

14. Hébert PC, Fergusson D, Blajchman M *et al.* Clinical outcomes following institution of the Canadian universal leukoreduction program for red blood cell transfusions. *JAMA* 2003; **289**: 1941–9.

15. Dodd RY. Pathogen inactivation: mechanisms of action and in vitro efficacy of various agents. *Vox Sang* 2002; **83** (suppl. 1): 267–70.

16. Aubuchon JP. Pathogen inactivation in cellular blood components: clinical trials and implications of introduction to transfusion medicine. *Vox Sang* 2002; **83** (suppl. 1): 271–5.

17. Williamson LM. Correcting haemostasis. *Vox Sang* 2004; **87** (suppl. 1): 51–7.

18. Robitaille N, Nuyt AM, Panagopoulos A, Hume HA. Exchange transfusion in the infant. In: Hillyer CD, Strauss RG, Luban NLC (eds) *Handbook of Pediatric Transfusion Medicine*, 1st edn. San Diego: Elsevier Academic Press, 2004, pp. 159–65.

19. Council of Europe. Red cells. In: *Guide to the Preparation, Use and Quality Assurance of Blood Components*, 11th edn. Germany: Council of Europe Publishing Strasbourg, 2005, pp. 89–116.

20. Tuman KJ. Tissue oxygen delivery: the physiology of anemia. *Anesthesiol Clin North Am* 1990; **8**: 451–69.

21. Hebert PC, Qun L, Biro GP. Review of physiologic mechanisms in response to anemia. *Can Med Assoc J* 1997; **156** (suppl.): S27–S40.

22. Hume HA, Kronick JB, Blanchette VB. Review of the literature on allogeneic red blood cells and plasma transfusion in children. *Can Med Assoc J* 1997; **156**: S41–S49.

23. Weiskopf RB. Do we know when to transfuse red cells to treat acute anemia? *Transfusion* 1998; **38**: 517–21.

24. Weiskopf RB, Viele MK, Feiner J *et al.* Human cardiovascular and metabolic response to acute, severe isovolemic anemia. *JAMA* 1998; **279**: 217–21.

25. British Committee for Standards in Haematology, Blood Transfusion Task Force. Transfusion guidelines for neonates and older children. *Br J Haematol* 2004; **124**: 433–53.

26. Roseff SD, Luban NLC, Manno CS. Guidelines for assessing appropriateness of pediatric transfusion. *Transfusion* 2002; **42**: 1398–413.

27. Simon TL, Alverson DC, Aubuchon J *et al.* Practice parameter for the use of red blood cell transfusions: developed by the Red Blood Cell Administration Practice Guideline Development Task Force of the College of American Pathologists. *Arch Pathol Lab Med* 1998; **122**: 130–8.

28. Expert Working Group. Guidelines for red blood cell and plasma transfusion for adults and children. *Can Med Assoc J* 1997; **156** (Suppl. 11).

29. Smith PJ, Ekert H. Evidence of stem-cell competition in children with malignant disease. A controlled study of hypertransfusion. *Lancet* 1976; **i**: 776–9.

30. Toogood IRG, Ekert H, Smith PJ. Controlled study of hypertransfusion during remission induction in childhood acute lymphocytic leukemia. *Lancet* 1978; **i**: 862–4.

31. Holzer BR, Egger M, Teuscher R *et al.* Childhood anemia in Africa: to transfuse or not transfuse? *Acta Tropica* 1993; **55**: 47–51.

32. Guay J, Hume H, Gauthier M, Tremblay P. Choc hémorragique. In: Lacroix J, Gauthier M, Beaufils F (eds) *Urgences et Soins Intensif Pédiatriques*. Montreal: Les Presses de l'Université de Montreal, 1994, pp. 73–87.

33. Soud T, Pieper P, Hazinski MF. Pediatric trauma. In: Hazinski MF (ed.) *Nursing Care of the Critically Ill Child*. St Louis, MO: Mosby Year Book, 1992.

34. American Heart Association in collaboration with International Liaison Committee on Resuscitation. Guidelines 2000 for Cardiopulmonary Resuscitation and Emergency

Cardiovascular Care: International Consensus on Science, Part 10: Pediatric Advanced Life Support. *Circulation* 2000; **102** (suppl. I): I291–I342.

35. Petz LD. Blood transfusion in acquired hemolytic anemias. In: Petz LD, Kleinman S, Swisher SN, Spence BK, Strauss RG (eds) *Clinical Practice of Transfusion Medicine*, 3rd edn. New York: Churchill Livingstone, 1996, pp. 469–99.

36. Telen MJ. Principles and problems of transfusion in sickle cell disease. *Semin Hematol* 2001; **38**: 315–23.

37. Ohene-Frempong K. Indications for red cell transfusion in sickle cell disease. *Semin Hematol* 2001; **38** (S1): 5–13.

38. Vichinsky EP, Haberkern CM, Neumayr L *et al*. A comparison of conservative and aggressive transfusion regimens in the perioperative management of sickle cell disease. *N Engl J Med* 1995; **333**: 206–13.

39. Ohene-Frempong K. Stroke in sickle cell disease: demographic, clinical, and therapeutic considerations. *Semin Hematol* 1991; **28**: 213–19.

40. Miller ST, Jensen D, Rao SP. Less intensive long-term transfusion therapy for sickle cell anemia and cerebrovascular accident. *J Pediatr* 1992; **120**: 54–7.

41. Cohen AR, Martin MB, Silber JH *et al*. A modified transfusion program for prevention of stroke in sickle cell disease. *Blood* 1992; **79**: 1657–61.

42. Adams RJ, McKie VC, Hsu L *et al*. Prevention of a first stroke by transfusions in children with sickle cell anemia and abnormal results on transcranial doppler ultrasonography. *N Engl J Med* 1998; **339**: 5–11.

42a. Adams RJ, Brambilla D. Optimizing Primary Stroke Prevention in Sickle Cell Anemia (STOP 2) Trial Investigators. Discontinuing prophylactic transfusions used to prevent stroke in sickle cell disease. *N Engl J Med* 2005; **353**: 2743–5.

43. Buchanan GR, Debaun MR, Quinn CT *et al*. Sickle cell disease. *Hematology (Am Soc Hematol Educ Program)* 2004; 35–47.

44. Vichinsky EP, Earles A, Johnson RA *et al*. Alloimmunization in sickle cell anemia and transfusion of racially unmatched blood. *N Engl J Med* 1990; **322**: 1617–21.

45. Aygun B, Padmanabhan S, Paley C, Chandrasekaran V. Clinical significance of RBC alloantibodies and autoantibodies in sickle cell patients who received transfusions. *Transfusion* 2002; **42**: 37–43.

46. Vichinsky EP, Luban NLC, Wright E *et al*. Prospective RBC phenotype matching in a stroke-prevention trial in sickle cell anemia: a multicenter transfusion trial. *Transfusion* 2001; **41**: 1086–92.

47. Castro O, Sandler G, Houston-Yu P, Rana S. Predicting the effect of transfusing only phenotype-matched RBCs to patients with sickle cell disease: theoretical and practical implications. *Transfusion* 2002; **42**: 684–90.

48. Jan K, Usami S, Smith JA. Effects of transfusion on the rheological properties of blood in sickle cell anemia. *Transfusion* 1982; **22**: 17–20.

49. Rackoff WR, Ohene-Frempong K, Month S *et al*. Neurologic events after partial exchange transfusion for priapism in sickle cell disease. *J Pediatr* 1992; **120**: 882–5.

50. King KE, Shirey RS, Lankiewicz MW *et al*. Delayed hemolytic transfusion reactions in sickle cell disease; simultaneous destruction of recipient's red cells. *Transfusion* 1997; **37**: 376–81.

51. Petz LD, Calhoun L, Shulman IA *et al*. The sickle cell hemolytic transfusion reaction syndrome. *Transfusion* 1997; **37**: 382–92.

52. Win N, Doughty H, Telfer P, Wild BJ, Pearson TC. Hyperhemolytic transfusion reaction in sickle cell disease. *Transfusion* 2001; **41**: 323–8.

53. Talano JA, Hillery CA, Gottschall JL, Baylerian DM, Scott JP. Delayed hemolytic transfusion reaction/hyperhemolysis syndrome in children with sickle cell disease. *Pediatrics* 2003; **111**: 661–5.

54. Cullis JO, Win N, Dudley JM, Kaye T. Posttransfusion hyperhemolysis in a patient with sickle cell disease: use of steroids and intravenous immunoglobulin to prevent further red cell destruction. *Vox Sang* 1995; **69**: 355–7.

55. Win N, Yeghen T, Needs M, Chen FE, Okpala I. Use of intravenous immunoglobulin and intravenous methylprednisolone in hyperhaemolysis syndrome in sickle cell disease. *Hematology (Am Soc Hematol Educ Program)* 2004; **9**: 433–6.

56. Piomelli S, Seaman C, Ackerman K *et al*. Planning an exchange transfusion in patients with sickle cell syndromes. *Am J Pediatr Hematol Oncol* 1990; **12**: 268–76.

57. Kim HC, Dugan NP, Silber JH *et al*. Erythrocytapheresis therapy to reduce iron overload in chronically transfused patients with sickle cell disease. *Blood* 1994; **83**: 1136–42.

58. Adams DM, Schultz WH, Ware RE, Kinney TR. Erythrocytapheresis can reduce iron overload and prevent the need for chelation therapy in chronically transfused pediatric patients. *J Pediatr Hematol Oncol* 1996; **18**: 46–50.

59. Hilliard LM, Williams BF, Lounsbury AE, Howard TH. Erythrocytapheresis limits iron accumulation in chronically transfused sickle cell patients. *Am J Hematol* 1998; **59**: 28–35.

60. Olivieri NF. The β-thalassemias. *N Engl J Med* 1999; **341**: 99–109.

61. Prati D. Benefits and complications of regular blood transfusion in patients with beta-thalassaemia major. *Vox Sang* 2000; **79**: 129–37.

62. Propper RD, Button LN, Nathan DG. New approaches to the transfusion management of thalassemia. *Blood* 1980; **55**: 55–60.

63. Cohen AR, Schmidt JM, Martin MB *et al*. Clinical trial of young red cell transfusions. *J Pediatr* 1984; **104**: 865–8.

64. Marcus RE, Wonke B, Bantock HM *et al*. A prospective trial of young red cells in 48 patients with transfusion-dependent thalassaemia. *Br J Haematol* 1985; **60**: 153–9.

65. Collins AF, Gonçalves-Digs C, Haddad S *et al*. Comparison of a transfusion preparation of newly formed red cells and standard washed red cell transfusions in patients with homozygous β-thalassemia. *Transfusion* 1994; **34**: 517–20.

66. Spanos T, Ladis V, Palamidou F *et al*. The impact of neocyte transfusion in the management of thalassaemia. *Vox Sang* 1996; **70**: 217–23.

67. Cohen AR, Galanello R, Pennell DJ *et al*. Thalassemia. *Hematoloy (Am Soc Hematol Educ Program)* 2004; 14–34.

68. Brecher M (ed.) *Technical Manual*, 14th edn. Bethesda, MD: American Association of Blood Banks, 2002, p. 556.

69. Michail-Merianou V, Pamphili-Panousopoulou L, Piperi-Lowes L *et al*. Alloimmunization to red cell antigens in thalassemia: comparative study of usual versus better match transfusion programs. *Vox Sang* 1987; **52**: 95–8.

70. Jayabose S, Tugal O, Ruddy R *et al*. Transfusion therapy for severe anemia. *Am J Pediatr Hematol Oncol* 1993; **15**: 324–7.

71. Berman B, Krieger A, Naiman JL. A new method for calculating volumes of blood required for partial exchange transfusion. *J Pediatr* 1979; **94**: 86–9.

72. Fosburg M, Dolan M, Propper R *et al.* Intensive plasma exchange in small and critically ill pediatric patients: techniques and clinical outcome. *J Clin Apheresis* 1983; **1**: 215–24.

73. Gorlin JB. Therapeutic plasma exchange and cytapheresis in pediatric patients. *Transfus Sci* 1999; **21**: 21–39.

74. Strauss RG. Neonatal anemia: pathophysiology and treatment. In: Wilson SM, Levitt JS, Strauss RG (eds) *Improving Transfusion Practice for Pediatric Patients*. Arlington, VA: American Association of Blood Banks, 1991, pp. 1–17.

75. Maier RF, Sonntag J, Walka M *et al.* Changing practices of red blood cell transfusions in infants with birth weight less than 1000 g. *J Pediatr* 2000; **136**: 220–4.

76. Brugnara C, Platt OS. Neonatal hematology: the neonatal erythrocyte and its disorders. In: Nathan DG, Orkin STT, Ginsberg D, Look AT (eds) *Hematology of Infancy and Childhood*, 6th edn. Philadelphia: Saunders, 2003, pp. 19–55.

77. Strauss RG. Blood banking issues pertaining to neonatal red blood cell transfusions. *Transfus Sci* 1999; **21**: 7–19.

78. Hume H. Red blood cell transfusions for preterm infants: the role of evidence-based medicine. *Semin Perinatol* 1997; **21**: 8–19.

79. Luban NL. Neonatal red blood cell transfusions. *Vox Sang* 2004; **87** (suppl. 2): 184–8.

80. Lin JC, Strauss RG, Kulhavy JC *et al.* Phlebotomy overdraw in the neonatal intensive care nursery. *Pediatrics* 2000; **106**: e19.

81. Miyashiro AM, dos Santos N, Guinsburg R *et al.* Strict red blood cell transfusion guideline reduces the need for transfusions in very-low-birth-weight infants in the first 4 weeks of life: a multicentre trial. *Vox Sang* 2005; **88**: 107–13.

82. Shannon KM, Keith JF, Mentzer WC *et al.* Recombinant human erythropoietin stimulates erythropoiesis and reduces erythrocyte transfusions in very low birth weight preterm infants. *Pediatrics* 1995; **95**: 1–8.

83. Fetus and Newborn Committee, Canadian Paediatric Society. RBC transfusions in newborn infants: revised guidelines. *Pediatrics and Child Health* 2002; **7**: 553–8.

84. Calhoun DA, Christenen RD, Edstrom CS *et al.* Consistent approaches to procedures and practices in neonatal hematology. *Clin Perinatol* 2000; **27**: 733–53.

85. Heddle NM, Kirpalani H, Whyte R *et al.* Identifying the optimal red cell transfusion threshold for extremely low birth weight infants: the premature in need of transfusion (PINT) study. *Transfusion* 2004; **44S**: 1A.

86. Luban NLC. Massive transfusion in the neonate. *Transfus Med Rev* 1995; **9**: 200–14.

87. Luban NLC, Strauss RG, Hume HA. Commentary on the safety of red cells preserved in extended-storage media for neonatal transfusions. *Transfusion* 1991; **31**: 229–35.

88. Strauss RG. Data-driven blood banking practices for neonatal RBC transfusions. *Transfusion* 2000; **40**: 1528–40.

89. Chambers LA. Evaluation of a filter-syringe set for preparation of packed cell aliquots for neonatal transfusion. *Am J Clin Pathol* 1995; **104**: 253–7.

90. Strauss RG, Villhauer PJ, Cordle DG. A method to collect, store and issue multiple aliquots of packed red blood cells for neonatal transfusions. *Vox Sang* 1995; **68**: 77–81.

91. Hall TL, Barnes A, Miller JR *et al.* Neonatal mortality following transfusion of red cells with high plasma potassium levels. *Transfusion* 1993; **33**: 606–9.

92. Manno CS, Hedberg KW, Kim HC *et al.* Comparison of the hemostatic effects of fresh whole blood, stored whole blood, and components after open heart surgery in children. *Blood* 1991; **77**: 930–6.

93. Mou SS, Giroir BP, Molitor-Kirsch A *et al.* Fresh whole blood versus reconstituted blood for pump priming in heart surgery in infants. *N Engl J Med* 2004; **351**: 1635–44.

94. Murphy RJC, Malhorta C, Sweet AY. Death following an exchange transfusion with hemoglobin SC blood. *J Pediatr* 1980; **96**: 110–12.

95. British Committee for Standards in Haematology Blood Transfusion Task Force. Guidelines for autologous donation: preoperative autologous donation. *Transfus Med* 1993; **3**: 307–16.

96. NHLBI. Transfusion alert: use of autologous blood. *Transfusion* 1995; **35**: 703–11.

97. Goodnough LT, Monk TG, Brecher ME. Autologous blood procurement in the surgical setting: lessons learned in the last 10 years. *Vox Sang* 1996; **71**: 133–41.

98. British Committee for Standards in Haematology Blood Transfusion Task Force. Guidelines for autologous transfusion. II. Perioperative haemodilution and cell salvage. *Br J Anaesth* 1997; **78**: 768–71.

99. Shander A, Rijhwani TS. Acute normovolemic hemodilution. *Transfusion* 2004; **44**: 26S–34S.

100. Etchason J, Petz L, Keeler E *et al.* The cost effectiveness of preoperative autologous blood donations. *N Engl J Med* 1995; **332**: 719–24.

101. Thompson HW, Luban NL. Autologous blood transfusion in the pediatric patient. *J Pediatr Surg* 1995; **30**: 1406–11.

102. Thomas MJ, Gillon J, Desmond MJ. Consensus conference on autologous transfusion. Preoperative autologous donation. *Transfusion* 1996; **36**: 633–9.

103. Moran MM, Kroon D, Tredwell SJ, Wadsworth LD. The role of autologous blood transfusion in adolescents undergoing spinal surgery. *Spine* 1995; **20**: 532–6.

104. Ridgeway S, Tai C, Alton P, Barnardo P, Harrison DJ. Pre-donated autologous blood transfusion in scoliosis surgery. *J Bone Joint Surg Br* 2003; **85**: 1032–6.

105. Tasaki T, Ohto H, Noguchi M, Abe R, Kikuchi S, Hoshino S. Autologous blood donation in elective surgery in children. *Vox Sang* 1994; **66**: 188–93.

106. Kemmotsu H, Joe K, Nakamura H, Yamashita M. Predeposited autologous blood transfusion for surgery in infants and children. *Pediatr Surg* 1995; **30**: 659–61.

107. Masuda M, Kawachi Y, Inaba S *et al.* Preoperative autologous blood donations in pediatric cardiac surgery. *Ann Thorac Surg* 1995; **60**: 1694–7.

108. Mayer MN, deMontalembert M, Audat F *et al.* Autologous blood donation for elective surgery in children weighing 8–25 kg. *Vox Sang* 1996; **70**: 224–8.

109. Haberkern M, Dangel P. Normovolemic hemodilution and intraoperative autotransfusion in children: experience with 30 cases of spinal fusion. *Eur J Pediatr Surg* 1991; **1**: 30–5.

110. Simpson MB, Georgopoulos G, Eilert RE. Intraoperative blood salvage in children and young adults undergoing spinal

surgery with predeposited autologous blood: efficacy and cost effectiveness. *J Pediatr Orthop* 1993; **13**: 777–80.

111. van Interson M, van der Waart FJ, Erdmann W, Trouwborst A. Systemic haemodynamics and oxygenation during haemodilution in children. *Lancet* 1995; **346**: 1127–9.

112. Siller TA, Dickson JH, Erwin WD. Efficacy and cost considerations of intraoperative autologous transfusion in spinal fusion for idiopathic scoliosis with predeposited blood. *Spine* 1996; **21**: 848–52.

113. Usher R, Shephard M, Lind J. The blood volume of the newborn infant and placental transfusion. *Acta Paediatr Scand* 1963; **52**: 497–512.

114. Yao AC, Lind J, Thasala R, Michelsson K. Placental transfusion in the premature infant with observation on clinical course and outcome. *Acta Paediatr Scand* 1969; **58**: 561–6.

115. Kinmond S, Aitchison TC, Holland BM, Jones JG, Turner TL, Wardrop CAJ. Umbilical cord clamping and preterm infants: a randomised trial. *Br Med J* 1993; **306**: 172–5.

116. McDonnell M, Henderson-Smart DJ. Delayed umbilical cord clamping in preterm infants: a feasibility study. *J Paediatr Child Health* 1997; **33**: 308–10.

117. Rabe H, Wacker A, Hulskamp G. A randomised controlled trial of delayed cord clamping in very low birth weight preterm infants. *Eur J Pediatr* 2000; **159**: 775–7.

118. Strauss RG, Mock DM, Johnson K *et al.* Circulating RBC volume, measured with biotinylated RBCs is superior to the Hct to document the hematologic effects of delayed versus immediate umbilical cord clamping in preterm neonates. *Transfusion* 2003; **43**: 1168–72.

119. Bifano EM, Dracker RA, Lorah K, Palit A. Collection and 28-day storage of human placental blood. *Pediatr Res* 1994; **36**: 90–4.

120. Ballin A, Arbel E, Kenet G *et al.* Autologous umbilical cord blood transfusion. *Arch Dis Child* 1995; **73**: F181–F183.

121. Surbek DV, Glanzmann R, Senn H-P. Can cord blood be used for autologous transfusion in preterm neonates? *Eur J Pediatr* 2000; **159**: 790–1.

122. Eichler H, Schaible T, Richter E. Cord blood as a source of autologous RBCs for transfusion to preterm infants. *Transfusion* 2000; **40**: 1111–17.

123. Brune T, Garritsen H, Hentschel R. Efficacy, recovery and safety of RBC from autologous placental blood: clinical experience in 52 newborns. *Transfusion* 2003; **43**: 1210–16.

124. Valderrabano F. Erythropoietin in chronic renal failure. *Kidney Int* 1996; **50**: 1373–91.

125. Vamvakas EC, Strauss RG. Meta-analysis of controlled clinical trials studying the efficacy of rHuEPO in reducing blood transfusions in the anemia of prematurity. *Transfusion* 2001; **41**: 406–15.

126. Rizzo JD, Lichtin AE, Woolf SH *et al.* Use of epoetin in patients with cancer: evidence-based clinical practice guidelines of the American Society of Clinical Oncology and the American Society of Hematology. *Blood* 2002; **100**: 2303–20.

127. Bohlius JF, Langensiepen S, Engert A, Schwarzer G, Bennett CL. Effectiveness of erythropoietin in the treatment of patients with malignancies: methods and preliminary results of a Cochrane review. *Best Pract Res Clin Haematol* 2005; **18**: 449–54.

128. Bokemeyer C, Aapro MS, Courdi A *et al.* EORTC guidelines for the use of erythropoietic proteins in anaemic patients with cancer. *Eur J Cancer* 2004; **40**: 2201–16.

129. Goldfinger D. Directed blood donations: pro. *Transfusion* 1989; **29**: 70–4.

130. Page PL. Directed blood donations: con. *Transfusion* 1989; **29**: 65–9.

131. Grindon AJ. Infectious disease markers in directed donors in the Atlanta region. *Transfusion* 1991; **31**: 872–3.

132. Starkey JM, MacPherson JL, Bolgiano DC *et al.* Markers for transfusion-transmitted disease in different groups of blood donors. *JAMA* 1989; **262**: 3452–4.

133. Petz L, Kanter MH, Pink J, Wylie B. Infectious disease markers in autologous and directed donations. *Transfus Med* 1995; **5**: 159–63.

134. Elbert C, Strauss RG, Barrett F *et al.* Biological mothers may be dangerous blood donors for their neonates. *Acta Haematol* 1991; **85**: 189–91.

135. Goldman M, Rémy-Prince S, Trépanier A, Décary F. Autologous donation error rates in Canada. *Transfusion* 1997; **37**: 523–7.

136. Strauss RG, Wieland MR, Randels MJ, Koerner TAW. Feasibility and success of a single-donor red cell program for pediatric elective surgery patients. *Transfusion* 1992; **32**: 747.

137. Strauss RG, Barnes A, Blanchette VS *et al.* Directed and limited-exposure blood donations for infants and children. *Transfusion* 1989; **30**: 68–72.

138. Smith JF, Ness PM, Moroff G, Luban NL. Retention of coagulation factors in plasma frozen after extended holding at 1–6 degrees C. *Vox Sang* 2000; **78**: 28–30.

139. O'Neill EM, Rowley J, Hansson-Wicher M, McCarter S, Rango G, Valeri CR. Effect of 24-hour whole-blood storage on plasma clotting factors. *Transfusion* 1999; **39**: 488–91.

140. Williamson LM, Allain JP. Virally inactivated fresh frozen plasma. *Vox Sang* 1995; **69**: 159–65.

141. Loirat C, Sonsino E, Hinglais N *et al.* Treatment of the childhood hemolytic uraemic syndrome with plasma. *Pediatr Nephrol* 1988; **2**: 279–85.

142. Rizzoni G, Claris-Appiani A, Edefonti A *et al.* Plasma infusion for hemolytic-uremic syndrome in children: results of a multicenter controlled trial. *J Pediatr* 1988; **112**: 284–90.

143. Stanworth SJ, Brunskill SJ, Hyde CJ, McClelland DB, Murphy MF. Is fresh frozen plasma clinically effective? A systematic review of randomised controlled trials. *Br J Haematol* 2004; **126**: 139–52.

144. Consensus Conference. Fresh-frozen plasma: indications and risks. *JAMA* 1985; **253**: 551–3.

145. Development Task Force of the College of American Pathologists. Practice parameter for the use of fresh-frozen plasma, cryoprecipitate, and platelets: fresh-frozen plasma, cryoprecipitate, and platelets administration practice guidelines. *JAMA* 1994; **271**: 777–81.

146. American Society of Anesthesiologists Task Force on Blood Component Therapy. Practice guidelines for blood component therapy. *Anesthesiology* 1996; **84**: 732–47.

147. British Committee for Standards in Haematology, Blood Transfusion Task Force. Guidelines for the use of fresh-frozen plasma, cryoprecipitate and cryosupernatant. *Br J Haematol* 2004; **126**: 11.

148. Monagle P, Chan A, Massicotte P, Chalmers E, Michelson AD. Antithrombotic therapy in children: the seventh ACCP conference on antithrombotic and thrombolytic therapy. *Chest* 2004; **126** (3 suppl.): 645S–687S.

149. Rosovsky R, Marks PW. Hematologic manifestations of systemic disease: liver and renal disease. Hoffman R, Benz EJ Jr, Shattil SJ *et al.* (eds) *Hematologic Principles and Practice*, 4th edn. Philadelphia: Elsevier Churchill Livingstone, 2005, pp. 2564–72.

150. Hambleton J, Leung LL, Levi M. Coagulation: consultative hemostasis. *Hematology (Am Soc Hematol Educ Program)* 2002; 335–52.

151. Levi M, de Jonge E, Meijers J. The diagnosis of disseminated intravascular coagulation. *Blood Rev* 2002; **16**: 217–23.

152. Hiippala ST, Myllylä GJ, Vahtera EM. Hemostatic factors and replacement of major blood loss with plasma-poor red cell concentrates. *Anesth Analg* 1995; **81**: 360–5.

153. Mannucci PM, Federici AB, Sirchia G. Hemostasis testing during blood replacement. A study of 172 cases. *Vox Sang* 1982; **42**: 113–23.

154. Hardy JF, Moerloose P, Samama M *et al.* Massive transfusion and coagulopathy: pathophysiology and implications for clinical management. *Can J Anesth* 2004; **51**: 293–310.

155. Andrew M, Paes B, Milner R *et al.* The development of the human coagulation system in the full-term infant. *Blood* 1987; **70**: 165–72.

156. Andrew M, Paes B, Milner R *et al.* Development of the coagulation system in the healthy premature infant. *Blood* 1988; **72**: 1651–7.

157. Northern Neonatal Nursing Initiative Trial Group. Randomised trial of prophylactic early fresh-frozen plasma or gelatin or glucose in preterm babies: outcome at 2 years. *Lancet* 1996; **348**: 229–32.

158. Mintz, PD. Rh immune globulin. In: Mintz PD (ed.) *Transfusion therapy clinical principle and practice*, 2nd edn. Bethesda, MD: AABB Press, 2005, pp. 429–31.

159. Gottschall J (ed.) Blood Transfusion Therapy: a Physician's Handbook, 8th edn. Bethesda, MD: AABB, 2005, p. 27.

160. Mannucio P, Duga S, Peyvandi F. Recessively inherited coagulation disorders. *Blood* 2004; **104**: 1243–52.

161. Pietersz RNL, Engelfriet CP, Reesink HW. International forum: evaluation of stored platelets. *Vox Sang* 2004; **86**: 203–23.

162. Hersh EM, Bodey GP, Nies BA, Freireich EJ. Causes of death in acute leukemi ten-year study of 414 patients from 1954–1963. *JAMA* 1965; **193**: 99–103.

163. Schiffer CA. Prophylactic platelet transfusion. *Transfusion* 1992; **32**: 295–8.

164. Stanworth SJ, Hyde C, Heddle N, Rebulla P, Brunskill S, Murphy MF. Prophylactic platelet transfusion for haemorrhage after chemotherapy and stem cell transplantation. *The Cochrane Collaboration* 2005; (1): CD004269.

165. Schiffer CA. Some aspects of recent advances in the use of blood cell components. *Br J Haematol* 1978; **39**: 289–94.

166. Hoak JC, Koepeke JA. Platelet transfusions. *Clin Haematol* 1976; **5**: 69.

167. Kelton JG, Blajchman MA. Platelet transfusions. *Can Med Assoc J* 1979; **121**: 1353–8.

168. Tomasulo PA, Lenes BA. Platelet transfusion therapy.

Menitove JE, McCarthy LJ (eds) *Hemostatic Disorders and the Blood Bank*. Arlington, VA: American Association of Blood Banks, 1984, pp. 63–89.

169. Pisciotto PT, Benson K, Hume H *et al.* Prophylactic versus therapeutic platelet transfusion practices in hematology and/or oncology patients. *Transfusion* 1995; **35**: 498–502.

170. Wong EC, Perez-Albuerne E, Moscow JA, Luban NL. Transfusion management strategies: a survey of practicing pediatric haematology/oncology specialists. *Pediatr Blood Cancer* 2005; **44**: 114–16.

171. Gaydos LA, Freireich EJ, Mantel N. The quantitative relation between platelet count and hemorrhage in patients with acute leukemia. *N Engl J Med* 1962; **266**: 905–9.

172. National Institutes of Health, Consensus Development Conference. Platelet transfusion therapy. *JAMA* 1987; **257**: 1777–80.

173. Gil-Fernandez JJ, Alegre A, Fernandez-Villalta MJ *et al.* Clinical results of a stringent policy on prophylactic platelet transfusion: nonrandomized comparative analysis in 190 bone marrow transplant patients from a single institution. *Bone Marrow Transplant* 1996; **18**: 931–5.

174. Gmür J, Burger J, Schanz U *et al.* Safety of stringent prophylactic platelet transfusion policy for patients with acute leukaemia. *Lancet* 1991; **338**: 1223–6.

175. Heckman KD, Weiner GJ, Davis CS *et al.* Randomized study of prophylactic platelet transfusion threshold during induction therapy for adult acute leukemia: 10,000/microL versus 20,000/microL. *J Clin Oncol* 1997; **15**: 1143–9.

176. Rebulla P, Finazzi G, Marangoni F *et al.* The threshold for prophylactic platelet transfusion in adults with acute myeloid leukemia. *N Engl J Med* 1997; **337**: 1870–5.

177. Wandt H, Frank M, Ehninger G *et al.* Safety and cost effectiveness of a 10×10^9/L for prophylactic platelet transfusions compared with the traditional 20×10^9/L trigger: a prospective comparative trial in 105 patients with acute myeloid leukemia. *Blood* 1998; **91**: 3601–6.

178. Sagmeister M, Oec L, Gmür J. A restrictive platelet transfusion policy allowing long-term support of outpatients with severe aplastic anemia. *Blood* 1999; **93**: 3124–6.

179. Klumpp TR, Herman JH, Gaughan JP *et al.* Clinical consequences of alterations in platelet transfusion dose: a prospective, randomized, double-blind trial. *Transfusion* 1999; **39**: 674–81.

180. Zumberg MS, del Rosario ML, Nejame CF *et al.* A prospective randomized trial of prophylactic platelet transfusion and bleeding incidence in hematopoietic stem cell transplant recipients: 10,000/microL versus 20,000/microL trigger. *Biol Blood Marrow Transplant* 2002; **8**: 569–76.

181. Schiffer CA, Anderson KC, Bennett CL. Platelet transfusion for patients with cancer: clinical practice guidelines of the American Society of Clinical Oncology. *J Clin Oncol* 2001; **19**: 1519–38.

182. British Committee for Standards in Haematology, Blood Transfusion Task Force. Guidelines for the use of platelet transfusions. *Br J Haematol* 2003; **122**: 10–23.

183. Bishop JF, Schiffer CA, Aisner J *et al.* Surgery in leukemia: a review of 167 operations on thrombocytopenic patients. *Am J Hematol* 1987; **26**: 147–55.

184. Doerfler ME, Kaufman B, Goldenberg AS. Central venous

catheter placement in patients with disorders of hemostasis. *Chest* 1996; **110**: 185–8.

185. Ray CE, Shenoy SS. Patients with thrombocytopenia: outcome of radiologic placement of central venous access devices. *Radiology* 1997; **204**: 97–9.

186. Howard SC, Gajjar A, Ribeiro RC *et al*. Safety of lumbar puncture for children with acute lymphoblastic leukemia and thrombocytopenia. *JAMA* 2000; **284**: 2222–4.

187. Feusner J. Platelet transfusion "trigger" for lumbar puncture. *Pediatr Blood Cancer* 2004; **43**: 793.

188. Veen JJ, Vora AJ, Welch JC. Lumbar puncture in thrombocytopenic children. *Br J Haematol* 2004; **127**: 234–5.

189. George JN, Woolf SH, Raskob GE *et al*. Idiopathic thrombocytopenic purpura: a practice guideline developed by explicit methods for the American Society of Hematology. *Blood* 1996; **88**: 3–40.

190. Cines DB, Blanchette VS. Immune thrombocytopenic purpura. *N Engl J Med* 2002; **346**: 995–1008.

191. Flordal PA, Sahlin S. Use of desmopressin to prevent bleeding complications in patients treated with aspirin. *Br J Surg* 1993; **80**: 723–4.

192. Sheridan DP, Card RT, Pinilla JC *et al*. Use of desmopressin acetate to reduce blood transfusion requirements during cardiac surgery in patients with acetylsalicylic-acid-induced platelet dysfunction. *Can J Surg* 1994; **37**: 33–6.

193. Herman JH, Benson K. Platelet transfusion therapy. Mintz PD (ed.) *Transfusion Therapy Clinical Principle and Practice*, 2nd edn. Bethesda, MD: AABB Press, 2005, pp. 335–53.

194. Addonizio VP. Platelet function in cardiopulmonary bypass and artificial organs. *Hematol Oncol Clin North Am* 1990; **4**: 145–55.

195. Campbell FW. The contribution of platelet dysfunction to post bypass bleeding. *J Cardiothorac Vasc Anesth* 1991; **5**: 8–12.

196. Simon TL, Aki BF, Murphy W. Controlled trial of routine administration of platelet concentrates in cardiopulmonary bypass surgery. *Ann Thorac Surg* 1984; **37**: 359–64.

197. Cheung PY, Sawicki G, Salas E *et al*. The mechanisms of platelet dysfunction during extracorporeal membrane oxygenation in critically ill neonates. *Crit Care Med* 2000; **28**: 2584–90.

198. Andrew M, Vegh P, Caco C *et al*. A randomized, controlled trial of platelet transfusion in thrombocytopenic premature infants. *J Pediatr* 1993; **123**: 285–91.

199. Murray NA, Howarth LJ, McCloy MP *et al*. Platelet transfusion in the management of severe thrombocytopenia in neonatal intensive care unit patients. *Transfus Med* 2002; **12**: 35–41.

200. Saxonhouse M, Slayton W, Sola MC. Platelet transfusions in the infant and child. In: Hillyer CD, Strauss RG, Luban NLC (eds) *Handbook of Pediatric Transfusion Medicine*, 1st edn. California: Elsevier Academic Press, San Diego, 2004, pp. 253–69.

200a. Kiefel V, Bassler D, Kroll H *et al*. Antigen-positive platelet transfusion in neonatal alloimmune thrombocytopenia (NAIT). *Blood* 2006 Jan 10; [Epub ahead of print].

201. Miguel L, Cid J. The clinical implications of platelet transfusions associated with ABO or Rh(D) incompatibility. *Transfus Med Rev* 2003; **17**: 57–68.

202. Josephson CD, Mullis NC, Van Demark C *et al*. Significant numbers of apheresis-derived group O platelet units have "high-titer" anti-A/A,B: implications for transfusion policy. *Transfusion* 2004; **44**: 805–8.

203. National Blood Transfusion Service Immunoglobulin Working Party. Recommendations for the use of anti-D immunoglobulin. *Prescribers J* 1991; **31**: 137.

204. Norol F, Bierling P, Roudot-Thoraval F *et al*. Platelet transfusion: a dose–response study. *Blood* 1998; **92**: 1448–53.

205. Tinmouth A, Tannock IF, Crump M *et al*. Low-dose prophylactic platelet transfusion in recipients of an autologous peripheral blood progenitor cell transplant and patients with acute leukemia: a randomized controlled trial with a sequential Bayesian design. *Transfusion* 2004; **44**: 1711–19.

206. Sensebé L, Giraudeau B, Bardiaux L *et al*. The efficiency of transfusing high doses of platelets in hematologic patients with thrombocytopenia: results of a prospective, randomized, open, blinded end point (PROBE) study. *Blood* 2005; **105**: 862–4.

207. Slichter SJ. Platelet transfusion: future directions. *Vox Sang* 2004; **87** (suppl. 2): 47–51.

208. Strauss RG. Low-dose prophylactic platelet transfusions: time for further study, but too early for routine clinical practice. *Transfusion* 2004; **44**: 1680–2.

209. Slichter SJ. Mechanisms and management of platelet refractoriness. In: Nance ST (ed.) *Transfusion Medicine in the 1990's*. Arlington, VA: American Association of Blood Banks, 1990, pp. 95–179.

210. Bock M, Muggenthaler KH, Schmidt U, Heim MU. Influence of antibiotics on posttransfusion platelet increment. *Transfusion* 1996; **36**: 952–4.

211. Alcorta I, Pereira A, Ordinas A. Clinical and laboratory factors associated with platelet transfusion refractorines case-control study. *Br J Haematol* 1996; **93**: 220–4.

212. Novotny VM. Prevention and management of platelet transfusion refractoriness. *Vox Sang* 1999; **76**: 1–13.

213. Petz LD, Garatty G, Calhoun L *et al*. Selecting donors of platelets for refractory patients on the basis of HLA antibody specificity. *Transfusion* 2000; **40**: 1446–56.

214. Rebula P, Morelati F, Revelli N *et al*. Outcomes of an automated procedure for the selection of effective platelets for patients refractory to random donors based on cross-matching locally available platelet products. *Br J Haematol* 2004; **125**: 83–9.

215. Delaflor-Weiss E, Mintz PD. The evaluation and management of platelet refractoriness and alloimmunization. *Transfus Med Rev* 2000; **14**: 180–96.

216. Shpilberg O, Glumenthal R, Sofer O *et al*. A controlled trial of tranexamic acid therapy for the reduction of bleeding during treatment of acute myeloid leukemia. *Leukemia Lymphoma* 1995; **19**: 141–4.

217. Lee EJ, Schiffer CA. Serial measurement of lymphocytotoxic antibody and response to nonmatched platelet transfusions in alloimmunized patients. *Blood* 1987; **70**: 1727–9.

218. Murphy MF, Metcalfe P, Ord J *et al*. Disappearance of HLA and platelet-specific antibodies in acute leukaemia patients alloimmunized by multiple transfusions. *Br J Haematol* 1987; **67**: 255–60.

219. Kickler T, Braine HG, Piantadosi S *et al*. A randomized, placebo-controlled trial of intravenous gammaglobulin in alloimmunized thrombocytopenic patients. *Blood* 1990; **75**: 313–16.

220. Bishton M, Chopra R. The role of granulocyte transfusions in neutropenic patients. *Br J Haematol* 2004; **127**: 501–8.

221. Brecher M (ed.). *AABB Technical Manual*, 14th edn. Bethesda MD: American Association of Blood Banks, 2002, p. 132.

222. Vamvakas EC, Pineda AA. Determinants of the efficacy of prophylactic granulocyte transfusions: a meta-analysis. *J Clin Apheresis* 1997; **12**: 74–81.

223. Hübel K, Carter RA, Liles WC, Dale DC *et al.* Granulocyte transfusion therapy for infections in candidates and recipients of HPC transplantation: a comparative analysis of feasibility and outcome for community donors versus related donors. *Transfusion* 2002; **42**: 1414–21.

224. Van Burik JH, Weisdorf DJ. Is it time for a new look at granulocyte transfusions? *Transfusion* 2002; **42**: 1393–5.

225. Nathan DG, Orkin SH, Ginsburg D, Look AT (eds). *Hematology of Infancy and Childhood*, 6th edn. Philadelphia: WB Saunders, 2003, Appendix 26, p. 1848.

226. Mohan P, Brocklehurst P. Granulocyte transfusions for neonates with confirmed or suspected sepsis and neutropenia. *Cochrane Database Syst Rev* 2003; (4): CD003956.

227. Rosenthal J, Healey T, Ellis R *et al.* A two-year follow-up of neonates with presumed sepsis treated with recombinant human granulocyte colony-stimulating factor during the first week of life. *J Pediatr* 1996; **128**: 135–7.

228. Stroncek DF, Leonard K, Eiber G *et al.* Alloimmunization after granulocyte transfusions. *Transfusion* 1996; **36**: 1009–15.

229. Wright DG, Robichaud KJ, Pizzo PA *et al.* Lethal pulmonary reactions associated with the combined use of amphotericin B and leukocyte transfusions. *N Engl J Med* 1981; **304**: 1185–9.

230. Weiss RA, Schoeneman M, Greifer I. Treatment of severe nephritic edema with albumin and furosemide. *NY State J Med* 1984; **84**: 384–6.

231. Luca A, Garcia-Pagan JC, Bosch J *et al.* Beneficial effects of intravenous albumin infusion on the hemodynamic and humoral changes after total paracentesis. *Hepatology* 1995; **22**: 753–8.

232. Gines A, Fernandez-Esparrach G, Monescillo A *et al.* Randomised trial comparing albumin, dextran 70, and polygeline in cirrhotic patients with ascites treated by paracentesis. *Gastroenterology* 1996; **111**: 1002–10.

233. Cochrane Injuries Group Albumin Reviewers. Human albumin administration in critically ill patients: stematic review of randomised controlled trials. *Br Med J* 1998; **317**: 235–40.

234. Wilkes Mm, Navickis RJ. Patient survival after human albumin administratio meta-analysis of randomized, controlled trials. *Ann Intern Med* 2001; **135**: 149–64.

235. Vincent JL, Navickis RJ, Wilkes MM. Morbidity in hospitalized patients receiving human albumin: A meta-analysis of randomized controlled trials. *Crit Care Med* 2004; **32**: 2029–38.

236. Finfer S, Bellomo R, Boyce N, French J, Myburgh J, Norton R. SAFE Study Investigators. A comparison of albumin and saline for fluid resuscitation in the intensive care unit. *N Engl J Med* 2004; **346**: 1061–6.

237. Alderson P, Bunn F, Lefebvre C, Li L, Roberts I, Schierhout G: Albumin Reviewers. Human albumin solution for resuscitation and volume expansion in critically ill patients. *The Cochrane Database Syst Rev* 2004, Issue 4: Art. No. CD001208.pub2.

238. Boldt J. Fluid choice for resuscitation of the trauma patient: a review of the physiological, pharmacological, and clinical evidence. *Can J Anaesth* 2004; **51**: 500–13.

239. Greenough A. Use and misuse of albumin infusions in neonatal care. *Eur J Pediatr* 1998; **157**: 699–702.

240. So KW, Fok TF, Ng PC, Wong WW, Cheung KL. Randomised controlled trial of colloid or crystalloid in hypotensive preterm infants. *Arch Dis Child* 1997; **761**: F43–F46.

241. Paul M, Dueck M, Joachim Herrmann H, Holzki J. A randomised, controlled study of fluid management in infants and toddlers during surgery: hydroxyethyl starch 6% (HES 70/0.5) vs lactated Ringer's solution. *Paediatr Anaesth* 2003; **12**: 603–8.

242. NIH Consensus Development Conference. Intravenous immunoglobulin: Prevention and treatment of disease. *JAMA* 1990; **264**: 3189–93.

243. Stiehn R. Appropriate therapeutic use of immunoglobulin. *Transfus Med Rev* 1996; **10**: 203–21.

244. Hughes RA, Raphael JC, Swan AV, Doorn PA. Intravenous immunoglobulin for Guillain–Barre syndrome. *Cochrane Database Syst Rev* 2004; (1): CD002063.

245. Romi F, Gilhus NE, Aarli JA. Myasthenia gravis: clinical, immunological, and therapeutic advances. *Acta Neurol Scand* 2005; **111**: 134–41.

246. Koller H, Kieseier BC, Jander S, Hartung HP. Chronic inflammatory demyelinating polyneuropathy. *N Engl J Med* 2005; **352**: 1343–56.

247. Subcommittee on Hyperbilirubinemia. Management of hyperbilirubinemia in the newborn infant 35 or more weeks of gestation. *Pediatrics* 2004; **114**: 297–316.

248. Skupski DW, Bussel JB. Alloimmune thrombocytopenia. *Clin Obstet Gynecol* 1999; **42**: 335–48.

249. Ohlsson A, Lacy JB. Intravenous immunoglobulin for suspected or subsequently proven infection in neonates. *Cochrane Database Syst Rev* 2004; (1): CD001239.

250. Preiksaitis JK, Brennan DC, Fishman J, Allen U. Canadian Society of Transplantation Consensus Workshop on cytomegalovirus management in solid organ transplantation final report. *Am J Transplant* 2005; **5**: 218–27.

251. Roche B, Samuel D. Treatment of hepatitis B and C after liver transplantation. Part 1, hepatitis B. *Transpl Int* 2005; **17**: 746–58.

252. Blanchette VS, Caraco M. Childhood acute immune thrombocytopenic purpura: 20 years later. *Semin Thromb Hemost* 2003; **29**: 605–17.

253. Savasman CM, Sandler SG. Serologic aspects of treating immune thrombocytopenic purpura using intravenous Rh immune globulin. *Immunohematology* 2001; **17**: 106–10.

33 | Hazards of transfusion

Naomi L.C. Luban and Edward C.C. Wong

There are many hazards to transfusion, some serious, others less serious and many undetected or poorly categorized. In the USA there is no established surveillance system for non-fatal transfusion events. In Europe and Canada, hemovigilance has become integrated into public health surveillance systems. Such systems provide important data on adverse outcomes, which provide opportunities for process improvement in all aspects of blood collection and administration. The ultimate goal of such systems is to use data on adverse events to reduce complications related to transfusion (Table 33.1). This chapter will review the more serious complications of blood component transfusion of importance to children with emphasis on recognition and prevention.

Table 33.1 Different types of adverse transfusion events.

Adverse event	Estimated risk
Serious	
Mistransfusion	1 in 14 000 to 1 in 19 000
ABO-incompatible transfusion	1 in 38 000
Death due to ABO-incompatible transfusion	1 in 1.8 million
Acute hemolytic transfusion reaction	1 in 12 000
Delayed hemolytic transfusion reaction	1 in 4000 to 1 in 12 000
Transfusion-related acute lung injury	1 in 2000 to 1 in 5000 (5–10% fatal)
Anaphylaxis	1 in 20 000 to 1 in 47 000
	1 in 1600 (platelets)
	1 in 23 000 (RBCs)
Graft-versus-host disease	1 in 1 million (Canada)
Posttransfusion purpura	1 in 143 000 to 1 in 294 000
Fluid overload	1 in 708 to 1 in 3200
	1 in 7000 to 1 in 15 000
Less serious	
Febrile nonhemolytic transfusion reaction	1 in 500
Allergic (urticaria)	1 in 250

Acute transfusion reactions

Acute hemolytic transfusion reactions

Acute hemolytic transfusion reactions (AHTRs) occur most often when a recipient with circulating preformed antibody is transfused with red blood cells containing the antigen to which the antibody developed. Most AHTRs are the result of transfusion of antibodies against the major blood group antigens, A or B. Due to the absence of preformed anti-A and -B, infants under 4 months of age are not at risk for AHTRs. Most ABO hemolytic transfusion reactions are a result of misidentifying the intended recipient of a unit of blood due to mislabelling of the specimen or misidentification of the patient at the time of transfusion; these reactions are therefore avoidable. Hemolytic transfusion reactions can also occur following the passive transfusion of isohemagglutinins found in ABO-incompatible plasma-containing platelet concentrates.[1,2] The severity of AHTRs is proportional to the rate and volume of transfused incompatible blood. When anti-A and -B binds to the C5–9 component of complement, intravascular RBC lysis occurs. The resultant interleukin (IL) inflammatory response is characterized by the generation of tumor necrosis factor (TNF)-α, IL-8, monocyte chemoattractant protein 1 (MCP-1), and the anaphylatoxins C3a and C5a, as well as the activation of Hageman factor.[3]

Nonimmune causes of acute hemolysis include those related to transfusion through mechanical devices and accessories like blood warmers, infusion devices, filters and catheters required to deliver blood and blood components, or to improper storage, exposure to hypoosmotic fluids, irradiation followed by storage of red blood cells and bacterial contamination.

Signs and symptoms of AHTRs include fever, chills, back and chest pain, nausea and shortness of breath. The patient may develop hypotension, vasoconstriction, ischemia and disseminated intravascular coagulation (DIC). Hypotension, microthrombi formation and hemoglobinuria may compromise renal blood flow precipitating acute renal failure.[4]

When an AHTR is suspected, the transfusion must be stopped immediately and a full transfusion reaction investigation should be initiated. A posttransfusion direct antiglobin test (DAT) may demonstrate the presence of antibody on the RBC surface. The blood unit/segment should be cultured. Life-threatening complications are due to renal injury, DIC and pulmonary involvement. Vital signs should be carefully monitored. Aggressive intravenous hydration is required to maintain intravascular volume and urine output. AHTRs are medical emergencies that are often associated with mortality; the highest rates (44%) have been seen in patients receiving the greatest volumes of incompatible blood.

Transfusion-related acute lung injury

Transfusion-related acute lung injury (TRALI), a clinical syndrome similar to adult respiratory distress syndrome (ARDS), is characterized by acute respiratory distress occurring 1–6 hours after transfusion of a plasma-containing blood component. TRALI is a serious adverse reaction to transfusion that may be under-recognized in pediatric patients.[5] There is usually fever, hypotension, bilateral pulmonary edema and severe hypoxemia with a normal central venous pressure. Chest radiography shows bilateral "white out" lung, i.e., pulmonary infiltrates without cardiac compromise. Patients with TRALI improve 2–3 days after the onset of symptoms, with aggressive respiratory support including oxygen and mechanical ventilation in the most severe cases.

Both HLA class I and class II and antigranulocyte antibodies have been implicated in TRALI reactions, but in about 10% or more cases,[5] no specific antibody specificity can be identified. Two different pathophysiologic mechanisms have been proposed to explain TRALI. The first is that donor leukocyte antibodies attach to corresponding antigens on recipient leukocytes, inducing activation and sequestration of neutrophils, endothelial damage and increased vascular permeability. The antibodies may also attach to corresponding antigen on the pulmonary endothelium with recruitment of granulocytes and subsequent endothelial cell damage. In one unusual case,[6] the transfusion of a nonleukodepleted blood product into a recipient with preexisting anti-HLA A2 antibodies produced TRALI.

The second mechanism involves neutrophil priming. In this two-hit model, surgery or infection primes the patient's neutrophils. The subsequent transfusion of stored red cell and/or platelet products with cytokines, IL6, IL8 and phosphatidylcholines then produces neutrophil sequestration.

TRALI has been reported rarely in children with malignancy (acute lymphoblastic leukemia),[5] those undergoing bone marrow transplantation,[7] with thalassemia undergoing chronic transfusion,[8] following cardiopulmonary bypass,[9] and recently in a mother–child designated donor pair.[10] Evaluation and confirmation of the phenomena is often difficult.[11] Methods to reduce the likelihood of TRALI include screening of donors for anti-white cell antibodies, deferral of donors with multiple pregnancies (and assumed anti-HLA and antineutrophil sensitization) and testing for lipid activators of neutrophils. None are practical. Leukodepletion of blood and blood products may or may not reduce the risk of TRALI.

Allergic reactions

Allergic transfusion reactions are the most common of all posttransfusion events. Allergy to soluble plasma proteins, drugs or other allergens may cause local reactions such as itching and urticaria or systemic symptoms such as bronchospasm or anaphylaxis. The severity of allergic reactions is not dose related; the patient who experiences urticaria during a transfusion will not develop anaphylaxis with continuation of the transfusion. Once established, most patients with allergic reactions respond to oral or parenteral antihistamines. For patients with a history of allergic reactions, pretreatment with an antihistamine may help to prevent recurrence. Severe allergic reactions with stridor or dyspnea are often associated with the development of anti-IgA antibodies in an IgA-deficient patient. Acute management includes intubation, oxygen and epinephrine (adrenaline). Management of such patients long term is often difficult and depends on confirmation of IgG and IgE anti-IgA antibodies.[12] Washed red blood cells and platelets and IgA-deficient plasma obtained from rare donor registries may be needed with premedication. Washing RBC or platelet concentrates will remove much of the plasma responsible for allergic reactions. Leukoreduction of cellular components will not decrease the incidence of allergic transfusion reactions.

Febrile reactions

Fever may be the first sign that a patient is receiving a component that is ABO incompatible or contaminated with bacteria, and such serious consequences must be considered when a patient develops fever during transfusion. A less serious but common adverse effect seen during transfusion of RBCs, platelets and plasma is the febrile nonhemolytic transfusion reaction (FNHTR), which complicates 0.5–2% of transfusions.[13] The risk for FNHTR is highest following the transfusion of platelets (1–3%) compared with red blood cells (0.5–6%). Although the traditional view holds that FNHTRs are due to the interplay of white blood cells (WBCs) contained in the components with preformed antileukocyte antibodies in the recipient, recent studies have demonstrated that pyrogenic cytokines, IL-1β, IL-6, IL-8 and TNF, in the plasma supernatant may induce prostaglandin E2 production in the thermoregulatory centers of the central nervous system. The intensity of the reactions correlates directly with the concentration of IL-1β and IL-6. FNHTRs are more common in individuals who have been previously transfused or pregnant, and are rare in infants with underdeveloped hypothalamic thermoregulatory centers. These reactions may make patients uncomfortable but are rarely associated with more serious problems. The incidence of FNHTRs can be reduced by removing leukocytes at the time of component collection (prestorage leukoreduction)[14] or by removing the plasma supernatant of platelets.[15,16] Leukoreduction by filtration of whole blood-derived platelets (platelet pools) at the time of transfusion may reduce but not prevent the reaction as the cytokines have already been released prior to the filtration. In such cases, plasma volume reduction or washing may be required.[16,17]

Massive transfusion

Massive transfusion, the replacement of a child's blood volume over a 6-hour period, may be needed for the replacement of massive blood losses due to trauma or coagulation defects.[10] The rapid infusion of large volumes of banked blood is also integral to several life-sustaining pediatric therapies such as extracorporeal membrane oxygenation (ECMO) and exchange transfusion. Certain hazards of massive transfusion occur secondary to the rapid rate of infusion of RBCs that have been stored in a refrigerator in anticoagulant/preservative solution for varying periods of time. Many of these hazards can be anticipated and avoided.

The adverse reactions associated with the rapid infusion of large volumes of cold, stored RBCs include:
- increased levels of extracellular potassium, which develop over the storage period of the RBC unit;
- poor function of the platelets contained in stored RBC components;
- progressively lowered levels of intraerythrocytic bisphosphoglycerate BPG (formerly known as 2,3 DPG);
- presence of citrate in the anticoagulant/preservative solution;
- metabolic consequences of the rapid infusion of a cold liquid.

Storage lesions

The storage of RBCs or whole blood in the liquid state results in biochemical derangements, which increase with storage time.

Hyperkalemia

Intracellular potassium leaks from the erythrocyte into the extracellular space. After 35 days of storage in citrate-phosphate-dextrose-adenine (CPDA-1), plasma K^+ concentrations reach 27.3 mmol/L on average. Storage in additive solution (AS-1) results in significantly less potassium leak. The risk of hyperkalemia is relatively insignificant in the routine administration of small volumes of RBC and whole blood. However, fatal cardiac dysrhythmia associated with hyperkalemia during neonatal exchange transfusion[18] and following the rapid intracardiac infusion of old RBCs has been reported.[19] Effective strategies for avoiding hyperkalemia-related dysrhythmias during massive transfusion include using RBCs that are < 5 days old or washed RBCs.[20] When whole blood is required and hyperkalemia is a concern, units should be < 5 days old, or reconstituted whole blood can be made by adding fresh frozen plasma (FFP) to washed stored RBCs.

Poor platelet function with increased storage time

The cold storage conditions that are ideal for RBCs are associated with poor *in vivo* platelet survival. The transfusion of large amounts of stored blood causes dilutional thrombocytopenia and does not provide viable platelets to participate in homeostasis. Platelet concentrates rather than whole blood are the preferred source for transfusion to thrombocytopenic, massively transfused patients who are hemorrhaging.

Low 2,3-diphosphoglycerate levels

The levels of intraerythrocyte 2,3 BPG affect the ability of RBCs to release oxygen at a given pH. After 2 weeks of storage, 2,3 BPG levels fall by > 50%, and reduced levels result in decreased ability to unload oxygen at the level of the tissues.[21] Although 2,3 BPG levels are gradually restored once red cells are transfused, the repletion of 2,3 BPG is such that even after 8 hours, only one-third of the metabolite is regenerated.

Anticoagulant/preservative solution

The anticoagulant/preservative solution used for whole blood collection contains citrate to bind ionized calcium and prevent coagulation of the donation. Unbound citrate is metabolized to bicarbonate. Massive transfusion of citrated blood components may cause the patient to become hypocalcemic, alkalotic or hypokalemic, and these states are observed more often in conjunction with plasma transfusion or exchange than with RBC transfusion. Patients with hypocalcemia complain of perioral paresthesia, twitching of the extremities and later, tetany. Children with hepatic or renal insufficiency who become hypocalcemic may develop hypotension or myocardial irritability. Some physicians routinely supplement calcium using 10% calcium gluconate (2 mL/kg/hr), particularly in the context of massive plasma transfusion or plasma exchange. Calcium is routinely administered for younger children undergoing plasma exchange or peripheral stem cell collections and for those with poor hepatic function because children can rarely warn staff of the signs of citrate toxicity. The dose used is 94 mg of calcium/100 mL of blood processed to a maximum of 2 g administered intravenously at a flow rate no greater than

120 mg/kg/h. When replacing calcium, serum ionized calcium levels should be monitored to avoid overreplacement.

Cold storage conditions

RBCs are stored in a refrigerator at 4–6°C. The rapid transfusion of components that have been stored in the cold can result in hypothermia and subsequent cardiac dysrhythmia/asystole. In adults, hypothermia-induced cardiac arrest is reported in half of those who receive 3 L or more of refrigerated blood at rates of 50–100 mL/min.[22] In infants, the transfusion of cold blood has been associated with apnea, hypotension and hypoglycemia. Blood warmers, devices which use either wet or dry heat, can raise the temperature of cold-stored RBCs to body temperature. The usefulness of such warmers is limited when large volumes of RBCs are required immediately. Microwave ovens should never be used to warm blood rapidly for transfusion because heating may be inconsistent and may cause *ex vivo* hemolysis.

Coagulopathy

Patients who require massive transfusion for treatment of severe hemorrhage are at risk for developing clinical and laboratory evidence of a coagulopathy. Coagulation abnormalities are due to dilution of circulating coagulation factors and platelets, local consumption of coagulation factors and DIC. The development of coagulopathy is strongly associated with the length of time during which a patient has been hypotensive. In the laboratory, the coagulopathy is characterized by thrombocytopenia, hypofibrinogenemia and prolongation of the prothrombin time (PT) and partial thromboplastin time (PTT). The patient demonstrates microvascular bleeding characterized by oozing from mucosal surfaces, sites of injury and venipuncture sites. Patients with severe tissue injury and profound hypotension are more likely to develop diffuse microvascular bleeding. The development of coagulopathy is strongly associated with mortality.[23] Careful assessment of the patient's clinical course in conjunction with coagulation testing allows the clinician appropriately to support patients with consumptive coagulopathy associated with massive transfusion with platelets, FFP and cryoprecipitate.

Bacterial contamination

Bacterial contamination of blood and blood products accounted for 10% of transfusion fatalities between 1985 and 1999 (reviewed in Ref. 24). The severity of the septic reaction is variable and dependent on the species of organism (Gram-negative greater then Gram-positive), the number of bacteria infused, the propagation rate of the bacteria and the clinical status of the recipient. Recipients who are immunosuppressed are at higher risk, whereas those on antibiotics may

be protected especially if the antibiotic is cidal to the organism. Severe reactions have been reported most frequently with platelets stored at room temperature but also with refrigerated cellular components, plasma, cryoprecipitate and albumin, in both allogeneic and autologous transfusion. Fever, chills, hypotension, oliguria and DIC have been reported. High fever or hypotension during a transfusion suggest a contaminated blood transfusion. Symptoms suggestive of either hemolytic transfusion reaction or TRALI with dyspnea and cough may occur. In a review of five clinical studies, platelet-associated bacteremia was less severe, with a mortality of 26%, compared with RBC-contaminated reactions, where a mortality of 71% was reported.[25] Implicated are Gram-positive organisms, including coagulase-negative staphylococci, *Bacillus* species, *Staphylococcus* and *Streptococcus* species for platelets. Cold-loving organisms such as *Yersinia enterocolitica*, cryophilic pseudomonads such as *Pseudomonas putida* and *P. fluorescens*, and *Enterobacter* spp., are most commonly identified as sources of RBC contamination.[26] Transfusion-associated babesiosis was reported in three of four infants in a New York hospital; *Babesia* has the same tick vector as *Borrelia burgdorferi*, the Lyme disease spirochete, which is known to survive in platelets stored at 20°C, RBCs stored at 4°C and FFP stored at –18°C, but has not yet been implicated in a transfusion outbreak.

Confirmation of a septic reaction mandates that cultures of the blood component and the recipient's blood grow the same organism.[27] The patient culture should be obtained from a different site (line) from where the unit was transfused. Confirmation can sometimes be difficult as the patient may be on antibiotics that are cidal to the organism, or the blood bag may have been discarded, making culture impossible.

Estimates of bacterial contamination of blood and blood products vary widely throughout the world. The prevalence of bacterial contamination is 0.002–1% for red blood cells and 0.04–10% for platelets.[24,27–30] There are multiple potential sources of blood component contamination, including unrecognized donor bacteremia and inadequate skin decontamination, which, in the case of pheresis donors, may be from a scarred phlebotomy site. Contamination can also occur during manufacturing of the blood bags or apheresis solutions used during collection. Pooling of products or contaminated water baths are other sources. The age of the product is also an important variable. Platelets older than 3 days and RBCs older than 21 days are more likely to be contaminated.[24,29,31]

Preventive measures to decrease the risks of transfusion-associated bacterial sepsis include extensive donor screening, vigorous skin decontamination and water-bath decontamination. Donor questioning about diarrhea and travel to endemic Lyme disease areas has been particularly helpful for *Yersinia* and *Borrelia*, respectively. In March 2004, US/blood collection facilities implemented a number of strategies to limit bacterial contamination of platelet concentrates. These included new requirements for phlebotomy arm preparation, institution of a diversion pouch where the initial 20–30 mL of the collection (where the maximal skin contamination source exists) is diverted, and a recommendation to use apheresis platelets. Additional methods to detect bacterial contamination of platelet units were implemented, including culture of the product, use of staining methods (Gram, acridine orange or Wright) and multiagent strips to measure pH and glucose. Feasibility studies for pretransfusion detection using endotoxin, RNA probes or polymerase chain reaction (PCR)-based methods have begun. Chemical or photochemical decontamination using psoralens hold promise, but are still being tested in clinical studies.[30,32]

Adverse reactions with delayed occurrence

Transfusion-associated alloimmunization

The most common delayed reactions to transfusion include those related to the immunologic consequences. The development of alloantibodies directed against foreign antigens present on the cellular elements of blood/blood components is called alloimmunization. Several factors influence the recipient's risk of becoming alloimmunized to erythrocyte, leukocyte or platelet antigens. Immunogenicity and dose of the foreign antigen, frequency and route of exposure, and the recipient's immune response to antigenic challenge are clearly determining factors. The short- and long-term clinical sequelae of alloimmunization depend on the antigen(s) involved.

Erythrocyte alloimmunization

RBC alloimmunization may occur when there is a genetic disparity in erythrocyte antigens between donor and recipient. The immunogenicity, or ability to stimulate an immune response, of most blood group antigens is poor. The blood group antigens Rh (Cc, D, Ee) and A and B are by far the most immunogenic. ABO antibodies, however, have been referred to as "naturally occurring" because they develop without an allogeneic red cell stimulus. ABO antibody production is stimulated by elements that are ubiquitous in nature, such as bacteria that possess substances similar to human A and B antigens. These antibodies (isohemagglutinins) can generally be detected in sera of infants by 3–6 months of age. The Rh system D antigen is the RBC antigen that is considered to be the most immunogenic in terms of antibody production as a result of exposure to foreign RBCs. Approximately 80% of RhD-negative recipients who receive a single 200-mL transfusion of RhD-positive red cells develop detectable anti-RhD antibodies within 2–5 months.[32,33] There has been some evidence that the minimum dose of RhD-positive red cells necessary for primary immunization is only 0.03 mL.[34] Therefore, it is easy to understand how the small numbers of RBCs present in a RhD-positive platelet concentrate could be sufficient to immunize a RhD-negative recipient. The relative immunogenicity or potency of other red cell antigens depends, in part, on the frequency with which the particular alloantibodies are encountered. More than half of the alloantibodies that result from transfusion and pregnancy are Rh antibodies (other than anti-RhD), with anti-Kell (anti-K) and anti-Duffy (anti-Fy^a) accounting for an additional 40%. Studies have indicated that the relative likelihood of blood-group antibody formation is as follows: RhD > K > RhE > Fy^a > Jk^a.[35]

The immunoglobulin subclasses IgG1 and IgG3 have greater affinity for Fc receptors on phagocytic cells and are more efficient at activating complement cells than IgG2 and IgG4; this accounts for the variability in the hemolysis that ensues, along with thermal range and antibody specificity.

Rates of immunization vary, with reported frequencies in hospital-based transfused populations ranging from 0.2 to 2.6%.[13,36] With the exclusion of the RhD antigen, alloimmunization to RBC antigens is approximately 1% per unit transfused. However, there is evidence that the immune response to blood group antigens is different depending on the patient population and the disease state for which the transfusion was given. Some individuals become immunized after a few transfusions, whereas others rarely become immunized and may be tolerized to transfusion despite repeated transfusions. The pathophysiology of alloimmunization is not clearly defined and may be due, in part, to the number of transfusions given, the heterogeneity of the donor/recipient population (in terms of expression of RBC antigens), concordant activation of antigen-presenting lymphocytes and whether certain immune response genes, yet to be determined, influence the response.

Neonates

Despite the frequent need for RBC transfusions, several studies provide evidence that RBC alloimmunization occurs only rarely in neonates transfused during the first 4 months of life. In one study, no unexpected RBC antibodies were detected in 53 premature infants who received a total of 683 RBC transfusions, with at least half being tested 5 months after birth.[37] Ludvigsen *et al.*[38] could detect no antibodies at least 3 weeks after the last transfusion in 90 full-term infants who received a total of 1269 transfusions with an average of 8.9 donor exposures/neonate. Other reports have supported the relative infrequency of alloantibody production directed against RBC antigens in neonates.[39,40] However, accurate transfusion histories could not be determined for all infants in these studies. There have been three reports of antibody formation in multiply transfused infants. Two cases involved development of allo-anti-E in infants at age 18 days and 11 weeks,[41,42] respectively, and the third was an infant who developed anti-K at 12 weeks.[43] The failure of newborns to initiate an immune response to foreign RBC antigens is probably multifactorial, and includes the immature immune status of the infant and inability of neonatal antigen-presenting cells to effectively prime self T-helper cells. Another contributing factor that may limit lymphocyte activation is the possibility that insufficient numbers of allogeneic lymphocytes are present in components prepared for neonates.[44]

Sickle-cell anemia

There have been several studies reporting extreme variability in the rates of alloimmunization for patients with sickle-cell anemia. The discrepancies can be attributed to whether all or only clinically significant antibodies were included in the analysis, whether pregnancy history was clearly delineated, and which population base was studied: children, adults or both. Reported rates of alloimmunization range from 5.7 to 36%.[45,46] The lower rate was reported in a group of 245 patients who had a median age of 10 years. In the largest prospective study of alloimmunization in patients with sickle-cell disease (SCD), 3047 patients were evaluated, of whom 1814 were transfused for an overall rate of RBC alloimmunization of 18.6%.[47] Alloimmunization rates were higher for patients with hemoglobin SS versus hemoglobin SC or (sickle-β⁺-thalassemia), reflecting lower transfusion rates in the latter group of patients. Patients transfused by the age of 10 years or younger had a lower rate of alloimmunization than those who were first transfused after the age of 10 years (9.6% vs. 20.7%, respectively). The majority (almost two-thirds) of the clinically significant antibodies that developed were in the Rh and Kell systems, with 17% of the immunized patients producing four or more antibodies. Vichinsky *et al.*[48] found a much higher rate of alloimmunization in chronically transfused black patients with SCD compared with transfused non-black patients with chronic hemolytic disorders; they suggested that the increased risk was related to the transfusion of racially discordant red cells. Luban,[49] reporting a study of 142 children with SCD, found a higher rate of alloimmunization in children of non-American Black descent versus American-born Afro-Americans, despite similar antigen phenotypes. The former group also developed more antibodies/child (3.17 vs. 1.25, respectively), perhaps due to differences in immune response genes.

Methods to reduce the risk of alloimmunization vary greatly. They include prevention by providing phenotypically matched red cells for all patients or matching only for those antigens that commonly cause alloimmunization. Other options include providing additional antigen matching only for patients who have become immunized, or providing antigen-matched blood only for patients who have a high likelihood of going on a chronic transfusion protocol.[50] When antigen-typed red-cell products are used preventively for sickle-cell patients, they are selected to be negative for Rhesus (D, C, E, c and e) and Kell (K and k) depending on the antigen typing of the patient. Additional typing for Kidd (Jkᵃ

and Jkᵇ), Duffy (Fyᵃ and Fyᵇ), the MNS system (M, N, S and s) and Lewis (Leᵃ and Leᵇ) may be performed. The use of racially matched blood has been suggested as a way to capitalize on variances in antigen frequencies between donors of European and African ethnicity.[51] A recent report on the race/ethnicity of ABO and RhD phenotypes in the USA provides more robust data than have been available to date.[52] In a single-institution study of 351 patients who received 8939 ABO- and RhD-matched units, 29.1% developed one blood group alloantibody. The authors calculated the percent of white donors that would be expected to match either a limited or extended protocol and concluded that extended matching was impractical.[53]

The development of autoantibodies in patients with SCD has been reported to occur more often in patients receiving chronic transfusion and in whom alloantibodies have developed.[54] The commonest autoantibodies observed have been cold-reacting antibodies, which although classified as clinically harmless, have caused considerable difficulties in cross-matching. Experimental evidence has shown that autoimmunization may develop after blood transfusion whether or not alloimmunization has occurred.[55]

The clinical outcome of RBC alloimmunization depends on the number and nature of the antibodies produced. Difficulty in finding compatible blood and an increased risk of delayed hemolytic transfusion reaction (DHTR) are two consequences of alloimmunization. DHTRs in patients with SCD pose additional problems in that they may often go unrecognized because the symptoms can mimic or induce a sickle-cell crisis.[56] This effect may be attributed in part to a low level of suspicion for DHTR or an inability clinically to separate the symptoms from SCD. A marked drop in hematocrit to levels lower than those before transfusion with reticulocytopenia has been observed in some patients with SCD experiencing a DHTR. This extreme decrease in hematocrit may be secondary to hemolysis of donor red cells in conjunction with suppression of erythropoiesis from transfusion. An alternative theory on the development of the extreme anemia is that autologous red cells are destroyed in concert with the transfused antigen-positive red cells; this is referred to as "bystander hemolysis."[55–57] Bystander hemolysis probably results from complement deposition and activation on autologous cells, which are subject to hemolysis. Therapy has included steroids, recombinant erythropoietin and intravenous immunoglobulin.[57]

Unique risks occur when there is concomitant alloantibody and autoantibody formation. First, the autoantibody can complicate the pretransfusion testing and mask the presence of coexisting alloantibodies. Secondly, the autoantibody may cause decreased survival of transfused cells. Thirdly, worsening hemolysis and volume overload may foster clinical deterioration. Close observation, steroid premedication and transfusing the smallest volume of red cells to maintain adequate oxygenation are advised.

Thalassemia

The reported incidence of clinically significant antibody production in children transfused for thalassemia has also been variable, ranging from 5.2 to 21.1%.[58] In certain areas of the world where there is heterogeneity of the donor population, higher rates are reported with autoantibody formation, as in SCD.[59] A consistent finding in most of these studies, however, is the association between the age at which transfusion is started and the risk of alloimmunization to RBC antigens.[60,61] As suggested in the CSSCD study,[47] patients who received initial transfusions before the age of 3 years were found to have a considerably lower incidence of alloimmunization.[60] The benefits of regular transfusion are complicated by transfusional iron overload, discussed in Chapter 5.

Leukocyte and platelet alloimmunization

Alloimmunization to leukocyte and platelet antigens may develop in multiply transfused recipients, or as a result of pregnancy or organ transplantation. Class I human leukocyte antigens (HLA-A, HLA-B) are major immunogens and are expressed on all nucleated cells as well as platelets. The class II antigens have a more limited distribution, and are found primarily on B lymphocytes, macrophages/monocytes, dendritic cells, activated T cells, and endothelial cells. Studies have indicated that WBC reduction of cellular components to levels $< 5 \times 10^6$/transfusion can diminish alloimmunization to HLA class I antigens (Table 33.2).[62,63] Ultraviolet irradiation has been shown to interfere with the function of antigen-presenting cells.[64–66] Studies evaluating the effectiveness of these technologies in reducing alloimmunization to platelet transfusion confirm effectiveness in adults. The Trial to Reduce Alloimmunization of Platelets (TRAP)[67] was a carefully controlled, multicenter, randomized trial that showed

that leukocyte-reduced platelets did not lower the incidence of refractoriness in pregnant women compared with controls, but halved the rate of alloantibody formation. Therefore, leukodepletion appears to eliminate primary sensitization but not secondary response.

Alloimmunization to transfused WBC antigens during infancy is rare. Studies have shown either no evidence of HLA antibodies associated with transfusion, whether or not attempts were made to leukocyte-reduce blood components, or transient detection of antibodies.[68,69] There is some evidence to suggest that alloantibodies directed against maternal blood cell antigens may develop as a result of intrauterine or perinatal exposure to these antigens. Passive transfer of IgG antibodies against HLA-, platelet- and granulocyte-specific antibodies to the neonate as a result of maternal alloimmunization is known to occur.[70,71]

The rate of HLA alloimmunization in older children and adults ranges from 30% to 70%.[72–74] The rates are related to the number of transfusions, type of transfusion, underlying disease and chemotherapeutic regimen. In a series of 100 children with malignant disorders (leukemia, lymphoma, Ewing sarcoma) who were receiving intensive transfusion support, 27% developed cytotoxic HLA antibodies. Persistence of HLA antibodies, despite continued transfusions, was observed in only 13% of the patients.[75] In contrast to patients with malignancy, in one study seven of eight patients with aplastic anemia developed alloantibodies. The difference in the rate of immunization is most likely due to the immunosuppressive effects of chemotherapy. Compared with HLA antigens, platelet-specific antigens do not appear to be as potent immunogenically; however, alloantibodies directed against various platelet antigen systems have been characterized in multitransfused patients.[76]

The clinical manifestations of alloimmunization to leukocyte and platelet antigens include febrile transfusion reactions, refractoriness to platelet transfusions, posttransfusion

Table 33.2 Blood component filters.

Generation	Pore size (μm)	Filter mechanism	Comment
First	170–260	Screen	Referred to as "clot" filter Used for all blood and blood components
Second	20–40	Micropore screen filter	Referred to as "microaggregate" filter Removes 75–90% of WBCs Only used for RBCs
Third	N/A	Adhesion, absorption	Referred to as "leukodepletion" filter Removes 99–99.9% of WBCs Used for cellular components including platelets collected by apheresis, platelet pools and RBCs
Fourth*	N/A	Adhesion, absorption, other	Under development

* Different manufacturers have variable claims about the degree of WBC removal and subsets of WBCs removed by their respective methods.

purpura (PTP) and TRALI. The latter is usually the result of passive transfusion of HLA-epitope-specific antibodies or leukoagglutinins directed against the recipient's antigen, which precipitates a chain of reactions that include cytokine release and complement activation. There has been, however, at least one report of a fatal pulmonary reaction in a multi-transfused child in whom antibody production was directed against donor leukocytes.[8]

Posttransfusion purpura

Posttransfusion purpura (PTP) is a rare manifestation of immune thrombocytopenia, first recognized by Shulman *et al.* in 1961.[77] This condition is characterized by the development of profound, but self-limiting, thrombocytopenia approximately 5–10 days after a blood transfusion in a recipient who has been previously exposed to platelet antigens through pregnancy or former transfusions. Alloantibodies are produced that destroy not only the transfused platelets, but the patient's own platelets. In the approximately 100 reported cases, the most commonly produced platelet antibody has been directed against the specific platelet antigen HPA-1a (PL^{A1}) located on glycoprotein IIIa (GpIIIa). Although the mechanism of autologous platelet destruction is unclear, several theories have been postulated, including:

- formation of a foreign antigen–antibody complex that binds to autologous platelets and mediates platelet destruction via a mechanism similar to that observed in drug purpura;[78]
- development of a second antibody with autoimmune specificity that reacts with HPA-1a-negative platelets;[78]
- transfused soluble platelet antigen in the donor plasma adsorbs to the recipient's platelets, thereby rendering them reactive with the alloantibody.[79]

PTP is a disease of adults, usually in their late 40s or older, occurring more frequently in females as a result of a previous pregnancy. The youngest patient reported to develop PTP was a 16-year-old female with no previous history of pregnancy.[80] While approximately 3% of the White population is negative for HPA-1a antigen and, therefore, at risk for development of PTP, far fewer than 3% of transfused individuals are affected. Part of the reason for this is that cases that are not clinically apparent may go unrecognized or a specific immune response gene may be necessary to produce anti-HPA-1a. There does appear to be a strong link between the Drw52 allele and the production of anti-HPA-1a alloantibody.[81] Packed RBCs and whole blood have been the components predominantly associated with the precipitation of PTP; however, platelets and plasma transfusion can also trigger the syndrome. Transfusion reactions, generally characterized by chills and fever, have frequently been reported in patients prior to or after the manifestation of PTP. Thrombocytopenia is usually severe, with platelet counts being $< 10 \times 10^9$/L. The duration of thrombocytopenia in untreated patients ranges from 7 to 48 days. In situations

where the patient is not bleeding or at risk of bleeding, careful observation may be all that is necessary. The most feared complication during the period of extreme thrombocytopenia is intracranial hemorrhage. Infusion of high-dose intravenous immunoglobulin (400–500 mg/kg/day for 10 days) has become the first line of therapy; however, this may require 3–4 days for a response. In severe cases of PTP, in the face of active bleeding, HPA-1a-negative platelets may provide transient benefit.[82] The efficacy of splenectomy, corticosteroids and plasma exchange for treatment of PTP has not been well established.

Transfusion-associated graft-versus-host disease

Graft-versus-host disease (GVHD) results from the engraftment of immunocompetent donor T lymphocytes into a recipient whose immune system is unable to reject them. It is a common sequela of bone marrow transplantation (BMT), but is also recognized as a rare risk associated with blood transfusion. Early reports of transfusion-associated (TA)-GVHD were in immunocompromised hosts. However, cases have been documented in immunocompetent transfusion recipients.[83]

Several factors play a role in the pathogenesis of TA-GVHD. Kinetic studies of donor leukocyte clearance after allogeneic transfusion have shown rapid clearance over the initial 2 days posttransfusion, followed by a transient increase in circulating donor leukocytes at 3–5 days prior to complete clearance by 7–10 days. It has been postulated that the transient increase represents an *in vivo* mixed lymphocyte reaction with activated donor T lymphocytes proliferating in an abortive GVHD.[84] By contrast, long-term chimerism (6 months to 1 year) has been observed in trauma patients who were transfused, and this has been postulated to be due to engraftment of stem cells.[85] It has been well recognized that immunocompetent T lymphocytes, capable of a proliferative response, must be present in the initial donor inoculum.

Virtually all cellular blood components have been implicated in reported cases of TA-GVHD. The syndrome has developed after transfusion of whole blood, red blood cells, platelets, fresh (nonfrozen) plasma and leukocytes harvested from both normal donors and donors with chronic myelocytic leukemia. The dosage of immunocompetent cells transfused is also important. Based on animal studies, a minimum dose of 1×10^7 cells/kg body weight is necessary to induce a "runting syndrome," and case studies suggest that a similar threshold is necessary to produce GVHD in humans.[86] However, there have been reports of fatal TA-GVHD occurring in children with severe combined immunodeficiency, in which a dose of only 8×10^4 lymphocytes/kg body weight were likely transfused.[87] The threshold number of viable cells necessary to produce a graft-versus-host reaction, therefore, may vary depending upon the immune status of the host as well as the antigenic similarity or disparity between donor and recipient. There must be sufficient disparity between donor and host histocompatibility antigens for the host to appear foreign to the donor and, therefore, to be capable of inducing antigenic stimulation. The host, on the other hand, must be incapable of mounting an immunologic reaction against the graft, either as a result of an immature or defective cellular immunity or host tolerance of the foreign cells. The latter scenario may occur when there exists donor homozygosity for an HLA haplotype, for which the recipient is haploidentical. In this setting the recipient's lymphocytes see only self antigens on the donor's cells. However, the homozygous donor cells see non-self antigens on the recipient's cells stimulating an alloreaction that can initiate GVHD.[88]

The immune response in GVHD is somewhat complex and is not completely understood. Two basic aspects involve (i) the afferent phase, in which recipient tissues stimulate T lymphocytes from the donor, which in turn undergo clonal proliferation and differentiation; and (ii) the efferent phase, in which donor effector cells damage recipient target tissues. The immunologic target is thought to be the host's major histocompatibility complex (MHC) antigens. In TA-GVHD, the recipient's B, T, epithelial and bone marrow stem cells become the main focus of attack. It was initially believed that the effector mechanism was the result of direct cytotoxicity by alloreactive donor T cells. The observation that the phenotype of many of the effector cells infiltrating target tissues was more consistent with natural killer (NK) cells than with mature T lymphocytes suggested a possible role for cytokines in the effector phase of GVHD. In this model, inflammatory cytokines, such as TNF-α and IL-1, released by host tissue damaged by chemotherapy, radiotherapy or infection, result in the increased expression of MHC and other adhesion molecules. This upregulation results in enhanced recognition of donor–recipient differences by alloreactive donor T cells present in the transfused component. The donor T cells then proliferate and secrete cytokines, in particular IL-2. Cytokine release in turn recruits additional donor T cells and macrophages, which are induced to secrete IL-1 and TNF-α. In this manner, the creation of a self-amplifying positive feedback loop eventually produces the clinical manifestations of GVHD.[89,90]

GVHD following blood transfusions manifests as an acute syndrome, the onset typically occurring within 4–30 days. The syndrome is characterized by involvement of the skin, liver, gastrointestinal tract and bone marrow. The initial clinical manifestations are usually a high fever occurring 8–10 days after the transfusion, followed within 24–48 hours by the appearance of a central maculopapular rash, which subsequently spreads to the extremities. In severe cases, the rash may progress to generalized erythroderma and desquamation. Additional clinical findings may include anorexia, nausea, vomiting and watery diarrhea with or without elevated liver enzymes and hyperbilirubinemia. Unlike GVHD following BMT, pancytopenia is a prominent finding in TA-GVHD. This typically results from the ability of the donor cells to recognize the recipient (host) marrow as antigenically foreign, leading to the destruction of stem cells and/or colony-forming units. In GVHD associated with BMT, the "host bone marrow" has been replaced by the donor's bone marrow, which, accordingly, is antigenically the same as the reacting donor lymphocytes. The development of bone marrow hypoplasia and aplasia associated with TA-GVHD places the patient at increased risk for hemorrhage or overwhelming infection. The duration of TA-GVHD is short, with the majority of patients dying within a few days to weeks (median time 21 days from onset), usually as a complication of marrow failure.[91] While immunosuppressive therapies such as prednisone, ciclosporin and antithymocyte globulin have been used to treat GVHD associated with BMT, this approach has not been effective for TA-GVHD, which is nearly uniformly fatal unless bone marrow or hematopoietic stem cell transplantation can be performed. A review of the clinical manifestation of TA-GVHD in neonates has shown that infants present later (median time of onset 28 days) with a slightly prolonged course. However, they have a similarly high rate of mortality.[92]

Diagnosis of TA-GVHD is usually based on the clinical presentation in conjunction with histologic findings on skin biopsy and supportive evidence of persistence of donor lymphocytes by cytogenetic, HLA or DNA analyses. Because there are several other clinical entities that may mimic TA-GVHD, including viral syndromes and drug reactions, it becomes important to make the correct diagnosis and to have an appreciation of those patients who are at greatest risk for TA-GVHD.

TA-GVHD has been reported in patients with several different clinical conditions. It has been difficult, however, to assess the risk of TA-GVHD for any particular group of patients for several reasons. First, the diagnosis may be difficult to make in the situation where there is a critically ill, multiply-transfused patient with infectious as well as other complications. Usually only severe cases are recognized, often only after death. Mild cases may go unrecognized. Secondly, because the development of TA-GVHD depends on several variables, including the number of viable T lymphocytes transfused, the extent of immune suppression in the patient, and the degree of HLA sharing between donor and recipient, each transfusion episode presents its own spectrum of risk. To assess the risk in any patient group, the number of blood components a particular category of patients will receive during the course of treatment must be taken into account. Finally, due to the high mortality rate, there are no prospective studies evaluating the risk of developing TA-GVHD in susceptible groups of patients.

Until recently, patients developing TA-GVHD all shared either a congenital or acquired deficiency of cell-mediated immunity. The first reported cases occurred in children with immunodeficiency syndromes involving a T-cell defect.[93]

Infants known either to have or who are suspected of having a congenital deficiency of T-cell function, including DiGeorge syndrome, Wiskott–Aldrich syndrome, severe combined immunodeficiency syndrome, reticular dysgenesis and purine nucleoside phosphorylase deficiency, are at risk. Infants with humoral immunodeficiency (B cell), however, are not. Another group of infants who appear to be at risk are those who receive intrauterine transfusions (IUT) and subsequently exchange transfusion. It has been postulated that the lymphocytes in the IUT may induce a state of nonspecific tolerance through exhaustion of fetal immune defenses, which then, with subsequent exchange transfusion, induces GVHD. Other occurrences of TA-GVHD in the neonatal setting are assumed to be related to the relative immunologic immaturity of the premature infant combined with transfusion of large volumes of fresh blood, such as may occur with exchange transfusion. Transfusion of maternal components, as occurs in the setting of neonatal alloimmune thrombocytopenia, has also been associated with TA-GVHD.

A transfusion from blood relatives or unrelated donors who share HLA haplotypes with the recipient is a risk factor whether in the setting of transfusion to a neonate, older child or adult with or without immunoincompetence. The risk of TA-GVHD in premature infants, with no other identifiable risk factors, as a result of routine small-volume transfusion is rare.[94] TA-GVHD has been reported in patients with hematologic malignancies and solid tumors, who have received cytotoxic chemotherapy, radiation treatment or both. Once again, the overall risk is difficult to assess, especially as therapeutic approaches to various malignancies become more intensive. The strong association, however, between Hodgkin disease of any stage and the development of TA-GVHD is believed to be the result of the intrinsic T-cell defects known to occur with this disease.[95] TA-GVHD in association with ablative chemotherapy and autologous BMT for solid tumors has also been reported. The doses of chemotherapy given render these patients severely immunocompromised. In these settings it is important to remember that components transfused during harvesting of either bone marrow or peripheral blood stem cells (which occurs before ablative therapy) may also potentially be implicated in the development of TA-GVHD. Viable allogeneic T lymphocytes contaminating the harvested component may be reinfused to the recipient, with the recipient's own stem cells, at a time when the recipient is aplastic and immunosuppressed. Patients with autoimmune diseases receiving fludarabine or other purine analogs are also at risk.[96]

There have been various clinical settings in which TA-GVHD has been reported to occur in patients presumed to be immunocompetent. While in a few cases no risk factors could be identified, the majority have been associated with transfusion of relatively fresh blood from an HLA-homozygous donor to a recipient who is a heterozygote for the donor's HLA haplotype. This is more likely to occur with transfusions from blood relatives, but has been reported to occur with unrelated donor transfusion.[97] Cardiac surgery, in association with the use of relatively fresh blood from either family donors or in the context of donor/recipient haplotype sharing, has been the clinical setting for most of the reported cases. The frequency of blood transfusion from an unrelated donor homozygous for an HLA haplotype for which the recipient is heterozygous depends on the HLA homogeneity of the population.[92,98]

No reports of patients with AIDS developing TA-GVHD have been published. An explanation for this apparent paradox, namely, why such an immunosuppressed group should not show signs of GVHD, is lacking. However, when an AIDS patient is transfused, the donor CD4 T lymphocytes may also become infected with human immunodeficiency virus (HIV) and thus are rendered unable to initiate the GVHD syndrome while intact CD8 T cells provide the host defense against GVHD.[99,100]

Table 33.3 reviews the indications for the use of irradiated blood and blood products. Because the treatment of TA-GVHD is almost always ineffective, efforts are directed at prevention and minimizing risk by reducing or inactivating

Table 33.3 Irradiation of blood components for prevention of transfusion-associated graft-versus-host disease.

Clearly established indications
Congenital cellular immune deficiency
  Confirmed
  Suspected
Hematopoietic stem cell transplantation
  Allogeneic
  Autologous
Neonate/fetus:
  Receiving intrauterine transfusion (IUT)
  Who has received IUT
  Weighing <1200 g
Any patient with Hodgkin disease
Any patient receiving blood from a biologic relative

Established but sometimes questioned
Any patient on high-dose chemotherapy, radiotherapy, or aggressive
  immunotherapy including fludarabine and other purine analogs
Recipients of HLA-matched, nonfamilial blood/blood products

Controversial
Solid organ transplantation recipients
Aplastic anemia not fitting category above
Neonates:
  Receiving exchange transfusion
  Receiving large-volume transfusion
  On extracorporeal membrane oxygenation

Not indicated
Human immunodeficiency virus
Pregnant women
Elderly patients

transfused donor lymphocytes. Methods available in blood banks for physically removing T lymphocytes (washing or filtration) do not provide effective prophylaxis against TA-GVHD. Current 3-log leukocyte depletion filters do not remove sufficient lymphocytes to prevent TA-GVHD. Inactivation of transfused lymphocytes by gamma irradiation of blood components remains the most effective method for inhibiting lymphocyte blast transformation and mitotic activity and hence preventing TA-GVHD. The recommended dose of irradiation is 25 Gy to the midplane of the component with a minimum of 15 Gy to any other region of the component.[13] The effect of this dose on platelet and granulocyte viability and function is not clinically significant. However, long-term storage of irradiated red cells at 4°C results in increased levels of potassium.[101] This may be of clinical concern if large volumes of blood need to be infused over a short period of time into patients who may be susceptible to the development of hyperkalemia, such as premature infants and patients with severe renal impairment.

Although not yet approved or licenced, photochemical inactivation methods using psoralens and similar photoactive compounds and UV irradiation may well be an alternative to gamma irradiation in the future.[102–104] Coupled with inhibition of viral and bacterial pathogens, such methods may reduce multiple transfusion risks.[105]

Transfusion-related immune modulation

Blood transfusion has been known to alter immune function since the observation in the 1970s of improved renal allograft survival in transfused patients. In addition, there have been several reports of decreased rates of recurrent spontaneous abortion and inflammatory bowel disease in transfusion recipients.[106–108] Recently, concern has developed over the immunosuppressive effects of transfusion and the potential clinical consequences, including increased rate of reactivation of viral infection, solid tumor recurrence and postoperative bacterial sepsis. Although the mechanism of the immunosuppressive effect of transfusion is poorly understood, it is probably related to a decrease in cell-mediated immunity. Observed effects include a shift from a T-helper (Th)1 to a Th2 immune response, decreased natural killer cell activity, decreased lymphocyte responses to mitogens, decreased cytoxic T-cell number and anergy to intradermal antigens, reversal in the CD4/CD8 ratio, increased number of HLA-DR-activated lymphocytes and lymphocyte blastogenesis. Although the role of the cellular elements of components versus plasma is also not clearly delineated, animal models suggest that soluble inflammatory mediators found in stored blood and not fresh blood enhanced tumor growth.[109,110] Furthermore, increased Fas/Fas ligand levels in stored blood, which may cause immune downregulation, is not observed in fresh blood or blood subject to prestorage leukoreduction.[111] The importance of both the cellular and noncellular facets of

transfusion-associated immune modulation is noted in a study of infants receiving washed, irradiated red cells in which infants were not observed to have the changes in cellular immunity associated with unwashed, nonirradiated red cells.[44]

Three randomized clinical trials have examined the effect of allogeneic transfusion on cancer recurrence.[112–114] Taken together, these studies failed to demonstrate an effect of allogeneic transfusion on tumor recurrence. However, a clinical trial examining the effect of leukoreduction on cancer recurrence has not been performed in the USA, and it remains a matter of debate whether leukoreduced products alter the risk of cancer recurrence.

Ten randomized clinical trials have examined the effect of transfusion on the rate of postoperative infections.[113–121] Comparison of these studies is difficult given differences in study design, use of buffy-coat-removed RBCs (used in Europe) in all but one study and the small numbers involved. Both beneficial and adverse effects on postoperative infections were reported in these clinical trials. In a meta-analysis of six of the studies, the relative risk associated with allogeneic transfusion was 0.94 (95% CI = 0.85–1.04, $P > 0.05$); however, using mathematical modeling, a study involving at least 3000 patients would be necessary to detect a 10% difference in postoperative infections in patients transfused with leukoreduced blood. Thus, the demonstration of a beneficial relationship between transfusion and the postoperative infection remains elusive despite more than 30 observation studies, which have demonstrated that perioperative transfusion is associated with increased postoperative infections.

Observations that transfusions in patients infected with HIV led to more rapid progression to AIDS and a higher death rate, suggested that transfusions resulted in immune suppression or viral reactivation. This was supported by *in vitro* studies of increased HIV expression in infected cells in culture using allogeneic leukocytes.[122] However, in a randomized clinical trial of non leuko reduced versus leukoreduced blood, there was no viral reactivation of HIV, cytomegalovirus (CMV), hepatitis B virus (HBV), hepatitis C virus (HCV), human T-cell lymphotropic virus I and II (HTLV-I/II) or human herpesvirus 8 (HHV-8).[123,124]

Transfusion-transmitted infections

Advances in blood donor screening have supported the concept that a zero-risk blood supply may be possible in the future. While the application of numerous serologic and molecular tests and more stringent donor questioning have improved blood safety, risks still remain. Some of these risks result from donors in the window period of infection, which is defined as that period during which a potential donor is infectious without detectable viral marker positivity. Nucleic acid tests (NAT) have improved or "closed" the window, contributing to reductions in residual risk. NATs based on viral protein using polymerase chain reaction are now part of the regular testing of blood donors in the USA, Canada and many other countries. Screening in the USA includes testing for HBV and HCV, HIV-1 and -2, HTLV-I and -II, syphilis and, in some centers, CMV, but many of these tests are antibody tests and therefore may miss active viremia. With NAT for HIV, the time of infection to detection has been reduced to 10 days. With NAT for HCV, there has been a reduction to 20 days.

Despite improvements in the questioning of donors, donors may still not be truthful about high-risk behaviors in which they engage.[125] New and emerging transfusion-transmitted diseases, such as Chagas disease, transfusion transmitted viruses (TTV) and hepatitis G and Epstein–Barr virus (EBV), continue to challenge transfusionists as some may result in transient illness or in asymptomatic infection. Other organisms have an exceedingly low or theoretical risk of disease; these include Creutzfeldt–Jakob disease (CJD), Lyme disease, HHV-8, parvovirus B19, ehrlichiosis and babesiosis.

The current estimates of the risk of transfusion-transmitted viral infection have been made possible through the Retroviral Epidemiology Donor Study and studies by the American Red Cross. Rates of seroconversion of large numbers of donors can be combined with estimates of the probability that blood was donated during a window period when donor testing would have been negative. Based on these studies, the current infectious risks in the USA are given in Table 33.4.

Hepatitis C virus

HCV is a single-stranded RNA virus belonging to the Flaviviridae family. It can be transmitted by cellular and noncellular blood and blood products, including intravenous immunoglobulin. The most notable characteristic of HCV is its persistence in host hepatocytes. Studies have found that 90% of posttransfusion non-A, non-B hepatitis is caused by HCV. Long-term follow-up of patients with posttransfusion hepatitis showed that approximately 70% of HCV-infected individuals develop chronic hepatitis.[126] The mechanism of persistence is probably due to the ability of the virus to mutate rapidly under immune pressure and to coexist as multiple mutants. These mutants have been termed "quasi-species" and they provide an excellent mechanism for the virus to escape the immune response.[127] In addition, HCV can persist in the liver in a dormant state by downregulating its replication to protect itself from immune clearance. While there may be an adequate humoral response to HCV, the neutralizing antibodies that develop rapidly become ineffective against emerging strains.[127]

First-generation screening tests for HCV were used in 1990 and were targeted against the c100–3 antigen. Second-generation screening assays were introduced in 1992 and were directed against multiple epitopes: c100–3 antigen, core protein designated c22–3 and an NS3 protein designated c33c; antibodies to the latter two epitopes appear earlier than anti-c100–3. Of HCV-infected individuals, 80% will develop specific antibody by 15 weeks from exposure and 100% by 6 months; in the majority of individuals, anti-HCV antibodies persist for very long periods. With the licencing of second-generation assays in March 1995, the incidence of transfusion-associated HCV declined from 5% in 1989 to < 1%. In the late 1990s NAT for HCV was instituted, resulting in a further reduction in residual risk to 1 in 1.9 million in the USA and 1 in 3.1 million in Canada.[128,129]

Acute posttransfusion hepatitis C infection is, in the majority of patients, asymptomatic and anicteric. The significance of infection with HCV lies in the propensity of the virus for persistent indolent infection. In both community-acquired and transfusion-associated HCV, the frequency of chronic hepatitis exceeds 60%, and that of persistent infection may exceed 90%.[130] Of those with chronic hepatitis, two-thirds develop chronic active hepatitis, cirrhosis and/or hepatocellular carcinoma (HCC). At least 20% of HCV-infected patients develop cirrhosis within two decades, and the risk for development of HCC is 1–5% after 20 years; once cirrhosis is established, the rate of development of HCC increases by 1–4% per year.[131] Patients with chronic HCV hepatitis can also present with a variety of extrahepatic manifestations thought to be of immunologic origin, including arthritis, lichen planus, glomerulonephritis, keratoconjunctivitis sicca and mixed cryoglobulinemia.

HCV infection in children can be divided into that acquired prenatally or perinatally or through transfusion of blood and blood products. The majority of data concerning posttransfusion HCV infection in children come from studies on multiply transfused hematology and oncology patients, neonates, and children who underwent cardiac surgery diagnosed before implementation of HCV screening.[132–135] In children treated for malignancy, the prevalence of HCV varies from 17 to 55% depending on the geographic area and detection method used. Ni *et al.* in Japan analyzed data from 61 children, most of whom had transfusion-dependent thalassemia, who were followed for 4 years. Twenty-six were HCV infected and of these 24 had elevated alanine aminotransferase (ALT), while only 10 of 34 noninfected patients had evidence of liver dysfunction. Six patients from each group had a liver biopsy. Five HCV-positive patients had evidence of portal fibrosis compared with two of the negative group. All specimens from both groups had evidence of hemochromatosis; iron overload is a known confounder of hepatic fibrosis and HCC development in adults. Similar degrees of liver damage were not seen in neonates and other children with malignancies. In neonates studied 35 years postexposure, minimal or no inflammatory activity was noted on liver biopsy.[132–136] Taken together, these studies suggest that chronic HCV infection may produce more severe liver damage in transfusion-dependent children than in those with malignancy and infants exposed during the neonatal period[132] or for open heart surgery.[135]

Table 33.4 Infectious risks of transfusion in USA, Canada and other countries.

Infectious agent/blood component	USA/other countries	Canada
HIV (with NAT)	1 in 2.1 million: repeat donors (USA)	1 in 4.7 million
	1 in 1 million: first-time donors (USA)	
HCV (with NAT)	1 in 1.9 million: repeat donors (USA)	1 in 3.1 million
	1 in 791 000: first-time donors (USA)	
HTLV	1 in 641 000	1 in 1.9 million
HBV	1 in 30 000 to 1 in 250 000 (USA)	1 in 31 000
	1 in 470 000 (France)	
Syphilis	Virtually nonexistent	
HAV	1 in 10 million	
Malaria	1 in 4 million	
Chagas disease	Extremely low	
CMV	Unknown	
WNV	Unknown	
Bacterial contamination		
Platelets*	1 in 1000 to 1 in 3000 (USA)	
	1 in 14 000 to 1 in 38 000 (France)	
Platelet fatality*	1 in 140 000	
RBCs	1 in 172 000 (France)	
	1 in 5 million (USA)	
	1 in 66 000 (NZ)	
RBC fatality	1 in 1 million (France)	
	1 in 8 million (USA)	

* Without pretransfusion culture of component.
CMV, cytomegalovirus; HAV, hepatitis A virus; HBV, hepatitis B virus; HCV, hepatitis C virus; HIV, human immunodeficiency virus; HTLV, human T-cell lymphotropic virus; NAT, nucleic acid test; RBC, red blood cell; WNV, West Nile virus.
Adapted with permission from Ref. 167.

Treatment of HCV is with interferon-α2b (IFN- α2b at 15 mg/kg/d), with or without ribavirin, 3 million units three times weekly for 6 or 12 months. Biochemical and virologic remission rates in treated children are poorly studied and side-effects are substantial. The current consensus among hepatologists is that patients with chronic active hepatitis or active cirrhosis on liver biopsy with compensated liver disease should be treated. Because patients with lower serum titers of HCV-RNA tend to have a more favorable response to therapy, the controversy lies in whether to treat HCV carriers with mild disease. Given that HCV is a chronic disease with significant morbidity and mortality, early intervention has significant appeal. In children, abnormal hepatic pathology is seen early in the disease while titers of HCV-RNA are lower; identification of recipients of HCV-positive blood should target neonatal and pediatric transfusion recipients so that therapy can be instituted early in the course of the disease.

Hepatitis G virus

Hepatitis G virus (HGV), and its strain variant GBV-C, are human flaviviruses. HGV/GBV-C is transmitted by transfusion of blood products and is found in 1–2% of eligible volunteer US blood donors; the occurrence is higher (3–14%) in Europe.[136] HGV/GBV-C can be detected by RNA PCR and by an antibody to the envelope region E2 of the virus. Anti-E2 is a recovery-phase antibody that is detectable only when HGV/GBV-C RNA has been cleared.[137] Studies have shown that the exposure rate among volunteer blood donors is three- to six-fold the rate of viremia. In high-risk groups such as hemophiliacs, intravenous drug users, homosexuals and prostitutes, the rate of exposure may be as high as 80–90%, with a viremia rate of 15–20%.[138,139] This large difference between exposure rates and active infection rates suggests that most of the HGV/GBV-C carriers eventually clear the virus. In the National Institutes of Health (NIH) prospective transfusion study, Alter *et al.*[138] found HGV/GBV-C RNA in 23% of patients with transfusion-associated non-A, non-B, non-C hepatitis. However, there was a dissociation between the subjects' ALT levels and the HGV/GBV-C RNA levels. This casts doubt on the causality of hepatitis by this agent and raises the possibility that it may be an "innocent bystander" virus. Among HCV-infected individuals, 10–20% are co-infected with HGV/GBV-C. Many studies have shown that HGV/GBV-C has no impact on the clinical course of HCV infection.[140] Also, response to interferon is identical in patients infected with HGV/GBV-C and HCV and in those infected with HCV alone.

There is evidence of HGV/GBV-C viremia in children, but the available literature on the subject is small. Vertical transmission from mother to infant has been demonstrated and preliminary data suggest persistent infection in those children without clinical or biochemical evidence of hepatitis.[141,142] HGV/GBV-C RNA has also been detected in multiply transfused children with chronic hepatitis B and C infection and has persisted after interferon-α therapy.[143–146]

As with other transfusion-transmitted viruses that are capable of causing persistent infection, there is no clear disease association, that the designation "hepatitis" virus may have been premature. More research is needed to evaluate the demographic and clinical characteristics of HGV/GBV-C infection, and to evaluate the association of HCV with aplastic anemia.[147]

Human immunodeficiency virus

Transfusion-transmitted HIV, from either plasma-derived clotting factor concentrate or blood and blood products, has brought the inherent mortality risk from transfusion to the forefront for clinician, patient and lay public. No other transfusion-transmitted disease has generated as much fear in the minds of patients and as much action on the part of regulatory agencies and manufacturers of plasma-derived products. Current testing of blood donors for anti-HIV-1 and -2 and HIV NAT has reduced the residual risk of HIV to 1 in 2 million in the USA and 1 in 4.7 million in Canada.[129,148] Since the implementation of HIV NAT testing in the USA, there have been two reported cases of HIV that occurred during the HIV window period. Of specific interest to pediatricians, one donor was an asymptomatic female recruited during a high-school blood drive.[149]

Studies of adults receiving blood and blood products demonstrated an infection peak in 1984 for individuals transfused. Clinical presentation occurred several years later, supporting a long incubation period.[150] The NHLBI-sponsored, multicenter Transfusion Safety Study (TSS) traced individuals who received known infected blood units over time. About 90% of the recipients seroconverted, while the other 10% remained PCR- and viral culture-confirmed uninfected. Variables associated with infectivity included the level of donor viremia at the time of donation, duration of refrigerator storage and type of blood component transfused; blood product manipulations that reduce WBC number (leukoreduction) or free virus (washing) were thought to decrease inoculum and therefore infectivity.[151]

While there are several published cases[152–3] and small cohort studies, only two studies have reported large numbers of children infected by transfusion. Jones *et al.*[154] described 212 cases reported to the Centers for Disease Control (CDC) from 1981 to 1987. The median age at HIV diagnosis was 4

years, with a range of 0.3–12.8 years. The median survival was 13.7 months, longer than the reported adult survival of 5.6 months. Of interest, 71% of cases were transfused in the first year of life. AIDS-associated illnesses were similar to those reported for perinatal transmission, except that there was less lymphoid interstitial pneumonitis and more encephalopathy. In a cohort study of infants transfused in Los Angeles (a high HIV-risk area of the USA) from 1980 to March 1987, 443 were traced and tested. Thirty-three had antibody to HIV and no other risk factor except for transfusion; 14 had unrecognized HIV infection and were identified through this lookback study. Estimates of the time interval from date of infection (birth) to date of HIV-related symptoms was on average 63 months (5.25 years) with a range of 3–95 months.[153]

The authors' studies involving transfused neonates and older children in an urban area demonstrate children presenting symptom-free as late as 9.5 years after transfusion.[156] It is therefore recommended that parents of adolescents and preadolescents who present with positive HIV screening tests be questioned about transfusion occurring before the introduction of HIV testing. Medical record reviews may be needed, as many families are unaware that transfusion was a routine part of neonatal supportive care. HIV-infected children from areas of the world where blood is purchased from commercial donors or where HIV testing is not routinely performed will probably continue to present as transfusion-associated cases.

Cytomegalovirus

CMV is a ubiquitous virus of the herpesvirus family that is harbored in WBCs. A significant proportion of blood donors (30–70%) are CMV seropositive, although there are regional differences that may in part be due to different donor demographics such as age, sex, race and socioeconomic status. Older age, female sex and lower socioeconomic status predispose to higher seroprevalence rates. Despite studies confirming that seropositive donors can transmit CMV to seronegative recipients, few have been able to document viremia in blood donors. This has led to the concept that both actively infected as well as latently infected donors can transmit CMV.

Three types of CMV infection are seen in the transfusion recipient: primary infection and two kinds of secondary infection, reactivation and reinfection. Primary infection occurs in a seronegative recipient of blood from a donor who is actively or latently infected. Patients are frequently symptomatic with a mononucleosis-like syndrome that is heterophile-negative. Viremia, viruria, an IgM-specific and then IgG-specific anti-CMV antibody response can be demonstrated. Reactivation occurs when a CMV-seropositive recipient is transfused with blood from either a CMV-seropositive or -seronegative donor. The donor leukocytes trigger an allograft reaction that reactivates the recipient's latent CMV. An IgG antibody titer rise and viral shedding may be found. Most of these infections are asymptomatic, except in immunocompromised hosts. Reinfection or coinfection occurs in a CMV-seropositive recipient of blood with a strain of CMV that differs from the strain that initially infected the recipient. An IgM and IgG response as well as viral shedding may be seen. The only way to distinguish reinfection from coinfection is to use molecular markers, wherein multiple strains of CMV may be identified in the coinfected recipient.

CMV infection may be asymptomatic and discovered only because of serial serologic tests, or it may produce significant morbidity and mortality. Certain select patient groups are at risk for the pneumonia, cytopenias, hepatitis, graft rejection, unexplained fever, and increased risk of bacterial and fungal infections associated with posttransfusion CMV:

• neonates, specifically those weighing < 1250 g who are seronegative and who require large amounts of blood (>50 mL);
• recipients of hematopoietic stem cell and solid-organ transplants;
• infants who receive intrauterine transfusions;
• other severely immunocompromised individuals.

Other immunocompromised patients, either seronegative or seropositive, do not appear to be at increased risk for mortality and morbidity from CMV.

The use of IgG-seronegative blood is considered to be the gold standard, despite the fact that most IgG-seropositive units are not infectious. Depending on the donor demographics in an area, such products are sometimes difficult to obtain. Donors with IgM-specific CMV antibody may transmit CMV more readily, as they are more likely to have acute viral infection and replication.[155] IgM antibody assays, however, are not well standardized. Hence, several different methods have been used to prevent or ameliorate posttransfusion CMV. Because the virus is probably harbored in WBCs, manipulations that can reduce or attenuate leukocyte cell number should reduce the risk of transmission. These methods include washing, freezing followed by washing, and filtration. The third-generation leukocyte-depletion filters have been shown to be effective in preventing primary CMV infection in neonates, adult patients with hematologic malignancies, and patients post-BMT.

A study by Bowden *et al.*[158] suggested equivalence between CMV seronegative and leukoreduced products when no more than 5×10^6 WBCs remained in the product in an at-risk BMT population. This study, its design and outcome, have been debated widely.[157] This study's conclusions of these studies' conclusions has been questioned. In a retrospective analysis of CMV-transmission in adult hematopoietic stem cell transplant (HSCT) patients, leukocyte-reduced RBC units, but not platelets, from CMV-positive donors transmitted CMV.[158] This phenomenon

could have resulted from collection of the unit during an infectious, high viremic period where plasma viremia occurred, or might have resulted from insufficient leukodepletion due to filter failure or failure to produce a product at less than 5×10^6 WBC.

Some oncologists argue that patients who may undergo HSCT regardless of donor and recipient serology should have blood and blood products manipulated to prevent new infection, reactivation or second strain infection. More routine use of prestorage leukodepletion filters that have undergone stringent quality control checks in the setting of blood centers and transfusion services adhering to good manufacturing practices, may well provide an acceptable product that does not depend on donor serostatus. A Canadian consensus conference,[159] American Association of Blood Banks (AABB) guidelines[13] and Food and Drug Administration (FDA) advisory committees are conflicted on the issue of seronegative/leukodepletion equivalency, which results in variable practices.

Gamma irradiation of blood to inhibit lymphocyte DNA replication will not prevent CMV infection. Many patients undergoing chemotherapy with or without transplantation receive irradiated blood for prevention of GVHD. Similarly, many patients who receive blood that is CMV seronegative or leukodepleted, receive CMV hyperimmune globulin or intravenous immunoglobulin with variable titers of CMV antibody and, in addition, may be receiving FFP for coagulopathies. They receive these plasma products to attenuate the development of graft-induced CMV or nosocomial acquisition of CMV. It is difficult to assess the serostatus of these individuals because of passive acquisition of CMV antibody. Tests for CMV early antigen, CMV, NAT or other molecular markers are necessary to establish posttransfusion CMV in these patients.

After establishing CMV serostatus before chemotherapy, many institutions use an algorithm that determines the nature of the CMV restrictions. CMV-seronegative and leukodepleted blood and blood products would then be provided to seronegative recipients on protocols that may result in HSCT and stem-cell rescue. The algorithm developed by the AABB is shown in Table 33.5.

Creutzfeldt-Jakob disease (CJD) and variant CJD (vCJD)

CJD occurs in one of several forms: sporadic, transmitted, familial and variant. CJD is characterized by the presence of the isoform of a prion protein (PRP^{SC}) that is resistant to cellular protease degradation. The abnormal prion causes spongiform degeneration, neuronal loss and progressive dementia. Case–control, lookback and autopsy studies failed to show a link between CJD and receipt of blood/blood components and derivatives until the summer of 2003. A potential case of vCJD associated with blood transfusion was documented, with an additional case reported in July 2004.[160]

Table 33.5 Recommendations of the American Association of Blood Banks (AABB) on use of CMV-safe blood.

Category	Clinical circumstance	CMV-seronegative blood (unmodified)	Leukocyte-reduced (LR) blood (CMV-unscreened)
I	CMV-positive patient	Not indicated	Not indicated
	CMV-negative patient	Not indicated	Not indicated
II	CMV-positive patient	Not indicated	Use of LR blood to prevent virus reactivation awaits further research
	CMV-negative patient	Either CMV-seronegative blood or LR blood is indicated	Either CMV-seronegative blood or LR blood is indicated
III	CMV-positive recipient	Not indicated	Not indicated
	CMV-negative recipient of CMV-positive organ	Not indicated	Not indicated
	CMV-negative recipient of CMV-negative organ	Either CMV-seronegative blood or LR blood is indicated	Either CMV-seronegative blood or LR blood is indicated
IV	CMV-positive recipient	Not indicated	Use of LR blood to prevent virus reactivation awaits further research
	CMV-negative recipient of CMV-positive organ	Either CMV-seronegative blood or LR blood is indicated	Either CMV-seronegative blood or LR blood is indicated
V	CMV-negative recipient of CMV-negative organ	Either CMV-seronegative blood or LR blood is indicated	Either CMV-seronegative blood or LR blood is indicated
	CMV-positive recipient	Either CMV-seronegative blood or LR blood is indicated	Either CMV-seronegative blood or LR blood is indicated
	CMV-negative recipient	Either CMV-seronegative blood or LR blood is indicated	LR blood may be slightly preferred to CMV-seronegative blood (passive CMV immunoglobulin)

Category I patients: general hospital patients and general surgery patients (including cardiac surgery); patients receiving chemotherapy that is not intended to produce severe neutropenia (adjuvant therapy for breast cancer, treatment of chronic lymphocytic leukemia, etc.); patients receiving corticosteroids (patients with immune thrombocytopenic purpura, collagen vascular diseases, etc.); full-term infants.

Category II patients: patients receiving chemotherapy that is intended to produce severe neutropenia (leukemia, lymphoma, etc.); pregnant patients; HIV-infected individuals.

Category III patients: solid organ allograft patients who do not require massive transfusion support.

Category IV patients: patients receiving allogeneic and autologous hematopoietic progenitor cell transplants.

Category V patients: low birthweight (<1200 g) premature infants.

The two cases developed despite the institution of donor deferrals, which includes donors who travel or reside in areas where bovine spongiform encephalopathy (BSE) epidemics have occurred. In the UK, no person who has ever received a blood transfusion can serve as a blood donor. An additional safeguard was mandated in Canada in the form of universal leukodepletion to reduce infectivity associated with the high concentrations of vCJD protein in peripheral white blood cells, especially lymphocytes. To date, no change in US or Canadian screening, deferral or testing for vCJD has been implemented.[161]

West Nile virus

West Nile virus (WNV) is an arthropod-borne virus transmitted via *Anopheles* mosquitoes between birds; humans are incidental hosts for this virus. The first cases of WNV via organ and blood transfusion were documented in 2002, with growing numbers of transfusion-related cases reported through 2004. In 20% of cases, infected humans, often the elderly and/or immunocompromised may develop severe flu-like symptoms and lymphadenopathy. Death occurs in 1 in 1000 infections. To reduce WNV transmission to patients, donor history questions are aimed at detecting symptomatic donors. Since August 2003, all blood products in the USA have been tested for WNV by NAT, in a unique nationwide clinical trial that took place in advance of test licensure. In 2003, when NAT was implemented, 1000 units were confirmed positive. Residual risk since implementation of WNV NAT cannot be established at this time. Twenty-three cases of transfusion-associated infection were investigated with six confirmed as of April 2004 and six still open. The 2005 summer season saw clusters of WNV in donors and additional recipient cases reported to CDC.

Other transfusion-transmitted organisms

Other transfusion-transmitted disorders include the parasites *Trypanosoma cruzi*, known to cause Chagas disease, and *Plasmodium* spp., the etiologic agents of malaria. *Babesia*, the intraerythrocytic protozoan parasite attributable to contact with infected tick vectors of the *Ixodes* group, has raised

Table 33.6 Prevention of some transfusion complications by leukocyte removal.

Established indications	Threshold level of WBC reduction to prevent the reaction
Febrile nonhemolytic transfusion reaction	5×10^8
Alloimmunization to class I HLA antigens	$<5 \times 10^6$
Infectious disease transmission by leukocytes	Unknown and dependent on virus in question. Plasma viremia may transmit disease, despite leukodepletion. See text
Graft-versus-host disease	Unknown. Gamma irradiation should be used
Transfusion-related acute lung injury (TRALI)	Passive transfer of antibody in plasma will not be attenuated by leukocyte removal

concerns. For these and other agents, only a handful of transfusion-transmitted cases have been reported. Control strategies have included instituting seasonal deferrals, regional testing and earmarking specific donor pools for leukocyte reduction (Table 33.6). As the endemic ranges of these agents expand, more extensive interventions, like donor testing and pathogen inactivation, will be required.[164]

Other emergency transfusion risks

TTV and hepatitis E are both viruses that are transfusion transmitted. TTV is highly associated with transfusion in areas endemic for TTV.[165] Hepatitis E, which is endemic in certain areas of the Near and Far East, has also been suspected of infrequent transfusion transmission.[166]

References

1. Angiolillo A, Luban NL. Hemolysis following an out-of-group platelet transfusion in an 8-month-old with Langerhans cell histiocytosis. *J Pediatr Hematol Oncol* 2004; **26**: 267–9.
2. Josephson CD, Mullis NC, Van Demark C *et al*. Significant numbers of apheresis-derived group O platelet units have "high-titer" anti-A/A,B: implications for transfusion policy. *Transfusion* 2004; **44**: 805–8.
3. Davenport RD, Streiter RM, Kunkel SL. Red cell ABO incompatibility and production of tumor necrosis factor-alpha. *Br J Haematol* 1991; **78**: 540–4.
4. Capon SM, Goldfinger D. Acute hemolytic transfusion reaction, a paradigm of the systemic inflammatory response: new insights into pathophysiology and treatment. *Transfusion* 1995; **35**: 513–20.
5. Silliman CC, Boshkov LK, Mehdizadehkashi Z *et al*. Transfusion-related acute lung injury: epidemiology and a prospective analysis of etiologic factors. *Blood* 2003; **101**: 454–62.
6. Bux J, Becker F, Seeger W *et al*. Transfusion-related acute lung injury due to HLA-A2-specific antibodies in recipient and NB1-specific antibodies in donor blood. *Br J Haematol* 1996; **93**: 707–13.
7. Leach M, Vora AJ, Jones DA *et al*. Transfusion-related acute lung injury (TRALI) following autologous stem cell transplant for relapsed acute myeloid leukemia: a case report and review of the literature. *Transfus Med* 1998; **8**: 333–7.
8. Wolf CF, Canale VC. Fatal pulmonary hypersensitivity reaction to HL-A incompatible blood transfusion: report of a case and review of the literature. *Transfusion* 1976; **16**: 135–40.
9. Nouraei SM, Wallis JP, Bolton D *et al*. Management of transfusion-related acute lung injury with extracorporeal cardiopulmonary support in a four-year-old child. *Br J Anaesth* 2003; **91**: 292–4.
10. Yang X, Ahmed S, Chandrasekaran V. Transfusion-related acute lung injury resulting from designated blood transfusion between mother and child: a report of two cases. *Am J Clin Pathol* 2004; **121**: 590–2.
11. Webert KE, Blajchman MA. Transfusion-related acute lung injury. *Transfus Med Rev* 2003; **17**: 252–62.
12. Gilstad CW, Kessler C, Sandler SG. Transfusing patients with anti-immunoglobulin Λ sub-class antibodies. *Vox Sang* 2002; **83**: 363.
13. Brecher ME (ed.) *Technical Manual*, 13th edn. Bethesda, MN: American Association of Blood Banks, 2003.
14. King KE, Shirey RS *et al*. Universal leukoreduction decreases the incidence of febrile nonhemolytic transfusion reactions to RBCs. *Transfusion* 2004: **44**: 25–9.
15. Heddle NM, Klama L, Meyer R, Thoman SK *et al*. A randomized controlled trial comparing plasma removal with white cell reduction to prevent reactions to platelets. *Transfusion* 1999; **39**: 231–8.
16. Heddle NM, Blajchman MA, Meyer RM *et al*. A randomized controlled trial comparing the frequency of acute reactions to plasma-removed platelets and prestorage WBC-reduced platelets. *Transfusion* 2002; **42**: 556–66.
17. Couban S, Carruthers J, Andreou P *et al*. Platelet transfusions in children: results of a randomized, prospective, crossover trial of plasma removal and a prospective audit of WBC reduction. *Transfusion* 2002; **42**: 753–8.
18. Scanlon JW, Krakaur R. Hyperkalemia following exchange transfusion. *J Pediatr* 198; **96**: 108–19.
19. Brown KA, Bissonnette B, McIntyre B. Hyperkalemia during rapid blood transfusion and hypovolemic cardiac arrest in children. *Can J Anaesth* 1990; **37**: 747–54.
20. Blanchette VS, Grey E, Hardie MJ *et al*. Hyperkalemia following exchange transfusion: Risk eliminated by washing red cell concentrates. *J Pediatr* 1993; **123**: 285.
21. Beutler E, Meul A, Wood LA. Depletion and regeneration of 2,3-diphosphoglyceric acid in stored red blood cells. *Transfusion* 1969; **9**: 109–15.
22. Boyan CP, Howland WS. Cardiac arrest and temperature of blood bank blood. *N Engl J Med* 1963; **183**: 58–60.

23. Phillips TF, Soulier G, Wilson RF. Outcome of massive transfusion exceeding two blood volumes in trauma and emergency surgery. *J Trauma* 1987; **27**: 903–10.

24. Blajchman MA. Bacterial contamination of cellular blood components: risks, sources and control. *Vox Sang* 2004; **87**: 98–103.

25. Goldman M, Blajchman M. Bacterial contamination. In: Popovsky M (ed.) *Transfusion Reactions*. Bethesda, MD: American Association of Blood Banks, 1996, pp. 126–58.

26. Wagner SJ, Moroff G, Katz AJ *et al.* Comparison of bacteria growth in single and pooled platelet concentrates after deliberate inoculation and storage. *Transfusion* 1995; **35**: 298–302.

27. Kuehnert MJ, Roth VR, Haley R *et al.* Transfusion-transmitted bacterial infection in the United States, 1998 through 2000. *Transfusion* 2001; **41**: 1493–9.

28. Perez P, Salmi LR, Follea G *et al.* BACTHEM Group; French Haemovigilance Network: Determinants of transfusion-associated bacterial contamination: Results of the French BACTHEM Case-Control Study. *Transfusion* 2001; **41**: 862–72.

29. Yomtovian R, Lazarus HM, Goodnough LT *et al.* A prospective microbiologic surveillance program to detect and prevent the transfusion of bacterially contaminated platelets. *Transfusion* 1993; **33**: 902–9.

30. Wagner S. Transfusion-related bacterial sepsis. *Curr Opin Hematol* 1997; **4**: 464–9.

31. Workshop on Bacterial Contamination of Platelets. Bethesda, MD: FDA, Center for Biologics Evaluation and Research, 1999. http://www.fda;gov/cber/minutes/workshop-min.htm.

32. Wagner, SJ. Transfusion-transmitted bacterial infection: risks, sources and interventions. *Vox Sang* 2004; **86**: 157–63.

33. Urbaniak SJ, Robertson AE. A successful program for immunizing Rh-negative volunteers for anti-D production using frozen/thawed blood. *Transfusion* 1981; **21**: 64–9.

34. Jakobowicz R, Williams L, Silberman F. Immunization of Rh negative volunteers by repeated injections of very small amounts of Rh positive blood. *Vox Sang* 1972; **23**: 376–81.

35. Issitt PD. *Applied Blood Group Serology*, 3rd edn. Miami: Montgomery Scientific, 1985, pp. 9–42.

36. Giblett ER. A critique of the theoretical hazard of inter- vs. intra-racial transfusion. *Transfusion* 1961; **1**: 233–8.

37. Floss AM, Strauss RG, Goeken N *et al.* Multiple transfusions fail to provoke antibodies against blood cell antigens in human infants. *Transfusion* 1986; **26**: 419–22.

38. Ludvigsen CW Jr, Swanson JL, Thompson TR *et al.* The failure of neonates to form red blood cell alloantibodies in response to multiple transfusions. *Am J Clin Pathol* 1987; **87**: 250–1.

39. Pass MA, Johnson JD, Shulman IA *et al.* Evaluation of a walking-donor blood transfusion program in an intensive care nursery. *J Pediatr* 1976; **89**: 646–51.

40. Rawls WE, Wong CL, Blajchman M *et al.* Neonatal cytomegalovirus infections: the relative role of neonatal blood transfusion and maternal exposure. *Clin Invest Med* 1984; **7**: 13–19.

41. Smith MR, Storey CG. Allo-anti-E in an 18-day-old infant [letter]. *Transfusion* 1984; **24**: 540.

42. DePalma L, Criss VR, Roseff SD *et al.* Presence of the red cell alloantibody anti-E in an 11-week-old infant. *Transfusion* 1992; **32**: 177–9.

43. Nurse GT. Directed donation and the developing world [letter]. *Transfusion* 1993; **33**: 90.

44. DePalma L, Duncan B, Chan MM *et al.* The neonatal immune response to washed and irradiated red cells: lack of evidence of lymphocyte activation. *Transfusion* 1991; **31**: 737–42.

45. Sarnaik S, Schornack J, Lusher JM. The incidence of development of irregular red cell antibodies in patients with sickle cell anemia. *Transfusion* 1986; **26**: 249–52.

46. Orlina AR, Unger PJ, Koshy M. Post-transfusion alloimmunization in patients with sickle cell disease. *Am J Hematol* 1978; **5**: 101–6.

47. Rosse WF, Gallagher D, Kinney TR *et al.* Transfusion and alloimmunization in sickle cell disease. *Blood* 1990; **76**: 1431–7.

48. Vichinsky EP, Earles A, Johnson RP *et al.* Alloimmunization in sickle cell anemia and transfusion of racially unmatched blood. *N Engl J Med* 1990; **322**: 1617–21.

49. Luban NLC. Variability in rates of alloimmunization in different groups of children with sickle cell disease: Effect of ethnic background. *Am J Pediatr Hematol Oncol* 1989; **11**: 314–19.

50. Aygun B, Padmanabhan S, Paley C *et al.* Clinical significance of RBC alloantibodies and autoantibodies in sickle cell patients who received transfusions. *Transfusion* 2002; **42**: 37–43.

51. Smith-Whitley K. Alloimmunization in patients with sickle cell disease. In: Herman J and Manno CS (eds) AABB Press, 2002, pp. 249–77.

52. Garratty G, Glynn SA, McEntire R. ABO and Rh(D) phenotype frequencies of different racial/ethnic groups in the United States. *Transfusion* 2004; **44**: 703–6.

53. Ambruso DR, Githens JH, Alcorn R *et al.* Experience with donors matched for minor blood group antigens in patients with sickle cell anemia who are receiving chronic transfusion therapy. *Transfusion* 1987; **27**: 94–8.

54. Castellino S, Combs M, Zimmerman S *et al.* Erythrocyte autoantibodies in paediatric patients with sickle cell disease receiving transfusion therapy: frequency, characteristics and significance. *Br J Haematol* 1999; **104**: 189–94.

55. Garratty G. Autoantibodies induced by blood transfusion. *Transfusion* 2004; **44**: 5–9.

56. King KE, Shirey RS, Lankiewicz MW *et al.* Delayed hemolytic transfusion reactions in sickle cell disease: Simultaneous destruction of recipients' red cells. *Transfusion* 1997; **37**: 376–81.

57. Petz LD, Calhoun L, Shulman IA *et al.* The sickle cell hemolytic transfusion reaction syndrome. *Transfusion* 1997; **37**: 382–92.

58. Sirchia G, Zanella A, Parravicini A *et al.* Red cell alloantibodies in thalassemia major. Results of an Italian cooperative study. *Transfusion* 1985; **25**: 110–12.

59. Ameen R, Al-Shemmari S, Al-Humood S *et al.* RBC alloimmunization and autoimmunization among transfusion-dependent Arab thalassemia patients. *Transfusion* 2003; **43**: 1604–10.

60. Spanos Th, Karageorga M, Ladis V *et al.* Red cell alloantibodies in patients with thalassemia. *Vox Sang* 1990; **58**: 50–5.

61. Michail-Merianou V, Pamphili-Panousopoulou L, Piperi-Lowes L *et al.* Alloimmunization to red cell antigens in thalassemia: Comparative study of usual versus better-match transfusion programmes. *Vox Sang* 1987; **52**: 95–8.

62. Seftel MD, Growe GH, Petraszko T *et al.* Universal prestorage leukoreduction in Canada decreases platelet alloimmunization and refractoriness. *Blood* 2004; **103**: 333–9.

63. Sirchia G, Rebulla P. Evidence-based medicine: the case for white cell reduction. *Transfusion* 1997; **37**: 543–9.

64. Deeg HJ, Sigaroudinia M. Ultraviolet B-induced loss of HLA class II antigen expression on lymphocytes is dose, time, and locus dependent. *Exp Hematol* 1990; **18**: 916–19.

65. Andreu G, Boccaccio C, Klaren J *et al.* The role of UV radiation in the prevention of human leukocyte antigen alloimmunization. *Transfus Med Rev* 1992; **6**: 212–24.

66. Blundell EL, Pamphilon DH, Fraser ID *et al.* A prospective, randomized study of the use of platelet concentrates irradiated with ultraviolet-B light in patients with hematologic malignancy. *Transfusion* 1996; **36**: 296–302.

67. Trial to Reduce Alloimmunization to Platelets (TRAP) Study Group. Leukocyte reduction and ultraviolet and irradiation of platelets to prevent alloimmunization and refractoriness to platelet transfusions. *N Eng J Med* 1997; **337**: 1661–9.

68. Strauss RG. Selection of white cell-reduced blood components for transfusions during early infancy. *Transfusion* 1993; **33**: 352–7.

69. Bedford-Russell AR, Rivers RPA, Davey N. The development of anti-HLA antibodies in multiply transfused preterm infants. *Arch Dis Child* 1993; **68**: 49–51.

70. Skacel PO, Stacey TE, Tidmarsh CEF *et al.* Maternal alloimmunization to HLA, platelet and granulocyte-specific antigens during pregnancy: its influence on cord blood granulocyte and platelet counts. *Br J Haematol* 1989; **71**: 119–23.

71. Elbert C, Strauss RG, Barrett F *et al.* Biological mothers may be dangerous blood donors for their neonates. *Acta Haematol* 1991; **85**: 189–91.

72. Dutcher JP, Schiffer CA, Aisner J *et al.* Long term follow up patients with leukemia receiving platelet transfusions: identification of a large group of patients who do not become alloimmunized. *Blood* 1981; **58**: 1007–11.

73. Lee EJ, Schiffer CA. Serial measurement of lymphocytotoxic antibody and response to nonmatched platelet transfusions in alloimmunized patients. *Blood* 1987; **70**: 1727–9.

74. Schiffer CA, Lichtenfeld JL, Wiernik PH *et al.* Antibody response in patients with acute nonlymphocytic leukemia. *Cancer* 1976; **37**: 2177–82.

75. Holohan TV, Terasaki PI, Deisseroth AB. Suppression of transfusion-related alloimmunization in intensively treated cancer patients. *Blood* 1981; **58**: 122–8.

76. Kickler T, Kennedy SD, Braine HG. Alloimmunization to platelet-specific antigens on glycoproteins IIb–IIIa and Ib/IX in multiply transfused thrombocytopenic patients. *Transfusion* 1990; **30**: 622–5.

77. Shulman NR, Aster RH, Leitner A *et al.* Immunoreactions involving platelets. V. Post-transfusion purpura due to a complement fixing antibody against a genetically controlled platelet antigen: A proposed mechanism for thrombocytopenia and its relevance in autoimmunity. *J Clin Invest* 1961; **40**: 1597–1620.

78. McFarland JG. Post-transfusion purpura. In: Popovsky MA (ed.) *Transfusion Reactions*, 2nd edn. Bethesda, MD. 2nd edition: AABB Press, 2001, pp. 187–212.

79. Kickler TS, Ness PM, Herman JH *et al.* Studies on the pathophysiology of post-transfusion purpura. *Blood* 1986; **68**: 347–50.

80. Chapman JF, Murphy MF, Berney SI *et al.* Post-transfusion purpura associated with anti-Bak^a and anti-PIA2 platelet antibodies and delayed haemolytic transfusion reaction. *Vox Sang* 1987; **52**: 313–17.

81. Valentin N, Vergracht A, Bignon J *et al.* HLA-Dw52a is involved in alloimmunization against PL A1 antigen. *Hum Immunol* 1990; **27**: 73–9.

82. Brecher ME, Moore SB, Letendre L. Post-transfusion purpura: the therapeutic value of PlA1-negative platelets. *Transfusion* 1990; **30**: 433–5.

83. Ohto H, Anderson KC. Survey of transfusion-associated graft-versus-host disease in immuno-competent recipients. *Transfus Med Rev* 1996; **10**: 31–43.

84. Lee TH, Donegan E, Slichter S *et al.* Transient increase in circulating donor leukocytes after allogeneic transfusions in immunocompetent recipients compatible with donor cell proliferation. *Blood* 1995; **85**: 1207–44.

85. Utter GH, Owings JT, Lee TH. Blood transfusion is associated with donor leukocyte microchimerism in trauma patients. *J Trauma* 2004; **57**: 702–7.

86. Ferrara JL, Cooke KR, Teshima T. The pathophysiology of graft-versus-host disease. *Inst J Hematol* 2003; **78**: 181–7.

87. Rubinstein A, Radl J, Cottier H. Unusual combined immunodeficiency syndrome exhibiting kappa-IgD paraproteinemia, residual gut immunity and graft versus host reaction after plasma infusion. *Acta Paediatr Scand* 1973; **62**: 365–72.

88. Wagner FF, Flegel WA. Transfusion associated graft-versus-host disease: risk due to homozygous HLA haplotypes. *Transfusion* 1995; **35**: 284–91.

89. Antin JG, Ferrara JLM. Cytokine dysregulation and acute graft-versus-host disease. *Blood* 1992; **80**: 2964–8.

90. Reddy P, Ferrara JL. Immunobiology of acute graft vs. host disease. *Blood Rev* 2003; **17**: 187–94.

91. Linden JV, Pisciotto PT. Transfusion-associated graft-versus-host disease and blood irradiation. *Transfus Med Rev* 1992; **2**: 116–23.

92. Ohto H, Anderson KC. Post-transfusion graft-versus-host disease in Japanese newborns. *Transfusion* 1996; **36**: 117–23.

93. Hathaway WE, Brangle RW, Nelson TL *et al.* Aplastic anemia and alymphocytosis in an infant with hypogammaglobulinemia: Graft-versus-host reaction? *J Pediatr* 1966; **68**: 713–22.

94. Strauss RG. Data-driven blood banking practices for neonatal RBC transfusions. *Transfusion* 2000; **40**: 1528–40.

95. Anderson KC, Weinstein HJ. Transfusion-associated graft-versus-host disease. *N Engl J Med* 1990; **323**: 315–21.

96. Leitman SF, Tisdale JF, Bolan CD *et al.* Transfusion-associated GVHD after fludarabine therapy in a patient with systemic lupus erythematosus. *Transfusion* 2003; **43**: 1667–71.

97. Shivdasani RA, Haluska FG, Dock NL *et al.* Graft-versus-host disease associated with transfusion of blood from unrelated HLA-homozygous donors. *N Engl J Med* 1993; **328**: 766–70.

98. Ohto H, Yasuda H, Noguchi M *et al.* Risk of transfusion-associated graft-versus-host disease as a result of directed donations from relatives. *Transfusion* 1992; **32**: 691–3.

99. Kruskall MS, Lee TH, Assmann SF *et al.* Survival of transfused donor white blood cells in HIV-infected recipients. *Blood* 2001; **98**: 272–9.

100. Pelszynski MM, Moroff G, Luban NLC *et al.* Effect of gamma irradiation of red blood cell units on T-cell inactivation as

assessed by limiting dilution analysis: implications for preventing transfusion-associated graft-versus-host disease. *Blood* 1994; **83**: 1683–9.

101. Anand AJ, Dzik WH, Imam A *et al.* Radiation-induced red cell damage: role of reactive oxygen species. *Transfusion* 1997; **37**: 160–5.

102. Grass JA, Wafa T, Reames A *et al.* Prevention of transfusion-associated graft-versus-host disease by photochemical treatment. *Blood* 1999; **93**: 3140–7.

103. Corash L, Lin L. Novel processes for inactivation of leukocytes to prevent transfusion-associated graft-versus-host disease. *Bone Marrow Transplant* 2004; **33**: 1–7.

104. Fast LD. The effect of exposing murine splenocytes to UVB light, psoralen plus UVA light, or gamma-irradiation on in vitro and in vivo immune responses. *Transfusion* 2003; **43**: 576–83.

105. Luban NLC. Prevention of transfusion-associated graft-versus-host disease by inactivation of T cells in platelet components. *Semin Hematol* 2001; **38** (4 suppl. 11): 34–45.

106. Clark DA, Gunby J, Daya S. The use of allogeneic leukocytes or IV IgG for the treatment of patients with recurrent spontaneous abortions. *Transfus Med Rev* 1997; **11**: 85–94.

107. Peters WR, Fry RD, Fleshman JW *et al.* Multiple blood transfusions reduce the recurrence rate of Crohn's disease. *Dis Colon Rectum* 1989; **32**: 749–53.

108. Williams JG, Hughes LE. Effect of perioperative blood transfusion on recurrence of Crohn's disease (letter). *Lancet* l989; **2**: 1524.

109. Blajchman MA, Dzik S, Vamvakas EC *et al.* Clinical and molecular basis of transfusion-induced immunomodulation: Summary of the proceedings of a state-of-the-art conference. *L Transfusion Med Rev* 2001; **15**: 108–35.

110. Vamvakas EC. White blood cell-containing allogeneic blood transfusion, postoperative infection and mortality: A meta-analysis of observational "before-and-after" studies. *Vox Sang* 2004; **86**: 111–19.

111. Puppo F, Ghio M, Contini P *et al.* Fas, Fas ligand, and transfusion immunomodulation. *Transfusion* 2001; **41**: 416–18.

112. Vamvakas, EC. Transfusion-associated cancer recurrence and postoperative infection: Meta-analysis of randomized, controlled clinical trials. *Transfusion* 1996; **36**: 175–86.

113. Busch O, Hop W, van Papendrecht M *et al.* Blood transfusion and prognosis in colorectal cancer. *N Engl J Med* 1993; **328**: 1372–6.

114. Houbiers JG, Brand A, van de Watering LM, *et al.* Randomised controlled trial comparing transfusion of leukocyte-depleted or buffy-coat-depleted blood in surgery for colorectal cancer. *Lancet* 1994; **344**: 573–8.

115. Heiss MM, Mempel W, Jauch KW *et al.* Beneficial effect of autologous blood transfusion on infectious complications after colorectal cancer surgery. *Lancet* 1993; **342**: 1328–33.

116. Jensen LS, Andersen AJ, Christiansen PM *et al.* Postoperative infection and natural killer cell function following blood transfusion in patients undergoing elective colorectal surgery. *Br J Surg* 1992; **79**: 513–16.

117. Jensen LS, Kissmeyer-Nielson P, Wolff B *et al.* Randomised comparison of leukocyte-depleted versus buffy-coat-poor blood transfusion and complications after colorectal surgery. *Lancet* 1996; **348**: 841–5.

118. van de Watering LM, Hermans J, Houbiers JG *et al.* Beneficial effects of leukocyte depletion of transfused blood on postoperative complications in patients undergoing cardiac surgery: A randomized clinical trial. *Circulation* 1998; **97**: 562–8.

119. Tartter PI, Mohandas K, Azar P *et al.* Randomized trial comparing packed red cell blood transfusion with and without leukocyte depletion for gastrointestinal surgery. *Am J Surg* 1998; **176**: 462–6.

120. Houbiers JG, van de Velde CJ, van de Watering LM *et al.* Transfusion of red cells is associated with increased incidence of bacterial infection after colorectal surgery: A prospective study. *Transfusion* 1997; **37**: 126–34.

121. Titlestad IL, Ebbesen LS, Ainsworth AP *et al.* Leukocyte-depletion of blood components does not significantly reduce the risk of infections complications. Results of a double-blinded, randomized study. *Int J Colorectal Dis* 2001; **16**: 147–53.

122. Wallis JP, Chapman CE, Orr KE *et al.* Effect of WBC reduction of transfused RBCs on postoperative infection rates in cardiac surgery. *Transfusion* 2002; **42**: 1127–34.

123. Busch MP, Lee T-H, Heitman J. Allogeneic leukocytes but not therapeutic blood elements induce reactivation and dissemination of latent human immunodeficiency virus type 1 infection: Implications for transfusion support of infected patients. *Blood* 1992; **80**: 2128–35.

124. Collier AC, Kalish LA, Bush MP *et al.* Leukocyte-reduced red blood cell transfusion in patients with anemia and human immunodeficiency infection: The Viral Activation Transfusion Study: A randomized controlled trial. *JAMA* 2001; **285**: 1592–601.

125. Asmuth DM, Kalish LA Laycock ME *et al.* Absence of HBV and HCV, HTLV-I and -II and human herpes virus-8 activation after allogeneic RBC transfusion in patients with advanced HIV-1 infections. *Transfusion* 2003; **43**: 451–8.

126. Williams AE, Thomson RA, Schreiber GB *et al.* Estimates of infectious disease risk factors in US blood donors. *JAMA* 1997; **277**: 967–72.

127. Shimitzu YK, Yoshikura H, Hijikata M *et al.* Neutralizing antibodies against hepatitis C virus and the emergence of neutralization escape mutant viruses. *J Virol* 1994; **68**: 1494–500.

128. Ogata NR, Alter HJ, Miller RH *et al.* Nucleotide sequence and mutation rate of the H strain of hepatitis C virus. *Proc Natl Acad Sci USA* 1991; **88**: 3392–6.

129. Dodd RY, Notarl IV, Stramer SL. Current prevalence and incidence of infectious disease markers and estimated window-period risk in the American Red Cross blood donor population. *Transfusion* 2002; **42**: 975–9.

130. Kleinman S, Chan P, Robillard P. Risk associated with transfusion of cellular blood components in Canada. *Transfus Med Rev* 2003; **17**: 120–62.

131. Alter M, Margolis HS, Krawczynski K *et al.* The natural history of community-acquired hepatitis C in the United States. The sentinel counties chronic non-A, non-B hepatitis study team. *N Engl J Med* 1992; **327**: 1899–905.

132. Tong MJ, El-Farra NS, Reikes AR *et al.* Clinical outcomes after transfusion-associated hepatitis C. *N Engl J Med* 1995; **332**: 1463–6.

133. Casiraghi MA, De Paschale M, Romano L *et al.* Long-term outcome (35 years) of hepatitis C after acquisition of infection

through mini transfusions of blood given at birth. *Hepatology* 2004; **39**: 90–6.

134. Strickland DK, Riely CA, Patrick CC *et al.* Hepatitis C infection among survivors of childhood cancer. *Blood* 2000; **95**: 3065–70.

135. Badizagen K, Jonas M, Ott MJ *et al.* Histopathology of the liver in children with chronic hepatitis C viral infection. *Hepatology* 1998; **28**: 1416.

136. Ni Y, Chang M, Lin K *et al.* Hepatitis C viral infection in thalassemic children: Clinical and molecular studies. *Pediatr Res* 1996; **39**: 323–8.

137. Vogt M, Lang T, Frosner G *et al.* Prevalence and clinical outcome of hepatitis C infection in children who underwent cardiac surgery before the implementation of blood-donor screening. *N Engl J Med* 1999; **341**: 866–70.

138. Alter HJ, Nakatsuji Y, Melpolder J *et al.* The incidence of transfusion-associated hepatitis G virus infection and its relation to liver disease. *N Engl J Med* 1997; **336**: 747–54.

139. Alter HJ. G-pers creepers, where'd you get those papers? A reassessment of the literature on the hepatitis G virus. *Transfusion* 1997; **37**: 569–72.

140. Stark K, Bienzle U, Hess G *et al.* Detection of the hepatitis G virus genome among injecting drug users, homosexual and bisexual men, and blood donors. *J Infect Dis* 1996; **174**: 1320–3.

141. Roth W, Waschk D, Marx S *et al.* Prevalence of hepatitis G virus and its strain variant, the GB agent in blood donations and their transmission to recipients. *Transfusion* 1997; **37**: 651–6.

142. Alter M, Gallagher M, Morris T *et al.* Acute non A–E hepatitis in the United States and the role of hepatitis G infection. *N Engl J Med* 1997; **336**: 741–6.

143. Fischler B, Lara C, Chen M *et al.* Genetic evidence for mother-to-infant transmission of hepatitis G virus. *J Infect Dis* 1997; **176**: 281–5.

144. Handa A, Jubran RF, Dickstein B *et al.* GB virus C/hepatitis G virus infection is frequent in American children and young adults. *Clin Infect Dis* 2000; **30**: 569–71.

145. Neilson J, Harrison P, Milligan DW *et al.* Hepatitis G virus in long-term survivors of haematological malignancy. *Lancet* 1996; **347**: 1632–3.

146. Kew MC, Kissianides C. HGV: hepatitis G virus or harmless G virus? *Lancet* 1996; **348** (suppl. II): 10.

147. Kudo T, Morishima T, Tsuzuki *et al.* Hepatitis G virus in immunosuppressed paediatric allograft recipients. *Lancet* 1996; **348**: 751.

148. Lopez-Alcorocho JM, Millan A, Garcia-Trevijano ER *et al.* Detection of hepatitis GB virus type C RNA in serum and liver of children with chronic viral hepatitis B and C. *Hepatology* 1997; **25**: 1258–60.

149. Kiem HP, Myerson D, Storb R *et al.* Prevalence of hepatitis G virus in patients with aplastic anemia. *Blood* 1997; **90**: 1335–6.

150. Busch MP, Kleinman SH, Nemo GJ. Current and emerging infectious risks of blood transfusions. *JAMA* 2003; **289**: 959–62.

151. Phelps R, Robbins K, Liberti T *et al.* Window-period human immunodeficiency virus transmission to two recipients by an adolescent blood donor. *Transfusion* 2004; **44**: 929–33.

152. Busch MD, Young MJ, Simpson SM *et al.* Risk of human immunodeficiency virus transmission by blood transfusion prior to implementation of HIV antibody screening in the San Francisco Bay area. *Transfusion* 1991; **31**: 4–11.

153. Kleinman SH, Niland JC, Azen SP *et al.* Prevalence of antibodies to human immunodeficiency virus type among blood donors prior to screening: the Transfusion Safety Study/NHLBI donor repository. *Transfusion* 1989; **29**: 572–80.

154. Jones DS, Byers RH, Bush TJ *et al.* Epidemiology of transfusion-associated acquired immunodeficiency syndrome in children in the United States, 1981 through 1989. *Pediatrics* 1993; **89**: 123–7.

155. Lieb LE, Mundy TM, Goldfinger D *et al.* Unrecognized human immunodeficiency virus type 1 infection in a cohort of transfused neonates: a retrospective investigation. *Pediatrics* 1995; **95**: 717–21.

156. Wayne C, Cornell M, O'Donnell R *et al.* Seroprevalence of HIV in a transfused pediatric cardiac cohort in a high prevalence area. *Transfusion* 1993; **33**: 544.

157. Lamberson HV, McMillan JA, Weiner LB *et al.* Prevention of transfusion-associated cytomegalovirus (CMV) infection in neonates by screening donors for IgM to CMV. *J Infect Dis* 1988; **157**: 820–3.

158. Bowden RA, Slichter SJ, Sayers M *et al.* A comparison of filtered leukocyte-reduced and cytomegalovirus (CMV) seronegative blood products for the prevention of transfusion-associated CMV infection after marrow transplant. *Blood* 1995; **86**: 3598–603.

159. Landaw EM, Kanter M, Petz LD. Safety of filtered leukocyte-reduced blood products for prevention of transfusion-associated cytomegalovirus infection [letter]. *Blood* 1996; **87**: 4910.

160. Nichols WG, Price T, Gooley T. Transfusion-transmitted cytomegalovirus infection after receipt of leukoreduced blood products. *Blood* 2003; **101**: 4195–200.

161. Fraser GA, Walker II, Canadian Blood and Marrow Transplant Group. Cytomegalovirus prophylaxis and treatment after hematopoietic stem cell transplantation in Canada: a description of current practices and comparison with Centers for Disease Control/Infectious Diseases Society of America/American Society for Blood and Marrow Transplantation guideline recommendations. *Biol Blood Marrow Transplant* 2004; **10**: 287.

162. UK reports potential case of transfusion-transmitted vCJD. *AABB Weekly Report* 2003; **9**(44): 1.

163. McCullough J, Anderson D, Brookie D. Consensus conference on vCJD screening of blood donors: report of the panel. *Transfusion* 2004; **44**: 675–83.

164. Zavizion B, Pereira M, de Melo Jorge M. Inactivation of protozoan parasites in red blood cells using INACTINE PEN110 chemistry. *Transfusion* 2004; **44**: 731–8.

165. Hsu HY, Ni YH, Chen HL *et al.* TT virus infection in healthy children, children after blood transfusions, and children with non-A to E hepatitis or other liver diseases in Taiwan. *J Med Virol* 2003; **69**: 66–71.

166. Matsubayashi K, Nagaoka Y, Sakata H *et al.* Transfusion-transmitted hepatitis E caused by apparently indigenous hepatitis E virus strain in Hokkaido, Japan. *Transfusion* 2004; **44**: 934–40.

167. Petrides M, Aubuchon JP. To transfuse or not transfuse: an assessment of issues and benefits in transfusion therapy 2nd edition. Mintz PD et al. AABB Press 2003, pp. 657–83.

34 Management of infection in children with bone marrow failure

Subarna Chakravorty and Ian M. Hann

During recent years, significant progress has been made in improving the outcome of children with malignancies; in the absence of new effective therapies, this has been mainly achieved by intensification of treatment using conventional drugs. However, such dosage intensification also increases the risk of infectious complications and can only proceed with improvements in supportive care in much the same way that heroic surgery requires advances in anesthesiology and intensive care methods. This chapter is not intended to deal with every possible infection or clinical manifestation of such, but rather to be a practical current guide to the management of infection. The last few years have seen major improvements in the development of hematopoietic growth factors, new antifungal agents and new antibiotics. Attempts are being made to identify good and poor risk factors for outcome of infection in order to facilitate shorter courses of antimicrobial agents.

Infections in neutropenic children

Comparison with adults

There are several large reviews of children with serious infections and neutropenia. The largest compared 759 children with 2321 adults admitted to four trials run by the European Organization for Research into the Treatment of Cancer (EORTC) International Antimicrobial Therapy Group (IATG).[1] This is the ideal way to look at patterns of infection and to determine whether risk factors predicting outcome can be identified. Children tended to have lower-risk disease with regard to outcome of infection compared with adults, despite common enrollment criteria within the EORTC centers, namely fever and neutropenia. Not surprisingly, the children had acute myeloid leukemia (AML) less frequently and acute lymphoblastic leukemia (ALL) more often, and proportionately more children were undergoing intensive therapy for solid tumors. The children had more upper

respiratory and fewer lower respiratory sites of infection. The incidence of bacteremia in these febrile neutropenic children was similar to that in the adults (22% vs. 24%), but pyrexia of unknown origin was more common in the younger patients (49% vs. 38% in adults) due to a lower incidence of clinically documented infections including pneumonias. The pattern of organisms causing bacteremia was also different, children experiencing more streptococcal species in blood cultures, whilst adults had more staphylococcal species. Most importantly, it was shown for the first time that the outcome in febrile neutropenic children was better, with an overall success rate for the initial empirical regimen of 66% versus 59% in adults. The mortality rate directly due to infection was only 1% in children compared with 4% in adults, and time to defervescence of temperature was shorter in the younger age group (median of 3 vs. 4 days).

Bone marrow transplant patients

One of the dramatic changes in practice over the last few years has been the introduction of unrelated donor or haploidentical allogeneic bone marrow transplants. Previously, such procedures were associated with an unacceptably high risk of rejection, graft-versus-host disease (GVHD) and infection. However, this picture has changed and a review from Minneapolis has looked at the pattern of late infection in these children.[2] The period after 7 weeks from the day of transplant was examined because the development of unrelated-donor bone marrow transplant (URD-BMT) has been associated with delayed infection problems, at least in part related to the prolonged immunosuppression (including high-dose steroids) and more frequent and severe GVHD. One hundred and fifty-one matched sibling donor (MSD) BMT procedures were compared with 98 URD-BMTs, of which 82 patients in the MSD group and 50 patients in the URD group were < 18 years of age. Of all the URD-BMT patients, 85% developed late infections compared with 68% in the MSD group. Two-thirds of infections occurred within the first 6 months and few after the first year, but URD-BMT patients were at risk for longer. About half of the infections were bacterial, evenly split between Gram-negative and Gram-positive organisms. Slightly more than one-third were viral and of these a third were due to cytomegalovirus (CMV), with the remainder due to herpes simplex (HSV), varicella zoster virus (VZV), respiratory syncytial virus (RSV) and influenza viruses. Eleven percent was due to fungi; in the URD-BMT group, half were due to *Candida* and a quarter to *Aspergillus*. About a third of these late infections were considered life-threatening, causing hypotension or requiring central venous pressure monitoring or mechanical ventilation. Blood and lungs were the commonest site of these life-threatening infections, occurring in 60% and 20% of cases respectively, and bacteria were implicated in nearly two-thirds of these infections, of which more than 80% were by Gram-negative organisms. A third of all late life-threatening bacterial infections were lethal. Life-threatening viral infections occurred in 13% of cases, and life-threatening fungal infections occurred in 24% of cases. In both groups there was an 80% mortality rate.

Children on antileukemic therapy

Deaths due to infection

A recent review of causes and risk factors for death in childhood ALL and AML unrelated to refractory leukemia, disease recurrence or second malignancy, between 1983 and 2002 within their own institution, was undertaken by the St Jude's Hospital researchers.[3] The estimated 10-year cumulative incidence of death was 2.9 ± 5.3% for ALL, and the estimated 5-year cumulative incidence of death was 7.6 ± 1.9% for patients with AML. For patients with ALL or AML, the incidence of death remained relatively constant during the time periods studied. Among 1011 patients in the ALL group, there were 36 deaths, of which 11 were due to infection during remission induction: eight fungal (five *Aspergillus* infections, two *Candida* infections and one other fungal infection), two viral (one patient had disseminated varicella and *Candida* infection) and one bacterial infection. There were 10 infection-related deaths during postremission chemotherapy, of which seven were due to proven or presumed bacterial sepsis: two *Pseudomonas*, two *E. coli* infections and three with septic shock with presumed bacterial infections. There were 23 infection-related deaths among the 260 children treated for AML, of which seven were at induction (six fungal infections – three *Aspergillus*, two *Candida* and one presumed fungal pneumonia – and one bacterial infection) and six were during postremission chemotherapy (all died due to fungal infections, of which five were due to *Aspergillus* and one due to presumed fungal pneumonia). Eighty percent of deaths in the ALL group were due to infections and nearly all non-leukemic deaths in AML were due to infections, the majority being due to *Aspergillus*.

Acute myeloid leukemia

Over the last decade, treatment for AML has become much more intensive and survival has dramatically improved. This has resulted in frequent infectious complications including overwhelming Gram-negative bacteremia and serious systemic fungal infections. A study conducted by the BFM group looks at the rate and nature of infections in children treated according to the AML-BFM-93 trial protocol,[4] and also serves as a good contemporary review of the problem. Overall, 855 infective episodes occurred in the 304 children studied, of which 61.2% (n = 523) episodes were classified as fever of unknown origin (FUO) and 32.1% (n = 275) had microbiologically documented infections. The remaining 6.7% of episodes were deemed to be infectious in origin on clinical grounds alone. Neutropenia was present in 74.1% of the episodes. Bloodstream infections occurred in 228 episodes, in which 252 isolates were identified (203 Gram-positive and 49 Gram-negative). Of the Gram-positive organisms isolated, the commonest was coagulase-negative *Staphylococcus* (80 episodes) followed by viridans group streptococci (VGS) (56 episodes). Infection with VGS was significantly higher during cycles of chemotherapy that included high dose cytarabine. Eighty percent of the bloodstream infections occurred when patients were neutropenic. Invasive fungal infections were probable or proven in 15 episodes, among which pulmonary aspergillosis was proven in five and suspected in five children, and invasive candidiasis was proven in two and suspected in three children. In 13.3% episodes (113 out of 855), pneumonia was diagnosed radiologically. Twenty patients died of infection-associated complications, most of them during early induction therapy (n = 11) giving an overall infection-related mortality of 6.6%. Children with Down syndrome were significantly overrepresented in this group (5/28 or 17.9% vs. 15/276 or 5.4%). Of the five children with Down syndrome, two had microbiologically proven pulmonary aspergillosis and one had an isolate of *Streptococcus pneumoniae* in the blood. Eighteen out of these 20 patients with fatal infections had radiologic signs of pneumonia; Gram-negative organisms (*Pseudomonas*) were isolated in five patients, Gram-positive in four (*Streptococcus*, *Enterococccus*, coagulase-negative *Staphylococcus*) and invasive aspergillosis was proven in four patients. Notably, six out of nine patients who died during consolidation had not achieved complete remission. It is important therefore to have a very low threshold for readmitting patients with AML, particularly with pulmonary symptoms, while maintaining a careful watch for invasive fungal infections.

Acute lymphoblastic leukemia

Children with ALL have a better prognosis overall and fewer serious infections than those with AML. However, it is all the more tragic when an eminently curable child dies of an infection induced principally by the antileukemic therapy. A review from the UK Acute Lymphoblastic Leukaemia (UKALL) trials run by the Medical Research Council[5] between 1985 and 1990, examined 1612 children who were entered into the UKALL X trial. Thirty-eight (2.3%) died during the first four induction weeks: 31 died from infections, of which 19 were due to bacteria, nine to fungi and three due to unknown infections. Gram-negative bacteria accounted for 12 cases, and seven were Gram-positive. Of the nine fungal infections, four involved *Aspergillus*, four were *Candida* and one was a *Mucor* infection. Thus, the message is that Gram-negative cover (which we believe should include an aminoglycoside as well as another agent; see below), as well as Gram-positive cover in a broad-spectrum empirical antibiotic regimen given immediately to these febrile neutropenic patients, remains essential. Also, the physician must remain wary of deep-seated fungal infections, especially *Aspergillus* affecting the lower and upper airways (including the paranasal sinuses, where it is frequently mistaken for viral or anerobic infections) and *Candida* involving the liver and spleen. The use of empirical amphotericin-based therapy must also be continued for patients who remain febrile after 3 or 4 days of broad-spectrum antibiotic therapy (see below).

Risk factors and prognostic factors with regard to outcome of infection

The UKALL X study showed clearly that children with Down syndrome and also girls with ALL are at increased risk of fatal infection. In addition, fatal infections occurred more frequently in patients with very high risk ALL receiving an allogeneic BMT in first remission.

There have been a number of other studies that have sought to predict who might be susceptible to serious infections and also, amongst those with fever, who will prove to have bacteremia.[6–8] The aim of these studies was to try to predict who can safely receive attenuated courses of antibiotics or even be treated at home or on experimental monotherapy antibiotic protocols. Apart from absolute neutropenia, the above studies identified other risk factors for bacteremia during febrile episodes, such as: the presence of hypotensive shock, C-reactive protein levels of > 90 mg/L, temperature > 39°C at the time of presentation, absolute monocytopenia of < 100/mm^3 and diagnosis of relapsed leukemia.

Based on the observed risk factors for bacteremia, Santolaya *et al.* from Santiago, Chile, conducted a trial of early hospital discharge followed by outpatient management versus continued hospitalization of children with cancer, fever and neutropenia who were deemed to be at low risk for invasive bacterial infection.[9] Low-risk children were randomly assigned after 24–36 hours of hospitalization to receive ambulatory or hospitalized treatment and monitored until the episode resolved. A total of 161 out of 390 febrile

neutropenic episodes were considered to be low risk, of which 149 were randomly assigned to ambulatory (*n* = 78) or hospital-based (*n* = 71) treatment. The outcome was favorable in 95% of ambulatory-treated patients and 94% of hospital-treated patients (*P* = NS). Of the eight patients with an unfavorable outcome (four in each group), seven children recovered completely with therapy modifications. One child died in intensive care with overwhelming *Pseudomonas* septicemia. No significant serious adverse effects of the drug treatments were reported. The mean cost of an episode was significantly lower in the ambulatory group (*P* = 0.003).

Patients with high temperature and persistent neutropenia and also those with hypovolemic shock are at highest risk of serious infection and these tend to be children with leukemia, especially those with AML, infants with ALL, other children receiving very intensive protocols for ALL and mature B-cell non-Hodgkin lymphoma, and following allogeneic BMT procedures.

Prophylaxis

Having defined the groups of patients who are susceptible to severe infection, it is of course logical to consider preventing such events. In fact this has proved to be a great deal more difficult than was ever envisaged. One of the overriding problems has been the difficulty of organizing large randomized trials. In this area, placebo-controlled and double-blind studies are undoubtedly the ideal because there is little evidence, with few exceptions, that anything works and the end points are open to observer prejudice, for example, the institution of therapeutic courses of antibiotics. In addition, it has not been possible to perform trials of prophylaxis with quinolone antibiotics, which are active in preventing Gram-negative infections in adults but which may carry a risk of arthropathy in children.[10]

Mouth care and oral nonabsorbable antibiotics

In real life, all mouth-care and oral nonabsorbable antibiotic (ONA) regimens are extremely difficult to manage in children. Although there have been many vogues for prevention of infection with ONA,[11,12] the regimens are often complex, usually very unpalatable and may cause diarrhea, and compliance is almost impossible without psychologic disturbance in children. It is therefore not surprising that evidence of the effectiveness of such regimens in preventing infection in young patients is lacking. With regard to mouth care, there is no doubt that this modality of therapy is important and certainly improves the tolerability of therapy,[11] although which mouthwashes should be used is unclear, with evidence that chlorhexidine causes discomfort, taste change and teeth staining.[12] Regular cleaning of teeth with soft toothbrushes that are changed every 2–3 weeks helps prevent systemic dissemination of oral pathogens.[13] Ideally, all patients should have regular dental checks in order to reduce the risk of infections, gum problems and mucositis. The use of fluconazole and aciclovir prophylaxis in high-risk (usually AML and BMT) patients has significantly improved this problem.

Fungal infections

The increasing use of unrelated BMT and severely myelotoxic chemotherapeutic agents in children has led to the inevitable rise in the prevalence of fungal infections, posing one of the greatest challenges of modern antileukemic therapies. The major issues in the management of fungal infections are prevention, diagnosis and treatment. Treatment of these infections is difficult, often involves unacceptable costs and toxicity and is frequently unsuccessful.

It is clear from several studies that not all patients undergoing chemotherapy require antifungal prophylaxis, and in one review, Prentice *et al.* have stratified the risk groups according to degree and duration of neutropenia, underlying disease and therapy used, use of corticosteroids and prior candidal colonization. The group most at risk are those with neutrophil counts of $< 0.1 \times 10^9/L$ for > 3 weeks or $< 0.5 \times 10^9/L$ for > 5 weeks, with chronic GVHD, undergoing unrelated or mismatched donor BMT, corticosteroid therapy of > 2 mg/kg for > 2 weeks, receiving high-dose cytarabine, or colonized by *Candida tropicalis*.[14]

The use of high-efficiency particulate air (HEPA) filter systems has undoubtedly reduced the risk of *Aspergillus* infection in high-risk patients.[15] Susceptible patients should be nursed in air-filtered rooms wherever possible, and avoid contact with spores from compost heaps and building sites, or food with a high spore content, such as pepper.

Three main oral drug prophylactic regimens have been tried. The original schedules contained frequent high-dose polyenes (nystatin and oral amphotericin) and these are still widely used, although the evidence for their efficacy is limited and they are often not well tolerated by children. A large multicenter trial in 502 children showed that once-daily oral fluconazole prophylaxis resulted in a significant reduction in invasive fungal infection: there were 2.1% in the fluconazole arm compared with 8.4% in the polyenes ($P = 0.002$).[16] This drug is palatable, and the once-daily usage is a major bonus; however, it should only be used in patients with a high risk of *Candida* infection, because of the danger of emergence of resistant species, e.g., *Candida cruzei*, and *Candida glabrata*, and because it will probably not prevent infection with other fungi such as *Aspergillus*. Another imidazole, itraconazole, may have greater efficacy in also preventing *Aspergillus* infections and has been recently investigated in a nonrandom open-labelled study of 103 children mainly undergoing allogeneic BMT. Although around 50% of the children did not complete their course of prophylaxis due to poor compliance or adverse effects, no proven systemic fungal infection occurred and about a quarter received intravenous amphotericin

due to antibiotic-resistant fevers.[17] Thus, this drug may be useful in very high-risk patients where compliance can be guaranteed via the nasogastric or intravenous route. However, it is hoped that the newer azoles such as voriconazole and the echinocandins may be more effective when tested in double-blind, placebo-controlled randomized trials.

Pneumocystis carinii infection

It has been known for 20 years that this infection can be prevented by co-trimoxazole prophylaxis.[18] What has been more uncertain is whether this antibiotic can prevent other infections.[19] In general, the prophylactic effect against bacterial infections is at best a weak one and thus co-trimoxazole is now used almost exclusively to prevent *Pneumocystis* infection. Reactions to it are very uncommon and other antibiotics and maneuvers, such as the use of inhaled pentamidine and oral dapsone, have a much shorter track record and may be more toxic and less effective. Patients at highest risk of *Pneumocystis* pneumonia are those undergoing allogeneic BMT, infants receiving intensive protocols for ALL, and other patients following induction therapy for ALL. Pentamidine inhalations and dapsone are usually reserved for children who do not tolerate co-trimoxazole and who are at continuing risk post-BMT or whilst receiving chemotherapy.

Antiviral prophylaxis

The most important preventive measure against viral infection is vaccination. Where vaccines are live or live-attenuated as with measles, the conventional policy is to rely upon herd immunity and vaccination of siblings and other child contacts. There is a continuing controversy over the prevention of VZV infections, which rarely cause fatal illnesses now that intravenous aciclovir can cure most infections and prompt use of zoster immune globulin (ZIG) following contact can prevent most serious episodes. However, the risk of infection is still quite high, with an approximate risk of 4.6 per 100 patient-years in children undergoing continuation therapy for ALL.[20] A recent report of a two-dose regime of live attenuated varicella zoster vaccine given to 17 children either on maintenance therapy for ALL or 3–6 months after the end of treatment for solid tumor found that 94% achieved seroconversion, one patient suffered from a mild self-limiting varicella-induced hepatitis, and no children suffered from herpes zoster at 27 months follow-up.[21] Often, the problem with vaccination is that the chemotherapy treatment schedule has to be interrupted for several weeks and mild skin reactions are relatively common. Currently, this is an unresolved issue, although cost–benefit analysis indicates that vaccination is likely to be safe and to reduce the need for painful intramuscular ZIG injections.

Several studies have shown that herpes simplex infections can be prevented in patients undergoing BMT procedures and treatment for leukemia.[22] As a consequence, most BMT patients are given oral aciclovir prophylaxis during the period of neutropenia. Longer periods of prophylaxis for a number of months may prevent some VZV infections but the risk period is long and there is clearly a problem with diminishing returns. In childhood, herpes simplex infections are uncommon other than in BMT patients, and it is usually not considered justified to use aciclovir prophylactically when there will be a long period of relatively low risk and thus the possibility of allowing the development of resistant viral strains.

CMV infection remains a significant cause of transplant-related mortality in high-risk children and preemptive treatment based on surveillance using a real-time polymerase chain reaction (PCR)-based assay or an antigenemia assay using the pp65 antigen is the mainstay of the current anti-CMV strategies.[23] Although aciclovir is usually ineffective in preventing CMV infections, there has been recent interest in the oral agent valaciclovir for CMV prophylaxis; this has been shown to be as effective and less toxic than standard prophylaxis using intravenous ganciclovir.[24,25]

Indwelling venous catheter sepsis

It is always assumed, although rarely proven, that many infections occurring in the modern era are caused or exacerbated by the now ubiquitous indwelling intravenous catheters. Thus, it would be good to prevent such infections. It is often forgotten that by far the most important means of preventing infection in any situation is by very careful handwashing. This is particularly true when handling intravenous catheters, and it is everyone's experience that problems with infection increase when there is inadequate or overpressurized nursing. The value of continuous staff and family education regarding aseptic techniques in handling catheters was shown serendipitously in a well-designed trial.[26] Children with central venous catheters were entered into a placebo-controlled double-blind study of adding broad-spectrum antibiotics to the flush solution. By doing the trial, as is often the case, the authors heightened awareness of the problem and reduced the incidence of infection to a level that made it impossible to assess the effectiveness or otherwise of the antibiotic flush. Their conclusion is to be commended: "staff education is essential and probably the most effective factor in preventing catheter-related sepsis." It should be added that educating the parents is just as important. A recent randomized prospective study compared the rate of catheter-related infections in patients with malignancies using a minocycline-rifampicin-impregnated silicone catheter versus conventional catheters and found a significant reduction of infections ($P = 0.003$) using the former, with no reported incidence of allergic reactions to the antibiotic-impregnated catheters.[27] This interesting development in the prevention of catheter-associated sepsis needs further evaluation.

Planned progressive antimicrobial therapy

Antibiotics

Over the last 25 years since early empirical antibiotic therapy first came into routine practice, there have been a multitude of attempts to modify protocols.[28] When choosing which antibiotic combination to use empirically for fever and neutropenia, it is absolutely essential to know about the local flora and fauna. Close liaison with microbiologists and infectious disease specialists is never more important than when making these decisions. One major consideration, for example, would be the existence of multiresistant organisms within an individual institution. Thus, the recommendations below must *not* be regarded as being cast in stone; they must be regularly reviewed and should be adapted to local circumstances. It is not the only possible approach but is based on the larger available studies (Fig. 34.1).

The principle involved is that the regimen must have excellent Gram-negative cover and efficacy, with a broad spectrum of cover against other organisms. A large number of studies have proven the efficacy of piperacillin–tazobactam along with an aminoglycoside (amikacin), including one involving 858 febrile episodes in neutropenic patients.[29] The EORTC IATG trials have led the way in large multicenter trials whereby the number of patient entries meets statistical criteria for meaningful end points. Several important advances were made with this approach, including the demonstration that single daily dosing of an aminoglycoside (amikacin given with ceftriaxone in this trial)[30] was as effective as multiple daily dosing of an aminoglycoside (with ceftazidime). This was subsequently reproduced in many other trials.[31,32] The conclusion of all these studies has been that once-daily aminoglycosides have a lower risk of nephrotoxicity, probably equivalent risk of ototoxicity and equivalent or possibly superior efficacy. There has not been a vast published experience in children, but where this has been examined, the above statements hold up.[33]

The EORTC IATG investigated the possibility of dropping the aminoglycoside after 3 days in combination with ceftazidime.[34] This approach was adopted as a "halfway house" because of the potential damage of single-agent therapy in high-risk neutropenic patients. Although this study concluded that it would be detrimental to discontinue the aminoglycoside early, there has been a great amount of recent interest in monotherapy in febrile neutropenia, and several studies using carbapenems (meropenem) or fourth-generation cephalosporins (cefipime, not available in the UK) show no striking differences between monotherapy and multidrug combinations.[35–37] The Infectious Diseases Society of America has recently published guidelines[38] for the use of antimicrobial agents in febrile neutropenic patients with cancer, but the reader is referred to Fig. 34.1 for the current practice in the UK in pediatric patients.

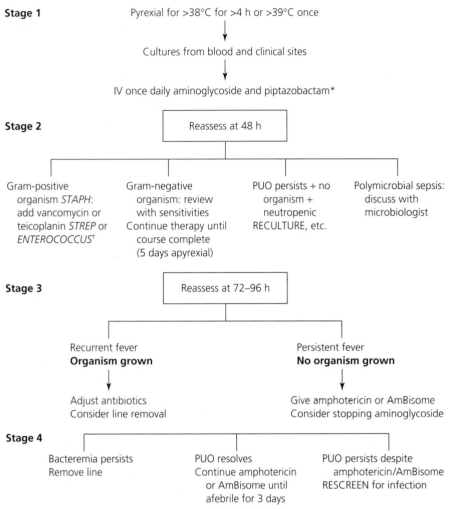

Stage 1

Pyrexial for >38°C for >4 h or >39°C once

↓

Cultures from blood and clinical sites

↓

IV once daily aminoglycoside and piptazobactam*

Stage 2

Reassess at 48 h

Gram-positive organism *STAPH*: add vancomycin or teicoplanin *STREP* or *ENTEROCOCCUS*†

Gram-negative organism: review with sensitivities Continue therapy until course complete (5 days apyrexial)

PUO persists + no organism + neutropenic RECULTURE, etc.

Polymicrobial sepsis: discuss with microbiologist

Stage 3

Reassess at 72–96 h

Recurrent fever **Organism grown**

Persistent fever **No organism grown**

Adjust antibiotics Consider line removal

Give amphotericin or AmBisome Consider stopping aminoglycoside

Stage 4

Bacteremia persists Remove line

PUO resolves Continue amphotericin or AmBisome until afebrile for 3 days

PUO persists despite amphotericin/AmBisome RESCREEN for infection

* If given i.v. piptazobactam within previous 2 weeks give ceftazidime and aminoglycoside. If ceftazidime-resistant organisms or ceftazidime within previous 2 weeks, give ciprofloxacin and aminoglycoside first.

† If on piptazobactam and aminoglycoside, review with sensitivities. If on ceftazidime or ciprofloxacin + aminoglycoside, add vancomycin or teicoplanin as in *Staph*. regimen.

Fig. 34.1 Planned progressive approach to infection in severely neutropenic children. PUO, pyrexia of unknown origin; i.v., intravenous.

The proposed planned progressive approach to therapy suggested in Fig. 34.1 contains a number of other features. An assessment on day 2 or 3 is valuable because this is the stage at which blood culture results become available. If Gram-positive organisms are grown and the patient is responding, it is reasonable to continue with the empirical regimen because in the EORTC studies such a policy was associated with a good outcome. However, the addition of vancomycin or teicoplanin in the presence of a microbiologically proven Gram-positive infection is an alternative approach. This does not mean that all patients with an inflamed central venous catheter exit site should be treated with an additional Gram-positive agent because there is only a poor correlation between this frequent clinical finding and the existence of serious Gram-positive infections; morover, extensive use of vancomycin in the empirical setting can lead to the rise of vancomycin-resistant organisms.[38]

If the patient is afebrile within 3–5 days of treatment, broad-spectrum antibiotics should be continued until the patient is afebrile for at least 5 days. If fever persists beyond 96 hours and no causative organism has been identified, empirical antifungal treatment with amphotericin is recommended (see below) and the patient needs to be reassessed and rescreened for infection, including further blood cultures and radiologic investigations.

Management of unresponsive fever and antifungal therapy

Children with persistent severe neutropenia frequently do

not respond to a wide variety of antimicrobial agents. It must, however, be remembered that the mortality in this situation is very low and defervescence often occurs only when the blood counts begin to recover and probably irrespective of what therapy is given. Thus, a panic-stricken approach to the problem is entirely unjustified, especially when it involves multiple agents that are potentially toxic, inefficacious and antagonistic. For example, the use of metronidazole should be reserved for high-risk situations, for example children with serious perineal problems or gastrointestinal fistulas, because anerobic infections are otherwise very rare in this situation. There is no justification for using this drug for every patient with diarrhea, sinusitis (where fungal infection is thus often consequently forgotten about) or oral mucositis. The most important point is regularly to repeat blood cultures and to look carefully for specific infections from a clinical standpoint. Another main strategy is to seek disseminated candidiasis in patients with splenomegaly (abdominal sonography) and aspergillosis in patients with rhinosinusitis (computed tomography, CT, of sinuses) and in those with suggestive clinical symptoms such as pleuritic pain or cough or with persistent pyrexia of unknown origin (PUO) or clinical deterioration (high-resolution chest CT).

Empirical antifungal therapy in antibiotic-resistant fevers in patients with malignancies and neutropenia has dramatically improved outcomes in a large number of patients, making it possible for many to undergo successful antineoplastic therapy.[39] Due to difficulties in diagnosis of fungal infection in patients with neutropenia, empirical antifungal therapy has now become the accepted clinical practice.[40] There have been a large number of recent additions to the antifungal armamentarium other than conventional amphotericin B, and these agents (liposomal amphotericin B, voriconazole and, more recently, caspofungin) have all been studied in the setting of empirical therapy in antibiotic-resistant fevers.[41–43] Currently available evidence suggests that both voriconazole and caspofungin are suitable alternatives to liposomal amphotericin B in the empirical treatment of antibiotic-resistant fevers in neutropenic patients, but further evaluation in terms of costs and clinical effectiveness along with evaluation of these agents in the pediatric population are needed. At present, AmBisome is the only drug licenced for empirical therapy in children.

With the emergence of new antifungal drugs, it is important to avoid overtreatment of persistent fevers with these significantly more expensive agents. One way to achieve this would be to improve laboratory diagnosis of invasive fungal infections, and current techniques such as the ELISA-based galactomannan assay and PCR assay for detection of invasive aspergillosis are being evaluated. The PCR-based technique on blood samples has been shown to carry a sensitivity of 63.6% and a specificity of 63.5% whereas the galactomannan assay although showing an impressive specificity of 98.9%, is only sensitive in 33.3% of cases.[44] When used on CT-based bronchoalveolar lavage fluid, the galactomannan assay showed a 100% sensitivity and specificity in diagnosing invasive pulmonary aspergillosis.[45] There is still a need to improve these tests to a level where they are as useful as they are in detecting cytomegalovirus infections because early presumptive therapy is crucial in treating such infections.

The role of secondary prophylaxis in patients undergoing high-risk procedures has been evaluated in a retrospective study using voriconazole with good results.[46] This, along with the use of granulocytes from granulocyte colony-stimulating factor (G-CSF)-stimulated donors[47] in patients with previous proven invasive fungal infection undergoing myeloablative chemotherapy or bone marrow transplants, need further evaluation.

The use of monocyte–macrophage growth factors to treat fungal infection is addressed below.

Viral infections and interstitial pneumonia

Most viral infections occur at times when patients are not neutropenic and thus this subject is not dealt with in great detail here. The only very effective antiviral agent is aciclovir, which is an active agent for herpes simplex and VZV infections. There is no really effective treatment for measles pneumonia or encephalitis, although various drugs such as interferons and ribavirin have been tried, along with intravenous immunoglobulin. More recently, adenovirus has emerged as a serious pathogen in immunocompromised patients such as those undergoing mismatched or unrelated BMT.[48] Children appear to be at greater risk of acquiring adenoviral infections in the BMT setting, and up to 27% of children[49] and 19.7% of adults[50] have been prospectively shown to acquire adenoviral infection 30–90 days post-BMT. Although cidofovir and ribavarin have been used to treat adenovirus infection, they have mostly proved to be unsuccessful in established disease. In the absence of an effective antiviral agent against adenoviral disease, attempts have been made to improve surveillance techniques by quantitative PCR assays, and to develop cellular therapies such as those using donor-derived adenovirus-specific cytotoxic T lymphocytes or using donor lymphocyte infusion and withdrawing immunosuppression upon detection of adenoviral infection on surveillance.[48]

CMV infection does occasionally occur in neutropenic children, sometimes with hepatitis or gastroenteric problems, but usually with an interstitial pneumonia (Fig. 34.2). The management of pneumonia is tricky and there is again a temptation to indulge in polypharmacy. Figure 34.2 provides a suggested plan of action, and there are some additional points worth emphasizing. First, it is most important to institute a thorough diagnostic search at an early stage. Secondly, with the proposed approach, it is now very rarely necessary to proceed to lung biopsy with the attendant risk of bleeding, pneumothorax, etc., because the patients usually respond

CAUSES
- *Pneumocystis carinii*
- Cytomegalovirus
- Measles (usually no preceding rash)
- Varicella zoster (rare)
- Fungal infections
- Mycoplasma, *Legionella*
- Common respiratory viruses: influenza, parainfluenza, adenovirus, RSV

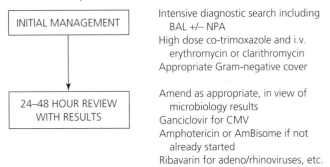

INITIAL MANAGEMENT

Intensive diagnostic search including BAL +/– NPA
High dose co-trimoxazole and i.v. erythromycin or clarithromycin
Appropriate Gram-negative cover

24–48 HOUR REVIEW WITH RESULTS

Amend as appropriate, in view of microbiology results
Ganciclovir for CMV
Amphotericin or AmBisome if not already started
Ribavarin for adeno/rhinoviruses, etc.
Consider lung biopsy

Fig. 34.2 Management plan for interstitial pneumonia.
BAL, bronchoalveolar lavage; NPA, nasopharyngeal aspirate; CMV, cytomegalovirus; RSV, respiratory syncytial virus.

to therapy or there is an answer from less invasive tests. Finally, *Pneumocystis carinii* pneumonia will often respond to high doses of co-trimoxazole with or without pentamidine. Nonresponders usually respond to steroid therapy; if not, moribund patients have been rescued by surfactant therapy.

Hematopoietic growth factors

Very few good clinical studies have been carried out with these new agents, and these have been reviewed.[51] It can be said that G-CSF reduces the duration of neutropenia and probably leads to a reduced number of febrile days and fewer days receiving antibiotics in adults and children undergoing BMT for nonmyeloid disorders. Their safety in children with myeloid disorders (i.e., mainly AML) is largely unproven, unlike in adults where several large, double-blind, placebo-controlled trials have shown that the use of G-CSF in adults postremission induction did not affect the overall and disease-free survival from AML but significantly improved neutrophil recovery, duration of fever, reduced parenteral antibiotic use and hospitalization.[52] A recent meta-analysis looked at 16 studies involving 1183 children,[53] and concluded that colony-stimulating factors (CSFs) in children with cancer, including those undergoing high-risk ALL protocols and solid tumors, reduced the rate of febrile neutropenia by 20% and decreased the duration of hospitalization by about 2 days. Prophylactic CSFs reduced the documented infection rates by 22% and amphotericin use by 50%. However, CSFs were not associated with a reduction in infection-related mortality. A number of trials are underway, and currently it is probably reasonable to reserve G-CSF therapy for patients

with an expected incidence of febrile neutropenia of > 40%[54] or those who would previously have been given granulocyte-rich transfusions. The latter have been abandoned in most centers because of their dubious efficacy, infection transmission risk and the associated severe logistic difficulties, apart from the rare situation of localizing infections not responding to antibiotics.

There is some evidence that macrophage CSF (M-CSF) may assist the response of severe systemic fungal infection to amphotericin.[55–57] This may be useful prophylactically or in patients who have failed to respond to amphotericin and its lipid formulations. This activity could be related to augmentation of the antifungal activity of monocytes, macrophages and neutrophils exposed to M-CSF and granulocyte–macrophage CSF (GM-CSF). In view of the life-threatening nature of these infections, this is a potentially important development and it is to be hoped that randomized trials in patients with systemic infections will be completed shortly.

Future developments

It is hoped that pharmaceutical companies will devise an answer to vancomycin-resistant enterococci because the macrolide antibiotics represent the last line of defense against methicillin-resistant *Staphylococcus aureus* and β-lactam-resistant enterococci.[58] It is probably only a matter of time before these defenses are more seriously breached. In fact, the main defense line is the human mucosal barrier, and the possibility of effective protective agents is at last on the horizon with the production of keratinocyte-derived growth factors. The ensuing years will hopefully see the completion of trials looking at a variety of "networked" cytokines, including mucosal protective agents, G-CSF and GM-CSF, and thrombopoietins. The biggest current challenge is the detection, prevention and treatment of fungal infections. We need even better agents and good randomized trials of prophylaxis and combination therapies in, for example, *Aspergillus* pneumonia and brain infection. Also coming to the horizon is the problem of adenovirus in the BMT setting, especially in the mismatched and unrelated BMTs, along with the need for quick, sensitive and effective methods of detection of the virus and development of effective therapies such as adoptive imunotherapies or development of newer viral agents. It should be an exciting era.

Conclusions

Clinicians can be forgiven for looking askance at the apparent cornucopia of antimicrobial agents that has been produced over recent years. What are the best agents, when should they be used, and why do they still fail? The fact is that there is still a lot to learn and there is a desperate need for better agents, including immunomodulatory agents, for example to prevent the development of invasive fungal infections. The suggestions made above for a planned progressive approach to the management of infections is an attempt to adopt a rational, calm and hopefully scientific approach to the problem.

References

1. Hann I, Viscoli C, Paesmans M, Gaya H, Glauser M. A comparison of outcome from febrile neutropenic episodes in children compared with adults: results from four EORTC studies. International Antimicrobial Therapy Cooperative Group (IATCG) of the European Organization for Research and Treatment of Cancer (EORTC). *Br J Haematol* 1997; **99**: 580–8.

2. Ochs L, Shu XO, Miller J *et al.* Late infections after allogeneic bone marrow transplantations: comparison of incidence in related and unrelated donor transplant recipients. *Blood* 1995; **86**: 3979–86.

3. Rubnitz JE, Lensing S, Zhou Y *et al.* Death during induction therapy and first remission of acute leukemia in childhood: the St. Jude experience. *Cancer* 2004; **101**: 1677–84.

4. Lehrnbecher T, Varwig D, Kaiser J, Reinhardt D, Klingebiel T, Creutzig U. Infectious complications in pediatric acute myeloid leukemia: analysis of the prospective multi-institutional clinical trial AML-BFM 93. *Leukemia* 2004; **18**: 72–7.

5. Wheeler K, Chessells JM, Bailey CC, Richards SM. Treatment related deaths during induction and in first remission in acute lymphoblastic leukaemia: MRC UKALL X. *Arch Dis Child* 1996; **74**: 101–7.

6. Santolaya ME, Alvarez AM, Becker A *et al.* Prospective, multicenter evaluation of risk factors associated with invasive bacterial infection in children with cancer, neutropenia, and fever. *J Clin Oncol* 2001; **19**: 3415–21.

7. Rackoff WR, Gonin R, Robinson C, Kreissman SG, Breitfeld PB. Predicting the risk of bacteremia in childen with fever and neutropenia. *J Clin Oncol* 1996; **14**: 919–24.

8. Lucas KG, Brown AE, Armstrong D, Chapman D, Heller G. The identification of febrile, neutropenic children with neoplastic disease at low risk for bacteremia and complications of sepsis. *Cancer* 1996; **77**: 791–8.

9. Santolaya ME, Alvarez AM, Aviles CL *et al.* Early hospital discharge followed by outpatient management versus continued hospitalization of children with cancer, fever, and neutropenia at low risk for invasive bacterial infection. *J Clin Oncol* 2004; **22**: 3784–9.

10. Alfaham M, Holt ME, Goodchild MC. Arthropathy in a patient with cystic fibrosis taking ciprofloxacin. *Br Med J* 1987; **295**: 699.

11. Carl W. Oral complications of local and systemic cancer treatment. *Curr Opin Oncol* 1995; **7**: 320–4.

12. Foote RL, Loprinzi CL, Frank AR *et al.* Randomized trial of a chlorhexidine mouthwash for alleviation of radiation-induced mucositis. *J Clin Oncol* 1994; **12**: 2630–3.

13. Kennedy HF, Morrison D, Tomlinson D, Gibson BE, Bagg J, Gemmell CG. Gingivitis and toothbrushes: potential roles in viridans streptococcal bacteraemia. *J Infect* 2003; **46**: 67–70.

14. Prentice HG, Kibbler CC, Prentice AG. Towards a targeted, risk-based, antifungal strategy in neutropenic patients. *Br J Haematol* 2000; **110**: 273–84.

15. O'Donnell MR, Schmidt GM, Tegtmeier BR *et al.* Prediction of systemic fungal infection in allogeneic marrow recipients: impact of amphotericin prophylaxis in high-risk patients. *J Clin Oncol* 1994; **12**: 827–34.

16. Ninane J. A multicentre study of fluconazole versus oral polyenes in the prevention of fungal infection in children with hematological or oncological malignancies. Multicentre Study Group. *Eur J Clin Microbiol Infect Dis* 1994; **13**: 330–7.

17. Foot AB, Veys PA, Gibson BE. Itraconazole oral solution as antifungal prophylaxis in children undergoing stem cell transplantation or intensive chemotherapy for haematological disorders. *Bone Marrow Transplant* 1999; **24**: 1089–93.

18. Hughes WT. Treatment and prophylaxis for *Pneumocystis carinii* pneumonia. *Parasitol Today* 1987; **3**: 332–5.

19. EORTC International Antimicrobial Therapy Project Group. Trimethoprim-sulfamethoxazole in the prevention of infection in neutropenic patients. *J Infect Dis* 1984; **150**: 372–9.

20. Buda K, Tubergen DG, Levin MJ. The frequency and consequences of varicella exposure and varicella infection in children receiving maintenance therapy for acute lymphoblastic leukemia. *J Pediatr Hematol Oncol* 1996; **18**: 106–12.

21. Leung TF, Li CK, Hung EC *et al.* Immunogenicity of a two-dose regime of varicella vaccine in children with cancers. *Eur J Haematol* 2004; **72**: 353–7.

22. Hann IM, Prentice HG, Blacklock HA *et al.* Acyclovir prophylaxis against herpes virus infections in severely immunocompromised patients: randomised double blind trial. *Br Med J* 1983; **287**: 384–8.

23. Leruez-ille M, Ouachee M, Delarue R *et al.* Monitoring cytomegalovirus infection in adult and pediatric bone marrow transplant recipients by a real-time PCR assay performed with blood plasma. *J Clin Microbiol* 2003; **41**: 2040–6.

24. Winston DJ, Yeager AM, Chandrasekar PH, Snydman DR, Petersen FB, Territo MC. Randomized comparison of oral valacyclovir and intravenous ganciclovir for prevention of cytomegalovirus disease after allogeneic bone marrow transplantation. *Clin Infect Dis* 2003; **36**: 749–58.

25. Ljungman P, de la Camera R, Milpied N *et al.* Randomized study of valacyclovir as prophylaxis against cytomegalovirus reactivation in recipients of allogeneic bone marrow transplants. *Blood* 2002; **99**: 3050–6.

26. Daghistani D, Horn M, Rodriguez Z, Schoenike S, Toledano S. Prevention of indwelling central venous catheter sepsis. *Med Pediatr Oncol* 1996; **26**: 405–8.

27. Hanna H, Benjamin R, Chatzinikolaou I *et al.* Long-term silicone central venous catheters impregnated with minocycline and rifampin decrease rates of catheter-related bloodstream infection in cancer patients: a prospective randomized clinical trial. *J Clin Oncol* 2004; **22**: 3163–71.

28. Gaya H, Fenelon LE. Planned progressive therapy: logical sequence of management of infection in the neutropenic patient. In: Jenkins JT, Williams JD (eds) *Infection and Haematology*. Oxford: Butterworth-Heinemann, 1994, pp. 145–63.

29. Cometta A, Zinner S, de Bock R *et al.* Piperacillin-tazobactam plus amikacin versus ceftazidime plus amikacin as empiric therapy for fever in granulocytopenic patients with cancer. The International Antimicrobial Therapy Cooperative Group of the European Organization for Research and Treatment of Cancer. *Antimicrob Agents Chemother* 1995; **39**: 445–52.

30. International Antimicrobial Therapy Cooperative Group of the European Organization for Research and Treatment of Cancer. Efficacy and toxicity of single daily doses of amikacin and ceftriaxone versus multiple daily doses of amikacin and ceftazidime for infection in patients with cancer and granulocytopenia. *Ann Intern Med* 1993; **119**: 584–93.

31. Hatala R, Dinh T, Cook DJ. Once-daily aminoglycoside dosing in immunocompetent adults: a meta-analysis. *Ann Intern Med* 1996; **124**: 717–25.

32. Barza M, Ioannidis JP, Cappelleri JC, Lau J. Single or multiple daily doses of aminoglycosides: a meta-analysis. *Br Med J* 1996; **312**: 338–45.

33. Viscoli C, Dudley M, Ferrea G *et al.* Serum concentrations and safety of single daily dosing of amikacin in children undergoing bone marrow transplantation. *J Antimicrob Chemother* 1991; **27** (suppl. C): 113–20.

34. EORTC International Antimicrobial Therapy Cooperative Group. Ceftazidime combined with a short or long course of amikacin for empirical therapy of gram-negative bacteremia in cancer patients with granulocytopenia. *N Engl J Med* 1987; **317**: 1692–8.

35. Meropenem Study Group of Leuven, London and Nijmegen. Equivalent efficacies of meropenem and ceftazidime as empirical monotherapy of febrile neutropenic patients. *J Antimicrob Chemother* 1995; **36**: 185–200.

36. Behre G, Link H, Maschmeyer G *et al.* Meropenem monotherapy versus combination therapy with ceftazidime and amikacin for empirical treatment of febrile neutropenic patients. *Ann Hematol* 1998; **76**: 73–80.

37. Bohme A, Shah PM, Stille W, Hoelzer D. Piperacillin/tazobactam versus cefepime as initial empirical antimicrobial therapy in febrile neutropenic patients: a prospective randomized pilot study. *Eur J Med Res* 1998; **3**: 324–30.

38. Hughes WT, Armstrong D, Bodey GP *et al.* 2002 guidelines for the use of antimicrobial agents in neutropenic patients with cancer. *Clin Infect Dis* 2002; **34**: 730–51.

39. Klastersky J. Antifungal therapy in patients with fever and neutropenia: more rational and less empirical? *N Engl J Med* 2004; **351**: 1445–7.

40. EORTC International Antimicrobial Therapy Cooperative Group. Empiric antifungal therapy in febrile granulocytopenic patients. *Am J Med* 1989; **86**: 668–72.

41. Walsh TJ, Teppler H, Donowitz GR *et al.* Caspofungin versus liposomal amphotericin B for empirical antifungal therapy in patients with persistent fever and neutropenia. *N Engl J Med* 2004; **351**: 1391–402.

42. Walsh TJ, Pappas P, Winston DJ *et al.* Voriconazole compared with liposomal amphotericin B for empirical antifungal therapy in patients with neutropenia and persistent fever. *N Engl J Med* 2002; **346**: 225–34.

43. Walsh TJ, Finberg RW, Arndt C *et al.* Liposomal amphotericin B for empirical therapy in patients with persistent fever and neutropenia. National Institute of Allergy and Infectious Diseases Mycoses Study Group. *N Engl J Med* 1999; **340**: 764–71.

44. Buchheidt D, Hummel M, Schleiermacher D *et al.* Prospective clinical evaluation of a LightCycler-mediated polymerase chain reaction assay, a nested-PCR assay and a galactomannan enzyme-linked immunosorbent assay for detection of invasive aspergillosis in neutropenic cancer patients and haematological stem cell transplant recipients. *Br J Haematol* 2004; **125**: 196–202.

45. Becker MJ, Lugtenburg EJ, Cornelissen JJ, Van Der SC, Hoogsteden HC, de Marie S. Galactomannan detection in computerized tomography-based broncho-alveolar lavage fluid and serum in haematological patients at risk for invasive pulmonary aspergillosis. *Br J Haematol* 2003; **121**: 448–57.

46. Cordonnier C, Maury S, Pautas C *et al.* Secondary antifungal prophylaxis with voriconazole to adhere to scheduled treatment in leukemic patients and stem cell transplant recipients. *Bone Marrow Transplant* 2004; **33**: 943–8.

47. Cesaro S, Chinello P, De Silvestro G *et al.* Granulocyte transfusions from G-CSF-stimulated donors for the treatment of severe infections in neutropenic pediatric patients with onco-hematological diseases. *Support Care Cancer* 2003; **11**: 101–6.

48. Leen AM, Rooney CM. Adenovirus as an emerging pathogen in immunocompromised patients. *Br J Haematol* 2005; **128**: 135–44.

49. Lion T, Baumgartinger R, Watzinger F *et al.* Molecular monitoring of adenovirus in peripheral blood after allogeneic bone marrow transplantation permits early diagnosis of disseminated disease. *Blood* 2003; **102**: 1114–20.

50. Chakrabarti S, Mautner V, Osman H *et al.* Adenovirus infections following allogeneic stem cell transplantation: incidence and outcome in relation to graft manipulation, immunosuppression, and immune recovery. *Blood* 2002; **100**: 1619–27.

51. Hann IM. Haemopoietic growth factors and childhood cancer. *Eur J Cancer* 1995; **31A**: 1476–8.

52. Heil G, Hoelzer D, Sanz MA *et al.* A randomised, double-blind, placebo controlled, phase III study of filgrastim in remission induction and consolidation therapy for adults with de novo acute myeloid leukemia. The International Acute Myeloid Leukemia Study Group. *Blood* 1997; **90**: 4710–18.

53. Sung L, Nathan PC, Lange B, Beyene J, Buchanan GR. Prophylactic granulocyte colony-stimulating factor and granulocyte–macrophage colony-stimulating factor decrease febrile neutropenia after chemotherapy in children with cancer: a meta-analysis of randomized controlled trials. *J Clin Oncol* 2004; **22**: 3350–6.

54. Lehrnbecher T, Welte K. Haematopoietic growth factors in children with neutropenia. *Br J Haematol* 2002; **116**: 28–56.

55. Roilides E, Sein T, Holmes A *et al.* Effects of macrophage colony-stimulating factor on antifungal activity of mononuclear phagocytes against *Aspergillus fumigatus*. *J Infect Dis* 1995; **172**: 1028–34.

56. Capetti A, Bonfanti P, Magni C, Milazzo F. Employment of recombinant human granulocyte–macrophage colony stimulating factor in oesophageal candidiasis in AIDS patients. *AIDS* 1995; **9**: 1378–9.

57. Peters BG, Adkins DR, Harrison BR *et al.* Antifungal effects of yeast-derived rhu-GM-CSF in patients receiving high-dose chemotherapy given with or without autologous stem cell transplantation: a retrospective analysis. *Bone Marrow Transplant* 1996; **18**: 93–102.

58. Rowe PM. Preparing for battle against vancomycin resistance. *Lancet* 1996; **347**: 252.

Secondary Problems

35 Hematologic effects of systemic disease and nonhematopoietic tumors

Angela Thomas

Introduction

Systemic disease can have both obvious and subtle effects on blood and bone marrow. Sometimes the clinician will be alerted to the disease because of these effects, whereas on other occasions the underlying disorder is known and the specific hematologic effects or complications are sought. Several different pathologic processes can contribute to the final picture, and drugs used to treat the conditions may also have predictable or idiosyncratic effects. Nonhematopoietic tumors are accompanied by an enormous range of hematologic abnormalities affecting peripheral blood and bone marrow; some are directly caused by the presence of a tumor within the tissue, some are secondary to the effects of the tumor, and others arise as a result of treatment. A pediatric hematologist has an important role in providing diagnostic help and support in the investigation and management of children with hematologic problems secondary to other disorders. Many of the conditions are covered in other chapters: disturbances of hemostasis are described in Chapter 29, and storage disorders are described in Chapter 36. The remaining disorders will be described either by the blood picture that they present, or the disease that they accompany depending on the likelihood of presentation.

Anemia of chronic disease

Anemia is the commonest hematologic manifestation of systemic disease and is the result of a number of contributing factors. It occurs in patients with a variety of chronic inflammatory and malignant conditions and can be complicated by bleeding, immune phenomena, nutritional deficiencies and other organ- or disease-specific features. Chronic inflammatory conditions may result from chronic infection such as tuberculosis or osteomyelitis or be secondary to connective tissue disorders such as systemic lupus erythematosus (SLE),

or chronic inflammatory bowel disease. Characteristically the red cells are normocytic and normochromic or mildly hypochromic and red-cell morphology is unremarkable; the reticulocyte count is normal or low. The anemia is usually mild, 2–3 g/dL below the lower normal limit for a given individual, and nonprogressive with the severity being related to the severity of the disease process. Serum iron, iron-binding capacity and transferrin saturation are reduced and serum ferritin is normal or raised. If a bone marrow aspirate has been performed, stainable reticuloendothelial iron is seen in the particles but with reduced numbers of sideroblasts reflecting defective incorporation of iron into hemoglobin. With prolonged severe inflammation or infection, the anemia becomes more marked and a microcytic, hypochromic picture can result. Associated features indicative of chronic inflammation such as neutrophilia, thrombocytosis and rouleaux formation may be present. In addition to hematologic tests, there may be low albumin, elevated fibrinogen and γ-globulin concentrations. It is not uncommon for a patient with anemia of chronic disease due to chronic inflammation or (less commonly in children) malignancy to develop iron-deficiency anemia. Indeed, iron deficiency is common in children, particularly toddlers and teenage girls (Chapter 5). The iron deficiency may well be a combination of dietary insufficiency coupled with gastrointestinal blood loss, which is seen particularly in inflammatory bowel disease or secondary to nonsteroidal antiinflammatory drugs or steroids used in the connective tissue disorders. Reduced serum ferritin unequivocally demonstrates iron deficiency but ferritin measurements may be in the normal range when chronic inflammatory conditions and iron deficiency coexist. Serum transferrin receptor measurements can help to tease apart the anemia of iron deficiency and chronic inflammatory conditions because high values are seen in the former but not in the latter, although this is not so discriminating in anemia secondary to malignancy.[1,2]

The anemia is multifactorial although the molecular and cellular mechanisms are not well understood. There is a moderately shortened erythrocyte lifespan, survival being reduced to the 60–90 day range, instead of the normal 90–120 days. This is possibly secondary to increased phagocytosis by macrophages and splenic activity.[3] There is also a defective marrow response to anemia, with only a one- to two-fold increase in erythropoiesis rather than the normal 6–8-fold response. This is not associated with an endogenous deficiency of erythropoietin (EPO), or its defective release but to the inhibitory activity of other cytokines. During an inflammatory response there is increased production of the cytokines tumor necrosis factor (TNF)-α and interleukin (IL)-1 derived from macrophages. IL-1 is one of the stimulators of interferon (IFN)-γ production by T lymphocytes, and both TNF-α and IFN-γ have been shown to suppress erythropoiesis.[4,5]

A third component of the problem is impaired release of iron from reticuloendothelial cells for use in the marrow, again possibly cytokine mediated; both TNF-α and IL-1 lead to reduced serum iron concentrations and a shift of iron into the storage form in the bone marrow.[5] However, the anemia of chronic disease cannot be attributed simply to iron-deficient erythropoiesis;[6] iron absorption from the gut remains normal or low.

It is important to explore any easily correctable component of anemia in any child simply assumed to have a low hemoglobin through chronic disease. The response to pharmacologic doses of EPO is variable but if the endogenous concentration is < 500 units/L, therapy can occasionally be clinically worthwhile particularly where the anemia is severe enough to warrant transfusion support.[7,8]

Renal disease

The anemia of chronic renal disease is thought to result from a combination of the anemia of chronic disease and erythropoietin deficiency leading to impaired red-cell production, and is more marked than anemia of chronic disease alone. Generally there is a 2 g/dL fall in hemoglobin for every 10 mmol/L rise in blood urea. There is hypoplasia of the erythroid precursors in the bone marrow with little or no interference with normal leukopoiesis or megakaryocytopoiesis although lymphopenia may occur.[9] The blood film characteristically shows normochromic, normocytic red cells, which may be spiculated (echinocytes or keratocytes); hypersegmented neutrophils may be seen. Red cell survival is variably reduced both in chronic and acute renal failure, and this may be exacerbated by hemodialysis. Blood loss during hemodialysis or secondary to defective platelet function seen in renal failure may result in iron deficiency. Treatment with recombinant EPO is highly effective and beneficial if given with care. It is expensive, however, and it is important to explore other correctable components of the anemia, for instance iron deficiency, before using it. Failure to respond to

EPO should provoke a search for compounding problems before dose escalation is considered.[10] It is interesting that the mild bleeding tendency commonly seen in chronic renal failure can be improved after correction of the anemia by EPO.[11]

Hemolytic–uremic syndrome

Hemolytic–uremic syndrome (HUS) is a combination of a microangiopathic hemolytic anemia, thrombocytopenia and acute renal failure. The thrombocytopenia is not associated with a disseminated consumptive coagulopathy, and tests of coagulation are usually normal or only mildly deranged. The platelet count may be modestly or profoundly reduced. Platelet survival is shortened, and platelet-aggregating activity has been found in the plasma of some affected children.[12] The disease occurs sporadically and in epidemics, and the majority of children have a prodromal illness of abdominal pain and bloody diarrhea.

The epidemic form of HUS is associated with infection by enteropathogenic Gram-negative bacteria, usually *Escherichia coli* serotype 0157:H7, which produce exotoxins similar to those produced by *Shigella dysenteriae* type I and collectively referred to as Shiga toxins. These toxins bind to cell receptors, identified as ceramide trihexoside, which are expressed to varying degrees in different tissues (being particularly prevalent in infant glomerular endothelial cells).[13]

Most infants eventually recover without sequelae. Overall, mortality is 5% and long-term severe morbidity is around 10%.[14] Older children have a greater chance of progressing to end-stage renal failure, and have a higher incidence of atypical HUS (that without prodromal diarrhea). It is more serious and has other distinguishing features including normal urine output, gross proteinuria, hypertension, a relapsing course and more severe changes on renal biopsy.[15]

Treatment is supportive with the addition of fresh frozen plasma (FFP) infusions or plasma exchange for severe cases. Platelet transfusions are seldom indicated except occasionally to cover the surgical insertion of dialysis catheters. As the mechanism producing the thrombocytopenia is *in vivo* aggregation, there are theoretical grounds for keeping such transfusions to a minimum to avoid further microvascular thrombosis.

Thrombotic thrombocytopenic purpura

Also known as Moschcowitz syndrome (after the first author to describe the disease in the early 1920s), this is a syndrome of often undetermined cause, although it has been reported following stem cell transplantation, particularly if the donor is unrelated,[16] and infection.[17] It chiefly affects young adults and is characterized by a pentad of features, which include the triad for HUS (microangiopathic hemolytic anemia, thrombocytopenia and renal dysfunction) with two additional features, fever and neurologic disturbances. There is no evidence that the disorder observed occasionally in children differs from that encountered in adults.[18] It is probable that thrombotic thrombocytopenic purpura (TTP) and HUS (at least the sporadic and atypical type of the latter, see above) represent a similar pathologic process, with TTP being the more serious multisystem form of the disorder. Congenital or acquired deficiency of the von Willebrand factor (vWF)-cleaving protease, ADAMTS-13, has been specifically associated with a diagnosis of TTP, although this is not found in all patients.[19] The clinical course of TTP is variable, but the disease is serious with a high mortality if untreated. Two-thirds of patients die within 3 months;[18] some patients pursue a chronic relapsing course.[20]

The majority of patients respond to empirical plasma exchange with FFP.[21] Based on the rationale that von Willebrand multimers may be involved in the pathogenesis of the disorder, some patients failing to respond have subsequently improved if cryosupernatant (i.e., plasma with cryoprecipitate and thus vWF removed) is used rather than whole plasma.[22]

Liver disease

Anemia

Hematologic abnormalities in liver disease can affect both the cellular components of the blood and the coagulation system; the latter is dealt with in Chapter 29. Chronic liver disease is associated with anemia that is mildly macrocytic and often accompanied by target cells mainly due to increased cholesterol in the membrane. Leucopenia and thrombocytopenia may be present if there is hypersplenism but the hypersegmented neutrophils of megaloblastic anemia will not be seen and the macrocytes will be round rather than oval. Contributing factors to the anemia may include blood loss from bleeding varices and consequent iron deficiency, and poor iron absorption.

Hemolysis

Chronic immune hepatitis can be associated with immune hemolysis. Acute alcohol intoxication on a background of chronic alcohol ingestion can result in acute hemolysis, Zieve syndrome, but this has not been described in children. Wilson disease is a rare liver-based disorder of copper metabolism that is recessively inherited. Copper accumulates in the liver, brain, kidney and cornea, giving characteristic Kayser–Fleischer rings seen by slit-lamp ophthalmoscopy. It can cause both acute hemolytic anemia with no morphologic abnormality and an acute Heinz body hemolytic anemia due to sudden release of copper from the liver. If a child presents with an unexplained episode of hemolysis, it is important to exclude Wilson disease because it is fatal if left untreated.

Acute liver disease

Acute viral hepatitis, usually seronegative, may be followed by aplastic anemia. Clinical features and liver histology suggest a central role for an immune-mediated mechanism.[23] Bone marrow transplantation from a matched sibling donor or antithymocyte globulin and ciclosporin are the treatments available.

Reye syndrome is characterized by acute encephalopathy and fatty liver degeneration that typically follows a few days after apparent resolution of an unremarkable febrile viral infection. It has been linked to the use of aspirin as an antipyretic, and for this reason the drug is not recommended for children. Hematologic changes are those of acute hepatic disruption, chiefly disturbances of coagulation with occasional disseminated consumption and thrombocytopenia.

Gastrointestinal disease

Inflammatory bowel disease

Iron-deficiency anemia due to inadequate intake or loss of iron through bleeding and anemia of chronic disease are often encountered in patients with inflammatory bowel disease (IBD), which includes both Crohn disease and ulcerative colitis. Crohn disease can also be associated with folate deficiency due to malabsorption or vitamin B_{12} deficiency if the terminal ileum is involved. The drug sulfasalazine, an antifolate agent, is used to treat both IBD and Crohn disease. Sulfasalazine can also cause oxidative hemolysis, with "bite cells," similar to those in glucose-6-phosphate dehydrogenase deficiency, seen on the blood film. When iron deficiency coexists with folate deficiency, there may be hypochromic microcytes in addition to macrocytes, or the blood features of iron deficiency may dominate. Hypersegmented neutrophils may suggest a double deficiency but can occur with iron deficiency alone. Iron deficiency is sometimes unmasked when the folate deficiency is treated: after an initial rise in hemoglobin there is no further improvement, and microcytic, hypochromic cells appear on the blood film. An eosinophilia can accompany IBD and a thrombocytosis is often seen in ulcerative colitis, a reactive basophilia can be seen.

Celiac disease

Celiac disease is a gluten-sensitive enteropathy resulting in villous atrophy in the small intestine. Iron and folate malabsorption are common in untreated celiac disease as the proximal small intestine is predominantly affected. Vitamin B_{12} deficiency is less common, as the terminal ileum is relatively spared, although when specifically sought has been reported in 41% of untreated patients.[24] In addition to the nutritional deficiencies, features of hyposplenism, such as Howell–Jolly bodies and Pappenheimer bodies, may be present due to the splenic atrophy that occurs in this disease. Dapsone, used to treat dermatitis herpetiformis which may occur in celiac disease, can cause an oxidative hemolysis.

Endocrine disorders

Thyroid disease

Hypothyroidism is associated with mild or (occasionally) moderate anemia that is normochromic and mildly macrocytic. In addition, there may be small numbers of irregularly contracted cells, and a basophilia may be seen.[25] Red cell survival is normal. Hyperthyroidism conversely is associated with an increase in red cell mass, although hemoglobin concentration is usually normal, and can be associated with a lymphocytosis, neutropenia and basopenia, although as basophils are so infrequent in normal blood this is not diagnostically helpful.

Adrenal and pituitary insufficiency

These give rise to a mild normochromic anemia and are associated with lymphocytosis, eosinophilia, monocytopenia and neutropenia. Anemia associated with hypofunction of the pituitary is partly due to target endocrine organ failure but also to growth hormone deficiency, which affects erythropoiesis directly via its paracrine growth-promoting mediator, insulin-like growth factor 1. EPO levels are increased and there is a direct stimulatory effect on erythroid cells.[26,27]

Heart disease

Congenital heart disease

Tissue hypoxia secondary to cyanotic congenital heart disease (CHD) stimulates erythropoietin production resulting in polycythemia. The blood film rarely shows polychromasia and nucleated red blood cells unless there is an acute-on-chronic hypoxic episode. Thrombocytopenia and platelet function defects are also recognized, and activation of the coagulation system has been demonstrated.[28] These hemostatic changes are described in detail in Chapter 29 along with those that occur in Noonan syndrome, in which CHD is a feature. Children with cyanotic CHD rarely have hemorrhagic problems unless they are undergoing surgery; paradoxically they are reported to be at risk of thrombotic complications. Phlebotomy has been recommended in this group of patients to improve cerebral circulation and theoretically reduce the risk of cerebral arterial thrombosis.[29] However, because the circulatory effects of phlebotomy are transient and because iron-deficient red cells are less deformable, phlebotomy-induced iron deficiency results in symptoms of hyperviscosity at a level of hematocrit lower than in those who are not iron deficient. Low-dose iron therapy can be effective in relieving the symptoms of hyperviscosity.[30,31] Phlebotomy should be reserved for the temporary relief of significant, intrusive hyperviscosity symptoms.[32] Cyanotic CHD can result in functional hyposplenism (see below) due to poor perfusion of the spleen.

DiGeorge syndrome

DiGeorge syndrome, or velocardiofacial syndrome, is a rare disorder characterized by a spectrum of thymic and parathyroid gland abnormalities, conotruncal cardiac defects, typical facial dysmorphism and chromosome 22q11.2 deletion. It can also be associated with hypocalcemia and lymphopenia with reduced T cells. There have been reports of graft-versus-host disease secondary to blood transfusion in infants with this syndrome, and there is an argument for giving neonates with suspected DiGeorge syndrome irradiated products until the immune status is known.[33,34]

Cardiac anomalies and hyposplenism

Cardiac anomalies, particularly situs inversus, may be associated with hyposplenism and thus the blood film may show Howell–Jolly bodies, Pappenheimer bodies, a lymphocytosis, monocytosis and platelets in the high normal or elevated range.

Lung disease

Hypoxia

Chronic hypoxia, which can arise from a variety of pulmonary disorders, may lead to a compensatory polycythemia. Occasionally, the increased hyperviscosity leads to decreased tissue blood flow. Acute hypoxia, such as may occur in severe pneumonia, gives a different picture, the blood film showing polychromasia and nucleated red blood cells, as the bone marrow tries to compensate rapidly for the fall in oxygen tension. Apart from these changes, the other hematologic manifestations of pulmonary disease are dependent on the disorder itself.

Pulmonary hemosiderosis

This term describes a number of rare childhood disorders where repeated intraalveolar microhemorrhages result in pulmonary dysfunction, hemoptysis and hemosiderin-laden macrophages being lost to the external environment through the gut by swallowing. A major feature is therefore anemia due to iron deficiency. There are primary and secondary causes, with the former being more common in children.

Apart from a primary idiopathic type, there is also a variant associated with hypersensitivity to cows' milk and one that occurs with a progressive glomerulonephritis (Goodpasture syndrome).

Loeffler syndrome

This is not a distinct clinical entity and probably represents an unusual allergic manifestation to a variety of antigens. It is characterized by transient widespread pulmonary infiltrates seen on radiography in association with a high eosinophil count. In the absence of an identifiable allergen (such as migrating parasites), the condition usually resolves after a few days or weeks. It is distinct from the rare hypereosinophilic syndrome, which is a chronic disorder of unknown cause involving higher counts (up to $100 \times 10^9/\text{L}$) and which may damage other organs, notably the heart.[35] Asthma and bronchoallergic fungal infections can also be accompanied by a mild eosinophilia.

Skin disease

Eczema

A mild eosinophilia may be seen with eczema. Severe eczema and psoriasis can be accompanied by a mild anemia that has features of the anemia of chronic disease. Wiskott–Aldrich syndrome is characterized by severe eczema, thrombocytopenia where the platelets are small, and immune dysfunction; it is discussed in Chapter 19.

Mast cell disease

Mast cells, which are found in peripheral tissue, play a central role in inflammatory and immediate allergic reactions; they are only rarely found in the peripheral blood. In mast cell disease, large numbers are found either in the skin (cutaneous mastocytosis) or internal organs, particularly the gastrointestinal tract (systemic mastocytosis). These cells can release histamine and heparin-like substances, which cause urticaria of the skin and a heparin-like coagulation defect that can cause significant hemorrhage.[36–38] Cutaneous mastocytosis is the commonest form in children presenting under the age of 2 years, either as a solitary mastocytoma or more usually as urticaria pigmentosa. It is a benign disease and may regress spontaneously in children.[39] Involvement outside the skin is unusual, with bone lesions being the commonest; bone marrow infiltration is rare.[40]

Connective tissue disease

Anemia of chronic disease is common amongst this group of disorders but certain diseases may have their own distinctive characteristics.

Systemic lupus erythematosus

Many hematologic changes in addition to anemia of chronic disease have been described in systemic lupus erythematosus (SLE). Autoantibodies to red cells, neutrophils or (most commonly) platelets result in peripheral destruction reflected by cytopenias and increased marrow precursors. The disease can present as an immune cytopenia, mimicking chronic immune thrombocytopenic purpura (ITP), although the serology may be different, with lupus-associated antiplatelet antibodies more commonly fixing complement.[41] As might be anticipated, thrombocytopenic babies can be born to mothers with SLE as they can to mothers with ITP if maternal antiplatelet antibodies cross the placenta. Therapy for SLE-associated thrombocytopenia is as for chronic ITP, and the problem tends to respond to steroids along with other manifestations of the disease. There is evidence that splenectomy is less likely to be successful than in "true" ITP,[42] and severe refractory cases are difficult to manage. The presence or otherwise of thrombocytopenia has no prognostic importance in terms of other manifestations and progress of the SLE.[43]

SLE may also be the cause of marrow aplasia, or selective granulocyte aplasia. Lymphopenia, with abnormalities of T-cell function proportional to disease activity, is common. Circulating antiphospholipid antibodies ("lupus anticoagulants"), seen in other conditions as well as SLE, are discussed in Chapter 29.

Systemic-onset juvenile rheumatoid arthritis

The anemia of chronic disease is often complicated by iron deficiency as a result of gastrointestinal blood loss from analgesics (particularly nonsteroidal antiinflammatory drugs) and steroids. The two causes can be difficult to distinguish as serum ferritin may be normal despite iron deficiency due to its being elevated as part of an acute-phase response. Response to oral iron is blunted, possibly due to high circulating concentrations of IL-6; however, parenteral iron has been recommended in children whose circulating transferrin receptor concentration is increased.[44] In the absence of iron deficiency, the anemia of rheumatoid arthritis can be corrected by erythropoietin.[45] As well as anemia, a modest secondary thrombocytosis is not uncommon. Neutrophilia, observed in flare-up of the disease, needs to be differentiated from secondary bacterial infections.

Of children with juvenile rheumatoid arthritis, 20% have splenomegaly, although not necessarily the triad of rheumatoid arthritis, splenomegaly and neutropenia described by Felty. Neutropenia may result from hypersplenism alone, or be immune-mediated with detectable antineutrophil IgG antibodies. It does not always resolve after splenectomy.

There is evidence in some patients for a granulocyte maturation arrest, with low levels of granulocyte colony-stimulating factor (G-CSF) activity.

Wegener granulomatosis

Wegener granulomatosis is a necrotizing granulomatous small vessel vasculitis and is rare in childhood. It preferentially involves the upper airways, lungs and kidneys and therefore presents with fever, cough, hemoptysis, epistaxis, nasal discharge, nodular pulmonary infiltrates and renal failure. Evidence suggests that there is an underlying autoimmune inflammatory process but with infections and environmental and genetic factors also contributing. Hematologic features variably include normochromic, normocytic anemia, red-cell fragmentation typical of microangiopathic hemolytic anemia, leukocytosis with neutrophilia and eosinophilia, and a secondary thrombocytosis. Introduction of combined treatment with cyclophosphamide and steroids has improved patient outcome although disease relapses are common as is the risk of long-term organ damage.[46]

Polyarteritis nodosa

This is rare in childhood and is a cause of eosinophilia. If renal disease is present or there is severe hypertension, a microangiopathic hemolytic anemia may result.

Red-cell fragmentation syndromes

These occur as a result of physical damage to red cells such as heat damage from burns, abnormal surfaces (e.g., prosthetic heart valves), mechanical damage in exercise-induced "march hemoglobinuria" and turbulent flow in severe valvular disease. Hemolysis can also be due to a microangiopathic hemolytic anemia (MAHA). This last condition is characterized by the triad of anemia, thrombocytopenia and red cell fragments and is caused by the shearing of red cells by damaged endothelium, fibrin deposition in capillaries or both. Sometimes, the first feature identified will be an unexplained thrombocytopenia, and a search for fragments may reveal the underlying syndrome. It can be due to the presence of large-vessel lesions and vascular malformations including giant hemangiomas (i.e., Kasabach–Merritt syndrome) and may be the first indication that such a lesion is present. A search for vascular malformations should include the mesentery and gut, where they may not be clinically detectable and can also result in gastrointestinal bleeding. MAHA is also seen in disseminated intravascular coagulation (DIC) accompanying sepsis or renal vein thrombosis and in pathologic processes involving the small vessels of the kidney including HUS and TTP (see above).

In red-cell fragmentation syndromes, the blood film shows microspherocytes, fragments and often polychromasia. If there is thrombocytopenia, large platelets may be seen. In childhood, the commonest cause is enteric infection with accompanying renal failure. In these cases, there is often a leukocytosis and neutrophilia and sometimes echinocytosis, probably reflecting the toxin-induced damage to the red cell contributing to the hemolysis. Hemolysis in microangiopathic and mechanical hemolytic anemias is intravascular and if severe and chronic can lead to iron deficiency from persistent hemoglobinuria.

Infection

The hematologic response to infection depends on the type of invading organism and the state of health of the patient prior to becoming infected. Serious or overwhelming infections can be associated with profound disturbances of hemostasis and DIC. Acute bacterial infections produce a neutrophilia, except where sepsis is overwhelming or in preterm neonates where a paradoxical neutropenia is common. An increase in the number of immature neutrophils (band or stab cells) is also seen, and an increased ratio of band cell to mature forms is a more reliable indicator of sepsis in the neonate than the absolute neutrophil count.[47]

Subacute or chronic bacterial sepsis (such as that due to *Salmonella*, *Brucella* or tuberculosis) tends to increase the number of monocytes. Virus infections can produce a transient neutrophilia as part of an acute-phase response, and subsequently, if they produce hematologic changes, tend to cause disturbances in the number and/or morphology of lymphocytes. Parasites, if they penetrate tissues, cause an eosinophilia. Infections with many different organisms can occasionally provoke inappropriate hemophagocytosis (so-called infection-associated hemophagocytic syndrome; see Chapter 15), whereas others can result in leukemoid reactions or transient erythroblastopenia. Specific organisms and infections of particular hematologic importance are considered in more detail below.

Transient erythroblastopenia of childhood

This is characterized by profound normochromic anemia with absent or grossly reduced reticulocytes in an otherwise well child. Often there is an associated thrombocytosis whereas white cells are unremarkable. The cause of transient erythroblastopenia of childhood is not proven but has been reported to follow toxic, allergic or infectious episodes. However, a study in 10 children failed to show any definite proof of a viral etiology.[48] Most patients recover within 1–2 months from diagnosis and many begin to recover by the time they present. Transient erythroblastopenia of childhood can be confused with Diamond–Blackfan anemia, and differentiating features are discussed in Chapter 2.

Leukemoid reaction

Leukemoid reactions may be myeloid or lymphoid and are secondary to some other, underlying disease, most commonly infection. Such a reaction reverses on treatment of the underlying condition but may be confused with leukemia. In Down syndrome, transient abnormal myelopoiesis may be seen but this is distinct from a leukemoid reaction.

Causes of myeloid leukemoid reactions include any strong stimulus to the bone marrow, particularly severe bacterial infection, malignant disease and tuberculosis. Toxic changes, such as toxic granulation in the neutrophils and relatively few myelocytes and myeloblasts compared with the total neutrophil count, favor a reactive etiology. Lymphoid leukemoid reactions are classically seen in whooping cough, where the lymphocyte count may reach $100 \times 10^9/L$, or in the self-limiting condition acute infectious lymphocytosis, which is probably due to coxsackievirus[49] and results in lymphocyte counts of $\leq 50 \times 10^9/L$. Because chronic lymphocytic leukemia is so rare in children, these diseases are rarely confused with each other.

Hemolysis

Infection can precipitate most forms of hemolysis including cold immune hemolysis, fragmentation syndromes, oxidant hemolysis and that secondary to parasitized red cells or toxin production.

Cold autoimmune hemolytic anemia

In this syndrome, the autoantibody attaches to the red cell mainly in the peripheral circulation where the blood temperature is cooler. The antibody, usually IgM, binds to the red cells best at 4°C and the severity of the hemolysis and consequent anemia depend upon the antibody titer, the affinity of the antibody for red cells, its ability to bind complement and its thermal amplitude. The antibody is nearly always directed at the I or i antigen on the red-cell surface. Both mycoplasma and Epstein–Barr virus infections have been associated with cold autoimmune hemolytic anemia (AIHA), which is usually transient. Clinical features, when present, are mainly due to hemolysis rather than to red cell agglutination in peripheral vessels. Agglutination is seen on the blood film, even in the absence of clinical features, and with varying numbers of spherocytes and a degree of polychromasia dependent on the severity of the hemolysis. The mean corpuscular volume (MCV), mean corpuscular hemoglobin (MCH) and mean corpuscular hemoglobin concentration (MCHC) are raised due to the presence of the agglutinates.

Paroxysmal cold hemoglobinuria

This rare syndrome can occur after viral infections, including measles, or less commonly as a late manifestation of syphilis, and results in acute intravascular hemolysis. The antibody, named the Donath–Landsteiner antibody, is an IgG and directed against the P blood group antigens. It binds to red cells in the cold but causes lysis with complement in the warm. Variable numbers of spherocytes and polychromasia are seen on the blood film.

Bacterial and parasitic infections

Clostridium welchii and *Cl. perfringens* septicemia can result in severe intravascular hemolysis characterized by the presence of microspherocytes on the blood film. The bacteria produce several hemolytic toxins, one of which exposes the Thomsen–Friedenreich cryptoantigen (or T-antigen).[50] Infection can follow penetrating wounds or peritonitis from a perforated viscus, or occur in immunosuppressed patients.[51,52]

Bartonellosis, malaria and babesiosis can all cause a hemolytic anemia. *Bartonella* organisms coat the red cells and result in their rapid removal from the blood, whereas malaria and *Babesia* colonize the red blood cells and cause their destruction. In addition, malaria also induces antibodies resulting in autoimmune hemolysis and increased destruction of the parasite-damaged red cells by the spleen. All of the organisms can be identified on correctly prepared and stained blood films, although in the later stages of bartonellosis the organisms leave the bloodstream. Heavy infestation with *Plasmodium falciparum* malaria parasites can cause severe acute intravascular hemolysis and acute tubular necrosis described as "blackwater fever." It can also cause cerebral malaria. In both conditions, small vessels are occluded with parasitized cells, with associated intravascular fibrin and perivascular hemorrhage. Immune-mediated thrombocytopenia without DIC is also common in malaria.

Specific infections

Visceral leishmaniasis (kala-azar)

Visceral leishmaniasis is transmitted by sandflies and can cause fever, pancytopenia, hepatosplenomegaly and, to a lesser extent, lymphadenopathy up to several years after exposure. It may be mistaken for a lymphoma. Bone marrow or splenic aspirates may show the parasites, so called Leishman–Donovan bodies, in and around the macrophages. Hemophagocytosis may also be seen.

Tuberculosis

Childhood tuberculosis is an increasing problem with the emergence of multidrug resistance and human immunodeficiency virus (HIV) coinfection. Tuberculosis produces several hematologic features including monocytosis, anemia of chronic disease or a myeloid leukemoid reaction (see above). Thrombocytopenia and pancytopenia have also been reported. Bone marrow involvement is rare, except in immunosuppressed patients, but when it does occur may result in a leukoerythroblastic film and granulomas in the bone-marrow biopsy.

Epstein–Barr virus

Primary infection by Epstein–Barr virus (EBV) causes infectious mononucleosis (IM), which is predominantly a disease of adolescents and young adults. Infection can occur in young children, where its presentation and clinical features may be mild so that EBV is not recognized as the cause. IM, commonly known as "glandular fever," presents with pharyngitis, fever, lymphadenopathy and hepatosplenomegaly. Rarely, there may be a generalized rash. The incidence of rash approaches 100% in patients given ampicillin, a strange, induced allergy that is almost pathognomonic for the disease. The same applies to the now more commonly used analogous antibiotic, amoxicillin.

EBV infects B lymphocytes but the characteristic atypical mononuclear cells seen on the blood film are mainly activated CD8+ T lymphocytes. These cells contribute to the lymphocytosis and leukocytosis seen in IM and are highly pleomorphic. They are large, with blue cytoplasm, and may have nucleoli. Where they abut other cells, their edges are typically "scalloped." They usually comprise > 25% of the total lymphocytes (commonly > 50%) in contrast to the "EBV-negative" IM-like syndromes. There may be accompanying neutropenia, which can be severe, and mild thrombocytopenia in about one-third of patients. Severe thrombocytopenia occurs in < 1% of patients and is probably of immune etiology; cold AIHA can occur (see above) with accompanying red-cell agglutination but often not overt hemolysis; spherocytes and polychromasia may be seen on the blood film to varying degrees.[53,54] Hemophagocytosis can occur, and rarely aplastic anemia some weeks after the primary infection.

The diagnosis is made by the typical hematology together with specific EBV serology. A widely used and reliable screening test detects heterophile red cell agglutinins, a feature of classical "glandular fever" noted by Paul and Bunnell in the 1930s. Unlike naturally occurring heterophile antibodies, the agglutinins seen in IM are not absorbed by guinea pig kidney. They are absorbed by ox red cells, and agglutinate sheep and horse red cells. These features are exploited in the popular "monospot" test of Lee and Davidshon, where sera are exposed to either guinea pig kidney or beef red cell stroma before being assessed for their potential to agglutinate horse red cells. Heterophile antibodies appear around the same time as the atypical lymphocytosis, or shortly thereafter, and peak around 2 weeks. They can persist for several months. They are not specific, and can occasionally arise in disorders other than IM, including acute leukemia and lymphoma.

There is no treatment of proven benefit in uncomplicated IM. The benefit of steroids, often used for symptomatic thrombocytopenia or severe hemolysis, is difficult to assess as both problems normally recover quickly with or without therapy. High-dose immunoglobulin has also been used.[55]

EBV infection in immunosuppressed patients

EBV infection in some individuals with cellular immune deficiency states can give rise to uncontrolled lymphoproliferative disorders. X-linked lymphoproliferative disease (Purtilo or Duncan syndrome) is a rare inherited inability to combat EBV infection where patients may die of progressive disease, occasionally associated with a virus-induced hemophagocytic syndrome.[56] They also suffer from marrow aplasia, hypogammaglobulinemia and lymphomas. Those on aggressive immunosuppressive therapy following solid organ transplants, recipients of allogeneic marrow grafts and patients with HIV infection can all develop polyclonal proliferation of B lymphocytes that carry the EBV genome and which in some instances progresses to a fatal clonal lymphoma. In marrow transplant patients, the problem usually involves donor-derived lymphocytes and occurs in recipients of mismatched T-cell-depleted marrow after treatment with T-cell antibodies for graft-versus-host disease. A later form of the disease may arise from host cells.[57]

Burkitt lymphoma

This is endemic in Africa, where it is the commonest cancer in children. It commonly presents with jaw lesions, extranodal abdominal involvement and ovarian tumors in girls. EBV has been identified in Burkitt cell culture but there is some evidence that *Plasmodium falciparum* malaria might interact with EBV in the etiology of this disease.[58,59]

Human immunodeficiency virus

HIV infection in children is covered in detail in Chapter 19. The direct hematologic (as opposed to the immunologic) effects of the virus can briefly be summarized as cytopenias due either to a direct effect on marrow stem cells resulting in decreased production or as a consequence of autoantibodies to blood cellular elements.[60,61] Hemostatic abnormalities that predispose patients to thromboembolism have also been recognized.[62]

Anemia in HIV-infected children is commonly due to many factors other than the virus. A study in Abidjan, where the prevalence of HIV infection in unselected children admitted to hospital was 8.2%, showed that the most frequent reason for admission in such patients was malnutrition; malaria can also coexist.[63] The virus can, however, result in an autoimmune hemolytic state in which the direct antiglobulin test is positive, although overt hemolysis is rare.[60,62] It can also cause reticulocytopenia.[60]

ITP is a common manifestation of HIV infection and can be the first sign of infection in otherwise apparently well children.[64] It can therefore be mistaken for simple ITP (see Chapter 23), although careful examination of the child with HIV will usually identify lymphadenopathy or hepatosplenomegaly. HIV testing of selected thrombocytopenic children, such as those in high-risk groups or those with ITP that does not resolve, should be considered. Neutropenia is not uncommon and may be immune mediated, but may also be compounded by reduced production due to antiretroviral therapy or co-trimoxazole. Highly active antiretroviral therapy (HAART) is being used successfully in children and allowing discontinuation of prophylactic medication for *Pneumocystis* pneumonia or opportunistic infections.[65]

Lymphomas and other HIV-associated malignancies arise less frequently in children than adults, although the number of children developing malignancies is increasing as they live longer and the number with HIV infection increases.[66]

Parvovirus B19

In normal individuals, acute infection by B19 parvovirus produces fifth disease (erythema infectiosum), which is characterized by facial erythema, giving a "slapped cheek" appearance and sometimes arthralgia/arthritis. It often goes unnoticed, and a study in Scotland has shown that by 20 years of age, 65% of people have antibodies to the virus.[67] The virus itself has a predilection for the P antigen on red cells and binds to erythroid precursors in the bone marrow, preventing their replication, and to a lesser extent, replication of the other cell lineages. In people whose red cells have a normal lifespan this has little clinical impact, but in those whose red cells have a shortened cell lifespan, such as a patient with sickle-cell disease or hereditary spherocytosis, this can result in an acute aplastic crisis characterized by a rapidly falling hemoglobin and the absence of a reticulocyte response. In immunocompromised individuals, infection can result in a pure red cell aplasia or prolonged pancytopenia,[68] which is also not infrequently seen in children on chemotherapy for leukemia,[69] suggesting that normal immunity is necessary for virus control. Because viral infection is prevalent in the population, therapeutic immune globulin preparations are a good source of anti-B19 antibodies, and IgG administration can lead to cure of anemia in the congenitally immunodeficient patient and to its amelioration in AIDS patients with persistent parvovirus infection.[70] Fetal infection with parvovirus B19 can lead to hydrops fetalis. It can also occasionally cause symptomatic pancytopenia in otherwise healthy children.[71]

TORCH infections

This is a miscellaneous group of congenital infections including *Toxoplasma*, rubella, cytomegalovirus (CMV), herpes simplex (HSV), HIV and syphilis. Although they are all very different diseases, the collective acronym is justified by certain common features: they can all cause neonatal anemia, thrombocytopenia (see also Chapter 22) and hepatosplenomegaly.

Kawasaki disease

Kawasaki disease is an acute multisystem vasculitic condition that occurs in children and is self-limiting. It is characterized by fever, bilateral nonexudative conjunctivitis, erythema of the lips and oral mucosa, rash and cervical lymphadenopathy. Coronary artery aneurysms or ectasia develop in approximately 15–25% of untreated children and may lead to ischemic heart disease or sudden death through coronary artery occlusion or rupture.[72] Treatment is based on the use of aspirin and intravenous immunoglobulin.[73] The most striking hematologic feature, apart from the marked neutrophilia and acute-phase response seen during the acute stage of the disease (up to 4 weeks), is a secondary thrombocytosis. This commonly arises during the second week of the illness and may persist into the subacute and convalescent phase, with counts commonly well in excess of $1000 \times 10^9/\text{L}$. There is some evidence that it is mediated through production of the acute-phase cytokine IL-6.[74]

Nutritional disorders

Hematinic deficiencies are described in Chapters 5 and 6, but brief consideration is given here to protein-calorie malnutrition, scurvy and anorexia nervosa, all of which can produce hematologic abnormalities.

Protein-calorie malnutrition

This all-embracing term covers malnutrition due to protein deficiency in the presence of adequate carbohydrate calorie intake (kwashiorkor); simple calorie deficiency (marasmus) and, as commonly occurs, a combination of the two. While primarily a problem of underdeveloped countries, malnutrition can also arise in children of strict vegetarians and can complicate some chronic diseases such as renal failure, malignancy and serious intestinal disorders.

Anemia is usual in children with severe protein deficiency. Uncomplicated, it is usually mild, normochromic and normocytic and appears to be due to reduced cell production despite adequate erythropoietin drive.[75] Frequently, concomitant iron or folate deficiency will complicate the picture. Protein-calorie malnutrition also predisposes children to infection, which is in part due to impaired leukocyte function.[76]

Scurvy

Scurvy (vitamin C deficiency) is rare, but is occasionally seen in children between the ages of 6 months and 2 years due to poor dietary intake and where fruit juices are boiled. Those affected become irritable and dislike being handled. The legs become tender and this can result in pseudoparalysis, where the child lies in a froglike pose. Purple spongy swellings appear around erupted teeth. Petechial, subperiosteal, orbital or subdural hemorrhages may arise, together with hematuria or melena. Mild anemia is common, probably due to extravasation of blood. The bleeding tendency is due to loss of vascular integrity with collagen deficiency.

Anorexia nervosa

Anorexia nervosa produces hematologic changes in its more advanced stages. As might be expected, these are similar to those seen in severe malnutrition and include macrocytosis,[77] mild anemia, neutropenia and thrombocytopenia. There is a predisposition to infection associated with neutropenia and the lower ranges of body mass index.[78] The marrow undergoes gelatinous change and occasionally can become severely hypoplastic.[79] Small numbers of irregularly contracted erythrocytes are seen, similar to those of hypothyroidism, possibly reflecting a disturbance in the composition of membrane lipids.[80]

Drugs

The list of candidate drugs causing hematologic side-effects is long. Certain drugs are associated with specific side-effects that may not be predictable but are well described; others occur in a dose-dependent fashion or are unpredictable. It should be assumed that any drug can cause a hematologic side-effect, particularly perhaps an immune-mediated thrombocytopenia, when such an effect occurs in a child for no other obvious reason. Myelosuppression affecting all cell lines is a dose-dependent side-effect of many antineoplastic agents (see Chapters 16, 20 and 21). Idiosyncratic marrow failure (aplasia) can also occur as an aberrant response to noncytotoxic drugs such as chloramphenicol and butazone (see Chapter 4), and can affect one cell line preferentially, such as the myeloid line with carbimazole. Drugs can also reduce the numbers of circulating blood cells by shortening their survival, either via an immune-mediated effect or through direct damage. Neutropenia is covered in Chapter 14. Drug-induced immune hemolytic anemia is discussed in Chapter 8, and red cell damage from oxidant drugs in Chapter 9. Two specific drug effects are mentioned below.

Sodium valproate, used in epilepsy, has a high incidence of drug-induced thrombocytopenia. In an early prospective study of 45 children, one-third had a measurable fall in their platelet count, one child reaching a nadir of 35×10^9/L.[81] Subsequent studies have confirmed this phenomenon, with several showing the occurrence of thrombocytopenia in 12–18%

of patients, with the platelet count inversely correlated with age and dose of sodium valproate but not duration of treatment.[82–84] It is not clear whether the thrombocytopenia is always or wholly immune-mediated; there is some evidence of defective platelet production.[85,86]

Heparin-induced thrombocytopenia

Heparin-induced thrombocytopenia (HIT) is of two types: HIT type I, which occurs soon after starting heparin and is a mild, transient, nonimmune disorder; and HIT type II, which is an immune-mediated thrombocytopenia that is severe and arises after 8–10 days of heparin.[87,88] HIT type II affects up to 3% of patients treated with unfractionated heparin; it is less frequent when low-molecular-weight heparins are used.[89] It is characterized by a fall in platelet count, not necessarily outside the normal range, platelet activation and consequent arteriovenous thromboembolism. Platelet activation is due to an antibody against a neoantigen formed by the heparin–platelet factor 4 complex.[88]

Heparin is not as frequently used in pediatrics as in adult medicine due to the lower incidence of thromboembolic disease. It is used, however, and all patients on intensive care invariably receive small but significant amounts from indwelling catheters and arterial lines. A study by Risch *et al.*[90] reports on 70 pediatric patients with HIT, the majority of whom were on intensive care. The diagnostic features and outcomes were similar to those seen in adults.

Patients receiving any form of heparin for longer than 5 days should have their platelet count measured. Any who develop a decreasing platelet count, unexplained thrombosis, or resistance to heparin anticoagulation should be tested for heparin-associated antibodies. Heparin should be withdrawn immediately and alternative anticoagulation instituted, even if thrombocytopenic. Danaparoid, lepirudin and argatroban appear to improve outcomes.[90]

Hematologic effects of nonhematopoietic tumors

The effects of cancer on peripheral blood and bone marrow are legion; some are characteristic but few are diagnostic by themselves. Even larger centers will see only perhaps 50 cases per year and these will be a mix of different tumors, with only a small number in even the most common diagnostic categories. Therefore, to build up a picture of typical findings requires collaboration, and this area is not well documented in the literature, except as incidental details in incidental case reports. This section concentrates on the common abnormalities of blood and bone marrow that are not directly caused by treatment, and also highlights some characteristic and other, less common, features of infiltrated bone marrow.

Peripheral blood abnormalities

Anemia, erythrocytosis, leukopenia, leukocytosis, thrombocytopenia, thrombocytosis, microangiopathic hemolysis and rouleaux have all been seen at presentation in children with cancer. No single pattern is restricted to any particular form of cancer but it is worth highlighting some of the typical findings in the peripheral blood.

Anemia of chronic disease

The anemia may be mild or severe and is often a concern to the treating physician. Characteristically it is normochromic and microcytic with normal or raised serum ferritin, low serum iron and rouleaux formation. The anemia is probably caused by the complex interaction of a variety of cytokines (see above) produced in response to the presence of a tumor; it may be associated with some degree of reactive thrombocytosis. In most children with cancer, anemia is not primarily due to marrow infiltration or bleeding. Even in those with disseminated disease, bone marrow infiltration is not the sole (or even, necessarily, the prime) cause of anemia. Concomitant iron deficiency is difficult to exclude by laboratory tests, and assessment of response to oral iron therapy is impractical in most children with cancer. If bone marrow aspirates are performed, iron stains will be helpful in showing whether stainable iron is present. In anemia of chronic disease, iron is present but there is poor incorporation into red blood cells, reflected by decreased numbers of sideroblasts; absent stainable iron is seen in the deficient state.

It is easier to appreciate the importance of anemia of chronic disorders if cancers that have not infiltrated the marrow are considered. Wilms tumor and hepatoblastoma stand out in this regard. Although both erythrocytosis and anemia are said to be features, albeit rare ones, of Wilms tumor,[91] the typical pattern is of mild or moderate anemia. In the last 55 consecutive children with Wilms tumor seen in three UK Children's Cancer Study Group (UKCCSG) centers (Newcastle, Edinburgh and Glasgow), the average hemoglobin was 10.7 g/dL (range 5.8–15.7 g/dL). The average MCV was 75.3 fL (range 64–91 fL). This excludes a single case of mesoblastic nephroma where the hemoglobin was 20.1 g/dL and MCV was 103.8 fL. Ferritin levels were measured in only six children, five of whom had an MCV of ≤ 70 fL, and were normal or raised in all six cases. It was not possible to estimate what contribution bleeding from the renal tract may have made to the usually mild anemia. Ferritin levels are rarely informative in determining the cause of microcytosis in children presenting with cancer; an iron stain of a bone marrow is more helpful. In 12 children with hepatoblastoma from the same UKCCSG centers (age range 3 weeks to 7 years), the average hemoglobin was 10.3 g/dL (range 5.5–15.6 g/dL) and MCV was 74 fL (range 61–89 fL). These two diseases are associated with lower MCVs than other neoplastic diseases. Hodgkin lymphoma is classically described as having a microcytic anemia at presentation. However, blood counts at presentation from 74 consecutive patients with Hodgkin lymphoma had an average MCV of 79.6 fL. Twenty patients were 17 years or older and, if excluded, the average MCV was 79.8 fL. Of the 46 children (age range 4–15 years) only 12 had an MCV below the normal range for age, and average hemoglobin for 45 children was 11.8 g/dL. Although anemia of chronic disorder does occur in neuroblastoma, frequent or marked microcytosis is less common. The only child with marked microcytosis (MCV < 70 fL) of 49 with widely disseminated neuroblastoma from two centers (Newcastle and Edinburgh) was found to have concomitant β-thalassemia trait. These examples of discrepancy between textbook descriptions of classical features and routine experience suggest that the "classical" picture may have been inordinately influenced by individual cases with "exciting" hematologic features; erythrocytosis, occasionally seen in Wilms tumor or mesoblastic nephroma (see above), is a rare condition in childhood and thus worthy of reporting while microcytosis is commonplace and of less interest.

Reactive thrombocytosis

A variety of stimuli and diseases can sometimes produce dramatically high platelet counts in children,[92] in some of whom elevated IL-6 levels may be a contributory factor.[93,94] Rebound during cancer treatment is one of the common causes, but thrombocytosis is not thought to be particularly common at presentation.[92] To some extent the frequency of thrombocytosis depends on its definition (see Chapter 24). Patients with Wilms tumor and hepatoblastoma provide a useful source of information about platelet counts. In the groups of patients from the three UKCCSG centers described above, the average platelet count in those with Wilms tumor was 383×10^9/L (range $91–885 \times 10^9$/L, including eight children with counts $> 500 \times 10^9$/L) and in those with hepatoblastoma it was 865×10^9/L (range $502–1674 \times 10^9$/L). Similar platelet counts may be found in some children with localized neuroblastoma, rhabdomyosarcoma, Ewing tumor and other cancers. Perhaps more surprising is the average platelet count of 244×10^9/L (range $44–839 \times 10^9$/L) for the last 49 cases of neuroblastoma with infiltrated bone marrow seen in two centers (as above), of whom eight had counts $> 400 \times 10^9$/L. Both sets of observations, in Wilms tumor, hepatoblastoma and disseminated neuroblastoma, suggest that other factors may influence the platelet count rather more than the presence (or absence) of marrow infiltration.

Neutrophilia and neutropenia

There is an even less consistent pattern in neutrophil counts at presentation. Moderate reactive neutrophilia seems to be as common as mild neutropenia, even in children with infiltrated marrows. Beyond awareness of potential infective risks, there is little of practical importance in the neutrophil count in most cases.

Microangiopathic hemolysis

Microangiopathic hemolytic anemia, manifest by red cell fragmentation with perhaps a degree of thrombocytopenia and either with or without derangements in coagulation, has been seen in a wide range of cancers. Acute promyelocytic leukemia is the most-recognized cause of DIC in childhood cancer. However, among the nonhematopoietic tumors no single type stands out. Minor red cell fragmentation or poikilocytosis is so common and nonspecific that it is of little value as a diagnostic pointer or in alerting hematologists (or clinicians) to a clinically important coagulopathy. However, fragments and thrombocytopenia may alert a hematologist to the presence of an otherwise unsuspected hemangioma.

Leukoerythroblastic blood film

The presence of circulating nucleated red blood cells and myelocytes immediately raises the possibility of bone marrow infiltration but this peripheral blood picture is not generally as striking in children as in adults with disseminated cancer. Leukoerythroblastic pictures may be associated with pancytopenia, isolated cytopenias and normal or raised white cell counts. A case can be made for examining the bone marrow in any child with such a picture at diagnosis, even if this is not one of the recommended initial investigations for the tumor, whatever the rest of the blood count indicates. However, a leukoerythroblastic picture is a poor diagnostic aid and should not be used to help discriminate between leukemia and nonhematopoietic cancer in cases where the initial differential diagnosis is broad; it is the bone marrow appearances that matter. Striking leukoerythroblastosis may occur in nonmalignant conditions such as infection or hemolytic anemia.

Circulating tumor cells

Circulating tumor cells are rarely seen in the peripheral blood of children with cancer. However, primitive cells that cannot be positively identified as either hematopoietic or nonhematopoietic cells are seen from time to time. Neuroblastoma,[95] medulloblastoma[96] and rhabdomyosarcoma[97] have all been mistaken for acute leukemia because of peripheral blood abnormalities and, in the case of the cited example of rhabdomyosarcoma, cerebrospinal fluid (CSF) and pleural fluid involvement. Such reports are sometimes used as examples of circulating tumor cells. Highlighting these rare cases may give an unrealistic impression of the typical child with cancer for at least two reasons. Firstly, such cells are extremely rare. Secondly, closer inspection of these three

published cases shows that very small numbers of circulating "blasts" ($0.03–0.12 \times 10^9$/L) were found, there were no distinctive features that could help distinguish between non-hematopoietic cells and normal or malignant hematopoietic precursors, and the striking blood abnormality was simply a leukoerythroblastic reaction. In none of these cases did the authors claim that the circulating blasts were necessarily tumor cells. The syndrome of carcinocythemia, in which clumps of tumor cells may be found in the blood, seems to be more common in adults and may reflect tumor emboli rather than circulating tumor cells.

Newer techniques, with sensitivities in the range of one malignant cell per $10^4–10^6$ normal cells, have identified circulating tumor cells in peripheral blood, for instance in neuroblastoma and Ewing sarcoma, and correlations with bone marrow findings and clinical outcome have been made.[98–101] Techniques include immunocytochemistry to detect disialoganglioside (GD2) and reverse transcription-PCR (RT-PCR) to detect tyrosine hydroxylase (TH) or GD2 synthase mRNA in neuroblastoma.[99,100] RT-PCR is used to detect the chimeric transcripts *EWS-FLI1* and *EWS-ERG* found in Ewing sarcoma and primitive neuroectodermal tumors (PNET).[101,102] The specificity of these markers has not been fully validated; false positives have been found using anti-GD2 by some workers,[103] and it might be important to combine information from both immunologic and molecular cytogenetic techniques. It is not perhaps surprising that these cells can be detected given the metastatic nature of these tumors and widespread disease at presentation or relapse. However, it is more important to determine the significance of these cells and whether quantitative analysis can help either to direct therapy or predict outcome. These techniques are being used to determine the level of residual disease in bone marrow specimens, peripheral blood and peripheral blood stem cell harvests, but it is important that this is correlated with clinical staging and outcome in rigorous well-designed clinical trials so that the importance of detecting such tumor cells can be ascertained.

Bone marrow abnormalities

Bone marrow specimens have been part of the staging procedure in certain children's cancers from the 1960s. From early studies[104,105] experience of the pattern of metastases and relapse has grown and has indicated those tumors in which there is a sufficiently high incidence of dissemination to warrant routine examination of the bone marrow at diagnosis. In most centers attention has focused on the small round-cell tumors: neuroblastoma, Ewing tumor, PNET and rhabdomyosarcoma. Accuracy of the primary diagnosis has steadily improved over the past 35 years but the adequacy of material gained from bone marrow specimens to determine disease involvement had not been clearly specified. It is only within the last 20 years that the routine practice of obtaining marrow from more than one site, and by both aspirate and trephine biopsy, has gained wider acceptance.[106] Apart from unique clinical circumstances, routine monitoring of bone marrow is virtually restricted to neuroblastoma, for which internationally agreed criteria for staging and assessment of response have been developed.[107,108] It is important that adequate specimens are obtained because crucial treatment decisions are made on the basis of the results.

The following section deals mainly with the appearances of infiltrated bone marrow and draws on both the scanty published data and collective personal experience.

Neuroblastoma

Neuroblastoma is the commonest malignant infiltrate of bone marrow of children after leukemia. In most cases its detection and correct identification present few problems; there is usually a strong clinical suspicion of the correct diagnosis, and a simple diagnostic test allows the detection of high levels of catecholamine metabolites in > 90% of patients with neuroblastoma. The simplicity of this test and its general reliability have probably contributed to the lack of vigor with which hematologists have studied the tumor cells because the diagnosis is often known at the time of examining the bone marrow. Despite the frequency with which neuroblastoma is seen by hematologists, only sporadic descriptions, as opposed to studies of frequency of infiltration, existed until Mills and Bird[109] described the "variability of the microscopic pattern of marrow infiltration," having studied both bone marrow aspirate smears and trephine biopsies from 48 new cases.

Cytology

In the current HR-NBL-1/ESIOP trial it is recommended that bone marrow smears are made at the bedside from freshly aspirated bone marrow. Unless the operator is very experienced, or has a "spreader" to help, the aspirated bone marrow is often put into ethylenediamine tetraacetate (EDTA) and cytologic preparations made later. This may introduce other artifacts and should not, if possible, be relied on as the sole or routine method of handling aspirated bone marrow. It can be difficult for the operator, however, as increasing numbers of aspirate specimens are needed for the different biologic and cytogenetic studies.

Superficially, individual neuroblasts often resemble lymphoblasts, and occasionally they may also have a few vacuoles. To help differentiate them from leukemic cells, it is important that the marrow smear is carefully examined under low power, when different and distinct patterns of infiltration are best seen. Mills and Bird describe three patterns: "clumps," "clumps and rosettes" and a "pseudoleukemic" pattern.[109] On examination of a marrow smear, different patterns may be found; none is mutually exclusive within an individual case, particularly if marrow aspirates

are obtained from more than one site. Neuroblasts have a tendency to adhere so strongly to each other that in the process of aspirating the marrow, which is often difficult to achieve, cells are often ripped apart from each other and from the tumor stroma and/or the reactive marrow fibrous tissue. This leaves numerous bare nuclei and often large amounts of cytoplasmic or stromal debris over the surface of the smear, as well as producing the more familiar clumps, doublets and intact single cells. However, it is important not to assume that bare nuclei on a smear are from neuroblastoma cells because they may be from other, nonmalignant, necrotic cells present in the marrow.

Mills and Bird[109] often found ball-like clumps, some with a central lumen, resembling rosettes. Others failed to find significant numbers of rosettes,[106] but one study showed that, provided the smears were examined carefully, rosettes were present in the majority of cases,[110] and large numbers of these structures were virtually diagnostic of neuroblastoma.

The partially fibrillar nature of the center of the rosettes strongly resembles earlier descriptions of neuroblastoma cytoplasm,[111] and the centers also stain strongly with UJ13A,[112] a monoclonal antibody to the neural cell adhesion molecule (NCAM), which reacts strongly with most neuroblastomas.[113] However, this antibody is not specific, and false positive reactions have been reported.[112,114] Although syncytia have often been described, it remains possible that they too are artifacts. Careful examination of rosettes on smears suggests that filamentous extensions of neuroblast cytoplasm extend into the centers of the rosettes, which may also contain secreted substances; together they may give the impression of multinucleate cells.

Bone marrow histology

Mills and Bird[109] also provided the first satisfactory descriptions and illustrations of the histologic features of neuroblastoma in the bone marrow, highlighting the prominent reticulin fibrosis. The range of appearances they described was confirmed shortly after in a larger study.[115]

From these two studies it is clear that the term "small round-cell tumor," when used to describe neuroblastoma within the bone marrow, can be very misleading. Tumor cells ranging in size from that of a lymphoblast to that of a megakaryocyte can be found, with variable amounts of fibrotic stroma. In some biopsies, fibrosis with few easily identifiable tumor cells predominates. In others, almost monomorphous sheets of tumor cells can be found. Both extremes can occur in different biopsies taken at the same time from the same patient. Occasionally, clear-cut differentiation to ganglion cells is obvious. The classic rosettes in histologic sections of the primary tumor in neuroblastoma are less often found in sections of the marrow than apparently similar structures on aspirate smears. This may reflect some degree of crush artifact in relatively small pieces of tissue or some effect of the tissue (i.e., bone marrow) in which the metastases have developed. It is also possible that the rosettes in aspirated bone marrow represent a cytologic manifestation of the classic rosette found in histologic preparations.

The extent of infiltration may vary between two simultaneous biopsies from different sites; in one there may be complete replacement of hematopoietic tissue, and in the other no evidence of tumor or a single, small, well-circumscribed cellular nodule. There is often marked discrepancy between the apparent tumor load inferred from the aspirate and biopsy appearances. Such variations highlight the patchy, nonuniform distribution of metastases within bone marrow and the futility of attempting to quantify infiltration of marrow as a simple percentage of aspirated cells. Despite studies carried out nearly 30 years ago,[106,116] it is only more recently that pediatric oncologists and hematologists have come to accept that single aspirates are inadequate for staging.[117,118] This growing appreciation has culminated in internationally agreed criteria for both staging and assessing response to treatment;[107,108] these recommend at least two aspirates and two trephine biopsies from two separate sites as part of the initial staging and also on each occasion that full reassessment of response is carried out. The exception to this general advice is that trephine biopsy, as opposed to aspirate, is recognized as being technically difficult in infants aged < 6 months; it could then remain an optional investigation. The current international high-risk neuroblastoma trial, HR-NBL-1/ESIOP of the Société Internationale d'Oncologie Pédiatrique (SIOP), specifies adequacy of trephine – at least 0.5-cm bone marrow core and preferably 1-cm cores from each posterior iliac crest – because treatment decisions with regard to failure of protocol and proceeding to peripheral blood stem cell rescue depend on the results. A study of adequacy of bone marrow biopsy in neuroblastoma has shown that central review of 605 specimens from 25 centers of the European Neuroblastoma Study Group assessed 25% as being inadequate,[119] a deterioration in performance from a study 3 years earlier, when 17% were assessed as inadequate. Despite the documented frequency of "inadequate" samples, one recent estimate of marrow involvement within some European centers showed that only 10% of children with stage 4 disease at presentation have no "conventionally" detectable tumor at presentation.[120] In the HR-NBL-1/ESIOP trial, biologic, immunocytochemical and molecular data on bone marrow aspirates taken at the same time as the trephines are being collected and hopefully will help to clarify the significance of minimal disease and the sensitivity of the standard bone marrow investigations.

Monitoring effects of treatment: restaging
The role of monitoring progress in treatment by attempting to measure the response of bone marrow metastases is still evolving. Once treatment has started it is difficult to find tumor cells in aspirated marrow, even from children with previously heavy infiltration. The trephine biopsy assumes even greater importance. There has only been one attempt to describe the range of histologic abnormalities in bone marrow of treated children.[115] Four main patterns emerged, which were graded 1 to 4.
- Grade 1: marrow without abnormal architecture, infiltrate or fibrous stroma, albeit often very hypocellular.
- Grade 2: marrow with similar features but with a pathologic increase in reticulin.
- Grade 3: marrow with distorted architecture, increased fibrous stroma and abnormal although not frankly malignant mononuclear cells.
- Grade 4: marrow with an obvious infiltrate of malignant cells.

This grading of bone marrow histology was offered as an alternative to the simple "yes or no" response to the question asked of the hematologist: is the marrow clear of disease? Apparent clearance of malignant cells does not equate with a normal marrow appearance. Whether such a grading system will prove to be clinically important remains to be seen. However, it was clear from the material examined in this study that histologic patterns identical to the posttreatment fibrotic picture could be found in children with infiltrated bone marrow who had not yet received any treatment. One small study[121] showed that the massive reticulin fibrosis and distorted architecture (grade 3 appearances), which often persisted after treatment, were most unlikely to be caused by the trauma of earlier biopsies. It also contrasted the persistence of abnormal fibrous tissue in treated neuroblastoma with the speed of resolution of fibrosis in B-precursor acute lymphoblastic leukemia. The hypothesis that such persisting fibrosis implies failure to eradicate all tumor from the bone marrow has not yet been effectively tested. The combination of fibrosis, unidentifiable mononuclear cells and, occasionally, ganglion-like cells also raises the possibility that differentiation may be taking place. Whether some of these cells can revert to aggressive neuroblastoma also remains unknown.

Immunocytochemical and molecular techniques
Accurate staging is most problematic in apparently limited stage disease (stages 1–3) and those rare children with stage 4 disease but without obvious marrow involvement. There have been many studies looking at the potential ability of immunologic tests to increase the sensitivity of detection of metastatic disease.[122–124] Unfortunately, there have been problems with specificity because one of the early monoclonal antibodies used, NCAM, was positive in osteoblasts and other tumors such as Ewing tumor, PNET, rhabdomyosarcoma, medulloblastoma, retinoblastoma and pinealblastoma. In addition, antibodies used in immunophenotyping leukemic cells, CD10, CD19 and terminal deoxynucleotidyl transferase (TdT) can be positive in other malignant or reactive conditions.[125] More recently, other monoclonal antibodies have been used, and a study by Swerts and colleagues[126] has compared flow cytometry and immunocytochemistry in detecting

residual neuroblastoma cells in material found negative by cytomorphologic examination. CD9, CD81, CD56, CD45 and GD2 antibodies were used, and 28 bone marrow (BM) samples, 12 biopsies and three peripheral blood stem cell (PBSC) preparations from 22 patients with neuroblastoma were assessed. Flow cytometric and immunocytochemical analyses showed residual neuroblastoma cells in 4 of the 28 BM samples. One PBSC and 20 BM samples were negative for both assays. Four BM and two PBSC were positive with immunocytochemistry but negative with flow analysis. There was a strong correlation between the two techniques, with immunocytochemistry being more sensitive. However, there are no clinical outcome data available and so the significance of the findings has not been determined.

Molecular tests have been developed targeting the TH gene. TH is the first enzyme in the pathway of catecholamine synthesis and is expressed by neuroblastoma cells. RT-PCR and real-time PCR have been used to examine the expression of TH mRNA in neuroblastoma. A study by Tchirkov and colleagues[98] looked at the significance of molecular quantification of minimal residual disease in metastatic neuroblastoma. Real-time PCR that allowed quantification of TH mRNA was performed on 165 BM, peripheral blood (PB) and PBSC samples from 30 children, and results correlated with disease status and patient survival. The levels of TH mRNA agreed well with clinical status and were significantly different across the groups, which included samples obtained from patients at diagnosis, after three cycles of chemotherapy, in complete or very good partial remission, and at relapse. Overall survival was significantly worse for patients with > 1000 TH copies in BM after initial chemotherapy ($P = 0.0075$).

Combinations of techniques may improve accuracy of minimal residual disease detection but will obviously increase expense and complexity. A study by Corrias and colleagues[100] has compared immunocytochemistry with routine cytomorphologic techniques and molecular tests using TH RT-PCR and also has data on outcome. The accuracy of different techniques was studied in 2247 evaluations from 247 patients with neuroblastoma; 561 BMs, 265 PB samples and 69 PBSC were analyzed, and immunocytochemistry using an anti-GD2 antibody gave the most accurate results. Positive results obtained by immunocytochemistry in BM and PB samples taken from stage 1, 2 and 3 patients at diagnosis correlated with an unfavorable outcome. No correlation was found between positive results obtained by immunocytochemistry or TH RT-PCR in BM, PB or PBSC samples from stage 4 patients. Patients who have a negative TH RT-PCR may still have localized deposits in bone marrow, shown using magnetic resonance imaging.[127]

Finally, TH RT-PCR has also been used to determine if PBSC preparations have been contaminated by neuroblastoma cells,[98,100,128] and to estimate tumor depletion in contaminated autografts using CD34 selection.[98] Positive results have correlated with a less favorable outcome in several studies,[98,128] with Tchirkov and colleagues,[98] showing that in 57% of cases PBSC harvests were contaminated by neuroblastoma cells, and at the level of > 500 TH copies survival was significantly decreased ($P = 0.003$).

Molecular and immunocytochemical tests are not yet routine, nor do they replace careful, expert scrutiny of bone marrow aspirates and trephines. However, they may find a place in conjunction with conventional techniques, for instance in those with apparently localized disease and for detecting disease in PBSC preparations.

Soft tissue sarcomas

Soft tissue sarcomas account for approximately 7% of malignant neoplasms in children, and include rhabdomyosarcoma, which is the commonest, and the Ewing family of tumors, namely Ewing sarcoma, primary neuroectodermal tumor of bone (PNET), soft tissue Ewing, and Askin tumor of the chest wall. Major progress in the accuracy of diagnosis and classification has been made by the identification of specific, recurring genetic alterations t(2;13)(q35;q14) and t(1;13)(p36;q14) in alveolar rhabdomyosarcomas, and t(11;22)(q24;q12) or t(21;22)(q22;q12) for the Ewing tumor family.[129]

Rhabdomyosarcoma

Marrow infiltration at presentation is thought to occur in 25–30% of cases.[105,130] Many have been thought to be embryonal rhabdomyosarcoma but more recent reports have been predominantly of alveolar rhabdomyosarcoma.

There may have been some difficulty with inaccurate diagnosis, but this has improved over the past 30 years with the addition of molecular techniques (see above). Disseminated alveolar rhabdomyosarcoma has in the past often been misdiagnosed as a hematologic or other form of cancer,[131–133] particularly those cases with occult primary tumors.

Rhabdomyosarcoma may be the commonest cause of disseminated nonhematopoietic cancer of children and adolescents in whom the primary tumor is hard to find, and although occasionally neuroblastoma can present in this way, there are the biochemical markers of elevated urinary catecholamine metabolites to help make the diagnosis.

Cytology

The cytologic features of alveolar rhabdomyosarcoma in the marrow are characteristic,[131,134] and along with the bone marrow histology are virtually diagnostic.[134] The study by Reid *et al.*[134] described features of alveolar rhabdomyosarcoma, and reported no cases of bone marrow invasion by embryonal rhabdomyosarcoma. In my experience, only one case of infiltration was due to embryonal rhabdomyosarcoma, and this was seen in the bone marrow trephine only. Appearances of marrow infiltration echo those described elsewhere,[131,134] including extensive invasion accompanied by bone marrow failure, and as noted can resemble leukemia. However, there is a tendency for the cells to clump, particularly noted in the trails of the bone marrow smears, but the clumping is not as prominent as in neuroblastoma, Ewing tumor or PNET. Vacuolation of cytoplasm is prominent, often peripherally placed in a rim of cytoplasm that stains darker than the main body of cytoplasm. The vacuoles may coalesce into elongated lakes, and on staining with periodic acid–Schiff (PAS) there is a striking positivity often corresponding to the position of the vacuoles. Multinucleate cells are commonly seen, including giant cells with up to 10 nuclei per cell, and these may be the result of tumor cells having ingested other tumor cells. The tumor cells may also ingest red cells or erythroblasts. However, this is not unique and has been seen in some cases of Ewing tumor as well as in histiocytic malignancy, mono-cytic leukemia and breast cancer, and therefore it is not specific for rhabdomyosarcoma. Nonetheless, this combina-tion of cytologic features is characteristic of rhabdomyosar-coma and should suggest the correct diagnosis. Bone marrow aspirates can also be analyzed for the molecular markers t(2;13)(q35;q14) and t(1;13)(p36;q14) specific to this tumor. There is some recent work indicating that rhabdomyosar-coma cells express chemokine and tyrosine kinase receptors that respond to stromal-derived factor and hepatocyte growth factor, modulating the metastatic behavior of the cells by directing them to the bone marrow and lymph nodes.[135]

Bone marrow histology

Reid and colleagues[134] give a thorough description of the bone marrow histologic features of metastatic rhabdomyosarcoma. This is important for two reasons: the first is that bone mar-row may provide the only tissue for diagnosis if the site of the primary is unknown; the second is the prognostic import-ance, several studies having shown that bone marrow infiltra-tion by rhabdomyosarcoma is associated with a significantly worse outcome.[136] Alveolar patterns of infiltration were found that are so characteristic that, once recognized, the correct diagnosis may be made even in children in whom no primary tumor can be found. Supportive evidence may also be found in the almost universal expression of desmin by the tumor cells and by detecting the translocation t(2;13). The overall rate of marrow infiltration in this study was similar to those reported elsewhere but all cases had alveolar patterns of bone marrow histology. This is different from other centers, in which embryonal rhabdomyosarcoma features strongly; for example, Ruymann *et al.*[130] reported that 12 of 30 cases with bone marrow infiltration had the embryonal subtype. This discrepancy may reflect the relatively small number of published cases investigated by both aspirates and trephine biopsies and the small number of cases reported from indi-vidual centers. Further experience of trephine biopsies and more uniform diagnostic criteria, with the help of other discriminators such as molecular markers, within the entire field of small round-cell cancers are needed to build up an accurate picture of the frequency of bone marrow dissemin-ation in rhabdomyosarcoma.[137]

Ewing tumor and primitive neuroectodermal tumor

The bone marrow is infiltrated in approximately 22–38% of cases of Ewing tumor and PNET.[138,139] Over half of those with bone marrow infiltration have evidence of metastases else-where. Studies emphasize the focal nature of bone marrow metastases and, as in neuroblastoma, highlight the need for examination of more than one site with both aspirates and biopsies as results from each investigation are often not concordant. Immunocytochemical stains have thus far been disappointing as an aid to diagnosis, apart from detecting the apparent lack of desmin positivity. However, molecular studies to detect the translocation t(11;22) or its rarer variant t(21;22), expressing the transcripts *EWS-FLI1* and *EWS-ERG* respectively, have shown that in apparently localized dis-ease, bone marrow micrometastases and circulating malig-nant cells can be detected, and predict poor outcome and systemic relapse.[101,140] Outcome of stem cell transplants may also be predicted by detection of malignant cells, both in the harvest and in the patient posttransplant.[141]

In general, tumor infiltration is less extensive than in neuroblastoma. The cells are approximately twice the size of small lymphocytes, can occur in clumps or smaller aggregates, and occasional rosettes are seen.[110] Cells may be vacuolated with a Burkitt lymphoma-like pattern and dis-tinct from rhabdomyosarcoma. The PAS reaction is often positive, being finely dispersed or showing block positivity. Phagocytosis of other cells is occasionally seen. Histology shows patchy infiltration with irregular groups of cells in a fibrous stroma; desmin stains are negative.

PNET is even rarer than Ewing sarcoma and hematologists/pathologists in any single center will rarely see this tumor infiltrating bone marrow. There are few descriptions of such cells but it appears that they may form clumps readily and have striking vacuolation, sometimes even more so than in Ewing tumor.[139]

Other tumors

There can scarcely be a cancer of childhood that has not been found to infiltrate bone marrow at some stage of the disease. No single center will ever see enough cases to obtain a com-prehensive and reliable in-house background of experience. Instead, occasional examples in atlases of hematology, the handing down of knowledge from hematologist to hema-tologist, and the opinions of other experienced microscopists must be relied upon. Involvement of the bone marrow by osteosarcoma, retinoblastoma, malignant germ-cell tumor and medulloblastoma has been reported. Disseminated osteosar-coma may present a virtually diagnostic picture of a marrow that is very difficult to aspirate and a trephine showing tumor cells embedded in a matrix of osteoid. The few aspirated cells should stain strongly positive for alkaline phosphatase.

Other tissues

Samples of tissue in fluids other than blood or bone marrow are often examined in hematology laboratories, due to the expertise in preparation of these fluids. Techniques include cell counting, cytospin preparation, special stains and flow cytometry. CSF, pleural effusions, ascites fluid and joint fluid may all be examined by a hematologist. Cytospin preparations can result in significant artifact, including a "flattening" effect and the displacement of granules to one side of the cell. In addition, normal nonhematopoietic cells present in, for example, pleural fluid or ascites can look malignant. Such cells are usually mesothelial lining cells or reactive macrophages. Where the fluid is infiltrated with malignant hematopoietic cells, the diagnosis is not usually too difficult as the mesothelial cells will be in the minority and supplementary immunophenotypic and cytogenetic analysis can be performed. However, problems in correctly identifying mesothelial cells may arise if nonhematopoietic malignant infiltration is suspected, not least because the number of malignant cells in effusions or ascites in such cases is often much lower than in cases of lymphoblastic or Burkitt lymphoma, and mesothelial cells are thus relatively more prominent; there may also be a scattering of lymphoid cells. Immunophenotypic analysis of these lymphoid cells is unhelpful and, at worst, confusing. Most will be T cells and as immunophenotyping does not discriminate between monoclonal or polyclonal proliferation, this might mislead the unwary into diagnosing a lymphoid malignancy. Molecular studies to show polyclonal T-cell infiltrates may not be readily available in many centers and may take too long to be immediately helpful to clinicians. Nonhematopoietic tumor cells have a tendency to clump but otherwise have no characteristic cytologic features. The pattern of vacuolation may be helpful in rhabdomyosarcoma but collective experience of such infiltration is not reported. Morphologic expertise is of great importance. Just as consultation with a histopathologist can be very helpful with interpretation of trephine specimens, so can discussion with an experienced cytopathologist in such cases.

Brain tumors and retinoblastoma are well known to involve the CSF although rarely at presentation (<1% of low-stage cases).[142] If extraglobal progression is found after enucleation, or other signs or symptoms of central nervous system involvement are present, both bone marrow and CSF examination should be carried out.

Conclusions

There are few descriptions of peripheral blood, bone marrow and other body fluid abnormalities in children with nonhematopoietic cancer. Reports of results with immunocytochemical and molecular techniques are much more common, but comparison with morphologic and histologic findings is not always made. It is tempting to equate positive results using the newer, possibly more sensitive techniques with clinical significance but more studies are needed to evaluate specificity, sensitivity and prognostic potential. These techniques are complex and expensive and are only available in a few specialized centers. It is therefore essential that they do not replace the conventional diagnostic and staging assessment of nonhematopoietic tumors. However, it is also incumbent upon hematologists to set diagnostic and investigative standards through collaboration with other centers and networks and to be rigorous in their description and recording of findings in this rare set of tumors.

Acknowledgments

I would like to thank Annette Weddell, data manager at the Royal Hospital for Sick Children, Edinburgh, and Jennifer Ferguson at the Royal Hospital for Sick Children, Glasgow, for retrieving the peripheral blood and bone marrow data on patients with nonhematopoietic tumors.

References

1. Fitzsimons EJ, Brock JH. The anaemia of chronic disease. *Br Med J* 2001; **322**: 811–12.
2. Lee EJ, Oh EJ, Park YJ, Lee HK, Kim BK. Soluble transferrin receptor (sTfR), ferritin and sTfR/log ferritin index in anemic patients with nonhematologic malignancy and chronic inflammation. *Clin Chem* 2002; **48**: 1118–21.
3. Lee G. The anaemia of chronic disease. *Semin Hematol* 1983; **20**: 61–80.
4. Krantz S. Pathogenesis and treatment of the anemia of chronic disease. *Am J Med Sci* 1994; **307**: 353–9.
5. Means RJ. Pathogenesis of the anemia of chronic disease. *Stem Cell* 1995; **13**: 32–7.
6. Cavill I, Ricketts C, Napier J. Erythropoiesis in the anaemia of chronic disease. *Scand J Haematol* 1977; **19**: 509–12.
7. Means RJ. Clinical application of recombinant erythropoietin in the anemia of chronic disease. *Hematol Oncol Clin North Am* 1994; **8**: 933–44.
8. Krantz S. Erythropoietin and the anemia of chronic disease. *Nephrol Dial Transplant* 1995; **10** (suppl. 2): 10–17.
9. Bain B. Quantitative changes in blood cells. In: Bain BJ (ed.) *Blood Cells: A Practical Guide*, 2nd edn. Oxford: Blackwell Science, 1995, pp. 160–83.
10. MacDougall I, Hutton R, Cavill I. Treating renal anaemia with recombinant human erythropoietin: practical guidelines and a clinical algorithm. *Br Med J* 1990; **300**: 655–9.
11. Moia M, Mannucci P, Vizzotto L, Casati S, Cattaneo M, Ponticelli C. Improvement in the haemostatic defect of uraemia

after treatment with recombinant human erythropoietin. *Lancet* 1987; **ii**: 1227–9.

12. Monnens L, van de Meer W, Langenhuysen C, van Munster P, van Oustrom C. Platelet aggregating factor in the epidemic form of haemolytic-uraemic syndrome of childhood. *Clin Nephrol* 1985; **15**: 14–17.

13. Rondeau E, Peraldi M-N. *Escherichia coli* and the hemolytic uremic syndrome. *N Engl J Med* 1996; **355**: 660–2.

14. Siegler R. The hemolytic uremic syndrome. *Pediatr Clin North Am* 1995; **42**: 1505–29.

15. Renaud C, Niaudet P, Gagnadoux M, Breyer M, Habib R. Haemolytic uraemic syndrome: prognostic factors in children over 3 years of age. *Pediatr Nephrol* 1995; **9**: 24–9.

16. Fuge R, Bird JM, Fraser A *et al.* The clinical features, risk factors and outcome of thrombotic thrombocytopenic purpura occurring after bone marrow transplantation. *Br J Haematol* 2001; **113**: 58–64.

17. Coppo P, Veyradier A, Durey MA *et al.* [Pathophysiology of thrombotic microangiopathies: current understanding.] *Ann Med Interne (Paris)* 2002; **153**: 153–66.

18. Sills R. Thrombotic thrombocytopenic purpura: I. Pathophysiology and clinical manifestations. *Am J Pediatr Hematol Oncol* 1984; **6**: 425–30.

19. Peyvandi F, Ferrari S, Lavoretano S, Canciani MT, Mannucci PM. von Willebrand factor cleaving protease (ADAMTS-13) and ADAMTS-13 neutralizing autoantibodies in 100 patients with thrombotic thrombocytopenic purpura. *Br J Haematol* 2004; **127**: 433–9.

20. Upshaw J. Congenital deficiency of a factor in normal plasma that reverses microangiopathic hemolysis and thrombocytopenia. *N Engl J Med* 1978; **298**: 1350–2.

21. Rock G, Shumak K, Buskard N *et al.* Comparison of plasma exchange with plasma infusion in the treatment of thrombotic thrombocytopenic purpura. *N Engl J Med* 1991; **325**: 393–7.

22. Rock G, Shumak K, Sutton D *et al.* Cryosupernatant as replacement fluid for plasma exchange in thrombotic thrombocytopenic purpura. *Br J Haematol* 1996; **94**: 383–6.

23. Lu J, Basu A, Melenhorst JJ, Young NS, Brown KE. Analysis of T-cell repertoire in hepatitis-associated aplastic anemia. *Blood* 2004; **103**: 4588–93.

24. Dahele A, Ghosh S. Vitamin B12 deficiency in untreated celiac disease. *Am J Gastroenterol* 2001; **96**: 745–50.

25. Wardrop C, Huthinson H. Red cell shape in hypothyroidism. *Lancet* 1969; **ii**: 1243.

26. Merchav S, Tatarsky I, Hochberg Z. Enhancement of erythropoiesis *in vitro* by human growth hormone is mediated by insulin-like growth factor. *Br J Haematol* 1988; **70**: 267–71.

27. Sohmiya M, Kato Y. Effect of long-term administration of recombinant human growth hormone (rhGH) on plasma erythropoietin (EPO) and haemoglobin levels in anaemic patients with adult GH deficiency. *Clin Endocrinol* 2001; **55**: 749–54.

28. Levin E, Wu J, Devine DV *et al.* Hemostatic parameters and platelet activation marker expression in cyanotic and acyanotic pediatric patients undergoing cardiac surgery in the presence of tranexamic acid. *Thromb Haemost* 2000; **83**: 54–9.

29. Kumor-Kurek M, Siudalska H. [Hematologic disorders in patients with cyanotic congenital heart disease.] *Pol Merkuriusz Lek* 1999; **7**: 82–4.

30. Perloff JK, Rosove MH, Child JS, Wright GB. Adults with cyanotic congenital heart disease: hematologic management. *Ann Intern Med* 1988; **109**: 406–13.

31. Gaiha M, Sethi HP, Sudha R, Arora R, Acharya NR. A clinico-hematological study of iron deficiency anemia and its correlation with hyperviscosity symptoms in cyanotic congenital heart disease. *Indian Heart J* 1993; **45**: 53–5.

32. Perloff JK, Marelli AJ, Miner PD. Risk of stroke in adults with cyanotic congenital heart disease. *Circulation* 1994; **89**: 911.

33. Brouard J, Morin M, Borel B *et al.* [Di George's syndrome complicated by graft versus host reaction.] *Arch Fr Pediatr* 1985; **42**: 853–5.

34. Wintergerst U, Meyer U, Remberger K, Belohradsky BH. [Graft versus host reaction in an infant with DiGeorge syndrome.] *Monatsschr Kinderheilkd* 1989; **137**: 345–7.

35. Weller P, Bubley G. The idiopathic hypereosinophilic syndrome. *Blood* 1994; **83**: 2759–79.

36. Smith T, Welch T, Allen J, Sondheimer J. Cutaneous mastocytosis with bleeding: probable heparin effect. *Cutis* 1987; **39**: 241–4.

37. Brett EM, Ong BH, Friedmann T. Mast-cell disease in children. Report of eleven cases. *Br J Dermatol* 1967; **79**: 197–209.

38. Hansen U, Wiese R, Knolle J. [Shock and coagulation disorders in systemic mastocytosis.] *Dtsch Med Wochenschr* 1994; **119**: 1231–4.

39. Arock M. [Mastocytosis, classification, biological diagnosis and therapy.] *Ann Biol Clin (Paris)* 2004; **62**: 657–69.

40. Azana J, Torrelo A, Mediero I, Zambrano A. Urticaria pigmentosa: a review of 67 pediatric cases. *Pediatr Dermatol* 1994; **11**: 102–6.

41. Dixon R, Rosse W, Ebbert L. Quantitative determination of antibody in idiopathic thrombocytopenic purpura. *N Engl J Med* 1975; **292**: 230–6.

42. Hall S, McCormick J, Griepp P, Michet C, McKenna C. Splenectomy does not cure the thrombocytopenia of systemic lupus erythematosus. *Ann Intern Med* 1985; **102**: 325–8.

43. Miller M, Urowitz M, Gladman D. The significance of thrombocytopenia in systemic lupus erythematosus. *Arthritis Rheumatol* 1983; **26**: 1181–6.

44. Cazzola M, Ponchio L, de-Benedetti F *et al.* Defective iron supply for erythropoiesis and adequate endogenous erythropoietin production in the anemia associated with systemic-onset juvenile chronic arthritis. *Blood* 1996; **87**: 4824–30.

45. Arndt U, Kaltwasser JP, Gottschalk R, Hoelzer D, Moller B. Correction of iron-deficient erythropoiesis in the treatment of anemia of chronic disease with recombinant human erythropoietin. *Ann Hematol* 2005; **84**: 159–66.

46. Frosch M, Foell D. Wegener granulomatosis in childhood and adolescence. *Eur J Pediatr* 2004; **163**: 425–34.

47. Zipursky A, Palko J, Milner R *et al.* The hematology of bacterial infections in premature infants. *Pediatrics* 1976; **57**: 839–53.

48. Skeppner G, Kreuger A, Elinder G. Transient erythroblastopenia of childhood: prospective study of 10 patients with special reference to viral infections. *J Pediatr Hematol Oncol* 2002; **24**: 294–8.

49. Grose C, Horwitz M. Characterization of an enterovirus associated with acute infectious lymphocytosis. *J Gen Virol* 1976; **30**: 347–55.

50. Seges RA, Kenny A, Bird GW, Wingham J, Baals H, Stauffer UG. Pediatric surgical patients with severe anaerobic infection: report of 16 T-antigen positive cases and possible hazards of blood transfusion. *J Pediatr Surg* 1981; **16**: 905–10.

51. Caya JG, Farmer SG, Ritch PS *et al*. Clostridial septicemia complicating the course of leukemia. *Cancer* 1986; **57**: 2045–8.

52. Becker RC, Giuliani M, Savage RA, Weick JK. Massive hemolysis in *Clostridium perfringens* infections. *Surg Oncol* 1987; **35**: 13–18.

53. Bowman HS, Marsh WL, Schumacher HR, Oyen R, Reihart J. Auto anti-N immunohemolytic anemia in infectious mononucleosis. *Am J Clin Pathol* 1974; **61**: 465–72.

54. Sharp A. Platelets, bleeding and haemostasis in infectious mononucleosis. In: Carter R, Penman H (eds) *Infectious Mononucleosis*. Oxford: Blackwell Scientific, 1969.

55. Duncombe A, Amos R, Metcalfe P, Pearson T. Intravenous immunoglobulin therapy in thrombocytopenic infectious mononucleosis. *Clin Lab Haematol* 1989; **11**: 11–15.

56. Purtilo DT. X-linked lymphoproliferative disease (XLP) as a model of Epstein–Barr virus-induced immunopathology. *Springer Semin Immunopathol* 1991; **13**: 181–97.

57. Gratama J. Epstein–Barr virus infections in bone marrow transplant recipients. In: Forman S, Blume K, Thomas E (eds) *Bone Marrow Transplantation*. Boston: Blackwell Scientific Publications, 1994.

58. van den Bosch CA. Is endemic Burkitt's lymphoma an alliance between three infections and a tumour promoter? *Lancet Oncol* 2004; **5**: 738–46.

59. Rochford R, Cannon MJ, Moormann AM. Endemic Burkitt's lymphoma: a polymicrobial disease? *Nat Rev Microbiol* 2005; **3**: 182–7.

60. Zon L, Groopman J. Hematologic manifestations of the human immunodeficiency virus. *Semin Hematol* 1988; **25**: 208–18.

61. Hilgartner M. Hematologic manifestations in HIV-infected children. *J Pediatr* 1991; **119**: S47–S49.

62. Saif MW. HIV-associated autoimmune hemolytic anemia: an update. *AIDS Patient Care STDS* 2001; **15**: 217–24.

63. Vetter KM, Djomond G, Zadi F *et al*. Clinical spectrum of human immunodeficiency virus disease in children in a West African city. Project RETRO-CI. *Pediatr Infect Dis J* 1996; **15**: 438–42.

64. Ellaurie M, Burns E, Bernstein L *et al*. Thrombocytopenia and human immunodeficiency virus in children. *Pediatrics* 1988; **82**: 905–8.

65. Nachman S, Gona P, Dankner W *et al*. The rate of serious bacterial infections among HIV-infected children with immune reconstitution who have discontinued opportunistic infection prophylaxis. *Pediatrics* 2005 Mar 16 [Epub ahead of print].

66. Serraino D, Franceschi S. Kaposi's sarcoma and non-Hodgkin's lymphomas in children and adolescents with AIDS. *AIDS* 1996; **10**: 643–7.

67. Prowse C, Dow B, Pelly SJ *et al*. Human parvovirus B19 infection in persons with haemophilia. *Thromb Haemost* 1998; **80**: 351.

68. Kurtzman G, Ozawa K, Cohen B, Hanson G, Oseas R, Young N. Chronic bone marrow failure due to persistent B19 parvovirus infection. *N Engl J Med* 1987; **317**: 287–94.

69. Mihal V, Dusek J, Hajduch M, Cohen B, Fingerova H, Vesely J. Transient aplastic crisis in a leukemic child caused by

70. Young NS. Parvovirus infection and its treatment. *Clin Exp Immunol* 1996; **104** (suppl. 1): 26–30.

71. van Horn D, Mortimer P, Young N *et al*. Human parvovirus-associated red cell aplasia in the absence of underlying hemolytic anemia. *Am J Pediatr Hematol Oncol* 1986; **8**: 235–9.

72. Newburger JW, Takahashi M, Gerber MA *et al*. Diagnosis, treatment, and long-term management of Kawasaki disease: a statement for health professionals from the Committee on Rheumatic Fever, Endocarditis, and Kawasaki Disease, Council on Cardiovascular Disease in the Young, American Heart Association. *Pediatrics* 2004; **114**: 1708–33.

73. Samuel J, O'Sullivan J. Kawasaki disease. *Br J Hosp Med* 1996; **55**: 91.

74. Gupta M, Noel GJ, Schaefer M, Friedman D, Bussel J, Johann-Liang R. Cytokine modulation with immune gamma-globulin in peripheral blood of normal children and its implications in Kawasaki disease treatment. *J Clin Immunol* 2001; **21**: 193–9.

75. Fondu R, Haga P, Halvorsen S. The regulation of erythropoiesis in protein-calorie malnutrition. *Br J Haematol* 1978; **38**: 29–36.

76. Selvaraj R, Bhat K. Metabolic and bactericidal activities in leukocytes in protein-calorie malnutrition. *Am J Clin Nutr* 1972; **25**: 166–74.

77. Keenan WJ. Macrocytosis as an indicator of human disease. *J Am Board Fam Pract* 1989; **2**: 252–6.

78. Devuyst O, Lambert M, Rodhain J, Lefebvre C, Coche E. Haematological changes and infectious complications in anorexia nervosa. *Q J Med* 1993; **86**: 791–9.

79. Bailly D, Lambin I, Garzon G, Parquet P. Bone marrow hypoplasia in anorexia nervosa: a case report. *Int J Eat Disord* 1994; **16**: 97–100.

80. Mant M, Faragher B. The haematology of anorexia nervosa. *Br J Haematol* 1972; **23**: 737–49.

81. Barr RD, Copeland SA, Stockwell ML, Morris N, Kelton JC. Valproic acid and immune thrombocytopenia. *Arch Dis Child* 1982; **57**: 681–4.

82. Ko CH, Kong CK, Tse PW. Valproic acid and thrombo-cytopenia: cross-sectional study. *Hong Kong Med J* 2001; **7**: 15–21.

83. Conley EL, Coley KC, Pollock BG, Dapos SV, Maxwell R, Branch RA. Prevalence and risk of thrombocytopenia with valproic acid: experience at a psychiatric teaching hospital. *Pharmacotherapy* 2001; **21**: 1325–30.

84. De Berardis D, Campanella D, Matera V *et al*. Thrombo-cytopenia during valproic acid treatment in young patients with new-onset bipolar disorder. *J Clin Psychopharmacol* 2003; **23**: 451–8.

85. Ganick DJ, Sunder T, Finley JL. Severe hematologic toxicity of valproic acid: a report of four patients. *Am J Pediatr Hematol Oncol* 1990; **12**: 80–5.

86. Gesundheit B, Kirby M, Lau W, Koren G, Abdelhaleem M. Thrombocytopenia and megakaryocyte dysplasia: an adverse effect of valproic acid treatment. *J Pediatr Hematol Oncol* 2002; **24**: 589–90.

87. Harenberg J, Jorg I, Fenyvesi T. Heparin-induced thrombocytopenia: pathophysiology and new treatment options. *Pathophysiol Haemost Thromb* 2002; **32**: 289–94.

88. Warkentin TE, Kelton JG. A 14 year study of heparin-induced thrombocytopenia. *Am J Med* 1996; **101**: 502–7.

89. Lubenow N. New developments in diagnosis and treatment of heparin-induced thrombocytopenia. *Pathophysiol Haemost Thromb* 2003–2004; **33**: 407–12.

90. Risch L, Fischer JE, Herklotz R, Huber AR. Heparin-induced thrombocytopenia in paediatrics: clinical characteristics, therapy and outcomes. *Intensive Care Med* 2004; **30**: 1615–24.

91. Altman AJ. Management of malignant solid tumors. In: Nathan DG, Oski FA (eds) *Hematology of Infancy and Childhood*, 4th edn. Philadelphia: WB Saunders, 1992, pp. 1384.

92. Vora AJ, Lilleyman JS. Secondary thrombocytosis. *Arch Dis Child* 1993; **68**: 88–90.

93. Frenkel EP. Southwestern internal medicine conference; the clinical spectrum of thrombocytosis and thrombocythemia. *Am J Med Sci* 1991; **301**: 69–80.

94. De Beneditti F, Martini A. Secondary thrombocytosis. *Arch Dis Child* 1993; **69**: 170–1.

95. Christenson WN, Ultmann JE, Mohos SC. Disseminated neuroblastoma in an adult presenting the picture of thrombocytopenic purpura. *Blood* 1956; **11**: 273–8.

96. Pollack ER, Miller HJ, Vye MV. Medulloblastoma presenting as leukemia. *Am J Clin Pathol* 1981; **76**: 98–103.

97. Nunez C, Abboud SL, Lemon NC, Kemp JA. Ovarian rhabdomyosarcoma presenting as leukemia. *Cancer* 1983; **52**: 297–300.

98. Tchirkov A, Paillard C, Halle P *et al.* Significance of molecular quantification of minimal residual disease in metastatic neuroblastoma. *J Hematother Stem Cell Res* 2003; **12**: 435–42.

99. Cheung IY, Sahota A, Cheung NK. Measuring circulating neuroblastoma cells by quantitative reverse transcriptase-polymerase chain reaction analysis. *Cancer* 2004; **101**: 2303–8.

100. Corrias MV, Faulkner LB, Pistorio A *et al.* Detection of neuroblastoma cells in bone marrow and peripheral blood by different techniques: accuracy and relationship with clinical features of patients. *Clin Cancer Res* 2004; **10**: 7978–85.

101. Avigad S, Cohen IJ, Zilberstein J *et al.* The predictive potential of molecular detection in the nonmetastatic Ewing family of tumors. *Cancer* 2004; **100**: 1053–8.

102. Delattre O, Zucman J, Melot T *et al.* The Ewing family of tumors: a subgroup of small-round-cell tumors defined by specific chimeric transcripts. *N Engl J Med* 1994; **331**: 294–9.

103. Mehes G, Luegmayr A, Ambros IM, Ladenstein R, Ambros PF. Combined automatic immunological and molecular cytogenetic analysis allows exact identification and quantification of tumor cells in the bone marrow. *Clin Cancer Res* 2001; **7**: 1969–75.

104. Delta BG, Pinkel D. Bone marrow aspiration in children with malignant tumors. *J Pediatr* 1964; **64**: 542–6.

105. Finklestein JZ, Ekert H, Isaacs H Jr, Higgins G. Bone marrow metastases in children with solid tumors. *Am J Dis Child* 1970; **119**: 49–52.

106. Franklin IM, Pritchard J. Detection of bone marrow invasion by neuroblastoma is improved by sampling at two sites with both aspirates and trephine biopsies. *J Clin Pathol* 1983; **36**: 1215–18.

107. Brodeur GM, Seeger RC, Barrett A *et al.* International criteria for diagnosis, staging and response to treatment in patients with neuroblastoma. *J Clin Oncol* 1988; **6**: 1874–81.

108. Brodeur GM, Pritchard J, Berthold F *et al.* Revisions of the international criteria for neuroblastoma diagnosis, staging and response to treatment. *J Clin Oncol* 1993; **11**: 1466–77.

109. Mills AE, Bird AR. Bone marrow changes in neuroblastoma. *Pediatr Pathol* 1986; **5**: 225–34.

110. Smith SR, Reid MM. Neuroblastoma rosettes in aspirated bone marrow. *Br J Haematol* 1994; **88**: 445–7.

111. Head DR, Kennedy PS, Goyette RE. Metastatic neuroblastoma in bone marrow aspirate smear. *Am J Clin Pathol* 1979; **72**: 1008–11.

112. Goldman A, Vivian G, Gordon I, Pritchard J, Kemshead J. Immunolocalization of neuroblastoma using radiolabeled monoclonal antibody. UJ 13A. *J Pediatr* 1984; **105**: 252–6.

113. Kemshead JT, Clayton J, Patel K. Monoclonal antibodies used for the diagnosis of the small round cell tumors of childhood. In: Kemshead JT (ed.) *Pediatric Tumors: Immunological and Molecular Markers*. Boca Raton, FL: CRC Press, 1989, pp. 31–45.

114. Reid MM. Detection of marrow infiltration by neuroblastoma in clinical practice: how far have we come? *Eur J Cancer* 1994; **30A**: 134–5.

115. Reid MM, Hamilton PJ. Histology of neuroblastoma involving bone marrow: the problem of detecting residual tumour after initiation of chemotherapy. *Br J Haematol* 1988; **69**: 487–90.

116. Savage RS, Hoffman GC, Shaker K. Diagnostic problems involved in detection of metastatic neoplasms by bone-marrow aspirate compared with needle biopsy. *Am J Clin Pathol* 1978; **70**: 623–7.

117. Bostrom B, Nesbit ME Jr, Brunning RD. The value of bone marrow trephine biopsy in the diagnosis of metastatic neuroblastoma. *Am J Pediatr Hematol Oncol* 1985; **7**: 303–5.

118. Favrot MC, Frappaz D, Maritaz O *et al.* Histological, cytological and immunological analyses are complementary for the detection of neuroblastoma cells in bone marrow. *Br J Cancer* 1986; **54**: 637–41.

119. Reid MM, Roald B. Adequacy of bone marrow trephine biopsy specimens in children. *J Clin Pathol* 1996; **49**: 226–9.

120. Reid MM, Pearson ADJ. Bone-marrow infiltration in neuroblastoma. *Lancet* 1991; **337**: 681–2.

121. Turner GE, Reid MM. What is marrow fibrosis after treatment of neuroblastoma? *J Clin Pathol* 1993; **46**: 61–3.

122. Oppedal BR, Storm-Mathisen I, Kemshead JT, Brandtzaeg P. Bone marrow examination in neuroblastoma patients: a morphologic, immunocytochemical, and immuno-histochemical study. *Hum Pathol* 1989; **20**: 800–5.

123. Carey PJ, Thomas L, Buckle G, Reid MM. Immunocytochemical examination of bone marrow in disseminated neuroblastoma. *J Clin Pathol* 1990; **43**: 9–12.

124. Reid MM, Malcolm AJ, McGuckin AG. Immunocytochemical detection of neuroblastoma in frozen sections of bone marrow trephine biopsy specimens. *J Clin Pathol* 1990; **43**: 334–6.

125. Longacre TA, Foucar K, Crago S *et al.* Hematogones: a multiparameter analysis of bone marrow precursor cells. *Blood* 1989; **73**: 543–52.

126. Swerts K, De Moerloose B, Dhooge C *et al.* Detection of residual neuroblastoma cells in bone marrow: comparison of flow cytometry with immunocytochemistry. *Cytometry B Clin Cytom* 2004; **61**: 9–19.

127. Takemoto C, Nishiuchi R, Endo C, Oda M, Seino Y. Comparison of two methods for evaluating bone marrow

metastasis of neuroblastoma: Reverse transcription-polymerase chain reaction for tyrosine hydroxylase and magnetic resonance imaging. *Pediatr Int* 2004; **46**: 387–93.

128. Burchill SA, Kinsey SE, Picton S *et al.* Minimal residual disease at the time of peripheral blood stem cell harvest in patients with advanced neuroblastoma. *Med Pediatr Oncol* 2001; **36**: 213–19.

129. Koscielniak E, Morgan M, Treuner J. Soft tissue sarcoma in children: prognosis and management. *Paediatr Drugs* 2002; **4**: 21–8.

130. Ruymann FB, Newton WA Jr, Ragab AH, Donaldson MH, Foulkes M. Bone marrow metastases at diagnosis in children and adolescents with rhabdomyosarcoma. A report from the intergroup rhabdomyosarcoma study. *Cancer* 1984; **53**: 368–73.

131. Etcubanas E, Peiper S, Stass S, Green A. Rhabdomyosarcoma, presenting as disseminated malignancy from an unknown primary site: a retrospective study of ten pediatric cases. *Med Pediatr Oncol* 1989; **17**: 39–44.

132. Maywald O, Metzgeroth G, Schoch C *et al.* Alveolar rhabdomyosarcoma with bone marrow infiltration mimicking haematological neoplasia. *Br J Haematol* 2002; **119**: 583.

133. Cheng L, Shah HO, Lin JH. Alveolar rhabdomyosarcoma with concurrent metastases to bone marrow and lymph nodes simulating acute hematologic malignancy. *J Pediatr Hematol Oncol* 2004; **26**: 696–7.

134. Reid MM, Saunders PWG, Bown N *et al.* Alveolar rhabdomyosarcoma infiltrating bone marrow at presentation: the value to diagnosis of bone marrow trephine biopsy specimens. *J Clin Pathol* 1992; **45**: 759–62.

135. Jankowski K, Kucia M, Wysoczynski M *et al.* Both hepatocyte growth factor (HGF) and stromal-derived factor-1 regulate the metastatic behavior of human rhabdomyosarcoma cells, but only HGF enhances their resistance to radiochemotherapy. *Cancer Res* 2003; **63**: 7926–35.

136. Carli M, Colombatti R, Oberlin O *et al.* European intergroup studies (MMT4-89 and MMT4-91) on childhood metastatic rhabdomyosarcoma: final results and analysis of prognostic factors. *J Clin Oncol* 2004; **22**: 4787–94.

137. Athale UH, Shurtleff SA, Jenkins JJ *et al.* Use of reverse transcriptase polymerase chain reaction for diagnosis and staging of alveolar rhabdomyosarcoma, Ewing sarcoma family of tumors, and desmoplastic small round cell tumor. *J Pediatr Hematol Oncol* 2001; **23**: 99–104.

138. Oberlin O, Bayle C, Hartmann O, Terrier-Lacombe MJ, Lemerle J. Incidence of bone marrow involvement in Ewing's sarcoma: value of extensive investigation of the bone marrow. *Med Pediatr Oncol* 1995; **24**: 343–6.

139. Reid MM. Hematologic effects of non-hemopoietic tumors. In: Lilleyman J, Hann I, Blanchette V (eds) *Pediatric Hematology*, 2nd edn. London: Churchill Livingstone, 1999, pp. 791–800.

140. Schleiermacher G, Peter M, Oberlin O *et al.* Increased risk of systemic relapses associated with bone marrow micrometastasis and circulating tumor cells in localized Ewing tumor. *J Clin Oncol* 2003; **21**: 85–91.

141. Yaniv I, Cohen IJ, Stein J *et al.* Tumor cells are present in stem cell harvests of Ewings sarcoma patients and their persistence following transplantation is associated with relapse. *Pediatr Blood Cancer* 2004; **42**: 404–9.

142. Pratt CB, Meyer D, Chenaille P, Crom DB. The use of bone marrow aspirations and lumbar punctures at the time of diagnosis of retinoblastoma. *J Clin Oncol* 1989; **7**: 140–3.

36   Lysosomal storage disorders

Brad T. Tinkle and Gregory A. Grabowski

Introduction

The lysosomal storage disorders (LSDs) are a group of more than 40 different diseases, the majority of which are caused by a deficiency of a lysosomal enzyme (Table 36.1). Most result from single gene mutations that alter an enzyme's amino acid sequence. However, several LSDs result from gene deficits that alter posttranslational modification of lysosomal enzymes with consequent defects in multiple enzymes. The pathogenesis of the LSDs derives from an inability to adequately degrade normal metabolites within lysosomes. The particular metabolites accumulate to abnormal levels (i.e., stores) within a variety of tissues or cell types giving rise to the clinical heterogeneity.

The incidence of LSDs, as a group, is roughly 1 in 7000 to 1 in 9000.[1,2] All but two LSDs are autosomal recessive. Thus, family histories are usually not informative. Fabry disease and mucopolysaccharidosis type II are X-linked, and familial recurrence is likely. The rarity and clinical variability of the LSDs makes recognition challenging and underdiagnosis likely. Moreover, essentially all LSDs manifest in childhood, thereby placing the pediatrician and/or pediatric hematologist at the cutting edge of their medical care. For many LSDs, an abnormal peripheral blood smear and/or characteristic bone marrow findings can be the first clue to diagnosis.

The significant morbidity and/or mortality associated with each LSD and the development of effective cell and enzyme replacement therapies have made recognition and accurate diagnosis essential. The marked clinical variability and, in some, phenotypic similarity to other LSDs makes differentiation among the LSDs challenging even for experienced physicians. For example, the mucopolysaccharidoses have significant clinical similarities including characteristic bony abnormalities (dysostosis multiplex), hepatosplenomegaly, neurologic impairment and coarse facial features. Although most of the LSDs have been characterized at the biochemical

and genetic levels, selecting the specific biochemical or genetic test can be daunting. Clinical insight can guide the selection of the proper tests to expedite the diagnosis. Fortunately, detailed history, physical examination, and a few simple tests can significantly focus the differential diagnosis.

Many patients afflicted by an LSD will present to the pediatric hematologist with hypersplenism, thrombophilia, anemia, and/or unusual bony abnormalities on radiography. Inclusion bodies within white blood cells or their precursors are observed in several of the LSDs, making a peripheral blood smear examination highly useful (Table 36.1). The cells of interest are best observed in the trail of the smear. Using standard staining methods, vacuolation may be present in lymphocytes or monocytes, and careful examination of the neutrophils and eosinophils can reveal typical inclusion bodies (e.g., Alder–Reilly bodies). Lymphocytic vacuolations are typically clear and well demarcated and can occur as small or large vacuoles of variable number. Monocyte vacuolation is best appreciated in smears from anticoagulated blood. Examination under polarized light may also be helpful and can reveal birefringent storage material. Additional stains or ultrastructural examination are not very useful in narrowing the diagnostic list but can be used as a supplement if initial testing does not define the LSD.

Bone marrow aspirates can be equally revealing and, indeed, may be essential in guiding further work-up. In the absence of a diagnostic peripheral smear (e.g., hereditary spherocytosis), children presenting with cytopenias or asymptomatic splenomegaly require a bone marrow biopsy with marrow aspiration to exclude infection, malignancy, or a LSD. Bone marrow aspirates for LSDs are best prepared from anticoagulated marrow samples as they are easy to spread, provide excellent cell type recognition, and cellular contents of lipids, carbohydrates and enzymes are preserved. Several stains to characterize storage materials should be considered including periodic acid–Schiff (PAS) for carbohydrates, lipid stains such as luxol fast blue and Sudan black, alcoholic basic

Table 36.1 The various types of lysosomal storage disorders and the characteristic cellular attributes.

Disease	Eponym/synonym	Enzyme deficiency/protein function	Characteristic cell types
Aspartylglucosaminuria		Aspartylglucosaminidase	Small lymphocytic vacuoles
Cholesteryl ester storage disease	Wolman disease	Lysosomal acid lipase	Foamy macrophage (rare); lymphocytic lipid inclusions; sea-blue histiocytes (rare)
		Cholesteryl ester storage disease	
Cystinosis		Lysosomal cystine transport protein	Cystine crystals within foam cells
Fabry disease	Fabry disease	α-galactosidase A	Foamy macrophages
Farber lipogranulomatosis	Farber disease	Acid ceramidase	Foamy macrophages
Fucosidosis		α-L-fucosidase	Foamy macrophages with hemophagocytosis; small lymphocytic inclusions; vacuolated plasma cells
Galactosialidosis types I and II		Protective protein for β-galactosidase and neuraminidase	Foamy macrophages (rare); vacuolated lymphocytes
Gaucher disease types I, II and III	Gaucher disease	Glucocerebrosidase	Gaucher cell
Globoid cell leukodystrophy	Krabbe disease	Galactocerebrosidase	
Glycogen storage disease II	Pompe disease	Acid α-glucosidase	Lymphocyte glycogen inclusions
G_{M1} gangliosidosis types I, II and III	Landing disease	β-galactosidase	Foamy macrophages (rare); coarsely vacuolated lymphocytes; abnormal granules of the eosinophils
G_{M2} gangliosidosis type I	Tay–Sachs disease	β-hexosaminidase A	
G_{M2} gangliosidosis type II	Sandhoff disease	β-hexosaminidases A and B	Foamy macrophages; vacuolated lymphocytes
G_{M2} gangliosidosis type AB	Tay–Sachs disease, AB variant	G_{M2}-activator	
α-mannosidosis types I and II		α-mannosidase	Foamy macrophages; vacuolated lymphocytes and plasma cells
β-mannosidosis		β-mannosidase	
Metachromatic leukodystrophy	Late infantile, juvenile, and adult forms	Arylsulfatase A	
Metachromatic leukodystrophy	Adult metachromatic leukodystrophy	Saposin B	
Mucolipidosis type I	Sialidosis types I/II	Neuraminidase/sialidase 1	Foamy macrophages; vacuolated lymphocytes; finely granulated neutrophils
Mucolipidosis types II and III	I-cell disease Pseudo-Hurler polydystrophy	N-acetylglucosamine-1-phosphotransferase	Small lymphocytic inclusions; vacuolated plasma cells
Mucolipidosis type III	Pseudo-Hurler polydystrophy	Phosphotransferase γ-subunit	Foamy macrophages; vacuolated plasma cells
Mucolipidosis type IV		Mitochondrial NADH dehydrogenase 5	Gasser cells (few); Alder–Reilly bodies
Mucopolysaccharidosis type I	Hurler, Hurler–Scheie and Scheie syndromes	α-L-Iduronidase	Gasser cells
Mucopolysaccharidosis type II	Hunter syndrome	Iduronate sulfatase	Gasser cells; vacuolated lymphocytes
Mucopolysaccharidosis type IIIA	Sanfilippo syndrome	Heparan N-sulfatase	Gasser cells
Mucopolysaccharidosis type IIIB	Sanfilippo syndrome	α-N-acetylglucosaminidase	Gasser cells
Mucopolysaccharidosis type IIIC	Sanfilippo syndrome	Acetyl-CoA:α-glucosaminide acetyltransferase	Foamy macrophages; vacuolated lymphocytes; finely granulated neutrophils
Mucopolysaccharidosis type IIID	Sanfilippo syndrome	N-acetylglucosamine 6-sulfatase	Gasser cells
Mucopolysaccharidosis type IVA	Morquio syndrome	Galactosamine-6-sulfatase	Gasser cells; Alder–Reilly bodies
Mucopolysaccharidosis type IVB	Morquio syndrome	β-Galactosidase	Gasser cells; Alder–Reilly bodies; lymphocytic vacuoles
Mucopolysaccharidosis type VI	Maroteaux–Lamy syndrome	Arylsulfatase B	Gasser cells; Alder–Reilly bodies
Mucopolysaccharidosis type VII	Sly syndrome	β-glucuronidase	Gasser cells; Alder–Reilly bodies
Mucopolysaccharidosis type IX		Hyaluronidase	Gasser cells
Multiple sulfatase deficiency	Mucosulfatidosis	Sulfatase modifying factor 1	Alder–Reilly bodies
Neuronal ceroid lipofuscinosis (NCL), CLN1	Santavuori disease	Palmitoyl-protein thioesterase 1	Lymphocyte granular osmiophilic deposits
Neuronal ceroid lipofuscinosis, CLN2	Jansky–Bielschowsky disease	Tripeptidyl-peptidase 1	Curvilinear lymphocyte inclusions
Neuronal ceroid lipofuscinosis, CLN3	Batten disease Vogt–Spielmeyer disease	Protein function not known[152]	Lymphocyte inclusions
Neuronal ceroid lipofuscinosis, CLN5	Late infantile NCL, Finnish variant	Protein function not known[153]	Curvilinear lymphocyte inclusions
Neuronal ceroid lipofuscinosis, CLN6	Late infantile NCL, early juvenile variant	ER-resident protein of unknown function[154]	Curvilinear lymphocyte inclusions
Neuronal ceroid lipofuscinosis, CLN8	Northern epilepsy	ER-resident protein of unknown function[155]	
Niemann–Pick disease types A and B	Niemann–Pick disease	Acid sphingomyelinase	Foamy macrophages; sea-blue histiocytes
Niemann–Pick disease type C1	Niemann–Pick disease	Niemann–Pick C1 protein	Foamy macrophages; occasional coarsely vacuolated lymphocytes; sea-blue histiocytes
Niemann–Pick disease type C2	Niemann–Pick disease	Epididymal secretory protein	Foamy macrophages; occasional coarsely vacuolated lymphocytes; sea-blue histiocytes
Pyknodysostosis		Cathepsin K	
Schindler disease types I and II	Schindler disease/Kanzaki disease	α-N-acetylgalactosaminidase	Small vacuoles in leukocytes
Sialic acid storage disease	Sialuria, Salla disease	Sialin	Foamy macrophages with hemophagocytosis; small lymphocytic inclusions

ER, endoplasmic reticulum.

Table 36.2 Effective therapies for the lysosomal storage disorders.

Storage disorder	HSCT[4]	ERT	Substrate reduction[156]
Aspartylglucosaminuria	Not effective		
Fabry disease		+	
Farber disease	Effective (few cases reported)		
Gaucher disease type I	Restricted use	+	+
Gaucher disease type II	Not effective		
Gaucher disease type III	Somatic improvement	+	
Hurler disease (MPS I)	Somatic improvement	+	
Hunter disease (MPS II)	Somatic improvement	+*	
I-cell disease	Effective (few cases reported)		
Krabbe disease	Effective		
α-mannosidosis	Clinical improvement		
Maroteaux–Lamy syndrome (MPS VI)	Clinical improvement (few cases reported)	+*	
Metachromatic leukodystrophy	Effective in some		
Morquio disease	Visceral improvement		
Niemann–Pick type A	Not effective		
Niemann–Pick type B	Effective		
Niemann–Pick type C	Somatic improvement		
Pompe disease		+	
Sandhoff disease			+
Sanfilippo (MPS III)	Not effective		
Sly disease (MPS VII)	Effective (few cases reported)		
Tay–Sachs disease			+
Wolman disease	Effective (few cases reported)		

* In clinical trials.
HSCT, hematopoietic stem cell transplant; ERT, enzyme replacement therapy.

fuschin, acid phosphatase and ferric hematoxylin for sphingomyelin. Polarized light microscopy may enhance the characterization of the storage material.

Management of the various LSDs is disease specific and includes hematopoietic stem cell transplantation (HSCT), enzyme reconstitution and substrate depletion approaches (Table 36.2). Supportive therapies continue to have essential roles. HSCT has specific therapeutic roles in selected LSDs, but the results are disease and organ-system specific, and timing of engraftment is critical.[3–5] The theory for use of HSCT suggests that the normal levels of lysosomal enzymes in derivatives of hematopoietic stem cells could supply the missing enzyme to deficient cells by secretion and reuptake. Thus, the lysosomal enzymes released within tissues from donor white blood cells would be taken up by the deficient host cells, and then delivered to the intracellular site of action (i.e., the lysosome). Consequently, the abnormally accumulated substrates diminish in serum, tissues and other bodily fluids. Improvement in hepatosplenomegaly and cytopenias is universal. Prevention, stabilization or improvement of neurologic function is variable and is highly dependent on the type of disease, severity, age of onset, and the timing of the HSCT as well as attendant complications.[6] Newer treatment modalities such as enzyme replacement therapy (ERT) and substrate inhibition are available for a limited number of LSDs but can effect substantial improvement in morbidity.[7] Comprehensive reviews of the LSDs are available.[8] Here, highlights of the hematologic findings in various LSDs and their therapies are presented.

Sphingolipidoses

The sphingolipidoses derive their name from the accumulation of complex lipids containing ceramide. Ceramide is composed of a sphingosine backbone covalently linked to fatty acid acyl chains of variable length, hence sphingolipid. Ceramide, an amino alcohol, can have covalent links to phosphate (sphingomyelin), glycoside (glycosphingolipids), or sulfated glycoside (sulfoglycosphingolipids) groups. The stepwise degradation of these sphingolipids occurs in the lysosomal compartment. Defective enzymatic activity at each step in this degradation pathway leads to accumulation of specific by-products and the distinctive storage material and phenotype. There are 10 well-recognized sphingolipidoses, of which only Gaucher disease and Niemann–Pick disease variants have significant frequencies and well-characterized hematologic findings.

Gaucher disease

Gaucher disease is the most common LSD and has an incidence in the general population of 1 in 57 000 to 1 in 86 000.[1,2] This disease is pan-ethnic, but the prevalence varies among different ethnic and demographic groups. Among Ashkenazi Jews, the prevalence is approximately 1 in 855, whereas among non-Jews in the Netherlands, a prevalence of 1 in 325 000 was found.[9] Gaucher disease results from the defective activity of acid β-glucosidase (glucocerebrosidase) and consequent accumulation of glucosylceramide (glucocerebroside) in tissue macrophages. Storage is most evident in tissue macrophages of the liver, spleen, bone marrow and lung.

Gaucher disease has been divided into three clinical phenotypes, which are distinguished by the absence (type 1) or presence and severity (types 2 and 3) of central nervous system (CNS) disease (see below). Diagnosis and classification of Gaucher disease is based on clinical features and established by biochemical or genetic testing. Acid β-glucosidase analyses are sensitive, generally available, and usually are conducted on leukocytes or cultured fibroblasts. The enzyme deficiency is generic and is the preferred method of diagnosis of affected patients. Carrier testing by enzyme analysis is not reliable. Genetic testing by allele-specific or total gene sequencing is available. More than 200 mutations have been identified. Genotype–phenotype correlations are limited, but may be useful in differentiating among the types.[10–14] Indeed, there is a continuum of clinical features between the phenotypes, particularly types 2 and 3, that is quantitative, namely more or less acute or progressive CNS disease. Between types 2 and 3, and type 1, the distinguishing feature is categorical, i.e., type 1 is defined as the absence of primary CNS involvement by Gaucher disease. This is not age dependent in that type 1 (previously termed adult) Gaucher disease can present at any age from early childhood to late adulthood.[15] The detection of a N370S allele in an affected patient has significant clinical utility because it is prognostic of type 1, nonneuronopathic Gaucher disease, in all cases to date.

In all variants of Gaucher disease, a distinctive hematologic feature is the presence of Gaucher cells in bone marrow and other tissues (Fig. 36.1). Gaucher cells are large tissue storage cells of macrophage lineage. The cytoplasm of these cells stains pale gray-blue with Giemsa, and they have eccentrically placed nuclei due to numerous large vacuoles.[16] The storage bodies are loose in appearance, stain weakly positive with PAS, are strongly acid phosphatase positive, and stain pale gray with lipophilic stains, namely Sudan black. These cells are not "foamy" in appearance. Morphologically similar "Gaucher-like" cells are observed in chronic granulomatous disease, thalassemia, multiple myeloma, Hodgkin disease,

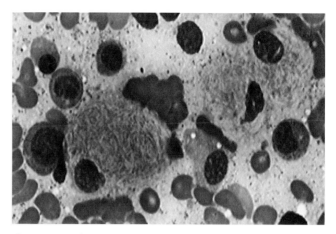

Fig. 36.1 Gaucher cell in a bone marrow aspirate of a patient with Gaucher type 1 disease (Giemsa stained). Note the "wrinkled tissue paper" appearance and eccentrically placed nucleus.

lymphoma, AIDS, and acute lymphoblastic leukemia but can be distinguished readily.[9,17] The Gaucher cells can be sufficiently abundant (near total replacement) in bone marrow to interfere with normal hematopoiesis in some individuals. Myelofibrosis and/or bone marrow failure occurs infrequently.[18,19]

Gaucher disease type 1 (nonneuronopathic)

Gaucher disease type 1 is the most common variant. In the International Collaborative Gaucher Group Registry, type 1 disease accounts for 90% of all cases.[20] The age of onset can vary from childhood to late adulthood, and the clinical severity varies from severe to indolent. Most data derive from affected patients of European ancestry and are heavily influenced by the ascertainment bias of the Ashkenazi-Jewish phenotypes. However, the clinical spectrum of type 1 variants is becoming increasingly broad with descriptions of patients from other demographic regions.

The most common presenting finding in affected patients is asymptomatic splenomegaly.[15,20,21] Derivative findings can include bleeding due to thrombocytopenia as a result of splenic sequestration, low-grade chronic consumptive coagulopathy secondary to intrasplenic activation,[22] bone marrow infiltration, and factor XI deficiency among Ashkenazi Jews.[23] In the pediatric population, anemia and thrombocytopenia are the most common hematologic findings.[24,25] Anemia is usually mild and due to splenic sequestration and bone marrow involvement. Also, many patients have an unexplained macrocytosis.

The skeletal manifestations include bone marrow infiltration with Erlenmeyer flask deformity from bone marrow expansion (50–61%), generalized bone mineral loss (universal), infarction (16–35%), and bone pain (20–66%).[25–29] The resultant osteopenia/osteoporosis and infarction can lead to pathologic and/or osteoporotic fractures accounting for some bone pain. About 50% of affected patients experience one or more episodes of bone crises characterized by fever, an increased sedimentation rate, and excruciating localized pain. Such episodes are more frequent among adolescents and young adults. The most frequently involved sites are along the femurs. These bone crises mimic osteomyelitis, which may need to be excluded by biopsy and culture.[30] About 50% of untreated affected children have growth retardation and shorter than expected final heights.[31,32]

Hepatosplenomegaly can be massive, with abdominal distension and pain (Fig. 36.2). The volumetric increase in these organs, particularly splenomegaly, can cause early satiety, nausea, dyspareunia and ligamentous pain. Hypersplenism develops in the majority. Splenic sizes can range from four to more than 70 times normal predicted volumes. Splenic infarction is common and occasionally presents acutely with pain, rigid abdomen, fever, metabolic acidosis and hyperuricemia. Splenic nuclide scans are helpful in differentiating old (cold) versus new (surrounding hot) infarcts in the presence of an acute abdomen. Hypersplenism with sequestration of platelets and red blood cells can lead to thrombocytopenia and anemia. Concurrent iron, folate, or vitamin B_{12} deficiencies should be excluded. Clinically significant liver dysfunction due to Gaucher disease alone is uncommon, despite significant hepatomegaly in 79% of affected patients.[15] Mild, persistent elevation of aspartate aminotransferase (also called serum glutamate oxaloacetate transaminase), alanine transaminase (also called serum glutamate pyruvate transaminase), and γ-glutamyl transferase can be found frequently.

Recommendations from expert panels are available for evaluation and monitoring of treated or untreated Gaucher disease type 1 patients.[20,24] Symptomatic management of Gaucher disease type 1 involves addressing concurrent complications such as the portal and pulmonary hypertension, as well as the bone manifestations. The skeletal manifestations are frequent and require pain management, physical therapy and orthopedic surgery. Concomitant ERT and bisphosphonate treatment improves bone mineral density, but has minor effects on focal cortical thinning of the long bones with significant marrow involvement.[33,34] Splenectomy, once the mainstay of treatment for the hypersplenism, now has utility limited to acute intervention for severe hypersplenism or infarction in the era of ERT.[35–37] HSCT should cure Gaucher disease type 1, but the attendant morbidity and mortality have severely limited its use especially given the efficacy and safety of ERT.[9]

ERT for Gaucher disease has been available since 1991.[38] The theory of ERT is to reconstitute the lysosomal enzyme levels sufficient to degrade stored substrate and maintain normal cellular metabolism.[39] Regular infusions of imiglucerase (Cerezyme, Genzyme Corp, Cambridge, MA) reverses many disease signs and symptoms.[40,41] The outcomes summary below is based on reports of treatment results from approximately 2000 affected patients.[20,42] Anemia shows a

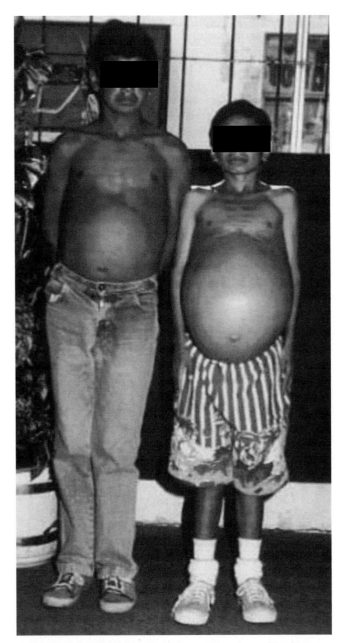

Fig. 36.2 Abdominal distension due to massive hepatosplenomegaly in Gaucher disease type 1. Clinical variability is evident among the siblings (aged 16 and 17 years) shown here.

rapid and sustained response within 6 months, eliminating the need for blood transfusions. Platelet counts respond more slowly, but within 12 months, normal platelet counts are achieved in splenectomized patients. This may take up to 5 years of continuous ERT in the nonsplenectomized patient. Spleen and liver sizes show major decreases within the first 1 to 3 years of ERT. Decreased bone pain and less frequent bone crises also occur in the majority of patients.[43] Normalization of growth rates and catch-up growth occurs in children with growth retardation.[44] Patients generally report greater energy, less pain, reduced dyspnea and improved quality of life. Detailed therapeutic goals are available.[20,35]

An alternative/supplementary approach to ERT is to reduce the flux of the offending substrate (e.g., glucosylceramide) through the lysosomes, by decreasing its synthesis, and therefore its delivery. This has been termed substrate depletion. Inhibitors of glucosylceramide synthase have been used and are approved for restricted use in Europe and the USA. The available agent is miglustat (*N*-butyldeoxynojirimycin, Zavesca), which has been clinically tested with promising results.[45–49] The agent is approved in the USA for use in affected patients who have medical indications for not receiving ERT.[50]

Gaucher disease type 2 (acute neuronopathic)

Gaucher disease type 2 is a rare variant comprising less than 1% of total cases.[51,52] This severe, rapidly progressive CNS disease has infantile onset of failure to thrive, organomegaly and neurologic symptoms. Oculomotor apraxia and/or strabismus occur from birth to 3–4 months of age. Opisthotonus, bulbar signs, limb rigidity and seizures develop within 6–7 months. Most infants die within the first 2 years of life, with a mean survival of 9 months.[53] No therapeutic intervention has had clear clinical benefit for the CNS disease.[54]

Gaucher disease type 3 (subacute neuronopathic)

The subacute neuronopathic variant, type 3, accounts for about 4–5% of total Gaucher disease in Europe and the USA.[20] Several variants of type 3 disease have been delineated and are distinguished clinically by the degree and progression of visceral and CNS manifestations.[55] Massive visceral disease with rapid progression and relatively static CNS disease or isolated eye findings are predominant in one variant whereas rapid progression of CNS disease with uncontrollable myoclonic seizures characterizes another variant. Additional variants with calcification of the aortic root and valves, and variable hydrocephalus have been described in Japan and the Middle East, but appear pan-ethnically.[56–61] Neurologic findings include variable presence and progression of decreased mental capacities, oculomotor apraxia, seizures, poor coordination and hypertonicity. Type 3 disease is distinguished from the type 2 by the neurologic manifestations in children > 1 year of age. The variants cannot be differentiated by enzyme testing. L444P homozygosity is highly associated, but not exclusively so, with neuronopathic variants.[62]

HSCT has improved the visceral disease in type 3 patients, but the effect on CNS resolution is not well established.[6,63] ERT has shown clear benefit for the visceral disease in type 3 patients, but the efficacy for CNS involvement is controversial.[64] Experimental studies in type 3 with miglustat are ongoing.[65]

Niemann–Pick disease

The group of disorders termed Niemann–Pick disease involves the accumulation of unesterified cholesterol or sphingomyelin in the lysosomes of tissue macrophages and other cell types. This group of diseases has a frequency of about 1 in 130 000.[2] Types A and B result from deficiencies of acid sphingomyelinase and the accumulation of sphingomyelin. The type C variant was originally thought to be due to sphingomyelinase deficiency but is now known to be the result of a defect in one of two genes involved in lipid/sterol trafficking.[66–68]

Niemann–Pick disease types A and B represent a clinical continuum due to the degree of acid sphingomyelinase deficiency. Their overall incidence is 1 in 248 000, but may be more frequent in those of Jewish ancestry.[2,69] The diagnosis is established in suspected patients by the deficiency of acid sphingomyelinase in leukocytes or cultured fibroblasts. The enzyme does not normally occur in plasma. Typically, the enzyme activity is < 5% of normal in type A (NPA), a severe neurologic variant, compared with somewhat higher levels in Niemann–Pick type B (NPB).[70]

In both variants, microcytic anemia can occur late in the clinical course. Peripheral blood smears reveal vacuolated lymphocytes, with the number of cells involved roughly correlated to clinical severity, that is, more in NPA than NPB. Use of special stains reveals a lack of demonstrable sudanophilic lipid or glycogen material. Bone marrow smears demonstrate "foamy" cells with numerous uniform vacuoles, often described as having a "honeycomb" appearance (Fig. 36.3). These "Niemann–Pick" cells are 25–75 μm in diameter, contain a single nucleus, and have a white birefringence unstained. Lipid droplets may appear yellowish under ultraviolet light. In addition, sea-blue histiocytes are often numerous. These macrophages are filled with numerous fine granulations that stain blue with Giemsa-type stains

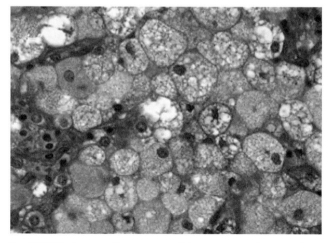

Fig. 36.3 The honeycomb appearance of the tissue macrophage seen here in the lung of a patient with Niemann–Pick type B (×63).

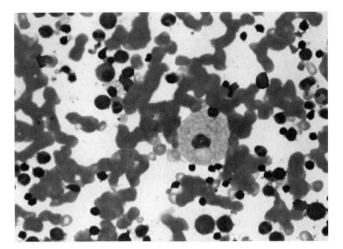

Fig. 36.4 Sea-blue histiocyte in the bone marrow of a patient with Niemann–Pick type B (×63). Compared with the sea-blue histiocyte seen in Niemann–Pick type C, it has a finer granular appearance.

(Fig. 36.4). The granulations contain ceroid or lipofuscin that has autofluorescence. They exhibit stable sudanophilia and stain positive with PAS. Sea-blue histiocytes are not specific for NPB disease and can be found infrequently in lecithin–cholesterol acyltransferase deficiency,[71] cholesteryl ester storage disease,[72] myelodysplastic syndromes,[73–75] and in people receiving total parenteral nutrition.[76–78] Sudan black staining reveals a reddish birefringence of the lamellar inclusions. Additional staining methods such as the Schultz reaction for cholesterol and ferric hematoxylin for sphingomyelin are positive.[79] The inclusions are poorly visualized with PAS and acid phosphatase reactions. Similar "foamy" cells are seen in cholesteryl ester storage/Wolman disease, lipoprotein lipase deficiency, and G_{M1} gangliosidosis but can be differentiated on specific staining. Importantly, liver biopsy shows involvement of the Kupffer cells and hepatocytes, unlike Gaucher disease in which storage is restricted to Kupffer cells. Diagnosis of NPA or NPB is based on clinical suspicion, the presence of foamy bone marrow storage cells, and deficient acid sphingomyelinase activity. Genetic testing is available for the three most common mutations, which are present in > 90% of NPA and NPB to date.

Niemann–Pick type A (infantile, acute neuronopathic)

Infants appear normal at birth but may develop prolonged jaundice. More specific findings associated with Niemann-Pick disease present at about 4–6 months of age. These children often manifest poor feeding, failure to thrive, protuberant abdomen, hepatosplenomegaly and cherry-red macula. Psychomotor delays with muscular weakness and hypotonia are noted usually before 6 months of age and follow a progressive neurodegenerative course. Storage in tissue macrophages leads to significant lymphadenopathy and bone marrow involvement, but no bony changes are

noted except osteoporosis. Infiltration of the lung alveoli can be visualized on chest X-ray in the minority of patients. Death commonly occurs before 2–3 years of age. Management is largely supportive.

Niemann–Pick disease type B (nonneuronopathic)

NPB displays a more variable phenotype than type A and, in comparison, represents a less severe clinical variant of acid sphingomyelinase deficiency. Importantly, affected patients lack primary CNS disease, although the presence of ataxia may represent the continuous spectrum between the A and B types.[69] NPB usually presents later in childhood with a protuberant abdomen due to splenomegaly with or without hepatomegaly. The liver involvement can result in cirrhosis, portal hypertension and ascites.[80,81] Less than 10% have cherry red macula and most live into adolescence or adulthood. Pulmonary interstitial and alveolar infiltration is extensive as seen by imaging techniques, but pulmonary function deficits are poorly documented (Fig. 36.3). In a few cases, continued infiltration can cause decreased diffusion capacity leading to respiratory compromise in late adolescence or adulthood.[82–88]

A single NPB patient underwent allogeneic transplantation at 3 years of age with resultant reduction of liver sphingomyelin levels.[89] The patient did not have CNS involvement at 3 years, but at 16 years posttransplant, a neurodegenerative course led to severe physical and mental deficiencies.[90]

Niemann–Pick disease type C

Niemann–Pick type C (NPC) variations are autosomal recessive disorders of lipid trafficking that have major CNS involvement.[91] The prevalence of this disorder is 1 in 150 000 to 1 in 211 000.[2,92] It exhibits genetic heterogeneity, with the involvement of two known genes, *NPC1* and *NPC2*. Nearly 95% of the > 100 mutations found to be associated with type C disease reside within *NPC1*.[92–94] The actions of the *NPC1* and *NPC2* gene products and their respective substrates are not well characterized but the decrease in acid sphingomyelinase and acid β-glucosidase are secondary effects.[95–97]

Peripheral blood lymphocytes may exhibit coarse vacuolization. Foamy macrophages and sea-blue histiocytes (Figs 36.5 and 36.6) are typically seen on bone marrow aspirate as well as in the liver, spleen, lymph nodes and lungs.[98] These storage cells have variably sized and shaped vacuoles that have a "ragged" appearance and do not have birefringence or sudanophilia.[99] The Schultz reaction for cholesterol is strongly positive, as is the acid phosphatase reaction. Diagnosis is made by the demonstration of intralysosomal accumulation of cholesterol by filipin staining or mutation analysis of the *NPC1* or *NPC2* genes; however, most affected patients have private mutations and DNA analysis is not available clinically.

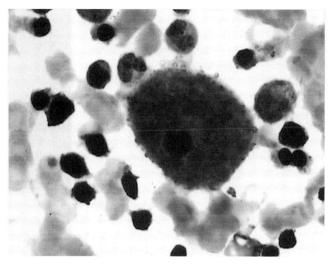

Fig. 36.5 Granulations seen in the bone marrow histiocyte in a patient with Niemann–Pick type C disease are typically very coarse.

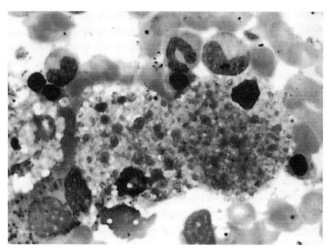

Fig. 36.6 In Niemann–Pick type C disease, the sea-blue histiocyte of the bone marrow stains very intensely and may be useful in differentiation from type B.

Clinically, the presentation is highly variable and patients may exhibit signs and symptoms at any time in life.[92,100–105] More than half will manifest prolonged neonatal jaundice.[106] About 10% develop cholestatic jaundice requiring liver transplantation.[106–109] Beyond the neonatal period, many affected patients will present with neuropsychiatric symptoms. About 90% of patients have splenomegaly with or without hepatomegaly, but the degree of splenic enlargement is less than in Niemann–Pick A/B disease. Early in the disease course, most will experience behavioral disturbances around school age. Vertical supranuclear gaze palsy, which is seen in nearly all affected individuals, may become evident at this time.[92] The course worsens with the onset of ataxia, dementia, oromotor dysfunction, dystonia, gelastic cataplexy, violent behavior and/or seizures. The neuropsychiatric features

often worsen with the onset of puberty. Progression to loss of motor control leads to a nonambulatory state. Death commonly occurs in late adolescence or young adulthood from CNS and pulmonary complications.

Therapy is symptomatic treatment.[110] Attempts to use liver transplantation and hydroxymethylglutaryl (HMG)-CoA reductase inhibitors failed to show clinical benefit.[92,107,111] HSCT in an affected 3 year old led to visceral improvement, but the neurologic status continued to decline.[112] Because of the secondary accumulation of glucosylceramide and gangliosides, a trial is underway using substrate depletion.[110]

Mucopolysaccharidoses

The mucopolysaccharidoses (MPS) constitute a group of disorders that result in the lysosomal accumulation of glycosaminoglycans (GAGs) in cells throughout the body. Clinically, MPS patients often present with coarsened facial features, skeletal manifestations, and joint limitations. Keratan, heparan and/or dermatan sulfate in the urine in excessive amounts is highly suggestive of one of the mucopolysaccharide disorders. Distinguishing these MPS variants depends on clinical acumen and enzymatic analyses.[113] The MPS variants are listed in Table 36.1, and those of significant frequency and/or hematologic importance are described in more detail.

Vacuolated lymphocytes with basophilic inclusions (Gasser cells) are observed in all types of MPS although they are more numerous in Sanfilippo syndrome (MPS III) and rare in Hurler syndrome (MPS IH). These inclusion bodies are metachromatic when stained with toluidine blue and are best visualized under oil immersion. Neutrophils can contain coarse basophilic inclusions and Alder–Reilly bodies, which are similar in appearance to toxic granules but are lilac-rose or brown colored (Fig. 36.7). Alder–Reilly bodies are seen in the absence of toxic changes. In Maroteaux–Lamy syndrome (MPS VI) and Sly syndrome (MPS VII), the majority of

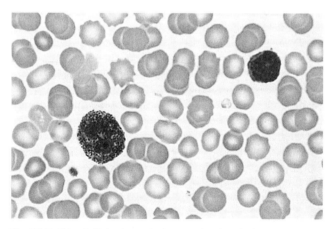

Fig. 36.7 Alder–Reilly body seen in the granulocytic series is common among the mucopolysaccharidoses.

neutrophils will contain Alder–Reilly bodies. These cells are also present in multiple sulfatase deficiency, a very rare disease. Bone marrow aspiration is usually not necessary, but Gasser-type cells as single- or multi-nucleated cells may occur. Bone marrow plasma cells demonstrate basophilic inclusions.

Mucopolysaccharidosis type I (Hurler, Hurler–Scheie, and Scheie syndromes)

Mucopolysaccharidosis type I (MPS I) results from the deficiency of α-L-iduronidase and has a prevalence ranging from 1 in 76 000 to 1 in 130 000.[1,2,114,115] The MPS I variants have a wide clinical spectrum: Hurler (MPS IH, severe), Hurler–Scheie (MPS IH/S, intermediate), and Scheie (MPS IS, attenuated) variants.

MPS IH often presents in the neonatal period with umbilical or inguinal hernias. Within the first year of life, affected patients exhibit coarsening of the facial features, macrocephaly, progressive corneal clouding, an enlarged tongue, hepatosplenomegaly, recurrent upper respiratory infections, deafness and growth deceleration. GAGs deposited in the heart valves and coronary arteries can predispose patients to myocardial infarction.[116,117] Skeletal manifestations include dysostosis multiplex with anterior hypoplasia of the vertebrae, enlarged diaphyses, hypoplastic epiphyses, and progressive thoracolumbar kyphosis with or without a gibbus deformity.[118] Global developmental delay is readily apparent by 12–24 months of age, with an achieved maximal functional age of 2–4 years before progressive deterioration. Life expectancy is less than 10 years of age and demise is usually related to respiratory insufficiency and/or cardiac valvular dysfunction.

Hurler–Scheie syndrome (MPS IH/S) has similar somatic involvement, but little or no neurologic signs or symptoms. MPS IH/S patients present with corneal clouding, joint stiffness, dysostosis multiplex, and deafness usually between 3 and 8 years of age. Mucopolysaccharide accumulation in the heart valve leaflets may necessitate valve replacement. Deposition of mucopolysaccharides in the meninges leads to pachymeningitis cervicalis, which may cause obstructive hydrocephalus. Those with Hurler–Scheie typically have a life expectancy of less than 25 years.

Scheie syndrome (MPS IS) is rare, and typically has onset in childhood with mild coarsening of the facial features and joint stiffness, and preservation of stature and intellect as well as a near-normal lifespan. The decreased range of motion and the development of carpal tunnel syndrome become a functional limitation later in life.[119] Patients have corneal clouding and some develop glaucoma, either of which may cause visual impairment. Much like Hurler–Scheie, cardiac valvular deposits can lead to valvular insufficiency requiring valve replacement.[120]

Treatment of MPS I involves symptomatic care as well as HSCT and ERT. These patients benefit from physical and occupational therapies for joint mobility and adaptations. Progressive tracheal stenosis occurs secondarily to glycosaminoglycan deposition, causing dyspnea and obstructive sleep apnea with many patients benefiting from tracheostomy.

Transplanted patients achieve and maintain normal leukocytic enzyme levels.[4,121–124] These patients experience improved cardiac function as well as decreased coronary artery and pulmonary accumulations.[4,116,125] The bony and neuropsychiatric complications remain problematic but promising results suggest steady gains over time.[6,126,127] Phase III clinical trials of ERT in MPS IH/S and MPS IS have shown marked reduction in urinary GAGs, decreased liver and spleen volumes, increased range of motion, and improved exercise tolerance.[128] Laronidase (Aldurazyme, Genzyme Corp.) was approved in the USA for use in MPS I in 2003.[50,129]

Gentamicin is being explored as a potential alternative or addition to ERT for the treatment of MPS IH. The antibiotic action of gentamicin is to inhibit mRNA translation into protein. However, gentamicin can be used to block nonsense-mediated decay, a cellular process used to recognize and degrade mRNA transcripts with premature stop codons. Research trials of gentamicin have restored α-L-iduronidate levels.[130] Although promising, this type of therapy is only potentially useful for Hurler patients with specific mutations.

Mucopolysaccharidosis type II (Hunter syndrome)

MPS II is an X-linked recessive disorder that occurs in 1 in 34 000 to 1 in 111 000 males and may be more common among people from the Pacific rim as well as those of Jewish descent.[1,2,114,115,131,132] There is significant phenotypic variation, with the majority of patients having CNS and visceral phenotypes. The deficiency of iduronidate sulfatase results in the accumulation of dermatan and heparan sulfate. The clinical features in the majority of patients are similar to MPS IH, with delayed development, short stature, macrocephaly, hydrocephalus, coarse facial features, hepatosplenomegaly, dysostosis multiplex, limited range of motion, deafness and chronic diarrhea, with the major difference being the lack of significant corneal clouding and a slower, progressive course.[133] Life expectancy is 10–15 years in the more severe variant. Survival into the fourth to sixth decades, with normal intellectual function, has been observed.[134]

HSCT has been performed in a number of patients.[3,6,135–140] Normal leukocytic enzyme levels are readily achieved in engrafted patients with demonstrable decrease in urinary mucopolysaccharides. Histologic clearance of stored substrate occurs in bone marrow and liver. Somatic improvement in the facial features, hepatomegaly, joint contractures and short stature has been seen in the majority with little or no improvement of the dysostosis multiplex or in sensorineural hearing loss. Improved quality of life occurs in many, but there is little neuropsychiatric benefit. Recommendations for patients to even undergo HSCT are controversial.[5,140,141] ERT is currently in phase III trials.[142]

Mucopolysaccharidosis type VI (Maroteaux–Lamy syndrome)

Maroteaux–Lamy syndrome results from arylsulfatase B deficiency and has an incidence ranging from 1 in 100 000 to 1 in 1 300 000.[1,2,114,115] Dermatan sulfate accumulates in most tissues throughout the body. The clinical features are very similar to MPS IH and MPS II syndromes (e.g., short stature, cloudy cornea, hepatomegaly, thickened skin, dysostosis multiplex and stiff joints) except that CNS involvement is not a feature of MPS VI. The cardiac valves can become thickened and calcified leading to pulmonary hypertension and heart failure.[143] Accumulation can occur in the meninges, as is seen in Hurler syndrome, resulting in obstructive hydrocephalus. Intelligence is usually normal. Death occurs in the second or third decade due to cardiac disease.

HSCT results in metabolic correction and somatic improvement.[6] There is variable benefit for the musculoskeletal system probably related to the age of transplantation, but no improvement in the corneal clouding.[3,6,144,145] Significant improvement in cardiac and pulmonary function has been observed.[4] ERT phase I/II trials are encouraging, based on the observations of reduced urinary glycosaminoglycan levels and clinical improvement.[146]

Wolman disease/cholesteryl ester storage disease

Wolman and cholesteryl ester storage disease (CESD) results from lysosomal acid lipase deficiency leading to abnormal fat stores in visceral organs and fat malabsorption. Wolman disease is rare, occurring in 1 in 528 000.[2] CESD appears less rare, and its true prevalence may be about 1 in 100 000 in some populations.[147] In Wolman disease, onset occurs in the neonatal period with severe failure to thrive, vomiting, diarrhea, hepatosplenomegaly and calcifications of the adrenal glands.[148] Anemia is usually seen in the first 1–2 months of life. Peripheral lymphocytes may contain intranuclear as well as intracytoplasmic vacuoles. Foam cells are usually evident in bone marrow aspirates after the first month of life and are also occasionally seen in the peripheral blood. Diagnosis is based on clinical concerns and confirmed by enzyme assay of lysosomal acid lipase activity in peripheral leukocytes or cultured fibroblasts. Death commonly occurs in the first year of life.

CESD represents a less severe phenotype with significant clinical variability. The most consistent findings are hepatomegaly and hypercholesterolemia.[149] Morbidity is related to liver function, which worsens over time and progresses to cirrhosis and fibrosis. Esophageal varices are uncommon but have been reported.[149] Bone marrow aspirates are usually normal but foam cells may be seen in those with a moderate–severe phenotype.

Management is symptomatic. Hypercholesterolemia has responded to HMG-CoA reductase inhibitors, cholestyramine and a low-cholesterol diet.[148,150] This approach has had no significant effects on hepatic progression. At least two Wolman disease patients have undergone HSCT with successful engraftment at several years follow up.[4,151] These patients demonstrate normal levels of lysosomal acid lipase and show no signs of clinical disease.

References

1. Poorthuis BJ, Wevers RA, Kleijer WJ *et al.* The frequency of lysosomal storage diseases in The Netherlands. *Hum Genet* 1999; **105**: 151–6.
2. Meikle PJ, Hopwood JJ, Clague AE *et al.* Prevalence of lysosomal storage disorders. *JAMA* 1999; **281**: 249–54.
3. Imaizumi M, Gushi K, Kurobane I *et al.* Long-term effects of bone marrow transplantation for inborn errors of metabolism: a study of four patients with lysosomal storage diseases. *Acta Paediatr Jpn* 1994; **36**: 30–6.
4. Krivit W. Allogeneic stem cell transplantation for the treatment of lysosomal and peroxisomal metabolic diseases. *Springer Semin Immunopathol* 2004; **26**: 119–32.
5. Krivit W, Shapiro EG. Bone marrow transplantation for storage diseases. In: Desnick RJ (ed.). *Treatment of Genetic Disease*. New York, Churchill Livingstone, 1991, pp. 203–21.
6. Krivit W. Stem cell bone marrow transplantation in patients with metabolic storage diseases. *Adv Pediatr* 2002; **49**: 359–78.
7. Grabowski GA, Hopkin RJ. Enzyme therapy for lysosomal storage disease: principles, practice, and prospects. *Annu Rev Genomics Hum Genet* 2003; **4**: 403–36.
8. Scriver CR, Beaudet AL, Valle D, Sly WS (eds). *The Metabolic and Molecular Bases of Inherited Diseases*, 8th edn. New York: McGraw-Hill, 2001.
9. Beutler E, Grabowski G. Glucosylceramide lipidosis: Gaucher disease. In: Scriver CR, Beaudet AL, Sly WS, Valle D (eds) *The Metabolic and Molecular Bases of Inherited Disease*, 8th edn. New York: McGraw-Hill, 2001, pp. 3635–68.
10. Zhao H, Bailey LA, Elsas LJ 2nd *et al.* Gaucher disease: in vivo evidence for allele dose leading to neuronopathic and nonneuronopathic phenotypes. *Am J Med Genet A* 2003; **116**: 52–6.
11. Sidransky E, Bottler A, Stubblefield B *et al.* DNA mutational analysis of type 1 and type 3 Gaucher patients: how well do mutations predict phenotype? *Hum Mutat* 1994; **3**: 25–8.
12. Orvisky E, Park JK, LaMarca ME *et al.* Glucosylsphingosine accumulation in tissues from patients with Gaucher disease: correlation with phenotype and genotype. *Mol Genet Metab* 2002; **76**: 262–70.
13. Park JK, Koprivica V, Andrews DQ *et al.* Glucocerebrosidase mutations among African-American patients with type 1 Gaucher disease. *Am J Med Genet* 2001; **99**: 147–51.
14. Koprivica V, Stone DL, Park JK *et al.* Analysis and classification

of 304 mutant alleles in patients with type 1 and type 3 Gaucher disease. *Am J Hum Genet* 2000; **66**: 1777–86.

15. Charrow J, Andersson HC, Kaplan P *et al*. The Gaucher registry: demographics and disease characteristics of 1698 patients with Gaucher disease. *Arch Intern Med* 2000; **160**: 2835–43.

16. Parkin JL, Brunning RD. Pathology of the Gaucher cell. *Prog Clin Biol Res* 1982; **95**: 151–75.

17. Florena AM, Franco V, Campesi G. Immunophenotypical comparison of Gaucher's and pseudo-Gaucher cells. *Pathol Int* 1996; **46**: 155–60.

18. Tsuboi K, Iida S, Kato M *et al*. Improvement of splenomegaly and pancytopenia by enzyme replacement therapy against type 1 Gaucher disease: a report of sibling cases. *Int J Hematol* 2001; **73**: 356–62.

19. Cohen IJ, Katz K, Freud E *et al*. Long-term follow-up of partial splenectomy in Gaucher's disease. *Am J Surg* 1992; **164**: 345–7.

20. Weinreb NJ, Aggio MC, Andersson HC *et al*. Gaucher disease type 1: revised recommendations on evaluations and monitoring for adult patients. *Semin Hematol* 2004; **41**: 15–22.

21. McLennan MK, Withers CE. Gaucher's disease involving the spleen. *Can Assoc Radiol J* 1992; **43**: 45–8.

22. Hollak CE, Levi M, Berends F *et al*. Coagulation abnormalities in type 1 Gaucher disease are due to low-grade activation and can be partly restored by enzyme supplementation therapy. *Br J Haematol* 1997; **96**: 470–6.

23. Seligsohn U, Zitman D, Many A *et al*. Coexistence of factor XI (plasma thromboplastin antecedent) deficiency and Gaucher's disease. *Isr J Med Sci* 1976; **12**: 1448–52.

24. Grabowski GA, Andria G, Baldellou A *et al*. Pediatric non-neuronopathic Gaucher disease: presentation, diagnosis and assessment. Consensus statements. *Eur J Pediatr* 2004; **163**: 58–66.

25. Zevin S, Abrahamov A, Hadas-Halpern I *et al*. Adult-type Gaucher disease in children: genetics, clinical features and enzyme replacement therapy. *Q J Med* 1993; **86**: 565–73.

26. Pastores GM, Wallenstein S, Desnick RJ *et al*. Bone density in Type 1 Gaucher disease. *J Bone Miner Res* 1996; **11**: 1801–7.

27. Beighton P, Goldblatt J, Sacks S. Bone involvement in Gaucher disease. *Prog Clin Biol Res* 1982; **95**: 107–29.

28. Bembi B, Ciana G, Mengel E *et al*. Bone complications in children with Gaucher disease. *Br J Radiol* 2002; **75** (suppl. 1): A37–A44.

29. Wenstrup RJ, Roca-Espiau M, Weinreb NJ *et al*. Skeletal aspects of Gaucher disease: a review. *Br J Radiol* 2002; **75** (suppl. 1): A2–A12.

30. Stowens DW, Teitelbaum SL, Kahn AJ *et al*. Skeletal complications of Gaucher disease. *Medicine (Baltimore)* 1985; **64**: 310–22.

31. Kaplan P, Mazur A, Manor O *et al*. Acceleration of retarded growth in children with Gaucher disease after treatment with alglucerase. *J Pediatr* 1996; **129**: 149–53.

32. Kauli R, Zaizov R, Lazar L *et al*. Delayed growth and puberty in patients with Gaucher disease type 1: natural history and effect of splenectomy and/or enzyme replacement therapy. *Isr Med Assoc J* 2000; **2**: 158–63.

33. McHugh K, Olsen EO, Vellodi A. Gaucher disease in children: radiology of non-central nervous system manifestations. *Clin Radiol* 2004; **59**: 117–23.

34. Wenstrup RJ, Bailey L, Grabowski GA *et al*. Gaucher disease: alendronate disodium improves bone mineral density in adults receiving enzyme therapy. *Blood* 2004; **104**: 1253–7.

35. Pastores GM, Weinreb NJ, Aerts H *et al*. Therapeutic goals in the treatment of Gaucher disease. *Semin Hematol* 2004; **41**: 4–14.

36. Coon WW. The spleen and splenectomy. *Surg Gynecol Obstet* 1991; **173**: 407–14.

37. Zimran A, Elstein D, Schiffmann R *et al*. Outcome of partial splenectomy for type I Gaucher disease. *J Pediatr* 1995; **126**: 596–7.

38. Barton NW, Brady RO, Dambrosia JM *et al*. Replacement therapy for inherited enzyme deficiency: macrophage-targeted glucocerebrosidase for Gaucher's disease. *N Engl J Med* 1991; **324**: 1464–70.

39. Grabowski GA, Barton NW, Pastores G *et al*. Enzyme therapy in type 1 Gaucher disease: comparative efficacy of mannose-terminated glucocerebrosidase from natural and recombinant sources. *Ann Intern Med* 1995; **122**: 33–9.

40. Hoppe H. Cerezyme – recombinant protein treatment for Gaucher's disease. *J Biotechnol* 2000; **76**: 259–61.

41. Heitner R, Arndt S, Levin JB. Imiglucerase low-dose therapy for paediatric Gaucher disease: a long-term cohort study. *S Afr Med J* 2004; **94**: 647–51.

42. Weinreb NJ, Charrow J, Andersson HC *et al*. Effectiveness of enzyme replacement therapy in 1028 patients with type 1 Gaucher disease after 2 to 5 years of treatment: a report from the Gaucher Registry. *Am J Med* 2002; **113**: 112–19.

43. Grabowski GA, Dulisse B, Charrow J, Weinreb N. The effect of enzyme therapy on bone crises and bone pain in type 1 Gaucher disease, a platform presentation at the American College of Medical Genetics Annual Meeting, March 2005, Dallas, TX.

44. Elstein D, Abrahamov A, Dweck A *et al*. Gaucher disease: pediatric concerns. *Paediatr Drugs* 2002; **4**: 417–26.

45. McCormack PL, Goa KL. Miglustat. *Drugs* 2003; **63**: 2427–34; discussion 2435–6.

46. Platt FM, Jeyakumar M, Andersson U *et al*. Inhibition of substrate synthesis as a strategy for glycolipid lysosomal storage disease therapy. *J Inherit Metab Dis* 2001; **24**: 275–90.

47. Cox TM, Aerts JM, Andria G *et al*. The role of the iminosugar N-butyldeoxynojirimycin (miglustat) in the management of type I (non-neuronopathic) Gaucher disease: a position statement. *J Inherit Metab Dis* 2003; **26**: 513–26.

48. Lachmann RH. Miglustat. Oxford GlycoSciences/Actelion. *Curr Opin Investig Drugs* 2003; **4**: 472–9.

49. Elstein D, Hollak C, Aerts JM *et al*. Sustained therapeutic effects of oral miglustat (Zavesca, N-butyldeoxynojirimycin, OGT 918) in type I Gaucher disease. *J Inherit Metab Dis* 2004; **27**: 757–66.

50. Hussar DA. New drugs of 2003. *J Am Pharm Assoc (Wash DC)* 2004; **44**: 168–206; quiz 207–10.

51. Fredrickson DS, Slaon HR. Glucosyl ceramide lipidoses: Gaucher's disease. In: Stanbury JB, Wyngaarden JB, Fredrickson DS (eds) *The Metabolic Basis of Inherited Disease*, 3rd edn. New York: McGraw-Hill, 1972, p. 730.

52. Tayebi N, Stone DL, Sidransky E. Type 2 Gaucher disease: an expanding phenotype. *Mol Genet Metab* 1999; **68**: 209–19.

53. Brady RO, Barranger JA. Glucosylceramide lipidosis: Gaucher's disease. In: Stanbury JB, Wyngaarden JB, Fredrickson DS, Goldstein JL, Brown MS (eds) *The Metabolic*

Basis of Inherited Disease, 3rd edn. New York: McGraw-Hill, 1983, pp. 842–56.

54. Bove KE, Daugherty C, Grabowski GA. Pathological findings in Gaucher disease type 2 patients following enzyme therapy. *Hum Pathol* 1995; **26**: 1040–5.

55. Patterson MC, Horowitz M, Abel RB *et al.* Isolated horizontal supranuclear gaze palsy as a marker of severe systemic involvement in Gaucher's disease. *Neurology* 1993; **43**: 1993–7.

56. Eto Y, Ida H. Clinical and molecular characteristics of Japanese Gaucher disease. *Neurochem Res* 1999; **24**: 207–11.

57. Inui K, Yanagihara K, Otani K *et al.* A new variant neuropathic type of Gaucher's disease characterized by hydrocephalus, corneal opacities, deformed toes, and fibrous thickening of spleen and liver capsules. *J Pediatr* 2001; **138**: 137–9.

58. Casta A, Hayden K, Wolf WJ. Calcification of the ascending aorta and aortic and mitral valves in Gaucher's disease. *Am J Cardiol* 1984; **54**: 1390–1.

59. Wilson ER, Barton NW, Barranger JA. Vascular involvement in type 3 neuronopathic Gaucher's disease. *Arch Pathol Lab Med* 1985; **109**: 82–4.

60. Chabas A, Cormand B, Grinberg D *et al.* Unusual expression of Gaucher's disease: cardiovascular calcifications in three sibs homozygous for the D409H mutation. *J Med Genet* 1995; **32**: 740–2.

61. George R, McMahon J, Lytle B *et al.* Severe valvular and aortic arch calcification in a patient with Gaucher's disease homozygous for the D409H mutation. *Clin Genet* 2001; **59**: 360–3.

62. Stone DL, Tayebi N, Orvisky E *et al.* Glucocerebrosidase gene mutations in patients with type 2 Gaucher disease. *Hum Mutat* 2000; **15**: 181–8.

63. Ringden O, Groth CG, Erikson A *et al.* Ten years' experience of bone marrow transplantation for Gaucher disease. *Transplantation* 1995; **59**: 864–70.

64. Vellodi A, Bembi B, de Villemeur TB *et al.* Management of neuronopathic Gaucher disease: a European consensus. *J Inherit Metab Dis* 2001; **24**: 319–27.

65. Schiffmann R, Brady RO. New prospects for the treatment of lysosomal storage diseases. *Drugs* 2002; **62**: 733–42.

66. Naureckiene S, Sleat DE, Lackland H *et al.* Identification of HE1 as the second gene of Niemann–Pick C disease. *Science* 2000; **290**: 2298–301.

67. Sleat DE, Wiseman JA, El-Banna M *et al.* Genetic evidence for nonredundant functional cooperativity between NPC1 and NPC2 in lipid transport. *Proc Natl Acad Sci USA* 2004; **101**: 5886–91.

68. Chikh K, Vey S, Simonot C *et al.* Niemann–Pick type C disease: importance of *N*-glycosylation sites for function and cellular location of the NPC2 protein. *Mol Genet Metab* 2004; **83**: 220–30.

69. Schuchman EH, Desnick R. Niemann–Pick disease types A and B: acid sphingomyelinase deficiencies. In: Scriver CR, Beaudet AL, Valle D, Sly WS (eds) *The Metabolic and Molecular Bases of Inherited Disease*, 8th edn. New York: McGraw-Hill, 2001, pp. 3589–610.

70. Graber D, Salvayre R, Levade T. Accurate differentiation of neuronopathic and nonneuronopathic forms of Niemann–Pick disease by evaluation of the effective residual lysosomal sphingomyelinase activity in intact cells. *J Neurochem* 1994; **63**: 1060–8.

71. Quattrin N, De Rosa L, Quattrin S Jr *et al.* Sea blue histiocytosis. A clinical cytologic and nosographic study on 23 cases. *Klin Wochenschr* 1978; **56**: 17–30.

72. Besley GT, Broadhead DM, Lawlor E *et al.* Cholesterol ester storage disease in an adult presenting with sea-blue histiocytosis. *Clin Genet* 1984; **26**: 195–203.

73. Howard MR, Kesteven PJ. Sea blue histiocytosis: a common abnormality of the bone marrow in myelodysplastic syndromes. *J Clin Pathol* 1993; **46**: 1030–2.

74. Kelsey PR, Geary CG. Sea-blue histiocytes and Gaucher cells in bone marrow of patients with chronic myeloid leukaemia. *J Clin Pathol* 1988; **41**: 960–2.

75. Mason BA, Bowers GR, Guccion JG *et al.* Sea-blue histiocytes in a patient with lymphoma. *Am J Med* 1978; **64**: 515–18.

76. Bigorgne C, Le Tourneau A, Vahedi K *et al.* Sea-blue histiocyte syndrome in bone marrow secondary to total parenteral nutrition. *Leukemia Lymphoma* 1998; **28**: 523–9.

77. Maier-Redelsperger M, Girot R. Sea-blue histiocytes in bone-marrow due to a long-term total parenteral nutrition including fat-emulsions. *Br J Haematol* 1997; **97**: 689.

78. Meiklejohn DJ, Baden H, Greaves M. Sea-blue histiocytosis and pancytopaenia associated with chronic total parenteral nutrition administration. *Clin Lab Haematol* 1997; **19**: 219–21.

79. Brady R. *Sphingomyelin Lipidosis: Niemann–Pick Disease*, 5th edn. New York: McGraw-Hill, 1983.

80. Tassoni JP Jr, Fawaz KA, Johnston DE. Cirrhosis and portal hypertension in a patient with adult Niemann–Pick disease. *Gastroenterology* 1991; **100**: 567–9.

81. Putterman C, Zelingher J, Shouval D. Liver failure and the sea-blue histiocyte/adult Niemann–Pick disease. Case report and review of the literature. *J Clin Gastroenterol* 1992; **15**: 146–9.

82. Minai OA, Sullivan EJ, Stoller JK. Pulmonary involvement in Niemann–Pick disease: case report and literature review. *Respir Med* 2000; **94**: 1241–51.

83. Gogus S, Gocmen A, Kocak N *et al.* Lipidosis with sea-blue histiocytes. Report of two siblings with lung involvement. *Turk J Pediatr* 1994; **36**: 139–44.

84. Ferretti GR, Lantuejoul S, Brambilla E *et al.* Case report. Pulmonary involvement in Niemann–Pick disease subtype B: CT findings. *J Comput Assist Tomogr* 1996; **20**: 990–2.

85. Gonzalez-Reimers E, Sanchez-Perez MJ, Bonilla-Arjona A *et al.* Case report. Pulmonary involvement in an adult male affected by type B Niemann–Pick disease. *Br J Radiol* 2003; **76**: 838–40.

86. Duchateau F, Dechambre S, Coche E. Imaging of pulmonary manifestations in subtype B of Niemann–Pick disease. *Br J Radiol* 2001; **74**: 1059–61.

87. Niggemann B, Rebien W, Rahn W *et al.* Asymptomatic pulmonary involvement in 2 children with Niemann–Pick disease type B. *Respiration* 1994; **61**: 55–7.

88. Nicholson AG, Wells AU, Hooper J *et al.* Successful treatment of endogenous lipoid pneumonia due to Niemann–Pick Type B disease with whole-lung lavage. *Am J Respir Crit Care Med* 2002; **165**: 128–31.

89. Vellodi A, Hobbs JR, O'Donnell NM *et al.* Treatment of Niemann–Pick disease type B by allogeneic bone marrow transplantation. *Br Med J* 1987; **295**: 1375–6.

90. Victor S, Coulter JB, Besley GT *et al.* Niemann–Pick disease: sixteen-year follow-up of allogeneic bone marrow

transplantation in a type B variant. *J Inherit Metab Dis* 2003; **26**: 775–85.

91. Patterson MC. A riddle wrapped in a mystery: understanding Niemann–Pick disease, type C. *Neurologist* 2003; **9**: 301–10.

92. Patterson MC, Vanier MT, Suzuki K *et al.* Niemann–Pick disease type C: A lipid trafficking disorder. In: Scriver CR, Beaudet AL, Valle D, Sly WS (eds) *The Metabolic and Molecular Bases of Inherited Disease*, 8th edn. New York: McGraw-Hill, 2001, pp. 3611–33.

93. Park WD, O'Brien JF, Lundquist PA *et al.* Identification of 58 novel mutations in Niemann–Pick disease type C: correlation with biochemical phenotype and importance of PTC1-like domains in NPC1. *Hum Mutat* 2003; **22**: 313–25.

94. Millat G, Chikh K, Naureckiene S *et al.* Niemann–Pick disease type C: Spectrum of HE1 mutations and genotype/phenotype correlations in the NPC2 group. *Am J Hum Genet* 2001; **69**: 1013–21.

95. Sturley SL, Patterson MC, Balch W *et al.* The pathophysiology and mechanisms of NP-C disease. *Biochim Biophys Acta* 2004; **1685**: 83–7.

96. Neufeld EB, Wastney M, Patel S *et al.* The Niemann–Pick C1 protein resides in a vesicular compartment linked to retrograde transport of multiple lysosomal cargo. *J Biol Chem* 1999; **274**: 9627–35.

97. Salvioli R, Scarpa S, Ciaffoni F *et al.* Glucosylceramidase mass and subcellular localization are modulated by cholesterol in Niemann–Pick disease type C. *J Biol Chem* 2004; **279**: 17674–80.

98. Elleder M, Nevoral J, Spicakova V *et al.* A new variant of sphingomyelinase deficiency (Niemann–Pick): visceromegaly, minimal neurological lesions and low in vivo degradation rate of sphingomyelin. *J Inherit Metab Dis* 1986; **9**: 357–66.

99. Gilbert EF, Callahan J, Viseskul C *et al.* Niemann–Pick disease type C. Pathological, histochemical, ultrastructural and biochemical studies. *Eur J Pediatr* 1981; **136**: 263–74.

100. Vanier MT, Millat G. Niemann–Pick disease type C. *Clin Genet* 2003; **64**: 269–81.

101. Lossos A, Schlesinger I, Okon E *et al.* Adult-onset Niemann–Pick type C disease. Clinical, biochemical, and genetic study. *Arch Neurol* 1997; **54**: 1536–41.

102. Grau AJ, Brandt T, Weisbrod M *et al.* Adult Niemann–Pick disease type C mimicking features of multiple sclerosis. *J Neurol Neurosurg Psychiatry* 1997; **63**: 552.

103. Maconochie IK, Chong S, Mieli-Vergani G *et al.* Fetal ascites: an unusual presentation of Niemann–Pick disease type C. *Arch Dis Child* 1989; **64**: 1391–3.

104. Manning DJ, Price WI, Pearse RG. Fetal ascites: an unusual presentation of Niemann–Pick disease type C. *Arch Dis Child* 1990; **65**: 335–6.

105. Shulman LM, David NJ, Weiner WJ. Psychosis as the initial manifestation of adult-onset Niemann–Pick disease type C. *Neurology* 1995; **45**: 1739–43.

106. Vanier MT, Wenger DA, Comly ME *et al.* Niemann–Pick disease group C: Clinical variability and diagnosis based on defective cholesterol esterification. A collaborative study on 70 patients. *Clin Genet* 1988; **33**: 331–48.

107. Gartner JC Jr, Bergman I, Malatack JJ *et al.* Progression of neurovisceral storage disease with supranuclear ophthalmoplegia following orthotopic liver transplantation. *Pediatrics* 1986; **77**: 104–6.

108. Rutledge JC. Progressive neonatal liver failure due to type C Niemann–Pick disease. *Pediatr Pathol* 1989; **9**: 779–84.

109. Jaeken J, Proesmans W, Eggermont E *et al.* Niemann–Pick type C disease and early cholestasis in three brothers. *Acta Paediatr Belg* 1980; **33**: 43–6.

110. Patterson MC, Platt F. Therapy of Niemann–Pick disease, type C. *Biochim Biophys Acta* 2004; **1685**: 77–82.

111. Patterson MC, Di Bisceglie AM, Higgins JJ *et al.* The effect of cholesterol-lowering agents on hepatic and plasma cholesterol in Niemann–Pick disease type C. *Neurology* 1993; **43**: 61–4.

112. Hsu YS, Hwu WL, Huang SF *et al.* Niemann–Pick disease type C (a cellular cholesterol lipidosis) treated by bone marrow transplantation. *Bone Marrow Transplant* 1999; **24**: 103–7.

113. Hall CW, Liebaers I, Di Natale P *et al.* Enzymic diagnosis of the genetic mucopolysaccharide storage disorders. *Methods Enzymol* 1978; **50**: 439–56.

114. Lowry RB, Applegarth DA, Toone JR *et al.* An update on the frequency of mucopolysaccharide syndromes in British Columbia. *Hum Genet* 1990; **85**: 389–90.

115. Nelson J. Incidence of the mucopolysaccharidoses in Northern Ireland. *Hum Genet* 1997; **101**: 355–8.

116. Braunlin EA, Rose AG, Hopwood JJ *et al.* Coronary artery patency following long-term successful engraftment 14 years after bone marrow transplantation in the Hurler syndrome. *Am J Cardiol* 2001; **88**: 1075–7.

117. Brosius FC 3rd, Roberts WC. Coronary artery disease in the Hurler syndrome. Qualitative and quantitative analysis of the extent of coronary narrowing at necropsy in six children. *Am J Cardiol* 1981; **47**: 649–53.

118. Spranger J. The systemic mucopolysaccharidoses. *Ergeb Inn Med Kinderheilkd* 1972; **32**: 165–265.

119. Hamilton E, Pitt P. Articular manifestations of Scheie's syndrome. *Ann Rheum Dis* 1992; **51**: 542–3.

120. Butman SM, Karl L, Copeland JG. Combined aortic and mitral valve replacement in an adult with Scheie's disease. *Chest* 1989; **96**: 209–10.

121. Whitley CB, Belani KG, Chang PN *et al.* Long-term outcome of Hurler syndrome following bone marrow transplantation. *Am J Med Genet* 1993; **46**: 209–18.

122. Vellodi A, Young EP, Cooper A *et al.* Bone marrow transplantation for mucopolysaccharidosis type I: experience of two British centres. *Arch Dis Child* 1997; **76**: 92–9.

123. Souillet G, Guffon N, Maire I *et al.* Outcome of 27 patients with Hurler's syndrome transplanted from either related or unrelated haematopoietic stem cell sources. *Bone Marrow Transplant* 2003; **31**: 1105–17.

124. Peters C, Shapiro EG, Krivit W. Neuropsychological development in children with Hurler syndrome following hematopoietic stem cell transplantation. *Pediatr Transplant* 1998; **2**: 250–3.

125. Braunlin EA, Stauffer NR, Peters CH *et al.* Usefulness of bone marrow transplantation in the Hurler syndrome. *Am J Cardiol* 2003; **92**: 882–6.

126. Hite SH, Peters C, Krivit W. Correction of odontoid dysplasia following bone-marrow transplantation and engraftment (in Hurler syndrome MPS 1H). *Pediatr Radiol* 2000; **30**: 464–70.

127. Staba SL, Escolar ML, Poe M *et al.* Cord-blood transplants from unrelated donors in patients with Hurler's syndrome. *N Engl J Med* 2004; **350**: 1960–9.

128. Wraith JE, Clarke LA, Beck M *et al.* Enzyme replacement therapy for mucopolysaccharidosis I: a randomized, double-blinded, placebo-controlled, multinational study of recombinant human alpha-L-iduronidase (laronidase). *J Pediatr* 2004; **144**: 581–8.

129. Alpha-L-iduronidase (laronidase; aldurazyme). *Med Lett Drugs Ther* 2003; **45**: 88.

130. Keeling KM, Bedwell DM. Clinically relevant aminoglycosides can suppress disease-associated premature stop mutations in the IDUA and P53 cDNAs in a mammalian translation system. *J Mol Med* 2002; **80**: 367–76.

131. Schaap T, Bach G. Incidence of mucopolysaccharidoses in Israel: is Hunter disease a "Jewish disease"? *Hum Genet* 1980; **56**: 221–3.

132. Young ID, Harper PS. Incidence of Hunter's syndrome. *Hum Genet* 1982; **60**: 391–2.

133. Neufeld EF, Muenzer J. The mucopolysaccharidoses. In: Scriver CR, Beaudet AL, Valle D, Sly WS (eds) *The Metabolic and Molecular Bases of Inherited Disease*, 8th edn. New York: McGraw-Hill, 2001, pp. 3421–52.

134. Hobolth N, Pedersen C. Six cases of a mild form of Hunter syndrome in five generations. Three affected males with progeny. *Clin Genet* 1978; **20**: 121.

135. McKinnis EJ, Sulzbacher S, Rutledge JC *et al.* Bone marrow transplantation in Hunter syndrome. *J Pediatr* 1996; **129**: 145–8.

136. Coppa GV, Gabrielli O, Cordiali R *et al.* Bone marrow transplantation in a Hunter patient with P266H mutation. *Int J Mol Med* 1999; **4**: 433–6.

137. Coppa GV, Gabrielli O, Zampini L *et al.* Bone marrow transplantation in Hunter syndrome. *J Inherit Metab Dis* 1995; **18**: 91–2.

138. Bergstrom SK, Quinn JJ, Greenstein R *et al.* Long-term follow-up of a patient transplanted for Hunter's disease type IIB: a case report and literature review. *Bone Marrow Transplant* 1994; **14**: 653–8.

139. Li P, Thompson JN, Hug G *et al.* Biochemical and molecular analysis in a patient with the severe form of Hunter syndrome after bone marrow transplantation. *Am J Med Genet* 1996; **64**: 531–5.

140. Vellodi A, Young E, Cooper A *et al.* Long-term follow-up following bone marrow transplantation for Hunter disease. *J Inherit Metab Dis* 1999; **22**: 638–48.

141. Peters C, Krivit W. Hematopoietic cell transplantation for mucopolysaccharidosis IIB (Hunter syndrome). *Bone Marrow Transplant* 2000; **25**: 1097–9.

142. Muenzer J, Lamsa JC, Garcia A *et al.* Enzyme replacement therapy in mucopolysaccharidosis type II (Hunter syndrome): a preliminary report. *Acta Paediatr Suppl* 2002; **91**: 98–9.

143. Tan CT, Schaff HV, Miller FA Jr *et al.* Valvular heart disease in four patients with Maroteaux–Lamy syndrome. *Circulation* 1992; **85**: 188–95.

144. Krivit W, Pierpont ME, Ayaz K *et al.* Bone-marrow transplantation in the Maroteaux–Lamy syndrome (mucopolysaccharidosis type VI). Biochemical and clinical status 24 months after transplantation. *N Engl J Med* 1984; **311**: 1606–11.

145. McGovern MM, Ludman MD, Short MP *et al.* Bone marrow transplantation in Maroteaux–Lamy syndrome (MPS type 6): status 40 months after BMT. *Birth Defects* 1986; **22**: 41–53.

146. Harmatz P, Whitley CB, Waber L *et al.* Enzyme replacement therapy in mucopolysaccharidosis VI (Maroteaux–Lamy syndrome). *J Pediatr* 2004; **144**: 574–80.

147. Schmitz G, Assmann G. Acid lipase deficiency: Wolman's disease and cholesteryl ester storage disease. In: Stanbury JB, Wyngaarden JB, Fredrickson DS, Goldberg M, Brown MS (eds) *The Metabolic Basis of Inherited Disease*, 6th edn. New York: McGraw-Hill, 1989, pp. 1623–44.

148. Assmann G, Seedorf U. Acid lipase deficiency: Wolman disease and cholesteryl ester storage disease. In: Scriver CR, Beaudet AL, Valle D, Sly WS (eds) *The Metabolic and Molecular Bases of Inherited Disease*, 8th edn. New York: McGraw-Hill, 2001, pp. 3551–72.

149. Pfeiffer U, Jeschke R. Cholesterylester-Speicherkrankheit. *Virchows Arch B* 1980; **33**: 17.

150. Ginsberg HN, Le NA, Short MP *et al.* Suppression of apolipoprotein B production during treatment of cholesteryl ester storage disease with lovastatin. Implications for regulation of apolipoprotein B synthesis. *J Clin Invest* 1987; **80**: 1692–7.

151. Krivit W, Peters C, Dusenbery K *et al.* Wolman disease successfully treated by bone marrow transplantation. *Bone Marrow Transplant* 2000; **26**: 567–70.

152. Phillips SN, Benedict JW, Weimer JM *et al.* CLN3, the protein associated with batten disease: Structure, function and localization. *J Neurosci Res* 2005; **79**: 573–83.

153. Vesa J, Chin MH, Oelgeschlager K *et al.* Neuronal ceroid lipofuscinoses are connected at molecular level: interaction of CLN5 protein with CLN2 and CLN3. *Mol Biol Cell* 2002; **13**: 2410–20.

154. Mole SE, Michaux G, Codlin S *et al.* CLN6, which is associated with a lysosomal storage disease, is an endoplasmic reticulum protein. *Exp Cell Res* 2004; **298**: 399–406.

155. Lonka L, Salonen T, Siintola E *et al.* Localization of wild-type and mutant neuronal ceroid lipofuscinosis CLN8 proteins in non-neuronal and neuronal cells. *J Neurosci Res* 2004; **76**: 862–71.

156. Butters TD, Mellor HR, Narita K *et al.* Small-molecule therapeutics for the treatment of glycolipid lysosomal storage disorders. *Philos Trans R Soc Lond B Biol Sci* 2003; **358**: 927–45.

Reference values

Paula S. Simpkin and Roderick F. Hinchliffe

The values of many hematologic variables change markedly in the first weeks and months of life and reference data are important to enable proper interpretation of laboratory results, both in infancy and until an age at which adult reference ranges can be applied.

Most reference data are affected to some degree by factors such as racial origin, diet, drug intake and the presence of subclinical illness. Other variables include the methodology and instrumentation used to obtain the data and the method of statistical analysis. Ideally, each laboratory would generate its own reference ranges from the population it serves, but this is rarely if ever practical. However, the following tables and figures (listed below) should prove useful in most circumstances.

Contents

Blood count variables: a summary (birth–18 years)   Table 37.1

Hematologic variables in healthy premature infants
Red cell values   Table 37.2
Hemoglobin values   Table 37.3
Neutrophil values   Tables 37.4 and Fig. 37.1
Platelet values   Figure 37.2
Coagulation screening tests, 24–29 weeks' gestation   Table 37.5
Coagulation factor levels, 30–36 weeks' gestation   Table 37.6
Coagulation inhibitor levels, 30–36 weeks' gestation   Table 37.7

Hematologic variables in term infants and older children

Red cells and associated variables
In the first year   Table 37.8
In African neonates   Table 37.9
4–18 years   Table 37.10
Reticulocytes in the first year   Table 37.11
Hemoglobins F and A$_2$ Tables 37.12 and 37.13
Methemoglobin   Table 37.14
Red cell enzymes   Table 37.15
Red cell morphology in term neonates   Figure 37.3
Iron and transferrin   Tables 37.16 and Fig. 37.4
Serum ferritin   Figure 37.5
Soluble transferrin receptor   Table 37.17
Zinc protoporphyrin   Table 37.18
Vitamin B$_{12}$, serum and red cell folate   Tables 37.19 and 37.20
Erythropoietin   Table 37.21
Red cell and plasma volume   Table 37.22

Red cell survival in term and preterm infants   Table 37.23
Bilirubin   Figure 37.6
Haptoglobin   Table 37.24

Normal white cell values
Neutrophils
At term   Figure 37.7
In the first month   Figure 37.8
Immature forms in the first month   Tables 37.25 and Fig. 37.9
In African neonates   Table 37.26
At 2, 5 and 13 months   Table 37.27
4–19 years   Table 37.28

Lymphocytes
In the first month   Table 37.29
In African neonates   Table 37.26
At 2, 5 and 13 months   Table 37.27
4–19 years   Table 37.28
Subsets   Table 37.30

Monocytes and eosinophils
In the first month   Table 37.29
At 2, 5 and 13 months   Table 37.27
4–19 years   Table 37.28

Basophils
At 2, 5 and 13 months   Table 37.27
4–19 years   Table 37.28

Progenitor cells   Table 37.31

Other hematologic variables

Normal values for hemostatic variables
Coagulation factor levels in healthy term infants   Table 37.32
Coagulation inhibitor levels in healthy term infants   Table 37.33
FDP-D dimer levels at birth   Table 37.34
PIVKA-II levels at birth   Figure 37.10
Platelet count throughout childhood   Table 37.35
PFA-100 closure time in children and adults   Table 37.36
Bleeding time in and children and adults   Table 37.37

Normal values for immunoglobulins
IgG, IgA, IgM, neonate to adult   Table 37.38
IgG subclasses, neonate to adult   Table 37.39
IgD, infants and children   Table 37.40
IgE, neonate to adult   Table 37.41

Normal values for the ESR in children   Table 37.42

Normal isohemagglutinin titers: birth to adult   Table 37.43

Table 37.1 Normal blood count values from birth to 18 years.

Age	Hemoglobin (g/dl)	RBC ($\times10^{12}$/l)	Hematocrit	MCV (fl)	WBC ($\times10^9$/l)	Neutrophils ($\times10^9$/l)	Lymphocytes ($\times10^9$/l)	Monocytes ($\times10^9$/l)	Eosinophils ($\times10^9$/l)	Basophils ($\times10^9$/l)	Platelets ($\times10^9$/l)
Birth (term infants)	14.9–23.7	3.7–6.5	0.47–0.75	100–125	10–26	2.7–14.4	2.0–7.3	0–1.9	0–0.85	0–0.1	150–450
2 weeks	13.4–19.8	3.9–5.9	0.41–0.65	88–110	6–21	1.5–5.4	2.8–9.1	0.1–1.7	0–0.85	0–0.1	170–500
2 months	9.4–130	3.1–4.3	0.28–0.42	84–98	5–15	0.7–4.8	33–10.3	0.4–1.2	0.05–0.9	0.02–0.13	210–650
6 months	10.0–13.0	3.8–4.9	0.3–0.38	73–84	6–17	1–6	3.3–11.5	0.2–1.3	0.1–1.1	0.02–02	210–560
1 year	10.1–13.0	3.9–5.1	0.3–0.38	70–82	6–16	1–8	3.4–10.5	0.2–0.9	0.05–0.9	0.02–0.13	200–550
2–6 years	11.0–13.8	3.9–5.0	0.32–0.4	72–87	6–17	1.5–8.5	1.8–8.4	0.15–1.3	0.05–1.1	0.02–0.12	210–490
6–12 years	11.1–14.7	3.9–5.2	0.32–0.43	76–90	4.5–14.5	1.5–8.0	1.5–5.0	0.15–1.3	0.05–1.0	0.02–0.12	170–450
12–18 years											
Female	12.1–15.1	4.1–5.1	0.35–0.44	77–94							
					4.5–13	1.5–6	1.5–4.5	0.15–1.3	0.05–0.8	0.02–0.12	180–430
Male	12.1–16.6	4.2–5.6	0.35–0.49	77–92							

Compiled from various sources. Red cell values at birth derived from skin puncture blood; most other data from venous blood.
MCV, mean corpuscular volume; RBC, red blood cell; WBC, white blood cell.

Table 37.2 Red blood cell (RBC) values (mean ± 1 SD) on the first postnatal day from 24 weeks' gestational age.

Gestational age (weeks)	24–25 (n = 7)	26–27 (n = 11)	28–29 (n = 7)	30–31 (n = 35)	32–33 (n = 23)	34–35 (n = 23)	36–37 (n = 20)	Term (n = 19)
RBC ($\times10^{12}$/l)	4.65 ± 0.43	4.73 ± 0.45	4.62 ± 0.75	4.79 ± 0.74	5.0 ± 0.76	5.09 ± 0.5	5.27 ± 0.68	5.14 ± 0.7
Hemoglobin (g/dl)	19.4 ± 1.5	19.0 ± 2.5	19.3 ± 1.8	19.1 ± 2.2	18.5 ± 2.0	19.6 ± 2.1	19.2 ± 11.7	19.3 ± 2.2
Hematocrit	0.63 ± 0.04	0.62 ± 0.08	0.60 ± 0.07	0.60 ± 0.08	0.60 ± 0.08	0.61 ± 0.07	0.64 ± 0.07	0.61 ± 0.074
MCV (fl)	135 ± 0.2	132 ± 14.4	131 ± 13.5	127 ± 12.7	123 ± 15.7	122 ± 10.0	121 ± 12.5	119 ± 9.4
Reticulocytes	6.0 ± 0.5	9.6 ± 3.2	7.5 ± 2.5	5.8 ± 2.0	5.0 ± 1.9	3.9 ± 1.6	4.2 ± 1.8	3.2 ± 1.4
Weight (g)	725 ± 185	993 ± 194	1174 ± 128	1450 ± 232	1816 ± 192	1957 ± 291	2245 ± 213	

Counts performed on heel-prick blood. MCV, mean corpuscular volume.
Reproduced with permission from Ref. 1.

Table 37.3 Hemoglobin values (g/dl, median and 95% range) in the first 6 months of life in iron-sufficient (serum ferritin ≥ 10 µg/l) preterm infants.

Age	Birthweight 1000–1500 g	Number tested	Birthweight 1501–2000 g	Number tested
2 weeks	16.3 (11.7–18.4)	17	14.8 (11.8–19.6)	39
1 month	10.9 (8.7–15.2)	15	11.5 (8.2–15.0)	42
2 months	8.8 (7.1–11.5)	17	9.4 (8.0–11.4)	47
3 months	9.8 (8.9–11.2)	16	10.2 (9.3–11.8)	41
4 months	11.3 (9.1–13.1)	13	11.3 (9.1–13.1)	37
5 months	11.6 (10.2–14.3)	8	11.8 (10.4–13.0)	21
6 months	12.0 (9.4–13.8)	9	11.8 (10.7–12.6)	21

All infants had an uncomplicated course in the first 2 weeks of life and none received exchange transfusion. Counts obtained from venous and skin-puncture blood.
Reproduced with permission from Ref. 2.

Table 37.4 Values for mature and immature neutrophils and the ratio of immature to total neutrophils in 24 infants < 33 weeks' gestation.

Age (hours)	Mature neutrophils (×10⁹/l)		Immature neutrophils (×10⁹/l)		Immature : total ratio	
	Median (range)	Mean	Median (range)	Mean	Median (range)	Mean
1 (*n* = 10)	4.64 (2.20–8.18)	4.57	0.11 (0–1.5)	0.30	0.04 (0–0.35)	0.09
12 (*n* = 17)	6.80 (4.0–22.48)	8.61	0.27 (0–1.6)	0.48	0.04 (0–0.21)	0.06
24 (*n* = 17)	5.60 (2.61–21.20)	7.64	0.14 (0–3.66)	0.47	0.03 (0–0.17)	0.05
48 (*n* = 20)	4.98 (1.02–14.43)	6.24	0.13 (0–2.15)	0.44	0.02 (0–0.17)	0.05
72 (*n* = 22)	3.19 (1.28–13.94)	4.63	0.16 (0–2.42)	0.38	0.3 (0–0.25)	0.05
96 (*n* = 21)	3.44 (1.37–16.56)	5.33	0.23 (0–3.95)	0.45	0.05 (0–0.37)	0.07
120 (*n* = 17)	3.46 (1.27–15.00)	4.98	0.25 (0–2.89)	0.44	0.05 (0–0.21)	0.07

Reproduced with permission from Ref. 3.

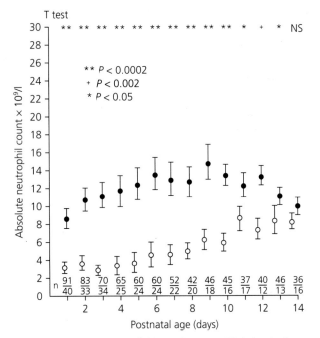

Fig. 37.1 Neutrophil count (×10⁹/l, bar indicates ± 1 SD) during the first 14 days of life in babies of appropriate weight for gestational age (•) and those who were small for gestational age (○). Reproduced with permission from Ref. 4.

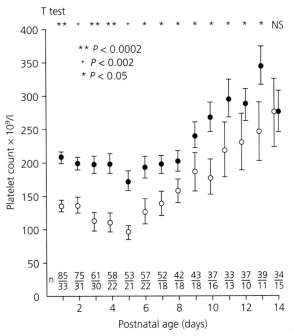

Fig. 37.2 Platelet count (×10⁹/l, bar indicates ± 1 SD) during the first 14 days of life in babies of appropriate weight for gestational age (•) and babies who were small for gestational age (○). Reproduced with permission from Ref. 4.

Table 37.5 Coagulation data (mean and 95% range) in 52 infants of 24–29 weeks' gestational age.

Birthweight (g)	992 (623–1489)
PT (s)	14.5 (11.7–21.6)
Adult mean PT (s)	11.6–12.1
PT ratio	1.2 (1–1.9)
APTT (s)	69.5 (40.6–101)*
Adult mean APTT (s)	30.5–32.5
APTT ratio	2.2 (1.3–3.3)
Fibrinogen (g/l)	1.35 (0.62–4.21)

* 6 values of > 100 s recorded as 101 s.
APTT, activated partial thromboplastin time; PT, prothrombin time.
Summarized from Ref. 5.

Table 37.6 Reference values for coagulation tests in healthy premature infants (30–36 weeks' gestation) during the first 6 months of life.

	Day 1		Day 5		Day 30		Day 90		Day 180		Adult	
	M	B	M	B	M	B	M	B	M	B	M	B
PT (s)	13.0	(10.6–16.2)*	12.5	(10.0–15.3)*†	11.8	(10.0–13.6)*	12.3	(10.0–14.6)*	12.5	(10.0–15.0)*	12.4	(10.8–13.9)
APTT (s)	53.6	(27.5–79.4)‡	50.5	(26.9–74.1)‡	44.7	(26.9–62.5)	39.5	(28.3–50.7)	37.5	(21.7–53.3)*	33.5	(26.6–40.3)
TCT (s)	24.8	(19.2–30.4)*	24.1	(18.8–29.4)*	24.4	(18.8–29.9)*	25.1	(19.4–30.8)*	25.2	(18.9–31.5)*	25.0	(19.7–30.3)
Fibrinogen (g/l)	2.43	(1.50–3.73)*†‡	2.80	(1.60–4.18)*†‡	2.54	(1.50–4.14)*†	2.46	(1.50–3.52)*†	2.28	(1.50–3.60)†	2.78	(1.56–4.00)
H (unit/ml)	0.45	(0.20–0.77)†	0.57	(0.29–0.85)‡	0.57	(0.36–0.95)†‡	0.68	(0.30–1.06)	0.87	(0.51–1.23)	1.08	(0.70–1.46)
FV (unit/ml)	0.88	(0.41–1.44)*†‡	1.00	(0.46–1.54)	1.02	(0.48–1.56)	0.99	(0.59–1.39)	1.02	(0.58–1.46)	1.06	(0.62–1~50)
FVII (unit/ml)	0.67	(0.21–1.13)	0.84	(0.30–1.38)	0.83	(0.21–1.45)	0.87	(0.31–1.43)	0.99	(0.47–1.51)*	1.05	(0.67–1.43)
FVIII (unit/ml)	1.11	(0.50–2.13)*†	1.15	(0.53–2.05)*†‡	1.11	(0.50–1.99)*†‡	1.06	(0.58–1.88)*†‡	0.99	(0.50–1.87)*‡	0.99	(0.50–1.49)
vWF (unit/ml)	1.36	(0.78–2.10)†	1.33	(0.72–2.19)†	1.36	(0.66–2.16)†	1.12	(0.75–1.84)*†	0.98	(0.54–1.58)*†	0.92	(0.50–1.58)
FIX (unit/ml)	0.35	(0.19–0.65)†‡	0.42	(0.14–0.74)†‡	0.44	(0.13–0.80)†	0.59	(0.25–0.93)	0.81	(0.50–1.20)†	1.09	(0.55–1.63)
FX (unit/ml)	0.41	(0.11–0.71)	0.51	(0.19–0.83)	0.56	(0.20–0.92)	0.67	(0.35–0.99)	0.77	(0.35–1.19)	1.06	(0.70–1.52)
FXI (unit/ml)	0.30	(0.08–0.52)†‡	0.41	(0.13–0.69)‡	0.43	(0.15–0.71)‡	0.59	(0.25–0.93)‡	0.78	(0.46–1.10)	0.97	(0.67–1.27)
FXII (unit/ml)	0.38	(0.10–0.66)‡	0.39	(0.09–0.69)‡	0.43	(0.11–0.75)	0.61	(0.15–1.07)	0.82	(0.22–1.42)	1.08	(0.52–1.64)
PK (unit/ml)	0.33	(0.09–0.57)	0.45	(0.28–0.75)†	0.59	(0.31–0.87)	0.79	(0.37–1.21)	0.78	(0.40–1.16)	1.12	(0.62–1.62)
HMWK (unit/ml)	0.49	(0.09–0.89)	0.62	(0.24–1.00)‡	0.64	(0.16–1.12)‡	0.78	(0.32–1.24)	0.83	(0.41–1.25)*	0.92	(0.50–1.36)
FXIIIa (unit/ml)	0.70	(0.32–1.08)	1.01	(0.57–1.45)*	0.99	(0.51–1.47)*	1.13	(0.71–1.55)*	1.13	(0.65–1.61)*	1.05	(0.55–1.55)
FXIIIb (unit/ml)	0.81	(0.35–1.27)	1.10	(0.68–1.58)*	1.07	(0.57–1.57)*	1.21	(0.75–1.67)	1.15	(0.67–1.63)	0.97	(0.57–1.37)
Plasminogen (CTA, unit/ml)	1.70	(1.12–2.48)†‡	1.91	(1.21–2.61)‡	1.81	(1.09–2.53)	2.38	(1.58–3.18)	2.75	(1.91–3.59)	3.36	(2.48–4.24)

All values are given as a mean (M) followed by lower and upper boundaries (B) encompassing 95% of the population. All factors except fibrinogen and plasminogen are expressed as unit/ml where pooled plasma contains 1.0 unit/ml. Plasminogen units are those recommended by the Committee on Thrombolytic Agents (CTA). Between 40 and 96 samples were assayed for each value for newborns.

* Values indistinguishable from those of adults.

† Measurements are skewed owing to a disproportionate number of high values. Lower limit, which excludes the lower 2.5% of the population, is given (B).

‡ Values different from those of full-term infants.

PT, prothrombin time; APTT, activated partial thromboplastin time; TCT, thrombin clotting time; vWF, von Willebrand factor; PK, prekallikrein; HMWK, high-molecular-weight kininogen.

Reproduced with permission from Ref 6.

Table 37.7 Reference values for inhibitors of coagulation in healthy premature infants (30–36 weeks' gestation) during the first 6 months of life.

	Day 1		Day 5		Day 30		Day 90		Day 180		Adult	
	M	B	M	B	M	B	M	B	M	B	M	B
ATIII (unit/ml)	0.38	(0.14–0.62)‡	0.56	(0.30–0.82)*	0.59	(0.37–0.81)‡	0.83	(0.45–1.21)‡	0.90	(0.52–1.28)‡	1.05	(0.79–1.31)
α_2-M (unit/ml)	1.10	(0.56–1.82)†‡	1.25	(0.71–1.77)*	1.38	(0.72–2.04)	1.80	(1.20–2.66)†	2.09	(1.10–3.21)†	0.86	(0.52–1.20)
α_2-AP (unit/ml)	0.78	(0.40–1.16)	0.81	(0.49–1.13)*	0.89	(0.55–1.23)†	1.06	(0.64–1.48)△	1.15	(0.77–1.53)	1.02	(0.68–1.36)
C1E-INH (unit/ml)	0.65	(0.31–0.99)	0.83	(0.45–1.21)	0.74	(0.40–1.24)†‡	1.14	(0.60–1.68)*	1.40	(0.96–2.04)†	1.01	(0.71–1.31)
α_1-AT (unit/ml)	0.90	(0.36–1.44)*	0.94	(0.42–1.46)‡	0.76	(0.38–1.12)‡	0.81	(0.49–1.13)*‡	0.82	(0.48–1.16)*	0.93	(0.55–1.31)
HCII (unit/ml)	0.32	(0.00–0.60)‡	0.34	(0.00–0.69)*	0.43	(0.15–0.71)	0.61	(0.20–1.11)†	0.89	(0.45–1.40)*†‡	0.96	(0.66–1.26)
Protein C (unit/ml)	0.28	(0.12–0.44)*	0.31	(0.11–0.51)*	0.37	(0.15–0.59)‡	0.45	(0.23–0.67)‡	0.57	(0.31–0.83)	0.96	(0.64–1.28)
Protein S (unit/ml)	0.26	(0.14–0.38)‡	0.37	(0.13–0.61)*	0.56	(0.22–0.90)	0.76	(0.40–1.12)‡	0.82	(0.44–1.20)	0.92	(0.60–1.24)

All values are expressed in unit/ml, where pooled plasma contains 1.0 unit/ml. All values are given as a mean (M) followed by lower and upper boundaries (B) encompassing 95% of the population. Between 40 and 75 samples were assayed for each value for newborns.

* Values indistinguishable from those of adults.

† Measurements are skewed owing to a disproportionate number of high values. Lower limit, which excludes the lower 2.5% of the population, is given (B).

‡ Values different from those of full-term infants.

ATIII, antithrombin III; α_2-M, α_2-macroglobulin; α_2-AP, α_2-antiplasmin; C1E-INH, C1 esterase inhibitor; α_1-AT, α_1-antitrypsin; HCII, heparin cofactor II.

Reproduced with permission from Ref 6.

Table 37.8 Normal hemoglobin (Hb) and red blood cell (RBC) values in the first year of life.

	0.5 months (n = 232)	1 month (n = 240)	2 months (n = 241)	4 months (n = 52)	6 months (n = 52)	9 months (n = 56)	12 months (n = 56)
Hb (g/dl)							
Mean	16.6	13.9	11.2	12.2	12.6	12.7	12.7
–2 SD	13.4	10.7	9.4	10.3	11.1	11.4	11.3
Hematocrit							
Mean	0.53	0.44	0.35	0.38	0.36	0.36	0.37
–2 SD	41	33	28	32	31	32	33
RBC (×10¹²/l)							
Mean	4.9	4.3	3.7	4.3	4.7	4.7	4.7
–2 SD, +2 SD	3.9–5.9	3.3–5.3	3.1–4.3	3.5–5.1	3.9–5.5	4.0–5.3	4.1–5.3
MCH (pg)							
Mean	33.6	32.5	30.4	28.6	26.8	27.3	26.8
–2 SD	30	29	27	25	24	25	24
MCV (fl)							
Mean	105.3	101.3	94.8	86.7	76.3	77.7	77.7
–2 SD	88	91	84	76	68	70	71
MCHC (g/dl)							
Mean	31.4	31.8	31.8	32.7	35.0	34.9	34.3
–2 SD	28.1	28.1	28.3	28.8	32.7	32.4	32.1

Values after the age of 2 months were obtained from an iron-supplemented group in whom iron deficiency was excluded. Counts performed on venous blood.
MCH, mean corpuscular hemoglobin; MCHC, mean corpuscular hemoglobin concentration; MCV, mean corpuscular volume.
Reproduced with permission from Ref. 7.

Table 37.9 Hemoglobin (Hb), hematocrit (Hct) and red blood cells (RBC) in term African neonates. Values are means ± 1 SD.

	Number tested	Hb (g/dl)	Hct	RBC (×10¹²/l)
Day 1	304	15.6 ± 2.0	0.450 ± 0.065	4.00 ± 0.67
Day 3	261	15.5 ± 2.1	0.442 ± 0.062	3.91 ± 0.61
Day 7	249	14.2 ± 2.3	0.413 ± 0.063	3.67 ± 0.55
Week 2	233	13.1 ± 1.9	0.391 ± 0.043	3.45 ± 0.56
Week 3	145	11.1 ± 1.8	0.356 ± 0.050	3.27 ± 0.47
Week 4	117	10.6 ± 1.6	0.325 ± 0.044	3.01 ± 0.48

Values are lower than those reported in neonates from Europe and North America, and may be intrinsic to this group. Other variables (RBC indices, reticulocytes) do not differ from those in other populations studied. Hb measured as oxyhemoglobin, Hct by centrifuged microhematocrit and RBC by hemocytometry using venous blood.
Summarized from Ref. 8.

Table 37.10 Red cell values (3rd to 97th centiles) derived from 2135 Irish schoolchildren.

Age (years)	Hb (g/dl)	RBC (x10^{12}/l)	Hematocrit	MCV (fl)	MCH (pg)	MCHC (g/dl)
Girls and boys						
4 + 5	11.0–13.6	3.93–4.99	0.32–0.40	75–87	25.4–29.6	32.9–35.7
6	11.1–13.8	3.93–4.98	0.32–0.40	76–87	25.6–30.7	32.9–35.6
7	11.3–14.2	3.98–5.05	0.33–0.41	75–87	25.4–30.7	33.2–35.7
8	11.5–14.2	4.00–5.11	0.33–0.41	77–89	26.3–31.7	33.1–36.4
9	11.9–14.5	4.08–5.04	0.34–0.41	76–89	26.2–31.2	33.3–35.8
10	11.9–14.5	4.12–5.06	0.34–0.42	77–90	26.5–30.9	33.2–35.7
11	12.1–14.5	4.13–5.19	0.35–0.42	78–89	25.9–31.2	33.1–35.7
12	12.1–14.7	4.16–5.17	0.35–0.43	77–90	26.3–30.9	32.7–35.7
Girls						
13 + 14	12.1–14.6	4.03–5.05	0.35–0.43	80–93	27.3–32.3	33.2–35.2
15–19	11.8–15.1	4.06–5.07	0.35–0.44	79–94	26.7–32.5	33.0–35.5
Boys						
13 + 14	12.4–15.6	4.33–5.42	0.36–0.45	79–91	26.9–31.8	33.4–35.4
15–18	13.2–16.6	4.46–5.61	0.38–0.49	79–92	26.9–31.9	33.5–35.2

MCH, mean corpuscular hemoglobin; MCHC, mean corpuscular hemoglobin concentration; MCV, mean corpuscular volume.
Summarized from Ref. 9.

Table 37.11 Reticulocyte counts (×10^9/l) in the first year of life in term infants.

Age	Reticulocytes
1 day	110–450
7 days	10–80
1 month	10–65
2 months	45–210
5 months	30–120
12 months	40–140

Data from various sources, based on microscope and flow cytometric counts.

Table 37.12 Percentage of hemoglobin F in the first year of life.

Age	Number tested	Mean	2 SD	Range
1–7 days	10	74.7	5.4	61–79.6
2 weeks	13	74.9	5.7	66–88.5
1 month	11	60.2	6.3	45.7–67.3
2 months	10	45.6	10.1	29.4–60.8
3 months	10	26.6	14.5	14.8–55.9
4 months	10	17.7	6.1	9.4–28.5
5 months	10	10.4	6.7	2.3–22.4
6 months	15	6.5	3.0	2.7–13.0
8 months	11	5.1	3.6	2.3–11.9
10 months	10	2.1	0.7	1.5–3.5
12 months	10	2.6	1.5	1.3–5.0
1–14 years and adults	100	0.6	0.4	–

HbF measured by alkali denaturation.
Reproduced with permission from Ref. 10.

Table 37.13 Percentage of hemoglobin A$_2$ in the first 2 years of life.

Age (months)	A			B			
	No. tested	Mean	SD	No. tested	Mean	SD	Range
Birth	16	0.4	0.2				
1	6	0.8	0.3	5	0.8	0.4	0.4–13
2	7	1.3	0.7	9	1.3	0.5	0.4–1.9
3	8	1.7	0.3	8	2.2	0.6	1.0–3.0
4	9	2.1	0.3	3	2.4	0.4	2.0–2.8
5	8	2.3	0.2				
5–6				15	2.5	0.3	2.1–3.1
6	8	2.5	0.3				
7–8	6	2.5	0.4				
7–9				22	2.7	0.4	1.9–3.5
9–10	6	2.5	0.4				
10–12				14	2.7	0.4	2.0–3.3
12	5	2.5	0.3				
13–16				13	2.6	0.5	1.6–3.3
17–20				13	2.9	0.4	2.1–3.6
21–24				15	2.8	0.4	2.0–3.6

Data derived from two studies: A (Ref. 11) measured by microcolumn chromatography and B (Ref. 12) measured by elution following electrophoresis.

Table 37.14 Methemoglobin levels in children and adults.

Subjects	Methemoglobin (g/dl)				Methemoglobin (% of total Hb)			
	No.	Mean	SD	Range	No.	Mean	SD	Range
Prematures, birth–7 days	29	0.43	0.07	0.02–0.83	24	2.3	1.26	0.08–4.4
Prematures, 7–72 days	21	0.31	0.19	0.02–0.78	18	2.2	1.07	0.02–4.7
Newborns, 1–10 days	39	0.22	0.17	0–0.58	25	1.5	0.81	0–2.8
Infants, 1 month–1 year	8	0.14	0.09	0.02–0.29	8	1.2	0.78	0.17–2.4
Children, 1–14 years	35	0.11	0.09	0–0.33	35	0.79	0.62	0–2.4
Adults, 14–78 years	30	0.11	0.09	0–0.28	27	0.82	0.63	0–1.9

Summarized from Ref. 13.

Table 37.15 Comparison of enzyme activities and glutathione content in newborn and adult red blood cells.

Enzyme	Activity in normal adult RBC in IU/g Hb (mean ± 1 SD at 37°C) (100%) activity	Mean activity in newborn RBC as percentage of mean in normal adult RBC
Aldolase	3.19 ± 0.86	140
Enolase	5.39 ± 0.83	250
Glucose phosphate isomerase	60.8 ± 11.0	162
Glucose 6-phosphate dehydrogenase	8.34 ± 1.59	174
WHO method	121 ± 2.09	
Glutathione peroxidase	30.82 ± 4.65	56
Glyceraldehyde phosphate dehydrogenase	226 ± 41.9	170
Hexokinase	1.78 ± 0.38	239
Lactate dehydrogenase	200 ± 26.5	132
NADH-methemoglobin reductase	19.2 ± 3.85 (at 30°C)	Increased
Phosphofructokinase	11.01 ± 2.33	97
Phosphoglycerate kinase	320 ± 36.1	165
Pyruvate kinase	15.0 ± 1.99	160
6-Phosphogluconate dehydrogenase	8.78 ± 0.78	150
Triose phosphate isomerase	211 ± 39.7	101
Glutathione	6570 ± 1040 nmol/g Hb	156

Percentage activity in newborn RBCs compared with mean adult (100%) values is presented with quantitative data from studies on adult RBCs. Newborn data from Ref. 14; quantitative date from Ref. 15.
Reproduced with permission from Ref. 16.

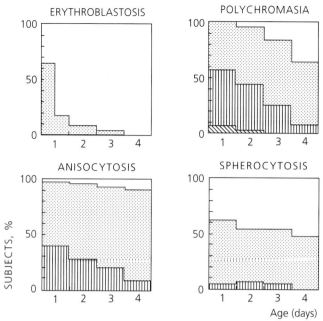

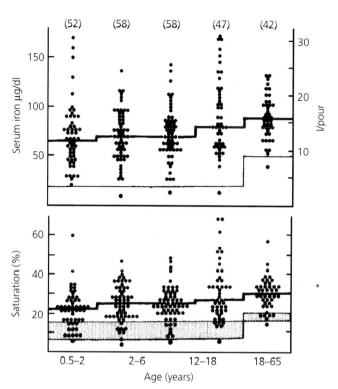

Fig. 37.3 Red blood cell morphology in the first 4 days of life in 138 healthy term infants. Findings are graded from normal (white area) to mild, moderate and marked change (the last only in the case of polychromasia). Erythroblastosis: mild, 1–2 cells/10–15 fields; moderate, 1–5 cells/100 WBC. Polychromasia: mild, 1 cell in every or every other field; moderate, 1–3 cells/field; marked, > 3 cells/field. Anisocytosis: mild, < 5 cells/field differ in size from normal; moderate, the variation is more marked. Spherocytosis: mild, 1 spherocyte in every or every other field; moderate, on average > 1 spherocyte/field. Reproduced with permission from Ref. 17.

Fig. 37.4 Normal values for serum iron and transferrin saturation in individuals with normal values of hemoglobin, mean corpuscular volume, serum ferritin and free erythrocyte protoporphyrin. The heavy horizontal lines indicate the median values, the lower lines the lower limit of the 95% range, and the stippled area an intermediate zone of overlap between iron-deficient and normal subjects. Numbers of subjects are given in parentheses. Reproduced with permission from Ref. 19.

Table 37.16 Values of serum iron, total iron-binding capacity (TIBC) and transferrin saturation from a group of 47 infants.

		Age (months)						
		0.5	1	2	4	6	9	12
Serum iron								
µmol/l	Median	??	??	16	15	14	15	14
	95% range	11–36	10–31	3–29	3–29	5–24	6–24	6–28
µg/dl	Median	120	125	87	84	77	84	78
	95% range	63–201	58–172	15–159	18–164	28–135	35–155	35–155
TIBC								
µmol/l	Mean ± SD	34 ± 8	36 ± 8	44 ± 10	54 ± 7	58 ± 9	61 ± 7	64 ± 7
µg/dl	Mean ± SD	191 ± 43	199 ± 43	246 ± 55	300 ± 39	321 ± 51	341 ± 42	358 ± 38
Transferrin saturation (%)								
	Median	68	63	34	27	23	25	23
	95% range	30–99	35–94	21–63	7–53	10–43	10–39	10–47

Not all infants were tested on each occasion, and those with Hb < 11 g/dl, MCV < 71 fL or serum ferritin < 10 µg/l were excluded. Reproduced with permission from Ref. 18.

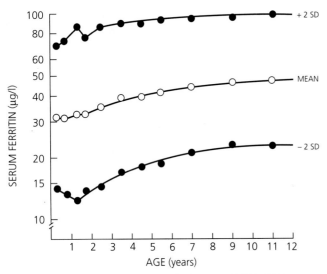

Fig. 37.5 Serum ferritin concentration (μg/l, mean ± 2 SD) in 3819 children aged 6 months to 12 years. Subjects with low hematocrit and evidence of increased iron absorption were excluded. Mean values for boys and girls were similar in each age group and there was no significant difference between blacks, whites and American Indians in age-matched samples. Ferritin measured by a two-site radioimmunometric assay. Reproduced with permission from Ref. 20.

Table 37.17 Reference limits for soluble transferrin receptor concentration (mg/l). Values in parentheses are confidence limits.

Age group	2.5% reference limit	97.5% reference limit
6 months to 4 years	1.5 (1.4–1.5)	3.3 (3.1–3.4)
4–10 years	1.3 (1.3–1.4)	3.0 (2.9–3.2)
10–16 years	1.1 (1.1–1.2)	2.7 (2.7–2.8)
>16 years	0.9 (0.9–1.0)	2.3 (2.2–2.4)

Reproduced with permission from Ref. 21.

Table 37.18 Red cell zinc protoporphyrin values (μmol/mol heme, 97.5th percentile) for females and males aged 0–17 years.

			Number studied	
Age groups	Males	Females	Males	Females
0–12 months	64	74	145	203
13–24 months	63	59	605	725
2–5 years	64	57	1926	1822
6–9 years	57	55	522	408
10–17 years	58	62	61	61
Total			3259	3219

Reproduced with permission from Ref. 22.

Table 37.19 Range of serum vitamin B_{12} (pmol/l) and serum folate (nmol/l) levels in childhood.

	Vitamin B_{12}		Folate	
Age (years)	Male	Female	Male	Female
0–1	216–891	168–1117	16.3–50.8	14.3–51.5
2–3	195–897	307–892	5.7–34.0	3.9–35.6
4–6	181–795	231–1038	5.1–29.4	6.1–31.9
7–9	200–863	182–866	5.2–27.0	5.4–30.4
10–12	135–803	145–752	3.4–24.5	2.3–23.1
13–18	158–638	134–605	2.7–19.9	2.7–16.3

Measured by radioimmunoassay in 1486 children (vitamin B_{12}) and 1368 children (folate).
Summarized from Ref. 23.

Table 37.20 Red cell folate levels (μg/l, mean and range) in the first year of life.

Age	Term infants ($n = 24$)	Preterm infants ($n = 20$)
Birth	315 (100–960)	689 (88–1291)
2–3 months		164 (26–394)
3–4 months	283 (110–489)	
6–8 months	247 (100–466)	299 (139–558)
1 year	277 (74–995)	

Obtained by microbiologic assay.
Summarized from Refs 24 and 25.

Table 37.21 Range of erythropoietin values (mIU/ml) in childhood.

Age (years)	Male	Female
1–3	1.7–17.9	2.1–15.9
4–6	3.5–21.9	2.9–8.5
7–9	1.0–13.5	2.1–8.2
10–12	1.0–14.0	1.1–9.1
13–15	2.2–14.4	3.8–20.5
16–18	1.5–15.2	2.0–14.2

Measured by enzyme-linked immunosorbent assay (ELISA) in 1122 children. Summarized from Ref. 26.

Table 37.22 Mean red cell, plasma and total blood volume (ml/kg) measurements in children.

Age	Red cell volume	Plasma volume	Total blood volume	Reference
Newborn	(43.4)	41.3	84.7	27
3 days	31*	51*	82*	28
	49†	44†	93†	28
1–7 days	37.9	(39.8)	77.7	29
1 week–30 months	29.5	(48.5)	78.0	29
3–11 months	(32.7)	46.0	78.7	30
3 months–1 year	23.3	(45.4)	68.7	29
1–2 years	24.1	(43.6)	67.7	29
1–3 years	(34.9)	47.9	82.8	30
2–4 years	22.9	(40.0)	62.9	29
3–5 years	(36.0)	48.4	84.4	30
4–6 years	26.7	(42.9)	69.6	29
5–7 years	(34.9)	48.9	83.8	31
6–8 years	23.3	(42.8)	66.1	29
7–9 years	(35.9)	47.8	83.7	30
8–12 years	25.9	(40.8)	667	29
9–11 years	(38.0)	48.5	86.5	30
11–13 years	(37.4)	46.4	83.8	30

Data in parentheses calculated from the measured variables.

* No placental transfusion at birth.

† Placental transfusion at birth.

Table 37.23 Red blood cell survival (T_{50} measured by ^{51}Cr) in term and premature infants.

	Number	Range (days)	Mean (days)
Term infants	10	17–25	22.8
	11	21–35	28
Premature infants	6	10–18	15.8
	6	9–20	15.2

Reproduced with permission from Refs 31 and 32.

Table 37.24 Serum haptoglobin concentration in preterm and term infants and in adults.

Age	Number tested	5th to 95th percentile reference limits for serum haptoglobin concentration (g/l)
1 month		
Preterm	75	0.12–0.85
Term	96	0.11–1.08
3 months		
Preterm	59	0.21–1.19
Term	96	0.21–1.65
6 months		
Preterm	33	0.39–2.62
Term	57	0.41–3.24
Adults	250	0.35–2.78

Measurements performed by nephelometry.

Summarized from Ref. 34.

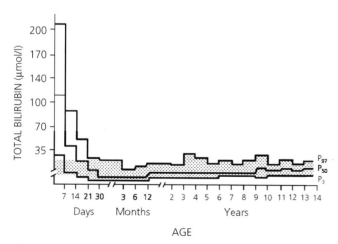

Fig. 37.6 Total bilirubin (µmol/l) measured in 2099 children. The 3rd, 50th and 97th percentiles and the adult normal range (stippled area) are shown. Reproduced with permission from Ref. 33.

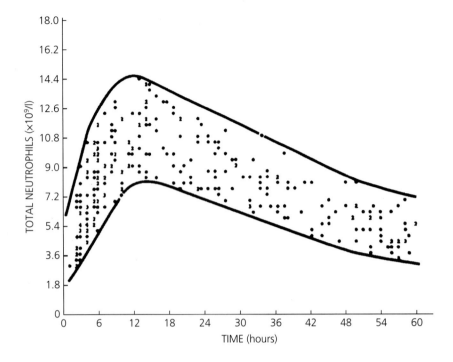

Fig. 37.7 Total neutrophil count (×10⁹/l, including band cells and earlier forms) in the first 60 hours of life. Each dot represents a single value and numbers represent the number of values at the same point. Data based on automated leukocyte count and 100-cell differential. Reproduced with permission from Ref. 35.

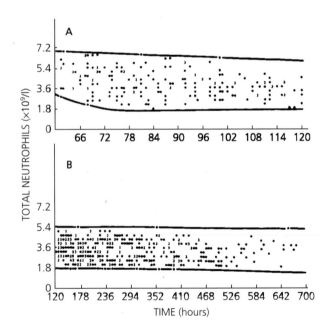

Fig. 37.8 Neutrophil count (×10⁹/l) between (A) 60–120 hours and (B) 120 hours to 28 days. Data obtained and expressed as in Fig. 37.7. Reproduced with permission from Ref. 35.

Table 37.25 Normal limits of the immature : total and immature : segmented granulocyte ratios in healthy neonates.

	Day 1	Day 7	Day 28	Reference
Immature : total	0.16	0.12	0.12	35
Immature : total (African)	0.22	0.21	0.18	36
Immature : segmented	0.3 (neonatal period)			37

Table 37.26 Mean and range of values for neutrophils, band forms and lymphocytes (×10⁹/l) in African neonates.

	Day 1	Day 7	Day 28
Neutrophils	5.67 (0.98–12.9)	2.01 (0.57–6.5)	1.67 (0.65–3.2)
Band forms	1.16 (0.16–2.3)	0.55 (0–1.5)	0.36 (0–0.39)
Lymphocytes	5.10 (1.4–8.0)	5.63 (2.2–15.5)	6.55 (3.2–9.9)

Data based on 100-cell differential count.
Summarized from Ref. 36.

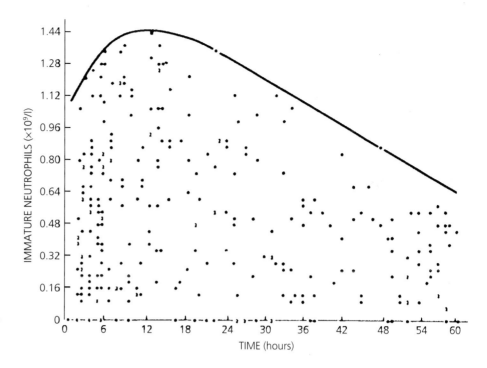

Fig. 37.9 Reference range for immature neutrophils (×10⁹/l) in the first 60 hours of life. Data obtained and expressed as in Fig. 37.7. Reproduced with permission from Ref. 35.

Table 37.27 Total and differential white cell count (×10⁹/l, mean and 95% range) from a cohort of children tested at 2, 5 and 13 months of age.

	2 months (*n* = 100)	5 months (*n* = 96)	13 months (*n* = 86)
Total WBC	8.9 (5.1–15.3)	10.0 (5.9–17.0)	9.7 (5.8–16.2)
Neutrophils	1.8 (0.7–4.8)	2.5 (1.1–5.8)	2.7 (1.0–7.7)
Lymphocytes	5.8 (3.3–10.3)	6.2 (3.3–11.5)	6.0 (3.4–10.5)
Monocytes	0.7 (0.4–1.2)	0.56 (0.25–1.27)	0.5 (0.2–0.92)
Eosinophils	0.3 (0.09–0.8)	0.32 (0.1–1.1)	0.2 (0.05–0.9)
Basophils	0.05 (0.02–0.13)	0.07 (0.02–0.2)	0.06 (0.02–0.13)

Reproduced with permission from Ref. 38.

Table 37.28 Differential leukocyte counts in children.

Age (years)	Number	Mean	3rd Centile	97th Centile	Age (years)	Number	Mean	3rd Centile	97th Centile
Neutrophils (×10⁹/l)					16	49	3.64	1.9	7.6
					17–19	45	3.62	1.8	5.8
Girls and boys									
4–5	133	3.57	1.7	7.6	*Boys*				
6	143	3.48	1.8	6.7	7	105	3.13	1.7	5.7
					8	90	3.36	1.7	6.0
Girls					9	112	3.16	1.7	6.5
7	72	3.38	2.0	5.8	10	131	3.04	1.7	5.9
8	82	3.75	1.8	8.0	11	130	3.22	1.7	5.8
9	96	3.31	1.6	6.2	12	118	2.84	1.5	4.7
10	87	3.45	1.8	6.5	13	50	2.91	1.7	5.9
11	107	3.37	1.6	6.2	14	40	2.79	1.6	4.8
12	97	3.28	1.7	5.8	15	33	3.26	1.8	6.3
13	70	3.56	1.8	7.2	16	13	2.90	1.9	5.5
14	60	3.68	2.1	7.1	17–18	17	2.82	1.7	4.5
15	58	3.64	1.7	6.7					

(continued p. 804)

Table 37.28 (cont'd)

Age (years)	Number	Mean	3rd Centile	97th Centile	Age (years)	Number	Mean	3rd Centile	97th Centile
Lymphocytes (×10⁹/l)					**Basophils (×10⁹/l)**				
Girls and boys					*Girls and boys*				
4–5	133	2.80	1.7	4.1	4–5	133	0.165	0.00	0.73
6	143	2.75	1.6	4.2	6	143	0.150	0.02	0.55
7	177	2.64	1.7	3.8	7	177	0.157	0.02	0.64
8	178	2.65	1.7	4.1	8	172	0.144	0.02	0.51
9	214	2.63	1.5	3.9	9	208	0.105	0.01	0.35
10	225	2.45	1.5	3.6	10	218	0.114	0.01	0.54
11	246	2.43	1.5	3.7	11	237	0.093	0.01	0.38
12	232	2.36	1.5	3.4	12	215	0.071	0.01	0.21
13	156	2.38	1.4	3.6	13	120	0.064	0.01	0.34
14	129	2.27	1.4	3.5	14	100	0.078	0.01	0.43
15	107	2.21	1.3	3.4	15	91	0.063	0.01	0.25
16	73	2.21	1.3	3.3	16	62	0.062	0.00	0.20
17–19	84	2.18	1.3	3.0	17–19	61	0.059	0.01	0.17
Girls					*Girls*				
7	72	2.72	1.7	4.1	4–5	52	0.136	0.00	0.45
8	82	2.78	1.8	4.4	6	63	0.152	0.02	0.55
9	96	2.67	1.7	4.0	7	72	0.155	0.02	0.61
10	87	2.58	1.7	3.8	8	82	0.160	0.02	0.60
Boys					9	96	0.114	0.02	0.46
7	105	2.58	1.7	3.7	10	87	0.146	0.01	0.54
8	96	2.53	1.6	3.9	11	107	0.087	0.02	0.34
9	118	2.60	1.5	3.9	17–19	44	0.065	0.01	0.17
10	138	2.37	1.4	3.6	*Boys*				
Eosinophils (×10⁹/l)					4–5	81	0.183	0.00	0.85
					6	80	0.148	0.02	0.55
Girls					7	105	0.158	0.02	0.70
4–5	67	0.28	0.05	0.95	8	90	0.129	0.01	0.44
6	75	0.30	0.08	0.90	9	112	0.098	0.01	0.34
7	99	0.35	0.09	1.07	10	131	0.092	0.01	0.43
8	96	0.33	0.08	0.95	11	130	0.098	0.01	0.41
9	100	0.31	0.07	1.03	17–18	17	0.042	0.01	0.10
10	124	0.32	0.06	0.84					
11	111	0.29	0.07	1.12	**Monocytes (×10⁹/l)**				
12	107	0.27	0.06	0.73	*Girls and boys*				
13	54	0.20	0.05	0.51	4–5	133	0.66	0.33	1.10
14	49	0.21	0.05	0.64	6	143	0.67	0.33	1.16
15	46	0.18	0.04	0.53	7	177	0.65	0.33	1.21
16	34	0.22	0.10	0.69	8	178	0.62	0.32	1.11
17–19	24	0.16	0.05	0.33	9	214	0.60	0.38	0.95
Boys					10	225	0.59	0.33	0.99
4–5	133	0.35	0.06	0.98	11	245	0.61	0.33	1.00
6	143	0.41	0.08	1.34	*Girls*				
7	177	0.43	0.10	1.49	12	97	0.62	0.37	1.00
8	172	0.37	0.08	1.03	13	70	0.63	0.40	0.95
9	208	0.40	0.08	1.20	14	60	0.62	0.37	1.10
10	218	0.35	0.07	0.91	15	58	0.64	0.38	1.08
11	237	0.34	0.07	1.03	16	49	0.66	0.32	0.97
12	215	0.33	0.06	0.87	17–19	44	0.67	0.36	1.05
13	120	0.26	0.07	0.74	*Boys*				
14	100	0.29	0.05	0.89	12	135	0.56	0.31	0.88
15	91	0.24	0.06	0.66	13	85	0.53	0.24	0.86
16	62	0.23	0.07	0.63	14	69	0.55	0.27	1.03
17–19	61	0.33	0.05	1.31	15	49	0.57	0.33	0.92
					16	25	0.48	0.23	0.84
					17–18	39	0.52	0.32	0.79

Summarized from Ref. 9.

Table 37.29 Normal values for lymphocytes, monocytes and eosinophils (×10⁹/l) from birth to 30 days of age based on a study of 393 infants.

		Age (hours)		
	Percentile	0–60	61–120	121–720
Lymphocytes	95	7.26	6.62	9.13
	50	4.19	8.66	5.62
	5	2.02	1.92	2.86
Monocytes	95	1.91	1.74	1.72
	50	0.6	0.53	0.67
	5	0	0	0.10
Eosinophils	95	0.84	0.81	0.84
	50	0.14	0.18	0.24
	5	0	0	0

Data based on 100-cell differential count.
Reproduced with permission from Ref. 39.

Table 37.30 Absolute counts (×10⁹/l), median and percentiles (5th to 95th percentiles) of T-cell (CD3), helper/inducer T-cell (CD4), suppressor/cytotoxic T-cell (CD8) and B-cell (CD19) lymphocytes and natural killer (CD15–56) cells in peripheral blood.

Age	N	CD19 B cells	CD3 T cells	CD3/CD4 T helper cells	CD3/CD8 T suppressor cells	CD15-56 natural killer cells
Neonatal	20	0.6 (0.04–1.1)	2.8 (0.6–5.0)	1.9 (0.4–3.5)	1.1 (0.2–1.9)	1.0 (0.1–1.9)
1 week–2 months	13	1.0 (0.6–1.9)	4.6 (2.3–7.0)	3.5 (1.7–5.3)	1.0 (0.4–1.7)	0.5 (0.2–1.4)
2–5 months	46	1.3 (0.6–3.0)	3.6 (2.3–6.5)	2.5 (1.5–5.0)	1.0 (0.5–1.6)	0.3 (0.1–1.3)
5–9 months	105	1.3 (0.7–2.5)	3.8 (2.4–6.9)	2.8 (1.4–5.1)	1.1 (0.6–2.2)	0.3 (0.1–1.0)
9–15 months	70	1.4 (0.6–2.7)	3.4 (1.6–6.7)	2.3 (1.0–4.6)	1.1 (0.4–2.1)	0.4 (0.2–1.2)
15–24 months	33	1.3 (0.6–3.1)	3.5 (1.4–8.0)	2.2 (0.9–5.5)	1.2 (0.4–2.3)	0.4 (0.1–1.4)
2–5 years	33	0.8 (0.2–2.1)	2.3 (0.9–4.5)	1.3 (0.5–2.4)	0.8 (0.3–1.6)	0.4 (0.1–1.0)
5–10 years	35	0.5 (0.2–1.6)	1.9 (0.7–4.2)	1.0 (0.3–2.0)	0.8 (0.3–1.8)	0.3 (0.09–0.9)
10–16 years	23	0.3 (0.2–0.6)	1.5 (0.8–3.5)	0.8 (0.4–2.1)	0.4 (0.2–1.2)	0.3 (0.07–1.2)
Adults	51	0.2 (0.1–0.5)	1.2 (0.7–2.1)	0.7 (0.3–1.4)	0.4 (0.2–0.9)	0.3 (0.09–0.6)

Data obtained by flow cytometry.
Summarized from Ref. 40.

Table 37.31 Normal progenitor cell numbers during development.*

Age	PB BFU-E	BM BFU-E	BM CFU-E	PB CFU-GM	BM CFU-GM	PB CFU-Meg	BM CFU-Meg
Fetus 18–20 weeks	75–1500			20–700		1–10	
Birth, term	40–100			10–200		5–20	
Adults	5–40	10–150	25–150	5–20	15–100	2–10	1–30

* Data are approximate ranges derived from various sources, and indicate numbers of progenitor cells per 10⁵ mononuclear cells plated.
PB, peripheral blood; BM, bone marrow; BFU-E, erythroid burst-forming unit; CFU-E, erythroid colony-forming unit; CFU-GM, granulocyte–macrophage colony-forming unit; CFU-Meg, megakaryocyte colony-forming unit.
Reproduced with permission from Ref. 41.

Table 37.32 Reference values for coagulation tests in the healthy full-term infant during the first 6 months of life.

	Day 1 (n)	Day 5 (n)	Day 30 (n)	Day 90 (n)	Day 180 (n)	Adult (n)
PT (s)	13.0 ± 1.43 (61)*	12A ± 1.46 (77)*†	11.8 ± 1.25 (67)*†	11.9 ± 1.15 (62)*	12.3 ± 0.79 (47)*	12.4 ± 0.78 (29)
APTT (s)	42.9 ± 5.80 (61)	42.6 ± 8.62 (76)	40.4 ± 7.42 (67)	37.1 ± 6.52 (62)*	35.5 ± 3.71 (47)*	33.5 ± 3.44 (29)
TCT (s)	23.5 ± 2.38 (58)*	23.1 ± 3.07 (64)†	24.3 ± 2.44 (53)*	25.1 ± 2.32 (52)*	25.5 ± 2.86 (41)*	25.0 ± 2.66 (19)
Fibrinogen (g/l)	2.83 ± 0.58 (61)*	3.12 ± 0.75 (77)*	2.70 ± 0.54 (67)*	2.43 ± 0.68 (60)*†	2.51 ± 0.68 (47)*†	2.78 ± 0.61 (29)
FII (unit/ml)	0.48 ± 0.11 (61)	0.63 ± 0.15 (76)	0.68 ± 0.17 (67)	0.75 ± 0.15 (62)	0.88 ± 0.14 (47)	1.08 ± 0.19 (29)
FV (unit/ml)	0.72 ± 0.18 (61)	0.95 ± 0.25 (76)	0.98 ± 0.18 (67)	0.90 ± 0.21 (62)	0.91 ± 0.18 (47)	1.06 ± 0.22 (29)
FVII (unit/ml)	0.66 ± 0.19 (60)	0.89 ± 0.27 (75)	0.90 ± 0.24 (67)	0.91 ± 0.26 (62)	0.87 ± 0.20 (47)	1.05 ± 0.19 (29)
FVIII (unit/ml)	1.00 ± 0.39 (60)*†	0.88 ± 0.33 (75)*†	0.91 ± 0.33 (67)*†	0.79 ± 0.23 (62)*†	0.73 ± 0.18 (47)†	0.99 ± 0.25 (29)
vWF (unit/ml)	1.53 ± 0.67 (40)†	1.40 ± 0.57 (43)	1.28 ± 0.59 (40)†	1.18 ± 0.44 (40)†	1.07 ± 0.45 (46)†	0.92 ± 0.33 (29)†
FIX (unit/ml)	0.53 ± 0.19 (59)	0.53 ± 0.19 (75)	0.51 ± 0.15 (67)	0.67 ± 0.23 (62)	0.86 ± 0.25 (47)	1.09 ± 0.27 (29)
FX (unit/ml)	0.40 ± 0.14 (60)	0.49 ± 0.15 (76)	0.59 ± 0.14 (67)	0.71 ± 0.18 (62)	0.78 ± 0.20 (47)	1.06 ± 0.23 (29)
FXI (unit/ml)	0.38 ± 0.14 (60)	0.55 ± 0.16 (74)	0.53 ± 0 13 (67)	0.69 ± 0.14 (62)	0.86 ± 0.24 (47)	0.97 ± 0.15 (29)
FXII (unit/ml)	0.53 ± 0.20 (60)	0.47 ± 0.18 (75)	0.49 ± 0.16 (67)	0.67 ± 0.21 (62)	0.77 ± 0.19 (47)	1.08 ± 0.28 (29)
PK (unit/ml)	0.37 ± 0.16 (45)†	0.48 ± 0.14 (51)	0.57 ± 0.17 (48)	0.73 ± 0.16 (46)	0.86 ± 0.15 (43)	1.12 ± 0.25 (29)
HMWK (unit/ml)	0.54 ± 0.24 (47)	0.74 ± 0.28 (63)	0.77 ± 0.22 (50)*	0.82 ± 0.32 (46)*	0.82 ± 0.32 (48)*	0.92 ± 0.22 (29)
FXIIIa (unit/ml)	0.79 ± 0.26 (44)	0.94 ± 0.25 (49)*	0.93 ± 0.27 (44)*	1.04 ± 0.34 (44)*	1.04 ± 0.29 (41)*	1.05 ± 0.25 (29)
FXIIIb (unit/ml)	0.76 ± 0.23 (44)	1.06 ± 0.37 (47)*	1.11 ± 0.36 (45)*	1.16 ± 0.34 (44)*	1.10 ± 0.30 (41)*	0.97 ± 0.20 (29)
Plasminogen (CTA, unit/ml)	1.95 ± 0.35 (44)	2.17 ± 0.38 (60)	1.98 ± 0.36 (52)	2.48 ± 0.37 (44)	3.01 ± 0.40 (47)	3.36 ± 0.44 (29)

All values expressed as mean ± 1 SD. All factors except fibrinogen and plasminogen are expressed as unit/mL where pooled plasma contains 1.0 unit/mL. Plasminogen units are those recommended by the Committee on Thrombolytic Agents (CTA). Note that longer or shorter APTT and TCT values may be obtained in newborns and infants using reagent combinations other than those used in this study.

* Values do not differ statistically from adult values.

† These measurements are skewed because of a disproportionate number of high values.

PT, prothrombin time; APTT, activated partial thromboplastin time; TCT, thrombin clotting time; vWF, von Willebrand factor; PK, prekallikrein; HMWK, high-molecular-weight kininogen.

Reproduced with permission from Ref. 42.

Table 37.33 Reference values for the inhibitors of coagulation in the healthy full-term infant during the first 6 months of life.

	Day 1 (n)	Day 5 (n)	Day 30 (n)	Day 90 (n)	Day 180 (n)	Adult (n)
ATIII (unit/ml)	0.63 ± 0.12 (58)	0.67 ± 0.13 (74)	0.78 ± 0.15 (66)	0.97 ± 0.12 (60)*	1.04 ± 0.10 (56)*	1.05 ± 0.13 (28)
α_2-M (unit/ml)	1.39 ± 0.22 (54)	1.48 ± 0.25 (73)	1.50 ± 0.22 (61)	1.76 ± 0.25 (55)	1.91 ± 0.21 (55)	0.86 ± 0.17 (29)
α_2-AP (unit/ml)	0.85 ± 0.15 (55)	1.00 ± 0.15 (75)*	1.00 ± 0.12 (62)*	1.08 ± 0.16 (55)*	1.11 ± 0.14 (53)*	1.02 ± 0.17 (29)
C1E-INH (unit/ml)	0.72 ± 0.18 (59)	0.90 ± 0.15 (76)*	0.89 ± 0.21 (63)	1.15 ± 0.22 (55)	1.41 ± 0.26 (55)	1.01 ± 0.15 (29)
α_1-AT (unit/ml)	0.93 ± 0.22 (57)*	0.89 ± 0.20 (75)*	0.62 ± 0.13 (61)	0.72 ± 0.15 (56)	0.77 ± 0.15 (55)	0.93 ± 0.19 (29)
HCII (unit/ml)	0.43 ± 0.25 (56)	0.48 ± 0.24 (72)	0.47 ± 0.20 (58)	0.72 ± 0.37 (58)	1.20 ± 0.35 (55)	0.96 ± 0.15 (29)
Protein C (unit/ml)	0.35 ± 0.09 (41)	0.42 ± 0.11 (44)	0.43 ± 0.11 (43)	0.54 ± 0.13 (44)	0.59 ± 0.11 (52)	0.96 ± 0.16 (28)
Protein S (unit/ml)	0.36 ± 0.12 (40)	0.50 ± 0.14 (48)	0.63 ± 0.15 (41)	0.86 ± 0.16 (46)*	0.87 ± 0.16 (49)*	0.92 ± 0.16 (29)

All values expressed in unit/mL as mean ± 1 SD.

* Values indistinguishable from those of adults.

ATIII, antithrombin III; α_2-M, α_2-macroglobulin; α_2-AP, α_2-antiplasmin; C1E-INH, C1 esterase inhibitor; α_1-AT, α_1-antitrypsin; HCII, heparin cofactor II.
Reproduced with permission from Ref. 42.

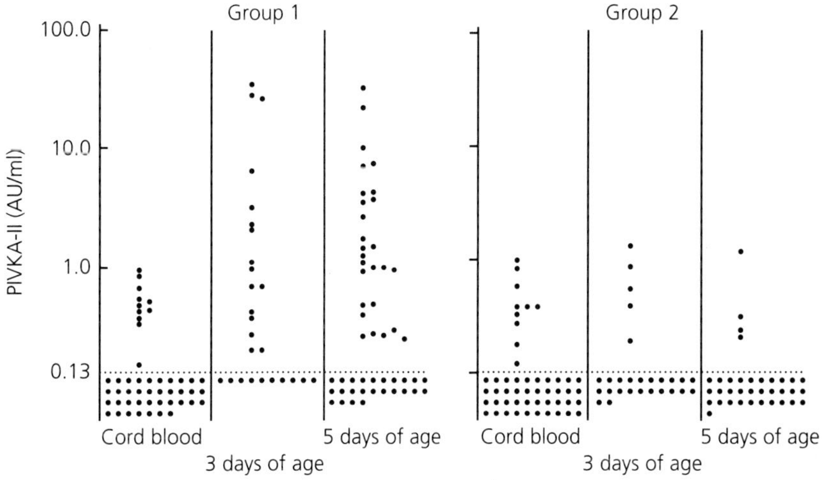

Fig. 37.10 PIVKA (protein induced by vitamin K absence or antagonism)-II levels in cord blood and blood samples obtained at 3 or 5 days of age. Group I did not receive vitamin K and Group 2 did. The dotted line indicates the lower limit of sensitivity of the assay. One arbitrary unit of PIVKA-II corresponds to one μg of purified prothrombin (Factor II). Reproduced with permission from Ref. 44.

Table 37.34 Concentrations of D-dimers in blood from 15 preterm infants and 45 born at full term.

Concentration of D-dimers (mg/l)	No. (%) of patients		
	Full term (*n* = 45)	Preterm (*n* = 15)	Total (*n* = 60)
<0.25	24 (53%)	7 (47%)	31 (52%)
0.25–0.5	14 (31%)	2 (13%)	16 (27%)
0.5–1	6 (13%)	2 (13%)	8 (13%)
1–2	1 (2%)	2 (13%)	3 (5%)
2–4	0	2 (13%)	2 (3%)

All D-dimer concentrations in the pregnant mothers were < 0.25 mg/l. Reproduced with permission from Ref. 43.

Table 37.35 Platelet count (×10⁹/l) during childhood.

Age	Both sexes	Girls	Boys
2 months	214–648 (*n* = 119)		
5 months	210–560 (*n* = 106)		
13 months	180–508 (*n* = 101)		
1–3 years	207–558 (*n* = 68)		
4–6 years		193–489 (*n* = 118)	205–450 (*n* = 159)
7–8 years		191–439 (*n* = 155)	194–420 (*n* = 202)
9–10 years		201–384 (*n* = 182)	174–415 (*n* = 258)
11–12 years		180–387 (*n* = 206)	178–382 (*n* = 274)
13–14 years		188–429 (*n* = 129)	183–370 (*n* = 157)
15–18 years		170–359 (*n* = 151)	189–374 (*n* = 116)

Data from our laboratory (2 months to 3 years, 95% range) and Ref. 11 (3rd to 97th centiles). Platelet counts are significantly lower at 5 months than at 2 months of age, and at 13 months than at 5 months (*P* < 0.001 for both). The fall in counts with age from 4 years is statistically significant, as are the overall higher values in girls than boys between 4 and 18 years (*P* < 0.0001 for both).

Table 37.36 PFA-100 closure times in healthy children and adults, and in children with hemophilia.

Subjects	Number	Age (years)	Closure times (s)	
			Col/Epi	Col/ADP
Healthy children				
21-gauge needle	30	2.5–17	82–165	70–110
23-gauge needle	27	5–17	91–142	77–112
Combined data	57	2.5–17	83–163	72–111
Healthy adults				
21-gauge needle	31	25–54	82–142	67–111
Healthy neonates	17	>37 weeks' gestational age	61–108	48–65
Hemophiliacs	11	6–18	109 ± 20	81 ± 13

All subjects had hemoglobin and platelets within normal reference limits for age.
Col/Epi, collagen/epinephrine membrane; Col/ADP, collagen/ADP membrane.
Reproduced with permission from Ref. 45.

Table 37.37 Bleeding time (min) in children and adults.

Subjects	Number	Mean	SD	Range
Children	36	4.6	1.4	2.5–8.5
Adults	48	4.6	12	2.5–6.5

Bleeding time performed using a template technique with incision 6 mm long and 1 mm deep and sphygmomanometer pressure 40 mmHg. Note that using this technique, bleeding times up to 11.5 min have been observed in apparently healthy children tested in our laboratory. Summarized from Ref. 46.

Table 37.38 Serum immunoglobulin levels in UK Caucasians (–2 SD, meridian, +2 SD by log-Gaussian).

Age		IgG (g/l)	IgA (g/l)	IgM (g/l)
	Cord	10.8 (5.2–18.0)	<0.02	0.1 (0.02–0.2)
Weeks	0–2	9.4 (5.0–17.0)	0.02 (0.01–0.08)	0.1 (0.05–0.2)
	2–6	7.1 (3.9–13.0)	0.05 (0.02–0.15)	0.2 (0.08–0.4)
	6–12	3.9 (2.1–7.7)	0.15 (0.05–0.4)	0.4 (0.15–0.7)
Months	3–6	4.6 (2.4–8.8)	0.2 (0.1–0.5)	0.6 (0.2–1.0)
	6–9	5.2 (3.0–9.0)	0.3 (0.15–0.7)	0.8 (0.4–1.6)
	9–12	5.8 (3.0–10.9)	0.4 (0.2–0.7)	1.2 (0.6–2.1)
Years	1–2	6.4 (3.1–13.8)	0.7 (0.3–1.2)	1.3 (0.5–2.2)
	2–3	7.0 (3.7–15.8)	0.8 (0.3–1.3)	1.3 (0.5–2.2)
	3–6	9.9 (4.9–16.1)	1.0 (0.4–2.0)	1.3 (0.5–2.0)
	6–9	9.9 (5.4–16.1)	1.3 (0.5–2.4)	1.2 (0.5–1.8)
	9–12	9.9 (5.4–16.1)	1.4 (0.7–2.5)	1.1 (0.5–1.8)
	12–15	9.9 (5.4–16.1)	1.9 (0.8–2.8)	1.2 (0.5–1.9)
	15–45	11 (6.0–16.0)	1.9 (0.8–2.8)	1.2 (0.5–1.9)
	>45	11 (6.0–16.0)	1.9 (0.8–4.0)	1.2 (0.5–2.0)

Determined in 53 males and 54 females above 15 years and in groups of at least 30 subjects for the other age groups.
Reproduced with permission from Ref. 47.

Table 37.39 Mean and 5th to 95th centile ranges (g/l) for IgG subclasses at various ages.

Age	IgG1	IgG2	IgG3	IgG4
Cord blood	4.7 (3.6–8.4)	2.1 (1.2–4.0)	0.6 (0.3–1.5)	0.2 (<0.5)
6 months	2.3 (1.5–3.0)	0.4 (0.3–0.5)	0.3 (0.1–0.6)	<0.1
2 years	3.5 (2.3–5.8)	1.1 (0.3–2.9)	0.4 (0.1–0.8)	<0.1
5 years	3.7 (2.3–6.4)	2.0 (0.7–4.5)	0.5 (0.1–1.1)	0.3 (<0.1–0.8)
10 years	5.2 (3.6–7.3)	2.6 (1.4–4.5)	0.7 (0.3–1.1)	0.4 (<0.1–1.0)
15 years	5.4 (3.8–7.7)	2.6 (1.3–4.6)	0.7 (0.2–1.2)	0.4 (<0.1–1.1)
Adult	5.9 (3.2–10.2)	3.0 (1.2–6.6)	0.7 (0.2–1.9)	0.5 (<0.1–1.3)

In adults IgG3 levels are higher in females than in males, and IgG4 higher in males than females. No sex difference is seen before the age of 15 years.
Reproduced with permission from Ref. 47.

Table 37.40 Serum IgD levels (g/l).

Number	Age	IgD
23	6 weeks to 19 months	<0.01–0.016
105	3–14 years	<0.01–0.036

Reproduced with permission from Ref. 48.

Table 37.41 Total serum IgE levels.*

Age	Median	95th centile
Newborn	0.5	5
3 months	3	11
1 year	8	29
5 years	15	52
10 years	18	63
Adult	26	120

* Data expressed in units in relation to the first British Standard for human serum IgE 75/502.
Reproduced with permission from Ref. 47.

Table 37.42 Erythrocyte sedimentation rate (mm/h) in healthy children.

Method	Number	Age (years)	Mean	Range	% > 20 mm/h
Wintrobe	245	4–11	12.0	1–41	9
	169	12–15	7.5	<1–34	7
Westergren	78	4–7	13	<1–55	
(read at 45 min)	153	8–14	10.5	1–62	

Summarized from Refs 49–51.

Table 37.43 Isohemagglutinin titers in relation to age.

Age	Mean (range)
Cord blood	0*
1–3 months	1 : 5[†] (0 to 1 : 10)
4–6 months	1 : 10[†] (0 to 1 : 160)
7–12 months	1 : 80[‡] (0 to 1 : 640)
13–24 months	1 : 80[‡] (0 to 1 : 640)
25–36 months	1 : 160[§] (1 : 10 to 1 : 640)
3–5 years	1 : 80 (1 : 5 to 1 : 640)
6–8 years	1 : 80 (1 : 5 to 1 : 640)
9–11 years	1 : 160 (1 : 20 to 1 : 640)
12–16 years	1 : 160 (1 : 10 to 1 : 320)
Adult	1 : 160 (1 : 10 to 1 : 640)

* Isohemogglutinin (IHA) activity is rarely detectable in cord blood.
† 50% of normal infants will not have IHA at this age.
‡ 10% of normal infants will not have IHA at this age.
§ Beyond this age all normal individuals have IHA with the exception of those of blood group AB.
Summarized from Ref. 52.

Acknowledgment

Sharon Barrott provided expert secretarial assistance.

References

1. Zaisov R, Matoth Y. Red cell values on the first postnatal day during the last 16 weeks of gestation. *Am J Hematol* 1976; **1**: 272–8.

2. Lundstrom U, Siimes MA, Dallman PR. At what age does iron supplementation become necessary in low-birth-weight infants? *Pediatr* 1977; **91**: 878–83.

3. Lloyd BW, Oto A. Normal values for mature and immature neutrophils in very preterm babies. *Arch Dis Child* 1982; **57**: 233–5.

4. McIntosh N, Kempson C, Tyler RM. Blood counts in extremely low birthweight infants. *Arch Dis Child* 1988; **63**: 74–6.

5. Seguin JH, Topper WH. Coagulation studies in very low-birthweight infants. *Am J Perinatol* 1994; **11**: 27–9.

6. Andrew M, Paes B, Milner R *et al.* Development of the coagulation system in the healthy premature infant. *Blood* 1988; **72**: 1651–7.

7. Saarinen UM, Siimes MA. Developmental changes in red blood cell counts and indices of infants after exclusion of iron deficiency by laboratory criteria and continuous iron supplementation. *J Pediatr* 1978; **92**: 412–16.

8. Scott-Emuakpor AB, Okola AA, Omene JA, Ukpe SI. Normal haematological values of the African neonate. *Blut* 1985; **51**: 11–18.

9. Taylor MRH, Holland CV, Spencer R, Jackson JF, O'Connor GI, O'Donnell JR. Haematological reference ranges for schoolchildren. *Clin Lab Haematol* 1997; **19**: 1–15.

10. Schröter W, Natz C. Diagnostic significance of hemoglobin F and A2 levels in homo- and heterozygous β-thalassaemia during infancy. *Helv Paediatr Acta* 1981; **36**: 519–25.

11. Galanello R, Melis MA, Ruggeri R, Cao A. Prospective study of red blood cell indices, hemoglobin A₂ and hemoglobin F in infants heterozygous for β-thalassaemia. *J Pediatr* 1981; **99**: 105–8.

12. Metaxotou-Mavromati AD, Antonopoulo HK, Laskari SS, Tsiarta HK, Ladis VA, Kattamis CA. Developmental charges in hemoglobin F levels during the first two years of life in normal and heterozygous β-thalassaemia infants. *Pediatrics* 1982; **69**: 734–8.

13. Kravitz H, Elegant LD, Kaiser E, Kagan BM. Methemoglobin values in premature and mature infants and children. *Am J Dis Child* 1956; **91**: 1–5.

14. Konrad PM, Valentine WM, Paglia DE. Enzymatic activities and glutathione content of erythrocytes in the newborn: comparison of red cells of older normal subjects and those with comparable reticulocytosis. *Acta Haematol* 1972; **48**: 193–201.

15. Beutler E. *Red Cell Metabolism*, 3rd edn. New York: Grime and Stratton, 1984.

16. Hinchliffe RF, Lilleyman JS (eds) *Practical Paediatric Haematology.* Chichester: John Wiley & Sons, 1987.

17. Hovi LM, Siimes MA. Red blood cell morphology in healthy fullterm newborns. *Acta Paediatr Scand* 1983; **72**: 135–6.

18. Koerper MA, Dallman PR. Serum iron concentration and transferrin saturation in the diagnosis of iron deficiency in children: normal developmental changes. *J Pediatr* 1977; **91**: 870–4.

19. Saarinen UM, Siimes MA. Developmental changes in serum iron, total iron-binding capacity, and transferrin saturation in infancy. *J Pediatr* 1977; **91**: 875–7.

20. Deinard AS, Schwartz S, Yip R. Developmental changes in serum ferritin and erythrocyte protoporphyrin in normal (non-anemic) children. *Am J Clin Nutr* 1983; **38**: 71–6.

21. Suominen P, Virtanen A, Lehtonen-Veromaa M *et al.* Regression-based reference limits for serum transferrin receptor in children 6 months and 16 years of age. *Clin Chem* 2001; **47**: 935–6.

22. Soldin P, Miller M, Soldin SJ. Pediatric reference ranges for zinc protoporphyrin. *Clin Biochem* 2003; **36**: 21–5.

23. Hicks JM, Cook J, Godwin ID, Soldin SJ. Vitamin B12 and folate. Pediatric reference ranges. *Arch Pathol Lab Med* 1993; **117**: 704–6.

24. Vanier TM, Tyas JF. Folic acid status in newborn infants during the first year of life. *Arch Dis Child* 1966; **41**: 658–65.

25. Vanier TM, Tyas JF. Folic acid status in premature infants. *Arch Dis Child* 1967; **42**: 57–61.

26. Krafte Jacobs B, Williams J, Soldin SJ. Plasma erythropoietin reference ranges in children. *J Pediatr* 1995; **126**: 601–3.

27. Gomez P, Coca L, Vargas C, Acebillo J, Martinex A. Normal reference-intervals for 20 biochemical variables in healthy infants, children and adolescents. *Clin Chem* 1984; **30**: 407–12.

28. Mollison PL, Veall N, Cutbush M. Red cell and plasma volume in newborn infants. *Arch Dis Child* 1950; **25**: 242–53.

29. Usher R, Shephard M, Lind J. The blood volume of the newborn infant and placental transfusion. *Acta Paediatr Scand* 1963; **52**: 497–512.

30. Sukarochana K, Parenzan L, Thalardas N, Kieselwelter WB. Red cell mass determinations in infancy and childhood, with the use of radioactive chromium. *J Pediatr* 1961; **59**: 903–8.

31. Russell SJM. Blood volume studies in health children. *Arch Dis Child* 1949; **24**: 88–98.

32. Foconi S, Sjolin S. Survival of Cr-labelled red cells from newborn infants. *Acta Paediatr* 1959; **48** (suppl. 117): 18–23.

33. Kaplan E, Hsu KS. Determination of erythrocyte survival in newborn infants by means of Cr-labelled erythrocytes. *Pediatrics* 1961; **27**: 354–61.

34. Kanakoudi F, Drossou V, Tzimouli V *et al.* Serum concentrations of 10 acute-phase proteins in healthy term and preterm infants from birth to age 6 months. *Clin Chem* 1995; **41**: 605–8.

35. Manroe BL, Weinberg AG, Rosenfeld CR, Browne R. The neonatal blood count in health and disease. I. Reference values for neutrophilic cells. *J Pediatr* 1979; **95**: 89–98.

36. Scott-Emuakpor AB, Okolo AA, Omene JA, Ukpe SI. Pattern of leukocytes in blood of healthy African neonates. *Acta Haematol* 1985; **74**: 104–7.

37. Zipursky A, Jaber HM. The haematology of bacterial infection in newborn infants. *Clin Haematol* 1978; **7**: 175–93.

38. Bellamy GJ, Hinchliffe RF, Crawshaw KC, Finn A, Bell F. Total and differential leucocyte counts in infants at 2, 5 and 13 months of age. *Clin Lab Haematol* 2000; **22**: 81–7.

39. Weinberg AG, Rosenfeld CR, Manroe BL, Browne R. Neonatal blood cell count in health and disease. II. Values for

lymphocytes, monocytes, and eosinophils. *J Pediatr* 1985; **106**: 462–6.

40. Comans-Bitter WM, de Groot R, van den Beemd R *et al.* Immunophenotyping of blood lymphocytes in childhood. *J Pediatr* 1997; **130**: 388–93.

41. Auerbach AD, Alter BP. Prenatal and postnatal diagnosis of aplastic anaemia. In: Alter BP (ed.) *Perinatal Haematology. Methods in Haematology*. Edinburgh: Churchill Livingstone, 1989, pp. 225–51.

42. Andrew M, Paes B, Milner R *et al.* Development of the human coagulation system in the full-term infant. *Blood* 1987; **70**: 165–72.

43. Hudson IRB, Gibson BES, Brownlie J, Holland BM, Turner TL, Webber RG. Increased concentrations of D-dimers in newborn infants. *Arch Dis Child* 1990; **65**: 383–4.

44. Motohara K, Endo F, Matsuda I. Effect of vitamin K administration on acarboxy prothrombin (PIVKA-II) levels in newborns. *Lancet* 1985; **ii**: 242–4.

45. Carcao MD, Blanchette VS, Dean JA *et al.* The platelet function analyzer (PFA-100): a novel *in-vitro* system for evaluation of primary haemostasis in children. *Br J Haematol* 1998; **101**: 70–3.

46. Buchanan GR, Holtkamp CA. Prolonged bleeding time in children and young adults with hemophilia. *Pediatrics* 1980; **66**: 951–5.

47. Ward AM, Sheldon J, Rowbottom A, Wild GD (eds) *Protein Reference Unit Handbook of Clinical Immunochemistry*, 8th edn. Sheffield: PRU Publications, 2004.

48. Buckley RH, Fiscus SA. Serum IgD and IgE concentrations in immunodeficiency diseases. *J Clin Invest* 1975; **55**: 157–65.

49. Hollinger N, Robinson SJ. A study of the erythrocyte sedimentation rate for well children. *J Pediatr* 1953; **42**: 304–19.

50. Osgood EE, Baker RL, Brownlee IE, Osgood MW, Ellis M, Cohen W. Total, differential and absolute leukocyte counts and sedimentation rates of healthy children four to seven years of age. *Am J Dis Child* 1939; **58**: 61–70.

51. Osgood EE, Baker RL, Brownlee IE, Osgood MW, Ellis M, Cohen W. Total, differential and absolute leukocyte counts and sedimentation rates for healthy children. Standards for children eight to fourteen years of age. *Am J Dis Child* 1939; **58**: 282–94.

52. Ellis EF, Robbins JB. In: Johnson TR, Moore WH (eds) *Children are Different: Developmental Physiology*. Columbus, OH: Ross Laboratories, 1978.

Index

Page numbers in **bold** represent tables, those in *italic* represent figures.

Aase–Smith syndrome 45
abdominal painful crisis 221
abetalipoproteinemia 269–71
ABO blood group system 151–2
  effect on factor VIII and von Willebrand
    factor **600**
  incompatibility 156, 162, 164
Abe–Letterer–Siwe disease *see* Langerhans
    cell histiocytosis
acanthocytes 269–71
acquired aplastic anemia 64–76
  clinical presentation 66
  diagnosis and laboratory evaluation
    67–8, *67*
  epidemiology 64
  etiology 64–5
  natural history 66–7
  pathophysiology 65–6
  treatment
    androgens and growth factors 71
    hematopoietic stem cell transplantation
      68–9, *69*
    immunosuppressive therapy 69, 70–1
    myelodysplastic syndrome 71–2
    paroxysmal nocturnal hemoglobinuria
      72
    supportive care 68
acute chest syndrome 222–3, *222*
acute hemolytic anemia 183
acute hemolytic transfusion reactions 724–5
acute hepatic necrosis 221
acute hepatic porphyria 198–204
  acute intermittent porphyria 199–202,
    200, 201
  ALAD deficiency porphyria 198–9
  hereditary coproporphyria 202
  treatment 203–4
  variegate porphyria 202–3

acute intermittent porphyria 199–202, **200,
    201**
acute lymphoblastic leukemia *see*
    lymphoblastic leukemia
acute myeloid leukemia 360–83, 409, 416
  classification 363–4, **364**
  clinical manifestations 362–3, *363*
  cytogenetics and molecular markers 364
  environmental risk factors **362**
  epidemiology 361–2, **361, 362**
  gene expression profiling 364–5
  genetic risk factors **361**
  incidence *361*
  late effects 374–5
  neutropenia in 726
  risk-group stratification and prognostic
    factors 365–7
    FLT3 marker 366–7
    good cytogenetics 365
    intermediate cytogenetics 365–6
    poor cytogenetics 366
  survival rates *360*
  therapy 367–74
    allogeneic HSCT 372–3, *372*
    AML BFM-93 trial 369, *369*
    CCG-2891 trial 369–71, *370*
    CNS prophylaxis 373
    Down syndrome 374
    extramedullary leukemia 373
    gemtuzumab ozogamicin 371
    historical overview 367
    MRC AML-10 and AML-12 trials
      367–9, *368*
    refractory/recurrent disease 374
    secondary leukemia 373–4
    supportive care 373
    targeted 371
acute splenic sequestration 220–1
acute transfusion reactions 724–8
  acute hemolytic 724–5
  allergic reactions 725

anticoagulant/preservative solution
    726–7
  bacterial contamination 727–8
  coagulopathy 727
  cold storage conditions 727
  febrile reactions 725–6
  massive transfusion 726
  storage lesions 726
  transfusion-related acute lung injury 725
adenosine deaminase
  deficiency 429–30
  overexpression **173, 174**, 186–7
adenosylcobalamin deficiency 110–11
adenylate kinase deficiency **174**
adhesion disorders 307–10
  acquired 310
  hyperimmunoglobulin E syndrome 309
  leukocyte adhesion deficiency 308
  Rac2 mutations 310
  Wiskott–Aldrich syndrome 309–10, **310**
ADP receptor antagonists **567**, 575
adrenal/pituitary insufficiency 760
adult metachromatic leukodystrophy 779
agammaglobulinemia, autosomal recessive
    forms 438
alanine dehydrogenase deficiency
    porphyria 198–9
albumin transfusion 715–16
Alder–Reilly bodies *785*
aldolase deficiency **173, 174**, 177
alemtuzumab 539
alkylating agents 464
allergic reactions to blood transfusion 725
alloimmune neonatal thrombocytopenia
    661–2
alloimmunization 293
  transfusion-associated 728
Alport syndrome **31**, 52, 512
amegakaryocytic thrombocytopenia 508,
    513
anaplastic large-cell lymphoma 490, **490**

androgens
  acquired aplastic anemia 64–76
  dyskeratosis congenita 31, 40
  Fanconi anemia 30, 31, 32, 37, 39
  Shwachman–Diamond syndrome 37–40
anemia
  acquired aplastic *see* acquired aplastic
    anemia
  of chronic disease 757–8, 767
  Diamond–Blackfan *see* Diamond–
    Blackfan anemia
  Fanconi *see* Fanconi anemia
  immune hemolytic 151–70
  iron deficiency 89
  iron-loading 97–8
  macroangiopathic 142–3
  megaloblastic *see* megaloblastic anemia
  microangiopathic hemolytic 142–3,
    517–18
  nonimmune neonatal 130–50
  pernicious 117
  red cell transfusion 699
  refractory 413
    with excess of blasts **408**, 413
    with ringed sideroblasts 94, **408**
    in transformation **408**, 413
  sickle cell disease 219
  sideroblastic 91–4
anhidrotic ectodermal dysplasia 436–7
ankyrin deficiency 263
anorexia nervosa 766
anthracyclines 464
antibody production defects 439
anti-CD20 monoclonal antibody 539
anti-CD52 monoclonal antibody 539
anticoagulant/preservative solutions, acute
    reaction to 726–7
anticoagulants 679–84
  low-molecular-weight heparin 681–2,
    681, *682*
  unfractionated heparin 679–81, **680**, **681**
  warfarin 682–4, *683*, **683**, **684**
antifolate drugs 118–19
antigen presentation 428, *428*
antigen processing 5
antigen recognition and heterogeneity
    426–8, *426*, *427*
  antigen presentation and lymphocyte
    activation 428, *428*
  B-lymphocyte development 427
  T-lymphocyte development 427
  variable domain gene rearrangement 427
antiglobulin test 153–4, *154*
antileukemic drugs 463–5, *463*
antimicrobial-induced platelet disorders
    575–6
antimicrobial peptides 305–6
antiphospholipid antibodies 636–7
antiplatelet antibodies 577

anti-Rh(D) immunoglobulin 537
antiviral prophylaxis 748–9
aorta-gonad mesonephros 4
apheresis 694
aplastic crisis 260
ascorbic acid 538
L-asparaginase 464
aspartylglucosaminuria 780
ataxia telangiectasia 435–6
ataxia telangiectasia-like disorder 436
atransferrinemia, congenital 147
autoimmune lymphoproliferative
    syndrome 434–5
autoimmune neonatal thrombocytopenia
    662–3
autosomal recessive hyper-IgM syndrome
    438
azathioprine 537–8

bacterial contamination of blood for
    transfusion 727–8
bacterial infections 327, 519
Barth syndrome **31**, 325
basopenia 332
basophilia 332
basophils 332
Batten disease 779
B-cell lymphoblastic leukemia 457–8
B-cell lymphoma 488–9, *491*
B-cells 5–6
  development 427
  disorders of function 437–8
  interactions with T-cells *428*
  reference values **805**
Bernard–Soulier syndrome 508–9, **508**, 566,
    567, 569
  clinical features 569
  heterozygotes 569
  laboratory diagnosis 569
  molecular genetics 569
  prenatal diagnosis 569
bilayer couple effect 256
birth asphyxia 518–19
blasT-cells, in myelodysplasia 407
bleeding time 565
  reference values **807**
blood component filters **730**
blood component therapy 605, 693–723
  albumin 715–16
  cryoprecipitate 715
  granulocytes 714–15
  immunoglobulins 716–17
  plasma 706–9
  platelets 709–13
  preparation 693–5
    anticoagulant/preservative solutions
      693–4, **694**
    apheresis 694
    pathogen reduction 695

prestorage leukocyte reduction 694–5,
    695
  whole blood donations 693
  red blood cells 696–706
  whole blood 695–6
  see also blood transfusion
blood count **793**
  sickle cell disease 213–30
blood film, sickle cell disease 215
blood group abnormalities 270–1
blood loss
  fetomaternal hemorrhage 133–5, **135**
  internal hemorrhage 136
  intraabdominal hemorrhage 136–7
  neonatal 133–7
    concealed hemorrhage before or during
      delivery 133–5, *134*, **135**
    iatrogenic blood loss 137
    obstetric accidents and malformations
      of cord/placenta 135–7, **136**
blood storage, clinical effects of 726, 727
blood transfusion
  acute transfusion reactions 724–8
    acute hemolytic 724–5
    allergic reactions 725
    anticoagulant/preservative solution
      726–7
    bacterial contamination 727–8
    coagulopathy 727
    cold storage conditions 727
    febrile reactions 725–6
    massive transfusion 726
    storage lesions 726
    transfusion-related acute lung injury
      725
  delayed transfusion reactions 728–40
    erythrocyte alloimmunization 728–30
    graft-versus-host disease 731–4
    immune modulation 734
    infection 734–40
    leukocyte and platelet
      alloimmunization 730–1
    posttransfusion purpura 731
    transfusion-associated
      alloimmunization 728
  neonates **148**
  sickle cell disease 225
  see also blood component therapy
blood volume **801**
Bloom syndrome 436
Bohr effect 233–4
bone and joint problems, sickle cell disease
    220
bone marrow
  congenital disorders 416
  lymphoblastic leukemia 454–6, **455**,
    456
  myelodysplastic syndromes 405–18,
    407

bone marrow abnormalities 768–72
  neuroblastoma 769–71
  soft tissue sarcomas 771–2
bone marrow disorders 520
bone marrow failure
  failure of red cell production 11–29
  genes associated with **31**
  inherited 30–63
    with predominantly anemia 44–8
    with predominantly neutropenia
      48–51
    with predominantly pancytopenia
      32–44
    with predominantly thrombocytopenia
      51–3
    unclassifiable/poorly classifiable 53
  management of infection 745–54
    neutropenia 745–7
    planned progressive antimicrobial
      therapy 749–52, *750, 752*
    risk/prognostic factors 747–9
bone marrow transplantation
  Diamond–Blackfan anemia 14–15
  immunodeficiency disorders 441–3
  myelodysplastic syndromes 412–13
  thalassemias 297
Bruton tyrosine kinase deficiency 325,
  437–8
Burkitt lymphoma 764
burst-forming unit erythroid 7, 13

candidiasis, in leukemia patients 453
cardiopulmonary bypass 633–5, **634**
  neonate 658–9
cardiopulmonary leukemia 454
cardiovascular drugs, and platelet disorders
  576
cardiovascular system, hemostatic
    complications 633–5
  cardiopulmonary bypass 633–5, **634**
  congenital heart disease 633
  extracorporeal membrane oxygenation
    635
cartilage-hair-hypoplasia syndrome 326,
  435
catalase deficiency 318
cation transport disorders 271–4, *272*
CD4 lymphocytopenia, idiopathic 431
CD40 ligand deficiency 433–4
celiac disease 759–60
central nervous system
  leukemia 452
  non-Hodgkin lymphoma 485
central venous access 591–2
cerebrovascular disease 223–4
Chédiak–Higashi syndrome 312–13, *312,*
  313, 325–6, 508, **508**, 511, **568**, 571
chemokines 6, **307**
chemotaxis, acquired disorders 310

cholecystectomy 242
cholesteryl ester storage disease 779, 787
chorea-acanthocytosis 270
chromatography 239
chronic granulomatous disease 315–16, *315,*
  315, 439–40
chronic mucocutaneous candidiasis 435
chronic myeloid leukemia 384–404
  biology 385–6, *386*
  clinical features 386, **386**
  diagnosis 387–9
    accelerated-phase disease 388–9, **389**
    blast crisis 389
    bone marrow 388
    cytogenetics 388
    peripheral blood 387–8
  differential diagnosis 389
  etiology 384
  examination 386
  future directions
    immunotherapy 399
    novel drugs 398–9, **398**
    stem cell transplantation 398
  management 390–8
    accelerated-phase disease 397–8
    allogeneic stem cell transplantation
      393–5
    blasT-cell crisis 397–8
    chronic-phase disease 390–7
    donor lymphocyte infusion 396, *396*
    imatinib 391–3, *391*, **392**
    interferon-a 396–7
    relapse 395–6
  molecular biology 384–6, *384, 385*
  natural history 384
chronic nonspherocytic hemolytic anemia
  184
chronic pulmonary disease 223
chronic pulmonary hemosiderosis 88
ciclosporin 538
clotting factor concentrates 588–91, *590*, **590**
coagulation data
  fetuses and newborns 643–4, **644, 645**
  reference values **794**
coagulation disorders 608–23
  acquired 624–42
    cardiovascular disease 633–5, 658–9
    developmental hemostasis 624–6, **625,**
      626
    disseminated intravascular coagulation
      626–8, 654–5
    evaluation of bleeding 626
    inhibitors of coagulation 635–7
    liver disease 630–1, 657–8
    liver transplantation 631–2
    metabolic disease 635
    neonate 654–9, **654**
    renal disease 632–3
    vitamin K deficiency 628–30, 655–7

bleeding symptoms in *609*
and developmental hemostasis 610
final common pathway of coagulation
    613–19
  factor V deficiency 615–16
  factor X deficiency 614–15
  fibrinogen abnormalities 617–19
  prothrombn deficiency 616–17
hemophilia 585–97
inherited 649–51, **649**
  hemophilia 649–51, *650*
  von Willebrand disease 651
multiple congenital deficiency states
    619–20
  combined deficiency of vitamin K-
    dependent factors 619–20
  combined factor V/factor VIII
    deficiency 619
prolonged activated partial
    thromboplastin time 611–13
  factor XI deficiency 612–13
  factor XII, prekallikrein and high-
    molecular-weight kininogen
    deficiency 612
prolonged prothrombin time 610–11
von Willebrand disease *see* von
    Willebrand disease
without associated screening test
    abnormalities 620–3
  Ehlers–Danlos syndrome 621–3, **622**
  factor XIII deficiency 620
  α_2-plasmin inhibitor deficiency 621
  plasminogen activator inhibitor-1
    deficiency 621
coagulation factors **608**
  inhibitors 645–6
  reference values **795, 806**
  neonate 644–6, **645**
  laboratory investigation **648**
  see also individual factors
coagulation tests, reference values **625, 795,**
  806
coagulopathy 727
cobalamin 105–6, *105, 106*
  acquired disorders of metabolism
    116–17, **116**
    malabsorption 117
    nitrous oxide 116
    nutrition 116
  deficiency 119, 147
  metabolism 107–8, *107*
  reference values **800**
  tests of absorption 120
  transport disorders 108–9
    Imerslund–Gräsbeck syndrome 108
    intrinsic factor deficiency 108
    transcobalamin 108
    transcobalamin II deficiency 108–9
  utilization disorders 109–12, *109*

cold agglutinin disease 158–9, *158*
  laboratory studies 158–9
  treatment 159
$\alpha_2\beta_1$ collagen receptor **567**
GpVI collage receptor **567**
colony-forming unit erythroid 7, 13
common gamma-chain deficiency 429
common lymphoid progenitor 3
common variable immunodeficiency 325, 438
complement cascade *312, 425*
complement system
  deficiencies 440
    management of 440–1
  disorders 311
  immune hemolysis 153
congenital amegakaryocytic
    thrombocytopenia **31**, 43–4
  cancer predisposition 43
  clinical features 43
  laboratory evaluation and diagnosis 43
  pathogenesis 43
  therapy and prognosis 44
congenital atransferrinemia 89
congenital dyserythropoietic anemias
    18–22, **19, 31**, 48, 143
  differential diagnosis 22
  modifiers of severity in 21–2
  type I 18–20, **31**
    clinical features 18
    electron microscopy 19
    inheritance and genetic 19
    laboratory findings 18–19
    management 19–20
  type II 20–1, **31**
    clinical features 20
    electron microscopy 20
    inheritance and genetics 20
    laboratory findings 20
    pathogenesis 20–1
    treatment 21
  type III 21, **31**
  unclassified 21
congenital erythropoietic porphyria 204–5
congenital heart disease 633
congenital Heinz body hemolytic anemia
    240–2
  genetics 241–2
  laboratory diagnosis 242
  pathogenesis 240–1
  treatment 242
congenital leukemia 520
congenital microcytic hypochromic anemia
    89
congenital sideroblastic anemia **31**, 48
congenital thrombotic thrombocytopenic
    purpura 143
connective tissue disease 761–2
contraception, sickle cell disease 217–18

Coombs test 153–4, *154*
coproporphyrinogen oxidase 202
corticosteroids
  ITP 537, **537**
  lymphoblastic leukemia 464
cranial bleeds in neonates **136**
Creutzfeldt–Jakob disease, transfusion-
    related 738–9
cryoprecipitate transfusion 715
CTLA-4-Ig 538–9
C-X-C chemokines 6
cyanotic congenital heart disease 519
cyclic neutropenia **31**, 50, 323
cyclooxygenase inhibitors 574–5
cyclophosphamide 538
cytogenetics
  lymphoblastic leukemia 456–7, **456**
  myelodysplastic syndromes 409–10, **410**
  non-Hodgkin lymphoma 487–8
cytokines 50
  therapy of MDS 412
cytologic tests of hemoglobin 237–8, *238*
cytomegalovirus **142**, 516
  transfusion-related 737–8, **739**
cytopenia, refractory 408–9

dactylitis 220
danazol 538
D-dimers **807**
deferiprone 296–7
deferoxamine *see* iron-chelating therapy
delayed transfusion reactions 728–40
  erythrocyte alloimmunization 728–30
  graft-versus-host disease 731–4
  immune modulation 734
  infection 734–40
  leukocyte and platelet alloimmunization
    730–1
  posttransfusion purpura 731
  transfusion-associated alloimmunization
    728
denaturation tests 238
dendritic cells 7
dense body deficiency 571
desmopressin
  hemophilia 590
  von Willebrand disease 604–5
Diamond–Blackfan anemia 11–15, **31**, 44–8,
    143
  cancer predisposition 45
  clinical features 11–12, **11**, *12*, 44–5, *45*
    hematological 44–5
    nonhematological 45
  differential diagnosis 17–18
  genetic aspects 46
  inheritance and genetics 12–13
  laboratory evaluation and diagnosis 12,
    46–7
  long-term prognosis 48

  pathogenesis 13, 46
  prognosis 15
  treatment 13–15, 47–8
    bone marrow transplantation 14–15
    hematopoietic stem cell transplantation
      47–8
    interleukin-3 14
    megadose methylprednisolone 14
    prolactin 14
    spontaneous remission 14
    steroids 13–14, *13*, 47
    transfusion 14, 47
DIDMOAD syndrome 93
diet, and iron status 86–7, **87**
differential white cell count **803–4**
DiGeorge syndrome 433, 760
diphosphoglycerate mutase deficiency **173**,
    179
disseminated intravascular coagulation
    142–3, 626–8
  clinical features 627
  etiology 626–7, **627**
  in infants 517
  laboratory diagnosis 627–8
  management 628
  neonate 654–5
  pathophysiology 627
DNA analysis *240*
DNA ligase defects 436
DNA repair defects 435–6
Down syndrome, abnormal myelopoiesis in
    415
drug-induced hematologic effects 766
  immune hemolytic anemias 160–1, *160*,
    161
  neutropenia 327
Dubowitz syndrome 44
Duncan disease 433
dyskeratosis congenita **31**, 40–2
  clinical features 40–1, *41*
    hematologic features 40
    nonhematologic features 40–1
  genetic aspects 41
  laboratory evaluation and diagnosis 42
  pathogenesis 41–2
  prenatal diagnosis 42
  therapy and prognosis 42–3
    androgens 42
    growth factors 42
    hematopoietic stem cell transplantation
      42–3
dyskerin 41

Ebstein syndrome **31**, 52
echinocytes 269–71
Eckstein syndrome **509**, 512
eczema 761
Ehlers–Danlos syndrome 621–3, **622**
electrophoresis 239

Embden–Meyerhof pathway 171, *172*, **173**
  disorders of 175–81
    aldolase deficiency 177
    diphosphoglycerate mutase deficiency 179
    enolase deficiency 179
    glucose phosphate isomerase deficiency 175–6
    hexokinase deficiency 175
    phosphofructokinase deficiency 176–7
    phosphoglycerate kinase deficiency 178–9
    phosphoglycerate mutase deficiency 179
    pyruvate kinase deficiency 179–81, **181**
    triosephosphate isomerase deficiency 177–8
embryonic hemoglobins *236*
endocrine disorders, hematologic effects 760
enolase deficiency **173**, **174**, 179
enzyme replacement 443
enzyme screening tests 173–4
eosinopenia 331–2
eosinophilia 332, *332*
  in lymphoblastic leukemia 458–9
  in MDS 416
eosinophils 331–2
  function 331
  normal range 331
  reference values **805**
  structure 331–2
epinephrine, defective response to 570
epipodophyllotoxin 465
Epstein–Barr virus 764
Epstein syndrome 509, 512, **567**, 574
erythrocytes *see* red cells
erythrocyte sedimentation rate **808**
erythroid cells 7–8
erythroid Krüppel-like factor 8
erythropoiesis, at birth 130
erythropoietic protoporphyria 206–7
erythropoietin 7, 705, **800**
  reference values **800**
essential thrombocytosis 551–4
  clinical and laboratory features 552–3, **552**
  familial forms **553**
  pathogenesis 551
  treatment options 553–4
Evans syndrome 157–8, 330
extracorporeal membrane oxygenation 635
extracorporeal perfusion 576–7
eye problems in sickle cell disease 224

FAB classification
  lymphoblastic leukemia **455**
  myelodysplastic syndromes 408, **408**, **409**

Fabry disease **779**, **780**
factor II *see* prothrombin
factor V
  combined factor V/factor VIII deficiency 619, 652–3
  deficiency 615–16
    clinical and laboratory features 615–16
    inheritance and prevalence 615
    neonate 652–3
    structure and function 615
    treatment 616
  inhibitors 636
factor VII deficiency 610–11
  clinical and laboratory features 611
  inheritance and prevalence 611
  neonate 652–3
  structure and function 610–11
  treatment 611
factor VIII
  combined factor V/factor VIII deficiency 619, 652–3
  deficiency *see* hemophilia
  inhibitors 635
factor IX
  deficiency *see* hemophilia
  inhibitors 635
factor X deficiency
  clinical and laboratory features 614–15
  inheritance and prevalence 614
  neonate 652–3
  structure and function 614
  treatment 615
factor XI deficiency 612–13, 614–15
  clinical and laboratory features 613
  inheritance and prevalence 612–13
  neonate 652–3
  structure and function 612
  treatment 613
factor XII deficiency 612
factor XIII deficiency 620
  clinical and laboratory features 620
  inheritance and prevalence 620
  neonate 653
  structure and function 620
  treatment 620
familial autosomal dominant nonsyndromic thrombocytopenia **31**
familial MDS 416
familial platelet disorder 52–3
familial thrombocytopenia with dyserythropoiesis 52
Fanconi anemia **31**, 32–7, 144, 416, 436, 513
  cancer predisposition 33
  clinical manifestations 32–3, *32*
    hematologic features 32
    nonhematologic features 32–3
  genetic aspects 33–4
  laboratory evaluation and diagnosis 35

  pathogenesis
    apoptosis 34
    chromosome breakage studies 34
    hematopoietic stem cell and progenitor phenotype 34
    mouse models 34
    protein complex 34
  prenatal diagnosis 35
  therapy and prognosis 35–7
    androgens 37
    gene therapy 37
    hematopoietic growth factors 36–7
    hematopoietic stem cell transplantation 35–6
Farber disease **779**, **780**
favism 184
Fechtner syndrome **31**, 52, 509, 512, **567**, 574
Felty syndrome 330
ferritin 83
  reference values *800*
ferrochelatase 206–7
fetal hemoglobin 235–6
fetal red cell membranes 259
fetomaternal hemorrhage 133–5, **135**
  clinical manifestations 133–4
  laboratory diagnosis 135
fetoplacental hemorrhage 135
fetus
  coagulation data 643–4, **645**
  hemoglobin 130
    diagnostic and therapeutic relevance 235–6
    reference values **797**
    structure and function 235
  iron status 85–6
fibrinogen abnormalities 617–19
  clinical and laboratory features 618
  inheritance and prevalence 617–18
  neonate 652
  structure and function 617
  treatment 618–19
fibrinolysis 646–7
fibrinolytic system, reference values **626**
flippase 256
floppase 256
folate 106–7, *106*
  inborn errors of metabolism 112–14
    glutamate formiminotransferase deficiency 114
    methylenetetrahydrofolate reductase deficiency 112–13
    methylenetetrahydrofolate reductase polymorphisms 113–14
  metabolism 107–8, *107*
  reference values **800**
  transport disorders 114–15
    cellular uptake defects 115
    cerebral folate deficiency 115

folate (*cont'd*)
    hereditary folate malabsorption
        114–15
folate deficiency 117–19, **117**, 147
    antifolate drugs 118–19
    excess utilization 118
    malabsorption 118
    nutrition 117–18
    pregnancy 118
    tissue effects 119
folic acid antimetabolites 464
follicular lymphoma 491, **492**
Fontan procedure 685
food-cobalamin malabsorption 117
fungal infections in bone marrow failure
        748
    treatment 750–1

gallstones 221
gastrointestinal disease, hematologic effects
        759–60
    celiac disease 759–60
    inflammatory bowel disease 759
Gaucher disease 635, **779**, **780**, 781–3, *781*,
        782
    type 1 (nonneuronopathic) 781–3
    type 2 (acute neuronopathic) 783
    type 3 (subacute neuronopathic) 783
gene therapy
    Fanconi anemia 37
    immunodeficiency disorders 443
giant hemangioma syndrome *see* Kasabach-
        Merritt syndrome
gigantoblasts 21
Glanzmann thrombasthenia **568**, 572–3
    clinical features 573
    heterozygotes 573
    laboratory diagnosis 573
    molecular genetics 573
    prenatal diagnosis 573
Glenn procedure 685
globin-chain structural abnormalities 140
glucose 6-phosphate dehydrogenase 171
    deficiency 139, **173**, **174**, 181–5, 316
        classification of variants **182**
        clinical signs and symptoms 183–4
        diagnosis 184
        malaria protection 182–3
        pathophysiology of hemolysis **183**
        treatment and prevention 185
glucose phosphate isomerase deficiency
        140, **173**, **174**, 175–6
glutamate formiminotransferase deficiency
        114
gamma-glutamycysteine synthetase **174**
glutamylcysteine synthetase **173**
glutathione metabolism disorders 317, **318**
glutathione peroxidase **318**
    deficiency 185

glutathione reductase **173**, **174**, **318**
    deficiency 185
glutathione synthesis deficiency 185
glutathione synthetase **173**, **174**, **318**
glycogen storage disease type Ib **31**, 325
glycophorin C deficiency 269
Goodpasture syndrome 88
GpIb-V-IX complex 508
GpIIb-IIIa antagonists 575
graft-versus-host disease 394–5, 469–70
    transfusion-related 731–4
granulation disorders 311–14
    acquired 310
    Chédiak–Higashi syndrome 311–13, *312*,
        312, 326, 508, **508**, 511, **568**, 571
    specific granule deficiency 313
granulocyte alloantigens 328–9
granulocytes
    in myelodysplasia **407**
    phagocytic receptors **312**
    reference values **802**
granulocyte-specific antigens 328
granulocyte transfusion 714–15
gray platelet syndrome **508**, 510, **568**, 572
growth problems in sickle cell disease
        217–18

Hallervorden–Spatz syndrome 95
hand-foot syndrome 220
Hand-Schüller–Christian disease *see*
        Langerhans cell histiocytosis
haptoglobin, reference values **801**
Hb Baltimore 242
Hb Barts 288
Hb Barts hydrops syndrome 291
Hb Constant Spring 244
Hb Hollandia 242
Hb Icaria 244
Hb Knossos 243
Hb Koya Dora 244
Hb Lepore 242
Hb Lepore Boston 242
HbM anomalies 246–7, **246**, **247**
Hb Monroe 244
Hb Seal Rock 244
heart disease
    hematologic effects 760
    and thrombosis 685–6
        mechanical prosthetic heart valves
            685–6
        prophylaxis 685
    see also cardiovascular system,
        hemostatic complications
Heinz bodies *238*
hemangioma 143
hematologic values at birth 130–1, **131**
    gestational age 131
    postnatal age 131
    quality of sample 131

site of sampling 131
    timing of cord clamping at birth 131
hematopoiesis
    neonates 130
    see also hematopoietic
hematopoietic growth factors 36–7, 660–1
    bone marrow failure 752
hematopoietic stem cells 3
    cryopreservation 390
hematopoietic stem cell transplantation
    acquired aplastic anemia 68–9, *69*
    alternative donor 69
    chronic myeloid leukemia 393–4, **393**
    congenital amegakaryocytic
        thrombocytopenia 43
    Diamond–Blackfan syndrome 47–8
    dyskeratosis congenita 42
    Fanconi anemia 35–6
    Kostmann syndrome 50
    matched sibling donor 68–9
    Shwachman–Diamond syndrome 40
    sickle cell disease 226
    survival *69*
    versus immunotherapy 71
heme biosynthesis *82*, 84–5, 197–8, *199*
hemochromatosis, hereditary 99
hemoglobin
    fetal 130
        diagnostic and therapeutic relevance
            235–6
        reference values **797**
        structure and function 235
    function 233–4, *233*
        heterotropic interactions of oxygen
            binding 233–4
        homotropic interactions of oxygen
            binding 233
    genetic control of synthesis 281–3, *282*
    identification 237–40
        chromatography 239
        cytologic tests 237–8, *238*
        denaturation tests 238
        DNA analysis *240*
        electrophoresis 239
        isoelectric focusing *239*
        mass spectrometry 239
        oxygen affinity 238
        routine hematology 237
        solubility test 238
        spectral analysis 238
    reference values **793**, **796**
    structure 231–3
        primary 231–2, *231*
        secondary 232
        tertiary and quaternary 232–3, *232*, *233*
    see also various Hb types
hemoglobin disorders 240–7
    congenital Heinz body hemolytic anemia
        240–2

decreased oxygen affinity 245–6
HbM anomalies 246–7, **246**, **247**
increased oxygen affinity 245
thalassemic variants 242–5, **243**, *244*
hemoglobinopathies
neonatal 140–1
globin-chain structural abnormalities 140
thalassemia syndromes 140–1
hemoglobin variants 234–7
adult hemoglobins
HbA2 235, **797**
HbA *234*
developmental changes 236–7, *236*
embryonic hemoglobins *236*
fetal hemoglobin
diagnostic and therapeutic relevance 235–6
reference values **797**
structure and function 235
hemolysis
infection-induced 763
microangiopathic 768
neonatal alloimmune 162–5
ABO incompatibility 164
minor blood group incompatibility 164–5
rhesus hemolytic disease of newborn 162–4, **164**
red cell transfusion 698
see also immune haemolytic anemias
hemolytic-uremic syndrome 517, 632–3, 758
hemophagocytic lymphohistiocytosis 353–5, 520
biology 353
clinical presentation *354*, **354**
genetic defects **353**
incidence and epidemiology 353–4
survival 355
treatment 354–5
hemophilia 583–97
clinical presentation 586, **586**, *587*
comprehensive care approach 594
diagnosis 586
differential diagnosis 586–7
genetics, carrier testing and genetic counseling 587–8
historical perspective 585
neonate 649–51, *650*
clinical features 649–50, *650*
diagnosis 650–1
management 651
perinatal management 650
social care 594–5
identification cards 594
leisure activities 594–5
school 594
vaccinations 594
transition to adult services 595

treatment 588–92
central venous access 591–2
complications 592–4
desmopressin 591
factor concentrates 588–91, **590**, *590*
type A and B 585–6
type C *see* factor XI deficiency
hemosiderin 83
hemosiderosis, pulmonary 760–1
hemostasis
developmental 624–6, **625**, **626**, 672
disorders of *see* coagulation disorders
neonate 643–9
bleeding problems 648–9, **648**
coagulation data 643–4, **644**, **645**
coagulation proteins 644–6
fibrinolysis 646–7
platelets 647–8
thrombin regulation 646
heparin
low-molecular-weight 681–2, **681**, *682*
unfractionated 679–81, **680**, **681**
heparin-induced platelet disorders 576
heparin-induced thrombocytopenia 519, 766
hepatic sequestration 221
hepatitis C, transfusion-related 745–6
hepatitis G, transfusion-related 736–7
hepatoerythropoietic porphyria 205–6
hereditary coproporphyria 202
hereditary elliptocytosis 138, 265–9
clinical syndromes 265–7
common hereditary elliptocytosis 265–6, *266*
hereditary pyropoikilocytosis 266
silent carrier 265
Southeast Asian ovalocytosis 266–7
spherocytic elliptocytosis 266
diagnosis 267
molecular genetics 267–9
glycophorin C deficiency 269
protein 4.1 mutations 268–9
spectrin mutations 267–8, *268*
pathophysiology 267
resistance to malaria 269
treatment 269
hereditary orotic aciduria 115–16
hereditary pyropoikilocytosis 138
hereditary spherocytosis 137–8, 259–65
clinical features 259–60
complications 260
differential diagnosis 261–2, *262*
laboratory diagnosis 260–1, *261*
molecular genetics 263–4
pathophysiology 262–3, *262*
treatment 264–5, *264*, *265*
Hermansky–Pudlak syndrome 511, **568**, 571
herpes simplex **142**, 516
hexokinase deficiency **173**, **174**, 175

hexose monophosphate shunt 171, *172*, **173**
disorders of 181–5
glucose 6-dehydrogenase deficiency 181–5
glutathione peroxidase deficiency 185
glutathione reductase deficiency 185
glutathione synthesis deficiency 185
high-density lipoprotein deficiency 274
high-moleculer-weight kininogen deficiency 612
histiocytic disorders 340–59
hemophagocytic lymphohistiocytosis 353–5
histiocytes and normal immune system 340–2, *342*
Langerhans cell histiocytosis 343–51
macrophage related (class II) histiocytoses 353–5
modern classification 342–3, **343**
non-Langerhans cell (class I) histiocytoses 351–3
Hodgkin disease 491–7
cell biology and pathology 492, **492**
clinical presentation 492–3
diagnostic investigations and staging
biopsy 493
blood tests 493, **494**
bone marrow studies 493
imaging 493
laparotomy 493
staging 494, **494**
epidemiology 492
etiology 492
long-term sequelae 497–8, **497**
educational and psychologic functioning 498
endocrine dysfunction 497–8
fertility 498
growth impairment 497
organ dysfunction 498
second tumors 497
prognostic features 494
treatment 494–7, **495**, **496**
relapsed disease 496–7
Hoyeraal–Hreidarsson syndrome 41, **437**
HSCT *see* hematopoietic stem cell transplantation
human immunodeficiency virus 444–5, 764–5
clinical staging **445**
manifestations 444–5
specific and adjuvant treatment 445
transfusion-related 737
transmission and prevention 444
Hunter syndrome **779**, **780**, 786–7
Hurler syndrome **779**, **780**, 786
Hurler–Scheie syndrome **779**, 786
hydration disorders 271–4, *272*
hydrocytosis 271, 273

hydrops fetalis 132
hydroxycarbamide 225–6, 242
hypercoagulable states 518–19
hyperhemolysis 219
hyper-IgM syndrome 325
hyperimmunoglobulin E syndrome 308–9
hypogammaglobulinemia 311
  transient of infancy 439
hyposplenism 445–6
hypoxia 760

iatrogenic blood loss in neonates 137
I-cell disease **780**
ICF syndrome **437**
idiopathic thrombocytopenic purpura
    526–47
  clinical course 530–2, *531*, **531**
  clinical features and diagnosis 529–32
  differential diagnosis 530, **530**, **531**
  history 526
  incidence 526–7, *527*
  management 532–6
    acute bleeding 533, **534–5**
    mild bleeding and long-term bleeding
      problems 533, **534–5**
    refractory disease 533
  new treatment options 538–9
  pathogenesis 527–9
    immune regulation 529, *529*, **529**
    platelet antigen and autoantibody
      527–8, **528**
    platelet destruction 528–9, *528*
  refractory, treatment 537–9
    ascorbic acid 538
    azathioprine 537–8
    cyclic high-dose methylprednisolone
      538
    cyclophosphamide 538
    danazol 538
    plasma exchange and protein A
      immunoadsorption 538
    splenectomy 538
    vinca alkaloids 537
  staging **530**
  standard treatment 536–7, **536**
    anti-Rh(D) immunoglobulin 537
    corticosteroids 537, **537**
    immunoglobulin 536, **536**
imatinib mesilate 391–3, *391*
  clinical trials
    in adults 391, **392**
    in children 391–2, **392**
  resistance 392–3, **392**
  treatment with 393
Imerslund–Gräsbeck syndrome 108
immune hemolytic anemias 151–70
  cold agglutinin disease 158–9, *158*
    laboratory studies 158–9
    treatment 159

drug-induced 160–1, *160*, **161**
  mechanisms of immune hemolysis 151–4
    antiglobulin test (Coombs test) 153–4,
      154
    complement system 153
    immunoglobulins **152**
    mononuclear phagocytic system 153
    red blood cell antigens 151–2
  neonatal alloimmune hemolysis 162–5
    ABO incompatibility 164
    minor blood group incompatibility
      164–5
    rhesus hemolytic disease of newborn
      162–4, **164**
  paroxysmal cold hemoglobinuria
    159–60
    laboratory investigations 159–60
    treatment 160
  paroxysmal nocturnal hemoglobinuria
    72, 165–6
  warm autoimmune hemolytic anemia
    155–8
    clinical course and prognosis 157
    clinical features 155
    Evans syndrome 157–8
    laboratory features 155–6
    treatment 156–7
immune neutropenia 327–30
  granulocyte antigens 327
  human neutrophil antigen system 327–9,
    328
  neonatal alloimmune neutropenia 329
  primary autoimmune neutropenia 329
  secondary immune neutropenias
    329–30
immunodeficiency 425–49
  acquired (secondary) immunodeficiency
    diseases 443–6
    HIV 1 and 2 444–5
    hyposplenism 445–6
  antigen recognition and heterogeneity
    426–8, *426*, *427*
    antigen presentation and lymphocyte
      activation 428, *428*
    B-lymphocyte development 427
    T-lymphocyte development 427
    variable domain gene rearrangement
      427
  innate immune system 425–6, *425*
  major histocompatibility complex 426
  primary immunodeficiency diseases
    428–43
    autoimmune lymphoproliferative
      syndrome 434–5
    B-cell function disorders 437–8
    chronic mucocutaneous candidiasis
      435
    combined immunodeficiency 432–4
    DNA repair defects 435–6

humoral immune defects 438–9
  IL-12-dependent IFN-gamma pathway
    defects 440
  phagocytic cell disorders 439–40
  plasma protein deficiencies 440–1
  short-limbed dwarfism 435
  T-cell and "combined"
    immunodeficiency 428–32, **429**
specific immunity 425
treatment 441–3
  blood products 442
  bone marrow transplantation 442–3
  support for families and patients 442
  supportive care 441–2
  treatment of infections 442
  vaccination 441, **441**
immunoglobulin A deficiency 438–9
immunoglobulins **152**
  in ITP 536, **536**
  reference values **808**
  replacement therapy 443
  structure *427*
  transfusion 715
immunoreceptor tyrosine-based activation
    motifs *see* ITAMS
immunotherapy
  acquired aplastic anemia 69–71, *70*
  chronic myeloid leukemia 399
  versus hematopoietic stem cell
    transplantation 71
inclusion bodies 237–8
incontinentia pigmenti 436–7
indwelling venous catheter sepsis 749
infantile pyknocytosis 138
infant leukemias 457
  treatment 467–8
infants, iron status 86
infections
  bone marrow failure 745–54
    neutropenia 745–7
    planned progressive antimicrobial
      therapy 749–52, *750*, *752*
    risk/prognostic factors 747–9
  hematologic effects 766–8
    Burkitt lymphoma 764
    Epstein–Barr virus 764
    hemolysis 763
    human immunodeficiency virus
      764–5
    Kawasaki disease 765
    leukemoid reactions 763
    parvovirus 765
    TORCH infections 765
    transient erythroblastopenia of
      childhood 762
    tuberculosis 763–4
    visceral leishmaniasis 763
  neonatal 141–2, **142**, 145–6
  and neutropenia 326–7

in sickle cell disease 218–19, **218**
transfusion-transmitted 734–40, **736**
    Creutzfeldt–Jakob diseaes 738–9
    cytomegalovirus 737–8, **739**
    hepatitis C virus 735–6
    hepatitis G virus 736–7
    human immunodeficiency virus 737
    West Nile virus 739
inflammatory bowel disease 759
innate immune system 305–6, 425–6, *425*
integrin α₂β₁ deficiency 570
interferon-α 396–7, 539
interleukin-3, Diamond–Blackfan anemia
    14
interleukin-7Ra deficiency 429
interleukin-12-dependent IFN-γ pathway,
    defects in 440
intrauterine infections 516
intrinsic factor deficiency 108
IPEX syndrome **437**
iron-chelating therapy 97, 293–7, *294*, **295**,
    296
    endocrine system 294
    growth 294
    liver disease 294
    management of 294–7, **295**, **296**
    optimal body iron *294*
iron deficiency 85–91, 146–7
    causes **87**, *88*
    diagnosis 87
    differential diagnosis 87–9
    effects of 89–90
        anemia 89
        growth and development 89–90
    etiology 85–7
        developmental factors 85–6
        dietary factors 86–7
    management 90–1
        clinical 90
        iron therapy 91
        prevention 90
    prevalence **90**
iron metabolism 85
    body iron distribution and turnover 81–3,
        81, 82
        ferritin and hemosiderin 83
        transferrin 81–2
        transferrin receptor 82–3
    body iron stores 83–4, *83*
        increased 84
        reduced 83–4
    heme synthesis *82*, 84–5
    inborn errors 147
    inherited disorders 89
    iron absorption 79–81
        bioavailability of dietary iron 80–1
        dietary iron content 79–80, **80**
        mucosal cell control 81
    red cell cycle *85*

iron overload 94–9, 293–4
    acute overdose 94–5
    chronic 95–7, **95**
        clinical effects 96–7, **97**
        etiology 95–6
        focal iron overload 96
        perinatal iron overload 96
    management 97–9
        iron chelation therapy 97
        iron-loading anemias 97–8
        transfusion therapy 98–9, **98**
iron, reference values *799*
isoelectric focusing *239*
ITAMS 4
ITP *see* idiopathic thrombocytic purpura

Jacobsen syndrome 510
JAK-3 deficiency 429
Jansky–Bielschowsky disease **779**
jaundice, neonatal 183
juvenile myelomonocytic leukemia 413–15
    biology 414
    clinical features 413
    cytogenetics **410**
    diagnosis 409, 413
    hematologic findings 413–14
    management 414–15
juvenile rheumatoid arthritis, systemic-
    onset 761–2
juvenile xanthogranulomatous disease
    351–3, *352*

Kanzaki disease **779**
Kasabach–Merritt syndrome 518, 664
Kawasaki diseaes 765
Kayser–Fleischer rings 759
killer inhibitory receptors 3
Kleihauer test 135, 237, *238*
Klippel–Feil anomaly 45
Kostmann syndrome 30, **31**, 48–50, 322, 416
    cancer predisposition 49
    classification 321–2, **321**
    clinical features 48–9
    common features 322
    genetic aspects 49
    laboratory features and diagnosis 49–50
    pathogenesis 49
    therapy and prognosis 50
Krabbe disease **779, 780**

lactose dehydrogenase deficiency **173, 174**
Landing disease **779**
Langerhans cell histiocytosis 343–51
    biology 343–4, *344*
    clinical presentation and therapy 345–51,
        346, *347–50*
    incidence and epidemiology 344–5
    survivors 151
large granular lymphocytic leukemia 330

lead toxicity 93
leg ulcers 222
leishmaniasis, visceral 763
leukemia 577
    acute myeloid 360–83
    chronic myeloid 384–404
    congenital 520
    infant 457
    juvenile myelomonocytic 413–15
    lymphoblastic 450–81
leukemoid reactions 763
leukocytes
    alloimmunization 730–1
    recruitment of 306–7, **307**
    removal from blood **740**
leukocyte adhesion deficiency 307–8
leukocyte endothelial adhesion **307**
leukoerythroblastic blood film 768
liver disease 270
    hematologic effects 757–77
    hemostatic complications 630–2
        hepatic failure 630–1
        liver transplantation 631–2
        neonate 657–8
    platelet aggregation in 576
liver transplantation 631–2
Loeffler syndrome 761
lung disease, hematologic effects 760–1
lymphoblastic leukemia 450–81
    aplastic/hypoplastic 459
    clinical characteristics 450–4, **450**,
        451
        cardiopulmonary 454
        central nervous system 452
        eye 453
        gastrointestinal 453
        genitourinary 452–3
        mediastinal masses 451–2
        skeletal 453
        skin 454
    complications 470–3, **472**
        bleeding 471
        central nervous system 472
        early 470–1
        gonadal 471 2
        growth 472
        infections 471
        late 471–3, **472**
        liver 472
        second malignancies 473
        thrombosis 471
    differential diagnosis **451**
    immunological classification **455**
    laboratory findings 454–9
        biological subsets 457–9
        bone marrow 454–6, **455, 456**
        cytomolecular genetics 456–7, **456**
        gene expression profiles 457
    neutropenia in 726–7

lymphoblastic leukemia (*cont'd*)
  prognostic factors 459–62, **459**
    cellular phenotype and genotype
      460–1
    clinical phenotype 459, *460, 461*
    minimal residual disease 462, **462**
    response to treatment 461–2
  supportive care 471
  treatment
    antileukemic drugs 463–5, *463*
    B-cell lymphoblastic leukemia 467
    bone marrow transplantation 469–70,
      470
    duration of 467
    infant leukemia 467–8
    intensive polychemotherapy 465–6
    newly diagnosed disease 462–8, *463*
    relapsed disease 468–9, **469**
lymphocytes
  reference values **805**
  see also B-cells; T-cells
lymphoid cells 3–6
lymphomas 482–503
  Hodgkin disease 491–7
  non-Hodgkin 482–91
  sequalae of therapy 497–8, **497**
lysosomal storage disorders 778–91, **779**
  mucopolysaccharidoses 785–7
    type I 786
    type II 786–7
    type VI 787
  sphingolipidoses 780–5
    Gaucher disease 781–3, *781, 782*
    Niemann–Pick disease 783–5, *783–5*
  treatment **780**
  Wolman disease/cholesteryl ester storage
    disease 787

macroangiopathic anemias 142–3
major histocompatibility complex 426
  class I deficiency 434
  class II deficiency 430–1
malaria **142**
malnutrition cycle *444*
mannose-binding lectin deficiency 440
mannose-binding protein deficiency 311
Maroteaux–Lamy syndrome **779, 780**, 785,
  787
mass spectrometry 239
mast-cell disease 761
maternal autoimmune thrombocytopenia
  515–16
maternal drug use 517
May–Hegglin anomaly **31**, 52, **509**, 511–12,
  567, 574
MDS *see* myelodysplastic syndromes
mediastinal masses 451–2
Mediterranean macrothrombocytopenia **31**,
  53

Mediterranean thrombocytopenia **509**,
  513–14
megakaryocyte/erythrocyte progenitor 3
megakaryocyte lineage cells 8
megakaryocytes, in myelodysplasia **407**
megaloblastic anemia 105–29, 260
  acquired disorders of cobalamin
    metabolism 116–17, **116**
    malabsorption 117
    nitrous oxide 116
    nutrition 116
  cobalamin 105–6, *105, 106*
    metabolism 107–8, *107*
  cobalamin transport disorders 108–9
    Imerslund–Gräsbeck syndrome 108
    intrinsic factor deficiency 108
    transcobalamin 108
    transcobalamin II deficiency 108–9
  cobalamin utilization disorders 109–12,
    109
  diagnosis 119–20
  folate 106–7, *106*
    metabolism 107–8, *107*
  folate deficiency 117–19, **117**
    antifolate drugs 118–19
    excess utilization 118
    malabsorption 118
    nutrition 117–18
    pregnancy 118
    tissue effects 119
  folate transport disorders 114–15
    cellular uptake defects 115
    cerebral folate deficiency 115
    hereditary folate malabsorption
      114–15
  hereditary orotic aciduria 115–16
  inborn errors of folate metabolism 112–14
    glutamate formiminotransferase
      deficiency 114
    methylenetetrahydrofolate reductase
      deficiency 112–13
    methylenetetrahydrofolate reductase
      polymorphisms 113–14
    thiamine-responsive 115
  treatment 120
metachromatic leukodystrophy **780**
metastatic neuroblastoma 520
methemoglobin, reference values **798**
methylcobalamin deficiency 112
methylenetetrahydrofolate reductase
  deficiency 112–13
  polymorphisms 113–14
methylmalonic acidurias 109–12
  adenosylcobalamin deficiency 110–11
  combined adenosylcobalamin and
    methylcobalamin deficiency 111–12
  methylcobalamin deficiency 112
  methylmalonyl-CoA mutase deficiency
    110

methylmalonyl-CoA mutase deficiency 110
methylprednisolone 538
  Diamond–Blackfan syndrome 14
microangiopathic hemolysis 768
microangiopathic hemolytic anemias 142–3,
  517–18
monocytes 6, 333, **333**
  in myelodysplasia **407**
  reference values **805**
monocytopenia 333
monocytosis 333, **333**
mononuclear phagocytes 153
Montreal platelet syndrome **31**, 53, **508**, 509,
  567
Morquio syndrome **779, 780**
Moschcowitz syndrome *see* thrombotic
  thrombocytopenic purpura
myelodysplastic syndromes 71–2, 405–22,
  577
  biology and pathogenesis 410–11
  cytogenetics 409–10, **410**
  investigations 406–9
    blood and bone marrow investigation
      406–8, **407**
    FAB classification 408, **408, 409**
    morphologic diagnosis of refractory
      cytopenias 408–9
  prognosis 411, *411*
  subtypes
    abnormal myelopoiesis in Down
      syndrome 415
    familial syndromes and congenital
      bone marrow disorders 416
    juvenile myelomonocytic leukemia
      413–15
    refractory anemia 413
    refractory anemia in transformation
      413
    syndromes with eosinophilia 416
    therapy-related syndromes 416–17
  treatment 411–13
    bone marrow transplantation 412–13
    chemotherapy 411–12
    cytokines and differentiating agents
      412
myeloid lineage 6–7
  clinical features 406
  history 405
  incidence and epidemiology 405–6, **406**
myelokathexis 50, 326
myeloperoxidase deficiency 316–17
myelopoiesis, transient abnormal 520
myeloproliferative disorders 577
MYH9-related disease 511, 574

NADPH oxidase *314*
natural killer cell deficiency 426
natural killer cells 3–4
  reference values **805**

necrotizing enterocolitis 519
NEMO signaling pathway defects 436–7
neonatal alloimmune neutropenia 329
neonatal alloimmune thrombocytopenia
    514–15
neonatal jaundice 183
neonatal red cell membranes 259
neonate
    acquired coagulation disorders 654–9,
       654
      cardiopulmonary bypass 658–9
      disseminated intravascular coagulation
       654–5
      liver disease 657–8
      vitamin K deficiency 655–7
    coagulation data 643–4, **644**
    cranial bleeds **136**
    enzyme activities **798**
    glutathione **798**
    granulocyte transfusion 714
    hematopoiesis 130
    hemoglobinopathies 140–1
    hemostasis 643–9
      bleeding problems 648–9, **648**
      coagulation data 643–4, **644, 645**
      coagulation proteins 644–6
      fibrinolysis 646–7
      platelets 647–8
      thrombin regulation 646
    inherited coagulation disorders 649–51,
       649
      hemophilia 649–51, *650*
      von Willebrand disease 651
    internal hemorrhage 136
    intraabdominal hemorrhage 136–7
    iron status 85–6
    nonimmune anemias *see* nonimmune
      neonatal anemias
    plasma transfusion 708–9, **708, 709**
    platelets
      function 562–4, **564**
      transfusion 712, **712**
    rare inherited bleeding disorders 652–4
      coagulation factor deficiencies 652–3
      combined deficiency of vitamin K-
        dependent coagulation factors 653–4
      factor XIII deficiency 653
      fibrinogen disorders 652
    red cells 130
      alloimmunization 728–9
      transfusion 702–4, **703**
    reference values **796**
    sickle cell disease 140, 216
    thrombocytopenia 659–64
      alloimmune 661–2
      autoimmune 662–3
      clinical features 660
      etiology and mechanisms 659–60, **660**
      hematopoietic growth factors 660–1

incidence 659
  inherited 663, **663**
    platelet transfusion therapy 660, **661**
nephrotic syndrome 632
Netherton syndrome **437**
neuroacanthocytosis 270–1
neuroblastoma 769–71
  metastatic 520
neutropenia **31**, 44, 767
  acquired 326–7, **326**
  bone marrow failure 745–7
    antileukemic therapy 746–7
    bone marrow transplant patients
      745–6
    comparison with adults 745
  congenital *see* Kostmann syndrome
  cyclic **31**, 50, 323
  definition 320
  drug-induced 327
  ELA2 mutations 323–4
  immune 327–30
  investigation of 330–1
  and nutritional deficiencies 330
  pathophysiologic mechanisms 321
  primary immunodeficiency disorders
    325–6
  severe chronic 321
  severe congenital 322
    clinical presentation 322
    treatment 322
    transformation to myelodysplastic
      syndrome and acute myeloid
      leukemia 323
  see also Kostmann syndrome
neutrophil function tests 318
neutrophilia 331, **331**, 767
neutrophils 6
  granule contents **312**
  hypersegmentation *119*
  kinetics 319–20, **321**
  maturation *320*
  normal structure and development
    318–19, *319*
  reference values *794*, **794**, *802*, **802**, *803*
Niemann–Pick disease *779*, *780*, 783–5,
    783–5
  type A (infantile, acute neuronopathic)
    784
  type B (nonneuronopathic) 784
  type C 784–5
Nijmegen breakage syndrome 436
nitrous oxide, and cobalamin metabolism
    116
nonhematopoietic tumors 766–73
  anemia of chronic disease 767
  bone marrow abnormalities 768–72
  circulating tumor cells 768
  leukoerythroblastic blood film 768
  microangiopathic hemolysis 768

neutrophilia and neutropenia 767–8
  reactive thrombocytosis 767
non-Hodgkin lymphoma 482–91
  classification 484, **484**
  clinical presentation
    abdominal primary 484–5, *485*
    CNS involvement 485
    localized disease 485
    mediastinal primary 485
  diagnostic investigations and staging
    485–7, **486**
    biopsy 486
    blood tests 486
    bone marrow studies 486
    gallium and positive emission
      tomography 486–7
    imaging 486
    lumbar puncture 486
    staging 486, **487**
  epidemiology 482
  etiology and cell biology 482–4, *483*
  prognostic factors
    cytogenetics 487–8
    site 487
    stage 487
    therapy 487
  treatment 488–91, **489**
    advanced stage B-cell 488–9
    advanced state T-cell 489–90
    anaplastic large-cell lymphoma 490,
      490
    disease following immunosuppression
      491
    follicular lymphoma 491
    high-dose chemotherapy with stem cell
      support 491
    large B-cell lymphoma 490
    localized disease 488
    peripheral T-cell lymphoma 490
    primary mediastinal B-cell lymphoma
      490–1
nonimmune neonatal anemias 130–50
  causes **132**
  classification 131–2, **132**
  diagnostic approach 132–3, **133**
  hematologic values at birth 130–1, **131**
    gestational age 131
    postnatal age 131
    quality of sample 131
    site of sampling 131
    timing of cord clamping at birth 131
  hematopoiesis in neonatal period 130
  hemolysis-induced 137–43
    hemoglobinopathies 140–1
    infections 141–2, **142**
    macroangiopathic and
      microangiopathic anemias 142–3
    red cell enzyme deficiencies 139–40
    red cell membrane disorders 137–9

nonimmune neonatal anemias (*cont'd*)
  impaired red cell production 143–7
    infection 145–6
    inherited disorders 143–4
    nutritional deficiencies 146–7
    physiologic anemia of infancy/
      prematurity 144–5
  management 147–8
    diagnosis 147
    preventive/prophylactic methods
      147–8
    transfusion **148**
  secondary to blood loss 133–7
    concealed hemorrhage before or during
      delivery 133–5, *134*, **135**
    iatrogenic blood loss 137
    obstetric accidents and malformations
      of cord/placenta 135–7, **136**
nonsyndromic myelokathexis **31**
Northern epilepsy **779**
Norwood procedure 685
nutritional deficiencies 146–7
  cobalamin deficiency 147
  folate deficiency 147
  inborn errors of iron metabolism 147
  iron deficiency 146–7
  and neutropenia 330
nutritional disorders, hematologic effects
  765–6

obstetric accidents 135–7, **136**
oculocutaneous albinism 511
Omenn syndrome 430
opsonization disorders 310–12
  acquired 312
  humoral disorders
    complement disorders 311
    hypogammaglobulinemias 311
    mannose-binding protein deficiency
      311
osteoporosis 520
oxidant scavenging disorders 317
oxidative metabolism disorders 313–17
  chronic granulomatous disease 315–16,
    315, **315**
  glucose-6-phosphate dehydrogenase
    deficiency 316
  myeloperoxidase deficiency 316–17
  oxidant scavenging 317
oxygen affinity of hemoglobin *233*, *238*
  decreased 245–6
  increased 245
oxymetholone 37

Paris–Trousseau syndrome **508**, 510
paroxysmal cold hemoglobinuria
  159–60
  laboratory investigations 159–60
  treatment 160

paroxysmal nocturnal hemoglobinuria 72,
  165–6
  clinical features 165–6
  diagnosis 166
  treatment 166
parvovirus 16, 17, **142**, 219, 765
PBG deaminase 199–202, **200**, **201**
Pearson syndrome **31**, 44, 144, 325
pernicious anemia 117
phagocyte function disorders
  ingestion 311–12, **312**
  investigation of 317–18
  opsonization 310–11, 312
  phagocyte numbers 318–30
phagocytic cell disorders 439–40
phagocytic leukocytes 6–7
phosphofructokinase deficiency **173**, **174**,
  176–7
phosphoglycerate kinase deficiency **173**,
  174, 178–9
phosphoglycerate mutase deficiency **173**,
  174, 179
photocutaneous porphyria
  congenital erythropoietic porphyria
    204–5
  erythropoietic protoporphyria 206–7
  hepatoerythropoietic porphyria 205–6
  porphyria cutanea tarda 205–6
physiologic anemia of infancy/prematurity
  144–5
placental infarction 520
placental malformations 135–7, **136**
plasma exchange 538
plasma protein deficiencies 440–1
plasma transfusion 706–9
  description and storage 706
  dosage and administration 709
  indications and contraindications 706–8
    congenital coagulation factor
      deficiencies 707–8
    disseminated intravascular coagulation
      707
    massive transfusion 707
    reversal of warfarin effect 707
    severe liver disease 707
  neonates 708–9, **708**, **709**
plasma volume **801**
α_2-plasmin inhibitor deficiency 621
plasminogen activator inhibitor-1 deficiency
  621
platelets
  aggregation 565
  alloimmunization 730–1
  counting 548–9
  destruction 528–9, *528*
  function 562, *563*
    neonates 562–4, **564**, 647–8
  reference values *794*
  stimulated production 549–50, *550*

transfusion 660, **661**, 709–13
  description and storage 709–10
  indications 710–12
  neonates 712, **712**
  platelet refractoriness 713
  product choice, dosage and
    administration 712–13
  see also thrombocytosis
platelet count, reference values **807**
platelet function disorders 562–82
  acquired 574–7, **575**
    acute leukemias and myelodysplastic
      syndromes 577
    antiplatelet antibodies 577
    drugs and other agents 574–6
    extracorporeal perfusion 576–7
    liver disease 576
    myeloproliferative disorders 577
    storage pool deficiency 577
    uremia 576
  clinical history 564–5, **564**
    bleeding 564–5
    gender and family history 565
    medical history 565
    medications 565
  clinical tests 565–6
    bleeding time 565
    blood smear 565
    platelet aggregation 565
  differential diagnosis 566, **566**
  inherited 566–74, **567–8**
    abnormalities of platelet coagulant
      activity 573–4
    adhesion defects 566, 569–70
    aggregation defects 572–3
    agonist receptor defects 570
    MYH9-related disease 574
    secretion defects 571–2
    signaling pathway defects 570–1
  normal platelet function 562, *563*
  physical examination 565
  platelet function in newborn 562–4, *564*
  treatment 577–8
    activated factor VII 578
    antifibrinolytic agents 578
    bone marrow transplantation 578
    desmopressin 578
    gene therapy 578
    platelet transfusion 578
Pneumocystis carinii 748
polyarteritis nodosa 762
polymorphonuclear neutrophils 6
Pompe disease **779**, **780**
porphyria 193–212
  acute hepatic 198–204
    acute intermittent porphyria 199–202,
      200, **201**
    ALAD deficiency porphyria 198–9
    hereditary coproporphyria 202

treatment 203–4
variegate porphyria 202–3
classification **193**
clinical signs and symptoms 193–7, **194**
cutaneous manifestations 196–7, **196**
neurovisceral manifestations 194–5,
195
diagnosis **197**
epidemiology 193
heme biosynthesis and pathway 197–8,
199
photocutaneous
congenital erythropoietic porphyria
204–5
erythropoietic protoporphyria 206–7
hepatoerythropoietic porphyria 205–6
porphyria cutanea tarda 205–6
uroporphyrinogen decarboxylase
205–6
prevalence **193**
porphyria cutanea tarda 205–6
postthrombotic syndrome 674
preeclampsia 516
pregnancy
folate deficiency 117–19
sickle cell disease 217–18
prekallikrein deficiency 612
priapism 222
procoagulants 644–5, **645**
progenitor cells, reference values **805**
prolactin, Diamond–Blackfan anemia 14
protein 4.1 mutations 268–9
protein 4.2 deficiency 264
protein A immunoadsorption 538
protein-calorie malnutrition 765
protein C deficiency 519
protein S deficiency 519
prothrombin deficiency 616–17
clinical and laboratory features 616–17
inheritance and prevalence 616
neonate 652–3
structure and function 616
treatment 617
prothrombin time, prolonged 610–11
prothrombotic disorders 684–5
acquired 685
congenital 684–5
protoporphyrinogen oxidase 202–3
protozoal infections 327
pseudo-Hurler polydystrophy **779**
pseudo-von Willebrand disease **508**, 509
puberty, iron status 86
purine antagonists 464
purine nucleoside phosphorylase deficiency
430
purpura, posttransfusion 731
pyrimidine 5′-nucleotidase deficiency **173**,
174, 186
pyrimidine antagonists 464

pyruvate kinase deficiency 139–40, **173**,
174, 179–81, **181**

Quebec syndrome **508**, 511, **568**, 572

Rac2 mutation 310
reactive thrombocytosis 554–7
clinical and laboratory features 554–7,
555, **556**
complications 557
indications for treatment 557
pathophysiology 554
red cells
adenosine deaminase 12
alloimmunization 728–30
antigens 151–2
enzyme deficiencies 139–40
glucose 6-phosphate dehydrogenase
deficiency 139
glucose phosphate isomerase deficiency
140
pyruvate kinase deficiency 139–40
failure of production 11–29
congenital dyserythropoietic anemias
18–22, **19**
red cell aplasia 11–18
impaired production 143–7
infection 145–6
inherited disorders 143–4
nutritional deficiencies 146–7
membrane 130
membrane disorders 137–9
hereditary elliptocytosis 138
hereditary pyropoikilocytosis 138
hereditary spherocytosis 137–8
infantile pyknocytosis 138
in myelodysplasia **407**
neonatal, half-life 130
reference values **796**, **797**
red cell aplasia 11–18
aplastic crisis 16–17
chronic acquired 17
Diamond–Blackfan anemia 11–15
differential diagnosis 17–18
transient erythroblastopenia of childhood
15–16
red cell count **793**
red cell cycle *85*
red cell enzymopathies 171–92
clinical findings 172–3, **174**
Embden–Meyerhof pathway disorders
175–81
aldolase deficiency 177
diphosphoglycerate mutase deficiency
179
enolase deficiency 179
glucosephosphate isomerase deficiency
175–6
hexokinase deficiency 175

phosphofructokinase deficiency 176–7
phosphoglycerate kinase deficiency
178–9
phosphoglycerate mutase deficiency
179
pyruvate kinase deficiency 179–81,
181
triosephosphate isomerase deficiency
177–8
epidemiology 172
hexose monophosphate shunt disorders
181–5
glucose 6-dehydrogenase deficiency
181–5
glutathione peroxidase deficiency
185
glutathione reductase deficiency 185
glutathione synthesis deficiency 185
laboratory information
analysis of intermediate metabolites
173
basic data 173
direct enzyme and DNA measurement
175
enzyme screening tests 173–4
metabolic intermediates **174**
prevalence **173**
red cell morphology 173
red cell nucleotide metabolism disorders
186–7
see also red cell metabolism
red cell fragmentation syndromes 762
red cell membrane abnormalities 255–80
disorders of hydration and cation
transport 271–4
echinocytes and acanthocytes 269–71
hereditary elliptocytosis 265–9
hereditary spherocytosis 259–65
membrane lipids 255–6
components 255
lipid renewal pathways 256
organization and dynamics 255–6
membrane proteins 256–9
components 256–8, *257*, **257**
fetal and neonatal membranes 259
membrane deformability 258–9
membrane transport 259
target-cells 271
red cell metabolism 130, 171–2, *172*
red cell nucleotide metabolism disorders
186–7
red cell survival **801**
red cell transfusion 696–706
autologous 704–5
blood group choice, dosage and
administration 701–2, **701**, **702**
description and storage 696, **697**
directed donations 705–6
erythropoietin 705

red cell transfusion (*cont'd*)
  indications for 696, 698–701, **698**
  limited-exposure blood donor programs
    705–6
  neonates 702–4, **703**
red cell volume **801**
reference values 792–810
  bleeding time **807**
  blood count **793**
  blood volume **801**
  coagulation **794**
  coagulation inhibitors **795, 806**
  coagulation tests **625, 795, 806**
  cobalamin **800**
  D-dimers **807**
  differential white cell count **803–4**
  enzyme activity and glutathione content
    798
  eosinophils **805**
  erythrocyte sedimentation rate **808**
  erythropoeitin **800**
  folate **800**
  granulocytes **802**
  hemoglobin **793**
  hemoglobin variants **707**
  immunoglobulins **808**
  lymphocytes **805**
  methemoglobin **798**
  monocytes **805**
  neutrophils 794, **794**, 802, *803*
  normal hemoglobin **796**
  plasma volume **801**
  platelet count **807**
  platelets *794*
  progenitor cells **805**
  red cells **796, 797**
  red cell count **793**
  red cell morphology *799*
  red cell survival **801**
  red cell volume **801**
  reticulocyte count **797**
  serum ferritin *800*
  serum haptoglobin **801**
  serum iron *799*
  serum transferrin *799*
  T-cells, B-cells and natural killer cells
    805
  total bilirubin *801*
  zine protoporphyrin **800**
refractory anemia 413
  with excess of blasts **408**
  with ringed sideroblasts 94, **408**
  in transformation **408**
renal disease
  hematologic effects 758–9
  hemostatic complications 632–3
    chronic renal failure 632
    hemolytic-uremic syndrome 632–3
    nephrotic syndrome 632

renal failure, in sickle cell disease 221–2
respiratory distress syndrome 519
reticular dysgenesis **31**, 44, 325, 430
reticulocyte count **797**
rhabdomyosarcoma 771
Rh deficiency syndrome 273–4
rhesus hemolytic disease of newborn
    162–4, **164**, 519
  diagnosis and management in neonate
    163
  prenatal management of Rh-sensitized
    pregnancy 162–3
  prevention of maternal Rh immunization
    162
rhesus system 152
rituximab 539
Rosai–Dorfman disease 355
rubella **142**
  congenital 516
RUNX1-thrombocytopenia-leukemia
    syndrome 511

Salla disease **779**
Sandhoff disease **779, 780**
Sanfilippo syndrome **779, 780**
Santavuori disease **779**
Scheie syndrome **779**, 786
Schilling test 120
Schimke immuno-osseous dysplasia 44,
    435
Schindler disease **779**
SCID *see* severe combined
    immunodeficiency
Scott syndrome **568**, 573–4
scurvy 765–6
Sebastian syndrome **31**, 52, **509**, 512, **567**,
    574
Seckel syndrome 44
severe combined immunodeficiency 325,
    428–32
  classification **429**
  clinical features and diagnosis 431–2
  lymphocyte metabolism defects 429–31
  with maternofetal engraftment 430
  signalling receptor defects 429
  X-linked 429
short-limbed dwarfism, and
    immunodeficiency 435
Shprintzen syndrome 433
Shwachman syndrome 435
Shwachman–Diamond syndrome **31**, 324,
    406, 416
  cancer predisposition 38
  clinical manifestations 37–8
    hematological features 37
    nonhematological features 37–8
  genetic aspects 38
  pathogenesis 38–9
  therapy and prognosis 39–40

  androgens 39–40
  hematopoietic stem cell transplantation
    40
  supportive care 39
sialidosis 779
sialuria 779
sickle cell disease 213–30
  definitive testing 215–16, **215**
  epidemiology 213–14, **214**
  laboratory features 215
  management 224–6
    blood transfusion 225
    experimental therapies **826**
    hematopoietic stem cell transplantation
      226
    hydroxycarbamide 225–6
    long-term surveillance 225
    pain management 225
  neonatal 140
  neonatal screening 216
  red cells
    alloimmunization 730
    transfusion 699–700
sickle cell trait 214
sickle solubility test 215
specific problems 217–24, **217**
  abdomen 220–1
  anemia 219
  bones and joints *220*
  cerebrovascular disease 223–4
  contraception and pregnancy 217–18
  eye disease 224
  growth and development 217
  infection 218–19, **218**
  leg ulcers 222
  priapism 222
  pulmonary manifestations 222–3, *222*
  renal manifestations 221–2
  vasoocclusive events 219–20
sickle test 238
sideroblastic anemias 91–4
  acquired 94
  classification **92**
  congenital 91–4
    diagnosis 92
    differential diagnosis 93–4
    etiology 91–2
    management 94
    molecular basis 92
  inherited 147
sideroblasts, ringed 93, 94
sinus histiocytosis with massive
    lymphadenopathy 355
sitosterolemia 274
skin disease, hematologic effects 761
Sly syndrome **779, 780**, 785
soft tissue sarcomas 771–2
solubility test 239

somatic gene therapy 443
spectral analysis 238
spectrin
  deficiency 263
  mutations 257–8, *268*
sphingolipidoses 780–5
  Gaucher disease 781–3, *781, 782*
  Niemann–Pick disease 783–5, *783–5*
splenectomy 242, 293
steroids, Diamond–Blackfan anemia 13–14,
  13
stomatocytosis 271, 273
  acquired 274
storage pool disease 571
  acquired 577
Swiss cheese appearance 19
syphilis **142**
systemic arterial thromboembolic events
  677–9, **677**
  classification 677–8
  clinical symptoms 677
  diagnosis 678
  epidemiology 677
  etiology 677
  outcomes 677
  treatment 678–9, **679**
systemic disease, hematologic effects
  757–77
  anemia of chronic disease 757–8
  connective tissue disease 761–2
  drugs 766
  endocrine disorders 760
  gastrointestinal disease 759–60
  heart disease 760
  infection 762–5
  liver disease 759
  lung disease 760–1
  nonhematopoietic tumors 766–73
  nutritional disorders 765–6
  red-cell fragmentation syndromes
    762
  renal disease 758–9
  skin disease 761
systemic lupus erythematosus 329, 761
systemic venous thromboembolism 673–7,
  673
  central venous line-related 674–5, *674*
  clinical systems 674
  diagnosis 675
  epidemiology 673
  etiology 673–4
  incidence 674
  treatment 675–7, *676*

target-cells 271
TAR syndrome 33, *45*, 52
Tay–Sachs disease **779, 780**
T-cell lymphoblastic leukemia 458
T-cell lymphoma 489–90

T-cells 3–4
  development 427
  interactions with B-cells *428*
  reference values **805**
testicular leukemia 452–3
thalassemias 281–301
  alpha-thalassemias 298
    clinical features 291
    pathophysiology 287–8
  beta-thalassemias
    clinical features 288–9
    intermediate forms *290*
    pathophysiology 287
  beta-thalassemia trait 289
  bone marrow transplantation 297
  classification **283**
  clinical management 293–7
    experimental approaches 297
    infective complications 293
    iron overload and iron-chelating
      therapy 293–7, *294*, **295, 296**
    red cell transfusions 293
    splenectomy 293
  db-thalassemia 290–1
  distribution 283–4, *284, 285*
  (egdb)o thalassemia 291
  genetic control of hemoglobin synthesis
    281–3, *282*
  HbE b thalassemia 298
  pathophysiology 284–8
    cellular pathology 286–8, *288*
    molecular pathology 284–6
  prenatal diagnosis 292
  red cells
    alloimmunization 730
    transfusion 700–1
  screening and prevention 291–2
  thalassemia intermedia 297–8
thalassemia syndromes 140–1
thalassemic hemoglobin variants 242–5,
  243, *244*
thiamine-responsive megaloblastic anemia
  115
thrombin, regulation in neonate 646
thrombocytopenia 507–25
  with absent radii 31, 51–2, **509**, 512–13
    cancer predisposition 51
    clinical features 51
    genetic aspects 51
    laboratory evaluation and diagnosis 52
    pathogenesis 51–2
    therapy and prognosis 52
  amegakaryocytic 508, 513
  with associated myeloid malignancies 31
  associated with radioulnar synostosis 53
  congenital 514–20
    infant factors 517–20
    maternal factors 514–17, **514**
    placental factors 520

with dyserythropoiesis **31**
heparin-induced 519, 766
history 507–8
inherited 508–14
  with dysfunctional platelets 508–11
  without dysfunctional platelets
    511–14
maternal autoimmune 515–16
Mediterranean **509**, 513–14
neonate 659–64
  alloimmune 514–15, 661–2
  clinical features 660
  etiology and mechanisms 659–60,
    660
  hematopoietic growth factors 660–1
  incidence 659
  inherited 663, **663**
  platelet transfusion therapy 660, **661**
pure genetic **509**, 513
with radioulnar dysostosis 31
thrombocytosis 548–61
  definition and classification 548
  diagnostic features 548–9, **549**
    counting of platelets 548–9
  essential 551–4
    clinical and laboratory features 552–3,
      552
    familial forms **553**
    pathogenesis 551
    treatment options 553–4
  reactive 554–7, 767
    clinical and laboratory features 554–7,
      555, 556
    complications 557
    indications for treatment 557
    pathophysiology 554
  stimulated platelet production 549–50,
    550
  symptoms 548
thromboembolic complications 672–90
  developmental hemostasis 672
  and heart disease 685–6
  prothrombotic disorders 684–5
    acquired 685
    congenital 684–5
  systemic arterial thromboembolic events
    677–9, **677**
  systemic venous thromboembolism
    673–7, **673**
  treatment
    anticoagulants 679–84
    thrombolytic therapy 684
thrombolytic agents, and platelet disorders
  576
thrombolytic therapy 684
thrombotic thrombocytopenic purpura
  517–18, 758–9
thromboxane A_2 receptor deficiency **567**,
  570

thymus transplants 443
thyroid disease 760
TORCH syndromes 516, 765
total iron binding capacity **799**
toxoplasmosis **142**, 516
transcobalamin 109
transcobalamin II deficiency 108–9
transferrin 81–2
  receptors 82–3
  reference values *799*
transfusion-related acute lung injury
    725
transient abnormal myelopoiesis 415
transient erythroblastopenia of childhood
    15–16, 762
  clinical features 15
  differential diagnosis 16
  etiology and pathophysiology 15–16
  hematologic findings 15
  treatment and prognosis 16
transient hypogammaglobulinemia of
    infancy 439
triosephosphate isomerase deficiency **173**,
    174, 177–8
trisomy syndromes 513
tuberculosis 763–4
twin-to-twin transfusion 135

umbilical cord
  blood 69
  clamping 131
  malformations 135–7, **136**
uremia 271
  platelet aggregation in 565
uroporphyrinogen decarboxylase 205–6
uroporphyrinogen III synthase 204–5

vaccination
  hemophilia 594
  immunodeficiency disorders 441, **441**
variegate porphyria 202–3
vasoocclusive events 219–20
V(D)J recombination defects 430
velocardiofacial syndrome 433
vinca alkaloids 464, 537
viral infections 326
vitamin B$_{12}$ *see* cobalamin
vitamin E, deficiency 270
vitamin K deficiency 628–30
  clinical features 629
  etiology 629
  laboratory diagnosis 629
  neonate 655–7
  prophylaxis 630, 656–7
  treatment 629–30
vitamin K-dependent coagulation factors,
    combined deficiency 619–20,
    653–4
Vogt–Spielmeyer disease **779**
von Willebrand disease 569–70, 598–607
  biosynthesis and function 598–9, *599*
  classification **598**, 600–3, **602**
    type 1 601–2
    type 2 **508**, 509, 602–3, *603*
    type 3 602
  clinical management 603–5
    adjunctive therapies 604
    blood component therapy 605
    desmopressin 604–5
  laboratory evaluation 599–600
    screening tests 599–600
    tests for vWF-FVIII complex 600, **600**,
    601

neonate 651
  clinical features 651
  diagnosis 651
  management 651
  platelet-type **567**
von Willebrand factor inhibitors 636

warfarin 682–4, *683*, **683**, **684**
warm autoimmune hemolytic anemia
    155–8
  clinical course and prognosis 157
  clinical features 155
  Evans syndrome 157–8
  laboratory features 155–6
  treatment 156–7
Wegener granulomatosis 762
Weibel–Palade bodies 599
West Nile virus, transfusion-related 739
WHIM syndrome **31**, 51, 326
whole blood transfusion 695–6
Wiskott–Aldrich syndrome 53, 309–10, **310**,
    432–3, 508, **508**, 510–11, **568**, 571–2
Wolman disease **779**, **780**

xerocytosis 272–3
X-linked agammaglobulinemia 325, 437–8
X-linked hyper-IgM syndrome 433–4
X-linked lymphoproliferative disease 433
X-linked thrombocytopenia **31**, **508**, 510
X-linked thrombocytopenia/
    dyserythropoietic anemia **508**
X-linked thrombocytopenia/thalassemia
    508

Zellweger syndrome 94
Zieve syndrome 759